Cardiological Society of India

CARDIOLOGY

Update 2018

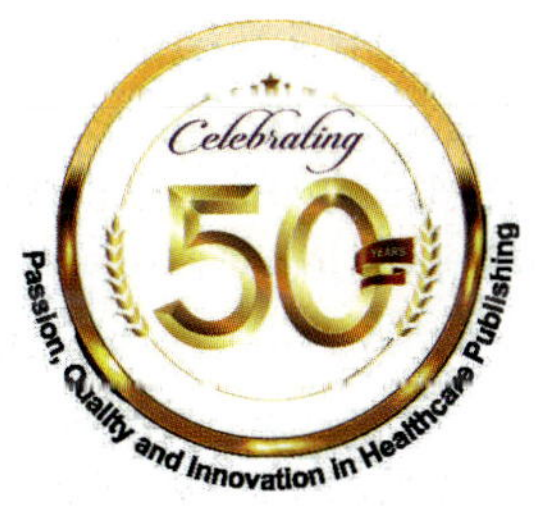

DISCLAIMER

Cardiological Society of India

CARDIOLOGY

Update 2018

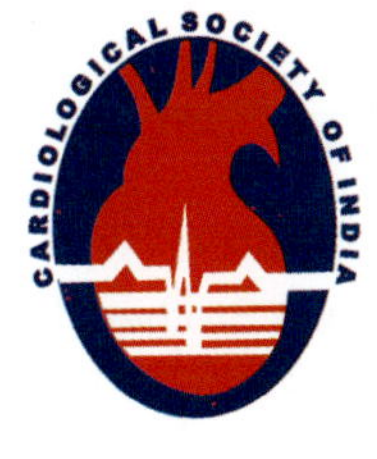

Editor-in-Chief

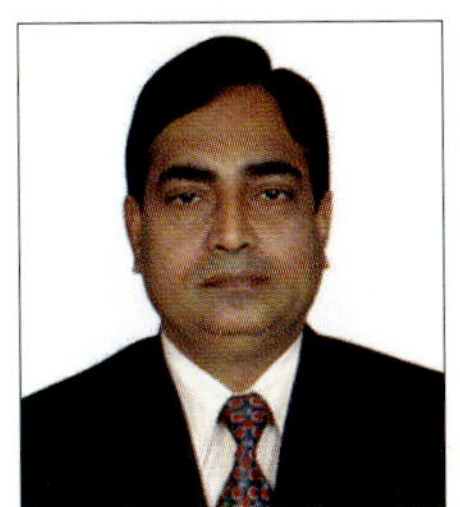

Kewal C Goswami MD DM
Professor
Department of Cardiology
All India Institute of Medical Sciences
New Delhi, India

Co-Editors

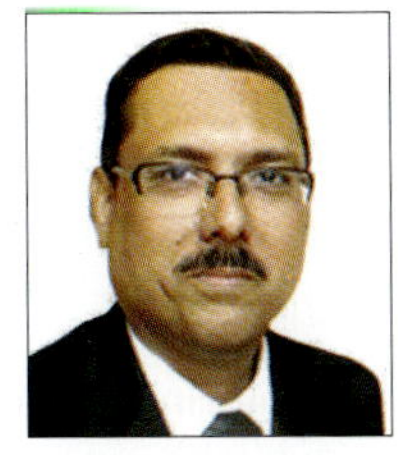

Rakesh Yadav MD DM
Professor
Department of Cardiology
All India Institute of Medical Sciences
New Delhi, India

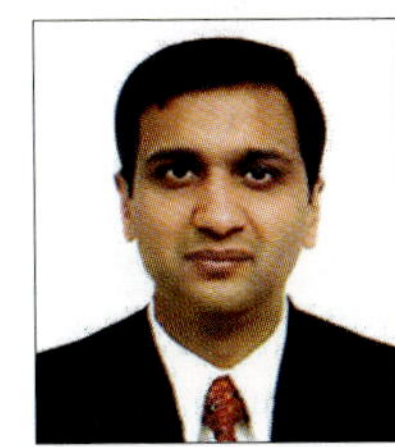

Nitish Naik MD DM
Professor
Department of Cardiology
All India Institute of Medical Sciences
New Delhi, India

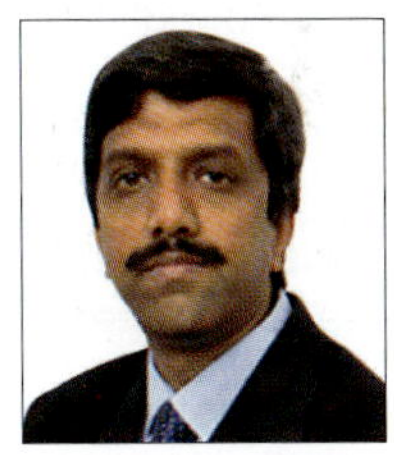

S Ramakrishnan MD DM
Professor
Department of Cardiology
All India Institute of Medical Sciences
New Delhi, India

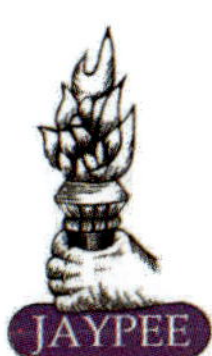

JAYPEE BROTHERS MEDICAL PUBLISHERS
The Health Sciences Publisher
New Delhi | London | Panama

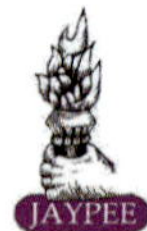

Jaypee Brothers Medical Publishers (P) Ltd

Headquarters

Jaypee Brothers Medical Publishers (P) Ltd
4838/24, Ansari Road, Daryaganj
New Delhi 110 002, India
Phone: +91-11-43574357
Fax: +91-11-43574314
Email: jaypee@jaypeebrothers.com

Overseas Offices

J.P. Medical Ltd
83 Victoria Street, London
SW1H 0HW (UK)
Phone: +44 20 3170 8910
Fax: +44 (0)20 3008 6180
Email: info@jpmedpub.com

Jaypee-Highlights Medical Publishers Inc
City of Knowledge, Bld. 235, 2nd Floor, Clayton
Panama City, Panama
Phone: +1 507-301-0496
Fax: +1 507-301-0499
Email: cservice@jphmedical.com

Jaypee Brothers Medical Publishers (P) Ltd
17/1-B Babar Road, Block-B, Shaymali
Mohammadpur, Dhaka-1207
Bangladesh
Mobile: +08801912003485
Email: jaypeedhaka@gmail.com

Jaypee Brothers Medical Publishers (P) Ltd
Bhotahity, Kathmandu, Nepal
Phone: +977-9741283608
Email: kathmandu@jaypeebrothers.com

Website: www.jaypeebrothers.com
Website: www.jaypeedigital.com

Inquiries for bulk sales may be solicited at: jaypee@jaypeebrothers.com

CSI Cardiology Update 2018 / Kewal C Goswami

First Edition: **2019**

ISBN: 978-93-5270-521-4

Printed at: Ajanta Offset & Packagings Ltd., Faridabad, Haryana

Dedicated to

Our parents, family, teachers, students and patients

CONTRIBUTORS

EDITOR-IN-CHIEF

Kewal C Goswami MD DM
Professor
Department of Cardiology
All India Institute of Medical Sciences
New Delhi, India

CO-EDITORS

Rakesh Yadav MD DM
Professor
Department of Cardiology
All India Institute of Medical Sciences
New Delhi, India

Nitish Naik MD DM
Professor
Department of Cardiology
All India Institute of Medical Sciences
New Delhi, India

S Ramakrishnan MD DM
Professor
Department of Cardiology
All India Institute of Medical Sciences
New Delhi, India

CONTRIBUTING AUTHORS

AK Pancholia MD FACC FESC FCSI MAMS
Head, Department of Medicine and Preventive Cardiology, Arihant Hospital
Indore, Madhya Pradesh, India

A Sreenivas Kumar MD DM FACC
Chief Cardiologist
Department of Cardiology
Citizens Hospital
Hyderabad, Telangana, India

Abhishek Gupta MD
Senior Resident
Department of Cardiology
GB Pant Institute of Post Graduate Medical Education and Research
New Delhi, India

Abhishek Roy MD
Post-Doctoral Trainee
Department of Cardiology
Narayana Health-Rabindranath Tagore International Institute of Cardiac Science
Kolkata, West Bengal, India

Aditya Kapoor MD DM FACC FESC FCSI FAPSC
Professor, Department of Cardiology
Sanjay Gandhi Postgraduate Institute of Medical Sciences
Lucknow, Uttar Pradesh, India

AJ Swamy MD DM
Senior Cardiologist
Department of Cardiology
Armed Forces Medical College
Pune, Maharashtra, India

Ajay K Sinha MD PhD FACC FESC FCSI FICC FAPSC
Director, Department of Cardiology
Paras HMRI Hospitals
Patna, Bihar, India

Ajay S Vamadevan MPH PhD
Deputy Director and Head
Health Systems Unit,
Centre for Chronic Disease Control
New Delhi, India

Akshay Mehta MD DM
Consultant Cardiologist
Department of Cardiology
Nanavati Super Speciality Hospital
Mumbai, Maharashtra, India

Amal K Banerjee MD DM FACC FESC FACP FAPSC FICC FCSI FICP
Consultant and Interventional Cardiologist
Kolkata

Ambuj Roy MD DM
Professor
Department of Cardiology
Cardiothoracic Centre
All India Institute of Medical Sciences
New Delhi, India

Ambukeshwar Singh MD DM
Consultant Cardiology
Divine Heart Hospital
Lucknow, Uttar Pradesh, India

Amit Gupta DNB MNAMS FRCP FIMSA DFID PGDD
Director and Head
Department of Diabetology
Center for Diabetes and Allied Sciences
Gurugram, Haryana, India

Amir Ahmadi MD
Assistant Clinical Professor
Mount Sinai Hospital
New York

Angelika Koljaja-Batzner MD
Klinikum Würzburg Mitte, Juliusspital
Schweinfurt, Germany

Anil Kumar Mehra MD
Director
Cardiac Catheterization Lab
Assistant Professor
Keck School of Medicine
University of Southern California
Los Angeles, California, USA

Anindya Mukherjee MD DM
Post-Doctoral Trainee
Department of Cardiology
NRS Medical College
Kolkata, West Bengal, India

Anjan Lal Dutta MD DM FACC
Clinical Director
Department of Cardiology
Peerless Hospital, Kolkata, West Bengal, India
Past President, National CSI

Ankur Jhavar MD
Postgraduate Medical Education
Department of Cardiology
Nanavati Super Speciality Hospital
Mumbai, Maharashtra, India

Anoop Jain DM
Senior Professor and Head
Department of Cardiology
Sawai Man Singh Hospital
Jaipur, Rajasthan, India

Anunay Gupta MD DM
Assistant Professor
Department of Cardiology
Vardhman Mahavir Medical College and Safdarjung Hospital
New Delhi, India

Aparna Jaswal MD DNB FHRS CCDS FACC FESC
Associate Director
Department of Electrophysiology
Fortis Escorts Heart Institute
New Delhi, India

Arka Chatterjee MD FACC FSCAI
Assistant Professor
Department of Medicine
University of Alabama at Birmingham
Birmingham, Alabama, USA

Arun Sharma MD
Senior Resident
Department of Cardiovascular Radiology and Endovascular interventions
All India Institute of Medical Sciences
New Delhi, India

Arunangshu Ganguly MD DNB MNAMS FESC FACC FSCAI
Senior Interventional Cardiologist
Chairman and MD Healthworld Hospitals
Durgapur, West Bengal, India

Arup Dasbiswas MD DM FIAE FCSI FICC FIAMS FICP FSCAI FACC FESC
Professor, DNBE (CCARDIO)
Department of Cardiology
Rabindranath Tagore International Institute of Cardiac Sciences
Kolkata, West Bengal, India

Ashish K Govil MD DM
Consultant Interventional Cardiologist
Department of Cardiology
Delhi Heart and Lung Institute
New Delhi, India

Ashish Tiwari MD FIPC
Senior Resident
Department of Cardiology
King George's Medical University
Lucknow, Uttar Pradesh, India

Ashok Goyal MD
Consultant Physician
Head and Director
Department of Internal Medicine
Bani Park Hospital
Jaipur, Rajasthan, India

Ashwat S Dhillon MD
Fellow
Department of Cardiology
Keck School of Medicine of the University of Southern California
Los Angeles, CA, USA

Ashwin B Mehta MD FACC FISE FICP
Director
Department of Cardiology
Jaslok Hospital and Research Centre
Mumbai, Maharashtra, India

Atul Mathur MD DM
Director Interventional Cardiology and Chief of Cardiac Cath Labs
Fortis Escorts Heart Institute
New Delhi, India

Auriom Kar MD DM
Post-Doctoral Trainee
Department of Cardiology
Nil Ratan Sircar Medical College
Kolkata, West Bengal, India

Avani Jain MD
Clinical Assistant
Intensive Care Unit
Choithram Hospital
Indore, Madhya Pradesh, India

Avik Karak MD
Senior Resident
Department of Cardiology
Medical College Kolkata
Kolkata, West Bengal, India

Avinash Verma MD DNB
Senior Consultant Cardiologist
Pushpawati Singhania Heart Institute
New Delhi, India

Aviraj Choudhary MD
Fellow
Department of Cardiology
Institute of Medical Sciences
Banaras Hindu University
Varanasi, Uttar Pradesh, India

Ayush Shukla MD DM
Consultant Cardiology
Department of Cardiology
Divine Heart Hospital
Lucknow, Uttar Pradesh, India

Balbir Singh MD DM FACC
Chairman
Electrophysiology and Pacing
Medanta Hospital
Gurugram, Haryana, India

Balram Airan MS Mch FIACS FIACTS FAMS
Chief Cardiac Surgeon and Head
Department of CTVS
Mahatma Gandhi University of Medical Sciences and Technology
Jaipur, Rajasthan, India

Binjo Vazhappilly MD DM
Cardiologist
Department of Cardiology
Westfort Hitech Hospital
Thrissur, Kerala, India

Biswaranjan Mishra MD DM FCSI FIAE FESC
Chief Consultant Cardiologist
Department of Cardiology
Max Diagnostic Centre
Cuttack, Odisha, Indi

BP Singh MD DM
Professor and Head
Department of Cardiology
Indira Gandhi Institute of Medical Sciences
Patna, Bihar, India

Brian Pinto MD DM
Chief Cardiologist
Cardiology
Holy Family Hospital and Research Centre
Mumbai, Maharashtra, India

C Raghu MD DM FACC FESC FSCAI
Director and Lead Cardiologist
Aster Prime Hospital
Hyderabad, Telangana, India

C Venkata S Ram MD MACP FACC FASH
Director
Apollo Institute for Blood Pressure Management
Apollo Blood Pressure Clinics
World Hypertension League/South Asia Office Apollo Hospitals
Hyderabad, Telangana, India
Texas Blood Pressure Institute
Dallas, Texas, USA

CB Meena MD DM
Senior Professor
Department of Cardiology
Sawai Man Singh Hospital
Jaipur, Rajasthan, India

Cherian Koshy MD DM
Associate Professor
Department of Cardiology
Pushpagiri Institute of Medical Sciences and Research Centre
Thiruvalla, Kerala, India

Chinar Patel MD
Smidt Heart Institute
Cedars-Sinai Medical Center
Los Angeles, USA

Chukwudi Nwagbara MBBS
Clinical Associate
Department of Interventional Cardiology
Indraprastha Apollo Hospitals
New Delhi, India

DS Gambhir MD DM FAMS FCSI FICC FCAPSC FSCAI FACC
Group Director
Department of Cardiology
Kailash Health Care Ltd.
Director
Kailash Hospital and Heart Institute
Noida, Uttar Pradesh, India

Debabrata Roy MD DM FACC FSCAI FESC
Senior Consultant Interventional Cardiologist
Department of Cardiology
Narayana Health-Rabindranath Tagore International Institute of Cardiac Science
Kolkata, West Bengal, India

Deepak Saha MD DNB FESC
Consultant
Department of Cardiology
Virinchi Hospital
Hyderabad, Telangana, India

Dev B Pahlajani MD FACC FSCAI
Head
Department of Cardiology
Breach Candy Hospital
Mumbai, Maharashtra, India

Dhiman Kahali MD Dip Card DM FSCAI FESC
Senior Consultant Interventional Cardiologist, Interventional Cardiology
BM Birla Heart Research Centre
Kolkata, West Bengal, India

Dinesh Gautam MD DM
Assistant Professor
Department of Cardiology
SMS Medical College
Jaipur, Rajasthan, India

Dinkar Bhasin MD
Senior Resident
Department of Cardiology
All India Institute of Medical Sciences
New Delhi, India

Dipak R Das MD DM
Assistant Professor
Department of Cardiology
Srirama Chandra Bhanja Medical College
Cuttack, Odisha, India

Dipak Sarma MD MRCP FRCPE FRCPI FCSI
Senior Consultant
Cardiology and Critical Care
Jorhat Christian Medical Centre Hospital
Jorhat, Assam, India

Dorairaj Prabhakaran MD DM MSc FRCP FNASc
Vice President
Research and Policy, Centre for Chronic Disease Control
Public Health Foundation of India (PHFI)
Gurgaon, Haryana, India

G Nagarjuna MD
Apollo Hospitals
Secunderabad, Telangana, India

G Vijayaraghavan MD DM FRCP FACC FAHA
Vice Chairman and Director
Department of Cardiology
Kerala Institute of Medical Sciences
Thiruvananthapuram, Kerala, India

GN Mahapatra MD DSc
Senior Consultant and Head
Department of Nuclear Medicine, SPECT-CT and PET-CT
Seven Hills Hospital
Mumbai, Maharashtra, India

GC Khilnani MD FCCP FAMS FICCM FICP FNCCP FISDA
Professor and Head
Department of Pulmonary Medicine and Sleep Disorders
All India Institute of Medical Sciences
New Delhi, India

Ganesh K Mani MCh MNAMS
Chairman
Department of Cardio Thoracic Vascular Surgery
Max Smart Super Speciality Hospital
New Delhi, India

Gautam Sharma MD DM
Professor
Department of Cardiology
All India Institute of Medical Sciences
New Delhi, India

Geetha Subramanian MD DM FISC FCSI FIAE FISE FMMC
Professor and Head
Department of Cardiology
Institute of Medical Sciences
Banaras Hindu University
Varanasi, Uttar Pradesh, India

George Joseph MD DM FCSI
Professor
Department of Cardiology
Christian Medical College
Vellore, Tamil Nadu, India

Gonzalo Luis Alonso Salinas MD PhD
Department of Cardiology
Hospital Ramón y Cajal.
Universidad de Alcalá
CIBERCV, Hospital Ramón y Cajal.
Madrid, Spain

HK Chopra MD DM FACC FAHA FESC FISCU FASE FCSI FIAE FIMSA FGSI FWHA FISU
Chief Cardiologist
Department of Cardiology
Moolchand Medcity
New Delhi, India

HS Isser MD DM
Professor
Department of Cardiology
Vardhman Mahavir Medical College and Safdarjung Hospital
New Delhi, India

Hardeep K Grewal MD
Consultant
Department of Cardiology
Medanta- The Medicity
Gurugram, Haryana, India

Harikrishnan S MD DM
Professor
Department of Cardiology
Sree Chitra Tirunal Institute for Medical Sciences and Technology
Trivandrum, Kerala, India

Harinder K Bali MD DM
Director
Department of Cardiology
Fortis Hospital
Mohali, Punjab, India

Harsh Wardhan MD DM
Head
Department of Cardiology
Primus Super Specialty Hospital
New Delhi, India

Harsha V Niraghatam MS
Senior President
Department of Cardiothoracic and Vascular Surgery
All India Institute of Medical Sciences
New Delhi, India

Hiteshi KC Chauhan MD
Associate Consultant
Department of Cardiology
Fortis Hospital
Mohali, Punjab, India

Hubert Seggewiss MD FESC
Consultant HOCM
Klinikum Würzburg Mitte, Juliusspital
Schweinfurt, Germany

Jagat Narula MD PhD MACC
Philip J and Harriet L Goodhart Chair of Cardiology
Zena and Michael A Wiener Cardiovascular Institute
Icahn School of Medicine
Mount Sinai, New York
Chief, Division of Cardiology
Luke's Hospital of Mount Sinai, New York
Director, Cardiovascular Imaging Program
Mount Sinai Health System, New York
Associate Dean
Arnhold Institute for Global Health
Mount Sinai, New York

J Shiv Kumar MD DM
Sr Consultant Cardiologist
Department of Cardiology
Apollo Hospitals
Secunderabad, Telangana, India

Jabir Abdullakutty MD DM FSCAI FACC FESC
Senior Consultant Cardiologist and Director of clinical research
Department of Cardiology
Lisie Hospital, Kochi, Kerala, India

Jagdish C Mohan MD DM FASE
Chairman, Department of Cardiology
Institute of Heart and Vascular Diseases
Jaipur Golden Hospital
New Delhi, India

Jayagopal P Balagopalan MD DM DNB FACC FSCAI FRCP(E)
Director and Interventional Cardiologist
Cardiology, Lakshmi Hospital
Palakkad, Kerala, India

Jayaraman Balachander MD DM
Senior Professor
Department of Cardiology
Jawaharlal Institute of Postgraduate Medical Education and Research
Puducherry, India

Jimmy George MD DM
Consultant Cardiologist
Department of Cardiology
Lisie Hospital
Kochi, Kerala, India

José Luis Zamorano MD PhD
Department of Cardiology
Hospital Ramón y Cajal.
Universidad de Alcalá
CIBERCV, Hospital Ramón y Cajal.
Madrid, Spain

Joseph Theodore MD DM
Assistant Professor
Department of Cardiology
Jawaharlal Institute of Postgraduate Medical Education and Research
Puducherry, India

JPS Sawhney DM FESC FACC
Chairperson
Department of Cardiology
Dharma Vira Heart Center
Sir Ganga Ram Hospital
New Delhi, India

Jugal Kishor Sharma MD FICP FACP FRCP (Glasgow and Edin) FACE FGSI FIMSA FIAMS FISH FDI
Medical Director and Senior Consultant
Internal Medicine Dibetes and Clinical Cardiology
Central Delhi Diabetes Centre
New Delhi, India

Julian Thottan MD DM
Cardiologist
Department of Cardiology
Westfort Hitech Hospital
Thrissur, Kerala, India

Kewal C Goswami MD DM
Professor
Department of Cardiology
All India Institute of Medical Sciences
New Delhi, India

K Tamilselvan MD DM
Assistant Professor
Department of Cardiology
Madras Medical College
Chennai, Tamil Nadu, India

K Venugopal MD DM
Professor
Department of Cardiology
Pushpagiri Institute of Medical Sciences and Research Centre
Thiruvalla, Kerala, India

Kailash K Goyal MD DM
Consultant Cardiologist
Department of Cardiology
Fathima Hospital
Kozhikode, Kerala, India

Kajal Ganguly MD DM FACC FESC FCSI FICP
Professor and Head
Department of Cardiology
Nil Ratan Sircar Medical College
Kolkata, West Bengal, India

Kamal K Sethi MD DM FHRS FACC FCSI FISE
Director
Department of Cardiology
Delhi Heart and Lung Institute
New Delhi, India
Chairman and Managing Director
Delhi Heart and Lung Institute
New Delhi, India

Kamaldeep Bansal MD
Fellow
Department of Cardiology
Institute of Medical Sciences
Banaras Hindu University
Varanasi, Uttar Pradesh, India

Kapil Kumawat MD DM CEPS CCDS
Senior Consultant Cardiologist
Department of Cardiology
Narayana Institute of Cardiac Sciences
Bangalore, Karnataka, India

Karishma Landge SRF
Senior Research Fellow
Department of Cardiology
All India Institute of Medical Sciences
New Delhi, India

Kevin Marzo MD FACC FSCAI
Chief of Cardiology
Department of Cardiology
NYU Winthrop Hospital
Mineola, NY USA

Kinjal Banerjee MD
Clinical Research Fellow
Cleveland Clinic, Cleveland, OH, USA

Kiran Gaur MSc PhD
Associate Professor
Statistics
Sri Karan Narendra College of Agriculture
Jaipur, Rajasthan, India

KK Aggarwal MD
Senior Consultant Cardiologist
Moolchand Hospital
President
Heart Care Foundation of India
Delhi, India

Krishnarpan Chatterjee MD DNB
Senior Resident
Department of Cardiology
Sanjay Gandhi Post Graduate Institute of Medical Sciences
Lucknow, Uttar Pradesh, India

Kushal Madan PhD FAHA
Cardiac Rehabilitation Consultant
Dharma Vira Heart Center
Sir Ganga Ram Hospital
New Delhi, India

Leah Raj MD
Fellow in Cardiology
Department of Cardiology
Keck School of Medicine of the University of Southern California
Los Angeles, CA, USA

Lekha Pathak MD DM SRCP
Director of Cardiology
Department of Cardiology
Nanavati Super Speciality Hospital
Mumbai, Maharashtra, India

MS Hiremath MD DM MNAMS
Director
Cathlab
Ruby Hall Clinic
Pune, India

M Sitaram DM MD FDSRCS FFDRCS
Cardiologist
Department of Cardiology
Apollo Hospitals
Secunderabad, Telangana, India

M Khalilullah MD DM
Director and Senior Consultant Cardiologist
The Heart Centre
New Delhi, India

Madhu Shukla Dip Card
Senior Clinical Associate
Department of Cardiology
Institute of Heart and Vascular Diseases
Jaipur Golden Hospital
New Delhi, India

Maki Ono MD
Clinical Fellow
Section of Cardiac Electrophysiology and Pacing
Department of Cardiovascular Medicine
Cleveland Clinic
Cleveland, Ohio, USA

Malay Acharya MD DM
Residential Medical Officer and Clinical Tutor
Department of Cardiology
NRS Medical College
Kolkata, West Bengal, India

Mandeep Bhargava MD DM
Director, Center for Ventricular Tachycardia
Section of Cardiac Electrophysiology and Pacing
Department of Cardiovascular Medicine
Cleveland Clinic
Cleveland, Ohio, USA

Manju Mani MS DA DNB
Director of Quality and Anaesthesiology
Department of Cardiac Surgery
Max Smart Super Speciality Hospital
New Delhi, India

Marina Pascual Izco MD PhD
Department of Cardiology
Hospital Ramón y Cajal
Universidad de Alcalá
Madrid, Spain

Mathew Samuel Kalarickal MD DM FACC FSCAI
Director, Cath Lab
Apollo Hospitals
Chennai, Tamil Nadu, India

Matthew I Tomey MD FACC
Assistant Professor
Medicine (Cardiology)
Icahn School of Medicine
Mount Sinai
New York, USA

Matthias Raschpichler MD
Smidt Heart Institute
Cedars-Sinai Medical Center
Los Angeles, USA

Md Abdul Azeez Asad MD DNB
Fellow
Department Interventional Cardiology
Apollo Hospital
Hyderabad, Telangana, India

Meenakshi MS MD DM
Fellow
Department Interventional Cardiology
Madras Medical Mission
Chennai, Tamil Nadu, India

Meghna Gupta MBBS
Physician
Department of Medicine
Kishori Ram Hospital and Diabetes Care Centre
Bhatinda, Punjab, India

Michael Valentine MD FACC
Senior Cardiologist
Stroobants Cardiovascular Center
Centra Health
Lynchburg, VA, USA

Milind Hote MS Mch
Professor
Department of CTVS
All India Institute of Medical Sciences
New Delhi, India

Mohanan Padinhare MD DM
Director and HOD
Department of Cardiology
Westfort Hitech Hospital
Thrissur, Kerala, India

Mohit D Gupta MD DM
Professor
Department of Cardiology
GB Pant Institute of Post Graduate Medical Education and Research
New Delhi, India

Mona Bhatia MD FRCR FSSCT FSCMR
Director and Head
Department of Imaging
Fortis Escorts Heart Institute
New Delhi, India

MP Girish MP MD DM
Professor
Department of Cardiology
GB Pant Institute of Post Graduate Medical Education and Research
New Delhi, India

Mrinal K Das MD DM FICP FICP FCSI
Consultant and Interventional Cardiologist
Department of Cardiology
BM Birla Heart Research Centre
Kolkata, West Bengal, India

Mullasari S Ajit MD DM FRCP
Director and Head
Department of Cardiology
Institute of Cardio Vascular Diseases
Madras Medical Mission hospital
Chennai, Tamil Nadu, India

Muzil Munshi DNB Resident
Cardiothoracic Surgery
Asian Heart Institute
Mumbai, Maharashtra, India

MV Padma Srivastava MD DM FAMS FNASc FIAN
Professor
Department of Neurology
All India Institute of Medical Sciences
New Delhi, India

Nagendra Boopathy Senguttuvan MD DM FACC FSCAI
Assistant Professor and Consultant
Department of Cardiology
Sri Ramachandra Medical College and Research Institute
Chennai, Tamil Nadu, India

Nakul Sinha MD DM
Senior Consultant and Chief Interventional Cardiologist
Cardiology
SAHARA and DIVINE Hospital
Lucknow, Uttar Pradesh, India

Narendra Kumar MD MSc PhD MCSE FCEP FRCP FACC FESC ECES
Consultant Electrophysiologist
Department of Cardiology
Paras HMRI Hospitals
Patna, Bihar, India

Narendra N Khanna MD DM FRCP (Lond, Edin and Glasg) FACC FESC FSCAI FCCP FAPSIC FIMSA FEISI FICC FIAMS FCSI FICP
Senior Consultant Interventional Cardiology
Cardiology and Vascular Interventions
Indraprastha Apollo Hospital
New Delhi, India

Naresh D Munot MD MRCP
Senior Registrar
Department of Cardiology
Bombay Hospital and Bombay Hospital Institute of Medical Sciences
Mumbai, Maharashtra, India

Naveen Garg MD DM DNB
Professor
Department of Cardiology
Sanjay Gandhi Post Graduate Institute of Medical Sciences
Lucknow, Uttar Pradesh, India

Neeraj A Desai MD
Consultant, Cardiology
Holy Family Hospital and Research Centre
Mumbai, Maharashtra, India

Neeraj Parakh MD DM MAMS FACC
Associate Professor
Department of Cardiology
All India Institute of Medical Sciences
New Delhi, India

Neha Maddali MD
Department of Cardiology
NYU Winthrop Hospital
Mineola, New York, USA

Neil Bardoloi MD DM FESC FACC
Managing Director and Head
Department of Cardiology
Excelcare Hospitals
Guwahati, Assam, India

Nihar Mehta MD DNB DNB Fellowship in Interventional Cardiology and Cardiovascular Imaging (South Korea)
Consultant Cardiologist
Department of Cardiology
Jaslok Hospital and Research Centre
Mumbai, Maharashtra, India

Nirav Kumar MD DNB
Associate Professor
Department of Cardiology
Indira Gandhi Institute of Medical Sciences Patna
Patna, Bihar, India

Niteen V Deshpande MD DM DNB FACC FESC
Director
Cath Lab
Cardiology
Spandan Heart Institute and Research Center
Nagpur, Maharashtra, India

Nitin Aggarwal MD DM
Consultant
Department of Cardiology
Sri Balaji Action Medical Institute
Rajiv Gandhi Cancer Institute And Research Centre
New Delhi, India

Nitin Modi DNB DM
Consultant
Department of Cardiology
CHL Hospital
Indore, Madhya Pradesh, India

Nitish Naik MD DM
Professor
Department of Cardiology
All India Institute of Medical Sciences
New Delhi, India

Nyal Borges MD
Department of Cardiology
Cleveland Clinic
Cleveland, Ohio, USA

Oussama Wazni MD
Section Head
Section of Cardiac Pacing and Electrophysiology
Department of Cardiovascular Medicine
Cleveland Clinic
Cleveland, Ohio, USA

OP Yadava MS DNB (General Surgery) DNB (CTVS) FIACS FICC FCSI
CEO and Chief Cardiac Surgeon
Department of Cardiology
National Heart Institute
New Delhi, India

PC Manoria MD DM FICA (USA) FESC (Europe) FIAMS
Director
Department of Cardiology
Manoria Heart and Critical Care Hospital
Bhopal, Madhya Pradesh, India

Pankaj Manoria MD DM FESC (Europe) FSCAI (USA) FICA (USA) FIAMS
Chief Intervention Cardiologist and Director
Cardiac Cath Lab
Manoria Heart and Critical Care Hospital
Bhopal, Madhya Pradesh, India

Panniyammakal Jeemon PhD MPH FRSPH FESC
Assistant Professor
Epidemiology
Sree Chitra Tirunal Institute for Medical Sciences and Technology
Trivandrum, Tamil Nadu, India

Parayoru K Asokan MD DM FRCP FICC FACC FSCAI FESC
Chief and Senior Consultant Cardiologist
Department of Cardiology
Fathima Hospital
Kozhikode, Kerala, India

Parneesh Arora MD DM
Principal Consultant Cardiology
Department of Cardiology
Fortis Hospital
Noida, Uttar Pradesh, India

Parth Parikh MD
Department of Cardiology
Cleveland Clinic, Cleveland
Ohio, USA

Pawan K Sharma MD FACC FSCAI
Assistant Professor
Department of Medicine
Division of Cardiology
Adjunct Assistant Professor
Department of Radiology and Imaging Sciences
University of Utah School of Medicine
Salt Lake City, Utah, USA

Pawan Tiwari MD DM
Assistant Professor
Department of Pulmonary Medicine and Sleep Disorders
All India Institute of Medical Sciences
New Delhi, India

Pintu Nahata MD DM (Cardio) FACC (USA) FSCAI (USA) FESC (Europe)
Professor and Head
Department of Cardiology
SP Medical College and HRMC Centre
Bikaner, Rajasthan, India

Prafulla G Kerkar MD DM DNB FACC FESC FSCAI FCSI
Professor and Head
Department of Cardiology
Seth GSMC and KEM Hospital
Mumbai, Maharashtra, India

Prakash Deedwania MD FACC FAHA FACP FASH FHFSA FESC
Professor
Department of Medicine
UCSF School of Medicine
San Francisco, California, USA

Praloy Chakraborty MD DM
Professor
Department of Cardiology
Vardhman Mahavir Medical College and Safdarjung Hospital
New Delhi, India

Pramod K Sharma MCh DNB
Senior Consultant Cardiac Surgery
Department of Cardiac Surgery
Max Smart Super Speciality Hospital
New Delhi, India

Pramod Sagar Arsikere MD
Senior Resident
Department of Cardiology
Sanjay Gandhi Postgraduate Institute of Medical Sciences
Lucknow, Uttar Pradesh, India

Pratap Chandra Rath MD DM
Head and Director, Apollo Hospitals
Hyderabad, Telangana, India

Pravesh Vishwakarma MD DM
Assistant Professor
Department of Cardiology
King George's Medical University
Lucknow, Uttar Pradesh, India

Pravin K Goel MD DM FACC
Professor and Head
Department of Cardiology
Sanjay Gandhi Post Graduate of Medical Sciences
Lucknow, Uttar Pradesh, India

Priya Jagia MD DNB
Professor
Department of Cardiovascular Radiology and Endovascular interventions
All India Institute of Medical Sciences
New Delhi, India

R Alagesan MD DM
Retired Professor
Department of Cardiology
Madras Medical College
Chennai, Tamil Nadu, India

Raj Makkar MD
Director, Interventional Cardiology and Cardiac Catheterization Laboratories
Assistant Director
Smidt Heart Institute
Cedars-Sinai Medical Center
Los Angeles, USA

Raj Pratap Singh MD DM
Senior Resident
Department of Cardiology
Sanjay Gandhi Postgraduate Institute of Medical Sciences
Lucknow, Uttar Pradesh, India

Raja Selvaraj MD DNB FCEP
Additional Professor and Head
Department of Cardiology
Jawaharlal Institute of Postgraduate Medical Education and Research
Puducherry, India

Rajan J Manjuran MD DM PGDHRM FCSI FACC
Emeritus Professor
Department of Cardiology
Pushpagiri Institute of Medical Sciences and Research Centre
Tiruvalla, Kerala, India

Rajdatt A Deore MD DM
Head
Department of Cardiology
AIMS Hospital
Pune, Maharashtra, India

Rajeev Bagarhatta MD DM
Senior Professor
Department of Cardiology
SMS Medical College
Jaipur, Rajasthan, India

Rajeev Gupta MD PhD
Chairman
Department of Preventive Cardiology and Internal Medicine
Eternal Heart Care Centre and Research Institute
Jaipur, Rajasthan, India

Rajeev Narang MD DM
Professor
Department of Cardiology
All India Institute of Medical Sciences
New Delhi, India

Rajesh A Dhopeshwarkar MD DM (AIIMS) FHRS CEPS
Consultant Interventional Cardiology and Electrophysiology
Department of Cardiology
Deenanath Mangeshkar Hospital
Pune, Maharashtra, India

Rajesh Khadgawat MD DM DNB MNAMS
Professor
Department of Endocrinology and Metabolism
All India Institute of Medical Sciences
New Delhi, India

Rajiv Agarwal MD DM
Senior Director
Department of Cardiology
Max Smart Super Speciality Hospital
New Delhi, India

Rajiv Bajaj MD DM
Consultant
Department of Cardiology
Batra Hospital
New Delhi, India

Rajnish Sardana MD DM
Chief
Cardiology, Pacing and Electrophysiology
Department of Cardiology
Jaypee Hospital
Noida, Uttar Pradesh, India

Rakesh Yadav MD DM
Professor
Department of Cardiology
All India Institute of Medical Sciences
New Delhi, India

Ramachandran Paramasivam MD DM
Fellow
Department of Interventional Cardiology
The Madras Medical Mission
Chennai, Tamil Nadu, India

Ramakanta Panda MCh
Vice Chairman and Managing Director
Chief of Cardiothoracic Surgery
Asian Heart Institute
Mumbai, Maharashtra, India

Ramakrishna Janapati MD DM
Consultant Cardiologist
Department of Cardiology
Citizens Hospital
Hyderabad, Telangana, India

Ramesh Daggubati MD FACC FSCAI
Associate Chief
Department of Cardiology
NYU Winthrop Hospital
Mineola, New York, USA

Ramu Adela PhD
Assistant Professor
Department of Pharmacology
National Institute of Pharmaceutical Education and Research
Guwahati, Assam, India

Ranjan Modi MD DM
Consultant Cardiologist
Department of Cardiology
Fortis Escorts Heart Institute
Okhla, New Delhi, India

Ranjit K Nath MD DM FESC FSCAI FACC
Professor and Head
Department of Cardiology
Dr Ram Manohar Lohia Hospital and PGIMER
New Delhi, India

Ravi R Kasliwal MD DM FASE FIMSA MNAMS
Chairman
Department of Clinical and Preventive Cardiology
Medanta - The Medicity
Gurugram, Haryana, India

Ravi V Prasad MD DM
Associate Professor
Department of Cardiology
Indira Gandhi Institute of Medical Sciences
Patna, Bihar, India

Richard Chazal MD
Medical Director
Heart and Vascular Institute
Fort Myers, Florida, USA

Rimpy Joseph MD DM DNB
Stroke Fellow
Department of Neurology
All India Institute of Medical Sciences
New Delhi, India

Rishi A Bhargava MD DM
Assistant Professor
Department of Cardiology
Seth GSMC and KEM Hospital
Mumbai, Maharashtra, India

Rishi Sethi MD DM FACC FESC FRCP FSCAI FAPSIC FCSI FISC MAMS
Professor
Department of Cardiology
King George's Medical University
Lucknow, Uttar Pradesh, India

Ritesh Kalwar MD
Consultant Physician
Department of General Medicine
Jorhat Christian Medical Centre Hospital
Jorhat, Assam, India

Rohit Bhatia MD DM DNB
Professor
Department of Neurology
All India Institute of Medical Sciences
New Delhi, India

Rohit Malhotra MD
Associate Professor
Department of Cardiovascular Medicine
University of Virginia Health System
Charlottesville, VA, USA

Roopa Salwan MD DM
Senior Director
Department of Cardiology
Max Super Speciality Hospital
New Delhi, India

Roopali Khanna MD DM FACC
Associate Professor
Department of Cardiology
Sanjay Gandhi Post Graduate Institute of Medical Sciences
Lucknow, Uttar Pradesh, India

SS Iyengar DM FRCP (E)
Consultant
Department of cardiology
Manipal Hospital
Bangalore, Karnataka, India

S Sivasankaran MD DM MNAMS
Professor
Cardiology
Sree Chitra Tirunal Institute for Medical Sciences and Technology
Trivandrum, Kerala, India

S Srikant MD
Senior Resident
Department of Cardiology
All India Institute of Medical Sciences
New Delhi, India

SS Chatterjee MD DM
Director
Department of Cardiology
Indira Gandhi Institute of Cardiology
Patna, Bihar, India

Sabarirajan Sokkaiyan MD
Registrar
Department of Cardiology
Kovai Medical Center and Hospital
Coimbatore, Tamil Nadu, India

Sachin Talwar MS MCh
Professor
Department of Cardiothoracic and Vascular Surgery
All India Institute of Medical Sciences
New Delhi, India

Sahil Sareen DM
Senior Resident
Department of Cardiology
Sawai Man Singh Hospital
Jaipur, Rajasthan, India

Sajith Pavitran MD DM
Cardiologist
Department of Cardiology
Apollo Hospitals
Secunderabad, Telangana, India

Saleha Noorain MD DNB
Cardiologist
Department of Cardiology
Manipal Hospital
Bangalore, Karnataka, India

Sameer Dani MD DM
Director
Department of Cardiology
Apollo Hospital
Ahmedabad, Gujarat, India

Samin Sharma MD
Director, Clinical and Interventional Cardiology President, Mount Sinai Heart Network
Dean of International Clinical Affiliations
Anandi Lal Sharma Professor of Medicine Icahn School

Samir Kapadia MD
Professor of Medicine
Director, Catheterization Laboratory
Cleveland Clinic
Cleveland, Ohio, USA

Sandeep Bansal MD DM
Professor and Head
Consultant, Department of Cardiology
Vardhman Mahavir Medical College and Safdarjung Hospital
New Delhi, India

Sandeep Seth MD DM
Professor
Department of Cardiology
All India Institute of Medical Sciences
New Delhi, India

Sandeep Singh MD DM
Professor
Department of Cardiology
All India Institute of Medical Sciences
New Delhi, India

Sanjay Mittal MD DM
Senior Director
Department of Clinical Cardiology and Research
Medanta - The Medicity
Gurugram, Haryana, India

Sanjay Shah MD DM
Director of Cardiology
Apex Heart Institute, Ahmedabad
Associate Professor
Department of Cardiology
Sheth VS General Hospital and
Smt NHL Municipal Medical College
Ahmedabad, Gujarat, India

Sanjeev Kumar MD
Assistant Professor
Cardiovascular Radiology and Endovascular Intervention
All India Institute of Medical Sciences
New Delhi, India

Sanjeev Sanghvi MD DM
Senior Professor
Department of Cardiology
Dr SN Medical College
Jodhpur, Rajasthan, India

Santanu Guha MD DM FACC FCSI FESC
Professor and Head
Department of Cardiology
Medical College Kolkata
Kolkata, West Bengal, India

Sarat Chandra MD DM FACC FESC FCSI
Consultant
Cardiology
Virinchi Hospital and Indo-US Hospital
Hyderabad, Telangana , India

Sarjun Basha SKM MD DNB
Consultant Cardiologist
Cardiology, Peacock Hospital
Tiruttani, Tamil Nadu, India

Satish K Kaushik MD DM FCSI FIAE FISC FACC
Patron Department of Cardiology
American International institute of Medical Sciences
Udaipur, Rajasthan, India

Satyanarayan Routray MD DM FACC
Professor
Department of Cardiology
Srirama Chandra Bhanja Medical College
Cuttack, Odisha, India

Satyavan Sharma MD DM FAMS FACC FESC FSCAI
Professor and Head
Department of Cardiology
Bombay Hospital Institute of Medical Sciences
Mumbai, Maharashtra, India

Satyendra Tewari MD DM FACC FSCAI FESC FAPSC FCSI FICC
Professor
Department of Cardiology
Sanjay Gandhi Postgraduate Institute of Medical Sciences
Lucknow, Uttar Pradesh, India

Saumitra Ray MD FRCP FCSI FICP FESC FACC
Professor
Department of Cardiology
Vivekananda Institute of Medical Sciences
Consultant Interventional Cardiologist
AMRI Hospitals and Woodland Hospital
Kolkata, West Bengal, India

Shantanu P Sengupta MD DNB FACC FASE
Heart Failure Specialist
Cardiology
Sengupta Hospital and Research Institute
Nagpur, Maharashtra, India

Sharad Agrawal MD DM MNAMS FICC FRCP FACC
Consultant Cardiologist and Honorary Senior Lecturer
Sunderland Royal Hospital
Sunderland, United Kingdom

Sharad Chandra DM FACC FESC FSCAI FAPSIC
Professor
Department of Cardiology
King George's Medical University
Lucknow, Uttar Pradesh, India

Sharad Kumar Parashar MD
Department of Medicine
Advance Institute of Medical Sciences
Bhopal, Madhya Pradesh, India

Shashank Jain DMRD DNB
Senior Resident
Department of Radiodiagnosis and Imaging
Fortis Escorts Heart Institute
New Delhi, India

Shashank R Joshi MD DM FICP FACP FACE FRCP (Lond, Glasg and Edin)
Consultant Endocrinologist
Department of Endocrinology
Joshi Clinic, Lilavati Hospital, Apollo Sugar Clinic and Bhatia Hospital
Mumbai, Maharashtra, India

Shishu Shankar Mishra MD FAIMS MCAM DoCM FCCP FIAE FICC FCSI
Professor and Director
Department of Cardiology
Hi-Tech Medical College
Bhubaneswar, Odisha, India
Director and Senior Consultant
Cardiologist Department of Cardiology
Med 'N' Heart Clinic
Cuttack, Odisha, India

Siddharthan Deepti MD DM
Assistant Professor
Department of Cardiology
All India Institute of Medical Sciences
New Delhi, India

Sohan K Sharma MD DM FSCAI (USA)
Assistant Professor
Department of Cardiology
SMS Medical College
Jaipur, Rajasthan, India

Sonia Arora DNHE
Consultant
Department of Diet and Nutrition
Kishori Ram Hospital and Diabetes Care Center and Pragma Hospital
Bathinda, Punjab, India

Soumik Chaudhuri MD DM
Consultant Cardiologist
Department of Cardiology
Peerless Hospital
Kolkata, West Bengal, India

Soumitra Kumar MD DM FCSI FACC FESC FSCAI FICC FIAE FICP
Professor and Head
Department of Cardiology
Vivekananda Institute of Medical Sciences
Kolkata, West Bengal, India

Soura Mookerjee MD DTM&H DM FACC FESC
Professor of Cardiology
North Bengal Medical College
Darjeeling , West Bengal, India

Sulthan R Salih MD
Senior resident in Cardiology
Department of Cardiology
Pushpagiri Institute of Medical Sciences and Research Centre
Tiruvalla, Kerala, India

Sumanta Chatterjee MD DM
Consultant Cardiologist
Department of cardiology
AMRI Hospitals
Kolkata, West Bengal India

Sundeep Mishra MD DM FACC FSCAI
Professor
Department of Cardiology
All India Institute of Medical Sciences
New Delhi, India

Sunil Modi MD DM FACC FICC FCSI
Senior Consultant Cardiologist
Apollo Heart Institute
Indraprastha Apollo Hospital
New Delhi, India

Sunil Sharma DNB FSCAI
Consultant
Department of Cardiology
CHL Hospital
Indore, Madhya Pradesh, India

Sunil Vanzara MCh CVTS MD
Consultant Surgeon
Cardiothoracic Surgery
Asian Heart Institute
Mumbai, Maharashtra, India

Suparna Rao MRCP (UK)
Clinical Associate
Department of Cardiology
Indraprastha Apollo Hospitals
New Delhi, India

Surender Deora MD DM
Associate Professor
Department of Cardiology
All India Institute of Medical Sciences
Jodhpur, Rajasthan, India

Surendra K Chutani DM
Consultant Cardiologist
Department of Cardiology
New York Presbyterian Hospital Center
New York, USA

Swati Mahajan MD
Senior Resident
Department of Cardiology
Dr SN Medical College
Jodhpur, Rajasthan, India

TK Mishra MD DM
Professor and Head
Department of Cardiology
MKCG Medical College
Brahmapur, Orissa, India

TS Kler MD DM FRCP FACC DSc (Honoris Causa)
Chairman
PSRI Heart Institute
New Delhi, India

Tarun Chakravarty MD
Smidt Heart Institute
Cedars-Sinai Medical Center
Los Angeles, USA

Tejas Patel MD DM FCSI FACC FSCAI FESC
Chairman and Chief Interventional Cardiologist
Apex Heart Institute, Ahmedabad
Professor and Head
Department of Cardiology
Sheth VS General Hospital and
Smt NHL Municipal Medical College
Ahmedabad, Gujarat, India

Thomas Alexander MD DM FACC
Head
Department of Cardiology
Kovai Medical Center and Hospital
Coimbatore, Tamil Nadu, India

Umesh C Samal MD FICC FIACM FACC FIAE FISE FISC FAPVS FEAC
Director
Cardiology - Heart Failure, Paras – HMRI Hospital Patna and Permanent Chief Trustee, ICC HFFI Patna
Patna, Bihar, India

Upendra Kaul MD DM FCSI FSCAI FAPSIC FACC FAMS
Executive Director and Dean
Department of Cardiology
Batra Hospital and Medical Research Center
New Delhi, India

VK Bahl MD DM
Professor and Head
Department of Cardiology
All India Institute of Medical Sciences
New Delhi, India

Vanita Arora MD DNB
Director and Head, Cardiac Electrophysiology Lab and Arrhythmia Services
Senior Consultant Cardiac Electrophysiologist and Interventional Cardiologist
Max Healthcare Super Speciality Hospital
New Delhi, India

Varun Gupta MS Masters in Thoracic Surgery
Research Associate
Thoracic Surgery
Lugenklinik Hemer
Hemer, North Rhine-Westphalia, Germany

Vidyut Jain MD FACC FSCAI FESC
Chairman and Consultant
Department of Cardiology
Choithram hospital and research center
Indore, Madhya Pradesh, India

Vijay Iyer MD PhD FACC FSCAI
Associate Professor
Department of Medicine
University at Buffalo
Buffalo, New York, USA

Vijay Kumar Chopra MD DM FACC
Director, Heart Failure Program
Medanta - The Medicity
Gurugram, Haryana, India

Vikas Singh MD DM FACC
Consultant Intervention Cardiologist
Department of Cardiology
Daksh Heart Care and 4A Heart Hospital
Patna, Bihar, India

Vikash Kumar MD
Fellow, Department of Cardiology
Sri Ramachandran Institute of Higher Education and Research
Chennai, Tamil Nadu, India

Vineeta Ojha DM
Assistant Professor
Cardiovascular Radiology and Endovascular Intervention
All India Institute of Medical Sciences
New Delhi, India

Vishnu VY MD DM
Assistant Professor
Department of Neurology
All India Institute of Medical Sciences
New Delhi, India

Vishwas Mohan Dip Card
Attending Cardiologist
Department of Cardiology
Max Hospital Saket
New Delhi, India

Vitull K Gupta MD FICP FCSI FACP
Professor and Unit Head
Department of Medicine
Aditya Institute of Management Studies and Research
Mumbai, Maharashtra, India

Consultant
Kishori Ram Hospital and Diabetes Care Centre
Bhatinda, Punjab, India

Vivek Singh Rathore MD
Resident, Department of Cardiology
BM Birla Heart Research Centre
Kolkata, West Bengal, India

Vivudh P Singh MD DM
Associate Consultant
Department of Interventional Cardiology, Fortis Escorts Heart Institute
New Delhi, India

Walid I Saliba MD
Director, EP Lab Director and Center for Atrial Fibrillation, Section of Cardiac Electrophysiology and Pacing
Department of Cardiovascular Medicine
Cleveland Clinic
Cleveland, Ohio, USA

PREFACE

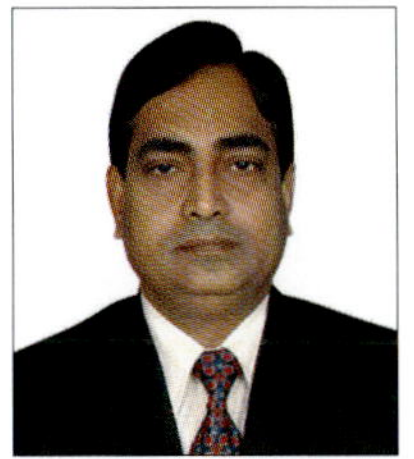

Editor-in-Chief
Kewal C Goswami MD DM
Professor
Department of Cardiology
All India Institute of Medical Sciences
New Delhi, India

I am pleased to offer *Cardiology Update – 2018* for release at the 70th Annual Conference of the Cardiological Society of India. As President – Elect of this august body I must remind our entire community that cardiovascular diseases remain the scourge of modern day life where the demands and pressures of a fast moving lifestyle are in direct conflict with human biological needs. Developing countries like ours are facing the brunt of this epidemic grappling with cardiovascular disease in ever younger populations at the peak of their productive lives, often nipping careers that are yet to find flight. Though considerable progress has been achieved in the understanding and treatment of cardiovascular diseases with an era of personalized medicine not too far distant in the future in the developed world, the cardiologist in countries like ours still faces challenges in knitting together a strategy that is realistic and affordable for his patient. Yet this strategy has to be scientifically robust and find peer acceptance across the entire community of cardiologists. Equally he is required to extend state of the art care for his other group of elite patients who can easily move across continents to seek contemporary care. This dual challenge is an enigmatic problem for which solutions will not be easy to define and implement. I hope readers of the book are motivated and spurred to greater ideas and loftier goals in helping our country tackle this menace of cardiovascular diseases.

With the burgeoning amount of information already available on the web and in print, colleagues often question me on the need for another textbook on cardiology. Indeed even I was flummoxed about whether I should indeed embark upon such a venture or whether this was an exercise in futility. Exhaustive texts are so easily available at the press of a button of your phone, tablet and laptop. However paradoxically, there are many textbooks of cardiology and even more journals, focused updates of relevant contemporary topics in everyday cardiology often do not find space in both textbooks as well as journals. Lengthy discourses in modern day cardiology textbooks (and subspecialty reviews in journals) often obfuscate bed side dilemmas of modern medicine and a litany of clinical trials published every other week sometimes create more questions that offering answers. This edition of *Cardiology Update – 2018* attempts to bring into sharp focus these very controversial yet relevant topics, with views from Indian experts that define approaches and color practices in our sphere of life. This reflects the theme of this years' 70th Annual Conference of Cardiological Society of India – Translating Recent Advances into Regional Needs. We hope this book is useful not only for residents in training, but also for general physicians and general cardiologists as well as for interventional cardiologists and electrophysiologists. A lot of effort was put in compiling topics that are relevant for everyday cardiology and find scant mention in available texts. Medicine is as much an art as it is a science. As many of these chapters are authored by leading subject experts in the country, we hope the reader is not only enriched with knowledge that is captured from an Indian standpoint, but also able to translate this into improving his/her practice, an important objective of this book (as well as the conference).

I am profusely thankful to the galaxy of reputed national and international faculty who have taken considerable time and effort to compile this edition of Cardiology Update. I recognize they have taken precious time out of their busy schedules to give their considered views on important issues on contemporary cardiology and appreciate their sincere efforts in making this book possible. I would also like to place on record my sincere gratitude for Jaypee Publishers in working tirelessly with the authors and compiling this book. Mankind Pharmaceuticals has been very kind to extend an unrestricted educational grant for the publication of this book and I am deeply grateful to them. I also extend my sincere thanks to the members of the entire Cardiological Society of India including its office bearers in offering constructive advice and guidance and being supportive in making this manuscript possible. I am also greatly indebted to my editorial team in painstakingly going through the numerous manuscripts.

I would be failing in my duty if I do not acknowledge my family including my wife and mother for putting up with my prolonged absences from home.

With warm personal regards

CONTENTS

SECTION 1: CORONARY ARTERY DISEASE RISK FACTORS

1. Smokeless Tobacco and Cardiovascular Disease 3

Surender Deora, Kewal C Goswami

Pharmacokinetics of smokeless tobacco 5
Smokeless tobacco and cardiovascular risk factors 5
Smokeless tobacco and cardiovascular disease 6
Health policy implications 6

2. Alcohol and Coronary Artery Disease: Fact versus Fiction 8

JPS Sawhney, Kushal Madan

Understanding "standard drink" 8
Alcohol and cardiovascular mortality 8
Alcohol and coronary artery disease 8
Alcohol and cardiovascular medications 9
Possible mechanisms for coronary artery disease protection by alcohol 9
Drinking patterns and coronary heart disease 9
Influence of age and sex on cardiovascular effects of alcohol 9
The genetics of alcohol and cardiovascular disease 10
Points to consider from the past studies 10
Alcohol and Indian population 11
Detrimental effects of alcohol intake 11
A word of caution 11

3. Vitamin D and Cardiovascular Disease: Indian Perspective 13

Ramu Adela, Rajesh Khadgawat

Assessment of vitamin D nutritional status 13
Vitamin D nutritional status in the world and in India 13
Vitamin D and nonskeletal effects 14
Vitamin D and cardiovascular diseases 14
Mechanism of vitamin D and proposed cardioprotection 15
Vitamin D and cardiovascular disease: evidences from observational studies 15
Vitamin D and cardiovascular disease: evidences from interventional studies 17
Indian studies 17

4. Hormone Replacement Therapy and Cardiovascular Diseases 20

Geetha Subramanian, Aviraj Choudhary, Kamaldeep Bansal

Menopause-induced changes in cardiovascular functions 20
Effects of hormone replacement therapy on coronary heart disease risk 21
Clinical studies of hormone replacement therapy and coronary heart disease 21

SECTION 2: LIPIDS AND DIET

5. Cholesterol and Coronary Artery Disease Controversy 27

Rajiv Bajaj

Cholesterol and coronary artery disease controversy 27
Functions of cholesterol 28
Early research on cholesterol 29
Diet and health 30
Present and future 31

6. Indian Dyslipidemia: Challenges in Management 32

Saumitra Ray, Sumanta Chatterjee

Indian epidemiological studies on dyslipidemia 32
Association between lipid levels and risk of heart disease in India 33
Laboratory parameters assessment 34
Inadequate management of dyslipidemia in India 34
Indian guideline recommendation on dyslipidemia management 34
Cardiovascular risk stratification of Indian patient 35
Treatment goal according to ASCVD risk stratification 35
Cardiovascular disease prevention: lipid targets 35
Lowering of low-density lipoprotein reduces risk of cardiovascular events 36
Drugs for management of dyslipidemia 36
Drugs for management of hypertriglyceridemia 36
Familial hypercholesterolemia in India 37
Dyslipidemia in type 2 diabetes and metabolic syndrome 37
Dyslipidemia in acute coronary syndrome 37
Dyslipidemia in moderate-to-severe chronic kidney disease 37
Dyslipidemia and stroke prevention 37
Safety assessment during pharmacotherapy in dyslipidemia 37

7. Indian Diet and Coronary Artery Disease 39

Abhishek Gupta, MP Girish, Mohit D Gupta

Prevalence of disease—is there underestimation of actual problem? 39
Diet and coronary artery disease: evidence 39
Indian diet 39
Contaminated vegetarianism 40
Oil consumption 40
Fruit and vegetables in Indian diet—more productions but less consumption 41
Antioxidants—do they have any role in our diet? 42
Protein source—Indian food/cuisine is high in carbs, starch, and fat 42
Susceptibility of Indians 43
Preventive measures to reduce this epidemic 43

8. Edible Oils: What is Right and What is Wrong? 46

Sonia Arora, Vitull K Gupta, Meghna Gupta

Composition of fats 46
Trans fatty acids or partially hydrogenated fatty acids 47

Cholesterol 48
What are edible oils? 48
What is right and what is wrong oil? 48
Characteristics of different oils 49
Choosing the right oil 50
Why rotation or blending is needed? 50

9. Statins and Diabetes **53**
Rajeev Bagarhatta, Sohan K Sharma, Dinesh Gautam
Pathophysiology of dyslipidemia in diabetes 53
Management of dyslipidemia in diabetes 53
New onset diabetes with statin 55

10. Statin Intolerance: Guide to Management **57**
Mrinal K Das
Definitions of statin intolerance 57
Types of statin intolerance 57
Anecdotal data 58
Clinical features 58
Evaluation of statin intolerance 59
Management 60
Alternative agents 61
Indian experience with statin-induced muscle symptom 62

11. Nonfasting Lipid Levels: Clinical Relevance and Implications for Practice **66**
Ajay K Sinha, Vikas Singh, Narendra Kumar
Rationale for requirement of a fasting sample 66
Emergence of nonfasting levels measurement 66
Lipid component measurement 67

SECTION 3: DIABETES AND HEART

12. Diabetes and Cardiovascular Disease: Implications of Recent Cardiovascular Outcome trials with Newer Anti-diabetic Drugs for Cardiovascular Protection **73**
Prakash Deedwania
Background 73
Therapeutic strategies for control of cardiovascular disease in diabetes 74
Role of antidiabetic (hypoglycemic) medications in cardiovascular protection 75

13. Diabetes Classification New Dimensions **79**
Jugal Kishor Sharma, Amit Gupta
Diabetes classification: history 79
Diabetes classification: why do we need a new classification system? 79
New proposed classification of diabetes 80

14. **Prevention of Coronary Artery Disease in Diabetes Mellitus** 83
Ranjan Modi, Sunil Modi
Lifestyle modification 83
Lipid-lowering therapy 84
Antithrombotic medications 86
Bariatric surgery 86
Future or what is in horizon 86

15. **Diabetes and Coronary Artery Disease: Prevalence and Mechanisms** 89
Satyanarayan Routray, Dipak R Das
Prevalence of diabetes and coronary artery disease 89
Diabetes and coronary artery disease: mechanisms 90

16. **Management of Diabetes in Heart Failure** 95
Shashank R Joshi
The problem 95
Screening for heart failure in type 2 diabetes mellitus 95
Glycemia control and heart failure: choice of antidiabetic therapies 96
Metformin 96
Sodium-glucose cotransporter 2 inhibitors 96
Dipeptidyl peptidase-4 inhibitors 97
Glucagon-like peptide-1 receptor agonists 97
Sulfonylureas 97
Thiazolidinediones 98
Insulin 98

SECTION 4: HYPERTENSION

17. **Epidemiology of Hypertension in India: The Real Scenario** 103
Rajeev Gupta, Kiran Gaur
Systematic reviews of epidemiological studies 103
Association of hypertension with macrolevel risk factors 110

18. **Primary Prevention of Hypertension** 113
Panniyammakal Jeemon, Dorairaj Prabhakaran
Classification of hypertension 113
The need for primary prevention of hypertension in India 113
Primary prevention 114
GAPS in knowledge and future research needs 116

19. **Cutoff for Hypertension: Implications of 2017 Guidelines for Indian Patients** 119
Rajeev Narang, S Srikant
Other highlights 121

20. Initial Choice of Drugs in Uncomplicated Hypertension: Not Monotherapy Anymore but Combination 123

C Venkata S Ram

Pharmacological treatment of hypertension 123
An abbreviated overview of drugs for initial combination therapy 125
Initial combination therapy not monotherapy is the answer for blood pressure control 126

21. Are ACE inhibitor and ARB Equal in Hypertension? 129

SS Chatterjee, Arka Chatterjee

Mechanism of action 129
Efficacy in reducing blood pressure 129
Efficacy for surrogate clinical outcomes 130
Effects in select patient subsets 130
Adverse effects and patient compliance 131
Cost-effectiveness 131

22. Diuretics as Antihypertensive in Elderly 133

Anunay Gupta, HS Isser

Issues with elderly population 133
Blood pressure goals and targets 133
Clinical trials in elderly population 134
Diuretics as first line antihypertensive drug 135

23. Treating Resistant Hypertension: Stepwise Approach 137

Binjo Vazhappilly, Julian Thottan, Mohanan Padinhare

Stepwise evaluation of resistant hypertension 137

24. Secondary Hypertension: When and How to Screen 142

Anjan Lal Dutta, Soumik Chaudhuri

Who to screen? 142
What to do before screening for secondary hypertension? 143
Conditions requiring reevaluation, after starting antihypertensive therapy 143
Role of ambulatory 24-hour blood pressure monitoring 144
Role of echocardiography in secondary hypertension 144
How to screen? 144
Uncommon causes of secondary hypertension 146
When secondary hypertension may present as resistant hypertension 147

25. Managing Low Diastolic Blood Pressure in Elderly Hypertensive 150

HK Chopra, AK Pancholia

Pathophysiology of the J-curve 150
Diastolic blood pressure control: how low is too low? Clinical trial evidences 151
Low diastolic blood pressure and atherosclerosis in elderly subjects 151
Isolated diastolic hypotension and incident heart failure in elderly 151

26. **Ambulatory Blood Pressure Monitoring—When to Order and How to Interpret?** 153
Rajan J Manjuran, Sulthan R Salih
History and relevance of ABPM 153
Procedure 153
Indications 154
Merits and drawbacks 157
Future directions 158

27. **Home Blood Pressure Monitoring: Current Status** 160
Vidyut Jain, Avani Jain
Review of literature 160

SECTION 5: CHRONIC CORONARY ARTERY DISEASE

28. **Best Method for Risk Stratification in CAD—Anatomy, Physiology, or Both** 167
Pawan K Sharma, Kewal C Goswami
Methods for risk stratification in CAD 167
Risk stratification using noninvasive methods 167
Risk stratification using invasive methods 169
Potential uses and limitations of the traditional syntax score 170

29. **Screening for Coronary Artery Disease in Asymptomatic Adults** 173
Pratap Chandra Rath, Md Abdul Azeez Asad
Rationale for screening 173
Screening tests 173
Anatomic (imaging) techniques 175
Other methods for the assessment of cardiovascular risk 176
Safety of screening tests 176

30. **Optimal Medical Management for Chronic Stable Angina in 2018** 179
Satyavan Sharma, Naresh D Munot
Lessons learnt from randomized trials 179
What constitutes optimal medical therapy? 180
Other drugs for angina 184

31. **Beta-Blockers in Chronic Stable Coronary Artery Disease: Current Status** 187
J Shiv Kumar, M Sitaram, Sajith Pavitran, G Nagarjuna
Incidence and prevalence 187
Pathophysiology of coronary artery disease 187
Pharmacotherapeutics of beta-blockers 188
Newer generations of beta-blockers 188
Adverse effects of beta-blockers 189
Guidelines for use of beta-blockers in angina 189

32. Revascularization in Chronic Stable Angina—Current Status **191**

Parneesh Arora, Upendra Kaul

Evidence from trials 191
Current approach to revascularization for SIHD 192
Indications for coronary angiography 192
Choice of revascularization PCI or coronary artery bypass grafting 192

33. Revascularization in Diabetes: Rational Choices in 2018 **198**

Rajiv Agarwal

Surgery or percutaneous coronary intervention 199
Freedom trial 199
Other randomized trials 199
Incomplete revascularization 200
Second-generation drug-eluting stents 200
Real world scenario 200
Registry data 200
Rational choice of revascularization strategy: evolving a consensus 200
New randomized trials needed 201
Comparison with medical therapy 201
Acute coronary syndromes 201
Type and duration of diabetes 201

34. Enhanced External Counterpulsation: Current Status **204**

Ashok Goyal

Enhanced external counterpulsion in coronary artery disease and heart failure treatment 204
Mechanism of action 205
Indications and contraindications 207
Enhanced external counterpulsion in extracardiac diseases 208

35. Cardiac Rehabilitation: The Road Less Travelled **210**

Satyendra Tewari, Raj Pratap Singh

Indications of cardiac rehabilitation 211
Inpatient cardiac rehabilitation 211
Barriers to cardiac rehabilitation in India 212

SECTION 6: ACUTE CORONARY SYNDROMES

36. Why Seek Vulnerable Coronary Plaques? **217**

Amir Ahmadi, Michael Valentine, Rick Chazal, Jagat Narula

What is a vulnerable plaque? 217
How is vulnerable plaque identified? 218
The quantitative extent of high-risk features 218
The number of adverse plaque characteristics 219
The evidence of plaque progression 219

37. Protecting Heart from Ischemia-Reperfusion Injury: Current Understanding **221**

Jabir Abdullakutty, Jimmy George

Mediators of myocardial reperfusion injury 221
Therapies to reduce ischemic injury 223
Reperfusion by primary percutaneous coronary intervention, thrombolysis, or both 223
Other therapies to reduce ischemic injury 223
Pharmacological interventions to reduce reperfusion injury 224

38. Risk Stratification in Unstable Angina/NSTEMI: A Current Approach **226**

Anoop Jain, CB Meena, Sahil Sareen

Epidemiology 226
Pathophysiology 226
Clinical and risk assessment 226
Noninvasive testing 228
Stratification of risk 228
Management 230

39. hs-cTroponin in Acute Coronary Syndrome: Current Status **235**

Amal K Banerjee

Clinical perspective 236
Clinical practice guidelines 236
Risk assessment and outcomes 237

40. Managing Acute Coronary Syndrome in Renal Dysfunction **240**

Parayoru K Asokan, Kailash K Goyal

Pathophysiology 240
Diagnosis of acute coronary syndrome in patients with renal dysfunction 240
Management 240

SECTION 7: ST-SEGMENT ELEVATION MYOCARDIAL INFARCTION

41. Burden and Outcome of STEMI in India **249**

Santanu Guha, Avik Karak

Preamble 249
Burden of cardiovascular diseases in India 249
Burden of cardiovascular disease risk factors 250
Determinants of cardiovascular disease in Indians 250
Epidemiology of STEMI in India 250
Outcome of STEMI 251

42. Choosing Fibrinolytics in STEMI: Economics over Efficacy? **256**

Mullasari S Ajit, Meenakshi MS

Importance of early revascularization 256
Pharmacoinvasive strategy 256

Fibrinolytic drugs—classification and comparison 257
Efficacy of fibrinolytics—based on trials 257
Choice of fibrinolytic in ST-elevation myocardial infarction 258

43. Routine PCI after IV Thrombolysis—Is it Ready for Prime Time? 260
Lekha Pathak, Ankur Jhavar
Strategy clock in STEMI 260
Treatment delay in STEMI 260
Reperfusion strategies 261

44. Revascularizing Nonculprit Artery in AMI: Uniform Strategy or Case-based Approach 265
Ranjit K Nath, Kewal C Goswami
Approach to the management of nonculprit lesions in STEMI 265

45. Improving Outcomes of Primary Percutaneous Coronary Intervention: Technical Aspects 271
Ambukeshwar Singh, Ayush Shukla, Nakul Sinha
Prehospital or patient preparation 271
Loading dose 271
Role of counseling 272
Angiography 272
Slow flow or no reflow 273
Deferred stenting 274

46. Late Presenters with STEMI: Which is the Best Strategy? 276
Soumitra Kumar
Risk stratification in latecomers after STEMI 276
Reperfusion PCI in latecomers with STEMI 277
Nonreperfusion options for late presenters with STEMI 278

47. Acute Coronary Syndrome in Elderly 281
Surender Deora, Kewal C Goswami
Challenges in elderly 281
Management 282
Medical management 282
Thrombolysis versus primary percutaneous coronary intervention 283
Cardiac rehabilitation 283

48. Right Ventricular Myocardial Infarction: An Update 286
Shishu Shankar Mishra, Biswaranjan Mishra
Definition 286
Incidence 286
Pathophysiology 286
Clinical presentation 287
Differential diagnosis 287

Management 289
Prognosis 290

49. Cardiogenic Shock in Myocardial Infarction: Optimal Approach **292**
Siddharthan Deepti, Sandeep Singh
Definitions 292
Incidence, temporal trends, and etiologies 292
Outcomes 292
Management 293

50. Optimizing STEMI Care—Developing Regional Networks **298**
Sabarirajan Sokkaiyan, Thomas Alexander
Magnitude of the problem 298
Developing regional STEMI networks—the STEMI India experience 299

SECTION 8: DUAL ANTIPLATELET THERAPY

51. Choice of Dual Antiplatelet Therapy in Acute Coronary Syndrome: Is There a Consensus? **305**
Hiremath MS, Deore RA
Aspirin 306
Ticlopidine 306
Clopidogrel 306
Prasugrel 308
Ticagrelor 308

52. Optimal Duration of Dual Antiplatelet Therapy after Acute Coronary Syndrome: Current Status **311**
Dhiman Kahali, Vivek Singh Rathore
Risk stratification tools for ischemia and bleeding risks 311
Type of P2Y12 inhibitor and timing of initiation 312
DAPT after percutaneous coronary intervention for ACS 313
DAPT in patients treated with CABG surgery for ACS 315
DAPT for patients with medically managed ACS 316
Resistance to drugs 317
Duration of DAPT after PCI in patients with peripheral artery disease 317

53. Switching Between DAPT Agents: The Right Strategy **320**
Harinder K Bali, Hiteshi KC Chauhan
Dual antiplatelet therapy clinical conundrum unraveled 320
Switching modalities 322
Switching between various oral P2Y12 Inhibitors 322
Switching between oral and intravenous P2Y12 inhibitors 329
Platelet function testing and switching of P2Y12 inhibitors 332
The way forward: what is the right strategy to switch DAPT? 332

54. **Management of Bleeding in Planned or Unplanned Surgery in a Patient on Dual Antiplatelet Therapy** 336

Sameer Dani

Dual antiplatelet therapy and pharmacology 336
Prevention of bleeding 337
Treatment of bleeding 339

SECTION 9: CORONARY INTERVENTION

55. **History and Evolution of Coronary Intervention** 345

Dev B Pahlajani, Akshay Mehta

Arrival of coronary angiography 347
New devices 349
History of fractional flow reserve, intravascular ultrasound, and optical coherence tomography 350

56. **Bifurcation Stenting: Optimal Strategy in 2018** 353

Ashwin B Mehta, Nihar Mehta

Definitions and classifications 353
Anatomical considerations 353
Relation between sizes of vessels: Murray's law and finet's law 355
Plaque shift versus carina shift 355
Threatened side branch morphologies: Preventing side branch occlusion 355
Stenting strategy in bifurcation lesions—one or two stents? 356
Tips and tricks 359

57. **Left Main Coronary Artery Stenting in 2018** 363

DS Gambhir

Stenting versus bypass surgery for left main coronary artery disease 363
Very long-term follow-up after left main coronary artery stenting 365
Current guidelines for left main coronary artery stenting 365
Selection of left main bifurcation stenting strategy 365
Role of adjust devices 366
Personal experience 368

58. **Current Update in the Treatment of Calcified Lesions** 370

Matthew I Tomey, Samin Sharma

Identification and classification of calcification 370
Patient and lesion selection 371
Wire selection 371
Modification of calcified lesions 371
Performance of atheroablation 373
Postatheroablation angioplasty and stenting 376
Comparative efficacy 376
Other devices 376

59. Protected Percutaneous Coronary Interventions: Treating the Complex Higher-risk Indicated Patients **379**

Mathew Samuel Kalarickal, Ramachandran Paramasivam

Complex high-risk indicated patients 379
CHIP PCI hospital 380
CHIP physician 380
Patient evaluation and procedure planning 380
Hemodynamic support devices 380
Post-procedure care 382
Current evidence 382

60. Ostial Coronary Lesions: Tips and Tricks for the Interventionist **384**

Pravesh Vishwakarma, Rishi Sethi

Morphology and histology 384
Diagnostic challenges 384
Selection of hardwares 385
Special techniques for ostial stent placement 388

61. Approach to Management of Chronic Total Occlusion **391**

Pravin K Goel, Roopali Khanna

Imaging of chronic total occlusion lesions 392
Predictors of chronic total occlusion-percutaneous coronary intervention success 392
Hybrid algorithm for chronic total occlusion-percutaneous coronary intervention 393
Chronic total occlusion-percutaneous coronary intervention techniques 393
Complications of chronic total occlusion-percutaneous coronary intervention 394

62. Hybrid Coronary Revascularization **396**

C Raghu

Benefits of coronary artery bypass grafting over percutaneous coronary intervention 396
Why percutaneous coronary intervention is preferred in practice? 396
In coronary artery bypass grafting, which is the preferred surgical conduit? 397
Which is better on-pump versus off-pump surgery? 397
Minimally invasive direct coronary artery bypass surgery 397
Robotic-assisted coronary artery bypass grafting 397
Endoscopic bypass grafting 397
Hybrid coronary revascularization 397
Hybrid outcomes 398

63. Should all Percutaneous Coronary Interventions be Radial Only? **400**

Tejas Patel, Surender Deora, Sanjay Shah

Background 400

64. Contemporary Coronary Stents: Implications for My Practice **404**

Neha Maddali, Kevin Marzo, Ramesh Daggubati

Design 405
Implications on clinical practice 407
Drug-eluting stent safety and efficacy in specific patient populations 408

65. **Fractional Flow Reserve and Instantaneous Wave-free Ratio—Which Should Be the Gold Standard?** **411**

Nagendra Boopathy Senguttuvan, Nitish Naik, Kewal C Goswami

Fractional flow reserve 411
Advantages of fractional flow reserve 412
Clinical utility of fractional flow reserve 413
Case study 414
Instantaneous wave-free pressure ratio 416
Comparison of invasive physiological indices to noninvasive physiology measured by positron emission tomography 416
Hybrid approach 417
Standalone instantaneous wave-free ratio approach 417
Merits and demerits 417

66. **Optical Coherence Tomography in Coronary Artery Disease: A Review** **419**

Ashwat S Dhillon, Leah Raj, Anil Kumar Mehra

Principles of optical coherence tomography 419
Preparation of imaging system and image acquisition 420
Optical coherence tomography interpretation in intracoronary imaging 420
Optical coherence tomography versus intravascular ultrasound 421
Correlation of optical coherence tomography with fractional flow reserve 422
Clinical utility of optical coherence tomography imaging 422
Stent selection (diameter and length) 423
Optimization after stent deployment 423

67. **Stem Cells in Cardiovascular Disease: Is there an indication?** **426**

Vijay Iyer

Challenges in cell therapy 426
Cell types and mechanisms 427
Clinical trials with stem cells 427
Nonischemic dilated cardiomyopathy 431
Future directions in cell therapy and lessons learned 431

68. **Future of Interventional Cardiology** **433**

VK Bahl, Dinkar Bhasin

Percutaneous mitral valve therapies 433

SECTION 10: INTERVENTION IN STRUCTURAL HEART DISEASE

69. **TAVR: Indications and Limitations in Clinical Practice** **443**

Tarun Chakravarty, Matthias Raschpichler, Chinar Patel, Raj Makkar

Eligibility for transcatheter aortic valve replacement 443
Transcatheter aortic valve replacement for degenerative bioprosthetic aortic valves 444
Current generation commercially available transcatheter aortic valve 445
Indications for transcatheter aortic valve replacement 445
Limitations of transcatheter aortic valve replacement 445

70. Imaging for Transcatheter Aortic Valve Implantation: Practical Aspects **448**

Kinjal Banerjee, Nyal Borges, Parth Parikh, Samir Kapadia

Planning phase 448
Planning phase: procedural planning 449
Procedure phase 451
Postprocedure follow-up 452

71. Alcohol Ablation for HOCM: Progress over the Past Two Decades **455**

Hubert Seggewiss, Angelika Koljaja-Batzner

Historical development of percutaneous septal ablation 455
Indication for septal ablation 455
Technique of septal ablation 456
Acute results and complications 458
Follow-up results 459

72. Percutaneous Management of Paravalvular Leak: Patient Selection and Outcomes **462**

A Sreenivas Kumar, Ramakrishna Janapati

Etiology of paravalvular leak 462
Clinical diagnosis 462
Imaging 462
Indications for paravalvular leak closure 465
Devices for percutaneous paravalvular leak closure 465
Technique of transcatheter paravalvular leak closure 465
Outcomes and complications of paravalvular leak closure procedures 467
Medical therapy 467

73. Left Atrial Appendage Closure Device for Stroke Prevention in Atrial Fibrillation **468**

Balbir Singh

Existing options of stroke prevention in atrial fibrillation 468
Rationale for left atrial appendage occlusion 468
Identifying the right patient for device closure 469
Intolerance or contraindications to oral anticoagulant or new oral anticoagulants 469
Device implantation 470
Postprocedural treatment 470
Clinical trial results 470
Discussion 470

SECTION 11: CARDIAC IMAGING

74. Utility of Echo in Assessment and Management of Functional Mitral Regurgitation **475**

Gonzalo Luis Alonso Salinas, Marina Pascual Izco, José Luis Zamorano

Mechanism and etiology of mitral regurgitation 475

Ultrasound assessment of functional mitral regurgitation 475
Management of functional mitral regurgitation 479

75. **Diastology Demystified** **481**
Jagdish C Mohan, Vishwas Mohan, Madhu Shukla
Physiology of diastole 482
Factors contributing to diastole 482
Significance of diastolic function 483
Left atrial volume and diastolic function/dysfunction 488
Mitral inflow velocities 490
Mitral inflow measurements 491
Mitral inflow: acquisition and feasibility 491
Mitral annular velocities 492
Practical tips 494
Pulmonary vein flow and diastolic function 496
Acquisition of pulmonary vein flow signals 498
Pulmonary vein flow parameters 499
Mitral flow propagation by color M-mode 499
Longitudinal strain, rotation, and untwisting rate by acoustic speckle tracking 500
Diastolic stress test 500
The new guidelines on diastolic function 501

76. **Echocardiographic Assessment of Right Ventricular Function** **503**
K Tamilselvan, R Alagesan
Anatomical and physiological basis for right ventricular echocardiography 503
Right ventricular chamber dimensions assessment 503
Right ventricular anterior wall thickness assessment 504
Assessment of right ventricular hemodynamics 504
Assessment of right ventricular systolic function 506
Right ventricular myocardial performance index 506
Tissue doppler imaging of right ventricular 507
Right ventricular strain imaging 507
Assessment of right ventricular diastolic function 509
Right ventricular wall motion assessment 509
Transesophageal echocardiography 509

77. **Longitudinal Strain Imaging: Is it a Clinical Tool? An Echocardiographic Appreciation** **511**
G Vijayaraghavan, S Sivasankaran
Definition 511
Longitudinal strain 511
Speckle tracking for strain imaging 512
Longitudinal strain imaging protocol 512
Ejection fraction and global longitudinal strain 513
Ischemic heart disease and regional strain 513
Infiltrative diseases: amyloidosis 514
Left ventricular endomyocardial fibrosis 515
Hypertrophic cardiomyopathy 515

Left bundle branch, cardiac failure, and cardiac resynchronization therapy 515
Myocarditis 515
Strain imaging in rare situations 517
Limitations of strain imaging 518

78. Three-Dimensional Echocardiography—Current Indications **521**
Hardeep K Grewal, Ravi R Kasliwal
Left ventricle assessment 521
Right ventricle assessment 524
Left atrial assessment 525
Three-dimensional strain of left ventricle 526
Left ventricle dyssynchrony analysis 526
Valve assessment 527
Transcatheter interventions for valvular heart disease 534

79. Intervention and Fusion Echocardiography **542**
Shantanu P Sengupta
Problems during structural heart disease interventions 542
Understanding fusion imaging 542
Interatrial septal defect closure 543
Mitral valve interventions 545
Aortic valve interventions 545

80. Interpreting a Nuclear Stress Test **548**
GN Mahapatra
Approach to interpretation 548

81. Myocardial Viability Assessment: How Do We Apply in Clinical Practice? **559**
Nagendra Boopathy Senguttuvan, Kewal C Goswami
Energy and ischemia 559
Revascularization 560
Modalities of viability testing 560
Role of viability testing in the management of ischemic cardiomyopathy 563
Future direction 565

82. Computed Tomography Coronary Angiography—Essentials for Cardiologists **566**
Priya Jagia, Arun Sharma
Conventional angiography or computed tomography coronary angiography 566

83. Current Indications for Cardiac Magnetic Resonance Imaging **572**
Mona Bhatia, Shashank Jain
Technical aspects of cardiac MRI 572
Indications and applications 573
Future developments 579

SECTION 12: CARDIOVASCULAR PHARMACOLOGY

84. Newer Antianginals **583**

Kewal C Goswami, Anunay Gupta

Ranolazine 583
Nicorandil 584
Ivabradine 584
Trimetazidine 585
Fasudil 585
Allopurinol 586
Endothelin receptor blockers 586
Testosterone 586
High-dose statins 586
Molsidomine 587
Investigational drugs 587

85. Newer Antihypertensives **588**

TK Mishra

Newer drugs for hypertension 588
Emerging molecules 590
Future prospects 591

86. Newer Agents for Dyslipidemia **593**

Iyengar SS, Saleha N

Ezetimibe 593
Proprotein convertase subtilisin/kexin type 9 inhibitors 594
Inclisiran 595
Microsomal triglyceride transfer protein inhibitor: lomitapide 596
Antisense oligonucleotide against apolipoprotein B—mipomersen 596
Bempedoic acid 596
Gemcabene 596
CAT-2054 597
Novel drugs targeting high-density lipoprotein cholesterol 597
What are the recommendations of the medical societies on new nonstatin medications? 598
Safety of very low low-density lipoprotein cholestrol 599
Highest risk-highest benefit strategy 599

87. Choosing Between NOACS Wisely: Are They all the Same? **601**

Sandeep Bansal, Anunay Gupta

Pharmacokinetics and pharmacodynamics differences 601
Major differences in trials 602
Compliance 604

88. Newer Antihyperkalemic Drugs **606**

AK Pancholia

Clinical manifestations of hyperkalemia 606
Therapy for hyperkalemia 607

89. Drug Interactions in Cardiology **612**

Arunangshu Ganguly

Incidence 612
Mechanism of drug–drug interaction 612

90. Unsuspected Drug Toxicity in Cardiology Practice **620**

Ashish Tiwari, Sharad Chandra

Cardiotoxicity of cytotoxic drugs 620

SECTION 13: HEART FAILURE

91. Heart Failure in India **627**

Sandeep Seth, Karishma Landge

Heart failure in India is reaching epidemic proportions 627
Causes 627
Severity of disease 627
Tackling the problem in India 628

92. Biomarkers for Heart Failure: Current Role and Relevance **631**

Anunay Gupta, Ambuj Roy

Natriuretic peptides: B-type natriuretic peptide and N-terminal prohormone B-type natriuretic peptide 631
Newer biomarkers 633

93. Practical Tips for using Beta-blockers, ACEI, ARBs, ARNI, Diuretics, Aldosterone Antagonists in Heart Failure **635**

Vijay Kumar Chopra, Sanjay Mittal

Beta-blockers 635
Angiotensin-converting enzyme inhibitor 636
Angiotensin receptor blockers 637
Angiotensin receptor neprilysin inhibitor 637
Diuretics 638
Aldosterone antagonists 638

94. HFpEF—How to Diagnose and Manage? **640**

Sanjeev Sanghvi, Swati Mahajan

Pathophysiology of HFpEF 640
Diagnosis of HFpEF 640
History and clinical examination 640

Investigations 642
Treatment 643

95. Heart Failure with Midrange Ejection Fraction—What is This? 647
Arup Dasbiswas
Clinical characteristics 647
Predictors and outcomes of heart failure with midrange ejection fraction 648

96. Monitoring Therapy in Heart Failure with Reduced Ejection Fraction 650
Soura Mookerjee
Trials of biomarker-guided therapy for heart failure 650
Multidisciplinary care approach to the management of heart failure patients 650
Remote monitoring of heart failure: tools and results 651

97. Stepwise Approach to Acute Decompensated Heart Failure 656
BP Singh, Ravi V Prasad, Nirav Kumar
Pathophysiology 656
Evaluation of the patient with acute decompensated heart failure 656
Relevant investigations 658
Management goals 658
Treatment of acute heart failure 658
Management of patients with cardiogenic shock 661

98. Advanced Heart Failure Therapies—An Overview 664
Rishi A Bhargava, Prafulla G Kerkar
Estimating prognosis in advanced heart failure 664
Advanced heart failure—treatment strategies 664
Advanced heart failure therapies—Indian scenario 669

99. Takotsubo Cardiomyopathy—An Update 671
Pintu Nahata
History 671
Diagnostic criteria 671
Epidemiology 671
Etiopathogenesis 671
Clinical features 672
Variant 673
Management 674
Prognosis 674

SECTION 14: SYNCOPE

100. Syncope: What is New? 679
Satish K Kaushik, Surendra K Chutani
The new or revised concepts 679

101. Tilt Table Testing in Syncope 682

Surender Deora, Kewal C Goswami

Pathophysiology of vasovagal syncope 682
Head-up tilt test 682
Response to head-up tilt test 683
Indications 684
Complications and contraindications 684
Future prospects 684

102. Implantable and External Loop Recorders: Indications in My Practice 686

Praloy Chakraborty

Patients with syncope 686
Patients with palpitations 688
Nonestablished indications 688

103. Sudden Death in Dilated Cardiomyopathy—What is New in 2018? 690

Kamal K Sethi, Ashish K Govil

Pathophysiology of dilated cardiomyopathy 690
Role of drug therapy in sudden cardiac death 690
Role of implantable cardioverter defibrillator 691
Risk stratification 693

104. Orthostatic Hypotension 696

Siddharthan Deepti, Kewal C Goswami

Definition 696
Epidemiology 696
Physiology of the normal orthostatic response 696
Etiology 698
Clinical presentation 700
Orthostatic testing and variants of orthostatic hypotension 700
Differential diagnosis 701
Management 701
Treatment 701

SECTION 15: ATRIAL FIBRILLATION

105. Stroke Prevention in Atrial Fibrillation: New Oral Anticoagulants 705

Sharad Agrawal

Epidemiology of stroke in atrial fibrillation 705
Risk stratification tools in atrial fibrillation 705
Antithrombotic management of atrial fibrillation 706
Current recommendations for antithrombotic therapy in atrial fibrillation 708

106. Catheter Ablation of Atrial Fibrillation 710

Dinkar Bhasin, Gautam Sharma

Advantages of maintaining sinus rhythm 710

Pathophysiology of atrial fibrillation 710
Indications for atrial fibrillation ablation 711
Technique for pulmonary vein isolation 711
Adjunctive ablation strategies 713
Complications of atrial fibrillation ablation 713
Outcomes 714

107. Postoperative Atrial Fibrillation: Clinical Correlates and Management **715**

Krishnarpan Chatterjee, Naveen Garg

Incidence and time course 715
Pathogenesis 715
Clinical manifestations and diagnosis 716
Prevention of atrial fibrillation and complications 716
Management 718
Anticoagulation 718

108. Managing Antithrombotics after Percutaneous Coronary Intervention in Atrial Fibrillation: Current Recommendations **721**

Sundeep Mishra

Why risk of thrombosis after percutaneous coronary intervention? 721
Why risk of stroke after onset of atrial fibrillation? 722
How to prevent thrombosis in patient undergoing percutaneous coronary intervention? 722
How to prevent stroke in a patient with atrial fibrillation? 724
How to balance risks and benefits in patient of atrial fibrillation undergoing percutaneous coronary intervention 727

109. Treatment of Atrial Fibrillation in Heart Failure: Is It Any Different? **732**

Rajesh A Dhopeshwarkar

Goals of treatment in atrial fibrillation 732
Challenges in device management in patients with atrial fibrillation and heart failure 735

110. Managing Atrial Fibrillation in Acute Myocardial Infarction **736**

Jayagopal P Balagopalan, Sarjun Basha

Predictors of atrial fibrillation in acute myocardial infarction 736
Management of atrial fibrillation in acute myocardial infarction 736

SECTION 16: VENTRICULAR ARRHYTHMIAS

111. Ventricular Arrhythmias in Acute Myocardial Infarction **741**

Rajesh A Dhopeshwarkar, Rakesh Yadav, Kewal C Goswami

Types of ventricular arrhythmias 741
Mechanism and pathogenesis of ventricular arrhythmias after acute myocardial infarction 741
Predictors of sustained ventricular tachycardia and ventricular fibrillation 741
Management of ventricular arrhythmias 743

112. Ventricular Arrhythmias and Sudden Death: Problems and Opportunities in Clinical Practice **746**

Kapil Kumawat

Mechanisms of ventricular arrhythmias and sudden cardiac death 746
Epidemiology 747
Therapies for ventricular arrhythmias and sudden cardiac death 747
Devices for treatment of ventricular arrhythmias and sudden cardiac death 748
Prevention, prediction, and treatment of VAS and SCD in specific disorders 749

113. Electrocardiography Clues in a Sudden Cardiac Death Survivor **756**

Ranjan Modi, Aparna Jaswal

Structural heart disease 757
Ischemic heart disease 758
Nonstructural heart disease: inherited 758
Nonstructural heart disease: noninherited 764
Electrocardiography-based tests 765
Common forms of sudden cardiac death 765
Multiple risk markers: cumulative risk 766
Importance of dynamic monitoring 767

114. Premature Ventricular Complex: When and How to Ablate? **771**

Joseph Theodore, Raja Selvaraj

When do premature ventricular complexes need to be treated? 771
To treat or not to treat a premature ventricular complex 771
How to treat? 772
Technique of premature ventricular complex ablation 772
Ablation of premature ventricular complexes 774
Outcomes 774

115. Epicardial Ventricular Tachycardia: Recognition and Approach **775**

Maki Ono, Walid I Saliba, Oussama Wazni, Mandeep Bhargava

Preoperative assessment and recognition 775
Approach to access the pericardial space 777
Mapping and ablation 778
Complications 779

116. Cardiopulmonary Resuscitation: What's New? **783**

Nitin Modi, Sunil Sharma

2015 American heart association guideline update
for cardiopulmonary resuscitation and emergency cardiovascular care 783

SECTION 17: CARDIAC IMPLANTABLE ELECTRONIC DEVICES

117. Improving Outcomes in Patients with Cardiac Resynchronization Therapy **791**

Rohit Malhotra

Patient selection 791
Preprocedure planning 794

118. CRT-D versus CRT-P—What should be the Standard of Care in Nonischemic Cardiomyopathy? **799**

TS Kler, Avinash Verma

Burden of sudden cardiac death in NICM 799
CRT-D in NICM—lack of benefit is consistent 800
Is the trail design at fault? 802
So which NICM patient needs icd or CRT-D? 802

119. ICD in HFrEF—When are They not Needed? **804**

Rajnish Sardana, Praloy Chakraborty

Early after myocardial infarction 804
Early after myocardial revascularization 805
Recent onset nonischemic cardiomyopathy 806

120. Leadless Pacemakers: Current Review and Future Directions **809**

Vanita Arora

Potential complications with conventional pacing system 809
Animal studies and technological advancements 809
Current leadless cardiac pacemakers 810
How the algorithm functions 813

SECTION 18: CARDIAC SURGERY

121. Time to Embrace Total Arterial Revascularization **819**

Ramakanta Panda, Sunil Vanzara

Reason for low atherosclerosis in arterial conduits 819
Types of arterial conduits 820
Indications and contraindications to use total arterial revascularization 820
Techniques of harvesting 821
Factors influencing graft patency 822
Comparative patency data of arterial grafts 823
Survival benefit 823
Discussion 825

122. Surgery in Acute Myocardial Infarction **831**

Ganesh K Mani, Pramod K Sharma, Manju Mani

Coronary artery bypass surgery after failed PCI 831
Outcome of surgery within 6 hours 832
Optimal timing of coronary artery bypass surgery in acute myocardial infarction 832
Operative strategy (arrested or beating heart?) 833
Personal experience 833

123. Recent Advances in Coronary Artery Bypass Graft **836**

OP Yadava

Minimally invasive CABG 837

Conduits—improving patency 837
On versus off-pump CABG 838
Hybrid myocardial revascularization 838
No option coronary artery disease 838
Quality initiatives 839
Miscellaneous 839

124. Redo Coronary Artery Bypass Grafting: Challenges and Outcomes **841**

Ramakanta Panda, Muzil Munshi

Incidence 841
Patient risk profile 842
Indications 842
Preoperative evaluation and planning 843
Technical aspects and challenges associated with redo coronary artery bypass grafting 845

125. LVAD—Should Indians Borrow to Afford Them? **852**

Sachin Talwar, Harsha V Niraghatam

Epidemiology 852
The Indian scenario 852
Protocol for management of heart failure in India 853
Heart transplantation versus VAD's for end stage heart failure 858
Pros and cons of LVADS in India 860

126. Heart Transplantation in India: Successes and Challenges **863**

Balram Airan, Milind Hote

Successes 863
Challenges 866
Roadmap for the future 869

SECTION 19: STROKE

127. Atrial Fibrillation and Stroke: An Update **873**

Rohit Bhatia, Rimpy Joseph

Epidemiology and global burden 873
Updated model for stroke mechanism in atrial fibrillation and concept of atrial cardiopathy 874
Atrial fibrillation detection in stroke 874
Stroke risk stratification scores 876
Are type of atrial fibrillation and duration of episodes predictive of stroke risk? 876
Serum biomarkers as predictors of stroke risk in atrial fibrillation? 877
Structural and functional markers of left atrial and left atrial appendage as stroke predictors in atrial fibrillation 877
Assessment of bleeding risk 878
Management strategies 878

128. Current Reperfusion Strategy in Acute Ischemic Stroke **887**

MV Padma Srivastava, Vishnu VY

Thrombolysis in acute ischemic stroke: "Time clock" 887
Recent advances in stroke thrombolysis 888
Next generation thrombolytic agent: tenecteplase 888
Endovascular therapy: "tissue clock" 889

129. Prevention of Stroke in Cardiac Patients **892**

Harsh Wardhan, Nitin Aggarwal

Definition of stroke and transient ischemic attack 892
Cardiac embolism and stroke 892
Stroke prevention in atrial fibrillation 893
Oral anticoagulants 894
Patent foramen ovale 895
Aortic arch disease 896
Myocardial infarction, left ventricular dysfunction, and heart failure 896
Dilated cardiomyopathy 897
Valvular heart disease 897

130. Stroke in Cath Lab **901**

Neeraj Parakh, Kewal C Goswami

Incidence 901
Mechanism and risk factors 901
Presentation 901
Evaluation 902
Treatment 902

SECTION 20: PERIPHERAL VASCULAR DISEASE

131. Varicose Veins: Interventional Approach **907**

Sanjeev Kumar, Vineeta Ojha

Anatomy and pathophysiology 907
Natural history 908
Classification 908
Indications for treatment 908
Treatment options for varicose veins 908
Interventional approach to management of varicose veins 909

132. Deep Vein Thrombosis: Controversies and Consensus **916**

Surender Deora, Kewal C Goswami

Evaluation and management of deep vein thrombosis 916

133. Renal Artery Stenosis: When and How to Intervene? **923**

George Joseph

Atherosclerotic renal artery stenosis 923

Fibromuscular dysplasia 927
Takayasu arteritis 928
Christian Medical College, Vellore Interventional Experience in Takayasu Arteritis Renal Artery Stenosis 929

134. Carotid Artery Stenting in 2018 932
Vivudh P Singh, Ranjan Modi, Atul Mathur
Management of carotid artery disease 932
Secondary prevention in asymptomatic patients 933
Tertiary prevention in recently symptomatic patients 934
Carotid artery stenosis versus carotid endarterectomy 935
Timing of interventions after onset of symptoms 935
Carotid artery stenting over carotid endarterectomy 936
Staged or synchronous bilateral carotid interventions 936
Carotid artery stenting technique 936
Complications 937
New aspects of 2017 guidelines added to the 2009 guidelines 939

135. Critical Limb Ischemia: Current Management 941
Narendra N Khanna, Chukwudi Nwagbara, Suparna Rao
Epidemiology and risk factors 941
Pathophysiology of critical limb ischemia 941
Clinical features 942
Classification 942
Differential diagnosis of leg pain on exertion 942
Evaluation of critical limb ischemia 943
Treatment of critical limb ischemia 945

SECTION 21: WOMEN AND HEART DISEASE

136. Coronary Artery Disease in Women: Unfair Assessment and Outcomes 957
Roopa Salwan
Risk factors for coronary artery disease 958
Pathophysiology of IHD in women 959
Assessment of ischemic heart disease in women 960
Clinical spectrum of ischemic heart disease 961
Indian data 962
Myocardial infarction with nonobstructive coronary arteries 962

137. Hypertension in Pregnancy—A Stepwise Approach 966
Cherian Koshy, K Venugopal
Classification of hypertensive disorders in pregnancy 966
Grading of hypertension (NICE guidelines) 966
Management 966
Investigations 967
Chronic hypertension 968

Timing of termination of pregnancy 968
Postpartum hypertension 969
Indian data 969

138. Peripartum Cardiomyopathy **970**
Abhishek Roy, Debabrata Roy
Physiology of normal pregnancy 970
Etiopathogenesis of peripartum cardiomyopathy 970
Clinical features 972
Diagnosis 972
Differential diagnosis 973
Management 973
Prognosis and follow-up 975
Counseling for future pregnancies 975

139. Mitral Stenosis in Pregnancy: The Last Straw on the Camel's Back! **978**
AJ Swamy, Deepak Saha, Sarat Chandra
Prevalence and incidence in India 978
Hemodynamic changes in pregnancy 978
Hemodynamics during labor and delivery 978
Pathophysiology of mitral stenosis during pregnancy 979
Percutaneous balloon mitral valvuloplasty 980
Surgical mitral valvoplasty/mitral replacement 980

140. Heart Failure in Pregnancy **983**
Kajal Ganguly, Anindya Mukherjee, Malay Acharya, Auriom Kar
Epidemiology 983
Physiology 983
Etiology and pathophysiology 983
Clinical presentation 985
Investigations 985
Differential diagnosis 985
Management principles 985
Treating reversible factors 986
Supportive measures 986
The mode of delivery 986
The puerperium and long-term management 986
Heart failure with preserved ejection fraction 987

SECTION 22: SYSTEMIC DISEASES AND HEART

141. Hypothyroidism and Heart **991**
Niteen V Deshpande
Effects of thyroid hormone on cardiovascular system 991
Cardiovascular manifestations 993
Hypothyroidism and heart failure 993

Effect of heart disease on thyroid function 994
Treatment of hypothyroidism and heart 994

142. Cardiorenal Syndrome: Current Update **997**
Dipak Sarma, Ritesh Kalwar
Definition 997
Classification 997
Link and pathophysiology 997
Biomarker in cardiorenal syndrome 998
Management 999

143. Anemia in Heart Failure **1002**
Umesh C Samal, Harikrishnan S
Epidemiology of anemia and iron deficiency in heart failure 1002
Pathogenesis of anemia in heart failure 1002
Consequences of anemia and iron deficiency in heart failure 1002
How to diagnose iron deficiency? 1003
Treatment of anemia and iron deficiency 1003

144. When to Screen and How to Manage OSA in Cardiology Practice **1005**
GC Khilnani, Pawan Tiwari
Extent of the problem 1005
Risk factors for obstructive sleep apnea 1005
Consequences and complications of obstructive sleep apnea 1006
Screening tools for obstructive sleep apnea 1006
Barriers in integrating OSA management in cardiology practice and solutions 1008
Diagnosis of obstructive sleep apnea 1008
Overview of management of obstructive sleep apnea 1009

SECTION 23: EMERGING ISSUES IN CARDIOLOGY

145. mCardiology: mHealth in Cardiology **1013**
Ambuj Roy, Ajay S Vamadevan
Need for technology 1013

146. Telemonitoring in Cardiology **1017**
Pramod Sagar Arsikere, Aditya Kapoor
Various applications of telecardiology

147. Executive Cardiac Checkup: Is it Really Needed? **1024**
Brian Pinto, Neeraj A Desai
Computed tomography coronary calcium scoring 1025

148. Cardiology and Ethics: Mission Impossible? **1028**
Raja Selvaraj, Jayaraman Balachander
Challenges specific to cardiology 1028

What can the cardiologist do? 1029
What should regulatory bodies do? 1030

SECTION 24: MISCELLANEOUS

149. Development of Cardiology and Interventions in India—An Insider's Glimpse **1033**

M Khalilullah

Implantable valves 1034
Left atrial appendage closure 1035
Interventional electrophysiology 1035

150. Evidence-based Medicine: Are Randomized Controlled Trials the Gold Standard? **1036**

Vitull K Gupta, Meghna Gupta, Varun Gupta

History of evidence-based medicine 1036
What is evidence-based medicine? 1036
Classification of evidence-based medicine 1037
Qualification of evidence 1037
Statistical measures in evidence-based medicine 1037
How do we actually practice evidence based medicine? 1037
Types of research study designs 1038
Limitations of evidence-based medicine 1038
Application of evidence-based medicine in developing countries like India 1038
Can evidence-based medicine be influenced? 1038
Pharma industry, research, and evidence-based medicine 1039
Are randomized controlled trials the gold standard? 1039

151. Erectile Dysfunction in a Cardiac Patient **1043**

Ranjit K Nath, Neil Bardoloi

Etiology 1043
Pathophysiologic basis of erectile dysfunction and cardiovascular disease 1043
Erectile dysfunction with established cardiovascular disease 1046
Erectile dysfunction and future cardiovascular events 1046
Erectile dysfunction with occult cardiovascular disease 1046
Workup for patients with erectile dysfunction and cardiovascular disease 1046
Management of erectile dysfunction and cardiovascular disease 1047

152. Noncardiac Surgery: How to "Clear" a Patient? **1050**

PC Manoria, Pankaj Manoria, Sharad Kumar Parashar

Ancillary preoperative cardiac testing: recommendations 1051
Elective noncardiac surgery in patients with prior percutaneous coronary intervention: timing and recommendations 1052
Anticoagulant therapy 1052
Preoperative evaluation in specific patients population: general considerations 1053
Perioperative arrhythmias 1053

153. How to Defend a Complaint in Cardiology 1055

KK Aggarwal

Defense argument no. 1 1055
Defense argument no. 2 1055
Defense argument no. 3 1055
Defense argument no. 4 1055
Defense argument no. 5 1056
Defense argument no. 6 1056
Defense argument no. 7 1056
Defense argument no. 8 1056
Defense argument no. 9 1056
Defense argument no. 10 1056
Defense argument no. 11 1057
Defense argument no. 12 1057
Defense argument no. 13 1057
Defense argument no. 14 1057
Defense argument no. 15 1058
Defense argument no. 16 1058
Defense argument no. 17 1058
Defense argument no. 18 1058
Defense argument no. 19 1058
Defense argument no. 20 1059
Defense argument no. 21 1059
Defense argument no. 22 1059
Defense argument no. 23 1059
Defense argument no. 24 1059
Defense argument no. 25 1060
Defense argument no. 26 1060

154. Sports and Heart Diseases 1061

Kewal C Goswami, Vikash Kumar, Nagendra Boopathy Senguttuvan

Types of exercise 1061
Cardiovascular response to exercise 1061
Benefits of exercise 1062
Risks of exercise 1062
Clinical problems in sports cardiology 1062
Screening abnormalities 1063

Index 1067

SECTION 1

Coronary Artery Disease Risk Factors

CHAPTER 1

Smokeless Tobacco and Cardiovascular Disease

Surender Deora, Kewal C Goswami

INTRODUCTION

Tobacco has been used by human beings since 600 AD.[1] Columbus came to know about tobacco from Caribbean and introduced it in Europe. It was introduced in India in early 1600 AD by Portuguese traders mainly as a barter commodity to trade Indian textiles.[2] The harmful effect of tobacco was also known since the Mughal era and the Jahangir, the Mughal emperor of India, had even passed orders to ban it.[3] The spiritual leader, Guru Gobind Singh, the 10th Sikh guru, prohibited smoking for the Sikh community. He said, "Wine is bad, Indian hemp (bhang) destroys one generation, but tobacco destroys all generations".[4] Not only in India, the king James I of England and Shah Abbas of Persia were aware of the harmful effect of tobacco. King James described tobacco smoking as "a custom loathsome to the eye, hateful to the nose, harmful to the brain, and dangerous to the lungs". Initially, it was mainly used by affluent class but gradually penetrated at all socioeconomic strata in various forms.

The term "smokeless tobacco" (SLT) mainly refers to chewing, spitting, sniffing unburned tobacco in one or the other form either alone or mixed with other constituents. The SLT is mainly obtained from *Nicotiana rustica* which contains more nitrosamines as compared to the tobacco for smoking obtained from *Nicotiana tabacum*. Mainly, it was consumed with betel quid (pan) for decades and later in the form of bidi (tobacco wrapped in dried leaves of special trees). Some people used for its presumed medicinal value which although has never been proved in any system of medicine being practiced in India.

The various forms and different names of SLT consumed in India are *Pan, Gutkha, Zarda, Naswar*, and *Mishri* or *Gul* (Table 1 and Figs. 1 to 3).

- *Pan* is a betel leaf containing mixture of tobacco, areca nuts, spices, and lime (to increase the bioavailability of nicotine)
- *Gutkha* is nothing but powdered form of scented tobacco, areca nut mixed with lime.
- *Zarda* is Indian chewing tobacco flavored with spices and flavored form of tobacco is also used in pan
- *Naswar* is a moist, powdered tobacco snuff consumed mostly in India, Pakistan, Afghanistan and neighboring countries. *Naswar* is snuffed in the floor of mouth, under

TABLE 1: Various types of smokeless tobacco

Common name	Ingredients
Gutkha	Tobacco, areca nut, condiments, flavoring agent
Khaini	Tobacco flakes, lime
Naswar	Tobacco, slaked lime, indigo, cardamom oil, menthol
Gul	Burned tobacco powder, molasses
Zarda	Boiled tobacco
Pan	Betel leaf, areca nut, tobacco, lime, spices
Moist snuff (US type)	Pulverized tobacco, fermented
Moist snuff or snus (Swedish type)	Pulverized tobacco, nonfermented

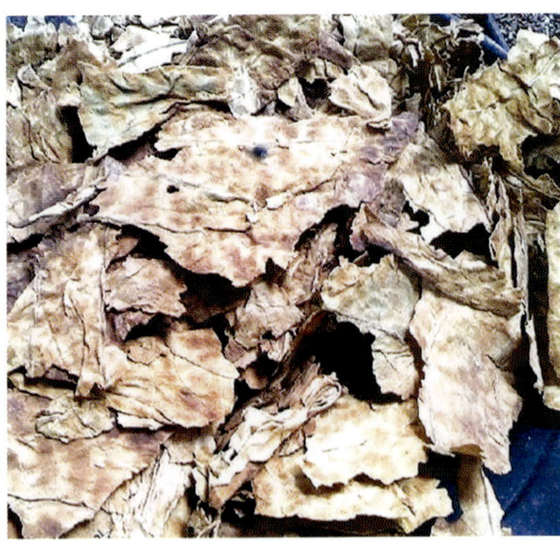
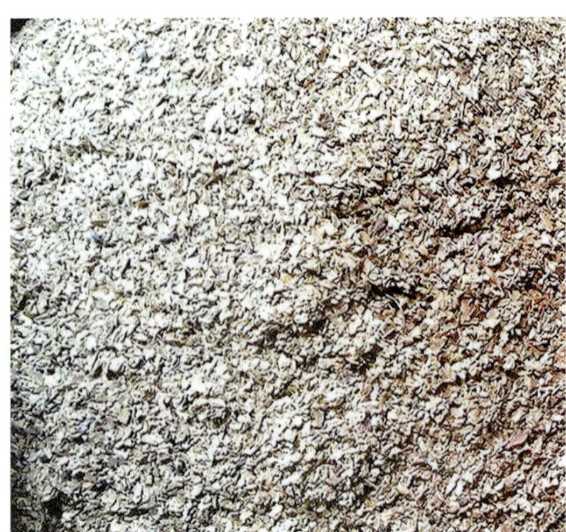

FIG. 1: Dried tobacco leaves and Zarda.

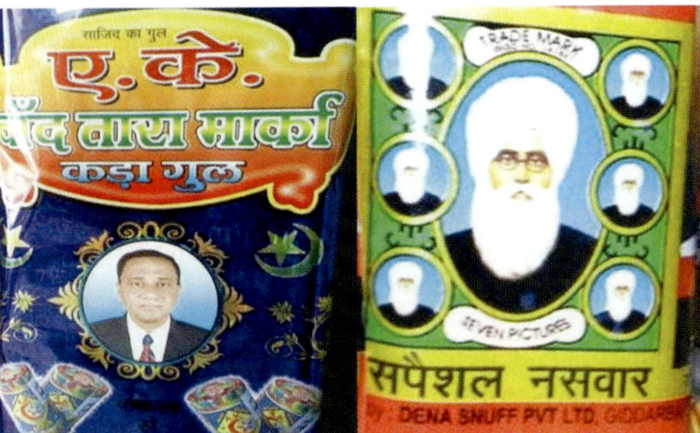

FIG. 2: Gul and Naswar in Indian market.

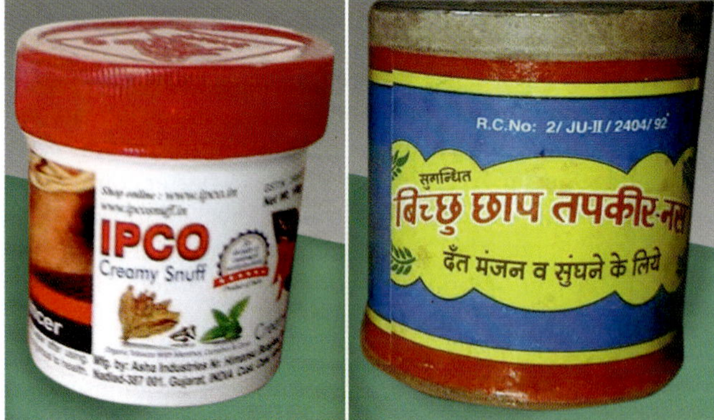

FIG. 3: Snuff and Tapkeer in Indian market.

the lower lip, or inside the cheek for prolong period to get desired effect

- *Mishri or Gul* is tobacco powder applied to teeth and gums with index fingers and used as dentifrices
- *Snuff* is a pulverized tobacco either fermented (US type) or nonfermented (Swedish type). The pattern of use of snuff is slightly different in these two countries where in Sweden it is placed under the upper lip and in United States between the lower gum and chin.[5] It is usually inhaled or snuffed into the nasal cavity, delivering a swift hit of nicotine. It is usually in the flavored form.

Smokeless tobacco is not only common in middle income and poor countries but is also quite commonly used as snuff in North America and in Europe mainly Sweden. Inhalation of tobacco or snuff is relatively less common in India as compared to western countries

There are more than 350 million populations globally using SLT with the majority living in Southeast Asian region.[6] The prevalence of SLT in this region is 1.3–38% in males and 4.6–27.9% in females.[7] India is one of the largest consumers of tobacco products both in number and relative share. The prevalence of tobacco use in Indian population more than 15 years age is 34.6% (47.9% males, 20.3% females) and is mainly consumed as SLT (49.3% males, 85.5% females).[8] The average age of initiation was 17.9 years similar to that of smoking.[9] It is specially increasing in younger children in India. A cross-sectional study in Delhi and Chennai (Project MYTRI) reported higher use of SLT in 6th grade students than 8th grade.[10] Tobacco use in any form accounts for 6 million deaths globally every year which is expected to increase 8 million by 2030. According to Tobacco Control Policy (TCP) Indian cohort survey, Gutkha was the most common form of SLT used in India followed by chewing of tobacco (Fig. 4).[11]

The association of tobacco consumption mainly in form of smoking and cardiovascular disease (CVD) is well established.[12] The historical trend of smoking and CVD in Unites states ran parallel in last century. The rate of smoking and CVD increased till first half of 20th century and later decreased gradually because increased awareness and well proven causation of various diseases.[13,14] The use of SLT which was common in middle income countries became gradually increased in developed countries as the trends for smoking decreased whereas the smoking and SLT both increased in developing countries especially Southeast Asia.[15] The main reason of increased use of SLT is because of its easy availability, lack of awareness of its harmful effect,

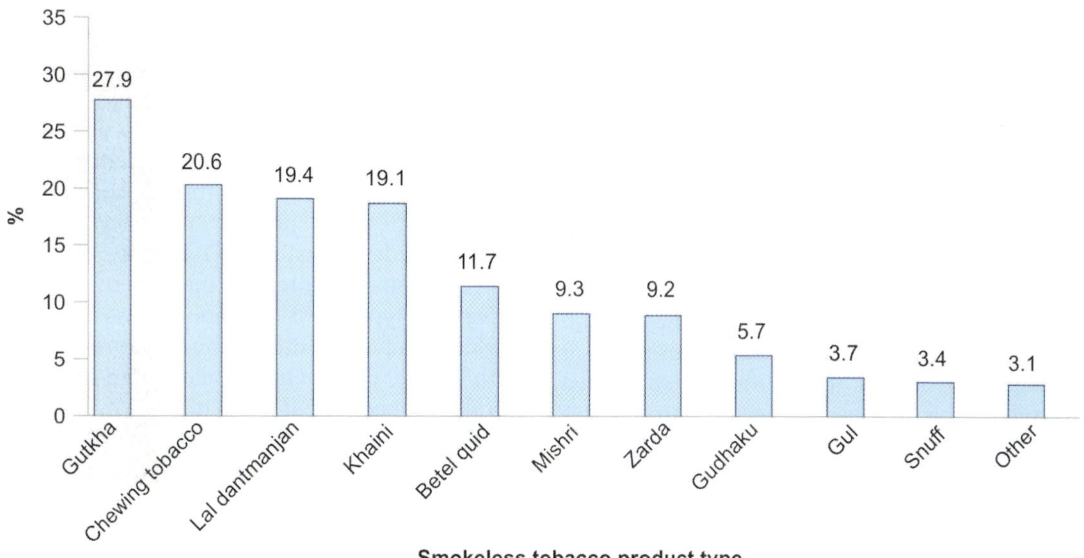

FIG. 4: Prevalence of smokeless tobacco used in India.

Source: Gravely S, Fong GT, Driezen P, et al. An examination of the effectiveness of health warning labels on smokeless tobacco products in four states in India: findings from the TCP India cohort survey. BMC Public Health. 2016;16:1246.

aggressive marketing by the companies, presumption of it being medicinal value, as mouth freshener, and dentifrices. Tobacco consumption is the most important preventable risk factor for premature death especially in young middle-aged adults.[16]

PHARMACOKINETICS OF SMOKELESS TOBACCO

Nicotine is the main constituent in tobacco causing addiction and most of its harmful effect. The level of nicotine in blood depends upon the concentration of tobacco in the product, its pH level, moisture level, and the size of tobacco cutting.[17,18] It is water- and lipid-soluble weak base and readily crosses the mucosa in unionized form. If the pH of the SLT is higher, i.e., if it is more alkaline then more nicotine remains in unionized form, hence more absorbed resulting in higher nicotine blood level.[19] The maximum level of nicotine is similar in both smoking and SLT but the level of nicotine is more sustained in SLT as compared to smoking where rapid peaks and troughs are seen.[20]

SMOKELESS TOBACCO AND CARDIOVASCULAR RISK FACTORS

Nicotine increases the blood pressure (BP) and heart rate (HR) by enhancing the release of dopamine, epinephrine, norepinephrine, vasopressin, etc. and activation of sympathetic nervous system. The long-term effect of SLT on BP depends on many factors including the type and amount of SLT used and level of physical activity. Increase in BP is not only because of nicotine but also because of high sodium content of the tobacco product and licorice in SLT. This has been proved by measuring the urinary sodium content in various types of SLT.[21] The licorice increases the sodium level by inhibiting the metabolism of mineralocorticoids and thus increases the BP. The acute effects of SLT causes increase in HR and BP which in one of the study shows increase by 19 beats/min of HR and by 21/14 mm Hg of BP.[22] In a population-based survey of more than 30,000 participants in Sweden, the chronic SLT users were more likely to have higher BP (>160/90 mm Hg).[23] More often it is the diastolic BP which is elevated as shown in a study of 135 middle aged healthy volunteers with ambulatory BP monitoring.[24] But in those who are physically active like baseball players, no significant elevation in BP and HR was noted in SLT users.[25] Use of tobacco has been shown to be associated with insulin resistance and incident diabetes. Higher serum level of insulin and fibrinogen was noted in SLT users as compared to non-users.[26] A prospective population-based study in middle aged Swedish men using snuff found significant risk of developing diabetes at follow-up of 10 years.[27] SLT has also been associated with abnormal lipid profile. A study conducted in Asians with regular tobacco chewing habits reported significantly high level of low-density lipoproteins cholesterol (LDL-C) and low level of high-density lipoproteins cholesterol (HDL-C).[28] Similarly, Tucker et al. in a population based study reported 2.5 times higher prevalence of hypercholesterolemia in SLT users.[29] Gupta et al. studied association between SLT and CV risk factors in a population based case control study in Bikaner region, India.[30] They found significant higher prevalence of hypertension, tachycardia, dyslipidemia and diabetes as compared to nontobacco users. All these studies were in isolation and in different regions of the globe where different types of SLT products with different tobacco content and other constituents were being used. The effect of SLT on vascular inflammation, atherosclerosis and thrombosis is still unclear and needs large studies with all types of SLT products.

SMOKELESS TOBACCO AND CARDIOVASCULAR DISEASE

Smokeless tobacco has been associated with various diseases including cancer of the oral cavity, esophagus, and pancreas.[31,32] It has also been associated with low birth weight, preterm or stillbirth.[30] The association of SLT with CVD is not very well established as it is for smoking.[33] Various studies in different regions of the world produced different results depending upon the type of SLT consumed and their level of chemical constituents. Apart from the Southeast Asian countries, the main consumer of SLT although in different forms is in Sweden and United States. The SLT consumed in India have high levels of tobacco-specific nitrosamines as compared to that present in moist snuff available in European market.[34,35] Also, the SLT available in India has varied methods of preparation, variable tobacco content and varied methods of using it which causes different effects as compared to SLT available in western countries. The meta-analysis by Boffetta and Straif calculated SLT-attributable fraction of CVD.[36] In their analysis, SLT use contributed 5.6% of fatal coronary heart disease (CHD) in Sweden and 0.5% in America. This meta-analysis included eight studies that evaluated the risk of fatal myocardial infarction and five studies that evaluated the risk of fatal stroke but this analysis did not include Asian studies. Three studies showed significant association of SLT and CV death (including stroke and CV death) but other studies did not show that strong association. But the overall cohort has shown positive association between CV death and SLT. The meta-analysis by Vidyasagaran et al. has shown increased risk of fatal ischemic heart disease (IHD) and stroke with SLT.[37] Another study by Gupta et al. also known as Mumbai cohort study the results was mixed. At follow-up of 5 years, SLT use was associated with significant fatal CV event in females but not in males.[38] The study including patients from India, China, and Taiwan has shown insignificant association of SLT and CV mortality in India but significant association in China and Taiwan.[39] The incidence of nonfatal stroke did not show an increased risk in SLT users but most of the studies with this end point have been conducted in Nordic region like Sweden.[40] The incidence of nonfatal IHD shows significant heterogeneity depending upon the geographical area of study. The studies conducted in Nordic region did not show an increased risk for nonfatal IHD but those from the Asian region showed a 40% increased risk.[41] No data available for this outcome from North American studies. There are limited data on the risk of CHD with different type of SLT products. Gupta et al. first time did a meta-analysis with different SLT products and risk of CHD.[42] They found a significant association between snuff use or snus (most commonly consumed in Europe) and fatal CHD. But there was no significant association between chewing tobacco (most commonly consumed in Asia) and fatal CHD which may be due to small studies and significant heterogeneity between the studies. This study also analyzed the fraction of fatal CHD attributable to SLT in different regions where it was found to be highest in Sweden (5%) followed by Southeast Asia (0.77%), and least in United States (0.14%).

HEALTH POLICY IMPLICATIONS

Smokeless tobacco has not received much focus among policy makers and researchers because it is presumed to be less harmful than smoked tobacco. It is also thought to be a regional rather than global problem although the most population in developing countries consumes SLT rather than cigarettes. The problem in policy making is lack of concrete evidence against SLT because of its various types and composition. Moreover, the pattern of consumption of the various types of SLT differs in these countries therefore all studies have not shown consistent results. SLT is found to be equally detrimental as compared to smoking at least in Indian subcontinent with little data available with us. The tobacco specific nitrosamine available in the Indian SLT is much higher and varied as compared to that available in Sweden and hence more injurious to health.[43] Therefore, the policy needs to be as strict as that for smoking tobacco. Cigarettes and Other Tobacco Products Act (COTPA) 2003 prohibits all type of advertisement of any type of tobacco products. India is a signatory of WHO Framework Convention on Tobacco control (FCTC) and MPOWER package and has implemented tobacco control awareness programs.[44] The impact of the FCTC is that the prevalence of smoking has declined in the countries who have strictly implemented it.[45] But it is difficult to assess the effect of these measures in controlling the SLT use because of the little available quality data.[46] Continuous government efforts, effective advocacy by NGOs, and inclusion of harmful effect of tobacco in all forms in school curriculum are some of the ways in dealing with this problem.

CONCLUSION

In India, SLT is the dominant form of tobacco used and is equally dangerous to health as smoked tobacco. It causes more sustained raised nicotine level in blood as compared to smoked tobacco and hence is more addictive. It causes raised BP, impaired blood sugar level and dyslipidemia and hence is prone to cause CVD. The available literature from the Indian subcontinent shows an association of SLT and increased risk of fatal IHD and stroke. A multipronged approach is needed for the control of all types of tobacco use so that the younger and productive population of the country remains healthy.

REFERENCES

1. Hughes JR. Nicotine related disorders. In: Sadock BJ, Sadock VI (Eds). Kaplan & Sadock's Comprehensive Textbook of Psychiatry, 7th edition. Philadelphia, Lippincott: Williams & Wilkins; 2000.
2. Gupta VM, Sen P. Tobacco: the addictive slow poison (editorial). Indian J Public Health. 2001;45:75-81.
3. Chattopadhayya A. Jahangir's interest in public health and medicine. Bull Inst Hist Med. Hyderabad. 1995;25:170-82.
4. Chattopadhayya A. Harmful effects of tobacco noticed in history. Bull Inst Hist Med, Hyderabad. 1993;23:53-8.
5. Asplund K. Smokeless tobacco and cardiovascular disease. Prog Cardiovasc Dis. 2003;45:383-94.
6. Sinha DN, Agarwal N, Gupta PC. Prevalence of smokeless tobacco use and number of users in 121 countries. Br J Med Med Res. 2015;9:1-20.

7. Geneva: WHO; 2011. WHO, editor. Global Status Report on Noncommunicable Diseases 2010.
8. Sinha DN, Palipudi KM, Rolle I, et al. Tobacco use among youth and adults in member countries of South- East Asia region: Review of findings from surveys under the Global Tobacco Surveillance System. Indian J Public Health. 2011;55:169-76.
9. International Institute for Population Sciences (IIPS), Ministry of Health and Family Welfare (MoHFW), Government of India (2010) Global Adult Tobacco Survey India report (GATS India), 2009–10. New Delhi: MoHFW, Government of India; Mumbai: IIPS.
10. Reddy KS, Perry CL, Stigler MH, et al. Differences in tobacco use among young people in urban India by sex, socioeconomic status, age, and school grade: assessment of baseline survey data. Lancet. 2006;367:589-94.
11. Gravely S, Fong GT, Driezen P, et al. An examination of the effectiveness of health warning labels on smokeless tobacco products in four states in India: findings from the TCP India cohort survey. BMC Public Health. 2016;16:1246.
12. Ezzati M, Lopez AD. Measuring the accumulated hazards of smoking: Global and regional estimates for 2000. Tob Control. 2003;12:79-85.
13. Nabel EG, Braunwald E. A tale of coronary artery disease and myocardial infarction. N Engl J Med. 2012;366:54-63.
14. Fuster V, Kelly BB; Board for Global Health. Promoting cardiovascular health in developing world: A critical challenge to achieve global health. Washington: Institute of Medicine;2010.
15. Gaziano TA, Bitton A, Anand S, et al. Growing epidemic of coronary heart disease in low- and middle-income countries. Curr Probl Cardiol. 2010;35:7-115.
16. World Health Organization. WHO Report on Global Tobacco Epidemic: Warning about Dangers of Tobacco. Geneva: World Health Organization; 2011.
17. Fant RV, Henningfield JE, Nelson RAet al. Pharmacokinetics and pharmacodynamics of moist snuff in humans. Tob Control. 1999;8:387-92.
18. Benowitz NL, Porchet H, Sheiner L, et al. Nicotine absorption and cardiovascular effects with smokeless tobacco use: Comparison with cigarettes and nicotine gum. Clin Pharmacol Ther 1988;44:23-8.
19. Hukkanen J, Jacob III P, Benowitz NL. Metabolism and disposition kinetics of nicotine. Pharmacol Rev. 2005;57:79-115.
20. Henningfield JE, Fant RV, Tomar SL. Smokeless tobacco: An addicting drug. Adv Dent Res. 1997;11:330-5.
21. Benowitz NL, Jacob P III, Yu L. Daily use of smokeless tobacco: Systemic effects. Ann Intern Med. 1989;111:112-6.
22. Westman E. Does smokeless tobacco cause hypertension? South Med J. 1995;88:716-20.
23. Bolinder GM, Ahlborg BO, Lindell JH. Use of smokeless tobacco: Blood pressure elevation and other health hazards found in a large-scale population survey. J Intern Med. 1992;232:327-34.
24. Bolinder G, de Faire U. Ambulatory 24-h blood pressure monitoring in healthy, middle-aged smokeless tobacco users, smokers, and nontobacco users. Am J Hypertens. 1998;11:1153-63.
25. Siegel D, Benowitz N, Ernster VL, et al. Smokeless tobacco, cardiovascular risk factors, and nicotine and cotinine levels in professional baseball players. Am J Public Health. 1992;82:417-21.
26. Eliasson M, Lundblad D, Hagg E. Cardiovascular risk factors in young snuff-users and cigarette smokers. J Intern Med. 1991;230:17-22.
27. Östenson CG, Hilding A, Grill V, et al. High consumption of smokeless tobacco ("snus") predicts increased risk of type 2 diabetes in a 10-year prospective study of middle-aged Swedish men. Scand J Public Health. 2012;40:730-7.
28. Khurana M, Sharma D, Khandelwal PD. Lipid profile in smokers and tobacco chewers – a comparative study. J Assoc Phys India. 2000;48:895-7.
29. Tucker LA. Use of smokeless tobacco, cigarette smoking, and hypercholesterolemia. Am J Public Health. 1989;79:1048-50.
30. Critchley JA, Unal B. Health effects associated with smokeless tobacco: A systematic review. Thorax. 2003;58:435-43.
31. Gupta BK, Kaushik A, Panwar RB, et al. Cardiovascular risk factors in tobacco-chewers: A controlled study. J Assoc Phys India. 2007;55:27-31.
32. Boffetta P, Hecht S, Gray N, et al. Smokeless tobacco and cancer. Lancet Oncol. 2008;9:667-75.
33. Mendis S, Puska P, Norrving B (Eds). Global Atlas on Cardiovascular Disease Prevention and Control. Geneva: World Health Organization, 2011.
34. Stepanov I, Hecht SS, Ramakrishnan S, et al. Tobacco specific nitrosamines in smokeless tobacco products marketed in India. Int J Cancer. 2005;116:16-19.
35. Osterdahl BG, Jansson C, Paccou A. Decreased levels of tobacco-specific N-nitrosamines in moist snuff on the Swedish market. J Agric Food Chem. 2004;52:5085-8.
36. Boffetta P, Straif K. Use of smokeless tobacco and risk of myocardial infarction and stroke: Systematic review with meta-analysis. BMJ. 2009;339:b3060.
37. Vidyasagaran AL, Siddiqi K, Kanaan M. Use of smokeless tobacco and risk of cardiovascular disease: A systematic review and meta-analysis. Eur J Prev Cardiol. 2016;23:1970-81.
38. Gupta PC, Pednekar MS, Parkin DM, et al. Tobacco associated mortality in Mumbai (Bombay) India. Results from the Bombay Cohort Study. Int J Epidemiol. 2005;34:1395-402.
39. Zhang L, Yang Y, Xu Z, et al. Chewing substances with or without tobacco and risk of cardiovascular disease in Asia: A meta-analysis. J Zhejiang Univ Sci 2010,11.081-9.
40. Hansson J, Pedersen NL, Galanti MR, et al. Use of snus and risk for cardiovascular disease: Results from the Swedish Twin Registry. J Intern Med. 2009;265:717-24.
41. Vendhan G, Vendhan K. Tobacco chewing and adult mortality: A case-control analysis of 22,000 cases and 429,000 controls, never smoking tobacco and never drinking alcohol, in South India. Asian Pac J Cancer Prev. 2015;16:1201-6.
42. Gupta R, Gupta S, Sharma S, et al. Risk of coronary heart disease among smokeless tobacco users: Results of systematic review and meta-analysis of global data. Nicotine Tob Res. 2018.
43. Stanfill SB, Connolly GN, Zhang L, et al. Global surveillance of oral tobacco products: Total nicotine, unionised nicotine and tobacco-specific N-nitrosamines. Tob Control. 2011;20:e2.
44. World Health Organization. WHO Report on Global Tobacco Epidemic: Warning about Dangers of Tobacco. Geneva: World Health Organization;2011.
45. Schotte K, et al. Implementation of key demand-reduction measures of the WHO Framework Convention on Tobacco Control and change in smoking prevalence in 126 countries: An association study. Lancet. 2017;2:e166-74.
46. Siddiqi K, Scammell K, Huque R, et al. Smokeless tobacco supply chain in South Asia: A comparative analysis using the WHO Framework Convention on Tobacco Control. Nicotine Tob Res. 2016;18(4):424-30.

CHAPTER 2

Alcohol and Coronary Artery Disease: Fact versus Fiction

JPS Sawhney, Kushal Madan

INTRODUCTION

There has been a lot of controversy around the use of alcohol in coronary artery disease (CAD). Many studies are in favor of wine as advantageous as compared to other alcoholic beverages. Some studies suggest that type of drink was not important. Heavy drinking is associated with increased mortality, hypertension, and cerebrovascular hemorrhage on the other end light-to-moderate consumption of alcohol is shown to be cardioprotective. How much drink is safe? In fact the definition of heavy, moderate and light drinking is not standardized. It must be known that definitions of a "standard drink" are variable by article and country thereby leading to imaginary facts rather than facts.

The purpose of this chapter is to explore the link between drinking alcohol and CAD. This chapter will put forward the facts associated with alcohol consumption and cardioprotective effects. So if someone does not drink already, is his heart a reason to start?

UNDERSTANDING "STANDARD DRINK"

A standard drink (or "unit of alcohol" in UK) is a notional drink that contains a specified fixed amount of pure alcohol (ethanol). Different countries define standard drinks differently. That means one standard drink always contains the same amount of alcohol regardless of the container size or the type of alcoholic beverage, but does not necessarily correspond to the typical serving size in the country in which it is served. For example, in the United States, a standard drink contains about 14 g of alcohol. The lowest number of grams of alcohol in Europe is in UK unit at 8 g and the highest in Austria at 20 g. In absolute terms, amounts of alcohol consumed less than 30 g per day is considered as light-moderate drinking and alcohol consumed more than 30 g/day is considered as heavy drinking.

ALCOHOL AND CARDIOVASCULAR MORTALITY

Epidemiological data indicate that there is a J-shaped curve to describe dose-response between alcohol intake and mortality, i.e., low-risk in light-to-moderate drinkers as compared to nondrinkers and highest risk among heavy drinkers. In a meta-analysis of 34 studies Di Castelnuovo et al. concluded that low levels of alcohol intake (1–2 drinks/day for women and 2–4 drinks/day for men) provided maximum protection (13–22% in women and 15–19% in men). On the other hand, alcohol intake more than two drinks per day in women and more than three drinks per day in men are associated with increased mortality.[2]

Gaziano et al. in a prospective cohort study, studied 89,299 men (age 40–84 years) from Physicians Health study, who were followed over 5.5 years for mortality.[3] They reported an L-shaped curve between light-to-moderate alcohol intake and cardiovascular (CV) mortality with decreased risk at 1 drink/week. It was also observed that there was decrease in CV mortality as compared with nondrinker even at more than or equal to two drinks per day.

Mukamal et al. studied 245,000 US adults and reported that alcohol intake of both light and moderate levels was associated with lower CV mortality compared with either heavy drinkers or nondrinkers.[4]

ALCOHOL AND CORONARY ARTERY DISEASE

Studies have reported that moderate consumption of alcohol is cardioprotective. Whether this cardioprotective effect is associated with lesser degree of coronary atherosclerosis was studied by Femia et al. in which association of alcohol with coronary atherosclerosis was assessed by coronary angiography in a large cohort of men (1,676) and women (465) from a coronary care unit.[5] It was concluded that in a selected high-risk population, moderate alcohol consumption was independently associated with less coronary atherosclerosis and lower risk for cardiac mortality. This conclusion cannot be extrapolated to the general population. To study the association between alcohol consumption and coronary atherosclerosis in asymptomatic subjects, study was performed on 1,795 individuals without coronary heart disease (CHD) using computerized tomography detected coronary calcium. It was concluded that the risk of extensive coronary calcification was 50% lower in individuals who consumed 1–2 alcoholic drinks per day than in nondrinkers.[6]

ALCOHOL AND CARDIOVASCULAR MEDICATIONS

Cardiovascular disease (CVD) patients are mainly taking lipid-lowering, antiplatelets or oral anticoagulant drugs. In such setting what are the interactions of alcohol and medications, how alcohol is metabolized or absorbed, whether alcohol affects the therapeutic effects of drugs, has not been sufficiently investigated. Moore et al. studied the risks of combined alcohol-medication use and reported that depending on type of medicine and amount of alcohol there could be aggravation of liver disease, dizziness, problems with coordination, insomnia, worsening of depression, and poor control of diabetes. Aspirin when combined with alcohol can raise the risk of gastrointestinal bleeding.[7]

However, more research is needed to determine the safety of alcohol consumption in combination with CV drugs.

POSSIBLE MECHANISMS FOR CORONARY ARTERY DISEASE PROTECTION BY ALCOHOL

It is hypothesized that moderate alcohol consumption reduces the risk of myocardial infarction (MI) through its effects on high-density lipoprotein cholesterol (HDLc), insulin sensitivity, thrombotic activity, and inflammation.

Effects on High-density Lipoprotein Cholesterol

Moderate alcohol intake is associated with increase in serum HDLc. This increase in HDLc is also associated with increase in apolipoproteins (A-I and A-II) which are the major HDL carrier proteins. According to Rimm et al. there will be 8 mg/dL increase in the plasma concentration of apolipoprotein A-I and a 16.8% reduction in CHD due to increased HDLc from 30 g alcohol per day.[8]

Antioxidant Effects

Alcohol intake may have antioxidant effect. There is a strong evidence from the observational studies that oxidation of low-density lipoprotein (LDL) is affected by the antioxidative effect of alcohol and thereby impeding the atherosclerotic process. It has been shown that grape-derived beverages are rich in nutritional polyphenolic antioxidants and hence have cardioprotective effects.[9,10]

Enhanced Insulin Sensitivity

Alcohol consumption is also associated with reduced insulin resistance and increased insulin sensitivity. This effect is probably due to suppressed fatty acid release from adipose tissue and elevation of adiponectin levels during the Krebs cycle of skeletal muscles, thereby facilitating glucose metabolism.[11,12]

Antithrombotic Effects

Alcohol promotes reduction in blood clotting and platelet aggregation, reduced levels of plasminogen activator inhibitor (PAI) activity, fibrinogen, plasma viscosity, von Willebrand factor and factor VII, and increased concentrations of tissue-type plasminogen activator (tPA) have been described.[13]

Anti-inflammatory Effects

Alcohol may confer cardioprotection by acting as an anti-inflammatory agent. Recent data show that alcohol consumption suppresses the production of proinflammatory cytokines such as tumor necrosis factor (TNF)-α, interleukin-5, interleukin-6, and C-reactive protein (CRP).[14]

DRINKING PATTERNS AND CORONARY HEART DISEASE

Not only choice of beverage but also the drinking pattern is an important factor of interest with respect to CAD and hypertension. Some of the studies mentioned in the report on moderate drinking from National Institute of Alcohol Abuse and Alcoholism assessed the differences between regular low per-occasion consumption and the same total weekly consumption all at once.[15] In fact, the pattern of alcohol drinking is not assessed by many studies, thereby making the comparison and conclusions difficult across the studies.

To assess the influence of drinking pattern and type of beverage (beer, red wine, white wine, and liquor) on risk of MI, Mukamal et al. studied 38,077 males who were free of CVD at baseline. There were 1,418 cases of MI during 12 years of follow-up once in every 4 years. As compared to men who consumed alcohol 3–4 or 5–7 days per week had decreased risks of MI as compared to those who consumed alcohol less than once per week. Also there was an inverse association between the risk of MI and four types of beverage, strongest for beer and liquor, intermediate for white wine, and weakest for red wine.[16]

The most favorable drinking pattern is regular daily or almost daily light drinking, with avoidance of clearly harmful binge drinking.[17]

INFLUENCE OF AGE AND SEX ON CARDIOVASCULAR EFFECTS OF ALCOHOL

Recent reviews suggest that alcohol consumption is mainly associated with a decreased risk of MI among men over 45 years of age and women over 55 years of age. To study whether the beneficial effect of alcohol is influenced by age, Hvidtfeldt et al. conducted a pooled analysis of eight prospective studies including 192,067 women and 74,919 men and showed an inverse relationship for both men and women for three age groups (≤50, 50–59, ≥60 years).[18] In a population-based study of 4,410 adults aged more than 65 years free of CVD at baseline, it was found that alcohol consumption was inversely associated with risk of CHD for men and women, and for different beverage types. Also it was concluded that moderate consumption (14 or more drinks/week) was associated with lowest risk of CHD.[19]

It has been reported that men and women have similar cardioprotective benefit especially in postmenopausal women. Nurse's health study,[20] studies from women's health initiative[21] and Swedish women's lifestyle and health study[22] have demonstrated an inverse relationship between moderate alcohol consumption and the risk of CAD and total mortality in women. But it is evident from the literature that women experience toxic effects of alcohol at approximately half the dose of men.[23] Overall evidence from epidemiological data indicates that alcohol consumption in women may be associated with an increased risk of breast cancer. Relative effect of moderate consumption of alcohol is lower than the increased risk of acquiring breast cancer especially for women with a family history of breast cancer. Although there has been a belief that alcohol enhances lactation but the scientific research does not support that alcohol consumption increases milk production but may actually decrease it.

THE GENETICS OF ALCOHOL AND CARDIOVASCULAR DISEASE

Alcohol dehydrogenase (ADH) catalyzes the oxidation of ethanol to acetaldehyde which is highly toxic affecting the myocardial structure and function. Any genetic variation in the activity of ADH enzyme can lead to excess acetaldehyde accumulation. Similarly cytochrome P450 2E1 (CYP2E1), is another enzyme which promotes conversion of ethanol to acetaldehyde.

Chen et al. identified a mitochondrial protein aldehyde dehydrogenase-2 (ALDH2) which plays an important role in alcohol metabolism.[24] ALDH2 activation is required for cardioprotection as it catalyzes the oxidation of acetaldehyde to a lesser toxic acetate. Therefore, it is the balance between the levels of ADH, CYP2E1, and ALDH activity that determines how much alcohol can be metabolized by liver, what are the byproducts and the underlying alcohol induced tissue injury including CVD.

The French Paradox

This term French paradox was first used in 1992 to describe the irony of the fact that in spite of high saturated fats in the diet, incidence of coronary events was less in French population. This was attributed to the fact that there was moderate consumption of red wine along with the meal.[25] Epidemiological studies indicate that the amount of alcohol consumed in France, i.e., 20–30 g/day can reduce risk of CHD by at least 40%.

Regular, moderate consumption of red wine has been associated with reduced CHD and mortality. Red wine has higher levels of polyphenols (flavonoids and nonflavonoids, which have antioxidant, antiendothelin-1, and antiplatelet effects) as compared with either forms of alcohol. But the cardioprotective effects are due to ethanol itself rather than a specific type of alcoholic beverage (wine, beer, and liquor). A differential cardioprotective effect of wine could be because wine is always consumed in moderation as compared to beer or liquor. Studies have shown equal protection from all types of alcohol suggesting that the specific alcoholic beverage is less important than the quantity and pattern of the alcohol intake.[26,27]

Two components to understand the pattern of drinking are frequency and binge drinking. Mukamal et al. in a cohort study of 1,935 MI patients followed up for 3.8 years showed that binge drinkers (even light binge drinkers) had 2-fold high-risk of mortality than drinkers who did not binge.[28] There is also an indication from the literature that more frequent drinking (several days/week or daily) is more beneficial as compared to occasional drinking.[29,30] Frequent drinking may also explain the so called "French Paradox." French people relate the beneficial effects of red wine to the frequency of drinking, i.e., every day with their meals.

POINTS TO CONSIDER FROM THE PAST STUDIES

- There have been no reported randomized controlled trials of alcohol consumption and CAD outcome data. This could be due to obvious ethical and logistical reasons
- *Errors in the past*: Shaper et al. in 1988 hypothesized the presence of systemic misclassification errors in the past studies associated with alcohol consumption and CHD.[31] According to Shaper et al. people decrease their alcohol consumption as they get older. Heavy drinkers tend to recue alcohol intake that have ischemic heart disease or high blood pressure. Inclusion of such population as abstainers might create bias which was not considered in past. Shaper's hypothesis was not further evaluated, but Fillmore et al. confirmed this and suggested that the cardiac protection by alcohol may have been overestimated.[32] They classified the misclassification errors:
    - Former drinker misclassification error, i.e., failure to eparate former drinkers from complete nondrinkers
    - Occasional drinker misclassification error, i.e., failure to separate occasional drinkers from complete non-drinkers.

  In their meta-analysis, they concluded that the few studies without this error (i.e., those that did not contaminate the abstainer category with occasional or former drinkers) show abstainers and "light" or "moderate" drinkers to be at equal risk for all-cause and CHD mortality.[33]
- As compared to heavy drinkers, moderate drinkers have a healthy lifestyle. It is presumed that heavy drinkers are likely to consume more tobacco, unhealthy diet and do less exercise and this unhealthy lifestyle could be the explanation for higher CV mortality in heavy drinkers

- Widespread belief that alcohol is beneficial in CAD could also induce selection bias in more recent studies
- Genetics can also influence the interindividual variations in the CV response to alcohol consumption.

ALCOHOL AND INDIAN POPULATION

There has been ample evidence from the literature to show that there exists a J- or U-shaped relation between alcohol consumption and CHD. That means CHD and mortality rates are lowest in light-to-moderate drinkers and highest among abstainers and heavy drinkers. However, there is paucity of data from India to support this concept. Limited data in Indians from the INTERHEART study, a case-control study of patients with incident acute MI, revealed that in South Asians alcohol consumption was not protective against CHD.[34] The odds ratio (OR) of having MI was 1.64 [95% confidence interval (CI) 1.21–2.27] among Indian alcohol users as compared to nonusers. Roy et al. conducted a surveillance study in ten industries across India to assess the CHD prevalence among 4,465 male subjects who were present or past alcohol users as compared to abstainers.[35] Consistent to INTERHEART study they did not observe any protective association between alcohol intake and the prevalence of CHD, rather suggested a possible harm of alcohol for coronary risk in Indian men, since there was significantly higher systolic blood pressure, diastolic blood pressure, and fasting blood sugar in alcohol users as compared to lifetime abstainers. The contradictory results could be due to differences in ethnicity, type of alcoholic beverage, and pattern of alcohol intake. The beneficial effect of moderate alcohol consumption is not a global finding because most of the research reported in literature is from western world where the climate, culture, and diet are so different from Asian countries. Similar to Indian population, it is reported that moderate alcohol does not confer cardioprotective effect on ischemic heart disease mortality among older Chinese population in Hong Kong.[36]

DETRIMENTAL EFFECTS OF ALCOHOL INTAKE

Alcohol abuse, binge drinking has all been associated with harmful effects such as hepatitis, liver cirrhosis, pancreatitis, hypertriglyceridemia, stroke, injuries, and accidents.[37] Corrao et al., in a meta-analysis of alcohol consumption and the risk of neoplasms and non-neoplastic disease, reported strong trends in risk for cancers of oral cavity, esophagus, and larynx.[38]

Ethanol at higher doses is associated with cardiotoxicity thereby developing alcoholic cardiomyopathy and heart failure.[39] Excessive alcohol uses can also precipitate cardiac arrhythmias typically atrial fibrillation.[40]

A WORD OF CAUTION

Alcohol is classified as a human carcinogen (class 1) by the International Agency for Research on Cancer, with a dose-related increase in prevalence of several cancers either exponentially (e.g., oral cavity and pharyngeal cancers) or linearly (e.g., esophageal and breast cancer), beginning at the level of the first to second drink per day.

Keeping this fact in mind it seems cardioprotective benefits are relatively less than increasing the risk of cancer.

The term "moderate drinking" is inappropriately used and should be avoided in scientific literature. Public health advocates suggest "nonharmful" or "drinking at low-risk" are more useful terms.

> Complete abstinence is easier than perfect moderation.
>
> **—St. Augustine**

CONCLUSION

Present available literature about the beneficial effects of alcohol is substantial and contradictory, so it is less likely to make a straightforward recommendation regarding the optimal limit of consumption of alcohol. Caution in making general recommendations is needed.

Based on the epidemiological and clinical evidence, as compared to nondrinkers, "moderate alcohol use" should not be interpreted as "healthy alcohol use" (Masters, 2003).

However, it is not suggested to initiate drinking if you do not already because alcohol certainly has well-established neurotoxic, hepatotoxic, and carcinogenic risks. There are safer and healthier ways to protect your heart.

Thus, we encourage people to discuss alcohol use with the physician and make an individualized decision about appropriate consumption.

REFERENCES

1. Deirdre M, Jean L. "Standard drink measures throughout Europe; peoples' understanding of standard drinks and their use in drinking guidelines, alcohol surveys and labelling" (PDF). Reducing Alcohol Related Harm. 2015. p. 8.
2. Di Castelnuovo A, Costanzo S, Bagnardi V, et al. Alcohol dosing and total mortality in men and women. Arch Intern Med. 2006;166:2437-45.
3. Gaziano JM, Gaziano TA, Glynn RJ, et al. Light-to-moderate alcohol consumption and mortality in the Physicians' Health Study enrollment cohort. J Am Coll Cardiol. 2000;35:96-105.
4. Mukamal KJ, Chen CM, Rao SR, et al. Alcohol consumption and cardiovascular mortality among U.S. adults, 1987 to 2002. J Am Coll Cardiol. 2010;55:1328-35.
5. Femia R, Natali A, L'Abbate A, et al. Coronary atherosclerosis and alcohol consumption: Angiographic and mortality data. Arterioscler Thromb Vasc Biol. 2006;26:1607-12.
6. Vliegenthart R, Oei HHS, van den Elzen APM, et al. Alcohol consumption and coronary calcification in a general population. Arch Intern Med. 2004;164:2355-60.
7. Moore AA, Whiteman EJ, Ward KT. Risks of combined alcohol/medication use in older adults. Am J Geriatr Pharmacother. 2007;5:64-74.
8. Rimm EB, Williams P, Fosher K, et al. Moderate alcohol intake and lower risk of coronary heart disease: Meta-analysis of effects on lipids and haemostatic factors. BMJ. 1999;319:1523-8.
9. van Golde PH, Sloots LM, Vermeulen WP, et al. The role of alcohol in the antilow density lipoprotein oxidation activity of red wine. Atherosclerosis. 1999;147:365-70.
10. Puddey IB, Croft KD, Abdu-Amsha Caccetta R, et al. Alcohol, free radicals and antioxidants. Novartis Found Symp. 1998;216:51-62.
11. Sierksma A, Patel H, Ouchi N, et al. Effect of moderate alcohol consumption on adiponectin, tumor necrosis factor-alpha, and insulin sensitivity. Diabetes Care. 2004;27:184-9.

12. Greenfield JR, Samaras K, Jenkins AB, et al. Moderate alcohol consumption, estrogen replacement therapy, and physical activity are associated with increased insulin sensitivity: Is abdominal adiposity the mediator? Diabetes Care. 2003;2:2734-40.
13. Hendriks, HF, Veenstra, J, Velthuis-te Wierik EJ, et al. Effect of moderate dose of alcohol with evening meal on fibrinolytic factors. BMJ. 1994;308:1003-6.
14. Albert MA, Glynn RJ, Ridker PM. Alcohol consumption and plasma concentration of C-reactive protein. Circulation. 2003;107:443-7.
15. Gunzerath L, Faden V, Zakhari S, et al. National Institute on Alcohol Abuse and Alcoholism report on moderate drinking. Alcohol Clin Exp Res. 2004;28:829-49.
16. Mukamal KJ, Conigrave KM, Mittleman MA, et al. Roles of drinking pattern and type of alcohol consumed in coronary heart disease in men. N Engl J Med. 2003;348:109-18.
17. Klatsky AL. Alcohol and cardiovascular diseases: Where do we stand today? J Intern Med. 2015;278:238-50.
18. Hvidtfeldt UA, Tolstrup JS, Jakobsen MU, et al. Alcohol intake and risk of coronary heart disease in younger, middle-aged, and older adults. Circulation. 2010;121:1589-97.
19. Mukamal KJ, Chung H, Jenny NS, et al. Alcohol consumption and risk of coronary heart disease in older adults: The Cardiovascular Health Study. J Am Geriatr Soc. 2006;54(1):30-7.
20. Stampfer MJ, Colditz GA, Willett WC, et al. A prospective study of moderate alcohol consumption and the risk of coronary disease and stroke in women. N Engl J Med. 1988;319:267-73.
21. Freiberg MS, Chang YF, Kraemer KL, et al. Alcohol consumption, hypertension, and total mortality among women. Am J Hypertens. 2009;22:1212-8.
22. Behrens G, Leitzmann MF, Sandin S, et al. The association between alcohol consumption and mortality: The Swedish women's lifestyle and health study. Eur J Epidemiol. 2011;26:81-90.
23. Baraona E, Abittan CS, Dohmen K, et al. Gender differences in pharmacokinetics of alcohol. Alcohol Clin Exp Res. 2001;25:502-7.
24. Chen CH, Budas GR, Churchill EN, et al. Activation of aldehyde dehydrogenase2 reduces ischemic damage to the heart. Science. 2008;321:1493-5.
25. Renaud S, de Lorgeril M. Wine, alcohol, platelets, and the French paradox for coronary heart disease. Lancet. 1992;339:1523-6.
26. Corder R, Mullent W, Khan NQ, et al. Red wine procyanidins and vascular health. Nature. 2006;444:566.
27. Ellison RC. Importance of pattern of alcohol consumption. Circulation. 2005;112:3818-9.
28. Mukamal KJ, Maclure M, Muller JE, et al. Binge drinking and mortality after acute myocardial infarction. Circulation. 2005;112:3839-45.
29. Britton A, Marmot M. Different measures of alcohol consumption and risk of coronary heart disease and all-cause mortality: 11-year follow-up of the Whitehall II Cohort Study. Addiction. 2004;99:109-16.
30. Mukamal KJ, Jensen MK, Gronbaek M, et al. Drinking frequency, mediating biomarkers, and risk of myocardial infarction in women and men. Circulation. 2005;112:1406-13.
31. Shaper AG, Wannamethee G, Walker M. Alcohol and mortality in British men: Explaining the U-shaped curve. Lancet. 1988;2:1267-73.
32. Fillmore KM, Kerr WC, Stockwell T, et al. Moderate alcohol use and reduced mortality risk: Systematic error in prospective studies. Addiction Res Theory. 2006;14:101-32.
33. Fillmore KM, Stockwell T, Chikritzhs T, et al. Moderate alcohol use and reduced mortality risk: Systematic error in prospective studies and new hypotheses. Ann Epidemiol. 2007;17:S16-23.
34. Joshi P, Islam S, Pais P, et al. Risk factors for early myocardial infarction in South Asians compared with individuals in other countries. JAMA. 2007;297:286-94.
35. Roy A, Prabhakaran D, Jeemon P, et al. Impact of alcohol on coronary heart disease in Indian men. Atherosclerosis. 2010;210:531-5.
36. Schooling CM, Sun W, Ho SY, et al. Moderate alcohol use and mortality from ischemic heart disease: A prospective study in older Chinese people. PLoS One. 2008;3:e2370.
37. Rehm J, Mathers C, Popova S, et al. Global burden of disease and injury and economic cost attributable to alcohol use and alcohol-use disorders. Lancet. 2009;373: 2223-33.
38. Corrao G, Bagnardi V, Zambon A, et al. A meta-analysis of alcohol consumption and the risk of 15 diseases. Prev Med. 2004;38:613-9.
39. Laonigro I, Correale M, Di Biase M, et al. Alcohol abuse and heart failure. Eur J Heart Fail. 2009;11:453-62.
40. Mukamal KJ, Tolstrup JS, Friberg J, et al. Alcohol consumption and risk of atrial fibrillation in men and women: The Copenhagen City Heart Study. Circulation. 2005;112:1736-42.

CHAPTER 3

Vitamin D and Cardiovascular Disease: Indian Perspective

Ramu Adela, Rajesh Khadgawat

INTRODUCTION

Vitamin D

Vitamin D, a secosteroid (steroid with open or broken ring), is fat-soluble vitamin involved in maintenance of calcium metabolism as well as musculoskeletal health. It exists in two forms, ergocalciferol (D2, from plant origin) and cholecalciferol (D_3, from animal origin). With limited sources in diet except for seafood, main source of vitamin D in humans is synthesis from cholesterol in epidermis by exposure to the UV radiation (sunlight). Exposure to sunlight for sufficient duration bring out chemical change in structure by opening a double bond which further initiates series of structural changes resulting in formation of cholecalciferol (also known as "Calciol"). Once formed, cholecalciferol, an inactive form, undergoes hydroxylation in liver and converted to 25-hydroxycholecalciferol [(25(OH)D) also known as "Calcidiol" or "Calcifediol"] which is further, hydroxylated in kidney to form active form of vitamin D, 1,25-dihydroxycholecalciferol [(1,25$(OH)_2$D) also known as "Calcidiol"]. Vitamin D receptors (VDRs) are intracellular receptors and found in all tissues of the body, including vascular smooth muscle, endothelium, and myocardium. The active metabolite 1,25$(OH)_2$D binds with the vitamin D receptor in cytoplasm in the targeted cell and form a heterodimeric complex (VDR-RXR) with retinoid receptor (RXR). Further VDR-RXR complex translocate to the nucleus where it binds with vitamin D responsive element (VDRE) in the DNA and exert its biological function through transcriptional regulation of targeted genes in targeted cells (Fig. 1).[1]

ASSESSMENT OF VITAMIN D NUTRITIONAL STATUS

Nutritional status of vitamin D is assessed by measuring serum levels of 25-hydroxyvitamin D. Although measurement of 1,25$(OH)_2$D, active form is also possible but measurement is cumbersome and at the same, not useful in providing nutritional status of vitamin D. One of the most debatable issues about vitamin D is cutoff used for defining vitamin D deficiency (VDD). Many societies suggest serum vitamin D levels between 12 and 20 ng/mL to define VDD; however, most widely used cutoff, all over the world is less than 20 ng/mL while levels between 20 and 30 ng/mL are considered as insufficient and levels more than 30 ng/mL is used to define vitamin D sufficiency. Further, levels of VDD (<20 ng/mL) are divided into severe (<5 ng/mL), moderate (5 ≤10), and mild VDD (10 ≤20 ng/mL).[2] These cutoffs are based on the physiological fact of occurrence of secondary hyperparathyroidism with decrease in vitamin D levels.

VITAMIN D NUTRITIONAL STATUS IN THE WORLD AND IN INDIA

High prevalence of VDD has been recognized very early at the start in 19th century (1920s) especially in causing rickets, which led to initiation of food fortification programs in most of the developed countries.[3] Over the years, vitamin D food fortification has resulted in improvement in vitamin D status of general population. However, errors in fortification (fortification of large amount of vitamin D by mistake) had raised concerns about these fortifications, which resulted in many countries converting universal fortification to optional fortification with vitamin D. Vitamin D food fortification program could not be started with wider success in our country.

In spite of food fortification, high prevalence of VDD has been reported all over the world, across all age groups and both sexes.[4,5] VDD is considered to be pandemic with report of widespread deficiency coming from every part of the world with maximum prevalence reported from Middle East and South Asian countries in spite of availability of sunlight throughout the year. Prevalence of VDD has been estimated to be approximately 30–60% in the general population.[6]

In spite of geographical location of India (located at 28° 36.8' N and 77° 12.5' E in the northern hemisphere of the

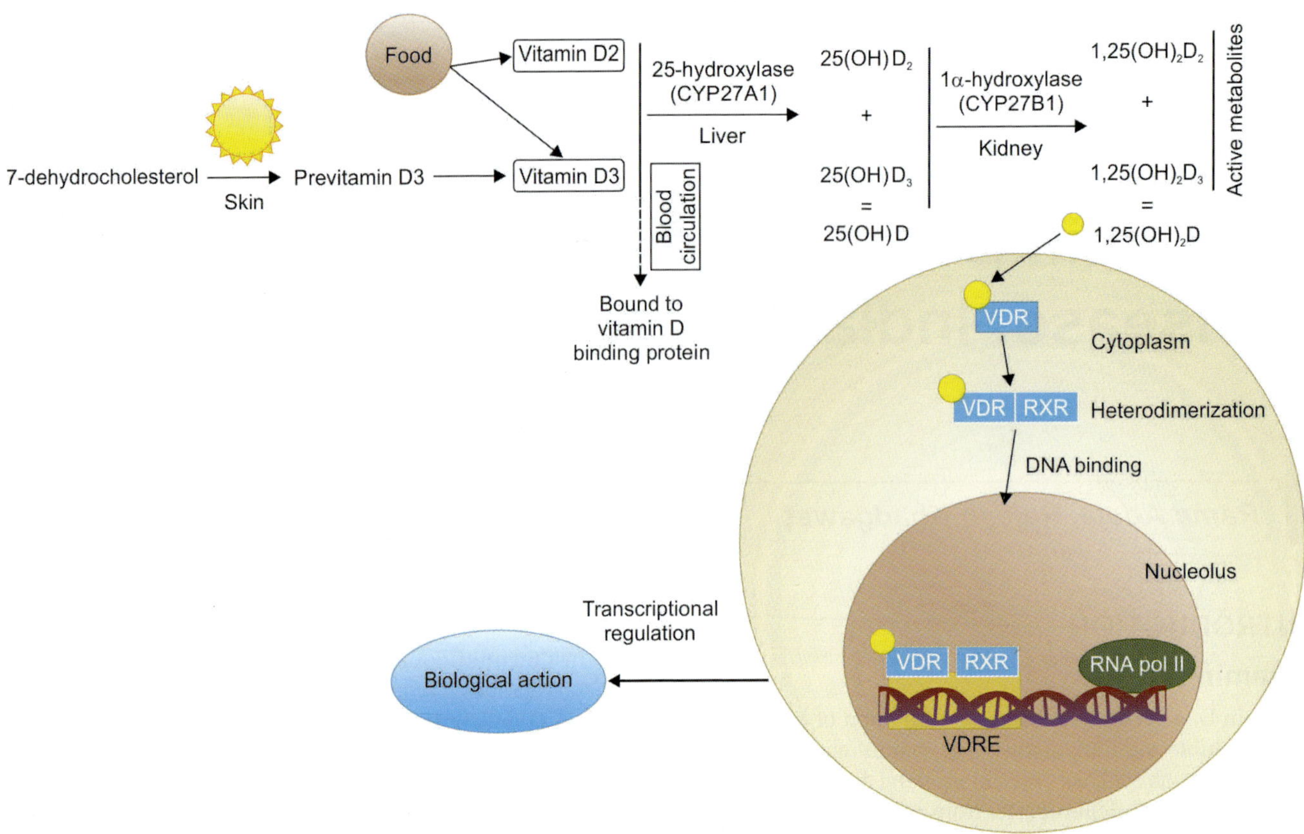

FIG. 1: Vitamin D synthesis, metabolism, and cellular action.

globe) which provides plenty of sunlight throughout the year, VDD was never a concern among Indians. Contrary to this assumption, high prevalence of VDD has been reported throughout the country for all age groups including neonates, infants, school going children, adolescents, adults, pregnancy, lactating women, and senior citizens. This is probably a result of poor sun exposure, dark skin complexion, atmospheric pollution, vegetarian foods habits, absence of food fortification with vitamin D, and poor intake of vitamin D supplements.[7] The most of the published studies on vitamin D status of general population report that very high prevalence to the extent of 70–95% using a cutoff of less than 20 ng/mL.

VITAMIN D AND NONSKELETAL EFFECTS

One of the major functions of vitamin D is maintenance of musculoskeletal health. However, over the years, association studies of levels of serum vitamin D with many chronic diseases has given a newer concept of role of vitamin D in nonskeletal diseases especially, noncommunicable diseases. Vitamin D has been reported to influence not only insulin sensitivity or resistance but also insulin secretion.[8] There are several studies, including data from the Framingham Heart Study,[9] demonstrating an inverse association between insulin resistance and serum 25-hydroxyvitamin D levels.

VITAMIN D AND CARDIOVASCULAR DISEASES

Vitamin D status has also been linked to cardiovascular (CV) risk factors, morbidity, and mortality.[10] VDD state has been shown to be associated with cardiovascular diseases (CVD) risk factors such as obesity, hypertension, hyperlipidemia, and diabetes mellitus. In a random sample of 6,784 subjects in the age group of 30–60 years, high serum levels of vitamin D was reported to be associated with lower incidence of metabolic syndrome and lipid profile favorable to CV health; however, no association between vitamin D level and blood pressure was found.[11] In one of the largest study, population-based sample of 16,603 men and women aged 18 years or older (Third National Health and Nutrition Examination Survey, 1988–1994). Subjects with CVD had a greater frequency of 25(OH)D deficiency (<20 ng/mL) than those without VDD. Even after adjustment of all CV risk factors, subjects with VDD had an increased risk of prevalent CVD with odds ratio 1.20.[12] Another large study of 18,225 US men (Health Professionals Follow-Up Study), low vitamin D status was found to be associated with increased risk of myocardial infarction (MI) as compared to subjects with vitamin D sufficiency.[13] Another data base study of 41,504 subjects, VDD was associated with highly significant (p <0.0001) increases in the prevalence of diabetes, hypertension, hyperlipidemia, and peripheral

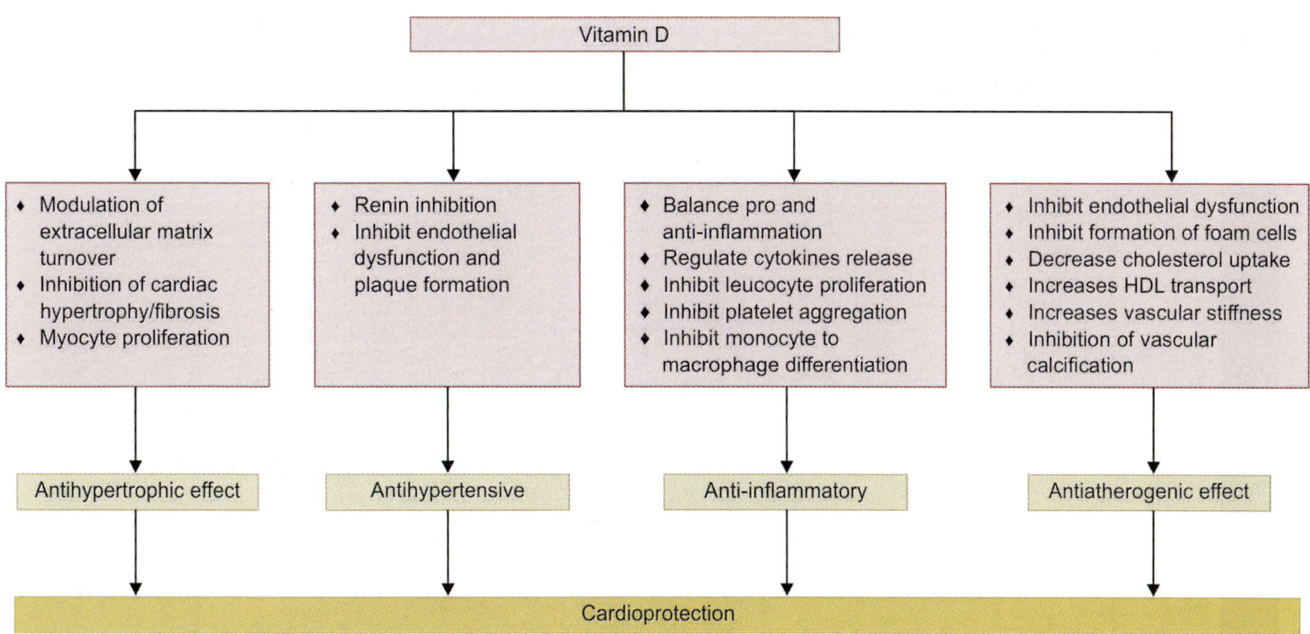

FLOWCHART 1: Proposed mechanisms for cardioprotection with vitamin D.

vascular disease. Serum vitamin D levels were also found to be significantly associated with coronary artery disease (CAD), MI, heart failure (HF), and stroke. Even in subjects without risk factors but with severe deficiency, also had increased likelihood of developing diabetes, hypertension, and hyperlipidemia.[14] In a recently published meta-analysis of 19 prospective studies with 66,000 participants, a linear and inverse association was found between circulating vitamin D level and risk of CVD.[15] Similarly, VDD has also been reported to be associated with subclinical markers of atherosclerosis like intima-media thickness (IMT), arterial stiffness, and coronary calcification.

MECHANISM OF VITAMIN D AND PROPOSED CARDIOPROTECTION

The exact mechanism of role of vitamin D in proposed cardioprotection has not been elucidated well. The most of the information is coming from individual studies assessing effect of vitamin D on cellular, molecular, and biochemical parameters associated with CVD. Vitamin D has shown to inhibit proliferation of vascular smooth muscle cells and increases calcification of smooth muscle cells.[16] It has also been shown to regulate the growth and proliferation of smooth muscle cells and cardiomyocytes. It has been reported to inhibit renin-angiotensin-aldosterone system (RAAS) and inhibit the endothelial dysfunction, the initiation step of plaque formation.[17] Similarly, vitamin D has also been found to be affecting the immune balance by suppressing proinflammatory and increasing anti-inflammatory cytokines and chemokines and inhibits endothelial dysfunction, leukocyte proliferation, cytokine release, and platelet aggregation the process involved in the atherosclerosis development.[18-21] It also shows antiatherogenic function by inhibiting the formation of foam cells, cholesterol uptake by the macrophages, and enabling high-density lipoprotein (HDL) transport.[22]

VITAMIN D AND CARDIOVASCULAR DISEASE: EVIDENCES FROM OBSERVATIONAL STUDIES

High prevalence of VDD has been reported from all ages in Indian population all across the country. Details of the Indian observational studies mentioned in table 1. Most of the studies reporting association between vitamin D and CAD had recruited patients admitted in hospital setting for management of CAD. Priya et al. reported high prevalence of VDD (80.4% using cutoff of <20 ng/mL) in North Indian hypertensive subjects in comparison to controls with 67.7%.[23] Another study reported VDD (<30 ng/mL) in 53.3% hypertensive pregnant women while only 3.3% healthy pregnant women without hypertension had VDD. In the same study, lower vitamin D levels were also found to be associated with hypertension disorders in pregnancy and circulatory cytokine and chemokine levels.[24] Cross-sectional studies have also reported higher prevalence of VDD in subjects with CAD patients and found to be independent predictor of CAD.[25-27] Multiple studies have also reported high prevalence VDD in patients admitted with MI patients.[28-30] Similarly, higher prevalence of VDD has also been reported in patients with ischemic stroke and is independent predictor of ischemic stroke.[31] Higher prevalence of VDD in patients with dilated cardiomyopathy has been reported and found to be correlated with cardiac function.[32]

TABLE 1: Indian studies exploring vitamin D status of subjects with coronary artery disease

Cardiovascular disease; reference	Study type and place	Study population and size	Outcome parameter assessed	Serum 25-hydroxyvitamin D level	Conclusion
Acute myocardial infarction (AMI)[28]	Observational study, Delhi	Healthy controls: 120 AMI cases: 120	Compared vitamin D status of AMI cases with healthy controls	Controls: 11.1 ng/mL Cases: 6.0 ng/mL	High prevalence of vitamin D deficiency among cases of acute MI as well as controls
AMI[29]	Observational study, Delhi	Control cases: 50 AMI cases: 50	Compared vitamin D status of AMI cases with healthy controls and correlation between FMD and vitamin D	Controls: 25.4 ng/mL AMI cases: 14.5 ng/mL	Majority of AMI cases were vitamin D deficient FMD was positively correlated with vitamin D
AMI[30]	Observational study, Bangalore	AMI: 314	Compared vitamin D deficiency among AMI patients	67.5% patients were vitamin D deficient and 16% were insufficient, 83.5% patient had abnormally low vitamin D	Vitamin D deficiency is common in patients with AMI
CAD[26]	Observational study, Uttar Pradesh	Control: 101 CAD: 140	Compared vitamin D status in CAD cases with controls	Controls: 28.8 ng/mL CAD: 18.2 ng/mL	Significantly low vitamin D levels observed in CAD Vitamin D deficiency was found to be an independent predictor of CAD
CAD[25]	Observational study, Andhra Pradesh	Healthy controls: 50 T2DM: 71 CAD: 28 T2DM + CAD: 38	Compared vitamin D status among study groups	Controls: 38.0 ng/mL T2DM: 32.0 ng/mL CAD: 30.8 ng/mL T2DM + CAD: 20.1 ng/mL	Low vitamin D levels observed in the T2DM, CAD and T2DM + CAD groups, compared to healthy controls
CAD[27]	Observational study, Chandigarh	Patients who underwent coronary angiography: 315	Compared vitamin D status of CAD patients with normal coronary artery	Normal coronary artery 11.3 ng/mL CAD: 14.1 ng/mL	Prevalence of vitamin D deficiency is very high in CAD, but it does not correlate with the angiographic severity of CAD
Hypertensive disorders in pregnancy[24]	Observational study, Hyderabad	Healthy pregnant: 30 Hypertension disorders in pregnancy: 30	Compared vitamin D status between the two groups	Healthy pregnant: 50.2 ng/mL Hypertension disorders in pregnancy: 28.64 ng/mL	Vitamin D levels decreased in severity of hypertensive disorders in pregnancy
Hypertension[23]	Observational study, Lucknow	Controls: 99 Hypertension cases: 102	Compared vitamin D status between the two groups	Controls: 33.5 ng/mL Hypertension cases: 15.1 ng/mL	Vitamin D deficiency is more prevalent with hypertension
Elderly subjects visiting cardiac checkup camp[47]	Observational study, Rajasthan	Control: 47 CAD: 53	Correlation between serum vitamin D level and cardiovascular morbidity	Vitamin D deficiency CAD: 28.30%; Controls: 25.53% Vitamin D insufficiency Cases: 49.05%; Controls: 23.40% Vitamin D sufficiency Cases: 22.64%; Controls: 51.04%	Vitamin D deficiency is common in elderly persons
Ischemic stroke[31]	Observational study, Hyderabad	Controls: 250 Ischemic stroke: 250	Compared vitamin D status between the two groups	Vitamin D deficiency Stroke cases: 48.8%; Controls: 31.6%	Vitamin D deficiency is an independently associated with ischemic stroke
Dilated cardiomyopathy (DCMP)[32]	Observational study, Lucknow	Controls: 60 DCMP: 56	Compared vitamin D status between the two groups	Controls: 28.2 ng/mL DCMP: 14.5 ng/mL	DCMP subjects had lower vitamin D levels than controls

FMD, flow-mediated dilatation; T2DM, type 2 diabetes mellitus; CAD, coronary artery disease; MI, myocardial infarction.

VITAMIN D AND CARDIOVASCULAR DISEASE: EVIDENCES FROM INTERVENTIONAL STUDIES

International Studies

Results of cross-sectional studies of association of vitamin D with CAD have not been verified in interventional studies with vitamin D. In a randomized, double-blind, placebo-controlled clinical trial of 5,108 community-residents aged 50–84 years, oral vitamin D in an initial dose of 200,000 IU, followed a month later by monthly doses of 100,000 IU, or placebo for a median of 3.3 years did not prevent CVD compared with placebo.[33] Another randomized trial, also did not show a reduction of mortality in patients with advanced HF received a daily vitamin D of 4,000 IU compared with placebo.[34] Study of 112 patients receiving 3,000 IU cholecalciferol daily for 20 weeks did not result in a significant reduction in blood pressure.[35] However, study with female subjects aged over 69 years who received vitamin D3 (800 IU) and calcium (1,200 mg) daily for 8 weeks' supplementation resulted in borderline yet significant decrease in systolic blood pressure ($p = 0.04$).[36] Witte et al. conducted a study on 229 chronic heart failure (CHF) and VDD [cholecalciferol (<20 ng/mL)]. Participants were allocated to 1-year of vitamin D supplementation (4,000 IU/daily) or placebo. The study showed improvement in cardiac function like LV ejection fraction and reversal of LV remodeling like LV end-diastolic diameter and LV end-systolic diameter.[37] Dalbeni et al. conducted a randomized double-blind placebo-controlled study on CHF patients, high-dose 800,000 IU (4,000 IU/daily) of cholecalciferol for 6 months. The study revealed that 25(OH)D levels and ejection fraction were increased and systolic blood pressure decreased after 6 months treatment.[38] Similarly, another research group reported that vitamin D supplementation (100,000 IU) in subjects with baseline vitamin D insufficiency did not improve CVD risk factors profile.[39] Tomson et al. reported data of vitamin D supplementation in BEST-D (Biochemical Efficacy and Safety Trial of vitamin D) double-blind randomized placebo-controlled trial (4,000 IU/day for 12 months) did not show any improvement on blood pressure, arterial stiffness, and cardiac function.[40] Another recently conducted single-center, double-blind, randomized, placebo-controlled study with vitamin D dosage of 2,800 IU per day did not show any favorable effect on lipid metabolism.[41] Chowdhury et al. conducted a meta-analysis with observational and interventional studies and concluded that in observational studies, serum 25(OH)D level was negatively associated with death due to CVD, cancer, and other causes; however, supplementation studies did not support role of vitamin D supplementation in improving clinical outcomes.[42] Recently, published systematic review with meta-analysis by using placebo-controlled randomized trials of at least 4 weeks of vitamin D supplementation, did not show any significant effect of vitamin D supplementation on CV function, i.e., flow-mediated dilatation (FMD), carotid-femoral pulse wave velocity.[43] Although, it would be difficult to compare results of these studies because of many limitations like lack of randomization, placebo-controlled design, use of hospital admitted population, small sample size, shorter duration of intervention, and absence of VDD in study subjects at baseline, but still most of the studies have not reported any significant positive impact on outcome parameters. Multiple meta-analyses published assessing effects of vitamin D supplementation in various CADs, suggest no beneficial role of vitamin D supplementation in established CAD. However, pooling of results of all intervention studies would be not very logistic as design, duration, and dose of supplementation of vitamin D is highly heterogeneous.

INDIAN STUDIES

The most of the studies published from India are of observational design with only three interventional studies have been conducted so far. Details of these studies are given in table 2.

Abid et al.[44] randomized 72 subjects with HF (NYHA class II or more) with vitamin D level less than 30 ng/mL into two groups, group I, subjects received cholecalciferol 60,000 IU weekly for 12 weeks while in group II, subjects received optimized medical therapy but not vitamin D. Although, there was a significant improvement in echocardiographic parameters, but the extent of change from baseline did not differ significantly between the two groups.

Narasimhan et al.[45] in an open label randomized controlled design, supplemented a single dose of 600,000 IU of cholecalciferol intramuscular injection in patients with ischemic stroke, and compared with patients who did not receive vitamin D. Using Scandinavian Stroke Scale (SSS) as outcome parameter, it was found that vitamin D supplemented group had significantly higher SSS than patient who did not receive. Even in supplemented group, higher scores were seen in subjects who had VDD at the time of screening in comparison to subjects who did not have. The sample size was small (30 in each group) and not double blind design but requires further exploration of results in larger studies.

Another recently published randomized, double-blind, placebo-controlled study,[46] effect of cholecalciferol supplementation on vascular function was assessed in 120 patients aged 18–70 years, with nondiabetic chronic kidney disease (CKD) stage 3–4 and VDD (≤20 ng/mL).

Intervention group received two oral doses of cholecalciferol (300,000 IU) at baseline and 8 weeks, compared with matching placebo. In comparison to placebo group, cholecalciferol supplementation significantly increased endothelium-dependent brachial artery flow-mediated dilation at 16 weeks. Intervention also led to significant favorable changes in pulse wave velocity and circulating interleukin (IL)-6 levels.

However, another interventional study, i.e., Indian Polypill study [The International Polycap Study 3 (TIPS-3)] which was initiated to study vitamin D supplementation effect on reducing major adverse CV events (ClinicalTrials.gov Identifier NCT01646437), is still ongoing.

TABLE 2: Indian studies assessing effect of vitamin D supplementation on cardiovascular outcomes

Cardiovascular disease, reference	Study type	Dose of vitamin D supplementation and frequency dosage	Duration of supplementation	Outcome parameters of intervention	Diseases groups and no. of subjects	Serum vitamin D levels before and after supplementation	Conclusion
Heart failure[44]	Nonrandomized	60,000 IU/ week	3 months	Association between vitamin D levels and echocardiographic parameters	Group 1: n = 38, vitamin D supplemented Group 2: n = 36, no supplementation	Before: Group 1: 18.14 ± 6.07 ng/mL Group 2: 20.48 ± 5.86 ng/mL After: Group 1: 34.7 ng/mL Group 2: 20.5 ng/mL	No improvement in left ventricular function, serum vitamin D levels increased following supplementation
Ischemic stroke[45]	Nonblinded and randomized, placebo	Single dose 600,000 IU	3 months	Stroke outcome	Group 1: n = 30, supplemented with vitamin D Group 2: n = 30 patients received placebo	Baseline: Group A: 17.98 ± 3.81 ng/mL Group B: 18.44 ± 4.69 ng/mL vitamin D levels were not measured after intervention	Improvement in the stroke outcome and EF and decreased systolic blood pressure
Cardiovascular risk in CKD[46]	Randomized, double-blind, placebo-controlled trial	300,000 IU at baseline and 8th weeks	16 weeks	Cardiovascular risks	Group 1: Placebo: 59 Group 2: Vitamin D: 58	Before: Group 1: 13.21 ng mL Group 2: 13.4 ng/mL After: Group 1: No change Group 2: 23.4 ng/mL	Increased endothelium-dependent brachial artery flow-mediated dilation and favorable changes in pulse wave velocity and circulating IL-6 levels

CKD, chronic kidney disease; IL-6, interleukin-6; EF, ejection fraction.

CONCLUSION

Based on the observation studies, association between VDD and CVD has been well reported. However, studies of supplementation of vitamin D did not show improvement in any of the clinical outcomes studied so far.

REFERENCES

1. Dusso AS. Kidney disease and vitamin D levels: 25-hydroxyvitamin D, 1,25-dihydroxy vitamin D, and VDR activation. Kidney Int Suppl. 2011;1:136-41.
2. Thacher TD, Clarke BL. Vitamin D insufficiency. Mayo Clin Proc. 2010;86: 50-60.
3. Ritu G, Gupta A. Fortification of foods with vitamin D in India. Nutrients. 2014;6:3601-23.
4. Holick MF. Evidence-based debate on health benefits of vitamin D revisited. Dermatoendocrinol. 2012:l4:183-90.
5. Holick MF, Binkley NC, Bischoff-Ferrari HA, et al. Guidelines for preventing and treating vitamin D deficiency and insufficiency revisited. J Clin Endocrinol Metab. 2012:97;1153-8.
6. Holick MF. The vitamin D deficiency pandemic and consequences for nonskeletal health: Mechanisms of action. Mol Asp Med. 2008;29:361-8.
7. Khadgawat R, Marwaha RK, Garg MK, et al. Impact of vitamin D fortified milk supplementation on vitamin D status of healthy school children aged 10–14 years. Osteoporos Int. 2013;24:2335-43.
8. Garg G, Kachhawa G, Ramot R, et al. Effect of vitamin D supplementation on insulin kinetics and cardiovascular risk factors in polycystic ovarian syndrome: A pilot study. Endocr Connect. 2015;4:108-16.
9. Cheng S, Massaro JM, Fox CS, et al. Adiposity, cardiometabolic risk, and vitamin D status: The Framingham Heart Study. Diabetes. 2010:59;242-8.
10. Al Mheid I, Quyyumi AA. Vitamin D and cardiovascular disease: Controversy unresolved. J Am Coll Cardiol. 2017:70;89-100.
11. Skaaby T, Nystrup L, Pisinger C, et al. Vitamin D status and changes in cardiovascular risk factors: A prospective study of a general population. Cardiology. 2012;123:62-70.
12. Kendrick J, Targher G, Smits G, et al. 25-hydroxyvitamin D deficiency is independently associated with cardiovascular disease in the third National Health and Nutrition Examination Survey. Atherosclerosis. 2009;205:255-60.
13. Giovannucci E, Liu Y, Hollis B, et al. 25-hydroxyvitamin D and risk of myocardial infarction in men: A prospective study. Arch Intern Med. 2008;168:1174-80.
14. Muhlestein JB. Relation of vitamin D deficiency to cardiovascular risk factors, disease status, and incident events in a general healthcare population. Am J Cardiol. 2010;106:963-8.
15. Pilz S, Tomaschitz A, Drechsler C, et al. Vitamin D supplementation: A promising approach for the prevention and treatment of strokes. Curr Drug Targets. 2011;12:88-96.
16. Wimalawansa SJ. Vitamin D and cardiovascular diseases: Causality. J Steroid Biochem Mol Biol. 2018;175:29-43.
17. Mozos I, Marginean O. Links between vitamin D deficiency and cardiovascular diseases. Biomed Res Int. 2015;2015:109275.

18. Verdoia M, Pergolini P, Rolla R, et al. Novara Atherosclerosis Study Group (NAS). Impact of high-dose statins on vitamin D levels and platelet function in patients with coronary artery disease. Thromb Res. 2017;150:90-5.
19. Verdoia M, Schaffer A, Sartori C, et al. Vitamin D deficiency is independently associated with the extent of coronary artery disease. Eur J Clin Invest. 2014;44:634-42.
20. van Etten E, Mathieu C. Immunoregulation by 1,25-dihydroxyvitamin D3: Basic concepts. J Steroid Biochem Mol Biol. 2005;97:93-101.
21. Silvagno F, De Vivo E, Attanasio A, et al. Mitochondrial localization of vitamin D receptor in human platelets and differentiated megakaryocytes. PLoS One. 2010;5:e8670.
22. Oh J, Riek AE, Darwech I, et al. Deletion of macrophage Vitamin D receptor promotes insulin resistance and monocyte cholesterol transport to accelerate atherosclerosis in mice. Cell Rep. 2015;10:1872-86.
23. Priya S, Singh A, Pradhan A, et al. Association of Vitamin D and essential hypertension in a North Indian population cohort. Heart India. 2017;5:7-11.
24. Adela R, Borkar RM, Mishra N, et al. Lower serum vitamin D metabolite levels in relation to circulating cytokines/chemokines and metabolic hormones in pregnant women with hypertensive disorders. Front Immunol. 2017;8:273.
25. Adela R, Borkar RM, Bhandi MM, et al. Lower vitamin D metabolites levels were associated with increased coronary artery diseases in type 2 diabetes patients in India. Sci Rep. 2016;6:37593.
26. Kumar M, Kumar G, Verma VK, et al. A study of association of vitamin D deficiency and coronary artery disease. Int J Res Med Sci. 2017;5:1765-70.
27. Dhibar DP, Sharma YP, Bhadada SK, et al. Association of vitamin D deficiency with coronary artery disease. J Clin Diagn Res. 2016;10:OC24-OC28.
28. Roy A, Lakshmy R, Tarik M, et al. Independent association of severe vitamin D deficiency as a risk of acute myocardial infarction in Indians. Indian Heart J. 2015;67:27-32.
29. Malik S, Giri S, Madhu SV, et al. Relationship of levels of Vitamin D with flow-mediated dilatation of brachial artery in patients of myocardial infarction and healthy control: A case-control study. Indian J Endocrinol Metab. 2016;20:684-9.
30. Karur S, Veerappa V, Nanjappa MC. Study of vitamin D deficiency prevalence in acute myocardial infarction. Int J Cardiol Heart Vessel. 2014;3:57-9.
31. Chaudhuri JR, Mridula KR, Alladi S, et al. Serum 25 hydroxyvitamin D deficiency in ischemic stroke and subtypes in Indian patients. J Stroke. 2014;16(1):44-50.
32. Priya S, Siddiqi Z, Karoli R, et al. Study of vitamin D status in patients with dilated cardiomyopathy at a teaching hospital in North India. J Cardiovasc Echogr. 2016;26:89-93.
33. Scragg R, Stewart AW, Waayer D, et al. Effect of monthly high-dose vitamin D supplementation on cardiovascular disease in the vitamin D assessment study: A randomized clinical trial. JAMA Cardiol. 2017;2:608-16.
34. Zittermann A, Ernst JB, Prokop S, et al. Effect of vitamin D on all-cause mortality in heart failure (EVITA): A 3-year randomized clinical trial with 4000 IU vitamin D daily. Eur Heart J. 2017;38:2279-86.
35. Larsen T, Mose FH, Bech JN, et al. Effect of cholecalciferol supplementation during winter months in patients with hypertension: A randomized, placebo-controlled trial. Am J Hypertens. 2012;25:1215-22.
36. Pfeifer M, Begerow B, Minne HW, et al. Effects of a short-term vitamin D3 and calcium supplementation on blood pressure and parathyroid hormone levels in elderly women. J Clin Endocrinol Metab. 2001;86:1633-7.
37. Witte KK, Byrom R, Gierula J, et al. Effects of Vitamin D on cardiac function in patients with chronic HF: The VINDICATE Study. J Am Coll Cardiol. 2016;67:2593-603.
38. Dalbeni A, Scaturro G, Degan M, et al. Effects of six months of vitamin D supplementation in patients with heart failure: A randomized double-blind controlled trial. Nutr Metab Cardiovasc Dis. 2014;24:861-8.
39. Kubiak JM, Thorsby PM, Kamycheva E, et al. Vitamin D supplementation does not improve CVD risk factors in vitamin D insufficient subjects. Endocr Connect. 2018;7(6):840-9.
40. Tomson J, Hin H, Emberson J, et al. Effects of vitamin D on blood pressure, arterial stiffness, and cardiac function in older people after 1 year: BEST-D (Biochemical Efficacy and Safety Trial of Vitamin D). J Am Heart Assoc.2017;6(10).
41. Schwetz V, Scharnagl H, Trummer C, et al. Vitamin D supplementation and lipoprotein metabolism: A randomized controlled trial. J Clin Lipidol. 2018;12(3):588-96.
42. Chowdhury R, Kunutsor S, Vitezova A, et al. Vitamin D and risk of cause specific death: Systematic review and meta-analysis of observational cohort and randomized intervention studies. BMJ. 2014;348:g1903.
43. Beveridge LA, Khan F, Struthers AD, et al. Effect of Vitamin D supplementation on markers of vascular function: A systematic review and individual participant meta-analysis. J Am Heart Assoc. 2018;7(11):e008273.
44. Abid MTK, Rabbani MU, Hasan A, et al. Vitamin D levels and its supplementation in patients of heart failure. J Indian Coll Cardiol. 2017;7:105-8.
45. Narasimhan S, Balasubramanian P. Role of vitamin D in the outcome of ischemic stroke: A randomized controlled trial. J Clin Diagn Res. 2017;11: CC06–CC10.
46. Kumar V, Yadav AK, Lal A, et al. A randomized trial of vitamin D supplementation on vascular function in CKD. J Am Soc Nephrol. 2017;28:3100-108.
47. Suthar OP, Mathur S, Gupta V, et al. Study of correlation of serum vitamin D levels with arterial stiffness and cardiovascular morbidity in elderly individuals of Western Rajasthan. J Assoc Phys India. 2018;60:18-22.

CHAPTER 4

Hormone Replacement Therapy and Cardiovascular Diseases

Geetha Subramanian, Aviraj Choudhary, Kamaldeep Bansal

INTRODUCTION

Cardiovascular disease (CVD) is one of the leading causes of death in women globally. In industrialized countries like UK, Northern Europe, and North America coronary heart disease (CHD) is the most common cause of death in women, whereas stroke is more common in Southern Europe. As cardiac events are very uncommon in premenopausal females which in itself shed the light over the protective influence of ovarian sex hormones inherent to menstruation cycle. After menopause however this protective influence begins to decrease and the risk for CVD tend to increase gradually equating itself to the male risk in eighths decade of life.[1,2] The estrogen deficiency that ensues after menopause is considered the main culprit in increasing the risk of CVD. Estrogen deficiency exerts its metabolic, hemodynamic, and vascular effects which influence the cardiac risk factors directly or indirectly. In some observational studies it has been shown that the hormone replacement therapy (HRT) in postmenopausal women had a lower rate of CVD and cardiac death than those not receiving HRT. However, randomized studies, Heart and Estrogen/progestin Replacement Study (HERS) and Women's Health Initiative (WHI) showed that HRT may actually increase the risk and events of CVD in postmenopausal women.

MENOPAUSE-INDUCED CHANGES IN CARDIOVASCULAR FUNCTIONS

Adverse changes in lipids and lipoproteins and in glucose and insulin metabolism accompany the onset of the menopause[3,4] encouraging the development of atheroma. There is also negative impact on vascular function, which results from the loss of ovarian hormones. As the female sex hormone concentration declines, there is a significant increase in the level of total cholesterol, low-density lipoprotein (LDL) cholesterol, and triglycerides whereas the high-density lipoprotein (HDL) cholesterol shows a declining trend. Indirect effects are also seen in alterations of blood pressure, obesity, body fat distribution, clotting factors, and glucose metabolism which are all independent risk factors for CVD as well. In 1976, the Framingham investigators reported a 2.6-fold higher incidence of cardiovascular events in age-matched postmenopausal women compared with premenopausal women.[5] Surgical menopause was associated with 2.7-fold higher risk of CHD compared with premenopausal women of the same age, and women with a natural menopause had 2.2-fold higher risk of CHD compared with premenopausal women of the same age.[5] Estrogen-deficient state in postmenopausal women can account for changes in the cardiovascular function.

Menopause shifts the overall balance toward atherogenic lipids and lipoprotein profiles. Lipoprotein(a) has been shown to have significantly increased in postmenopausal patients which is an important marker of cardiac risk.[6,7] Elevated levels of lipoprotein(a) has been associated with premature atherosclerosis, stroke, and myocardial infarction in various case control studies.[8-10] Further the role of coagulation factors, anticoagulation substances, and a balance between fibrinolytic and antifibrinolytic elements of the blood play a major role in development of atherogenic plaque. Elevated levels of fibrinogen and factor VII in postmenopausal than in premenopausal women of the same age has been shown in various population-based studies.[11-13] Also increased incidences of thromboembolic phenomenon[14] and CHD[15] have been found in congenital deficiencies of the coagulation inhibitors antithrombin III, protein C, and protein S. Increased plasma concentrations of plasminogen activator inhibitor-1 (PAI-1) and tissue plasminogen activator (tPA) antigen ultimately causes a reduced function of fibrinolytic system and increases the chances of CHD (Box 1).[16,17]

BOX 1 Various prothrombotics increase in menopausal state

- Lipoprotein(a)
- Fibrinogen
- Factor VII
- Plasminogen activator inhibitor-1
- Tissue plasminogen activator

EFFECTS OF HORMONE REPLACEMENT THERAPY ON CORONARY HEART DISEASE RISK

The administration of HRT induces variable amount of significant metabolic changes in women's body. The actual effect of administered therapy depends upon a number of factors like type of steroid used, dose of steroid, mode of administration, duration of therapy, and most importantly patients response is also individual. Estrogen substantially lowers the LDL cholesterol in turn lowering the total cholesterol and this effect is more evident by oral route of administration rather than transdermal route.[18] Other protective roles (Box 2) of estrogen include increasing the levels of HDL cholesterol particularly the HDL2 subfraction. Similarly, it also lowers the levels of lipoprotein(a) an important cardiovascular risk marker. The most notorious particles causing atherosclerosis are the small and dense LDL particles because of their capacity to get retained in the arterial wall leading to production of foam cells and generating atheromatous plaques. Oral HRT increases the overall clearance of small LDL particles from the circulation and is thus protective against CVD.[19] These benefits are however not observed with transdermal route of HRT.[20] Endogenous triglycerides are another important CVD risk parameter which is also influenced by the dose, route, and duration of HRT. Thus, transdermal estrogen decline triglyceride levels but oral estrogens increase their level because of first-pass metabolism.[18,21]

Addition of progestogens to HRT does not lower LDL. By increasing hepatic lipase activity androgenic progestogens such as norgestrel, attenuate the HDL-raising effect of estrogen.[21] While certain nonandrogenic progestogens, such as dydrogesterone, do not attenuate estrogen-induced increases in HDL[22] others, such as medroxyprogesterone acetate (MPA), have negative impact on estrogen-induced increases in HDL. Levonorgestrel being an androgenic progestogen decreases triglyceride levels by reducing the secretion of very LDL. Increase in triglycerides induced by oral estrogens is not prevented by addition of C21 progestogens. Thus, dual estrogen/progestogen HRT can increase HDL and triglycerides, or it can decrease triglycerides, but at the same time causes a decrease, or no increase, in HDL. Which change in lipid profile is more important in terms of CHD benefit remains unknown. In certain situations, it has been postulated that the some HRT regimens can benefit more than others.

BOX 2 Important cardiovascular benefits of estrogens

- Reduces atherosclerosis
- Increases HDL cholesterol
- Lowers LDL cholesterol
- Prevents platelet aggregation
- Promotes coronary artery vasodilatation
- Decreases lipoprotein(a) and inhibits LDL cholesterol oxidation

HDL, high-density lipoprotein; LDL, low-density lipoprotein.

Estrogen affects the metabolism and levels of insulin as well. The dynamics of glucose and insulin concentrations in postmenopausal women changes, usually improving insulin resistance after oral administration of 17-estradiol whereas, estradiol when given transdermally does not exert much effects.[23] In contrast, raised insulin levels and impair glucose tolerance have been linked with alkylated estrogens such as ethinylestradiol, and conjugated equine estrogens (CEE).[24] Addition of progesterone to HRT regime affects insulin metabolism as androgenic progesterones produce more insulin resistance whereas nonandrogenic progesterones does not have much effects. Oral estrogen reduces certain prothrombotic clotting factors like fibrinogen and factor VII, and also reduces the antifibrinolytic factor PAI-1, still producing increase in thrombogenesis.[25] A continuous combined transdermal HRT resulted in a significant decrease in factor VIIc, and an increase in fibrinolytic activity. Estradiol also exerts beneficial effects in terms of CVD by maintaining endothelial function and reducing angiotensin converting enzyme activity which has been reported with both oral and transdermal HRT.[26]

CLINICAL STUDIES OF HORMONE REPLACEMENT THERAPY AND CORONARY HEART DISEASE

Observational studies done worldwide have consistently shown that HRT is associated with a reduced incidence of CHD and total mortality in postmenopausal women. Five randomized controlled trials (RCTs) which have used total mortality and morbidity as end point was conducted (Box 3). Out of five, three were secondary prevention trials[27-29] and two were primary prevention.[30-32] RCTs conducted on HRT failed to show any beneficial effect on CHD and mortality in postmenopausal women. In contrary to RCT, observational studies have shown a 30–50% reduction in CHD and total mortality when analyzed among all women regardless of age. This difference between observational studies and RCTs is best exemplified within the WHI that evaluated HRT in both an observational cohort and in RCTs. The WHI observational study arm conducted in 53,054 women showed a 50% reduction in CHD in women who used estrogen + progestin (E+P) in contrast with women who do not. Whereas in RCT arm, the risk of CHD was increased 18% in women on combined CEE 0.625 mg + MPA 2.5 mg relative to

BOX 3 Randomized control trials for hormone replacement therapy in coronary artery disease

Secondary prevention trials:

- HERS (Heart and Estrogen/Progestin Replacement Study)
- ESPRIT (Estrogen in the Prevention of Reinfarction Trial)
- PHASE (Papworth HRT Atherosclerosis Study)

Primary prevention trials:

- WHI-EP (Women's Health Initiative Estrogen + Progestin Trial)
- WHI-E (Women's Health Initiative Estrogen Trial)

HRT, hormone replacement therapy.

placebo in the Women's Health Initiative estrogen-progestin (WHI-EP) trial.[30] This difference in clinical outcomes between observational studies and RCTs is mostly because of the different characteristics of the cohorts. In observational studies, women who used HRT were relatively young (30–60 years old), had recent menopause, were thin [approximate body mass index (BMI) of 25 kg/m^2] and were having typical menopausal symptoms for which HRT initiated. HRT in these patients was continued for longer periods (10–40 years). On the other hand, in RCTs women who used HRT were much older (>90% of women older than 55 years) and on average more than 10 years beyond menopause (average 13–23 years). Patients having predominant menopausal symptoms were excluded from RCT arm. Mean duration of HRT (1–6.8 years) in RCT arm was also considerably less than that of the HRT users in observational studies. Also, women in RCT arm were overweight (approximate BMI of 29 kg/m^2). It has been shown that the characteristics of women in RCTs were markedly different from those studied in observational studies. Thus, accounting for the discordance of the HRT effects on CHD and mortality from observational studies compared to RCTs among women regardless of age.

Although, in RCTs the effect of HRT on CHD over all ages is null, these trials also showed that there are beneficial effects of HRT on CHD according to the timing of initiation of HRT relative to age and menopause.[33] The largest RCT WHI had shown that compared to placebo, women who were randomized to CEE + MPA within 10 years of menopause had a 12% decrease in CHD events whereas women between 10 and 20 years after menopause had a 23% increased risk of CHD and women more than 20 years after menopause had a 66% increased risk of CHD ($p = 0.05$).[34] In WHI trial, only one-third were less than 60 years old and less than 5% were within a few years of menopause, representing the subgroup of women found in observational studies who had reduction in CHD with HRT. Whereas, older women (>60 years old) who were given HRT many years after menopause (>10 years) thus not representing the women in observational studies had increased risk of CHD with HRT. The standard dose of estrogen used for relief of vasomotor symptoms in women aged around 50 years may be inappropriately high for women some 15–20 years older.[27] The enormous data available after meta-analysis of RCTs emphasize that young postmenopausal women who started HRT in close proximity to menopause have reduced CHD and total mortality. These results are also in accordance with the results seen in observational studies where almost all the women started HRT in close proximity to menopause, typically within 6 years. Large RCTs (HERS and WHI-EP), observational studies, arterial imaging studies, and case-control studies consistently showed reduction in CHD risk with prolonged HRT use (>6 years).

Majority of adverse outcomes associated with HRT as shown in WHI and other RCTs are rare (<1 event per 1,000 treated women).[35] Younger women who started on HRT had lower adverse outcome as compared to older women who started on HRT later. Adverse effects like stroke and venous thromboembolism are rare and having incidence similar to commonly prescribed drugs. In WHI, the breast cancer risk differ with CEE alone associated with a reduction in breast cancer risk[36] and combined CEE + MPA associated with an increased risk,[37] the magnitude of risk seen with statin therapy is comparable to that of CEE + MPA therapy.[35]

CONCLUSION

The combined data from various RCTs and observational studies indicate that the effect of postmenopausal HRT on CHD and total mortality is influenced by the timing of initiation (age and time since menopause) and the duration of therapy (>6 years of use). The adverse events associated with HRT are rare (<1 additional event per 1,000 women) and even rarer in younger age women (<60 years or within 5 years of menopause). The adverse risk with estrogen alone is quite rare. In women with confirmed CHD, HRT should not be initiated for preventing future cardiovascular events. Women who are already taking HRT for noncardiac conditions, if develops CVD, can continue to take it if they are stable. If HRT is to be given for the sole purpose of preventing future cardiovascular events in postmenopausal women who do not have pre-existing CHD post should be considered only after a careful risk assessment. At present, the indications for HRT use are relief of menopausal symptoms, maintenance of quality of life and prevention of osteoporosis. Prevention of CHD has never been a licensed indication. It is, however, clearly possible to use appropriate HRT regimens safely in women at increased risk of CHD or with established disease. Patient preference as well as noncardiovascular risks and benefits should guide any decision regarding such therapy. In the final analysis, the difference in CHD and total mortality outcomes between observational studies and RCTs is reflected by the differences in the study design and the characteristics of the populations studied. In fact, data from RCTs and more than 40 consistent observational studies indicate that the young postmenopausal women with menopausal symptoms who use HRT for long periods of time have lower rates of CHD and total mortality than comparable postmenopausal women who do not use HRT.

REFERENCES

1. Speroff L. Quality of life issues in the management of the menopause. In: Popkin D, Peddle L, eds. Women's Health Today. New York: Parthenon. 1994:271-90.
2. Nabulsi A, Folsom A, White A, et al. Association of HRT with various cardiovascular risk factors in post-menopausal women. N Engl J Med. 1993;328:1069-75.
3. Stevenson J, Crook D, Godsland I. Influence of age and menopause on serum lipids and lipoproteins in healthy women. Atherosclerosis. 1993;98:83-90.
4. Walton C, Godsland IF, Proudler AJ, et al. The effects of the menopause on insulin sensitivity, secretion and elimination in non- obese, healthy women. Eur J Clin Invest. 1993;23:466-73.
5. Gordon T, Kannel WB, Hjortland MC, et al. Menopause and coronary heart disease. The Framingham study. Ann Intern Med. 1978;89:157-61.
6. Schriewer H, Assman G, Sandkamp M. The relationship of Lp(a) to risk factors of coronary heart Westfalia. J Clin Chem Clin Biochem. 1984;22:591-6.

7. Bruschi F, Meschia M, Soma MR, et al. Lp(a) levels in perimenopausal years: A population study [abstract]. Symposium on Women's Health in Menopause, September 1993, Milan, Italy.
8. Armstrong V, Cremer P, Eberle E. The association between serum Lp(a) concentrations and angiographically assessed coronary atherosclerosis. Atherosclerosis. 1986;62:249-57.
9. Zenker G, Koeltringer P, Bone G. Lipoprotein(a) as a strong indicator for cerebrovascular disease. Stroke. 1986;17:942-5.
10. Hajjar K, Gavish D, Breslow JL, et al. Lipoprotein(a) modulation of endothelial cell surface fibrinolysis and its potential role in atherosclerosis. Nature. 1989;339:303-4.
11. Meade T, Haines A, Imeson J, et al. Menopausal status and haemostatic variables. Lancet. 1983;1:22-4.
12. Folsom AR, Wu KK, Davis CE, et al. Population correlates of plasma fibrinogen and factor VII: Putative cardiovascular risk factors. Atherosclerosis. 1991;91:191-205.
13. Meilahn EN, Kuller LH, Matthews KA, et al. Hemostatic factors according to menopausal status and use of HRT. Ann Epidemiol. 1992;2:445-55.
14. Allaart CF, Briet E. Familial venous thrombophilia. In: Bloom AL, Forbes CD, Thomas DP, et al., eds. Haemostasis and Thrombosis, 3rd edition. Edinburgh: Churchill Livingstone, 1994:1349-60.
15. Meade TW, Cooper J, Miller GJ, et al. Antithrombin III and arterial disease. Lancet. 1991;337:850-1.
16. Scarabin PY, Bonithon-Kopp C, Bara L, et al. Relationship between plasminogen activator inhibitor activity and menopausal status. Fibrinolysis. 1990;4:233-6.
17. Gebara OCE, Mittleman MA, Sutherland P, et al. Association between increased estrogen status and increased fibrinolytic potential in the Framingham offspring study. Circulation. 1995;91:1952-8.
18. Godsland IF. Effects of postmenopausal hormone replacement therapy on lipid, lipoprotein, and apolipoprotein (a) concentrations: Analysis of studies published from 1974–2000. Fertil Steril. 2001;75:898-915.
19. van der Mooren MJ, de Graaf J, Demacker PN, et al. Changes in the low-density lipoprotein profile during 17 beta-estradiol-dydrogesterone therapy in postmenopausal women. Metabolism. 1994;43:799-802.
20. Stevenson JC, Oladipo A, Manassiev N, et al. Randomized trial of effect of transdermal continuous combined hormone replacement therapy on cardiovascular risk markers. Br J Haematol. 2004;124:802-8.
21. Crook D, Cust MP, Gangar KF, et al. Comparison of transdermal and oral estrogen-progestin replacement therapy: Effects on serum lipids and lipoproteins. Am J Obstet Gynecol. 1992;166:950-5.
22. Crook D, Godsland IF, Hull J, et al. Hormone replacement therapy with dydrogesterone and 17 beta-oestradiol: Effects on serum lipoproteins and glucose tolerance during 24-month follow up. Br J Obstet Gynaecol. 1997;104:298-304.
23. Spencer CP, Godsland IF, Cooper AJ, et al. Effects of oral and transdermal 17 beta-estradiol with cyclical oral norethindrone actetate on insulin sensitivity, secretion, and elimination in postmenopausal women. Metabolism. 2000;49:742-7.
24. Spellacy WN, Buhi WC, Birk SA. The effects of estrogens on carbohydrate metabolism: glucose, insulin and growth hormone studies on one hundred and seventy-one women ingesting premarin, mestranol, and ethinyl estradiol for six months. Am J Obstet Gynecol. 1972;114:378-92.
25. Winkler UH. Menopause, HRT and cardiovascular disease: A review of haemostaseological findings. Fibrinolysis. 1992;6 Suppl 3:5-10.
26. Proudler AJ, Cooper A, Whitehead M, et al. Effect of oestrogen only and oestrogen-progestogen replacement therapy upon circulating angiotensin I-converting enzyme activity in postmenopausal women. Clin Endocrinol. 2003;58:30-5.
27. Hulley S, Grady D, Bush T, et al. Randomized trial of estrogen plus progestin for secondary prevention of coronary heart disease in postmenopausal women. JAMA. 1998;280:605-13.
28. Clarke SC, Kelleher J, Lloyd-Jones H, et al. A study of hormone replacement therapy in postmenopausal women with ischemic heart disease: The Papworth HRT Atherosclerosis Study. BJOG. 2002;109:1056-62.
29. Cherry N, Gilmour K, Hannaford P, et al. Oestrogen therapy for the prevention of reinfarction in postmenopausal women: A randomized placebo controlled trial. Lancet. 2002;360:2001-8.
30. Rossouw JE, Anderson GL, Prentice RL, et al. Writing Group for the Women's Health Initiative Investigators. Risks and benefits of estrogen plus progestin in healthy postmenopausal women: Principal results from the Women's Health Initiative randomized controlled trial. JAMA. 2002;288:321-33.
31. Manson JE, Hsia J, Johnson KC, et al. Estrogen plus progestin and the risk of coronary heart disease. N Engl J Med. 2003;349:523-34.
32. Anderson GL, Limacher M, Assaf AR, et al. Women's Health Initiative Steering Committee. Effects of conjugated equine estrogen in postmenopausal women with hysterectomy: The Women's Health Initiative randomized controlled trial. JAMA. 2004;291:1701-12.
33. Hodis HN, Mack WJ, Lobo R. What is the cardioprotective role of hormone replacement therapy? Curr Atheroscl Rep. 2003;5:56-66.
34. Rossouw JE, Prentice RL, Manson JA, et al. Postmenopausal hormone therapy and risk of cardiovascular disease by age and years since menopause. JAMA. 2007;297:1465-77.
35. Hodis HN, Mack WJ. Postmenopausal hormone therapy in clinical perspective. Menopause. 2007;14:944-57.
36. Stefanick ML, Anderson GL, Margolis KL, et al. Effects of conjugated equine estrogens on breast cancer and mammography screening in postmenopausal women with hysterectomy. JAMA. 2006;295:1647-57.
37. Chlebowski RT, Hendrix SL, Langer RD, et al. Influence of estrogen plus progestin on breast cancer and mammography in healthy postmenopausal women: The Women's Health Initiative randomized trial. JAMA. 2003;289:3243-53.

SECTION 2

Lipids and Diet

CHAPTER 5

Cholesterol and Coronary Artery Disease Controversy

Rajiv Bajaj

INTRODUCTION

Our understanding of diseases of civilization and modern lifestyle have undergone a sea change over the last 50 years. Cholesterol has become synonymous with heart attacks. There is widespread anxiety about good and bad cholesterol. Cholesterol dictates current food preferences.

CHOLESTEROL AND CORONARY ARTERY DISEASE CONTROVERSY

Diseases of Civilization and Modern Lifestyle

Over the last 50 years, cholesterol has become synonymous with heart attacks. There is widespread anxiety about good and bad cholesterol. Cholesterol dictates current food preferences. Alcohol is often recommended for raising high-density lipoprotein (HDL) cholesterol. Butter and eggs are feared. Before the war, glucose was blamed for diabetes, obesity, atherosclerosis, cancer, and all other diseases of modern lifestyle.[1] These diseases were called saccharine diseases.[2] The original connotation of modern lifestyle was adopting agriculture, living on crops rich in glucose, being prone to glucose diseases.

Medical journals, textbooks, and conferences emphasize cholesterol, but some landmark research work and a few popular books oppose this view. Clearly, both sides cannot be entirely right or wrong. When we weigh the evidence for and against cholesterol, and look at its chemistry, we can discern its role, and the cause of confusion.

Cholesterol Hypothesis

Cholesterol has been implicated in pathogenesis of atherosclerosis because of rabbit experiments, cholesterol in atheroma, premature coronary artery disease (CAD) in familial hypercholesterolemia (FH), population studies of blood lipids, efficacy of statins or PCSK9 inhibitors; and diet studies like Oslo Diet-Heart Study and Lifestyle Heart Study (Dean Ornish).

Rabbits are herbivores, and plants do not contain cholesterol. Unlike rabbits, omnivores tolerate high-cholesterol diets. Their natural diet contains animal products, and excess cholesterol can be excreted in bile.

Cholesterol is suspected because of its presence in atheromas. Low-density lipoprotein (LDL) reaches wherever there is tissue damage and cell multiplication. Serum cholesterol levels therefore fall after infarction, stroke, fracture, sepsis, burns, and cancers. Low-grade vascular injury and inflammation attracts circulating LDL to vessel walls, their association is akin to that of wounds and bandages.

Familial hypercholesterolemia predisposes to atherosclerosis. There are fewer hepatic LDL receptors in FH, and the catabolism of LDL is slow. When Framingham statisticians found no relation between circulating cholesterol level and infarctions in their population, younger men were divided into cholesterol quartiles after excluding older men and all women. The highest quartile was a distillate of premature infarctions due to FH. This is the epidemiological evidence that implicates cholesterol.

Circulating lipids levels correlate with atherosclerotic risk because LDL and HDL levels change with diet. These changes are largely caused by dietary carbohydrates, as these are converted into triglycerides, VLDL, and then small dense LDL by body. Diets rich in unsaturated fatty acids do shift cholesterol from blood stream to cell membranes, but this is related to cholesterol's role in structural strength, not to atherosclerosis.

PURE and Other Contradictory Studies

Two recent studies have raised concerns about low-fat, low-cholesterol diet (LFLC) for preventing heart disease, and reopened an old controversy that was never fully resolved. PURE, a large prospective cohort study[3] identified a strong positive correlation between carbohydrate content of diet and hard end points. PREDIMED, both initial and recent revised versions, too showed that adding nuts and olive oil is better than a LFLC diet. Initial diet trials had repeatedly raised similar concerns. In anticoronary club trial, and Minnesota Coronary Survey,[4] mortality was higher with LFLC diet. These results had even precipitated a change in design of subsequent diet studies of 1970s. Multiple risk factor intervention trial (MRFIT), WHO factories study, and many others, therefore employed multiple preventive measures simultaneously. Thus the treatment arm stopped smoking, controlled blood pressure with antihypertensive drugs, exercised, and adopted LFLC diet. Despite a design that maximally favored the LFLC diet, these trials too, were negative. Curiously, lessons from the preceding diet trials began to hit their authors' blind spots. MRFIT blamed antihypertensive drugs for killing the LCFC diet group, and WHO factories study opined that stopping smoking is lethal! Later, the randomized Harvard's nurses' health study reported that increasing fruits, vegetables, olive oil, whole grains, and decreasing red meats, butter, sugar, etc. did not protect the heart. Currently, these randomized controlled trials are discounted, and fruits and vegetables are vigorously promoted based on statistical association found in inter heart case-control survey.

The studies that implicate dietary cholesterol are fewer. Oslo is a small *post-hoc* subanalysis of a negative trial, Ornish's even smaller trial could not be reproduced in subsequent studies, Lyon's heart study[5] a single center publication claimed 80% reduction in events with Mediterranean diet. Like its daughter, Indo-Mediterranean study, it crumbled under scrutiny. The celebrated diet was regular food cooked in canola margarine, and India's mustard oil version lost all its raw data to termites.

Nevertheless, there is a definite association between cholesterol and atherosclerosis, and biochemistry clarifies its role.

FUNCTIONS OF CHOLESTEROL

All nucleated animal cells synthesize cholesterol. In addition, dietary cholesterol is absorbed, and delivered to liver. Eating cholesterol does not affect blood levels in humans, since synthesis and excretion are regulated. Requirements increase in illnesses and during cell multiplication.

Animals have cholesterol for the same reason that plants have cellulose. Cholesterol stabilizes cell membranes, provides structural strength, and regulates membrane permeability.

Circulating lipoproteins have immune functions. They adsorb, internalize and isolate circulating bacterial endotoxins and all other injurious fat soluble debris, and deliver these to liver for catabolism. Liver secretes fresh, buoyant, cholesterol-rich LDL, and removes old, toxin-laden small dense LDL (sdLDL). LDL is not a blood pollutant, it is body's blood and tissue cleansing device.

Soluble Nutrients and Very-low-density Lipoprotein Synthesis

After digestion, water-soluble nutrients like amino acids go via portal vein to the liver; insoluble nutrients like triglycerides and cholesterol form chylomicrons, and directly enter general circulation.

The foremost health difference between modern and primitive diets is in their glucose content. Modern crops like sugarcane, grains, and tubers contain mostly glucose. Blood levels of glucose and amino acids are tightly regulated. Excess amounts, and all miscellaneous soluble nutrients like pentose, organic acids, alcohols, etc. are mostly converted to triglycerides, enter circulation as very low density lipoproteins (VLDL). Although conversion of dietary glucose to triglycerides prevents hyperglycemia, VLDL does not adsorb endotoxins efficiently. VLDL is LDL that has been reassigned to transport of soluble calories from intestine to liver to adipose cells. VLDL becomes sdLDL. LDL is not homogenous; assorted particles are collectively measured as LDL. Fresh LDL from liver is healthy, VLDL remnants, and aged-LDL require elimination by liver.

Thus, the body sends fats directly into blood stream as chylomicrons, and converts all soluble nutrients including milk and fruit to triglycerides before permitting them to enter the circulation.

Lipoproteins

Triglycerides of food reaches tissues in chylomicrons (apolipoprotein B48). Depleted chylomicrons (remnants) containing dietary cholesterol, fat soluble vitamins, etc. are internalized by hepatocytes. Fasting chylomicronemia occurs when peripheral lipase activity is diminished (e.g., obese, alcoholic diabetics), and produces severe hypertriglyceridemia. High levels of circulating remnants promote atherosclerosis. This happens in rabbit experiments, and rarely in humans (broad beta disease). Genetic chylomicron clearance disorders are aggravated by high-fat diets.

Very-low-density lipoprotein and LDL (apolipoprotein B100) are synthesized in liver. On a natural "forest" diet, the triglycerides come from food (animal fat), and glucose is manufactured in liver. Synthesis of triglycerides in liver is meagre. Blood level of VLDL and sdLDL is low. Liver secretes cholesterol-rich large LDL.

Modern livers are kept busy synthesizing triglycerides from glucose, secreting VLDL and removing VLDL remnants. This predisposes to fatty liver, and elevates blood VLDL and sdLDL.

Apolipoprotein A is secreted by intestine and liver. It interacts with circulating lipoproteins and tissues, adsorbs lipids, and delivers them to LDL and to liver. It is a mop for toxins and a mobile service station for plasma lipoproteins. Its levels therefore vary inversely with VLDL levels.

Theories of Atherosclerosis

According to cholesterol theory synthesis of LDL by liver is excessive, and this is due to fat or cholesterol in diet. High levels of LDL clog the arteries. This theory ignores the role of glucose in VLDL synthesis, the formation of sdLDL from VLDL, and does not explain the absence of atherosclerosis in primitive tribes, (targets for primordial prevention), presence in ancient Egyptians; equivocal mortality benefits of second line antilipid drugs and exercise.

Endothelial injury by hypertension, cigarette smoke, uremic toxins, hyperhomocysteinemia, pollutants, etc. leads to local inflammatory response. Glucose too, causes endothelial injury. It is a reactive aldehyde. It glycosylates numerous proteins like hemoglobin, endothelial adhesion protein, etc. Injury leads to inflammation and healing. Arteries, like other tissues, have stereotyped response to diverse injuries. Chronic low-grade endothelial injury leads to atherosclerosis.

Ancient Egyptians were wheat and barley farmers, they had adopted the modern, glucose-rich diet. Neel and many others have shown that glucose-naive populations are very susceptible to glucose injury. (Neel conclusively disproved his own "thrifty gene" hypothesis).

Statins deplete hepatic cholesterol. This increases hepatic LDL receptors, and sdLDL uptake. Thus, statins and PCSK9 inhibitors help by removing toxic sdLDL. Low hepatocyte cholesterol marginally depresses VLDL synthesis, and therefore raises blood sugar. Removal of old, spent, toxin-laden small dense LDL is helpful, removal of fresh buoyant LDL cannot be. Fanciful and illogical extrapolations of "LDL targets" are advocated for "eradicating atherosclerosis" despite evidence that aggressive LDL lowering increases nonvascular adverse events.

Advantages and Disadvantages of Glucose

Glucose is the explosive, emergency fuel for phagocytosis, sprinting, and anoxic tissues. Natural diet has very little glucose, the liver synthesizes it. Blood levels are 50–80 mg, rising moderately in fever, injury, and other emergencies.

Carbohydrates increase serum insulin and somatomedins, they are growth factors. Lactose produces rapid growth in breast-fed infants. Human body size is diminutive without cooking (pygmies), small with cooked natural diet, gigantic in glucose fed modern humans as it is in farmed animals.

When rice and flour entered India, physicians documented that they cause diabetes (*madhumai*).[1] Carbohydrate reduction was standard treatment for thousands of years. Current advice is riddled with contradictions. Fats are curtailed, forcing diabetics to take a high-glucose diet. Whole grains are recommended for lowering glycemic index, though they cannot match the spectacularly low glycemic index of fats. Voglibose and sodium-glucose cotransporter-2 (SGLT2) inhibitors are prescribed for blocking absorption of glucose by intestines and kidneys, though fat is the one that is feared.

Rapid weight loss occurs in type 1 diabetes because low blood insulin promotes catabolism of body fat. Conversely, hyperinsulinemia promotes fat synthesis. Carbohydrate restriction is therefore effective in obesity, calorie counting is not.

Cancer cells have damaged genes. They lack the complex organization essential for oxidative phosphorylation, are prone to cell death. On a high-glucose diet, they survive by anaerobic glycolysis and cause cancer. *In vitro* cancer cell lines require glucose and insulin, and glucose PET (positron emission tomography) scanning locates various cancers.

A simple rule has long existed, if diabetes predisposes to any condition, its cause is probably dietary glucose. Glycosylation of lens causes cataracts; joint cartilage, osteoarthritis; advanced glycated-end products, dementia.

The long list of modern diseases needs further additions like glaucoma, hypothyroidism. Diabetic mothers get eclampsia, dystocia, cesarean sections; their babies macrosomia, growth retardation, congenital defects. Even many cardiac arrhythmias may be due to altered autonomic function. Do autoimmune diseases, allergies, and many infectious diseases result from abnormal immune responses to innocuous environmental chemicals and microbes?

Lipid Profile

Absolute risk estimation is needed for calculating sensitivity, specificity and receiver operator curves. Lipidology emphasizes relative risk. Sensitivity, specificity, etc. are never calculated. The various risk calculators combine all risk factors like age, diabetes, tobacco apart from lipids, to separate 20% 10 year risk from 10%. Even this modest achievement is suspect.

There are equally significant inverse relationships between serum cholesterol and neuropsychiatric problems, cancers, and even lifespan.

Remnant chylomicrons (B48), fresh LDL from liver, spent LDL, and VLDL, are all measured together as LDL. Atherogenic spent particles are lumped together with healthful fresh LDL.

Low-density lipoprotein is emphasized; triglycerides are discounted, though LDL changes are downstream effects of triglyceride synthesis in liver. High triglycerides and low HDL are the commonest findings in diabetes and infarctions ("atherogenic dyslipidemia"). The obvious triglyceride/HDL ratio, which is automatically the most robust, is ignored.

EARLY RESEARCH ON CHOLESTEROL

The cholesterol saga started immediately after England won World War-2 and "dissolved" the Empire.[6] Diagnosis of myocardial infarctions had increased with availability of electrocardiogram (ECG). In USA, this was projected as an epidemic of heart disease. Government announced grand investment in research for rapid action against "the number one killer", as "its cause was unknown". A Harvard doctor prepared a list of all known and suspected associations like diabetes, smoking, etc., and an observational study began in Framingham. Decades were consumed in prospectively obtaining "p" values for already listed associations. This was then projected as extensive research, which lamentably, "failed to find the cause, but identified risk factors". The weak association between cholesterol and infarctions appeared very late, and only by excluding all women, and most men from analysis. This toehold triggered relentless campaigning on dangers of cholesterol. Diabetes had the strongest association, but it was discounted for another decade. These decades of cholesterol education gradually obscured the common knowledge that dietary glucose causes diabetes.

The original promises of world class research under the guidance of leading authorities and reputed medical bodies were renegaded. Start-ups like American Heart Association were handed over reins and finance to dominate. At Framingham, a group of statisticians worked under a single, unknown, and disillusioned internist for 6 years. Kannel, a young war veteran next became the sole medical expert of the haloed Framingham Study. He is hailed as "father of prevention"! The treatment research limb of the government's war against heart disease was shifted to Bethesda, over 400 miles away. It kept busy conducting lengthy trials of cholesterol. Their negative results were vigorously massaged to obtain some favorable p values. Those negative studies are still quoted as evidence in favor of cholesterol hypothesis.

Even as Framingham and National Institute of Health (NIH) began their slow charade, an army strongman started marketing dietary cholesterol as the cause of heart disease. Ancel keys had no background of research or heart diseases, but he was an old friend of the government, he had helped to slash costs of feeding US soldiers by developing and summarily approving the infamous K ration. He imposed cholesterol as the cause of heart problems, concealing or trashing all research that suggested the opposite, and showcasing his six and seven countries Studies. Both were fudged and silly. After his retirement his juniors exposed his duplicity by publishing his large randomized trial that showed the opposite of what he preached, a trial he had deliberately buried.[4] Immediately, almost on cue, Ornish, a Californian nonentity with unreliable data, became the messiah of preventing heart disease by reducing fat in diet. In Europe, a single obscure author claimed stupendous benefits of "Mediterranean Diet", spawning the humbug of "Indo-Mediterranean Diet".

Cholesterol lobby promotes weak statistical associations a causal, projects unreliable studies, but buries strong studies, biochemistry and physiology. Till recently, Inter Heart emphasized that over 90% of the risk is "accounted for" by conventional risk factors, and asserted that these, therefore, cause atherosclerosis. PURE study implicates carbohydrates. By analogy, if studies are conducted of why cars breakdown, we may discover many risk factors like number of dents, presence of carburetor, absence of GPS, tampered mileometer, age and financial status of owner, etc. and these may identify 95% of all cars that stop. Old cars tend to breakdown after running hundred thousand miles. To "discover" this we require analysis of car mileage; not complex statistics.

DIET AND HEALTH

To understand food, we must focus on nutrients that enter the body after digestion and absorption. Speed of assimilation matters less; physical appearances, antioxidants, etc. are mostly irrelevant. Biochemically, logical guidance about food has been replaced by charts that curtail fat and cholesterol, optimize blood lipids, and glorify obscure trace substances. Confusion abounds: (1) Indigestible items (fiber) have been declared healthy. (2) Almonds, honey, bottle gourds, pomegranates, etc. are ascribed mystical health effects. (3) Jargons like "junk foods", empty calories, fast food, anti-oxidants abound. (4) Very similar foods are ascribed opposite health effects, e.g., apples healthy, mangoes unhealthy; almonds good; and cashew bad.

Cooking oils have spawned an elaborate pseudoscience. All triglycerides are nutritionally almost identical, providing nine glucose-free calories per gram. Their glycerol is identical. Unsaturated fatty acids decrease phospholipid bilayer rigidity, necessitating cholesterol redistribution from blood to cell membranes. On a diet rich in unsaturated fatty acids, cholesterol shifts out of plasma, and serum levels are transiently depressed. Though projected as barometers of heart health, these shifts are irrelevant to atherosclerosis.

Beliefs about dietary sodium are equally illogical. Glomeruli filter over 1,200 g of salt daily, of which over 99.5% is reabsorbed in tubules. Glomerular and tubular functions are under exquisite, independent and multiple controls. Beliefs that 4 g of salt daily is healthy, seven is dangerous, amounts to believing that if glomeruli filter 1,252 g salt daily, and tubules reabsorb 1,250, it is healthy, but altering these loads by even 0.1% is deleterious.

Modified Heart Healthy Diet

Since, glucose toxicity is important in atherosclerosis and health, current diet recommendations can be modified. Food should provide calories and all essential nutrients in adequate quantities. Vitamin B12 and iron require special attention in vegetarians. The diet should be palatable and affordable.

Adults: Basic rules are: do not be scared of eating; calorie counting is not needed for calories that come from fat; fats are healthier than glucose, especially in sedentary lifestyle; high-fat, low-glucose diet is good for heart; quantity of fats should be increased, quality (olive oil, cold pressed oils, cows ghee, walnuts, etc.) adds more expense than value; trans-fats of vanaspati ghee, margarine, bakery, sometimes eatery or party food, should be avoided; high protein is not very good, so consider protein a nutrient, not fuel; reduce glucose by curtailing sugar, jaggery, and by increasing fat in food; restrict glucose to amounts that can be stored as glycogen. Thus, physically active people may increase starchy foods, but match their intake to their expenditure from day-to-day, perhaps from meal-to-meal. These rules will prevent heart disease, cancers, various surgeries, and ensure longevity.

Poor man's heart healthy diet would have liberal amounts of cheap fats; (refined vegetable oil, palm oil, palm oil saturated fraction), starch titrated to activity levels, cheapest vegetables and animal foods (eggs, and milk), small multiple meals, and frugality of sugar, jaggery, and total calories to avoid hyperinsulinemia.

Ovo-lacto vegetarians should think of animal foods as healthy, reduce sugar and increase fat. There can be no single diet for children. Those planned for sumo wrestling, basketball, equestrian jobs, etc. would require tailored diets from conception to adulthood. Geriatric diets should be palatable, and easy to digest. Instead of adding years to life, emphasis should be on enjoyment and affordability. Since a long life would be almost invariable, society will have to keep seniors happy and affordable, address legal rights and protection during long second childhoods.

Benefits of Low Fat, Low Cholesterol Diets

Cholesterol education, like animal rights and agriculture department's food pyramid, makes social sense. Carbohydrates make us large. Six feet humans are now common. Forest tribals are much smaller.

Cholesterol is present in animals, it is absent in plants. Cholesterol education leads to descending down in the food chain, from animal foods to plant foods. It greatly reduces the costs of feeding the population, the manpower and hectares required for production of food. It releases surplus manpower for urbanization, infrastructure, and businesses. Massive urbanization is possible; a world populated by dependent, compliant city folk. Exercise is essential for preserving health on a glucose-rich diet. The body has limited capacity for storing glycogen. In sedentary lifestyle, muscles contain glycogen and are insulin resistant. This predisposes to metabolic syndrome, diabetes, obesity, and thrombosis. Exercise depletes muscle glucose and improves insulin sensitivity, though it also increases wear and tear. The need for rest is equally important for health, but it is now seldom mentioned, even to patients discharged after myocardial infarction, congestive heart failure or major surgery. There are numerous publications on value of exercise in heart failure, but not of rest. Thus, cholesterol education leads to gigantic, hard-working, city dwellers maintained on cheap food; to a productive, docile, innocent workforce. The cholesterol myth fuels our prosperity.

PRESENT AND FUTURE

Structural integrity of cell membranes and isolation of lipophilic toxins from blood stream are vital functions of cholesterol. Cholesterol occurs in atheromas because it reaches wherever there is tissue injury. A high-glucose diet engages hepatocytes in triglyceride synthesis, and toxin clearance slows. Excessive dietary glucose can cause many other direct harmful effects, glycosylation of proteins, hyperinsulinemia. Reducing glucose in diet, SGLT2 inhibitors, or even exercise, may provide greater benefit than mere reduction of toxic sdLDL with drugs.

Medical establishments, governments, and media have not resolved the cholesterol controversy. Clearly, some higher power enforces the confusion. Its rise soon after the Empire won the war, and the proactive role of the United States government, suggests that above the three branches of modern states, are other, bigger powers. The cholesterol myth is kept alive by an all-powerful, but invisible, super-government. If doctors were paid well for knowledge, scientifically sound opinions, longevity of their patients, and very little for ordering or conducting hi-tech procedures, the cholesterol myth would collapse. The myth is deliberately kept alive by financial clout, and by other invisible influences.

Sodium-glucose cotransporter-2 trials can be expected to show benefits for arteries, veins, myocardium, dementia, cataracts, glaucoma, autoimmune diseases, cancers, glomeruli, etc. They will simultaneously show adverse effects on renal tubules and urinary tracts from excess urinary glucose, and little effect on dental caries, dyspepsia, and constipation. These trials may bring home the message of glucose toxicity, ending the cholesterol era. But will the next generation have the skills to make the post cholesterol world a better place than our prosperous, financially governed, global human farm?

CONCLUSION

Animals cell membranes contain cholesterol, it makes us flexible and mobile. Plants use cellulose. LDL and HDL work together like mop and pail for cleaning the circulation of endotoxins, cellular debris, etc. Fresh LDL and HDL are therefore both good, and old lipoproteins are bad because they contain endotoxins. High glucose diets change LDL to VLDL, and this becomes small dense LDL, which is atherogenic. Glucose is a reactive aldehyde that causes glycosylation of endothelial adhesion proteins. Glucose, smoke, etc. cause endothelial dysfunction, inflammation, and adhesion and deposition of small dense LDL causing atherosclerosis. High levels of old LDL or old HDL (familial hypercholesterolemia, alcohol, torcetrapib) predispose to atherosclerosis, and statins help by clearing small dense LDL from blood.

REFERENCES

1. Gary Taubes. The Carbohydrate Hypothesis. in Good Calories, Bad Calories. Anchor Books. 2007; pp. 89-204.
2. TL Cleave. Conception of a Single 'Saccharine Disease' in The Saccharine Disease. Bristol John Wright & Sons. 1974 chapter 2.
3. Dehghan M, Mente A, Zhang X, et al. Associations of fats and carbohydrate intake with cardiovascular disease and mortality in 18 countries from five continents (PURE): a prospective cohort study. Lancet. 2017;390(10107):2050-62.
4. Frantz ID, Dawson EA, Ashman PL, et al. Test of effect of lipid lowering by diet on cardiovascular risk. The Minnesota Coronary Survey. Arteriosclerosis. 1989;9(1):129-35.
5. de Lorgeril M, Salen P, Martin JL, et al. Mediterranean diet, traditional risk factors, and the rate of cardiovascular complications after myocardial infarction: final report of the Lyon Diet Heart Study. Circulation. 1999;99:779-85.
6. James Le Fanu. The Rise and Fall of Heart Disease. in The Rise and Fall of Modern Medicine. Little Brown & Co. Ltd., pp. 361-38.

CHAPTER 6

Indian Dyslipidemia: Challenges in Management

Saumitra Ray, Sumanta Chatterjee

INTRODUCTION

Abnormal values of lipoprotein lipids such as high total cholesterol (TC), low-density lipoprotein (LDL) cholesterol, very-low-density lipoprotein (VLDL) cholesterol, and triglycerides (TG) and low high-density lipoprotein (HDL) cholesterol are important coronary heart disease (CHD) risk factors. Many trials have shown that raised-LDL cholesterol (LDL-C) is the most common risk factor which leads to initiation and progression of coronary atherosclerosis. Robust data are available that show that lowering its levels can regress and stabilize atherosclerotic vascular disease.[1] Therefore, management of dyslipidemia is of paramount importance to reduce cardiovascular disease (CVD). In 2013, the National Heart, Lung, and Blood Institute (NHLBI), the American College of Cardiology (ACC), and the American Heart Association (AHA), released a joint guideline focusing on the risk of atherosclerotic cardiovascular disease (ASCVD). However, as evident by various studies, dyslipidemia in Indian population is characterized by low HDL cholesterol (HDL-C) and high TG. High TC and LDL-C are less common in Indian patients. Moreover, there are significant lifestyle, genetic, socioeconomic, and cultural differences in Indians versus European population. All these factors demand different treatment approaches for optimal management of dyslipidemia and CVD. Also, prevalence and the pattern of various risk factors that decides the category of CV risk differ from European population and therefore, risk assessment score varies. Apart from this, economical constraints on healthcare expenditure and delayed availability of newer agents also leads to different treatment approaches amongst treating physicians. Moreover, the side effect profile of the drugs used to treat dyslipidemia, notably statins, also varies from the European to the Indian population. No evidence-based Indian guidelines for dyslipidemia management considering all these factors have been developed and therefore, Indian physicians are forced to follow international guidelines for their patients. Hence, there is a need for adapting international guidelines for Indian patients through expert consensus for guiding Indian physicians. Though Indian guidelines for the management of dyslipidemia are not currently available, a consensus statement on the management of dyslipidemia in Indian subjects was published in 2014. And that is why it is a challenge to manage dyslipidemia in India especially in the absence of India-specific guidelines.[2,3]

INDIAN EPIDEMIOLOGICAL STUDIES ON DYSLIPIDEMIA

Heterogeneous data were showing an increasing secular trend in TC levels, but in view of various limitations and biases in data, robustness of this trend could not be confirmed. Prevalence of dyslipidemia in India is not adequately documented. However, India Heart Watch study was a big epidemiological survey of urban middle class subjects from 11 major cities of India. Prevalence in men and women, respectively were, TC more than 200 mg/dL in 25.1% (men) and 24.9% (women), LDL-C more than 130 mg/dL in 16.3% (men) and 15.1% (women) and more than 100 mg/dL in 49.5% (men) and 49.7% (women), HDL-C less than 40 mg/dL (men) and less than 50 mg/dL (women) in 33.6% and 52.8%, TC:HDL-C ratio is more than or equal to 4.5 in 29.4% and 16.8% and TG is more than or equal to 150 mg/dL in 42.1% and 32.9% (Fig. 1).[4]

India is undergoing a rapid epidemiological transition with increasing population, economic prosperity, urbanization and aging with associated risk factor transition. Adverse lifestyles such as greater smoking and tobacco use, change in nutritional habits with greater intake of unhealthy diets and increasing sedentary lifestyle are also responsible factors for development of CHD.[5] In the Jaipur Heart Watch (JHW) studies (six in number), 20-year mean cholesterol and other lipid parameters were evaluated. Total 712 people of 20–59 years were evaluated in JHW-1, 558 in JHW-2, 374 in JHW-3, 887 in JHW-4, 530 in JHW-5, and 1,100 in JHW-6.

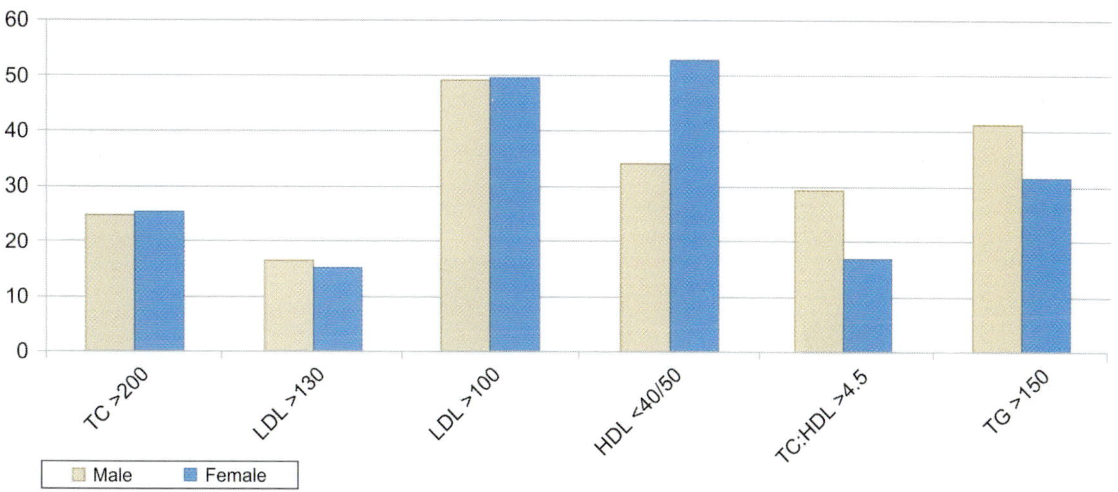

HDL, high-density lipoprotein; LDL, low-density lipoprotein; TC, total cholesterol; TG, triglyceride.

FIG. 1: Prevalence (%) of dyslipidemia in India Heart Watch multisite study, N = 6,123.

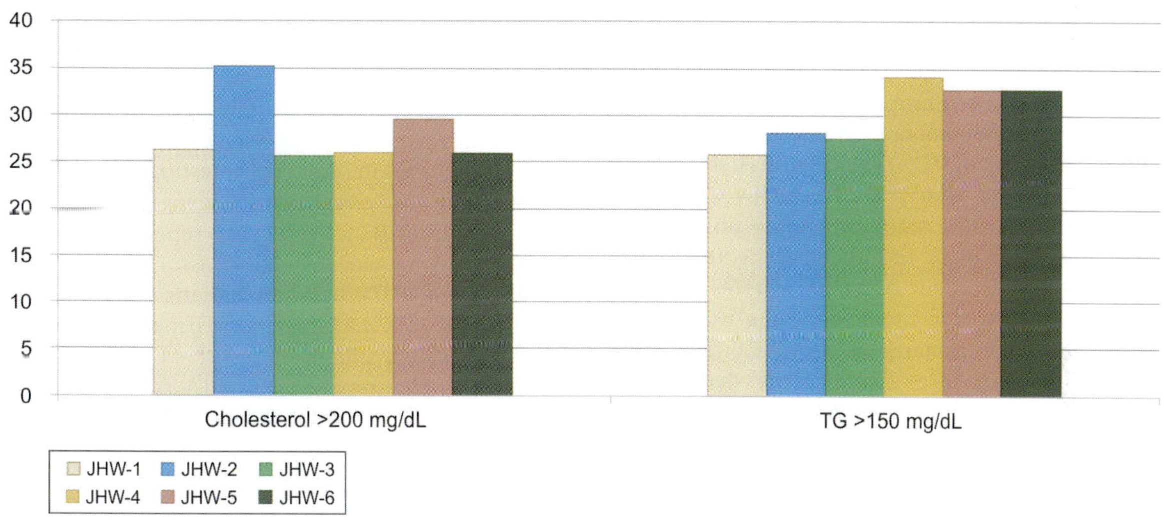

JHW, Jaipur Heart Watch; TG, triglyceride.

FIG. 2: Twenty-year trends in prevalence of hypercholesterolemia and hypertriglyceridemia among urban subjects in Jaipur Heart Watch.

There was high prevalence of overweight, hypertension, and lipid abnormalities. Age- and sex-adjusted trends showed significant increases in mean body mass index (BMI), fasting glucose, TC, HDL-C, and TG (quadratic and log-linear regression, $p < 0.001$). There was increase in overweight and obesity ($p < 0.05$) and hypertriglyceridemia but insignificant changes were observed in truncal obesity, hypertension, hypercholesterolemia and diabetes (Fig. 2).[5]

ASSOCIATION BETWEEN LIPID LEVELS AND RISK OF HEART DISEASE IN INDIA

In the INTERHEART study, relative importance of different lipid components in acute coronary syndrome is highlighted in which South Asian population was showing highest risk of myocardial infarction (MI) with high cholesterol level.[6]

In India, there are limited studies available which have prospectively evaluated importance of various cholesterol lipoproteins. In one study, done in the pre-statin era, a linear relationship of increasing TC levels with increasing mortality in various age-groups was observed (Fig. 3).[7]

Familial hypercholesterolemia (FH) is an important coronary risk factor with varying prevalence from 1:200 to 1:500 globally. It is commonly seen in young patients who have a history of MI. Many studies show that there is a relatively low prevalence of mild to moderate hypercholesterolemia in both population- and hospital-based subjects in India.[8]

A panel of Indian experts felt that QRISK®2 risk calculator for estimating CV risk in Indian subset of dyslipidemia is more appropriate than ASCVD risk score developed for the Americans.[3]

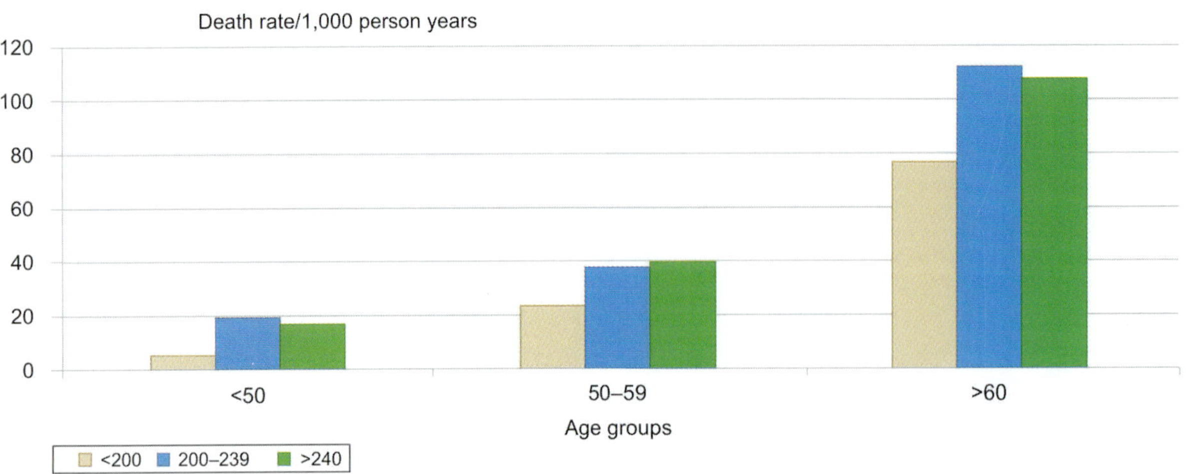

FIG. 3: Prospective study of association of cholesterol levels with cardiovascular mortality with preexisting coronary heart disease in India.

LABORATORY PARAMETERS ASSESSMENT

Assessment of lipid profile is crucial to assess CV risk and to decide on the treatment. Traditionally, assessments are done in fasting state. European Society of Cardiology (ESC) dyslipidemia guideline opined that both fasting and nonfasting assessment of TC, LDL-C, and HDL-C shows similar levels, whereas higher TG levels (by 27 mg/dL) are observed in nonfasting state depending on time and composition of the last meal. In Indian setting, this is even more due to higher content of carbohydrates in meal. The increase in TG levels in nonfasting state was seemed important as TGs are considered as strong CV risk factors for Asian Indians and is a characteristic dyslipidemic component in Indians.[9,10] Nonfasting assessments were considered helpful so that overcrowding of laboratory in morning will be reduced and patients' preference to perform lipid assessment increases. However, nonfasting lipid assessment has disadvantage of unclear evidence on time of assessment after meal (whether 1 h, 1.5 h, 2 h, and so), meal load or composition before assessment, and nonfasting cut-off levels for each of lipid components. Thus, fasting lipid assessment is still the gold standard, to be performed whenever feasible with nonfasting assessment reserved for those with CV risk assessments, in diabetic patients, distant residence patients (first-hand opportunity to screen for dyslipidemia with follow-up fasting evaluation at 3 months). It was suggested that for a LDL-centric management, i.e., when physicians treating dyslipidemia has kept the target of achieving LDL-C to a goal irrespective of the other lipid levels, a nonfasting measurement may prove equally useful.[3] This was also recommended by the European atherosclerosis society and European federation of clinical chemistry and laboratory medicine.

European Society of Cardiology recommended apolipoprotein B (ApoB) as an alternative marker for risk assessment especially in those with elevated TGs.[11] However, ApoB is expensive for Indian setting. Hence, it was suggested that ApoB should not form a part of routine dyslipidemia management in Indian setting.[3]

Lipoprotein-a [Lp(a)] was advised by ESC guideline as marker for estimation in patients with history of premature CV disease in family and in those with borderline CV risk. Routine Lp(a) estimation is felt to be inappropriate in Indian setting. Further, as Lp(a) estimation techniques are not validated in most laboratories in India, Lp(a) testing is liable to technical errors giving false positive or false negative results. A recent evaluation from Banerjee et al.[12] reported nonsignificantly higher trend for elevated Lp(a) association with ischemic heart disease (IHD) in Asian Indians [odds ratio (OR) 2.0] and Chinese (OR 4.8) than non-Hispanic Whites (OR 1.4). Lp(a) assessment should be restricted to premature (at age <40 years) or recurrent CVD, FH, history of premature CVD in family, and borderline high risk of CV disease.[3]

INADEQUATE MANAGEMENT OF DYSLIPIDEMIA IN INDIA

Epidemiological studies of hypercholesterolemia and dyslipidemia are important for developing strategies for prevention of CHD. In Indian Heart Watch study awareness about dyslipidemia and its consequences among dyslipidemic population was in 17.5% men and 13.2% women and statins was given to 7.5% men and 6.7% women, while control to targets of TC less than 200 mg/dL was in 4.5% men and 3.7% women (Fig. 4).[1] The PURE study also found low use of secondary prevention drugs and healthy lifestyle practices in low income countries including India. A study has also reported that availability of statins is no longer a problem, still the use is low in India.[4]

INDIAN GUIDELINE RECOMMENDATION ON DYSLIPIDEMIA MANAGEMENT

Management of dyslipidemia is a difficult task as not only the prevalence of dyslipidemia is constantly increasing, particularly at a younger age, but also the pattern of dyslipidemia

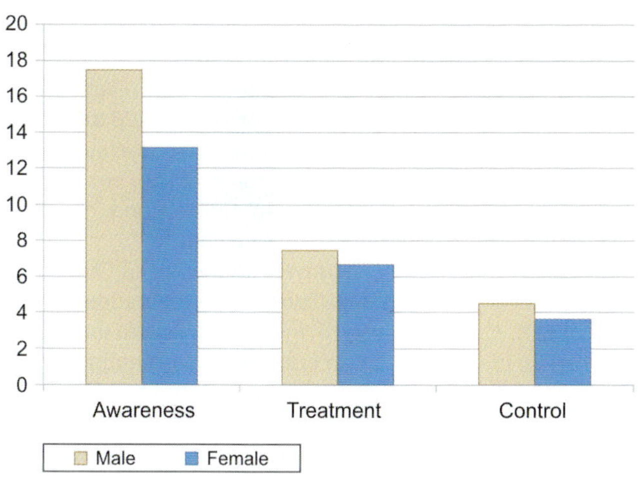

FIG. 4: Hypercholesterolemia awareness, treatment, and control among urban adults in India. (percentage prevalence): Indian Heart Watch Study.

is also different as compared to the Western populations. Furthermore, overall awareness about dyslipidemia and prevention of ASCVD, cultural beliefs, socioeconomic conditions, etc. are also different. For these reasons, there is a need to formulate a guideline recommendation for dyslipidemia and coronary artery disease (CAD) prevention for Indian patients which can be best suited for Indian conditions as well.

CARDIOVASCULAR RISK STRATIFICATION OF INDIAN PATIENT

Cardiovascular risk stratification is very much important for primary and secondary prevention of CAD, especially in high ASCVD score patients who do not have prior history of MI or any vascular condition. This is required to cater the appropriate statin to appropriate patients. This avoids both under treatment and over treatment with statins. Moreover, the awareness of the risk of ASCVD improves patients' health behaviors and improve the compliance to treatment (Table 1).[13-15]

TREATMENT GOAL ACCORDING TO ASCVD RISK STRATIFICATION

This outline recommends target goal of lipid levels and thresholds for statin therapy initiation based on risk categories (Table 2). It should be noted that therapeutic lifestyle change is also recommended in all individuals who have LDL-C or non-HDL-C values above the desired goals, and preferably in everyone regardless of their cholesterol levels.[15]

CARDIOVASCULAR DISEASE PREVENTION: LIPID TARGETS

European Society of Cardiology recommends cessation of tobacco use, healthy diet, body weight maintenance, physical activity (moderate-vigorous 2.5–5 h per week), blood pressure, and glycemic control (HbA1c <7%).[11] However, healthy diet is one of the most deficient means in CV disease prevention in India. Reducing carbohydrate intake was suggested. Indian Council of Medical Research National Institute of Nutrition Research recommends visible fat intake of 50 g per person per day. It is suggested to limit the use of coconut oil, vanaspati, and animal fats on the account of high amount of saturated fatty acids present in these sources. Further, it is advised to avoid olive oil for cooking in India as it has lower smoking point and may get denatured at cooking temperatures (deep frying) employed in routine.[3] In India, lower waist circumference (WC) cut-off for males (<90 cm) and females (<80 cm) are recommended contrasting to ESC

TABLE 1: Atherosclerotic cardiovascular disease risk categories in Indians

Risk category	Conventional risk markers	Nonconventional risk markers
Very high-risk	• Pre-existing ASCVD • DM with end organ damage or 2 or more major ASCVD risk factors • FHH	• None
High-risk (>15% risk of ASCVD death/MI/stroke over 10 years)	• 3 or more major ASCVD risk factors • DM other than above category • CKD stage 3B or 4 • FH (except FHH) • LDL >190 mg/dL/ heavy smoker/ strong family history of premature ASCVD	• CAC score >300 A • Carotid plaque (nonstenotic) • Lp(a) >50 mg/dL
Moderate-risk (5–15% risk of ASCVD death/MI/stroke over 10 years)	• 2 major ASCVD risk factors	• CAC score 100–299 • Raised carotid IMT/ aortic PWV • Lp(a) 20–49 mg/dL • Metabolic syndrome
Low-risk (<5% risk of ASCVD death/MI/stroke over 10 years)	• 0–1 major ASCVD risk factor	• None

ASCVD, atherosclerotic cardiovascular disease; CKD, chronic kidney disease; CAC, coronary artery calcium; DM, diabetes mellitus; FHH: familial homozygous hypercholesterolemia; LDL, low-density lipoprotein; MI, myocardial infarction; PWV, pulse wave velocity; IMT, intima media thickness; Lp(a), lipoprotein(a).

TABLE 2: Treatment goals and statin initiation according to atherosclerotic cardiovascular disease risk categories

Risk category	Treatment goal		Initiation of drug therapy	
	LDL mg/dL	Non-HDL mg/dL	LDL mg/dL	Non-HDL mg/dL
Very high-risk	<50	<80	>50	>80
High-risk	<70	<100	>70	>100
Moderate-risk	<100	<130	>100	>130
Low-risk	<100	<130	>130	>160

HDL, high-density lipoprotein; LDL, low-density lipoprotein.

recommendation of less than 94 cm and less than 82 cm, respectively.[11] Also, BMI cut-off was opined to be less than 23 kg/m^2 against ESC recommendation of 20–25 kg/m^2.[3] Alcohol was not found to be cardiac friendly for Indian population as opposed to most other ethnic groups.

LOWERING OF LOW-DENSITY LIPOPROTEIN REDUCES RISK OF CARDIOVASCULAR EVENTS

Low-density lipoprotein is a major culprit for development of atherosclerosis and causes CAD. Many studies have shown that as much as low LDL is better for CV event reduction. In a meta-analysis of 175,000 participants in 27 randomized trials of statins, the Cholesterol Treatment Trialists, (CTT) collaborators found that a reduction of 1 mmol/L (38.7 mg/dL) in LDL-C levels produced a 21% reduction in major vascular events over 5 years, irrespective of age, sex, base line LDL-C levels and presence or absence of vascular disease.[16]

DRUGS FOR MANAGEMENT OF DYSLIPIDEMIA

Statins remain the cornerstone for treatment of dyslipidemia. Statins are recommended in highest recommended or tolerated dose to reach the goal lipid levels and was agreed unanimously by the panel. However, panel identified three potential statins—(1) atorvastatin, (2) rosuvastatin, and (3) pitavastatin for clinical use in India. Descriptive studies in India have reported maximum utilization of atorvastatin and rosuvastatin to large extent (over 95% of prescriptions) than other statins.[17]

In the JUPITER trial, 106 people with no prior ASCVD or diabetes with baseline LDL-C less than or equal to 130 mg/dL and high sensitivity C-reactive protein more than or equal to 2 mg/L were treated with rosuvastatin 20 mg/d. The median LDL-C level attained was 55 mg/dL, as compared to 108 mg/dL at baseline. Those who achieved LDL-C less than 50 mg/dL had 65% reduction in the risk of major CV events and 46% reduction in total mortality. Approximately, 23% of the subjects reached LDL-C level of less than 40 mg/dL. In a *post hoc* analysis, no adverse effects were seen in this group.[18]

The ESC recommends use of ezetimibe, bile acid sequestrant, and cholesterol absorption inhibitors in a sequential manner as additional agents if the goal is not reached with statin alone. In cases with very high-risk who failed to achieve treatment goal, addition of proprotein convertase subtilisin/kexin type 9 (PCSK9) inhibitors should be considered. Panel suggested when lipid goals are not reached, causes of secondary dyslipidemia should be ruled out.[11]

In the IMPROVE-IT (Improved Reduction of Outcomes: Vytorin Efficacy international Trial), with ACS patients mean level of LDL-C was 69.9 mg/dL in the simvastatin group and 53.2 mg/dL in the simvastatin ezetimibe combination group. The median follow-up was for 7 years. Primary endpoint of CV death, MI, hospitalization for unstable angina, coronary revascularization (>3 days), or stroke occurred in 34.7% of the simvastatin group and 32.7% of the simvastatin plus ezetimibe group. The absolute risk reduction was 2% (numbers needed to treat-50) and relative risk reduction was 6.4% (hazard ratio 0.936; CI 0.887–0.988; p = 0.016). There was no safety signal.[19]

As per experts, to achieve LDL-C target, statins are first-line agents. In India, rosuvastatin (5–40 mg), atorvastatin (10–80 mg), and pitavastatin (1–4 mg) may be used as first choice. In case of failure to achieve goal LDL-C with statin alone, add ezetimibe (10 mg) as second agent followed by bile acid sequestrant, and cholesterol absorption inhibitors as needed. A combination of statin (in lower doses—e.g., atorvastatin 40 mg instead of 80 mg or rosuvastatin 20 mg instead of 40 mg) with ezetimibe may be considered in patients who have significant adverse effects with statins or who are diabetic or at high CV risk.

DRUGS FOR MANAGEMENT OF HYPERTRIGLYCERIDEMIA

The ESC recommended that statin should be given to all high-risk patients with TG more than 200 mg/dL and addition of fenofibrate to statin to be considered if target TG of less than 200 mg/dL is not reached with statin alone.[11] The risk of CV disease morbidity and mortality is increased significantly in case where estimated glomerular filtration (eGFR) is less than 15 mL/min/1.73 m^2. Using fenofibrate with statin thus demands lower dosage (75 mg/day) of fenofibrate. Further, reported prevalence of chronic kidney disease (CKD) in Indians is 17.2% with further increase in diabetic subset (18.8%) suggests significant burden of CKD. Panel opined that when eGFR is less than 60 mL/min/1.73 m^2, dose of fenofibrate should not be increased. In patients who have TGs more than 200 mg/dL, panel recommends use of fenofibrate in a low-dose with caution in CKD cases and strict implementation of lifestyle modification as a treatment strategy. In CAD cases, who have LDL-C less than 70 mg/dL with TG more than 200 mg/dL and HDL-C less than 35 mg/dL, panel suggested use of fenofibrate (75 mg/day) in addition to statin. Use of higher dose needs monitoring of eGFR in patients. Where fibrate is contraindicated or not tolerated, there is some evidence of biochemical benefit with saroglitazar, a dual PPAR agonist. This is safe in combination with statin but there is no evidence of its clinical outcome benefit.[12,20]

FAMILIAL HYPERCHOLESTEROLEMIA IN INDIA

Familial hypercholesterolemia, a common genetic disease not diagnosed, especially in Asian countries.[21] In India, sporadic case reports of FH are available in literature. However, the panel felt there is need to prospectively screen patients for FH and suggested use of clinical criteria for screening of FH in India. Panel stressed on assessing arcus cornealis before the age of 45 years especially in upper cornea as simple tool to start screening FH. In association with raised LDL-C (>250 mg/dL), these criteria can provide a clue to the diagnosis of FH. Genetic screening may be positive in ~ 60% cases which were classified as definite FH by clinical criteria. Target LDL-C in FH recommended by ESC guidelines is less than 100 mg/dL and less than 70 mg/dL without or with CVD, respectively. In high risk cases or in those with CVD or statin intolerance, PCSK9 inhibitor is recommended as treatment.[11]

DYSLIPIDEMIA IN TYPE 2 DIABETES AND METABOLIC SYNDROME

The ESC guidelines recommend non-HDL-C is less than 130 mg/dL and less than 100 mg/dL in high-risk and very high risk cases, respectively. In treating dyslipidemia, statins are recommended in all type 1 diabetes and in presence of microalbuminuria and/or renal disease irrespective of baseline LDL-C. LDL-C is less than 70 mg/dL (primary) and non-HDL-C is less than 100 mg/dL (secondary) are recommended in type 2 diabetes and CVD/CKD as well as in patients aged more than 40 years without CVD but with one or more CVD risk factor. Further, LDL-C is less than 100 mg/dL (primary) and non-HDL-C more than 130 mg/dL (secondary) is advised in type 2 diabetes without any risk factor and/or evidence of target organ damage.[11]

DYSLIPIDEMIA IN ACUTE CORONARY SYNDROME

The ESC recommends early high-dose statin for all cases with ACS and undergoing percutaneous coronary intervention (PCI) despite normal baseline LDL-C levels. Addition of ezetimibe and PCSK9 inhibitors should be considered, if LDL-C target is not reached with statin alone. In statin-intolerant cases, the latter two may be used alone or in combination. A goal LDL-C is less than 70 mg/dL or 50% reduction from the baseline value. Re-evaluation at 4–6 weeks is recommended. A loading of high-dose statin before elective PCI or in patients with non-ST elevation ACS should be considered when patients is are already receiving statins. Panel suggested when baseline LDL-C is less than 100 mg/dL in any ACS patients, a target should be 50% reduction from baseline. When the target of less than 50 mg/dL is desirable and is not achieved with statin alone, addition of ezetimibe may be considered.[11]

DYSLIPIDEMIA IN MODERATE-TO-SEVERE CHRONIC KIDNEY DISEASE

The ESC guidelines identified that CKD stage 3–5 are high or very high-risk for CV disease. Statin with or without ezetimibe is recommended in nondialysis-dependent CKD. In dialysis-dependent CKD cases without any CV disease, statins are not to be used. Statin, ezetimibe, or their combination should be continued at the time of dialysis initiation in all and especially in CV disease cases. Amongst two statins commonly used in India, atorvastatin dose was advised as 20 mg/day by NICE guidelines for primary or secondary prevention of CVD in CKD cases. These guidelines further advocate consultation of nephrologist if eGFR is less than 30 mL/min/1.73 m^2 and higher dose of atorvastatin is to be used. But, as recommended by ESC guidelines and opined by the panel, any dose of statin may be initiated to achieve the target LDL-C is less than 70 mg/dL.[11]

DYSLIPIDEMIA AND STROKE PREVENTION

For primary prevention of stroke, statin treatment is recommended to achieve desired goals in high-risk and very high CV risk cases. For secondary prevention of stroke, intensive statin treatment is recommended by ESC guidelines. ESC guidelines recommend high-dose statin for both primary as well as secondary stroke prevention.[11]

SAFETY ASSESSMENT DURING PHARMACOTHERAPY IN DYSLIPIDEMIA

In consideration of safety of statins, ESC guidelines recommend liver enzyme assessment especially alanine aminotransferase (ALT), at baseline, and once 8–12 weeks post-treatment or after increase in dose. Routine monitoring with ALT, thereafter is not recommended during therapy. If elevation of liver enzymes is over 3 times the upper limit of normal (ULN), reduce the dose or stop the drug and recheck liver enzymes in 4–6 weeks. Reintroduction should be cautiously done after ALT has returned to normal with lower dose at the start and then gradual increase with enzymes monitoring. Persistent elevation in enzymes excludes lipid lowering therapy as a culprit for liver damage. With regards to muscle damage, guideline recommends creatine kinase (CK) assessment at baseline. If elevation of CK is 4x ULN, do not start treatment. Routine monitoring is not necessary except when patients complain of myalgia. Elevation of CK during therapy to 10x ULN demands discontinuation of drug and bimonthly monitoring of CK and renal function. Asymptomatic CK elevation to less than 10x ULN, continue treatment and monitor CK bimonthly whereas in symptomatic elevation of CK to less than 10x ULN, discontinue treatment, monitor CK and restart at lower dose after CK is normalized. Panel agreed to these recommendations and suggested for cautious use of statins in cases of hypothyroidism and vitamin D deficiency.[11]

CONCLUSION

Cardiovascular disease is a major disease burden in India and as it is observed more commonly in young population compared to western population. Dyslipidemia is perhaps the most important risk factor for CVD, particularly for premature CVD. LDL-C is the primary target; but TGs and non-HDL-C can be considered for intervention in patients with grossly deranged levels. LDL-C less than 70 mg/dL is target for all ASCVD cases with optional reduction to less than 50 mg/dL in very high-risk cases. Optional lipid targets that can be considered in India include HDL-C less than 40 mg/dL and TGs less than 150 mg/dL (<100 mg/dL in very high-risk cases).

Statins are first-line drugs for dyslipidemia. Rosuvastatin, atorvastatin, and pitavastatin are commonly used in India. Ezetimibe should be second agent to statin to achieve the desired lipid targets. Low-dose statin in combination with ezetimibe may be considered in patients with significant statin related side effects. Addition of fenofibrate should be considered to statin to lower TGs less than 200 mg/dL, but with close follow-up for liver and kidney derangement.

For treatment of FH, statin, and ezetimibe combination is the primary treatment in India until PCSK9 inhibitors become readily available for clinical use.

In diabetes with high CV risk, LDL-C goal is less than 70 mg/dL. Combination of modest dose statin with ezetimibe should be considered to control dyslipidemia in diabetes.

In acute coronary syndrome and in patients undergoing PCI, LDL-C goal is less than 70 mg/dL with optional lowering to less than 50 mg/dL in very high-risk cases. High-dose statin with addition of ezetimibe, if necessary, is suggested to achieve these lipid targets.

In nondialysis dependent CKD, statin ± ezetimibe is advised to achieve LDL-C goal of less than 70 mg/dL, eGFR should guide the dosing choice. Use of high-dose statin in those with eGFR less than 30 mL/min/1.73 m^2 requires consultation with nephrologist. For primary and secondary stroke prevention, high-dose statins are advised. Follow-up monitoring is advised every 12 weeks till goals are reached and then annually. Liver function assessment at baseline and post-treatment (after 4–6 weeks) should be done. CK levels should be assessed in patients with myopathy or in those at high-risk of muscle damage.

REFERENCES

1. Gupta R, Rao R, Misra A, et al. Recent trends in epidemiology of dyslipidemias in India. Indian Heart J. 2017; 69:382-92.
2. Chandra KS, Bansal M, Nair T, et al. Consensus statement on management of dyslipidemia in Indian subjects. Indian Heart J. 2014;66(Suppl 3):S1-51.
3. Ray S, Sawhney JP, Das M K, et al. Consensus document on management of dyslipidemia in Indian patients: Adaptation of 2016 ESC/EAS Guidelines. Accepted for publication in IHJ. 2016.
4. Guptha S, Gupta R, Deedwania P, et al. Cholesterol lipoproteins, triglycerides and prevalence of dyslipidemias among urban Asian Indian subjects: a cross sectional study. Indian Heart J. 2014;66:280-8.
5. Patel V, Chatterji S, Chisholm D, et al. Chronic diseases and injuries in India. Lancet. 2011;377:413-28.
6. Karthikeyan G, Teo KK, Islam S, et al. Lipid profile, plasma apolipoproteins, and risk of a first myocardial infarction among Asians: an analysis from the INTERHEART Study. J Am Coll Cardiol. 2009;53:244-53.
7. Gupta R, Mohan I, Narula J. Trends in coronary heart disease epidemiology in India. Ann Global Health. 2016;82:307-15.
8. Gidding SS, Hegele RA, Cuchel MA, et al. On behalf of the International Society Severe Familial Hypercholesterolemia Panel: defining severe familial hypercholesterolaemia and the implications for clinical management: a consensus statement from the International Atherosclerosis Society Severe Familial Hypercholesterolemia Panel. Lancet Diab Endocrinol. 2016;4:850-61.
9. Singh AK, Singh R. Triglyceride and cardiovascular risk : A critical appraisal. Indian J Endocrinol Metabol. 2016;418-28.
10. Chen A, Tseng C. The Role of triglyceride in cardiovascular disease in Asian patients with type 2 diabetes - A systematic review. Rev Diabet Stud. 2013;10(2-3):101-9.
11. Catapano AL, Graham I, De Backer G, et al. 2016 ESC/EAS Guidelines for the management of dyslipidaemias. Eur Heart J. 2016;37(39):2999-3058.
12. Banerjee D, Wong EC, Shin J, et al. Racial and Ethnic Variation in Lipoprotein (a) Levels among Asian Indian and Chinese Patients. J Lipids. 2011.
13. Bovet P, Perret F, Cornuz J, et al. Improved smoking cessation in smokers given ultrasound photographs of their own atherosclerotic plaques. Prev Med. 2002; 34:215-20.
14. Wyman RA, Gimelli G, McBride PE, et al. Does detection of carotid plaque affect physician behavior or motivate patients? Am Heart J. 2007;154:1072-7.
15. Iyengar SS, Puri R, Narasingan SN. Lipid Association of India Expert Consensus Statement on Management of Dyslipidemia in Indians 2016: Part 1. JAPI. 1st March, 2016.
16. Mihaylova B, Emberson J, Blackwell L, et al. The effects of lowering LDL cholesterol with statin therapy in people at low risk of vascular disease: Meta-analysis of individual data from 27 randomised trials. Lancet. 2012;380:581-90.
17. Mohapatra S. Prescription patterns of hypolipidaemic drugs in a tertiary care teaching hospital of southern India. J Clin Diagnostic Res. 2014;8: 2012-4.
18. Hsia J, MacFadyen JG, Monyak J, et al. Cardiovascular event reduction and adverse events among subjects attaining low-density lipoprotein cholesterol <50 mg/dl with rosuvastatin. The JUPITER trial (justification for the use of statins in prevention: An intervention trial evaluating rosuvastatin). J Am Coll Cardiol. 2011; 57:1666-75.
19. Cannon CP, Blazing MA, Giugliano RP, et al. Ezetimibe added to statin therapy after acute coronary syndromes. N Engl J Med. 2015; 372:2387-97.
20. Ashfaq F, Goel PK, Sethi R, et al. Lipoprotein (a) levels in relation to severity of coronary artery disease in north Indian patients. Heart Views. 2013;14(1): 12-6.
21. Brinton E, Moriarty P, McGowan M, et al. Familial hypercholesterolemia. Med Roundtable Cardiovasc Ed. 2014;4:e8-17.

CHAPTER 7

Indian Diet and Coronary Artery Disease

Abhishek Gupta, MP Girish, Mohit D Gupta

"Food is more powerful than any pill. The food that we eat can make us fat or thin"

INTRODUCTION

Cardiovascular diseases (CVDs), especially coronary heart disease (CHD), are epidemic in India. The World Health Organization (WHO) and Global burden of disease study also have highlighted increasing trends in years of life lost (YLLs) and disability-adjusted life years (DALYs) from CHD in India. In India, studies have reported increasing CHD prevalence over the last 60 years, from 1% to 9–10% in urban populations and less than 1% to 4–6% in rural populations.[1]

This increase has been largely attributed to rapid westernization. Westernization has made food calorie rich and convenient for the common man, but because of the various ethnic, epigenetic reasons, and the high prevalence of sarcopenic adiposity, Indians are vulnerable to adverse effects of these dietary changes.

The present article attempts to provide, evidenced based strategies for a cardioprotective diet in Indian context.

PREVALENCE OF DISEASE—IS THERE UNDERESTIMATION OF ACTUAL PROBLEM?

Coronary heart disease is a major cause of mortality and morbidity all over the world. While the prevalence and mortality due to CHD is declining in the developed nations there has been an alarming increase over the past two decades in the prevalence of CHD and cardiovascular mortality in India and other South Asian countries.[1]

India is in a phase where it is going through an epidemiologic transition whereby the burden of communicable diseases has declined slowly, but that of noncommunicable diseases (NCD) has risen rapidly, thus leading to a dual burden.

The prevalence of ischemic heart disease (IHD) has increased sevenfold to about 14% by 2013. Similarly, it is more than quadrupled in rural areas, from 1.7 to 7.4% between 1970 and 2013.[2]

The Global Burden of Disease study estimate of age-standardized CVD death rate of 272 per 100,000 population in India is higher than the global average of 235 per 100,000 population. Some aspects of the CVD epidemic in India are particular as its accelerated build up, the early age of disease onset in the population, and the high case fatality rate.[2] The higher case fatality among Indians following acute coronary syndrome (ACS) could result in the underestimation of actual problem.

DIET AND CORONARY ARTERY DISEASE: EVIDENCE

Global disease burden of CVD is increasing across the globe including India, which is experiencing a rapid health transition. Diet and nutrition have been extensively investigated as risk factors for major CVDs in various studies like The INTERHEART study, The Lyon Diet Heart Study, The Framingham and offspring Study;[3] these studies are conducted within and across populations, to link several nutrients, minerals, food groups, and dietary patterns with an increased or decreased risk of CVD.[3-5]

INDIAN DIET

Diversity of Indian Diet—Is It Sufficient to make us Healthy?

India has a rich and highly varied cuisine, and its various diets are strongly related to social identity, religion, and other cultural factors, as well as local agricultural practices and availability of diverse foods. Indian food is paradoxically considered strongly vegetarian, but it is actually lacking in vegetable content rather, is centered on wheat, in the north, and rice, in the south with daal being the second most important element. One can have an entire South Indian vegetarian meal without encountering even a single vegetable. The most important vegetable that is consumed

TABLE 1: Westernized diet and risk patterns

	Evidence	Conclusion
Dietary pattern with added fats, fried food, eggs, organ, and processed meats, and sugar-sweetened beverages (Southern dietary pattern)	There was a 56% increase in cardiac events over 6 years with the Southern pattern, which was eaten more frequently by residents of the Stroke Belt who were male, black, smokers, less educated, physically inactive, and overweight or obese.[7]	A dietary pattern characteristic of the Southern United States (animal products and sweets) was associated with greater hazard of CHD, and is more common in overweight, Southern black men with lower levels of education and economic status

CHD, coronary heart disease.

is highly starchy aloo. Whatever amount of greens is taken is deeply fried which kills its nutrient content.[5]

Westernization of Indian Diet

The prevalence of CVDs increased by threefold in India as compared to west by the turn of 20th century[6] which is attributed to rapid westernization. Westernization is correlated with increase in consumption of sugar, salt, high fat dairy products, eggs, red meat, and oils with their trans-fat content (Table 1).

Various methods of improving the taste and prolonging the shelf life of food substances like salting, refining, hydrogenation, and frying increases the energy density of the food materials. The harmful components of the westernized diet are because of in its energy density and its ability to have a long shelf-life.

CONTAMINATED VEGETARIANISM

Vegetarianism prevalent in India is aptly criticized as the contaminated vegetarianism, consuming large amounts of fried foods, excess of salt, sugar, and ghee. Hence, the protective components in the vegetarian diet are considerably lacking in our diet.

Cholesterol and Diet

Since, cholesterol can be synthesized in the body, all recommendations advice to restrict dietary cholesterol consumption to be less than 300 mg/day, which is the average amount found in an ordinary egg yolk.

In typical omnivorous diets, the relationship of intake of cholesterol in low doses and blood cholesterol is linear. At higher cholesterol intakes, the relationship is curvilinear; changes in dietary cholesterol have less of an effect on serum cholesterol.

The also the magnitude of the effect differs from one person to another, largely from differences in the baseline diet as well as genetically determined intestinal cholesterol absorptive capacity (Table 2).

OIL CONSUMPTION

Oil is a cooking medium which makes food more palatable. The water content of food gets replaced by the oil, which makes the food energy dense (Fig. 1).

TABLE 2: Dietary cholesterol in India diet

	Evidence	Conclusion
Dietary cholesterol	Meta-analysis including 27 studies using prepared diets and assessing effect on cholesterol[8]	Added dietary cholesterol increases serum cholesterol; the effect is greatest when baseline intake is low Each 100-mg increment in dietary cholesterol increases TC by 2.2 mg/dL and increases the TC:HDL ratio by 0.02 units

HDL, high-density lipoprotein; TC, total cholesterol.

The invisible fat content of the cereals and pulses contribute to 3–5% of their weight. The person who consumes at least one nonvegetarian dish a day does not require additional oil in his diet. The invisible fat content of the Indian diet almost matches the daily requirement of 40–60 g/day. Therefore, only vegans and people involved in heavy manual labor requires up to one to two table-spoons of oil and that too only if they are unable to consume the recommended daily need of 30 g of nuts.[9]

The beneficial effect of fish and marine products in Indian diet is marred by the widespread deep-frying habit which oxidizes the cholesterol and transforms lipid contents making them more atherogenic.

Myth of Polyunsaturated Fatty Acid

Polyunsaturated fats contain essential fatty acids (FA), but have a short shelf-life, and thermal instability. It is better to use them as spreads or as seasoning. Most of refined oils with high polyunsaturated fatty acid (PUFA) can degrade easily at high temperatures to toxic component like free-radicals, trans-fats and malondialdehyde which are atherogenic, hence oil which are stable at high temperature like ghee, coconut oil, unrefined oil with high smoke point like mustard oil should be preferred for frying.

Widely advertised ω-6-polyunsaturated (mainly linoleic acid) cooking oils like sunflower oil, may not be heart friendly, since the prostaglandins derived from such oils are more thrombogenic than the ω-3-polyunsaturated oils (mainly ALNA) like canola, soybean, and rapeseed oil, so in diet n-6 to n-3 ratio should not be more that 5-10:1. There is also evidence, that if we keep n-6 FA intake lesser, n-3 FA can be converted into long chain n-3 FA like [2-ethylhexanoic acid (EHA) and dehydroepiandrosterone (DHEA)].[15]

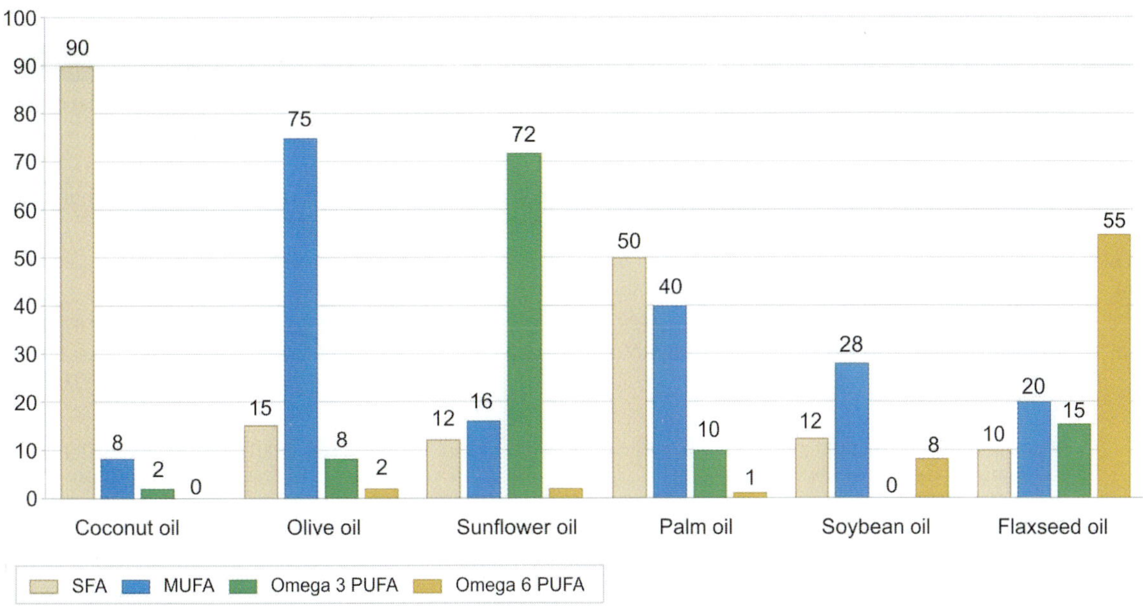

MUFA, monounsaturated fatty acids; PUFA, polyunsaturated fatty acids; SFA, saturated fatty acids.

FIG. 1: Various fraction of fatty acids in different oils.

Which Oil to be Preferred for Cooking?

The sterol for the plant kingdom is ergosterol and any plant product, therefore can be labelled as cholesterol free. Solid fats (at room temperature), including coconut oil and palm oil, have deleterious effects on atherosclerotic cardiovascular disease (ASCVD) risk factors. Liquid vegetable oils have beneficial effects on lipids and lipoproteins. As noted, they decrease low-density lipoprotein cholesterol (LDL-C).

The evidence base for olive oil [monounsaturated fatty acids (MUFAs) rich] is the most comprehensive, with clear evidence for a benefit in ASCVD risk reduction. As olive oil is expensive and out of reach for most of Indian population other alternative with equal benefit is mustard oil (MUFA rich).

Replacement with MUFAs or n-6 PUFAs lowered fasting serum total cholesterol (–8.4% and –9.2%, respectively), LDL-C (–11.3% and –13.6%), and total cholesterol to high-density lipoprotein cholesterol (HDL-C) ratio (–5.6% and –8.5%) ($p \leq 0.001$).

The sterol for the animal kingdom is cholesterol and the recognition of oxidized cholesterol as an atherogenic moiety made the fats and oils of animal origin unacceptable choice as a cooking medium (Table 3).

Controversies on Saturated Fatty Acids—Are They Really Bad? What should be Optimal Replacement Fatty Acid?

Saturated fatty acid (SFA)-rich foods (e.g., meat, butter, and cheese) increase LDL-C, HDL-C, and decreases triglycerides. Unsaturated fatty acids (for example, vegetable oils and fatty fish) decreases the amount of LDL-C and triglycerides in the blood and raises HDL-C.[16]

A recent meta-analysis of observational studies suggest that saturated fat intake is not associated with CVD, ischemic stroke, type 2 diabetes mellitus and all-cause mortality. In particular, a diet high in stearic acid appears to lower levels of unhealthy LDL-C.[17]

Available evidence from adequately controlled randomized trials suggest replacing SFA with mostly n-6 PUFA is unlikely to reduce CHD events, CHD mortality or total mortality.[18]

FRUIT AND VEGETABLES IN INDIAN DIET—MORE PRODUCTIONS BUT LESS CONSUMPTION

The WHO recommends a daily intake of at least 400 g (or five daily servings with an average serving size of 80 grams) of fruits and vegetables, excluding potatoes, cassava, and other starchy tubers to prevent diet-related chronic diseases and micronutrient deficiencies. But according to the India's Phytonutrient Report (2016) notes that Indians consume quite less than the norms.[19] Lifestyle factors such as long working hours and junk food consumption and other factors like high costs, lack of availability of the product throughout the year were some of the reasons attributed to low consumption.

Dark green vegetables reduces arterial stiffness and blood pressure, because of inorganic nitrate, which undergoes salivary bacterial conversion to nitrite, followed by gastrointestinal acidification to nitrous oxide (NO).[20]

TABLE 3: Summary of types of oils, content, and current evidence

	Evidence	Conclusion
Canola oil (MUFA-rich)	Canola oil reduces LDL-C but has no effect on HDL-C, lipid peroxidation, inflammation. But there are no data on CVD outcomes[10]	Canola oil can be used as plant-based oil that is rich in unsaturated fat, to replace other fats
Coconut oil (SFA-rich)	Many Reviews have shown definite cholesterol-raising effect of coconut oil. There are no data on CVD outcomes[11]	Because coconut oil is rich in SFA, its use is not recommended
Sunflower oil (PUFA-rich)	Sunflower oil reduces LDL-C with no clear effect on HDL-C when replaced with other fats/oils[12]	Sunflower oil is rich in MUFAs and PUFAs so can be used to replace other fats
Olive oil (MUFA-rich)	In the PREDIMED, a Mediterranean diet supplemented with extra-virgin olive oil reduced incident CVD by 30% compared with a lower-fat control diet	Extra-virgin (unrefined) olive oil is rich in MUFA and polyphenols and there is consistent evidence of its beneficial effect on CVD risk markers and CVD morbidity and mortality
Palm-oil (SFA-rich)	Meta-analysis of RCTs comparing palm oil to other vegetable oils demonstrates a cholesterol-raising effect[13]	Of all vegetable oils, palm oil is among the highest in SFAs and, consequently, increases risk of CHD. Consumption should be discouraged
Mustard oil (MUFA-rich)	Collaborative study with USA, AIIMS, and St. Johns Medical College, Bangalore has proved that use of mustard oil as cooking medium reduces the risk of coronary heart disease by almost 70% in comparison to sunflower oil[14]	Mustard oil is healthier than olive oil because it does not has trans FA, has low saturated fat and high in MUFA and PUFA such as ω-3FA and stable at high temperature which makes it ideal cooking oil and even deep frying oil

AIIMS, All India Institute of Medical Sciences; CHD, coronary heart disease; CVD, cardiovascular disease; FA, fatty acids; LDL-C, low-density lipoprotein cholesterol; HDL-C, high-density lipoprotein cholesterol; MUFA, monounsaturated fatty acids; PUFA, polyunsaturated fatty acids; RCTs, randomized controlled trials; SFA, saturated fatty acids.

ANTIOXIDANTS—DO THEY HAVE ANY ROLE IN OUR DIET?

Antioxidant phytochemicals like flavonoids are richly concentrated in blueberries, strawberries, raspberries, red cabbage, red radishes, and eggplant (purple vegetables) and have potent anti-inflammatory properties.

Multiple subsequent randomized controlled trials (RCTs) of antioxidant supplements reported either neutral or negative results, including the GISSI trial of vitamin E, the Physicians Health Study of beta-carotene, and the National Institutes of Health (NIH)—AARP Diet and Health study of multivitamin supplementation (Table 4).

A process known as hormesis is hypothesized to explain the neutral or negative effects of excess antioxidant supplementation. Hormesis is a biphasic dose response to a stressor (toxic chemical, thermal, or radiological) in which a substance is beneficial at low doses but harmful at higher doses. Low doses of oxidant stressors induce endogenous antioxidant production that seems to be protective (Table 4).[21]

TABLE 4: Vegetables and fruits in diet: Current evidence

	Evidence	Conclusion
Green-leafy vegetables	In the NHS and the HPFS it was found that 3 servings/ day of green leafy vegetables, combined with a low carbohydrate diet results in a 24% reduced risk of CVD[20]	Green-leafy vegetables (three servings daily) reduce the risk of incident T2DM and CVD
Antioxidant-rich fruits and vegetables	NHS II evaluated the relationship between anthocyanin intake and the risk of myocardial infarction during an 18-year follow-up[21]	A 32% reduced risk of myocardial infarction was observed in those with the highest vs. lowest quintile of anthocyanin intake (especially blueberries and strawberries)

CVD, cardiovascular disease; HPFS, Health Professional's Follow-up Study; NHS, Nurses' Health Study; T2DM, type 2 diabetes mellitus.

PROTEIN SOURCE—INDIAN FOOD/CUISINE IS HIGH IN CARBS, STARCH, AND FAT

If we look at veg high proteins—paneer/cottage cheese, milk, nuts are expensive. Second-grade vegetarian proteins are dals/lentils, green leafy vegetables are relatively cheap. Nonvegetarian proteins are eggs, chicken, fish which again are expensive (Table 5). Common Indian can't afford to consume them every day. So, carbs—roti/bread and rice—are consumed more to fill up your stomach.

TABLE 5: Role of protein from plant sources

	Evidence	Conclusion
Protein from plant sources	Participants from the Nurses' Health Study were studied from 1980 to 2012 and the Health Professionals Follow-up Study were studied from 1986 to 2012	Plant protein intake was associated with lower cardiovascular mortality (HR: 0.88 per 3% energy increment)[22]

HR, hazard ratio.

TABLE 6: Role of nuts in diet

	Evidence	Conclusion
Nuts	The PREDIMED RCT demonstrated that a high vegetable fat Mediterranean diet supplemented with mixed nuts at 30 g/day for 5 years, reduced CVD incidence by 30% compared with a lower-fat control diet[23]	Nuts are rich source of nutrients and also heart friendly and have favorable effect on fatty acid profile

CVD, cardiovascular disease; RCT, randomized controlled trial.

Concepts like "feed your children with more rotis only then they will get healthy" make our diet highly imbalanced.

Nuts—Do They Still have Bad Rap in Nutrition Circle?

While it is true that nuts are relatively energy dense, meaning that they contain a relatively high number of calories per unit weight. But they are actually an important part of a healthy diet. This paradox is because of satiating effect of nuts combined with incomplete digestion and reduction in metabolizable energy (Table 6).

Juices—Are They Really Elixir of Health in Present World?

Juicing of fruits and vegetables has gained popularity in modern world due to its ease and convenience. However, the process of juicing concentrates calories, which makes it much easier to ingest excessive energy. Though, phytochemical nutrients, such as lycopene, exhibit greater bioavailability in a liquid form versus the whole food, the clinical benefit of the same has not been proven yet. Hence, until more evidence come juicing primarily reserved for situations when daily intake of vegetables and fruits is inadequate.[24]

Gluten-free Diet—Are They Really Beneficial in Providing Weight Loss?

Gluten-free diet comprises of rich amount of fruits and vegetables, legumes and dried beans, lean protein sources, nuts and seeds, low-fat dairy or nondairy alternatives of calcium and vitamin D, and healthy fats, including ω-3-fatty acids. There is no evidence that avoidance of gluten in diet by normal population will result in weight loss. There is limited information about CV outcomes benefit of this dietary pattern.[25]

Dairy Products—Are They Enough to Meet Vitamin B12 Requirement?

Milk is an essential food item in Indian diet. The RDA of milk for Indian vegetarians is 300 g/day as compared to 200 g/day for nonvegetarians. In addition to milk, 80 g of meat, eggs or fish will provide rest of necessary vitamin B12. Although this recommended level of milk in lacto-vegetarians intake will provide adequate quantities of protein (0.4 g), calcium (360 mg), vitamin A, many B vitamins, and minerals, but it will be deficient in vitamin B12 (0.45 μg as against the RDA of 1.0 μg).

Cow's milk is a good source of vitamin B12, with 100 g of the milk containing 0.5–1.0 μg of vitamin B12. One glass of cow's milk (250 g) provides 2.5 μg of vitamin B12, adequate to meet the RDA for an adult man. But, it has been shown that the dilution with water, storage or boiling (all of which are common household practices) may reduce vitamin B12 to 2.1 μg (21% decrease).[26]

SUSCEPTIBILITY OF INDIANS

Small Body Frames

Salt and sugar are easily absorbed and get distributed in the total body water. Therefore, the amount consumed per drink/meal, per day needs to be matched with the body water content. The usual content of sugar in Indian diet in often high, which necessities an intense insulin response to maintain euglycemia. Such diet which is high in sugar, when consumed by children may not have any immediate clinical manifestations, but led to early onset of dysglycemia in adult life.[27]

Postprandial Metabolic Issues

Postprandial lipid abnormalities and oxidant stress are preventable components of dietary modification. Insulin response of food depends upon route, i.e., enteral versus par enteral and race. Indians have more intense plasma insulin levels in response to an oral glucose load compared to Europeans.[28]

Sarcopenic Adiposity

Sarcopenic adiposity refers to the situation of less muscle mass and more adipose tissue for the same body mass index, which is a risk factor for the premature onset of cardiovascular risk factors. Smaller body volume of Indians necessitates a hyper insulinemic response which is further intensified by the insulin resistance caused by sarcopenic adiposity. This vicious cycle of intense hyperinsulinemia is a reason for the early onset of all the risk factors at a low body mass index in Indians noted in various studies (Flowchart 1).[29]

PREVENTIVE MEASURES TO REDUCE THIS EPIDEMIC

- Try to reduce intake of fried fast-food and processed foods
- Try to include variety of oils (extra virgin olive oil, canola, peanut, unrefined mustard oil) and foods containing natural fats (nuts, seeds, avocado, olives, soy, fish) in your diet. And use oil rich in SFA as ghee for deep frying which is common in India
- Emphasize on low-fat or nonfat dairy products
- Increase the amount and variety of plant foods consumed—eat more unrefined vegetables, fruits, and

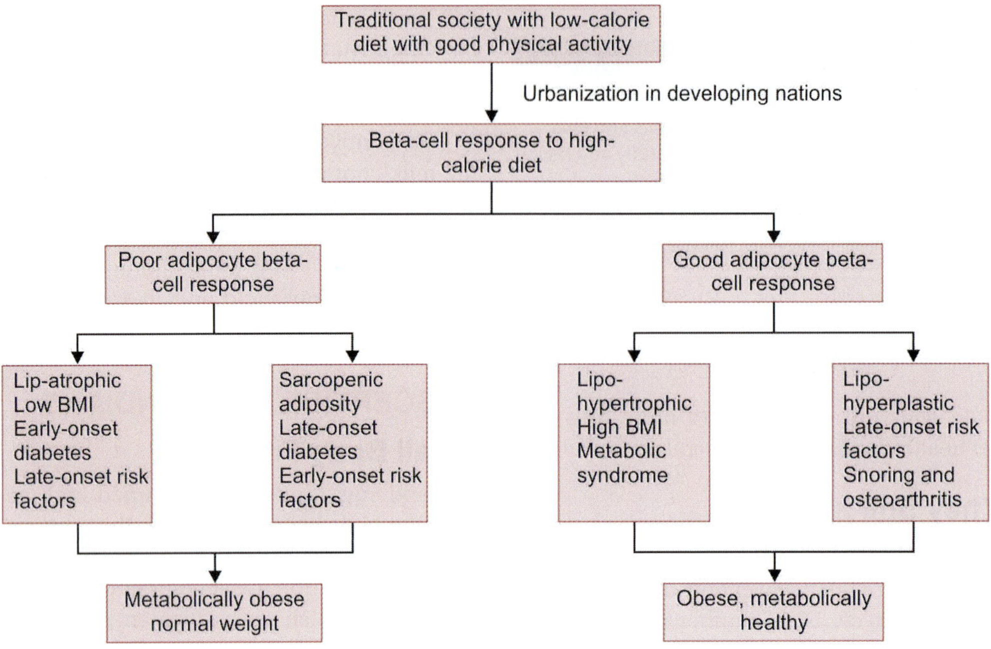

BMI, body mass index.

FLOWCHART 1: The spectrum of body response to diet and physical activity.

wholegrain cereals. Reduce intake of refined sources of carbohydrates with higher glycemic indices

- Increase consumption of legumes (like baked beans, soybeans, lentils and tofu) in your diet
- Have a handful of a variety of raw, unsalted nuts on most days of the week, especially walnuts and almonds
- Eat oily fish at least once per week
- Check consumption of alcohol less than two drinks per day
- Avoid visible fat in your meal
- Avoid added salt in your food
- The increased consumption of high-salt, high-SFA, high-energy processed foods promoted by large industries led to detrimental effect on cardiovascular health. There is a need to address these concerns and find sustainable solutions
- The production of oils for mass consumption, with respect to SFA, MUFA and PUFA content as well as preferential pricing of low-SFA oils are areas of policy which need early attention and action.

CONCLUSION

Choose your food wisely and stay healthy

Things to be included:

- MUFA-rich oil like mustard oil and olive oil
- Daily serving of nuts
- Green leafy vegetables and fruits
- Plant-based proteins
- Blueberries and strawberries
- Southern diets (added fats and oils, fried foods, eggs, organ and processed meats, sugar-sweetened drinks).

Things to be avoided:

- Coconut oil and palm oil rich in SFA
- Juicing should be avoided
- Animal based protein should be restricted
- Antioxidant supplement have no clear benefit
- Gluten free diet as a diet to reduce weight.

REFERENCES

1. Gupta R, Gupta KD. Coronary heart disease in low socioeconomic status subjects in India: an evolving epidemic. Indian Heart J. 2009;61:358e67.
2. Institute of Health Metrics and Evaluation. GBD Profile: India. http:/ www.healthdata.org/sites/default/files/country_profiles/GBD/country_report_india.pdf [Accessed August 2018].
3. Yusuf S, Hawken S, Ôunpu S, et al. Effect of potentially modifiable risk factors associated with myocardial infarction in 52 countries (the INTERHEART study): case-control study. Lancet. 2004;364:937.
4. Dorairaj P, Panniyammakal J, Ambuj R. Cardiovascular diseases in India current epidemiology and future directions. Circulation. 2016;133:1605-20.
5. Vecchio MG, Paramesh EC, Paramesh H, et al. Types of food and nutrient intake in India: a literature review. Indian J Pediatr. 2014;81(1):17-22.
6. Gupta R, Mishra A, Pais P, et al. Correlation of regional cardiovascular disease mortality in India with lifestyle and nutritional factors. Int J Cardiol. 2006;108:291-300.
7. Shikany JM, Safford MM, Newby PK, et al. Southern dietary pattern is associated with hazard of acute coronary heart disease in the reasons for geographic and racial differences in stroke (REGARDS) study. Circulation. 2015;132:804-14.
8. Hopkins PN. Effects of dietary cholesterol on serum cholesterol: a meta-analysis and review. Am J Clin Nutr. 1992;55:1060-70.
9. Dawber TR, Nickerson RJ, Brand FN, et al. Eggs, serum cholesterol and coronary heart disease. Am J Clin Nutr. 1982;36:617-25.
10. Lin L, Allemekinders H, Dansby A, et al. Evidence of health benefits of canola oil. Nutr Rev. 2013;71:370-85.
11. Eyres L, Eyres MF, Chisholm A, et al. Coconut oil consumption and cardiovascular risk factors in humans. Nutr Rev. 2016;74:267-80.
12. Bester D, Esterhuyse AJ, Truter EJ, et al. Cardiovascular effects of edible oils: a comparison between four popular edible oils. Nutr Res Rev. 2010;23:334-48.

13. Chen BK, Seligman B, Farquhar JW, et al. Multi-Country analysis of palm oil consumption and cardiovascular disease mortality for countries at different stages of economic development: 1980–1997. Global Health. 2011;7:45.
14. Vijayakumar M, Vasudevan DM, Sundaram KR, et al. A randomized study of coconut oil versus sunflower oil on cardiovascular risk factors in patients with stable coronary heart disease. Indian Heart J. 2016;68(4):498-506.
15. Burr ML. Lessons from the story of n-3 fatty acids. Am J Clin Nutr. 2000; 7:397-8.
16. Yasuda S, Shimokawa H. Potential usefulness of fish oil in the primary prevention of acute coronary syndrome. Eur Heart J. 2010;31:15-6.
17. Adkins Y, Kelley DS. Mechanisms underlying the cardioprotective effects of omega-3 polyunsaturated fatty acids. J Nutr Biochem. 2010;21:781-92.
18. Calder PC. N-3 polyunsaturated fatty acids and inflammation: from molecular biology to the clinic. Lipids. 2003;38:343-52.
19. http://icrier.org/pdf/India_Phytonutrient_Report_Ex_summary.pdf [Accessed August 2018].
20. Joshipura KJ, Hung HC, Li TY, et al. Intakes of fruits, vegetables and carbohydrate and the risk of CVD. Public Health Nutr. 2009;12:11.
21. Cassidy A, Mukamal KJ, Liu L, et al. High anthocyanin intake is associated with a reduced risk of myocardial infarction in young and middle-aged women. Circulation 2013;188-96.
22. Song M, Fung TT, Hu FB, et al. Association of animal and plant protein intake with all-cause and cause-specific mortality. JAMA Intern Med. 2016;176:1453-63.
23. Estruch R, Ros E, Salas-Salvadó J, et al.; PREDIMED Study Investigators. Primary prevention of cardiovascular disease with a Mediterranean diet [Published correction appears in N Engl J Med. 2014;370:886.
24. Böhm V, Bitsch R. Intestinal absorption of lycopene from different matrices and interactions to other carotenoids, the lipid status, and the antioxidant capacity of human plasma. Eur J Nutr. 1999;38:118-25.
25. El-Chammas K, Danner E. Gluten-free diet in nonceliac disease. Nutr Clin Pract. 2011;26:294-9.
26. Bor MV, et al. Daily intake of 4 to 7µg dietary vitamin B-12 is associated with steady concentrations of vitamin B-12-related biomarkers in a healthy young population. Am J Clin Nutr. 2010;91:571-7.
27. Yoon KH, Lee JH, Kim JW, et al. Epidemic of obesity and type 2 diabetes in Asia. Lancet. 2006;368:1681-8.
28. Misra A, Wasir JS, Vikram NK. Carbohydrate diets, postprandial hyperlipidaemia abdominal obesity: a recipe for atherogenic disaster. Indian J Med Res. 2005;121:5-8
29. Joshi SR, Parikh RM. India - Diabetes capital of the world: Now heading towards hypertension. J Assoc Physicians India. 2007;55:323-4.

CHAPTER 8

Edible Oils: What is Right and What is Wrong?

Sonia Arora, Vitull K Gupta, Meghna Gupta

INTRODUCTION

During the past decades, the world, particularly the developing countries like India have witnessed rapid changes in diets and lifestyles. General improvement in the standard of living has been accompanied by unhealthy dietary patterns and insufficient physical activity resulting in increased prevalence of lifestyle and diet-related chronic diseases worldwide. WHO states that by 2020 the place of the largest causes of death and disability will be occupied by cardiovascular diseases (CVDs) and prevalence of obesity, type 2 diabetes mellitus (T2DM) and hypertension (HTN) which are considered to be chronic diseases related to the diet and lifestyle is also increasing.

Diet includes foods and nutrients which provide energy and are essential for normal metabolism, physiologic and biochemical processes, growth and physical well-being. Diet essentially comprises of macronutrients like proteins, carbohydrates, fats, and micronutrients like vitamins and minerals which are required in small quantities. Triglycerides (TGs) are components of fat comprising of esters of alcohol glycerol and fatty acid (FA) chains. Generally, the words "lipids", "oils", and "fats" are used interchangeably. Fats that are liquid at room temperature are called "oils" and generally have unsaturated or short FA chains. Word "fats" broadly means solid fats at room temperature and word "lipids" include all oils and fats in general. Fat supplies more than double the calories as compared to carbohydrate or protein making it an important dietary component with concentrated source of energy. Fat intake gives taste to diet, is metabolically important constituent of the body, helps absorption of fat soluble vitamins A, D, E, and subcutaneous fat helps insulates the body.

COMPOSITION OF FATS[1]

Fats or lipids consist of FAs which are of two types as discussed here.

Saturated Fatty Acids

Saturated fatty acids (SFAs) are saturated with hydrogen atoms as carbon atoms have no double bonds in the fatty acid chain comprising of lauric acid, palmitic acid, and stearic acid which provide stability to saturated fats (SFs) and are usually solid at room temperature because single bonds between the carbon atoms are more stable than double bonds. Fat intake increases total cholesterol (TC) and low-density lipoprotein (LDL) cholesterol which is an important risk factor for cardiovascular diseases (CVDs), certain cancer and also impairs insulin sensitivity. SFAs are present in milk products (cream, ghee, butter, khoya, and paneer), animal tallow, palm oil, coconut products, and oil, etc. Results of ecological studies investigating the relation of coronary heart disease (CHD) to dietary intake of SFs suggested that development of CHD was related to higher intake of total fat content and SFs. In a study, it was seen that percentage of calories intake comprising of SFs was correlated strongly with coronary death rates in several defined populations in seven countries.[2]

Moreover correlation between the CHD incidences was weaker when compared to percentage of calories from total fat. Analysis of follow-up data from Nurses' Health Study showed that a 5% of calories from SF were associated with 17% more risk of CHD as compared to ingestion of equivalent percentage of calories from carbohydrates. Dietary intake of short- and medium-chain SFAs was shown to have insignificant CHD risk where as small CHD risk was observed with intakes of longer-chain SFAs.[3] Different SFAs have different effects on plasma lipid and lipoprotein levels that increase total plasma cholesterol and LDL cholesterol levels were observed with SFAs containing 12–16 carbon atoms.[4]

Unsaturated Fatty Acids

Unsaturated fatty acids (USFAs) comprise of monounsaturated fatty acids (MUFA) and polyunsaturated fatty acids (PUFA). MUFA contain one double bonds and PUFA contain more than one double bonds within the fatty acid chain.

Monounsaturated Fatty Acids

Lipid peroxidation occurs to a lesser degree in MUFA as compared to PUFA as MUFA contain one double bond only, e.g., oleic acid, erucic acid. Studies have shown decrease in total mortality and CHD deaths with increased intake of MUFA.[5] It is suggested that MUFAs are useful because it helps decrease free cholesterol by promoting cholesterol esterification in liver, promote receptor-mediated LDL uptake, lower LDL, and increase high-density lipoprotein (HDL). Recent evidence stresses on exploring the role of SFA, PUFA, and MUFA ratio in diet and intake of individual fat components as they influence LDL/HDL ratio and lipoprotein metabolism. Dietary sources of MUFA include almonds, peanuts, fruits like olives and avocados, olive oil, rice bran oil (RBO), groundnut oil, canola oil, and mustard oil.

Polyunsaturated Fatty Acids

Polyunsaturated fatty acids have a carbon–carbon double bond in a final N-6 position and are prone to lipid peroxidation because it has greater number of double bonds. Examples are linoleic acid, linolenic acid, arachidonic acid, eicosapentaenoic acid (EPA), and docosahexaenoic acid (DHA). Dietary sources include invisible fats present in pulses and cereals, sunflower oil has 50% PUFAs, corn oil 60%, cottonseed 50%, and safflower oil contain 70% PUFAs.

Results of another study suggested a substantial reduction in CHD risk when trans fat (TF) were replaced by polyunsaturated fat in the diet or other foods high in trans fatty acids (TFAs).[6]

Omega-3 and Omega-6 Fatty Acids

Omega-3 [α-linolenic acid (ALA), N-3] and omega-6 (linoleic acid) fatty acids are unsaturated "essential fatty acids" (EFAs) because human metabolism cannot create them.

Omega-6 Fatty Acids (Linoleic Acid, N-6)

At N-6 position there is double bond between carbon–carbon atoms and more number of double bonds make omega-6 fatty acids more prone to lipid per oxidation. Omega-6 fatty acids (N-6) are also important for health. PUFA intake decreases LDL and increases insulin sensitivity. A study concluded that a significantly lower incidence of type 2 diabetes mellitus (T2DM) was associated with higher intake of N-6 and substantial reduction of CHD risk was observed when long chain SFs was replaced by polyunsaturated fat.[7] But the beneficial effect of N-3 is reduced by intake of more quantity of N-6. Dietary sources include invisible fat in cereals and pulses, margarine, safflower oil corn oil, sunflower oil, kardi oil, etc.

Omega-3 Fatty Acids(Alpha-Linolenic Acid, N-3)

N-3 consists of double bond at N-3 carbon atom and is precursors to anti-inflammatory products in the body. Dietary sources include legumes, green leafy vegetables, citrus fruits, nuts, and fish, especially fatty fish. Mustard oil has 6–11% of N-3, canola/rapeseed 7%, hemp oil 20%, flax (linseed) oil has 55%, the richest plant-based source. Hemp and flax oils are not commonly used as table or cooking oil. Most of the N-3 available from plant sources is in form of ALA. Decrease platelet aggregation and formation of proaggregatory thromboxane A_2 was observed when dietary consumption of ALA was increased.[8] Several epidemiologic studies showed that increase in linolenic acid intake was associated with a decreased risk of CHD mortality[9,10] but in these studies other dietary factors like dietary vitamins, other fats, vegetables, and folate were not adequately adjusted. Based on strong data to support favorable effect of N-3 on prevention of CVD, it was suggested that diet rich in N-3 can be beneficial.[11] Evidence suggested that the protective effects of fish oil based N-3 may involve multiple mechanisms, like decreasing TG levels, reducing platelet aggregation, antiarrhythmic effects, improving endothelial dysfunction so decreasing atherosclerosis as well as improving endothelial-dependent vasomotor function.[12]

Omega 6 (N-6) to Omega 3 (N-3) Ratio

Balanced ratio of N-6 and N-3 is important for efficient body functions. N-6 and N-3 are converted into biological active components by competing for the common enzymes so when one component is consumed more than the other, it leads to imbalance in the metabolism of N-6 and N-3 gradually affecting several metabolic processes. Recommendations suggest that level of adequate intake of N-6 and N-3 depends on several factors like age, gender, and life style, etc. and several organizations have recommended different ratios like N-6:N-3 of 4:1 (Institute of Medicine) 5:4 (World Health Organization) and several suggest that ratio near 1:1 may be considered as optimal ratio.[13] Several foods are good sources of both N-6 and N-3 and ratio may be different like N-6:N-3 ratio is 4:1 in walnuts, 1689:1 in almonds. In green leafy vegetables the ratio is less than 1, so to improve the ratio several food combinations are suggested to get the ratio of at least 10 to 1. The best N-6:N-3 ratio was found in mustard oil (1.2:1) and canola oil (2.2:1) and adverse ratio was found in olive oil (12.84), corn oil (46.01), and peanut butter (225.63).

TRANS FATTY ACIDS OR PARTIALLY HYDROGENATED FATTY ACIDS

Incomplete hydrogenation of vegetable oils results in formation of TFs and complete hydrogenation results in formation of SFs. TFs may confer texture to food and structural stability. Lamb and beef contain small quantity of natural TFAs. A review suggested that even low consumption of 1–3% of total calorie intake of TFs leads to increased risk of coronary artery disease (CAD) and TFs are more dangerous to CV health than any other macronutrient even on a per-calorie basis.[14] Increased intake of TFs can increase the risk of CVD because it can lead to increase in LDL, TGs, lipoprotein (a) and decrease in HDL adversely affecting metabolism of EFA and prostaglandins promoting thrombogenesis and insulin resistance.[12] In a land mark study, it was found that the risk of CAD nearly doubled with 2% increase in intake of TF calories and to produce similar risk of CAD about 15%

increase in SF calories were required. It was found that risk of CHD decreased by more than half (53%) by replacing 2% of food energy from TFAs with nontrans unsaturated fats.[3] Sources of TFs include dalda and vanaspati ghee, margarines, baked foods, readymade mithais and processed foods, and ready to eat snacks.

CHOLESTEROL

Cholesterol, an essential component of animal life, is found in animal fats including dairy products and nonvegetarian foods. Chemically cholesterol is a waxy sterol of fat. Very small amount of cholesterol is present in plants so generally plant oils are devoid of cholesterol. It is thought that absorption of cholesterol from intestine is decreased by phytosterols, a plant product because both phytosterols and cholesterol compete with each other for absorption in intestine. It is recommended to restrict the cholesterol consumption to less than 200 mg by decreasing animal fat consumption. Adverse effects of increased consumption of cholesterol are because it increases TC and LDL[15] but the adverse effects are relatively less as compared to increased consumption of SFAs and TFAs[16] and different individuals responded very differently to the effects of dietary fats.[17] Cholesterol broadly is of two types, LDL and HDL. LDL is considered as "bad cholesterol" responsible for atherosclerosis and CAD where as HDL is "good cholesterol" help prevent and retard progression of atherosclerosis.

Ghani

Ghani is a traditional method of oil processing in India in which oilseeds and subsequently the expressed oil are held in a scooped circular pit in the exact centre of a circular mortar made of stone or wood with a stout, upright pestle descending from a top curved or angled piece, permitting the pestle to rotate as the animal moves in a circular ambit, exerting lateral pressure on the upper chest of the pit, first pulverizing the oilseed and then crushing out its oil. There are regional variations in ghani design in India like large granite ghanis of Southern India (capacity 35–40 kg), wooden ghani of Western India (capacity 8–15 kg), Bengal ghani (capacity 5–10 kg), and Punjab ghanis (small capacity with a short pestle). Sesame, rapeseed, mustard, coconut, groundnut, and safflower oils were produced from mild ghani crushing and oils produced are known as "Kachi Ghani ka Tel".

Cold Pressed Oils

Cold pressed oils are called when ancient methods of hydraulic press is used to produce oils and oils such produced are in natural state retaining natural odor, taste, color, flavor, and nutrition. This process avoids exposing the oil to chemical solvents or high temperatures during extraction.

Refined Oils

Refined oil are produced using mechanical and chemical extraction methods from seeds and vegetable products and these methods affect taste, destroy antioxidants, generate free radicals and are more susceptible to turn rancid but refined oils are relatively pure.

Unrefined Oils

Oils which are extracted from seeds or other vegetable material by exerting continuous pressure at high temperature of 200–250 °C are called unrefined oils and these are different from "cold pressed" oils called "expeller pressed" oils. Unrefined oils retain antioxidants, other nutrients, and flavor; so these oils are considered better and recommended for use.

Rancidity

Rancidity is the term used for development of unpleasant odor or flavor in fats and oils. Rancidity is classified according to the method of its production like hydrolytic, oxidative, and ketonic.

Smoke Point or Flash Point

Smoke point is the temperature at which decomposition and nutritional degradation of fats or oils occur resulting in formation of glycerol, free fatty acids (FFA), and bluish smoke giving an unpleasant and disagreeable flavor to the food. So, it is an important factor while selecting the oils required for heating that is use oils with higher smoke point for deep frying. Different oils have different smoke points depending on the origin and refinement of oils.

Flash point is the temperature much higher than the smoke point at which the vapors from oil can ignite when mixed with air. Dietary fat studies showed that when heated PUFA containing oils like soya, canola, sunflower, and corn oil degrade easily to toxic compounds.

WHAT ARE EDIBLE OILS?

Fatty acids triesters with glycerol which are in liquid form at room temperature are the class of lipids known as oils and are generally found in both plants and animals. TGs that are solid or semisolid at room temperature are classified as fats and occur predominantly in animals. Any material which has an oily or greasy feel and cannot be mixed with water is called "oil". Edible oils include oils used for cooking which involves heat as well as used in food preparation and flavoring not involving heat, such as salad dressings and bread dips.

WHAT IS RIGHT AND WHAT IS WRONG OIL?

Out of numerous available oils, which oil is the right oil or the wrong oil to use depends on the purpose of their use like cooking, deep frying, shelf-life of oil or other specific qualities or flavor determine the preference for use of that oil. More important is the health benefits which depend on fat composition of various oils, ratio between SFA, MUFA, and PUFA.

CHARACTERISTICS OF DIFFERENT OILS[18]

Mustard Oil

It is economical, vegetarian oil with characteristic pungent aroma and hot nutty taste, popularly used in East and North India containing 70% MUFA (42% erucic and 12% oleic acid), 22% PUFA (10% N-3 and 12% N-6), and 8% SFAs. Evidence suggests that mustard oil, which was previously thought to be harmful because of high erucic acid content, is now considered as one of the best as it has near ideal N-6:N-3 ratio of 6:5 and contains low SFAs and high MUFAs and PUFAs along with high amount of antioxidants. "Kachi Ghani" or cold-pressed mustard oil retains the natural properties and nutritional values of mustard. Studies indicate a dose-dependent benefit of intake of vegetables or use of mustard oil on ischemic heart disease (IHD) risk. The risk was lower with the use of mustard oil for frying as compared to the use of sunflower oil and risk decreased by about 70% when cooking medium was mustard oil.[19,20]

Rapeseed Oil (Canola Oil)

It is produced from plant belonging to *Brassica* family which is related to mustard plant and is known as "canola oil" after the term "Canadian oil". It has high MUFA and low SFA (<7%) contents with favorable N-3 levels and considered health oil by various associations and organizations.[21]

Olive Oil

As the name indicates olive oil is extracted from olives and considered to be the best oil as it has 75% MUFA and numerous useful antioxidants (hydroxytyrosol). High levels of MUFA and antioxidants (oleuropein or tyrosol) are present in extra virgin or virgin olive oil which is produced by minimum processing and intake of MUFA is known to decrease LDL and increase HDL, exerts anti-inflammatory, antithrombotic, antihypertensive and vasodilatory effect which may decrease CAD risk.[13,22] Epidemiological evidence suggests that antioxidants (oleuropein or tyrosol) have beneficial effect against some cancers, increases arterial elasticity, and decreases risk of stroke and IHD.[23] Big disadvantage is its unfavorable N-6:N-3 ratio.

Soyabean Oil

This oil is one of the most commonly used cooking oils which is rich in USFAs (51% linoleic acid, 23% oleic acid, and 7–10% α-linolenic acid) and 10% palmitic acid and 4% stearic acid (SFAs). Soyabean oil should be used fresh because it tends to turn rancid earlier. It is suggested that to achieve the combination of high PUFA and MUFA contents by combining the oils rich in MUFA or PUFA like olive oil, mustard oil or groundnut oil to achieve optimum health benefits.

Rice Bran Oil

It is produced from rice husk and germ and contain 47% MUFA, 33% PUFA, and 20% SFA making it oil with most favorable constituents rich in phytosterols, γ-oryzanol, and vitamin E. Vitamin E and γ-oryzanol are powerful antioxidant and help in prevention of IHD.[24] Phytosterols helps to decrease absorption of cholesterol absorption imparting health benefits. Its mild flavor and high smoke point (254°C) makes it useful for deep frying. Only disadvantage is unfavorable N-6:N-3 ratio of 23:1.

Sunflower Oil

It is a good cooking medium with clean taste and has high PUFA, low SAFs and low TFs with high contents of waxes, carotenoids, lecithin, and tocopherols. Sunflower oil has high levels of N-6 and unfavorable N-6:N-3 ratio of 120:1. More over evidence of health benefits of high N-6 intake is limited.

Cottonseed Oil

It is economical, stable for frying, has long shelf-life because of natural rancid-free property and contains 18% MUFA, 52% PUFA with naturally occurring SFAs (myristic, palmitic, stearic acids) thereby called as "naturally hydrogenated" oil. Its very high SFA and very low MUFA contents make its health benefits controversial.[25] Moreover because of excessive use of agrichemicals, cottonseeds and so cottonseed oil tends to contain high levels of pesticides, which may cause adverse health effects. It is commonly used in various types of processed and snack foods.

Corn Oil

Germ of corn is used to extract corn oil (Maize oil) which contains 55% PUFA, 30% MUFA, and 15% SFA. It is cheap and because of high smoke point useful for frying purposes. Its increased level of N-6 as compared to N-3 may cause or predispose to some disease and depression.

Groundnut Oil

Groundnut oil has a pleasant taste, high smoke point and contains 56% MUFA (oleic acid), 26% PUFA (linoleic acid), and 8% SFA (palmitic acid) which makes it cardiac friendly oils because it rich in MUFA and a balanced oil.

Safflower Oil

Safflower oil has high smoke point favorable for frying and contains low SFAs (6%), low MUFA (13%), and high PUFA (76%). It is not considered healthy oil because its consumption may decrease TC, LDL as well as HDL cholesterol. Other disadvantage is that PUFA may turn rancid or toxic on exposure to high temperatures.

Palm Oil

Fruits of palm are used to extract palm oil which is economical and has high smoke point making it favorable for frying.

Cardiac benefits of palm oil are controversial as it contains 48% SFAs and unfavorable N-6:N-3 ratio of 20:1. Palm oil was shown to be unsafe substitute for TF in the food industry as it can lead to adverse changes in LDL cholesterol and apolipoprotein B levels like changes done by TAs.[26] Red palm variety of palm oil is rich in carotenes like coenzyme Q10, glycolipids tocotrienols, tocopherols, and phytosterols.

Coconut Oil

Coconut oil is a plant fat extracted from coconut fruit and contains high levels of SFAs (90%) very little PUFA, MUFA, no cholesterol, vitamin E, vitamin K, and minerals such as iron. Coconut oil is primary oil used by tropical people and its SFAs consist of lauric acid which differs from SFAs of animal origin. SFAs in coconut oil mostly consist of the medium chain TGs and may not impart same risks as other SFAs.[26] Lauric acid is responsible for increasing HDL levels and thereby increases TC.

Sesame Oil ("Til ka Tel")

Sesame oil is a vegetable oil extracted from the seeds of sesame plant, one of the oldest plants used for the extraction of oil. In developing countries like India, less expensive and manual methods like hot water flotation, bridge presses, ram presses, the ghani process or small-scale expeller are used to extract oils whereas in advanced countries expeller press, larger-scale oil extraction machines, or by pressing followed by chemical solvent extraction are used. Cold pressing is popular method because it avoids chemical solvents or high temperature exposure during oil extraction and traditional methods like ghani help retain the pleasant taste, nutrients, and flavor. It is used as edible oil and for various other health benefits like skin care, hair care, anti-aging characteristics, alternative medicine, traditional massages, etc. Sesame oil is composed of almost equal amount of MUFAs (39% oleic acid) and PUFAs (41% linoleic acid) with remaining amount composed of SF (8% palmitic acid and 5% stearic acid). It is rich in vitamin K. It has high smoke points and it is least prone to turn rancid due to presence of natural antioxidants, such as sesamol. Sesame oil is most popular in states of Karnataka, Andhra Pradesh, and Tamil Nadu.

Linseed or Flaxseed Oil (Alsi ka Tel)

Linseed oil is an edible oil which is colorless to yellowish obtained by pressing or sometimes followed by solvent extraction from the dried, ripened seeds of the flax plant (*Linum usitatissimum*). Raw cold-pressed linseed oil is easily oxidized and rapidly becomes rancid generating an unpleasant odor, unless refrigerated, has a short shelf-life of only a few weeks making it less desirable for use as cooking oil. It is composed of 9–10% of SFAs (6% palmitic and 4% stearic), about 20% MUFAs (mainly 20% oleic acid), and more than 70% PUFAs (70% α-linolenic fatty acid). Several studies suggested that primary benefit of flaxseed oil is because of ALA and it exerts dose-dependent effects on inflammatory mediators and markers.[27]

Numerous studies analyzing epidemiological investigations and experimental data have shown the ability of increased omega-3 fatty acid intake to help regulate and reduce blood pressure in hypertension and diet low in SFs and rich in monounsaturated and polyunsaturated fats from flaxseed has been demonstrated to combat CVD.[28] Healthy properties are related to anti-inflammatory, antioxidant, anticarcinogenic activities and to the lowering of cholesterol, the decrease of CVD and the prevention of diabetes. Linseed oil is a drying oil that is, it can polymerize into a solid form, due to which it is used with combinations of other oils, resins or solvents as an impregnator, drying oil finish or varnish in wood finishing, as a pigment binder in oil paints, as a plasticizer and hardener in putty and in the manufacture of linoleum.

Butter

Butter is from animal source with high contents of cholesterol and SFAs. Butter can increase total, LDL and HDL cholesterol and its low smoke point makes is unfavorable for deep frying.

Ghee

Ghee is made by clarifying butter which has high smoke point making it favorable for frying.

Vanaspati Ghee

Vanaspati ghee is made by hydrogenation of refined vegetable oil. Hydrogenation increases TFAs, makes it less likely to turn rancid, more stable, increases shelf-life, but it does not contain bioactive compounds, natural vitamins or antioxidants and because of low smoke point it is not favored for deep frying. It is considered to be responsible for development of IHD because of its adverse lipid profile.

CHOOSING THE RIGHT OIL

Properties of cooking oil like fatty acid contents, micronutrients, shelf-life, smoke point, etc. are helpful in selection of right cooking oil. Among the available cooking oils, none of it fulfills the recommended profile because if oil has high MUFA which is desirable, it may not have desired N-6:N-3 ratio or appropriate ratio of MUFA, PUFA, or SFAs. So, it is recommended to rotate or blend the oils like mustard oil, groundnut oil, canola oil, RBO, etc. to achieve the desired lipid contents.

WHY ROTATION OR BLENDING IS NEEDED?

Evidence suggests that CV health is greatly influenced by dietary fat profile and type of fat affects the lipid profile of the individual increasing or decreasing the CVD risk. TC and LDL cholesterol are increased with increased intake of SFs. Intake of PUFA greatly reduces the CVD risk as compared to MUFA.[2] Intake of TFAs formed during partial hydrogenation of fat, increase LDL cholesterol, and decrease HDL cholesterol.[29] CVD protection is imparted by both N-6 and N-3. N-6 predominantly lowers LDL cholesterol and N-3 lowers TGs. N-3 is cardioprotective through various mechanisms like vasodilation, antiarrhythmic effect, anti-inflammatory effects, improves endothelial function, decreased platelet aggregation and reduces collagen deposition.[30] That is why it is important to have optimum composition of these fats to achieve health and cardioprotective effects. Numerous health and dietary bodies have issued guidelines suggesting various recommendations regarding fatty acid intake. Guidelines for prevention of CVD have suggested 8–10% SFAs of total calories, 5–8% PUFAs, and rest of the total calories are constituted by MUFA with ratio of PUFA:SFA to be about 0.8:1 and for PUFA comprising of both omega-6 and omega-3 in ratio 5:10.[4] Favorable ratio of SFA:MUFA:PUFA comes out to be 1:1.5:1 if maximum amount of total fat intake is taken into consideration.[31] American Heart Association (AHA) cardioprotective recommendations include intake of less than7% of saturated fat, less than 1% TF of total calorie consumption and less than 300 mg cholesterol per day. AHA suggests an important role of oils and fats in total dietary fat intake.[32] Evidence suggests that different lipid components have different favorable and adverse health effects. Even blending two cooking oils cannot fulfill the recommended ratio of different lipid components for favorable health and CVD effects, necessitating the need to blend more than two cooking oils to achieve desired lipid contents for health benefits.

CONCLUSION

In this present era of consumerism, people are exposed to different type of edible oils glorified with tall health claims and benefits, advertizing various cooking oils with attractive slogans, highlighting presence or absence of different lipid contents to influence people's choice of cooking oils. This chapter discusses various lipid contents, their harms and health benefits, desired composition of different lipid contents and composition of different edible or cooking oils in an attempt to demystifying the fancy statements for all the people. Out of the discussed edible oils, none of the oils fulfill the recommended criteria of lipid contents but two oils rapeseed and mustard oil which have high PUFA and MUFA, low SFA content and highest N-3:N-6 ratio seems to be imparting most health and CVD benefits. Evidence suggests use of ghee and butter as a cooking oil should be limited and use of reheated fats and oils should be avoided. Since none of the available cooking oils fulfill the criteria of various lipid contents, it is desirable to blend or rotate different cooking oils like mustard oil, groundnut oil, canola oil, and RBO with favorable lipid contents and limit the use of visible fat content for achieving desired favorable CV and overall health benefits.

REFERENCES

1. Bockisch M. Fats and Oils Handbook. Champaign, IL: AOCS Press. 1998; pp. 95-6.
2. Keys AB. Seven countries: a multivariate analysis of death and coronary heart disease. Cambridge, MA: Harvard University Press; 1980.
3. Hu FB, Stampfer MJ, Manson JE, et al. Dietary saturated fat and their food sources in relation to the risk of coronary heart disease in women. Am J Clin Nutr. 1999;70(6):1001-8.
4. Kris-Etherton PM, Yu S. Individual fatty acids on plasma lipids and lipoproteins: human studies. Am J Clin Nutr. 1997;65(5 Suppl):1628S-44S.
5. Jacobs D, Blackburn G, Higgins M, et al. Report of the conference on low blood cholesterol: mortality associations. Circulation. 1992;86(3):1046-60.
6. Hu FB, Stampfer MJ, Manson JE, et al. Dietary fat intake and risk of coronary heart disease in women. N Engl J Med. 1997;337(21):1491-9.
7. Abeywardena MY, McLennan PL, Charnock JS. Differential effects of dietary fish oil on myocardial prostaglandin I2 and thromboxane A2 production. Am J Physiol. 1991;260(2 Pt 2):H379-85.
8. Dolecek TA. Epidemiological evidence of relationships between dietary polyunsaturated fatty acids and mortality in the multiple risk factor intervention trial. Proc Soc Exp Biol Med. 1992;200(2):177-82.
9. Pietinen P, Ascherio A, Korhonen P, et al. Intake of fatty acids and risk of coronary heart disease in a cohort of Finnish men. The alpha-tocopherol, beta-carotene cancer prevention study. Am J Epidemiol. 1997;145(10):876-87.
10. Connor WE. Alpha-linolenic acid in health and disease. Am J ClinNutr. 1999; 69(5):827-8.
11. Newman WP, Middaugh JP, Propst MT, et al. Atherosclerosis in Alaska natives and non-natives. Lancet. 1993;341(8852):1056-7.
12. Joshi S, Joshi SR. Medicine Update 2013: Chapter 140. pp. 638-45.
13. Cicero AF, Gaddi A. Rice bran oil and gamma-oryzanol in the treatment of hyperlipoproteinaemias and other conditions. Phytother Res. 2001;15(4):277-86.
14. Mozaffarian D, Katan MB, Ascherio A, et al. Trans fatty acids and cardiovascular disease. N Engl J Med. 2006;354(15):1601-13.
15. Clarke R, Frost C, Collins R, et al. Dietary lipids and blood cholesterol: quantitative meta-analysis of metabolic ward studies. BMJ. 1997;314(7074):112-7.
16. Howell WH, McNamara DJ, Tosca MA, et al. Plasma lipid and lipoprotein responses to dietary fat and cholesterol: a meta-analysis. Am J Clin Nutr. 1997;65(6):1747-64.
17. Kris-Etherton P, Daniels SR, Eckel RH, et al. Summary of the scientific conference on dietary fatty acids and cardiovascular health: conference summary from the nutrition committee of the American Heart Association. Circulation. 2001;103(7):1034-9.
18. Mishra S, Manchanda SC. Cooking oils for heart health. J Prevent Cardiol. 2012;1(3):122-31.
19. Brown J, Thill DC, Brown AP, et al. Gene transfer between canola (Brassica napus L.) and related weed species. Ann Appl Biol. 1996;129(3):513-22.
20. De Lorgeril M, Salen P. The Mediterranean-style diet for the prevention of cardiovascular diseases. Public Health Nutr. 2006;9(1A):118-23.
21. Bester D, Esterhuyse Truster EJ, van Rooyen J. Cardiovascular effects of edible oils: a comparison between four popular edible oils. Nutr Res Rev. 2010;23:334-48.
22. Turner R, Etienne N, Alonso MG, et al. Antioxidant and anti-atherogenic activities of olive oil phenolics. Int J Vitam Nutr Res. 2005;75(1):61-70.
23. Sonestedt E, Ericson U, Gullberg B, et al. Do both heterocyclic amines and omega -6 polyunsaturated fatty acids contribute to incidence of breast cancer in post-menopausal women of Malmo diet and cancer cohort? Int J Cancer. 2008;123(7):1637-43.
24. Berquin IM, Min Y, Wu R, et al. Modulation of prostate cancer genetic risk by omega-3 and omega-6 fatty acids. J Clin Invest. 2007;117(7):1866-75.
25. Tarrago-Trani MT, Phillips KM, Lemar LE, et al. New and existing oils and fats used in products with reduced trans-fatty acid content. J Am Diet Assoc. 2006;106(6):867-80.
26. Marina AM, Che Man YB, Amin I. Virgin coconut oil: emerging functional food oil. Trends Food Sci Technol. 2009;20(10): 481-7.

27. Shim YY, BoGui PG, Arnison YW, et al. Flaxseed (Linum usitatissimum L.) bioactive compounds and peptide nomenclature: A review. Trends Food Sci Technol. 2014:38(1);5-20.
28. Rodriguez-Leyva D, Dupasquier CM, McCullough R, et al. The cardiovascular effects of flaxseed and its omega-3 fatty acid, alpha-linolenic acid. Can J Cardiol. 2010;26:489-96.
29. Temme EH, Mensink RP, Hornstra G. Comparison of the effects of diets enriched in lauric, palmitic, or oleic acids on serum lipids and lipoproteins in healthy women and men. Am J Clin Nutr. 1996;63(6):897-903.
30. Ascherio A, Rimm EB, Giovannucci EL, et al. Dietary fat and risk of coronary heart disease in men: cohort follow-up study in the United States. BMJ. 1996;313(7049):84-90.
31. Judd JT, Clevidence BA, Muesing RA, et al. Dietary trans fatty acids: effects of plasma lipids and lipoproteins of healthy men and women. Am J Clin Nutr. 1994;59(4):861-8.
32. Lichtenstein AH, Ausman LM, Carrasco W, et al. Hydrogenation impairs the hypolipidemic effect of corn oil in humans. Aterioscler Thromb. 1993;13(2): 154-61.

CHAPTER 9

Statins and Diabetes

Rajeev Bagarhatta, Sohan K Sharma, Dinesh Gautam

INTRODUCTION

In diabetes, clinical atherosclerotic cardiovascular diseases (ASCVD) like coronary artery disease (CAD), stroke, and peripheral artery disease is common due to increased tendency of generalized atherosclerotic macrovascular disease process.[1] ASCVD is the leading cause of morbidity and most common cause of mortality in diabetes and accounts for nearly 52% of deaths in type 2 diabetes (T2D) and 44% in type 1 diabetes (T1D).[2]

Although diabetes itself is risk factor for CVDs, other coexisting conditions like smoking, hypertension, dyslipidemia, premature CAD in family members, presence of albuminuria and chronic kidney disease are also important risk factors that need to be systematically addressed annually in all patients of diabetes. Among above mentioned risk factors dyslipidemia is common in diabetes. It consists of low high-density lipoprotein (HDL), increased triglycerides (TGs), and postprandial lipemia. Even if lipid profile is within normal range in diabetics functionally abnormal lipids like small dense low density lipoprotein (sdLDL) and dysfunctional HDL are not uncommon.

It is well-known fact now that besides glucose control global risk factors modifications like cessation of smoking, adequate blood pressure control, and cholesterol lowering prevent or slow progression of CVDs in diabetes.[2] Since, dyslipidemia is a major contributor of this CV mortality and morbidity, its control is important target to be addressed.

PATHOPHYSIOLOGY OF DYSLIPIDEMIA IN DIABETES

The management of dyslipidemia in diabetes essentially requires the understanding of the pathophysiology of lipid derangement in diabetes.

The lipid abnormalities in T2D consists of high TGs, decreased HDL cholesterol, and presence of sdLDL cholesterol and it leads to accelerated atherosclerosis. In T1D increased TGs are common, but HDL cholesterol is normal or high if hyperglycemia or albuminuria is present. In addition to above mentioned quantitative lipid abnormalities functional dysfunction of all lipoproteins is seen in diabetes. In diabetes because of insulin deficiency or resistance abnormal function of various intermediary enzymes leads to hypertriglyceridemia, low or dysfunctional HDL, and sdLDL (Fig. 1). Insulin deficiency or resistance activates hormonal sensitive lipase in centrally distributed adipose tissues which leads to increase release of nonesterified fatty acids (NEFAs) from stored TGs. High level of NEFAs in circulation results in increased uptake by liver and in turn hepatic TG overproduction and increased secretion of apolipoprotein B100. Both TG overproduction and increased apolipoprotein B100 secretion result in increased secretion of very-low-density lipoprotein (VLDL) that are rich in TGs and further catabolism of VLDL is also impaired leading to increased VLDL concentration in circulation.[3]

Decreased activity of lipoprotein lipase located on vascular endothelial cells in insulin deficiency or resistance contributes to postprandial lipemia. Circulating LDL can participate in cholesteryl ester transfer protein (CETP)-mediated exchange of its cholesterol esters for TGs rich lipoproteins viz. chylomicrons and VLDL which generates TGs rich and cholesterol esters depleted LDL particles by lipoprotein lipase action, produces sdLDL that is more atherogenic.[4]

The process of reverse cholesterol transport from peripheral tissues is important function of HDL, but because of CETP-mediated exchange of core lipids is increased and HDL cholesterol is also TG rich. It further converts into small, dysfunctional HDL particles due to increased hepatic lipase activity in diabetes and it is no more protective.

MANAGEMENT OF DYSLIPIDEMIA IN DIABETES

In lipid management of diabetes, an important tool of treatment includes lifestyle intervention and drug

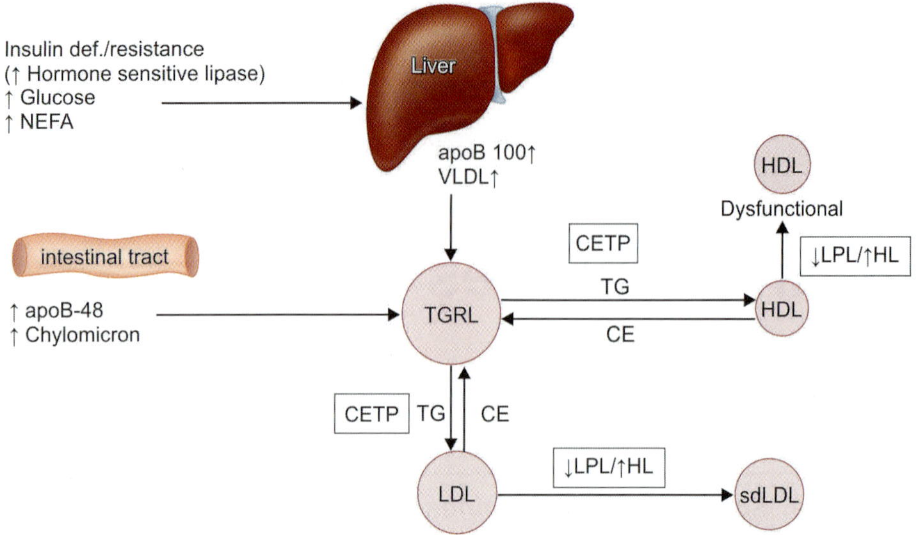

apo, apolipoprotein; CE, cholesteryl ester; CETP, cholesteryl ester transfer protein; HDL, high-density lipoprotein; HL, hepatic lipase; LDL, low-density lipoprotein; LPL, lipoprotein lipase; NEFA, nonesterfied fatty acid; sd-LDL, small dense-low-density lipoprotein; TG, triglyceride; TGRL, triglyceride-rich lipoprotein.

FIG. 1: Effects of diabetes on triglyceride-rich lipoproteins, HDL,and LDL. Increased avalability of glucose and nonesterified fatty acids in the liver leads to decreased degradation of apoB100 and increased secretion of VLDL. In the post prandial state, apoB-48 and chylomicrons are produced at a higher rate in the intestinal tract. Both liver derived VLDL and intestinal derived chlyomicrons contribute to overabundance of triglyceride-rich lipoproteins in blood. CETP facilitates the exchange of triclyceride and cholesteryl esters between triglyceride rich lipoprotein and LDL as well as HDL. Subsequently triglyceride-rich LDL and HDL are hydrolyzed by hepatic lipase leads to production of small dense LDL and dysfunctional HDL.

treatment. Among drugs, statin is the only drug recommended in diabetic dyslipidemia. Fibrates and niacin are not recommended in standard guidelines.[5-7] If the LDL cholesterol is still high (≥70 mg/dL) on maximally tolerated statin dose, ezetimibe and proprotein convertase subtilisin/kexin type 9 (PCSK9) inhibitors can be added.

Monitoring of Lipid Profile Status

For adult with diabetes and not on lipid lowering drugs, fasting lipid profile should be estimated at the initial evaluation and repeated every 5-year or more frequently if required, in patients with age less than 40 years. The patients of more than or equal to 40 years with diabetes are usually on guideline directed statin therapy, hence the lipid profile estimation should be done before starting the patient on statin and 4–12 weeks after initiation or change of the dosing of the drug and yearly thereafter.

Lifestyle Modification

The modification of lifestyle entails motivation of the patients for increased physical activity, weight loss, and above all medical nutrition therapy. Emphasis should be laid on decreased intake of saturated fats, trans-fats, and cholesterol while encouraging the patients for increased intake of viscous fibers (e.g., legumes, citrus fruits, and oats), omega-3 fatty acids, and plant sterols. These nutritional interventions are customized keeping the associated medical conditions, lipid status, type of diabetes, and patient's age in mind. In subjects with high TGs (≥150 mg/dL) and low HDL cholesterol (<40 mg/dL for males and <50 mg/dL for females), a good control of sugar has a beneficial effect on the plasma lipid status.

Initiation of Statin Therapy as per Risk Stratification

It is beyond doubt that because of increased prevalence of lipid derangements, T2D patients have higher incidence of clinical ASCVD and statin therapies in this subgroup of patients as per multiple clinical trials and meta-analysis of over 18,000 patients have shown significant reduction in CVD events and CAD-related mortality.[8-12]

In agreement with these recommendations statins form the drug of choice for cardio protection. As mentioned in Tables 1 and 2), there are two statin dosing intensities that are to be used in clinical practice.

It is known that the reduction with statin therapy in the coronary heart disease deaths and nonfatal myocardial infarction is maximum in patients with the highest number of risk factors but at the same time the statin therapy has overall benefit in patients with diabetes who are having a moderate or low-risk of CVD.[13]

The diabetic patients are risk stratified as per the presence or absence of documented clinical ASCVD and are respectively advised to receive secondary or primary prevention therapy. It is obvious that patients with clinical ASCVD are at higher risk and warrant high-intensity statin therapy as documented in multiple large randomized clinical studies.[14]

TABLE 1: Statins and additional drug treatment in diabetic patients*

Age	Clinical ASCVD◊	Recommended treatment¶
<40 years	No Yes	No statin required# High-intensity statin: Add ezetimibe or PCSK 9 inhibitors if LDL cholesterol ≥70 mg/dL despite maximally tolerated statin dose
≥40 years	• No • Yes	• Moderate-intensity statin† • High-intensity statin: Add ezetimibe or PCSK 9 inhibitors if LDL cholesterol ≥70 mg/dL despite maximally tolerated statin dose

*In addition to lifestyle modification.

¶maximally tolerated dose of statin to be used, if patients not able to tolerate intended intensity.

◊Clinical ASCVD include coronary artery disease, stroke, and peripheral artery disease. Other cardiovascular risk factors include smoking, high blood pressure, LDL cholesterol ≥100 mg/dL, albuminuria, chronic kidney disease, and family history of premature ASCVD.

#Moderate-intensity statin can be started after discussing the risk-benefits and patient preference if above mentioned other cardiovascular risk factors are present.

†High-intensity statin can be started after discussing the risk-benefits and patient preference if above mentioned other cardiovascular risk factors are present.

ASCVD, atherosclerotic cardiovascular disease; LDL, low density lipoprotein; PCSK9, proprotein convertase subtilisin/kexin type 9.

TABLE 2: Intensity of various statins

• High intensity statin therapy (reduces LDL cholesterol by ≥50%) once daily	• Moderate-intensity statin therapy (reduces LDL cholesterol by 30–50%) once daily
• Atorvastatin 40–80 mg • Rosuvastatin 20–40 mg	• Atorvastatin 10–20 mg • Rosuvastatin 5–10 mg • Simvastatin 20–40 mg • Lovastatin 40 mg • Pitavastatin 2–4 mg

LDL, low-density lipoprotein.

In the era of more costly lipid lowering drugs it becomes all the more essential to target these therapies only to high CV risk patients and hence, there are many risk factors calculators available though none of them is perfect.[15]

The commonly used American College of Cardiology or American Heart Association CVD risk calculator to estimate 10-year clinical ASCVD risk is incomplete because it does not accounts for duration of diabetes or presence of other complications like albuminuria.[15]

Primary Prevention

Moderate-intensity statin is recommended for primary prevention in patients of more than or equal to 40 years of age.[13,16] The intensity of therapy needs to be escalated, if there are additional CV risk factors present. However, for the population more than 75 years, which has not been represented much in primary prevention trials, the recommendation is for at least moderate-intensity statin therapy after discussing the risk benefit with the patients.[9,11,12]

For patients less than 40 years of age the statin treatment approaches remain same irrespective of type 1 or type 2 diabetes, especially in the presence of CV risk factors.[16] After discussing the risk benefits with the patient's moderate-intensity statin therapy is recommended for patients under the age of 40 years and/or who have T1D with other CV risk factors.[17]

Secondary Prevention

As per the results of cholesterol treatment trialists' collaboration which involved 26 statin trials comparing high versus moderate-intensity statin, high-intensity statin treatment is recommended for all patients of diabetes with clinical ASCVD as this treatment strategy reduced nonfatal CV event rates significantly.[9]

The addition of nonstatin LDL lowering agents like ezitimibe[18] and PCSK9 inhibitors[14] is recommended for patients with ASCVD who are already on maximally tolerated doses of statin therapy and LDL cholesterol is still more than 70 mg/dL. Other combination therapies like statin/fibrates and statin/niacin have not been shown to provide additional CV benefit over statin alone[5-7] and hence not recommended.

NEW ONSET DIABETES WITH STATIN

The role of statins is clearly established for primary and secondary prevention in reduction of further CV events in all high risk patients including diabetic ones. But there is a small increase in risk of incident diabetes in patients whose blood sugars are previously normal (over 5 years of follow-up, 1.2% of participants on placebo developed diabetes and 1.5% on rosuvastatin developed diabetes).[19] The CV events rate reduction far outweighs the risk of incident diabetes with statin use. A meta-analysis of 13 randomized statins trials showed an odds ratio of 1.09 for new diagnosis of diabetes, so that treatment of 255 patients with statin for 4 years resulted in an additional one case of diabetes while at the same time, it prevented 5.4 CV events in these patients.[19,20]

CONCLUSION

Diabetes is a strong risk factor for CVD outcome and dyslipidemia further aggravates the risk, so its management in diabetes is an important entity. Lipid profile assessment is essential in all patients of diabetes and also to assess adherence, response to therapy, and adverse effects. High-intensity statins are recommended at all ages in the presence of clinical ASCVD. As a primary prevention in patients less than 40 years and more than 75 years of age statins should be started after discussing risk benefits to the patients along with assessment of CV risk factors. Primary prevention is mandatory in patients between 40 years and 75 years of age with intensity of statin depending on CV risk factors.[21]

REFERENCES

1. Huang D, Refaat M, Mohammedi K, et al. Macrovascular complications in patients with diabetes and prediabetes. BioMed Res Int. 2017;1-10.
2. Morrish NJ, Wang SL, Stevens LK, et al. Mortality and causes of death in the WHO multinational study of vascular disease in diabetes. Diabetologia. 2001;44(2):S14-21.
3. Verges B. Pathophysiology of diabetic dyslipidaemia: where are we? Diabetologia. 2015;58:886-99.
4. Krauss RM. Lipids and lipoproteins in patients with type 2 diabetes. Diabetes Care. 2004;27:1496-504.
5. Ginsberg HN, Elam MB, Lovato LC, et al. ACCORD Study Group. Effects of combination lipid therapy in type 2 diabetes mellitus. N Engl J Med. 2010;362:1563-74.
6. Boden WE, Probstfield JL, Anderson T, et al. AIM-HIGH Investigators. Niacin in patients with low HDL cholesterol levels receiving intensive statin therapy. N Engl J Med. 2011;365:2255-67.
7. Landray MJ, Haynes R, Hopewell JC, et al. HPS2-THRIVE Collaborative Group. Effects of extended-release niacin with laropiprant in high risk patients. N Engl J Med. 2014;371:203-12.
8. Mihaylova B, Emberson J, Blackwell L, et al. Cholesterol treatment trialists' (CTT) Collaborators. The effects of lowering LDL cholesterol with statin therapy in people at low risk of vascular disease: meta-analysis of individual data from 27 randomised trials. Lancet. 2012;380:581-90.
9. Baigent C, Keech A, Kearney PM, et al. Cholesterol Treatment Trialists' (CTT) Collaborators. Efficacy and safety of cholesterol-lowering treatment: prospective meta-analysis of data from 90,056 participants in 14 randomised trials of statins. Lancet. 2005;366:1267-78.
10. Sever PS, Poulter NR, Dahlöf B, et al. Reduction in cardiovascular events with atorvastatin in 2,532 patients with type 2 diabetes: Anglo- Scandinavian Cardiac Outcomes Trial–lipid-lowering arm (ASCOT-LLA). Diabetes Care. 2005;28:1151-7.
11. Colhoun HM, Betteridge DJ, Durrington PN, et al.; CARDS investigators. Primary prevention of cardiovascular disease with atorvastatin in type 2 diabetes in the Collaborative Atorvastatin Diabetes Study (CARDS): multicentre randomized placebo-controlled trial. Lancet. 2004;364:685-96.
12. Kearney PM, Blackwell L, Collins R, et al. Cholesterol Treatment Trialists' (CTT) Collaborators. Efficacy of cholesterol-lowering therapy in 18,686 people with diabetes in 14 randomised trials of statins: a meta-analysis. Lancet. 2008;371:117-25.
13. Taylor F, Huffman MD, Macedo AF, et al. Statins for the primary prevention of cardiovascular disease. Cochrane Database Syst Rev. 2013;1:CD004816.
14. Sabatine MS, Giugliano RP, Keech AC, et al.; FOURIER Steering Committee and Investigators. Evolocumab and clinical outcomes in patients with cardiovascular disease. N Engl J Med. 2017;376:1713-22
15. Bohula EA, Morrow DA, Giugliano RP, et al. Atherothrombotic risk stratification and ezetimibe for secondary Prevention. J Am Coll Cardiol. 2017;69:911-21.
16. Collins R, Armitage J, Parish S, et al. Heart protection study collaborative group. MRC/BHF Heart protection study of cholesterol lowering with simvastatin in 5963 people with diabetes: a randomised placebo-controlled trial. Lancet. 2003;361:2005-16.
17. de Ferranti SD, de Boer IH, Fonseca V, et al. Type 1 diabetes mellitus and cardiovascular disease: a scientific statement from the American Heart Association and American Diabetes Association. Circulation. 2014;130:1110-30.
18. Cannon CP, Blazing MA, Giugliano RP, et al.; IMPROVE-IT Investigators. Ezetimibe added to statin therapy after acute coronary syndromes. N Engl J Med. 2015;372:2387-97.
19. Ridker PM, Pradhan A, MacFadyen JG, et al. Cardiovascular benefits and diabetes S102 Cardiovascular Disease and Risk Management Diabetes Care Volume 41, Supplement 1, January 2018 risks of statin therapy in primary prevention: an analysis from the JUPITER trial. Lancet. 2012;380:565-71.
20. Sattar N, Preiss D, Murray HM, et al. Statins and risk of incident diabetes: a collaborative meta-analysis of randomised statin trials. Lancet. 2010;375:735-42.
21. Matthew CR, George B, Andrew JM, et al. American diabetes association, cardiovascular disease and risk management: Standards of medical care in diabetes 2018. Diabetes Care. 2018;41(Suppl. 1):S86-104.

CHAPTER 10

Statin Intolerance: Guide to Management

Mrinal K Das

INTRODUCTION

In spite of the highly established beneficial effects of reduction of low-density lipoprotein (LDL)-cholesterol in atherosclerotic coronary heart disease (CHD),[1,2] the application of lipid-lowering therapy has become a challenging issue because of the increased internet-based awareness and concerns of the patients over probable side effects and potential toxicity of 3-hydroxy-3-methylglutaryl-coenzyme (HMG coenzyme) reductase inhibitors, otherwise known as statins. This can result in poor adherence to statin therapy and ultimately discontinuation.[3,4] It is very important for patients with high and very high cardiovascular (CV) risk, since discontinuation of statins for 4–6 weeks may cause instability of the atheroma plaque[5] and thereby increasing the risk of CV adverse events.[6] Therefore, there is a clinical need to ascertain the correct interpretation of the symptoms and signs presented by the patients after the statin therapy as well as developing approaches and therapies for such events so that the benefit of lipid-lowering therapy is continued. The present article will attempt on these aspects of perceived adverse effects of statin therapy otherwise also called "Statin Intolerance" (SI) and highlight the available remedial measures in the light of present information and knowledge.

DEFINITIONS OF STATIN INTOLERANCE

The definition of statin intolerance has evoked great deal of interest amongst clinicians and thus generating debate[7] over the years. The following are the various definitions given by different lipid organizations available till date.

National Lipid Association (NLA) defined SI in late 2014, as an inability to tolerate at least two statins—one at the lowest starting daily dose and another at any daily dose—due to either disturbing symptoms (real or perceived) or abnormal laboratory findings that are temporally associated with statin therapy. They are reversible after withholding statin.[4]

International Lipid Expert Panel (ILEP) definition added to the above text the subsidence of symptoms or changes in biomarkers or even significant improvement after either dose reduction or stopping the medicine. Symptoms or alteration in biomarkers are however not attributable to drug-drug interactions and predisposed conditions which have the propensity to increase the risk of statin intolerance.[8]

European Atherosclerosis Society (EAS) offered clinically oriented definition of SI by inserting the assessment of statin-associated muscle symptoms (SAMS) which included the characteristics of muscle symptoms, elevated creatine kinase (CK) levels and their temporal association with starting statin therapy, and suspension of the therapy and rechallenge.[9]

Canadian Consensus Working Group update, in 2016, defined SI as a clinical syndrome, not induced by drug interactions or risk factors for untreated intolerance and manifested by significant adverse symptoms and/or abnormal biomarker level that prevent the long-term treatment and adherence. These need to be documented by challenge (starting the medicine)/dechallenge (reduction of the dosage of medicine)/rechallenge (restarting the same medicine), as per the appropriateness, using at least two statins, including the commonly used atorvastatin and rosuvastatin. There should also be the documentation of the failure of maintenance of therapeutic goals, as recommended by the national guidelines.[10]

TYPES OF STATIN INTOLERANCE

Partial

There is inability to tolerate a suitable dose of a statin based on patient's CV risk as in acute coronary syndromes (ACS) there is intolerance of either atorvastatin at a dose of 40–80 mg or rosuvastatin at 20–40 mg dose. It can appear with temporal associations between symptoms and treatment onset or increased dose usually within 3–6 months.

Complete

Intolerance is when clinically apparent variety of side effects impairing organ function and/or quality of life after intake of any statin at any dose with or without associated laboratory findings.[7]

ANECDOTAL DATA

Statins are considered the most prescribed CV drugs,[11] both for dyslipidemia[12] as well as for patients with stable coronary artery disease (SCAD), ACS, cerebrovascular accident (CVA), hypertension, diabetes mellitus (DM), and chronic kidney disease (CKD) no matter whether there is dyslipidemia or not.[13] The beneficial effects of statins in both primary and secondary prevention[14-16] are the most talked about topic in both medical scientific forum and a topic of conjecture by the even unscientific social media. There has been 21% decrease in cardiovascular disease (CVD) mortality and morbidity achieved by lowering LDL-C by 1.0 mmol/L (38.7 mg/dL).[17]

The Cholesterol Treatment Trialists (CTT) collaboration showed 12% reduction in all-cause mortality per mmol/L reduction in LDL-C and significant reductions in myocardial infarction (MI) or coronary death (23%), the need for coronary revascularization (24%), and in fatal or nonfatal stroke (17%) after 5 years of statin therapy.[18] However, statin discontinuation rates over 50% after 1-year is quite high, even among patients with CHD.[3,19] The medical fraternity has enough evidence to project the ill-effects of statin nonadherence attributed to SI, increasing the risk for recurrent MI and CHD.[6,20] Mancini et al.[21] observed 70–80% of statin-treated patients being tolerant to treatment, and 20–30% to be statin intolerant. Definite evidence of SI was found in about 5–6% of patients.[21] Banach et al.[22,20] with a step-by-step approach yielded a diagnosis of complete statin intolerance in 2–3% of patients only. There have been few recent reports from Indian workers regarding the statin intolerance. Bharadwaj et al.[23] observed older women to be more vulnerable to SAMs especially those with multiple comorbidities and established polypharmacy. Myalgia was dose-dependent in those individuals and so they found that many physicians started with low dose of statin with subsequent up-titration as per tolerance.

Wander et al.[24] in the first-ever survey amongst 404 Indian physicians using statin mentioned that 92% respondents reported statin intolerance in the range of 2–20% in their clinical practice. Most of them (39%) reduced the dose of statin, followed by stopping statin and restarting at lower dose (34%). Use of alternate statin was done by 22.3% and using nonstatin by 10.9% respondents.

So number-wise, the incidence of statin intolerance is not very significant and hence proper caution is required before labeling the patient in order to impart the benefit of statin therapy.

CLINICAL FEATURES

Statin intolerance is not simply the occurrence of symptoms in general, but rather the symptoms that are perceived as unacceptable.[25] However, to correlate that negative symptoms causally to statins is often difficult to ascertain. Usually symptoms (more than 75%) are more likely to be due to statins if the complaints occur within the first 3 months of starting statin and disappear after stopping the medicine and reoccurring after resuming the same.[26,27]

Statins-specific adverse effects are shown in table 1.

TABLE 1: Incidence of statin-induced adverse features

Adverse effect	Percentage of patients	Markers (Present/ Absent)	Reference
Myalgia	3–5%	CK	27–29
Myopathy	0.1–0.2%	CK	27–29
Myonecrosis	0.0016%/year	CK	27–29,48
Diabetes mellitus	9–27%	Blood sugar, HbA1c	27–30
Hepatotoxicity	1%	ALT	14, 27

CK, creatine kinase; ALT, alanine aminotransferase; HbA1C, hemoglobin A1c.

Statin-Associated Muscle Symptoms

Statin-associated muscle symptoms are the most common side effects of statins with resultant discontinuation. They could be myalgia, muscle stiffness and tenderness, cramps, and loss of muscle power with severity ranging from mild to severe.[8,28] Based on the findings, classification of SAMS was done as follows[29]: (1) Myalgia, (2) Myopathy, (3) Myositis, and (4) Myonecrosis or Rhabdomyolysis.

The percentage of patients with muscle symptoms since 1993–2010 as per the trials carried out during the index years.[30]

The prevalence of SAMS is around 3–5% in randomized controlled trials including patients with dyslipidemia[31] and up to 20% in observational studies.[32,33] The European Atherosclerosis Society (EAS) consensus paper reported a SAMS prevalence as high as 29%.[9] The USAGE (Understanding Statin Use in America and Gaps in Education) study on current and previous users of statin via an internet-based study showed that SAMS occurred in 60% of current and 25% of previous users.[34] STOMP (Effect of Statins on Skeletal Muscle Function and Performance) study, a randomized, double-blind, placebo-controlled trial, found overall incidence of 5% of SAMS with myalgia in 9.4% of patients receiving atorvastatin and 4.6% of subjects on placebo.[35] Table 2 is depicted to ascertain the likelihood of SAMS.

Myalgia is defined as muscle pain or flu-like symptoms (heaviness, tenderness, stiffness, aches, or cramps) with normal CK levels. NLA recommends that the SAMS Clinical Index (SAMSCI) score, the greatest score (3 points) for the typical large muscle symmetric (e.g., bilateral) aches, 2 points for bilateral aches of the smaller distal or proximal musculature, and 1 point for asymmetric, nonuniform symptoms.[29] The SAMSCI score helps to confirm statin-related myalgia and to exclude the nocebo effect—psychologically conditioned symptoms as a result of expectations due to achieved knowledge of drug-related side effects. As per EAS

TABLE 2: Likelihood of SAMS

SAMS less likely		SAMS more likely
• Unilateral • No pattern in distribution • Tingling, twitching, shooting, nocturnal cramps or joint pain	Nature of symptoms	• Bilateral • Large muscle groups (e.g., thighs, buttocks, • calves, shoulder girdle) • Muscle ache, weakness, soreness, stiffness, • cramping, tenderness or general fatigue
• Onset before statin initiation • Onset >12 weeks after statin initiation	Timing of symptoms	• Onset 4–6 weeks after statin initiation • Onset after statin dosage increase
Nonstatin causes of muscle symptoms including: • Conditions, e.g., hypothyroidism, polymyalgia rheumatic vitamin D deficiency • Unaccustomed/heavy physical activity • Medicines e.g., glucocorticoids, antipsychotics, • Immunosuppressant or antiviral agents	Other considerations	**Risk factors for SAMS including:** • Medicine or food interactions • High-dose statin therapy • History of myopathy with other • Lipid-modifying medicines • Regular vigorous physical activity • Impaired hepatic or renal function • Substance abuse (e.g., alcohol, opioids, cocaine) female, low BMI
	CK levels	• Elevated (>ULN; but may also be normal) • Elevated CK levels decrease after statin ceased

SAMS, statin-associated muscle symptoms; BMI, body mass index; CK, creatine kinase; ULN, upper limit of normal.

consensus paper on SAMS, above cut-off point value of 4, muscle symptoms seem to be more attributable to statin therapy.[9]

Myopathy is weakness of the muscle occurring with normal or elevated CK.[36] Predisposing conditions for myopathy are age more than 75 years, female sex, renal and hepatic dysfunction, hypothyroidism, alcohol abuse, excessive physical exertion, genetic susceptibility, perioperative period, and concurrent use of drugs inhibiting the metabolism of statins (clarithromycin, erythromycin, azole antifungals, diltiazem, verapamil, amiodarone, fibrates particularly gemfibrozil, cyclosporin, clopidogrel, sulfonamides, and red yeast rice).[8,28,37] Low levels of vitamin D and coenzyme Q10 (CoQ10) might also increase the risk of statin intolerance.[38,39] The term does not necessarily connote symptoms or any degree of CK elevation. Muscle biopsy also suggests some myopathic statin-induced abnormalities that may be present in the context of normal CK levels.[35]

Myositis is muscle inflammation associated with symptoms like tenderness, CK elevation, and leukocyte infiltration into muscle tissue.

Myonecrosis is always associated with muscle damage and elevation of serum CK.[36] The most serious form of myonecrosis is rhabdomyolysis in which muscle breakdown is responsible for a massive release of CK and myoglobin, with dangerous complications viz., myoglobinuria and acute kidney injury (AKI).[36] Fortunately, it is very rare (incidence of 1.6 per 100,000 patient-years). Rhabdomyolysis usually occurs in genetically predisposed cases or where is drug–drug interaction.[40]

The risk of developing new onset DM are more in prediabetics with insulin resistance, overweight, high blood pressure, high triglycerides, low high-density lipoprotein cholesterol (HDL-C), hyperglycemia, and duration and intensity of statin therapy. However, benefits associated with statin therapy outweigh the risk of developing DM for high and very high-risk patients.[37,41-43] In JUPITER (The Justification for the Use of Statins in Prevention: an Intervention Trial Evaluating Rosuvastatin) trial during a follow-up period of up to 5 years, there was CV mortality benefits of statin exceeding the diabetes hazard, even in those having higher chance of developing diabetes. To circumvent the risk of new onset DM during statin therapy, it is prerogative of the treating physician to advise the patients to exercise, lose weight, stop smoking, and reduce caloric intake avoiding saturated and trans-fats.

EVALUATION OF STATIN INTOLERANCE

List of the routine biomarkers along with the novel or experimental biomarkers for ready reckoning is shown in table 3.

The most widely used serum marker is the serum CK level,[44] but it is inadequate as a diagnostic marker and nonspecific as levels are not always associated with myopathy.[45] One must remember that CK levels can also be elevated by exercise in a dose-independent manner[34] and by drug interactions, genetic variants, CoQ10 deficiency, and vitamin D deficiency.[46]

Routine liver function analyses are no longer recommended as the diagnostic yield is low and cost prohibitive.[47] Statin induced rise in aminotransferase levels is rare, mild, dose-related, and not related to reduction in LDL-C. They are usually temporary, and may to return to baseline levels after 2–4 weeks.[48,49] Persistent elevation of alanine aminotransferase (ALT) more than three upper limit of normal (ULN) were observed in more than 1% of patients treated with statins. There was correlation with more than 0.5% rate for moderate-dose rosuvastatin and at slightly

TABLE 3: List of the routine and novel biomarkers for statin-induced myopathy

Serial No.	Name
1.	Creatinine phosphokinase (CK)
2.	Aspartate aminotransferase (AST)
3.	Fatty acid binding protein 3 (FABP3)
4.	Myosin light chain 1 (MLC1)
5.	Skeletal muscle troponin I (sTnI)
6.	Myosin light chain 3 [MYL3 (S3)]
7.	CK isoform M (CKM)
8.	Phosphorus magnetic resonance spectroscopy (31P-MRS)
9.	MicroRNAs (miRNAs;133a/b and 499-5p)
10.	Complex genomic and lipidomic analyses: increased expression of arachidonic acid 5-lipoxygenase activating protein, phospholipase C, numerous species of phosphatidylethanolamine, selective pools of long-chain triglycerides, and phosphocholine ether

higher rates (about 1%) with all doses of atorvastatin or simvastatin 80 mg.[48] Interestingly, ALT elevations often improve even when statin therapy is continued. It is worth remembering that the use of statins prevents about 33% of major CVD events vis-à-vis placebo, and may cause serious liver disease only in 1/1,000,000 [number needed to harm (NNH) is 1 million]. Still between 10% and 30% of patients do not receive statins because of fear of hepatotoxicity.[8,22]

Lactate dehydrogenase is another early marker which might predict and diagnose statin intolerance and myopathy,[47] however, its clinical utility in cases of statin-induced myopathy warrants validation.[50]

Fatty acid-binding protein 3 (FABP3) and myosin light chain 1 (MLC1) could be other futuristic biomarkers of skeletal muscle toxicity.[50,51] Similarly, skeletal muscle troponin I (sTnI), myosin light chain 3 [MYL3 (S3)], CK isoform M (CKM), and FABP3 versus CK for drug-induced skeletal muscle injury, were found to outperform CK (Burch et al.).[52] When used in conjunction with CK, sTnI, MYL3, CKM, and FABP3 individually and collectively improved diagnostic sensitivity and specificity and diagnostic certainty, for skeletal muscle injury and responded in a sensitive manner to low levels of novel skeletal muscle injury degeneration/necrosis in rats. CKM showed the highest correlation ($r = 0.47$, $p < 0.0001$), followed by FABP3 ($r = 0.52$, $p < 0.0001$), MYL3 ($r = 0.48$, $p < 0.0001$), sTnI ($r = 0.47$, $p < 0.0001$), aspartate transaminase (AST; $r = 0.46$, $p < 0.0001$), and CK ($r = 0.32$, $p < 0.0001$).[52] These findings suggest that sTnI, MYL3, CKM, and FABP3 are suitable for voluntary use, in conjunction with CK, in experimental studies in rats to monitor statin-induced muscle injury and for the potential translational use in early clinical trials to ensure patient safety.[52] Dobkin[53] suggested the functional assessment of hip-flexor and abductor performance.

Phosphorus magnetic resonance spectroscopy (31P-MRS) study by Wu et al.[54] for the evaluation of the kinetics of recovery exercise phosphocreatine found that patients on statin therapy for 4 weeks had prolonged metabolic recovery time in the calf despite no change in serum CK levels.[54] However, there were several shortcomings like cost, dependence of renal dysfunction, rapid clearance, heterogeneous response depending on the type of myotoxicants in general.[47,55]

Complex genomic and combined lipidomic analyses have been tried, but were found to have difficulty to perform and interpret routinely in clinical practice.

Two microRNAs (miRNAs 133a/b and 499-5p) were assessed and miR-133a/b was found to be sensitive and specific markers of cardiac and skeletal muscle toxicity[56]; miR-499-5p was more applicable in statin-induced muscle injury in the marathon runners.[57] Thus, though the new biomarkers for statin-induced myopathy are on the horizon, most cannot be commonly used or recommended because of either the complex methodology or costs. Further works are highly warranted to ascertain their sensitivity and specificity.[47]

MANAGEMENT

The basic principle in the management of SI is to attempt with all vigor to not allow patients to discontinue the statin. All the stake holders should be convinced about the data that there is not only increased chance of developing plaque instability after statin discontinuation, but also there may be rebound inflammation after about 4–6 weeks of stopping statin. Since prevention is always better than cure, so the approach should start with the prevention. The following steps are apt from the preventive points of view.

Pretreatment Assessment

- Assess risk [(e.g., elderly, prior muscle pains, familial hypercholesterolemia (FH) of myopathy, renal disease, DM, hypothyroidism]
- Consider exogenous factors (e.g., statin dose, alcohol use, drug-drug interactions, excessive grapefruit juice use)
- Measure baseline CK, ALT, thyroid-stimulating hormone (TSH), and creatinine.

Counseling

- To inform the patients that statins are very well tolerated in most people
- To inform the patients about muscular symptoms and when to discontinue.

Monitoring

Check CK/ALT when monitoring lipid-lowering efficacy:

- At 6–8 weeks after starting or with dose increase and then every 6–12 months
- Avoid severe exercise for several days prior to testing.

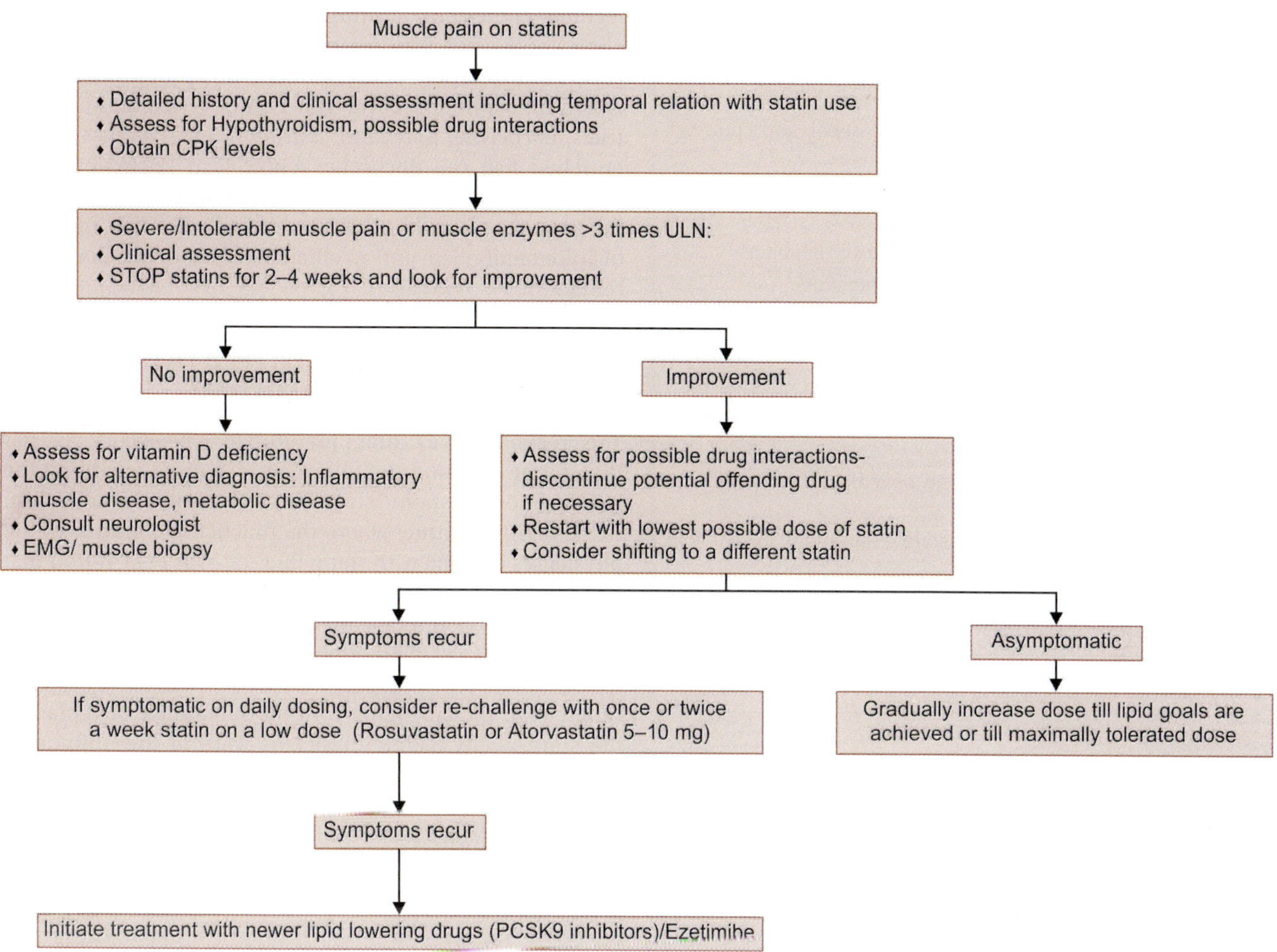

CK, creatine kinase; EMG, electromyography; LDL-C, low-density lipoprotein cholesterol; ULN, upper limit of normal.

FLOWCHART 1: Algorithm for the evaluation of statin-induced muscle disease.

Flowchart 1 depicts the algorithm for the management of SAMS.[58-60]

ALTERNATIVE AGENTS

There is a huge list of alternative agents to take care of statin intolerance as depicted in box 1. All these drugs or agents are not having the same potency to reduce the LDL-C. However, many of them may be considered for add-on therapy, which may alter the residual risk. Ezetimibe monotherapy was used limitedly in less than 5–10% patients since there was no United States Food and Drug Administration (US FDA) recommendations and restricted reimbursement in Europe.[61] Use of proprotein convertase subtilisin/kexin type 9 (PCSK9) is also used in very limited number of patients because of the cost involvement. Evolocumab and alirocumab underwent several phase II and phase III clinical trials in high-risk CV patients. Cohort included patients with statin intolerance FH. Evolocumab significantly reduced LDL-C by approximately 60–65%, having favorable effects on other lipid parameters and lipoprotein(a). It is well tolerated as a single agent or in combination with statins alone, or statins plus ezetimibe. The therapy did not demonstrate major side effects like SAMs or new onset DM, or neurocognitive disorders. The effectiveness and safety of evolocumab in a pooled analysis was comparable in patients with or without type 2 DM (T2DM) and did not differ between T2DM subgroups.[62-74]

Statin and other currently available drug combination have limited capacity to lower LDL-C in patients at high CV risk leaving a condition called residual risk. Bempedoic acid (ETC-1002) is a new star in the block acting through adenosine triphosphate-citrate lyase inhibition. The efficacy of combination of statins and bempedoic acid has been evaluated in a randomized controlled trial (NCT02072161).[75-78] Monacolins such as policosanols and bergamot inhibit HMG-CoA reductase, and red yeast rice extract (*Monascus purpureus*) contains a variety of monacolins.[79] Berberine and red yeast rice combination

BOX 1 Second-line statin alternatives[90]

Currently available agents:
- Cholesterol absorption inhibitors (Ezetimibe)
- Bile acid sequestrants (colesevelam, colestipol, and cholestyramine)
- Niacin
- Fibrates
- PCSK9 (proprotein convertase subtilisin/kexin) inhibitors
- Cholesteryl ester transfer protein (CETP) inhibitors
- Bempedoic acid (ETC-1002)

Nonpharmacological approaches:
- To reduce intake of saturated and trans fats
- To choose monounsaturated and polyunsaturated fats
- Mediterranean diet
- Plant extracts: Sugar cane-derived policosanols, and artichoke leaf extracts, red rice yeast
- Nutraceutical combination berberine, astaxanthin, CoQ10, folic acid
- Acid ethyl ester (AMR101)
- Chokeberry flavonoid extract
- Spirulina
- Viscous fiber

significantly improved different lipid fraction levels [i.e., lowered total cholesterol, LDL-C, and triglyceride levels ($p < 0.001$ for all) and increased HDL-C concentration ($p < 0.001$)] after treatment for 16 weeks.[80] Armolipid Plus, with ingredients of natural substances like red yeast rice, policosanol, and berberine combined with folic acid, astaxanthin, and CoQ10 having complementary lipid-lowering properties, had lower risk of statin intolerance like situation because of low doses of its active ingredients—low enough not to be associated with untoward effects but high enough to exert therapeutic effects in combination with other complementary substances.[81] Spirulina, a filamentous, water blue-green microalga (Cyanobacterium)[82] with lipid lowering in one meta-analysis[83] of seven randomized controlled trials demonstrated significant reduction of total cholesterol (–46.76 mg/dL; $p < 0.001$), LDL-C (–41.32 mg/dL; $p < 0.001$), triglycerides (–44.23 mg/dL; $p < 0.001$), and elevated levels of HDL-C (6.06 mg/dL; $p = 0.001$). Indian spice turmeric (*Curcuma longa L.*) has curcumin, a natural dietary polyphenol responsible for the yellow color of the analgesic, has antioxidant[84] and anti-inflammatory properties which may help in taking care of SAMS by preventing and reducing muscular fatigue. Curcumin is safe to consume, even at dosages of up to 8–12 g daily.[85] It blocks the inflammatory pathway of the nuclear factor, inhibits muscular atrophy, and help in rejuvenating muscle fibers after injuries.[86] It has also lipid-modifying properties and may serve as an adjunctive therapy in SAMS, with added benefit of reduction of LDL-C possibly at a lower statin dose.[87] It has the potentiality to modulate the biomarkers of HDL functionality by increasing apolipoprotein AI (apo-AI) and lecithin-cholesterol acyltransferase (LCAT) and decreasing cholesteryl ester transfer protein (CETP), paraoxonase-1 (PON1), myeloperoxidase (MPO), and lipoprotein-associated phospholipase A2 (Lp-PLA2).[88] In some human trials, berberine, polydatin, marine n-3 PUFAs, n-3 PUFA-enriched fish oil, docosahexaenoic acid (DHA)-enriched canola oil and quercetin-3-O-b-D glucoside demonstrated the capacity to lower PCSK9 levels, an important regulator of lipid metabolism and an efficient target for plasma LDL-C reduction.[89]

INDIAN EXPERIENCE WITH STATIN-INDUCED MUSCLE SYMPTOM

The recent survey amongst Indian physicians as per Wander et al. found the following responses regarding the management of statin intolerance[24] as shown in table 4. In ACCORDANCE study where the practicing behavior of the physicians in India with statin therapy, Das et al. found that when patients complained of myalgia and had a CK less than four times upper limit of normal (4X ULN), most of the physicians (56.29%) preferred to discontinue statin for 6 weeks and then rechallenge with the same statin at low dose rather than rechallenging with the same dose or replacing the statin. Only 3.66% physicians were of the opinion of discontinuing statin completely.[91] Figure 1 shows the physicians' preferred treatment choices for statin-induced myalgia or rise in CK less than four times ULN in that study.

CONCLUSION

Statins or HMG coenzyme reductase inhibitors are the most prescribed medicine in the modern times and the cornerstone in the therapy of atherosclerotic CHD. But, at times, it is associated with adverse effects in the form of statin-induced muscle symptoms or SAMs, new onset DM or hepatic disorder. This syndrome is called SI, which limits the achievement of therapeutic LDL goal. This in turn results in the instability of the atheroma plaque that might increase the morbidity and mortality associated with CAD. However, the condition can be challenged, dechallenged, and rechallenged starting with lower dose of the same drug or different drug. In extreme and definite cases, one may have to take recourse to nonstatin therapeutic measures. It is the prerogative of the

TABLE 4: Preferred options for management of statin intolerance

Preferred strategy	Percent Responders
Reducing statin dose	39%
Stopping statin and restarting at lower dose	34.5%
Using alternative statin	22.3%
Using nonstatin drugs	10.9%
Lifestyle modification	1.4%

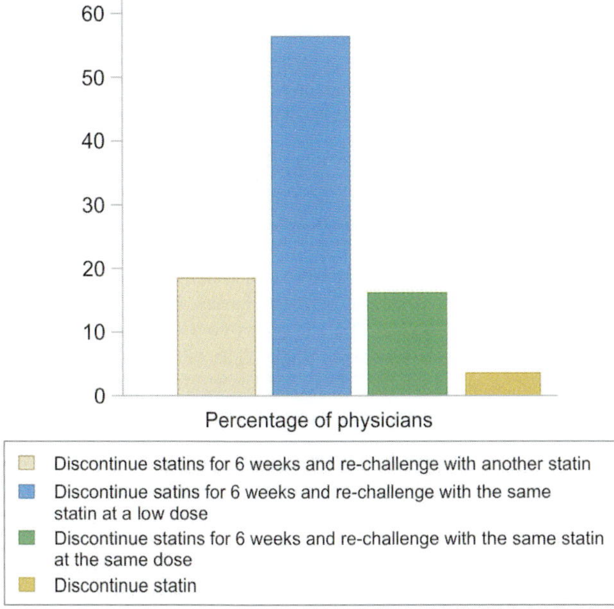

FIG. 1: Physician practice preferences for patients with statin induced muscle symptoms and creatine kinase levels <4 times normal.

treating physicians to convince the patient as well as himself or herself that this is a very rare condition that can be tackled appropriately and give the benefit of continuation of the therapy.

REFERENCES

1. Serban MC, Banach M, Mikhailidis DP. Clinical implications of the IMPROVE-IT trial in the light of current and future lipid lowering treatment options. Expert Opin Pharmacother. 2016;17:369-80.
2. Sampson UK, Fazio S, Linton MF. Residual cardiovascular risk despite optimal LDL cholesterol reduction with statins: the evidence, etiology, and therapeutic challenges. Curr Atheroscler Rep. 2012;14:1-10.
3. Banach M, Serban MC. Discussion around statin discontinuation in older adults and patients with wasting diseases. J Cachexia Sarcopenia Muscle. 2016;7:396-9.
4. Jacobson TA, Ito MK, Maki KC, et al. National Lipid Association recommendations for patient-centered management of dyslipidemia: Part 1—executive summary. J Clin Lipidol. 2014;8:473-88.
5. Banach M, Serban C, Sahebkar A, et al. Impact of statin therapy on coronary plaque composition: a systematic review and meta-analysis of virtual histology intravascular ultrasound studies. BMC Med. 2015;13:229.
6. Serban MC, Colantonio LD, Manthripragada AD, et al. Statin intolerance and risk of coronary heart events and all-cause mortality following myocardial infarction. J Am Coll Cardiol. 2017;69:1386-95.
7. Algharably EA, Filler I, Rosenfeld S, et al. Statin intolerance—a question of definition. Expert Opin Drug Saf. 2017;16:55-63.
8. Banach M, Rizzo M, Toth PP, et al. Statin intolerance—an attempt at a unified definition. Position paper from an International Lipid Expert Panel. Expert Opin Drug Saf. 2015;14:935-55.
9. Stroes ES, Thompson PD, Corsini A, et al. Statin-associated muscle symptoms: impact on statin therapy—European Atherosclerosis Society consensus panel statement on assessment, aetiology and management. Eur Heart J.2015;36:1012-22.
10. Mancini GB, Baker S, Bergeron J, et al. Diagnosis, prevention, and management of statin adverse effects and intolerance: Canadian Consensus Working Group Update (2016). Can J Cardiol. 2016;32:S35-65.
11. Raju SB, Varghese K, Madhu K. Management of statin intolerance. Indian J Endocrinol Metab. 2013;17:977-82.
12. Bosomworth NJ. Approach to identifying and managing atherogenic dyslipidemia: A metabolic consequence of obesity and diabetes. Can Fam Physician. 2013;59:1169-80.
13. Banach M, Mikhailidis DP, Kjeldsen SE, et al. Time for new indications for statins? Med Sci Monit. 2009;15:MS1-5.
14. Stone NJ, Robinson JG, Lichtenstein AH, et al. 2013 ACC/AHA guideline on the treatment of blood cholesterol to reduce atherosclerotic cardiovascular risk in adults: A report of the American College of Cardiology/American Heart Association Task Force on Practice Guidelines. J Am Coll Cardiol. 2014;63:2889-934.
15. Hobbs FD, Banach M, Mikhailidis DP, et al. Is statin-modified reduction in lipids the most important preventive therapy for cardiovascular disease? A pro/con debate. BMC Med. 2016;14:4.
16. Colantonio LD, Bittner V, Reynolds K, et al. Association of serum lipids and coronary heart disease in contemporary observational studies. Circulation. 2016;133:256-64.
17. Cholesterol Treatment Trialists' (CTT) Collaboration, Baigent C, Blackwell L, et al. Efficacy and safety of more intensive lowering of LDL cholesterol: A meta-analysis of data from 170,000 participants in 26 randomised trials. Lancet. 2010;376:1670-81.
18. Baigent C, Keech A, Kearney PM, et al. Efficacy and safety of cholesterol-lowering treatment: Prospective meta-analysis of data from 90,056 participants in 14 randomised trials of statins. Lancet. 2005;366:1267-78.
19. Jackevicius CA, Mamdani M, Tu JV. Adherence with statin therapy in elderly patients with and without acute coronary syndromes. JAMA. 2002;288:462-7.
20. Banach M, Stulc T, Dent R, et al. Statin non-adherence and residual cardio-vascular risk: there is need for substantial improvement. Int J Cardiol. 2016; 225:184-96.
21. Mancini GB, Baker S, Bergeron J, et al. Diagnosis, prevention, and management of statin adverse effects and intolerance: proceedings of a Canadian Working Group Consensus Conference. Can J Cardiol. 2011;27:635-62.
22. Banach M, Rizzo M, Toth PP, et al. Statin intolerance—an attempt at a unified definition. Position paper from an International Lipid Expert Panel. Arch Med Sci. 2015;11:1-23.
23. Bharadwaj S, Selvarajah S, Schneider EB. Muscular effects of statins in the elderly female: A review. Clin Interv Aging. 2013;8:47-59.
24. Wander GS, Jadav UM, Chemburkar A, et al. Lipid management in India: A nationwide cross sectional physician survey. Lipids Health Dis. 2017;16:130.
25. Stulc T, Ces˘ka R, Gotto AM Jr. Statin intolerance: the clinician's perspective. Curr Atheroscler Rep. 2015;17:69.
26. Parker BA, Capizzi JA, Grimaldi AS, et al. Effect of statins on skeletal muscle function. Circulation. 2013;127:96-103.
27. Ridker PM, Pradhan A, MacFadyen JG, et al. Cardiovascular benefits and diabetes risks of statin therapy in primary prevention: an analysis from the JUPITER trial. Lancet. 2012;380:565-71.
28. Banach M, Jankowski P, Jo´z´wiak J, et al. PoLA/CFPiP/PCS guidelines for the management of dyslipidaemias for family physicians 2016. Arch Med Sci. 2017;13:1-45.
29. Rosenson RS, Baker SK, Jacobson TA, et al. An assessment by the Statin Muscle Safety Task Force: 2014 update. J Clin Lipidol. 2014;8:S58-71.
30. Ganga HV, Slim HB, Thompson PD. A systematic review of statin-induced muscle problems in clinical trials. Am Heart J. 2014;168:6-15.
31. Bays H. Statin safety: An overview and assessment of the data-2005. Am J Cardiol. 2006;97:6C-26C.
32. Joy TR, Hegele RA. Narrative review: Statin-related myopathy. Ann Intern Med. 2009;150:858-68.
33. Grundy SM. Can statins cause chronic low-grade myopathy? Ann Intern Med. 2002;137:617-8.
34. Cohen JD, Brinton EA, Ito MK, et al. Understanding Statin Use in America and Gaps in Patient Education (USAGE): An internet-based survey of 10,138 current and former statin users. J Clin Lipidol. 2012;6:208-15.
35. Phillips PS, Haas RH, Bannykh S, et al. Statin-associated myopathy with normal creatine kinase levels. Ann Intern Med. 2002;137:581-5.
36. Thompson PD, Clarkson PM, Rosenson RS, et al. An assessment of statin safety by muscle experts. Am J Cardiol. 2006;97:69C-76C.
37. Authors Task Force Members, Catapano AL, Graham I, et al. ESC/EAS guidelines for the management of dyslipidaemias: The task force for the management

of dyslipidaemias of the European Society of Cardiology (ESC) and European Atherosclerosis Society (EAS) developed with the special contribution of the European Association for Cardiovascular Prevention & Rehabilitation (EACPR). Atherosclerosis. 2016;2016(253):281-344.
38. Michalska-Kasiczak M, Sahebkar A, Mikhailidis DP, et al. Analysis of vitamin D levels in patients with and without statin-associated myalgia—a systematic review and meta-analysis of 7 studies with 2420 patients. Int J Cardiol. 2015;178:111-6.
39. Banach M, Serban C, Sahebkar A, et al.; Lipid and Blood Pressure Meta-Analysis Collaboration Group. Effects of coenzyme Q10 on statin-induced myopathy: A meta-analysis of randomized controlled trials. Mayo Clin Proc. 2015;90:24-34.
40. Vrablik M, Zlatohlavek L, Stulc T, et al. Statin-associated myopathy: From genetic predisposition to clinical management. Physiol Res. 2014;63(Suppl 3):S327-34.
41. Barylski M, Nikolic D, Banach M, et al. Statins and new-onset diabetes. Curr Pharm Des. 2014;20:3657-64.
42. Banach M, Malodobra-Mazur M, Gluba A, et al. Statin therapy and new-onset diabetes: Molecular mechanisms and clinical relevance. Curr Pharm Des. 2013;19:4904-12.
43. Banach M, Mikhailidis DP. Statin therapy and new-onset diabetes: An attempt at recommendations. Expert Rev Endocrinol Metab. 2013;8:213-6.
44. Di Stasi SL, MacLeod TD, Winters JD, et al. Effects of statins on skeletal muscle: A perspective for physical therapists. Phys Ther. 2010;90:1530-42.
45. Kearns AK, Bilbie CL, Clarkson PM, et al. The creatine kinase response to eccentric exercise with atorvastatin 10 mg or 80 mg. Atherosclerosis. 2008;200:121-5.
46. Deichmann RE, Lavie CJ, Asher T, et al. The interaction between statins and exercise: mechanisms and strategies to counter the musculoskeletal side effects of this combination therapy. Ochsner J. 2015;15:429-37.
47. Muntean DM, Thompson PD, Catapano AL, et al. Statin-associated myopathy and the quest for biomarkers: Can we effectively predict statin-associated muscle symptoms? Drug Discov Today. 2017;22:85-96.
48. Davidson MH, Robinson JG. Safety of aggressive lipid management. J Am Coll Cardiol. 2007;49:1753-62.
49. Alsheikh-Ali AA, Maddukuri PV, Han H, et al. Effect of the magnitude of lipid lowering on risk of elevated liver enzymes, rhabdomyolysis, and cancer: Insights from large randomized statin trials. J Am Coll Cardiol. 2007;50:409-18.
50. Tonomura Y, Mori Y, Torii M, et al. Evaluation of the usefulness of biomarkers for cardiac and skeletal myotoxicity in rats. Toxicology. 2009;266:48-54.
51. Vaklavas C, Chatzizisis YS, Ziakas A, et al. Molecular basis of statin-associated myopathy. Atherosclerosis. 2009;202:18-28.
52. Burch PM, Greg Hall D, Walker EG, et al. Evaluation of the relative performance of drug-induced skeletal muscle injury biomarkers in rats. Toxicol Sci. 2016;150:247-56.
53. Dobkin BH. Underappreciated statin-induced myopathic weakness causes disability. Neurorehabilit Neural Repair. 2005;19:259-63.
54. Wu JS, Buettner C, Smithline H, et al. Evaluation of skeletal muscle during calf exercise by 31-phosphorus magnetic resonance spectroscopy in patients on statin medications. Muscle Nerve. 2011;43:76-81.
55. Tonomura Y, Matsushima S, Kashiwagi E, et al. Biomarker panel of cardiac and skeletal muscle troponins, fatty acid binding protein 3 and myosin light chain 3 for the accurate diagnosis of cardiotoxicity and musculoskeletal toxicity in rats. Toxicology. 2012;302:179-89.
56. Calvano J, Achanzar W, Murphy B, et al. Evaluation of microRNAs-208 and 133a/b as differential biomarkers of acute cardiac and skeletal muscle toxicity in rats. Toxicol Appl Pharmacol. 2016;312:53-60.
57. Min PK, Park J, Isaacs S, et al. Influence of statins on distinct circulating microRNAs during prolonged aerobic exercise. J Appl Physiol. 2016;120: 711-20.
58. Stroes ES, Thompson PD, Corsini A, et al. Statin-associated muscle symptoms: impact on statin therapy-European Atherosclerosis Society consensus panel statement on assessment, aetiology and management. Eur Heart J. 2015;36:1012-22.
59. Therapeutic Guidelines (eTG). Pharmacological management of dyslipidaemia. Melbourne: Australian Therapeutic Guidelines, 2012.
60. Kopecky S, Baum S, Foddy JM, et al. Insight into statin intolerance. Clin Cardiol. 2015;38(9):520-6.
61. Patel J, Martin SS, Banach M. Expert opinion: The therapeutic challenges faced by statin intolerance. Expert Opin Pharmacother. 2016;17:1497-507.
62. Sattar N, Preiss D, Robinson JG, et al. Lipid-lowering efficacy of the PCSK9 inhibitor evolocumab (AMG 145) in patients with type 2 diabetes: a meta-analysis of individual patient data. Lancet Diabetes Endocrinol. 2016;4:403-10.
63. Robinson JG, Nedergaard BS, Rogers WJ, et al. Effect of evolocumab or ezetimibe added to moderate- or high-intensity statin therapy on LDL-C lowering in patients with hypercholesterolemia: the LAPLACE-2 randomized clinical trial. JAMA. 2014;311:1870-82.
64. Preiss D. Should we worry about raised triglycerides: the controversy continues. In: 51st EASD Annual Meeting, Stockholm, Sweden; 2015.
65. Sattar N, Preiss D, Blom D, et al. Evaluation of the one-year efficacy, safety and glycaemic effects of evolocumab (AMG 145) in 4,802 subjects with, at high risk for, or at low risk for, diabetes mellitus. In: 51st EASD Annual Meeting, Stockholm, Sweden; 2015.
66. Stein EA, Giugliano RP, Koren MJ, et al. Efficacy and safety of evolocumab (AMG 145), a fully human monoclonal antibody to PCSK9, in hyperlipidaemic patients on various background lipid therapies: Pooled analysis of 1359 patients in four phase 2 trials. Eur Heart J. 2014;35:2249-59.
67. Toth PP, Descamps O, Genest J, et al. Pooled safety analysis of evolocumab in over 6000 patients from double-blind and open label extension studies. Circulation. 2017;135:1819-31.
68. Nissen SE, Stroes E, Dent-Acosta RE, et al. Efficacy and tolerability of evolocumab vs ezetimibe in patients with muscle-related statin intolerance: The GAUSS-3 randomized clinical trial. JAMA. 2016;315:1580-90.
69. Giugliano RP, Desai NR, Kohli P, et al. Efficacy, safety, and tolerability of a monoclonal antibody to proprotein convertase subtilisin/kexin type 9 in combination with a statin in patients with hypercholesterolaemia (LAPLACE-TIMI 57). Lancet. 2012;380:2007-17.
70. Robinson JG, Rogers WJ, Nedergaard BS, et al. Rationale and design of LAPLACE-2: A phase 3, randomized, double-blind, placebo-and ezetimibe-controlled trial evaluating the efficacy and safety of evolocumab in subjects with hypercholesterolemia on background statin therapy. Clin Cardiol. 2014;37: 195-203.
71. Dragan S, Serban MC, Banach M. Proprotein convertase subtilisin/kexin 9 inhibitors: an emerging lipid-lowering therapy? J Cardiovasc Pharmacol Ther. 2015;20:157-68.
72. Kotani K, Banach M. Lipoprotein(a) and inhibitors of proprotein convertase subtilisin/kexin type 9. J Thorac Dis. 2017;9:E78-82.
73. Momtazi AA, Banach M, Pirro M, et al. PCSK9 and diabetes: is there a link? Drug Discov Today. 2017;22:883-95.
74. Banach M, Rizzo M, Nikolic D, et al. Intensive LDL-cholesterol lowering therapy and neurocognitive function. Pharmacol Ther. 2017;170:181-91.
75. Katsiki N, Nikolic D, Montalto G, et al. The role of fibrate treatment in dyslipidemia: An overview. Curr Pharm Des. 2013;19:3124-31.
76. Nikolic D, Mikhailidis DP, Davidson MH, et al. ETC-1002: A future option for lipid disorders? Atherosclerosis. 2014;237:705-10.
77. Penson P, McGowan M, Banach M. Evaluating bempedoic acid for the treatment of hyperlipidaemia. Expert Opin Invest Drugs. 2017;26:251-9.
78. Ballantyne CM, McKenney JM, MacDougall DE, et al. Effect of ETC-1002 on serum low-density lipoprotein cholesterol in hypercholesterolemic patients receiving statin therapy. Am J Cardiol. 2016;117:1928-33.
79. Heber D, Yip I, Ashley JM, et al. Cholesterol-lowering effects of a proprietary Chinese red-yeast-rice dietary supplement. Am J Clin Nutr. 1999;69:231-6.
80. Trimarco B, Benvenuti C, Rozza F, et al. Clinical evidence of efficacy of red yeast rice and berberine in a large controlled study versus diet. Med J Nutr Metab. 2011;4:133-9.
81. Barrios V, Escobar C, Cicero AF, et al. A nutraceutical approach (Armolipid Plus) to reduce total and LDL cholesterol in individuals with mild to moderate dyslipidemia: Review of the clinical evidence. Atheroscler Suppl. 2017;24:1-15.
82. Thengodkar RR, Sivakami S. Degradation of chlorpyrifos by an alkaline phosphatase from the cyanobacterium spirulina platensis. Biodegradation. 2010;21:637-44.

83. Serban MC, Sahebkar A, Dragan S, et al. A systematic review and meta-analysis of the impact of Spirulina supplementation on plasma lipid concentrations. Clin Nutr. 2016;35:842-51.
84. Panahi Y, Sahebkar A, Parvin S, et al. A randomized controlled trial of anti-inflammatory effects of curcumin in patients with chronic sulphur mustard-induced skin complications. Ann Clin Biochem. 2012;49:580-8.
85. Sahebkar A. Curcuminoids for the management of hypertriglyceridaemia. Nat Rev Cardiol. 2014;11:123.
86. Epstein J, Sanderson IR, MacDonald TT. Curcumin as a therapeutic agent: The evidence of in vitro, animal and human studies. Br J Nutr. 2010;103: 1545-57.
87. Sahebkar A, Sabon N, Pirro M, et al. Curcumin: An effective adjunct in patients with statin-associated muscle symptoms? J Cachexia Sarcopenia Muscle. 2017;8:19-24.
88. Ganjali S, Blesso CN, Banach M, et al. Effects of curcumin on HDL functionality. Pharmacol Res. 2017;119:208-18.
89. Momtazi AA, Banach M, Pirro M, et al. Regulation of PCSK9 by nutraceuticals. Pharmacol Res. 2017;120:157-69.
90. Fitchet DH, Hegele RA, Verma S. Cardiology patient page. Statin intolerance. Circulation. 2015;131:e389-391.
91. Das MK, Ingole S, Hajare A, et al. Practicing behaviour of Indian physicians for the management of dyslipidemia versus 2016 ESC/EAS Guidelines for the Management of Dyslipidemia: ACCORDANCE Study, 2018(In Press).

CHAPTER 11

Nonfasting Lipid Levels: Clinical Relevance and Implications for Practice

Ajay K Sinha, Vikas Singh, Narendra Kumar

INTRODUCTION

Dyslipidemia is one of the most common risk factors for ischemic heart disease (IHD). Multiple studies focusing on conventional, nontraditional, and various novel risk factors of IHD have recognized dyslipidemia as a significant risk factor.[1] Lipid profile is the screening test for dyslipidemia where the total cholesterol (TC), triglycerides (TGs), high-density lipoprotein cholesterol (HDL-C), and low-density lipoprotein cholesterol (LDL-C) levels are tested. One of the challenges with lipid profile measurement is the need for sample collection exclusively in fasting state.[2,3] This is inconvenient to the patient and promotes noncompliance. Rationale for utilizing nonfasting lipid profiles in clinical practice are more accurate view of 24-hour lipids, time, and cost-efficiency, as well as endorsement by many societies including the American Heart Association.

RATIONALE FOR REQUIREMENT OF A FASTING SAMPLE

Postprandial changes in lipoprotein composition are known to occur, particularly the increase in TGs concentration which directly correlates with the meal fat and carbohydrate content.

The calculation of LDL-C using the Friedewald equation is significantly affected by the increased levels of TG.

Treatment goals are often based on the use of fasting samples for lipid measurement in many clinical trials and epidemiological studies.

Since, most people tend to eat food several times during the day, the postprandial state tends to predominate over a 24-hour duration. Therefore, generally, the lipid component of blood serum or plasma is obtained after 8 hours of fasting. The values obtained might not reflect accurate levels of the lipoprotein concentrations or the plasma lipid in the sample and may not be reliable risk marker for cardiovascular disease (CVD).[4,5] In addition, recent evidence has demonstrated that nonfasting TG concentrations are a better predictor of future coronary events compared to fasting TG, in both men and women. Hence, there is an urgent need to review the information available on the subject considering all pros and cons.

EMERGENCE OF NONFASTING LEVELS MEASUREMENT

There is a gap in scientific evidence to support superiority of fasting lipid profile compared to nonfasting one during evaluation of the overall CV risk assessment. In the last decade, scientific guidelines around the globe have encouraged the use of routine nonfasting lipid profiles. There has been paradigm shift in understanding fasting versus nonfasting lipid profile in certain countries, notably Denmark where standard clinical practice is for nonfasting lipid testing. As per the scientific guidelines issued from the Danish Society of Clinical Biochemistry recommending the use of random nonfasting lipid profiles as the benchmark for all laboratories in Denmark, and simultaneously suggesting physicians to reevaluate the TG levels in the fasting state when the nonfasting values are over 350 mg/dL (4 mmol/L).[6,7] In 2014, the National Institute for Health and Care Excellence (NICE) guidelines have also supported the use of nonfasting lipid measurement. The nonfasting lipid measurements simplifies the blood sampling for patients, general practitioners, laboratories, and hospital clinicians, and also improves patient compliance for testing for lipid.[8-10] There are some caveats that limit the wider adoption of nonfasting lipid estimation, including the following:

- Fasting lipid profile measurement is believed to provide more standardized measurement
- Nonfasting lipid profiles make calculation of LDL-C via the Friedewald equation invalid
- As fasting has been the clinical standard, it is unclear what values should be flagged as abnormal when using nonfasting rather than fasting plasma lipid profile.

LIPID COMPONENT MEASUREMENT

Total cholesterol, HDL-C, and TGs are measured directly. However, LDL-C can either be measured directly or calculated by the Friedewald equation, e.g., if TGs are 400 mg/dL (4.5 mmol/L) [by the formula—total cholesterol minus HDL-C minus TGs/2.2 (all in mmol/L), or minus TGs/5 with values in mg/dL].[11] Direct measurement of LDL-C is ideally preferred at TG concentrations more than or equal to 4.5 mmol/L (400 mg/dL).

Can Nonfasting Values be a Reliable Marker of Cardiovascular Diseases?

Often, the Friedewald equation is applied for fasting lipid profile and when the LDL-C is calculated using this formula with TG level of 400 mg/dL (4.5 mmol/L) is similar to LDL-C measured using either nonfasting and fasting lipid values. Therefore, there is no strong reason for a fasting sample for LDL measurement if TGs are not significantly raised.

Remnant cholesterol is another marker which is a significant causal risk factor for CVD and has been studied in detail. It is calculated as total cholesterol minus LDL-C minus HDL-C, using nonfasting or fasting lipid profiles.[12-14]

Non-HDL-C is calculated as total cholesterol minus HDL-C and is equivalent to LDL-C, remnant cholesterol, and lipoprotein(a) [Lp(a)] cholesterol combined. Several consensus papers and guidelines have supported the use of non-HDL-C for CVD risk prediction and does not require a fasting sample. Guidelines from ATP III and the Canadian Cardiovascular Society (CCS) have endorsed non-HDL-C as a secondary target for treatment of hyperlipidemia as it does not get altered by nonfasting condition.

For an accurate CVD risk prediction, additional measurement of Lp(a) is desirable. Whenever a patient is being screened for CV risk, Lp(a) should be ideally measured once for sure.[15] Due to the variation of Lp(a) levels up to 10% in any individual, its determination should be preferably included in all lipid profile estimations.

Triglyceride concentration increase during a fat tolerance test.[16] However, the increase in plasma TGs observed after usual food ingestion is not usually observed during a fat tolerance test.[17,18] As the Friedewald equation is used for calculation of LDL levels, which includes the TG concentration, thus estimated LDL is thought to be affected significantly by diet consumption. Although, the calculated LDL and directly measured cholesterol values are equivalent using both fasting and nonfasting samples. A modification of this formula may be used[19] when chylomicrons are high, which may be fairly accurate.

Several randomized cholesterol-lowering trials have used fasting level measurements, and for aliasing with evidence-based medicine, fasting blood sampling has often been the standard in day-to-day CV risk assessment. However, three major statin trials and plenty of population-based studies used random, nonfasting blood sampling, providing acceptable evidence to challenge the traditional practice of usage of fasting samples. Several large-scale registries and population-based studies including diabetic population from pediatric population to adult, both in female and male have now confirmed that plasma lipids and lipoproteins change only little with one's habitual food intake.[20] It applies to the most of individuals, but rarely some exhibit out of the box response.

How Much is the Difference Between Fasting and Nonfasting Samples?

During comparison of fasting with nonfasting lipid profile clinical studies, only little raised plasma TGs and insignificantly lesser total and LDL lipid levels were observed, with no change in HDL-C values. Such nonsignificant and transient changes in cholesterol levels seem to be clinically insignificant. Although, Langsted et al. observed a transient decrease in LDL lipid estimates of 23 mg/dL (0.6 mmol/L) after 1–3 hours of a meal consumption by a diabetic. It assumes clinical significance[21] especially when it is used as an argument to withhold statins for a patient. The maximal mean changes after 1–6 hours after a meal is considered to be clinically insignificant at +26 mg/dL (0.3 mmol/L) for TGs, 8 mg/dL (20.2 mmol/L) for total cholesterol, 8 mg/dL (20.2 mmol/L) for LDL-C, +8 mg/dL (0.2 mmol/L) for calculated remnant cholesterol, and 8 mg/dL (20.2 mmol/L) for calculated non-HDL-C, while concentrations for HDL-C, apolipoprotein A1, apolipoprotein B, and Lp(a) remained unchanged.[20,22] Interestingly, the reduction in LDL and total cholesterol levels at 1–3 hours after the last meal intake measured with and without diabetes became statistically nonsignificant after adjusting for plasma albumin concentration as a marker of fluid intake.

Is There Anything Against the Nonfasting Samples?

Several clinical studies have attributed marginal decrease in plasma LDL lipid level liberal fluids ingestion for nonfasting samples. This leads to changes although insignificant misclassification of CV risk, which, therefore, will lead to error in initiation of lipid therapy. Although this is associated with small risk, associated mostly with diabetics and is not a universal finding across the clinical studies.[21]

Nonfasting sample can possibly sometimes confuse the differentiation between familial hypercholesterolemia and congenital variants of high TGs. Pediatric population have highly variable plasma cholesterol levels and thus, necessitating for a fasting second sample for an accurate diagnosis of a lipid disorder needing drug therapy. Fasting is less critical for first-stage screening but may be more important when trying to establish a phenotypic diagnosis of genetically determined dyslipidemias.

Switching Your Practice Pattern from Fasting to Nonfasting Samples? Certain Facts to Keep in Mind

The lower LDL lipid levels observed especially in diabetics 1–6 hours after typical food intake needs to be kept in mind when using nonfasting cholesterol estimates to decide either

TABLE 1: When to use fasting and nonfasting blood samples for evaluating the plasma cholesterol profile

Patients for lipid profile testing	
Nonfasting	**Fasting**
• Initial lipid profile testing in any patient	• Nonfasting triglycerides 5 mmol/L (440 mg/dL)
• In children and elderly	• Known hypertriglyceridemia followed in lipid clinic
• For cardiovascular risk assessment	• Recovering from hypertriglyceridemic pancreatitis
• Patients admitted with acute coronary syndrome[a]	• Starting medications that cause severe hypertriglyceridemia
• In diabetic patients[b] (due to hypoglycemic risk)	• Additional laboratory tests are requested that require fasting[c] or morning samples (e.g., fasting glucose[c], therapeutic drug monitoring)
• Patients on stable drug therapy	
• If preferred by the patient	

[a]Repeated lipid profile testing is needed later as acute coronary syndrome lowers lipid concentrations.

[b]Diabetic hypertriglyceridemia may be masked by fasting.

[c]In many countries, fasting blood sampling is restricted to very few analytes besides lipid profiles: one example is fasting glucose; however, in many countries, even fasting glucose measurement is being replaced by measurement of hemoglobin A1c without the need to fast.

to start a statin or even modify its dosage. Interestingly, since the observed reduction in LDL lipid level is due to hemodilution and liberal water intake rather than to diet intake, a similar LDL reduction is likely to occur when using fasting lipid profiles with no restrictions on fluid intake.

Since statin therapy is decided not just on numerical value of plasma cholesterol in both European and US guidelines but rather on a person's comprehensive CV risk that includes the presence of CVD, familial hypercholesterolemia, and diabetes. Therefore, minor changes in the cholesterol level estimation to nonfasting conditions from fasting will affect only a few individuals regarding the decision to start a statin or not.

CONCLUSION

We mostly remain in the nonfasting state, reflecting "our habitual physiological status". Blood samples typically measured after 8–12 hours of fasting have been the standard for assessing the plasma lipid profile. Postprandial effects do not appear to diminish, and rather may in fact enhance the strength of the associations between plasma lipid, lipoprotein, and apolipoprotein concentrations and risk of CVD. A meta-analysis from the Emerging Risk Factors Collaboration suggested that nonfasting non-HDL-C and nonfasting calculated LDL-C were superior to fasting measurements for predicting CV risk.[23] Several prospective clinical studies have observed significant associations for nonfasting lipids, apolipoproteins, and lipoproteins with future risk of CVD. Therefore, numerous landmark statin therapy clinical trials have used nonfasting lipids for inclusion criteria and simultaneously for observing the therapeutic efficacy of lipid-lowering therapy. Such observations suggest that nonfasting blood level estimations is not only highly practical and effective but also advantageous in estimating cholesterol driven CVD risk and treatment responses.

A simple and practical approach recommendation to improve compliance of patients are to advice nonfasting cholesterol estimation for most individuals, while fasting sample may be considered for individuals with nonfasting plasma TG 440 mg/dL (5 mmol/L). Fasting can be a barrier to population screening, is unpopular with children, is often unsuitable for patients with diabetes, and counters the use of point-of-care testing, and fasting requirements can add to the overall costs of lipid testing. Nonfasting tests are also used to assess other metabolic disorders, such as hemoglobin A1c in diabetes.

Nonfasting and fasting measurements of the lipid profile must be viewed as complementary and not mutually exclusive.

A joint consensus statement from the European Atherosclerosis Society and European Federation of Clinical Chemistry and Laboratory Medicine summarized the practical utility of the fasting and nonfasting samples (Table 1).

Therefore, it is appears that the main reason for measuring lipid levels in the fasting rather than the nonfasting state is simply a custom worldwide; and due to this, the fasting requirement has been applied in almost all randomized lipid-lowering trials.

REFERENCES

1. Mendis S, Puska P, Norrving B. Global atlas on cardiovascular disease prevention and control. Geneva: World Health Organization; 2011.
2. Abideen ZU. To fast or not to fast? Choosing the best for serum lipid profile. J Pak Med Stud. 2013;3:101-2.
3. Mora S, Rifai N, Buring JE, et al. Fasting compared with nonfasting lipids and apolipoproteins for predicting incident cardiovascular events. Circulation. 2008;118:993-1001.
4. Rifai N, Warnick GR. Lipids, lipoproteins, apolipoproteins, and other cardiovascular risk factors. In: Burtis CA, Ashwood ER, Bruns DE (Eds). Tietz Textbook of Clinical Chemistry and Molecular Diagnostics. Philadelphia: Elsevier Health Sciences; 2012.
5. Simundic AM, Cornes M, Grankvist K, et al. Standardization of collection requirements for fasting samples: for the Working Group on Preanalytical Phase (WG-PA) of the European Federation of Clinical Chemistry and Laboratory Medicine (EFLM). Clinica Chimica Acta. 2014;432:33-7.
6. Nordestgaard BG, Hilsted L, Stender S. Plasma lipids in non-fasting patients and laboratory labeling values. Ugeskrift for læger. 2009;171:??.
7. Langsted A, Nordestgaard BG. Nonfasting lipids, lipoproteins, and apolipoproteins in individuals with and without diabetes: 58 434 individuals from the Copenhagen General Population Study. Clin Chem. 2011;57:482-9.
8. Watts GF, Cohn JS. Whither the lipid profile: feast, famine, or no free lunch? Clin Chem. 2011;57:363-5.
9. Gaziano JM. Should we fast before we measure our lipids? Arch Intern Med. 2012;172:1705-6.

10. Khera AV, Mora S. Fasting for lipid testing: is it worth the trouble? Arch Intern Med. 2012;172:1710-2.
11. Friedewald WT, Levy RI, Fredrickson DS. Estimation of the concentration of low density lipoprotein cholesterol in plasma, without use of the preparative ultracentrifuge. Clin Chem. 1972;18:499-502.
12. Varbo A, Benn M, Tybjaerg-Hansen A, et al. Remnant cholesterol as a causal risk factor for ischemic heart disease. J Am Coll Cardiol. 2013;61:427-36.
13. Varbo A, Benn M, Tybjaerg-Hansen A, et al. Elevated remnant cholesterol causes both low-grade inflammation and ischemic heart disease, whereas elevated low-density lipoprotein cholesterol causes ischemic heart disease without inflammation. Circulation. 2013;128:1298-309.
14. Nordestgaard BG, Varbo A. Triglycerides and cardiovascular disease. Lancet. 2014;384:626-35.
15. Kamstrup PR, Tybjaerg-Hansen A, Steffensen R, et al. Genetically elevated lipoprotein(a) and increased risk of myocardial infarction. JAMA. 2009;301: 2331-9.
16. Mihas C, Kolovou GD, Mikhailidis DP, et al. Diagnostic value of postprandial triglyceride testing in healthy subjects: a meta-analysis. Curr Vasc Pharmacol. 2011;9:271-80.
17. Klop B, Cohn JS, vanOostrom AJ, et al. Daytime triglyceride variability in men and women with different levels of triglyceridemia. Clin Chim Acta. 2011;412:2183-9.
18. Sidhu D, Naugler C. Fasting time and lipid levels in a community-based population: a cross-sectional study. Arch Intern Med. 2012;172:1707-10.
19. Martin SS, Blaha MJ, Elshazly MB, et al. Comparison of a novel method vs the Friedewald equation for estimating low density lipoprotein cholesterol levels from the standard lipid profile. JAMA. 2013;310:2061-8.
20. Steiner MJ, Skinner AC, Perrin EM. Fasting might not be necessary before lipid screening: a nationally representative cross-sectional study. Pediatrics. 2011;128:463-70.
21. Lund SS, Jensen T. Using nonfasting lipids—hemodilution or convenience? Clin Chem. 2011;57:1336-8.
22. Langsted A, Kamstrup PR, Nordestgaard BG. Lipoprotein(a): fasting and nonfasting levels, inflammation, and cardiovascular risk. Atherosclerosis. 2014;234:95-101.
23. Emerging Risk Factors Collaboration, Di Angelantonio E, Sarwar N, et al. Major lipids, apolipoproteins, and risk of vascular disease. JAMA. 2009;302:1993-2000.

SECTION 3

Diabetes and Heart

CHAPTER 12

Diabetes and Cardiovascular Disease: Implications of Recent Cardiovascular Outcome trials with Newer Anti-diabetic Drugs for Cardiovascular Protection

Prakash Deedwania

INTRODUCTION

Diabetes mellitus (DM) and coronary heart disorders (CHDs) are two of the most common noncommunicable diseases that are leading cause of death and disability in India. Diabetes increases the risk of most cardiovascular disorders (CVDs) by 2- to 4-fold and its presence in those with preexisting CVD is one of the most powerful predictors of adverse clinical outcome. It is important to note that although DM is considered as predominantly a metabolic condition primarily due to glycemic control perturbations it is now well recognized that most diabetic patients develop CVD and CV events are the leading cause of death and disability in DM. It is therefore essential that cardiologist be familiar with the implications of diabetes in their patients with DM and provide comprehensive therapeutic strategies to reduce the risk of CV events in their diabetic patients. Comprehensive CV risk reduction in DM should be focused on aggressive management of glycemic status, blood pressure (BP), lipids, as well as use of antithrombotic agents, and therapeutic lifestyle modification including recommendations for regular physical activities and prudent dietary modifications. In this chapter the primary focus will be centered on the clinical implications of the recent CV outcome trials (CVOTs) with a large number of newer antidiabetic drugs that have provided very encouraging and exciting data regarding their safety and in several cases cardioprotective efficacy in diabetic with preexisting CVD as well as those at high risk of future CV events.

BACKGROUND

Diabetes has reached epidemic proportions throughout the world. It is estimated that the number of cases of diabetes worldwide among adults 20 years or older is about 410 million and the prevalence is increasing with the number of cases projected to increase to over 640 million by the year 2040.[1]

The top three countries with the highest numbers of people with diabetes in are India, China, and the US. The greatest relative increases will occur in India, sub-Saharan Africa and the Middle East while the greatest absolute increase in the number of people with diabetes will be in India. India has the dubious distinction of being called as the "diabetes capital" of the world and is home to nearly 75 million cases of diabetes with a prevalence of 8.7% among the adult population.[1,2] The recent data from the Global Burden of Disease (GBD) the overall prevalence of DM increased by 66% between 1990–2016 from 3 to 5%, whereas age-standardized prevalence increased by 30% from 4.6 to 6%.[2] Also, the GBD data reveal that the number of deaths and DALYs due to DM have nearly tripled during the period from 1990–2016. These data also pointed out that DM significantly contributed to the causation of CHD, strokes, CKD, and peripheral artery disease (PAD). The factors responsible for these dramatic increases are increasing body mass index (obesity), dietary factors, and lack of regular physical activity.

It is now well recognized that CV frequently coexist with DM and CV events are the leading cause of death and disability in patients with DM. Individuals with diabetes have a 2- to 4- increase in the risk of cardiovascular disease (CVD) as compared to normal individuals (Fig. 1); there is also a higher case fatality rate in individuals with diabetes. CVD accounts

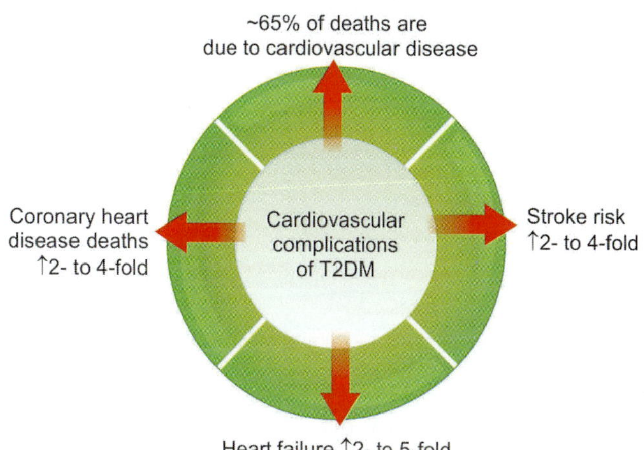

T2DM, type 2 diabetes mellitus.

FIG. 1: Showing the risk of cardiovascular events in diabetes mellitus.

for 60–75% of deaths in persons with DM. Much of the morbidity and mortality is from atherosclerotic coronary artery disease, cerebrovascular disease leading to stroke, congestive heart failure (CHF), PAD, and sudden cardiac death.

THERAPEUTIC STRATEGIES FOR CONTROL OF CARDIOVASCULAR DISEASE IN DIABETES

As mentioned earlier treatment strategies focused on the reduction of CVD and CV events in DM should consist of comprehensive risk reduction strategy which should be comprised of aggressive management of glycemic status, BP, lipids, as well as use of antithrombotic agents, and therapeutic lifestyle modification including recommendations for regular physical activities and prudent dietary modifications (Table 1).[3] Although, a number of studies in last two decades have demonstrated significant CV protection with the use of BP control, as well as lipid lowering therapy with statins in patients with DM the results of glucose lowering therapies with the traditional hypoglycemic agents have been rather disappointing.[4] Although, several trials conducted during the past decade evaluated the benefit of intensive glucose control with the available antidiabetic drugs these trials have generally failed to show significant benefit in reducing the risk of macrovascular events [such as myocardial infarction (MI) or stroke] despite demonstrating significant reductions in microvascular events such as diabetic nephropathy, retinopathy, and neuropathy (Table 2). The precise reason for the failure to achieve significant reduction in CV events

TABLE 1: Describing the multifactorial approaches for cardiovascular risk reduction in diabetes

Goals for risk-factor management in diabetes		
Risk factor	**Goal of therapy**	**Reference**
Cigarette smoking	Complete cessation	ADA
Blood pressure (with proteinuria)	<130/80 mm Hg <125/75 mm Hg	ACC/AHA 2017, ADA JNC 7, ADA
LDL-C	<100 mg/dL <70 mg/dL in high risk	2014 ACC/AHA guidelines, ADA 2018
Triglycerides 200–499 mg/dL	Non-HDL-C <130 mg/dL Triglyceride <150 mg/dL	2014 ACC/AHA guidelines, ADA 2018
Prothrombotic state	Low-dose aspirin therapy (patients with CHD and other high-risk patients)	ADA
Glucose	HbA1c <7%	ADA
Overweight and obesity (BMI ≥25 kg/m^2)	Lose 10% of body weight in a year	OEI
Physical inactivity	Excercise prescription dependent on patient status	ADA
Adverse nutrition	Diets lower in sturated fat and lower glycemic index (when necessary with caloric concentration)	A2014 ACC/AHA guidelines, ADA 2018 AHA

ACC/AHA, American College of Cardiology/American Heart Association; ADA, American Diabetes Association; BMI, body mass index; HDL, high-density lipoprotein; CHD, coronary heart disorders; LDL, low-density lipoprotein; OEI, obesity education initiative.

TABLE 2: Showing impact of intensive glucose lowering drugs on micro- and macrovascular events in diabetes

Intensive glucose control trials			
	A1c goals	**Microvascular complications**	**Macrovascular complications**
DCCT/EDIC Type 1 Diabetes	<6.05%	IT reduced overall microvascular complications	Trend toward lower risk of CVD events with IT 10-year post-trial follow-up: significant reductions in CVD outcomes and risk of nonfatal MI, stroke, or CVD death with IT
UKPDS Type 2 Diabetes	(used FPG goals)	Relationship between glucose control and microvascular complications extended into range of normal A1c, with no glycemic threshold	16% reduction in CV complications with IT
Advance Type 2 Diabetes	≤6.5% (IT) Local guidelines (CT)	IT significantly reduced overall microvascular complications	No significant reduction in CV outcomes with IT
VADT Type 2 Diabetes	<6.0% (IT) Planned separation of 1.5% (CT)	No significant reduction in microvascular complications with IT	
Accord Type 2 Diabetes	<6.0% (IT) 7.0–7.0% (CT)	Terminated glycemic control study because of increased mortality in patients receiving IT with A1c <6%	

ACCORD, Action to control cardiovascular risk in diabetes; CVD, cardiovascular disorders; DCCT/EDIC, Diabetes Control and Complications Trial/Epidemiology of Diabetic Interventions and Complications; UKPDS, UK, Prospective Diabetes Study; VADT, Veterans' Affairs Diabetes Trial; MI, myocardial infarction; IT, intensive therapy; CT, conventional therapy; FPG, fasting plasma glucose.

remains to be established, it has been suggested that the lack of favorable effect on CV events might be related to adverse effects of resultant hypoglycemia with the use of multiple hypoglycemic agents to achieve intensive glycemic control.

However, the scenario has changed dramatically with the recent introduction of several newer classes of hypoglycemic agents which have been tested in large prospective randomized clinical trials in patients with either preexisting CVD or those at high risk of CVD. These CVOTs have been conducted based on the 2008 Food and Drug Administration (FDA) mandate to demonstrate safety of all newer hypoglycemic agents prior to seeking approval. The following review is a concise synthesis of these new trial data from CVOTs for the clinical cardiologist as the clinicians must familiarize themselves with these drugs as they will become important part of therapeutic armamentarium for diabetic patients with pre-existing CVD or at future risk of CVD as evidenced by recent approval by the FDA of several of these agents for CV protection.

ROLE OF ANTIDIABETIC (HYPOGLYCEMIC) MEDICATIONS IN CARDIOVASCULAR PROTECTION

Hypoglycemic drugs, through various mechanisms of action lower blood glucose and effectively reduce microvascular target end-organ damage like retinopathy, nephropathy, and neuropathy.[4] However, there did not appear to be a strong and convincing relationship between the lowering of blood sugar [as evidenced by glycated hemoglobin (HbA1c) reduction] and reduction in CV events with the traditional drugs.[5-8] Additionally, some of the beneficial effects are mitigated by episodes of hypoglycemia that were associated increased risk of CV events and cardiac as well as all-cause mortality.[9-12]

The increased risk of heart failure (HF) and concerns about MI with the use of thiazolidinediones (rosiglitazone and pioglitazone) led to heightened awareness of potentially harmful CV effects of these otherwise effective hypoglycemic drugs and has resulted in drastic reduction in their clinical use. In response to the concerns of increased CV risk, the FDA and other regulatory agencies mandated all new diabetes drugs to demonstrate CV safety.[13-15] Since, the primary use of a hypoglycemic drug is to control blood glucose (as demonstrated by lowering HbA1c), it was required that all new drugs would be approved for marketing only after adequately powered RCTs could demonstrate that such treatment would not be associated with unacceptably high rates of CV events in the phase-3 clinical trials (upper bound of the 95% confidence interval for major adverse CV event not to exceed 1.8). Postapproval, a phase-4 CV safety outcome trial in high-risk patients (with pre-existing CVD) would need to further demonstrate a CV event rate not exceeding the upper bound of the 95% confidence interval of 1.3. A minimum of 2-year follow-up data would be required with independent adjudication of CV outcomes.

As a result of this mandate, the last half-decade has seen a steady stream of CV safety trials in patients with pre-existing CVD or those at risk of CVD (Fig. 2). And, although, these CVOTs were designed to demonstrate safety, some of the trials have shown unprecedented CV benefit in secondary prevention of CV events and related outcomes (Fig. 2). It is therefore critical for the cardiologist to familiarize with these newer therapies and results of these CVOTs so that they can prescribe the appropriate drugs for their diabetic patients with CVD or at risk of CVD to provide maximum CV protection and reduce the risk of future CV events. The following is a review of the newer hypoglycemic agents tested in the recent CVOTs.

Large CV Outcomes Trials in Diabetes

Study	SAVOR	EXAMINE	TECOS	CAROLINA	CARMELINA
DPP-4-inhibitors	saxagliptin	alogliptin	sitagliptin	linagliptin	linagliptin
Comparator	plac[illegible]	placeb[illegible]	placeb[illegible]	sulfonylurea	placebo
n	NEUTRAL	NEUTRAL	NEUTRAL	6,000	8,300
Results	2013	2013	2015	2017	2017

Study	EMPA-REG	CANVAS	DECLARE	VERTIS CV Study
SGLT-2 inhibitors	empagliflozin	canaglifl[illegible] CV BENEFIT	dapagliflozin	ertugliflozin
Comparator	pla[illegible] CV BENEFIT	[illegible]ebo	placebo	placebo
n	[illegible]	4,300	22,200	8,000
Results	2015	2017	2019	2019

Study	LEADER	ELIXA	SUSTAIN 6	EXSCEL	REWIND
GLP-1 RA	liraglutide	lixisenatide	semaglutide	exenatide LR	dulaglutide
Comparator	plac[illegible] CV BENEFIT	pl[illegible] NEUTRAL	[illegible] CV BENEFIT	[illegible] NEUTRAL	placebo
n	[illegible]	[illegible],000	[illegible],000	[illegible],400	8,300
Results	2015	2015	2016	2017	2019

GLP-1, glucagon-like-peptide 1; DPP-4, dipeptidyl peptidase-4; SGLT-2, sodium-glucose co-transporter 2.

FIG. 2: Showing summary of recent cardiovascular (CV) outcome trials with newer antidiabetic agents.

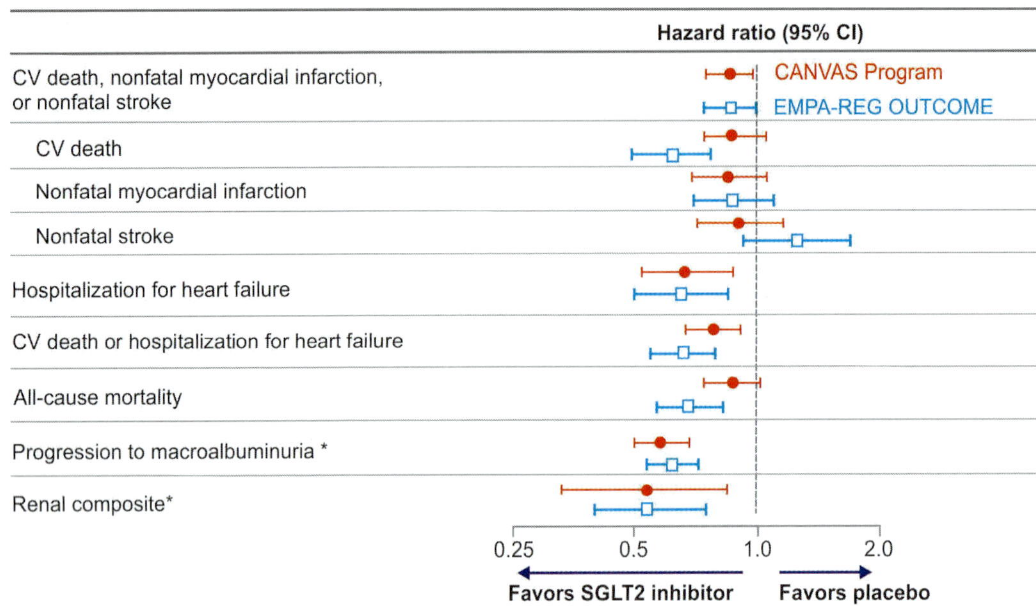

*CANVAS Program endpoints comparable with EMPA-REG OUTCOME.

CI, confidence interval; CV, cardiovascular; SGLT2, sodium-glucose co-transporter 2.

FIG. 3: Showing comparison of the EMPA-REG and CANVAS trials on major cardiovascular and renal outcomes.

Dipeptidyl Peptidase-4 Inhibitors

Dipeptidyl peptidase 4 (DPP-4) inhibitors prolong the activity of glucagon-like-peptide 1 (GLP-1) the gastric-inhibitory-peptide, and other incretins by preventing their breakdown.[16] The agents in this class have modest HbA1c reductions, but their appeal lies in that they do not cause hypoglycemia or weight gain.[16] Three DPP-4 inhibitors namely saxagliptin, alogliptin, and sitagliptin have been tested in CVOTs (SAVOR-TIMI 53, EXAMINE, and TECOS, respectively).[17-19] None were found to increase adverse CV events, CV mortality, or all-cause mortality (Tables 1 and 2). Neither was there a signal of CV benefit.

Heart failure hospitalizations were, however, a concern with this class of drugs. SAVOR-TIMI 53 showed an unexpected 27% increased risk of HF` hospitalizations (3.5% vs. 2.8%) with saxagliptin. This adverse effect was not initially apparent with alogliptin in the main report of the EXAMINE study. But a subsequent *post-hoc* analysis suggested increased HF hospitalizations (2.2% vs. 1.3%) in patients without a history of HF [hazard ratio (HR) 1.76 (1.07–2.90)] but no increase in those with pre-existing HF [1.00 (0.71–1.42)].[20] In 2015, the FDA issued a safety warning for the risk of HF risk with saxagliptin and alogliptin.[21] No signal of increased HF hospitalizations was seen with sitagliptin in TECOS.

Sodium-glucose Co-transporter 2 Inhibitors

Sodium-glucose co-transporter 2 (SGLT2) is a low affinity, high capacity sodium-glucose co-transporter in the proximal renal tubules and is responsible for glucose reabsorption. SGLT2 inhibitors are orally administered drugs that block this receptor, thereby, preventing glucose reabsorption into the blood stream and facilitating elimination of glucose in the urine (glycosuria). As a result, these agents also have a diuretic effect and promote weight and BP reduction by sodium and water loss.[22]

EMPA-REG OUTCOME trial evaluated the CV effects of 10 mg or 25 mg of empagliflozin added to standard therapy in diabetic patients with known CVD and demonstrated impressive results.[23] The primary composite outcome of CV death, MI, and stroke occurred less frequently with empagliflozin (10.5% compared to 12.1% in the placebo group; p = 0.04 for superiority) (Fig. 3). This difference was largely driven by significantly lower CV death in the treatment group (3.7% vs. 5.9%; p < 0.001) without significant differences in MI or stroke rates. All-cause death was also reduced with empagliflozin (5.7% vs 8.3%; p <0.001). Most interestingly, empagliflozin reduced HF admissions by 35% (2.7% vs. 4.1%; p = 0.002). This was a major paradigm shift from the previous hypoglycemic medications that either had no effect or increased HF hospitalizations (rosiglitazone, saxagliptin). Also, the beneficial CV effects of empagliflozin appeared much earlier than GLP-1 analogs like liraglutide suggesting a prominent hemodynamic rather than anti-atherosclerotic mechanism of action. The robustness of HF outcomes in the EMPA-REG OUTCOME trial have been debated due to the lack of cardiac function and biomarker assessment (**such as brain natriuretic peptide**) which are otherwise a norm in most HF trials. Additionally, in subgroup analysis, HF hospitalizations were statistically significantly reduced in patients without HF at baseline but not in those with HF.[24] Trials specifically evaluating HF outcomes are now underway.[25] Regardless, **prior to these findings, no glucose-lowering drug had shown an improvement in HF outcomes in patients with diabetes.**

Canagliflozin was the second SGLT2 inhibitor to undergo a CV safety trial (CANVAS)[26] and consistent with results of EMPA-REG OUTCOME, showed reduction in HF hospitalization (5.5% vs. 8.7%) (Fig. 3). Canagliflozin was shown to be superior to placebo in reducing the primary combined outcome of CV death, MI, and stroke (26.9% vs. 31.5%; p = 0.02), but did not improvement any of these outcomes individually. However, the reduction in the HF related outcome was identical to that observed with empagliflozin in the EMPA-REG OUTCOME trial.

Apart from CV benefits modulated through osmotic diuresis, reduction in weight, arterial stiffness, and left ventricular afterload, and overall modulation of the cardiorenal axis, SGLT2 inhibitors also reduce the progression of renal disease and delay the need for dialysis.[25,27] This is a major advantage in diabetic patients where renal disease is an important cause of progressive morbidity and mortality.

Prescribing physicians must be cognizant of some known adverse effects of SGLT2 inhibits. Since SGLT2 inhibitors act by inducing glycosuria, superficial genital mycotic infections (especially in women and uncircumcised men) are more common with their use. Their use can also be associated with increased risk of UTIs and diabetic ketoacidosis (rare). Increased amputation and bone fractures with canagliflozin in the CANVAS trial are also concerning. The FDA has issued a warning to avoid canagliflozin in patients that may be at a higher risk for amputations.[28]

Glucagon-like Peptide 1 Analogs

Glucagon-like peptide 1 analogs are a class of injectable hypoglycemic drugs that activate the endogenous GLP-1 receptor. They promote glucose-dependent insulin release, inhibit glucagon secretion, and delay gastric emptying.[29]

Lixisenatide, liraglutide, semaglutide, and most recently exenatide have been tested in CVOTs (ELIXA[30], LEADER[31], SUSTAIN-6[32], and EXSCEL[33] respectively) while dulaglutide is currently being tested (REWIND).[34] It is apparent from the results of the published trials that the benefits of GLP1 analogs may not be a class effect. While LEADER and SUSTAIN-6 were able to demonstrate CV event reduction, the results of ELIXA not as encouraging, and EXCEL showed no benefit.

ELIXA showed a neutral CV effect of shorter-acting lixisenatide (daily injection) added to standard therapy in diabetic patients who had an MI or unstable angina episode in the preceding 6 months. The positive results of the subsequent LEADER trial came as a surprise. Not only was liraglutide (daily injection) noninferior to placebo, it was superior in reducing the primary composite outcome of CV death, MI, and stroke (13% vs. 14.9% in placebo; p = 0.01). The reduction in the primary endpoint was driven by significantly lower CV mortality (4.7% vs. 6%; p = 0.007). Moreover, liraglutide reduced all-cause mortality as well (8.2% vs. 9.6%; p = 0.02). While there was numerical reduction in MI and stroke rates, this did not reach statistical significance. SUSTAIN-6, which had similar inclusion criteria as LEADER (Table 1), also showed composite CV event reduction (6.6% vs. 8.9%; p = 0.02) with semaglutide (weekly injection), which was driven by a significant reduction in strokes (1.6% vs 2.7%; p = 0.04) rather than CV mortality or MI.

Neither liraglutide nor semaglutide had a significant effect on HF admissions, suggesting a different mechanism of action than SGLT2 inhibitors. Though not completely understood, it has been postulated that these drugs may have more of an antiatherothrombotic effect. Other positive effects like BP lowering, weight reduction, and avoidance of hypoglycemia may contribute to improved CV outcomes.[35]

As mentioned, the CV benefits of GLP-1 agonists are not consistent across this class of medications. The recently published EXSCEL trial comparing exenatide weekly injection to placebo in diabetic patients, majority (73%) of whom had preexisting did not show a signal for benefit in any of the CV outcomes.[33] Results of the REWIND trial evaluating CV outcomes with dulaglutide (weekly injection) are expected in 2018.[34]

Gastrointestinal side effects, driven by delayed gastric emptying, are an important consideration while prescribing GLP1 agonists and may be a reason for nonadherence or discontinuation of the medication.

CONCLUSION AND FUTURE DIRECTION

The current global epidemic of DM with the attendant CVD poses a big challenge to health and quality of life of large populations. India is in the midst of the epidemic of DM and CHD with an increasing number of individuals being affected by these disorders in the prime of their careers. With this perspective, the current understanding of DM as a vascular as well as metabolic disorder is very important. Although, in the past glucose control with the traditional hypoglycemic agents including insulin failed to result in any significant CV benefit the recent CVOTs have provided clinicians with a new set of antidiabetic drugs with proven CV benefit in patients with diabetes and CVdiseased. New medications like empagliflozin and liraglutide improve not only CV mortality but also all-cause mortality in diabetic patients with CVD. The FDA has approved both empagliflozin and liraglutide to reduce the risk of CV death in adults with diabetes and CVD. It is important to keep in mind that these drugs in all of the CVOTs were used in addition to metformin as the baseline therapy in all patients so the clinician must still consider metformin as the first-line antidiabetic medication in most patients, if it is well tolerated. Additionally, SGLT2 inhibitors like empagliflozin and canagliflozin reduce HF hospitalizations. If the results of the ongoing trials with empagliflozin in HF patients prove their utility these drugs can be considered as additional choice for the treatment of CHF patients.

As many cardiac patients will present with coexisting DM it is critical for the clinician to understand the therapeutic strategies to reduce the risk of future CV events in such patients. As stated earlier, this can only be achieved with a comprehensive risk factor management (ABCDE approach) consisting of glycemic control (HbA1c <7%), BP control (<130/85 mm Hg), cholesterol lowering therapy with statins (LDL-C <70), dietary modification (low glycemic index foods with low saturated fat and caloric restriction, exercise on a regular basis (>30 minutes × 5 times/week).

There is an immediate need for clinicians to embrace the evidence and switch from traditional diabetes medications to newer therapies with proven CV benefit. Physician education and increasing awareness of these persuasive clinical trial results will increase their comfort level in making this transition to provide cardioprotective therapy in their patients with diabetes and CVD and those at high risk of future CV events.[35]

REFERENCES

1. IDF. (2015). IDF Diabetes Atlas, 7th edition (2015). [online]. Available from https://www.idf.org/e-library/epidemiology-research/diabetes-atlas/13-diabetes-atlas-seventh-edition.html [Accessed August, 2018].
2. Tripathy JP. Burden and risk factors of diabetes and hyperglycemia in India: findings from the Global Burden of Disease Study 2016. Diabetes Metab Syndr Obes. 2018;11:381-7.
3. Gaede P, Valentine WJ, Palmer AJ, et al. Cost-effectiveness of intensified versus conventional multifactorial intervention in type 2 diabetes: results and projections from the Steno-2 study. Diabetes Care. 2008;31:1510-5.
4. Intensive blood-glucose control with sulphonylureas or insulin compared with conventional treatment and risk of complications in patients with type 2 diabetes (UKPDS 33). UK Prospective Diabetes Study (UKPDS) Group. Lancet. 1998;352:837-53.
5. Wong MG, Perkovic V, Chalmers J, et al. Long-term Benefits of Intensive Glucose Control for Preventing End-Stage Kidney Disease: ADVANCE-ON. Diabetes Care. 2016;39:694-700.
6. Turnbull FM, Abraira C, Anderson RJ, et al. Intensive glucose control and macrovascular outcomes in type 2 diabetes. Diabetologia. 2009;52:2288-98.
7. Gerstein HC, Miller ME, Ismail-Beigi F, et al. Effects of intensive glycaemic control on ischaemic heart disease: analysis of data from the randomised, controlled ACCORD trial. Lancet. 2014;384:1936-41.
8. Hayward RA, Reaven PD, Wiitala WL, et al. Follow-up of glycemic control and cardiovascular outcomes in type 2 diabetes. N Engl J Med. 2015;372:2197-206.
9. Gerstein HC, Miller ME, Byington RP, et al. Effects of intensive glucose lowering in type 2 diabetes. N Engl J Med. 2008;358:2545-59.
10. Lago RM, Singh PP, Nesto RW. Congestive heart failure and cardiovascular death in patients with prediabetes and type 2 diabetes given thiazolidinediones: a meta-analysis of randomised clinical trials. Lancet. 2007;370:1129-36.
11. Home PD, Pocock SJ, Beck-Nielsen H, et al. Rosiglitazone evaluated for cardiovascular outcomes—an interim analysis. N Engl J Med. 2007;357:28-38.
12. Nissen SE, Wolski K. Effect of rosiglitazone on the risk of myocardial infarction and death from cardiovascular causes. N Engl J Med. 2007;356:2457-71.
13. US Department of Health and Human Services, Food and Drug Administration. (2008). Guidance for industry: diabetes mellitus—evaluating cardiovascular risk in new antidiabetic therapies to treat type 2 diabetes. [online]. Available from http://www.fda.gov/downloads/drugs/guidancecomplianceregulatoryinformation/guidances/ucm071627.pdf [Accessed August, 2018].
14. European Medicines Agency. (2012). Guideline on clinical investigation of medicinal products in the treatment or prevention of diabetes mellitus. [online]. Available from http://www.ema.europa.eu/docs/en_GB/document_library/Scientific_guideline/2012/06/WC500129256.pdf [Accessed August, 2018].
15. Hiatt WR, Kaul S, Smith RJ. The cardiovascular safety of diabetes drugs—insights from the rosiglitazone experience. N Engl J Med. 2013;369:1285-7.
16. Zhong J, Maiseyeu A, Davis SN, et al. DPP4 in cardiometabolic disease: recent insights from the laboratory and clinical trials of DPP4 inhibition. Circ Res. 2015;116:1491-504.
17. Scirica BM, Bhatt DL, Braunwald E, et al. SAVOR-TIMI 53 Steering Committee and Investigators. Saxagliptin and cardiovascular outcomes in patients with type 2 diabetes mellitus. N Engl J Med. 2013;369:1317-26.
18. White WB, Cannon CP, Heller SR, et al. EXAMINE Investigators. Alogliptin after acute coronary syndrome in patients with type 2 diabetes. N Engl J Med. 2013;369:1327-35.
19. Green JB, Bethel MA, Armstrong PW, et al. TECOS Study Group. Effect of sitagliptin on cardiovascular outcomes in type 2 diabetes. N Engl J Med. 2015;373:232-42.
20. Zannad F, Cannon CP, Cushman WC, et al. EXAMINE Investigators. Heart failure and mortality outcomes in patients with type 2 diabetes taking alogliptin versus placebo in EXAMINE: a multicentre, randomised, double-blind trial. Lancet. 2015;385:2067-76.
21. FDA. (2014). FDA Drug Safety Communication: FDA adds warnings about heart failure risk to labels of type 2 diabetes medicines containing saxagliptin and alogliptin. [online]. Available from https://www.fda.gov/downloads/Drugs/DrugSafety/UCM493965.pdf [Accessed August, 2018].
22. Abdul-Ghani MA, Norton L, Defronzo RA. Role of sodium-glucose cotransporter 2 (SGLT 2) inhibitors in the treatment of type 2 diabetes. Endocr Rev. 2011;32:515-31.
23. Zinman B, Wanner C, Lachin JM, et al. EMPA-REG OUTCOME Investigators. Empagliflozin, cardiovascular outcomes, and mortality in type 2 diabetes. N Engl J Med. 2015;373:2117-28.
24. Fitchett D, Zinman B, Wanner C, et al. Heart failure outcomes with empagliflozin in patients with type 2 diabetes at high cardiovascular risk: results of the EMPA-REG OUTCOME trial. Eur Heart J. 2016;37:1526-34.
25. ClinicalTrials.gov. (2017). EMPagliflozin outcomE tRial in Patients With chrOnic heaRt Failure With Reduced Ejection Fraction (EMPEROR-Reduced). [online]. Available from https://clinicaltrials.gov/ct2/show/NCT03057977 [Accessed August, 2018].
26. Neal B, Perkovic V, Mahaffey KW, et al. CANVAS Program Collaborative Group. Canagliflozin and Cardiovascular and Renal Events in Type 2 Diabetes. N Engl J Med. 2017;377:644-57.
27. Wanner C, Inzucchi SE, Lachin JM, et al. EMPA-REG OUTCOME Investigators. Empagliflozin and Progression of Kidney Disease in Type 2 Diabetes. N Engl J Med. 2016;375:323-34.
28. FDA. (2017). FDA Drug Safety Communication: FDA confirms increased risk of leg and foot amputations with the diabetes medicine canagliflozin (Invokana, Invokamet, Invokamet XR). [online]. Available from https://www.fda.gov/Drugs/DrugSafety/ucm557507.htm?source=govdelivery&utm_medium=email&utm_source=govdelivery [Accessed August, 2018].
29. Gupta A, Jelinek HF, Al-Aubaidy H. Glucagon like peptide-1 and its receptor agonists: Their roles in management of Type 2 diabetes mellitus. Diabetes Metab Syndr. 2017;11:225-30.
30. Pfeffer MA, Claggett B, Diaz R, et al. ELIXA Investigators. Lixisenatide in patients with type 2 diabetes and acute coronary syndrome. N Engl J Med. 2015;373:2247-57.
31. Marso SP, Daniels GH, Brown-Frandsen K, et al. Liraglutide and cardiovascular outcomes in type 2 diabetes. N Engl J Med. 2016;375:311-22.
32. Marso SP, Bain SC, Consoli A, et al. SUSTAIN-6 Investigators. Semaglutide and cardiovascular outcomes in patients with type 2 diabetes. N Engl J Med. 2016;375:1834-44.
33. Holman RR, Bethel MA, Mentz RJ, et al. EXSCEL Study Group. Effects of Once-Weekly Exenatide on Cardiovascular Outcomes in Type 2 Diabetes. N Engl J Med. 2017;377:1228-39.
34. Gerstein HC, Colhoun HM, Dagenais GR, et al. Design and baseline characteristics of participants in the Researching cardiovascular Events with a Weekly INcretin in Diabetes (REWIND) trial on the cardiovascular effects of dulaglutide. Diabetes Obes Metab. 2018 Jan;20(1):42-9.
35. Nassif ME, Kosiborod M. Are we ready to Bell the Cat?: A call for Cardiologists to Embrace Glucose-Lowering Therapies Proven to Improve Cardiovascular Outcomes .Circulation 2018;138: 4-6.

CHAPTER 13

Diabetes Classification New Dimensions

Jugal Kishor Sharma, Amit Gupta

INTRODUCTION: DIABETES A JOURNEY FROM ANTIQUITY TO 21ST CENTURY

Diabetes mellitus is known to mankind since antiquity with the first mention of the disease dated as early as 1500 BC. However the first clinical description was given by Sushruta 1000 years later.[1] Over the centuries diabetes has seen many changes with respect to its origin, pathophysiology, diagnosis, classification, management, and complications and a plethora of literature is available on diabetes. Some of the milestones in history of diabetes are worth remembering. These milestones may be as trivial as someone noticing that ants were attracted to urine of patients with diabetes (Ancient Indian Literature) to the more complex ones like identification of islets of Langerhans by Paul Langerhans in 1869[2] in pancreas and path breaking discovery of insulin in November 1921 by Banting and Best.[3] In 21st century diabetes has become a global challenge and can truly be called as a disease without borders.

TABLE 1: American Diabetes Association classification of diabetes (2017)

Type of diabetes	Pathophysiology
Type 1 diabetes	• Autoimmune β-cell destruction-absolute insulin deficiency
Type 2 diabetes	• Progressive loss of β-cell function along with insulin resistance
Gestational diabetes mellitus	• Associated with pregnancy
Miscellaneous	• MODY (maturity onset diabetes of young/monogenic diabetes) • LADA (latent autoimmune diabetes of adults) • Neonatal diabetes • Diseases of exocrine pancreas/fibro-calcific pancreatic diabetes (FCPD) • Drug or chemical induced diabetes

DIABETES CLASSIFICATION: HISTORY

First attempt to standardize the nomenclature and definition of diabetes was made in 1979 by a consensus statement given by National Diabetes Data Group[4] which was also endorsed 1 year later by World Health Organization (WHO). Based on the consensus diabetes was divided into two major types viz. insulin-dependent diabetes mellitus (IDDM) and noninsulin-dependent diabetes mellitus (NIDDM). This classification because of its inherent limitations added to the confusion. The classification and diagnostic criteria were again revised in 1997 and diabetes was classified into four types.[5] The American Diabetes Association (ADA) classifies diabetes as described in ADA standards of care 2017[6] into four types (Table 1).

A systematic review "Incorrect and Incomplete Coding and Classification of Diabetes: a Systematic Review" published in 2010 in Diabetic Medicine[7] drew attention to the implications for the incorrect and incomplete classification of diabetes. Stone MA et al. highlighted the often seen dilemma of differentiating between type 1 and type 2 diabetes mellitus especially in young patients. It also brought to the notice that there were consistent failures in recognizing other clinical subtype like maturity onset diabetes of young (MODY) and latent autoimmune diabetes of adults (LADA).[8]

DIABETES CLASSIFICATION: WHY DO WE NEED A NEW CLASSIFICATION SYSTEM?

Traditionally diabetes is classified into two types: type 1 and type 2. Type 1 and type 2 diabetes most likely only represent two extremes of hyperglycemia with multiple possibilities in between ranging from MODY, LADA, ketosis-prone diabetes (KPD), Fibrocalcific pancreatic diabetes (FCPD), gestational diabetes mellitus (GDM), Neonatal diabetes, and various secondary forms of diabetes.[9] There is enough evidence to consider Alzheimer's disease (AD) as type 3 diabetes characterized by insulin deficiency and insulin resistance leading to Alzheimer's type neurodegeneration with selective involvement of brain.[10] Glaucoma, an irreversible cause of blindness is also called as diabetes of brain and researchers say its type 4 diabetes.[11]

Diabetes results from interplay between genetic and environmental factors, while genetics determines susceptibility to the disease, the environment (lifestyle factors, physical activity, infections, obesity, and nutrition) plays a vital role in shaping the clinical phenotype of the patient with diabetes. Most of us have seen and experienced in our clinical settings that all diabetic patients are not alike. Some of the patients respond well to even low doses of medications and remain stable for decades while others do not respond even to multiple drugs including insulin and in such patient's disease progresses rapidly with development of multiple complications, earlier than that predicted by natural history of diabetes.

There is no perfect classification system for diabetes and current classification systems are not adequate. Diabetes is one of the diseases which has grown at a tremendous pace over the last few decades and poses a significant threat to human health. Diabetes is a chronic progressive disease and is associated with systemic complications. There have been several recent advances in the management of diabetes and its complications but yet there are challenges and unmet needs as we are not yet able to slow the progression of the disease or accurately predict the complications. There are challenges with the diagnosis as well as its management. Diabetes is a heterogeneous disease and current classification schemes do not seems to fulfill the requirement of an ideal classification system. An ideal classification system may be the one which serves as a guiding tool to both the researchers as well as clinicians. It must also address the patient centric issues like therapeutic education, evaluation of outcome with focus on prevention of the complications. It shall also help the clinicians to design the best management plan for the patient while incorporating current guidelines-based best practices. Nonetheless diagnostic criteria for diabetes are also based on single entity, i.e., glucose. This heterogeneity of diabetes warrants a new approach to classify diabetes which can be more meaningful to the patients, researchers, and clinicians.

NEW PROPOSED CLASSIFICATION OF DIABETES

In 2016, an article titled "The Time Is Right for a New Classification System for Diabetes: Rationale and Implications of the β-Cell-Centric Classification Schema" published in Diabetes Care, Stanley et al. emphasized on β-cell centric classification.[12] They proposed that all types of diabetes originate in abnormal β-cells which are further influenced by environmental, genetic, and immune components. The β-cell stress, abnormal β-cell function or losses of β-cells by more than dozen factors are central to development of diabetes. Though Stanley et al. could rationally explain the need for revision and reclassification they only urgently called for the review of the current diabetes mellitus classification system toward the consensus on a new and hopefully more useful and meaningful system.

Recently a paper published in Lancet by Ahlqvist Emma, et al. suggested novels subgroups of adult onset diabetes and their association with outcomes which can serve as a powerful tool for deciding treatment and identifying individuals who are at greater risk of developing complications.[13] The new classification of diabetes suggested by the authors was based on unsupervised data driven cluster analysis of six commonly measured variables in four separate population groups from Finland and Sweden. The variables consisted of glutamate decarboxylase antibodies (GADA), age at onset, body mass index (BMI), glycated hemoglobin (HbA1c), homeostatic model assessment 2 estimates of β-cell function, and insulin resistance were compared metabolically, genetically, and clinically. The study identified five clusters of patients with diabetes which were replicable. Based on the study adult onset diabetes can be classified into five types. These types are severe autoimmune diabetes (SAID), severe insulin deficiency diabetes (SIDD), severe insulin resistance diabetes (SIRD), mild obesity-related diabetes (MORD), and mild age-related diabetes (MARD) (Table 2).

TABLE 2: New proposed classification of diabetes

Type of diabetes	Autoantibody GAD	BMI	Metabolic control	Insulin deficiency or resistance (HOMA-β and HOMA-IR)
SAID	Positive	Low BMI	Poor	Insulin deficiency
SIDD	Negative	Low BMI	Poor	Insulin deficiency
SIRD	Negative	High BMI	Poor	Severe insulin resistance
MORD	Negative	High BMI	Modest metabolic derangements	Mild or no insulin resistance
MARD	Negative	Variable BMI	Modest metabolic derangements	Mild or no insulin resistance

BMI, body mass index; GAD, glutamic acid decarboxylase; HOMA-β, homeostatic model assessment for beta-cell function; HOMA-IR, homeostatic model assessment for insulin resistance; MARD, mild age-related diabetes; MORD, mild obesity-related diabetes; SAID, severe autoimmune diabetes; SIDD, severe insulin deficiency diabetes; SIRD, severe insulin resistant diabetes.

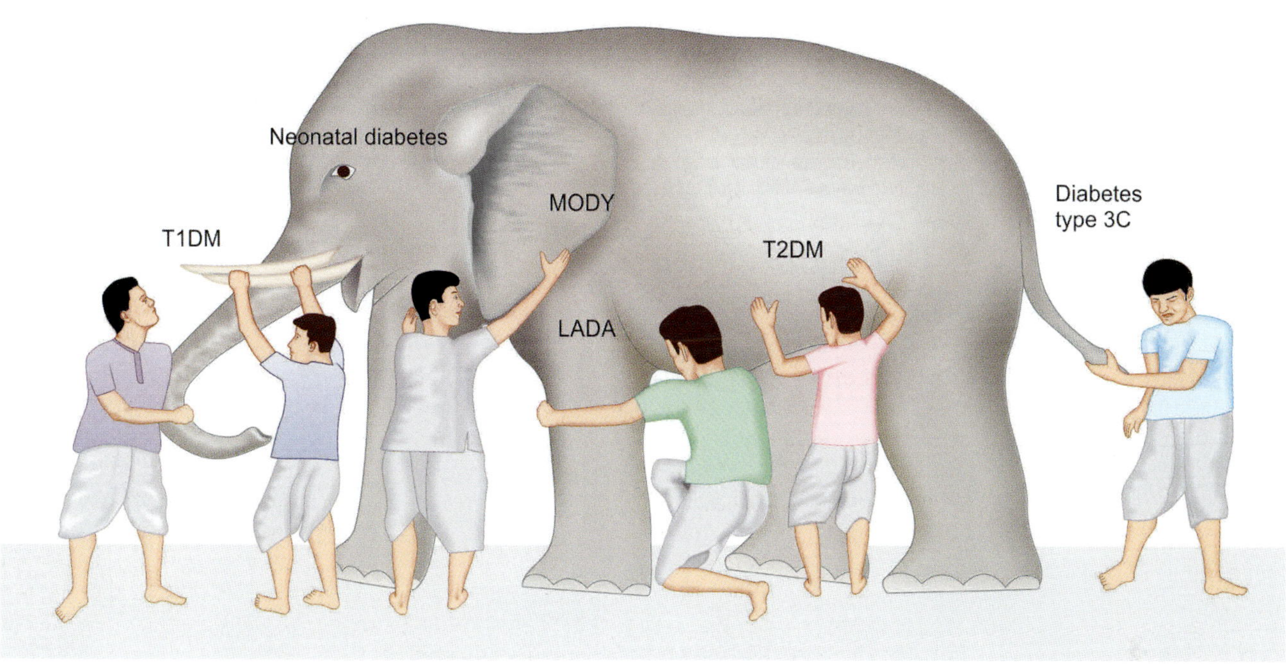

TIDM, type 1 diabetes mellitus; T2DM, type 2 diabetes mellitus; MODY,maturity onset diabetes of young; LADA, latent autoimmune diabetes of adults.

FIG. 1: Figure draws an analogy for diabetes classification to errors made in identification of an elephant by a group of blind men: A story from Hindu Upnishads.

The above proposed classification appears more realistic and is based on commonly measured variables in a patient with diabetes. The study also highlighted the fact that clustering of patients in above-mentioned groups can help predict risk of complications. The authors pointed that patients classified as severe autoimmune diabetes and severe insulin deficiency diabetes were younger at onset, were more prone to ketoacidosis as well as carried higher risk of future diabetic retinopathy. Patients with severe insulin resistance diabetes were at higher risk of developing diabetic nephropathy[14] and end stage renal disease (a known fact with insulin resistance). Risk of cardiovascular (CV) complications like stroke and myocardial infarction was similar in all age groups after adjusting for age and sex. What is apparent from this classification is that a reorganization of patients with diabetes in to such groups can be more useful for the clinicians and it will also aid researchers because of its replicability. A patient can be selected for more aggressive treatment in SIRD while a patient with only MARD or MORD can benefit more with a less intensive regimen. Also there is a possibility that low-risk groups may require less frequent hospital visits and more flexibility in care plan, leading to decreased cost of treatment.

The limitations of the above study are that it was limited only to Scandinavian population. Whether it will hold true or not for other ethnic populations remains to be seen. Other notable limitations are that study cannot confirm causes of five different type of diabetes and remains silent about overlap or changeover from one form to the other form of diabetes as well as there is lack of data on established risk factor like blood pressure and lipid profile. Nevertheless, it reestablishes the fact that time has really arrived to look at diabetes from several other perspectives.

CONCLUSION

The future trends in diabetes will undoubtedly be dominated by genetics, biomarkers, precision medicine, and use of technology in management of diabetes. Development of drugs targeting new sites for management of diabetes to improve the existing standard of care for our diabetic patients will also be at forefront. A newer classification scheme for diabetes is need of the hour. We also call upon the researchers to look at the Indian data for a more practical classification system.

REFERENCES

1. King KM, Rubin G. A history of diabetes: From antiquity to discovering insulin. Br J Nurs. 2003;12(18):1091-5.
2. Sakula A. Paul Langerhans (1847-1888): A centenary tribute. J R Soc Med. 1988;81(7):414.
3. Nutrition classics. The Journal of Laboratory and Clinical Medicine, Vol. VII, 1922: The internal secretion of the pancreas. By FG Banting, CH Best. Nutr Rev. 1987;45(4):55-7.
4. National Diabetes Data Group. Classification and diagnosis of diabetes mellitus and other categories of glucose intolerance. Diabetes. 1979;28(12):1039-57.
5. Alberti KG, Zimmet PF. Definition, diagnosis and classification of diabetes mellitus and its complications. Part 1: Diagnosis and classification of diabetes mellitus. Provisional report of a WHO consultation. Diabetic Med. 1998;15(7):539-53.
6. Marathe PH, Gao HX, Close KL. American Diabetes Association Standards of Medical Care in Diabetes 2017. J Diabetes. 2017;9(4):320-4.
7. Stone MA, Stefinovic JC, Wilkinson J, et al. Incorrect and incomplete coding and classification of diabetes: A systematic review. Diabetic Med. 2010;27(5):491-7.
8. Groop L, Tuomi T, Rowley M, et al. Latent autoimmune diabetes in adults (LADA)—more than a name. Diabetologia. 2006;49(9):1996-8.

9. Tuomi T, Santoro N, Caprio S, et al. The many faces of diabetes: A disease with increasing heterogeneity. The Lancet. 2014;383(9922):1084-94.
10. De la Monte SM, Wands JR. Alzheimer's disease is type 3 diabetes—evidence reviewed. J Diabetes Sci Technol. 2008;2(6):1101-13.
11. Faiq MA, Dada R, Saluja D, et al. Glaucoma–Diabetes of the brain: A radical hypothesis about its nature and pathogenesis. Med Hypotheses. 2014;82(5):535-46.
12. Schwartz SS, Epstein S, Corkey BE, et al. The time is right for a new classification system for diabetes: Rationale and implications of the β-cell–centric classification schema. Diabetes Care. 2016;39(2):179-86.
13. Ahlqvist E, Storm P, Käräjämäki A, et al. Novel subgroups of adult-onset diabetes and their association with outcomes: A data-driven cluster analysis of six variables. Lancet Diabetes Endocrinol. 2018;6(5):361-9.
14. Pan J, Wang YG. Insulin resistance and diabetic nephropathy. Med Recapitulate. 2008;11:039.

CHAPTER 14

Prevention of Coronary Artery Disease in Diabetes Mellitus

Ranjan Modi, Sunil Modi

INTRODUCTION

Diabetes mellitus (DM) is a principal risk factor for cardiovascular disease (CVD). Diabetes induced macrovascular disorders are retinopathy, nephropathy, peripheral vascular disease (PVD), stroke, and coronary artery disease (CAD). Evidence suggest that although hyperglycemia, contribute to myocardial damage after ischemic events, it is clearly not the only factor. Both prediabetes and presence of metabolic syndrome, in normoglycemic patients can increase the risk of CVD.[1-4]

Targeting individual risk factors reduces atherosclerotic cardiovascular disease (ASCVD) or CAD risk in DM, but simultaneously treating multiple risk factors may reduce cardiovascular (CV) event risk more than when treated individually. The Steno-2 study which showed a statistically and clinically significant 53% reduction in the primary composite CV event end point.

Cardiovascular risk differences between intensive and conventional therapy were studied after 1 year.[5] The number needed-to-treat was 5 over 7.8 years to achieve this magnitude of ASCVD risk reduction. The Steno-2 trial was not designed to identify which interventions were most effective, but use of statin and antihypertensive drugs may have accounted for much of the CV benefit.

The BARI-2D trial (Bypass Angioplasty Revascularization Investigation in Type 2 Diabetes) evaluated multiple interventions and their secondary analysis which all supported the fact that concurrent risk factor control lowers total mortality and the composite of death, myocardial infarction (MI), and stroke in patients with type 2 DM and established coronary heart disease (CHD).[6]

The BARI-2D trial demonstrated that control of multiple risk factors improved CV outcomes. Though achievement of treatment goals in DM care have improved over time, currently only a small percentage of world population with type 2 DM reach the recommended goals for glycated hemoglobin (HbA1c), blood pressure (BP), and low-density lipoprotein (LDL) cholesterol.[7]

Prevention of CAD in DM by addressing risk factors individually from clinical trials of lifestyle modification, lipid lowering, BP-lowering, aspirin therapy, and glucose-lowering therapies is presented here.

LIFESTYLE MODIFICATION

Appropriate lifestyle modifications have been shown to stabilize glycemic control and prevent and decrease CVD risk factors.

In a 4-year study, the Look AHEAD (Action for Health in Diabetes) research group examined the effects of lifestyle modifications on CVD risk factors.[8] Participants were divided into a "diabetes support and education group" (DSE, the control group) and an "intensive lifestyle intervention group" (ILI).[8] The ILI group was told to adhere to a 1,200–1,800-calorie diet and 175 minutes of physical activity each week. Risk factors evaluated at the end of the study were weight, fitness, HbA1c, BP, LDL-C,high-density lipoprotein (HDL)-C, and triglyceride (TG) levels. All CVD risk factors measured in Look AHEAD study were decreased in members of ILI except LDL-C levels which were greater in ILI than DSE.[8] The study evaluated the need for diabetes treatment in ILI versus DSE group and demonstrated the decrease in number of patients in ILI group over 4 years.

The specific American Diabetes Association (ADA) lifestyle recommendations and goals required for decreasing the risk of CVD include moderate weight loss, (i.e., 7–10% of body weight per year) and dietary modification.[9] The dietary guidelines recommend that only 25–35% of total daily calories should come from fat which should consist mainly of monounsaturated and polyunsaturated fats, proportion of saturated fats should be <7% of the total calorie intake with cholesterol intake reduced to <200 mg/day and a fiber intake of at least 14 g per 1,000 calories. Physical activity as well is an important lifestyle intervention for decreasing CVD risk with addition to diet restriction. Patients should be encouraged to achieve at least 150 minutes of moderate-intensity aerobic activity, or at least 90 minutes of vigorous aerobic activity in a week.

Smoking is another modifiable risk factor of CVD. Patients who smoke should be counseled and advised to quit as soon as possible to reduce the incidence of CV events.

LIPID-LOWERING THERAPY

Clinically, dyslipidemia is highly correlated with atherosclerosis, and up to 97% of diabetics are dyslipidemic.[10] In addition to the characteristic pattern of increased TG and decreased HDL found in diabetics, abnormalities are also seen in the structure of the lipoprotein particles. The predominant form of LDL is the small, dense form. Small dense LDL particles are more atherogenic than large LDL particles because they can more easily penetrate and form stronger attachments to the arterial wall, and they are more susceptible to oxidation. Because less cholesterol is carried in the core of small LDL particles than in the core of large particles, subjects with predominantly small LDL particles have higher numbers of particles at comparable LDL cholesterol levels.[11]

There is convincing evidence that the use of lipid lowering therapy and statins reduce ASCVD event rates in DM; part of this benefit is attributed to the pleomorphic anti-inflammatory effects of statins.[12-14] Patients with DM between the ages of 40 and 75 years have been identified as one of the four principal groups to benefit from statins therapy in the recent American College of Cardiology or American Heart Association (ACC/AHA) guidelines. The guidelines recommend treatment with a moderate or a high intensity statin for individuals with ≥7.5% 10-year risk of CVD.[15] In those <40 or >75 years of age, guidelines recommend individualizing statin therapy based on the benefits of ASCVD risk reduction versus the potential for adverse effects, interactions with other drugs, and patient preference.[15]

Cholesterol Treatment Trialist (CTT) collaboration meta-analysis showed that 39 mg/dL (1 mmol/L) lowering of LDL in high-risk individuals by statins reduces coronary mortality by 19%[16] and major vascular events by 21%, irrespective of prior history of vascular disease, gender, age, body mass index (BMI), baseline BP, smoking status, glomerular filtration rate (GFR), cholesterol, or predicted annual risk of major vascular events.[17]

The CARDS trial (Collaborative Atorvastatin Diabetes Study), assessed patients of type 2 DM, with mean baseline LDL cholesterol of 117 mg/dL (3.0 mmol/L) randomized to atorvastatin 10 mg daily or placebo. The primary CV composite outcome (time to first occurrence of acute CHD event, coronary revascularization, or stroke) showed a 37% reduction for atorvastatin compared to placebo group.

The TNT (Treating to New Targets) study which included patients with DM and CHD who were randomized to atorvastatin 10 mg versus 80 mg daily examined whether lowering LDL cholesterol below the threshold recommended at the time (100 mg/dL, 2.59 mmol/L) would result in greater CV risk reduction.[18] There was a 25% reduction in major CV events (composite of CHD death, nonfatal non-procedure-related MI, resuscitated cardiac arrest and fatal or nonfatal stroke) after a median of 4.9 years of treatment. This study provides further evidence for more aggressive LDL-lowering to reduce ASCVD in DM.

Statins and Development of Diabetes Mellitus

Statins may interfere with β-cell insulin secretion either by decreasing Ca^{2+}-dependent insulin secretion or by interfering with isoprenylation of guanosine triphosphate-binding proteins.[19] Statin inhibition of isoprenoid biosynthesis may lead to lower expression of insulin signaling proteins in adipocytes and to reduced glucose transporter expression or translocation.

Although, various trials and meta-analysis have shown clear benefits of statins to reduce CV events and mortality in patients with or at risk for ASCVD[16,17] statins can also modestly accelerate the development of DM in individuals with pre-existing risk factors.[20]

Meta-regression analysis of large trials showed that one additional case of DM resulted from treating 225 patients with statins for 4 years, whereas 5.4 vascular events were prevented over same period of time.

The risk of statin associated diabetes appears to be related to potency[21] and dose[22] of statin and may be slightly higher in women.[23]

Majority of professional bodies advise that considering the many treatments available for diabetes and the important magnitude of CV risk reduction by statins, provider should not avoid using statins when indicated solely because of concern for risk of developing diabetes.

Non-statin Lipid Lowering

Although, statins are effective in reducing ASCVD risk in DM, residual CV risk remains[18,24] and further lowering of lipids may be of value. Although many studies in past did not demonstrate, other pharmacological class agents provide additional benefit, the IMPROVE-IT trial (Improved Reduction of Outcomes: Vytorin Efficacy International Trial) supports use of a non-statin LDL-lowering strategy to further lower CV risk.[25] Ezetimibe lowered LDL cholesterol further by 24% despite the relatively low baseline concentrations, which was an unexpectedly potent effect. In the trial 27% of the study population had DM, and there was heterogeneity in response with a greater 14% CV benefit among those with DM. Thus the trial supported the hypothesis that further lower LDL targets may be beneficial to reduce residual ASCVD risk in patients with DM.

The unanswered question is whether targeting high TG and or low HDL and small LDL particle size will result in further benefits.

Lipid arm of ACCORD trial (Action to Control Cardiovascular Risk in Diabetes)[26] examined fenofibrate versus placebo on a background of simvastatin therapy, and the FIELD (Fenofibrate Intervention and Event Lowering in Diabetes) trial,[27] involved fenofibrate monotherapy versus placebo. Inclusion in the ACCORD-lipid substudy as well as in the FIELD study did not require high TG and low HDL cholesterol levels, a group which might benefit most from fibrate therapy.[26] Results of both ACCORD and FIELD trials were similar.

In ACCORD trial, although there was no difference in annual rate of primary composite outcome of major adverse cardiac events (MACE) for the fenofibrate as compared to placebo, prespecified subgroup analysis revealed 29% fewer events in those with baseline TG more than 204 mg/dL and HDL less than 34 mg/dL (14% fewer events in FIELD study in similar subgroup).

Although total of four such studies consistently demonstrate favorable effects of fibrates in the subgroup of patients with the specific lipid phenotype of high TG and low HDL,[24-28] further studies are needed to prove this benefit.

The addition of niacin on top of statin in (Atherothrombosis Intervention in Metabolic Syndrome with low HDL/High Triglycerides: Impact on Global Health Outcome) AIM-HIGH trial[29] and in (Heart Protection Study 2-Treatment of HDL to Reduce the Incidence of Vascular Events) HPS2-THRIVE trial[30] has not shown any further benefit and raising HDL with the use of cholesteryl ester transfer protein (CETP) inhibitors has also not shown any benefit in CV risk reduction.

LDL-lowering with Proprotein Convertase Subtilisin or Kexin Type 9 Inhibition

The latest class of LDL lowering medications consists of monoclonal antibodies to proprotein convertase subtilisin/kexin type 9 (PCSK9) present in hepatocytes. PCSK9 binds to and targets the LDL receptor for degradation.[31] PCSK9 inhibitors prevent the degradation of the LDL receptors, thereby leading to increased removal of LDL cholesterol from the circulation. Individuals with loss of function of PCSK9 mutations have lower LDL cholesterol levels and lower CHD incidence.[32] On the other hand gain of function mutations lead to most cases of familial hypercholesterolemia with elevated LDL cholesterol concentrations and resulting early ASCVD. Statins upregulate PCSK9, a potential reason that LDL cholesterol lowering with statins reaches a plateau.[33]

Although PCSK9 inhibition has a potent and durable effect to lower LDL, the currently available trials are exploratory and preliminary as far as beneficial effects on CV outcomes are concerned. Furthermore such effects in diabetic population remain uncertain and will need more research and data.

Blood Pressure Control

The age-adjusted prevalence of hypertension is higher in adults with DM as compared to those without DM, with higher rates seen in older persons.[34]

Elevated BP has shown to increase the risk of both micro- and macrovascular disease in DM,[35] and BP control reduces the risk of death and both micro- and macrovascular complications.[36]

In diabetics, every 10 mm of systolic BP lowering reduces all—cause mortality by 13%, CV events by 11% and stroke events by 27%.

In general, antihypertensive drug class does not affect the overall results and rather it is BP lowering per se which confers clinical benefit. However, there are differences between particular drugs and individual CV endpoints. For example, diuretics were associated with 17% lower relative risk of heart failure [mainly driven by (Antihypertensive and Lipid-Lowering Treatment to Prevent Heart Attack Trial) ALLAHAT trial], and angiotensin receptor blockers (ARB's) are associated with a lower risk of heart failure and mortality [mainly driven by (Losartan Intervention for Endpoint reduction in hypertension study) LIFE trial]. In contrast calcium channel blockers are associated with a higher relative risk of heart failure but a lower risk of stroke.

The benefits of renin-angiotensin-aldosterone system (RAAS) inhibitors to control BP in diabetics over other antihypertensive has been observed in (Appropriate Blood Pressure Control in Diabetes) ABCD trial[37] (Heart Outcomes Prevention Evaluation) HOPE trial[38] and in LIFE trial[39] and on the basis of these data, current guidelines from AHA or American Diabetes Association (ADA)[40] propose that RAAS blockade with an angiotensin-converting enzyme (ACE) inhibitor or ARB should be used first in the treatment of hypertension in DM.[41]

As far as the effect of standard versus more intensive BP lowering in individuals with DM is concerned,[42] a recent meta-analysis including three trials with a total of 7,312 adults with type 2 DM and hypertension were followed up for 2 to 5 years.[43] Intensive reduction of systolic BP to 130 mm Hg or lower or diastolic BP to 80 mm Hg or lower was associated with a 35% decrease in risk for stroke and a trend for reduced mortality as compared with a standard systolic BP target of 140–160 mm Hg and diastolic BP target of 85–100 mm Hg.

The recent AHA guidelines for CV risk reduction[15] recommend a BP goal of <140 mm Hg and <90 mm Hg for systolic and diastolic BP, respectively. The guidelines also recommend that initial therapy should include an ACE inhibitor or ARB for renal protection. The next choice could be to include a thiazide diuretic or calcium channel blocker. In the recently published (Systolic Blood Pressure Intervention Trial) SPRINT trial patients without DM, it would be reasonable to consider targeting BP <120/80 in individuals with DM, especially in the presence of renal disease or increased risk for stroke.

Glycemic Control

Although there are multiple mechanisms contributing to hyperglycemia in diabetes, progressive β-cell failure is a key aspect in the natural history of type 2 DM[44-46] leading to gradual worsening hyperglycemia and rising HbA1c.[47,48]

Considering the fact that 85% of patients with established DM take glucose-lowering medications and ASCVD in the form of MI and stroke accounts for up to 80% mortality in type 2 DM[49] it is desirable that medications to manage hyperglycemia must not adversely impact CV risk factors or increase ASCVD, and ideally should reverse atherosclerosis and lower CV risk. However, many antidiabetic medications have no beneficial effects on CV risk or actually may exacerbate CV disease or deteriorate CV risk factors.[50-57]

Intensive glycemic control reduces relative risk of nonfatal MI and CHD events by about 15%, although it has no effect of intensive glycemic control on all-cause mortality in meta-analysis of the multiple randomized trials targeting different intensity of glycemic control.[58]

In recent decades, several clinical trials have investigated the effect of intensive treatment of hyperglycemia on CV risk reduction. When intensive treatment of hyperglycemia is initiated early in patients with short duration of diabetes and low CV risk, with target glycosylated hemoglobin levels below 7%, significant CV benefits can be achieved. However the same does not hold true when tight glycemic control is targeted in older patients with history of long duration of DM and higher CV risk profile.

This early protection is postulated to result from a mechanism known as "metabolic memory," which means that the effect of the early glycemic exposure is remembered later in target organs resulting in long-term deleterious or protective effects. Epigenetic changes and intracellular metabolic changes resulting in oxidative stress, lowgrade inflammation, and endothelial dysfunction are the mechanisms considered to be involved in this process.

ANTITHROMBOTIC MEDICATIONS

The ADA and AHA, in the year 2007, jointly recommended that in patients with DM who are at increased CV risk, low-dose aspirin (acetylsalicylic acid, 75–162 mg/day) should be used as a primary prevention strategy.[59]

After this recommendation, the Japanese Primary Prevention of Atherosclerosis With Aspirin for Diabetes, JPAD)[60] and the (Prevention of Progression of Arterial Disease and Diabetes) POPADAD[61] trials raised doubts about the efficacy of low-dose aspirin in patients with DM. In the light of those results, the ADA, AHA, and American College of Cardiology Foundation (ACCF) convened to review and synthesize available evidence and updated recommendation in 2009.[59]

During the evaluation to determine the updated recommendations, the joint committee considered not only the benefits of aspirin for preventing CAD, but also the known problem of gastrointestinal bleeding with daily administration of aspirin.

The joint committee concluded that low-dose aspirin (75–162 mg/day) for CVD prevention is "reasonable" for adults with DM who have no history of vascular disease but who are at increased risk of CVD (10-year risk >10%) and are not at increased risk of bleeding.[62]

The committee added that aspirin should not be recommended for CVD prevention if patients are at low-risk of CVD (10-year risk <5%), noting that the potential adverse effects of bleeding are higher than the potential benefits. Low-dose aspirin "might be considered" for CVD prevention in patients with diabetes who are at intermediate risk of CVD (10-year >5–10%).[62]

The joint committee also stated that all modifiable CVD risk factors should be addressed and optimally managed for patients using aspirin. Helping patients reach their individual CV goals through such management will decrease their 10-year CVD risk, meaning that fewer patients with DM may need to continue taking aspirin in the long-term.

BARIATRIC SURGERY

Bariatric surgery induces substantial and sustained weight loss[63] and remission or improvement in type 2 DM in 40–85% of patients, hypertension in 28–75% of patients, and dyslipidemia in 70–90% of patients.[64]

The rates of improvement in obesity comorbidities vary based on both the specific procedure performed and under lying patient characteristics. Together, these metabolic improvements may lead to reduced ASCVD risk and event rates. Various observational cohort studies suggest that bariatric surgery versus usual care may be associated with reduced number of CV deaths and lower incidence of CV events in obese adults,[65] as well as reduced incidence of MI in obese individuals with type 2 DM.[66] In patients who have had bariatric surgery for obesity management, total mortality rates appear 30–40% lower[63] and may be more prominent in those with DM at the time of surgery,[67] although survival benefit effects may take years to manifest.

Thus, for patients with DM and BMI more than 35 kg/m^2 who have undergone appropriate medical and psychological evaluation, who understand the risks, lifestyle changes, and monitoring involved with bariatric surgery, have medical, social, and psychological support, bariatric surgery may be recommended when performed by an experienced bariatric surgeon at a bariatric center of excellence.

FUTURE OR WHAT IS IN HORIZON

A number of new approaches to treat DM are under development which may provide molecules with dual benefit of glycemic control as well as of CV risk reduction. In the meanwhile, CV outcome trials will provide useful information on CV safety of use of antidiabetic drugs in patients with established heart disease or in those at high-risk for CV events. The recent trials showing convincing CV benefits of using sodium-glucose co-transporter-2 (SGLT-2) inhibitors is significant and requires more trials to show their consistent benefits.

CONCLUSION

Cardiovascular disease remains the principal cause of death and disability among patients with DM, in whom CAD typically occurs 14.6 years earlier with greater severity, and with more diffuse distribution than in individuals without DM.

Reducing the ASCVD burden and preventing CAD in diabetes is a major clinical condition that should be given priority to reduce premature deaths, to improve quality of life and lessen economic burdens of associated morbidities.

The long-term treatment of DM is difficult and challenging because of diverse goals to control metabolic derangements and to simultaneously reduce CV risks. DM clearly exacerbates mechanism of atherosclerosis and heart failure which are not adequately modulated by focusing solely on glycemic control. Fortunately, aggressive management of other CV risk factors particularly lowering LDL and controlling BP provides substantial CV risk reduction.

Further investigations are required on potential benefits and risks of new glucose lowering therapies and optimal timings of (early/prolonged) glucose targeting interventions. Evidence for a more effective antiplatelet regimen than aspirin in moderate-to-high risk diabetic patients without ischemic heart disease (IHD) is necessary. Recommended BP goals are not fully evidence based, and the role of new potent PCSK9 inhibitors and of those drugs addressing TG and HDL need further studies. Another unaddressed issue is the risk benefit ratio of polypharmacy required in optimizing control of multiple CV risk factors resulting into reduced drugs compliance and risk of drug-drug interactions.

REFERENCES

1. Muhlestein JB, Anderson JL, Horne BD, et al. Effect of fasting glucose levels on mortality rate in patients with and without diabetes mellitus and coronary artery disease undergoing percutaneous coronary intervention. Am Heart J. 2003;146(2):351-8.
2. Thrainsdottir IS, Aspelund T, Thorgeirsson G, et al. The association between glucose abnormalities and heart failure in the population-based Reykjavik study. Diabetes Care. 2005;28(3):612-6.
3. Neilson C, Lange T. Blood glucose and heart failure in nondiabetic patients. Diabetes Care. 2005;28(3):607-11.
4. Glucose tolerance and mortality: comparison of WHO and American Diabetic Association diagnostic criteria. The DECODE study group. European Diabetes Epidemiology Group. Diabetes Epidemiology: Collaborative analysis of Diagnostic criteria in Europe. Lancet. 1999;354(9179):617-21.
5. Gaede P, Vedel P, Larsen N, et al. Multifactorial intervention and cardiovascular disease in patients with type 2 diabetes. N Engl J Med. 2003;348(5):383-93.
6. Bittner V, Bertolet M, Barraza Felix R, et al. Comprehensive cardiovascular risk factor control improves survival: The BARI 2D trial. J Am Coll Cardiol. 2015;66(7):765-73.
7. Ali MK, Bullard KM, Saaddine JB, et al. Achievement of goals in U.S. diabetes care, 1999-2010. N Engl J Med. 2013;368(17):1613-24.
8. The Look AHEAD Research Group, Wing RR. Long-term effects of a lifestyle intervention on weight and cardiovascular risk factors in individuals with type 2 diabetes mellitus: four-year results of the Look AHEAD trial. Arch Intern Med. 2010;170(17):1566-75.
9. Basevi V, Di Mario S, Morciano C, et al. Comments on: American Diabetes Association. Standards of medical care in diabetes—2011. Diabetes Care. 2011;34(Suppl 1):S11-61.
10. Fagot-Campagna A, Rolka DB, Beckles GL, et al. Prevalence of lipid abnormalities, awareness and treatment in US adults with diabetes. Diabetes. 2000;49(Suppl 1):A78.
11. Rosenson RS. Clinical role of LDL and HDL subclasses and apolipoprotein measurement. ACC Curr J Rev. 2004:33-7.
12. Satoh M, Tabuchi T, Itoh T, et al. NLRP3 inflammasome activation in coronary artery disease: results from prospective and randomized study of treatment with atorvastatin or rosuvastatin. Clin Sci (Lond). 2014;126(3):233-41.
13. Yilmaz A, Reiss C, Weng A, et al. Differential effects of statins on relevant functions of human monocyte-derived dendritic cells. J Leukoc Biol. 2006;79(3):529-38.
14. Moutzouri E, Tellis CC, Rousouli K, et al. Effect of simvastatin or its combination with ezetimibe on Toll-like receptor expression and lipopolysaccharide-induced cytokine production in monocytes of hypercholesterolemic patients. Atherosclerosis. 2012;225(2):381-7.
15. Stone NJ, Robinson JG, Lichtenstein AH, et al. 2013 ACC/AHA guideline on the treatment of blood cholesterol to reduce atherosclerotic cardiovascular risk in adults: a report of the American College of Cardiology/American Heart Association Task Force on Practice Guidelines. Circulation. 2014;129(25 Suppl 2):S1-45.
16. Baigent C, Blackwell L, Emberson J, et al. Efficacy and safety of more intensive lowering of LDL cholesterol: a meta-analysis of data from 170,000 participants in 26 randomized trials. Lancet. 2010;376(9753):1670-81.
17. Kearney PM, Blackwell L, Collins R, et al. Efficacy of cholesterol-lowering therapy in 18,686 people with diabetes in 14 randomized trials of statins: a meta-analysis. Lancet. 2008;371(9607):117-25.
18. Shepherd J, Barter P, Carmena R, et al. Effect of lowering LDL cholesterol substantially below currently recommended levels in patients with coronary heart disease and diabetes: The Treating to New Targets (TNT) study. Diabetes Care. 2006;29(6):1220-6.
19. Kostapanos MS, Liamis GL, Milionis HJ, et al. Do statins beneficially or adversely affect glucose homeostasis? Curr Vasc Pharmacol. 2010;8(5):612-31.
20. Ridker PM, Danielson E, Fonseca FA, et al. Rosuvastatin to prevent vascular events in men and women with elevated C-reactive protein. N Engl J Med. 2008;359(21):2195-207.
21. Carter AA, Gomes T, Camacho X, et al. Risk of incident diabetes among patients treated with statins: population based study. BMJ. 2013;346:f2610.
22. Preiss D, Seshasai SR, Welsh P, et al. Risk of incident diabetes with intensive-dose compared with moderate dose statin therapy: a meta-analysis. JAMA. 2011;305(24):2556-64.
23. Culver AL, Ockene IS, Balasubramanian R, et al. Statin use and risk of diabetes mellitus in postmenopausal women in the Women's Health Initiative. Arch Intern Med. 2012;172(2):144-52.
24. Collins R, Armitage J, Parish S, et al. MRC/BHF heart protection study of cholesterol lowering with simvastatin in 5,963 people with diabetes: a randomized placebo-controlled trial. Lancet. 2003;361(9374):2005-16.
25. Cannon CP, Blazing MA, Giugliano RP, et al. Ezetimibe added to statin therapy after acute coronary syndromes. N Engl J Med. 2015;372(25):2387-97.
26. Ginsberg HN, Elam MB, Lovato LC, et al. Effects of combination lipid therapy in type 2 diabetes mellitus. N Engl J Med. 2010;362(17):1563-74.
27. Keech A, Simes RJ, Barter P, et al. Effects of long-term fenofibrate therapy on cardiovascular events in 9,795 people with type 2 diabetes mellitus (the FIELD study): randomized controlled trial. Lancet. 2005;366(9500):1849-61.
28. Bezafibrate Infarction Prevention (BIP) study. Secondary prevention by raising HDL cholesterol and reducing triglycerides in patients with coronary artery disease. Circulation. 2000;102(1):21-7.
29. Boden WE, Probstfield JL, Anderson T, et al. Niacin in patients with low HDL cholesterol levels receiving intensive statin therapy. N Engl J Med. 2011;365(24):2255-67.
30. Landray MJ, Haynes R, Hopewell JC, et al. Effects of extended-release niacin with laropiprant in high-risk patients. N Engl J Med. 2014;371(3):203-12.
31. Seidah NG, Prat A. The biology and therapeutic targeting of the proprotein convertases. Nat Rev Drug Discov. 2012;11(5):367-83.
32. Benn M, Nordestgaard BG, Grande P, et al. PCSK9 R46L, low-density lipoprotein cholesterol levels, and risk of ischemic heart disease: 3 independent studies and meta-analyses. J Am Coll Cardiol. 2010;55(25):2833-42.
33. Sabatine MS, Giugliano RP, Keech AC, et al. Evolocumab and clinical outcomes in patients with cardiovascular disease. N Engl J Med. 2017;376(18):1713-22.
34. Keenan NL, Rosendorf KA, Centers for Disease Control and Prevention (CDC). Prevalence of hypertension and controlled hypertension—United States, 2005-2008. MMWR Suppl. 2011;60(1):94-7.
35. Authors/Task Force Members, Ryden L, Grant PJ, et al. ESC Guidelines on diabetes, pre-diabetes, and cardiovascular diseases developed in collaboration with the EASD: the Task Force on diabetes, pre-diabetes, and cardiovascular diseases of the European Society of Cardiology (ESC) and developed in collaboration with the European Association for the Study of Diabetes (EASD). Eur Heart J. 2013;34(39):3035-87.
36. Tight blood pressure control and risk of macrovascular and microvascular complications in type 2 diabetes: UKPDS 38. UK Prospective Diabetes Study Group. BMJ. 1998;317(7160):703-13.
37. Estacio RO, Jeffers BW, Hiatt WR, et al. The effect of nisoldipine as compared with enalapril on cardiovascular outcomes in patients with non-insulin-dependent diabetes and hypertension. N Engl J Med. 1998;338(10):645-52.

38. Heart Outcomes Prevention Evaluation Study Investigators. Effects of ramipril on cardiovascular and microvascular outcomes in people with diabetes mellitus: results of the HOPE study and MICRO-HOPE substudy. Heart Outcomes Prevention Evaluation Study Investigators. Lancet. 2000;355(9200):253-9.
39. Lindholm LH, Ibsen H, Dahlof B, et al. Cardiovascular morbidity and mortality in patients with diabetes in the Losartan Intervention For Endpoint reduction in hypertension study (LIFE): a randomized trial against atenolol. Lancet. 2002;359(9311):1004-10.
40. Fox CS, Golden SH, Anderson C, et al. Update on prevention of cardiovascular disease in adults with type 2 diabetes mellitus in light of recent evidence: a Scientific Statement from the American Heart Association and the American Diabetes Association. Circulation. 2015;132(8):691-718.
41. American Diabetes Association. Cardiovascular disease and risk management. Diabetes Care. 2016;39(Suppl 1):S60-71.
42. Hansson L, Zanchetti A, Carruthers SG, et al. Effects of intensive blood pressure lowering and low-dose aspirin in patients with hypertension: principal results of the Hypertension Optimal Treatment (HOT) randomized trial. HOT Study Group. Lancet. 1998;351(9118):1755-62.
43. McBrien K, Rabi DM, Campbell N, et al. Intensive and standard blood pressure targets in patients with type 2 diabetes mellitus: systematic review and meta-analysis. Arch Intern Med. 2012;172(17):1296-303.
44. Weyer C, Bogardus C, Mott DM, et al. The natural history of insulin secretory dysfunction and insulin resistance in the pathogenesis of type 2 diabetes mellitus. J Clin Invest. 1999;104(6):787-94.
45. Knowler WC, Pettitt DJ, Saad MF, et al. Diabetes mellitus in the Pima Indians: incidence, risk factors and pathogenesis. Diabetes Metab Rev. 1990;6(1):1-27.
46. Leahy JL. Natural history of beta-cell dysfunction in NIDDM. Diabetes Care. 1990;13(9):992-1010.
47. Intensive blood-glucose control with sulfonylureas or insulin compared with conventional treatment and risk of complications in patients with type 2 diabetes (UKPDS 33). UK Prospective Diabetes Study (UKPDS) Group. Lancet. 1998;352(9131):837-53.
48. Schultz TA, Lewis SB, Davis JL, et al. Effect of sulfonylurea therapy and plasma glucose levels on hemoglobin A1c in type II diabetes mellitus. Am J Med. 1981;70(2):373-8.
49. Morrish NJ, Wang SL, Stevens LK, et al. Mortality and causes of death in the WHO Multinational Study of Vascular Disease in Diabetes. Diabetologia. 2001;44 (Suppl 2):S14-21.
50. Freed MI, Ratner R, Marcovina SM, et al. Effects of rosiglitazone alone and in combination with atorvastatin on the metabolic abnormalities in type 2 diabetes mellitus. Am J Cardiol. 2002;90(9):947-52.
51. Del Prato S, Pulizzi N. The place of sulfonylureas in the therapy for type 2 diabetes mellitus. Metabolism. 2006;55(5 Suppl 1):S20-7.
52. Singh S, Loke YK, Furberg CD. Long-term risk of cardiovascular events with rosiglitazone: a meta-analysis. JAMA. 2007;298(10):1189-95.
53. van Wijk JP, de Koning EJ, Martens EP, et al. Thiazolidinediones and blood lipids in type 2 diabetes. Arterioscler Thromb Vasc Biol. 2003;23(10):1744-9.
54. Schernthaner G, Chilton RJ. Cardiovascular risk and thiazolidinediones—what do meta-analyses really tell us? Diabetes Obes Metab. 2010;12(12):1023-35.
55. Currie CJ, Poole CD, Evans M, et al. Mortality and other important diabetes-related outcomes with insulin versus other antihyperglycemic therapies in type 2 diabetes. J Clin Endocrinol Metab. 2013;98(2):668-77.
56. Eurich DT, Simpson S, Senthilselvan A, et al. Comparative safety and effectiveness of sitagliptin in patients with type 2 diabetes: retrospective population based cohort study. BMJ. 2013;346:f2267.
57. Holden SE, Currie CJ. Mortality risk with sulfonylureas compared to metformin. Diabetes Obes Metab. 2014;16(10):885-90.
58. Ray KK, Seshasai SR, Wijesuriya S, et al. Effect of intensive control of glucose on cardiovascular outcomes and death in patients with diabetes mellitus: a meta-analysis of randomized controlled trials. Lancet. 2009;373(9677):1765-72.
59. Pignone M, Alberts MJ, Colwell JA, et al. Aspirin for primary prevention of cardiovascular events in people with diabetes: a position statement of the American Diabetes Association, a scientific statement of the American Heart Association, and an expert consensus document of the American College of Cardiology Foundation. Diabetes Care. 2010;33(6):1395-402.
60. Ogawa H, Nakayama M, Morimoto T, et al. Low-dose aspirin for primary prevention of atherosclerotic events in patients with type 2 diabetes: a randomized controlled trial [published online ahead of print November 9, 2008]. JAMA. 2008;300(18):2134-41.
61. Belch J, MacCuish A, Campbell I, et al. The prevention of progression of arterial disease and diabetes (POPADAD) trial: factorial randomized placebo controlled trial of aspirin and antioxidants in patients with diabetes and asymptomatic peripheral arterial disease. BMJ. 2008;337:a1840.
62. Duez H, Lewis GF. Feinglos MN, Bethel MA (Eds.). Fat Metabolism in Insulin Resistance In: Type 2 diabetes mellitus: An Evidence-Based Approach to Practical Management. Durham, NC: Humana Press. 2009; pp. 49-74.
63. Sjöström L, Lindroos AK, Peltonen M, et al. Lifestyle, diabetes, and cardiovascular risk factors 10 years after bariatric surgery. N Engl J Med. 2004;351(26):2683-93.
64. Vetter ML, Cardillo S, Rickels MR, et al. Narrative review: effect of bariatric surgery on type 2 diabetes mellitus. Ann Intern Med. 2009;150(2):94-103.
65. Adams TD, Gress RE, Smith SC, et al. Long-term mortality after gastric bypass surgery. N Engl J Med. 2007;357(8):753-61.
66. Romeo S, Maglio C, Burza MA, et al. Cardiovascular events after bariatric surgery in obese subjects with type 2 diabetes. Diabetes Care. 2012;35(12):2613-7.
67. Arterburn DE, Olsen MK, Smith VA, et al. Association between bariatric surgery and long-term survival. JAMA. 2015;313(1):62-70.

CHAPTER 15

Diabetes and Coronary Artery Disease: Prevalence and Mechanisms

Satyanarayan Routray, Dipak R Das

INTRODUCTION

The association between diabetes mellitus (DM) and coronary artery disease (CAD) is very strong despite the fact that there are wide ethnic and geographical variations in their prevalence. The protective female gender effect is lost in diabetic subjects and indeed women with DM are possibly more prone to develop CAD than men with DM.[1] It was established in the "Organisation to Assess Strategies for Ischemic Syndromes study" (OASIS) that diabetic subjects without prior CAD had a similar risk as nondiabetic subjects with prior CAD, with poorer prognosis seen in diabetic subjects after a clinical event.[2] DM was described as a cardiovascular disease (CVD) equivalent according to National Cholesterol Education Program (NCEP) guidelines. Metabolic abnormalities due to DM have been found to predispose to vascular changes, leading to atherosclerotic endpoints.[3] In addition to CV risk factors seen in nondiabetic subjects, diabetic specific risk factors also contribute to CAD.[4] Furthermore, DM and CAD develop at an earlier age in Indians and associated complications are more as compared to Caucasians.[5-8] The reasons for this heightened CAD risk in Indians is not entirely clear, but is thought to be mainly due to high prevalence of insulin resistance and related atherogenic risk factor in this population.[5,6] It is also likely that factors associated with urban lifestyle or migration such as high calorie diet and lack of physical activity further enhance the underlying insulin resistance and consequently CAD. Not surprisingly, there seems to be a lack of relative decline in CAD rates in diabetics in India as compared to the West.[9,10]

PREVALENCE OF DIABETES AND CORONARY ARTERY DISEASE

The first systematic nationwide study on prevalence of DM in India was performed by the Indian Council of Medical Research (ICMR) task force on DM. The prevalence was reported to be 2.1% in urban and 1.5% in rural populations.[11] From these modest rates in early nineties, the prevalence has sky rocketed to the current alarmingly high rates of approximately 20% in urban and 10% in rural populations suggested by some authors.[12] The methods to acquire data for assessing the prevalence of CAD in diabetics has not been uniform across the world. The parameters to substantiate CAD have been nonhomogenous, thereby creating a lot of confusion. There is no prevailing consensus among researchers as to whether electrocardiography (ECG) or echocardiogram (ECHO) or radionuclide studies or angiographic evidence should be mandatory for substantiating CAD in DM. The specific data regarding prevalence of CAD in DM in Indians have been sparse. Evidence indicates that the prevalence of CAD is rapidly increasing in India, particularly in the urban areas. In the 1970s, prevalence of CAD was 1% in urban India.[13] By 1990, the prevalence of CAD reported by Chadha et al. in Delhi was 9.7%.[14] The increase in prevalence of CAD in urban and rural population suggested from a meta-analysis based on meta-analysis of the CAD prevalence based on the surveys conducted since 1990 was 9-fold and 2-fold, respectively.[15] CVD is the most common cause of death in diabetics and atherosclerosis accounts for almost 80% of all diabetic mortality.[16] Presence of DM increases the risk of CVD 2–4 folds. Type 2 DM represents more than 90% of the diabetic population in India. However, type 1 DM also has an independently higher risk of CVD and their disease develops at younger age. A striking increase in the risk of a first or recurrent myocardial infarction (MI) is reported in diabetics as compared with nondiabetics.

Haffner et al. in a population based study in Finland with follow-up period of 7 years showed that a diabetic patient without a history of MI has almost same risk for a first MI as a nondiabetic subjects who has already sustained MI.[17] Considering these, American Diabetic Association made recommendations to treat diabetic subjects as though they already have established CAD. All the manifestations of CAD are at least 2-fold more common in patients with DM than in nondiabetic individuals. Conversely, the prevalence of DM in CAD is approximately 20%.[16,17] There is evidence from Indian data that CAD is more common in diabetic subjects.

TABLE 1: Prevalence of coronary artery disease in different types of clinic or population-based studies

Author	Year	Clinic/ population (pop)	State/city	Percentage
Chaddha	1990	Pop	Delhi	9.7
Raman Kutty	1993	Pop	Kerala	7.4
Mohan	1995	Clinic	Chennai	17.8
Gupta	1995	Pop	UP	7.9
Ramachandran	1998	Pop	Chennai	14.3
Ramachandran	1999	Clinic	Chennai	11.4
Mohan	2001	Pop	Chennai	21.4
Gupta	2002	Pop	Rajasthan	8.2
ICMR	1984–87	Pop	Multicentric	8.1, 4.7 (F)
Pathak	2002	Pop	Ahmedabad	20.2
Agrawal	2004	Pop	Bikaner	19.3
Gupta	2001	Pop	Surat	19

South Indian studies by Mohan et al. and Ramachandran et al. in Chennai showed a prevalence of DM varying from 12% to 16%. MV Diabetes Center, Madras conducted a study to assess the prevalence of CAD was assessed in a large cohort of 6,597 noninsulin-dependent diabetes mellitus (NIDDM) patients.[10] Overall 17.8% of patients had CAD. Its prevalence was not significantly different in males and females. The Chennai Urban Population Study (CUPS) reported that overall CAD prevalence to be 11%, of which 12% was diabetic. Among these 21.4% had CAD, more than the double that of nondiabetics. All these data suggest that the epidemic of type 2 DM and CAD has already assumed alarming proportions and urgent measures are needed to stem it. The prevalence of CAD in different types of clinic or population-based studies conducted in India among diabetics is presented in table 1.

The registry data has created a new era and modality of information regarding prevalence of DM and CAD. OASIS registry 1 and 2 data have found out the age-adjusted prevalence of DM to be 39.1% in non-ST-elevation acute coronary syndrome (NSTE-ACS) patients in India.[18] The multicentric CREATE registry which included 20,468 patients of ACS recruited from 89 centers spanning 50 cities in India had documented the overall prevalence of DM to be 30.4% [ST-elevation myocardial infarction (STEMI)—26.9%, NSTEMI—35.8%].[19] As all recent statistics point out to a marked increase in DM worldwide, one can anticipate rising trends in prevalence of CAD associated with DM in India as well.

DIABETES AND CORONARY ARTERY DISEASE: MECHANISMS

Type 1 and type 2 DM are both independent and significant causative factor for CAD, stroke and peripheral arterial disease. Out of all hospitalizations due to complications of DM, more than 75% are attributable to CVD. Exposure of tissues to hyperglycemia in long-term is currently considered as the principal mechanism for pathogenesis of complications of DM.[20,21] Hyperglycemia leads to a lot of alterations in vascular tissues, which ultimately induce accelerated atherosclerosis. Presently, three principal mechanisms are suggested to explain most of the pathological changes found in vasculature of diabetic patients:

1. Nonenzymatic glycation of proteins and lipids
2. Protein kinase C (PKC) activation
3. Oxidative stress.

Importantly, these mechanisms are not independent (Fig. 1). For example, hyperglycemia-induced oxidative stress promotes the formation of advanced glycation end products (AGEs) and PKC activation.[22,23]

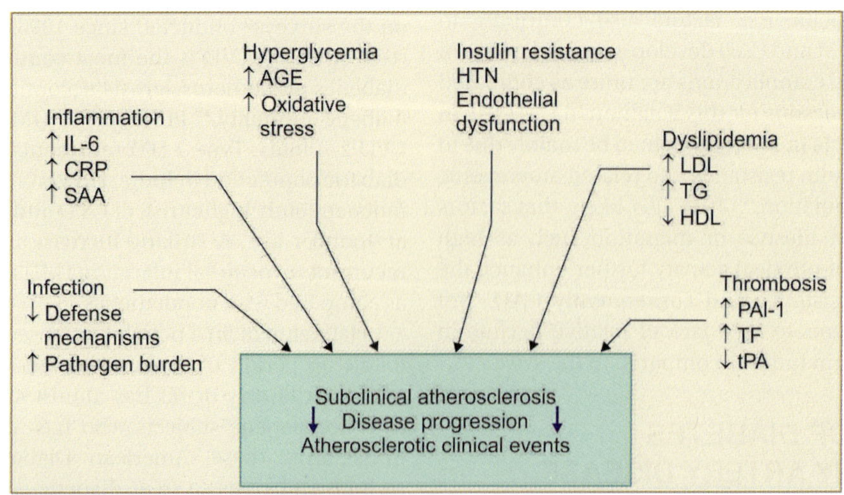

AGEs, advanced glycation end products; CRP, C-reactive protein; CHD, coronary heart disease; HDL, high-density lipoprotein; HTN, hypertension; IL-6, interleukin-6; LDL, low-density lipoprotein; PAI-1, plasminogen activator inhibitor-1; SAA, serum amyloid A; TF, tissue factor; TG, triglycerides; tPA, tissue plasminogen activator.

FIG. 1: Mechanism by which diabetes mellitus leads to coronary artery disease.

Source: Biondi-Zoccai GG, Abbate A, Liuzzo G, et al. Atherothrombosis, inflammation, and diabetes. J Am Coll Cardiol. 2003;41(7):1071-7.

Advanced Glycation End Products

Hyperglycemia often leads to progressive and irreversible cell dysfunction. Exact mechanism is not clear for these findings, but it has been found that cellular alterations may continue, even after return of normoglycemia (memory effect). Hence, long-term rather than short-term metabolic changes are crucial to the pathogenesis of CAD in DM. The proteins or lipoproteins present in the arterial wall react nonenzymatically with glucose, which is a key mechanism for enhanced atherosclerosis in DM. This is called as browning or Maillard reaction. Chemically reversible early glycosylation of glucose with reactive amino groups of circulating or vessel wall proteins produces Schiff bases, which later on gets modified to form more stable Amadori products. Schiff bases reach equilibrium levels in hours, whereas Amadori products reach in weeks. After a complex series of chemical rearrangements, early glycosylation products are changed over to AGE. AGE-protein adducts, once formed are virtually irreversible. With aging, AGEs continuously accumulate on long-lived vessel wall proteins at an accelerated rate in DM. Glucose concentration and time of exposure mainly determine the degree of nonenzymatic glycation. The tissue microenvironment redox potential is another critical factor to the formation of AGEs is situations in which the local redox potential has been shifted to favor oxidant stress, AGEs formation increases substantially.[24] The atherosclerotic process is accelerated by AGEs leading to different manifestations of CAD by diverse mechanism, which can be classified as nonreceptor dependent (Box 1) and receptor-mediated (Box 2).

Nonreceptor-mediated Mechanisms

Changes in molecular conformation of proteins are induced by AGEs which decrease their degradative capacity, alter enzymatic activity and interfere with receptor recognition (Box 1). Thus, changes in the normal physiology of proteins that are relevant to atherogenesis, may enhance CAD in DM.

BOX 1 Atherosclerosis promoting effects of advanced glycation end products: nonreceptor mediated mechanisms

- Extracellular matrix:
  - Collagen cross linking
  - Enhanced synthesis of extracellular matrix components
  - Trapping of LDL in the subendothelium
  - Glycosylated subendothelial matrix quenches nitric-oxide
- Functional alterations of regulatory proteins:
  - Basic fibroblast growth factor glycosylation reduces its heparin binding capacity and its mitogenic activity on endothelial cells
  - Inactivation of the complement regulatory protein CD59
- Lipoprotein modifications:
  - Glycosylated LDL
  - Reduced LDL recognition by cellular LDL receptors
  - Increased susceptibility of LDL to oxidative modification

LDL, low-density lipoprotein.

BOX 2 Atherosclerosis promoting effects of advanced glycation end products: receptor mediated mechanisms

- Promoting inflammation:
  - Secretion of cytokines such as TNF-α, IL-1
  - Chemotactic stimulus for monocyte-macrophages
- Induction of cellular proliferation:
  - Stimulation of PDGF and IGF-1 secretion from monocytes and possibly SmC
- Endothelial dysfunction:
  - Increased permeability of EC monolayers
  - Increased procoagulant activity
  - Increased expression of adhesion molecules
  - Increased intracellular oxidative stress

TNF-α, tumor necrosis factor alpha; IGF-1, insulin-like growth factor 1; IL-1, interleukin-1; PDGF, platelet-derived growth factor; SmC, somatomedin-C.

The most well-known example is interference of the normal physiology of the low-density lipoprotein (LDL) particle. Elevated level of AGEs have been found in clinical studies on LDL obtained from patients of DM compared with normal individuals.[25,26] The process of glycosylation affects both the phospholipid and apolipoprotein B (ApoB) components of LDL, which functionally alters the LDL clearance and make them more vulnerable to oxidative modifications. LDL glycosylation is increased in correlation with glucose levels, and AGE-ApoB levels are up to 4-fold higher in diabetic patients. Significant impairment of LDL-receptor-mediated uptake is produced by glycosylation of ApoB, thereby reducing the *in vivo* clearance of LDL compared to native LDL. Several studies have demonstrated that degradation of glycated LDL is impaired in cultured human fibroblasts (which possess LDL receptor) compared with normal LDL. This impairment is proportional to the extent of glycation. Human monocyte-derived macrophages in contrast to fibroblasts, recognize glycated LDL preferentially to native LDL. The uptake of glycated LDL by these cells, however, is not mediated by the LDL receptor pathway, but by a high-capacity, low-affinity receptor pathway. A nonspecific (scavenger) receptor presents on human macrophages also preferentially recognizes these glycated LDL. The recognition of glycated LDL by the scavenger receptor pathway is thought to be instrumental in accumulation of cholesteryl esters intracellularly. This process promotes atherosclerotic plaque progression and various manifestations of CAD.[26,27]

Increased susceptibility of LDL to oxidative modification induces atherogenesis. Glycation makes the LDL more vulnerable to oxidative modification, which is considered a critical initiating step. AGE-LDL formation and oxidation is found to be directly proportional to glucose concentration, which has been found to be inhibited by the AGE formation inhibitor aminoguanidine. Change in normal function of the complement regulatory protein is another mechanism. When the membrane attack complex (MAC) of complement gets deposited in blood vessels, it stimulates proliferation of fibroblasts and smooth muscle cells. This leads to release of growth factors such as fibroblast growth factor and platelet derived-growth factor (PDGF) from MAC-targeted endothelium. Cells express the regulatory membrane protein complement defense 59 (CD59), which limits complement activation and MAC formation. There is increased sensitivity of the endothelium in patients of DM to MAC-induced release of growth factors and cytokines. This is also attributed to glycation of the complement regulatory protein CD59 producing its inactivation.[27,28]

Receptor-mediated Mechanisms

The AGE receptor (RAGE), a member of the immunoglobulin superfamily of receptors, has been demonstrated in various types of cells involved with the process of atherosclerosis including endothelial cells, monocyte-derived macrophages, and smooth muscle cells (Box 2). The macrophage RAGE system is closely linked to AGE turnover. It represents a mechanism that responds to raising AGE levels with aging and degrades senescent proteins. In diabetic vasculature, cells expressing increased levels of RAGE are often proximal to areas in which AGEs are abundant. AGE interaction with RAGE on endothelial cells results in the induction of oxidative stress and consequently of the transcription factor nuclear factor kappa-light-chain-enhancer of activated B cells (NF-κB) and vascular cell adhesion molecule 1 (VCAM-1). In addition, engagement of AGEs with their specific receptors results in reduced endothelial barrier function leading to increased permeability of endothelial cell monolayers. The interaction of AGEs with RAGE-bearing endothelial cells can thus mediate initiating events in atherogenesis, which leads to catastrophic features of CAD. Increased endothelial permeability can cause enhanced lipid entry into the subendothelium. Enhancement of adhesive interactions of monocytes with the endothelial surface can subsequently result in transendothelial migration. Binding of soluble AGEs to RAGE-bearing monocytes induces chemotaxis, followed by mononuclear infiltration through an intact endothelial monolayer. Pathological studies of human atherosclerotic plaques showed infiltration of RAGE-expressing cells in the expanded intima. Monocyte-macrophage system interact with AGEs resulting in the production of mediators such as tumour necrosis factor-α, interleukin-1, PDGF, and insulin growth factor-I, which play a pivotal role in the pathogenesis of atherosclerosis. Binding of AGE-modified proteins to RAGE is associated with increased cellular proliferation in smooth muscle cells. This growth-promoting effects mediated by the RAGE are likely to be cytokine or growth-factor mediated. Under conditions of enhanced tissue AGE deposition, receptor-mediated interaction of AGE-proteins with vascular wall cells promotes the migration of inflammatory cells into the plaque with the subsequent release of growth-promoting cytokines.

Park and associates demonstrated the potential role of RAGE in the atherogenic process in DM. The induction of DM using streptozotocin resulted in atherosclerosis of increased severity compared to euglycemic ApoE controls in mice models. The atherosclerotic process extended distally in the aorta and major arteries. Vascular lesions developed more rapidly with the formation of more complex lesions (extensive monocyte infiltration, fibrous caps, etc.). Especially at sites of vascular lesions it was evident that increased expression of RAGE and the presence of AGEs in the vessel wall. Blocking the AGE-RAGE interaction by a modified domain of RAGE produced a striking suppression of lesions in diabetic mice. The lesions got arrested at the fatty streak stage and there was a large reduction in complex lesions. These effects were not dependent on glucose and lipid levels.[25-28]

Protein Kinase C

Cells in which glucose transport is mostly independent of insulin bear the brunt of metabolic effects of hyperglycemia. The resulting intracellular hyperglycemia has been linked to the activation of the PKC system and subsequent development of complications of DM. Elevated ambient glucose concentrations activate PKC by augmenting the production of diacylglycerol (DAG). This crucial endogenous cellular cofactor for PKC activation is generated from products of glycolysis such as dihydroxyacetone phosphate and glyceraldehyde-3-phosphate. Such elevated concentration of DAG leading to activation of PKC in the vasculature can be maintained long term.

Protein kinase C constitutes a family of approximately 12 isoforms of serine and threonine kinases. Despite several PKC isoforms getting expressed in vascular tissue, there is a preferential activation of PKC β2 in the aorta, heart, and retina, and PKC β1 in the glomeruli in the rat model of DM. The PKC system is widely distributed in cells and is instrumental in the transcription of several growth factors, and their signal transduction. PKC activation in several studies has been attributed to modulate growth rate, DNA synthesis, and growth factor receptor turnover in vascular smooth muscle cells (SMC). PKC activation is induced by hyperglycemia, thereby increasing PDGF-β receptor expression on smooth muscle cells and other vascular cells (e.g., endothelial cells, monocyte-macrophages). Activation of PKC stimulates the formation of transforming growth factor-β (TGF-β), which is the key growth factor for regulation of extracellular matrix formation by activating gene expression of proteoglycans and collagen and reducing the synthesis of proteolytic enzymes that break down matrix proteins, which has a key pathogenetic role in ACS. Enhanced expression of TGF-β is incriminated in capillary basement membrane thickening, which is one of the early structural abnormalities detected in almost all tissues in DM.[28,29]

Oxidative Stress

Oxidative stress has been incriminated as a powerful mechanism for accelerated atherosclerosis in diabetics. Hyperglycemia can induce oxidative stress through various pathways. Hyperglycemia induced intracellular reactive oxygen species (ROS), generated by the mitochondrial electron transport chain is one important mechanism leading to increased superoxide production.

Besides that, two other mechanisms have been postulated to explain how hyperglycemia induces increased ROS formation. Transition metal-catalyzed autoxidation of free glucose is one of those. Glucose itself starts the autoxidation process and free radical production producing superoxide anion (O_2^-) and hydrogen peroxide (H_2O_2) through this reaction. Another mechanism is autoxidation of protein-bound Amadori products catalyzed by transition metals, which produces superoxide and hydroxyl radicals and highly reactive dicarbonyl compounds (see glycoxidation).

Hyperglycemia may weaken natural antioxidant mechanisms. In healthy individuals, free radicals are rapidly eliminated by antioxidants such as vitamin C, vitamin E, and reduced glutathione. Decrease in glutathione content, as well as reduced vitamin E have been reported in patients of DM. Tissue and plasma levels of vitamin C are 40–50% lower in diabetics compared with nondiabetic subjects. Hyperglycemia-induced oxidant stress has close pathogenic link with two dominant mechanisms of vascular damage, namely AGEs formation and PKC activation as suggested by researchers.[28,30]

Glycoxidation

Some AGEs are generated by combined processes of oxidation and glycation and hence, known as glycoxidation products. The amount of oxidative stress and mechanism of formation is unique for each AGE. Protein-based AGEs are irreversible, so it has been postulated that they might serve as a biomarker for the long-term oxidative stress of DM on various tissues. AGE epitopes interact with the RAGE present on cell surface to release oxygen radicals by upregulating oxidative stress response genes. Thus, hyperglycemia not only enhances both AGEs formation and oxidative stress, it also facilitates interactions between glycation and oxidation mechanisms. On the long run, this contributes synergistically to the formation of AGEs, oxidative stress, and diabetic complications like CAD. Strong correlations have been found between levels of glycoxidation products in skin collagen and the severity of renal, retinal, and vascular disease in DM.[23,30]

Oxidative Stress and Protein Kinase C Activation

Activation of DAG-PKC can be produced by oxidants produced in the setting of hyperglycemia in vascular tissues in patients of DM. Indirect evidence to substantiate such concept has been gathered from several studies demonstrating antioxidants such as vitamin E can inhibit PKC activation probably by decreasing DAG levels.[28]

CONCLUSION

To conclude, DM and CAD are variously termed as "deadly duo" and "partners in crime". A study of their prevalence and mechanisms will definitely provide critical insights into these 21st century's alarming global pandemics. This may provide impetus to young and vibrant minds to explore new field of research in future, which can provide path-breaking strategies for countering this double menace.

REFERENCES

1. Gu K, Cowie CC, Harris MI. Diabetes and decline of heart disease mortality in US adults. JAMA. 1999;281(14):1921-7.
2. Malmberg K, Yusuf S, Gerstein HC, et al. Impact of diabetes on long term prognosis in patients with CAD: Results of OASIS. Circulation. 2000;102(9):1014-9.
3. Third report of NCEP on treatment of high blood cholesterol in adults (ATP III). JAMA. 2001;285(19):2486-97.
4. Hurst RT, Lee RW. Increase incidence of CAD in type 2 diabetes. Ann Intern Med. 2003;139(10);824-34.
5. Mather HM, Chaturbedi N, Fuller JH, et al. Mortality and morbidity from diabetes in South Asians and Europeans: 11-year follow-up of the Southall Diabetes Survey, London, UK. Diabet Med. 1998;15(1):53-9.
6. Joshi P, Islam S, Pais P, et al. Risk factors for early myocardial infarction in South Asians compared with individuals in other countries. JAMA. 2007;297(3):286-94.
7. Goyal A, Yusuf S. The burden of cardiovascular disease in the Indian subcontinent. Indian J Med Res. 2006;124(3):235-44.
8. McKeiguie PM, Shah B. Relationship of insulin resistance to high prevalence of cardiovascular disease in South Asians. Lancet. 1991;337:382-6.
9. Gammon BD, Gunarathne A. It's time to reappraise recruitment of South Asians to clinical trials. BMJ. 2008;336(7634):46.
10. Ramachandran A, Snehalatha C. Current scenario of diabetes in India. J Diabetes. 2017;1(1):18-28
11. Ramachandran A, Snehalatha C. Rising prevalence of NIDDM in an urban population in India. Diabetologia. 1997;40(2):232-7.
12. Reddy KS, Yusuf S. Emerging epidemic of cardiovascular disease in developing countries. Circulation. 1998;97(6):596-601.
13. Chadha SL, Radhakrishnan S, Ramachandran K, et al. Epidemiological study of coronary heart disease in urban population of Delhi. Indian J Med Res. 1990;92:424-30.
14. Gupta R, Gupta VP. Meta-analysis of coronary heart disease prevalence in India. Indian Heart J. 1996;48(3):241-5.
15. Kannel WB. Metabolic risk factors for coronary heart disease in women: perspective from the Framingham Study. Am Heart J. 1987;114(2):413-9.
16. Haffner SM, Letho S, Rönnemma T, et al. Mortality from coronary heart disease in subjects with type 2 diabetes and in nondiabetic subjects with and without prior myocardial infarction. Am J Med. 1998;339(4):229-34.
17. Mohan V, Premalatha G, Sastry NG. Ischaemic heart disease in south Indian NIDDM patients—a clinic based study on 6,597 NIDDM patients. Int J Diab Dev Countries. 1995;15:64-7.
18. Yusuf S, Flather M. Lessons learnt from OASIS 1 and 2. IHJ. 2005;57(3):217-25.
19. Xavier D, Pais P, Devereaux PJ, et al. Treatment and outcomes of acute coronary syndromes in India (CREATE): a prospective analysis of registry data. Lancet. 2008;371(9622):1435-42.
20. Laakso M. Hyperglycemia and cardiovascular disease in type 2 diabetes. Diabetes. 1999;48(5):937-42.
21. Grundy SM, Benjamin IJ, Burke GL, et al. Diabetes and cardiovascular disease: a statement for healthcare professionals from the American Heart Association. Circulation. 1999;48(5):937-42.
22. Nathan DM, Genuth S, Lachin J, et al.; Diabetes Control and Complications Trial Research Group. The effect of intensive treatment of diabetes on the development and progression of long-term complications in insulin-dependent diabetes mellitus. N Engl J Med. 1993;329(14):977-86.
23. Nishikawa T, Edelstein D, Du XL, et al. Normalizing mitochondrial superoxide production blocks three pathways of hyperglycaemic damage. Nature. 2000;404(6779):787-90.
24. Brownlee M, Cerami A, Vlassara H. Advanced glycosylation end products in tissue and the biochemical basis of diabetic complications. N Engl J Med. 1988;318(20):1315-21.

25. Schmidt AM, Yan SD, Wautier JL, et al. Activation of receptor for advanced glycation end products: a mechanism for chronic vascular dysfunction in diabetic vasculopathy and atherosclerosis. Circ Res. 1999;84(5):489-97.
26. Bowie A, Owens D, Collins P, et al. Glycosylated low density lipoprotein is more sensitive to oxidation: implications for the diabetic patient? Atherosclerosis. 1993;102(1):63-7.
27. Vlassara H, Bucala R, Striker L. Pathogenic effects of advanced glycosylation: biochemical, biologic, and clinical implications for diabetes and aging. Lab Invest. 1994;70(2):138-51.
28. Feener EP, King GL. Vascular dysfunction in diabetes mellitus. Lancet. 1997;350 Suppl 1):SI9-13.
29. Koya D, King GL. Protein kinase C activation and the development of diabetic complications. Diabetes. 1998;47(6):859-66.
30. Baynes JW. Role of oxidative stress in development of complications in diabetes. Diabetes. 1991;40(4):405-12.

CHAPTER 16

Management of Diabetes in Heart Failure

Shashank R Joshi

THE PROBLEM

The coexistence of heart failure (HF) and type 2 diabetes mellitus (T2DM) represents a multidimensional challenge, in the epidemiological, pathological, as well as clinical aspects. Hyperglycemia and insulin resistance in T2DM are well-recognized pathological mechanisms for the development of diabetic cardiomyopathy and resultant clinical HF.[1] Each 1% rise in the hemoglobin A1c (HbA1c) level is known to impose a 15% increased risk of developing HF.[2]

As observed in the Framingham Heart Study, diabetes mellitus (DM) is associated with 1.8-fold increased risk of HF in men, and 3.8-fold increased risk in women.[3] HF is also known to be among the most common early clinical manifestations of cardiovascular disease (CVD) in T2DM. One out of every seven patients of T2DM, without known CVD, develops HF over the ensuing 5–6 years.[4]

Heart failure and T2DM share a bidirectional clinico-pathological relationship. Patients with HF demonstrate a more than twofold greater odds of new-onset T2DM. Further, the development of DM also increases the mortality risk in HF by 2.5-fold.[5] Coexistence of DM and HF incrementally worsens the quality of life.[6] Further, chronic kidney disease (CKD) may complicate the clinical picture of DM as well as HF. These pathologically interrelated comorbidities frequently coexist, and significantly increase the risk of cardiovascular (CV) mortality.[7] The modifiable risk-factors for HF including obesity, hypertension, coronary artery disease, and anemia, commonly coexist in T2DM and need to be addressed for optimum holistic management of HF in T2DM.[8]

The Trivandrum Heart Failure Registry of patients hospitalized for HF, suggested DM to be present in over half of the hospitalized patients. Importantly, less than a quarter of these patients received guideline-based medical treatment. As expected, the registry did suggest significantly greater 90-day mortality in these patients not receiving optimum HF therapy, as compared to the optimally managed patients.[9] The PINNACLE India Quality Improvement Program (PIQIP) registry also reflected a similar lack of optimum guideline-directed medical therapy in Indian patients of HF.[10]

SCREENING FOR HEART FAILURE IN TYPE 2 DIABETES MELLITUS

The diagnosis of HF in T2DM depends on assessments of clinical signs and symptoms, electrocardiography (ECG), N-terminal pro-brain natriuretic peptide (NT-proBNP) level, as well as confirmatory echocardiography. While the assessments of signs and symptoms as well as ECG are recommended for every patient of T2DM, the optimum diagnosis of HF may be missed in the absence of echocardiography. Boonman de-Winter et al. suggested a simple screening tool based on a validated risk-score derived from the patient history and physical examination, as summarized in table 1.[11] As validated in a T2DM population in the Netherlands, this clinical screening approach demonstrated optimum sensitivity (70.8%), specificity (79.0%), negative

TABLE 1: Clinical screening tool for heart failure in type 2 diabetes mellitus

Clinical criterion	Score
Age >75 years	1
History of ischemic heart disease*	1
History of transient ischemic attack or stroke	1
Dyspnea or fatigue	2
Reported ankle edema or nocturia	1
Claudication-related complaints	1
Pulmonary crepitations, elevated JVP, peripheral edema, and/or hepatomegaly	1

If the total score is more than 3 points, the patient should be referred for echocardiography.

*Prior myocardial infarction/angina pectoris/coronary artery bypass graft and/or PCI

JVP, jugular venous pressure; PCI, percutaneous coronary intervention.

predictive value (87.6%), and positive predictive value (56.4%). If the overall score is more than 3, the patient should be referred for echocardiography to confirm the diagnosis of HF. The association between this clinical screening tool and confirmatory echocardiography was strong. Further, the incremental improvement of screening was marginal, when ECG and NT-proBNP were considered in addition to this clinical screening tool. Thus, in resource-limited settings, this clinical screening tool may be of relevance in timely screening for HF in T2DM.

Further, a systematic meta-analysis of Matsushita et al. has suggested an incremental value in predicting HF risk, based on albuminuria, as well as estimated glomerular filtration rate (eGFR).[12] Both these assessments independently improve the screening efficiency of HF in T2DM, and should be considered in all patients.

GLYCEMIA CONTROL AND HEART FAILURE: CHOICE OF ANTIDIABETIC THERAPIES

While the optimum management of T2DM, from an HF perspective, remains an area of immense scientific scope and interest, our understanding has evolved mainly with the serendipitous experiences, as well as some focused research in this area. Certain antidiabetic agents like thiazolidinediones (TZDs) and saxagliptin have demonstrated clear worsening of HF-related outcomes, whereas agents like sodium-glucose cotransporter 2 inhibitors (SGLT2i) agents have suggested promising leads. The evidence with other agents remains either insufficient or equivocal. While the jury is out regarding the choice of most glucose-lowering therapies and HF outcomes in T2DM, priority must be given to an individualized patient-centric approach for optimum holistic management of T2DM.

METFORMIN

As per the legally approved prescribing information, metformin is associated with the risk of lactic acidosis, in patients with HF. However, the clinical experience of metformin over the decades, suggests a possibly favorable risk-benefit balance, for glycemia control in T2DM with HF. Robust evidence from well-conducted randomized controlled trials is not currently available for metformin; however, the ongoing research will evolve our understanding in this regard, which is presently based on evidence from observational studies.

A recently published meta-analysis of 17 observational studies evaluated the use of metformin in patients of T2DM with CKD, HF, or chronic liver disease. In all these comorbidities, metformin use was associated with a significant and meaningful reduction in the risk of all-cause mortality. Further, the risk of readmissions for congestive heart failure (CHF) was also meaningfully reduced in patients with prior HF or CKD.[13] Another review of nine observational studies, performed in patients of T2DM and HF, suggested a significant 20% reduction in mortality with metformin, as compared to controls; the studies included in this review mostly compared metformin with sulfonylureas. Further, the use of metformin in patients with HF did not suggest an increase in the risk of lactic acidosis.[14] Mechanism-based studies on metformin have demonstrated inconsistent findings for plausible cardiovascular effects, in relation to cardiac function.[15-18] The European Society of Cardiology (ESC) guidelines suggest metformin as a safe option for glycemia control in patients of T2DM with HF.[19]

SODIUM-GLUCOSE COTRANSPORTER 2 INHIBITORS

The SGLT2i agents have demonstrated promising HF outcomes in patients of T2DM. These agents have a mild glucose-mediated diuretic effect; however, they are different from classical diuretic agents, in multiple ways. The SGLT2i agents demonstrate a more predominant effect on the interstitial fluid volume as compared to blood volume, unlike the classical diuretics. This may be associated with less profound implications on rebound mechanisms, like activation of the renin-angiotensin-aldosterone system (RAAS), as well as more meaningful implications on clinical outcomes related to HF.[20] Some of the SGLT2i agents have demonstrated robust cardiovascular protection in well-conducted studies. EMPA-REG OUTCOME study of empagliflozin, evaluated the CV outcomes in patients of T2DM with CVD (including significant coronary artery disease, peripheral arterial disease, myocardial infarction, or stroke). Empagliflozin demonstrated significant improvements in CV outcomes on top of standard of care, including 14% reduction in the risk of major adverse CV events (composite of CV death, myocardial infarction, and stroke), 38% risk reduction in CV death, and 32% relative reduction in all-cause death. Particularly, 35% reduction in the risk of hospitalizations for HF was also observed with empagliflozin, as assessed in the secondary analysis.[21] Further, the CV protective effects of empagliflozin were evident consistently, irrespective of the baseline HbA1c level, irrespective of the control of major CV risk-factors, and early and sustainably over the course of therapy.[21,22] Furthermore, empagliflozin reduced the risk of hospitalizations for HF consistently, across the spectrum of 5-year risk of HF at baseline, in this study.[23] A small study involving patients of T2DM with CVD and heart failure with preserved ejection fraction (HFpEF), demonstrated improvement in cardiac structure (left ventricular mass index) and function (early lateral annular tissue Doppler velocity), with the use of empagliflozin over 16 weeks.[24] At present, empagliflozin is the only oral antidiabetic agent, which is approved for reduction in the risk of CV death in patients of T2DM with CVD, and is also recommended by the ESC guidelines for preventing or delaying the onset of HF and prolonging life.[19]

The Canagliflozin Cardiovascular Assessment Study (CANVAS) program of canagliflozin, involving patients of T2DM with high CV risk, also demonstrated a 14% reduction in the risk of major adverse CV events with canagliflozin. In the secondary analysis, hospitalizations for HF were reduced by 33% in patients receiving canagliflozin.[25] However, significant reductions in CV mortality and all-cause mortality were not observed with canagliflozin, in either the patients with known history of atherosclerotic CVD, or in those with multiple CV risk-factors.[25] Till date, the data from prospective CV outcomes trials for the SGLT2i class are available only for empagliflozin and canagliflozin. The real-world observational studies have suggested possible benefit of SGLT2i agents on the HF outcomes in T2DM, as compared to other glucose-lowering drugs.[26] The limitations of observational studies must be considered during clinical decision making, as certain observations in these observational studies have been discordant with those in the randomized controlled trials of the CANVAS program.[27]

The DECLARE-TIMI 58, VERTIS CV, CREDENCE, EMPEROR, EMPERIAL, EMPA-VISION, EMPA-Kidney, DAPA-HF, DAPACARD, and DAPA-CKD are few of the ongoing trials that may provide further elaborate insights into CV and renal outcomes with the SGLT2i agents, in patients with or without T2DM. The currently available evidence suggests that the SGLT2i agents hold promise in terms of improving the HF outcomes, in patients with T2DM. The evidence for SGLT2i agents, in patients with advanced HF, is currently limited. Clinical discretion is essential when these agents are combined with loop diuretic agents; as appropriate, the dose of loop diuretic agent may be reduced. Dehydration should be avoided in patients receiving SGLT2i agents. These agents are not recommended for glycemia control, in patients with moderate-to-severe CKD (eGFR level of <45 mL/min/1.73 m^2).

DIPEPTIDYL PEPTIDASE-4 INHIBITORS

The evidence, regarding possible HF risk associated with the use of dipeptidyl peptidase-4 inhibitor (DPP4i) agents, has been evolving. The SAVOR-TIMI 53 study demonstrated significant 27% increased risk of hospitalizations for HF, associated with saxagliptin; this risk was more prominent in patients with increased levels of natriuretic peptide levels at baseline, prior history of HF, and background CKD.[28] The EXAMINE trial of alogliptin demonstrated a 19% nonsignificant increase in the risk of hospitalizations for HF, associated with alogliptin use.[29] In the TECOS trial of sitagliptin, no increase in the risk of HF-related hospitalizations or deaths was observed, in patients receiving sitagliptin.[30] A meta-analysis of these three studies suggested a nonsignificant, 14% numerically increased risk of HF-related hospitalizations with moderate heterogeneity, with DPP4i agents in comparison to placebo.[31]

The CV safety meta-analysis of linagliptin did not suggest increased risk of HF events.[32] The VIVIDD trial assessed vildagliptin in patients with heart failure with reduced ejection fraction (HFrEF). Vildagliptin was not associated with significant increase in left ventricular ejection fraction. However, the left ventricular end-diastolic volume was significantly increased in patients receiving vildagliptin.[33] The evidence on hard clinical CV outcomes with teneligliptin is presently under evaluation. Teneligliptin may cause QT interval prolongation in patients with arrhythmia, severe bradycardia or its history, patients with CHF, low-serum potassium, congenital prolonged QT syndrome, history of torsades de pointes, or patients using antiarrhythmic drugs.

A meta-analysis of good quality studies of DPP4i agents, demonstrated significant 13% increased risk of hospitalizations for HF with these agents. The evidence does not address whether this increased risk is a class effect for the DPP4i agents.[34]

In March 2018, a warning note was added to the prescribing information of all the DPP4i agents, for considering the risks and benefits of DPP4i agent prior to initiating treatment in patients at risk for HF, such as those with a prior history of HF and a history of renal impairment, and to observe these patients for signs and symptoms of HF during therapy. Patients must be advised of the characteristic symptoms of HF and to immediately report such symptoms. If HF develops, the DPP4i agent should be discontinued. If the available evidence is considered on face value, a conclusive evidence of increased risk of HF is presently available only for saxagliptin, among the DPP4i agents.

GLUCAGON-LIKE PEPTIDE-1 RECEPTOR AGONISTS

The glucagon-like peptide-1 receptor agonists (GLP-1RAs) are known to increase the heart rate. In patients of T2DM with CVD, liraglutide has demonstrated significant reduction in major adverse CV events, as well as CV mortality, in the LEADER trial.[35] Liraglutide is also indicated for reduction in CV events, beyond glycemia control, in patients of T2DM with CVD. However, the CV benefits evident with liraglutide are more likely to be based on antiatherosclerotic mechanisms. In terms of the HF-related outcomes, the GLP-1RA agents have not demonstrated a clinical benefit.[36] More importantly, liraglutide use had been associated with a nonsignificant trend of increase in death or hospitalization for HF, in patients of HFrEF, in the FIGHT study.[37] In another study involving patients of HFpEF, liraglutide therapy had been associated with increased heart rate by 6 beats/min, and significantly increased risk of serious cardiac events.[38]

The evidence suggests clinical consideration of possible increase in the heart rate with the use of GLP-1RA agents, in the management of T2DM with HF. Further, there is no evidence to suggest clinical benefit of these agents on HF-related outcomes.

SULFONYLUREAS

The available evidence based on observational studies, suggests a possibly increased risk of CV events and mortality, associated with the use of sulfonylureas.[39] The risk of HF with metformin and sulfonylureas was compared in an observational study of propensity matched groups. The use of sulfonylureas was associated with significant 30% increased risk for hospitalizations for HF, as compared to metformin. These findings were consistently observed in patients with or without prior HF.[40] In another propensity matched analysis of an observational registry database, DPP4i agents as well as TZDs were associated with lower risk of hospitalizations for HF, as compared to sulfonylureas.[41] The Bypass Angioplasty Revascularization Investigation 2 Diabetes (BARI 2D) was a randomized controlled trial, involving patients of T2DM and significant coronary artery disease. In this study, the insulin-provision therapy group (sulfonylureas and/or insulin) was associated with a similar incidence of HF events, as compared to insulin-sensitization therapy group (metformin and/or TZD).[42] The ongoing CAROLINA trial, for assessing the CV outcomes with linagliptin or glimepiride, as second-line therapies in T2DM, will provide further insights on CV outcomes with sulfonylureas.

Overall, the evidence, on possibly increased risk of HF events with the use of sulfonylureas, has been inconclusive. Limited evidence from observational studies suggests possibly increased risk for HF events associated with sulfonylurea use, in comparison to metformin, DPP4i agents, and TZDs. However, the subanalysis of a randomized controlled trial might suggest a possible benefit of doubt, in favor of a safe HF profile of these agents.

THIAZOLIDINEDIONES

The prescribing information of pioglitazone includes a warning statement related to the occurrence or exacerbation of congestive HF. Patients receiving TZDs should be closely monitored for the signs and symptoms of HF. If the development of HF is suspected, TZDs should be discontinued and HF should be managed as per the standards of care. TZDs are not recommended in patients with symptomatic HF, and are absolutely contraindicated in patients with established the New York Heart Association (NYHA) class III or IV HF.

The PROactive study assessed the CV outcomes with pioglitazone, in patients of T2DM with macrovascular complications.[43] In this trial, pioglitazone was associated with significantly increased risk of hospitalizations due to HF, but not in the rate of mortality due to HF. Further, the RECORD trial also demonstrated a 2.1-fold increased risk of death or hospitalization due to HF, in patients receiving rosiglitazone. An increased risk of fatal HF outcomes was observed with the use of rosiglitazone in this trial.[44]

INSULIN

Insulin hormone has a strong propensity for sodium and fluid retention, which may facilitate the pathological development of HF. The clinical evidence of possibly increased risk of HF outcomes with the use of insulin is presently limited, and inconclusive. In patients of T2DM with HF, evidence from randomized controlled trials and observational studies suggests an increased risk for HF-related hospitalizations, and mortality outcomes, associated with insulin use.[45] The effects of intensive glycemia control with insulin were assessed in patients of myocardial infarction and hyperglycemia, in the two DIGAMI studies; both these studies suggested contradictory outcomes for insulin, in terms of improvement in survival.[46,47] The ORIGIN trial of insulin glargine suggested a neutral effect on the risk of hospitalizations for HF. The effect of higher doses of insulin glargine was not evaluated in the ORIGIN study.[48] Among the short-acting insulin, the observational evidence is presently limited to make any conclusive inference.[49] In patients with advanced diabetes or comorbid diseases, the use of insulin may be unavoidable, regardless of the limited evidence on the possible increased risk of HF.

CONCLUSION

The importance of comprehensive management of T2DM, from a HF perspective, cannot be understated. HF is one of the most common manifestations of T2DM, and occurs early in the course of disease. Following guideline-directed medical therapy for HF is essential to improve outcomes. Our evidence-based understanding, on the possible influences of antidiabetic therapies on HF outcomes, has been evolving over time. At present, the evidence suggests a clearly increased risk of HF-related outcomes, with agents like saxagliptin and TZDs. SGLT2i agents have demonstrated a clinical promise in improving HF-related outcomes. The evidence regarding most of the other classes of agents on HF outcomes has been limited, inconsistent, or inconclusive. In the individualized patient-centric approach for the management of T2DM, the available evidence (with apposite strengths and limitations) on the HF outcomes with different agents should be considered to support clinical decision making.

REFERENCES

1. Jia G, DeMarco VG, Sowers JR. Insulin resistance and hyperinsulinaemia in diabetic cardiomyopathy. Nat Rev Endocrinol. 2016;12(3):144-53.
2. Erqou S, Lee CT, Suffoletto M, et al. Association between glycated haemoglobin and the risk of congestive heart failure in diabetes mellitus: systematic review and meta-analysis. Eur J Heart Fail. 2013;15(2):185-93.
3. Qazi MU, Malik S. Diabetes and Cardiovascular Disease: Insights from the Framingham Heart Study. Global Heart. 2013;8(1):43-8.
4. Shah AD, Langenberg C, Rapsomaniki E, et al. Type 2 diabetes and incidence of cardiovascular diseases: a cohort study in 1·9 million people. Lancet Diabetes Endocrinol. 2015;3(2):105-13.
5. Romero SP, Garcia-Egido A, Escobar MA, et al. Impact of new-onset diabetes mellitus and glycemic control on the prognosis of heart failure patients: a propensity-matched study in the community. Int J Cardiol. 2013;167(4):1206-16.
6. Fujita B, Lauten A, Goebel B, et al. Impact of diabetes mellitus on quality of life in patients with congestive heart failure. Qual Life Res. 2012;21(7):1171-6.
7. Pálsson R, Patel UD. Cardiovascular complications of diabetic kidney disease. Adv Chronic Kidney Dis. 2014;21(3):273-80.
8. Thomas MC. Type 2 diabetes and heart failure: challenges and solutions. Curr Cardiol Rev. 2016;12(3):249-55.
9. Harikrishnan S, Sanjay G, Anees T, et al. Clinical presentation, management, in-hospital and 90-day outcomes of heart failure patients in Trivandrum, Kerala, India: the Trivandrum Heart Failure Registry. Eur J Heart Fail. 2015;17(8):794-800.
10. Pokharel Y, Wei J, Hira RS, et al. Guideline-Directed Medication Use in Patients With Heart Failure With Reduced Ejection Fraction in India: American College of Cardiology's PINNACLE India Quality Improvement Program. Clin Cardiol. 2016;39(3):145-9.
11. Boonman-de Winter LJ, Rutten FH, et al. Efficiently screening heart failure in patients with type 2 diabetes. Eur J Heart Fail. 2015;17(2):187-95.
12. Matsushita K, Coresh J, Sang Y, et al. Kidney measures beyond traditional risk factors for cardiovascular prediction: A collaborative meta-analysis. Lancet Diabetes Endocrinol. 2015;3(7):514-25.

13. Crowley MJ, Diamantidis CJ, McDuffie JR, et al. Clinical outcomes of metformin use in populations with chronic kidney disease, congestive heart failure, or chronic liver disease: a systematic review. Ann Inter Med. 2017;166(3):191-200.
14. Eurich DT, Weir DL, Majumdar SR, et al. Comparative safety and effectiveness of metformin in patients with diabetes and heart failure: systematic review of observational studies involving 34,000 patients. Circ Heart Fail. 2013;6(3):395-402.
15. van der Meer RW, Rijzewijk LJ, de Jong HW, et al. Pioglitazone improves cardiac function and alters myocardial substrate metabolism without affecting cardiac triglyceride accumulation and high-energy phosphate metabolism in patients with well-controlled type 2 diabetes mellitus. Circulation. 2009;119(15):2069-77.
16. Rena G, Lang CC. Repurposing metformin for cardiovascular disease. Circulation. 2018;137(5):422-4.
17. Lexis CP, van der Horst IC, Lipsic E, et al. Effect of metformin on left ventricular function after acute myocardial infarction in patients without diabetes: the GIPS-III randomized clinical trial. JAMA. 2014;311(15):1526-35.
18. Leung M, Wong VW, Hudson M, et al. Impact of Improved Glycemic Control on Cardiac Function in Type 2 Diabetes Mellitus. Circ Cardiovasc Imaging. 2016;9(3):e003643.
19. Ponikowski P, Voors AA, Anker SD, et al. 2016 ESC Guidelines for the diagnosis and treatment of acute and chronic heart failure: The Task Force for the diagnosis and treatment of acute and chronic heart failure of the European Society of Cardiology (ESC). Developed with the special contribution of the Heart Failure Association (HFA) of the ESC. Eur J Heart Fail. 2016;18(8):891-975.
20. Hallow KM, Helmlinger G, Greasley PJ, et al. Why do SGLT2 inhibitors reduce heart failure hospitalization? A differential volume regulation hypothesis. Diabetes Obes Metab. 2018;20(3):479-87.
21. Zinman B, Wanner C, Lachin JM, et al. Empagliflozin, cardiovascular outcomes, and mortality in type 2 diabetes. N Engl J Med. 2015;373(22):2117-28.
22. Inzucchi SE, Fitchett D, Wanner C, et al. Does baseline HbA1c or change in HbA1c predict the reduction in cardiovascular death with empagliflozin? Results from EMPA-REG Outcome. Diabet Med. 2018;35(1):11-1.
23. Fitchett D, Butler J, van de Borne P, et al. Effects of empagliflozin on risk for cardiovascular death and heart failure hospitalization across the spectrum of heart failure risk in the EMPA-REG Outcome trial. Eur Heart J. 2017;39(5):363-70.
24. Verma S, Garg A, Yan AT, et al. Effect of Empagliflozin on Left Ventricular Mass and Diastolic Function in Individuals With Diabetes: An Important Clue to the EMPA-REG OUTCOME Trial? Diabetes Care. 2016;39(12):e212-3.
25. Mahaffey KW, Neal B, Perkovic V, et al. Canagliflozin for primary and secondary prevention of cardiovascular events: results from the CANVAS program (Canagliflozin Cardiovascular Assessment Study). Circulation. 2018;137(4):323-34.
26. Kosiborod M, Cavender MA, Fu AZ, et al. Lower Risk of Heart Failure and Death in Patients Initiated on Sodium-Glucose Cotransporter-2 Inhibitors Versus Other Glucose-Lowering Drugs Clinical Perspective: The CVD-REAL Study (Comparative Effectiveness of Cardiovascular Outcomes in New Users of Sodium-Glucose Cotransporter-2 Inhibitors). Circulation. 2017;136(3):249-59.
27. Suissa S. Lower risk of death with SGLT2 inhibitors in observational studies: real or bias? Diabetes Care. 2018;41(1):6-10.
28. Scirica BM, Braunwald E, Raz I, et al. Heart Failure, Saxagliptin, and Diabetes Mellitus: Observations from the SAVOR-TIMI 53 Randomized Trial. Circulation. 2015;132(15):e198.
29. Zannad F, Cannon C, Cushman W, et al. Alogliptin in patients with type 2 diabetes after acute coronary syndromes: heart failure outcomes and cardiovascular safety in heart failure patients. J Am Coll Cardiol. 2014;63(12 Suppl):A117.
30. McGuire DK, Van de Werf F, Armstrong PW, et al. Association Between Sitagliptin Use and Heart Failure Hospitalization and Related Outcomes In Type 2 Diabetes Mellitus: Secondary Analysis of a Randomized Clinical Trial. JAMA Cardiol. 2016;1(2):126-35.
31. Schernthaner G, Cahn A, Raz I. Is the use of DPP-4 inhibitors associated with an increased risk for heart failure? Lessons from EXAMINE, SAVOR-TIMI 53, and TECOS. Diabetes Care. 2016;39 Suppl 2:S210-8.
32. Rosenstock J, Marx N, Neubacher D, et al. Cardiovascular safety of linagliptin in type 2 diabetes: a comprehensive patient-level pooled analysis of prospectively adjudicated cardiovascular events. Cardiovasc Diabetol. 2015;14(1):57.
33. Levelt E, McCann GP, Schneider JE, et al. Effects of Vildagliptin on Ventricular Function in Patients with Type 2 Diabetes Mellitus and Heart Failure. JACC Heart Fail. 2018;6(5):443-4.
34. Verma S, Goldenberg RM, Bhatt DL, et al. Dipeptidyl peptidase-4 inhibitors and the risk of heart failure: a systematic review and meta-analysis. CMAJ Open. 2017;5(1):E152-77.
35. Marso SP, Daniels GH, Brown-Frandsen K, et al. Liraglutide and cardiovascular outcomes in type 2 diabetes. N Engl J Med. 2016;375(4):311-22.
36. Bethel MA, Patel RA, Merrill P, et al. Cardiovascular outcomes with glucagon-like peptide-1 receptor agonists in patients with type 2 diabetes: a meta-analysis. Lancet Diabetes Endocrinol. 2018;6(2):105-13.
37. Margulies KB, Hernandez AF, Redfield MM, et al. Effects of Liraglutide on Clinical Stability Among Patients With Advanced Heart Failure and Reduced Ejection Fraction: A Randomized Clinical Trial. JAMA. 2016;316(5):500-8.
38. Jorsal A, Kistorp C, Holmager P, et al. Effect of liraglutide, a glucagon-like peptide-1 analogue, on left ventricular function in stable chronic heart failure patients with and without diabetes (LIVE)—a multicentre, double-blind, randomised, placebo-controlled trial. Eur J Heart Fail. 2017;19(1):69-77.
39. Azoulay L, Suissa S. Sulfonylureas and the risks of cardiovascular events and death: a methodological meta-regression analysis of the observational studies. Diabetes Care. 2017;40(5):706-14.
40. Roumie CL, Min JY, McGowan LD, et al. Comparative safety of sulfonylurea and metformin monotherapy on the risk of heart failure: a cohort study. J Am Heart Assoc. 2017;6(4):e005379.
41. Fadini GP, Saragoni S, Russo P, et al. Intraclass differences in the risk of hospitalization for heart failure among patients with type 2 diabetes initiating a dipeptidyl peptidase-4 inhibitor or a sulphonylurea: Results from the OsMed Health-DB registry. Diabetes Obes Metab. 2017;19(10):1416-24.
42. BARI 2D Study Group, Frye RL, August P, et al. A randomized trial of therapies for type 2 diabetes and coronary artery disease. N Engl J Med. 2009;360(24):2503-15.
43. Dormandy JA, Charbonnel B, Eckland DJ, et al. Secondary prevention of macrovascular events in patients with type 2 diabetes in the PROactive Study (PROspective pioglitAzone Clinical Trial In macroVascular Events): a randomised controlled trial. Lancet. 2005;366(9493):1279-89.
44. Home PD, Pocock SJ, Beck-Nielsen H, et al. Rosiglitazone evaluated for cardiovascular outcomes in oral agent combination therapy for type 2 diabetes (RECORD): a multicentre, randomised, open-label trial. Lancet. 2009;373(9681):2125-35.
45. Cosmi F, Shen L, Magnoli M, et al. Treatment with insulin is associated with worse outcome in patients with chronic heart failure and diabetes. Eur J Heart Fail. 2018;20(5):888-95.
46. Malmberg K, Rydén L, Efendic S, et al. Randomized trial of insulin-glucose infusion followed by subcutaneous insulin treatment in diabetic patients with acute myocardial infarction (DIGAMI study): effects on mortality at 1 year. J Am Coll Cardiol. 1995;26(1):57-65.
47. Mellbin LG, Malmberg K, Norhammar AF, et al. Prognostic implications of glucose-lowering treatment in patients with acute myocardial infarction and diabetes: experiences from an extended follow-up of the Diabetes Mellitus Insulin–Glucose Infusion in Acute Myocardial Infarction (DIGAMI) 2 Study. Diabetologia. 2011;54(6):1308-17.
48. Gerstein HC, Bosch J, Dagenais GR, et al. Basal insulin and cardiovascular and other outcomes in dysglycemia. N Engl J Med. 2012;367(4):319-28.
49. Svensson AM, Miftaraj M, Franzén S, et al. Clinical effects, cardiovascular and renal outcomes associated with rapid-acting insulin analogs among individuals with type 2 diabetes: a nation-wide observational cohort study. Clin Diabetes Endocrinol. 2017;3(1):5.

SECTION 4

Hypertension

CHAPTER 17

Epidemiology of Hypertension in India: The Real Scenario

Rajeev Gupta, Kiran Gaur

INTRODUCTION

High blood pressure (BP) is the most important risk factor for global morbidity and mortality. The latest iteration of global burden of disease (GBD) study has reported that high systolic BP, poor diet, and tobacco use are the most important risk factors for mortality and morbidity.[1] GBD has estimated that more than 11% of global deaths are due to hypertension.[1] In India also, it has emerged as the most important risk factor for deaths and disability.[2] According to reports from World Health Organization (WHO),[3] GBD study,[4] and non-communicable disease risk factor collaboration (NCDRiSC)[5] the prevalence of hypertension is increasing globally and currently more than one billion people have hypertension (defined as systolic BP ≥140 mm Hg and/or diastolic BP ≥90 mm Hg). NCDRiSC study reported that number of adults with raised blood pressure increased from 594 million in 1975 to 1.3 billion in 2015, with the increase largely in low-income and middle-income countries.[5] This article reviews status of hypertension prevalence in India using systematic reviews of previous epidemiological studies, two recent large nationwide surveys and GBD study estimates for determining absolute burden of hypertension in India.

SYSTEMATIC REVIEWS OF EPIDEMIOLOGICAL STUDIES

In India, multiple reviews of previous studies have been conducted. All have reported a significant and increasing burden of hypertension.[6-9] This increase has been reported in both urban and rural areas in India. In the mid-1950s, Indian urban population-based epidemiological studies used older WHO criteria for diagnosis (known hypertension or BP >160 mm Hg systolic and/or 95 mm Hg diastolic) and reported hypertension prevalence of 1.2–4.0%.[6] Since, then prevalence of hypertension in Indian cities has been steadily increasing from 3.0–4.5% in early 1960's to 11.0–15.5% in mid-1990's.[6] Although rural populations in India generally have lower prevalence of hypertension there has been a significant increase in these populations from less than 1% in early 1960's to 5–7% in late 1990's.[6,7]

Systolic BP ≥140 mm Hg and/or diastolic BP ≥90 mm Hg is the currently accepted diagnostic threshold for hypertension worldwide, although the 2017 American College of Cardiology (ACC) and American Heart Association (AHA) hypertension guidelines have proposed a lower threshold.[10] Many prevalence studies of hypertension defined by current criteria have been performed in the present century in India. These studies have been performed in urban (Table 1) as well as rural (Table 2) populations.[9] Most of the studies are regional. There are only a few multi-centric studies in the country. All these studies reveal a greater prevalence of hypertension in urban populations.[9] However, recent studies report that hypertension is increasing more rapidly in the rural populations and there is an urban rural convergence in its prevalence.[9] These studies also show that almost a third of adult Indian population has high BP. This is similar to other parts of the developing world and only slightly lower than the developed countries.[3]

Reviews have reported that that there are large regional differences in hypertension prevalence in India as shown in tables 1 and 2. Anchala et al. performed a meta-analysis of recent hypertension prevalence studies in India and reported significant differences in hypertension in various zones of the country with greater prevalence in northern, eastern, and north-eastern regions of the country.[8]

Some years ago, we recommended that periodic surveys in India such as national family health surveys (NFHS), national statistical survey organization surveys (NSSOS), and district level household surveys (DLHS) should focus on hypertension screening.[9] Government of India, under the national program for control of cardiovascular diseases, stroke, diabetes, and cancer initiated a large project of opportunistic screening in India.[11] More than 50 million adults were screened and it was reported that 6.2% participants were suffering from diabetes while hypertension was

TABLE 1: Hypertension (BP >140 and/or 90 mm Hg) prevalence studies in urban populations

First Author	Year Reported	Place	Age Group	Sample Size	Prevalence (%)
Gupta R	1995	Jaipur	≥20	2212	30.9
Anand MP	2000	Mumbai	30–60	1662	34.0
Gupta R	2002	Jaipur	≥20	1123	33.4
Shanthirani CS	2003	Chennai	≥20	1262	21.1
Gupta PC	2004	Mumbai	≥35	88653	47.9
Prabhakaran D	2005	Delhi	20–59	2935	30.0
Reddy KS	2006	Multisite	20–69	19973	27.2
Mohan V	2007	Chennai	≥20	2350	20.0
Kaur P	2007	Chennai	18–69	2262	27.2
Yadav S	2008	Lucknow	≥30	1746	32.2
Gupta R	2012	National	≥35	2616	48.2
Prince MJ	2012	Chennai	≥60	1000	60.0
Gupta R	2012	Jaipur	≥20	739	32.1
Joshi SR	2012	Multisite	49(mean)	15662	46.0
Gupta R	2013	Multisite	≥20	6106	31.5
Bhagyalaxmi A	2013	Gujarat	15–64	1805	29.0
Bhansali A	2014	Multisite	>20	14059	26.3
Gupta R	2017	Multisite	35–70	15846	38.6
Tripathy JP	2017	Punjab	35–70	5127	40.4

BP, blood pressure.

TABLE 2: Hypertension prevalence studies in rural populations

First Author	Year Reported	Place	Age Group	Sample Size	Prevalence (%)
Gupta R	1994	Rajasthan	≥20	3148	16.9
Kusuma	2004	Andhra	≥20	1316	21.0
Hazarika NC	2004	Assam	≥30	3180	33.3
Krishnan	2008	Haryana	15–64	2828	9.3
Todkar SS	2009	Maharashtra	≥20	1297	7.2
Bhardwaj R	2010	Himachal	≥18	1092	35.9
By Y	2010	Karnataka	≥18	1900	18.3
Kinra S	2010	Multisite	20–69	1983	20.0
Gupta R	2012	Multisite	>35	4624	31.5
Prince MJ	2012	Tamilnadu	>65	1000	29.0
Kaur P	2012	Tamilnadu	25–64	10463	21.4
Kokiwar PR	2012	Tamilnadu	>30	924	19.0
Dutta A	2012	West Bengal	>18	1186	24.7
Borah PK	2012	Assam	>30	916	55.6
Haddad S	2012	Kerala	18–96	1660	23.5
Bansal SK	2012	Uttarakhand	>18	968	28.9
Meshram II	2012	Kerala	>20	4193	40.0
Bhagyalaxmi A	2013	Gujarat	15-64	1684	15.4
Gupta R	2017	Multisite	35-70	17577	26.3
Tripathy JP	2017	Punjab	35-70	5127	40.0

in 5.5%. These numbers are clearly an underestimate and much lower that the government sponsored (Indian Council of Medical Research) studies[12] as well as recent national studies[13,14] reviewed later.

Recent reviews of various local and regional hypertension epidemiological studies in India have reported that hypertension is present in 25–30% urban and 10–20% rural subjects in India.[7-9] However, there are large regional variations in its prevalence and these rates may be not truly representative. Multisite studies that evaluated hypertension prevalence using similar tools in various regions of the country are few. These studies are limited to male industrial workers,[15] lower socioeconomic status women,[16] middle class urban men and women,[17] urban and rural men and women at a few locations in the country,[18-21] and rural men and women.[22] Hypertension prevalence in these studies varies from 15 to 20% in rural and 20 to 35% in adult participants in these studies (Fig. 1). However, all these studies lack national representativeness.

Anchala et al[8] performed a meta-analysis of all hypertension epidemiology studies in India using studies from Medline, Web of Science, and Scopus databases from 1950 to 30 April 2013. These sites were searched for 'prevalence, burden, awareness, and control of BP or hypertension (≥140 mm Hg systolic BP and/or ≥90 mm Hg diastolic BP) among Indian adults of more than or equal to 18 years of age. Of the total 3,047 articles, 142 were included. Overall prevalence for hypertension in India was calculated as 29.8% (95% confidence interval (CI): 26.7–33.0). Significant differences in hypertension prevalence were noted between rural and urban regions [rural: 27.6% (23.2–32.0) and urban: 33.8% (29.7–37.8); p = 0.05]. Regional estimates for the prevalence of hypertension were, in rural populations: north 14.5% (13.3–15.7), east 31.7% (30.2–33.3), west 18.1% (16.9–19.2), and south 21.1% (20.1–22.0); and for urban: north 28.8% (26.9–30.8), east 34.5% (32.6–36.5), west 35.8% (35.2–36.5), and south 31.8% (30.4–33.1), respectively. Greater hypertension prevalence was observed in eastern regions of the country. It was concluded that we need more studies to detect true prevalence of hypertension in the country.

National Family Health Survey-4

Fourth NFHS was focused on obtaining multiple adult socioeconomic, demographic, and lifestyle factors using a nationally representative sample.[13] For the first time, this survey also determined hypertension prevalence among young men and women in India using a representative sampling across the country.[2] This survey was implemented in both urban and rural areas.[23,24] A uniform sample design was adopted in all the districts. The primary sampling units for rural areas were villages and for urban locations the census enumeration blocks. The field agencies were given a list of selected sampling units for each state or union territories that were selected for the fieldwork. NFHS-4 was designed to provide information on various demographic

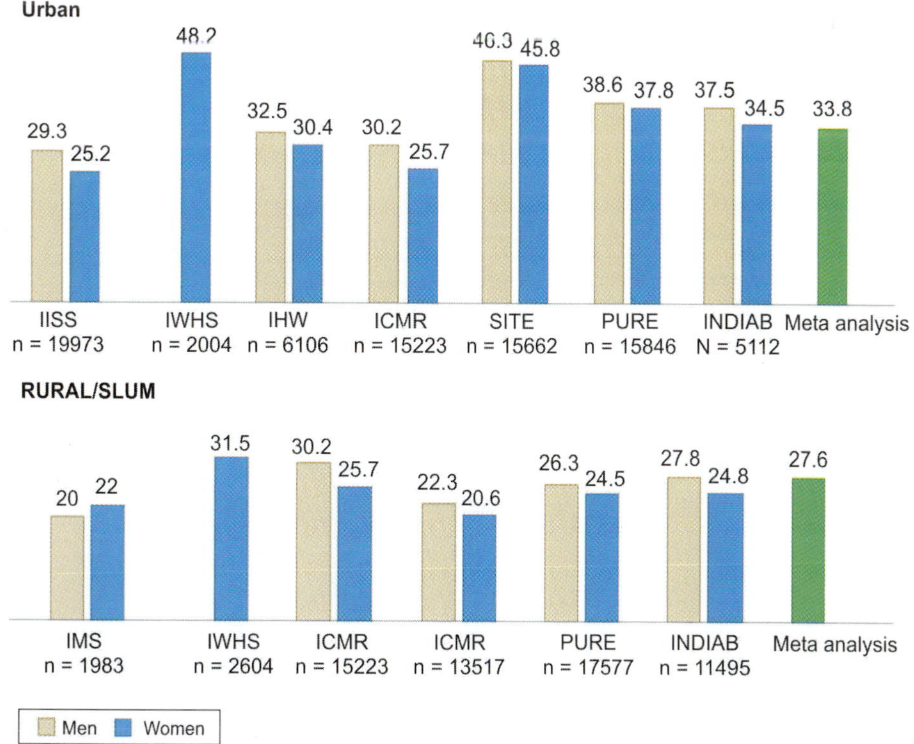

FIG. 1: Recent multisite studies of hypertension prevalence in Indian urban and rural populations. Study acronyms: IISS Indian Industrial Surveillance Study[15]; IWHS India Women Health Study[16]; IHW India Heart Watch[17]; ICMR Indian Council of Medical Research Study[18]; SITE Study for Investigation of Twin Epidemic[19]; INDIAB Indian Diabetes Study[20]; PURE Prospective Urban Rural Epidemiology Study[21]; IMS India Migration Study[22]; and Meta-analysis by Anchala et al.[8]

parameters and other family welfare and health indicators by background characteristics at the national and state level and, for the first time, at the district level also. Because of need to report health indicators at the district level, the NFHS-4 sample size was increased to 571,660 households, as compared with 109,041 households in NFHS-3. NFHS-4 adopted a two-stage sampling design in rural and urban areas of each district of India.[22] This survey ultimately interviewed 601,509 households, 699,686 women, and 103,525 men from 28,583 primary sampling units composed of villages in rural areas and census enumeration blocks in urban areas in 640 districts of the country. The domain of clinical, anthropometric, and biochemical testing in NFHS-4 included random blood glucose and BP measurements with estimates to be reported at the district level for women aged 15–49 years and men aged 15–54 years. All these components in the field were evaluated using portable equipment. An automatic and battery-operated BP instrument was used. Only medical or other personnel with specific training on the procedures were involved. NFHS-4 was conducted in two phases, and each phase covered almost an equal number of states or groups of states and union territories. Detailed methodology of BP measurement are available at NFHS-4 website[13] and has been reported earlier.[24]

We have obtained the hypertension prevalence data from the NFHS-4 website and prevalence in various states among men and women is reported in table 3. The sample sizes are population proportionate and data shows that there are significant differences in prevalence of hypertension in different states of the country. Accordingly, the prevalence is much greater in the southern, north eastern and north western states of the country and is significantly greater in men as compared to women (Table 3). Of the 33 states that are represented in table 3, hypertension prevalence of more than 15% is observed in 8/33 (24.2%) states and low prevalence (<5%) is observed in 6/33 (18.2%) states. Other states have a medium prevalence 5–15%.

TABLE 3: Hypertension prevalence (%) in young men (15–54 years) and women (15–49 years) in national family health survey (NFHS-4)

State (alphabetic)	Sample size	Hypertension (known or BP ≥140/90 mm Hg)		
		Men	Women	Total
Andaman & Nicobar	3219	27.9	9.0	18.5
Andhra Pradesh	11826	16.2	10.0	13.1
Arunachal Pradesh	16224	21.6	15.0	18.3
Assam	32307	19.6	16.0	17.8
Bihar	51243	9.4	5.9	7.7
Chandigarh	866	13.5	9.3	11.4
Chhattisgarh	28701	12.7	8.8	10.8
Delhi	6586	4.2	7.6	5.9
Goa	2457	13.2	8.5	10.9
Gujarat	28506	13.0	9.7	11.4
Haryana	25032	16.8	9.2	13.0
Himachal Pradesh	12114	21.9	12.1	17.5
Jammu & Kashmir	29384	13.7	11.6	12.7
Jharkhand	32866	12.2	7.8	10.0
Karnataka	30034	15.4	9.7	12.6
Kerala	12897	9.5	6.8	8.2
Madhya Pradesh	72313	10.9	7.9	9.4
Maharashtra	33957	15.9	9.1	12.5
Manipur	15342	20.4	11.4	15.9
Meghalaya	10347	10.4	9.9	10.2
Mizoram	13896	17.9	9.8	13.9
Nagaland	12230	23.1	16.0	19.6
Odisha	37930	12.5	9.0	10.8
Punjab	22511	21.8	13.2	17.5
Pondicherry	4618	15.1	9.1	12.1

Continued

Continued

State (alphabetic)	Sample size	Hypertension (known or BP ≥140/90 mm Hg)		
		Men	Women	Total
Rajasthan	47857	12.4	6.9	9.7
Sikkim	6096	27.3	16.5	21.9
Tamilnadu	33614	15.5	8.3	11.9
Telangana	8625	18.2	10.1	14.2
Tripura	5623	13.6	12.6	13.1
Uttarakhand	19290	17.2	9.6	13.4
Uttar Pradesh	110600	10.1	7.6	8.9
West Bengal	20057	12.4	10.3	11.4
Total	**799228**			

BP, blood pressure.

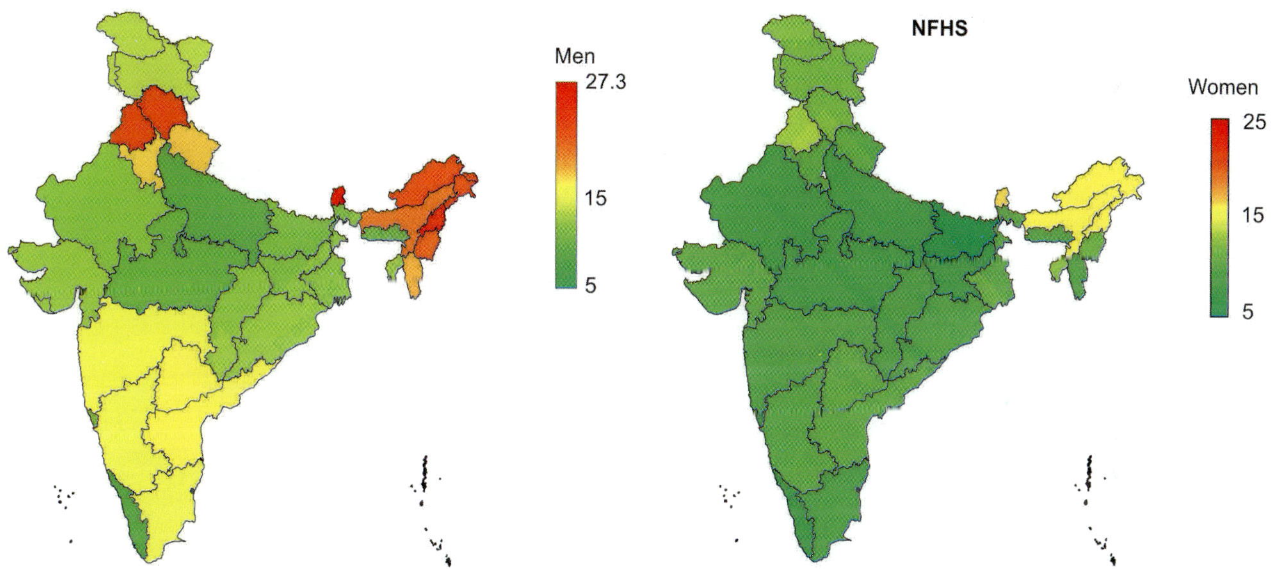

NFHS, national family health surveys.

FIG. 2: Heat map showing hypertension prevalence in various states of India in NFHS-4 study.

Country-level prevalence of hypertension in NFHS-4 among the younger age individuals is 13.6% in men, 8.8% in women and 11.3% overall.[13] The prevalence is significantly greater in urban as compared to rural locations: men 15.1% versus 12.6%, women 9.6% versus 8.5% ($p < 0.01$). The urban-rural differences are not as large as reported in the regional studies (Fig. 1).

Heat map showing prevalence of hypertension in various states of India is shown in figure 2. This shows that the highest prevalence of hypertension is in northern and north-eastern Indian states of the country that include Punjab, Himachal Pradesh, Assam, and north-eastern states. The prevalence is moderate in western and southern Indian states while the lowest prevalence is observed in central Indian states extending from Rajasthan in the west to Bihar in the east.

Limitations of the NFHS-4 study have been reported earlier.[24] A major shortcoming of the NFHS program is the exclusion of middle and older age adults. It is well-known that hypertension prevalence increases with age.[10] Exclusion of this high prevalence group has led to lower prevalence in this study as compared to previous regional and national studies in India. On the other hand, prospective studies collaboration has reported that intervention at younger age is associated with greater benefit in terms of vascular protection and reduction of cardiovascular mortality and morbidity.[25] Therefore, these data are important and convey an important message to healthcare policy-makers and providers.

District Level Household Survey-4 and Annual Health Surveys

Government of India along with the Registrar General of India have recently developed a robust method to estimate various cardiovascular risk factors in all states of the country.[26] Measurement of BP and data on hypertension prevalence is being obtained since the year 2012. Geldsetzer et al., pooled data from two large household surveys in India—DLHS-4 and annual health survey (AHS) which were undertaken between 2012 and 2014.[14] The data obtained are representative at the district level and jointly cover 29 states of India. Data from two states, Gujarat and Jammu & Kashmir - are not available.

Results of this study have been published recently.[14] In this study, of the 1,320,555 adults, 53.1% were women. The crude prevalence of hypertension reported in the study is 25.3% (95% CI 25.0–25.6%) with greater prevalence in men (27.4%, CI 27.0–27.7%) compared to women (23.6%, CI 23.3–23.8%). Age-standardized prevalence is significantly greater in men (24.5%, CI 24.2–24.9%) as compared to women (20.0%, CI 19.7–20.3%). The prevalence is greater in urban than rural participants. The age-standardized prevalence ranged from 13.5% (CI 12.2–14.9%) among women in Chhattisgarh to 43.5% (CI 38.3–48.9%) among men in Daman and Diu.

The study also reported that hypertension is common even among the younger age groups participants (18–25 years) with prevalence of 12.1% (CI 11.8–12.5%). There was positive association of socioeconomic status with hypertension prevalence although being in the richest versus poorest household income was associated with only a small difference (rural 4.15% and urban 3.47%). This suggests convergence of urban-rural and a rich-poor difference in hypertension prevalence in India as has been reported earlier.[9] This study also reported significant differences in prevalence of hypertension across the Indian states with age-adjusted prevalence varying from 18.0 to 41.6% as shown in table 4 and figure 3. This study concluded that there is a

TABLE 4: Hypertension prevalence in adult men and women in district level household survey (DLHS-4)

	Men (%)	Women (%)	Total (%, weighted average)
Andaman & Nicobar Island	37.2	26.3	32.1
Andhra Pradesh	28.3	20.7	24.5
Arunachal Pradesh	27.7	21.4	24.7
Assam	21.3	16.8	19.1
Bihar	20.2	20.8	20.5
Chandigarh	41.8	31.3	37.0
Chhattisgarh	17.1	13.5	15.3
Daman & Diu	43.5	36.3	40.8
Goa	32.9	26.4	29.7
Haryana	28.1	20.3	24.5
Himachal Pradesh	38.5	30.8	34.7
Jharkhand	24.7	18.8	21.8
Karnataka	25.5	21.0	23.3
Kerala	41.4	33.0	37.0
Madhya Pradesh	19.9	16.7	18.3
Maharashtra	28.2	21.8	25.1
Manipur	25.7	17.6	21.7
Meghalaya	22.9	18.3	20.6
Mizoram	24.5	14.8	19.7
Nagaland	39.6	31.8	35.8
NCT of Delhi	27.9	22.4	25.4
Odisha	17.2	15.6	16.4
Puducherry	27.3	17.6	22.4
Punjab	41.4	29.4	35.7
Rajasthan	23.7	16.5	20.2
Sikkim	36.2	30.4	33.5
Tamil	27.7	18.8	23.3
Telangana	26.5	19.6	23.1
Tripura	22.4	18.8	20.6
Uttar Pradesh	20.5	18.2	19.4
Uttarakhand	32.2	22.3	27.4
West Bengal	22.6	21.0	21.8

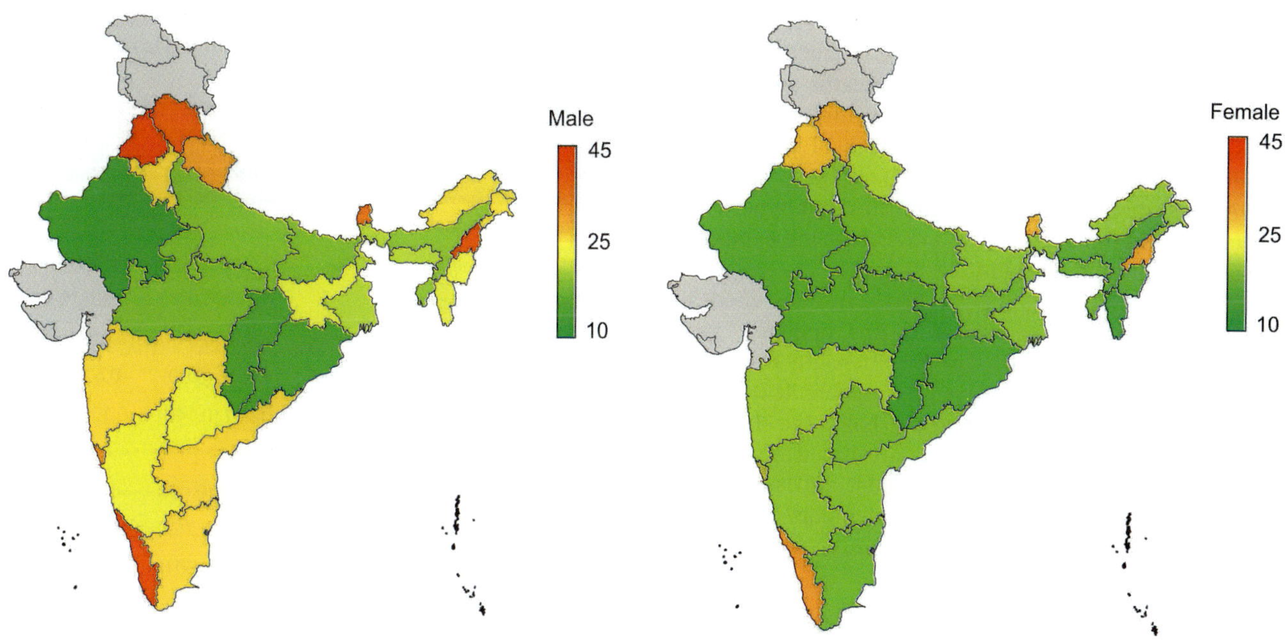

DLHS, district level household survey.

FIG. 3: Hypertension prevalence in various states of India in DLHS study.

TABLE 5: Increasing trends in deaths and disability adjusted life years (DALYs) due to high systolic blood pressure in India (Global Burden of Diseases Study 2016)

	1990	1995	2000	2005	2010	2016
Deaths						
Absolute numbers (thousands)	784.7	885.3	1005.0	1153.6	1385.6	1634.7
Death Rate/100,000	90.8	92.7	95.9	101.3	113.1	124.2
% of total deaths	8.9	9.9	10.8	12.2	14.4	16.7
DALYs						
Absolute numbers (millions)	20.9	23.4	26.2	29.3	34.4	39.4
DALY Rate/100,000	2415	2451	2497	2576	2807	3000
% of total DALYs	3.9	4.4	5.0	5.7	7.0	8.5

high prevalence of hypertension across all socioeconomic groups in India. The prevalence of hypertension is high even among the young age individuals. This is similar to previous studies from sub-national and regional studies in India.[8] This study concludes that this epidemiological evidence of high hypertension prevalence in India should prompt central and state governments in India towards increased efforts on hypertension detection, treatment, and control.[27]

There is a significant correlation of state-level hypertension prevalence among NFHS-4 and DLHS studies in both men (r = 0.55, p = 0.004) and women (r = 0.35, p = 0.077). This suggests that high BP at younger age, as observed in NFHS-4, has tracked into older age participants in DLHS, especially in men. This has important implications for primordial prevention of hypertension[10] in India and suggests that policies for reducing salt and fat consumption and promoting fruit and vegetable intake in India should begin at younger age groups in all regions of the country.

Global Burden of Diseases Study

The GBD study group has been estimating mortality and morbidity from various diseases of multiple risk factors for the last two decades.[1] Since the year 2010, the investigators have estimated various risk factors from 1990 onwards and calculated their impact on health.[28] High BP is the most important of disease burden and the current estimate from GBD 2016 suggest that more than 12% of global deaths are attributable to this risk factor.[1] Estimated data on deaths and disability adjusted life years (DALYs) or India are available at the GBD website.[29]

Table 5 shows trends in deaths and DALYs attributed to high systolic BP for India. High systolic BP led to 784,700 deaths in 1990 which more than doubled to 16,347,000 deaths in 2016, an increase of 108.3%. The death rate increased from 90.8 per 100,000 in 1990 to 124.2 per 100,000 in 2016, an increase by 36.8%. Similarly, absolute number of DALYs lost increased from 20.86 million in 1990 to 39.41 million in 2016 (increase by 88.9%) and DALYs per 100,000 increased from 2,415 in 1990 to 3,000 in 2016, an increase by 24.2%. These increases in deaths and DALYs in India are in contrast to high-income countries, where these rates are declining.[29] Absolute number of patients with hypertension is not available for India but increasing trends in DALYs and other parameters confirms that hypertension is increasing in the country and is one of the most important cause of deaths and disability.[2]

In 2016, GBD study for the first time estimated sub-national (state-level) causes of deaths and risk factors in India.[30] However, details of hypertension and related morbidity and mortality are not yet available. It is expected that future iterations of GBD study shall have these data. However, as GBD study estimates are based on synthesis of real-time data from various national and sub-national studies, it is expected that the study shall report similar state-level differences as highlighted in the present review.

ASSOCIATION OF HYPERTENSION WITH MACROLEVEL RISK FACTORS

Reasons for increasing hypertension in India are multiple. These include individual factors such as unhealthy lifestyle factors including sedentary habits, unhealthy diet (high-calorie, high-unrefined carbohydrate, high-fat, high-salt, and high-alcohol intake, etc.), stress, overweight, obesity, abdominal obesity and insulin resistance, and various genetic factors. Complex interplay of these is involved in pathogenesis of hypertension.[31] All these factors are well-known and are not highlighted in the present review. Factors specific to South Asian and Indians have been highlighted earlier and include overweight and obesity especially abdominal adiposity, diabetes, smoking and alcohol consumption, nutrition transition, and sedentary lifestyles.[32]

Data on association of hypertension with various social, economic, developmental, and other social determinants of health are sparse in India. A previous review has highlighted important of epidemiological transition in India in increasing prevalence of hypertension.[33] There is evidence that urban-rural differences in hypertension are decreasing and there is an urban-rural convergence.[9] Similar data are reported in the DLHS study also.[14] To determine association of prevalence of hypertension in different states in India with various social factors we performed a macrolevel analysis.

We used data on hypertension prevalence available from the DLHS (Table 4) and correlated it with various social factors. These factors include state-level human development index (HDI, derived from income, education, and fertility statistics),[34] social development index (SDI, derived from multiple socioeconomic factors),[35] urbanization index (UI, ratio of urban to rural population in a state),[36] epidemiological transition index (ETI, ratio of communicable to non-communicable disease mortality),[30] and healthcare quality index (HQI, availability of healthcare facilities at primary care).[37] We calculated Pearson's correlation coefficient (r) for each of these variables using state-level data of these socioeconomic

TABLE 6: Correlation of hypertension prevalence in Indian states with various socioeconomic and lifestyle indicators (Pearson's r)

	State level hypertension prevalence (DLHS)	
	Men	Women
Socioeconomic factors		
Human Development Index	0.620 (0.001)	0.558 (0.003)
Social Development Index	0.739 (0.001)	0.603 (0.010)
Urbanization Index	0.432 (0.014)	0.338 (0.058)
Epidemiological Transition Index	-0.646 (0.00)	-0.621 (0.001)
Healthcare Quality Index	0.262 (0.148)	0.127 (0.488)
Lifestyle factors		
Smoking/Tobacco use	-0.511 (0.008	-0.399 (0.043)
Alcohol intake	0.061 (0.767)	0.120 (.0559)
Overweight/Obesity (BMI >25 kg/m^2)	0.629 (0.001)	0.570 (0.002)
Numbers in parentheses are p value		

BMI, body mass index; DLHS, District Level Health Survey.

factors and hypertension prevalence (DLHS). The results are shown in table 6.

In both men and women, there is a positive association of HDI and SDI with hypertension prevalence at a macrolevel suggesting that these factors are important. These findings are also similar to results from 11-city India Heart Watch study where we reported that hypertension prevalence was greater in states with greater HDI and SDI.[38] There is a weak positive association (insignificant) with urbanization suggesting that urban-rural differences in hypertension prevalence in India are disappearing and it is likely that hypertension would be more common in rural areas of India in the near future. This would be, then, similar to hypertension epidemiology in high- and middle-income countries where it is more common in rural areas.[3,4] Significant association of hypertension with state-level prevalence of obesity (body mass index >25 kg/m^2) (Table 6) confirms internal consistency of the data.

We also performed correlation of hypertension prevalence (DLHS) with health quality index as published by the National Institution for Transforming India (NITI Aayog), Government of India (Fig. 4). No significant correlation is observed of hypertension prevalence with availability of primary healthcare in men (R^2 = 0.06) or in women (R^2 = 0.01). It is expected that states with greater hypertension prevalence would have better primary care. However, the data (Fig. 4) show that states with high prevalence of hypertension have similar quality of primary healthcare as those with low prevalence. Moreover, the health index has been developed with focus on mother and child healthcare and a better index needs to be developed that also focuses on chronic healthcare delivery, important for hypertension control. Better hypertension control in India needs focus on strengthening primary care in the country[3,39] and clearly more effort is required in India to upgrade primary care services for better hypertension control.[39,40]

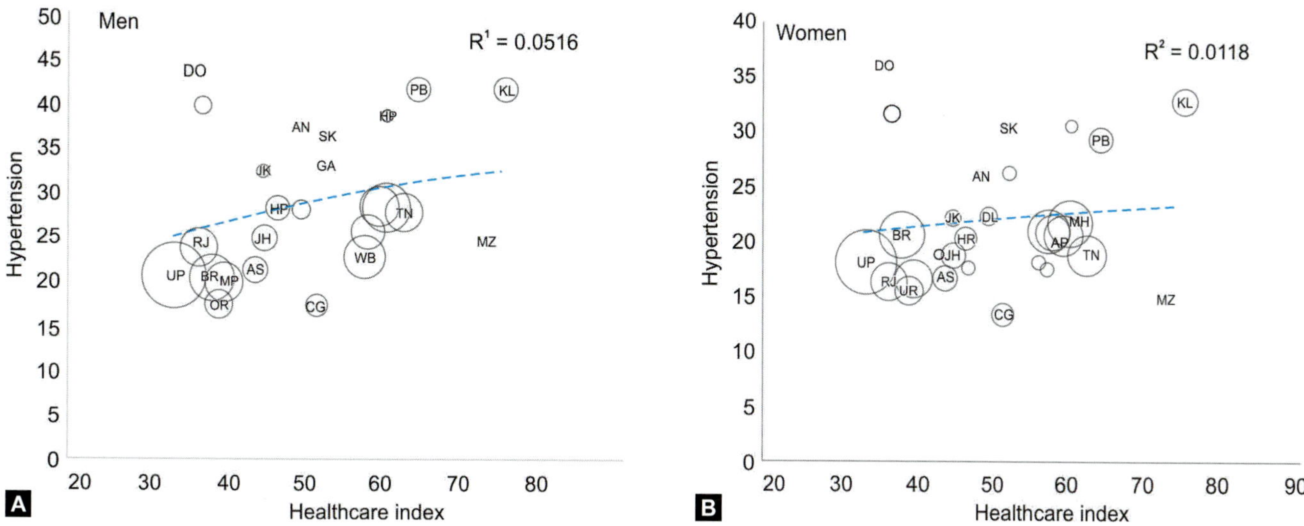

FIG. 4: Correlation of hypertension prevalence with healthcare quality index in men and women in various Indian states.

CONCLUSION

In conclusion, this review highlights that hypertension is the most important risk factor for disease burden in India.[2] Previous meta-analysis have reported increasing trends in hypertension in India.[6,7] High prevalence of hypertension has been reported in both urban and rural locations in the country.[8] However, these epidemiological studies have been mostly single or multi-site studies which have failed to provide national data. Two recent studies have used proper nationwide sampling and uniform tools to determine the true prevalence of hypertension in India. Fourth NFHS evaluated hypertension prevalence in younger men and women and reported hypertension in 13.8% men (15–54 years) and 8.8% women (15–49 years) with an overall prevalence of 11.3%. More representative data from DLHS and AHS reported hypertension in 25.3% with a greater prevalence in men (27.4%) as compared to women (20.0%). Hypertension is more in urban areas. The GBD study reports that hypertension associated mortality and morbidity in India is high and increasing. Our review shows that social determinants of hypertension are important and states with greater human and social development and urbanization (HDI, SDI, UI) have more hypertension. This is in contrast to developed countries, such as USA, where hypertension is more in less developed states.[41] This review also shows poor association of hypertension with healthcare availability. This suggests that primary healthcare system in the country needs to be ramped-up for better hypertension control in the country.

REFERENCES

1. Emmanuela G. Ashkan A. Amanuel AA, et al. Global, regional, and national comparative risk assessment of 84 behavioral, environmental and occupational, and metabolic risks or clusters of risks, 1990-2016: a systematic analysis for the Global Burden of Disease Study 2016. Global Health Metrics. 2017;390:1345-1422.
2. Gupta R, Xavier D. Hypertension: the most important non-communicable disease risk factor in India. Indian Heart J. 2018;70:565-72.
3. World Health Organization. Global Status Report on Non-Communicable Diseases 2014. Geneva: World Health Organization. 2014.
4. Farouzanfar MH, Ng M, Biryukov S, et al. Global burden of hypertension and systolic blood pressure of at least 110 to 115 mmHg, 1990-2015. JAMA. 2017;317:15-182.
5. NCD Risk Factor Collaboration (NCD-RiSC). Worldwide trends in blood pressure from 1975 to 2015: a pooled analysis of 1479 population-based measurement studies with 19.1 million participants. Lancet. 2017;389:37-55.
6. Gupta R, Al-Odat NA, Gupta VP. Hypertension epidemiology in India: Meta-analysis of fifty-year prevalence rates and blood pressure trends. J Hum Hypertens. 1996;10:465-472.
7. Gupta R. Trends in hypertension epidemiology in India. J Hum Hypertens. 2004;18:73-8.
8. Anchala R, Kannuri NK, Pant H, et al. Hypertension in India: a systematic review and meta-analysis of prevalence, awareness, and control of hypertension. J Hypertens. 2014; 32:1170-7.
9. Gupta R. Convergence in urban-rural prevalence of hypertension in India. J Hum Hypertens. 2016;30:79-82.
10. Carey R, Whelton P, 2017 ACC/AHA Guideline Writing Committee. Prevention, detection, evaluation, and management of high blood pressure in adults: Synopsis of the 2017 American College of Cardiology/American Heart Association Hypertension Guideline. Ann Intern Med. 2017; 2018;168(5):351-8.
11. Ministry of Health and Family Welfare. (2016). National Programme for Prevention and Control of Cancer, Diabetes, Cardiovascular Disease and Stroke (NPCDCS). [online] Available from https://mohfw.gov.in/about-us/departments/departments-health-and-family-welfare/national-programme-prevention-and-control-cancer-diabetes-cardiovascular-disease. [Accessed August, 2018].
12. Shah B, Mathur P. Surveillance of cardiovascular risk factors in India: the need and the scope. Indian J Med Res. 2010;132:634-42.
13. National Family Health Survey, India. (2009). About NFHS. [online] Available from http://rchiips.org/nfhs/abt.html. [Accessed August, 2018].
14. Geldsetzer P, Manne-Goehler J, Theilmann M, et al. Diabetes and hypertension in India: a nationally representative study of 1.3 million adults. JAMA Intern Med. 2018;178(3):363-72.
15. Reddy KS, Prabhakaran D, Chaturvedi V, et al. Methods for establishing a system for cardiovascular diseases in Indian industrial populations. Bull WHO. 2006;84:461-9.
16. Gupta R, Pandey RM, Misra A, et al. High prevalence and low hypertension awareness, treatment and control in Asian Indian women. J Hum Hypertens. 2012;26:585-93.
17. Gupta R, Deedwania PC, Achari V, et al. Normotension, prehypertension and hypertension in Asian Indians: prevalence, determinants, awareness, treatment and control. Am J Hypertens. 2013;26:83-94.

18. Shah B, Mathur P. Surveillance of cardiovascular risk factors in India: the need and the scope. Indian J Med Res. 2010;132:634-42.
19. Joshi SR, Saboo B, Vadivale M, et al. Prevalence of diagnosed and undiagnosed diabetes and hypertension in India: results from the Screening India's Twin Epidemic (SITE) study. Diabetes Technol Ther. 2012;14:8-15.
20. Bhansali A, Dhandhania VK, Mohan D, et al. Prevalence of and risk factors for hypertension in urban and rural India: the ICMR INDIAB study. J Hum Hypertens. 2015; 29:204-9.
21. Gupta R, Kaur M, Islam S, et al. Association of household wealth, educational status and social capital with hypertension awareness, treatment and control in South Asia. Am J Hypertens. 2017;30:373-81.
22. Kinra S, Bowen LJ, Lyngdoh T, et al. Sociodemographic patterning of non-communicable disease risk factors in rural India: a cross sectional study. BMJ. 2010; 341:c4974.
23. Ram F, Paswan B, Singh SK, et al. National family health survey-4 (2015-16). Econ Pol Weekly. 2017;52(16):66-70.
24. Gaur K, Mohan I, Gupta R. Syndemic of obesity, hypertension and hyperglycemia among 15-49 year olds in Rajasthan: district-level data from National Family Health Survey-4. RUHS J Health Sciences. 2017;2:54-64.
25. Prospective Studies Collaboration. Age-specific relevance of usual blood pressure to vascular mortality: a meta-analysis of individual data for one million adults in 61 prospective studies. Lancet. 2002;360:1903-13.
26. Government of India. (2015). District Level Household and Facility Survey. [online] Available from https://data.gov.in/resources/hypertension-age-18-years-and-above-dlhs-iv. [Accessed August, 2018].
27. Kanaya A. India's call to action: prioritize chronic cardiovascular disease. JAMA Intern Med. 2018;178:373-4.
28. IHME measuring what measures. (2018). Global Burden of Disease Study 2015. Health data. [online] Available from http://ghdx.healthdata.org/gbd-data-tool. [Accessed August 2018].
29. IHME measuring what measures. (2018). Global Burden of Diseases Study 2016. GBD Results tool. [online] Available from http://ghdx.healthdata.org/gbd-results-tool. [Accessed August 2018].
30. India State-Level Disease Burden Collaborators. Nations within a nation: variations in epidemiological transition across the states in India 1990-2016, in the Global Burden of Disease Study. Lancet. 2017;390:2437-60.
31. Hall ME, Hall JE. Pathogenesis of hypertension. In: Bakris GL, Sorrentino MJ (Eds). Hypertension: A Companion to Braunwald's Heart Disease, 3rd Edition. Philadelphia: Elsevier; 2018. pp. 33-51.
32. Joseph P, Gupta R, Yusuf S. Hypertension in South Asians. In: Bakris GL, Sorrentino MJ (Eds). Hypertension: A Companion to Braunwald's Heart Disease, 3rd edition. Philadelphia: Elsevier; 2018. pp. 27-32.
33. Gupta R, Gupta KD. Coronary heart disease in low socioeconomic status subjects in India: An evolving epidemic. Indian Heart J. 2009;61:358-67.
34. Government of India. (2015). Human development index and its components by states. [online] Available from https://data.gov.in/catalog/human-development-index-and-its-components-states. [Accessed August 2018].
35. Banerjee K. Social development index 2010. In: Mohanty M (Ed) India Social Development Report 2010. New Delhi: Oxford University Press; 2011. pp. 259-93.
36. Census of India. Rural urban distribution. Available at: http://censusindia.gov.in/Census_Data_2001/India_at_glance/rural.aspx. [Accessed August, 2018].
37. NITI Aayog (2018). Health. [online] Available from: http://social.niti.gov.in/health-index. [Accessed August, 2018].
38. Gupta R, Sharma KK, Gupta BK, et al. Geographic epidemiology of cardio-metabolic risk factors in urban middle-class residents in India: A cross sectional study. J Global Health. 2015;5:104-11.
39. Gupta R, Yusuf S. Towards better hypertension control in India. Indian J Med Res. 2014;139:657-60.
40. Freiden TR, Jaffe MG. Saving 100 million lives by improving global treatment of hypertension and reducing cardiovascular disease risk factors. J Clin Hypertens. 2018;20:208-11.
41. Whelton PK, Carey RM, Aronow WS, et al. 2017 ACC/AHA/AAPA/ABS/ ACPM/AGS/APhA/ASH/ASPC/NMA/PCNA guideline for the prevention, detection, evaluation and management of high blood pressure in adults: executive summary. J Am Coll Cardiol. 2018; 71:2199-269.

CHAPTER 18

Primary Prevention of Hypertension

Panniyammakal Jeemon, Dorairaj Prabhakaran

INTRODUCTION

Hypertension is one of the leading risk factor for cardiovascular disease (CVD) and a major contributor to global mortality and disability.[1] Annually, approximately over ten million deaths are attributable to hypertension.[2] The low- and middle-income countries (LMIC) bear disproportionately higher burden of hypertension in absolute numbers[3] due to a rapid increase in prevalence and the sheer size of its population. For example, LMICs contribute to nearly two-thirds of the mortality attributable to hypertension, globally.[3] The rising burden of hypertension in LMIC is also reflected in the rising population level mean blood pressure (BP) especially in the South Asian and sub-Saharan population.[4]

Despite progress in recent decades in prevention, detection, and treatment of high BP, hypertension remains an important global public health challenge. Hypertension is said to be a disease paradoxes. It is easy to detect but diagnosis rates are dismal, easy to treat but treatment rates are disappointing and several potent drugs are available but control rates are abysmal. For example, numerous meta-analyses have unequivocally demonstrated that treating and effectively lowering BP is associated with reductions in cardiovascular events and mortality.[5] However, treatment and control rates of hypertension are abysmally poor at the population level in LMIC.[6] Additionally, various studies conducted in LMIC suggest that hypertension onset occurs relatively early in life,[7] often associated with clustering of multiple CVDs risk factors,[8] and lead to premature cardiovascular events such as heart attacks and stroke.

Reducing the population level BP is an effective strategy in addressing the burden of hypertension. Although, pharmacological treatment is effective in reducing BP in the hypertensive group, its impacts on population mean BP reduction is limited. Primordial and primary prevention are key strategies for population-wide reduction in average BP. For example, more than half of the reduction in CVD mortality in developed countries is attributed to improvements in population level risk factors such as tobacco use, cholesterol, and BP control.[9]

CLASSIFICATION OF HYPERTENSION

The seventh report of the Joint National Committee on prevention, detection, evaluation, and treatment of high BP (JNC VII report) define hypertension as a confirmed elevation of systolic or diastolic BP (≥140 mm Hg or ≥90 mm Hg, respectively).[10] The cut-off will be based on the mean of two or more properly measured seated BP readings on each of two or more office visits. However, based on observational data, CVD risk begins to accrue at lower systolic BP (SBP) value of 115 mm Hg.[11] Lifestyle modifications in the context of delaying the onset of hypertension in individuals with systolic or diastolic BP (SBP or DBP) less than 140/90 mm Hg is largely referred to as primary prevention. The JNC VII report recommends individuals with SBP in the range of 120–139 mm Hg or DBP 80–90 mm Hg engage in health-promoting lifestyle modifications to prevent the development of hypertension and CVD.[10] Additionally, lifestyle modification is also recommended as concurrent treatment for patients with hypertension.

THE NEED FOR PRIMARY PREVENTION OF HYPERTENSION IN INDIA

Data on annual incidence of hypertension in Indian population are scarce. In a longitudinal follow-up study conducted in a representative sample from two cities of India (Delhi and Chennai), the average SBP increased by 2.6 mm Hg and one in six developed hypertension.[12] The estimated impact of 2.6 mm Hg rise in average BP on hypertension prevalence is large as it can double the current prevalence rate of 30% over a period of 10 years. The most susceptible group to develop hypertension is the least privileged, lesser educated, and from the lowest socioeconomic strata.[12] This will have important ramifications at the population level, due to lesser likelihood of treatment affordability. Additionally, there is a tendency to ignore treatment options among the above mentioned group due to asymptomatic nature of hypertension and could potentially lead to devastating health consequences. The impact of a major cardiovascular event due to uncontrolled hypertension on household economy is substantial as it takes away potentially productive life years and probable bankruptcy due to huge out of pocket payments for treatment.

PRIMARY PREVENTION

Primary prevention of hypertension provides an avenue to interrupt and prevent the continuing costly cycle of managing hypertension and its complications. In order to achieve the UN sustainable development goal (SDG) of one-third reduction in premature CVD mortality by 2030, concerted efforts must be undertaken not only in earlier detection and treatment of hypertension, but also in implementation of primary prevention strategies.[13] Primary prevention focuses on preserving good health by removing the precipitating causes or potential determinants of poor health. The larger goal of primary prevention efforts in hypertension is to curtail the growing incidence of hypertension in India.

There are two main approaches in the primary prevention of hypertension. The first one is known as the population-based approach of involving the general population. The main objective of the population wide approach is to bring down the average BP at the population level (Fig. 1). It is based on the principal that majority of the population falls under the middle portion of the blood pressure distribution, and majority of the adverse events occur among individuals in the middle of the BP distribution. Therefore, a minor reduction in the average BP shifts the population distribution curve toward the left and saves the population from potentially devastating adverse events. For example, Cook et al. based on their findings from the Framingham Heart Study, reported that a 2 mm Hg reduction in the population average of DBP for white United States residents aged 35–64 years would result in a 17% reduction in the prevalence of hypertension, a 14% decrease in the risk of stroke and transient ischemic attacks, and a 6% reduction in the risk of coronary heart disease.[14] The second approach is a targeted approach among high-risk individuals who are prone to develop hypertension. Given the high propensity for development of hypertension in older population, individuals from the low socioeconomic group, those who are currently consuming alcohol, those who are with moderately elevated BP, overweight and dysglycemic individuals,[12] targeting these subgroups for prevention of hypertension may provide greater yield. Higher risk older adults are more likely to be successful with lifestyle interventions than young adults with lower risk. However, prevention strategies targeted earlier in life provide the greatest long-term probability for overall risk reduction and burden of BP-related complications in the community.

Interventions for Primary Prevention of Hypertension

There is no convincing evidence of a J-shaped relationship or a "threshold" below which the relationship between level of BP and high-risk of cardiovascular and renal diseases is observed.[15] Therefore, the benefits of shifting the distribution

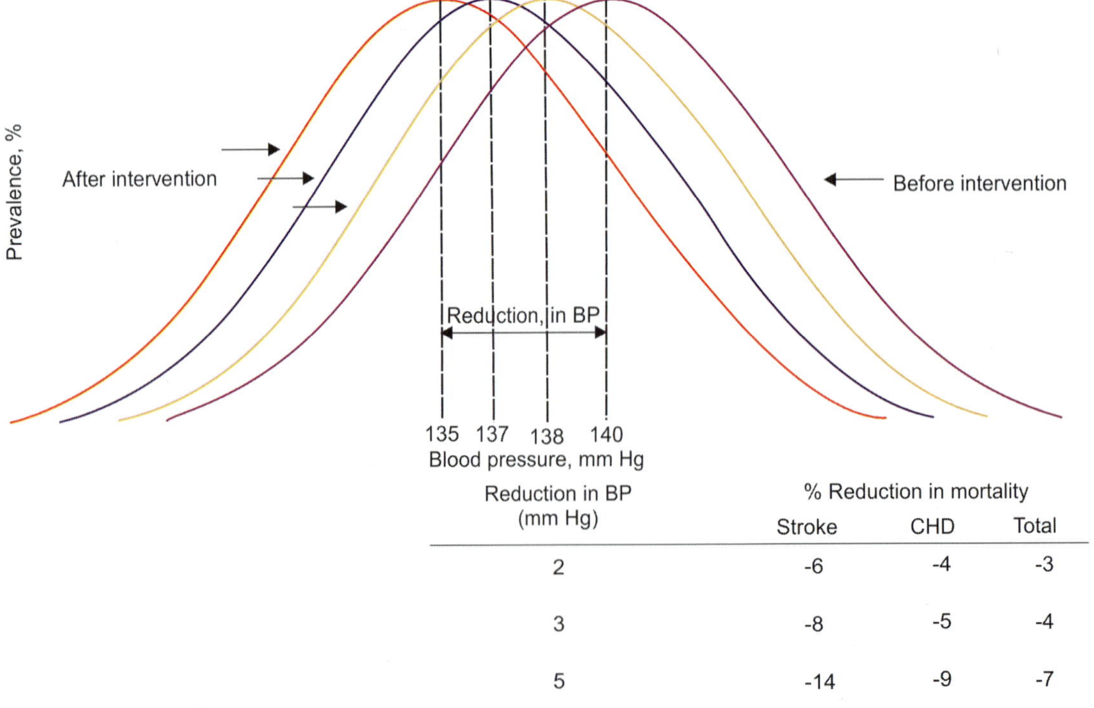

Reduction in BP (mm Hg)	% Reduction in mortality: Stroke	CHD	Total
2	-6	-4	-3
3	-8	-5	-4
5	-14	-9	-7

BP, blood pressure; CHD, coronary heart disease.

FIG. 1: Pictorial representation of shift of population level blood pressure distribution after primary prevention intervention.

TABLE 1: Recommendations for prevention of hypertension

Strategy	Detailed recommendation
Physical exercise	For nonhypertensive individuals to reduce the possibility of becoming hypertensive, accumulation of 30–60 min of moderate intensity dynamic exercise (e.g., walking, jogging, cycling, or swimming) 4–7 days per week in addition to the routine activities of daily living are recommended. There is no incremental benefit for higher intensities of exercise
Weight reduction	Multi-disciplinary approaches that includes dietary modification, increased physical activity and behavioral interventions are useful in reducing weight. Maintenance of health body weight with body mass index in the range of 18.5–24.9 and waist circumference <90 cm for men and <80 cm for women are recommended for nonhypertensive individuals to prevent hypertension. Lifestyle modification in combination with moderate intensity physical exercise is effective in reducing the body weight up to 6–7% of the baseline levels
Alcohol consumption	Healthy adults should avoid alcohol consumption or at least limit alcohol consumption to <2 drinks per day, and consumption should not exceed 14 standard drinks per week for men and 9 standard drinks per week for women. One standard drink is considered to be equivalent of 13.6 g or 17.2 mL of ethanol or approximately 44 mL (1.5 Oz) of 80-proof (40%) spirits, 355 mL (12 Oz) of 5% beer, or 148 mL (5 Oz) of 12% wine
Dietary recommendations	A DASH diet that is rich in fruits, vegetables, low-fat dairy products, dietary and soluble fiber, whole grains, and protein from plant sources that is reduced in saturated fat and cholesterol is recommended for prevention of hypertension. In India millets which were traditional diets are rich in fiber and should be encouraged. Even locally available, seasonal and inexpensive fruits and vegetables are helpful in reducing and maintaining optimal blood pressure
Sodium intake	No more than 2.4 g sodium (<6 g sodium chloride) is generally recommended as daily dietary intake
Potassium intake	Potassium supplementation is not recommended. However, dietary sources rich in potassium are effective in reducing blood pressure especially in a high sodium environment. These include fruits and vegetables
Calcium and magnesium supplementation	Both calcium and magnesium supplementation are not recommended for prevention of hypertension
Stress management	Relaxation techniques and Yoga-based interventions are recommended for primary prevention of hypertension based on evidence from multiple small studies carried out largely in the United Kingdom
Tobacco use	Though the influence of smoking/tobacco is limited in chronic hypertension, abstinence from tobacco is recommended as a broader primary prevention strategy
Enhancing access to appropriate facilities	Enhancing access to appropriate facilities such as green space, parks, walking trails, bike paths, etc. are effective in encouraging physical activity and reducing blood pressure
Fish oil supplementation	Evidence on fish oil supplementation on blood pressure reduction is equivocal and therefore not recommended as a strategy for primary prevention of hypertension
Herbal or botanical supplements	Available evidence is not sufficient to make recommendation on any of the herbal or botanical supplements for blood pressure reduction

DASH, Dietary Approaches to Stop Hypertension.

curve of population level BP toward the left with lower average BP far outweigh any potential risk associated with lowering average BP, even in normotensive individuals. The key strategies for primary prevention of hypertension are described in table 1.

Sodium Reduction

Sodium reduction is unequivocally the most efficient primary prevention intervention at the population level for hypertension.[16] On an average, 1.7 g/day reduction of average salt intake may result in 2 and 1 mm Hg reduction in SBP and DBP, respectively. No more than 2.4 g sodium or 6 g sodium chloride (just under a teaspoon of salt) is generally recommended as daily dietary intake. It has been estimated that moderated reduction in salt intake at the population level among middle-aged Indians may be sufficient enough to avert nearly 400,000 CVD events [myocardial infarctions (MIs) and stroke] and 81,000 deaths (5% reduction) over a period of 10 years.[17] Lower intake of dietary sodium reduces the risk of CVD, especially in those who are also overweight.

Potassium Supplementation

Potassium supplementation is considered as another useful strategy for BP reduction in both hypertensive and normotensive individuals.[18] A daily dietary intake of more than 3.5 g/day of potassium is generally recommended.[19] The benefits of potassium supplementation is observed to be larger in persons with high dietary sodium intake.[20] The preferred strategy to increase potassium intake is to consume foods rich in potassium (apart from fruits and vegetables sweet potato, navy bean, and yogurt are rich in potassium) rather than supplements. However, recent guidelines do not support supplementation of potassium.[21]

Weight Reduction

Several epidemiological studies suggest that weight gain is associated with increased risk of hypertension.[22,23] Similarly, randomized controlled trials also demonstrate that weight loss is associated with reduction in BP.[24] A sustained weight loss of 4.4 kg or more can reduce SBP and DBP by 5.0 and 7.0 mm Hg, respectively.[24]

Moderate Alcohol Consumption

Alcohol consumption is known as the most important modifiable risk factor for hypertension.[25] The relationship between high alcohol intake (typically three or more drinks per day) and elevated BP has been documented in many epidemiologic studies. A dose-dependent reduction in BP with reduction in alcohol consumption is reported in individuals who consume alcohol on a regular basis.[25] Available data suggest no cardiovascular protection among Indians even if they consume up to two standard drinks per day.[26] Additionally, isolated binge drinking (consuming more than four drinks in a row per occasion), a form of drinking associated with increased risk of heart disease,[27] is very common in Indians and it is extremely harmful.

Physical Activity

Inverse relationship between physical activity levels and BP has been reported from several epidemiological studies.[28-31] Regular aerobic physical activity for at least 30 min/day for at least 5 days of the week has been recommended for primary prevention of hypertension. Simple interventions such interruption of prolonged sitting time is also found to be effective in reducing BP.[32-34]

Dietary Pattern

The dietary approaches to stop hypertension (DASH) diet which is rich in fruits, vegetables, dietary, and soluble fiber, and low-fat dairy products but reduced in saturated and total fat is demonstrated to be effective in reducing mean BP in both hypertensive and nonhypertensive individuals.[35] The national high BP education program coordinating committee[36] for the primary prevention of hypertension recommends consumption of a diet rich in fruits, vegetables, and low-fat dairy products and reduced in saturated and total fats.

Comprehensive Lifestyle Modifications

Impact of lifestyle interventions on SBP is summarized in table 2. Clinical trials data suggest that comprehensive lifestyle modification interventions are effective in bringing down both SBP and DBP (Fig. 2)[37] in individuals with SBP in the range of 120–159 mm Hg and DBP in the range of 80–86 mm Hg. Similar reduction in BP has been documented in studies conducted in real life settings in India. For instance,

TABLE 2: Impact of lifestyle modification interventions on systolic blood pressure*

Modification	Effect on SBP reduction (range)
Weight reduction	5–20 mm Hg/10 kg weight loss
Adopt DASH eating plan	8–14 mm Hg
Dietary sodium restriction	2–8 mm Hg
Physical activity	4–9 mm Hg
Moderation of alcohol consumption	2–4 mm Hg

DASH, Dietary Approaches to Stop Hypertension; SBP, systolic blood pressure.

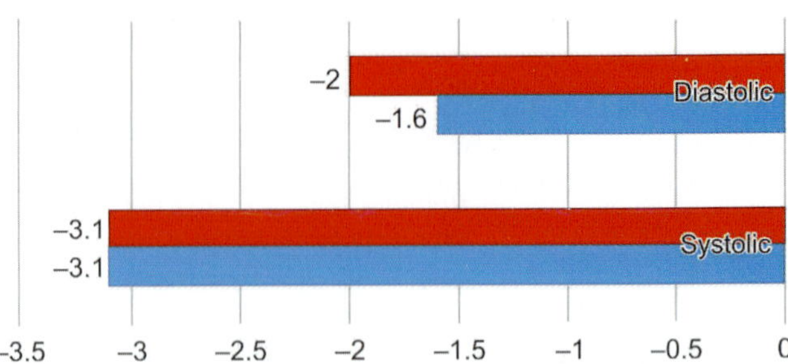

FIG. 2: Blood pressure reduction in multicomponent behavioral interventions. Blue bars indicate blood pressure reduction in individuals randomized to an established multi-component intervention (weight loss, reduced sodium intake, reduce alcohol consumption, and increased physical activity) and red bars indicate blood pressure reduction in individuals randomized to multicomponent intervention plus the Dietary Approaches to Stop Hypertension diet versus advice only.

a worksite-based intervention program implemented in India with both population-wide and high-risk approach was effective in bringing down both SBP and DBP to 5% of the baseline average BP.[8,38] Such intensive approaches may be useful in shifting the population distribution curve of BP toward the left and effectively bringing down the number of individuals with moderately elevated BP. Since, a large proportion of adverse cardiovascular events would occur in individuals belonging to the middle of the distribution curve of BP at the population level, comprehensive interventions may have the potential to delay such events.

Innovative Models in Primary Prevention of Hypertension

Task sharing strategy of involving frontline health workers has great potential for scale up of community-based intervention activities for primary prevention of hypertension at the national level. The DISHA study[39] is one of the largest community-based cluster randomized trial in India designed to test the effectiveness of "task sharing" interventions in shifting the population distribution of BP toward the left side of the distribution curve. Advent of mHealth technologies also opens the door to reach out to mass population lifestyle interventions targeting primary prevention of hypertension.

GAPS IN KNOWLEDGE AND FUTURE RESEARCH NEEDS

There are several pressing research needs in the primary prevention of hypertension. They are: (A) Early life influences (first thousand days) on BP and potential strategies to minimize risk in early life; (B) Physical and behavioral factors that influence BP during childhood and adolescence; (C) Testing alternative strategies of implementing lifestyle intervention at scale in community settings and identifying barriers to implementation; (D) Identifying the impact of novel strategies of improving physical fitness and reducing sedentary time such as high-intensity interval training and breaking the sitting time every 20 minutes, etc.; (E) Efficacy and effectiveness of specific dietary interventions, such as increased dietary protein or dietary fiber intake, and other modifications of whole diets in the prevention of hypertension; (F) Characterizing phenotypic, genetic, epigenetic, and metabolomic predictors of response to interventions for prevention of hypertension.

CONCLUSION

Comprehensive lifestyle interventions and policy interventions on salt restrictions have high potential of shifting the population distribution of BP toward the left of the distribution curve. Furthermore, several studies both epidemiological and randomized controlled trials suggest that the positive lifestyle changes for prevention of hypertension can be sustained over long periods. The BP-lowering effects of positive lifestyle changes observed is almost equivalent to the effect size observed in some of the drug trials in hypertension. Policy response on restricting the salt use is highly desirable and cost effective in the Indian settings. Despite several barriers to implementation, potential for health benefits makes primary prevention of hypertension an important national priority in India.

REFERENCES

1. Poulter NR, Prabhakaran D, Caulfield M. Hypertension. Lancet. 2015;386(9995):801-12.
2. Collaborators GBDRF, Forouzanfar MH, Alexander L, et al. Global, regional, and national comparative risk assessment of 79 behavioural, environmental and occupational, and metabolic risks or clusters of risks in 188 countries, 1990-2013: a systematic analysis for the Global Burden of Disease Study 2013. Lancet. 2015;386(10010):2287-323.
3. Arima H, Barzi F, Chalmers J. Mortality patterns in hypertension. J Hypertens. 2011;29 (Suppl 1):S3-7.
4. Danaei G, Finucane MM, Lin JK, et al. National, regional, and global trends in systolic blood pressure since 1980: systematic analysis of health examination surveys and epidemiological studies with 786 country-years and 5.4 million participants. Lancet. 2011;377(9765):568-77.
5. Law MR, Morris JK, Wald NJ. Use of blood pressure lowering drugs in the prevention of cardiovascular disease: meta-analysis of 147 randomised trials in the context of expectations from prospective epidemiological studies. BMJ. 2009;338:b1665.
6. Anchala R, Kannuri NK, Pant H, et al. Hypertension in India: a systematic review and meta-analysis of prevalence, awareness, and control of hypertension. J Hypertens. 2014;32(6):1170-7.
7. Gupta R, Misra A, Vikram NK, et al. Younger age of escalation of cardiovascular risk factors in Asian Indian subjects. BMC Cardiovasc Disord. 2009;9:28.
8. Jeemon P, Prabhakaran D, Goenka S, et al. Impact of comprehensive cardiovascular risk reduction programme on risk factor clustering associated with elevated blood pressure in an Indian industrial population. Indian J Med Res. 2012;135(4):485-93.
9. Unal B, Critchley JA, Capewell S. Explaining the decline in coronary heart disease mortality in England and Wales between 1981 and 2000. Circulation. 2004;109(9):1101-7.
10. Chobanian AV, Bakris GL, Black HR, et al. Seventh report of the Joint National Committee on Prevention, Detection, Evaluation, and Treatment of High Blood Pressure. Hypertension. 2003;42(6):1206-52.
11. Karmali KN, Lloyd-Jones DM. Global Risk Assessment to Guide Blood Pressure Management in Cardiovascular Disease Prevention. Hypertension. 2017;69(3):e2-9.
12. Prabhakaran D, Jeemon P, Ghosh S, et al. Prevalence and incidence of hypertension: Results from a representative cohort of over 16,000 adults in three cities of South Asia. Indian Heart J. 2017;69(4):434-41.
13. Jamison DT, Alwan A, Mock CN, et al. Universal health coverage and intersectoral action for health: key messages from Disease Control Priorities, 3rd edition. Lancet. 2018;391(10125):1108-20.
14. Cook NR, Cohen J, Hebert PR, et al. Implications of small reductions in diastolic blood pressure for primary prevention. Arch Intern Med. 1995;155(7):701-9.
15. Whelton PK. Epidemiology of hypertension. Lancet. 1994;344(8915):101-6.
16. He FJ, Li J, Macgregor GA. Effect of longer term modest salt reduction on blood pressure: Cochrane systematic review and meta-analysis of randomised trials. BMJ. 2013;346:f1325.
17. Basu S, Stuckler D, Vellakkal S, et al. Dietary salt reduction and cardiovascular disease rates in India: a mathematical model. PLoS One. 2012;7(9):e44037.
18. Aburto NJ, Hanson S, Gutierrez H, et al. Effect of increased potassium intake on cardiovascular risk factors and disease: systematic review and meta-analyses. BMJ. 2013;346:f1378.
19. Whelton PK, He J, Appel LJ, et al. Primary prevention of hypertension: clinical and public health advisory from The National High Blood Pressure Education Program. JAMA. 2002;288(15):1882-8.
20. Whelton PK, He J, Cutler JA, et al. Effects of oral potassium on blood pressure. Meta-analysis of randomized controlled clinical trials. JAMA. 1997;277(20):1624-32.
21. Daskalopoulou SS, Rabi DM, Zarnke KB, et al. The 2015 Canadian Hypertension Education Program recommendations for blood pressure measurement, diagnosis, assessment of risk, prevention, and treatment of hypertension. Can J Cardiol. 2015;31(5):549-68.
22. Zhao Y, Liu Y, Sun H, et al. Association of long-term dynamic change in body weight and incident hypertension: The Rural Chinese Cohort Study. Nutrition. 2018;54:76-82.
23. Yang G, Shu XO, Gao YT, et al. Impacts of weight change on prehypertension in middle-aged and elderly women. Int J Obes (Lond). 2007;31(12):1818-25.
24. Stevens VJ, Obarzanek E, Cook NR, et al. Long-term weight loss and changes in blood pressure: results of the Trials of Hypertension Prevention, phase II. Ann Inter Med. 2001;134(1):1-11.
25. Roerecke M, Kaczorowski J, Tobe SW, et al. The effect of a reduction in alcohol consumption on blood pressure: a systematic review and meta-analysis. Lancet Public Health. 2017;2(2):e108-20.
26. Roy A, Prabhakaran D, Jeemon P, et al. Impact of alcohol on coronary heart disease in Indian men. Atherosclerosis. 2010;210(2):531-5.
27. More deaths from heart disease in scotland on mondays may relate to binge drinking. BMJ 2000;320(7229):E.
28. von Kanel R. Accumulation of 30 min of moderately intense physical activity is a clinically meaningful treatment to reduce systolic blood pressure in prehypertension. J Hum Hypertens. 2008;22(7):444-6.
29. Park S, Rink L, Wallace J. Accumulation of physical activity: blood pressure reduction between 10-min walking sessions. J Hum Hypertens. 2008;22(7):475-82.
30. Maximova K, O'Loughlin J, Paradis G, et al. Declines in physical activity and higher systolic blood pressure in adolescence. Am J Epidemiol. 2009;170(9):1084-94.
31. Reaven PD, Barrett-Connor E, Edelstein S. Relation between leisure-time physical activity and blood pressure in older women. Circulation. 1991;83(2):559-65.
32. Mainsbridge C, Ahuja K, Williams A, et al. Blood pressure response to interrupting workplace sitting time with non-exercise physical activity: Results of a 12-month Cohort Study. J Occup Environ Med. 2018.
33. Chastin SFM, De Craemer M, De Cocker K, et al. How does light-intensity physical activity associate with adult cardiometabolic health and mortality? Systematic review with meta-analysis of experimental and observational studies. Br J Sports Med. 2018.
34. Chastin SF, Egerton T, Leask C, et al. Meta-analysis of the relationship between breaks in sedentary behavior and cardiometabolic health. Obesity (Silver Spring) 2015;23(9):1800-10.
35. Appel LJ, Moore TJ, Obarzanek E, et al. A clinical trial of the effects of dietary patterns on blood pressure. DASH Collaborative Research Group. N Engl J Med. 1997;336(16):1117-24.

36. National High Blood Pressure Education Program Working Group report on primary prevention of hypertension. Arch Intern Med. 1993;153(2):186-208.
37. Appel LJ, Champagne CM, Harsha DW, et al. Effects of comprehensive lifestyle modification on blood pressure control: main results of the PREMIER clinical trial. JAMA 2003;289(16):2083-93.
38. Prabhakaran D, Jeemon P, Goenka S, et al. Impact of a worksite intervention program on cardiovascular risk factors: a demonstration project in an Indian industrial population. J Am Coll Cardiol. 2009;53(18):1718-28.
39. Jeemon P, Narayanan G, Kondal D, et al. Task shifting of frontline community health workers for cardiovascular risk reduction: design and rationale of a cluster randomised controlled trial (DISHA study) in India. BMC Public Health. 2016;16:264.
40. Stamler R. Implications of the INTERSALT study. Hypertension. 1991;17(1 Suppl):I16-20.
41. Kaplan NM, Opie LH. Controversies in hypertension. Lancet. 2006;367(9505): 168-76.

CHAPTER 19

Cutoff for Hypertension: Implications of 2017 Guidelines for Indian Patients

Rajeev Narang, S Srikant

INTRODUCTION

Diagnosis of hypertension (HT) has altered considerably over recent years. Two main factors that have led to this change are publication of newer studies showing lower thresholds for diagnosis of HT and wide adoption of digital blood pressure (BP) recording instruments. The first provides scientific basis for altering the practice while second compels change due to practical considerations.

Digital BP instruments have become cheaper and widely available. They now provide more accurate, reliable, and reproducible readings. A number of studies have compared these instruments with traditional sphygmomanometer and found favorable results. Majority of these automated BP measuring devices use oscillometric technique. The British and Irish Hypertension Society lists many models which they have tested and found reliable (https://bihsoc.org/bp-monitors/).

A large proportion of patients in urban settings have digital BP recording instrument at home. This provides an opportunity to measure BP with several advantages. One is that, it is measured in home setting, hence avoiding the stress of hospital or clinic visit and eliminating white-coat HT phenomenon. Second is that multiple readings are possible over a period of one or more days providing information similar or even superior in some respects to ambulatory BP monitoring. The patients should hence be encouraged to invest in a good oscillometric BP monitoring instrument and record BP at home. They should also note these readings in a diary and bring it to clinic at time of visit. The frequency of BP recording will vary according to the situation. For stable patients once a week recording may be sufficient while those starting on new or altered therapies should measure it daily, so that lesser or greater than desired effect is picked-up early. Recording of BP by patients themselves also necessitates patient education in this regard. The cut offs for diagnosis are largely based on clinic visits rather than home settings. In addition, they do not consider normal variation in BP that is very common. Considering all data and taking into account normal variation of BP, it seems reasonable to educate patients to keep upper cutoff as 140 mm Hg. Regarding upper cutoff of diastolic BP, it is reasonable to educate patients that diastolic pressure above 90 mm Hg, if recorded on more than two occasions, indicates need for increase in dosage of medication. In recent years, emphasis has been shifting towards targeting mainly systolic BP, rather than diastolic. There are very few patients in whom diastolic BP remains elevated, when systolic pressure has come down to normal. Recent studies have also targeted systolic BP as preferred method of titrating therapy.

It is important to inform patient regarding lower cutoffs also. Patients recording their BP at home often get alarmed when lower than usual readings are obtained. Presence of symptoms should be ascertained in these patients. More severe symptoms include giddiness, dizziness, presyncope, or syncope. The symptoms are often postural as when patient get out of bed in the morning. The symptoms may be mild or subtle as fatigue, listlessness, and lack of energy.

Low systolic BP often leads to giddiness, dizziness, pre-syncope, and syncope, especially in elderly persons. Patients should be educated that they need to reduce their BP medication, if systolic BP falls to less than 110 mm Hg. Low diastolic BP is a complaint most often made by elderly persons who have isolated systolic HT as a result of stiffening and reduced compliance of major blood vessels. Asymptomatic low diastolic BP has not been documented to have any deleterious effects in studies of BP control. There is some evidence that incidence of open-angle glaucoma may be increased, if patients who have diastolic BP lower than 60 mm Hg.

Wide adoption of self-recording of BP by digital instruments also provide an opportunity of self-management of BP by patients. For this, patient should be prescribed at least one drug in small dose which they can up or down-titrate. For example, patients may be advised to take amlodipine 2.5 mg twice a day initially. If on home monitoring BP is found to be low, this can be reduced to once a day or omitted altogether.

On the other hand, if the systolic or diastolic BP continues to be high, this can be up-titrated to 5 mg twice a day. Patients should also be educated regarding maximum dose that can be taken. Similar instructions can be given with other agents, e.g., telmisartan (20 mg) or hydrochlorothiazide (12.5 mg).

In 2017, American Heart Association updated the HT guidelines.[1] The major change was that systolic BP of 130 mm Hg or more or diastolic of 80 mm Hg or more is considered HT and needs to be controlled (Tables 1 and 2). Hence, persons with systolic BP of 130–140 mm Hg and/or diastolic 80–90 mm Hg are now classified as hypertensive, while they were earlier classified as prehypertensive by Joint National Committee (JNC) 7 criteria.[2] This re-labels a large number of people as having elevated BP and warranting life style changes. The 2017 guideline also emphasizes individualized cardiovascular risk assessment. They use 10-year cardiovascular disease (CVD) risk calculation to decide on treatment threshold.[3] This will also mean that most elderly patients would get treated with medications earlier. Use of a risk calculator for BP treatment may over-estimate risk in many individuals and perhaps lead to over-medication. Whether a CVD risk calculator can decide when to treat HT is debatable.

Basic question is whether intensive treatment of HT is better than less aggressive approach. Although systolic blood pressure intervention (SPRINT) trial showed it to be beneficial, ACCORD and secondary prevention of small subcortical strokes (SPS3) trials did not find significant benefit.[4-6] SPRINT trial found that in patients (N = 9,361) at high risk of CVD without history of stroke or diabetes, intensive BP control (systolic <120 mm Hg) improved cardiovascular outcomes and overall survival compared to standard therapy (target systolic BP 135–139 mm Hg). Some serious adverse events were modestly increased. In ACCORD study, 4,733 patients with diabetes at higher risk of cardiovascular events were studied. Intensive BP control (target systolic BP <120 mm Hg) did not reduce adverse events [rates of nonfatal myocardial infarction (MI), nonfatal stroke, or cardiovascular mortality] when compared with standard BP control (target systolic BP <140 mm Hg). In SPS3 study, 3,020 patients with recent lacunar stroke were studied. It was found that target systolic BP less than 30 mm Hg did not reduce incident stroke when compared to higher-target systolic BP control (140–150 mm Hg).

However, the probability (P) value (0.08) did indicate a trend towards reduction. Greater emphasis seems to have been given to the SPRINT data in 2017 guidelines.

Another aspect is that stage-1 HT becomes a very narrow range and normal variability of BP may make a person in and out of this stage (Fig. 1). It is common these days for patients to record BP at home with oscillometric devices and to bring to the clinic a chart of those readings, some of which may be in stage 1 and others in elevated BP range.

Narrowness of stages may make this classification difficult to implement.

American College of Physicians has set the threshold for treatment at 150 mm Hg for average risk older (>60 years) people.[7] It was estimated that this new guideline would classify almost 46% of middle-aged Americans as hypertensive as compared to 32% as per the previous guidelines.[8]

Additionally, the prevalence of high BP is expected to triple among men under age of 45 years, and double among women under 45 years of age and would result in almost 20 million of them getting started on medication. Other major guideline-making associations like the American College of Physicians/National Institute for Health and Care Excellence (NICE)/ European Society of Cardiology (ESC) have not as yet accepted this guideline.

TABLE 1: Controlled reading of blood pressure for different stages

Category	Blood pressure (2 or more readings taken on 2 or more occasions)
Normal	SBP <120 and DBP <80 mm Hg
Elevated	SBP 120–129 and DBP <80 mm Hg
Hypertension	SBP >130 or DBP >80 mm Hg
Stage 1	SBP 130–139 or DBP 80–89 mm Hg
Stage 2	SBP ≥140 or DBP ≥90 mm Hg

DBP, diastolic blood pressure; SBP, systolic blood pressure.

TABLE 2: Treatment for different group of blood pressure stages

Group	Treatment (goal for everyone is <130/80 mm Hg)
"Elevated" BP (SBP 120–129 and DBP <80 mm Hg)	Lifestyle modification (non-pharmacological therapy)
Stage-1 hypertension (SBP 130–139 and DBP 80–89 mm Hg) • Without known clinicalatherosclerotic cardiovascular disease and • 10-year cardiovascular risk <10% (According to the ACC/AHA calculator)	Lifestyle modification; re-assessment after 3–6 months
Stage-1 hypertension (SBP 130–139 and DBP 80–89 mm Hg) • With known clinicalatherosclerotic cardiovascular disease or • 10-year cardiovascular risk ≥10% (According to the ACC/AHA calculator)	Lifestyle modification and drug therapy; reassess in one month
Stage-2 hypertension (SBP ≥140 mm Hg or (DBP ≥90 mm Hg)	Lifestyle modification and drug therapy (consider two agents from different classes); reassess in 1 month

ACC, American college of cardiology; AHA, American heart association; DBP, diastolic blood pressure; SBP, systolic blood pressure.

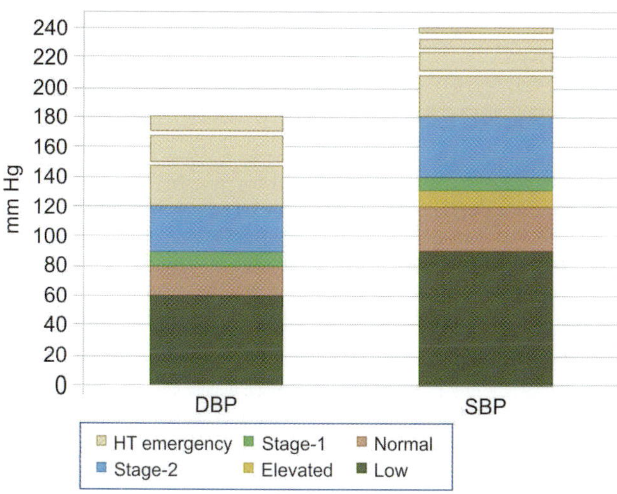

DBP, diastolic blood pressure; HT, hypertension; SBP, systolic blood pressure.

FIG. 1: Stage-1 and stage-2 of blood pressure.

OTHER HIGHLIGHTS

Other highlights of these guidelines include:

Screen for Other Risk Factors

Screen for risk factors like smoking, diabetes, dyslipidemia, obesity, wrong diet, stress, and sleep-apnea.

Investigations

Basic testing for HT includes fasting blood glucose, blood cell count, lipids, metabolic panel, thyroid-stimulating hormone, urinalysis, and electrocardiogram with optional echocardiogram, uric acid, and urinary albumin-to-creatinine ratio.

Screening for Secondary Causes

The screening for secondary causes of HT is necessary for new-onset or uncontrolled HT in adults including drug-resistant (≥3 drugs), abrupt onset, age less than 30 years, target organ damage [cerebral vascular disease, retinopathy, left ventricular hypertrophy, heart failure, coronary artery disease (CAD), chronic kidney disease (CKD), peripheral artery disease, albuminuria].

Screening includes testing for CKD, Reno vascular disease, primary aldosteronism, obstructive sleep-apnea, drug-induced HT, and alcohol-induced HT. Others include pheochromocytoma, Cushing's syndrome, congenital adrenal hyperplasia, hypothyroidism, hyperthyroidism, and aortic coarctation.

Treatment

Non-pharmacologic Therapy

Weight loss, sodium restriction, and potassium supplementation, increased physical activity, restrict alcohol. Use of medications is recommended in patients with clinical CVD and an average systolic BP greater than or equal to 130 mm Hg or a diastolic BP greater than or equal to 80 mm Hg. Use of medication is also recommended for a systolic BP greater than or equal to 140 mm Hg or a diastolic BP greater than or equal to 90 mm Hg.

Targets

For adults with confirmed HT and known CVD or 10-year atherosclerotic cardiovascular disease (ASCVD) event risk of 10% or higher, a BP target of less than 130/80 mm Hg is recommended. For adults with confirmed HT, but without additional markers of increased CVD risk, a BP target of less than 130/80 mm Hg is recommended as reasonable.

Principles of Drug Therapy

Initial therapy includes thiazide diuretics, calcium channel blocker (CCBs) and angiotensin-converting enzyme (ACE) inhibitors or angiotensin receptor blocker (ARBs). Two first-line drugs of different classes are recommended with stage-2 HT. The primary change in recommendations regarding pharmacologic therapy is the elimination of beta- blockers from first-line therapy for patients with primary HT. For adults with confirmed HT and known stable CVD or greater than or equal to 10% 10-year ASCVD risk, a BP target of less than 130/80 mm Hg is recommended.

The strategy is to first follow standard treatment guidelines for CAD, heart failure with reduced ejection fraction (HFrEF), previous MI, and stable angina, with the addition of other drugs as needed to further control BP. In heart failure with preserved ejection fraction (HFpEF) with symptoms of volume overload, diuretics should be used to control HT, following which ACE inhibitors or ARBs and beta-blockers should be titrated to systolic BP less than 130 mm Hg. Treatment of HT with an ARB can be useful for prevention of recurrence of atrial fibrillation.

Chronic Kidney Disease

Blood pressure goal should be less than 130/80 mm Hg. In those with stage-3 or higher CKD or stage 1 or 2 CKD with albuminuria (>300 mg/day), treatment with an ACE inhibitor is reasonable to slow progression of kidney disease. An ARB is reasonable, if an ACE inhibitor is not tolerated. In adults with acute intracranial hemorrhage and systolic BP greater than 220 mm Hg, it may be reasonable to use intravenous drug infusion to lower systolic BP. In acute ischemic stroke, BP should be lowered slowly to less than 185/110 mm Hg prior to thrombolytic therapy.

Diabetes Mellitus

Antihypertensive drug treatment should be initiated at BP greater than or equal to 130/80 mm Hg with a treatment goal of less than 130/80 mm Hg. In adults with diabetes mellitus (DM) and HT, all first-line classes of antihypertensive agents (i.e., diuretics, ACE inhibitors, ARBs, and CCBs) are useful and effective. ACE inhibitors or ARBs may be considered in the presence of albuminuria.

Age-related Issues

Although the new guideline lowers the blood-pressure goal for people over 65 years of age, it suggests that 30-year-olds and 80-year-olds should have the same goal. Treatment of HT is recommended for adults (≥65 years of age), with an average systolic BP greater than or equal to 130 mm Hg with systolic BP treatment goal of less than 130 mm Hg. In addition, the new guideline does not consider isolated systolic HT, which is a major problem among many people over 70 years of age. For older adults (≥65 years of age) with HT and a high burden of comorbidity and/or limited life expectancy, clinical judgment, patient preference, is reasonable for decisions regarding intensity of BP lowering and choice of antihypertensive drugs.

CONCLUSION

The new guidelines in 2017 have mainly reset the treatment threshold to 130/80 mm Hg. Most part of the guidelines summate the current knowledge on drug therapy and disease management along with promotion of team-based system approaches for better diagnosis and management. Rather than advocate a specific target for all adults, the focus should be on choosing BP targets that allow for "a choice based on a patient's risk profile, susceptibility to harms, and treatment preferences".

REFERENCES

1. Whelton PK, Carey RM, Aronow WS, et al. ACC/AHA/AAPA/ABC/ACPM/AGS/APhA/ASH/ASPC/NMA/PCNA Guideline for the prevention, detection, evaluation, and management of high blood pressure in adults: A Report of the American College of Cardiology/American Heart Association Task Force on Clinical Practice Guidelines. Hypertension. 2018;71(6):1269-1324.
2. Chobanian AV, Bakris GL, Black HR, et al. The Seventh report of the joint national committee on prevention, detection, evaluation, and treatment of high blood pressure: The JNC 7 report. JAMA. 2003;289(19):2560-72.
3. ASCVD Risk Estimator Plus (2017). Estimate risk. [online] Available from tools.acc.org/ASCVD- Risk-Estimator-Plus/. [Accessed August, 2018].
4. Wright JT, Williamson JD, Whelton PK, et al. A Randomized Trial of Intensive versus Standard Blood-Pressure Control. N Engl J Med. 2015;373(22):2103-16.
5. ACCORD Study Group, Cushman WC, Evans GW, et al. Effects of intensive blood-pressure control in type 2 diabetes mellitus. N Engl J Med. 2010;362(17):1575-85.
6. SPS3 Study Group, Benavente OR, Coffey CS, et al. Blood- pressure targets in patients with recent lacunar stroke: the SPS3 randomised trial. Lancet Lond Engl. 2013;382(9891):507-15.
7. Qaseem A, Wilt TJ, Rich R, et al. Pharmacologic treatment of hypertension in adults aged 60 years or older to higher versus lower blood pressure targets: A clinical practice guideline from the American college of physicians and the American academy of family physicians. Ann Intern Med. 2017;166(6):430-7.
8. Muntner P, Carey RM, Gidding S, et al. Potential U.S. Population Impact of the 2017 ACC/AHA High Blood Pressure Guideline. J Am Coll Cardiol. 2018;71(2):109-18.

CHAPTER 20

Initial Choice of Drugs in Uncomplicated Hypertension: Not Monotherapy Anymore but Combination

C Venkata S Ram

INTRODUCTION

Systemic hypertension is a major risk factor for premature mortality and excessive morbidity. Despite numerous advances in our understanding of the pathophysiology, disease implications, and effective drug therapy, hypertension remains uncontrolled in a majority of patients. In other words, patients with hypertension remain "hypertensive" even under medical care. Although hypertension is a precursor of chronic disease burden punctuated by acute events, effective blood pressure (BP) control prevents the complication rate. A number of studies have clearly shown that controlling hypertension saves lives. Hence, there is unmistakable evidence that elevated BP (by any definition) should be treated.

The American guidelines[1] define hypertension as a BP level more than 130/80 mm Hg (Table 1) whereas the Europeans[2,3] have retained the old definition, i.e., a BP level more than 140/90 mm Hg (Table 2). Although the American and European definitions of hypertension differ, the therapeutic BP goal is the same, i.e., less than 130/80 mm Hg in both the reports (Table 3). Whether we apply American or European definition, hypertension is rampant in India. Studies have shown that hypertension prevalence in India is escalating in the urban and rural populations alike.[4] Uncontrolled hypertension imposes tremendous and a formidable disease burden in India.[5-8] It is obligatory then to detect hypertension early and restore the BP to normal level without needless procrastination. Unless we control hypertension persuasively, our citizens (including the young) are vulnerable to develop coronary artery disease (CAD), congestive heart failure (CHF), chronic kidney disease (CKD), end-stage renal disease (ESRD), cerebrovascular disease (CeVD), dementia, peripheral vascular disease (PVD), and die prematurely.

This chapter is restricted to the management of hypertension and not on the ways and means to detect hypertension. Hence, the commentary below will focus only on treatment aspects of hypertension. Whereas, pharmacological treatment is required for most patients with hypertension, the value of lifestyle modifications is incontrovertible. The first step in the management of hypertension always should be advocate salt restriction, physical activity, normal body weight, and avoidance of tobacco and alcohol in excess. These hygienic recommendations form the foundation of hypertension treatment principles.

PHARMACOLOGICAL TREATMENT OF HYPERTENSION

The primary goal of antihypertensive therapy is to reduce cardiovascular morbidity and mortality. There are excellent outcome data and observations demonstrating the drug treatment reduces the complications in hypertension.[9,10] The cardiovascular disease (CVD) risk reduction from

TABLE 1: Blood pressure categories

Systolic, diastolic blood pressure (mm Hg)	JNC 7	2017/ACC/AHA	Indian Hypertension Guidelines
<120 and <80	Normal BP	Normal BP	Optimal
120–129 and <80	Prehypertension	Elevated BP	Normal
130–139 or 80–89	Prehypertension	Stage 1 hypertension	High normal
140–159 or 90–99	Stage 1 hypertension	Stage 2 hypertension	Stage 1 hypertension
≥160 or ≥100	Stage 2 hypertension	Stage 2 hypertension	Stage 2 hypertension

ACC, American College of Cardiology; AHA, American Heart Association; JNC, Joint National Committee.

TABLE 2: European classification of office BP and definitions of hypertension grade

Category	Systolic (mm Hg)		Diastolic (mm Hg)
Optimal	<120	and	<80
Normal	120–129	and/or	80–84
High normal	130–139	and/or	85–89
Grade 1 hypertension	140–159	and/or	90–99
Grade 2 hypertension	160–179	and/or	100–109
Grade 3 hypertension	≥180	and/or	≥110
Isolated systolic hypertension	≥140	and	<90

TABLE 3: New goal for blood pressure levels

Hypertension	BP goal is the same
ESC/ESH >140/90 mm Hg	>130/80 mm Hg
ACC/AHA >130/80 mm Hg	
Definitions differ but the goal blood pressure is same	

ACC, American College of Cardiology; AHA, American Heart Association; ESH, European Society of Hypertension; ESC, European Society of Cardiology.

antihypertensive drug treatment is directly proportional to the level of BP reduction rather than a specific drug class.[11,12] However, different drug classes provide unique and important benefits over and beyond BP control in patients with comorbidities.[13,14] It is evident that lower the BP, the better is the survival and disease prevention. Hence, it is important to achieve the goal BP less than 130/80 mm Hg in most patients with hypertension.

Within the large spectrum of available antihypertensive drugs, the preferred initial choice of therapy depends on factors such as the cost, tolerability, adherence, age, and comorbidities such as diabetes, CKD, CAD, CeVD, CHF, etc. The doctors should select the drug(s) upon consideration of these factors. American guidelines proposed diuretics, calcium channel blockers (CCBs), angiotensin-converting enzyme inhibitors (ACEIs), and angiotensin receptor blockers (ARBs) for the initial therapy of hypertension whereas the Europeans have restored β-blockers to the list as primary agents.

While a number of studies have shown the efficacy of monotherapies to control hypertension in the short term, nearly all the major outcome trials have utilized combination therapy to achieve and maintain target BP levels (Fig. 1). Until recently, various guidelines recommended initiating therapy with one drug and adding other drugs in sequence (so called stepped care approach). This sequential monotherapy has been shown to be effective in the prevention of hypertension-related complications. However, the stepped-care strategy has also demonstrated that monotherapy may be sufficient in only 30–40% of patients whereas with dual or triple drug combinations, the BP control rate is close to 90% or even higher.[15,16] Furthermore, response to monotherapy takes time at the risk of nonadherence, and patients are exposed to long periods of elevated BP levels. It makes sense, therefore, to initiate therapy with dual drug combination to claim BP control early and to assure patient compliance. Thus, we are moving fast to implement initial combination therapy (instead of monotherapy) to control hypertension. There may be instances like doubtful hypertension, white coat hypertension, frail, elderly, and acute intercurrent illness, where monotherapy may be the right choice but for a vast majority, initiating combination therapy is strongly recommended by the latest guidelines. Thus, the consideration in 2018 is not which antihypertensive drug initially but which combination? The author strongly recommends initiating with combination therapy for the following reasons:

- Safe
- Effective and tolerated
- Required
- Timely control of BP

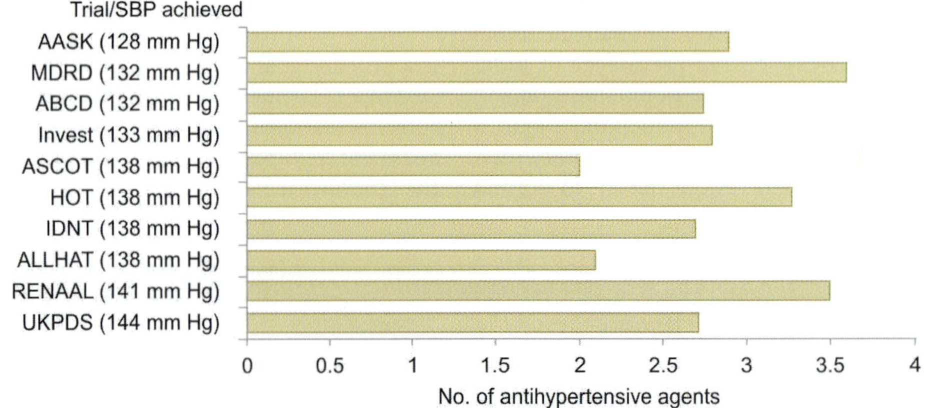

SBP, systolic blood pressure.

FIG. 1: Blood pressure control usually requires combination therapy.

- Patient satisfaction
- Positive clinical outcomes.

AN ABBREVIATED OVERVIEW OF DRUGS FOR INITIAL COMBINATION THERAPY

Diuretics

Diuretics are among the first generation of drugs shown to lower the BP level in patients with hypertension. All the guidelines have consistently recommended diuretics as an essential component of antihypertensive therapy. And there are excellent outcome data from clinical trials using diuretics as a part and parcel of therapy. The initial mechanism of BP reduction by diuretics is natriuresis, but the long-term BP control is via a reduction in the systemic vascular resistance (SVR). Diuretics are also less expensive than other classes of antihypertensive drugs.

For uncomplicated hypertension, a thiazide or a thiazide-type diuretic (chlorthalidone, indapamide) are preferred. In patients with CKD and CHF, loop diuretics are to be chosen. The traditional biochemical and metabolic side effects of diuretics can be minimized by using a low-dose; however, occasional monitoring of electrolytes and renal function is necessary. The American guidelines[1] have identified chlorthalidone as a "preferred" diuretic due to its long duration of action whereas the European guidelines[2,3] suggest a thiazide or a thiazide-type diuretic like chlorthalidone and indapamide. With judicious utilization of low-dose diuretic therapy (as a part of combination therapy), one can expect a significant reduction in the BP levels.

Beta-Blockers

Beta-blockers were widely used for the treatment of hypertension for many decades. However, their popularity weaned with the meta-analyses showing that atenolol-based treatments offered no target organ protection (TOP).[17,18] Hence, recent guidelines (except European) have downgraded β-blockers as secondary, not primary drugs for hypertension (Table 4). Beta-blockers should still be considered for compelling indications such as CAD, compensated CHF, and sympathetic overdrive situations. The documented benefits of β-blockers ensure that this class of drugs will continue to be useful in selected situations.

TABLE 4: Primary drugs for hypertension

US	European
Diuretics	Diuretics
CCBs	CCBs
ARBs	ARBs
ACEIs	ACEIs
	β-blockers

CCB, calcium channel blocker; ARB, angiotensin receptor blocker; ACEIs, angiotensin-converting enzyme inhibitors.

Cardioselective β-blockers and vasodilating β-blockers are well tolerated and less likely to cause the traditional β-blocker side effects like depression, erectile dysfunction, and metabolic aberrations. Hence, it is preferable to consider metoprolol, nebivolol, bisoprolol, and carvedilol instead of atenolol and propranolol. Like any drug class, β-blockers are best applied in clinical practice taking into account the indications and contraindications. Vast clinical experience in India endorses the utility of β-blockers in the treatment of hypertension.

Calcium Channel Blockers

Calcium channel blockers are extremely reliable drugs to treat hypertension. Either as monotherapy or as a part of multidrug regimen, CCBs have become a highly useful class of drugs with proven efficacy and positive clinical outcomes. Evidence-based recommendation for CCBs is on the basis of dihydropyridine CCBs. The molecular mechanisms of various CCBs may differ slightly but the main site of their action is mediated by the inhibition of L-type voltage-dependent calcium channels. Although the first clinically useful CCB is nifedipine, bulk of new evidence is obtained from amlodipine and other newer drugs in the class.

Studies have demonstrated that CCBs (by lowering the BP level) reduce hypertension-related cardiovascular complications; they also have been shown to cause regression of left ventricular hypertrophy (LVH), prevent experimental atherosclerosis, and reduce proteinuria (in combination with ACEIs or ARBs). When given in proper doses, CCBs are effective irrespective of age, gender, ethnicity, and comorbid conditions. In combination with other antihypertensive drugs, CCBs are of considerable value in the treatment and prevention of resistant hypertension.

Outcome studies ranging from the earlier Syst-Eur to the recent FEVER and ACCOMPLISH[19] have all attested to the safety, utility, and the value of CCBs in the treatment of hypertension. Guidelines consistently recommend CCBs as primary drugs to treat hypertension.

Angiotensin-converting Enzymes Inhibitors

The renin–angiotensin–aldosterone system (RAAS) plays a pivotal role in BP regulation and in the pathophysiology of hypertension, particularly in the progression of target organ damage (TOD). The blockade of the RAAS, therefore, has become a meaningful pathway to lower the BP and to offer TOP. ACEIs as the name implies reduce the formation of angiotensin-II and thus, inhibit its vasoconstrictor actions. In addition, ACEIs also promote the functions of vasodilatory kinins. ACEIs (usually) in combination with a diuretic lower the BP in patients with hypertension. With the possible exception of captopril and lisinopril, other ACEIs are prodrugs which are converted into active compounds in the body. Some ACEIs like ramipril and perindopril have a greater affinity for tissue ACE. To what extent, this tissue affinity is responsible for TOP is not known.

Angiotensin-converting enzyme inhibitors have been recommended in the recent guidelines for initial treatment of hypertension. Although they may occasionally suffice as monotherapy, the efficacy of ACEIs for BP reduction is most expressed in combination with a diuretic. The fall in BP in response to ACEI is not accompanied by reflex tachycardia as these drugs also inhibit the sympathetic nervous system (SNS) to some extent. The efficacy of ACEIs is offset in the presence of high salt intake or with the concomitant use of nonsteroidal anti-inflammatory drugs (NSAIDs). Recent outcome trials like ASCOT-BPLA[20] and ACCOMPLISH[19] have further signified the therapeutic role of ACEIs (in combination with CCBs). A number of ACEIs ranging from benazepril to trandolapril are available for BP control but the outcome trials are limited to captopril, enalapril, perindopril, and ramipril. While one can start with a low dose of an ACEI, it is essential to apply optimal doses used in outcome trials.

Renin-angiotensin-aldosterone system blockade in general (including ACEIs) is particularly indicated in patients with atherosclerotic vascular disease, diabetes, renal dysfunction, metabolic syndrome, left ventricular dysfunction, and CHF. ACEIs may cause cough and rarely angioneurotic edema, and are contraindicated in pregnancy.

Angiotensin Receptor Blockers

Angiotensin receptor blockers have now become the central piece of the pharmacological blockade of the RAAS for the management of hypertension and comorbidities. As the name implies, the principal locus of ARB is inhibition of the angiotensin receptors (AT1R) located in the cardiovascular system and other organs such as the kidney, brain, and the adrenal gland. Angiotensin receptor blockers also attenuate the activity of SNS to some extent. It is argued that for BP reduction, ARBs are slightly superior to ACEIs. Like ACEIs, the BP lowering efficacy of ARBs is potentiated in combination with a diuretic. All the ARBs ranging from azilsartan to valsartan are effective in the treatment of hypertension and comorbidities. They differ in terms of duration action, renal or hepatic exertion, and outcome trials. The fundamental action of ARB is via the blockade of the AT1R but drugs like azilsartan have additional pathways of vasodilation, i.e., promoting the vasodilatory Ang 1-7.[21] It remains to be seen whether these ancillary mechanisms offer an advantage for TOP.

A number of studies with ARBs have ratified their benefits in patients with CVD, CeVD, diabetes, metabolic syndrome, and CKD. Thus, both ACEIs and ARBs appear to furnish similar TOP. However, the ability of ARBs to preserve renal function is persuasive and impelling. RAAS blockade, in general, improves endothelial function and suppresses reactive oxygen species and vascular inflammation. Certain differential effects of ARBs are emerging beyond BP control. For example, losartan has a modest uricosuric effect and telmisartan has an effect on PPARγ which may exert favorable metabolic effects. And azilsartan augments Ang 1-7 which may increase its potency and duration of action.

The efficacy of ARBs for BP control is enhanced when used in conjunction with diuretics or CCBs. The side effects and tolerability profile of ARBs is superior to ACEIs. The combination of ACEIs and ARBs is not useful and may even be detrimental in terms of potential adverse renal consequences. Pregnancy is an absolute contraindication for the use of ARBs. Cough and angioneurotic edema are less likely to occur with ARBs in comparison to ACEIs.

INITIAL COMBINATION THERAPY NOT MONOTHERAPY IS THE ANSWER FOR BLOOD PRESSURE CONTROL

The old stepped-care approach for the pharmacological treatment of hypertension is steadily being replaced with treat to target BP goals promptly to avoid exposure to persistently elevated BP levels. The earlier concept of initial monotherapy was based on the pharmacological observations but not on the outcome data. It is abundantly clear and well accepted now that in a majority of patients with hypertension, multiple drugs are required to achieve and maintain normotension. Hypertension guidelines do not propose therapeutic strategies based on the mechanisms of BP elevation. Instead, the preeminent goal of antihypertensive therapy is to achieve normotension. And to accomplish this purpose, combinations of drugs interrupts the diverse pathophysiological mechanisms of hypertension. Apart from lowering the BP level, the prescribed therapy should also counter the pathophysiological mechanisms of hypertension and TOD. These parameters dictate and mandate initiating combination therapy for hypertension, not monotherapy anymore. Combining two classes of drugs produces a synergistic effect on BP reduction (Fig. 2) whereas incremental doses of monotherapy has a ceiling effect on BP while increasing the dose dependent adverse effects (Fig. 3). The era of initial and sequential monotherapy is (rightly) now replaced by initial combination therapy.[22-24] Combination therapy can be in the form of separate drugs or fixed dose combination (FDC) or fixed pill combination (FPC). Studies have convincingly demonstrated that a FDC or FPC is to be preferred to promote and sustain patient adherence. The key to unlock the problem of hypertension control in the community is to promote adherence to prescribed therapy. Combination therapy produces a greater

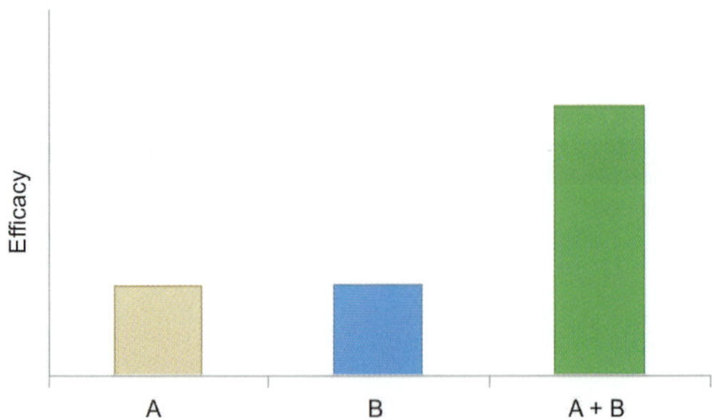

FIG. 2: Synergistic effects of combination therapy on efficacy.

effect on BP reduction while attenuating the side effects of the component drugs.

The latest American and European hypertension guidelines resolutely recommend initial combination therapy (Fig. 4). And it is the right logic. This approach is urgently germane to India which is under the wrath of uncontrolled hypertension and its devastating consequences. It is timely and appropriate for India to accept and welcome the notion of initial combination therapy for effective and prompt BP control. And as stated earlier, FDC or FPC is preferable over separate components to secure adherence to therapy. Examples of rational combinations are illustrated in boxes 1 and 2.

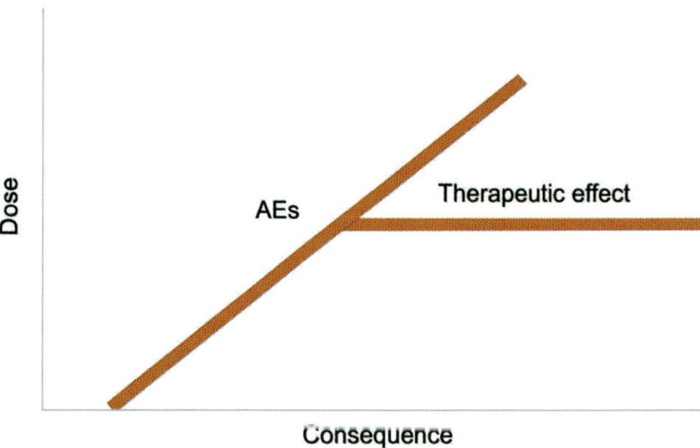

AEs, adverse effects.

FIG. 3: Monotherapy has a ceiling effect on blood pressure reduction.

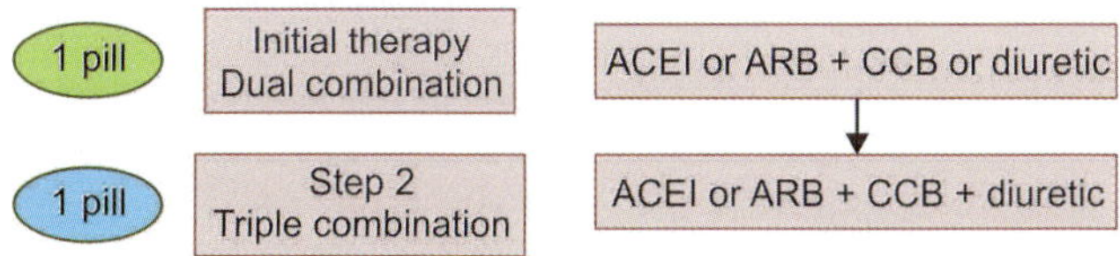

ARB, angiotensin receptor blocker; ACEIs, angiotensin-converting enzyme inhibitors; CCB, calcium channel blocker.

FIG. 4: Dual or triple combination therapy: new guidelines.

BOX 1 Examples of preferred combinations

- LVH: RAAS blocker + CCB
- Albuminuria: RAAS blocker plus other drugs
- Renal dysfunction: RAAS blocker plus other drugs
- CHF: RAAS blocker + diuretic ± CCB ± mineralocorticoid
- Diabetes/metabolic syndrome: RAAS blocker + CCB ± diuretic
- Systolic hypertension: CCB or diuretic or both
- Peripheral artery disease: RAAS blocker + CCB
- CAD: Beta-blocker + RAAS blocker ± CCB
- Cerebrovascular disease: CCB plus other drugs

CCB, calcium channel blocker; CHF, congestive heart failure; LVH, left ventricular hypertrophy; RAAS, renin–angiotensin–aldosterone system; CAD, coronary artery disease.

BOX 2 Acceptable dual drug combinations

- RAAS blocker + CCB
- RAAS blocker + diuretic
- Beta-blocker + diuretic
- CCBs + diuretic
- Beta-blocker + DHP CCB

Unacceptable combination

- ACEI + ARB

Acceptable triple drug combination

- Any nonduplicating combination from dual-drug choices
- Preferable → RAAS blocker + DHP CCB + Diuretic

ARB, angiotensin receptor blocker; ACEIs, angiotensin converting enzyme inhibitors; CCB, calcium channel blocker; DHP, dihydropyridine; RAAS, renin–angiotensin–aldosterone system.

The current platform for therapeutic discourse is not which monotherapy for hypertension but which combination? The elements of combination, to some extent, are governed by so-called "compelling" indications such as CAD, CHF, diabetes, CKD, etc. The combination therapy is also a foolproof concept that it eliminates factors which were previously considered such as age, racial background, salt-sensitivity volume, and comorbidities in the choice of initial monotherapy. Therefore, combination therapy is both user and patient friendly.

The time has come to treat hypertension with initial combination therapy replacing the traditional monotherapy. A large number of randomized clinical trials (RCTs) have demonstrated the value and necessity of combination therapy in achieving goal BP levels in a timely manner and in providing significant TOP. And admirable meta-analyzes have cogently affirmed the clinical benefits of optimal dose combination therapies in the treatment of hypertension and in the prevention of its complications. The evidence to implement initial combination therapy is well grounded and relevant particularly to the Indian scenario in order to improve BP control rates in an enduring fashion.

ACKNOWLEDGMENT

The author thanks the secretarial and editorial assistance provided by Ms Madhavi Nagaraj in the preparation of this chapter.

REFERENCES

1. Whelton PK, Carey RM, Aronow WS, et al. 2017 ACC/AHA/AAPA/ABS/ACPM/AGS/APhA/ASH/ASPC/NMA/PCNA guideline for the prevention, detection, evaluation and management of high blood pressure in adults: executive summary. J Am Coll Cardiol. 2018;71:2199-269.
2. Williams B, Mancia G, Barcelona I, et al. 2018 ESC/ESH guidelines for the management of arterial hypertension presented at the 28th European meeting on hypertension and cardiovascular protection. Barcelona. 2018.
3. Williams B, Mancia G, Barcelona I, et al. 2018 ESC/ESH guidelines for the management of arterial hypertension. J Hypertens, in press. 2018.
4. Singh M, Kotwal A, Mittal C, et al. Prevalence and correlates of hypertension in a semi-rural population of South India. J Hum Hypertens. 2018;32:66-74.

5. Anchala R, Kannuri NK, Pant H, et al. Hypertension in India: a systematic review and meta-analysis of prevalence, awareness, and control of hypertension. J Hypertens. 2014;32:1170-77.
6. Gupta R, Pandey RM, Misra A, et al. High prevalence and low hypertension awareness, treatment and control in Asian Indian women. J Hum Hypertens. 2012;26:585-93.
7. Pednekar MS, Gupta R, Gupta PC. Association of blood pressure and cardiovascular mortality in India: Mumbai Cohort Study. Am J Hypertens. 2009;22:1076-84.
8. Wander GS, Ram CVS. Global Impact of 2017 American Heart Association/American College of Cardiology, Hypertension Guidelines. A Perspective from India. Circulation. 2018;137:549-50.
9. Psaty BM, Lumley T, Furberg CD, et al. Health outcomes associated with various antihypertensive therapies used as first-line agents: a network meta-analysis. JAMA. 2003;289:2534-44.
10. Blood Pressure Lowering Treatment Trialists' Collaboration. Effects of different blood-pressure-lowering regimens on major cardiovascular events: results of prospectively-designed overviews of randomised trials. Lancet. 2003;362:1527-35.
11. Staessen JA, Wang J-W, Thijs L. Cardiovascular protection and blood pressure reduction: a meta-analysis. Lancet. 2001;358:1305-15.
12. Blood Pressure Lowering Treatment Trialists' Collaboration. Effects of ACE inhibitors, calcium antagonists, and other blood-pressure-lowering drugs: results of prospectively designed overviews of randomised trials. Lancet. 2000;355:1955-64.
13. Blood Pressure Lowering Treatment Trialists' Collaboration. Blood pressure-dependent and independent effects of agents that inhibit the renin-angiotensin system. J Hypertens. 2007;25:951-8.
14. Staessen JA, Wang J-G, Thijs L. Cardiovascular prevention and blood pressure reduction: a quantitative overview updated until 1 March 2003. J Hypertens. 2003;21:1055-76.
15. Law MR, Wald NJ, Morris JK, et al. Value of low dose combination treatment with blood pressure lowering drugs: analysis of 354 randomised trials. BMJ. 2003;326:1427-31.
16. Wald DS, Law M, Morris JK, et al. Combination therapy versus monotherapy in reducing blood pressure: meta-analysis on 11,000 participants from 42 trials. Am J Med. 2009;122:290-300.
17. Carlberg B, Samuelsson O, Lindholm LH. Atenolol in hypertension: is it a wise choice? Lancet. 2004;364:1684-9.
18. Lindholm LH, Carlberg B, Samuelsson O. Should β blockers remain first choice in the treatment of primary hypertension? A meta-analysis. Lancet. 2005;366:1545-53.
19. Jamerson K, Weber MA, Bakrias GL, et al. Benazepril plus amlodipine or hydrochlorothiazide for hypertension in high risk patients. N Engl J Med. 2008;359:2417-28.
20. The CAFÉ Investigators, for the Anglo-Scandinavian Cardiac Outcomes Trial (ASCOT) Investigators. Differential impact of blood pressure-lowering drugs on central aortic pressure and clinical outcome. Principal results of the Conduit Artery Function Evaluation (CAFÉ) Study. Circulation. 2006;113:1213-25.
21. Kurtz TW, Kajiya T. Differential pharmacology and the benefit/risk of azilsartan compared to other sartans. Vascular Health and Risk Management. 2012;8:133-43.
22. Gradman AH, Basile JN, Carter BL. Combination therapy in hypertension. JASH. 2010;4:42-50.
23. Wald DS, Law M, Morris JK, et al. Combination therapy versus monotherapy in reducing blood pressure: meta-analysis of 11,000 participants from 42 trials. Am J Med. 2009;122:290-300.
24. Egan M, Bandyopadhyay D, Shaftman SR, et al. Initial monotherapy and combination therapy and hypertension control the first year. Hypertension. 2012;59:1124-31.

CHAPTER 21

Are ACE inhibitor and ARB Equal in Hypertension?

SS Chatterjee, Arka Chatterjee

INTRODUCTION

The era of renin-angiotensin system (RAS) blockade began with the introduction of the first angiotensin-converting enzyme (ACE) inhibitor captopril in 1971.[1] Since then the class of drug has rapidly become a staple for a host of cardiovascular disease (CVD) states. Losartan, the first angiotensin receptor blocker (ARB), became available in 1995.[2] Both these classes of drugs are used for similar indications; however, ARBs are generally considered alternatives for ACE inhibitors in case of drug intolerance. We examine the relevant data supporting the use of these agents for hypertension and in hypertension with compelling indications.

MECHANISM OF ACTION

Both ACE inhibitors and ARBs have a similar mechanism of action, albeit affecting the RAS at different levels (Fig. 1). ACE inhibitors stop the conversion of angiotensin I to angiotensin II, thus reducing the effects of activated angiotensin II type 1 receptors. These varied effects include vasoconstriction, sodium or water retention, sympathetic activation, etc. Also, ACE inhibition retards the breakdown of bradykinin, thus increasing vasodilation. However, the adverse effects of ACE inhibitors are also secondary to increased bradykinin, i.e., cough, angioedema, etc. ACE inhibition also reduces the angiotensin II type 2 receptor activation which has also been postulated to increase vasodilatory effects. On the other hand, ARB agents specifically block activation of type 1 receptors which thus precludes the additional effects of ACE inhibitors on type 2 receptors and bradykinin.

EFFICACY IN REDUCING BLOOD PRESSURE

Multiple aggregated studies have tried to answer the question of variability in different agents for ACE inhibitors and ARBs and whether there is an incremental reduction in

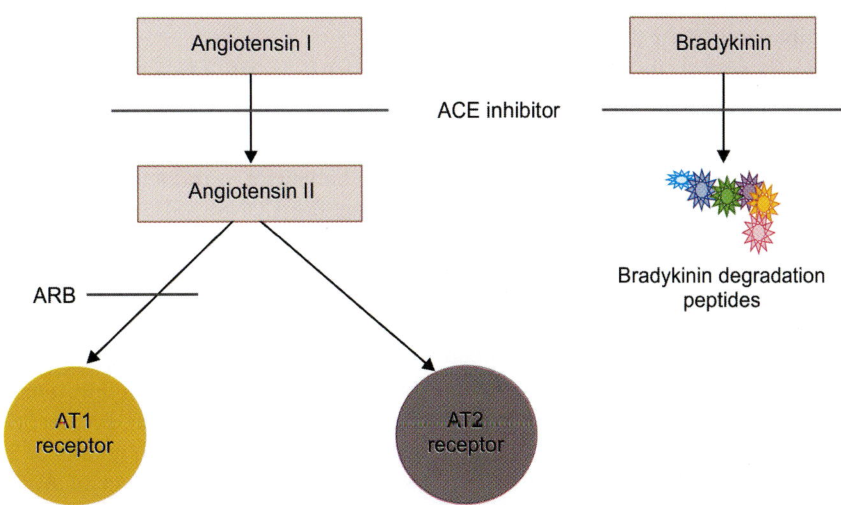

ACE, angiotensin-converting enzyme; ARB, angiotensin receptor blocker.

FIG. 1: ACE inhibitors and ARBs affect the RAS at different levels.

blood pressure (BP) for one over the other. Pooling 12,954 patients from 92 double blind randomized trials, Heran et al. concluded that the trough BP reduction was –8/–5 mm Hg for both ACE inhibitors.[3] The same trough BP reduction was found in a pooled analysis of 13,451 patients from 46 trials.[4] Using ambulatory BP as an outcome, the reduction of BP with ACE inhibitors and ARBs has been estimated to be –12.9/–7.7 mm Hg and –13.3/–7.8 mm Hg, respectively.[5] However, newer ARBs may produce greater BP reduction than ACE inhibitors. In a randomized study of 884 patients, azilsartan 40 and 80 mg doses produced higher reduction in trough BP (20.6 ± 0.95 and 21.2 ± 0.95 mm Hg) as compared to 10 mg dose of ramipril (12.2 ± 0.95 mm Hg).[6] Olmesartan has also been shown to be more efficacious than perindopril whether it is used for monotherapy or in combination with amlodipine.[7,8]

EFFICACY FOR SURROGATE CLINICAL OUTCOMES

The goal of treating hypertension is in preventing cardiovascular (CV) events and other target organ pathology. Thus, it is more important to see how these two different RAS blockers fare specifically in terms of prevention of deleterious events.

Overall Mortality

There are no dedicated head-to-head trials comparing ACE inhibitors and ARBs in hypertensive patients without concomitant CVD or other comorbidities. In individual trials investigating patients at higher risk of CVD outcomes (e.g., HOPE), ACE inhibitors (enalapril) showed mortality reduction but it should be noted that less than 50% patients were truly hypertensive.[9] Vark et al. performed a large meta-analysis which only included trials where the sample population comprised at least two-thirds hypertensive patients being randomized to RAS blockade versus placebo.[10] There was a definite reduction in overall mortality. However, the effect was driven by trials using ACE inhibitors only with no significant reduction seen in the pooled ARB trials. Conflicting results were obtained when the same question was examined in the REACH cohort, in which more than 90% patients were classified as hypertensive. In a propensity matched analysis, ARB use was shown to have better mortality outcome (11.6% vs. 12.6%, p = 0.005).[11]

Prevention of Cardiovascular Events

In the REACH cohort, a composite outcome of CV mortality, myocardial infarction (MI), stroke or other CV hospitalization was lower for patients using ARB as compared to ACE inhibitors.[11] However, contradictory results have also been reported, as in a meta-analysis of 108,212 patients by Savarese et al.[12] ACE inhibitors significantly reduced the composite outcome of CV mortality, MI or stroke by a margin of 14.9%. ARB use, although still significantly protective, had a lower reduction of 7%. While ACE inhibitors were found to be protective for MI, stroke and new onset heart failure (HF) individually also, ARBs were not found to be protective for MI or HF. A more recent network meta-analysis again showed equivalence for both classes with no difference in the risk reduction for CV mortality, MI or stroke.[13] In patients who have had a stroke, ARB does not appear to be protective against a second stroke as shown by the results of the PROFESS study.[14]

Prevention of Nephropathy

No difference in proteinuria or albuminuria was noted in a meta-analysis including 17 studies looking into this question.[15] Telmisartan and ramipril were found to have similar effects on the trajectories of renal function in patients included in the ONTARGET study. There was no difference in a composite outcome comprising dialysis, a doubling in serum creatinine and death. However, ramipril seemed to protect against worsening of glomerular filtration rate slightly better than telmisartan. The question of nephropathy or albuminuria becomes even more important for diabetic patients and in this group too, there does not seem to be a difference in efficacy of both classes. In a large network meta-analysis, Catala-Lopez et al. have shown comparable CV and renal outcomes.[16]

EFFECTS IN SELECT PATIENT SUBSETS

Patients with hypertension frequently have comorbidities which dictate therapy choices. Thus, it is useful to review the evidence for ACE or ARB use in these select patient subsets with compelling indications.

Patients with Coronary Artery Disease

There is no sizeable data suggesting a major benefit for either class in patients with CAD but no HF or left ventricular dysfunction. In fact, in the CAMELOT trial, outcomes with enalapril were poorer than those with amlodipine. However, there is a wealth of data in head-to-head trials comparing patients at higher risk of CV events with similar reduction in MI for both ACE and ARB which can be extrapolated to this population also.[17]

Patients with Heart Failure

The HF population is the most well studied with respect to actions of RAS blockade. Both the classes have been proven to be beneficial in reducing overall mortality in this patient subset. The CONSENSUS study established this finding for ACE inhibitors with enalapril while the CHARM study with candesartan was definitive in this respect for ARBs.[18-20] While enalapril produced a 31% 1-year mortality reduction in NYHA class IV HF patients, candesartan either added to enalapril or on its own also reduced mortality in similar patients. Along with mortality reduction, enalapril and candesartan also appeared to reduce recurrent admissions in these patients.[18,21] Based on the results of SAVE, AIR, and TRACE studies, the protective effect of ACE inhibitors in patients who have HF after a MI is well established.[22] Interestingly, in a network meta-analysis spanning multiple decades, Burnett et al. suggest ACE inhibitors but not ARBs provide mortality benefit in these patients as monotherapy and incremental benefit when used in combination with beta blockers or mineralocorticoid receptor antagonists.[23] While this analysis was weighted toward ACE inhibitors just because of the increased time period of follow up for the same compared to ARB, some authors do believe that there is an incremental benefit with ACE inhibitors likely attributable to the increase in other vasoactive mediators and AT2 receptor activation.[24]

ADVERSE EFFECTS AND PATIENT COMPLIANCE

Both classes of drugs are reasonably well tolerated. The most common adverse effect in patients taking ACE inhibitors is dry cough.[25] ACE inhibitors have been estimated to produce cough in 11.48% patients in a pooled analysis.[26] Out of these, just under a quarter end up stopping ACE inhibitors. Angioedema is rarer, happening in about 0.3–0.7% patients.[27,28] About a fifth of angioedema instances may lead to fatalities and there is a predilection for more African-American patients to have angioedema.[29,30] However, in comparison, ARBs are much better tolerated and have remarkably lower discontinuation rates.[31] In fact, in pooled analyzes, it is suggested that ARBs have lower discontinuation rates than placebo.[32]

COST-EFFECTIVENESS

While any analysis for cost-effectiveness is dictated by geographical variations in availability of generic versions of drugs in various markets and many other factors, some analyzes have actually found ARBs to be more efficacious in the long run, especially in diabetic nephropathy patients.[33] Fixed dose combinations incorporating ARBs with other agents may help also with patient compliance and also control patient cost.

CONCLUSION

The only way to differentiate the efficacy of ACE inhibitors and ARBs would be to run head-to-head randomized trials for each population of interest. However, with the wealth of data already available regarding both these classes' efficacy in improving CV outcomes, it is doubtful that a large trial will be formulated soon. There is no good evidence to support choosing one specifically over the other; however, ACE inhibitors are definitely worse when it comes to adverse effects and needing replacement of drug. Angioedema, although very rare, can be fatal in patients taking ACE inhibitors.

Thus, both are still very favorable first-line antihypertensives with the adverse effect profile weighing the scales mildly toward ARB.

REFERENCES

1. Ondetti MA, Rubin B, Cushman DW. Design of specific inhibitors of angiotensin-converting enzyme: new class of orally active antihypertensive agents. Science. 1977;196(4288):441-4.
2. Crozier I, Ikram H, Awan N, et al. Losartan in heart failure. Hemodynamic effects and tolerability. Losartan Hemodynamic Study Group. Circulation. 1995;91(3):691-7.
3. Heran BS, Wong MM, Heran IK, et al. Blood pressure lowering efficacy of angiotensin converting enzyme (ACE) inhibitors for primary hypertension. Cochrane Database Syst Rev. 2008;(4):CD003823.
4. Heran BS, Wong MM, Heran IK, et al. Blood pressure lowering efficacy of angiotensin receptor blockers for primary hypertension. Cochrane Database Syst Rev. 2008;(4):CD003822.
5. Messerli FH, Makani H, Benjo A, et al. Antihypertensive efficacy of hydrochlorothiazide as evaluated by ambulatory blood pressure monitoring: a meta-analysis of randomized trials. J Am Coll Cardiol. 2011;57(5):590-600.
6. Bonner G, Bakris GL, Sica D, et al. Antihypertensive efficacy of the angiotensin receptor blocker azilsartan medoxomil compared with the angiotensin-converting enzyme inhibitor ramipril. J Hum Hypertens. 2013;27(8):479-86.
7. Omboni S, Malacco E, Mallion JM, et al. Twenty-four hour and early morning blood pressure control of olmesartan vs. ramipril in elderly hypertensive patients: pooled individual data analysis of two randomized, double-blind, parallel-group studies. J Hypertens. 2012;30(7):1468-77.
8. Ruilope LM, SS Investigators. Fixed-Combination Olmesartan/Amlodipine Was Superior to Perindopril + Amlodipine in Reducing Central Systolic Blood Pressure in Hypertensive Patients With Diabetes. J Clin Hypertens (Greenwich). 2016;18(6):528-35.
9. Heart Outcomes Prevention Evaluation Study Investigators, Yusuf S, Sleight P, et al. Effects of an angiotensin-converting-enzyme inhibitor, ramipril, on cardiovascular events in high-risk patients. N Engl J Med. 2000;342(3):145-53.
10. van Vark LC, Bertrand M, Akkerhuis KM, et al. Angiotensin-converting enzyme inhibitors reduce mortality in hypertension: a meta-analysis of randomized clinical trials of renin-angiotensin-aldosterone system inhibitors involving 158,998 patients. Eur Heart J. 2012;33(16):2088-97.
11. Potier L, Roussel R, Elbez Y, et al. Angiotensin-converting enzyme inhibitors and angiotensin receptor blockers in high vascular risk. Heart. 2017;103(17):1339-46.
12. Savarese G, Costanzo P, Cleland JG, et al. A meta-analysis reporting effects of angiotensin-converting enzyme inhibitors and angiotensin receptor blockers in patients without heart failure. J Am Coll Cardiol. 2013;61(2):131-42.
13. Ricci F, Di Castelnuovo A, Savarese G, et al. ACE-inhibitors versus angiotensin receptor blockers for prevention of events in cardiovascular patients without heart failure - A network meta-analysis. Int J Cardiol. 2016;217:128-34.
14. Yusuf S, Diener HC, Sacco RL, et al. Telmisartan to prevent recurrent stroke and cardiovascular events. N Engl J Med. 2008;359(12):1225-37.
15. Xu R, Sun S, Huo Y, et al. Effects of ACEIs Versus ARBs on Proteinuria or Albuminuria in Primary Hypertension: A Meta-Analysis of Randomized Trials. Medicine (Baltimore). 2015;94(39):e1560.
16. Catalá-López F, Macías Saint-Gerons D, González-Bermejo D, et al. Cardiovascular and Renal Outcomes of Renin-Angiotensin System Blockade in Adult Patients with Diabetes Mellitus: A Systematic Review with Network Meta-Analyses. PLoS Med. 2016;13(3):e1001971.
17. Messerli FH, Bangalore S. Angiotensin Receptor Blockers Reduce Cardiovascular Events, Including the Risk of Myocardial Infarction. Circulation. 2017;135(22):2085-7.
18. Granger CB, McMurray JJ, Yusuf S, et al. Effects of candesartan in patients with chronic heart failure and reduced left-ventricular systolic function intolerant to angiotensin-converting-enzyme inhibitors: the CHARM-Alternative trial. Lancet. 2003;362(9386):772-6.
19. McMurray JJ, Ostergren J, Swedberg K, et al. Effects of candesartan in patients with chronic heart failure and reduced left-ventricular systolic function taking angiotensin-converting-enzyme inhibitors: the CHARM-Added trial. Lancet. 2003;362(9386):767-71.
20. Group CTS. Effects of enalapril on mortality in severe congestive heart failure. Results of the Cooperative North Scandinavian Enalapril Survival Study (CONSENSUS). N Engl J Med. 1987;316(23):1429-35.
21. Investigators S, Yusuf S, Pitt B, et al. Effect of enalapril on survival in patients with reduced left ventricular ejection fractions and congestive heart failure. N Engl J Med. 1991;325(5):293-302.

22. Flather MD, Yusuf S, Køber L, et al. Long-term ACE-inhibitor therapy in patients with heart failure or left-ventricular dysfunction: a systematic overview of data from individual patients. ACE-Inhibitor Myocardial Infarction Collaborative Group. Lancet. 2000;355(9215):1575-81.
23. Burnett H, Earley A, Voors A, et al. Thirty Years of Evidence on the Efficacy of Drug Treatments for Chronic Heart Failure With Reduced Ejection Fraction: A Network Meta-Analysis. Circ Heart Fail. 2017;10(1).
24. Packer M, McMurray JJV. Importance of endogenous compensatory vasoactive peptides in broadening the effects of inhibitors of the renin-angiotensin system for the treatment of heart failure. Lancet. 2017;389(10081):1831-40.
25. Law MR, Wald NJ, Morris JK, et al. Value of low dose combination treatment with blood pressure lowering drugs: analysis of 354 randomised trials. BMJ. 2003;326(7404):1427.
26. Bangalore S, Kumar S, Messerli FH. Angiotensin-converting enzyme inhibitor associated cough: deceptive information from the Physicians' Desk Reference. Am J Med. 2010;123(11):1016-30.
27. Makani H, Messerli FH, Romero J, et al. Meta-analysis of randomized trials of angioedema as an adverse event of renin-angiotensin system inhibitors. Am J Cardiol. 2012;110(3):383-91.
28. Banerji A, Blumenthal KG, Lai KH, et al. Epidemiology of ACE Inhibitor Angioedema Utilizing a Large Electronic Health Record. J Allergy Clin Immunol Pract. 2017;5(3):744-9.
29. Slater EE, Merrill DD, Guess HA, et al. Clinical profile of angioedema associated with angiotensin converting-enzyme inhibition. JAMA. 1988;260(7):967-70.
30. Dean DE, Schultz DL, Powers RH. Asphyxia due to angiotensin converting enzyme (ACE) inhibitor mediated angioedema of the tongue during the treatment of hypertensive heart disease. J Forensic Sci. 2001;46(5):1239-43.
31. Bangalore S, Fakheri R, Toklu B, et al. Angiotensin-Converting Enzyme Inhibitors or Angiotensin Receptor Blockers in Patients Without Heart Failure? Insights From 254,301 Patients From Randomized Trials. Mayo Clin Proc. 2016;91(1):51-60.
32. Thomopoulos C, Parati G, Zanchetti A. Effects of blood-pressure-lowering treatment in hypertension: 9. Discontinuations for adverse events attributed to different classes of antihypertensive drugs: meta-analyses of randomized trials. J Hypertens. 2016;34(10):1921-32.
33. Stafylas PC, Sarafidis PA, Grekas DM, et al. A cost-effectiveness analysis of angiotensin-converting enzyme inhibitors and angiotensin receptor blockers in diabetic nephropathy. J Clin Hypertens (Greenwich). 2007;9(10):751-9.

CHAPTER 22

Diuretics as Antihypertensive in Elderly

Anunay Gupta, HS Isser

INTRODUCTION

Hypertension is a common problem in elderly (age older than 60–65 years). Hypertension increases with age, affecting approximately 66% of the elderly population (aged ≥65 years). As life expectancy increases number of elderly needing antihypertensive medications is expected to increase. Elderly patients have a higher absolute risk of cardiovascular (CV) events, compared to younger individuals with the same risk factor profile. A number of placebo-controlled clinical trials have demonstrated that blood pressure (BP) control reduces CV events in elderly patients, even in those aged older than 80 years. Five-year number needed to treat (NNT) estimates indicate that fewer than 100 older people needed to be treated to prevent one event. Despite advances in medical care, hypertension control rates remain low, especially in the elderly population. In India, prevalence of hypertension was 42.7% in elderly (aged more than 60 years) population, was significantly higher in age group more than 80 years (61%) and females (48%).[1] Elderly individuals usually have isolated systolic hypertension (ISH) with normal diastolic pressures.[2] Most of the recent guidelines suggest that the amount of BP reduction is major determinant of reduction in CV risk in both younger and older patients rather the choice of antihypertensive drug. Even though antihypertensive drugs choice is well-guided today, BP target is still a subject of debate in view of 2017 guidelines of hypertension.[3] This chapter reviews diuretics as antihypertensive agent in elderly patients.

ISSUES WITH ELDERLY POPULATION

Elderly patients are more likely to have ISH—systolic blood pressure (SBP) more than or equal to 140 mm Hg; diastolic blood pressure (DBP) less than 90 mm Hg, more than 65% of hypertensive patients aged older than or equal to 60 years and more than 90% of those aged older than 70 years have ISH.[2] There is a linear increase in both SBP and DBP up to sixth decade of life after which SBP continues to increase while there is a gradual decline in DBP.[4] Various pathophysiological mechanisms associated with ISH are increase in arterial stiffness from arteriosclerosis, endothelial dysfunction, elastin calcifications, increased salt sensitivity and increased sympathetic activity.[4] Aggressive treatment of ISH may also lead to fall in DBP and DBP less than 70 mm Hg especially less than 60 mm Hg have been shown to be associated with increased risk of stroke and coronary heart disease (CHD) in a *post hoc* analysis of SHEP (Systolic Hypertension in the Elderly Program) trial.[5] Similarly in recently published analysis of landmark SPRINT (Systolic Blood Pressure Intervention Trial) trial it was seen that in patients with isolated hypertension when diastolic pressure fell to less than 55 mm Hg, the hazards of increased CV events were at least 25% higher relative to 70 mm Hg.[6] Both thiazide-like diuretics and calcium channel blockers (CCBs) are considered as first-line drugs in ISH. β-blockers should be avoided in this population. Elderly patients frequently have associated comorbidities such as diabetes mellitus, chronic kidney disease, cerebrovascular accident, and parkinsonism which influence the choice of antihypertensive drugs. Elderly population are at risk of postural hypotension leading to falls and injuries. These characteristics must be considered while choosing antihypertensive drugs for this population.

BLOOD PRESSURE GOALS AND TARGETS

Hypertension is one of the primary risk factors for myocardial infarction (MI), stroke, heart failure (HF), renal failure, and most other adverse vascular events in the older population. Eighth Joint National Committee (JNC 8) published in 2014 recommended that in population aged 60 years or older, initiate treatment to lower BP at SBP of 150 mm Hg or higher or DBP of 90 mm Hg or higher and treat to a goal SBP <150 mm Hg and goal DBP <90 mm Hg.[7] These pressure goals are not supported by all other guidelines and societies. According to European Society of Hypertension (ESH)/European Society of Cardiology (ESC) 2013 guidelines,[8] the minority report from the 2013 JNC 8 guidelines,[9] the 2013 Canadian Hypertension Education Program guidelines,[10] the 2011 UK guidelines,[11] the 2014 American Society of Hypertension (ASH)/International Society of Hypertension guidelines,[12] a BP below 140/90 mm Hg has been recommended in elderly between 60 and 79 years of age. In adults aged 80 years and older, a BP below 150/90 mm Hg has been recommended by these guidelines, with a target goal of less than 140/90 mm Hg considered in those with diabetes mellitus or chronic kidney disease. However, 2017 guidelines for high BP in adults have redefined hypertension as SBP more than 130 mm Hg and diastolic BP more than 80 mm Hg.[3]

CLINICAL TRIALS IN ELDERLY POPULATION

The Medical Research Council (MRC) trial randomized 4,396 patients aged 65–74 to atenolol 50 mg daily; hydrochlorothiazide 25 mg or 50 mg plus amiloride 2.5 mg or 5 mg daily. Mean follow-up was 5.8 years. Primary outcome was strokes, coronary events, and deaths from all causes. After adjusting for baseline characteristics the diuretic group had significantly reduced risks of stroke [31% (3–51%) p = 0.04], coronary events [44% (21–60%), p = 0.0009], and all cardiovascular CV events [35% (17–49%), p = 0.0005] compared with the placebo group. The β-blocker group showed no significant reductions in these endpoints. The reduction in strokes was seen predominantly in nonsmokers taking the diuretics. Thus, in the MRC trial in elderly patients hydrochlorothiazide and amiloride reduced the risk of stroke, whereas β-blockers failed to reduce the risk of stroke despite a similar lowering of BP.[13]

The SHEP trial was another trial which supported use of diuretics in this population.[14] Total 4,736 persons aged 60 years and above with average SBP of 170 mm Hg and average DBP of 77 mm Hg were randomized to chlorthalidone (12.5–25 mg/day) versus placebo, other drugs added were atenolol (25–50 mg/day) with average follow-up of 4.5 years. Stroke was the primary endpoint. Significant improvement in BP was accomplished in the treatment group compared with the group receiving placebo (SBP, 143 mm Hg vs. 155 mm Hg, respectively), leading to significant reduction in stroke (36%), coronary artery disease (CAD; 27%), chronic heart failure (CHF; 55%, 81% in those with previous MI). In a *post hoc* analysis of SHEP trial, it was seen that decrease in DBP of more than 5 mm Hg was associated with increased risk for stroke [relative risk (RR): 1.14; 95% confidence interval (CI): 1.05–1.22], for CHD (RR: 1.08; 95% CI: 1.00–1.16), and for cardiovascular disease (CVD) (RR: 1.11; 95% CI: 1.05–1.16).[5]

The Antihypertensive and Lipid-Lowering Treatment to Prevent Heart Attack Trial (ALLHAT) trial included 42,418 patients (mean age, 67 years) with hypertension and at least one other risk factor for CAD.[15] Total 57.5% of the participants were aged more than 65 years; therefore, this study is considered a study in the elderly. The patients were randomized to a treatment group with a thiazide-type diuretic (chlorthalidone 12.5–25 mg/day), a CCB (amlodipine 2.5–10 mg/day), an ACE-inhibitor (lisinopril 10–40 mg/day), or an alpha-blocker (doxazosin). The doxazosin component of the study was terminated early because of a 25% greater incidence of combined CVD events compared with the chlorthalidone arm. At 5 years of follow-up 68.2% patients in chlorthalidone arm 66.3% patients in amlodipine arm and 61.2% patients in lisinopril arm have achieved BP goal of less than 140/90 mm Hg. There were no differences in the primary outcome of fatal or nonfatal coronary events and no mortality difference between the CCB, angiotensin-converting enzyme (ACE) inhibitor, and diuretic groups. The diuretic treatment group had lower HF rates compared with the CCB group [relative risk (RR): 1.33; 95% confidence interval (CI): 1.18–1.49] and lower combined CV outcomes (RR: 1.13; 95% CI: 1.06–1.20), strokes (6.3% vs. 5.6%; RR: 1.15; 95% CI: 1.02–1.30) and HF (RR: 1.20; 95% CI: 1.09–1.34) compared with the ACE-inhibitor group. This trial established that chlorthalidone was superior to doxazosin, lisinopril, and amlodipine in preventing HF in a subanalysis of ALLHAT, chlorthalidone was superior to other agents in preventing HF in patients with the metabolic syndrome and also in patients with diabetes. Even after adjustment for BP, the difference in risk of stroke and HF between treatment arms was statistically significant.

The Hypertension in the Very Elderly Trial (HYVET) trial was published in 2008 and recruited more than 3,800 elderly patients (patients aged ≥80 years; mean, 83.6 years) with systolic hypertension, diastolic hypertension, or ISH. Patients were randomly assigned to take indapamide (thiazide-like diuretics) (sustained release, 1.5 mg) or matching placebo. The ACE-inhibitor perindopril (2 mg or 4 mg), or matching placebo, was added if necessary to achieve the target BP of 150/80 mm Hg. The primary end point of the trial was fatal or nonfatal stroke. Significant reduction in mean BP was achieved in the treatment group (143/78 mm Hg vs. 158/84 mm Hg) at 2 years. The target BP was reached in 19.9% of patients in the placebo group and in 48.0% in the active-treatment group ($p < 0.001$). At 2 years, 25.8%, 23.9%, and 49.5% of patients in the active-treatment group were receiving indapamide alone, indapamide and perindopril (2 mg), and indapamide and perindopril (4 mg), respectively. The study was stopped early as a result of significant reductions in fatal stroke (6.5% in the active group vs. 10.7% in the placebo group) and all-cause mortality (47.2% in the active group, 59.6% in the placebo group). This trial showed that diuretics indapamide use in "Hypertension in the Very Elderly", reduced the rate of HF by 64%.[16]

The only one exception was the ANBP2 study (Second Australian National Blood Pressure Study), a prospective, randomized, open-label study with blinded assessment of endpoints in 6,083 subjects with hypertension who were 65–84 years of age and received health care at 1,594 family practices. Subjects were followed for a median of 4.1 years, and the total numbers of cardiovascular events in the two treatment groups were compared. Treatment with an ACE inhibitor in older subjects was found to be better than treatment with diuretic agents, despite similar reductions of BP.[17] There were 695 CV events or deaths from any cause in the ACE-inhibitor group (56.1 per 1,000 patient-years) and 736 CV events or deaths from any cause in the diuretic group (59.8 per 1,000 patient-years; the HR for a CV event or death with ACE-inhibitor treatment was 0.89 (95% confidence interval, 0.79–1.00); p = 0.05). Among male subjects, the HR was 0.83 (95 % CI, 0.71- 0.97; p = 0.02); among female subjects, the hazard ratio was 1.00 (95% CI,: 0.83–1.21; p = 0.98); the p value for the interaction between sex and treatment-group assignment was 0.15. The rates of nonfatal CV events and MIs decreased with ACE-inhibitor treatment, whereas a similar number of strokes occurred in each group (although there were more fatal strokes in the ACE-inhibitor group). But design of the ANBP2 study was less rigorous than other studies, it was a prospective, randomized, open-label, blinded-endpoint (PROBE) study that is prone to bias. In the ANBP2 study, 83% of the participants received their assigned treatment, only 58% of participants were randomly assigned to an ACE inhibitor, and 62% of those assigned to a diuretic were still receiving assigned treatment at the end of the study.[17]

DIURETICS AS FIRST-LINE ANTIHYPERTENSIVE DRUG

Diuretics have been recommended as first-line antihypertensive agent in elderly according to JNC 7 guidelines.[18] Mechanism attributing to fall of BP initially seen with diuretics is due to the reductions in extracellular fluid and plasma volumes. The persistent antihypertensive effects seen later are due to fall in systemic resistance.

Which Diuretic to be Used?

Among all available diuretics only thiazide diuretics have been evaluated as first-line drug for treatment of hypertension. Chlorthalidone and indapamide (thiazide-like diuretics) are significantly more potent antihypertensive agents than hydrochlorothiazide, (thiazide-type diuretic) at similar dose levels. Chlorthalidone and indapamide have more longer (>24 h) duration of action compared to thiazide which may be responsible for more hypokalemia seen with chlorthalidone.[18] Use of sodium restricted diet along with thiazide diuretics contribute to more BP lowering and reduce the risk of hypokalemia.[19]

Thiazide Diuretics: When to Use and When not to Use?

If patient with hypertension and osteoporosis; thiazide-like diuretics have advantages over ACE inhibitors, angiotensin receptor blockers, and CCBs because these drugs stimulate distal tubular reabsorption of calcium, leading to a decrease in urinary calcium excretion. Hence, thiazide diuretics may have a beneficial effect on bone mineral density. In a recently published *post hoc* analysis of the ALLHAT trial the rates of hip or pelvic fractures among patients treated with thiazide-like diuretics, ACE-inhibitors, and CCBs were compared, chlorthalidone had significantly fewer hip or pelvic fractures as compared with those assigned either lisinopril or amlodipine (1.3% vs. 1.7%).[20]

Thiazides reduce the excretion of calcium as discussed above and uric acid and therefore increase their plasma levels. They should be avoided in patients with gout.[21] They increase potassium and magnesium excretion, leading to hypokalemia and hypomagnesemia. Diuretics have been implicated to increase blood glucose levels, which has been shown to be related to hypokalemia.[22] It was seen in SHEP trial that each 0.5 mEq/L decrease in serum potassium during the 1st year of treatment was associated with a 45% higher adjusted diabetes risk.[23] Thiazide-induced diabetes can be prevented by potassium supplementation or combination with ACE-inhibitor or potassium-sparing diuretics.[24]

Diuretics cause increased cholesterol and triglyceride levels along rise in low-density lipoprotein cholesterol. The rise in cholesterol was dose dependent and greater in blacks. A reduction in the high-density lipoprotein cholesterol levels was seen in patients with diabetes.[25] Whether these effects in lipid profile will have adverse effect is not well-known due to short-term follow-up of most of the trials.

CONCLUSION

Thiazide-type diuretics are inexpensive safe and effective antihypertensives in elderly. Thiazide-like diuretics are as effective as other antihypertensive drugs in elderly and very elderly population as supported by multiple large randomized control trials. British Hypertension Society recommended that diuretics and CCBs should be first-line drugs in hypertensive patients aged more than 55 years. Thiazide-type diuretics prevent HF and stroke in hypertensive patients, and may be superior to other agents in preventing new-onset HF. Diuretics reduced the risk of CHD and all-cause mortality. Chlorthalidone and indapamide should be preferred over thiazide. The benefit of diuretics as first-line antihypertensive drugs should be weighed against side effects such as risk of new onset diabetes, electrolyte imbalance and derangement in lipid profile.

REFERENCES

1. Sheth AM, Jadav PA. Prevalence and factors affecting hypertension among old age population in rural area. Int J Commun Med Pub Health. 2016;3(7):1866-71.
2. Franklin SS, Jacobs MJ, Wong ND, et al. Predominance of isolated systolic hypertension among middle-aged and elderly US hypertensives: analysis based on National Health and Nutrition Examination Survey (NHANES) III. Hypertens Dallas Tex 1979. 2001;37(3):869-74.
3. Whelton PK, Carey RM, Aronow WS, et al. 2017 ACC/AHA/AAPA/ABC/ACPM/AGS/APhA/ASH/ASPC/NMA/PCNA Guideline for the Prevention, Detection, Evaluation, and Management of High Blood Pressure in Adults: Executive Summary: A Report of the American College of Cardiology/American Heart Association Task Force on Clinical Practice Guidelines. Hypertens Dallas Tex 1979. 2018;71(6):1269-324.
4. Bavishi C, Goel S, Messerli FH. Isolated Systolic Hypertension: An Update After SPRINT. Am J Med. 2016;129(12):1251-8.
5. Somes GW, Pahor M, Shorr RI, et al. The role of diastolic blood pressure when treating isolated systolic hypertension. Arch Intern Med. 1999;159(17):2004-9.
6. Khan NA, Rabkin SW, Zhao Y, et al. Effect of Lowering Diastolic Pressure in Patients With and Without Cardiovascular Disease: Analysis of the SPRINT

(Systolic Blood Pressure Intervention Trial). Hypertens Dallas Tex 1979. 2018;71(5):840-7.
7. James PA, Oparil S, Carter BL, et al. 2014 evidence-based guideline for the management of high blood pressure in adults: report from the panel members appointed to the Eighth Joint National Committee (JNC 8). JAMA. 2014;311(5):507-20.
8. Mancia G, Fagard R, Narkiewicz K, et al. 2013 ESH/ESC Guidelines for the management of arterial hypertension: the Task Force for the management of arterial hypertension of the European Society of Hypertension (ESH) and of the European Society of Cardiology (ESC). J Hypertens. 2013;31(7):1281-357.
9. Wright JT, Fine LJ, Lackland DT, et al. Evidence supporting a systolic blood pressure goal of less than 150 mm Hg in patients aged 60 years or older: the minority view. Ann Intern Med. 2014;160(7):499-503.
10. Hackam DG, Quinn RR, Ravani P, et al. The 2013 Canadian Hypertension Education Program recommendations for blood pressure measurement, diagnosis, assessment of risk, prevention, and treatment of hypertension. Can J Cardiol. 2013;29(5):528-42.
11. Krause T, Lovibond K, Caulfield M, et al. Management of hypertension: summary of NICE guidance. BMJ. 2011;343:d4891.
12. Weber MA, Schiffrin EL, White WB, et al. Clinical practice guidelines for the management of hypertension in the community: a statement by the American Society of Hypertension and the International Society of Hypertension. J Clin Hypertens Greenwich Conn. 2014;16(1):14-26.
13. MRC trial of treatment of mild hypertension: principal results. Medical Research Council Working Party. Br Med J Clin Res Ed. 1985;291(6488):97-104.
14. Prevention of stroke by antihypertensive drug treatment in older persons with isolated systolic hypertension. Final results of the Systolic Hypertension in the Elderly Program (SHEP). SHEP Cooperative Research Group. JAMA. 1991;265(24):3255-64.
15. ALLHAT Officers and Coordinators for the ALLHAT Collaborative Research Group. The Antihypertensive and Lipid-Lowering Treatment to Prevent Heart Attack Trial. Major outcomes in high-risk hypertensive patients randomized to angiotensin-converting enzyme inhibitor or calcium channel blocker vs diuretic: The Antihypertensive and Lipid-Lowering Treatment to Prevent Heart Attack Trial (ALLHAT). JAMA. 2002;288(23):2981-97.
16. Beckett NS, Peters R, Fletcher AE, et al. Treatment of hypertension in patients 80 years of age or older. N Engl J Med. 2008;358(18):1887-98.
17. Wing LM, Reid CM, Ryan P, et al. A comparison of outcomes with angiotensin-converting-enzyme inhibitors and diuretics for hypertension in the elderly. N Engl J Med. 2003;348:583-92.
18. Peterzan MA, Hardy R, Chaturvedi N, et al. Meta-analysis of dose-response relationships for hydrochlorothiazide, chlorthalidone, and bendroflumethiazide on blood pressure, serum potassium, and urate. Hypertens Dallas Tex 1979. 2012;59(6):1104-9.
19. Ram CV, Garrett BN, Kaplan NM. Moderate sodium restriction and various diuretics in the treatment of hypertension. Arch Intern Med. 1981;141(8):1015-9.
20. Puttnam R, Davis BR, Pressel SL, et al. Association of 3 Different Antihypertensive Medications with Hip and Pelvic Fracture Risk in Older Adults: Secondary Analysis of a Randomized Clinical Trial. JAMA Intern Med. 2017;177(1):67-76.
21. Pascual E, Perdiguero M. Gout, diuretics and the kidney. Ann Rheum Dis. 2006;65(8):981-2.
22. Plavinik FL, Rodrigues CI, Zanella MT, et al. Hypokalemia, glucose intolerance, and hyperinsulinemia during diuretic therapy. Hypertens Dallas Tex 1979. 1992;19 (Suppl):II26-9.
23. Shafi T, Appel LJ, Miller ER, et al. Changes in serum potassium mediate thiazide-induced diabetes. Hypertens Dallas Tex 1979. 2008;52(6):1022-9.
24. Jeunemaitre X, Charru A, Chatellier G, et al. Long-term metabolic effects of spironolactone and thiazides combined with potassium-sparing agents for treatment of essential hypertension. Am J Cardiol. 1988;62(16):1072-7.
25. Kasiske BL, Ma JZ, Kalil RS, et al. Effects of antihypertensive therapy on serum lipids. Ann Intern Med. 1995;122(2):133-41.

CHAPTER 23

Treating Resistant Hypertension: Stepwise Approach

Binjo Vazhappilly, Julian Thottan, Mohanan Padinhare

INTRODUCTION

Resistant hypertension (rHTN) is defined as blood pressure (BP) that remained above goal despite the concurrent use of three antihypertensive agents of different classes including a diuretic at optimal dosages and whose BP is controlled with four or more medications.[1] Prevalence of rHTN varies from 2 to 40% depending on how rHTN was defined and they generally do not incorporate detailed information regarding medication dosing, treatment adherence, appropriate use of diuretics, and other clinical factors that may affect BP.

STEPWISE EVALUATION OF RESISTANT HYPERTENSION

Resistant hypertension is a diagnosis by exclusion. First, the accuracy of BP measurements using optimal technique needs to be established. Errors should be minimized by avoiding common pitfalls like improper patient positioning, inappropriate cuff size, poor timing of measurements, and equipment-related errors.

Out-of-Office Blood Pressure Monitoring

Since the prevalence of white coat hypertension (WCH) in patients with suspected rHTN based on office BP measurements is very high, 24 hours ambulatory blood pressure monitoring (ABPM) should be part of the routine work-up. The importance of 24-hour ABPM to rule out WCH in the setting of suspected rHTN is demonstrated by de la Sierra et al.[2] This study showed roughly one-third of patients labeled as rHTN by office BP measurement had WCH. Clinical signs suggestive of WCH are high office BP values without signs of target organ damage and the presence of symptoms associated with hypotension (i.e., dizziness, fatigue, and blurring) that may be related to antihypertensive overtreatment.

When ABPM is not feasible, home BP monitoring may be substituted and has been shown to correlate closely with daytime ABPM readings although it will not provide information about nocturnal patterns. Automated office measurements can reduce the white coat effect but will miss masked hypertension. Thus, even in the setting of goal office measurements, it might be useful to pursue ABPM when disproportionate target organ damage is present (Flowchart 1).

Rule Out Secondary Hypertension

The absence of a night-time drop (dipping of >10% relative to the daytime BP) or any increase of BP during night time ("reverse nocturnal dipping") is often associated with secondary hypertension.[3] The most common causes of secondary hypertension are obstructive sleep apnea (OSA), renal parenchymal and/or vascular disease, and primary aldosteronism (PA).

Nondipping or reverse dipping associated with a history of snoring, daytime sleepiness, and morning headache should prompt to suspect OSA. Screening for OSA can easily be done by assessing daytime sleepiness using a questionnaire (Epworth screening questionnaire) and by sleep study to assess apnea–hypopnea index.

Screening for renal parenchymal disease should be performed by urine analysis, serum creatinine concentration, and renal ultrasound if required. Renal artery stenosis (RAS) should be suspected in patients with abrupt progression of the severity of hypertension or recent renal function deterioration [particularly after therapy with angiotensin-converting enzyme (ACE)-inhibitors or angiotensin-receptor blockers (ARB)] or patients presenting with flash pulmonary edema (i.e., Pickering syndrome).

Clinical signs of PA are not very specific. Hyperaldosteronism is classically associated with metabolic alkalosis and hypokalemia. Hypokalemia is present in only approximately 40% of the patients with confirmed PA. Screening can be done by plasma aldosterone–renin ratio (ARR) after adequately preparing the patient (Table 1).

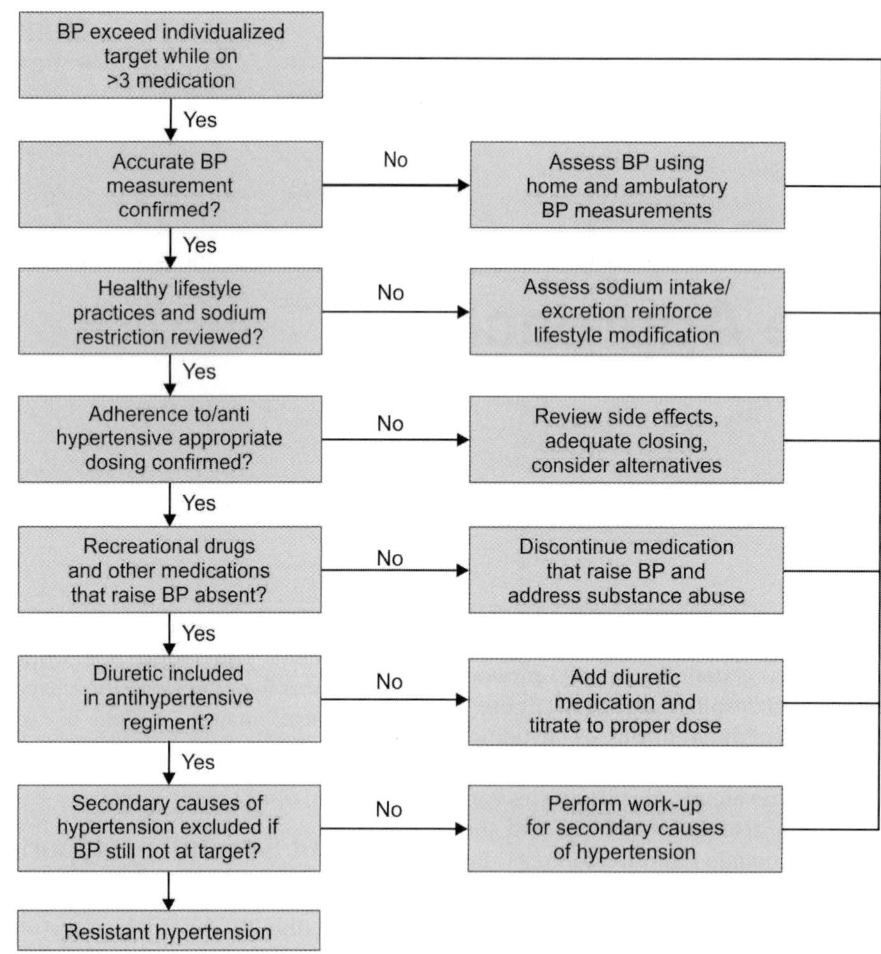

BP, blood pressure.

FLOWCHART 1: Systematic approach to patients with suspected resistant hypertension.

Evaluate the Presence of Vascular Remodeling

In patients with true rHTN vascular remodeling is likely to be present. The gold standard method to noninvasively assess arterial stiffness is the measurement of carotid-femoral pulse wave velocity (PWV). Alternatively, pulse pressure (PP) is a valid and widely available proxy of vascular stiffness.[4] PWV more than 10 m/s,[5] 24 hours PP more than or equal to 63 mm Hg or central PP more than 55 mm Hg suggests vascular remodeling.[6] The absence of increased arterial stiffness suggests the presence of pseudoresistance, and we should search for poor treatment adherence, lifestyle factors known to increase arterial BP, and drugs interfering with the antihypertensive treatment.

Poor Treatment Adherence

Nonadherence deserves special attention to identify and address adherence barriers effectively. Around 50% of the patients with apparent resistance were not taking their medication as prescribed, when adherence is assessed by urine analysis.[7]

In another study among patients with rHTN, 10% were completely nonadherent, and 52% were partially or completely nonadherent.[8] Several strategies have been proposed to assess and improve therapy adherence, including the measurement of drug concentrations in serum or urine, the use of pillboxes recording every opening event, and specific counseling programs. Performing 24 hours ABPM immediately after the patient has taken his or her antihypertensive drugs in the presence of a nurse or physician is an easy way to assess the effect of the prescribed medication.

Check Lifestyle Factors

Obesity, excessive salt intake, and alcohol consumption are frequently associated with rHTN. In hypertensive population, weight loss is associated with modest BP reduction (i.e., systolic/diastolic BP reduction of 2/1 mm Hg per kg of body weight loss). Excessive sodium consumption (>6 g sodium chloride/day) is a major contributor to treatment resistance, particularly when associated with increased arterial stiffness. The BP-lowering effect of decreased sodium consumption is

TABLE 1: Potential causes of secondary hypertension

Cause	Diagnostic testing
Evaluate in all patients	
• Parenchymal kidney disease	• Basic blood chemistry, including creatinine, sodium, potassium, bicarbonate; urinalysis with microscopic examination, urine protein-to-creatinine and/or albumin to creatinine ration kidney ultrasound
Secondary causes to be considered	
• Renal artery stenosis ○ Atherosclerotic ○ Fibromuscular dysplasia • Obstructive sleep apnea • High aldosterone states: ○ Primary hyperaldosteronism – Adrenal adenoma – Bilateral adrenal hyperplasia ○ Secondary hyperaldosteronism – Renal artery stenosis – Renin-secreting tumor ○ Glucocorticoid remediable aldosteronism • Crushing syndrome • Congenital adrenal hyperplasia • Apparent mineralocorticoid excess • Liddle syndrome • Gordon syndrome • Pheochromocytoma • Hyper-or hypothyroidism • Aortic coarctation	• Kidney ultrasound with duplex Doppler, magnetic resonance imaging, computed tomography angiography • Conventional angiography • Berlin questionnaire, overnight oximetry, polysomnography. Serum sodium and potassium concentration, serum aldosterone concentration-to-plasma renin activity ratio, BP response to mineralocorticoid receptor antagonist, genetic testing • Dexamethasone suppression test, 25-urine cortisol excretion, and salivary cortisol • Clinical diagnosis: ○ Clinical diagnosis, aldosterone and rennin levels, and electrolytes ○ Clinical diagnosis, family history, aldosterone and renin levels, and serum electrolytes ○ Plasma-free metanephrines, 24-h urine metanephrines, and catecholamines ○ Thyroid stimulating hormone ○ BP measurements in both arms and legs, echocardiogram, thoracic CTA or MRA

CTA, computed tomography angiogram; MRA, magnetic resonance angiography; BP, blood pressure.

particularly marked in "salt-sensitive" patients with HT (i.e., Africans and East Asians, obese, and elderly of all ethnicities).[9]

Acute alcohol intake increases BP by centrally mediated sympathetic activation. Chronic heavy alcohol intake (>60 g/day ethanol) increases BP even in normotensive subjects. Interventions targeting simultaneously several lifestyle modifications (i.e., weight loss, lower salt, and alcohol consumption) are more effective than interventions targeting each of these factors sequentially.

BOX 1 Substances that can raise blood pressure

- Nonsteroidal anti-inflammatory drugs (NSAIDs)
- Anabolic steroids
- Antidepressants:
  - Monoamine oxidase inhibitors
  - Selective serotonin reuptake inhibitor
  - Selective norepinephrine uptake inhibitors
- Calcineurin inhibitors:
  - Cyclosporin
  - Tacrolimus
- Glucocorticoids
- Erythropoietin
- Contraceptives:
  - Estrogen containing
  - Progesterone containing
- Sympathomimetics
  - Vascular endothelial growth factor (VEGF) inhibitors
  - Tyrosine kinase inhibitors
- Others:
  - Anabolic steroids, caffeine, cocaine, ethanol (in excess)

Drugs and Other Medications

Several substances and drugs can induce arterial hypertension or interfere with antihypertensive medications. Common that can raise BP is given in box 1.

Treatment Approach for Treatment-resistant Hypertension

Renin–angiotensin–aldosterone system (RAAS) activation plays an important role in the pathophysiology of hypertension. In accordance with guidelines, first step in the treatment of rHTN should be with the combination of A (ACE-inhibitor or ARB) with C [calcium channel blockers (CCB)] plus D (thiazide-like diuretic, i.e., chlorthalidone or indapamide) at the maximal tolerated dosage. This combination acts on different BP regulatory systems in a way that both activated and counter-regulatory mechanisms are inhibited. It promote natriuresis and vasodilation and "A" inhibits the RAAS and the sympathetic nervous system (SNS) activated by "C + D".[10] RAAS activation is often absent in elderly patients and in patients of African origin.[11] In patients with moderate-to-severe impairment of renal function [i.e., glomerular filtration rate (GFR) ≤45 mL/min/1.73 m^2], a shift from a thiazide (-like) to a loop diuretic should be considered.

If the patient under "A + C + D" is still hypertensive a clinical evaluation to determine whether sodium and water retention (search for peripheral edema, increased urinary sodium excretion, increased left ventricular (LV) filling pressures, etc.) or sympathetic activation and increased arterial stiffness (increased average heart rate on 24 hours

ABPM and increased PWV or PP) predominate. If volume expansion predominates, spironolactone (25–50 mg/day) or eplerenone (50–100 mg/day in the case of gynecomastia with spironolactone) should be added.[12,13] In the case of increased SNS activity and/or arterial stiffness, an α-blocker (i.e., doxazosin) that may have favorable effects on BP and vascular remodeling should be added.[14-16] If persistent volume expansion present, add a long-acting loop diuretic (i.e., torasemide) in addition to thiazide. If persistent sympathetic overactivity is suspected, adding a β-blocker with vasodilator properties (i.e., nebivolol which is also NO donor) or a combined α/β-blocker (i.e., carvedilol and labetalol) should be considered.[17] In the case of increased arterial stiffness, aldosterone antagonists have been shown to have favorable effects on BP and vascular remodeling.[18]

Device-based Interventions

Attenuation of exaggerated activity of the SNS represents the aim of device-based interventions [i.e., carotid baroreceptor stimulation and renal denervation (RDN)] for the treatment of rHTN. Carotid baroreceptor stimulation decreases central neural sympathetic outflow through electrical activation of this sympathoinhibitory reflexogenic area. RDN decreases sympathetic overactivity by ablation of renal sympatho-excitatory afferents. Carotid baroreceptor stimulation significantly decreases resting heart rate, whereas RDN has no detectable effect on this variable.

Carotid Baroreceptor Stimulation

In humans with rHTN, baroreceptor stimulation has been found to decrease 24-hour ambulatory BP by 10/6 mm Hg at 4-month follow up.[19] Another study showed that unilateral right-sided carotid baroreceptor stimulation may be more effective than left-sided or bilateral stimulation in lowering office BP in patients with rHTN.[20] The main disadvantages of this technique are the need for surgical implantation and the lack of data on its effectiveness on cardiovascular (CV) events. The BP-lowering effect of baroreceptor stimulation may be attenuated in rHTN associated with hyperaldosteronism.[21] It should be considered only after documented failure of adequate drug treatment, and the implantation of the device should be performed by experienced surgeons in selected hypertension centers (class IIb, level C).[22]

Catheter-based Renal Denervation

Renal denervation was found to be an effective treatment for rHTN in early trials. However, these results were not confirmed by the Symplicity Hypertension-3 study which failed to show significant BP reduction compared with sham treatment, casting doubts on the efficacy of RDN.[23,24] SPYRAL HTN-OFF MED trial a multicenter, international trial randomly assigned 80 patients from the United States, Europe, Japan, and Australia who were either drug naïve or had discontinued their antihypertensive medications to either renal denervation (n = 38) or sham control (n = 42). Patients were followed for up to 3 months and the primary endpoint was change in 24-hour blood pressure at the end of the follow-up period. Drug surveillance was done to ensure patient compliance with absence of antihypertensive medication.

Results showed a significant decrease from baseline to 3 months in office and 24-hour ambulatory blood pressure in the renal denervation group, while no significant changes were noted in the sham control group. Researchers highlighted that the mean difference between the groups favored renal denervation for 3 months change in both office and 24-hour BP. There were no major adverse events reported in either group.

This novel trial[25] differs substantially from previous renal denervation trials in terms of the hypertensive population enrolled, the renal denervation technique used, and the absence of concomitant antihypertensive medications. It was postulated that identification of specific subsets of patients who could potentially benefit from RDN, or clinical features that may help to predict outcomes after the procedure, might be of importance.

CONCLUSION

Various steps in identifying and managing rHTN can be concluded as follows:

- Accurate BP measurement by optimal techniques
- Identify individuals with WCH and masked hypertension by out-of-office BP measurement preferably ABPM
- Screen for secondary causes and treat if present
- Confirm guideline-directed medications in optimal doses and its strict adherence
- Check confounding lifestyle factors (obesity, salt intake, and alcohol consumption) and minimize them
- Identify and avoid substances and drugs that interfere with antihypertensive medications
- Add aldosterone antagonist/α-blocker/β-blocker with vasodilator properties/combined α- and β-blocker depending on patient's scenario
- Device-based intervention may be beneficial in selected patients.

REFERENCES

1. Calhoun DA, Jones D, Textor S, et al. Resistant hypertension: Diagnosis, evaluation, and treatment: A scientific statement from the American Heart Association Professional Education Committee of the Council for High Blood Pressure Research. Circulation. 2008;117:e510-26.
2. de la Sierra A, Segura J, Banegas JR, et al. Clinical features of 8295 patients with resistant hypertension classified on the basis of ambulatory blood pressure monitoring. Hypertension. 2011;57:898-902.
3. Rimoldi SF, Scherrer U, Messerli FH. Secondary arterial hypertension: When, who, and how to screen? Eur Heart J. 2014;35:1245-54.
4. Laurent S, Cockcroft J, Van Bortel L, et al. Expert consensus document on arterial stiffness: methodological issues and clinical applications. Eur Heart J. 2006;27:2588-605.
5. Mattace-Raso F, Hofman A, Verwoert GC, et al. Determinants of pulse wave velocity in healthy people and in the presence of cardiovascular risk factors: 'Establishing normal and reference values'. Eur Heart J. 2010;31:2338-50.
6. Ott C, Schmid A, Toennes SW, et al. Central pulse pressure predicts BP reduction after renal denervation in patients with treatment-resistant hypertension. Euro Interv. 2015;11:110-6.

7. Jung O, Gechter JL, Wunder C, et al. Resistant hypertension? Assessment of adherence by toxicological urine analysis. J Hypertens. 2013;31:766-74.
8. Tomaszewski M, White C, Patel P, et al. High rates of non-adherence to antihypertensive treatment revealed by high-performance liquid chromatography-tandem mass spectrometry (HP LC-MS/MS) urine analysis. Heart. 2014;100:855-61.
9. Vollmer WM, Sacks FM, Ard J, et al. Effects of diet and sodium intake on blood pressure: Subgroup analysis of the DASH-sodium trial. Ann Intern Med. 2001;135:1019-28.
10. Sever PS, Messerli FH. Hypertension management 2011: Optimal combination therapy. Eur Heart J. 2011;32:2499-506.
11. Eide IK, Torjesen PA, Drolsum A, et al. Low-renin status in therapy-resistant hypertension: A clue to efficient treatment. J Hypertens. 2004;22:2217-26.
12. Chapman N, Dobson J, Wilson S, et al. Effect of spironolactone on blood pressure in subjects with resistant hypertension. Hypertension. 2007;49:839-45.
13. Vaclavik J, Sedlak R, Plachy M, et al. Addition of spironolactone in patients with resistant arterial hypertension (ASPIRANT): A randomized, double-blind, placebo-controlled trial. Hypertension. 2011;57:1069-75.
14. Chapman N, Chang CL, Dahlof B, et al. Effect of doxazosin gastrointestinal therapeutic system as third-line antihypertensive therapy on blood pressure and lipids in the Anglo-Scandinavian Cardiac Outcomes Trial. Circulation. 2008;118:42-8.
15. Chapman N, Chen CY, Fujita T, et al. Time to re-appraise the role of alpha-1 adrenoceptor antagonists in the management of hypertension? J Hypertens. 2010;28:1796-803.
16. Komai N, Ohishi M, Moriguchi A, et al. Low-dose doxazosin improved aortic stiffness and endothelial dysfunction as measured by noninvasive evaluation. Hypertens Res. 2002;25:5-10.
17. Mann SJ. Drug therapy for resistant hypertension: Simplifying the approach. J Clin Hypertens (Greenwich). 2011;13:120-30.
18. Duprez DA. Aldosterone and the vasculature: Mechanisms mediating resistant hypertension. J Clin Hypertens (Greenwich). 2007;9:13-18.
19. Heusser K, Tank J, Engeli S, et al. Carotid baroreceptor stimulation, sympathetic activity, baroreflex function, and blood pressure in hypertensive patients. Hypertension. 2010;55:619-26.
20. de Leeuw PW, Alnima T, Lovett E, et al. Bilateral or unilateral stimulation for baroreflex activation therapy. Hypertension. 2015;65:187-92.
21. Lohmeier TE, Liu B, Hildebrandt DA, et al. Global- and renal-specific sympatho-inhibition in aldosterone hypertension. Hypertension. 2015;65:1223-30.
22. Mancia G, Fagard R, Narkiewicz K, et al. 2013 ESH/ESC guidelines for the management of arterial hypertension: The Task Force for the Management of Arterial Hypertension of the European Society of Hypertension (ESH) and of the European Society of Cardiology (ESC). Eur Heart J. 2013;34:2159-219.
23. Bhatt DL, Kandzari DE, O'Neill WW, et al. A controlled trial of renal denervation for resistant hypertension. N Engl J Med. 2014;370:1393-401.
24. Lobo MD, Sobotka PA, Pathak A. Interventional procedures and future drug therapy for hypertension. Eur Heart J. 2016;38:1101-11.
25. Townsend RR, Mahfoud F, Kandzari DE. Catheter-based renal denervation in patients with uncontrolled hypertension in the absence of antihypertensive medications (SPYRAL HTN-OFF MED): A randomised, sham-controlled, proof-of-concept trial. Lancet. 2017;11:2160-70.

CHAPTER 24

Secondary Hypertension: When and How to Screen

Anjan Lal Dutta, Soumik Chaudhuri

INTRODUCTION

Essential hypertension is the cause of the vast majority of cases of arterial hypertension. Approximately 5–10% of adults with hypertension have secondary hypertension.[1] Secondary hypertension is defined as increased systemic blood pressure (BP) due to an identifiable cause (Box 1). Secondary forms are less common and screening for them can be expensive and laborious and hence it is not cost-effective to perform complete evaluations for all secondary causes in each and every patient. At the same time, one should be aware of the fact that secondary hypertension may be "cured" if a correctable cause can be detected in time. Thus, early detection and treatment are important to minimize/prevent irreversible changes in the systemic vasculature which may give rise to persistent hypertension with a poor long-term outcome.[2,3]

WHO TO SCREEN?

Look for a secondary cause of hypertension while evaluating *all* patients with hypertension.

However, only *test* for secondary hypertension, if indicated based on this comprehensive evaluation.

BOX 1 Causes of secondary hypertension

Renal

- Renovascular hypertension
  - Fibromuscular dysplasia
  - Atheromatous renal artery stenosis
- Other causes
  - Polycystic kidney disease
  - Renal tumors (Wilms tumor, renal cell carcinoma)
  - Renal segmental hypoplasia (Ask-Upmark kidney)

Endocrine

- Adrenal causes
  - Primary hyperaldosteronism (Conn's syndrome)
  - Pheochromocytoma
  - Congenital adrenal hyperplasia (17α-hydroxylase deficiency, 11β- hydroxylase deficiency)
  - Glucocorticoid-remediable aldosteronism
- Other endocrine causes
  - Hyperparathyroidism
  - Hyperthyroidism
  - Hypothyroidism
  - Neurogenic hypertension
  - Acromegaly

Other causes

- Obstructive sleep apnea
- Hormonal contraceptives
- Drugs: alcohol, nasal decongestants with adrenergic effects, nonsteroidal anti-inflammatory drugs, monoamine oxidase inhibitors (MAOIs), adrenoreceptor stimulants, buspirone, carbamazapine, bromocriptine, St John's wort
- Neurologic disorders (Binswanger's disease)
- Licorice (when consumed in excessive amounts)
- Scleroderma
- Neurofibromatosis
- Pregnancy
- Heavy alcohol use
- Steroid use
- Nicotine use
- Malformed aorta
- Aortic valve disease
- Coarctation of the aorta
- Atherosclerosis
- Anemia
- Fever
- White coat hypertension
- Perioperative hypertension

General Characteristics Suggestive of Secondary Hypertension (Box 2)

- *Age:* The most common causes of hypertension in prepubertal children are renal parenchymal or vascular disease and coarctation of aorta.[4] Patients in the 2nd, and especially 3rd, decade of life, who are otherwise healthy and without obvious risk factors or strong familial history of hypertension, are prime candidates for secondary form of screening. In the elderly population with coronary artery disease and any other form of atherosclerosis, the presence of severe hypertension can point towards risk factors suggestive of a secondary type like renal artery stenosis (RAS)
- *Habitus:* Body habitus can be an important clue in identifying some specific subgroup of patients who present with secondary hypertension. Resistant hypertension in an overweight patient should lead us to look for hypothyroidism, obstructive sleep apnea (OSA)[5] or Cushing's syndrome
- *Atherosclerosis:* Significant RAS (≥50%) is present in up to one-third (~30%) of patients who have atherosclerotic disease and hypertension.[6,7] The following features are suggestive of RAS—deterioration of a previously adequately controlled hypertension, nondipping pattern on ambulatory blood pressure monitoring (ABPM) and a resistant form of hypertension
- *Hypertension pattern:* The following group of patients should be screened for a secondary form—significant hypertension at initial presentation (>180/110 mm Hg), poorly/inadequately controlled resistant hypertension or hypertensive urgencies or emergencies.[8] A 10% nighttime drop of BP, as compared to the daytime value (in ABPM), is normal; its absence should arouse suspicion of secondary forms of hypertension such as OSA.[9,10]

WHAT TO DO BEFORE SCREENING FOR SECONDARY HYPERTENSION?

Rule out the following conditions:

- *Pseudohypertension:* Pseudohypertension is defined as cuff diastolic BP at least 15 mm Hg higher than a simultaneously measured intra-arterial BP. It is predominantly found in aged patients and present with persistently high BP but surprisingly do not have corresponding end-organ damage. Their arteries are highly calcified, and hence rigid, requiring increased cuff pressure to compress the artery, resulting in spuriously elevated readings. The Osler's maneuver may help in differentiating this entity but its reproducibility is low.[11,12]
- *Pseudoresistance:* Incorrect methods of measurement of BP (also known as pseudoresistance) can result in falsely increased BP up to 15 mm Hg.[13] The most common sources of error include choosing a smaller-than-appropriate sized cuff and take the BP immediately after an activity or exertion, without allowing the patient to rest for a minimum of 5 minutes.
- *White coat hypertension:* This is a phenomenon in which patients exhibit a BP level above the normal range in a clinical setting, though they do not exhibit it in other settings. It is believed that the phenomenon is due to anxiety experienced during a clinic visit. White coat hypertension is a frequent cause of pseudoresistance with a prevalence of about 20–30%.[14] The 24-hour ABPM is a valuable tool to assess the likelihood of secondary hypertension.
- *Poor patient adherence:* Poor patient adherence to therapy is widespread reaching about 40% in patients with newly diagnosed hypertension.[15] This could be due to medication adverse effects, complicated dosing, inadequate patient education or simply the cost of medication. The physician may at times also be the one to blame by failing to optimize therapy to reach target BP control.
- *Drug related:* There are a number of medications which may also lead to treatment resistance.[16] The most common are nonsteroidal anti-inflammatory drugs and glucocorticoids. They act via pathways favoring retention of fluid and sodium and can raise systolic BP by 4–5 mm Hg, especially in hypertensive patients.[17] Some drugs increase BP via activation of the sympathetic nervous system and include amphetamines, phenylpropanolamine, cocaine and phenylephrine, among others. Other common drugs that may lead to secondary hypertension include—licorice, oral contraceptive pills, monoamine oxidase inhibitors, cyclosporine A, vascular endothelial growth factor inhibitors, tyrosine kinase inhibitors and alcohol.

BOX 2 Clinical characteristics suggestive of secondary hypertension

- Resistant hypertension (140/90 mm Hg despite three antihypertensive drugs including a diuretic)
- Early onset of hypertension (i.e., <30 years) in patients without other risk factors (i.e., family history, obesity, etc.)
- Increased BP in prepubertal children
- Severe hypertension (180/110 mm Hg) or hypertensive emergencies
- Sudden increase of BP in a previously stable patient
- Nondipping or reverse dipping during 24-hour ambulatory BP monitoring
- Presence of target organ damage (i.e., left ventricular hypertrophy, hypertensive retinopathy, etc.)

CONDITIONS REQUIRING REEVALUATION, AFTER STARTING ANTIHYPERTENSIVE THERAPY

The presence of a few clinical or biochemical responses, after starting antihypertensive therapy, may suggest the presence of secondary hypertension. A reevaluation should be considered if there is:

- *Significant deterioration of renal function after initiation of an angiotensin-converting enzyme (ACE) inhibitor* (RAS, especially bilateral)

- *Significant hypokalemia with low doses of diuretics* (suggestive of mineralocorticoid excess, especially primary aldosteronism).

ROLE OF AMBULATORY 24-HOUR BLOOD PRESSURE MONITORING

Ambulatory BP monitoring is generally regarded as the most accurate method currently to monitor BP.[10] Ambulatory BP should be considered in patients with suspected secondary hypertension as it allows us to evaluate treatment compliance, rule out white coat hypertension and assess for dipping status. Chamber-based BP measurements are primarily targeted to differentiate hypertensive patients from nonhypertensive subjects and hence have diagnostic values, whereas reference values for 24-hour ABPM are based on response-oriented thresholds and are therefore lower than clinical values (Table 1).[1,18,19] Reverse nocturnal dipping, especially when associated with tachycardia, is suggestive of secondary forms like RAS or OSA.[20]

ROLE OF ECHOCARDIOGRAPHY IN SECONDARY HYPERTENSION

Echocardiography can be a very useful tool in the armory, in patients with secondary hypertension. Left ventricular hypertrophy (LVH) should always be sought for, in hypertensive patients and values incongruous with duration of hypertension may lead us to actively look for secondary causes such as renovascular hypertension or primary aldosteronism.[21] In patients with OSA, LVH is a quite common and is usually associated with left atrial enlargement and right ventricular hypertrophy.[22] In a young hypertensive adult, echocardiography is the investigation of choice for screening coarctation of the aorta.

HOW TO SCREEN?

We shall now discuss how to screen for and diagnose some of the common causes of secondary hypertension (Flowchart 1).

TABLE 1: Thresholds values for office, home and ambulatory blood pressure measurement

Category	Systolic (mm Hg)	Diastolic (mm Hg)
Office and home blood pressure measurements		
Office BP	≥140	≥90
Home BP	≥135	≥85
Ambulatory BP measurements		
24-hour	≥130	≥80
Daytime (or awake)	≥135	≥85
Night-time (or awake)	≥120	≥70

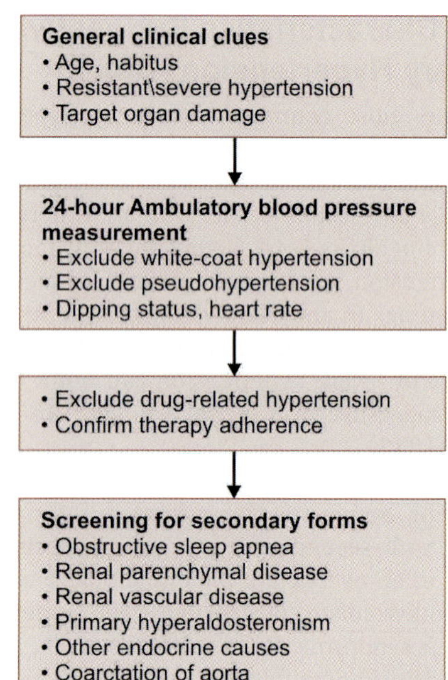

FLOWCHART 1: Screening for secondary hypertension.

Obstructive Sleep Apnea

Obstructive sleep apnea has been recognized as one of the most common causes for secondary hypertension.[5,23] The prevalence is about 2–30% and increases with age, plateauing at 55–65 years. It is clinically characterized by recurrent episodes of obstructive apneas (complete cessation of breathing) and hypopneas (slow and shallow breathing) and is caused by partial collapse of the upper airways during sleep. The severity of OSA is classified based on the apnea-hypopnea index (AHI)—number of apneas plus hypopneas per hour of sleep.[24] Possible pathways to explicate the rise in BP in OSA, include increased sympathetic nervous system activity and modified renin-angiotensin-aldosterone system (RAAS) hemodynamics[25,26] due to recurrent nocturnal hypoxemia. Moreover, hypoxemia has been associated with systemic endothelial dysfunction[27,28] even in the absence of traditional cardiovascular risk factors,[29] possibly mediated by excessive oxidative stress.[30,31] Several studies have shown a decrease in nocturnal,[32] or in both nocturnal and daytime BP,[32,33] after successful continuous positive airway pressure therapy of OSA.

Medical History

- Snoring
- Excessive daytime sleepiness (narcolepsy)
- Morning headaches
- Lack of concentration
- Irritability
- Increased frequency of motor vehicle accidents.

Clinical Features

- Narrow upper airway (Large neck, macroglossia)
- 24-hour ABPM (Non-dipper, tachycardia or bradycardia)

- Left ventricular hypertrophy
- Cor pulmonale
- Pulmonary hypertension
- Central obesity
- Pedal edema.

How to Screen?

Screening Questionnaire (e.g., Epworth's) followed by polysomnography.

- AHI 5–15: Mild OSA
- AHI 15–30: Moderate OSA
- AHI more than 30: Severe OSA.

Renal Artery Stenosis

Renal artery stenosis has a bimodal pattern of etiology. In the younger subgroup, i.e., less than 40 years of age, fibromuscular dysplasia of the renal artery is the most common cause. Imaging plays a very important role in diagnosis and suspected patients should be screened with a quick and inexpensive Doppler ultrasound. Renal angiography remains the gold standard for confirmation. As fibromuscular dysplasia is generally present in multiple sites, other vascular beds should also be evaluated.[34] In older adults and aged patients, the most common cause of renovascular disease is atherosclerotic disease.[34] The prevalence of RAS in a general set of hypertensive patients is anywhere between 1% and 8%[35,36] but in the presence of generalized atherosclerosis, it can go up to as high as 25–35%.[37] The presence of the following features in an adult patient would raise suspicion of RAS:

- Rapid and inappropriate deterioration of renal function with angiotensin receptor blockers (ARB) or ACE inhibitor
- Decompensation in a previously well-controlled smoker or diabetic, hypertensive patient
- Abdominal bruit
- Atherosclerosis (in multiple vascular beds)
- Pickering syndrome (Flash pulmonary edema in the presence of bilateral RAS).[38,39]

If screening confirms significant RAS, renal angiography with hemodynamic assessment to detect a significant translesional gradient should be considered.[40] After percutaneous (or surgical) treatment of RAS, as long as BP and renal function (GFR) remain stable and well-controlled, no further examinations are necessary. Otherwise, renal perfusion or vessel patency should be assessed with duplex ultrasonography or magnetic resonance imaging (MRI).

Medical History

- Smoking
- Diabetes mellitus
- Atherosclerotic disease
- Worsening of renal function with ACE inhibitor or ARB
- Pickering syndrome-flash pulmonary edema.

Clinical and Laboratory Features

- 24-hour ABPM (Severe hypertension, reverse nocturnal dipping)
- Coronary artery disease
- Left ventricular hypertrophy
- Flash pulmonary edema
- Impaired renal function
- Secondary hyperaldosteronism
- Abdominal bruits
- Peripheral vascular disease.

How to Screen?

Duplex sonography or computed tomography (CT) scan or MRI as initial screening investigation.

- *No stenosis:* No further investigation
- *Stenosis/ambiguous result*: Renal angiography and hemodynamic assessment.

Is there Really any Use of Screening for Atherosclerotic Renal Artery Stenosis?

Despite there being substantial improvement in imaging techniques over the past decade, doubts still linger whether intervention in atherosclerotic RAS (with angioplasty) actually results in any tangible mortality benefits. There are a number of studies which have compared conservative medical therapy versus revascularization and similar rates of cardiovascular events, renal episodes and death was seen in both these groups.[41] Furthermore, it is difficult to establish a linear cause-effect relationship between atherosclerotic RAS and hypertension, and currently available tests lack enough sensitivity or specificity to truly predict how much of the rise in BP can be attributed to stenosis. Unsurprisingly, the true contribution of RAS to hypertension can only be acknowledged in the postoperative phase, once the BP stabilizes to normal levels (or does not!).[42] Prolonged hypertension, with poor renal function, and advanced nephrosclerosis is thus a poor candidate to select for revascularization.

There is one specific subgroup known as the Pickering syndrome, and is characterized by recurrent bouts of flash pulmonary edema, in the presence of bilateral RAS.[38,39] Emergent revascularization can indeed prove to be the difference between life and death in this situation. Nevertheless, most randomized trials have showed very poor-to-insignificant benefits of revascularization in patients of RAS.

However, the advent of catheter-based renal denervation for the management of resistant hypertension has definitely upped the enthusiasm and vigor in this field and more subjects are actively being screened for RAS. Nonetheless, the data at this time is simply not adequate to evaluate the long-term benefits of renal denervation on BP (SYMPLICITY HTN 2 and 3) and more studies are required to confirm whether this novel technique will truly be a game changer or not, in the management of resistant hypertension.[42]

Primary Hyperaldosteronism

Primary hyperaldosteronism, also referred to as Conn syndrome, is a condition where there is an inappropriately high plasma aldosterone level, which is independent of the feedback loop of renin-angiotensin system and cannot be suppressed by sodium loading. It is characterized by:

- Hypertension
- Increased aldosterone secretion from the adrenal glands
- Decreased plasma renin activity ((PRA).

The prevalence of primary hyperaldosteronism is between 1.4% and 23%,[43] with a higher prevalence in resistant hypertensives. The common causes for primary aldosteronism are:

- Idiopathic hyperaldosteronism
- Aldosterone-secreting adenoma
- Idiopathic adrenal hyperplasia
- Rarely, glucocorticoid-remediable aldosteronism.

Medical History

- Fatigue
- Muscle weakness
- Polyuria, polydipsia
- Constipation.

Clinical Features

- 24-hour ABPM (Severe hypertension, decreased nocturnal dipping)
- Hypokalemic symptoms
- Left ventricular hypertrophy
- Myocardial fibrosis
- Muscle weakness.

Laboratory Findings

- *Blood:* Aldosterone ↑
  - Renin ↓
  - K^+↓
  - Na^+↓
  - Mg^{2+}↓
  - Metabolic alkalosis.
- *Urine:* Aldosterone ↑
  - K^+↑
  - Na^+↓
  - Metabolic acidosis.

How to Screen?

Screen for the following three parameters (Table 2):

1. Aldosterone-renin ratio (ARR)
2. Plasma renin activity
3. Plasma aldosterone concentration (PAC).
   - If PRA ↑, PAC ↑, ARR→: Consider secondary hyperaldosteronism
   - If PRA ↓, PAC ↓, ARR→: Consider other causes
   - If PRA↓, PAC ↑, ARR↑: Investigate further by:
     - *Confirmatory tests:* Sodium loading, captopril suppression tests
     - *Imaging:* CT/MRI scanning
     - Adrenal vein sampling for lateralization.

TABLE 2: Aldosterone-renin ratio cut-off values for the diagnosis of primary aldosteronism

Plasma aldosterone concentration (PAC)	Plasma renin activity (PRA)		Direct renin concentration (DRC)	
	ng/ mL h	pmol/ L min	mU/L	ng/L
ng/dL	> 27	> 2.1	> 3.3	> 5.4
pmol/ L	>750	> 59	> 90	> 150

Conversion factor: Aldosterone 1 ng/dL→27.7 pmol/L. Conversion factor PRA 1 ng/mL h → 1 pmol/L min divided by 12.8. Conversion factor: PRA 1 ng/mL h → DRC 1 mU/L divided by 8.2. Conversion factor: PRA 1 ng/mL h → 1 DRC ng/L divided by 5.2.

UNCOMMON CAUSES OF SECONDARY HYPERTENSION

Renal Parenchymal Disease

- It has a prevalence of 2–10%[4]
- Most common cause of secondary hypertension in children and also a common cause in adults[44]
- Signs and symptoms:
  - Loss of adequate BP control
  - History of diabetes mellitus
  - History of smoking
  - Generalized atherosclerosis
  - Previous renal failure/nocturia
  - Edema, loss of muscle mass
- Screen with urinalysis (Protein, erythrocytes, leucocytes)
- Measurement of serum creatinine is an initial screening tool
- Diagnosis should be done with renal ultrasound.

Cushing's Syndrome

- Rare syndrome with prevalence of less than 1%.[45]
- Typical age range is 25–45 years; affects women 3–8 times more than men[46]
- Sign and symptoms include:
  - Hypertension is very common (>80%)
  - Obesity
  - Facial plethora
  - Buffalo hump
  - Hirsutism
  - Purple striae on abdomen
- Diagnosis by positive results in at least two of the following tests:
  - 24-hour urinary cortisol (>55 µg/24 h)
  - Low dose dexamethasone suppression test (1.8 µ/dL)
  - Late evening salivary cortisol
- Specificity of these tests is 84–96% in obese patients with positive features.

Thyroid Disorders

- Prevalence of 1–3%[47]
- Both hyper- and hypothyroidism have been associated with arterial hypertension.
- In hypothyroidism, diastolic BP is particularly elevated since low cardiac output is compensated by peripheral vasoconstriction to maintain adequate tissue perfusion

- In contrast, hyperthyroidism is associated with increased cardiac output and predominately systolic BP elevation
- Signs and symptoms:
  - *Hyperthyroidism*: Palpitations, weight loss, heat intolerance, exophthalmos, tachycardia
  - *Hypothyroidism*: Bradycardia, weight gain, fatigue, muscle weakness
- Thyroid-stimulating hormone (TSH) levels are most useful in screening for thyroid disorders.

Pheochromocytoma

- *Prevalence*: 0.2% of hypertensive patients
- The clinical features are due to paroxysmal rises in plasma levels of catecholamines and are characterized by the classical "5 Ps":[48]
  - Paroxysmal hypertension
  - Perspiration
  - Palpitation
  - Pounding headache
  - Pallor.
- Pheochromocytoma screening is to be considered when one or more of the following parameters are present:
  - Hypertension (resistant) with features of increased adrenergic drive (the "5 Ps")
  - Adrenal mass with features suggestive of a pheochromocytoma including, but not limited to, size more than 4 cm with hemorrhagic or cystic changes).
  - Family history of pheochromocytoma
  - Presence of genetic syndromes which have a known association with pheochromocytoma (von Hippel-Lindau syndrome, multiple endocrine neoplasia II, von Recklinghausen's disease (Type 1 neurofibromatosis), familial carotid body tumors).
- *Screening tests* for pheochromocytoma include:
  - Measurement of plasma free-metanephrine or urinary fractionated metanephrine levels
  - 24-hour catecholamine levels in urine
- If screening is positive, imaging with abdominal/adrenal MRI or CT is indicated
- If abdominal imaging is negative, scintigraphic localization with 123I-metaiodobenzylguanidine (MIBG) or additional imaging (i.e., whole body MRI or others) is indicated.

Coarctation of Aorta

- Aortic coarctation is the second most common cause of hypertension in children and young adults
- It is characterized by constriction of the lumen of the aorta usually near the ligamentum arteriosum
- Some of the common symptoms include pounding headaches, claudication of legs, muscle cramps and nose bleeds
- The presence of hypertension, with difficult to palpate femoral pulses, should raise a suspicion of coarctation. Other common findings include posterior ribs notching on a chest X-ray (due to collateral circulation) and systolic murmurs in the precordial area or the back
- The investigation of choice for screening is echocardiography. Other alternatives include MRI or CT scans[49]
- Percutaneous balloon angioplasty is as efficacious as early surgical repair[50]
- As per the latest guidelines,[51,52] patients with coarctation of aorta should undergo follow-up every 2 years in centers which handle specialized care for congenital heart disease, especially in older subjects. Follow-up should include echocardiography and measurement of BP along with imaging modalities like MRI scanning. Subjects with prolonged hypertension should undergo lifelong follow-up.

WHEN SECONDARY HYPERTENSION MAY PRESENT AS RESISTANT HYPERTENSION

- Some patients, especially middle-aged or elderly ladies, with hyperaldosteronism (*Adrenal hyperplasia, not Conn syndrome*) may not respond to conventional antihypertensive agents. The ARR may or may not be deranged in them and the only clue sometimes may be an unprovoked level of low potassium (~3 mEq/L). These patients tend to respond well to a therapeutic trial of mineralocorticoid receptor antagonists
- Some patients of OSA may not be obese. They have a history of snoring at night and present with increased daytime fatigue as a primary symptom, and not necessarily narcolepsy. The diagnosis of OSA is not readily made in them and they are regarded as resistant hypertension patients
- When an elderly male patient, previously well-controlled on antihypertensive agents, tends to suddenly decompensate, with or without flash pulmonary edema, consider atherosclerotic RAS.

CONCLUSION

Secondary hypertension accounts for a very small subset of hypertensive patients (<10%). It is thus neither practical nor cost-effective to screen for secondary causes in all patients and should only be considered when the index of clinical suspicion is high. On a more ominous note, even with diagnosis and appropriate therapy of the cause of hypertension, BP seldom ever returns to baseline levels. This could hint at either irreversible vascular remodeling occurring before adequate treatment is initiated or the presence of attendant essential hypertension as well.

It is, thus, imperative to diagnose and treat subjects of secondary hypertension in a timely manner and ameliorate reversible causes. This prevents long-term, irreversible changes in the systemic vasculature and decreases the risk of developing persistent hypertension and significant end organ damage. The initial evaluation of all patients with hypertension should include consideration of the possibility of secondary hypertension but screening and testing for secondary hypertension should be based on the presence of suggestive clinical clues.

REFERENCES

1. Mancia G, Fagard R, Narkiewicz K, et al. 2013 ESH/ESC Guidelines for the management of arterial hypertension: The Task Force for the management of arterial hypertension of the European Society of Hypertension (ESH) and of the European Society of Cardiology (ESC). Eur Heart J. 2013;34:2159-219.
2. Streeten DH, Anderson GH Jr, Wagner S. Effect of age on response of secondary hypertension to specific treatment. Am J Hypertens 1990;3:360-5.
3. Muiesan ML, Rizzoni D, Salvetti M, et al. Structural changes in small resistance arteries and left ventricular geometry in patients with primary and secondary hypertension. J Hypertens. 2002;20:1439-44.
4. Arar MY, Hogg RJ, Arant BS Jr, et al. Etiology of sustained hypertension in children in the southwestern United States. Pediatr Nephrol. 1994;8:186-9.
5. Pedrosa RP, Drager LF, Gonzaga CC, et al. Obstructive sleep apnea: the most common secondary cause of hypertension associated with resistant hypertension. Hypertension. 2011;58:811-7.
6. Garovic VD, Textor SC. Renovascular hypertension and ischemic nephropathy. Circulation. 2005;112:1362-74.
7. Leertouwer TC, Pattynama PM, van den Berg-Huysmans A. Incidental renal artery stenosis in peripheral vascular disease: a case for treatment? Kidney Int. 2001;59:1480-3.
8. Borgel J, Springer S, Ghafoor J, et al. Unrecognized secondary causes of hypertension in patients with hypertensive urgency/emergency: prevalence and co-prevalence. Clin Res Cardiol. 2010;99:499-506.
9. Davies CW, Crosby JH, Mullins RL, et al. Case-control study of 24 hour ambulatory blood pressure in patients with obstructive sleep apnoea and normal matched control subjects. Thorax. 2000;55:736-40.
10. Pickering TG, Shimbo D, Haas D. Ambulatory blood-pressure monitoring. N Engl J Med. 2006;354:2368-74.
11. Messerli FH, Ventura HO, Amodeo C. Osler's maneuver and pseudohypertension. N Engl J Med. 1985;312:1548-51.
12. Belmin J, Visintin JM, Salvatore R, et al. Osler's maneuver: absence of usefulness for the detection of pseudohypertension in an elderly population. Am J Med. 1995;98:42-49.
13. Pickering TG, Hall JE, Appel LJ, et al. Recommendations for blood pressure measurement in humans and experimental animals: part 1: blood pressure measurement in humans: a statement for professionals from the Subcommittee of Professional and Public Education of the American Heart Association Council on High Blood Pressure Research. Circulation. 2005;111:697-716.
14. Mazzaglia G, Mantovani LG, Sturkenboom MC, et al. Patterns of persistence with antihypertensive medications in newly diagnosed hypertensive patients in Italy: a retrospective cohort study in primary care. J Hypertens. 2005;23:2093-100.
15. Verdecchia P, Schillaci G, Borgioni C, et al. White coat hypertension and white coat effect. Similarities and differences. Am J Hypertens. 1995;8:790-8.
16. Grossman E, Messerli FH. Drug-induced hypertension: an unappreciated cause of secondary hypertension. Am J Med. 2012;125:14-22.
17. Izhar M, Alausa T, Folker A, et al. Effects of COX inhibition on blood pressure and kidney function in ACE inhibitor-treated blacks and hispanics. Hypertension. 2004;43:573-7.
18. Kikuya M, Hansen TW, Thijs L, et al. Diagnostic thresholds for ambulatory blood pressure monitoring based on 10-year cardiovascular risk. Circulation. 2007;115:2145-52.
19. O'Brien E, Parati G, Stergiou G, et al. European Society of Hypertension position paper on ambulatory blood pressure monitoring. J Hypertens. 2013;31:1731-68.
20. Verdecchia P, Angeli F, Borgioni C, et al. Ambulatory blood pressure and cardiovascular outcome in relation to perceived sleep deprivation. Hypertension. 2007;49:777-83.
21. Rossi GP, Sacchetto A, Pavan E, et al. Remodeling of the left ventricle in primary aldosteronism due to Conn's adenoma. Circulation. 1997;95:1471-8.
22. Cloward TV, Walker JM, Farney RJ, et al. Left ventricular hypertrophy is a common echocardiographic abnormality in severe obstructive sleep apnea and reverses with nasal continuous positive airway pressure. Chest. 2003;124:594-601.
23. Logan AG, Perlikowski SM, Mente A, et al. High prevalence of unrecognized sleep apnoea in drug-resistant hypertension. J Hypertens. 2001;19:2271-7.
24. Iber C, Ancoli-Israel S, Chesson A, et al. The AASM Manual for the Scoring of Sleep and Associated Events: Rules, Terminology and Technical Specifications, 1st Edition. Westchester, IL: American Academy of Sleep Medicine; 2007.
25. Calhoun DA, Nishizaka MK, Zaman MA, et al. Aldosterone excretion among subjects with resistant hypertension and symptoms of sleep apnea. Chest. 2004;125:112-7.
26. Goodfriend TL, Calhoun DA. Resistant hypertension, obesity, sleep apnea, and aldosterone: theory and therapy. Hypertension. 2004;43:518-24.
27. Ip MS, Tse HF, Lam B, et al. Endothelial function in obstructive sleep apnea and response to treatment. Am J Respir Crit Care Med. 2004;169:348-53.
28. Rimoldi SF, Rexhaj E, Pratali L, et al. Systemic vascular dysfunction in patients with chronic mountain sickness. Chest. 2012;141:139-46.
29. Bruno RM, Rossi L, Fabbrini M, et al. Renal vasodilating capacity and endothelial function are impaired in patients with obstructive sleep apnea syndrome and no traditional cardiovascular risk factors. J Hypertens. 2013;31:1456-64.
30. Bailey DM, Rimoldi SF, Rexhaj E, et al. Oxidative-nitrosative stress and systemic vascular function in highlanders with and without exaggerated hypoxemia. Chest. 2013;143:444-51.
31. Becker HF, Jerrentrup A, Ploch T, et al. Effect of nasal continuous positive airway pressure treatment on blood pressure in patients with obstructive sleep apnea. Circulation. 2003;107:68-73.
32. Logan AG, Tkacova R, Perlikowski SM, et al. Refractory hypertension and sleep apnoea: effect of CPAP on blood pressure and baroreflex. Eur Respir J. 2003;21:241-7.
33. Suzuki M, Otsuka K, Guilleminault C. Long-term nasal continuous positive airway pressure administration can normalize hypertension in obstructive sleep apnea patients. Sleep. 1993;16:545-9.
34. Slovut DP, Olin JW. Fibromuscular dysplasia. N Engl J Med. 2004;350:1862-71.
35. Kalra PA, Guo H, Kausz AT, et al. Atherosclerotic renovascular disease in United States patients aged 67 years or older: risk factors, revascularization, and prognosis. Kidney Int. 2005;68:293-301.
36. Rimoldi SF, de Marchi SF, Windecker S, et al. Screening renal artery angiography in hypertensive patients undergoing coronary angiography and 6-month follow-up after ad hoc percutaneous revascularization. J Hypertens. 2010;28:842-7.
37. Textor SC, Lerman L. Renovascular hypertension and ischemic nephropathy. Am J Hypertens. 2010;23:1159-69.
38. Messerli FH, Bangalore S, Makani H, et al. Flash pulmonary oedema and bilateral renal artery stenosis: the Pickering syndrome. Eur Heart J. 2011;32:2231-5.
39. Rimoldi SF, Yuzefpolskaya M, Allemann Y, et al. Flash pulmonary edema. Prog Cardiovasc Dis. 2009;52:249-59.
40. Mangiacapra F, Trana C, Sarno G, et al. Translesional pressure gradients to predict blood pressure response after renal artery stenting in patients with renovascular hypertension. Circ Cardiovasc Interv. 2010;3:537-42.
41. Cooper CJ, Murphy TP, Cutlip DE, et al. Stenting and medical therapy for atherosclerotic renal-artery stenosis. N Engl J Med. 2014 Jan 2;370(1):13-22.
42. Schmieder RE, Redon J, Grassi G, et al. ESH position paper: renal denervation—an interventional therapy of resistant hypertension. J Hypertens. 2012;30:837-41.
43. Funder JW, Carey RM, Fardella C, et al. Case detection, diagnosis, and treatment of patients with primary aldosteronism: an endocrine society clinical practice guideline. J Clin Endocrinol Metab. 2008;93:3266-81.
44. Whaley-Connell AT, Sowers JR, Stevens LA, et al. CKD in the United States: Kidney Early Evaluation Program (KEEP) and National Health and Nutrition Examination Survey (NHANES) 1999-2004. Am J Kidney Dis. 2008;51:S13-20.
45. Newell-Price J, Bertagna X, Grossman AB, et al. Cushing's syndrome. Lancet. 2006;367:1605-17.
46. Nieman LK, Biller BM, Findling JW, et al. The diagnosis of Cushing's syndrome: an Endocrine Society Clinical Practice Guideline. J Clin Endocrinol Metab. 2008;93:1526-40.
47. de Leeuw PW, Postma CT, Kroon AA. Treatment of atherosclerotic renal artery stenosis: time for a new approach. JAMA. 2013;309:663-4.

48. Young WF Jr. Adrenal causes of hypertension: pheochromocytoma and primary aldosteronism. Rev Endocr Metab Disord. 2007;8:309-20.
49. Weber HS, Cyran SE. Endovascular stenting for native coarctation of the aorta is an effective alternative to surgical intervention in older children. Congenit Heart Dis. 2008;3:54-9.
50. Baumgartner H, Bonhoeffer P, De Groot NM, et al. ESC Guidelines for the management of grown-up congenital heart disease. Eur Heart J. 2010;31:2915-57.
51. Messerli FH, Nachbur B, Senn A, et al. Hypertension in coarctation of the abdominal aorta. Schweiz Med Wochenschr. 1973;103:307-8.
52. Stewart AB, Ahmed R, Travill CM, et al. Coarctation of the aorta life and health 20-44 years after surgical repair. Br Heart J. 1993;69:65-70.

CHAPTER 25

Managing Low Diastolic Blood Pressure in Elderly Hypertensive

HK Chopra, AK Pancholia

INTRODUCTION

Prevention of cardiovascular disease (CVD) by reduction of systolic blood pressure (SBP) and diastolic blood pressure (DBP) by antihypertensive drugs is the primary goal. However, several reports, but not all, have shown that, in hypertensive subjects treated with drugs, low DBP is frequently associated with increased mortality.[1] It is very difficult to evaluate this finding because it is difficult in epidemiological studies to assess a J-shaped association with mortality apart from that in humans, the decrease of DBP is related to both the aging process[2] and the result of drug treatment, making the net drug effect quite difficult to define. Apart from that isolated systolic hypertension (ISH) is difficult to treat and aggressive treatment may lead to excessive lowering of DBP. In subjects more than 50 years of age with advanced renal failure,[3] the increased aortic stiffness and low DBP were independent predictors of cardiovascular (CV) risk. DBP is a component of pulse pressure (PP), increased PP is the main hemodynamic consequence of increased aortic stiffness. In a population of 16,913 subjects followed for 13 years,[4] low DBP alone was a significant predictor of CV and non-CV mortality among persons aged more than 50 years (most >70 years). However, the evaluation of the underlying pathophysiological mechanisms was limited, particularly regarding hemodynamic parameters (Fig. 1).

There are problems related to the new guidelines, as ACC/AHA guideline 2017[5] has reduced the BP targets further to 130/80 mm Hg in elderly and the use of antihypertensive drugs to reduce SBP to that target may lead to further lowering of DBP and leading to further damage. There are increased chances that by reducing patients' SBP down to 120 mm, which is a target, recommended by recent clinical trials, the DBP falls so low that will lead more harm. According to the recent SPRINT trial,[6] there is recommendation for the intensive lowering of SBP for some high-risk patients, the physicians should not look at driving down SBP in isolation without considering implications of lowering the DBP.

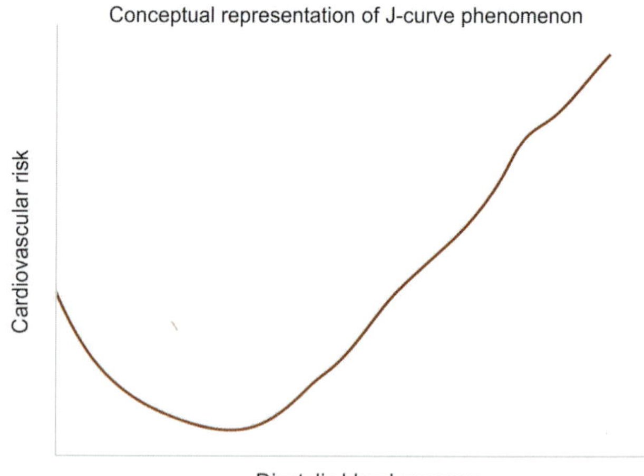

FIG. 1: J-curve concept.

PATHOPHYSIOLOGY OF THE J-CURVE

Four potential pathophysiological mechanisms have been proposed to explain the existence of a J-curve. First, the J-curve is suggestive of more severe underlying chronic illness, which there by increases mortality.[7] Second, low DBP could also be a marker of cardiac function. Indeed, in the population of North Karelia,[4] especially in patients more than 70 years of age, the DBP-mortality relation was considered as a direct main result of cardiac failure. Third, the J-curve reflects increased arterial stiffness suggestive of advance vascular disease and of increased mortality.[8,9,10] Fourth, low DBP may reduce coronary perfusion during the diastole, especially in subjects with coronary heart disease.[11] Even in the absence of evident contractile dysfunction in older subjects, subendocardial myocardial dysfunction may exist.[12] The frail elderly with a high burden of CV disease, even in the absence of evident severe coronary heart disease, in a nonhypertrophied fibrotic heart, oxygen delivery may be impaired in the case of DBP less than 60 mm Hg and further could impair subendocardial contractility.

DIASTOLIC BLOOD PRESSURE CONTROL: HOW LOW IS TOO LOW? CLINICAL TRIAL EVIDENCES

Isolated diastolic hypotension (IDH) is a relatively uncommon complication of antihypertensive therapy that may complicate the therapy in elderly. Elderly persons more often have ISH with a wide PP and normal or sometimes even low diastolic pressure. A large number of studies, notable amongst them the Systolic Hypertension in the Elderly Program (SHEP),[13] have demonstrated the substantial benefits of treating this form of hypertension, but DBP lowering is an inevitable problem in treating these patients. This reality leads us to some important questions: At what point in the treatment of ISH does the potential harm of low DBP outweigh the benefit of lowering SBP? Is the increased event rate associated with diastolic hypotension a result of treatment, or is it seen even in placebo treated patients? In order to address these issues, investigators reanalyzed the data from the SHEP trial.[14] The researchers observed a higher incidence of CVD events in patients with ISH whose DBP were lowered to less than 70 mm Hg. Furthermore, it was observed that the relative risk of CV events nearly doubled in those patients whose DBP were reduced to below 55 mm Hg. However, there were some problems with the data because, again, the number of patients with DBP less than 55 mm Hg were small and on careful analysis of this study it was observed that even levels of 45 mm Hg were not harmful. These phenomena were noted in the treatment arm but not the placebo arm. It is unclear whether the increase in the event rate associated with low DBP in the treatment arm was a direct consequence of diastolic hypotension or instead due to unmasking of subclinical disease that was manifested by antihypertensive therapy. Therefore, it can be concluded for patients whose DBP levels fall to about 55–60 mm Hg should be carefully monitored and other CV risk factors should be treated more aggressively in this subset of patients.

Based on these results the recommendation is to treat patients with ISH to lower SBP to less than 140 mm Hg, as recommended by the Seventh Report of the Joint National Committee on Prevention, Detection, Evaluation, and Treatment of High Blood Pressure[7] or less than 130 mm by recent ACC/AHA guideline.[5] However, caution should be exercised in patients whose DBP is around 56–60 mm Hg since at this point the risk may approach benefit. In this subset of patients, it would be prudent to offer aggressive control of other CV risk factors.

LOW DIASTOLIC BLOOD PRESSURE AND ATHEROSCLEROSIS IN ELDERLY SUBJECTS

The Rotterdam Study

This study demonstrated a J-shaped relationship between DBP and the common carotid artery intima-media thickness. The J-shaped curve was most noticeable in patients with relatively high PP. It has been suggested that an increased intima-media thickness of the common carotid artery may not reflect atherosclerosis and may, at least in part, be a reflection of an adaptive response of the vessel wall to changes in shear and tensile stresses.[15] Still, increased intima-media thickness of the common carotid artery has consistently been associated with elevated CV risk factor levels,[16,17] prevalent CVD[17] and atherosclerosis elsewhere in the arterial system.[18-20]

In addition, progression of the common carotid artery intima-media thickness over time has been associated with risk factors for atherosclerosis,[21] and the increased intima-media thickness has been demonstrated to be a strong predictor of myocardial infarction.[22] The Cardiovascular Health Study[23] included 2,189 subjects who were not receiving antihypertensive treatment and were free from CVD. The study demonstrated that for all levels of SBP, there existed a continuous inverse association between DBP and the intima-media thickness of the common carotid artery, with no evidence of a J-shaped relationship. In another study of older individuals with and without ISH,[24] it was observed that a DBP below 75 mm Hg was a strong marker for carotid atherosclerotic plaques. This association was limited to the subset of subjects with ISH only. The fall of DBP is because of reduced arterial compliance of the aorta and large arteries, that is, in turn has been associated with atherosclerotic abnormalities.[25,26] As a consequence, a considerable proportion of older subjects with a relatively low DBP may have existing vascular damage (i.e., increased arterial stiffness and atherosclerosis), in particular, those with a relatively high PP.

ISOLATED DIASTOLIC HYPOTENSION AND INCIDENT HEART FAILURE IN ELDERLY

Recent analysis demonstrates that IDH was an independent risk factor for incident heart failure (HF) among community-dwelling older adults, which was similar in magnitude to the effect of ISH on incident HF in this cohort. It has been demonstrated that the effect of IDH on incident HF was homogeneous across a wide spectrum of older adults, including those with SBP more than 140 mm Hg. Although, diastolic hypotension has been shown to be associated with adverse CV outcomes.[25]

Isolated diastolic hypotension is also primarily a manifestation of impaired aortic compliance associated with aging, which results in an increased SBP and a reduced DBP, thereby leading to a wide PP.[27] As a result of this there can be an increased afterload and myocardial oxygen demand leading in turn to myocardial ischemia and subsequent systolic and diastolic dysfunction.[28,29] In frail older adults poor outcomes associated with a DBP less than 60 mm Hg have been reported to be independent of aortic compliance and left ventricular ejection fraction.[30] Hypertension or uncontrolled SBP is unlikely to explain the association between IDH and incident HF, because the association persisted after excluding those with SBP more than 140 mm Hg. Further studies, are needed to explain the detailed mechanisms by which IDH is associated with incident HF. Poor outcomes have been observed with a low DBP in patients with hypertension and coronary artery, excessive DBP reduction should be avoided in these patients.[31] A DBP 60 mm Hg may be a reasonable value to maintain in older adults with ISH. Future hypertension guidelines need to focus on optimal DBP parameters for older adults receiving antihypertensive therapy.

CONCLUSION

Isolated systolic hypertension is very common in elderly population. Some patients with ISH may be treated to the level that uncovers the subclinical disease and some may even be over treated. In older patients who are treated for ISH, a DBP of less than 70 mmHg (and especially <60 mm) recognizes a high-risk group that deserve special monitoring and even more aggressive treatment for other CV risk factors. Recent hypertension guidelines have reduced the target further creating a real challenge for physicians in treating hypertension in elderly. Further studies are needed to determine whether such an intensive drop in DBP and associated increase risk of CVD events could be prevented by more careful titration of antihypertensive therapy while maintaining the SBP control.

REFERENCES

1. Messerli FH, Mancia G, Conti R, et al. Dogma disputed: can aggressively lowered blood pressure in hypertensive patients with coronary artery disease be dangerous. Ann Intern Med. 2006;144:884-93.
2. Franklin SS, Larson MG, Khan SA, et al. Does the relation of blood pressure to coronary heart disease risk change with aging? The Framingham Heart Study. Circulation. 2001;103:1245-9.
3. Blacher J, Guerin A, Pannier B, et al. Impact of aortic stiffness on survival in end-stage renal disease. Circulation. 1999;99:2434-9.
4. Tuomilehto J, Ryynanen OP, Koistinen A, et al. Low diastolic blood pressure and mortality in a population-based cohort of 16913 hypertensive patients in North Karelia, Finland. J Hypertens. 1998;16:1235-42.
5. Whelton PK, Carey RM, Aronow WS, et al. 2017 ACC/AHA/AAPA/ABC/ACPM/AGS/APhA/ASH/ASPC/NMA/PCNA Guideline for the Prevention, Detection, Evaluation, and Management of High Blood Pressure in Adults.
6. Wright JT Jr, Williamson JD, Whelton PK, et al. SPRINT Research Group. A randomized trial of intensive versus standard blood-pressure control. N Engl J Med. 2015;373(22):2103-16.
7. Boshuizen HC, Izaks GJ, van Burin S, et al. Blood pressure and mortality in elderly people aged 85 and older: community based study. BMJ. 1998;316: 1780-4.
8. Benetos A, Rudnichi A, Safar M, et al. Pulse pressure and cardiovascular mortality in normotensive and hypertensive subjects. Hypertension. 1998;32: 560-4.
9. Blacher J, Protogerou AD, Safar ME. Cardiovascular risk and the macrocirculation. In: Safar ME (ed). Macro- and Microcirculation in Hypertension. London, UK: Lippincott Williams & Wilkins; 2005. p. 83-97.
10. Kannel WB, Wilson PWF, Nam BH, et al. A likely explanation for the J-curve of blood pressure cardiovascular risk. Am J Cardiol. 2004;94:380-4.
11. Cruickshank JM. Coronary blood flow reserve and the J curve relation between diastolic blood pressure and myocardial infarction. BMJ. 1988;297:1227-30.
12. Lumens J, Delhaas T, Arts T, et al. Impaired subendocardial contractile myofiber function in asymptomatic aged humans, as detected using MRI. Am J Physiol. 2006;291:H1573-9.
13. H Mitchell Perry. SHEP study group. JAMA. 2000:284;465-71.
14. Somes GW, Pahor M, Shorr RI, et al. The role of diastolic blood pressure when treating isolated systolic hypertension. Arch Intern Med. 1999;159(17):2004-9.
15. Stary HC, Blankenhorn DH, Chandler B, et al. A definition of the intima of human arteries and of its atherosclerosis-prone regions. Arterioscler Thromb Vasc Biol. 1992;12:120-34.
16. Heiss G, Sharett AR, Barnes R, et al. Carotid atherosclerosis measured by B mode ultrasound in populations: associations with cardiovascular risk factors in the ARIC Study. Am J Epidemiol. 1991;134:250-6.
17. O'Leary DH, Polak JF, Kronmal RA, et al. Distribution and correlates of sonographically detected carotid artery disease in the Cardiovascular Health Study. Stroke. 1992;23:1752-60.
18. Bots ML, Witteman JCM, Grobbee DE. Carotid intima-media wall thickness in women with and without atherosclerosis of the abdominal aorta. Atherosclerosis. 1993;102:99-105.
19. Polak JF, O'Leary DH, Kronmal RA, et al. Sonographic evaluation of the carotid artery atherosclerosis in the elderly: relationship of disease severity to stroke and transient ischemic attack. Radiology. 1993;188:363-70.
20. Bots ML, Hofman A, Grobbee DE. Common carotid intima-media thickness and lower extremity arterial atherosclerosis: the Rotterdam Study. Arterioscler Thromb Vasc Biol. 1994;14:1885-91.
21. Salonen R, Salonen JT. Progression of carotid atherosclerosis and its determinants: a population-based ultrasonography study. Atherosclerosis. 1990;81: 33-40.
22. Salonen JT, Salonen R. Ultrasonographically assessed carotid morphology and the risk of coronary heart disease. Arterioscler Thromb Vasc Biol. 1991;11: 1245-9.
23. Psaty BM, Furberg CD, Kuller LH, et al. Isolated systolic hypertension and subclinical cardiovascular disease in the elderly: initial findings from the Cardiovascular Health Study. JAMA. 1992;268:1287-91.
24. Sutton-Tyrell K, Alcorn HG, Wolfson SK, et al. Predictors of carotid stenosis in older adults with and without isolated systolic hypertension. Stroke. 1993;24: 355-61.
25. Hirai T, Sasayama S, Kawasaki T, et al. Stiffness of systemic arteries in patients with myocardial infarction: a noninvasive method to predict severity of coronary atherosclerosis. Circulation. 1989;80:78-86.
26. Arnett DK, Evans GW, Riley WA. Arterial stiffness: a new cardiovascular risk factor. Am J Epidemiol. 1994;140:669-82.
27. Bots ML, Mulder PGH, Hofman A, et al. Reproducibility of carotid intima-media thickness measurements: The Rotterdam Study. J Clin Epidemiol. 1994;47:921-30.
28. Rose GA, Blackburn H, Gillum RF, et al. Cardiovascular Survey Methods. Geneva, Switzerland: World Health Organization; 1982.
29. WHO Collaborating Centre for Drug Statistics Methodology. Anatomical Therapeutic Chemical (ATC) Classification. Oslo, Norway: World Health Organization; 1992.
30. Stary HC, Blankenhorn DH, Chandler B, et al. A definition of the intima of human arteries and of its atherosclerosis-prone regions. Arterioscler Thromb Vasc Biol. 1992;12:120-34.
31. Wendelhag I, Olov G, Wikstrand J. Arterial wall thickness in familial hypercholesterolaemia: ultrasound measurement of intima-media thickness in the common carotid artery. Arterioscler Thromb Vasc Biol. 1992;12:70-7.

CHAPTER 26

Ambulatory Blood Pressure Monitoring—When to Order and How to Interpret?

Rajan J Manjuran, Sulthan R Salih

INTRODUCTION

Systemic hypertension (SH) is the most important cardiovascular (CV) risk factor leading to significant morbidity and mortality worldwide.[1-5] The 2010 Global Burden of Disease Study identified hypertension as the main cause of morbidity accounting for 7% of global disability-adjusted life years.[6] Classically, hypertension has been measured and evaluated using blood pressure (BP) measurement taken in the office setting—OBP. Although it measures the BP reading at the point in time, this reading cannot account for observer technique, variability of BP and may be falsely elevated or falsely reduced and will not be indicative of the BP throughout the day and night. The BP recorded by a physician is generally higher than that recorded by a nurse.[7] These shortcomings can be overcome by the use of home BP monitoring (HBPM) and ambulatory BP monitoring (ABPM). The advantages of ABPM far outweigh the convenience and availability of OBP. HBPM has few advantageous over ABPM in that it can detect BP readings over longer period of time and involves the patient with his hypertension management. But ABPM can record nighttime BP and monitor variations in BP over short time, say 24–48 hours. This is a short review of ABPM and the rational for its use in daily practice.

HISTORY AND RELEVANCE OF ABPM

The idea that OBP is not the true BP is as old as 1940s. Ayman and Goldshine, in 1940, instructed 34 of their hypertensive patients to record BP at home, either themselves or by family members.[8] In all these 34 patients followed up for an average of 21 visits, the BP recorded outside the office was around 50 mm Hg systolic and 25 mm Hg diastolic less than the OBP. The credit for development of ABPM must go to Maurice Sokolow (1911–2002), an internist from San Francisco. He noticed near normal life expectancy in many of his hypertensive patients. In 1962, he and his colleagues developed the first semiautomatic ABPM device. There was a BP cuff that was manually inflated like in the sphygmomanometer, and the Korotkoff sounds were recorded on a tape recorder. He demonstrated the variability of BP during the day and lack of correlation with OBP. He also demonstrated correlation between ABPM and higher event rate over a 10-year period in patients whose OBP were similar and is considered a landmark trial in hypertension.[9] Higher ABPM values have been correlated with more subclinical end organ damage.[10] Based on the SYST-EUR study on patients with isolated systolic hypertension,[11] the Dublin study,[12] and the PAMELA population study,[13] Mancia et al.[14] derived a relationship curve which show that the CV events and mortality have a steeper relationship with ABPM than OBP and hence can predict these events earlier. The prediction of events is significant even after adjusting for OBP values.[15] This higher predictability of events can be due to the higher number of readings that are obtained. Thus, it increases the reliability and reproducibility compared to OBP. Currently, the ABPM monitors are of much smaller in size and use more accurate oscillometric technique of recording and digital storage of the readings.

PROCEDURE

Ambulatory BP monitoring is done using recorders that automatically records BP at set intervals for a set duration of time (Fig. 1). These can record BP during routine daily activities of the patient. The present day ABPM use oscillometric method for BP recording. The monitors are small and light weight so that they can be carried around with ease. A BP cuff is wrapped around the patients arm and is connected to the monitor which is worn using a belt around the waist or the shoulder. The cuff inflates and deflates to record BP. The patient is instructed to stop moving, not to talk, to keep his arm still at heart level and not to exert while BP is being recorded. The patients are advised to maintain a diary of events throughout the day which can be correlated with the ABPM readings.

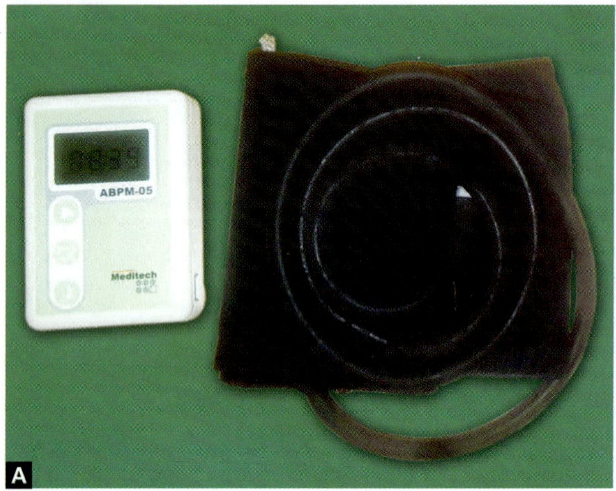

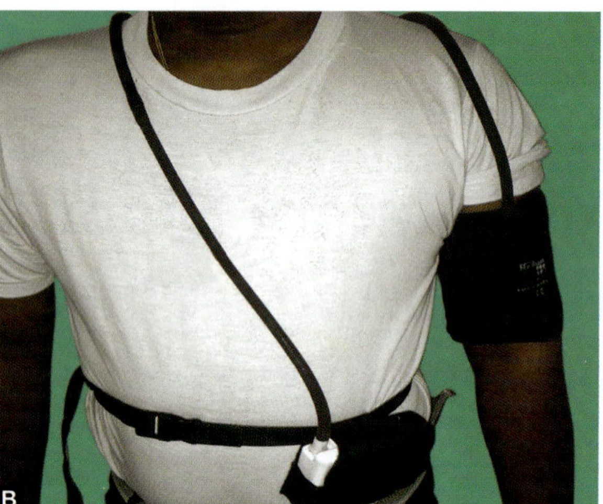

FIG. 1: (A) Ambulatory blood pressure monitor (ABPM) device and cuff; (B) ABPM device connected to the patient.

The monitors are programed to record BP at intervals of 15–30 minutes during the daytime and 30 minutes to 1 hour during the nighttime. The nighttime is set according to the routine sleep-on and sleep-off time of the patient. These recordings are then downloaded on to computer and analyzed. The BP readings are grouped into 24-hour, daytime and nighttime mean. The sleep-on time and sleep-off time can be adjusted after recording is over. Usually, the nighttime is set from 10 pm to 6 am.

There are a large number of ABPM equipment in the market. These devices have to be validated based on internationally accepted protocols. European Society of Hypertension (ESH) International protocol for the validation of BP measuring devices of 2010 is the commonly used protocol.[16] The device must record BP within 5 mm Hg of a mercury sphygmomanometer reading. The software for analysis is also important and recommendations have been included in the 2013 ESH Position paper on ABPM.[17]

For an ABPM recording to be valid it has to have at least 70% of the expected BP recordings. There must be at least 20 valid BP readings in the daytime and 7 valid reading in the nighttime. Not meeting of these criteria can result in ABPM recording not indicating the true mean day and nighttime recordings. In patients, with irregular rhythm like atrial fibrillation, ABPM cannot be relied.

INDICATIONS

The most common indications for ABPM are:

- Suspected white-coat hypertension; treated or untreated
- Suspected masked hypertension; treated or untreated
- Patients with a high risk of future cardiovascular events (even if clinic BP is normal)
- Identifying abnormal 24-hour BP patterns:
  - Dipping status
  - Daytime hypertension
  - Siesta dipping or postprandial hypotension
  - Nocturnal hypertension.
- Assessment of treatment:
  - Assessing 24-hour BP control
  - Identifying true resistant hypertension
  - Assessing morning hypertension and morning BP surge
  - Screening and follow up of obstructive sleep apnea
  - Assessing short-term BP variability
  - Identifying ambulatory hypotension
  - Assessing endocrine hypertension
  - Evaluation of medication-related symptoms.

Definition of Hypertension using ABPM, Normal, and Abnormal Patterns

The 2017 American College of Cardiology/American Heart Association (ACC/AHA) hypertension guidelines and 2013 European Society of Cardiology/European Society of Hypertension (ESC/ESH) guidelines defined hypertension using ABPM as given in Table 1.[18,19]

The main advantage of ABPM is the nighttime BP recordings. Normally, nighttime BP readings (both systolic and diastolic) are lower than the daytime readings. Based on the nocturnal dip of BP patients can be classified as follows:

- *Normal dippers:* The mean nighttime BP must be 10–20% lower than the average daytime BP to be called normal nocturnal dipping (Figs. 2 and 3). Dippers may also be defined by a mean night or mean day BP ratio less than

TABLE 1: ACC/AHA and ESC/ESH guidelines defined hypertension as follows

	Systolic BP (mm Hg)	Diastolic BP (mm Hg)
24-hour mean	≥130	≥80
Day-time mean (awake time)	≥135	≥85
Nighttime mean (sleep time)	≥120	≥70

ACC/AHA, American College of Cardiology/American Heart Association; ESC/ESH, European Society of Cardiology/European Society of Hypertension.

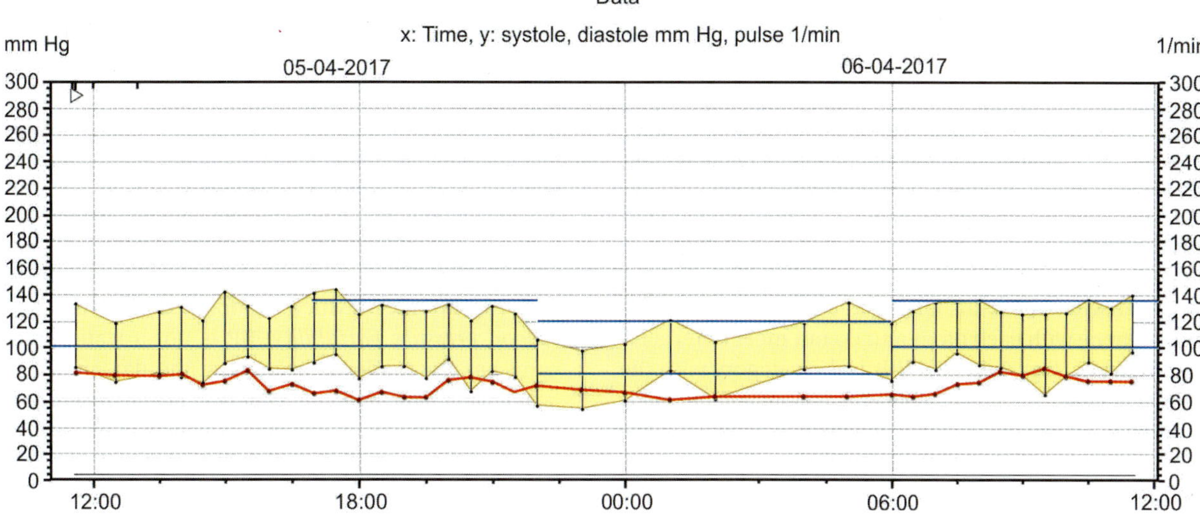

FIG. 2: Normal ambulatory blood pressure monitor record. The 24-hour, daytime and nighttime mean blood pressures are normal with 15% dipping at night.

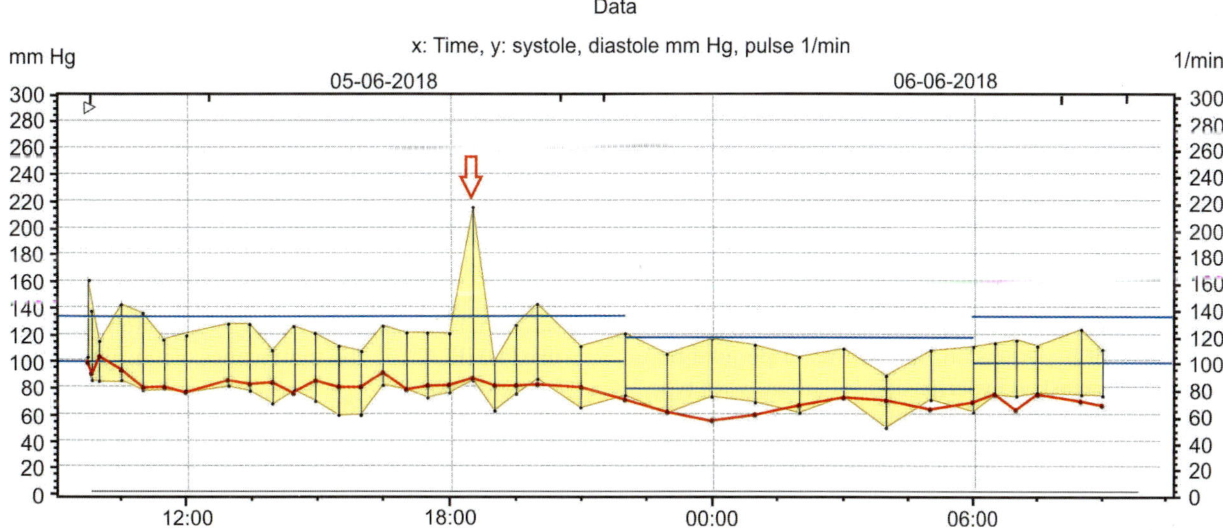

FIG. 3: Normal ambulatory blood pressure monitor record. The 24-hour, the day time and nighttime, mean blood pressures (BPs) are normal. Three is 10–15% dipping of nocturnal BP. There is a single abnormal BP reading of 220/80 mm Hg which is a wrong reading. This is excluded from analysis to avoid wrong results (red arrow). There are adequate number of BP readings to consider this report as valid. We can also suspect a white coat effect because the first BP recording is above the normal threshold.

or equal to 0.9. These are patients with lowest CV risk compared to the other categories based on dipping status.

- *Nondippers:* The mean nighttime BP is lower than daytime BP, but the magnitude of reduction is less than 10% (Fig. 4). In these individuals, there is higher incidence left ventricular hypertrophy, ventricular arrhythmias, and major CV events compared to normal dippers.[20-23] An increase in CV mortality has also been shown in nondippers in the Ohasama[24] and PAMELA[25] studies. On the renal side, these patients have been shown to have greater risk of albuminuria, lower glomerular filtration rate and impaired sodium excretion.[26-29] More strokes, silent cerebral infarcts, and lower brain matter volume has also been shown to be associated with nondipping.[30-32] All these show the higher end organ damage with nondipping status. Hence, not only just daytime BP control but also adequate fall in BP at night is needed to reduce morbidity and mortality associated with SH.
- *Reverse-dippers or night BP risers*: Contrary to the normal dipping pattern, mean BP at night is higher than the daytime mean BP (Fig. 5). Cardiovascular events are highest in this group, even higher than the nondippers.[33] In these, patients a four times CV mortality risk has been shown in the Ohasama study.[24] Majority of these patients have either obstructive sleep apnea or diabetes mellitus (DM). Better control of the causative factor may ameliorate the mortality risk and convert these patients to either a nondipper or dipper.

- *Hyperdippers or extreme dippers*: The mean nighttime BP is greater than or equal to 20% lower than the mean daytime BP. Most studies could not find associations between extreme dippers and outcomes, usually due to the low prevalence. But extreme dipping is not benign. Mild cognitive impairment and silent cerebrovascular disease has been shown to be higher in extreme dippers.[34-36]

There exist various phenotypes of patients based on their OBP and ABPM.

- *Normotension:* An individual is said to be a true normotensive if both his OBP and ABPM values are in concordance with each other and do not meet criteria for hypertension (Figs 2 and 3). This is the category with the lowest CV risk.
- *Sustained hypertension*: An individual is said to have sustained hypertension if both his OBP and ABPM are in concordance and meet criteria for hypertension. They have higher CV morbidity and mortality as has been shown in large trials based on OBP.[1-6]
- *White coat hypertension:* Also called isolated clinic hypertension. An individual is said to have white coat hypertension if his OBP readings are diagnostic of hypertension but ABPM values are normal. Although previously considered benign, these patients have been shown to have a higher risk of all-cause mortality in a recent study.[37] Also patients with white coat hypertension are more likely to progress to sustained hypertension and hence the need for early intervention and lifestyle modification.[38] Incidence of new onset DM is also higher in these patients.[39]
- *Masked hypertension*: An individual is said to have masked hypertension if his OBP values are normal, but ABPM is diagnostic of hypertension. About 10% of population is said to have masked hypertension.[13] Patients with type 2 diabetes mellitus have higher prevalence of masked hypertension.[40-42] They have higher CV morbidity and mortality compared to normotensives. A recent study showed these patients have the highest risk and a stronger correlation with all cause and CV mortality than sustained hypertension.[37] They also have a higher progression to sustained hypertension and DM.[38,39]
- *Nocturnal hypertension*: An individual is said to have isolated nocturnal hypertension if his OBP is normal and ABPM shows elevated nighttime mean BP with normal daytime mean BP (Fig. 4). These patients also have higher CV events compared to normal population.

There are other additional parameters that can be measured with ABPM which cannot be done with OBP.

- *Blood pressure variability:* BP is not a static parameter and has fluctuations throughout the day and night and over weeks to months. Although not a true measure of BP variability (BPV), ABPM gives enough readings to suggest an increased variability in BP over short-term period (Fig. 6). BP variability over short- and long-term have been independently associated with higher CV risk and renal damage.[43-50] Increased BPV over the short-term period has been shown to increase subclinical organ damage[50,51]
- *Morning BP rise*: There is a rise of BP in the early morning hours starting a few minutes before waking to a few minutes after waking (Fig. 5). Number of stroke and myocardial infarctions have been noted to be more frequent in this period. Rise in heart rate, cortisol and other parameters have also been implicated other than BP rise.[52-54] This morning rise of BP is regarded as a physiological phenomenon although there have been some studies which show association of adverse events with excessive morning rise of BP.[55-57] But these findings have not been validated in large population based studies like PAMELA.[50, 58] The significance of morning BP surge is hence debated.
- *Blood pressure load*: It is defined as the percentage of readings in the ABPM report that are above the threshold value for that time period, daytime or nighttime. It is

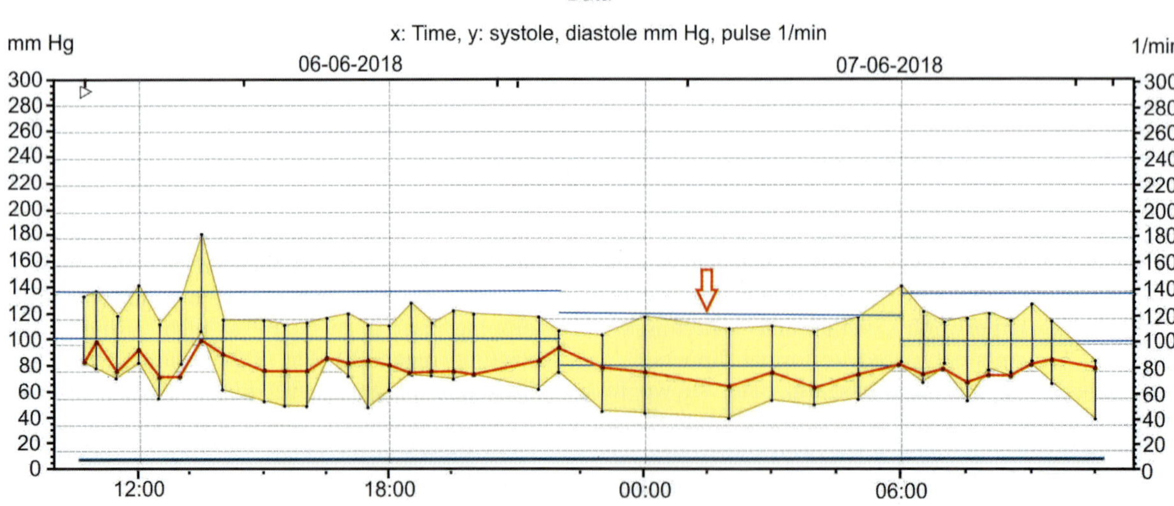

FIG. 4: Ambulatory blood pressure monitor record showing a normal daytime mean blood pressure (BP) with <10% fall in nocturnal BP (red arrow) which indicates nondipping. The nighttime mean BP is above the threshold for hypertension suggestive of isolated nocturnal hypertension.

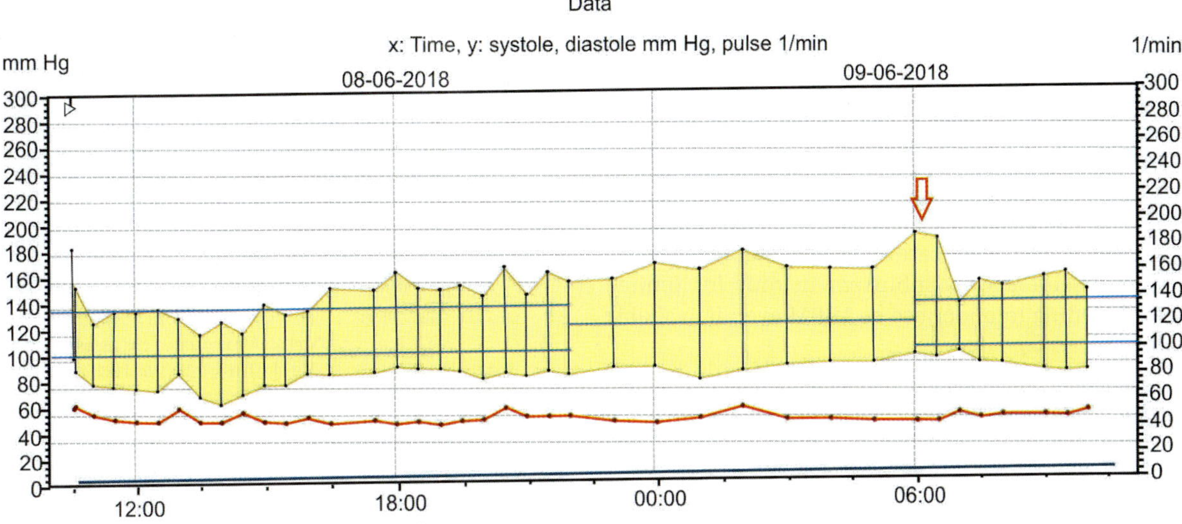

FIG. 5: Ambulatory blood pressure monitor record showing sustained hypertension with reverse dipping pattern. Also note the blood pressure surge in the morning (red arrow).

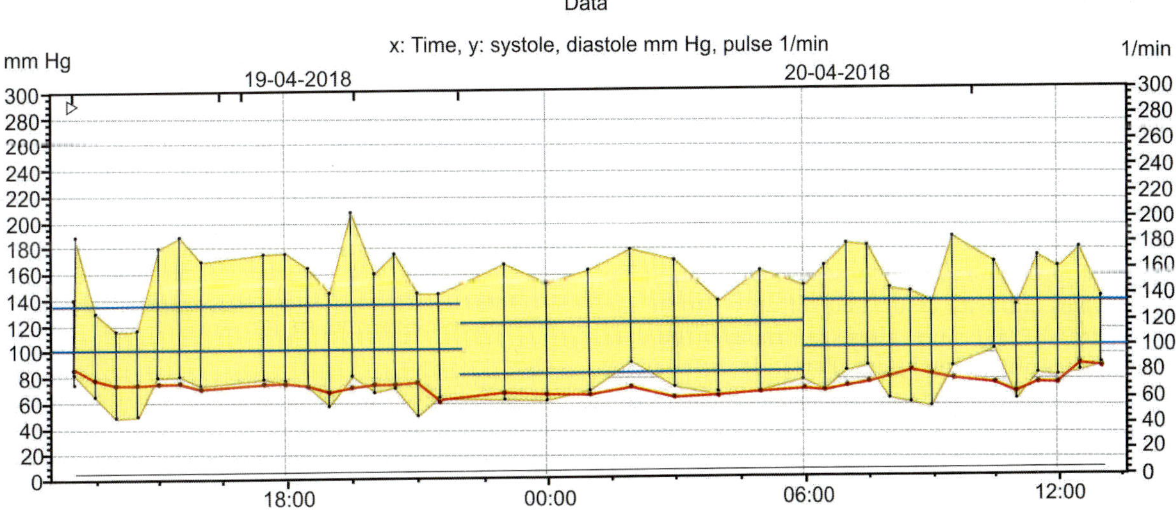

FIG. 6: Ambulatory blood pressure monitor record showing sustained hypertension with nondipping pattern and blood pressure variability.

an indicator of the time for which the patient stays hypertensive. But it is a poor indicator as it does not reflect the magnitude of hypertension and individual BP readings cannot be compared to the mean time period threshold. These shortcomings have more or less been addressed with BP variability.

- *Postprandial hypotension*: It is also called Siesta dipping. Fall in BP after meals can be documented with ABPM. This is recognized if the patients maintain a diary of events throughout the monitoring period.
- *Ambulatory hypotension*: Although not the ideal method, ABPM can provide readings to suggest that a patient has an ambulatory hypotension. Like postprandial hypotension, recognition of ambulatory hypotension requires the maintenance of diary of events.

MERITS AND DRAWBACKS

In addition to the above-mentioned merits of stratifying risks better and identification of special categories of hypertension, some more merits need to be mentioned. It can avoid unnecessary drug treatment of white coat hypertension. It can also help individualize the treatment for each patient. For the evaluation of duration of drug effect ABPM is ideal as it can record nighttime BP. Also placebos are said to have negligible effect on ABPM results.[59]

Although ABPM has a lot of merits it is not without drawbacks. There have not been large randomized trials making use of ABPM for the CV outcomes. ABPM requires a special BP monitor which is able to record the BP at set intervals and there is a need for a computer to analyze the data. This increases the cost of the procedure and reduces the widespread availability. But the cost factors become favorable in the long run. The BP recordings obtained in patients of irregular heart rhythms especially atrial fibrillation are not reliable. Some patients complain of disturbed sleep due to the recurrent inflation and deflation of the BP cuff, which may in turn lead to elevated nighttime readings. Compared to HBPM there is no active participation of patient in the management of hypertension. Most countries with healthcare based on insurance there is no reimbursement or reimbursement only for limited indications leading to under use of ABPM even if available and indicated.

FUTURE DIRECTIONS

As discussed above, OBP is largely insufficient in predicting events and treating hypertension. ABPM is here to stay and future guidelines may be entirely based on ABPM than OBP, hence providing the best prognosis for patients. With gaining popularity and huge impact of ABPM, various organizations have started maintaining registries based on ABPM. An ABPM-based registry will give a better outlook and provide more data for optimizing the use of ABPM. With the emergence of central aortic blood pressure measurement (CAABPM) noninvasively using cuff-based methods with greater accuracy, the next direction ABPM might take is the CAABPM. There has been an integration of mobile devices into the health monitoring, like the apple watch being able to detect subclinical atrial fibrillation. Wireless bluetooth-based BP monitors have been released and with slight programmability these can also double up as ABPM devices and with associated software can be the future compact ABPM devices. These can transfer the data to a mobile device and be analyzed, alleviating the need for a computer. With Wi-Fi based printing, using mobile device based ABPM, the cost of a computer and space occupied can be saved.

CONCLUSION

At present OBP is the accepted method of recording BP and is correlated with CV morbidity and mortality. However, ABPM which records the BP during day and night is a superior method of BP assessment and has been better correlated with morbidity and mortality, including end organ damage, compared to OBP. Various patterns of BP variations during night have been recognized by ABPM and each has its own prognostic significance. ABPM is the only technique which can detect white coat and masked hypertension. ABPM can guide the choice and timing of antihypertensive drug administration. The drawback of ABPM is the lack of large randomized trials using the technique, the cost and lack of easy availability. With the refinement of technology and greater acceptance by the treating physicians, ABPM in the near future will be the accepted method of BP recording for evaluation and management of a patient of systemic hypertension.

REFERENCES

1. Kannel WB, Wolf PA. Framingham study insights on the hazards of elevated blood pressure. JAMA. 2008;300:2545.
2. Kannel WB, Wolf PA, Verter J, et al. Epidemiologic assessment of the role of blood pressure in stroke. The Framingham study. JAMA. 1970;214:301-10.
3. Kannel WB, Dawber TR, McGee DL. Perspectives on systolic hypertension. The Framingham study. Circulation. 1980; 61:1179-82.
4. Redon J, Tellez-Plaza M, Orozco-Beltran D, et al. Impact of hypertension on mortality and cardiovascular disease burden in patients with cardiovascular risk factors from a general practice setting. J Hypertens. 2016;34:1075-83.
5. Lawes CMM, Vander Hoorn S, Rodgers A, et al. Global burden of blood-pressure-related disease, 2001. Lance. 2008;371:1513-8.
6. Lim SS, Vos T, Flaxman AD, et al. A comparative risk assessment of burden of disease and injury attributable to 67 risk factors and risk factor clusters in 21 regions, 1990–2010: a systematic analysis for the Global Burden of Disease Study 2010. Lancet. 2012;380:2224-60.
7. Little P, Barnett J, Barnsley L, et al. Comparison of agreement between different measures of blood pressure in primary care and daytime ambulatory blood pressure. BMJ. 2002;325:254.
8. Ayman G. Blood pressure determinations by patients with essential hypertension: The difference between clinic and home readings before treatment. Am J Med Sci. 1940;20:465-74.
9. Perloff D, Sokolow M, Cowan R. The prognostic value of ambulatory blood pressures. JAMA. 1983;249:2792-8.
10. Mancia G, Parati G. Ambulatory blood pressure monitoring and organ damage. Hypertension. 2000;36:894-900.
11. Staessen JA, Thijs L, Fagard R, et al. Predicting cardiovascular risk using conventional vs ambulatory blood pressure in older patients with systolic hypertension. Systolic Hypertension in Europe Trial Investigators. JAMA. 1999;282:539-46.
12. Dolan E, Stanton A, Thijs L, et al. Superiority of ambulatory over clinic blood pressure measurement in predicting mortality: The Dublin Outcome study. Hypertension. 2005;46:156-61.
13. Mancia G, Sega R, Bravi C, et al. Ambulatory blood pressure normality: results from the PAMELA study. J Hypertens. 1995;13:1377-90.
14. Mancia G, Verdecchia P. Clinical value of ambulatory blood pressure: Evidence and limits. Circ Res. 2015;116:1034-45.
15. Clement DL, De Buyzere ML, De Bacquer DA, et al. Prognostic value of ambulatory blood-pressure recordings in patients with treated hypertension. N Engl J Med. 2003;348:2407-15.
16. O'Brien E, Atkins N, Stergiou G, et al. European Society of Hypertension International Protocol revision 2010 for the validation of blood pressure measuring devices in adults. Blood Press Monit. 2010;15:23-38.
17. O'Brien E, Parati G, Stergiou G, et al. European Society of Hypertension position paper on ambulatory blood pressure monitoring. J Hypertens. 2013; 31:1731-68.
18. Whelton PK, Carey RM, Aronow WS, et al. 2017 ACC/AHA/AAPA/ABC/ACPM/AGS/APhA/ASH/ASPC/NMA/PCNA Guideline for the Prevention, Detection, Evaluation, and Management of High Blood Pressure in Adults: Executive Summary: A Report of the American College of Cardiology/American Heart Association Task Force on Clinical Practice Guidelines. Hypertension. 2018;71: 1269-324.
19. Mancia G, Fagard R, Narkiewicz K, et al. 2013 ESH/ESC Guidelines for the management of arterial hypertension. Eur Heart J. 2013;34: 2159-219.
20. Rizzoni D, Muiesan ML, Montani G, et al. Relationship between initial cardiovascular structural changes and daytime and nighttime blood pressure monitoring. Am J Hypertens. 1992;5:180-6.
21. Verdecchia P, Schillaci G, Guerrieri M, et al. Circadian blood pressure changes and left ventricular hypertrophy in essential hypertension. Circulation. 1990;81:528-36.
22. Palatini P, Penzo M, Racioppa A, et al. Clinical relevance of nighttime blood pressure and of daytime blood pressure variability. Arch Intern Med. 1992;152:1855-60.
23. Schillaci G, Verdecchia P, Borgioni C, et al. Association between persistent pressure overload and ventricular arrhythmias in essential hypertension. Hypertension. 1996;28:284-9.

24. Ohkubo T, Imai Y, Tsuji I, et al. Relation between nocturnal decline in blood pressure and mortality. The Ohasama Study. Am J Hypertens. 1997; 10:1201-7.
25. Sega R, Facchetti R, Bombelli M, et al. Prognostic value of ambulatory and home blood pressures compared with office blood pressure in the general population: follow-up results from the Pressioni Arteriose Monitorate e Loro Associazioni (PAMELA) Study. Circulation. 2005;111:1777-83.
26. Bianchi S, Bigazzi R, Baldari G, et al. Diurnal variations of blood pressure and microalbuminuria in essential hypertension. Am J Hypertens. 1994;7: 23-9.
27. Redon J, Liao Y, Lozano J V, et al. Ambulatory blood pressure and microalbuminuria in essential hypertension: role of circadian variability. J Hypertens. 1994;12:947-53.
28. Fujii T, Uzu T, Nishimura M, et al. Circadian rhythm of natriuresis is disturbed in nondipper type of essential hypertension. Am J Kidney Dis. 1999;33:29-35.
29. Bankir L, Bochud M, Maillard M, et al. Nighttime blood pressure and nocturnal dipping are associated with daytime urinary sodium excretion in African subjects. Hypertension. 2008;51:891-8.
30. Shimada K, Kawamoto A, Matsubayashi K, et al. Diurnal blood pressure variations and silent cerebrovascular damage in elderly patients with hypertension. J Hypertens. 1992;10: 875-8.
31. Schwartz GL, Bailey KR, Mosley T, et al. Association of ambulatory blood pressure with ischemic brain injury. Hypertension. 2007;49:1228-34.
32. Nagai M, Hoshide S, Ishikawa J, et al. Ambulatory blood pressure as an independent determinant of brain atrophy and cognitive function in elderly hypertension. J Hypertens. 2008;26:1636-41.
33. Verdecchia P, Porcellati C, Schillaci G, et al. Ambulatory blood pressure. An independent predictor of prognosis in essential hypertension. Hypertension. 1994;24:793-801.
34. Shimada K, Kawamoto A, Matsubayashi K, et al. Silent cerebrovascular disease in the elderly. Correlation with ambulatory pressure. Hypertension. 1990;16:692-9.
35. Guo H, Tabara Y, Igase M, et al. Abnormal nocturnal blood pressure profile is associated with mild cognitive impairment in the elderly: the J-SHIPP study. Hypertens Res. 2010;33:32-6.
36. Kario K, Matsuo T, Kobayashi H, et al. Nocturnal fall of blood pressure and silent cerebrovascular damage in elderly hypertensive patients. Advanced silent cerebrovascular damage in extreme dippers. Hypertension. 1996;27:130-5.
37. Banegas JR, Ruilope LM, de la Sierra A, et al. Relationship between Clinic and Ambulatory Blood-Pressure Measurements and Mortality. N Engl J Med. 2018;378:1509-20.
38. Mancia G, Bombelli M, Facchetti R, et al. Long-Term Risk of Sustained Hypertension in White-Coat or Masked Hypertension. Hypertension. 2009;54:226-32.
39. Mancia G, Bombelli M, Facchetti R, et al. Increased long-term risk of new-onset diabetes mellitus in white-coat and masked hypertension. J Hypertens. 2009;27:1672-78.
40. Eguchi K, Ishikawa J, Hoshide S, et al. Masked Hypertension in Diabetes Mellitus: A Potential Risk. J Clin Hypertens. 2007;9:601-7.
41. Leitão CB, Canani LH, Kramer CK, et al. Masked hypertension, urinary albumin excretion rate, and echocardiographic parameters in putatively normotensive type 2 diabetic patients. Diabetes Care. 2007;30:1255-60.
42. Franklin SS, Thijs L, Li Y, et al. Masked hypertension in diabetes mellitus: treatment implications for clinical practice. Hypertension. 2013;61:964-71.
43. Parati G, Ochoa JE, Salvi P, et al. Prognostic value of blood pressure variability and average blood pressure levels in patients with hypertension and diabetes. Diabetes Care. 2013;36(Suppl 2): S312-24
44. Mancia G, Bombelli M, Facchetti R, et al. Long-Term Prognostic Value of Blood Pressure Variability in the General Population: Results of the Pressioni Arteriose Monitorate e Loro Associazioni Study. Hypertension. 2007;49:1265-70.
45. Manios E, Tsagalis G, Tsivgoulis G, et al. Time rate of blood pressure variation is associated with impaired renal function in hypertensive patients. J Hypertens. 2009;27:2244-8.
46. Frattola A, Parati G, Cuspidi C, et al. Prognostic value of 24-hour blood pressure variability. J Hypertens. 1993;11:1133-7.
47. Parati G, Pomidossi G, Albini F, et al. Relationship of 24-hour blood pressure mean and variability to severity of target-organ damage in hypertension. J Hypertens. 1987;5:93-8.
48. Mancia G, Parati G, Hennig M, et al. Relation between blood pressure variability and carotid artery damage in hypertension: baseline data from the European Lacidipine Study on Atherosclerosis (ELSA). J Hypertens. 2001;19:1981-9.
49. Mancia G, Parati G. The role of blood pressure variability in end-organ damage. J Hypertens Suppl. 2003;21:S17-23.
50. Sega R, Corrao G, Bombelli M, et al. Blood pressure variability and organ damage in a general population: results from the PAMELA study (Pressioni Arteriose Monitorate E Loro Associazioni). Hypertension. 2002;39:710-4.
51. Sander D, Kukla C, Klingelhöfer J, et al. Relationship between circadian blood pressure patterns and progression of early carotid atherosclerosis: A 3-year follow-up study. Circulation. 2000;102:1536-41.
52. Elliott WJ. Circadian variation in the timing of stroke onset: a meta-analysis. Stroke. 1998;29:992-6.
53. Muller JE, Ludmer PL, Willich SN, et al. Circadian variation in the frequency of sudden cardiac death. Circulation. 1987;75:131-8.
54. Dodt C, Breckling U, Derad I, et al. Plasma epinephrine and norepinephrine concentrations of healthy humans associated with nighttime sleep and morning arousal. Hypertension. 1997;30:71-6.
55. Metoki H, Ohkubo T, Kikuya M, et al. Prognostic significance for stroke of a morning pressor surge and a nocturnal blood pressure decline: The Ohasama Study. Hypertension. 2006;47:149-54.
56. Kario K, Ishikawa J, Pickering TG, et al. Morning hypertension: The strongest independent risk factor for stroke in elderly hypertensive patients. Hypertens Res. 2006;29:581-7.
57. Giles TD. Circadian rhythm of blood pressure and the relation to cardiovascular events. J Hypertens. 2006;24:S11-6.
58. Verdecchia P, Angeli F, Mazzotta G, et al. Day-night dip and early-morning surge in blood pressure in hypertension: Prognostic implications. Hypertension. 2012;60:34-42.
59. Mancia G, Omboni S, Parati G, et al. Lack of placebo effect on ambulatory blood pressure. Am J Hypertens. 1995;8:311-5.

CHAPTER 27

Home Blood Pressure Monitoring: Current Status

Vidyut Jain, Avani Jain

INTRODUCTION

Hypertension is the most common preventable cause of cardiovascular diseases and cerebrovascular events. Home blood pressure monitoring (HBPM) is the self-monitoring system that can be adopted into the care for patients with hypertension.[1] A growing body of evidence supports that the recording of blood pressure (BP) at home or outside clinic provides more accurate information and there by prediction of future events. Till recent the gold standard for these predictions used to be 24-hour ambulatory blood pressure monitoring (ABPM) that measures daytime and nighttime pressures.[2] The objective of this paper is to perform a systematic review of the available evidence on the usefulness of HBPM in the diagnosis and treatment of hypertension.

REVIEW OF LITERATURE

In last two decades, many studies have analyzed the clinical usefulness of ABPM as a valuable technique that significantly improves the management of hypertensive patients.[1] However, because of its cost, the need for trained clinic staff, and the interference with patients' usual activities, ABPM is currently recommended in only selected cases.[1,2]

Regarding HBPM, only in the last decade convincing evidences has been available. Observations in many studies published in 2008, and onward created great interest in clinical application of this method of BP monitoring.[3]

In the present era, discussion on the application of HBPM in clinical practice can be focused on: (1) diagnostic value in hypertension, i.e., white coat and masked hypertension; (2) usefulness in assessing the antihypertensive drug efficacy and adjusting the dose and different molecules; (3) management of hypertension, especially regarding compliance with treatment and percentage of hypertension control rate; (4) comparison with other modalities, i.e., ABPM. Some other area of interest can be used of HBPM in special populations (children, patients with chronic kidney disease). Analysis of HBPM data can be further informative for prediction of target-organ damage, morbidity, or mortality pattern in different subgroup.

Diagnostic Capability of HBPM

In last two decades, various studies assessed the diagnostic accuracy of HBPM comparing it with ABPM highlighting sensitivity and specificity. Data are presented in table 1.

TABLE 1: Analysis of study for diagnostic performance of home blood pressure monitoring as compared to ambulatory monitoring as the reference method

Study	Number	Subject	Diagnosis	Specificity	Sensitivity
Nesbitt et al.[5] 1977	199	Untreated	Hypertension	84	93
Sterigiou[6] 1998	189	Treated	White coat HBP	57	85
Comas[7] 1999	58	Treated	White coat HBP	84	82
Agarwal 2006[9]	104	Hemodialysis	hypertension	80	84
Stergiou et al.[8] 2008	133	Untreated	Hypertension	74	76
Shinmo et al.[10] 2009	229	Untreated	Hypertension	100	79
Serigiou et al.[4] 2010	44	Treated	Resistant hypertension	93	63
Masding et al.[11] 2009	55	Untreated	Diabetes II	100	79

HBP, home blood pressure.

In earlier studies which compared HBPM with ambulatory or office BP measurements in the diagnosis of sustained, white coat, or masked hypertension utilized mainly aneroid devices, but recent studies used validated oscillometric devices. Emphasis of these studies was on several advantages of home compared to office measurements, including the detection of the white-coat and the masked hypertension phenomena in clinical practice.[2,3]

Table 1 shows various studies comparing the sensitivity-specificity and diagnostic accuracy of HBPM, office, and ambulatory BP as reference in untreated, treated, as well as subjects with diabetes type 2, chronic renal failure, or hemodialysis, and children and adolescents.[4-6] Apparently, moderate agreement was seen between two methods of BP monitoring with higher specificity and lower sensitivity and positive predictive value. HBPM can easily detect masked hypertension and white coat hypertension as much as ABPM which is accepted as standard tool for the same. HBPM analysis was similar in the different populations included in these studies particularly in children and adolescents. HBPM appears to have considerable more potential in the assessment of elevated BP in children, and may prove an important tool when further data will be available.[12]

HBPM in Treated Hypertension

The main application of HBPM is its use in the long-term follow-up of treated hypertension. In SHEAF (Self-measurement of blood pressure at Home in the Elderly: Assessment and Follow-up)[13] study where 4,939 elderly treated hypertensive were followed for 3.1 years and data showed that even in apparently office controlled BP masked hypertension was present in about 42% thus exposing them to high risk (hazard ratio of 2.06) while comparing them with patients with low office and home BP in another group of patient with white coat reaction this risk was low (hazard ratio was 1.18). Thus, HBPM can better analyze the cardiovascular risk.[14]

HBPM for Treatment Adjustment

A comparative analysis of studies involving randomized controlled antihypertensive treatment adjustment based on home versus clinic or ambulatory BP is discussed.[15-20] Larger BP decline was noted in HBPM group in two trials.[21,22]

The difference in BP values in untreated and treated subjects was significant in home BP group. There by it is presumed that HBPM can offer more appropriate direction in management of drug therapy.

In another study termed THOP, which enrolled 400 subjects with elevated office BP to decide about therapeutic management based upon office or home BP where in monitoring was done for 1 year for outcome emphasized that adjustment based on HBPM required less intensive drugs.[23]

In HOMERUS study, 160 patients with hypertension were included for treatment adjustment. It has similar observation to that reported in THOP that for the same target of BP based on HBPM requirement of drugs was less after 1 year follow-up as compared with ambulatory BP.[24]

In a study reported by Zarnike which included 98 subjects to titrate therapy based on either ambulatory BP or home BP reading having high daytime diastolic BP with intention to attain the goal of diastolic BP of 80 mm Hg or less, no significant difference was observed in two groups at 6 months follow-up.[20]

HBPM in the Assessment of Antihypertensive Drug Effects

To find out the utility of HBPM for analyzing efficacy of medication used for BP control meta-analysis of 30 studies involving 6,794 subjects showed that antihypertensive treatment reduces home BP by approximately 20% less than office BP.[24] The paradox observed may be due to the difference in baseline BP levels. Thus, larger decline in mean pressure may be due to white coat and placebo effect.[21,22]

Early morning rise in BP is nowadays believed to have significant impact in outcome of BP trials.[25] The stress is on to evaluate the relationship of either BP value on target organ damage and it is postulated that home BP is more relevant to clinic BP and equivalent to ambulatory BP in predicting the long-term outcome.[26] It has been noted in many studies that home BP measurements gives us more reliable information on treatment-induced changes in BP.[27-32] Other important observation is that the morning:evening home BP ratio provides information on action and duration of antihypertensive drugs as the trough:peak ratio assessed by 24-hour ABPM.[33,34]

In assessment of effect of antihypertensive drug Zamke further reported larger BP decline in group of patient comparing with central BP with HBPM.[20] In another study by Niranen in patient with daytime diastolic BP of 86–110 mm Hg studied for 6 months similar decline was noted both ambulatory and HBPM group.[19] In a published report by Verberk et al. of 364 patient treated for hypertension comparing central with HBPM for 12 months, higher effect in HBPM was seen.[23]

In a study of 206 hypertensive patients the effect of treatment on left ventricular wall thickness was assessed by monitoring their BP by office, HBPM and ambulatory BP methods for 1 year and it was observed that office BP monitoring in predicting left ventricular hypertrophy was less informative.[26]

HBPM in the Assessment of Resistant Hypertension

Ambulatory blood pressure monitoring is considered to be better for the evaluation and management of patients with resistant hypertension.[1] However, a small study provides a direct comparison with ambulatory monitoring and confirmed the usefulness of home BP in resistant hypertension (Table 1). Now both American and European guidelines have also included resistant hypertension is an indication for HBPM.

HBPM and Hypertension Control

A meta-analysis of 18 randomized controlled trials (RCTs) including 2,714 hypertensive subjects allocated to HBPM or to usual care showed a significant 10% greater chance of reaching the BP target with home monitoring.[34] This difference though small, yet if applied in the entire population of hypertensive subjects, is expected to have an important impact on cardiovascular disease prevention.

In an RCT in 441 uncontrolled hypertensive patients, from general practice, HBPM resulted in a small but significant improvement of BP at 6 months, with no additional cost; this benefit was sustained after a year.[35] Report from J-Home study which included 2,363 hypertensive patients, highlights that 33–46% of patients had better control of their BP adjusted on HBPM the same stand true for patient with chronic kidney diseases where the accurate monitoring BP is needed for diagnosis and treatment.[36]

In an another challenging telemedicine study, 111 subjects with uncontrolled BP on single drug therapy were trained to self-monitor their home BP and self-titrate drug treatment after informing the monitoring center. Most of them were compliant, i.e., 78% in this 8-week program, 80% were satisfied. BP was well controlled in 71% by self-titrating and a significant decline in home BP was achieved.[37]

Many evidences and data are available from recently published studies which have testified the utility of HBPM for initial diagnosis, control of BP, and long-term control of BP. The wide application of this method in the management of hypertension in clinical practice has been endorsed by recent American and European guidelines.[2,3]

Home BP monitoring requires patient to be well informed, some patient may overuse the device, and prone to anxiety and more fluctuation and have tendency to titrate the dose of drug every day and resulting into poor net control of BP. Detection of excessive BP-lowering effect of antihypertensive drugs in patients with white coat phenomenon can help in avoidance of over treatment. Similarly under treatment seen in patient with masked hypertension can be better judged.[38]

Role of HBPM in Clinical Practice

The available evidence justifies the significant role of HBPM in decision making in hypertensive patients. The ABPM and HBPM despite their similarities, assess different aspects of the BP profile. Regarding the application of HBPM in the diagnosis of hypertension, particularly in cases with diagnostic disagreement with office measurements (white-coat or masked hypertension) remains good choice. A modified version of this strategy has been suggested which allows treatment decisions to be made on the basis of home measurements in subjects with home BP less than 125/75 mm Hg (no drug therapy) or greater than 135/84 mm Hg (initiation of drug therapy), whereas in intermediate home BP values, ambulatory BP can be helpful.[39]

The detection of masked hypertension often poses controversies in terms of who are the subjects to be screened. Many patients with borderline office BP levels, or elevated office BP normalized on repeat.

Blood pressure measurement, as anxiety factor, is reduced. The other group likely to benefit are those at high total cardiovascular risk and all treated hypertensive. Home BP monitoring is also useful in order to solve the discrepancies of diagnosis of office and home measurements (white coat or masked hypertension).[40]

Home blood pressure monitoring can be considered as the optimal method for the long-term follow-up and adherence for drug management because of its wider availability and easy affordability as compared to ABPM.[3,41] The evidence shows that hypertension control rates also improves by implementing HBPM all treated hypertensives.[2,3] A statement by the American Heart Association and the American Society of Hypertension endorsed that, as it is the case with home monitoring of glucose in diabetes, HBPM device may be prescribed by healthcare providers,[2] but it should be assured that patient should not take treatment decisions exclusively on the basis of home BP measurements. Many studies have shown that hypertensive patients observe over and under report their home BP values.[42]

CONCLUSION

In the present era value of both HBPM and ABPM remains extremely useful in hypertension management, with some overlap of their clinical indications. However, because of the important scientific advancement taking place in the field of HBPM, it may be expected that the number of HBPM applications and indications will be increasing, making this approach more acceptable over other methods. Further studies on HBPM with prognostic stratification of hypertensive patients are needed to increase its utility. Finally, automated BP measuring devices combining the functionalities and advantages of both ABPM and HBPM will yield more useful data for better management of hypertension.

REFERENCES

1. O'Brien E, Asmar R, Beilin L, et al. European Society of Hypertension recommendations for conventional, ambulatory and home blood pressure measurement. J Hypertens. 2003;21:821-48.
2. Lovibond K, Jowett S, Barton P, et al. Cost-effectiveness of options for the diagnosis of high blood pressure in primary care: a modelling study. Lancet. 2011;378:1219-30.
3. Parati G, Stergiou GS, Asmar R, et al. European society of hypertension guidelines for blood pressure monitoring at home: a summary report of the Second International Consensus Conference on Home Blood Pressure Monitoring. J Hypertens. 2008;26:1505-26.
4. Stergiou GS, Bliziotis IA. Home blood pressure monitoring in the diagnosis and treatment of hypertension. Am J Hypertens. 2011;24:123-34.
5. Nesbitt SD, Amerena JV, Grant E, et al. Home blood pressure as a predictor of future blood pressure stability in borderline hypertension. The Tecumseh Study. Am J Hyperten. 1997;10:1270-80.
6. Stergiou GS, Zourbaki AS, Skeva I, et al. White coat effect detected using self-monitoring of blood pressure at home comparison with ambulatory blood pressure. Am J Hypertens.1998;11(7):820-27.
7. Comas A, González-Nuevo JP, Plaza F, et al. Home self-monitoring of arterial pressure: identification of the white coat reaction. Aten Primaria. 1999;24:5-11.
8. Stergiou GS, Nasothimiou E, Giovas P, et al. Diagnosis of hypertension in children and adolescents based on home versus ambulatory blood pressure monitoring. J Hypertens. 2008;26:1556-62.

9. Agarwal R, Andersen MJ, Bishu K, et al. Home blood pressure monitoring improves the diagnosis of hypertension in hemodialysis patients. Kidney Int. 2006;69:900-6.
10. Shimbo D, Kuruvilla S, Haas D, et al. Preventing misdiagnosis of ambulatory hypertension: algorithm using office and home blood pressures. J Hypertens. 2009;27:1775-83.
11. Masding MG, Jones JR, Bartley E, et al. Assessment of blood pressure in patients with type 2 diabetes: comparison between home blood pressure monitoring, clinic blood pressure measurement and 24-h ambulatory blood pressure monitoring. Diabet Med. 2001;18:431-7.
12. Stergiou GS, Karpettas N, Kapoyiannis A, et al. Home blood pressure monitoring in children and adolescents: a systematic review. J Hypertens. 2009;27:1941-7.
13. Mallion JM, Genes N ,Vaur L, et al. Blood pressure levels, risk factors and antihypertensive treatments; Lessons from SHEAF study. J Hum Hpertens. 2001;15(12):841-848.
14. Bobrie G, Chatellier G, Genes N, et al. Cardiovascular prognosis of "masked hypertension" detected by blood pressure self-measurement in elderly treated hypertensive patients. JAMA. 2004;291:1342-9.
15. Broege PA, James GD, Pickering TG. Management of hypertension in the elderly using home blood pressures. Blood Press Monit. 2001;6:139-44.
16. Staessen JA, Den Hond E, Keary L, et al. Treatment of hypertension based on home or office blood pressure (THOP) trial investigators. Antihypertensive treatment based on blood pressure measurement at home or in the physician's office: a randomized controlled trial. JAMA. 2004;291:955-64.
17. Verberk WJ, Kroon AA, Lenders JW, et al. Home versus office measurement, reduction of unnecessary treatment study investigators. Self-measurement of blood pressure at home reduces the need for antihypertensive drugs: a randomized, controlled trial. Hypertension. 2007;50:1019-25.
18. Tobe SW, Hunter K, Geerts R, et al. Canadian Hypertension Society. IMPPACT: Investigation of medical professionals and patients achieving control together. Can J Cardiol. 2008;24:205-8.
19. Niiranen TJ, Kantola IM, Vesalainen R, et al. A comparison of home measurement and ambulatory monitoring of blood pressure in the adjustment of antihypertensive treatment. Am J Hypertens. 2006;19(5):468-74.
20. Zarnke KB, Feagan BG, Mahon JL, et al. A randomized study comparing a patient-directed hypertension management strategy with usual office-based care. Am J Hypertens. 1997;10:58-67.
21. McManus RJ, Mant J, Bray EP, et al. Telemonitoring and self-management in the control of hypertension (TASMINH2): a randomised controlled trial. Lancet. 2010;376(9736):163-72.
22. Staessen JA, Den Hond E, Celis H, et al. Treatment of Hypertension Based on Home or Office Blood Pressure (THOP) Trial Investigators. Antihypertensive treatment based on blood pressure measurement at home or in the physician's office: a randomized controlled trial. JAMA. 2004;291:955-64.
23. Verberk WJ, Kroon AA, Lenders JW, et al. Home versus office measurement, reduction of unnecessary treatment study investigators. Self-measurement of blood pressure at home reduces the need for antihypertensive drugs: a randomized, controlled trial. Hypertension. 2007;50:1019-25.
24. Ishikawa J, Carroll DJ, Kuruvilla S, et al. Changes in home versus clinic blood pressure with antihypertensive treatments: a meta-analysis. Hypertension. 2008;52:856-64.
25. Pickering TG. Morning hypertension. J Clin Hypertens (Greenwich). 2007;9: 224-8.
26. Mancia G, Zanchetti A, Agabiti-Rosei E, et al. Ambulatory blood pressure is superior to clinic blood pressure in predicting treatment-induced regression of left ventricular hypertrophy. SAMPLE Study Group. Study on Ambulatory Monitoring of Blood Pressure and Lisinopril Evaluation. Circulation. 1997;95:1464-70.
27. Ménard J, Serrurier D, Bautier P, et al. Crossover design to test antihypertensive drugs with self-recorded blood pressure. Hypertension. 1988;11:153-9.
28. Mengden T, Binswanger B, Weisser B, et al. An evaluation of self-measured blood pressure in a study with a calcium-channel antagonist versus a beta blocker. Am J Hypertens. 1992;5:154-60.
29. Vaur L, Dubroca I, Genès N, et al. Superiority of home blood pressure measurements over office measurements for testing antihypertensive drugs. Blood Press Monit. 1998;3:107-114.
30. Imai Y, Ohkubo T, Chonan K, et al. Usefulness of home blood pressure measurements in assessing the effect of treatment in a single-blind placebo-controlled open trial. J Hypertens. 2001;19:179-85.
31. Beitelshees AL, Gong Y, Bailey KR, et al. Comparison of office, ambulatory, and home blood pressure antihypertensive response to atenolol and hydrochlorothiazide. J Clin Hypertens. 2010;12:14-21.
32. Ménard J, Chatellier G, Day M, et al. Self-measurement of blood pressure at home to evaluate drug effects by the trough: peak ratio. J Hypertens Suppl. 1994;12:S21-5.
33. Stergiou GS, Efstathiou SP, Skeva II, et al. Comparison of the smoothness index, the trough: peak ratio and the morning: evening ratio in assessing the features of the antihypertensive drug effect. J Hypertens. 2003;21(5):913-20.
34. Cappuccio FP, Kerry SM, Forbes L, et al. Blood pressure control by home monitoring: meta-analysis of randomised trials. BMJ. 2004;329:145.
35. McManus RJ, Mant J, Roalfe A, et al. Targets and self-monitoring in hypertension: randomised controlled trial and cost effectiveness analysis. BMJ. 2005;331:493.
36. Obara T, Ohkubo T, Asayama K, et al. J-HOME Study Group. Home blood pressure measurements associated with better blood pressure control: the J-HOME study. J Hum Hypertens. 2008;22:197-204.
37. Agarwal R, Light RP. Chronobiology of arterial hypertension in hemodialysis patients: implications for home blood pressure monitoring. Am J Kidney Dis. 2009;54:693-701.
38. Rogers MA, Small D, Buchan DA, et al. Home monitoring service improves mean arterial pressure in patients with essential hypertension. A randomized, controlled trial. Ann Intern Med. 2001;134:1024-32.
39. Bobrie G, Postel-Vinay N, Delonca J, et al. Self-measurement and self-titration in hypertension: a pilot telemedicine study. Am J Hypertens. 2007;20:1314-20.
40. Pickering TG, White WB, Giles TD, et al. When and how to use self (home) and ambulatory blood pressure monitoring. J Am Soc Hypertens. 2010;4:56-61.
41. McGowan N, Padfield PL. Self-blood pressure monitoring: a worthy substitute for ambulatory blood pressure? J Hum Hypertens. 2010;24(12):801-6.
42. Myers MG. Reporting bias in self-measurement of blood pressure. Blood Press Monit. 2001;6:181-3.

SECTION 5

Chronic Coronary Artery Disease

CHAPTER 28

Best Method for Risk Stratification in CAD—Anatomy, Physiology, or Both

Pawan K Sharma, Kewal C Goswami

INTRODUCTION

The prevalence of cardiovascular diseases, especially coronary artery disease (CAD), is increasing in India like an epidemic and has become an important public health problem. The disease of circulatory system is the number one cause of mortality amongst the top eight registered causes of death. In 2015, the diseases of circulatory system was responsible for 33.2% of all the registered deaths with males accounting for 32.8% and females being 33.9%. Out of these, ischemic heart disease was listed in 26.9% as the cause of death. The diseases of pulmonary circulation and other heart diseases were responsible for 45.3% of deaths.

The age distribution of diseases of circulatory system was 19.1% between ages 25 and 34 years, 27.3% between ages 35 and 44 years, 35.6–45.6% for age of more than or equal to 45 years and 25.2% for population of more than or equal to70 years of age.[1]

This data suggests that almost 75% of deaths occur in the younger working age group leading to massive economic burden on the society. In the INTERHEART study, 8 common risk factors explained more than 90% of acute myocardial infarctions (MIs) in South Asian and Indian patients.[2] These risk factors were dyslipidemia, smoking or tobacco use, hypertension, diabetes, abdominal obesity, lack of physical activity, less intake of fruits and vegetables, and psychological stress. The interventions to prevent and treat heart disease could be very cost effective because most of the deaths occur in the younger working age group. A vast number of patients are seen in the medical centers or hospitals for treatment of CAD. Therefore, in addition to primary prevention, the secondary prevention by identifying appropriate risk stratification and revascularization strategies can play a significant role in preventing morbidity and mortality.

In the outpatient settings, various stress tests can be helpful in defining the extent of ischemia and coronary risks and decide whether medical therapy is optimal or patient should be referred for revascularization. While in the catheterization laboratory, the risks involved in treating severe CAD by percutaneous coronary intervention (PCI) can be assessed by various risk scores and the most commonly used risk score now a days is the SYNTAX score (SS).

In order to standardize the severity and extent of CAD, the SS was developed in 2006 as part of the SYNTAX (Synergy between PCI with Taxus and Cardiac Surgery) trial.[3] The SS can be useful in predicting adverse ischemic events in patients undergoing PCI.[4-6]

METHODS FOR RISK STRATIFICATION IN CAD

Noninvasive Methods

- Exercise treadmill test (ETT)
- Myocardial perfusion SPECT study
- Stress echocardiography
- Coronary calcium score assessment
- Coronary computed tomography (CTA) angiography without or with fractional flow reserve (FFR).

Invasive Methods (in the Catheterization Laboratory)

- Invasive coronary angiography
- Invasive coronary angiography with FFR.

RISK STRATIFICATION USING NONINVASIVE METHODS

If a patient is having symptoms suggesting acute coronary syndrome, then he should directly go to the catheterization laboratory for defining the coronary anatomy and possible revascularization. If a patient has no symptoms or has mild symptoms but CAD is suspected, then the risk can be assessed by noninvasive testing which would help to decide the need for medical therapy or invasive coronary angiography.

Exercise Treadmill Test

Treadmill test is most commonly used for assessing the exercise capacity of an individual with interpretable baseline ECG. The exercise tolerance is measured in metabolic equivalents (METs). One MET unit is defined as the energy expenditure at rest equivalent to an oxygen uptake of about 3.5 mL O_2/min/kg body weight. The sensitivity of ETT has been reported between 65 and 70%.[7] Although, ETT helps in identifying high risk patients who may have severe CAD, but the leads showing ST depression do not localize the site of ischemia or the culprit vessel and do not assess the extent of myocardial ischemia.

Myocardial Perfusion SPECT Study

The risk of cardiac mortality is considered low if less than 1%, intermediate 1–3%, and high-risk more than 3% per year. A normal myocardial perfusion SPECT study (MPS) means a low-risk for cardiac events.[8] The risk of having cardiac events increases with worsening of perfusion abnormalities.[9] Therefore, patients with normal myocardial perfusion study or with mild abnormalities on the perfusion study can be treated medically without having any anatomical assessment by angiography. On the other hand, patients with significantly extensive and severe defects are considered at high-risk for having cardiac events and should be referred for coronary angiography and possible revascularization. Similarly, patient with mild perfusion abnormalities but certain high risk features still should be referred for coronary angiography. These high-risk features include poor left ventricular systolic function,[10] transient ischemic dilatation,[11] increased lung uptake, and diabetes,[12] atrial fibrillation,[13] those having pharmacological stress test,[14] high pretest probability of CAD,[15,16] very abnormal stress ECG.[17]

If patients have normal or mild ischemia, the medical therapy as initial treatment strategy has been shown to have better survival than referring patients for revascularization. When there is moderate-to-severe ischemia as defined by more than 10% of the total myocardial ischemia, the revascularization has a better survival benefit over the medical therapy. This supports the finding that myocardial perfusion study can help stratify the risks of revascularization versus medical therapy in individual patients.[18]

Stress Echocardiogram

Based on 16-segment analysis, the stress echo helps to locate and define the extent of wall motion abnormality predicting the culprit vessel causing the ischemia. On an average, the sensitivity of stress echo is around 84% and specificity is about 87%.[19]

Coronary Calcium Score

The coronary calcium score is useful in risk stratification of asymptomatic patients with intermediate clinical risk but it does not provide much prognostic value in patients with known CAD. Although, 95% of patients having first MI have abnormal coronary calcium score but still about 5% people can have MI without having any coronary artery calcification.[20] If the coronary calcium score is more than 400 and patient is free of symptoms, the patient can be referred for stress testing to assess the risk. In asymptomatic patients with coronary calcium score less than 100, no further testing is warranted. However, if the coronary calcium score is between 100 and 400 and patient has risk factors such as metabolic syndrome, diabetes, chest pain, advanced age, the stress test may be useful.[21] It appears that patients with high calcium score but normal myocardial perfusion study are at low-risk in the short-term but may be at higher risk in the long-term. Therefore, aggressive medical therapy with statins is recommended in this population.[22]

Coronary Computed Tomography Angiogram

Sometimes, the MPS is normal in patients with significant multi vessel disease due to balanced ischemia. Therefore, it may be replaced by the coronary CTA because the coronary CTA will more likely be abnormal in patients who would need some revascularization. If coronary CTA is normal, then aggressive medical therapy would be appropriate. If the coronary CTA shows severe CAD, then patient can be directly referred for coronary angiography.

If the results of coronary CTA are equivocal for any severe disease or if it clearly shows severe disease but the anatomy is not suitable for any kind of revascularization, then the patient can be referred for stress myocardial perfusion testing to assess for extent of ischemia before considering revascularization. The stress MPS can also be considered in patients with very dense calcification because coronary CTA is not very helpful in such situations.

On the other hand, coronary CTA may be useful in patients with questionable MPS results or if there is discrepancy between the clinical picture and ECG changes during stress and MPS results.

It is possible that with increasing role of coronary CTA, the MPS may be limited to patients with equivocal CTA or to assess the extent of ischemia in patients with known CAD.

It is, therefore, suggested that the noninvasive assessment of coronary anatomy by coronary CTA has a complimentary role to the physiological assessment with myocardial stress testing and FFR.

Anatomical SYNTAX Score Derived from Coronary Computed Tomography Angiogram (Developed in 2013)

Coronary CTA is a noninvasive method to obtain similar information about coronary anatomy as invasive angiography. Overall, a good correlation has been found between the SS calculated by coronary CTA and the invasive coronary angiography. Coronary CTA can risk stratify patients by the presence and severity of obstructive disease along with the presence of nonobstructive coronary plaque. Patients with absence of obstructive coronary disease and coronary plaque have a very low-risk of coronary events (<0.3% annual risk).[23]

Mortality and coronary event rates increase as number of vessels with obstructive disease or total plaque burden increases.[24]

Noninvasive Functional SYNTAX Score (Developed in 2015)

Coronary CTA technique is useful in generating a three-dimensional (3D) coronary tree for a specific patient. By using the computer generated fluid dynamics, blood flow in the vascular bed can be simulated and a noninvasive FFR can be calculated. This FFR derived from CT, i.e., FFR_{CT} has shown to have a high correlation with invasive FFR.[25] The coronary CTA technique can be very useful in calculating a noninvasive functional SYNTAX score (fSS) by recalculating the SS counting only the ischemia-producing lesions with FFR_{CT} less than 0.80. In some cases, the FFR_{CT} cannot be calculated due to image artifacts, extensive coronary calcification or prior revascularization with metallic stents. Overall, the FFR_{CT} can be performed in more than 85% of cases.[26] This noninvasive way of calculating FFR_{CT} provides a combined anatomical and physiological risk stratification before an invasive procedure is undertaken. On the other hand, FFR_{CT} also has the potential advantage of calculating fSS after the invasive coronary angiography without needing a pressure wire.

RISK STRATIFICATION USING INVASIVE METHODS

Risk Scores

The first risk score described in 1977 was the Duke Jeopardy Score[26] which was validated in 1985.[27] It demonstrated that by estimating the myocardium at risk on the basis of the particular location of coronary artery stenosis gave more prognostic information than the number of diseased arteries involved. The prognostic ability of this score was significantly improved by including the degree of coronary artery stenosis and by attributing a higher score to the disease of the left anterior descending artery than to other coronary arteries.

Later on, depending on the type of lesion, another classification was proposed which was designed as a guide to estimate the possibility of successful balloon angioplasty and its possible complications.[28,29] Lesions were classified as types A, B, or C, based on the angiographic characteristics such as lesion length, tortuosity, calcification, thrombus, bifurcation, total occlusion. The success rate of balloon angioplasty with type A lesions was more than 85%, type B: 60–85%, and type C: less than 60%. In addition to predicting outcomes after balloon angioplasty, it also predicted the outcomes whether patient received bare-metal stent[30] or drug-eluting stent.[31]

The SYNTAX Score

Based on the number, location, complexity and functional impact of obstructive lesions noted on invasive coronary angiography, the SS was developed in 2006 and provides a standardized coronary artery tree. The distributions of the coronary arteries are mapped based on the ARTS (Arterial Revascularization Therapies Studies) investigators' modification of coronary tree segments.[32,33] The amount of jeopardized myocardium depends on the fraction of blood supplied to the left ventricle by each coronary segment.[34] A clinically significant lesion is defined as a diameter narrowing of more than or equal to 50% in vessels with a minimum diameter of more than or equal to 1.5 mm. The sum of individual lesion scores gives the final SS which is purely an anatomical tool and is described as low 0–22, intermediate 23–32, or high more than 32.[4]

Prognostic Value of SYNTAX Score

The SYNTAX trial showed that in patients with multi vessel and/or left main (LM) CAD,[4] at 1 year follow-up, major adverse cardiovascular and cerebrovascular events (MACCE), which included all-cause death, MI, stroke, and target vessel revascularization (TVR), were significantly lower in the coronary artery bypass graft (CABG) group (12.4%) compared with the PCI group (17.8%, p = 0.002). At 1 year, MACCE rates progressively increased in patients with higher SS who were treated with PCI. Even the 5 year follow-up results of the SYNTAX trial showed that CABG was associated with significantly lower MACCE rates in patients with SS more than 32 and between 23 and 32 compared with the PCI cohort.[35]

It has been noted that SS more than 34 is associated with significantly higher rates of ischemic events in patients undergoing PCI for unprotected LM than in those undergoing CABG. These results suggest that CABG should be considered in patients with higher SS with multi vessel is ease and in patients with unprotected LM CAD.[36] Similarly, in patients with Non ST-segment elevation acute coronary syndrome and ST-segment elevation MI, patients in the upper tertile of SS had significantly higher rates of ischemic events than did patients in the lower 2 tertiles. At 1 year, the SS was an independent predictor of all-cause death, cardiac death, and MI.[37-39]

In contrast to patients undergoing PCI, SS seems not to influence clinical outcomes after CABG. Both mortality and composite ischemic outcomes in patients undergoing CABG are independent from SS.[4,40,41]

Various Risk Scores Derived from SYNTAX Score

Since, SS is purely an anatomical score and it does not take into account the effect of clinical factors, patients with equivalent scores may have different short- and long-term outcomes, depending on the presence of comorbidities.[42] To overcome these limitations and to improve the predictive ability of SS, different clinical-based scores have been combined with SS. These are global risk classification (GRC), clinical SYNTAX score (cSS), logistic clinical SS, fSS, residual SYNTAX score (rSS), CABG SYNTAX score, and SYNTAX score II (SS II).

Global Risk Classification (Developed in 2010)

The GRC is a combination of SS and Euro SCORE (European System for Cardiac Operative Risk Evaluation). The GRC showed a net reclassification improvement of 26% in patient undergoing PCI for LM CAD.[43] Additionally, GRC can identify a low-risk cohort of patients that could be safely treated with PCI.[44]

Clinical SYNTAX Score (Developed in 2010)

The cSS is determined by multiplying the SS with the modified ACEF (age, creatinine clearance, and ejection fraction) score. The cSS has a better discriminatory power for 5-year mortality and MACE than either SS alone or modified ACEF score did.[45] However, the main limitations of cSS is that it has a poor discriminative power for ischemic outcomes in the lower 2 tertiles and that its prognostic performance is poorer for pooled patients with double- and triple-vessel CAD than for patients with only triple vessel CAD.[45]

Logistic Clinical SYNTAX Score (Developed in 2011)

The logistic cSS variables were selected on the basis of logistic regression coefficients, thus developing score charts for individual risk assessment. This score had substantial improvement in the predictive ability for 1-year all-cause death compared with SS.[46]

Functional SYNTAX Score (Developed in 2011)

The anatomically severe lesion may not be physiologically significant when assessed by FFR, therefore, fSS was proposed which incorporated FFR with SS. The fSS reclassified 32% of patients from the high to medium risk SS whereas 59% of the cases were reclassified from medium-risk to the low-risk group.[47] The fSS was also associated with better inter- and intra-observer reproducibility.

Residual SYNTAX Score (Developed in 2012)

Since, incomplete revascularization is associated with an increased risk of adverse ischemic outcomes after PCI in patients with high SS,[36] the rSS was proposed to quantify residual CAD after PCI. The rSS calculation is similar to SS, except that it is calculated after PCI. The rSS is an independent predictor of all cause death, cardiac mortality, MI, unplanned revascularization, and MACE at 1 year.[48]

Coronary Artery Bypass Graft SYNTAX Score (Developed in 2013)

The original SS can be used only for native CAD and not for patients with CABG, therefore, CABG SS was developed.[49] First the baseline SS of native vessels is calculated and then points are subtracted depending on the graft functionality and final CABG SS is calculated. The major limitation of this score is that it does not take into consideration the type of graft used. The study suggests higher all cause death and MACE in patients with high CABG SS but larger studies are needed to validate its prognostic capabilities.

SYNTAX Score II (Developed in 2012)

The SS II combines anatomical SS with patient's clinical characteristics and the anatomical presence of unprotected LM coronary disease. These clinical characteristics include the age, creatinine clearance, left ventricular ejection fraction, peripheral vascular disease, female sex, and chronic obstructive pulmonary disease. This score predicts the 4 years all-cause mortality in patients with LM/multi vessel CAD and helps making a decision between CABG or PCI in such patients. A nomogram for SS II has also been proposed for bedside application.[50]

POTENTIAL USES AND LIMITATIONS OF THE TRADITIONAL SYNTAX SCORE

The traditional SS can be used as a standardized tool is assessing the extent and severity of CAD in a uniform fashion and enrolling patients in randomized controlled trials. It may help clinicians to decide the most appropriate revascularization modality (PCI vs. CABG). It may also help predict procedural outcomes, especially when discussing with patients and their relatives regarding potential outcomes associated with a given revascularization strategy.[51]

The SS has a major limitation that it is purely an angiographic score and does not take into account the role of comorbidities for risk stratification of patients undergoing PCI. Secondly, the SS has significant inter-observer variability commonly noted on visual estimation of vessel stenosis. Similar to any angiographic assessment, the SS does not identify vulnerable plaques or predict coronary plaque burden. SS does not predict the effect of viable or nonviable myocardium beyond the stenosis. The SS cannot appreciate the major differences in the operator skills and experience in dealing with complex procedures, the effect of new revascularization techniques or availability of various devices.

CONCLUSION

In patients with normal or mild ischemia on stress study, the medical therapy has better survival and should be tried first. High-risk patients with large area of myocardium at risk (>10% myocardium) should be referred for coronary angiography and will benefit from revascularization strategy. In asymptomatic patients with coronary calcium score less than 100, no further cardiac work up is needed whereas asymptomatic patients with coronary calcium score more than 400 should be referred for myocardial perfusion stress for risk stratification.

The SS II which involves the combination of anatomical and physiological variables along with clinical comorbidities represents a significant improvement in predicting the prognosis and procedural outcomes of revascularization strategies such as PCI or CABG in today's clinical practice.

With improvements in coronary CTA techniques and computer models, the calculation of fSS with the possibility of determining FFR noninvasively[52] may have a significant effect in predicting prognosis of different revascularization strategies. The newly developed technique of calculating CTA-derived SS provides an accurate assessment of patient's coronary tree prior to cardiac catheterization. Furthermore, the physiological assessment by calculating the FFR_{CT} with the calculation of the noninvasive fSS will allow for an individualized risk stratification of CAD without unnecessarily undergoing invasive coronary angiography.

Thus, the integration of coronary anatomy and physiology with the comorbidities offers a personalized risk stratification of CAD to help the physicians in the decision making process for an appropriate revascularization strategy.

REFERENCES

1. Registrar General of India. (2015). Report on Medical Certification of Cause of Death 2015, New Delhi India: Office of the Registrar General. [online] Available from www.censusindia.gov.in [Accessed August 2018].
2. Joshi PP, Islam S, Pais P, et al. Risk factors for early myocardial infarction in South Asians compared with individuals in other countries. JAMA. 2007;297:286-94.
3. Sianos G, Morel MA, Kappetein AP, et al. The SYNTAX score: an angiographic tool grading the complexity of coronary artery disease. Euro Intervention. 2005;1:219-27.
4. Serruys PW, Morice MC, Kappetein AP, et al. for the SYNTAX Investigators. Percutaneous coronary intervention versus coronary artery bypass grafting for severe coronary artery disease. N Engl J Med. 2009;360:961-72.
5. Capodanno D, Di Salvo ME, Cincotta G, et al. Usefulness of the SYNTAX score for predicting clinical outcome after percutaneous coronary intervention of unprotected left main coronary artery disease. Circ Cardiovasc Interv. 2009;2:302-8.
6. Valgimigli M, Serruys PW, Tsuchida K, et al. Cyphering the complexity of coronary artery disease using the SYNTAX score to predict clinical outcome in patients with three-vessel lumen obstruction undergoing percutaneous coronary intervention. Am J Cardiol. 2007;99:1070-81.
7. Gianrossi R, Detrano R, Mulvihill D, et al. Exercise-induced ST depression in the diagnosis of coronary artery disease: a meta-analysis. Circulation. 1989; 80: 87-98.
8. Hachamovitch R, Shaw L, Berman DS. Methodological considerations in the assessment of noninvasive testing using outcomes research: pitfalls and limitations. Prog Cardiovasc Dis. 2000;43:215-30.
9. Berman DS, Abidov A, Kang X, et al. Prognostic validation of a 17 segment score derived from a 20 segment score for myocardial perfusion SPECT interpretation. J Nucl Cardiol. 2004;11:414-23.
10. Sharir T, Germano G, Kang X, et al. Prediction of myocardial infarction versus cardiac death by gated myocardial perfusion SPECT: risk stratification by the amount of stress-induced ischemia and the poststress ejection fraction. J Nucl Med. 2001;42:831-37.
11. Abidov A, Bax JJ, Hayes SW, et al. Transient ischemic dilation ratio of the left ventricle is a significant predictor of future cardiac events in patients with otherwise normal myocardial perfusion SPECT. J Am Coll Cardiol. 2003;42:1818-25.
12. Berman DS, Kang X, Hayes SW, et al. Adenosine myocardial perfusion single-photon emission computed tomography in women compared with men: impact of diabetes mellitus on incremental prognostic value and effect on patient management. J Am Coll Cardiol. 2003;41:1125-33.
13. Santos MM, Abidov A, Hayes SW, et al. Prognostic implications of myocardial perfusion SPECT in patients with atrial fibrillation [abstract]. J Nucl Med. 2002;43 (suppl):98P.
14. Hachamovitch R, Berman DS, Shaw LJ, et al. Incremental prognostic value of myocardial perfusion single photon emission computed tomography for the prediction of cardiac death: differential stratification for risk of cardiac death and myocardial infarction. Circulation. 1998;97:535-43.
15. Poornima IG, Miller TD, Christian TF, et al. Utility of myocardial perfusion imaging in patients with low risk treadmill scores. J Am Coll Cardiol. 2004;43:194-9.
16. Hachamovitch RHS, Friedman JD, Cohen I, et al. Is there a referral bias against revascularization of patients with reduced LV ejection fraction? Influence of ejection fraction and inducible ischemia on post-SPECT management of patients without a history of CAD. J Am Coll Cardiol. 2003;42:1286-94.
17. Hachamovitch R, Berman DS, Kiat H, et al. Value of stress myocardial perfusion single photon emission computed tomography in patients with normal resting electrocardiograms: an evaluation of incremental prognostic value and cost-effectiveness. Circulation. 2002;105:823-29.
18. Hachamovitch RHS, Cohen I, Germano G, et al. Inducible ischemia is superior to EF for identification of short-term survival benefit with revascularization vs. medical therapy [abstract]. Circulation. 2002;106:II-523.
19. Roger VI, Pellikka PA, Oh JK, et al. Stress echocardiography, Part I. Exercise echocardiography: Techniques, implementation, clinical applications, and correlations. Mayo Clin Proc. 1995;70:5.
20. Pohle K, Ropers D, Maffert R, et al. Coronary calcification in young patients with first, unheralded myocardial infarction: a risk factor matched analysis by electron beam tomography. Heart. 2003;89:625-8.
21. Berman DS, Wong ND, Gransar H, et al. Relationship between stress-induced myocardial ischemia and atherosclerosis measured by coronary calcium tomography. J Am Coll Cardiol. 2004;44:923-30.
22. Berman DS, Gransar H, Rozanski A, et al. Does coronary calcium add incremental value for predicting cardiac events when myocardial perfusion SPECT is normal [abstract]? Circulation. 2004;110:III-561-2.
23. Min JK, Dunning A, Lin FY, et al. Age and sex related difference in all-cause mortality risk based on coronary computed tomography angiography findings results from the international multicenter CONFIRM (Coronary CT angiography evaluation for clinical outcome: an International multicenter registry) of 23854 patients without known coronary artery disease. J Am Coll Cardiol. 2011;58:849-60.
24. Hadamitzky M, Taubert S, Deseive S, et al. Prognostic value of coronary computed tomography angiography during 5 years of follow up in patients with suspected coronary artery disease. Eur Heart J. 2013;34:3277-85.
25. Norgaard BL, Leipsic J, Gaur S, et al. Diagnostic performance of noninvasive fractional flow reserve derived from coronary computed tomography angiography in suspected coronary artery disease: the NXT trial (Analysis of Coronary Blood Flow Using CT Angiography: Next Steps). J Am Coll Cardiol. 2014;63:1145-55.
26. Dash H, Johnson RA, Dinsmore RE, et al. Cardiomyopathic syndrome due to coronary artery disease. I: Relation to angiographic extent of coronary disease and to remote myocardial infarction. Br Heart J. 1977;39:733-9.
27. Califf RM, Phillips HR 3rd, Hindman MC, et al. Prognostic value of a coronary artery jeopardy score. J Am Coll Cardiol. 1985;5:1055-63.
28. Ryan TJ, Faxon DP, Gunnar RM, et al. Guidelines for percutaneous transluminal angioplasty: a report of the American College of Cardiology/ American Heart Association Task Force on Assessment of Diagnostic and Therapeutic Cardiovascular Procedures (Subcommittee on Percutaneous Transluminal Coronary Angioplasty). J Am Coll Cardiol. 1988;12:529-45.
29. Ellis SG, Vandormael MG, Cowley MJ, et al. Coronary morphologic and clinical determinants of procedural outcome with angioplasty for multivessel coronary disease: implications for patient selection. Circulation. 1990;82:1193-202.
30. Kastrati A, Schomig A, Flezi S, et al. Prognostic value of the modified American College of Cardiology/ American Heart Association stenosis morphology classification for long-term angiographic and clinical outcome after coronary stent placement. Circulation. 1999;100:1285-90.
31. Khattab AA, Hamm CW, Senges J, et al. Prognostic value of the modified American College of Cardiology/ American Heart Association lesion morphology classification for clinical outcome after sirolimus- eluting coronary stent placement (results of the prospective multicenter German Cypher Registry). Am J Cardiol. 2008;101:477-82.
32. Austen WG, Edwards JE, Frye RL, et al. A reporting system on patients evaluated for coronary artery disease: report of the Ad Hoc Committee for Grading of Coronary Artery Disease, Council on Cardiovascular Surgery, American Heart Association. Circulation. 1975;51:5-40.
33. Serruys PW, Unger F, van Houts BA, et al. The ARTS study (Arterial Revascularization Therapies Study) Semin Interv Cardiol. 1999;4:209-19.
34. Leaman DM, Brower RW, Meester GT, et al. Coronary artery atherosclerosis: severity of the disease, severity of angina pectoris and compromised left ventricular function. Circulation. 1981;63:285-99.
35. Mohr FW, Morice MC, Kappetein AP, et al. Coronary artery bypass graft surgery versus percutaneous coronary intervention in patients with three-vessel disease and left main coronary disease: 5 year follow-up of the randomized, clinical SYNTAX trial. Lancet. 2013;381:629-38.
36. Capodanno D, Capranzano P, Di Salvo ME, et al. Usefulness of SYNTAX score to select patients with left main coronary artery disease to be treated with coronary artery bypass graft. J Am Coll Cardiol Intv. 2009;2:731-8.

37. Palmerini T, Genereux P, Caixeta A, et al. Prognostic value of the SYNTAX score in patients with acute coronary syndromes undergoing percutaneous coronary intervention: analysis from the ACUITY (Acute Catheterization and Urgent Intervention Triage StrategY) trial. J Am Col Cardiol. 2011;57:2389-97.
38. Magro M, Nauta S, Simsek C, et al. Value of the SYNTAX score in patients treated by primary percutaneous coronary intervention for acute ST-elevation myocardial infarction: the MI SYNTAX score study. Am Heart J. 2011;161:1771-81.
39. Garg S, Sarno G, Serruys PW, et al. Prediction of 1 year clinical outcomes using the SYNTAX score in patients with acute ST-segment elevation myocardial infarction undergoing primary percutaneous coronary intervention: a substudy of the STRATEGY (Single High-Dose Bolus Tirofiban and Sirolimus-Eluting Stent Versus Abciximab and Bare Metal Stent in Acute Myocardial Infarction) and MULTISTRATEGY (Multicenter Evaluation of Single High-Dose Bolus Tirofiban Versus Abciximab With Sirolimus- Eluting Stent or Bare Metal Stent in Acute Myocardial Infarction Study) trials. J Am Coll Cardiol Intv. 2011;4:66-75.
40. Mohr FW, Rastan AJ, Serruys PW, et al. Complex coronary anatomy in coronary artery bypass graft surgery: impact of complex coronary anatomy in modern bypass surgery? Lessons Learned from the SYNTAX trial after two years. J Thorac Cardiovasc Surg. 2011;141:130-40.
41. Lemesle G, Bonello L, de Labriolle A, et al. Prognostic value of the Syntax score in patients undergoing coronary artery bypass grafting for three-vessel coronary artery disease. Catheter Cardiovasc Interv. 2009;73:612-7.
42. Romagnoli E, Burzotta F, Trani C, et al. EuroSCORE as predictor of in-hospital mortality after percutaneous coronary intervention. Heart. 2009;95:43-8.
43. Capodanno D, Miano M, Cincotta G, et al. EuroSCORE refines the predictive ability of SYNTAX score in patients undergoing left main percutaneous coronary intervention. Am Heart J. 2010;159:103-9.
44. Serruys PW, Farooq V, Vranckx P, et al. A global risk approach to identify patients with left main or 3-vessel disease who could safely and efficaciously be treated with percutaneous coronary intervention: the SYNTAX Trial at 3 years. J Am Coll Cardiol Intv. 2012;5:606-17.
45. Garg S, Sarno G, Garcia-Garcia HM, et al. A new tool for the risk stratification of patients with complex coronary artery disease: the clinical SYNTAX score. Circ Cardiovasc Interv. 2010;3:317-26.
46. Farooq V, Vergouwe Y, Raber L, et al. Combined anatomical and clinical factors for the long-term risk stratification of patients undergoing percutaneous coronary intervention: the logistic clinical SYNTAX score. Eur Heart J. 2012;33:3098-104.
47. Nam CW, Mangiacapra F, Entjes R, et al. Functional SYNTAX score for risk assessment in multivessel coronary artery disease. J Am Coll Cardiol. 2011;58:1211-8.
48. Genereux P, Palmerini T, Caixeta A, et al. Quantification and impact of untreated coronary artery disease after percutaneous coronary intervention: the residual SYNTAX (Synergy Between PCI with Taxus and Cardiac Surgery) score. J Am Coll Cardiol. 2012;59:2165-74.
49. Farooq V, Girasis C, Magro M, et al. The CABG SYNTAX Score- an angiographic tool to grade the complexity of coronary disease following coronary artery bypass graft surgery: from the SYNTAX Left Main Angiographic (SYNTAX-LE MANS) substudy. Euro Intervention. 2013;8:1277-85.
50. Farooq V, van Klaveren D, Steyerberg EW, et al. Anatomical and clinical characteristics to guide decision making between coronary artery bypass surgery and percutaneous coronary intervention for individual patients: development and validation of SYNTAX score II. Lancet. 2013;381:639-50.
51. Singh M, Rihal CS, Gersh BJ, et al. Twenty-five-year trends in in-hospital and long-term outcome after percutaneous coronary intervention: a single-institution experience. Circulation. 2007;115:2835-41.
52. Koo BK, Erglis A, Doh JH, et al. Diagnosis of ischemia-causing coronary stenoses by noninvasive fractional flow reserve computed from coronary computed tomographic angiograms: results from the prospective multicenter DISCOVER-FLOW (Diagnosis of Ischemia-Causing Stenoses Obtained Via Noninvasive Fractional Flow Reserve) study. J Am Coll Cardiol. 2011;58:1989-97.

CHAPTER 29

Screening for Coronary Artery Disease in Asymptomatic Adults

Pratap Chandra Rath, Md Abdul Azeez Asad

INTRODUCTION

Cardiovascular disease (CVD), particularly coronary artery disease (CAD), is the most important cause of death in the world. Screening asymptomatic individuals for CAD for preventive management is therefore important prior to the development of adverse events [myocardial infarction (MI), sudden cardiac arrest] that have significant morbidity and mortality.[1]

RATIONALE FOR SCREENING

Advanced CAD can exist with minimal or no symptoms, with sudden and rapidly progressive manifestations. The initial manifestation of CAD in as many as 30% patients is an acute MI, unstable angina, or sudden cardiac death (SCD). The rationale for early detection of CAD is that it might allow identification of persons at elevated risk of major adverse cardiac events (MACEs) so that appropriate intervention, either as medical therapy (aggressive lipid lowering) for risk factors or coronary revascularization therapy, can be given to improve their prognosis. Other reasons for screening include detection of CAD in certain high-risk occupations (e.g., pilots, bus drivers, etc.) where an acute event could endanger large numbers of people. Also, individuals with higher risk of coronary heart disease (CHD) who are initiating an exercise program might benefit from screening.[2]

SCREENING TESTS

The available screening tests can be divided into invasive [e.g., coronary artery angiography (CAG)] or noninvasive and functional or anatomic.

Though catheter-based CAG is the gold standard for detection of CAD, it is relatively expensive and is associated with a minor but definite risk of serious complications like atheroembolism, bleeding, MI, arrhythmias, renal failure due to iodinated contrast media, stroke, and death. Hence, for the detection of CAD in asymptomatic individuals, noninvasive techniques are usually preferred.[3]

Functional or stress testing provides physiologic evidence of clinically significant coronary artery stenoses by demonstrating the effects of diminished coronary flow reserve (CFR) on symptoms, electrocardiogram (ECG) changes, myocardial perfusion defects on scintigraphy or positron emission tomography (PET), or regional wall motion abnormalities on echocardiography.[3]

The following tests are available for the noninvasive diagnosis of CHD and are summarized in table 1:

- Exercise ECG
- Echocardiography using either exercise or pharmacologic stress
- Radionuclide myocardial perfusion imaging (rMPI) using either exercise or pharmacologic stress and imaging with either single photon emission computed tomography (SPECT) or PET
- Cardiac magnetic resonance (CMR) imaging
- Coronary computed tomography (CT), either for detection of coronary artery calcifications (CAC) or for assessing coronary artery stenosis with coronary computed tomography angiography (CCTA)
- Hybrid imaging, using either SPECT/CT, PET/CT, or PET/magnetic resonance imaging (MRI).

Electrocardiogram at Rest and Stress

The ECG at rest may show prior coronary ischemia by means of changes, such as prominent Q-wave and T-wave inversion. However, its sensitivity is very low.[4]

Twenty-four hours ambulatory ECG can increase the diagnostic efficiency in detecting ECG signs of transient ischemia, but its sensitivity for CAD is low (19–62%).[5]

Electrocardiogram during exercise showed sensitivity and specificity of 68% and 77%, respectively, in CAD diagnosis in a meta-analysis[6] with approximately 24,000 patients who underwent conventional CAG and stress ECG. Higher

TABLE 1: Screening methods for detecting asymptomatic coronary artery ischemia

Screening methods	Detection of prevalent coronary heart disease (CHD)	Comments
	Functional tests	
Resting electrocardiogram (ECG)	Low sensitivity and specificity	Widely available, low cost
Exercise ECG	Moderate sensitivity (45–61%) and specificity (70–90%)	Widely available, low cost
Stress echocardiography: 1. Exercise stress echo 2. Pharmacologic stress echo (dobutamine, adenosine, and dipyridamole)	The sensitivity and specificity are satisfactory (80–85%) Able to assess left ventricular (LV) function and valvular abnormalities	Low cost, widely available Operator dependent Difficulty in interpreting the images in obese persons
Radionuclide single proton emission computed tomography (SPECT), myocardial perfusion imaging (MPI)	Good sensitivity (80–90%) and specificity (75–90%) The most widely used test to assess silent myocardial ischemia	Moderate to high cost Widely available High negative predictive value (95%) Image quality affected by body habitus and large breasts Screening of asymptomatic patients not prognostically useful unless high-risk patients are selected
Myocardial perfusion imaging (MPI) with positron emission tomography (PET)	High sensitivity for myocardial viability studies Accurate global and regional measurements of myocardial perfusion, blood flow, and function at stress and rest in a single study	Better image quality because of higher spatial resolution, less scattered, and fewer attenuation artifacts Lower radiation exposure than SPECT Costly, not universally available
	Anatomical tests	
Coronary artery calcium score (CAC)	CAC more prevalent in people with diabetes than nondiabetes Closely associated with total coronary artery atherosclerotic plaque burden Predicts incident ischemia, CHD morbidity and mortality	Moderate to high cost No differentiation between obstructive and nonobstructive CHD Up to 25% of patients have minimal or no CAC at the time of screening
Multidetector row computed tomography (MRCT) angiography	High sensitivity (83–99%) and specificity (93–98%)	Good sensitivity, specificity, and negative predictive value. High radiation doses High cost
Magnetic resonance imaging (MRI)	Good sensitivity (83–90%) and specificity (72–84%) Delayed gadolinium hyperenhancement linked to increased risk of major cardiovascular events Not adequately investigated	Able to assess myocardial structure and function and characterize ischemic, inflammatory and various types of cardiomyopathies High cost

sensitivity was found when CAD affects three arteries. The positive predictive value of the ECG per year in predicting CAD is estimated to be 70%.[7] However, this test is often inconclusive and inappropriate due to physical disability, vascular, and neuropathic changes or resting ECG changes.

Stress Echocardiography

This noninvasive test detects motion abnormalities of the heart during exercise or pharmacological stress (dobutamine) and provides information about the size and location of the ischemic area, as well as left ventricular (LV) function.[4] In asymptomatic diabetic patients, the sensitivity and specificity for CAD diagnosis are, respectively, 81% and 85%.[8] A 3-year follow-up of asymptomatic diabetic patients with negative stress ECGs showed probability of a CV event lower than 2% every year. Limitations include difficulty in interpreting the images in obese and chronic obstructive pulmonary disease (COPD) patients and interobserver variability. The use of intravenous ultrasound contrast agents can improve endocardial border delineation and hence diagnostic accuracy.[3]

Radionuclide Myocardial Perfusion Imaging

Stress testing (exercise or pharmacologic using adenosine or dipyridamole) combined with either SPECT or PET is more sensitive for the diagnosis of CAD, in both people with and without diabetes.[9,10] This can suggest location of lesion, extent of myocardial ischemia, and LV function[4] with better sensitivity (80–90%) and specificity (75–90%) when compared with stress ECG and a high negative predictive value (95%).[11,12]

Radionuclide myocardial perfusion imaging has an important role in the diagnosis of silent myocardial ischemia and risk stratification of diabetic patients with suspected CAD. Detection of ischemia in asymptomatic diabetes (DIAD) study reported any perfusion defect or LV function abnormality in about 22% of asymptomatic diabetics.[13]

The prevalence of asymptomatic LV dysfunction [ejection fraction (EF) <50%] is 6% in men and 0.8% in women of the general population. Transient ischemic dilation (TID), defined as the apparent presence of LV dilation on post stress relative to rest images, has been linked to increased CVD risk.[14] The left ventricular shape index (LVSI), derived as the ratio of maximum 3-D short- and long-axis LV dimensions, for end-systole and end-diastole, has been shown to be an independent predictor of congestive heart failure (CHF) hospitalization.[15]

Limitations of SPECT include high cost and poor diagnostic image quality in obese patients, as well as in women and men with large breasts. Also, global reductions in myocardial perfusion, such as in the setting of left main or three-vessel CHD, can result in underestimation of ischemic burden.[3]

Positron emission tomography provides better image quality with higher spatial resolution, less scatter, and fewer attenuation artifacts and lower radiation. Myocardial perfusion imaging with PET allows accurate global and regional measurements of myocardial perfusion, myocardial blood flow, and function at stress and rest in a single study session. Fluorodeoxyglucose (18F-FDG) PET imaging has high sensitivity for the detection of hibernating or viable myocardium.[16] Coronary flow reserve (CFR = stress divided by rest myocardial blood flow) assessed by PET integrates the effects of focal stenosis, diffuse disease, and coronary microvascular function.[16]

ANATOMIC (IMAGING) TECHNIQUES

Cardiac Magnetic Resonance Imaging

This test provides an accurate means of assessing myocardial structure and function and enables characterization of the range of myocardial diseases from ischemic to inflammatory and various types of cardiomyopathy. Delayed gadolinium enhancement CMR is a marker of prior MI in patients with unsuspected CAD and has been linked with a 4-fold increased risk of MACE and a 7-fold increased risk of mortality.[17]

Coronary Artery Calcium Score

Coronary artery calcium (CAC) is a noninvasive method that detects the amount of calcium in the coronary artery,[4] using multidetector row CT or electron beam tomography. Agatston et al.[18] developed a CAC algorithm based on calcification density of the plaques. In nondiabetic persons, the CAC score threshold at which the prevalence of ischemia increases substantially is more than 400 Agatston units,[19] with lower thresholds in diabetic patients. The Multi-Ethnic Study of Atherosclerosis (MESA), with 6,814 patients without known CAD, concluded that the inclusion of the CAC in the coronary disease risk factors improved risk stratification for CAD.[20] However, Qu et al. did not find a significant association between coronary events and CAC in 269 individuals with diabetes mellitus (DM) followed up for 6 years.[21]

Coronary Artery Calcium Score Limitations

Coronary artery calcium exposes the patient to ionizing radiation. The average effective dose ranges from 0.7 to 1.8 mSv, around ten times the effective dose of a chest X-ray. Kim et al.[22] studied the lifetime excess cancer risk due to radiation exposure from a single examination at the age of 40 years and showed that for a median dose of 2.3 mSv, this risk reached 9 cancers per 100,000 men and 28 cancers per 100,000 women.

Multislice Computed Tomography Angiography

Computed tomography angiography (CTA) is a relatively simple and noninvasive method to visualize the coronary artery and detect the degree of stenosis (Fig. 1). It also provides information about the composition of the plaques, the presence of remodeling, and extension of coronary lesions.[4]

When compared to invasive angiography, multislice computed tomography (MSCT) with 64 rows of detectors, demonstrated high sensitivity (between 83 and 99%), specificity (93–98%) and negative predictive value (99%) in a total of 542 patients in nine studies.[23] However, MSCT is not able to provide functional information. Any benefit of CT angiography to identify patient subgroups for different treatment strategies remains unproven and is thus not currently routinely recommended.[24]

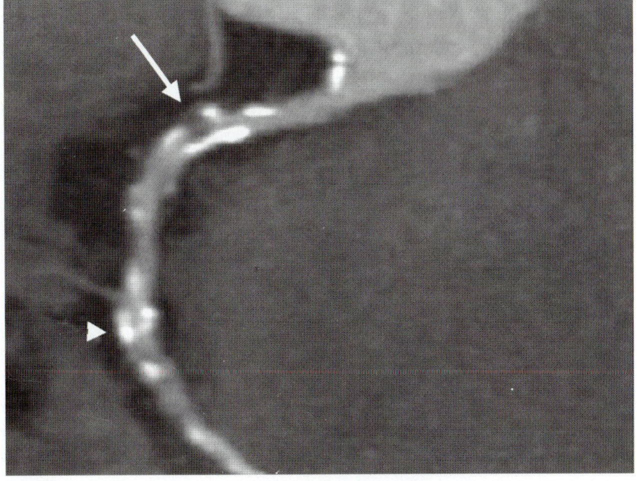

FIG. 1: Image of coronary computed tomography-angiography showing calcified plaques in right coronary artery.[32]

TABLE 2: Testing in asymptomatic patients at risk for stable coronary artery disease: 2013 European Society of Cardiology guidelines on the management of stable coronary artery disease

Recommendations	Class[a]	Level[b]
In asymptomatic adults with hypertension or diabetes a resting ECG should be considered for CV risk assessment	IIa	C
In asymptomatic adults at intermediate-risk (see SCORE for definition of intermediate-risk—www.heartscore.org) measurement of carotidintima-media thickness with screening for atherosclerotic plaques by carotid ultrasound, measurement of ankle-brachial index or measurement of coronary calcium using CT should be considered for CV risk assessment	IIa	B
In asymptomatic adults with diabetes, 40 years of age and older, measurement of coronary calcium using CT may be considered for CV risk assessment	IIb	B
In asymptomatic adults without hypertension or diabetes a resting ECG may be considered	IIb	C
In intermediate-risk asymptomatic adults (see SCORE for definition of intermediate—risk-www.heartscore.org), (including sedentary adults considering starting a vigorous exercising program), an exercise ECG may be considered for CV risk assessment partiularly when attention is paid to non-ECG markers such as exercise capacity	IIb	B
In asymptomatic adults with diabetes or asymptomatic adults with a strong family history of CAD or when previous risk assessment testing suggests high-risk of CAD, such as a coronary artery calcium score of 400 or greater stress imaging tests (MPI, stress echocardiography, and perfusion CMR) may be considered for advance CV risk assessment	IIb	C
In low- or intermediate-risk (based on SCORE) asymptomatic adults stress imaging tests are not indicated for further CV risk assessment	III	C

[a]Class of recommendation.
[b]Level of evidence.

CAD, coronary artery disease; CMR, cardiac magnetic resonance; CT, computed tomography; CV, cardiovascular; MPI, myocardial perfusion imaging; SCORE, systematic coronary risk evaluation.

OTHER METHODS FOR THE ASSESSMENT OF CARDIOVASCULAR RISK

Ankle-Brachial Index

Ankle-brachial index (ABI) is cost-effective, and can be done at the patient's bedside. Fowkes et al.[25] reported, in a meta-analysis of 48,294 healthy individuals, that a low ABI (≤0.9) was associated with increased 10-year CV mortality. However, a recent double blind randomized controlled trial did not find any improvement in outcomes after a mean follow-up of 8.2 years.[26]

High-Sensitivity C-Reactive Protein

A large meta-analysis[27] has shown that C-reactive protein (CRP) predicted vascular death in 160,039 individuals without known vascular disease after adjustment for age and sex. However, it predicted nonvascular death, e.g., death from cancer to the same extent. Recent European Society of Cardiology (ESC)[28] and American College of Cardiology/American Heart Association (ACC/AHA)[29] guidelines did not recommend high-sensitivity CRP (hs-CRP) measurement in asymptomatic low- or high-risk individuals (class III, level B).

Lipoprotein-associated Phospholipase A2

This is an enzyme expressed by inflammatory cells in atherosclerotic plaques and a marker of vascular inflammation. Tsimikas et al.[30] showed a significant relationship between lipoprotein-associated phospholipase A2 (Lp-PLA2) activity and incident CVD, but only a modest increase in C-statistic, from 0.717 to 0.737 ($p = 0.31$), compared to established risk factors alone.

Carotid Intima-Media Thickness

The measurement of the average thickness of the intima-media thickness (IMT) of the carotid artery aids in the stratification of CV risk.[31] However, the technique is not standardized with considerable variability in the IMT measurements between observers.

The ESC recommends measuring IMT by ultrasound to identify subclinical cases of CVD.[28] ACC/AHA 2013 guidelines have not recommended for or against carotid IMT (CIMT) measurement in asymptomatic individuals (Table 2).

SAFETY OF SCREENING TESTS

Unfavorable effects of screening tests include discomfort during the test, risks related to the screening test per se (e.g., allergic reactions, long-term radiation effects, or injury of coronary vessels during CAG), false-positive test results (with further unnecessary investigations), and false reassurances due to false negatives, and overdiagnosis.

Current Recommendations for Screening in Asymptomatic Adults

AHA/ACC 2013 Guideline on the Assessment of Cardiovascular Risk: A Report of the American College of ACC/AHA Task Force on Practice Guidelines

Assessment of CAC

IIb recommendation among individuals for whom a risk-based treatment decision is uncertain after formal risk estimation.

Recommendation 1

If, after quantitative risk assessment, a risk-based treatment decision is uncertain, assessment of one or more of the following—family history, hs-CRP, CAC score, or ABI—may be considered to inform treatment decision making. The National Heart, Lung, and Blood Institute (NHLBI) grade E (expert opinion); ACC/AHA class of recommendation (COR): IIb, level of evidence (LOE): B.

Recommendation 2

Routine measurement of CIMT is not recommended in clinical practice for risk assessment. NHLBI grade N (no recommendation for or against); ACC/AHA COR III: no benefit, LOE: B.

CONCLUSION

In asymptomatic individuals, a variety of tests are available for screening for CAD, including functional and anatomical imaging as well as new biomarkers. However, the use of these tests has not translated into net clinical outcomes and hence their utility must be limited, after careful consideration in patients with intermediate to high-risk for CAD. These are not indicated and therefore must be avoided as a routine strategy in low-risk individuals.

REFERENCES

1. Degrell P, Sorbets E, Feldman LJ, et al. Screening for coronary artery disease in asymptomatic individuals: why and how? Arch Cardiovasc Dis. 2015;108(12):675-82.
2. Douglas PS. (2017). Screening for coronary heart disease. [online] Available from https://www.uptodate.com/contents/screening-for-coronary-heart-disease.
3. Konstantinos M, Stavros L. Cardiovascular screening for the asymptomatic patient with diabetes: more cons than pros. J Diabetes Res. 2017;2017.
4. Tavares CA, Wajchjenberg BL, Rochitte C, et al. Screening for asymptomatic coronary artery disease in patients with type 2 diabetes mellitus. Arch Endocrinol Metab. 2016;60(2):143-51.
5. Chiariello M, Indolfi C, Cotecchia MR, et al. Asymptomatic transient ST changes during ambulatory ECG monitoring in diabetic patients. Am Heart J. 1985;110(3):529-34.
6. Gianrossi R, Detrano R, Mulvihill D, et al. Exercise-induced ST depression in the diagnosis of coronary artery disease. A meta-analysis. Circulation. 1989;80(1):87-98.
7. Bacci S, Villella M, Villella A, et al. Screening for silent myocardial ischaemia in type 2 diabetic patients with additional atherogenic risk factors: applicability and accuracy of the exercise stress test. Eur J Endocrinol. 2002;147(5):649-54.
8. Elhendy A, van Domburg RT, Poldermans D, et al. Safety and feasibility of dobutamine-atropine stress echocardiography for the diagnosis of coronary artery disease in diabetic patients unable to perform an exercise stress test. Diabetes Care. 1998;21(11):1797-802.
9. Kang X, Berman DS, Lewin H, et al. Comparative ability of myocardial perfusion single-photon emission computed tomography to detect coronary artery disease in patients with and without diabetes mellitus. Am Heart J. 1999;137(5):949-57.
10. Budoff MJ, Raggi P, Beller GA, et al. Noninvasive cardiovascular risk assessment of the asymptomatic diabetic patient: The Imaging Council of the American College of Cardiology. JACC Cardiovasc Imaging. 2016;9(2):176-92.
11. Vanzetto G, Ormezzano O, Fagret D, et al. Long-term additive prognostic value of thallium-201 myocardial perfusion imaging over clinical and exercise stress test in low to intermediate risk patients: study in 1,137 patients with 6-year follow-up. Circulation. 1999;100(14):1521-7.
12. Anand DV, Lim E, Hopkins D, et al. Risk stratification in uncomplicated type 2 diabetes: prospective evaluation of the combined use of coronary artery calcium imaging and selective myocardial perfusion scintigraphy. Eur Heart J. 2006;27(6):713-21.
13. Wackers FJ, Young LH, Inzucchi SE, et al. Detection of silent myocardial ischemia in asymptomatic diabetic subjects: the DIAD study. Diabetes Care. 2004;27(8):1954-61.
14. Weiss AT, Berman DS, Lew AS, et al. Transient ischemic dilation of the left ventricle on stress thallium-201 scintigraphy: a marker of severe and extensive coronary artery disease. J Am Coll Cardiol. 1987;9(4):752-9.
15. Abidov A, Slomka PJ, Nishina H, et al. Focal stress induced LV geometry changes independently predict presence of the angiographically significant CAD in patients undergoing myocardial perfusion SPECT. J Am Coll Cardiol. 2005;45:15A.
16. Sarikaya I. Cardiac applications of PET. Nucl Med Commun. 2015;36(10):971-85.
17. Budoff MJ, Raggi P, Beller GA, et al. Noninvasive cardiovascular risk assessment of the asymptomatic diabetic patient: The Imaging Council of the American College of Cardiology. JACC Cardiovasc Imag. 2016:9(2):176-92.
18. Agatston AS, Janowitz WR, Hildner FJ, et al. Quantification of coronary artery calcium using ultrafast computed tomography. J Am Coll Cardiol. 1990;15(4):827-32.
19. He ZX, Hedrick TD, Pratt CM, et al. Severity of coronary artery calcification by electron beam computed tomography predicts silent myocardial ischemia. Circulation. 2000;101(3):244-51.
20. Bild DE, Bluemke DA, Burke GL, et al. Multi-ethnic study of atherosclerosis: objectives and design. Am J Epidemiol. 2002;156(9):871-81.
21. Qu W, Le TT, Azen SP, et al. Value of coronary artery calcium scanning by computed tomography for predicting coronary heart disease in diabetic subjects. Diabetes Care. 2003;26(3):905-10.
22. Kim KP, Einstein AJ, Berrington de González A. Coronary artery calcification screening: estimated radiation dose and cancer risk. Arch Intern Med. 2009;169(13):1188-94.
23. Burgstahler C, Beck T, Reimann A, et al. Diagnostic accuracy of multislice computed tomography for the detection of coronary artery disease in diabetic patients. J Diabetes Complications. 2007;21(2):69-74.
24. Wolk MJ, Bailey SR, Doherty JU, et al. ACCF/AHA/ASE/ASNC/HFSA/HRS/SCAI/SCCT/SCMR/STS 2013 multimodality appropriate use criteria for the detection and risk assessment of stable ischemic heart disease: a report of the American College of Cardiology Foundation Appropriate Use Criteria Task Force, American Heart Association, American Society of Echocardiography, American Society of Nuclear Cardiology, Heart Failure Society of America, Heart Rhythm Society, Society for Cardiovascular Angiography and Interventions, Society of Cardiovascular Computed Tomography, Society for Cardiovascular Magnetic Resonance, and Society of Thoracic Surgeons. J Am Coll Cardiol. 2014;63(4):380-406.
25. Fowkes FG, Murray GD, Butcher I, et al. Ankle brachial index combined with Framingham Risk Score to predict cardiovascular events and mortality: a meta-analysis JAMA. 2008;300(2):197-208.
26. Fowkes FG, Price JF, Stewart MC, et al. Aspirin for prevention of cardiovascular events in a general population screened for a low ankle brachial index: a randomized controlled trial. JAMA. 2010;303:841-8.
27. Kaptoge S, Di Angelantonio E, Lowe G, et al. C-reactive protein concentration and risk of coronary heart disease, stroke, and mortality: an individual participant meta-analysis. Lancet. 2010;375(9709):132-40.
28. Perk J, De Backer G, Gohlke H, et al. European guidelines on cardiovascular disease prevention in clinical practice (version 2012). The Fifth Joint Task Force of the European Society of Cardiology and Other Societies on Cardiovascular Disease Prevention in Clinical Practice (constituted by representatives of nine societies and by invited experts). Eur Heart J. 2012;33(13):1635-701.

29. Goff DC Jr, Lloyd-Jones DM, Bennett G, et al. 2013 ACC/AHA guideline on the assessment of cardiovascular risk: a report of the American College of Cardiology/American Heart Association Task Force on Practice Guidelines. Circulation. 2014;129(25 Suppl 2):S49-73.
30. Tsimikas S, Willeit J, Knoflach M, et al. Lipoprotein-associated phospholipase A2 activity, ferritin levels, metabolic syndrome, and 10-year cardiovascular and non-cardiovascular mortality: results from the Bruneck study. Eur Heart J. 2009;30(1):107-15.
31. Cuspidi C, Lonati L, Macca G, et al. Cardiovascular risk stratification in hypertensive patients: impact of echocardiography. J Hypertens. 2001;19(3): 375-80.
32. Accuracy of dual-source CT coronary angiography: first experience in a high pre-test probability population without heart rate control. Scheffel H, Alkadhi H, Plass A, Vachenauer R, Desbiolles L, Gaemperli O, Schepis T, Frauenfelder T, Schertler T, Husmann L, Grunenfelder J, Genoni M, Kaufmann PA, Marincek B, Leschka S. Eur Radiol. 2006 Dec; 16(12): 2739-2747.

CHAPTER 30

Optimal Medical Management for Chronic Stable Angina in 2018

Satyavan Sharma, Naresh D Munot

INTRODUCTION

In clinical practice, the terms stable ischemic heart disease (SIHD), stable coronary artery disease (SCAD), and stable angina (SA) are used interchangeably. The pathological process underlying SIHD is an atheromatous plaque that obstructs or gradually narrows epicardial coronary arteries.

Typical SA presents with a retrosternal discomfort (constriction, pain, pressure, heaviness or burning) related to effort or mental stress, which is transient, and responds either to rest, nitrates, or disappearance of the precipitating factors. The discomfort is due to more than 70% narrowing of one or several of the major coronary arteries or more than 50% of the left main coronary artery. Microvascular dysfunction and coronary vasospasm may aggravate the impairment of coronary flow. The Canadian Cardiovascular Society (CCS) has proposed a specific system for grading of angina, which has gained widespread acceptance.[1]

This chapter aims to focus on the role of Optimal Medical Management or Therapy (OMT) in today's practice.

LESSONS LEARNT FROM RANDOMIZED TRIALS

The management of SIHD consists of medical therapy (MT), percutaneous coronary intervention (PCI) or coronary artery bypass grafting (CABG).

The earlier trials compared MT to CABG and subsequently there have been multiple randomized trials which compared contemporary techniques. From earlier trials, it was apparent that MT was associated with low event rates (Table 1). A meta-analysis of 12 trials of stenting versus MT indicates that the initial improvement in relief of angina with PCI over MT is not sustained in the current era of MT.[2] In addition, no randomized trial or meta-analysis has demonstrated a reduction in death or myocardial infarction (MI) with PCI vs. MT for SIHD.

TABLE 1: Cardiac death rates on medical therapy with different extents of coronary artery disease

Extent of CAD	Annual mortality with medical therapy (%)
1-vessel	1.4
2-vessel	2.4
1-vessel >95% proximal LAD	3.4
2-vessel >95% proximal LAD	4.2
3-vessel	4.2
3-vessel >95% in at least 1	5.4
3-vessel >75% proximal LAD	6.6
3-vessel >95% proximal LAD	8.2

CAD, coronary artery disease; LAD, left anterior descending.

Source: Modified from Mark DB, Nelson CL, Califf RM, et al. Continuing evolution of therapy for coronary artery disease. Initial results from the era of coronary angioplasty. Circulation. 1994;89:2015-25.[21]

The findings of the most debated contemporary trial, "COURAGE" (Clinical Outcomes Utilizing Revascularization and Aggressive Drug Evaluation) comparing OMT versus OMT plus PCI, indicated that as an initial medical strategy in patients with SIHD, PCI did not reduce death, MI or other major cardiovascular (CV) adverse events when added to OMT.[3] The patients in the COURAGE trial were symptomatic at baseline and had appreciable clinical comorbidity, a high prevalence of myocardial ischemia, and extensive angiographic coronary artery disease (CAD). Subgroup analysis of the COURAGE trial[3] revealed consistency among clinical groups and found no difference between PCI plus OMT versus OMT alone in patients with multivessel CAD, low ejection fraction (EF), class II or class III angina or diabetes. During an extended follow up of 15 years, there was no difference in survival between an initial strategy with PCI plus OMT versus OMT alone in patients with SIHD[4] as shown in table 2.

TABLE 2: Mortality in subjects on optimal medical therapy with percutaneous coronary intervention (PCI) versus without PCI on extended follow-up of COURAGE trial[4]

Mortality	With PCI	Without PCI
7 years	7.6% (85)	8.3% (95)
15 years	24.7% (284)	24.4%(277)

OMT, optimal medical therapy; PCI, percutaneous coronary intervention.

Two imaging substudies from the COURAGE trial provided discordant results between noninvasive assessment of ischemia and the potential benefits of revascularization.[5,6] The discordance of these two substudies supports the equipoise regarding whether the extent and severity of myocardial ischemia are favorably affected by PCI. The question whether PCI can reduce the risk for CV death or MI in selected patients at higher risk for ischemia remains under investigation. ISCHEMIA trial is underway and is designed to answer this question.

Fractional flow reserve (FFR)-guided PCI strategy plus best available MT was also compared with best available MT alone in the FAME-2 trial.[7] Findings from both the COURAGE and FAME-2 studies show that PCI reduces ischemia and need for further revascularization. Neither the FAME-2 nor the COURAGE showed a reduction in the incidence of death or MI with PCI. Based on data from randomized trials, it appears reasonable to pursue a strategy of initial MT for patients with SIHD and CCS class I or II and to reserve revascularization for those with severe symptoms, symptoms despite OMT, or with high-risk features.

The Bypass Angioplasty Revascularization Investigation 2 Diabetes (BARI 2D) trial tested treatment strategies for patients with SIHD and diabetes.[8] The hypothesis was that a strategy of prompt revascularization (either surgical or percutaneous) will reduce long-term rates of death and CV events as compared to MT. A strategy of prompt coronary revascularization in patients who have been treated with intensive MT for diabetes and SIHD did not significantly reduce the rate of death or any other major CV event.

In the recently published ORBITA (Objective Randomised Blinded Investigation with optimal medical Therapy of Angioplasty in stable angina) trial,[9] in patients with medically treated angina, PCI did not improve exercise time by more than that of a placebo procedure.

WHAT CONSTITUTES OPTIMAL MEDICAL THERAPY?

Given the impressive results of MT in multiple trials, a question arises as to what should be called as an OMT. In the COURAGE trial, MT comprised not only of antianginal medication, but also agents which modify atherosclerosis (Table 3). It is also important to realize that a high percentage of patients achieved guideline-directed targets. The excellent results of COURAGE are attributed to large number of drugs and extraordinary achievement of targets. In true sense, OMT involves antianginal and atherosclerosis modifying drugs and strict adherence to guideline-directed targets for risk factor control. In COURAGE, these were achieved for low-density lipoprotein (LDL), glycated hemoglobin (HbA1c), and systolic and diastolic BP in a significant percentage of patients at 5 years of follow-up (Table 4). There were high rates of adherence to the regimen of diet, regular exercise, and smoking cessation.

TABLE 3: Medications used in COURAGE trial[3]

Medication	OMT plus PCI (n = 1,149)	OMT alone (n = 1,138)
ACEI or ARB	717 (62%)	734 (65%)
Statins plus other antilipids	1,081 (94%)	1,108 (97%)
Aspirin	1,097 (96%)	1,077 (95%)
Beta-blockers	975 (85%)	1,008 (89%)
Calcium channel blockers	459 (40%)	488 (43%)
Nitrates	714 (62%)	825 (72%)

ACEI, angiotensin-converting enzyme inhibitor; ARB, angiotensin receptor blocker; OMT, optimal medical therapy; PCI, percutaneous coronary intervention.

TABLE 4: Guideline-directed targets achieved in COURAGE trial[3]

Target achieved at 5-year follow-up	Percentage
LDL cholesterol <85 mg/dL	70%
Systolic BP <130 mm Hg	65%
Diastolic BP <85 mm Hg	94%
HbA1c <7.0%	45%

HbA1c, glycated hemoglobin; LDL, low-density lipoprotein; BP, blood pressure.

In the light of above data, it is obvious that comprehensive management of SA involves many aspects and will be discussed under the following headings:

- Treatment of coexisting conditions that precipitate or worsen angina
- Management of coronary risk factors
- Interventions for secondary prevention including life style changes
- Pharmacotherapy for angina.

Treatment of Coexisting Conditions that Precipitate or Worsen Angina

Medical conditions like anemia, marked weight gain, occult thyrotoxicosis, fever, infections, and tachycardia can increase myocardial demand or reduce delivery and can contribute to onset of angina or exacerbation of SA. Identification and treatment of these conditions is important.

Management of Coronary Risk Factors

Lifestyle interventions can potentially prevent more than 90% of all cardiovascular disease (CVD) deaths. Nine risk factors accounted for 90% of the risk for MI in men and 94% of the risk in women in the INTERHEART study.[10] The factors were abnormal lipids, smoking, hypertension (HT), diabetes, abdominal obesity, psychosocial factors, low consumption of fruit and vegetables, alcohol consumption, and lack of physical activity.

Management of Dyslipidemia

Dyslipidemia should be managed according to lipid guidelines with pharmacological and lifestyle interventions. The 2013 American College of Cardiology/American Heart Association (ACC/AHA) guidelines for cholesterol management advocate high-intensity statin therapy in all patients with established ischemic heart disease and less than 75 years of age, in the absence of contraindications, with less emphasis on LDL target goals.[11] Other interventions (fibrates, resins, nicotinic acid, and ezetimibe) may lower LDL cholesterol, but no benefit in clinical outcomes has been reported for these alternatives.

Cigarette Smoking

Smoking remains one of the most important risk factors for CAD. It can aggravate angina and also add in the progression of atherosclerosis. Smoking cessation lessens the risk of coronary events and all strategies for smoking cessation should be adopted in smokers. Nicotine replacement therapy is safe and should be considered in individual cases.

Hypertension

Epidemiological links between increased blood pressure (BP) and CAD severity and mortality are well established. HT predisposes to vascular injury, accelerates the development of atherosclerosis, increases myocardial O_2 demand, intensifies ischemia in patients with preexisting obstructive CAD, and predisposes to atrial fibrillation (AF). BP control is an essential component of the management of patients with SA with a goal of less than 130/80 mm Hg according to the 2017 ACC/AHA guidelines.[12]

Management of Diabetes Mellitus

Diabetes mellitus (DM) is a strong risk factor for CV complications, increases the risk of progression of coronary disease and should be managed carefully, with good control of HbA1c to below 7.0% generally and 6.5–6.9% on an individual basis. Glucose control should be based on individual considerations, depending on the patient's characteristics including age, presence of complications, and diabetes duration.

Obesity

Obesity is usually associated with a constellation of other risk factors and can be associated with an increased risk of death in CAD. Weight reduction in overweight and obese people is recommended in order to achieve favorable effects on BP, dyslipidemia and glucose metabolism.

Diet

A healthy diet reduces CVD risk. Energy intake should be limited to the amount of energy needed to maintain (or obtain) a healthy weight—that is, a BMI less than 23 kg/m^2.

Physical Activity

Clinical practice guidelines for prevention of CVD recommend more than 150 minutes of moderate intensity or more than 60–75 minutes of vigorous exercise each week. Guidelines on secondary prevention of SIHD have recommended similar levels of regular moderate or vigorous exercise.[13] A large scale study, STABILITY,[14] from 39 countries in patients with SIHD demonstrated that low volumes of physical activity are associated with large risk reductions for CV and all-cause mortality. Increasing volume of physical activity yields additional health benefits.

Interventions for Secondary Prevention Including Lifestyle Changes

The objectives and different means for prevention of secondary events are described in table 5.

Aspirin

Aspirin remains the cornerstone of pharmacological prevention of arterial thrombosis. The benefits of aspirin in reducing vascular events, MI, and sudden death have been documented in several studies and meta-analysis. Administration of aspirin daily is advisable in patients with SIHD and no contraindication to this drug. Dosing at 75–162 mg daily appears to have comparable effects on secondary prevention as 160–320 mg daily and is associated with a lower bleeding risk. Thus, aspirin 75–162 mg daily is preferred for secondary prevention in absence of coronary stenting.[15]

Clopidogrel, a thienopyridine derivative, may be substituted for aspirin in patients with aspirin hypersensitivity or those who cannot tolerate aspirin.

Angiotensin-converting Enzyme Inhibitor and Angiotensin Receptor Blockers

The beneficial effects of angiotensin-converting enzyme inhibitors (ACEIs) or angiotensin receptor blockers (ARBs) include reductions in left ventricular hypertrophy, vascular hypertrophy, progression of atherosclerosis, plaque rupture, and thrombosis. These drugs are not beneficial for the treatment of angina; however, they have benefits in reducing the risk for future ischemic events.

Angiotensin-converting enzyme inhibitors should be prescribed in patients with SIHD who have DM, HT, reduced (≤40%) left ventricular ejection fraction (LVEF), chronic kidney disease (CKD), or other vascular disease unless contraindicated.[15] Those patients who cannot tolerate ACEIs are candidates for ARBs.

TABLE 5: Prevention of secondary events

Objectives	Measures
• Reduce plaque progression • Stabilize plaque • Prevent thrombosis	• Aspirin • Statins • ACEI or ARBS • Lifestyle modification

ACEI, angiotensin-converting enzyme inhibitor; ARB, angiotensin receptor blocker.

Statins

Patients with documented CAD are regarded as being at very high risk and should be treated with statins. The treatment target is LDL-C less than 70 mg/dL and/or more than 50% reduction if the target level cannot be reached.

Antioxidants

According to current evidence, there is no basis for recommending supplemental folate, vitamin E, vitamin C, or beta carotene for the purpose of improving CV outcomes.

Lifestyle Changes

Certain changes in lifestyle can be useful in reducing episodes of angina. It is useful to counsel about dietary habits, physical activity, and types of work the patient can do.

Pharmacotherapy for Angina

Antianginal drugs are classified as first- or second-line drugs. There are also certain drugs which are not commonly used or are investigational (Box 1).

First-line Antianginal Drugs

First-line antianginal drugs alter the hemodynamics and can cause significant changes in the heart rate (HR) and BP. These include nitrates, β-blockers, and calcium channel blockers (CCBs). These drugs reduce anginal symptoms and prolong exercise duration and/or time to ST-segment depression on the electrocardiogram (ECG). Frequently, a combination of these drugs is necessary for symptom control. None of these drugs has been shown to be disease modifying. The first-line drugs are briefly discussed below.

Nitrates

Nitrates act by different mechanisms. The main mechanism is venodilatation, causing preload reduction and resultant relief in angina. They also cause arteriolar dilatation.

Glyceryl trinitrate (GTN), isosorbide dinitrate (IDN), and isosorbide-5-mononitrate (IMN) are the commonly used nitrates. They can be used via sublingual, oral, sustained oral, oral spray, transdermal patch, buccal, and intravenous route.

For quick relief, short-acting nitrates (GTN and IMN) are given sublingually and can be repeated every 5 minutes till complete relief of pain or maximum of 4–5 tablets. GTN spray (nitrolingual) can also be used for quick relief and the dose is 0.4 mg per spray. The long-acting nitrates used for angina prophylaxis are nitroglycerine, IDN, and IMN.

On prolonged administration, tolerance can develop to nitrates, and the same can be prevented by dosing free intervals. Common side effects include headaches, tachycardia, facial flushing, hypotension, and syncope. Coadministration of nitrates with a phosphodiesterase-5 inhibitor or alcohol can cause hypotension and should be avoided. Left ventricular outflow obstruction in hypertrophic cardiomyopathy can be worsened by nitrates.

BOX 1 Classification of antianginal drugs

First-line drugs:
- Beta-blockers
- Calcium channel blockers:
  - Dihydropyridine, e.g. amlodipine
  - Nondihydropyridine, e.g. verapamil, diltiazem
- Nitrates

Second-line drugs:
- Ranolazine
- Nicorandil
- Trimetazidine
- Ivabradine

Other drugs:
- Molsidomine
- Allopurinol
- Others (L-arginine, Bosentan, GLP-1 mimetics, etc.)

Beta-blockers

Beta-blockers lower the HR, prolong diastolic filling, and improve the myocardial blood flow. They also reduce the cardiac output, and inhibit renin release, thus lowering BP and systolic wall stress. Beta-blockers are the standard of care after episodes of myocardial ischemia and in patients with heart failure (HF) with low EF. Mostly β1 selective agents like metoprolol tartrate (short acting) or succinate (long-acting), bisoprolol, and carvedilol, with additional α-antagonist activity are preferred. Nebivolol, a highly selective β1 blocker, has additional nitrate like properties by generating nitric oxide and is preferred in elderly and in patients with chronic obstructive pulmonary disease.

Side effects and contraindications to β-blockers are summarized in table 6. Abrupt withdrawal of β-blockers after prolonged administration can precipitate angina. Withdrawing the drug should be done in a stepwise manner over the course of 2–3 weeks. The β-blockers may mask the clinical signs of hyperthyroidism and precipitate thyroid storm with abrupt discontinuation.

Calcium Channel Blockers

All CCBs (nondihydropyridine and dihydropyridine) have similar antianginal efficacy, cause epicardial vasodilatation, and are specifically useful in relieving vasospastic angina. Nondihydropyridine CCBs additionally reduce myocardial

TABLE 6: Side effects and contraindications to beta-blockers

Side effects	Contraindications

• Increased insulin resistance
• Hampers exercise tolerance
• Depressive symptoms
• Sexual dysfunction
• Raynaud's phenemenon
• Aggravates peripheral arterial disease
	• Relative:
	  ○ Diabetes (masks hypoglycemia symptoms)
	  ○ Chronic obstructive pulmonary disease
	• Absolute:
	  ○ Severe bronchospasm
	  ○ Advanced atrioventricular block
	  ○ Sick sinus with bradycardia
	  ○ Untreated pheochromocytoma

oxygen demand via negative inotropic and chronotropic action, whereas dihydropyridine CCBs improve bioavailability of nitric oxide and improve endothelial function.

Pedal edema, constipation, headache, and dizziness are common side effects. Ankle edema is due to increased capillary hydrostatic pressure from arteriolar dilatation. Nondihydropyridine CCBs can cause bradycardia and heart blocks. They may also precipitate or worsen congestive HF in those with systolic dysfunction. CCBs inhibit lower esophageal sphincter function and can cause gastroesophageal reflux.

There can be drug interactions with CCBs due to inhibition of hepatic microsomal enzymes. They may raise levels of statins and other drugs. Magnesium supplements may enhance the actions of CCBs by antagonizing calcium.

Second-line Antianginal Drugs

Many patients with chronic angina remain symptomatic despite receiving the combination of two or more first-line drugs at maximum tolerated dosages. Most of these drugs except nicorandil do not lower the BP. Table 7 summarizes important characteristics of second-line drugs. A brief discussion of each agent is described here.

Ranolazine

The antianginal efficacy of ranolazine has been established in the MARISA, CARISA, MERLIN-TIMI 36, ERICA, and TERISA trials.[16] Ranolazine was approved by the United States Food and Drug Administration (FDA) in 2006 for management of chronic SA. Ranolazine inhibits the late inward sodium current and prevents intracellular calcium overload and diastolic relaxation failure. It prolongs the QT interval and is contraindicated in patients with congenital or acquired long-QT syndrome. An ECG should be obtained at baseline and follow-up to evaluate the drug's effect on QT interval. Ranolazine clearance is reduced in renal insufficiency and it is contraindicated in severe renal failure or moderate-to-severe hepatic impairment. Initial dose of ranolazine is 500 mg twice daily. For patients who remain symptomatic, 1,000 mg twice daily may be used. At very high doses of up to 2,000 mg/day, syncope and postural hypotension can occur due to α-adrenergic receptor blockade.

Ivabradine

Heart rate reduction is a recognized strategy for preventing myocardial ischemia and angina pectoris in patients with stable CAD. Ivabradine, by lowering the HR, has been shown to increase exercise capacity and reduce anginal frequency and severity. Ivabradine blocks transmembrane f-channels and disrupts I_f ion current flow. This blockade and disruption prolong diastolic depolarization and slow sinoatrial node firing, which in turn lowers the HR in a dose-dependent manner.

Post hoc analyses of a randomized trial have suggested that ivabradine might improve CV outcomes such as death, MI, or hospitalization for HF in patients with stable disease.[17] However, data from SIGNIFY trial[18] fail to confirm these findings. While ivabradine improved angina in patients with CCS class II angina or higher taking OMT, there was a concern about an increase in the risk of CV death and nonfatal MI. The use of ivabradine in patients with SA who do not have clinical HF is not recommended.

The common side effects include bradycardia, transient visual disturbances (phosphenes), and AF. Other adverse effects include first-degree atrioventricular block, headache, dizziness, uncontrolled BP, and ventricular extrasystoles.

Ivabradine has been approved by US FDA for reducing risk of hospitalization for HF in stable chronic HF patients with low EF (<35%), who are in sinus rhythm but not for angina. On the other hand, the European Medicines Agency (EMA) has also approved ivabradine for chronic SA in individuals not tolerating β-blockers.

Trimetazidine

Trimetazidine inhibits fatty acid β-oxidation and increases glucose utilization by myocardium, thereby preventing reduction of adenosine triphosphate (ATP) levels after hypoxia or ischemia and preserving ionic pump function. It also decreases free radical generation and prevents intracellular calcium overload and acidosis. Trimetazidine increases work capacity and delays the ECG changes and symptoms during exercise. As it has no effect on HR and BP, it can be used as an add-on drug with the first-line "hemodynamic" drugs.

The EMA has approved trimetazidine as an add-on drug in patients poorly controlled with first-line drugs. The US FDA has not approved the drug.

TABLE 7: Characteristics of second-line antianginal drugs

Drug	Mechanism of action	Dose	Contraindications	Major adverse effects
Ivabradine	Decrease pacemaker activity in sinus node	5–7.5 mg bd	Severe liver disease, low heart rate, and allergy	Visual disturbances
Nicorandil	Opening K^+ channels	20 mg bd	Low blood pressure and CCF	Oral, intestinal, and perianal ulceration
Ranolazine	Inhibition of Na^+ channels	500–2,000 mg daily	Liver cirrhosis	Nausea, dizziness, and QT prolongation
Trimetazidine	Inhibition of reduction of ATP, stimulation of glucose consumption by myocardium	20 mg tds or 35 mg bd	Pregnancy, breastfeeding, allergy, Parkinson's disease, tremors, movement disorder, seizures, and severe renal failure	Gastric discomfort, headache, and movement disorders

bd, twice a day; tds, thrice a day; CCF, congestive cardiac failure; ATP, adenosine triphosphate.

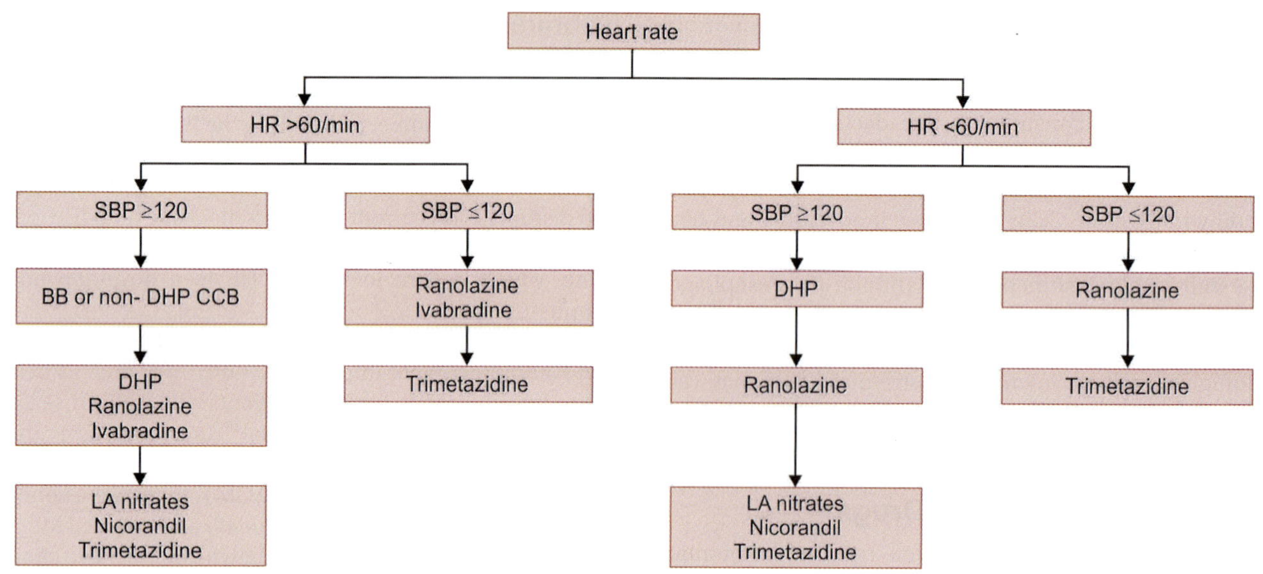

BB, β-blocker; CCB, calcium channel blocker; DHP, dihydropyridine; HR, heart rate; SBP, systolic blood pressure.

FLOWCHART 1: A tailored therapeutic approach for initiating therapy.[22]

Nicorandil

Nicorandil opens the ATP-sensitive potassium channels, with additional nitric oxide donor action, effectively leading to direct coronary dilatation. It prevents angina and myocardial ischemia by its vasodilator action on systemic and coronary vessels. It does not cause tachyphylaxis or impair endothelial function.

The European Society of Cardiology (ESC) guidelines state "For second-line treatment it is recommended to add long-acting nitrates or ivabradine or nicorandil or ranolazine, according to HR, BP, and tolerance (IIa—B)" and may be considered in patients with microvascular angina with refractory symptoms (IIb—B). The National Institute for Health and Clinical Excellence (NICE) in the UK also recommends nicorandil for these purposes. Nicorandil is EMA—but not FDA—approved.

OTHER DRUGS FOR ANGINA

Molsidomine dilates venous capacitance vessels (reducing preload), dilates coronary arterial segments, exerts a platelet stabilizing effect by inhibiting thromboxane, and has a nitric oxide-donating effect. It has been available in Europe since 1977 but has not been approved by the US FDA.

Allopurinol, a xanthine oxidase inhibitor, is also antianginal. Allopurinol 600 mg/day increased times to ST-segment depression and to chest pain.[19] In optimally treated SCAD patients, allopurinol reduced vascular oxidative stress, while in HF patients it conserved ATP.

L-Arginine, Bosentan, GLP-1 mimetics and DPP-4 analogues, Mildronate, Fasudil, Estrogen/Progesterone are other investigational drugs for angina and at present do not have a role in clinical practice.

How to Choose the Appropriate Antianginal Drug?

The guidelines do not provide any suggestions to guide choice within each step or among steps. A systematic therapeutic approach, tailored to individual profiles [BP, HR, diabetes, and left ventricle (LV) systolic function] and drug characteristics is necessary. Flowchart 1 describes an initial approach for selecting drugs for MT of chronic SA. Table 8 details the drug combinations which should be avoided during treatment of angina.

Stable Angina and Hypertension

In patients with SA, who require antihypertensive treatment, ESC guidelines suggest the use of renin-angiotensin system blockers, β-blockers, CCBs, and long-acting nitrates for symptomatic relief. These drugs, in addition to BP control, also present additional benefits in terms of symptom relief and favorable prognosis. The BP threshold levels in such patients have already been discussed.

TABLE 8: Drug combinations to be avoided or used with caution

Drug combination	Reason
Ivabradine + ranolazine + nicorandil*	No safety data
Ivabradine + nondihydropyridine CCBs *	Significant HR reduction
Beta-blockers + nondihydropyridine CCBs^	Significant HR reduction

*To be avoided
^Can be used with caution
CCB, calcium channel blocker; HR, heart rate.

Stable Angina and Heart Rate

There is robust evidence suggesting that increased HR in patients with CAD is harmful, since it increases myocardial oxygen demand leading to ischemia and anginal symptoms. Current ESC guidelines recommend the use of HR lowering agents such as β-blockers, nondihydropyridine CCBs, and ivabradine in order to decrease HR. Excessive HR reduction is not advisable, since it may lead to chronotropic incompetence-related symptoms. The SIGNIFY trial[18] showed an increased risk of CV events and AF in patients with an excessive decrease in HR and ignited a debate about the HR threshold. Recently, a threshold level of 60 beats/min (except for ivabradine, which should not be initiated in HRs <70 beats/min) has been suggested. The use of drugs in patients with low HR is tricky and drugs with minimal or no HR effects are advised.

Atrial fibrillation may aggravate angina symptoms since it increases HR and thus myocardial oxygen consumption. Hence, in patients with SA and AF, HR lowering antianginal drugs such as β-blockers and nondihydropyridine CCBs should be preferred.

Diabetes with Stable Angina

The presence of DM leads to more extensive vascular disease and a more severe ischemic burden (both anginal and silent). When treating DM with angina, drugs that have a positive or at least a neutral metabolic profile have to be preferred. The use of β-blockers in diabetics has been debated given the higher incidence of new onset DM or worsening of the glycemic profile in these patients. It seems that these unfavorable effects are limited to the majority of the nonvasodilating β-blockers. In effect, vasodilating β-blockers present a favorable metabolic profile since they improve insulin sensitivity and they do not cause deleterious effects on lipid profile.

Ranolazine is an antianginal drug with favorable effects in reduction of HbA1c levels and may be preferred in patients with angina and DM for symptomatic relief.

Left Ventricular Systolic Function and Stable Angina

A large majority of HF cases with reduced EF are linked to CAD. In the subgroup of patients with HF and SA, it is preferable to administer drugs that not only reduce anginal symptoms, but also improve prognosis.

On the basis of the MERIT-HF, COPERNICUS, COMET, CIBIS-II studies, β-blockers, particularly metoprolol, carvedilol, and bisoprolol, are recommended for the long-term management of patients with angina and LV systolic dysfunction.[20] Beta-blockers reduce angina, delay HF, reduce the rate of rehospitalizations, and improve prognosis. Ivabradine is also useful in reducing angina and HF hospitalizations. Nitrates have a useful role, combining vasodilating and antianginal effect.

CONCLUSION

As highlighted in the manuscript, the therapy of SA should include aggressive treatment of risk factors, lifestyle modifications, and medications. The aim of therapy is preventing angina and reducing adverse CV outcomes. Therapy should be initiated with one or two first-line drugs, namely a β-blocker or CCB. Nitrates may be added for acute episodes of angina and prophylaxis. Ranolazine, nicorandil, and ivabradine can be used as add-on therapy. Addition of an ACEI or ARB is advised in those with HT, DM, CKD, previous MI and reduced LVEF less than or equal to 40%. The final choice of drugs should be individualized depending on patient profile and safety considerations.

REFERENCES

1. Kaul P, Naylor CD, Armstrong PW, et al. Assessment of activity status and survival according to the Canadian Cardiovascular Society angina classification. Can J Cardiol. 2009;25(7):e225-231.
2. Bangalore S, Pursnani S, Kumar S, et al. Percutaneous coronary intervention versus optimal medical therapy for prevention of spontaneous myocardial infarction in subjects with stable ischemic heart disease. Circulation. 2013;127(7):769-81.
3. Boden WE, O'Rourke RA, Teo KK, et al. COURAGE Trial Research Group. Optimal medical therapy with or without PCI for stable coronary disease. N Engl J Med. 2007;356:1503.
4. Sedlis SP, Hartigan PM, Teo TT, et al. Effect of PCI on long-term survival in patients with stable ischemic heart disease. N Engl J Med. 2015;373:1937.
5. Shaw LJ, Berman DS, Maron DJ, et al. Optimal medical therapy with or without percutaneous coronary intervention to reduce ischemic burden: results from the Clinical Outcomes Utilizing Revascularization and Aggressive Drug Evaluation (COURAGE) trial nuclear substudy. Circulation. 2008;117:1283-91.
6. Shaw LJ, Weintraub WS, Maron DJ, et al. Baseline stress myocardial perfusion imaging results and outcomes in patients with stable ischemic heart disease randomized to optimal medical therapy with or without percutaneous coronary intervention. Am Heart J. 2012;164:243-50.
7. De Bruyne B, Pijls NH, Kalesan B, et al. Fractional flow reserve-guided PCI versus medical therapy in stable coronary disease (FAME 2). N Engl J Med. 2012;367:991.
8. Chaitman BR, Hardison RM, Adler D, et al. Bypass Angioplasty Revascularization Investigation 2 Diabetes (BARI 2D) Study Group. The Bypass Angioplasty Revascularization Investigation 2 Diabetes randomized trial of different treatment strategies in type 2 diabetes mellitus with stable ischemic heart disease: impact of treatment strategy on cardiac mortality and myocardial infarction. Circulation. 2009;120(25):2529.
9. Al-Lamee R, Thompson D, Dehbi HM, et al. Percutaneous coronary intervention in stable angina (ORBITA): a double-blind, randomised controlled trial. Lancet. 2018;391:31.
10. Yusuf S, Hawken S, Ounpuu S, et al. Effect of potentially modifiable risk factors associated with myocardial infarction in 52 countries (the INTERHEART study): case-control study. Lancet. 2004;364:937.
11. Stone NJ, Robinson JG, Lichtenstein AH, et al. 2013 ACC/AHA guideline on the treatment of blood cholesterol to reduce atherosclerotic cardiovascular risk in adults: a report of the American College of Cardiology/American Heart Association Task Force on Practice Guidelines. Circulation. 2014;129:S1.
12. Whelton PK, Carey RM, Aronow WS, et al. 2017 ACC/AHA/AAPA/ABC/ACPM/AGS/APhA/ASH/ASPC/NMA/PCNA Guideline for the Prevention, Detection, Evaluation, and Management of High Blood Pressure in Adults: A Report of the American College of Cardiology/American Heart Association Task Force on Clinical Practice Guidelines. Hypertension. 2018;71:e13.
13. Montalescot G, Sechtem U, Achenbach A, et al. 2013 ESC guidelines on the management of stable coronary artery disease. The Task Force on the management of stable coronary artery disease of the European Society of Cardiology, Eur Heart J. 2013;34:2949.
14. Stewart RAH, Held C, Hadziosmanovic N, et al.; on behalf of STABILITY investigators. Physical activity and mortality in patients with stable coronary heart disease. J Am Coll Cardiol. 2017;70(14):1689-700.
15. Smith SC Jr, Benjamin EJ, Bonow RO, et al. AHA/ACCF Secondary Prevention and Risk Reduction Therapy for Patients with Coronary and other Atherosclerotic

Vascular Disease: 2011 update: a guideline from the American Heart Association and American College of Cardiology Foundation. Circulation. 2011;124: 2458-73.

16. Arnold SV, McGuire DK, Spertus JA, et al. Glucose-lowering medications and angina burden in patients with stable coronary disease: results from the Type 2 diabetes Evaluation of Ranolazine In subjects with chronic Stable Angina (TERISA) Trial. Am Heart J. 2015;170:753.
17. Fox K, Ford I, Steg PG, et al. Ivabradine for patients with stable coronary artery disease and left-ventricular systolic dysfunction (BEAUTIFUL): a randomised, double-blind, placebo-controlled trial. Lancet. 2008;372:807.
18. Fox K, Ford I, Steg PG, et al. Ivabradine in stable coronary artery disease without clinical heart failure (SIGNIFY trial). N Engl J Med. 2014;371:1091.
19. Noman A, Ang DS, Ogston S, et al. Effect of high-dose allopurinol on exercise in patients with chronic stable angina: a randomised, placebo controlled crossover trial. Lancet. 2010;375:2161.
20. Hjalmarson A, Goldstein S, Fagerberg B, et al. Effects of controlled-release metoprolol on total mortality, hospitalizations, and well-being in patients with heart failure: the Metoprolol CR/XL Randomized Intervention Trial in congestive heart failure (MERIT-HF). MERIT-HF Study Group. JAMA. 2000;283:1295.
21. Mark DB, Nelson CL, Califf RM, et al. Continuing evolution of therapy for coronary artery disease. Initial results from the era of coronary angioplasty. Circulation. 1994;89:2015-25.
22. Manolis AJ, Poulimenos LE, Ambrosio G, et al. Medical treatment of stable angina: a tailored therapeutic approach. Int J Cardiol. 2016;220:445-53.

CHAPTER 31

Beta-Blockers in Chronic Stable Coronary Artery Disease: Current Status

J Shiv Kumar, M Sitaram, Sajith Pavitran, G Nagarjuna

INTRODUCTION

Coronary artery disease (CAD) is a major cause of death and disability all over the world. CAD is typically a chronic disease with progression over a period of years or decades.[1]

Angina pectoris remains a major presenting symptom among patients of CAD, with numerically more patients of chronic stable CAD attending cardiology clinics than myocardial infarction (MI) (8.3% vs. 2.8%).[2]

Among the various remedies available for angina pectoris nitrates, β-blockers, calcium channel blockers (CCB) and angiotensin-converting enzyme inhibitors (ACEIs) and β-blockers have retained their important position because of their predictable response and their safety profile in different clinical situations.

The introduction of a new range of β-blockers with additional pharmacological properties has ensured the β-blockers their place in the prescriptions for CAD in years to come.

INCIDENCE AND PREVALENCE

The 2016 heart disease and stroke statistics update of American Heart Association (AHA) reports that 15.5 million adults (6.2% of adult population) have CAD, including 7.6 million (2.8%) with MI and 8.2 million (3.3%) with angina pectoris. These estimates of CAD increase with age in both sexes. An individual's risk factor burden translated in to marked differences in life time risk of CAD and these differences are consistent across all races in both cohorts.[2]

It is well known that despite paucity of symptoms, the extent of nonobstructive CAD is associated with worse prognosis, compared with adults without CAD.

The incidence of CAD and CAD mortality has been steadily decreasing in the USA and other Western countries, while the incidence of CAD is increasing alarmingly in Southeast Asian countries including India. With the increasing average lifespan of individuals across the globe, the global burden of chronic stable CAD is poised to increase sharply in future, with predictable concerns about spiraling costs of public health care.

PATHOPHYSIOLOGY OF CORONARY ARTERY DISEASE

Atherosclerosis is a chronic inflammatory process triggered by accumulation of cholesterol containing low-density lipoprotein (LDL) particles in the arterial wall. Major etiological factors include hyperlipidemia, hypertension, diabetes, and cigarette smoking—all of which are thought to initiate and promote vascular inflammation.

Atherosclerotic disease of the epicardial coronary arteries has been recognized as the cause of angina pectoris for more than two centuries, and sudden thrombotic occlusion of an epicardial coronary artery has been well established as the cause of acute MI for more than 100 years.

However, the epicardial arteries are only one segment of the arterial circulation. They give rise to myriads of smaller blood vessels, and arterioles which constitute the coronary microcirculation—the main site of regulation of myocardial blood flow.

The coronary arteries are classified as three components:

1. Proximal conductance vessels (500 μm to 3–5 mm)
2. Intermediate (periarteriolar vessels 100–500 μm)
3. Distal (arteriolar vessels <100 μm).

The cardiac pump is an aerobic organ that requires continuous perfusion with oxygenated blood to generate the adenosine triphosphate (ATP), the vital substrate for ventricular contraction.[1] The role of coronary circulation is to provide an adequate match between myocardial oxygen demand and supply. The integrated coronary response to increase in oxygen demand is an excellent example of autoregulation in regional blood flow in human body.[3]

It consists of:

- Metabolic vasodilators
- Periarteriolar autoregulation
- Flow mediated, endothelium-dependent vasodilatation

- Extravascular tissue pressure
- Neurohumoral control.

Small arteries and arterioles are richly innervated by both sympathetic and parasympathetic nerve terminals that play an important role of regulation of coronary blood flow.

Neural and biohumoral regulation of the coronary microcirculation has been receiving increasing attention in the recent years and the effect of sympathetic overactivity over the coronary microcirculation has been the focus of renewed interest.

Sympathetic nervous system in the heart controls the circulatory adaptation in coronary bed through the following pathways:

- Beta 1-adrenoceptors mediated chronotropic, inotropic, and dromotropic effects
- Beta 2-adrenoceptors mediated vasodilatation of smaller coronary arterioles
- Alpha 1-adrenoceptors causing vasoconstriction in coronary vessels constriction
- Alpha 2 vasoconstriction in microcirculation.

This paradoxic vasoconstriction in smaller coronary arteries and microcirculation is believed to help preserve flow in the vulnerable inner layer of left ventricle (LV) especially during exercise.

Parasympathetic neural response over coronary arteries is one of uniform vasodilatation.

Nitric oxide (NO) production and release are the main mechanism of endothelium mediated vasodilatation.

Defective release of NO might be the etiological factor in patients with chest pain and normal coronaries as well as in patients with chronic stable angina.

Myocardial oxygen demand is the ultimate determinant of clinical outcomes and the importance of the supply versus demand equation in the coronary vascular bed is well recognized.

Myocardial oxygen demand is based on three factors namely: (1) heart rate (HR), (2) ventricular systolic pressure, and (C) LV size. Of these, HR and systolic LV pressure seem to be the key determinants of oxygen consumption of the heart and the double product [HR × systolic blood pressure (SBP)] is considered to be a reliable index of the same. These variables increase the workload of the LV and also increase the wall stress in the LV, indirectly increasing the resistance to coronary filling.[4]

Drugs that reduce the HR and BP thus aid in improving the LV function by reducing the LV wall stress and improving diastolic coronary blood flow.

PHARMACOTHERAPEUTICS OF BETA-BLOCKERS

Beta-adrenoceptors are G protein coupled transmembrane proteins. Their main antianginal action lies in the intracellular part of the β-receptor that is coupled to the G protein complex Gs (stimulating) and Gi (inhibitory). Agonists bind to the ligand site and stimulate the β-adrenergic receptors (β_1, β_2, and β_3 subtypes). This binding triggers adenylyl cyclase to convert cyclic ATP to cyclic AMP which acts as a second messenger initiating a cascade of events that are organ dependent. Interaction with Gs complex mediates positive inotropic and chronotropic actions while interaction with Gi complex may mediate the antiapoptotic effect of β_2 receptors.

Beta-blockers exert several cardioprotective effects. Despite the action of β_1 inhibition in blocking coronary vasodilation, there is overall benefit in coronary circulation because of the slowing of the HR and prolonging the diastole (the main period of coronary flow). In addition, by reducing cardiac output and by inhibition on renin release from the juxtaglomerular cells, β-blockers lower the BP and thus reduce systolic heart stress.[5]

The main mechanisms of protection of ischemic myocardium by β-blockers have been tabulated in box 1.

NEWER GENERATIONS OF BETA-BLOCKERS

Beta-blockers have remained as the main stay in treatment of CAD and their utility has been further enhanced by the synthesis of β-blockers with selective action on the β-receptors.

Although the β-blockers as a group have similar therapeutic effects, their pharmacological properties are markedly different. The classification of β-blockers and their individual properties are outlined in table 1.[6]

Beta-blockers exert their antianginal effect mostly by their action of β_1 receptor inhibition. Selective β_1-blockers (like atenolol, bisoprolol, metoprolol, and nebivolol) have minimal effect on β_2-receptors localized in bronchial muscle and thus may be preferable in patients with chronic obstructive airway disease or bronchial asthma. However, these drugs become less selective at higher doses and may begin to block β_2-adrenoceptors in the tracheobronchial tree causing bronchospasm. Furthermore β_1 selective blockers should be used with caution in patients with peripheral vascular disease.

The vasodilator activity of some of the newer generation of β-blockers is achieved through two pathways:

BOX 1 Possible mechanisms of protection of ischemic myocardium by beta-blockers

- Reduction in myocardial oxygen demands via:
  - Negative inotropic action
  - Reduction of heart rate
  - Blood pressure decrease
- Increase of coronary blood flow via:
  - Increase in diastolic perfusion time by reducing heart rate
  - Augmentation of collateral blood flow
  - Redistribution of blood flow to ischemic areas
- Alterations in the myocardial substrate utilization
- Decrease the microvascular damage
- Stabilization of the cell and lysosomal membranes
- Shift the oxyhemoglobin dissociation curve to the right
- Inhibition of the platelet aggregation
- Protection of myocardial cell against catecholamine-induced transmembrane potassium shifts

TABLE 1: Classification and physiological actions of β-adrenergic receptors and β-blockers used in angina pectoris

Drug	ISA	Plasma half-life (h)	Lipid soluble	Plasma protein binding (%)	Dosage for angina (mg)
Non-cardioselective					
Propranolol (inderal)	–	8–11	+++	90	80–320
Nadolol Penbutolol	–	20–24	0	98	40–80
Sotalol	–	7–8	0	5	80–240 BID
Timolol	–	4–5	+	60	10 mg/BID
Cardioselective					
Acebutolol Atenolol	++ –	8–13 6–7	0 0	15 10	400–1,200 50–200 QD
Bisoprolol Metoprolol	– –	9–12 3–7	+ +	30 12	10 mg/QD 50–200/BID
Vasodilatory (nonselective)					
Labetalol Pindolol Carvedilol	– β_1, β_2 –	6–8 4 6	+++ + +	90 55 95	300–600 2.5–7.5 12.5–25
Selective					
Nebivolol	–	6–10	++	98	2.5–10

1. Combined β- and α-adrenergic receptor blockade (labetalol and carvedilol).
2. Direct vasodilator activity through activation of NO synthase and release of NO (nebivolol).

Carvedilol may also ameliorate myocardial ischemic effects by different mechanisms:

- Inhibition of monocyte adhesion to endothelium
- Scavenging oxygen free radicals
- Protection of endothelial function
- Direct vasodilation
- Inhibition of LDL protein oxidation.

Nebivolol has greater selectivity for β_1-receptors than all other β-blockers. The NO potentiating vasodilatory effect of nebivolol is unique among β-blockers and at doses below 10 mg/day does not inhibit the increase in HR normally seen with exercise.[7,8]

ADVERSE EFFECTS OF BETA-BLOCKERS

- Negative metabolic effects:
  - Increase in insulin resistance and predisposition to diabetes
  - Weight gain
  - Worsening of glycemic control.
- Bradycardia and heart block
- Worsening of peripheral vascular disease and Raynaud's phenomena
- Bronchospasm.

In a meta-analysis of clinical trial experiences over 20 years, it was proven that β-blockers provide equal reduction of angina and cardiovascular (CV) adverse events compared to CCBs or nitrates.[8]

Beta-blockers in CAD with LV dysfunction needs special mention in view of increasing benefits noted in this subset.[9]

The Cardiac Insufficiency Bisoprolol Study (CIBIS) trial (1994) showed 32% reduction in all-cause mortality in New York Heart Association class III and IV patients of ischemic and nonischemic cardiomyopathy treated with β-blockers.[10]

The Metoprolol CR/XL Randomized Intervention Trial in Congestive Heart Failure (MERIT-HF) trial (2002) established the role of β-blockers in patients with heart failure where 34% reduction in mortality was noted in patients taking metoprolol versus placebo.[11]

The Carvedilol Post-Infarct Survival Control in LV Dysfunction (CAPRICORN) (2001) trial was the only large randomized clinical trial where patients of recent MI and LV dysfunction were studied in the era of reperfusion and the subjects followed up for 1.3 years showed significant reduction in CV mortality in the group treated with carvedilol.[12]

The Carvedilol Prospective Randomized Cumulative Survival (COPERNICUS) trial (2001) showed that in CAD patients with reduced EF (as low as <25%) carvedilol reduced 12 months mortality figures by 38% and risk of death or hospitalization by 31%.[13]

GUIDELINES FOR USE OF BETA-BLOCKERS IN ANGINA

American Heart Association has made the following recommendations in 2012 regarding β-blockers in treatment of stable ischaemic heart disease.[14]

AHA recommendations

Class I

- Beta-blocker therapy should be continued for 3 years in all patients with normal LV function after MI or ACS (264-266) (level of evidence B)

- Beta-blockers therapy should be used in all patients with LV systolic dysfunction (EF 40%) with heart failure or prior MI, unless contraindicated (level of evidence A).

Class II

BB may be considered as chronic therapy for other CAD patients (level of evidence C).

The European Society of Cardiology (ESC) guidelines have noted that β-blockers may be protective in patients with stable angina but without support of firm placebo-controlled clinical trials. It was pointed out that a recent retrospective study (REACH registry)[15] found that the risk of CV events was not lowered in CAD patients without prior MI despite using β-blockers. In summary it was mentioned that there was evidence for prognostic benefits from the use of β-blockers in post-MI patients or in heart failure and that extrapolation from these data suggested that β-blockers may be the first-line antiangina therapy in stable CAD patients without contraindications.[16]

ESC Recommendations for Beta-blockers

- For angina relief class: 1, level A
- For asymptomatic patients with large area of ischemia (>10%): class IIb level C.

CONCLUSION

Beta-adrenergic blockade has always remained the first-line of treatment for patients with chronic stable angina along with nitrates. The symptomatic relief from angina and reduction of recurring ischemic events even in the face of mild-to-moderate LV dysfunction, will continue to make this class of drugs a front line management choice. However, the reduction in mortality is seen only in the post-MI angina group of patients. There are new additions to subclasses of β-blockers with additional therapeutic benefits, but the clinician is well advised to be conversant with a few of the proven agents and their side effects rather than change drugs frequently.

REFERENCES

1. Lopez AD, Mathers CD, Ezzati M, et al. Global Burden of Disease and Risk Factors. New York: Oxford University Press; 2006.
2. Mojaffarian D, Benjamin EJ, Go AS, et al. Heart Disease and Stroke Statistics-2016, Update: A report from the American Heart Association. Circulation. 2016;133:e38-360.
3. Morrow DA, Gersh BJ, Braunwald E. Chronic coronary artery disease. In: Zipes DP, Libby P, Bonow RO, Braunwald E (Eds). Braunwald's Heart Disease, 7th edition. Philadelphia: WB Saunders; 2005.
4. Sedehi D, Cigorroa JE. Precipitants of Myocardial Ischemia. In: de Lemos JA, Omland T (Eds). Chronic Coronary Artery Disease: A Companion to Braunwald's Heart Disease, 1st edition. Philadelphia, PA: Elsevier 2018. pp. 69-78.
5. Opie LH, Yusuf S. Beta blocking agents. In: Opie H, Gersh BJ (Eds). Drugs for the Heart, 5th edition. Philadelphia: WB Saunders; 2001. pp 1-32.
6. Schroeder JS, Frishman WH, Parker JD, et al. Pharmacological options for treatment of ischemic disease. In: Antman M, Sabatine MS (Eds). Cardiovascular Therapeutics: A Companion to Braunwald's Heart Disease, 4th edition. Philadelphia: Elsevier; 2013. pp. 83-1305.
7. Frishman WH. Alpha and beta-adrenergic blocking drugs. In: Frishman WH, Sonemblick EH, Sica DA, (Eds). Cardiovascular Pharmacotherapeutics, 2nd edition. New York: McGraw Hill; 2003. pp 67-97.
8. Irfan A, Hirsch GA. Beta-blocker therapy in patients with stable coronary artery disease. Am Coll Cardiol. 2015.
9. Goldberger JJ, Bonow RO, Cuffe M, et al. Effect of beta blocker dose on survival after myocardial infarction. J Am Coll Cardiol. 2015;66:1431-41.
10. The Cardiac Insufficiency Bisoprolol Study II (CIBIS-II): a randomised trial. Lancet. 1999;353:9-13.
11. Effect of metoprolol CR/XL in chronic heart failure: Metoprolol CR/XL Randomised Intervention Trial in Congestive Heart Failure (MERIT-HF). Lancet. 1999;353:2001-7.
12. Dangie HJ. Effect of Carvedilol on outcome after myocardial infarction in patients with left ventricular dysfunction: the CAPRICORN randomised trial. Lancet. 2001;357:1385-90.
13. Packer M, Fowler MB, Roecker EB, et al. Carvedilol Prospective Randomised Cumulative Survival (COPERNICUS) stydy. Circulation. 2002;106:2194-9.
14. Andersson C, Shilane D, GO A.S, Beta Blocker therapy and cardiac events among patients with newly diagnosed coronary heart disease J Am Coll Cardiol, 2014; 64:247-252.
15. Bangalore S, Steig G, Deedwania P, et al. Beta-blocker use and clinical outcomes in stable outpatients with and without coronary artery disease. JAMA. 2012;308:1340-9.
16. Montalescot G, Sechtem U, et al. 2013 ESC guidelines on the management of stable coronary artery disease: the Task Force on the management of stable coronary artery disease of the European Society of Cardiology. Eur Heart J. 2013;34:2949-3003.

CHAPTER 32

Revascularization in Chronic Stable Angina—Current Status

Parneesh Arora, Upendra Kaul

INTRODUCTION

Chronic stable angina (CSA) also labeled as stable coronary artery disease (CAD) or stable ischemic heart disease (SIHD)[1] refers to patients with angina, its equivalent, or no symptoms who experience episodes of reversible myocardial supply demand mismatch, in absence of acute myocardial infarction (MI) or unstable angina. Nearly 300,000 percutaneous coronary interventions (PCIs) are performed annually in patients with SIHD in USA alone[2] and probably numbers in India would be much higher. As per National Interventional Council (NIC) registry for 2011, 22.3% of 152,332 PCI were for SIHD.[3] Data from randomized trials conflicts with current practice which is probably based on premise that wherein, epicardial stenosis is the cause of angina, ischemia, myocardial infraction, and death and these can be prevented by revascularization. This was probably outcome of landmark angiography-based studies which documented natural history of epicardial CAD and its adverse impact of survival.[4] Other studies correlating abnormal exercise stress test findings with presence of obstructive CAD[5] added fuel to the fire.

However, the trials subsequently did not bear out initial enthusiasm and need to be considered in order to understand current approach to patients with SIHD.

EVIDENCE FROM TRIALS

The proof whether PCI affects hard outcomes over medicine comes from randomized trials.

Prevention of Death and Myocardial Infarction

Trials comparing optimal medical therapy (OMT) to PCI, consistently showed disappointing result. The first trial to be done was ACME[6] trial (Angioplasty Compared to Medicine) in 1992 in 212 patients which though reported improvement in angina (64% vs. 54%) and exercise tolerance, but did not reduce mortality or MI. Subsequently, MASS[7] (Medicine, Angioplasty, or Surgery Study) included high-risk patients, with proximal left anterior descending (LAD) artery stenosis was negative for reduction of mortality and MI. RITA-2[8] (Second Randomized Intervention Treatment of Angina) a large trial of 1,000 patients, death or MI were less frequent with medical therapy then PCI (3.3% vs. 6.3% $p = 0.02$). Angina improved more with PCI with 16.5% absolute excess of grade 2 or worse angina in the medical therapy group at 3 months ($p < 0.001$).

In the stent era, MASS II[9] trial involving 611 patients with SIHD and proximal LAD stenosis, medical therapy reduced composite end point of cardiac mortality, MI, or refractory angina compared to PCI.

The landmark COURAGE[10] (Clinical Outcomes Utilizing Revascularization and Aggressive Drug Evaluation) trial compared initial strategy of PCI with protocol mandated OMT, with OMT alone in 2,287 patients with angina or objective evidence of ischemic and significant CAD (>70% stenosis). Crossover from OMT to PCI for refractory angina was permitted. After 4.6 years, there was no difference in death or nonfatal MI between two groups with 30% crossover from OMT group to percutaneous transluminal coronary angioplasty (PTCA). A meta-analysis in 2012[11] also did not show improvement in survival [odds ratio (OR) 0.98; 95% confidence interval (CI): 0.83–1.15] or in MI (combined OR 1.12; 95% CI: 0.93–1.34).

High-risk Subgroups

- *Diabetes mellitus*: The BARI 2D[12] trial of 2,368 patients with type 2 diabetes mellitus and stable CAD did not show any difference in mortality or major adverse cardiac events (MACE) at 5 years between PCI with medical management versus intensive medical management group. Subgroup analysis for amount of jeopardized myocardium, number of diseased vessels, numbers of lesions, proximal LAD disease, abnormal left ventricular function, prior revascularization, presence of total occlusion was also negative indicating the events are not prevented by PCI

- *Proximal LAD*: In COURAGE trial MACE were more in patients with proximal LAD stenosis more than 90%, however, PTCA did not improve these outcomes (p = 0.79)[13]
- *Three vessel CAD and low ejection fraction*: Again in COURAGE trial though survival was reduced in this subgroups of patients, however there was no benefit from initial PTCA and OMT compared to OMT alone.[14]

Hemodynamic Assessment of Significance of Epicardial Stenosis

With disappointing results from previous anatomy-based trials, tools to assess hemodynamic significance of epicardial CAD were developed. The hypothesis was that probably replacing oculostenotic reflex with ischemic PCI reflex, would lead to improved outcomes. Fractional flow reserve (FFR) is one such method and cut-off of FFR less than 0.8 was suggested for hemodynamically significant stenosis.

The FAME[16] (Fractional Flow Reserve versus Angiography for Multivessel Evaluation) trial randomized 1,005 patients to angiography-guided PTCA or FFR-guided PTCA. FFR-guided PTCA was associated with fewer PTCA and reduction in end point of death, MI or revascularization at 2 years. However, FAME-2[17] trial which randomized 888 patients to initial PCI + medical therapy against medical therapy alone did not show any difference in death, or MI at 2 years following. The subsequent analysis after excluding events in first 7 days, cited balance in favor of PCI group for reduction of MI. The criteria for diagnosis periprocedural MI were however questioned. The trial was terminated prematurely because composite end point favored FFR groups driven solely by urgent revascularization which was also criticized because of confounding factors.

In the recently published ORBITA[18] (Percutaneous Coronary Intervention in Stable Angina) trial 200 patients with ischemic symptoms having more than 70% single vessel stenosis were randomized to PCI (105 patients) and placebo procedure (95 patients), FFR was 0.69. There was no significant difference in primary end point of exercise time increment between groups at 6 weeks. In a subsequent analysis however it was shown that the stress echocardiography findings did improve in patients undergoing PCI and patients with lower FFR values benefitted more.[19]

CURRENT APPROACH TO REVASCULARIZATION FOR SIHD

Primary to understanding the current approach to SIHD is to understand that ischemia can result from dysfunction anywhere along vascular delivery conduit from aorta to microvasculature. This will help not only in selecting appropriate medical therapy for patients but also to select patients who would benefit from revascularization. Assessment of hemodynamic severity of stenosis in coronary artery is an integral part of selecting patients for intervention.

Assessment of Hemodynamic Severity of Epicardial Stenosis

- Fractional flow reserve is defined as ratio of mean distal coronary pressure to mean aorta pressure and requires induction of maximum hyperemia with pharmacological agents most common being adenosine. Incorporating stenosis severity, myocardial territory and viability, collateral perfusion, FFR can assess functional significance of a coronary stenosis. There is overall an acceptable correlation with noninvasive functional testing.[20] The cut-off value of 0.80 has been validated in multiple prospective randomized trial.[21] Trials with FFR-based revascularization and their outcomes are shown in table 1[22]
- Instant wave-free ratio (iFR) has been introduced as an alternative for FFR. This offers drug-free index of stenosis severity with accuracy comparable to FFR[23] and does not require induction of hyperemia. Instant wave-free ratio-guided revascularization has been proven to be noninferior to FFR-guided revascularization for MACE at 1 year follow up in two large randomized multicenter trials.[24,25]

INDICATIONS FOR CORONARY ANGIOGRAPHY

Current indications for coronary angiography for patients with SIHD as per American College of Cardiology are mentioned in table 2.[26]

CHOICE OF REVASCULARIZATION PCI OR CORONARY ARTERY BYPASS GRAFTING

- *Percutaneous coronary intervention versus coronary artery bypass grafting (CABG) overall*: Out of all trials available, the only large randomized trial comparing CABG and drug-eluting stents (DES) in current era is the SYNTAX Trial[27] (SYNergy between percutaneous coronary interventions with TAXus and cardiac surgery). In this trial patients were randomized to receive either DES or CABG. MACE of death, stroke, MI or repeat revascularization during 3 years after randomization occurred in 20.2% of CABG patients and 28.0% PCI with DES patients ($p < 0.001$), largely driven by less MI and less repeat revascularization in CABG group. At 5 years follow-up MACE was 26.9% for CABG and 37.3% for PCI ($p < 0.0001$) and combined endpoint of death, stroke and MI were also lower in CABG group ($p = 0.03$). Complexity of CAD was scored in the trial (SYNTAX score) with low score (<22) including less complicated, 23–32 indicating intermediate, and more than 33 indicating complicated anatomy. At 12 months MACE was same for CABG and

TABLE 1: Fractional flow reserve-based intervention trials and outcomes

Study name	Year	Size	Trial design	Clinical presentation	FFR cut-off	Outcomes
DEFER	2001	325 patients at 14 medical centers	Prospective, randomized	Stable chest pain and an intermediate stenosis without objective evidence of ischemia	0.75	No benefit stenting a nonischemic stenosis
FAME	2009	1,005 patients at 20 medical centers	Prospective, randomized	Multivessel CAD	0.80	Routine measurement of FFR in patients with multivessel CAD who are undergoing PCI with drug-eluting stent significantly reduces MACE at 1 year
FAME 2	2012	888 patients at 28 medical centers	Prospective, randomized	Stable CAD and hemodynamically significant stenoses	0.80	FFR-guided PCI with drug-eluting stent + OMT vs. OMT alone decreased the rate of urgent revascularization. In FFR negative lesions, OMT alone resulted in excellent outcomes, regardless of the angiographic appearance of the stenoses
Muller et al.	2011	730 patients at 1 Belgium center	Observational, nonrandomized study	Angiographically intermediate isolated proximal LAD stenosis	0.80	Medical treatment is associated with favorable long-term clinical outcomes in angiographically equivocal lesions nonischemic by FFR
Mayo Registry	2013	7,358 patients at the Mayo Clinic	Retrospective registry	Patients undergoing PCI, excluding STEMI or cardiogenic shock	<0.75 → PCI 0.75–0.80 → operator discretion >0.8 → OMT	FFR-guided treatment strategy is associated with a favorable long-term outcome with decreased MACE
Van Belle et al. (R3F)	2014	1,075 patients at 20 centers in France	Prospective observational study	Angiographically ambiguous lesion	0.80	FFR during diagnostic angiography is safe and associated with reclassification of the revascularization decision in about half of the patients
RIPCORD	2014	200 patients at 10 centers in the United Kingdom	Prospective observational study	Stable angina	0.8	FFR has an important influence both on which coronary arteries have significant stenosis and on patient management
DANAMI-3-PRIMULTI	2015	627 patients at two centers in Europe	Prospective randomized controlled trial	Patients with STEMI and multivessel disease who had undergone primary PCI of an infarct-related coronary artery	0.80	Complete-staged revascularization during the index admission, guided by FFR reduces the risk of future events, driven by fewer repeat revascularizations
Compare-Acute	2017	885 at 24 centers in Europe and Asia	Prospective randomized controlled trial	Patients with STEMI and multivessel disease who had undergone primary PCI of an infarct-related coronary artery	0.80	FFR-guided complete revascularization of noninfarct-related arteries in the acute setting resulted in lower MACE, driven by decreased revascularization
IRIS-FFR	2017	5,846 patients	Prospective registry	Patients with at least one coronary lesion	0.75	FFR ≤0.75: The risk of MACE was significantly lower in revascularized lesions than in deferred lesions Lesions with FFR ≥0.76, the risk of MACE was not significantly different between deferred and revascularized lesions

CAD, coronary artery disease; FFR, fractional flow reserve; IRIS, Interventional Cardiology Research Incooperation Society; LAD, left anterior descending; MACE: major adverse cardiac events; OMT: optimal medical therapy; PCI: percutaneous coronary intervention; STEMI: ST-elevation myocardial infarction.

TABLE 2: Indications for coronary angiography in patients with stable ischemic heart disease

Class	Indication	Level of evidence
I (indicated)	Patients with SIHD who have survived sudden cardiac death or potentially life-threatening ventricular arrhythmia should undergo coronary angiography to assess cardiac risk	B
	Patients with SIHD in whom symptoms and signs of heart failure develop should be evaluated to determine whether coronary angiography should be performed for risk assessment	B
	Coronary angiography is recommended for patients with SIHD whose clinical characteristics and results of noninvasive testing indicate a high likelihood of severe ischemic heart disease and when the benefits are deemed to exceed risk	C
II (good supportive evidence)	Coronary angiography is reasonable to further assess risk in patients with SIHD who have depressed LV function (EF <50%) and moderate-risk criteria on noninvasive testing with demonstrable ischemia	C
	Coronary angiography is reasonable to further assess risk in patients with SIHD and inconclusive prognostic information after noninvasive testing or in patients for whom noninvasive testing is contraindicated or inadequate	C
	Coronary angiography for risk assessment is reasonable for patients with SIHD who have unsatisfactory quality of life because of angina, have preserved LV function (EF >50%), and have intermediate-risk criteria on noninvasive testing	C

EV, ejection fraction; LV, left ventricle; SIHD, stable ischemic heart disease.

PCI for low SYNTAX score, but was higher in PCI group with intermediate or high score. At 3 years follow-up the mortality rate was greater in subjects with three-vessel CAD treated with DES than those with CABG. It seems reasonable to conclude that for complex and diffuse CAD, CABG scores over PCI but for uncomplicated or less complicated anatomy survival rate is same.

- *Percutaneous coronary intervention versus coronary artery bypass grafting for left main coronary artery disease*: In SYNTAX trial after excluding patients who underwent surgery because of complex disease, 705 patients with unprotected left main disease were randomized to PCI or CABG. Majority had low SYNTAX scores. At 1 year rates of all-cause death and MACE score were similar.[27] Repeat revascularization was more common in PCI group than in CABG (11.8% vs. 6.5%), but stroke was more common in CABG group (2.7% vs. 0.3%). At 5 years follow-up MACE rates did not differ for low or intermediate SYNTAX scores, but for high SYNTAX scores MACE was higher for PCI group (46.5% vs. 29.7%, p = 0.003). In PRECOMBAT (Premier of Randomized Comparison of Bypass Surgery Versus Angioplasty Using Sirolimus-Eluting Stent in Patients With Left Main Coronary Artery Disease) study of 600 patients composite endpoint of death, MI or stroke at 2 years was same (4.4% vs. 4.7%) for PCI versus CABG but target lesion revascularization was more often required in PCI group (9.0% vs. 4.2%).[28]

The above randomized trials suggest that major clinical outcomes in selected patients with left main CAD are similar with CABG and PCI at 1–2 years follow-up but repeat revascularization rates are higher after PCI than after CABG

- *Percutaneous coronary intervention or coronary artery bypass grafting in diabetes mellitus*: A comprehensive meta analyses of 8 trials in patients with diabetes mellitus and multivessel CAD establishes the superiority of CABG over PCI in this subset of patients. At 5 years or longest follow-up, patients with diabetes mellitus randomized to CABG, had lower all-cause mortality rate than those randomized to PCI with DES or bare metal stents (RR 0.67%; 95% CI: 0.52–0.86; p = 0.002).[29] Patients with diabetes should receive guideline indicated medical therapy and revascularization should be considered in those with symptoms impacting quality of life. Current indications for CABG and PCI are mentioned in table 3.

Based on above evidence flowchart 1 shows suggests algorithm for approach to revascularization to improve survival and flowchart 2 shows the algorithm for revascularization to improve symptoms.

CONCLUSION

Chronic stable angina or SIHD needs to be viewed as a syndrome where ischemia may result from pathology anywhere from epicardial stenosis to resistance vessels. Hence, if mechanism can be identified then selecting appropriate patients for revascularization would be possible. This is essential because despite multiple trials there is no evidence that strategy of initial revascularization especially routine PCI scores over medical therapy as far as hard cardiovascular outcomes are concerned. If at all there is evidence for survival benefit of patients it is for CABG where indicated. Compared to CABG, in select patients, PCI may offer similar outcomes at least in intermediate follow-up (around 5 years). Strategies for hemodynamic assessment like FFR and iFR may help in deciding which patients may have comparable results for PCI versus CABG as well as which patients can be continued on OMT.

TABLE 3: Guidelines for coronary artery bypass grafting and percutaneous coronary intervention in stable ischemic heart disease[30,31]

Anatomic setting	Class	Recommendation	Levels of evidence
Unprotected left main			
CABG	I		B
PCI	IIa	For SIHD when both of the following are present: • Anatomic conditions associated with a low-risk for PCI procedural complications and a high likelihood of a good long-term outcome • Clinical characteristics that predict a significantly increased risk for adverse surgical outcomes	B
	IIb	For SIHD when both of the following are present: • Anatomic conditions associated with a low to intermediate risk for PCI procedural complications and an intermediate to high likelihood of a good long-term outcome • Clinical characteristics that predict increased risk for adverse surgical outcomes (e.g., STS-predicted operative mortality >2%)	B
	III	For SIHD in patients (vs. performing CABG) with unfavorable anatomy for PCI and who are good candidates for CABG	B
Three-vessel coronary artery disease with or without proximal left anterior descending coronary artery disease			
CABG	I		B
PCI	IIa	It is reasonable to choose CABG over PCI in patients with complex three-vessel CAD (e.g., SYNTAX score 222) who are good candidates for CABG	B
	IIb		B
Two-vessel coronary artery disease with proximal left anterior descending coronary artery disease			
CABG	I	–	B
PCI	IIb	–	B
Two-vessel coronary artery disease without proximal left anterior descending coronary artery disease			
CABG	IIa	With extensive ischemia	B
PCI	IIb	Without extensive ischemia	C
	IIb		B
One-vessel proximal left anterior descending coronary artery disease			
CABG	IIa	With LIMA	B
PCI	IIb		B
One-vessel coronary artery disease without proximal left anterior descending coronary artery disease			
CABG	III	Harm	B
PCI	III	Harm	B
Left ventricular dysfunction			
CABG	IIa	EF of 35–50%	B
	IIb	EF <35% without significant left main disease	B
PCI	N/A	Insufficient data	
Survivors of sudden cardiac death with presumed ischemia-mediated ventricular tachycardia			
CABG	I	–	B
PCI	I	–	C

CABG, coronary artery bypass grafting; CAD, coronary artery disease; EF, ejection fraction; LIMA, left internal mammary artery; N/A, not applicable; PCI, percutaneous coronary intervention; SIHD, stable ischemic heart disease; STS, Society of Thoracic Surgeons; SYNTAX, SYNergy between PCI with TAXus and Cardiac Surgery.

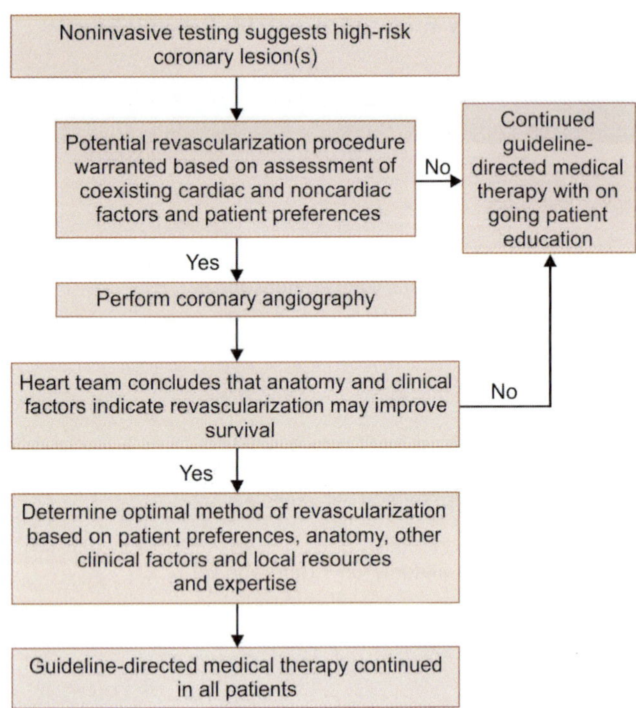

FLOWCHART 1: Suggested algorithm for revascularization[30] to improve survival.

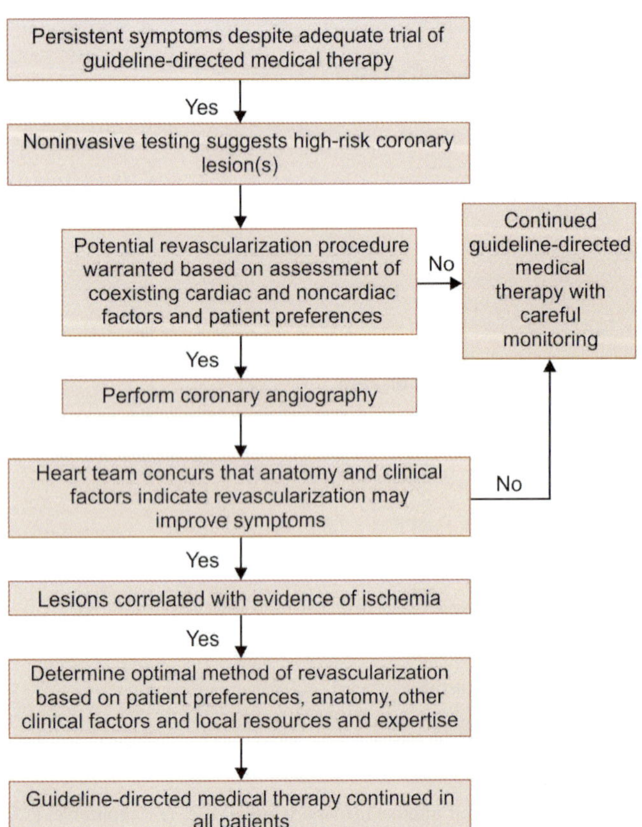

FLOWCHART 2: Suggested algorithm to improve symptoms.[30]

REFERENCES

1. Fihn SD, Gardin JM, Abrams J, et al. 2012 ACCF/AHA/ACP/AATS/PCNA/SCAI/STS guideline for the diagnosis and management of patients with stable ischemic heart disease: A report of the American College of Cardiology Foundation/American Heart Association Task Force on Practice Guidelines, and the American College of Physicians, American Association for Thoracic Surgery, Preventive Cardiovascular Nurses Association, Society for Cardiovascular Angiography and Interventions, and Society of Thoracic Surgeons. J Am Coll Cardiol. 2012;60:e44-164.
2. Dehmer GJ, Weaver D, Roe MT, et al. A contemporary view of diagnostic cardiac catheterization and percutaneous coronary intervention in the United States: a report from the CathPCI Registry of the National Cardiovascular Data Registry, 2010 through June 2011. J Am Coll Cardiol. 2012;60:2017-31.
3. Mardikar HM, Ramakrishnan S, Mishra S, et al. Report on Indian coronary intervention data for the year 2011 – National Interventional Council. Indian Heart J. 2013;65(5):518-21.
4. Jones WB, Riley CP, Reeves TJ, et al. Natural history of coronary artery disease. Bull N Y Acad Med. 1972;48:1109-25.
5. Hultgren H, Calciano A, Platt F, et al. A clinical evaluation of coronary arteriography. Am J Med. 1967;42:228-47.
6. Parisi AF, Folland ED, Hartigan P. A comparison of angioplasty with medical therapy in the treatment of single-vessel coronary artery disease. Veterans affairs ACME investigators. N Engl J Med. 1992;326:10-6.
7. Hueb WA, Bellotti G, de Oliveira SA, et al. The Medicine, Angioplasty or Surgery Study (MASS): A prospective, randomized trial of medical therapy, balloon angioplasty or bypass surgery for single proximal left anterior descending artery stenoses. J Am Coll Cardiol. 1995;26:1600-5.
8. Coronary angioplasty versus medical therapy for angina: the second Randomised Intervention Treatment of Angina (RITA-2) trial. RITA-2 trial participants. Lancet. 1997;350:461-8.
9. Hueb W, Soares PR, Gersh BJ, et al. The Medicine, Angioplasty, or Surgery Study (MASS-II): A randomized, controlled clinical trial of three therapeutic strategies for multivessel coronary artery disease: one-year results. J Am Coll Cardiol. 2004;43:1743-51.
10. Boden WE, O'Rourke RA, Teo KK, et al. Optimal medical therapy with or without PCI for stable coronary disease. N Engl J Med. 2007;356:1503-16.
11. Stergiopoulos K, Brown DL. Initial coronary stent implantation with medical therapy vs medical therapy alone for stable coronary artery disease: meta-analysis of randomized controlled trials. Arch Intern Med. 2012;172:312-9.
12. Frye RL, August P, Brooks MM, et al. A randomized trial of therapies for type 2 diabetes and coronary artery disease. N Engl J Med. 2009;360:2503-15.
13. Mancini GB, Bates ER, Maron DJ, et al. Quantitative results of baseline angiography and percutaneous coronary intervention in the COURAGE trial. Circ Cardiovasc Qual Outcomes. 2009;2:320-7.
14. Mancini GB, Hartigan PM, Bates ER, et al. Prognostic importance of coronary anatomy and left ventricular ejection fraction despite optimal therapy: Assessment of residual risk in the clinical outcomes utilizing revascularization and aggressive drug evaluation trial. Am Heart J. 2013;166:481-7.
15. Mitchell JD, Brown DL. Harmonizing the Paradigm With the Data in Stable Coronary Artery Disease: A Review and Viewpoint. J Am Heart Assoc. 2017;6(11). pii: e007006.
16. Tonino PA, De Bruyne B, Pijls NH, et al. Fractional flow reserve versus angiography for guiding percutaneous coronary intervention. N Engl J Med. 2009;360:213-24.
17. De Bruyne B, Fearon WF, Pijls NH, et al. Fractional flow reserve-guided PCI for stable coronary artery disease. N Engl J Med. 2014;371:1208-17.
18. Al-Lamee R, Thompson D, Dehbi HM, et al. Percutaneous coronary intervention in stable angina (ORBITA): a double-blind, randomised controlled trial. Lancet. 2018;391(10115):31-40.
19. Al-Lamee R, Howard JP, Matthew J Shun-Shin, et al. Fractional Flow Reserve and Instantaneous Wave-Free Ratio as Predictors of the Placebo-Controlled Response to Percutaneous Coronary Intervention in Stable Single-Vessel Coronary Artery Disease: Physiology-Stratified Analysis of ORBITA. Circulation. 2018;138: in print.
20. Christou MA, Siontis GC, Katritsis DG, et al. Meta-analysis of fractional flow reserve versus quantitative coronary angiography and noninvasive imaging for evaluation of myocardial ischemia. Am J Cardiol. 2007;99:450-6.

21. Shlofmitz E, Jeremias A. (2017). FFR in 2017: Current Status in PCI Management. [online] Available from http://www.acc.org/latest-in-cardiology/articles/2017/05/25/08/34/ffr-in-2017-current-status-in-pci-management.
22. Rioufol G, Mewton N, Rabilloud M, et al. Functional testing underlying revascularization: The FUTURE trial. Presented at American Heart Association Scientific Sessions 2016 on November 14, 2016.
23. Ahn JM, Park DW, Shin ES, et al. Fractional flow reserve and cardiac events in coronary artery disease: Data from a prospective IRIS-FFR Registry (Interventional Cardiology Research Incooperation Society Fractional Flow Reserve). Circulation. 2017;136(24):2393-4.
24. Götberg M, Christiansen EH, Gudmundsdottir IJ, et al. Instantaneous wave-free ratio versus fractional flow reserve to guide PCI. N Engl J Med. 2017;376:1813-23.
25. Davies JE, Sen S, Dehbi HM, et al. Use of the instantaneous wave-free ratio or fractional flow reserve in PCI. N Engl J Med. 2017;376:1824-34.
26. Fihn SD, Blankenship JC, Alexander KP, et al. 2014 ACC/AHA/AATS/PCNA/SCAI/STS Focused Update of the Guideline for the Diagnosis and Management of Patients With Stable Ischemic Heart Disease. Circulation. 2014;130:1749-67.
27. Serruys PW, Morice MC, Kappetein AP, et al. Percutaneous Coronary Intervention versus Coronary-Artery Bypass Grafting for Severe Coronary Artery Disease. N Engl J Med. 2009;360:961-72.
28. Morice MC, Serruys PW, Kappetein AP, et al. Outcomes in patients with de novo left main disease treated with either percutaneous coronary intervention using paclitaxel-eluting stents or coronary artery bypass graft treatment in the Synergy Between Percutaneous Coronary Intervention with TAXUS and Cardiac Surgery (SYNTAX) trial. Circulation. 2010;121(24):2645-53.
29. Park SJ, Kim YH, Park DW, et al. Randomized Trial of Stents versus Bypass Surgery for Left Main Coronary Artery Disease. N Engl J Med. 2011;364:1718-27.
30. Verma S, Farkouh ME, Yanagawa B, et al. Comparison of coronary artery bypass surgery and percutaneous coronary intervention in patients with diabetes: a meta-analysis of randomized controlled trials. Lancet Diabetes Endocrinol. 2013;1(4):317-28.
31. Fihn SD, Gardin JM, Abrams J, et al. 2012 ACCF/AHA/ACP/AATS/PCNA/SCAI/STS guideline for diagnosis and management of patients with stable ischemic heart disease. A report of the American College of Cardiology foundation/American heart association task force on practice guidelines. J Am Coll Cardiol. 2012;60(24):2564-603.

CHAPTER 33

Revascularization in Diabetes: Rational Choices in 2018

Rajiv Agarwal

SUMMARY

The outcome of coronary revascularization in diabetic patients is undeniably worse than that in nondiabetics regardless of the modality chosen. Large randomized trials have looked at the choice between coronary artery bypass grafting (CABG) and percutaneous coronary intervention (PCI) in diabetic patients including BARI, BARI 2D, ARTS II, CARDia, VA-CARDS, and BEST besides the SYNTAX and FREEDOM trial. They all suggest that in stable multivessel disease with diabetes, CABG offers superior outcome as compared to PCI including approximately 30% mortality benefit with CABG. There is lower incidence of angina and repeat revascularization and also fewer hard endpoints like recurrent myocardial infarction (MI) and mortality with CABG. Stroke, however, occurs more frequently after CABG than with PCI. Coronary revascularization guidelines, therefore, recommend CABG over PCI for stable multivessel disease in diabetic patients as a class I recommendation.

The SYNTAX trial looked at anatomical complexity of coronary disease and suggested that in the low-risk tertile (SYNTAX score ≤22), diabetic multivessel disease patients did as well with PCI, even with the now obsolete Taxus stent, as with CABG.

The randomized trials do not represent the full spectrum of diabetic patients undergoing revascularization as often patients with weak hearts, repeat procedures and comorbidities are excluded. In many such patients in the real world, PCI may be chosen over CABG with a reasonable expectation of faster recovery and less procedure-related morbidity even at the cost of more incomplete revascularization. There is also a strong patient preference for less invasive treatment by PCI rather than CABG, provided results can be assured. Registry data also documents the marked preference for PCI over CABG even in multivessel diabetics in clinical practice despite better results with surgery. Hence, the continuing search to define the subsets, if any, of multivessel diabetic patients who can safely be offered PCI.

The results of PCI are continually improving with second-generation drug-eluting stents (DES) performing better than the first generation. In a network meta-analysis of diabetic patients, second-generation DES had equivalent outcome to CABG.

The heart team is useful in evolving consensus here. Diabetes alone cannot lead to a reflexive recommendation of CABG for revascularization. Decisions should be guided by data including accounting for both coronary anatomy (SYNTAX score) and clinical factors to predict mortality by SYNTAX-II. Recent data suggests that with modern techniques including the above and fractional flow reserve (FFR) guidance, PCI outcomes are better than historical controls and comparable to CABG even in the diabetic patient.

There is urgent need for a new randomized trial using contemporary techniques of PCI and CABG. We need to be forward looking but vigilant against hype.

INTRODUCTION

Approximately 20–30% of patients admitted with acute coronary syndromes (ACS) have diabetes mellitus (DM), mostly type 2 diabetes (T2DM).[1] Diabetes increases the risk of developing coronary artery disease (CAD) and has been called a CAD risk equivalent.[2] An individual with diabetes has the same coronary disease risk as a person with prior MI. The prognosis of a diabetic with MI is worse than that of a nondiabetic. This is especially true in long-standing diabetics and those on insulin therapy. Coronary atherosclerosis is more extensive in diabetic patients, with faster disease progression, more diffuse disease, more left main involvement and poorer outcomes with any revascularization treatment as compared to patients without diabetes.[3] Diabetic patients have increased platelet reactivity and impaired responsiveness to clopidogrel which can be a problem following coronary stents.[4] Diabetic patients also tend to have more restenosis after balloon angioplasty and bare metal stents than nondiabetics.[5,6]

SURGERY OR PERCUTANEOUS CORONARY INTERVENTION

Coronary revascularization is a key component of the management of the patient with diabetes and is the focus of this paper. The outcome of coronary revascularization in diabetic patients is undeniably worse than that in nondiabetics regardless of the modality chosen. The more important question is how to revascularize these patients—mainly the choice between percutaneous coronary intervention (PCI) and coronary artery bypass grafting (CABG). A survival advantage at 5 years of CABG over PCI in diabetic patients was demonstrated as early as 1996 in a subgroup analysis of the diabetic patients in the Bypass Angioplasty Revascularization Investigation (BARI) trial.[7] No such survival difference was seen in the overall trial. This superiority of CABG over PCI in diabetic patients was due to lower cardiac mortality, was confined to those surgical patients receiving at least one internal mammary artery graft[8] and was maintained at 7 years and 10 years.[9,10] Although this trial compared plain balloon angioplasty with CABG, yet the difference in outcomes has persisted till date despite the improvement in technology and techniques including the introduction of bare metal stents[11] and first-generation drug-eluting stents (DES).[12] Particularly noteworthy is the persisting mortality benefit with CABG as compared to PCI in diabetic patients in the large FREEDOM (Future REvascularization Evaluation in patients with DIabetes mellitus: Optimal management of Multivessel disease) trial.[12]

FREEDOM TRIAL

The FREEDOM trial of 2012 is the largest and most contemporary randomized controlled trial (RCT) which focused exclusively on diabetic patients. It showed superior outcomes with CABG than with PCI in all subgroups. All-cause death and also MI were significantly less with CABG than with PCI, while stroke rate and repeat revascularization were increased with CABG.

Guidelines

Coronary revascularization guidelines therefore recommend CABG over PCI for stable multivessel disease in diabetic patients as a class I recommendation.[13-15] However, CABG in diabetics may be associated with considerable morbidity related to infections, sternal and leg wound problems, renal insufficiency, etc. Patients also increasingly prefer the rapid recovery, and less invasive nature of PCI.

OTHER RANDOMIZED TRIALS

Numerous randomized trials have been conducted on diabetic patients with stable CAD comparing the outcomes of PCI with CABG.[8,12,16-24] The problem is in being able to compare similar patients who are representative of the whole group because, traditionally, patients with multivessel disease with less anatomical complexity have been offered PCI whereas patients with more complex disease including diffuse disease and chronic total occlusions (CTOs) have been offered CABG.

One approach, which was used in the Bypass Angioplasty Revascularization Investigation 2 Diabetes (BARI-2D)[16] trial of 2009, randomized diabetic patients with multivessel disease between early revascularization and intensive medical therapy with a nonrandomized assignment to a PCI or CABG stratum based on clinical and angiographic data. The CABG stratum had more extensive and complex disease. This trial failed to demonstrate a benefit of PCI over medical therapy and we shall discuss this later. The CABG stratum showed improvement in the composite endpoint of death or MI or stroke over medical therapy. BARI-2D, therefore, offers an indirect comparison of the results of CABG and PCI in disparate patient groups.

Reasons offered for better results with CABG range from an inherent advantage over PCI by virtue of bypassing mild nonculprit lesions to the presence of more complex disease in the CABG stratum, thereby allowing the emergence of an advantage of revascularization over medical therapy.[17] CABG bypasses not just the critical lesion but also associated milder lesions which may progress in future. Indeed, after PCI with current stents that have low restenosis rates, repeat ischemic events happen more often at nontreated sites which had mild or no disease on initial angiogram.[18] This suggests that CABG may have an inherent theoretical advantage over lesion specific treatment by PCI, especially in diabetic patient with multivessel disease.

Other randomized trials have directly compared PCI and CABG in patients deemed eligible for both procedures. While rigorous, this method also excludes many patients who are eligible for only one procedure. The large randomized trials include ARTS II, CARDia, VA-CARDS, and BEST besides the SYNTAX (SYNergy between percutaneous coronary intervention with TAXus and cardiac surgery) and FREEDOM trial.[19-25,12] They all suggest that in stable multivessel disease with diabetes, CABG offers superior outcome as compared to PCI including approximately 30% mortality benefit with CABG. This benefit is driven not only by lower incidence of angina and repeat revascularization but also fewer hard endpoints like recurrent MI and mortality. Stroke, however, occurs more frequently after CABG than with PCI. The difference between CABG and PCI may emerge only on longer term follow-up. Thus, in one meta-analysis there was no difference in the rates of MI and death at 1 year but at 5 years, CABG came out significantly ahead.[26] Other meta-analyses with varying criteria and even patient level analysis of data have also shown CABG to be superior.[27-29] It may therefore be argued that even in the less complex patients where both procedures are possible, CABG is superior to PCI in diabetics.

SYNTAX Trial

The SYNTAX trial assessed the complexity of multivessel disease by angiography using an anatomical SYNTAX score and divided patients into low, intermediate and high risk tertiles.[23] Diabetics did worse overall than nondiabetics regardless of the method of revascularization. CABG performed better overall than PCI. However, in the low-risk tertile (SYNTAX score ≤22), the results of PCI and CABG were comparable both in the diabetic and nondiabetic subgroup at 1 year and 5 years.[24,25] This was based on numerically lower rates of death, MI and cerebrovascular accident but significantly higher repeat revascularization with PCI than with CABG.

Thus, there exists a subgroup of diabetic multivessel disease patients with low anatomical complexity in whom PCI, even with the now obsolete Taxus stent, performs as well as CABG. The limitations of subgroup analysis are however well known and the equally large FREEDOM trial could not identify such a low risk group for PCI.[12]

INCOMPLETE REVASCULARIZATION

Anatomical, technical and clinical factors may lead to incomplete revascularization in patients with multivessel disease. This may be more so in PCI where some lesions may be left untreated due to CTOs, lesion complexity or even contrast load. In one large meta-analysis of multivessel disease, incomplete revascularization occurred in 56% of PCI versus 25% of CABG patients.[30] Incomplete revascularization was associated with an adverse impact on long-term survival, and MI with more repeat revascularization. In clinical practice, most physicians are unwilling to leave incomplete revascularization in a large viable left anterior descending (LAD) territory and this may impact choice of therapy.

SECOND-GENERATION DRUG-ELUTING STENTS

The results of the randomized trials may be outdated with the current improvement in technology from plain balloon angioplasty to bare metal stent to DES.[31] Even the often quoted FREEDOM trial used first-generation DES. Contemporary second-generation DES have thinner struts, better geometry, better polymer and drugs than first-generation DES. This contributes to better initial outcomes, less restenosis, and less repeat procedures with second-generation DES as compared to first generation. In a network meta-analysis of diabetic patients, second-generation DES had equivalent outcome to CABG.[32] However, RCTs directly comparing second-generation DES with CABG are needed to confirm that PCI has indeed caught up with surgery.

REAL WORLD SCENARIO

Beyond the need for better technology, it should also be remembered that the topline results of the randomized trials do not fully reflect clinical realities. The trials enroll selected patients and most often exclude patients with severe left ventricular dysfunction, left main disease, recent ACS, prior revascularization and significant comorbidities including renal failure. In many such patients in the real world, PCI may be chosen over CABG with a reasonable expectation of faster recovery and less procedure related morbidity even at the cost of more incomplete revascularization. There is also a strong patient preference for less invasive treatment by PCI rather than CABG provided results can be assured. Hence, the continuing search to define the subsets, if any, of multivessel diabetic patients who can safely be offered PCI.

REGISTRY DATA

Real world practices are best assessed by registry data. In the BARI, those patients who refused randomization in the main trial were enrolled in a registry in which physicians chose the method of revascularization. Twice as many patients were offered PCI as compared to CABG based on clinical factors. PCI fared as well as CABG even in diabetics unlike the main trial out to 7 years. Thus with proper selection, PCI in diabetics may be as safe as surgery and more acceptable to patients and physicians.[33] These were, however, stable lower risk patients who were BARI eligible.

Another registry covering the province of British Columbia, Canada at the time of the FREEDOM trial found that 63% of diabetic patients undergoing revascularization were characterized as ACS rather than stable ischemic heart disease (SIHD).[34] Again, PCI was chosen twice as often as CABG. However, CABG patients in this report did significantly better than those offered PCI. Patients offered PCI were older and had more left ventricular dysfunction, which may have influenced the outcome. Thus, the real world preference for PCI is completely missed in the RCTs although CABG may be underutilized in practice.

Another nationwide registry from Sweden enrolled all type 1 diabetics who were offered multivessel revascularization over a 19-year period. It also highlighted the preference of PCI over CABG in multivessel diabetic patients in practice.[35] PCI patients were sicker with more advanced age, female gender, poorer renal function, more prior MI and stroke and other comorbidities and longer duration of diabetes than CABG patients. However, surgical patients had better long-term outcome partly due to imbalance in baseline factors. The preference for PCI over CABG increased markedly from the early to the late years of the study. This certainly reflects physician and patient preference for a less invasive procedure in sicker patients. Thus, in the real world, multivessel diabetic patients may be offered PCI rather than CABG at two ends of the spectrum, viz., either if they are thought to have less anatomical complexity or if they have high clinical risk.

RATIONAL CHOICE OF REVASCULARIZATION STRATEGY: EVOLVING A CONSENSUS

Is real world practice, which often chooses PCI over CABG in multivessel diabetics, rational or an example of therapeutic anarchy? Should we offer PCI over CABG to selected diabetic patients with multivessel disease despite higher incidence of incomplete revascularization? Does the lesion independent nature of CABG confer an irreducible advantage despite improvement in PCI treatment of individual lesions?

The heart team is useful in evolving consensus here but should not be deciding merely by competing expert opinions.

A randomized trial to capture the entire clinical spectrum and validate this approach is difficult. More science is needed.

The SYNTAX and FREEDOM trials are already outdated as they compared conventional PCI with first-generation DES. A rational choice of procedure must account for high clinical risk and use the best available technology.

SYNTAX-II Score and Trial

The anatomical SYNTAX score has been upgraded to the SYNTAX-II score by incorporating those clinical variables which impacted outcomes in the SYNTAX trial database and predicting 4-year mortality on this basis.[36] Factors like age, gender, renal function, ejection fraction, peripheral vascular disease and chronic obstructive pulmonary disease were found to impact outcomes. The performance of the SYNTAX-II score has been validated in multiple studies.[37] Interestingly, once the SYNTAX score was calculated, presence of diabetes no longer influenced the relative benefit of CABG and PCI. Thus, diabetes alone cannot lead to a reflexive recommendation of CABG for revascularization.

The recently published SYNTAX-II trial compared the outcomes of contemporary PCI with matched controls from SYNTAX trial in *de novo* three-vessel disease.[38] Overall, the heart team chose PCI in 454 out of 708 patients that were screened. Decision-making was guided by the SYNTAX-II score and the procedure was guided by FFR and intravascular ultrasound. With these advances, along with a heart team approach and contemporary strategies for CTOs, there was a 42% improvement in 1-year outcomes of PCI from SYNTAX-I to SYNTAX-II trial (MACCE 17.4 vs. 10.6%). This was driven by a significant decline in MI, definite stent thrombosis and repeat revascularization. SYNTAX-II patients with diabetes did as well as those without diabetes. Exploratory analysis also suggests that the 1-year outcome of contemporary PCI from SYNTAX-II matches that of a CABG subgroup from SYNTAX trial. These findings need to be confirmed over the longer term as differences in outcome might emerge at 5 years, but are potentially practice changing.

NEW RANDOMIZED TRIALS NEEDED

There is urgent need for a new randomized trial using contemporary techniques of PCI and CABG in order to better inform choice of revascularization strategy in the contemporary era in diabetics and even those without diabetes. Of course, technology keeps changing and outcome data takes time to accrue, so in each timeframe, we need to be forward looking but vigilant against hype.

COMPARISON WITH MEDICAL THERAPY

The second controversial area is the need to demonstrate superiority over medical therapy in SIHD patients in order to recommend revascularization. The negative results of the BARI-2D trial when comparing PCI and medical therapy in stable low risk patients are mentioned above.[16] The Clinical Outcomes Utilizing Revascularization and Aggressive Drug Evaluation (COURAGE) trial shows similar results.[39] A nuclear substudy of COURAGE suggests that patients with significant documented ischemia may derive benefit from revascularization, but this finding is controversial.[40] The more recent sham-controlled ORBITA trial looked at a low risk single vessel disease population with no left ventricular dysfunction and found no improvement in exercise capacity with PCI compared to medical therapy at 6 weeks.[41] All these trials suffer from a high rate of subsequent revascularization in the medical arm. In ORBITA, once the randomized trial was over, fully 85% of patients in the medical arm underwent PCI, thus preventing longer follow-up and calling the conclusions into question.[42] However, one may conclude that asymptomatic or even mildly symptomatic patients can be offered initial intensive medical management with revascularization reserved for significant symptoms. The still on-going International Study of Comparative Health Effectiveness with Medical and Invasive Approaches (ISCHEMIA) trial may offer further answers although it is already mired in controversy due to late modification of primary endpoint and the lack of sham controls.[43] Recent improvements in medical therapy including drugs like ranolazine, trimetazidine and ivabradine in addition to statins, angiotensin-converting enzyme inhibitors or angiotensin receptor blockers and beta-blockers need to be acknowledged. Newer antidiabetic drugs, including the SGLT2 inhibitors, offer the potential for further cardiovascular event reduction but are beyond the scope of this chapter.[44,45] The impact, if any, on outcomes of medical therapy versus revascularization is unknown.

ACUTE CORONARY SYNDROMES

There is a paucity of randomized data on revascularization strategy in diabetic patients with ACS who turn out to have multivessel disease. This group constitutes the majority of patients undergoing revascularization in diabetes with a preference for PCI in clinical practice despite better outcomes in selected patients with CABG.[34] Culprit vessel intervention alone may be the favored strategy in unstable patients with multivessel intervention in the same sitting being reserved for cardiogenic shock and also simple lesions in stable patients.

TYPE AND DURATION OF DIABETES

Data is also limited on the influence of the type and duration of diabetes on the relative outcomes of PCI and CABG. The Swedish registry mentioned earlier suggests that CABG is superior to PCI in both type I and type II diabetes.[35] Insulin treated patients did worse than those on oral drugs in the FREEDOM trial, but this may be due to more advanced disease in patients taking insulin.[46] It may be noted that when patients were randomized between insulin provision and insulin sensitization in the BARI-2D study, there was no difference in outcome except more hypoglycemia with insulin.[16]

CONCLUSION

The heart team approach as adopted in many centers has gone a long way in improving the patient's access to information about both procedures. In such a scenario, patient preference will assume greater importance as the patient has to decide the importance he/she attaches to cost, invasiveness of approach, rapidity of recovery, and chance of repeat procedures, besides the data about lesser mortality but more stroke with CABG. An expanding group of lower risk patients may choose PCI over CABG even in presence of diabetes.

Pending the availability of more data, the heart team should recognize that revascularization decisions in diabetic multivessel disease are complex. Where there is equipoise and both procedures are anatomically feasible, the heart team should counsel patients accordingly. A formal calculation of SYNTAX score (upgraded to clinical SYNTAX-II) may be used in addition to expert opinion. Inclusion of functional data by FFR may further improve outcomes of PCI, and even reduce the number of lesions treated and stents used as is being studied in the FAME 3 (Fractional flow reserve versus Angiography for Multivessel Evaluation) trial.[46] The recent presentation of the SYNTAX-III revolution data using CT-derived FFR has shown a roadmap for further improvement of rational decision making even in surgical patients.[47,48]

REFERENCES

1. Luscher TF, Creager MA, Beckman JA, et al. Diabetes and vascular disease: pathophysiology, clinical consequences, and medical therapy: Part II. Circulation. 2003;108:1655-61.
2. Haffner SM, Lehto S, Ronnemaa T, et al. Mortality from coronary heart disease in subjects with type 2 diabetes and in non-diabetic subjects with and without prior myocardial infarction. N Engl J Med. 1998;339:229-34.
3. Marso SP, Mercado N, Maehara A, et al. Plaque composition and clinical outcomes in acute coronary syndrome patients with metabolic syndrome or diabetes. JACC Cardiovasc Imaging. 2012;5:S42-52.
4. Angiolillo DJ, Jakubowski JA, Ferreiro JL, et al. Impaired responsiveness to the platelet P2Y12 receptor antagonist clopidogrel in patients with type 2 diabetes and coronary artery disease. J Am Coll Cardiol. 2014;64:1005-14.
5. Stein B, Weintraub WS, Gebhart SSP, et al. Influence of diabetes mellitus on early and late outcome after percutaneous transluminal coronary angioplasty. Circulation. 1995;91:979-89.
6. Elezi S, Kastrati A, Pache J, et al. Diabetes mellitus and the clinical and angiographic outcome after coronary stent placement. J Am Coll Cardiol. 1998;32:1866-73.
7. The BARI Investigators. The Bypass Angioplasty Revascularization Investigation (BARI) Investigators. Comparison of coronary bypass surgery with angioplasty in patients with multivessel disease. N Engl J Med. 1996;335:217-25.
8. The BARI Investigators. Influence of Diabetes on 5-Year Mortality and Morbidity in a Randomized Trial Comparing CABG and PTCA in Patients with Multivessel Disease. The Bypass Angioplasty Revascularization Investigation (BARI). Circulation. 1997;96:1761-9.
9. The BARI Investigators. Seven-Year Outcome in the Bypass Angioplasty Revascularization Investigation (BARI) By Treatment and Diabetic Status. J Am Coll Cardiol. 2000;35:1122-9.
10. The BARI Investigators. The Final 10-Year Follow-Up Results from the BARI Randomized Trial. J Am Coll Cardiol. 2007;49:1600-6.
11. Wilson SR, Vakili BA, Sherman W, et al. Effect of diabetes on long-term mortality following contemporary percutaneous coronary intervention: analysis of 4,284 cases. Diabetes Care. 2004;27:1137-42.
12. Farkouh ME, Domanski M, Sleeper LA, et al. Strategies for multivessel revascularization in patients with diabetes for the FREEDOM Trial Investigators. N Engl J Med. 2012;367:2375-84.
13. Windecker S, Kolh P, Alfonso F, et al. 2014 ESC/EACTS guidelines on myocardial revascularization. Eur Heart J. 2014;35:2541-619.
14. Levine GN, Bates ER, Blankenship JC, et al. 2011 ACCF/AHA/SCAI guideline for percutaneous coronary intervention. J Am Coll Cardiol. 2011;58:e44-122.
15. Fihn SD, Blankenship JC, Alexander KP, et al. 2014 ACC/AHA/AATS/PCNA/SCAI/STS focused update of the guideline for the diagnosis and management of patients with stable ischemic heart disease: a report of the American College of Cardiology/American Heart Association Task Force on Practice Guidelines. Circulation. 2014;130:1749-67.
16. BARI-2D Study Group. A randomized trial of therapies for type 2 diabetes and coronary artery disease. N Engl J Med. 2009;360:2503-15.
17. Ikeno F, Brooks MM, Nakagawa K, et al. SYNTAX Score and Long-Term Outcomes: The BARI-2D Trial. J Am Coll Cardiol. 2017;69:395-403.
18. Cutlip DE, Chhabra AG, Baim DS, et al. Beyond Restenosis Five-Year Clinical Outcomes From Second-Generation Coronary Stent Trials. Circulation. 2004;110:1226-30.
19. Onuma Y, Wykrzykowska JJ, Garg S, et al. 5-Year follow-up of coronary revascularization in diabetic patients with multivessel coronary artery disease: insights from ARTS (arterial revascularization therapy study)-II and ARTS-I trials. JACC Cardiovasc Interv. 2011;4:317-23.
20. Kapur A, Hall RJ, Malik IS, et al. Randomized comparison of percutaneous coronary intervention with coronary artery bypass grafting in diabetic patients. 1-year results of the CARDia (Coronary Artery Revascularization in Diabetes) trial. J Am Coll Cardiol. 2010;55:432-40.
21. Kamalesh M, Sharp TG, Tang XC, et al. Percutaneous coronary intervention versus coronary bypass surgery in United States veterans with diabetes. J Am Coll Cardiol. 2013;61:808-16.
22. Park SJ, Ahn JM, Kim YH, et al. Trial of everolimus-eluting stents or bypass surgery for coronary disease. N Engl J Med. 2015;372:1204-12.
23. Mohr FW, Morice MC, Kappetein AP, et al. Coronary artery bypass graft surgery versus percutaneous coronary intervention in patients with three-vessel disease and left main coronary disease: 5-year follow-up of the randomised, clinical SYNTAX trial. Lancet. 2013;381:629-38.
24. Banning AP, Westaby S, Morice MC, et al. Diabetic and nondiabetic patients with left main and/or 3-vessel coronary artery disease: comparison of outcomes with cardiac surgery and paclitaxel-eluting stents. J Am Coll Cardiol. 2010;55:1067-75.
25. Kappetein AP, Head SJ, Morice MC, et al. Treatment of complex coronary artery disease in patients with diabetes: 5-year results comparing outcomes of bypass surgery and percutaneous coronary intervention in the SYNTAX trial. Eur J Cardiothorac Surg. 2013;43:1006-13.
26. Fanari Z, Weissa SA, Zhang W, et al. Meta-analysis of three randomized controlled trials comparing coronary artery bypass grafting with percutaneous coronary intervention using drug-eluting stenting in patients with diabetes. Interact Cardiovasc Thorac Surg. 2014;19:1002-7.
27. Verma S, Farkouh ME, Yanagawa B, et al. Comparison of coronary artery bypass surgery and percutaneous coronary intervention in patients with diabetes: a meta-analysis of randomised controlled trials. Lancet Diabetes Endocrinol. 2013;1:317-28.
28. DeLuca G, Schaffer A, Verdoia M et al. Meta-analysis of 14 trials comparing bypass grafting vs drug-eluting stents in diabetic patients with multivessel coronary artery disease. Nutr Metab Cardiovasc Dis. 2014;24:344-54.
29. Mancini GBJ, Farkouh ME, Brooks MM. Medical Treatment and Revascularization Options in Patients with Type 2 Diabetes and Coronary Disease. J Am Coll Cardiol. 2016;68:985-95.
30. Garcia H, Sandoval Y, Roukoz H, et al. Outcomes After Complete Versus Incomplete Revascularization of Patients with Multivessel Coronary Artery Disease. A Meta-Analysis of 89,883 Patients Enrolled in Randomized Clinical Trials and Observational Studies. J Am Coll Cardiol. 2013;62:1421-31.
31. Kassimis G, Bourantas CV, Tushar R, et al. Percutaneous coronary intervention vs. cardiac surgery in diabetic patients. Where are we now and where should we be going? Hellenic J Cardiol. 2017;58:178-89.
32. Bangalore S, Toklu B, Feit F. Outcomes with Coronary Artery Bypass Graft Surgery versus Percutaneous Coronary Intervention for Patients with Diabetes

Mellitus. Can Newer Generation Drug-Eluting Stents Bridge the Gap? Circ Cardiovasc Interv. 2014;7:518-25.
33. Feit F, Brooks MM, Sopko G. Long-Term Clinical Outcome in the Bypass Angioplasty Revascularization Investigation Registry Comparison With the Randomized Trial. Circulation. 2000;101:2795-802.
34. Ramanathan K, Abel JG, Park JE, et al. Surgical Versus Percutaneous Coronary Revascularization in Patients with Diabetes and Acute Coronary Syndromes. J Am Coll Cardiol. 2017;70:2995-3006.
35. Nyström T, Sartipy U, Franzén S, et al. PCI versus CABG in patients with type 1 diabetes and multivessel disease. J Am Coll Cardiol. 2017;70:1441-51.
36. Farooq V, van Klaversen D, Steyerberg E, et al. Anatomical and clinical characteristics to guide decision making between coronary artery bypass surgery and coronary intervention for individual patients: development and validation of the SYNTAX score II. Lancet. 2013;381:639-50.
37. Cavalcante R, Sotomi Y, Mancone M, et al. Impact of the SYNTAX scores I and II in patients with diabetes and multivessel coronary disease: a pooled analysis of patient level data from the SYNTAX, PRECOMBAT, and BEST trials. Eur Heart J. 2017;38:1969-77.
38. Escaned J, Collet C, Ryan N, et al. Clinical outcomes of state-of-the-art percutaneous coronary revascularization in patients with de novo three vessel disease: 1-year results of the SYNTAX II study. Eur Heart J. 2017;38:3124-34.
39. Boden WE, O'Rourke RA, Teo KK, et al. Optimal Medical Therapy with or without PCI for Stable Coronary Disease. N Engl J Med. 2007;356:1503-16.
40. Shaw LJ, Berman DS, Maron DJ, et al. Optimal medical therapy with or without percutaneous coronary intervention to reduce ischemic burden: results from the Clinical Outcomes Utilizing Revascularization and Aggressive Drug Evaluation (COURAGE) trial nuclear substudy. Circulation. 2008;117:1283-91.
41. Al-Lamee R, Thompson D, Dehbi HM, et al. Percutaneous coronary intervention in stable angina (ORBITA): a double-blind, randomised controlled trial. Lancet. 2018;391:31-40.
42. Controversies in interventional cardiology I: interventional management in stable coronary artery disease. Presented at Society for Cardiovascular Angiography and Interventions, 2018. San Diego, CA: SCAI; 2018.
43. Rajkumar CA, Nijjer SS, Cole GD. Moving the Goalposts Into Unblinded Territory: The Larger Lessons of DEFER and FAME 2 and Their Implications for Shifting End Points in ISCHEMIA. Circ Cardiovasc Qual Outcomes. 2018;11:e004665.
44. Zinman B, Wanner C, Lachin JM, et al. Empagliflozin, Cardiovascular Outcomes, and Mortality in Type 2 Diabetes. N Engl J Med. 2015;373:2117-28.
45. Neal B, Perkovic V, Mahaffey KW, et al. Canagliflozin and Cardiovascular and Renal Events in Type 2 Diabetes. N Engl J Med. 2017;377:644-57.
46. Dangas GD, Farkouh ME, Sleeper LA, et al Long-Term Outcome of PCI versus CABG in Insulin and Non–Insulin-Treated Diabetic Patients. Results from the FREEDOM Trial. J Am Coll Cardiol. 2014;64:1189-97.
47. Zimmermann FM, De Bruyne B, Pijls NH, et al. Rationale and design of the Fractional Flow Reserve versus Angiography for Multivessel Evaluation (FAME) 3 Trial: a comparison of fractional flow reserve-guided percutaneous coronary intervention and coronary artery bypass graft surgery in patients with multivessel coronary artery disease. Am Heart J. 2015;170:619-26.
48. Serruys PW. SYNTAX III Revolution: non-invasive Heart Team assessment of multivessel coronary disease with coronary CT angiography. Presented at EuroPCR 2018. Paris: EuroPCR; 2018.

CHAPTER 34

Enhanced External Counterpulsation: Current Status

Ashok Goyal

INTRODUCTION

Cardiovascular diseases particularly coronary artery disease (CAD) is currently a leading cause of death in India and is rapidly presenting as an epidemic, resulting in 23% of total and 32% of adult deaths in 2010–2013. Using more stringent criteria (clinical ± Q waves), the prevalence varies from 1 to 2% in rural populations and 2–4% in urban populations.[1] Heart failure (HF) incidence has also reached epidemic proportions with 5.7 million patients in USA, 10 million in Europe, and 20 million in Asia, and is the most frequent cause of emergency visits and hospitalization in the elderly population, accounting for 5–10% of all hospital admissions and an estimated 50% mortality at 5 years.[2]

The CAD patients with refractory angina and HF have imposed a great challenge for their treatment due to: (1) high morbidity and mortality, (2) increased cost burden because of repeated emergency department (ED) visits or hospitalization, (3) high rate of stent restenosis or graft occlusion, and (4) high risk of repeat revascularization procedures.

Optimal medical therapy (OMT) and invasive revascularization, i.e., percutaneous coronary interventions (PCI: balloon angioplasty or stent implantation) and coronary artery bypass surgery (CABG), are the most widely used treatment modalities, but neither of these treatment modalities provide a complete cure of this progressive disease with its causative mechanisms still persisting even after treatment. Further, the role of standard revascularization procedures in chronic stable angina (CSA) is not well understood and still under investigation and debate. Furthermore, during or after revascularization procedures, myocardial infarction (MI) remains a common entity due to distal micro-thromboembolism leading to myonecrosis, coronary spasm, arrhythmias, or hypotension.[3] Despite many advances in OMT and invasive revascularization procedures, a significant number of patients suffering from chronic refractory angina pectoris with or without underlying HF could not be successfully managed, and are left to suffer with their symptoms of restricted activities to anticipate a reduced life expectancy.

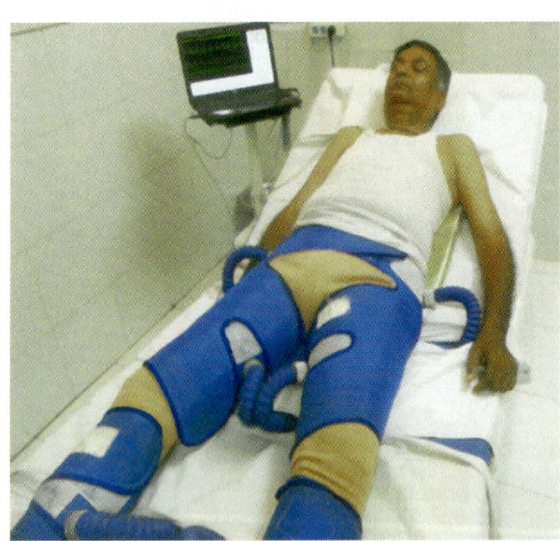

FIG. 1: Enhanced external counterpulsation machine. Consisting of a patient bed attached to an air compressor unit, computerized control panel, three sets of cuffs wrapped around the caves, thighs, and buttocks of the patient.

Enhanced external counterpulsation (EECP) therapy with a different mode of action consists of a bed with attached air compressor and computerized control panel that involves the electrocardiography (ECG)—gated sequential inflation or deflation of three sets of cuffs wrapped around the lower extremities (i.e. calf, thigh, buttock), which produces hemodynamic effects similar to those of an intra-aortic balloon pump (IABP) (Fig. 1).

ENHANCED EXTERNAL COUNTERPULSION IN CORONARY ARTERY DISEASE AND HEART FAILURE TREATMENT

Enhanced external counterpulsation was carefully reviewed in the 2012—Stable Ischemic Heart Disease (SIHD) guideline, but the comments received after the guideline's publication prompted a re-examination of the existing literature in 2014.[4] The efficacy of EECP in treating SIHD has been evaluated in several randomized controlled trials (RCTs) and nonrandomized, observational, prospective trials and registry studies, which documented significant and long-term clinical benefit from EECP therapy in patients of CSA.

The MUST-EECP (Multicenter Study of Enhanced External Counterpulsation) was landmark prospective, blind study that randomly assigned 139 patients of CSA with positive exercise stress test. Patients were subjected to either full dose EECP or to sham (placebo) method with minimal pressures. The study showed a significant increase in exercise time post-EECP from baseline (426 ± 20 s to 470 ± 20 s, $p < 0.001$) versus the sham group without active counterpulsation (432 ± 22 s to 464 ± 22 s, $p < 0.03$) and significant improved time for more than or equal to 1 mm ST-segment depression on stress testing in the EECP group (337 ± 18 s to 379 ± 18 s, $p < 0.002$) compared with placebo (326 ± 21 s to 330 ± 20 s, $p < 0.74$). These effects were maintained 12 months after EECP treatment.[5] Additional RCTs were published in 2009 by Buschmann et al.[6] and in 2010 by Gloeker et al.[7] comparing intracoronary and collateral blood flow rates by angiography in patients treated with EECP against those treated with sham procedure, and proved that collateral flow index increased significantly in the EECP-treated group compared with sham-treated group. Another small unblinded RCT published in 2011 by Bondesson et al.[8] in patients with refractory angina—Canadian Cardiovascular Society (CCS) class III being randomized to EECP and no-EECP groups. Mean CCS angina class was significantly improved in EECP group but not in no-EECP group. However, data from RCTs on long-term outcomes are lacking.

International EECP Patient Registry (IEPR) enrolled 7,500 patients from more than 90 centers and their results have demonstrated the symptomatic clinical benefit by at least one functional angina class with improvement in exercise tolerance, myocardial perfusion, and antianginal drug requirement[9,10] which might be maintained for up to 5 years in patients with favorable initial clinical response. About 86% of IEPR patients completed the 35-hour treatment, designated as EECP responders and the remaining as EECP nonresponders. At 5 years, major adverse cardiovascular events (death, acute MI, new or redo- CABG or PCI) were significantly lower among EECP responders (23%) compared to nonresponders (86%). EECP responders also have significant post-therapy improvement in perfusion defects on radionuclide stress tests performed to the same cardiac work load and double product.[11-13]

Percutaneous coronary interventions candidates suitable for and treated with EECP had 1-year major event rates comparable to patients receiving elective PCI. These results suggested that EECP, a noninvasive procedure, could be used as a first-line treatment keeping invasive revascularization reserved for EECP failures, or in high-risk patients with SIHD.[14] However, it warrants a need of a randomized controlled study to ascertain the efficacy of EECP combined with drug therapy as a first-line treatment in select patients with SIHD.

Soren et al.[15,16] have evaluated the safety and efficacy of EECP therapy in patients with refractory angina and severe left ventricular dysfunction [ejection fraction (EF) <35%] and found a significant and persistent reduction in angina severity: 72% improved from severe angina to no or mild angina and 52% stopped using nitroglycerin with significantly decreased ED visits and hospitalizations.

However, many studies on EECP therapy were not double blind, and lack good control groups because of technical and ethical limitations.

MECHANISM OF ACTION

Despite favorable findings, the mechanism(s) for the clinical effectiveness of EECP in CAD and HF patients remains largely unknown. Recent (2016) systemic review and meta-analysis of the available literature (5 RCTs and 1 prospective studies between 1992 and 2007) focused on the effect of EECP on the measurement of myocardial perfusion, and concluded that the standard EECP therapy (35 1-hour sessions) significantly increased myocardial perfusion and left ventricular function in CAD patients [pooled weighted mean differences (WMD) = statistical index: −0.19; 95% confidence interval (CI): −0.38 to 0.00; $p = 0.049$ with no significant publication bias—Begg's $p = 0.091$; Egger's $p = 0.282$].[17] However, EECP is expected to work through several pathways affecting each other (Flowchart 1).

The hemodynamic effects of EECP has been assessed through both noninvasive and invasive techniques and found to be similar to those of IABP for diastolic augmentation and systemic vascular resistance. However, the right atrial pressure, pulmonary capillary wedge pressure, and cardiac index increased during EECP in contrast to IABP, suggesting that EECP increases venous return, raises cardiac preload, and increases cardiac output. Further, in contrast to IABP, the EECP therapy is thought to provide permanent effects on the heart, because the resulting increase in coronary artery perfusion pressure may enhance coronary collateral development or increase flow through existing collaterals[18,19] (Fig. 2).

Endothelium plays an integral part in vascular homeostasis, and its dysfunction leads to decreased nitric oxide—a potent vasodilator, antiproliferative, anti-inflammatory molecule, and increased endothelin-1—a potent vasoconstrictor, mitogenic, proinflammatory molecule. Prospective and randomized controlled studies [20,21] predicted EECP in CAD patients, through its sheer stress, leads to a significant increase in plasma nitric oxide levels and decrease in plasma endothelin-1 levels. These studies showed significant increase in flow-mediated dilatation of peripheral arteries, and thereby improving coronary blood flow in EECP treated patients.

Braith et al.[21] in their randomized controlled study in 42 symptomatic CAD patients (28 by active-EECP and 14 by sham EECP) showed EECP treatment-mediated significant reduction in proinflammatory cytokines, vascular cell

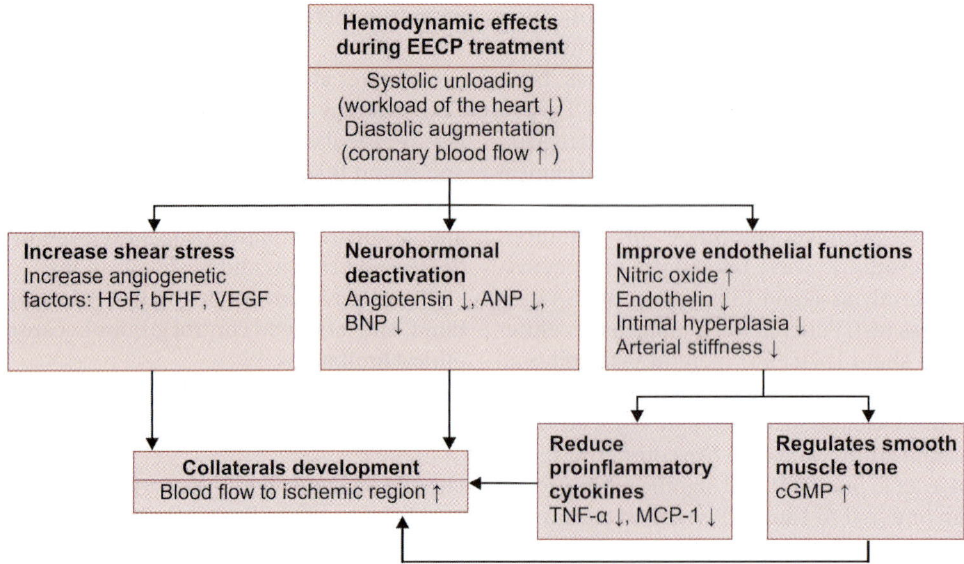

ANP, atrial natriuretic peptide; bFHF, basic fibroblast growth factor; BNP, brain-type natriuretic peptide; cGMP, cyclic guanosine monophosphate; HGF, hepatocyte growth factor; MCP-1, monocyte chemotactic protein-1; TNF, tumor necrosis factor; VEGF, vascular endothelial growth factor.

FLOWCHART 1: Mechanisms of enhanced external counterpulsation (EECP) therapy. Possible mechanisms responsible for the clinical benefit associated with EECP therapy. Acute hemodynamic and neurohormonal changes, prolonged stimulus to increase sheer stress which promotes endothelial function improvement is thought to promote myocardial collateralization via opening of latent conduits, arteriogenesis, and angiogenesis.

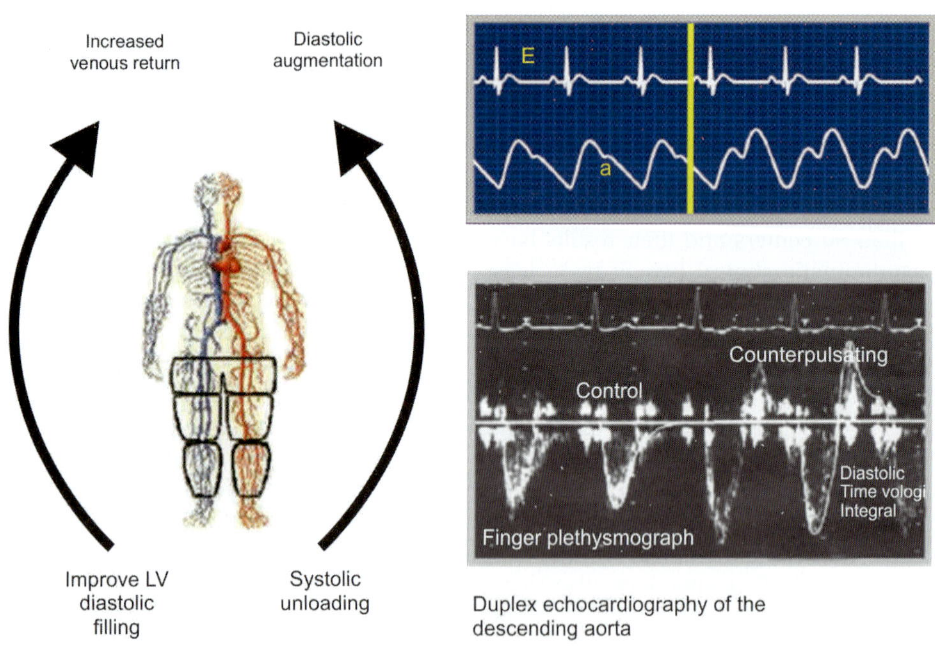

EECP, enhanced external counterpulsation; LV, left ventricular.

FIG. 2: Acute hemodynamic effects of enhanced external counterpulsation therapy. Right upper corner: Showing the ECG tracing and finger plethysmogram. As soon as the device turned on (yellow line) diastolic augmentation starts. Right lower corner: Showing the diastolic augmentation by echocardiography. E (ECG), electrocardiogram; a, aortic notch.

With permission from: Soran O. The role of enhanced external counterpulsation therapy in the management of coronary artery disease. Angina Pectoris. 1998:137-58.

adhesion molecule-1, high-sensitivity C-reactive protein (HS-CRP), and lipid peroxidation marker (8-isoprostane platelet growth factor 2α) in active-EECP as compared to sham EECP group.

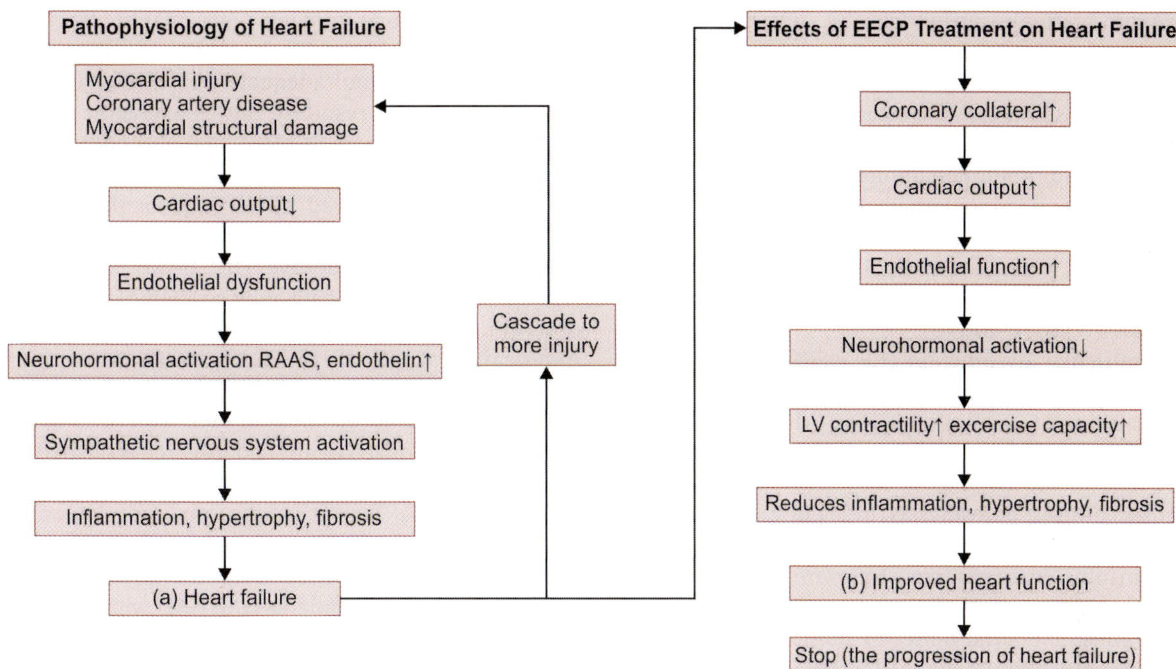

LV, left ventricular; RAAS, renin-angiotensin-aldosterone system.

FLOWCHART 2: Enhanced external counterpulsation (EECP) in heart failure. (a) Pathophysiology of heart failure starting with some form of injury to the heart muscle and cascading down to heart failure and leading back to more myocardial injury; (b) EECP stops the path back to more myocardial injury and reduces the negative remodelling effects of heart failure, thereby improving heart function.

Vascular shear stress is a known stimulus for angiogenesis leading to coronary collateral development and recruitment by increasing vascular endothelial growth factors (VEGFs), fibroblast growth factors, and platelet-derived growth factors. EECP treatment in CAD patients through its shear stress effects has shown to increase plasma levels of these growth factors.[22]

As illustrated the pathophysiology of HF in flowchart 2, HF is not a single organ disease but a systemic disease. HF usually starts with some form of injury to the myocardium, reducing the ability of the heart to effectively eject blood, decreasing the cardiac output, leading to endothelial dysfunction and activating the neurohormonal [Renin-Angiotensin-Aldosterone System (RAAS) and endothelin] and sympathetic nervous system, which in turn leads to myocardial hypertrophy, fibrosis, inflammatory injury, and further atherosclerosis. This chain reaction continues and cascades to worsening of HF.

Enhanced external counterpulsation is a treatment methodology that deals with every aspect of the deteriorating effects leading to HF. There is ample scientific evidence that EECP promotes coronary collateral circulation providing more blood supply to ischemic regions of the heart to improve cardiac output. The improved cardiac function increases blood flow velocity, and the sheer stress on the endothelium promotes the release of circulating endothelial progenitor cells and improve endothelial function. This in turn reduces neurohormonal or sympathetic activation, inflammatory reaction, arterial wall stiffness, intimal hyperplasia, myocardial hypertrophy and fibrosis, thereby lowering vascular resistance and decelerating the deteriorating effects so as to stop the progression of HF.

INDICATIONS AND CONTRAINDICATIONS

United States Food and Drug Administration (US FDA) has approved EECP therapy for: (1) refractory angina pectoris not responding to OMT or not amenable to invasive revascularization procedures, and (2) congestive HF. The following group of patients of angina or angina equivalent with or without HF may be benefitted from EECP therapy (Table 1).

TABLE 1: Indications and contraindications of enhanced external counterpulsation in patients of coronary artery disease and heart failure

Indications	Contraindications
Abnormal coronary artery anatomy	Aortic insufficiency
Restenosis of stents or grafts	Arrhythmias
Noncardiac morbid conditions	Severe uncontrolled hypertension
Unwillingness for invasive revascularization	Deep vein thrombosis
Stable heart failure	Aortic aneurysm
LV dysfunction—moderate-to-severe	Recent cardiac catheterization
–	Coagulopathy prothrombin time—INR >2.5
–	Pregnancy

INR, international normalized ratio; LV, left ventricular.

- Coronary anatomy unsuitable for invasive revascularization, e.g., diffuses atherosclerosis or congenital anomalies
- Restenosis of stents or grafts after invasive revascularization and redo revascularization is not possible
- Advanced comorbid conditions of noncardiac origin (lungs, liver, and kidney) or advanced age that increases the risk of invasive revascularization procedures.
- On OMT, not willing for additional invasive revascularization procedures
- Stable HF (NYHA II and III)
- Left ventricular dysfunction (EF <35%) due to cardiomyopathy—ischemic or idiopathic.

Enhanced external counterpulsation therapy may be somewhat uncomfortable due to the high pressure sequential compressions of the cuffs as it can cause skin abrasions, ecchymoses, bruises, paresthesias, or leg or waist pains. It is not recommended in the following conditions (Table 1):

- Aortic insufficiency (moderate to severe)—as the regurgitation would prevent diastolic augmentation
- Arrhythmias like atrial flutter or fibrillation and ventricular premature contractions (if frequent)—as these may interfere with EECP system triggering
- Hypertension (BP > 180/110 mm Hg)—as the augmented diastolic pressure may exceed safe limits
- Deep vein thrombosis (DVT) is an absolute contraindication—as it may cause pulmonary thromboembolism (PTE)
- Aortic aneurysm (>4 mm) or dissection—as diastolic pressure augmentation may be detrimental
- Cardiac catheterization from femoral route (2 weeks)—as there may be risk of bleeding from the site of arterial puncture
- Coagulopathy (prothrombin time—international normalized ratio >2.5)—as it may cause bruises in the legs
- Pregnancy—as the effects of EECP therapy on the fetus have not been studied.

ENHANCED EXTERNAL COUNTERPULSION IN EXTRACARDIAC DISEASES

Several research publications have revealed the potential uses of EECP in the treatment of various extracardiac disease like cardiac syndrome X (nonobstructive CAD),[23] ischemic strokes,[24-26] erectile dysfunction,[27,28] and hepatorenal syndrome.[29] New studies do explore the role of EECP therapy in primary and secondary prevention of CAD in persons who are prone to have CAD due to the presence of multiple risk factors like diabetes, hypertension, obesity, dyslipidemia, and tobacco user.

CONCLUSION

Several clinical trials[30-32] in last two decades have suggested that EECP is truly and rather only noninvasive, efficacious, safe, cost-effective, and OPD-based therapy in improving angina pectoris, long-term left ventricular functions, exercise capacity and quality of life in CAD and HF patients that have failed to respond adequately to OMT, PCI, or CABG. Its positive clinical response rate is averaging 70–80% and sustained up to 5 years or more, and also complements the invasive revascularization.

It has been approved by US FDA for the management of refractory angina—chronic stable (class IIb—level of evidence B) and congestive HF. However, due to large and quality scientific data now available, and as per the description of the rating or evidence levels defined by American College of Cardiology and American Heart Association guidelines, it is believed that EECP has earned a Class IIa treatment recommendation with level of evidence A.[33] More randomized controlled research is needed for more confirmatory mechanism of action and long-term effects of EECP therapy. Recent studies, may provide an array of hope to ascertain the efficacy of EECP—a truly noninvasive treatment combined with drug therapy, as a first-line treatment in selected patients with CAD with or without HF, keeping invasive revascularization reserved for EECP failures, or high-risk patients.

REFERENCES

1. Gupta R, Mohan I, Narula J. Trends in coronary heart disease epidemiology in India. An Glob Health. 2016;82(2):307-15.
2. Huffman MD, Prabhakaran DR. Heart failure: Epidemiology and prevention in India. Natl Med J India. 2010;23(5):283-8.
3. Lansky AJ, Stone GW. Periprocedural myocardial infarction. Cir Cardiovasc Interv 2010;3(6):602-10.
4. Jacobs AK, Anderson JL, Halperin JL. The evolution and future of ACC/AHA clinical practice guidelines: a 30-year journey. J Am Coll Cardiol. 2014;64(13):1373-84.
5. Arora RR, Chou TM, Jain D, et al. The multicenter study of enhance external counterpulsation (MUST-EECP): effect of EECP on exercise-induced myocardial ischemia and anginal episodes. J Am Coll Cardiol. 1999;33(7):1833-40.
6. Buchmann EE, Utz W, Pagonas N, et al. Improvement of fractional flow reserve and collateral flow by treatment with external counterpulsation (Art.Net.-2 Trial). Eur J Clin Invest. 2009;39(10):866-75.
7. Gloekler S, Meier P, de Marchi SF, et al. Coronary collateral growth by external counterpulsation: a randomized controlled trial. Heart. 2010;96(3):202-7.
8. Bondesson SM, Edvinsson ML, Pettersson T, et al. Reduced peripheral vascular reactivity in refractory angina pectoris: Effect of enhanced external counterpulsation. J Geriatr Cardiol. 2011;8:215-23.
9. Arora RR, Chou TM, Jain D, et al. Effects of enhanced external counterpulsation on health-related quality of life continue 12 months after treatment: A substudy of the multicentre study of enhanced external counter pulsation. J Investig Med. 2002;50(1):25-32.
10. Bagger JP, Hall RJ, Koutroulis G, et al. Effect of enhanced external counterpulsation on dobutamine-induced left ventricular wall motion abnormalities in severe chronic angina pectoris. Am J Cardiol. 2004;15;93(4):465-7.
11. Lawson WE, Hui JCK, Cohn PF. Long-term prognosis of patients with angina treated with enhanced external counterpulsation: Five-years follow-up study. Clin Cardiol. 2000;23:254-8.
12. Lawson WE, Hui JC, Kennard ED, et al. IEPR Investigators. Predictors of benefit in angina patients one year after completion of enhanced external counterpulsation: initial responders to treatment versus non responders. Cardiology. 2005;103(4):201-6.
13. Loh PH, Cleland JG, Louis AA, et al. Enhanced external counterpulsation in the treatment of chronic refractory angina: a long-term follow-up outcome from the International Enhanced External Counterpulsation Patient Registry. Clin Cardiol. 2008;31(4):159-64.

14. Holubkov R, Kennard ED, Foris JM, et al. Comparison of patients undergoing Enhanced External Counterpulsation and Percutaneous Coronary Intervention for Stable Angina Pactoris. Am J Cardiol. 2002;89:1182-6.
15. Soren O, Kennard ED, Kfoury AG, et al. Two-year clinical outcomes after enhanced external counterpulsation (EECP) therapy in patients with refractory angina pectoris and left ventricular dysfunction (Report from the International EECP Patient Registry). Am J Cardiol. 2006;97:17-20.
16. Soren O, Kennard ED, Bart BA, et al. Impact of enhanced external counterpulsation treatment on emergency department visits and hospitalizations in refractory angina patients with left ventricular dysfunction. Congest Heart Fail. 2007;13(1):36-40.
17. Qin X, Deng Y, Wu D, et al. Does enhanced External counterpulsation (EECP) significantly affect myocardial ?: A systematic review & meta-analysis. PloS One 2016;11(4): e0151822.
18. Taguchi I, Ogawa K, Kanaya T, et al. Effects of enhanced external counterpulsation on hemodynamics and its mechanism. Circ J. 2004;68(11):1030-4.
19. Michaels AD, Tacy T, Teitel D, et al. Invasive left ventricular energetic during enhance external counterpulsation. Am J Ther. 2009;16(3):239-46.
20. Schechter M, Matetzky S, Feinberg MS, et al. External counterpulsation therapy improves endothelial function in patients with refractory angina pectoris. J Am Coll Cardiol. 2003;42(12):2090-5.
21. Braith RW, Conti CR, Nichols WW, et al. Enhance external counterpulsation improves peripheral artery flow mediated dilatation in patients with chronic angina: a randomized sham-controlled study. Circulation. 2010;122:1612-20.
22. Resnick N, Collins T, Atkinson W, et al. Platelet-derived growth factor B chain promoter contains a cis-acting shear-stress-responsive element. Proc Natl Acad Sci USA. 1993;90(10):4591-5.
23. Bonetti PO, Gadasalli SN, Lerman A, et al. Successful treatment of symptomatic coronary endothelial dysfunction with enhanced external counterpulsation. Mayo Clin Proc. 2004;79:690-2.
24. Alexandrov AW, Ribo M, Wong KS, et al. Perfusion augmentation in acute stroke using mechanical counterpulsation- phase IIa: Effect of external counterpulsation on middle cerebral artery mean flow velocity in five healthy subjects. Stroke. 2008;39:2760-4.
25. Wenhua L, Jinghao H, Xiangyan C, et al. Predictors of good functional outcome in counterpulsation-treated recent ischaemic stroke patients. BMJ Open. 2013;3(6). pii:e002932.
26. Li X, Wenhua L, Jinghao H, et al. Enhancing cerebral perfusion with external counterpulsation after ischaemic cerebral perfusion. J Neurol Neurosurg Psychiatry. 2014;10:1136.
27. Lawson WE, Hui JC, Kennard ED. Effect of enhanced external counterpulsation on medically refractory angina patients with erectile dysfunction. Int J Clin Pract. 2007;61:757-62.
28. El-Sakka AI, Morsy AM, Fagih BL, et al. Enhanced external counterpulsation in patients with coronary artery disease-associated erectile dysfunction. Part-II: impact of disease duration and treatment courses. J Sex Med. 2007;4;1448-53.
29. Werner D, Tragner P, Wawer A, et al. Enhanced external counterpulsation: a new technique to augment renal function in liver cirrhosis. Nephrol Dial Transplant. 2005;20:920-6.
30. Stys TP, Lowson WE, Hui JC, et al. Effects of enhanced external counterpulsation on stress radionuclide coronary perfusion and exercise capacity in chronic stable angina pectoris. Am J Cardiol. 2002;89(7):822-4.
31. Pettersson T, Bondesson S, Cojocaru D, et al. One year follow-up of patients with refractory angina pectoris treated with enhanced external counterpulsation. BMC Cardiovasc Disord. 2006;6:28.
32. Braverman DL. Enhanced external counterpulsation: an innovative physical therapy for refractory angina. PM R. 2009;1(3):268-76.
33. Piscione F. Angina pectoris. In: Innasimuthu AL, Budzyński J, Soran O (Eds). The Role of Enhanced External Counterpulsation Therapy in Management of Coronary Artery Disease. London, UK: InTech Publishers; 2011. pp. 137-58.
34. Soran O. The role of enhanced external counterpulsation therapy in the management of coronary artery disease. Angina Pectoris. 1998:137-58.

CHAPTER 35

Cardiac Rehabilitation: The Road Less Travelled

Satyendra Tewari, Raj Pratap Singh

INTRODUCTION

Cardiac rehabilitation (CR) is defined as comprehensive long-term programs involving medical evaluation, prescribed exercise, cardiac risk factor modification, education, and counseling, designed to limit the physiological and psychological effect of cardiac illness, reduce the risk of sudden death (approximately 10%) or reinfarction, control cardiac symptoms, and enhance the psychological and vocational status of the individual patient.[1] CR is a process where cardiac patient in partnership with a multidisciplinary team is encouraged and supported to achieve and maintain optimal physical and psychosocial health.[2] CR is an umbrella term that covers various facets of a holistic and comprehensive cardiac care and encompasses all measures used to help people with heart disease to return to active life and prevent recurrence of events (Fig. 1).

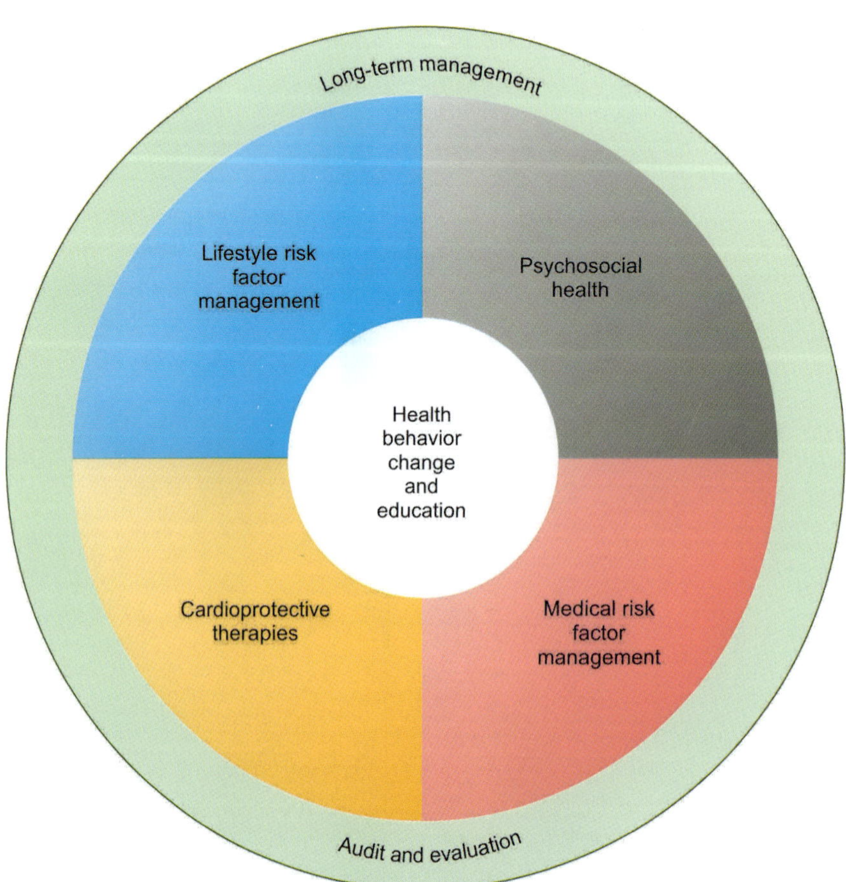

FIG. 1: Comprehensive approach to cardiac rehabilitation.[3]

Cardiac rehabilitation has been studied in multiple randomized controlled trials (RCTs), observational and cohort studies.[4] These as well as multiple meta-analysis and systematic reviews have shown that structured CR leads to decreased mortality,[5] morbidity, myocardial infarction and hospital admissions,[6] early mobility and return to work and routine activity, improvement in quality of life, physical fitness and psychosocial wellbeing, and decreased symptoms of depression.[5,7-10] Despite such robust evidence of multitude of benefits proper CR is available only to minority of patients and it remains a road less travelled. The American Heart Association (AHA) scientific statement on exercise and acute CV events noted that risk of major cardiovascular event is one event in 60,000–80,000 hours of supervised exercise.[11,12]

The goal of CR is to enable cardiac patients to lead a fulfilling life by maximizing their physical, psychological, and social functioning. This is achieved by:

- Introducing and encouraging behavior that minimize the risk of further cardiac events
- Facilitating and shortening the period of recovery after an acute cardiac event
- Promoting strategies for achieving recommended goals for prevention of cardiovascular disease (CVD)
- Developing and maintaining skills for long-term behavior change and self-management
- Promoting appropriate use of health and community services
- Improving compliance with treatment and exercise advised

INDICATIONS OF CARDIAC REHABILITATION

- Acute coronary syndrome [ST-elevation myocardial infraction (STEMI) or non-STEMI or unstable angina]
- Chronic stable angina
- Compensated heart failure
- Postcoronary angioplasty
- Postpacemaker, intracardiac defibrillator implantation
- Postcardiac surgery like coronary artery bypass grafting or valvular surgery
- Left ventricular assist device therapy
- Heart or other organ transplant
- Patients at high risk of cardiac events, e.g., diabetes, hyperlipidemia, and hypertension
- Peripheral vascular disease.

From the given list of indications it is clear that there can be varied conditions requiring CR and patient with each one of them may differ. Thus there is a heterogeneity and hence the rehabilitation program has to be tailored according to the need of patient (one size does not fit all). It is also important to understand that in order to implement CR correctly one needs to have a multidisciplinary team involving the specialist (cardiologist), trained nursing staff, people specially trained for providing out of hospital education and nutrition and exercise advice with support from family members and local physician. It is of utmost importance that the CR services meet the need of patient and family members of patient should be encouraged to participate in CR program.

Traditionally four phases of CR have been described:[13,14]

- *Phase 1:* (Inpatient) Usually lasts during the duration of hospitalization. It consists of a gradual, progressive exercise and education program and improves patient's understanding of disease and preventive efforts to slow the progression of disease
- *Phase 2:* (Postdischarge) Graded physical activity and behavior modification aimed at weight loss, healthy eating, smoking cessation, and other factors to reduce disease risk
- *Phase 3:* (Outpatient exercise program) Lasts 6–12 months. Consists of supervised exercise programs that can be performed at home or in a community service facility with continuous emphasis on risk factor reduction
- *Phase 4:* Indefinite duration maintenance phase.

INPATIENT CARDIAC REHABILITATION

In current era the hospitalization durations continue to decrease therefore there is often not sufficient time for to address all aspects of CR. Nevertheless CR should begin soon after admission. Inpatient CR consists of providing information, reassurance and counseling, mobilization guidelines, appropriate discharge planning, and referral to outpatient CR, and primary care physician in a clear simple understandable form. Patient and family should be informed regarding nature of disease, prognosis, prospective treatment, importance of medications and compliance, resumption of physical activity, modification of risk factors, and psychosocial issues. The aim of mobilization program is a progressive increase in physical activity and can start as early as first day. It should balance the risks of premature activity with the deleterious effects of bed rest. Early mobilization improves self-confidence. The protocols vary according to hospital practices and age, frailty, presence of comorbidity, and current medical condition. For example, after coronary angioplasty mobilization may be achieved in a single days whereas in patient of heart failure it may be much slower.

A six-stage progression of mobilization has been developed:[15]

1. Go to toilet and shower in wheel chair, sit in chair for meals, do arm and leg exercises. Supported by ward staff in these processes
2. Shower in a wheelchair while remaining seated, do arm and leg exercises, walk slowly for 1–2 minutes twice a day
3. Patient to shower on their own while seated on the wheelchair, walk to the toilet as necessary. Walk slowly for 2–3 minutes twice a day
4. Walk at an easy pace for 3–4 minutes twice a day. In addition, patient may walk around room as much as they like
5. Walk for 4–5 minutes twice a day. Climb one flight of stairs with the supervision of the nurse or physiotherapist
6. Walk for up to 10 minutes twice a day. Climb two flights of stairs with the supervision of the nurse or physiotherapist.

The progression through these stages varies according to patient status. Close watch for symptoms should be kept and brought immediately to notice of treating physician. Every patient should also be seen by a clinical nutritionist or dietitian, anthropometric measurements made, and full risk profile recorded. At discharge the patient and family should be counseled regarding medications, compliance, symptoms of deterioration, and importance of continuing CR. Patient should be provided with information about local community resources and patient support group. A communication to local physician and if possible CR coordinator or physiotherapist should be made for continuing supervised exercise and rehabilitation in postdischarge period.

Postdischarge Period

May vary from 2 to 6 weeks. Patient contact can be made by home visits or telephone by rehabilitation team. Patient has clear instructions on his or her individualized exercise prescription. Initially walking on level ground is prescribed. Initially, the intensity of exercise is maintained at about 4 metabolic equivalents (METs) and heart rate should not exceed 20 beats/minutes above their resting heart rate. If tolerated well then walking distance is progressively increased to 3–5 km. Patient should be followed up in outpatient department (OPD) for symptoms and assessment of anthropometry and behavioral therapy regarding lifestyle changes and risk factor modifications. Also the food diaries should be given to patients to complete at home.

Outpatient Cardiac Rehabilitation

Structure outpatient CR is aimed at developing a lifelong approach for cardiovascular prevention. Usually last up to 1-year after discharge. Patient can exercise at home or CR facilities without monitoring but with supervised and structured exercise programs. Low to moderate intensity exercises corresponding to 60–75% of maximum heart rate initially followed by addition of resistance exercises if appropriate is the norm. Aerobic exercises like jogging, cycling, rowing, and treadmill are preferred. A warm up of 15 minutes followed by exercise session for 30–35 minutes followed by cooldown of 10 minutes is reasonably good.[16] Food diaries should be collected and reviewed with areas for improvement highlighted. Patients can attend nutrition talks if available. The patients should be counseled regarding continuing preventive measures (e.g., reduce weight, decrease salt, stop smoking, control hypertension, etc.) and supportive things like mindful meditation. Various scales can be used to analyze the performance of patient and improvement of symptoms, e.g., six-minute Walk Test, Seattle Angina Questionnaire, Minnesota Living with Heart Failure, Special Activity Questionnaire, Depression, Anxiety, and Stress Scale, and Borg Scale for Perceived Exertion.

Maintenance Phase

This phase continues lifelong. Patient continues to exercise unsupervised and continues dietary and lifestyle modification with periodic OPD visits at local or specialty centre. Continuing ongoing preventive measures is an integral part of CR and should continue indefinitely.

It is clear that CR requires a coordinated effort of lots of people like patient, family members, treating cardiologist, nutritionist, nurse, physiotherapist, local physician, etc. It becomes difficult for busy centers. Therefore in developed countries there is a concept of CR teams and there is a person designated as rehabilitation coordinator who coordinates a team of various professionals in providing CR services. At some places there are specific CR centers providing professional exercise, nutritional and psychosocial services under single roof. Despite proven role and robust evidence participation in CR programs is poor with average of 20–50% in developed countries. The situation in developing countries is abysmal where CR remains the road not travelled.

BARRIERS TO CARDIAC REHABILITATION IN INDIA

- Lack of any structured and coordinated CR program at most of centers
- Overburdened tertiary center hospitals
- Poor referral for CR
- Physician inertia; few physicians or cardiologist endorse and effectively counsel regarding the need of proper CR
- Poor patient adherence, leading to low enrolment and high dropout rate
- Multiple morbidities, leading to poor functional capacity
- Poor exercise habits
- Patient compliance with medication and abstinence from tobacco is poor
- Problems with transport and geographical barriers
- Poor social support
- Lack of leave from work to attend center-based sessions
- Lack of availability of nutritionist and physiotherapist trained for CR
- *Geographical constraints:* Availability of services is poor in many geographical areas and transportation to urban centers cost time and money. CR otherwise is also best provided locally.

What can be done to improve the situation? As treating cardiologists the onus lies on us to put things on right track. Cardiologist and his team should counsel regarding the disease, its nature, prognosis, importance of preventive measures, exercise, and compliance with medications. In hospital dietary advice and exercise counseling also helps. It is important to dissipate information and educate medical, paramedical staff as well as patient and relatives regarding the concept and benefits of CR. Local physician is at an advantage to provide CR services as he is more accessible to the patient and able to see and monitor his progress frequently. The habit of referring the patient back to local general practitioner should be encouraged because since CVD are a major burden to society government should take steps to set up CR services and promote the concept of prevention (both primary and secondary).

Cardiac rehabilitation is thus an amalgamation of various efforts that one can do to promote and preserve cardiovascular health. In view of current epidemic of CVD it needs to be emphasized and adopted widely. We may be practicing it in some form or other things need to be put together to make a coordinated effort so that CR no more remains a road less travelled.

REFERENCES

1. Wenger NK, Froelicher ES, Smith LK, et al. Cardiac rehabilitation as secondary prevention. Agency for Health Care Policy and Research and National Heart, Lung, and Blood Institute. Clin Pract Guidel Quick Ref Guide Clin. 1995(17):1-23.
2. Scottish Intercollegiate Guidelines Network (SIGN). Guideline 57, Cardiac Rehabilitation; 2002.
3. British Association for Cardiovascular Prevention and Rehabilitation. BACPR standards and core components for cardiovascular disease prevention and rehabilitation 2012, 2nd edition. UKBACPR, 2012. [online] Available from www.bacpr.com/resources/46C_BACPR_Standards_and_Core_Components_2012.pdf.
4. Dalal HM, Doherty P, Taylor RS. Cardiac rehabilitation. BMJ. 2015;351:h5000.
5. Anderson L, Oldridge N, Thompson DR, et al. Exercisebased cardiac rehabilitation for coronary heart disease: Cochrane systematic review and meta-analysis. J Am Coll Cardiol. 2016;67(1):1-12.
6. Sagar VA, Davies EJ, Briscoe S, et al. Exercise-based rehabilitation for heart failure: systematic review and meta-analysis. Open Heart. 2015;2:e000163.
7. Hammill BG, Curtis LH, Schulman KA, et al. Relationship between cardiac rehabilitation and long-term risks of death and myocardial infarction among elderly medicare beneficiaries. Circulation. 2010;121(1):63-70.
8. Milani RV, Lavie CJ. Impact of cardiac rehabilitation on depression and its associated mortality. Am J Med. 2007;120(9):799-806.
9. Pahor M, Guralnik JM, Ambrosius AT, et al. Effect of structured physical activity on prevention of major mobility disability in older adults. The LIFE Study Randomized Clinical Trial. JAMA. 2014;311(23):2387-96.
10. O'Connor CM, Whellan DJ, Lee KL, et al. Efficacy and safety of exercise training in patients with chronic heart failure HF-ACTION randomized controlled trial. JAMA. 2009;301(14):1439-50.
11. Leon AS, Franklin BA, Costa F, et al. Cardiac rehabilitation and secondary prevention of coronary heart disease: an American Heart Association scientific statement from the Council on Clinical Cardiology (Subcommittee on Exercise, Cardiac Rehabilitation, and Prevention) and the Council on Nutrition, Physical Activity, and Metabolism (Subcommittee on Physical Activity), in collaboration with the American association of Cardiovascular and Pulmonary Rehabilitation. Circulation. 2005;111(3):369-76.
12. Smith SC Jr, Benjamin EJ, Bonow RO, et al. AHA/ACCF Secondary Prevention and Risk Reduction Therapy for Patients With Coronary and Other Atherosclerotic Vascular Disease: 2011 Update. Circulation. 2011;124:2458-73.
13. McLaughlin M A. Rehabilitation of the patient with coronary artery disease. In: Fuster V, Harrington RA, Narula J, Eapen ZJ (Eds). Hurst's The Heart, 14 edition. McGraw Hill: New York; 2017. pp. 1173-85.
14. Fuster V, O'Rourke RA, Walsh RA, et al. Hursts's the Heart, 13th edition. New York: McGraw-Hill; 2011.
15. Recommended framework for cardiac rehabilitation '04, National heart foundation of Australia and Australian cardiac rehabilitation association.
16. American College of Sports Medicine. ACSM's guidelines for exercise testing and prescription. Philadelphia: Lippincott William and Wilkins; 2005.

SECTION 6

Acute Coronary Syndromes

CHAPTER 36

Why Seek Vulnerable Coronary Plaques?

Amir Ahmadi, Michael Valentine, Rick Chazal, Jagat Narula

WHAT IS A VULNERABLE PLAQUE?

The plaques associated with acute coronary events including sudden death, myocardial infarction and unstable angina in a majority of cases result from acute coronary thrombosis secondary to plaque rupture.[1] In about a fourth of cases eroded surface of the plaques leads to thrombotic occlusion of the coronary lumen. Whereas the latter occurs predominantly in young smoking women, the common garden variety of the plaque rupture-related acute events are associated with abundance of coronary risk factors and more likely to occur in older men and postmenopausal women.

The ruptured plaques carry distinct histopathological characteristics. These plaques reveal large plaque burden owing to huge necrotic core that is associated with substantial extraluminal growth (or positive remodeling). The expansive growth of the plaque is limited by the maximal stretch capability of the medial smooth muscle cell layer and at that time the plaque growth results in rapid strangulation of the luminal patency. Due to the significant inflammatory component and hence heightened cytokine milieu and collagenolysis and elastolysis, these plaques are left with attenuated fibrous caps, usually <55 μm in thickness. Thin fibrous caps are amenable to high shear stress due to hemodynamic perturbances and disrupt to expose thrombogenic, tissue factor-rich necrotic cores to lumen. These characteristic plaque features [or high-risk plaque (HRP) features] could be seen with plaque rupture regardless of the degree of luminal stenosis. The angina-producing stable plaques, on the other hand do not usually carry large plaque burden or necrotic core, and are more likely to be constrictively (negatively) remodeled due to collagen/fibrous excess, even though they may be luminally critically occlusive.

It has been tacitly believed that the plaques with these definitive HRP features (i.e., large plaque and necrotic core burden, positive remodeling and thin inflamed fibrous caps) if still have the intact fibrous caps, should be considered vulnerable to rupture. The pathological studies have demonstrated that the lipid-rich plaques carrying fibrous caps of thinner than 85 μm are pathognomonic of vulnerable plaques. It is therefore important to identify vulnerable plaques with the expectation that the acute events could be prevented. Such a thinking could be of paramount clinical value because a simple relief of luminal stenosis does not prevent acute events (Fig. 1).

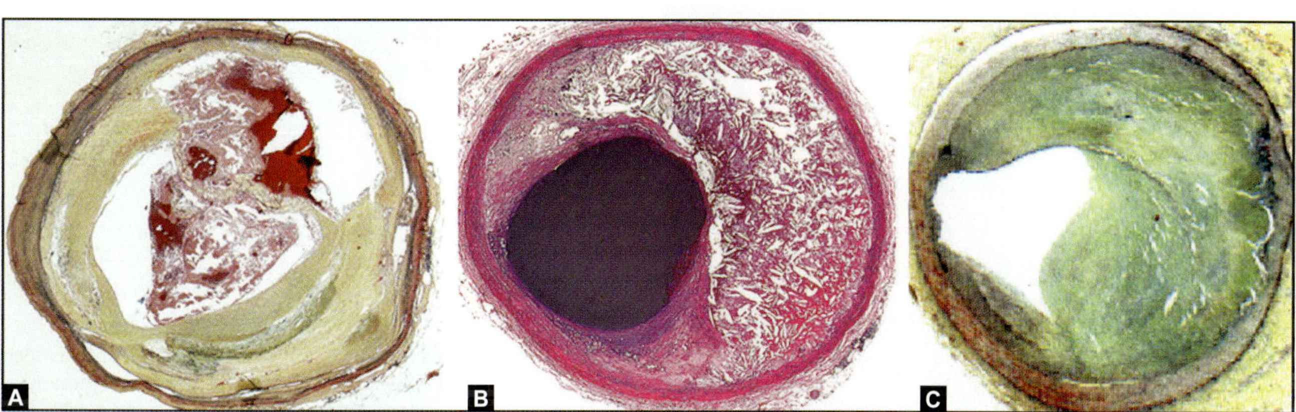

FIG. 1: Histopathologic characteristics **A,** Plaque rupture; **B,** High-risk plaque; **C,** Stable coronary lesion.

HOW IS VULNERABLE PLAQUE IDENTIFIED?

The intracoronary imaging strategies including intravascular ultrasound (IVUS) and optical coherence tomography (OCT) have confirmed the histopathological characteristics of vulnerable plaques *in vivo*. Whereas IVUS has demonstrated the presence of large plaque burden, echolucent necrotic core, and positive remodeling, the OCT has successfully mapped the fibrous cap thickness *in vivo*. However, the noninvasive imaging with computed tomography angiography (CTA) offers the most convenient basis of identification of the HRP characteristics (Fig. 2). These features in the CTA terminology have been called adverse plaque characteristics (APCs) owing to their association with poor prognostic outcomes.[2-4] Two CTA plaque characteristics have demonstrated the best association with clinical outcomes up to 10 years of follow-up. These two features include the existence of low-attenuation plaques with less than 30 Hounsfield unit density (LAP, <30 HU) which represents IVUS-verified necrotic core and positive remodeling (PR, >110%); by presence of these characteristic such plaques have been referred to as 2-feature-positive plaques (2-FPP) and are found to be associated with lesions responsible for acute coronary events; 22.5% of 2-FPP resulted in an acute event over a 2-year follow-up. On the other hand, 2-feature-negative plaques (2-FNP) were associated with benign outcomes with less than 0.5% of them resulting in acute events. Multiple other features have been suggested as the APC including circumferential necrotic cores (napkin-ring sign) and spotty calcification. The positive predictive value of HRP characteristics is increased based on the magnitude and number of HRP features and dynamicity of the HRP (see below).

THE QUANTITATIVE EXTENT OF HIGH-RISK FEATURES

The larger the necrotic core volume and the more expansive the positive remodeling, higher is the likelihood of rupture of the high-risk plaque.[3] The eventful HRP demonstrated two-fold greater expansive remodeling compared to the HRP that did not produce acute coronary events; eventful HRP demonstrated 126% remodeling against 113% remodeling of uneventful HRP. The LAP volume was 20 mm^3 in eventful plaques compared to 1.1 mm^3 in the HRP which did not result in acute coronary events. Napkin rings are circumferential large necrotic cores and although infrequent they are closely associated with future events. Further, not only that the quantitatively greater APCs are associated with the events, greater the APC sooner occurs the event. It is therefore expected that larger data would allow us to define more accurate quantitative thresholds for identifying HRP likely to result in major adverse coronary events.

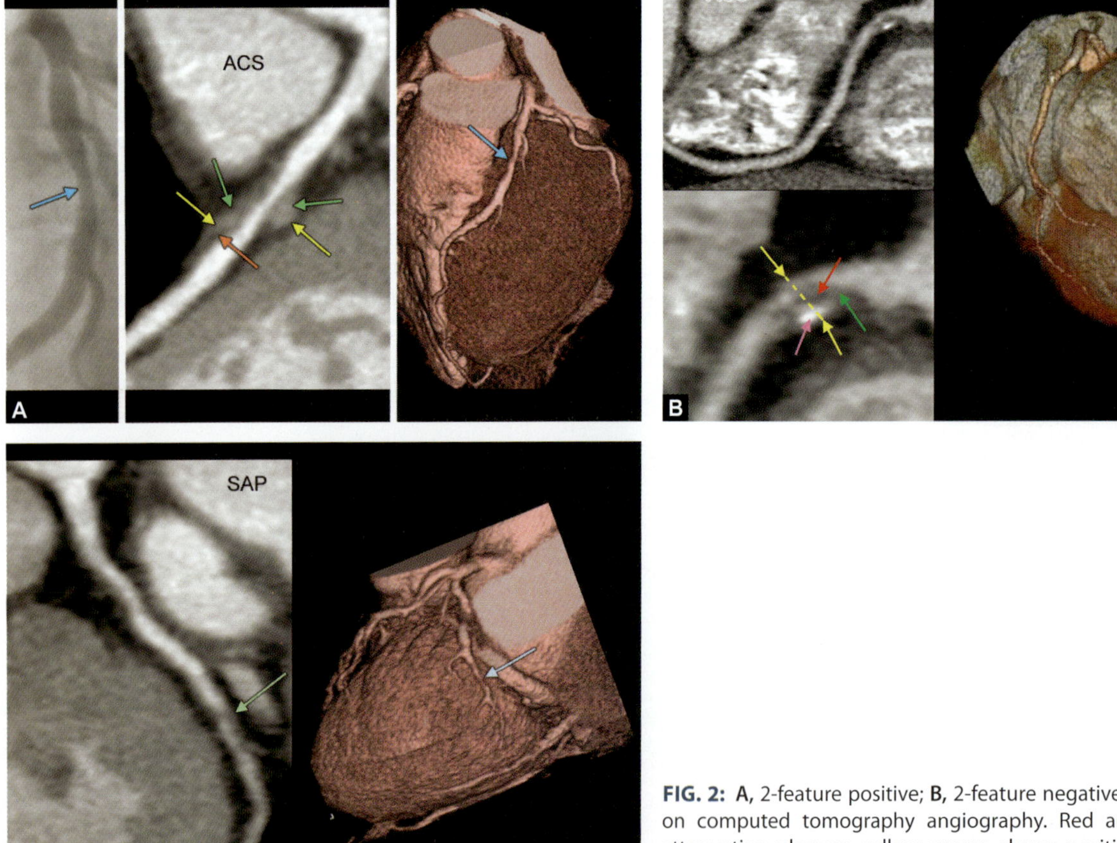

FIG. 2: A, 2-feature positive; **B,** 2-feature negative; **C,** Plaques as seen on computed tomography angiography. Red arrows suggest low-attenuation plaques, yellow arrows shows positive remodeling, and green arrows point to fibrous plaque component.

THE NUMBER OF ADVERSE PLAQUE CHARACTERISTICS

Similar to quantitatively greater APC dose, it has been proposed that the greater number of APCs may contribute to improve positive predictive value of plaque characteristics. Recent CTA studies have revealed progressively superior outcome prediction with addition of increasing number of APCs. Similarly, the landmark PROSPECT (Providing Regional Observations to Study Predictors of Events in the Coronary Tree) study revealed higher plaque burden, IVUS-verified thin fibrous cap and more severe luminal obstruction as the three important determinants of adverse outcomes over 3.4 years in nonculprit vessels in 697 patients undergoing primary percutaneous coronary interventions.[5] Whereas, the absence of all three APCs had a high negative predictive value with only 0.3% adverse events, one, two, and three features showed vessel-specific adverse events in 4.8%, 10.5%, and 18.2% instances. Even though there is increasingly superior positive predictive value for the increasing number of APCs, the number of patients with greater number of APCs becomes significantly smaller.

THE EVIDENCE OF PLAQUE PROGRESSION

Although, it has been tacitly believed that only minimally obstructive HRP are associated with adverse outcomes, a review of those studies suggest that the previous angiograms of the fateful patients were far removed from the index event between 6 and 18 months and information about the plaque behavior in the interim was not available. Those studies which had the angiograms done incidentally within 3–6 months of the fateful events revealed significantly luminally stenotic coronary lesions.[6] Similar data were available from the PROSPECT study[5] which demonstrated almost doubling of the luminal stenosis in the culprit HRP over the follow-up of 3.5 years. In the pathological analysis of almost 300 plaques, it was demonstrated that 95% of the plaques that resulted in an acute event demonstrated more than 50% cross-sectional vascular area involvement. Therefore, it is becoming increasingly clear that the plaques must progress or enlarge (often causing significant luminal occlusion) before they are ready to rupture and result in an acute event. This phenomenon was observed in serial computed tomography (CT) angiograms of a large number of patients wherein the plaque progression[4] was the most important determinant of adverse outcome (Fig. 3). We have also observed that a few plaques that are able to result in an event in spite of relatively mild luminal stenosis harbor huge necrotic cores and could contribute to the hemodynamic turbulence in the luminal flow.[7]

CONCLUSION

The CT angiographic features of the HRP are well established. It is our considered opinion that all CT angiograms should always be reported with comprehensive plaque characterization and where possible, fractional flow reserve. A greater

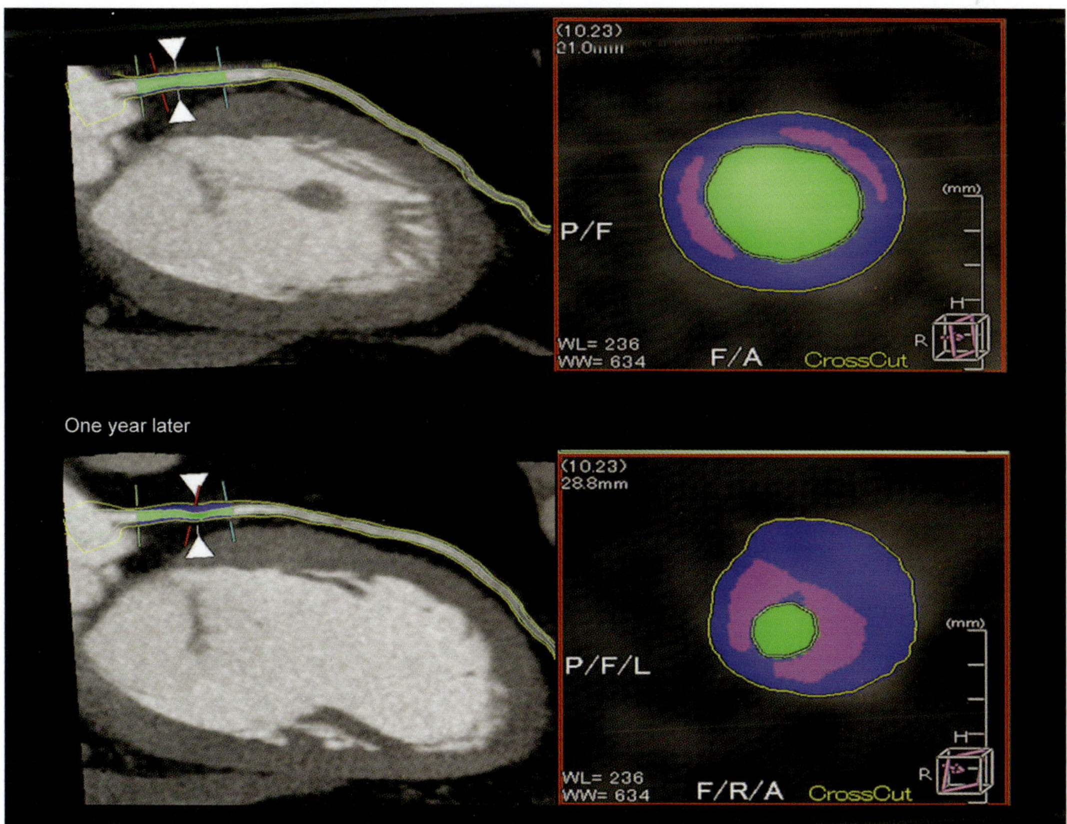

FIG. 3: Serial computed tomography angiography performed at 1-year interval, demonstrates progression of low-attenuation plaques. Patient developed acute coronary event a few weeks after the second scan.

magnitude of HRP features, large number of APCs and plaque progression over time are associated with greater likelihood of major adverse cardiac events. It has also become evident that large lipid rich plaques may be as strong a determinant of abnormal fractional flow reserve as luminal stenosis.

REFERENCES

1. Narula J, Nakano M, Virmani R, et al. Histopathologic characteristics of atherosclerotic coronary disease and implications of the findings for the invasive and noninvasive detection of vulnerable plaques. J Am Coll Cardiol. 2013;61:1041-51.
2. Motoyama S, Kondo T, Sarai M, et al. Multislice computed tomographic characteristics of coronary lesions in acute coronary syndromes. J Am Coll Cardiol. 2007;50(4):319-26.
3. Motoyama S, Sarai M, Harigaya H, et al. Computed tomographic angiography characteristics of atherosclerotic plaques subsequently resulting in acute coronary syndrome. J Am Coll Cardiol. 2009;54:49-57.
4. Motoyama S, Ito H, Sarai M, et al. Plaque characterization by coronary computed tomography angiography and the likelihood of acute coronary events in mid-term follow-up. J Am Coll Cardiol. 2015;66:337-46.
5. Stone GW, Maehara A, Lansky AJ, et al. A prospective natural-history study of coronary atherosclerosis. N Engl J Med. 2011;364:226-35.
6. Ahmadi A, Leipsic J, Blankstein R, et al. Do plaques rapidly progress prior to myocardial infraction? The interplay between plaque vulnerability and progression. Cric res. 2015;117:99-104.
7. Ahmadi A, Stone GW, Leipsic J, et al. Association of coronary stenosis and plaque morphology with fractional flow reserve and outcomes. JAMA Cardiol. 2016;1:350-7.

CHAPTER 37

Protecting Heart from Ischemia-Reperfusion Injury: Current Understanding

Jabir Abdullakutty, Jimmy George

INTRODUCTION

Ischemic heart disease is the leading cause of death worldwide.[1] In patients with myocardial infarction (MI), the treatment of choice for reducing acute myocardial ischemic injury and limiting MI size is timely and effective myocardial reperfusion using either thrombolytic therapy or primary percutaneous coronary intervention (PPCI).[1-3] However, the process of reperfusion can itself induce cardiomyocyte death, known as myocardial reperfusion injury, for which there is still no effective therapy. Therefore, novel therapeutic strategies are required to protect the heart against ischemia or reperfusion injury, preserve myocardial function, prevent heart failure, and improve clinical outcomes in patients with ischemic heart disease.[4]

Myocardial infarction is usually caused by narrowing of the coronary artery due buildup of an atheromatous plaque and its subsequent rupture. Reperfusion is mandatory to salvage the ischemic myocardium; however this is accompanied by considerable changes in the mitochondrial permeability transition pore (mPTP) opening, generation of reactive oxygen species (ROS), bioavailability of nitric oxide (NO), intracellular distribution of Ca^{2+} and Na^{+}, and pH. Paradoxically, reperfusion itself can actually cause cardiomyocyte death and subsequent irreversible myocardial injury, a phenomenon termed "ischemia reperfusion injury (IRI)".[5,6]

The absence of nutrients and oxygen in the myocardium leads to a series of changes within the myocardium. The oxidative phosphorylation, leading to mitochondrial membrane depolarization, adenosine triphosphate (ATP) depletion, and inhibition of myocardial contractile function is largely affected with the lack of oxygen supply.[7] This process is fastened by the breakdown of all available ATP, as the F1F0-ATPase functions in reverse to maintain the mitochondrial membrane potential, resulting in hydrolysis of ATP and an increase in mitochondrial inorganic phosphate. Cellular metabolism switches to anaerobic glycolysis, in the absence of oxygen resulting in the lactate accumulation, which reduces intracellular pH less than 7.0. Activation of the Na^{+}-H^{+} ion exchanger occurs with intracellular accumulation of protons, which removes protons from the cell in exchange for Na^{+} entry. The reduction of ATP during ischemia halts function of the $3Na^{+}$-$2K^{+}$ ATPase, thereby increasing the intracellular Na^{+} overload. In response, the reverse activation of the $2Na^{+}$ Ca^{2+} ion exchanger results in intracellular Ca^{2+} overloading as the cell tries to remove Na^{+}.[8,9]

Myocardial ischemic conditioning is referred to an intervention that protects the heart from ischemia or reperfusion injury. This conditioning may be provided before (preconditioning), during (perconditioning) or after the prolonged ischemic insult (postconditioning).[8]

The term "reperfusion injury" has been used for many decades to describe those events associated with reperfusion, some may be transient, (e.g., ventricular arrhythmias, myocardial stunning, and so on) and others permanent, (e.g., death induced by reperfusion, known as lethal reperfusion injury).[9]

MEDIATORS OF MYOCARDIAL REPERFUSION INJURY

Oxidative Stress

There is a burst of oxidative stress during the initial phase of myocardial reperfusion. This oxidative stress imparts myocardial injury and cardiomyocyte death. Therefore, antioxidant therapy was considered for prevention of such injury. However, studies have reported mixed results with antioxidant therapy in prevention of myocardial reperfusion injury.[8]

Intracellular Calcium Overload

We have already mentioned about the Ca^{2+} overload occurring at the time of acute myocardial ischemia. This is exacerbated during myocardial reperfusion due to disruption of the plasma membrane, damage to the sarcoplasmic reticulum, and mitochondrial re-energization. Re-energization allows the entry of Ca^{2+} into the mitochondria via the Ca^{2+} uniporter due to the recovery of the mitochondrial membrane potential. The entry of Ca^{2+} induces the opening of the mPTP. Literature shows that pharmacologic antagonists of the sarcolemmal Ca^{2+}channel or the mitochondrial Ca^{2+} uniporter administered at the onset of myocardial reperfusion may reduce MI size by up to 50%.[10]

The Rapid Restoration of Physiological pH at the Time of Reperfusion

The intracellular pH which decreased to less than 7.0 during acute myocardial ischemia is restored to physiological pH during reperfusion by the activation of the Na^+-H^+ exchanger as well as the Na^+-HCO^- symporter and by the washout of lactate. This pH shift contributes to mPTP opening and cardiomyocyte rigor hypercontracture in the early phase of reperfusion. Therefore, myocardial reperfusion injury may be reduced by the slow normalization of physiologic pH at the time of myocardial reperfusion. This may be achieved via the pharmacologic inhibition of the Na^+-H^+ exchanger or by slowing the process of myocardial reperfusion.[11,12]

The Mitochondrial Permeability Transition Pore: An Important Target for Cardioprotection

Many of the above proponents of myocardial reperfusion injury appear to converge on the mPTP. The opening of mPTP, a nonselective channel of the inner mitochondrial membrane, causes depolarization of mitochondrial membrane and uncoupling of oxidative phosphorylation. This leads to ATP depletion and cell death. It has been shown that the mPTP is closed during acute ischemia. The mPTP opens during reperfusion in response to mitochondrial Ca^{2+} and phosphate overload, oxidative stress and relative ATP depletion, and rapid pH correction. Small and large animal MI models has shown that prevention of mPTP opening by mPTP inhibitors such as cyclosporin A at the onset of myocardial reperfusion reduce MI size by 40–50% (Fig. 1).[11]

Inflammation: Guilty Mediator or Innocent Bystander

The contributory role of inflammatory response accompanying an acute MI in the pathogenesis of reperfusion injury is largely unclear. Different strategies aimed at reducing inflammation during reperfusion have shown significant

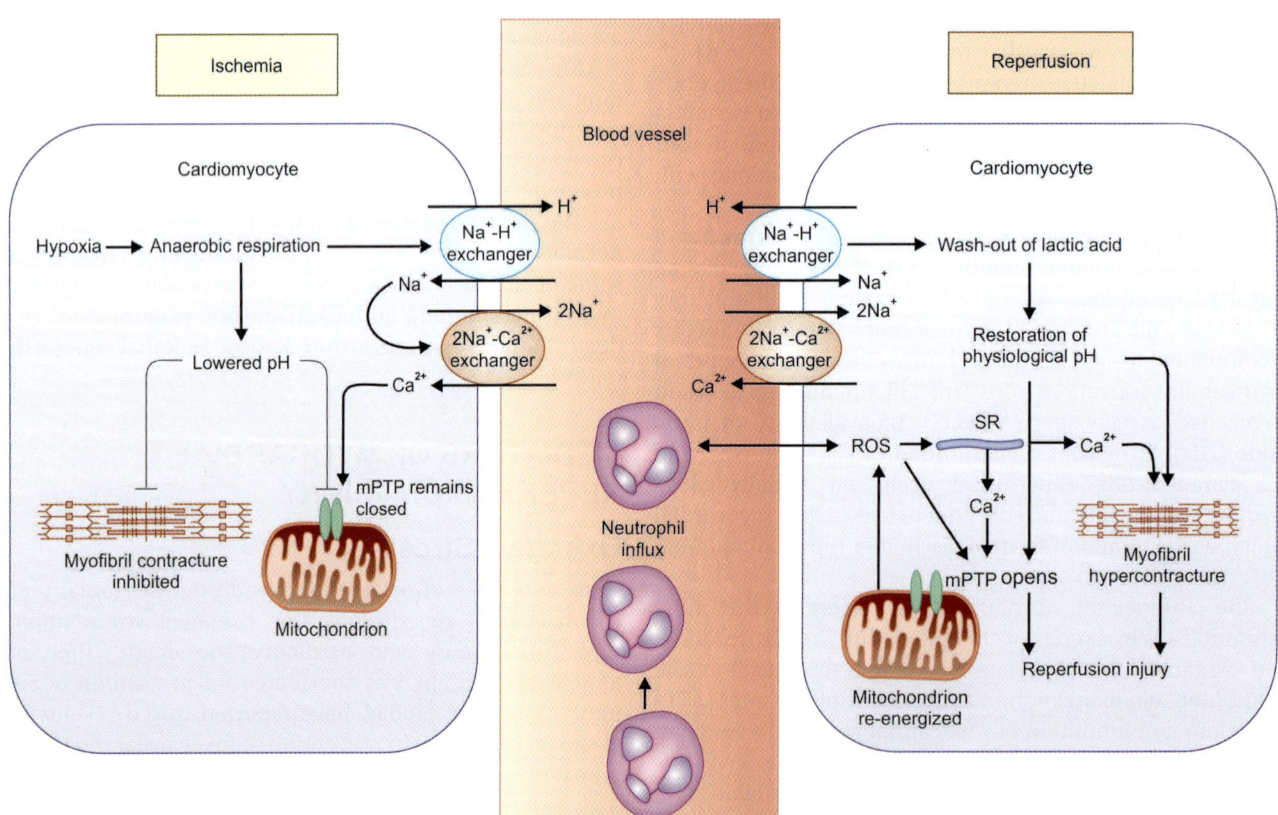

mPTP, mitochondrial permeability transition pore; ROS, reactive oxygen species; SR, sarcoplasmic reticulum.

FIG. 1: Schematic illustrating the main proponents of acute myocardial infarction.

reduction in MI size in experimental studies. But these results could not be reciprocated in clinical studies.[13,14]

THERAPIES TO REDUCE ISCHEMIC INJURY

There were four landmark studies that changed the course of ST-elevation myocardial infarction (STEMI) treatment and led to the development of strategies to reduce ischemic injury. These studies along with their findings are listed below:

- The demonstration of a spatial progression of necrosis during an infarction—Reimer et al.,[4] subjected anesthetized dogs to coronary occlusion of varying duration. They reported the progression of a wave front of myocardial necrosis from the central subendocardial layers with severe ischemia, to the less ischemic lateral boundaries and the subepicardium
- The demonstration of the reduced infarct size with reperfusion—Maroko et al., and Ginks et al.,[15] demonstrated that the myocardial can be salvaged by reperfusion within 3 hours after coronary occlusion ("time is muscle")
- The demonstration that coronary thrombosis is present in most cases of ongoing STEMI by DeWood et al.
- The administration of intracoronary thrombolytics (streptokinase) by Chazov et al. and later, in a larger group of patients, by Rentrop et al.[4,15]

REPERFUSION BY PRIMARY PERCUTANEOUS CORONARY INTERVENTION, THROMBOLYSIS, OR BOTH[16-19]

Reperfusion is considered to be the most effective therapy for the management of ischemic injury during STEMI. Pharmacological, mechanical, and combined reperfusion techniques have evolved over the years, and their efficacy has been greatly advanced by the development of adjunctive therapies. The use of lytic agents in placebo-controlled trials was crucial in the elucidation of the benefits of sustained reperfusion. The GISSI-1 trial was the first large-scale trial that demonstrated a substantial reduction in mortality by reperfusion with intravenous administration of thrombolytic agents.[16] During the early days, PCI for STEMI (primary angioplasty) was described as a rescue intervention in cases with unsuccessful thrombolysis and as an adjunctive therapy to thrombolysis. Angiogram was performed to evaluate the coronary anatomy and residual stenosis. It was only in 1983 that the use of primary angioplasty as an alternative to thrombolysis was acknowledged. Many studies comparing PCI and thrombolysis successfully demonstrated that timely PCI by an experienced team is superior to in-hospital thrombolytic therapy. Newer guidelines propose the use of thrombolytic therapy in patients who cannot get timely PCI. The planned PCI can be delayed until 3–24 hours after lytic administration. This approach differs from the facilitated approach, in which PCI is performed as soon

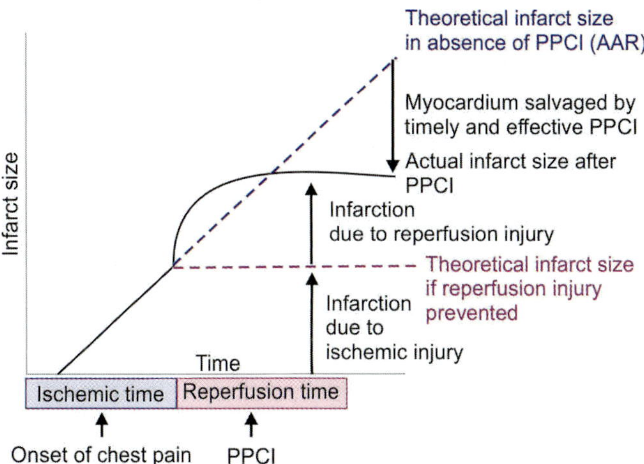

AAR, area at risk; PPCI, primary percutaneous coronary intervention.

FIG. 2: Illustrates the individual contributions of acute myocardial ischemic injury and myocardial reperfusion injury to final myocardial infarction (MI) size (expressed in arbitrary units) in ST-elevation MI patients up to 24 hours following primary percutaneous coronary intervention.

as the patient arrives at the PCI center.[17,20,21] The STREAM (Strategic Reperfusion Early After Myocardial Infarction) trial showed that prehospital administration of the thrombolytic tenecteplase in patients who could not get PCI within 1 hour resulted in rates similar to standard primary PCI for the composite end points of death, shock, congestive heart failure, or reinfarction at 30 days. One-year mortality rates in both groups were almost identical (Fig. 2).[22]

OTHER THERAPIES TO REDUCE ISCHEMIC INJURY

The mechanisms by which ongoing ischemic cascade that can be attempted slowing have been on investigation for long. Several randomized trials about various drugs have been tested, i.e., able to reduce oxygen consumption have. Among them, β-blockers are mainly studied in many STEMI trials, and there is no conclusive evidence of reduction in infarct size was noted, bringing the cardioprotective potential of β-blockers in STEMI into question. Majority of trials on β-blockers were done on nonreperfusion patients. Metoprolol compared with others have found to be having greater capacity in decreasing reperfusion injury.

Hypothermia has been well-established in reducing progression of ischemic damage in animal models of STEMI, but its clinical application of hypothermia has been limited. CHILL-MI (Rapid Endovascular Catheter Core Cooling combined with cold saline as an Adjunct to Percutaneous Coronary Intervention for the Treatment of Acute Myocardial Infarction) trial included patients scheduled for PCI. The subjects were randomly divided into two groups, i.e., standard care or a rapid cooling protocol (infusion of cold saline plus endovascular cooling device). A measured by cardiovascular magnetic resonance (CMR), hypothermia did not reduce infarct size, despite achievement of the target temperature.[23]

Nonpharmacological Interventions to Reduce Reperfusion Injury[24]

In nonpharmacological interventions the first major development was "ischemic preconditioning" described by Murry et al.[25] who, in 1986, reported that performing short duration cycles of ischemia and reperfusion before a prolonged coronary artery occlusion with reperfusion could considerably reduce final infarct size in dogs. Given that total ischemic time was unaltered by this intervention, this study suggested that there was more to limiting infarct size than a shorter duration of ischemia.[24,25]

The second breakthrough was the description of "ischemic postconditioning" by Zhao et al. in 2003. They showed that performing short duration episodes of ischemia and reperfusion immediately after reflow following prolonged ischemia could decrease the final infarct size in dogs by 30–40%. This effect was more unexpected than preconditioning, because the intervention was applied after reflow. Therefore, it has no connection to the duration of ischemia or any associated event and must be related to the prevention of events occurring after reperfusion.[26,27]

PHARMACOLOGICAL INTERVENTIONS TO REDUCE REPERFUSION INJURY

Cyclosporine-A

Cyclosporine-A has its mode of action as a postconditioning agent. It acts by inhibiting the opening of the mPTP channel. Piot et al. in his study of 58 patients randomized to receive a single bolus of cyclosporine-A or placebo immediately before PCI. There was significant increase in the area of reperfusion as observed.[28]

Metoprolol

Beta-blockers have been tested in various STEMI trials in 70s and 80s with no concrete cardioprotective effect. But majority of these trials were before the reperfusion era. Preclinical data from the pig model of infarction demonstrated that intravenous (IV) metoprolol very significantly reduces infarct size when administered before reperfusion.[29] The reduction in reperfusion injury rather than of reduced myocardial oxygen consumption, the mechanism responsible for this infarct-limiting effect is proposed to be related to a reduction in reperfusion injury due to the effect of metoprolol on circulating cells (neutrophils or platelets) rather than cardiomyocytes. This preclinical evidence led to the METOCARD-CNIC (Effect of Metoprolol in Cardioprotection during an Acute Myocardial Infarction) trial. The trial included 270 anterior STEMI patients undergoing PCI who were randomly divided into two groups, i.e., early IV metoprolol or control before reperfusion. Infarcts, measured by CMR, were significantly smaller in the IV metoprolol group, six-month CMR follow-up of more than 200 patients showed that the IV metoprolol group had a fewer proportion of lower left ventricular (LV) ejection. The encouraging results from the METOCARD-CNIC trial appear to contradict findings from the much larger COMMIT (ClOpidogrel and Metoprolol in Myocardial Infarction Trial). In this trial, STEMI patients undergoing thrombolysis were randomized to early IV metoprolol followed by oral metoprolol or matching placebo. The COMMIT showed significantly reduced rates of reinfarction and ventricular fibrillation in response to early IV metoprolol, but there was no infarct size reduction and had an excess cardiogenic shock, resulting in a net neutral effect on mortality.[30]

Glucose Modulators

Sodi-Pallares had proposed use of glucose to protect cardiomyocytes from energy depletion during MI.[30] Combine administration of glucose-insulin-potassium (GIK) during ongoing MI has been tested in several trials. The IMMEDIATE (Immediate Myocardial Metabolic Enhancement during Initial Assessment and Treatment in Emergency Care) trial included patients with suspected acute coronary. The subjects were randomized to GIK or placebo groups during transfer to the hospital. In the subgroup of patients presenting with STEMI, GIK significantly reduced CMR-evaluated infarct size. Lonborg et al. randomized 172 STEMI patients to receive IV injection of the glucagon-like peptide-1 (GLP-1) analog exenatide or placebo. Myocardial salvage on CMR was significantly higher in the exenatide group.[31]

Abciximab

Glycoprotein IIb or IIIa inhibitors reduce thrombotic events by their potent effect on platelets and platelet leukocyte aggregates implicated in ischemia-reperfusion (I/R) injury. The INFUSE-AMI (Intracoronary Abciximab and Aspiration Thrombectomy in Patients with Large Anterior Myocardial Infarction) trial recruited 452 anterior wall STEMI patients undergoing PCI to test the effect of abciximab and/or thrombectomy on infarct size, as evaluated by CMR. Thrombus aspiration had no effect on infarct size, but intracoronary administration of abciximab significantly reduced infarct size.[32,33]

REFERENCES

1. Braunwald E, Kloner RA. Myocardial reperfusion: a double-edged sword? J Clin Invest. 1985;76(5):1713-9.
2. Piper HM, Garcia-Dorado D, Ovize M. A fresh look at reperfusion injury. Cardiovasc Res. 1998;38(2):291-300.
3. Yellon DM, Hausenloy DJ. Myocardial reperfusion injury. N Engl J Med. 2007;357(11):1121-35.
4. Reimer KA, Lowe JE, Rasmussen MM, et al. The wavefront phenomenon of ischemic cell death. 1. Myocardial infarct size versus duration of coronary occlusion in dogs. Circulation. 1977;56(5):786-94.
5. Avkiran M, Marber MS. Na(+)/H(+) exchange inhibitors for cardioprotective therapy: progress, problems and prospects. J Am Coll Cardiol. 2002;39(5):747-53.
6. Hearse DJ, Humphrey SM, Chain EB. Abrupt reoxygenation of the anoxic potassium-arrested perfused rat heart: a study of myocardial enzyme release. J Mol Cell Cardiol. 1973;5(4):395-407.
7. Zweier JL, Flaherty JT, Weisfeldt ML. Direct measurement of free radical generation following reperfusion of ischemic myocardium. Proc Natl Acad Sci U S A. 1987;84(5):1404-7.
8. Smith RA, Hartley RC, Murphy MP. Mitochondria-targeted small molecule therapeutics and probes. Antioxid Redox Signal. 2011;15(12):3021-38.

9. Herzog WR, Vogel RA, Schlossberg ML, et al. Short-term low dose intracoronary diltiazem administered at the onset of reperfusion reduces myocardial infarct size. Int J Cardiol. 1997;59(1):21-7.
10. Miyamae M, Camacho SA, Weiner MW, et al. Attenuation of postischemic reperfusion injury is related to prevention of [Ca2+]m overload in rat hearts. Am J Physiol. 1996;271(5 Pt 2):H2145-53.
11. Bar FW, Tzivoni D, Dirksen MT, et al. Results of the first clinical study of adjunctive CAldaret (MCC-135) in patients undergoing primary percutaneous coronary intervention for ST-elevation Myocardial Infarction: the randomized multicenter CASTEMI study. Eur Heart J. 2006;27(21):2516-23.
12. Cohen MV, Yang XM, Downey JM. The pH hypothesis of postconditioning: staccato reperfusion reintroduces oxygen and perpetuates myocardial acidosis. Circulation. 2007;115(14):1895-903.
13. Shanmuganathan S, Hausenloy DJ, Duchen MR, et al. Mitochondrial permeability transition pores as a target for cardioprotection in the human heart. Am J Physiol Heart Circ Physiol. 2005;289(1):H237-42.
14. Ma XL, Tsao PS, Lefer AM. Antibody to CD-18 exerts endothelial and cardiac protective effects in myocardial ischemia and reperfusion. J Clin Invest. 1991;88(4):1237-43.
15. Ginks WR, Sybers HD, Maroko PR, et al. Coronary artery reperfusion. II. Reduction of myocardial infarct size at 1 week after the coronary occlusion. J Clin Invest 1972;51(10):2717-23.
16. Effectiveness of intravenous thrombolytic treatment in acute myocardial infarction. Gruppo Italiano per lo Studio della Streptochinasi nell'Infarto Miocardico (GISSI). Lancet. 1986;1(8478):397-402.
17. GUSTO Investigators. An international randomized trial comparing four thrombolytic strategies for acute myocardial infarction. N Engl J Med. 1993;329(10):673-82.
18. Van De Werf F, Adgey J, Ardissino D, et al. Single-bolus tenecteplase compared with frontloaded alteplase in acute myocardial infarction: the ASSENT-2 double-blind randomized trial. Lancet. 1999;354(9180):716-22.
19. Hartzler GO, Rutherford BD, McConahay DR, et al. Percutaneous transluminal coronary angioplasty with and without thrombolytic therapy for treatment of acute myocardial infarction. Am Heart J. 1983;106(5 Pt 1):965-73.
20. Pinto DS, Frederick PD, Chakrabarti AK, et al. Benefit of transferring ST-segment-elevation myocardial infarction patients for percutaneous coronary intervention compared with administration of onsite fibrinolytic declines as delays increase. Circulation. 2011;124(23):2512-21.
21. Armstrong PW, Gershlick AH, Goldstein P, et al. Fibrinolysis or primary PCI in ST-segment elevation myocardial infarction. N Engl J Med. 2013;368(15):1379-87.
22. Sinnaeve PR, Armstrong PW, Gershlick AH, et al. STEMI patients randomized to a pharmacoinvasive strategy or primary PCI: the STREAM 1-year mortality follow-up. Circulation. 2014;130:1139-45.
23. Erlinge D, Gotberg M, Lang I, et al. Rapid endovascular catheter core cooling combined with cold saline as an adjunct to percutaneous coronary intervention for the treatment of acute myocardial infarction. The CHILL-MI trial: a randomized controlled study of the use of central venous catheter core cooling combined with cold saline as an adjunct to percutaneous coronary intervention for the treatment of acute myocardial infarction. J Am Coll Cardiol. 2014;63(18):1857-65.
24. Zahger D, Yano J, Chaux A, et al. Absence of lethal reperfusion injury after 3 hours of reperfusion. A study in a single-canine-heart model of ischemia-reperfusion. Circulation. 1995;91(12):2989-94.
25. Murry CE, Jennings RB, Reimer KA. Preconditioning with ischemia: a delay of lethal cell injury in ischemic myocardium. Circulation. 1986;74(5):1124-36.
26. Przyklenk K, Bauer B, Ovize M, et al. Regional ischemic 'preconditioning' protects remote virgin myocardium from subsequent sustained coronary occlusion. Circulation. 1993;87(3):893-9.
27. Botker HE, Kharbanda R, Schmidt MR, et al. Remote ischemic conditioning before hospital admission, as a complement to angioplasty, and effect on myocardial salvage in patients with acute myocardial infarction: a randomized trial. Lancet. 2010;375(9716):727-34.
28. Piot C, Croisille P, Staat P, et al. Effect of cyclosporine on reperfusion injury in acute myocardial infarction. N Engl J Med. 2008;359(5):473-81.
29. Ibanez B, Cimmino G, Prat-Gonzalez S, et al. The cardioprotection granted by metoprolol is restricted to its administration prior to coronary reperfusion. Int J Cardiol. 2011;147(3):428-32.
30. Chen ZM, Pan HC, Chen YP, et al. Early intravenous then oral metoprolol in 45,852 patients with acute myocardial infarction: randomized placebo-controlled trial. Lancet. 2005;366(9497):1622-32.
31. Sodi-Pallares D, Testelli MR, Fishleder BI, et al. Effects of an intravenous infusion of a potassium glucose-insulin solution on the electrocardiographic signs of myocardial infarction: a preliminary clinical report. Am J Cardiol. 1962;9:166-81.
32. Stone GW, Maehara A, Witzenbichler B, et al. Intracoronary abciximab and aspiration thrombectomy in patients with large anterior myocardial infarction: the INFUSE-AMI randomized trial. JAMA. 2012;307(17):1817-26.
33. White SK, Frohlich GM, Sado DM, et al. Remote ischemic conditioning reduces myocardial infarct size and edema in patients with ST-segment elevation myocardial infarction. JACC Cardiovasc Interv. 2015;8(1 Pt B):178-88.

CHAPTER 38

Risk Stratification in Unstable Angina/NSTEMI: A Current Approach

Anoop Jain, CB Meena, Sahil Sareen

INTRODUCTION

Ischemic heart disease (IHD) may manifest clinically as either chronic stable angina or an acute coronary syndrome (ACS).[1] The spectrum of ACS includes ST-segment elevation myocardial infarction (STEMI), and the non-ST elevation acute coronary syndrome (NSTE-ACS). The latter consists of non-STEMI (NSTEMI) and unstable angina (UA), which have indistinguishable clinical presentations at the initial evaluation.

Several features help to differentiate ACS from chronic stable angina, including (1) sudden onset of symptoms at rest (or with minimal exertion) that lasts at least 10 minutes unless treated promptly; (2) severe pain, pressure, or discomfort in the chest; and (3) an accelerating pattern of angina that develops more frequently, with greater severity, or that awakens the patient from sleep. The 12-lead electrocardiogram (ECG) and markers of myocardial necrosis are essential tools in distinguishing between the three types of ACS. Patients with typical symptoms without persistent (>20 min continuously) ST-segment elevation in at least two contiguous electrocardiographic leads, but with elevation of myocardial biomarkers more than 99th percentile of normal, are classified as having NSTEMI. Patients without typical symptoms and serial negative markers of myocardial necrosis are classified as having UA, a diagnosis that carries a better prognosis.

EPIDEMIOLOGY

Cardiovascular diseases (CVDs) have now become the leading cause of mortality in India.[2] A quarter of all mortality is attributable to CVD. Ischemic heart disease and stroke are the predominant causes and are responsible for more than 80% of CVD deaths. The Global Burden of Disease Study estimate of age-standardized CVD death rate of 272 per 100,000 population in India is higher than the global average of 235 per 100,000 population.

Some aspects of the CVD epidemic in India are particular causes of concern, including its accelerated buildup, the early age of disease onset in the population, and the high case fatality rate.[2]

The fraction of ACS attributed to NSTEMI continues to increase, while that for STEMI is declining, for several reasons: (1) wider use of preventive measures, such as aspirin, statins, and smoking cessation; (2) aging of the population, with greater prevalence of diabetes and chronic kidney disease (CKD) and lower rates of smoking; and (3) broader use of troponin assays with higher sensitivity for myocardial necrosis, which shifts the diagnosis from UA to NSTEMI.[3]

PATHOPHYSIOLOGY

The pathogenesis of NSTE-ACS involves four processes operating singly or in various combinations: (1) disruption of an unstable atheromatous plaque, which may be driven at least in part by inflammation;[4] (2) coronary arterial vasoconstriction; (3) gradual intraluminal narrowing of an epicardial coronary artery caused by progressive atherosclerosis or restenosis after stenting; and (4) oxygen supply–demand mismatch (Fig. 1).[4]

Activation of the coagulation cascade and platelets play central roles in the formation of thrombus following plaque disruption.

CLINICAL AND RISK ASSESSMENT

Initial risk assessment is made clinically, based on the history, risk factors for coronary artery disease, clinical assessment (including the heart rate and blood pressure).[5,6]

The ECG is recommended by the clinical guidelines as a first-line test that should be performed immediately. The ECG has good specificity (97%), but poor sensitivity (28%) in ACS.[7] This assessment is of pivotal importance since cardiac biomarkers are usually unavailable initially. The most common abnormalities on the 12-lead ECG are

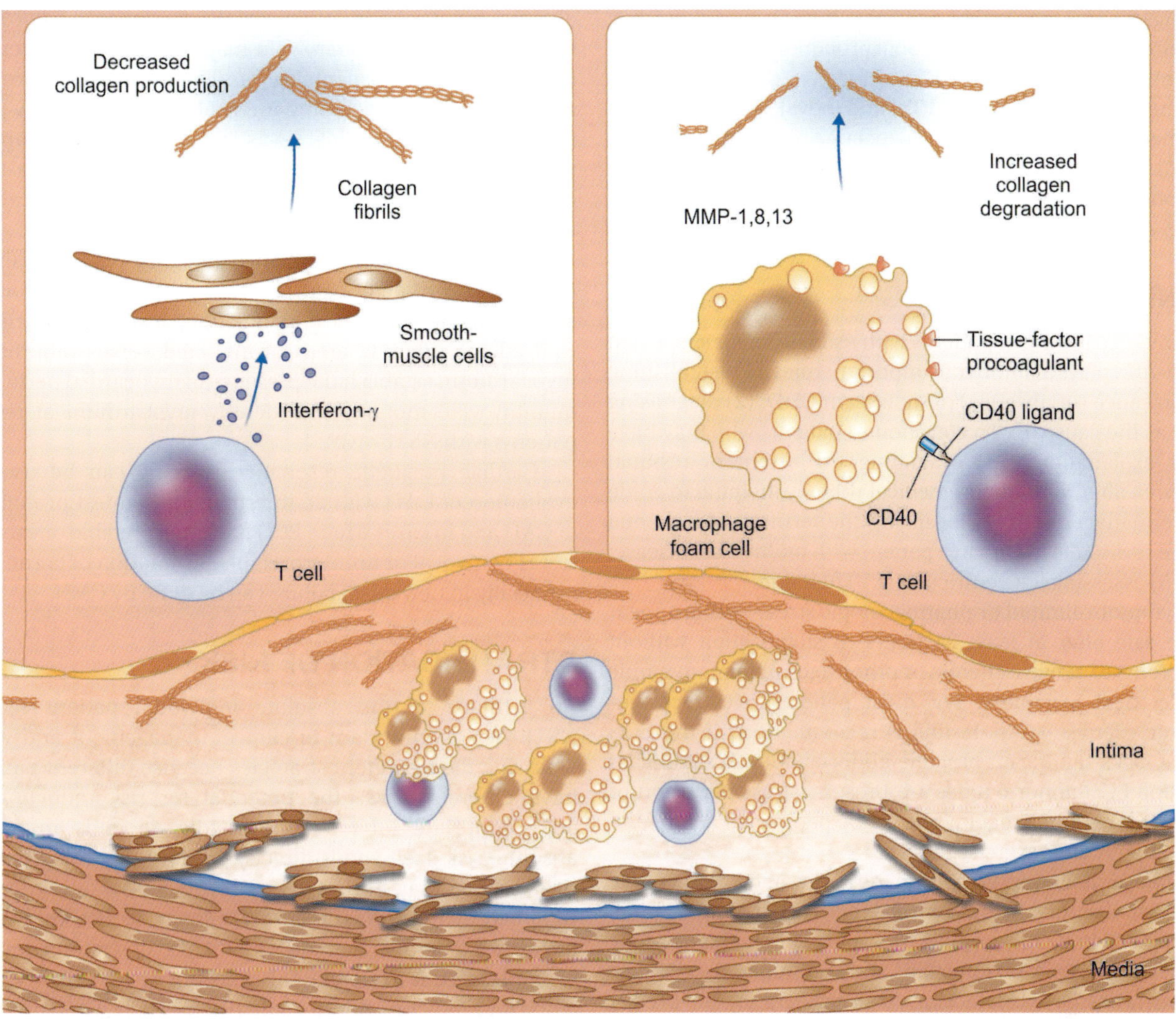

FIG. 1: Inflammatory pathways involved in rupture and thrombosis in coronary arteries: An atheromatous plaque is shown at the bottom of the figure depicting a central lipid core containing macrophage foam cells (in yellow) and T cells (in blue). Arterial smooth muscle cells (red) are the source of arterial collagen (triple helical structures). T cells are activated and produce cytokines, which inhibit the production of the new, interstitial collagen. T cells may also activate macrophages in the intima by expressing CD40 ligand. This inflammatory signaling causes overproduction of matrix metalloproteinases, which catalyze the initial rate-limiting step in collagen breakdown (top right). These consequences of inflammatory cascade contribute to the instability of the plaque's fibrous cap.

ST-segment depression and T wave inversion, which are more likely to be present while the patient is symptomatic. Greater degrees of ST-segment depression predict poorer outcomes. Deep (>0.2 mV) T wave inversions are compatible with, but not necessarily diagnostic of, NSTE-ACS, whereas isolated T wave inversions of lesser magnitude are not particularly helpful given their low specificity. More than half of patients with definite NSTE-ACS may have normal or nondiagnostic ECGs.

Cardiac-specific troponins I (cTnI) and T (cTnT) are the biomarkers of choice to identify myocardial necrosis, thus distinguishing between NSTE-ACS and UA. Since the sensitivities of different troponin assays in clinical practice vary, the consensus recommendation is to define MI by an elevation in cTnI or cTnT more than 99th percentile of the normal range of the specific assay used[8] with a typical temporal rise and fall occurring in a patient with a clinical presentation consistent with ACS. As high-sensitivity troponin (hsTn) assays[8] that can detect ultralow concentrations of troponin in approximately 90% of healthy individuals become increasingly available, consideration of the clinical context of a troponin elevation will become even more important in avoiding misdiagnosis and improper triage in management of patients. Several other biomarkers may be useful to determine prognosis and help guide care. Of these, the natriuretic peptides [i.e. brain natriuretic peptide (BNP) and N-terminal pro-BNP] have been most widely used in patients with NSTE-ACS. Similarly, C-reactive protein (CRP), a marker of inflammation, is elevated following NSTE-ACS, and the degree of elevation correlates with long-term cardiovascular (CV) outcomes. Other promising novel biomarkers in diagnosis of ACS include chemokine ligand-5 and ligand-18,[9] interleukin-6,[10] heart-type fatty acid-binding protein,[11] pentraxin,[12] midregional proadrenomedullin,[13] and copeptin.[13]

The combination of hs-cTn and novel biomarkers has also been investigated. In a prospective observational study of 478 patients, the combination of hs-cTn and copeptin demonstrated significantly higher sensitivity to identify NSTE-ACS than a repeat hs-cTn.[14]

NONINVASIVE TESTING

Noninvasive testing in patients with established or suspected NSTE-ACS plays a number of important roles: (1) establishing the presence (or absence) of significant CHD; (2) diagnosing CHD as the cause of cTn elevation in patients who may have other explanations; (3) evaluating the extent of residual ischemia after initiation of medical therapy, helping to guide future management; (4) localizing the territory of ischemia before revascularization in a patient with multivessel disease; and (5) assessing left ventricular (LV) function.

Symptom-limited or pharmacologic stress testing appear to be safe after at least 24 hours of stabilization without symptoms of active ischemia or other signs of hemodynamic or electrical instability. For most patients, electrocardiographic exercise stress testing is recommended if the ECG at rest lacks significant baseline abnormalities. If significant baseline ECG abnormalities are present, stress perfusion or echocardiographic imaging should be performed before and immediately after exercise.

Echocardiography is useful in the assessment of LV systolic and diastolic function and can also identify left atrial dilation, functional mitral regurgitation, tricuspid annular plane systolic excursion, diastolic dysfunction, and ventricular mechanical dyssynchrony. Speckle tracking echocardiography can predict patients of NSTE-ACS with acute coronary occlusion who may benefit from an early revascularization strategy.[15]

Coronary CT angiography (CCTA) has been proposed as a modality to improve the early management of NSTE-ACS patients. In a large study involving 1,000 patients at nine hospitals in the United States, CCTA facilitated the exclusion of a diagnosis of ACS, increasing discharge from the emergency department and reducing length of stay.[16] Three large randomized trials have shown that CCTA compared to standard evaluation expedites the triage of patients presenting with chest discomfort in the ED, thereby shortening length of stay.[16-18] The appropriate indications according to a study[19] include an ECG which is negative or indeterminate for myocardial ischemia, low-intermediate pretest likelihood by risk stratification tools, a TIMI risk score of 0–2 (low risk) or a HEART score less than 3, more than or equal to 1 negative troponin value, including point-of-care assays and equivocal or inadequate previous functional testing during index ED or within previous 6 months. It is also appropriate for evaluation of cardiac mass (suspected tumor or thrombus, or of a pericardial condition (pericardial mass, constrictive pericarditis, or complications of cardiac surgery). Evaluation of pulmonary vein anatomy prior to invasive radiofrequency ablation for atrial fibrillation can also be done via a coronary CT. Noninvasive coronary vein mapping prior to placement of biventricular pacemaker and noninvasive coronary arterial mapping, including internal mammary artery prior to repeat cardiac surgical revascularization are also appropriately assessed by CCTA, although for this intra- and extracardiac structural and functional assessment, cardiac magnetic resonance (CMR) is found to be better.

Cardiac magnetic resonance imaging (CMRI) using a rapid-scan protocol can provide precise measurements of ventricular volumes and function, evaluate ventricular wall edema, identify areas of infarcted versus hibernating myocardium, establish the presence of myocardial perfusion, quantify wall motion, and identify myocardium at risk in patients with NSTE-ACS.[20]

Cardiac magnetic resonance imaging can be used in evaluation of CAD with an intermediate pre-test probability of CAD and in cases where ECG is uninterpretable or exercise test is equivocal or uninterpretable. Evaluation of coronaries especially in new onset failure can be done by CMR.

STRATIFICATION OF RISK

An estimate of the absolute individual patient risk of NSTE-ACS is important in clinical management and when assessing the treatment strategies because different patients have different risks. The potential for risk reduction by an appropriate intervention broadly depends upon the absolute risk itself and is directly proportional to it. A single risk variable may not provide a reliable assessment of risk. In practice, there has been a tendency to use this single factor like a cardiac marker for patient risk stratification, for example, serum troponin. This may not be accurate enough alone for predicting the absolute risk specially when used in a qualitative manner.

For example, when compared to a well-validated risk scoring system (GRACE21), that uses multiple risk factors, a large proportion of troponin positive patients had low to medium risks and vice versa (Fig. 2).[21]

Therefore, a number of risk scoring systems have been developed to predict short- and medium-term outcome in patients with acute coronary syndromes. Fourteen observational studies[21-34] were identified that assessed the utility of various risk scores.

TIMI Risk Score

A 7-point score for patients with acute coronary syndromes derived by summing the presence of each of these factors (1 point for each) (Table 1):[22]

- Age more than 64 years
- More than three coronary risk factors
- Prior coronary angiographic coronary obstruction
- ST-segment deviation
- More than two angina events within 24 hours
- Use of aspirin within 7 days
- Elevated levels of cardiac biomarkers (e.g., troponin).

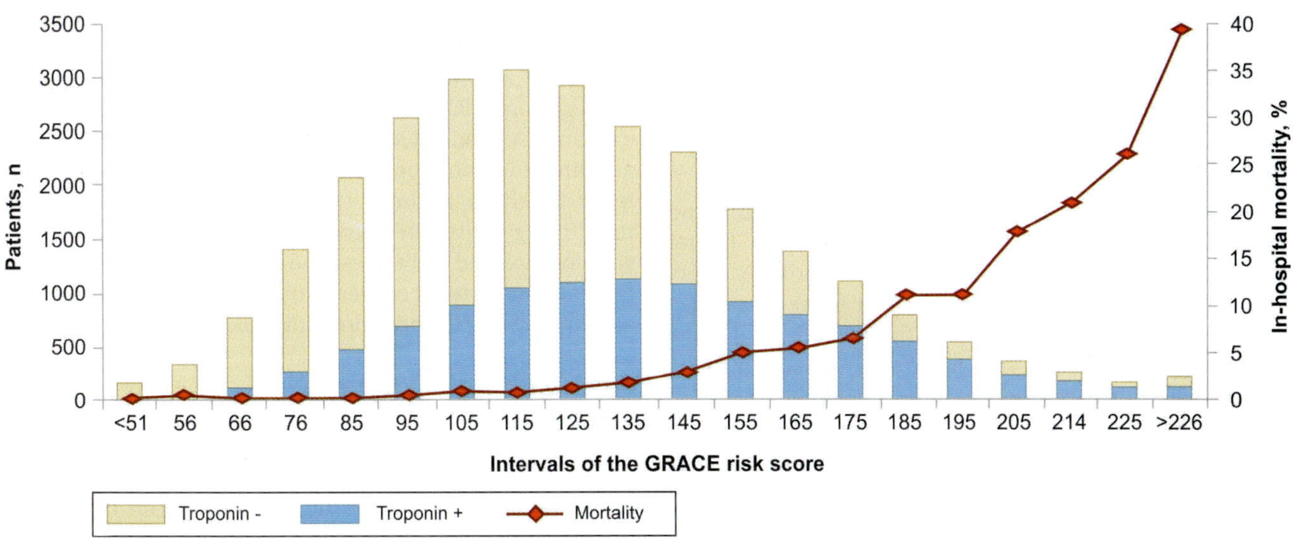

FIG. 2: Bar chart describes the distribution of (left axis) troponin positive (red bars) and troponin negative (yellow bars) patients according to category of GRACE risk score (ranging from 51 to 226) among 27,406 patients with non-ST elevation acute coronary syndrome in the GRACE registry. The blue curve (right axis) depicts the observed hospital mortality rates.

TABLE 1: TIMI risk score

TIMI score	14-day adverse cardiac event rate (%)
0/1	4.7
2	8.3
3	13.2
4	19.9
5	26.2
6/7	40.9

TABLE 2: GRACE risk score

GRACE score	Risk category	In-hospital deaths (%)	Postdischarge to 6 months (% of deaths)
<109	Low risk	<1	<3
109–140	Intermediate risk	1–3	3–8
>140	High risk	>3	>8

GRACE Risk Score

According to some studies, the GRACE risk score provides the most accurate stratification of risk both on admission and at discharge (Table 2).[35,36]

Variables used in the GRACE 2.0 risk calculation include age, systolic blood pressure, pulse rate, serum creatinine, Killip class at presentation, cardiac arrest at admission, elevated cardiac biomarkers and ST deviation. If the Killip class or serum creatinine values are not available, a modified score can be calculated by adding renal failure and use of diuretics, respectively.

One of the limitations of the GRACE score is its non-adoption in daily practice probably due to lack of awareness by medical and nursing staff, a lack of access to the on-line website, and lack of time in a busy department since the creatinine and troponin blood results are required before the score can be completed.

PURSUIT Risk Score

The PURSUIT risk score for death at 30 days was derived from the RCT of the same name (N = 9461; NSTE-ACS).[29] It includes variables like age, sex, (Canadian Cardiovascular Society (CCS)-class in previous 6 weeks, heart rate, systolic blood pressure (SBP), rales, and ST-segment depression at presentation.

Other risk scores include PREDICT, AMIS, EMMACE, SRI (simple risk score), and comparative studies have been undertaken to compare these aforementioned risk scores against one another. In the MINAP database (N = 100,686), the PURSUIT, GRACE, SRI, and EMMACE risk scores showed similarly high discrimination in predicting the likelihood of death.[30]

GRACE Risk Score versus PURSUIT Risk Score

Two studies of populations with non ST-segment elevation ACS showed no significant difference in discriminatory performance between the GRACE and PURSUIT risk scores for predicting in-hospital and one year mortality.[23-28] Similarly, GRACE and PURSUIT risk scores have been found to have a better discrimination for 1 year mortality than TIMI risk score.[28]

The various risk models reviewed use different components to make up their systems, and none is clearly superior, although PURSUIT, GRACE, and PREDICT seem to have better discrimination than TIMI for mortality.

Bleeding Risk

Various pharmacological agents (such as antithrombin and antiplatelet drugs) and coronary revascularization [either percutaneous coronary intervention (PCI) or coronary artery bypass graft (CABG) surgery] are known to be associated with some treatment hazards (particularly bleeding complications), which for the individual patient must be balanced against any potential treatment benefits.

Major bleeding events are associated with increased mortality in NSTE-ACS.[37,38] The can rapid risk stratification of unstable angina patients suppress adverse outcomes with early implementation of the ACC/AHA guidelines (CRUSADE) bleeding risk score was developed from a cohort of 71,277 NSTE-ACS patients (derivation cohort) and further validated in a cohort of 17,857 patients (validation cohort) from the same registry.[39] The CRUSADE bleeding risk score considered baseline patient characteristics (i.e., female gender, history of diabetes, history of peripheral vascular disease or stroke), admission clinical variables (i.e., heart rate, systolic blood pressure, signs of heart failure) and admission laboratory values (i.e., hematocrit, calculated creatinine clearance) to estimate the patient's likelihood of an in-hospital major bleeding event.

The acute catheterization and urgent intervention triage strategy (ACUITY) bleeding risk score was derived from a pooled cohort of 17,421 patients with ACS (both NSTE-ACS and STEMI) recruited in the ACUITY and harmonizing outcomes with revascularization and stents in acute myocardial infarction (HORIZONS-AMI) trials.[37]

CRUSADE and ACUITY scores have reasonable predictive value for major bleeding in ACS patients undergoing coronary angiography, with CRUSADE found to be the most discriminatory.[40] However, in patients medically treated or on oral anticoagulants, the predictive value of these scores is not established.

MANAGEMENT (BOX 1)

General Measures

After the initial evaluation and a directed history with physical examination is done, an ECG should be performed within 10 minutes of arrival. Blood specimens for cTn or, if possible, hsTn assay should be obtained and a second assay can be performed after 3–6 hours of the first test. Patients with elevated cTn or new ST-segment abnormalities or deemed to be at moderate or high risk based on a validated risk score should be admitted to a specialized cardiovascular intensive care unit (ICU). Patients with UA but without elevated cTn and ischemic electrocardiographic changes should be admitted to a monitored bed, preferably in a CV step-down unit.[1] In these settings, continuous electrocardiographic monitoring with telemetry should be present. Patients should be placed on bed rest and inhaled oxygen provided to patients with arterial oxygen saturation (SaO_2) less than 90% and those with HF and pulmonary rales.

BOX 1 Management of non-ST elevation acute coronary syndrome

- General measures
- Anti-ischemic therapy
- Antithrombotic therapy
- Intervention
- Rehabilitation

Anti-ischemic Therapy

Rationale

Beta-blockers

Beta-adrenergic receptor blockers decrease heart rate, blood pressure, and contractility, resulting in a reduction in myocardial oxygen demand. These effects are primarily the result of competitive antagonism of the β1 cardiomyocyte receptors. The evidence supporting their clinical benefit is largely derived from earlier studies in patients with acute MI before the current era of reperfusion therapy for STEMI. The findings have been extrapolated to include patients with UA and NSTEMI (Table 3).[41]

Nitrates

Therapy with nitrates exerts beneficial effects by decreasing preload and LV end-diastolic volume, thereby reducing myocardial oxygen demand. Nitrates also dilate both normal and diseased coronary arteries, an action that potentially increases both antegrade and collateral coronary blood flow. Typically, nitrates are used in patients with ACS who have hypertension or HF and in those with continued angina.

Calcium Channel Blockers (CCBs)

CCBs may cause vasodilation, reduce heart rate, or decrease myocardial contractility. Because these effects occur to a variable extent with the various CCBs, there is not a class effect. The American College of Cardiology/American Heart

TABLE 3: Class of drugs and their role in NSTE-ACS

Class of drug	Role in NSTE-ACS
Beta blockers	Decreased mortality
Nitrates	No benefit on mortality
Calcium channel blockers	No clear benefit on mortality or reinfarction
Nicorandil	Decreases arrhythmias and transient ischemia
Trimetazidine	Decreases short-term mortality
Ranolazine	Decreases recurrent ischemia and arrhythmias
Cyclosporine (inhibitor of mitochondrial permeability transition pore)	Reduces infarct size in small studies[42]

NSTE-ACS, non-ST elevation acute coronary syndrome.

TABLE 4: Antiplatelet and anticoagulation treatment summary for non-ST elevation acute coronary syndrome

<table>
<tr><th colspan="2">Initial treatment</th></tr>
<tr><td colspan="2">DAPT and anticoagulant therapy:
1. Aspirin (COR I, LOE A)
2. P2Y12 inhibitor, clopidogrel or ticagrelor (COR I, LOE B)
3. Anticoagulant:
Enoxaparin (COR I, LOE B) or fondaparinux (COR I, LOE B) or bivalirudin (for invasive strategy, COR I, LOE B)
4 Can consider GP IIB/IIIa receptor inhibitors in high-risk patients stratified to early invasive strategy (Eptifibatide or tirofiban; COR IIb, LOE B)</td></tr>
<tr><th colspan="2">During hospitalization</th></tr>
<tr><td>Medically treated patients:
1. Aspirin (COR I, LOE A)
2. P2Y12 inhibitor, either ticagrelor or clopidogrel (COR I, LOE B)
3. Anticoagulant:
Enoxaparin (COR I, LOE B) or UFH (COR I, LOE B) or fondaparinux (COR I, LOE B)</td><td>PCI-treated patients:
1. Aspirin (COR I, LOE A)
2. P2Y12 inhibitor, clopidogrel ticagrelor or prasugrel (COR I, LOE B)
3. Anticoagulant:
Enoxaparin (COR I, LOE B) or UFH (COR I, LOE B) or fondaparinux (CORI LOE B) or bivalirudin
4. Can consider GBIIb/IIIa receptor inhibitors in high-risk patients not adequately pretreated with clopidogrel (COR I, LOE A) or in high-risk patients adequately pre-trated with clopidogrel (COR IIa, LOE B)</td></tr>
<tr><th colspan="2">Long-term treatment</th></tr>
<tr><td>Medically treated patients:
1. Aspirin indefinitely (CORI, LOE A)
2. P2Y12 inhibbitor, clopidogrel or ticagrelor for up to 12 months (COR I, LOE B)</td><td>PCI-treated patients:
1. Aspirin indefinitely (COR I, LOE A)
2. P2Y12 inhibitor clopidogrel or ticagrelor or prasugrel for at least 12 months (COR I, LOE B)</td></tr>
</table>

Association (ACC/AHA) UA/NSTEMI guidelines recommend that for patients with continuing or frequent ischemia in whom a β-blocker cannot be given, a nondihydropyridine CCB should be administered (COR I, LOE B) in the absence of clinically significant LV dysfunction or other contraindications. It is reasonable to give a nondihydropyridine CCB (COR IIa, LOE C) to patients with recurrent ischemia after β-blockers and nitrates have been fully used.

Other Agents

Trimetazidine is also a piperazine derivative that shifts myocardial metabolism from fatty acid oxidation to more oxygen-efficient glucose oxidation pathways, thus reducing ischemia without measurable changes in the heart rate-blood pressure product. Nicorandil is a drug that activates ATP-sensitive K^+ channels and dilates peripheral and coronary arterioles. This K^+ channel function is also postulated to induce cardiac protection via an ischemic preconditioning-like effect. Cardiac ischemia is associated with alterations in intracellular sodium and calcium concentrations, leading to arrhythmias, decreased contractility, and myocyte death. Ranolazine preserves intracellular ATP levels, improves myocardial function, and limits the extent of ischemic myocardial necrosis. Its role in patients with ACS is less well defined than its demonstrated usefulness in some patients with chronic stable angina.

Antithrombotic Therapy

Antiplatelet and anticoagulation treatment summary for NSTE-ACS according to 2014 AHA/ACC guidelines is as shown in table 4.

About 10% of patients who are admitted with NSTE-ACS require long-term treatment with oral anticoagulants for various reasons, such as atrial fibrillation, prior venous thromboembolism, and mechanical heart valves.[43] The combination of antiplatelet and anticoagulant treatment, either as dual or as triple therapy, increases the bleeding risk three- to fourfold as compared to warfarin monotherapy.[43] In patients with NSTE-ACS receiving DAPT who had been receiving prior oral anticoagulation, it is reasonable to transition to a parenteral anticoagulant at or shortly after presentation (i.e., once therapeutic anticoagulation has waned). If immediate angiography is required, radial access is the preferred choice because it may reduce the risk of access site bleeding. After the procedure, the duration of triple therapy should be minimized.

In one study[44] participants with atrial fibrillation undergoing PCI with placement of stents, who were administred either low-dose rivaroxaban plus a P2Y12 inhibitor for 12 months or very-low-dose rivaroxaban plus DAPT for 1, 6, or 12 months were associated with a lower rate of clinically significant bleeding than was standard therapy with a vitamin K antagonist plus DAPT for 1, 6, or 12 months. The three groups had similar efficacy rate.

Predictive value of the HAS-BLED (Hypertension, Abnormal renal/liver function, Stroke, Bleeding history or predisposition, Labile international normalized ratio, Elderly, Drugs or alcohol use) score for clinical outcomes has been investigated in patients with and without atrial fibrillation[45] (Flowchart 1).

The HAS-BLED scoring system is similar to the GRACE and CRUSADE systems but better than TIMI system to

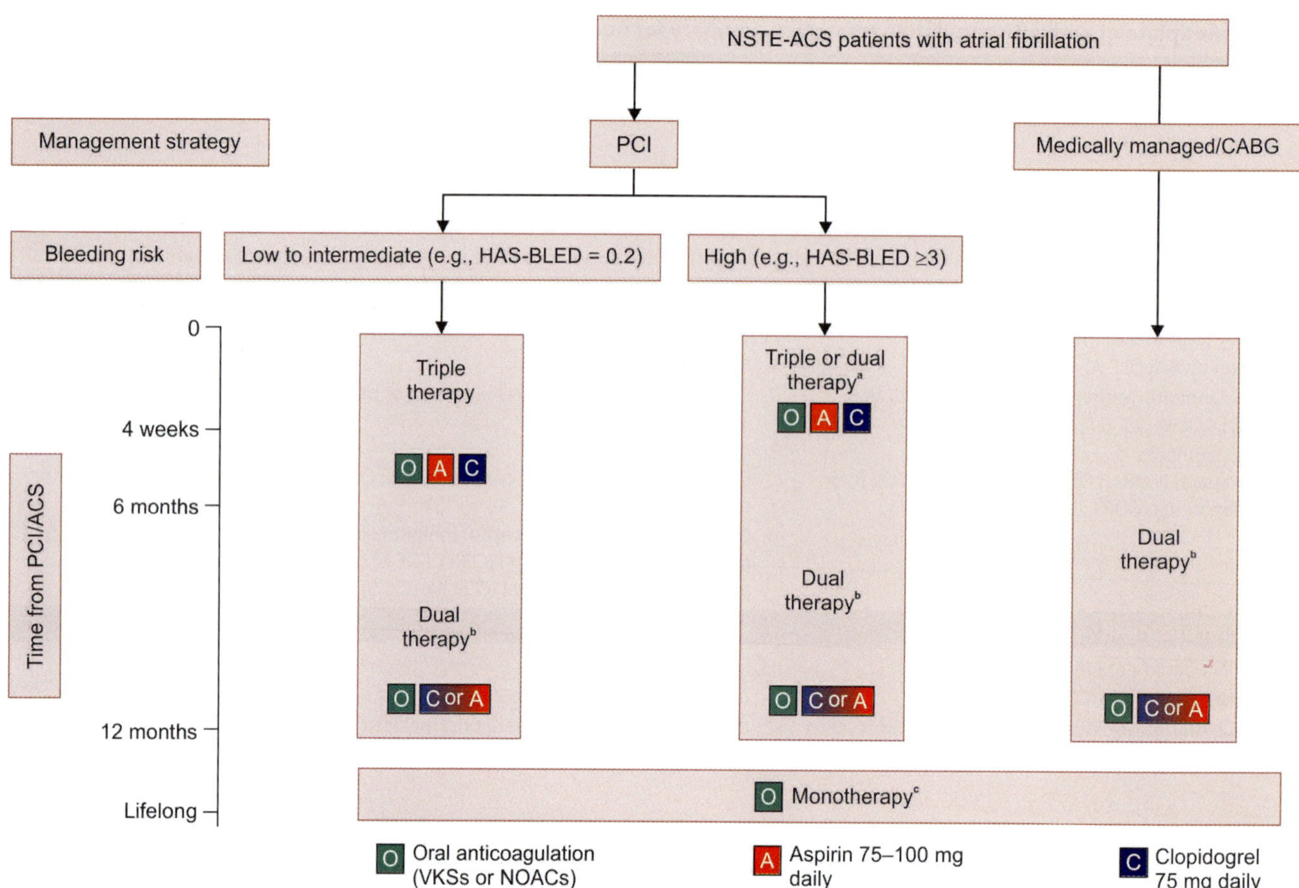

PCI, percutaneous coronary intervention; CABG, coronary artery bypass graft.

FLOWCHART 1: Antithrombotic strategies in patients with non-ST elevation acute coronary syndrome (NSTE-ACS) and nonvalvular atrial fibrillation (AF).

predict long-term survival outcomes in patients with NSTEMI without atrial fibrillation.[45] However, HAS-BLED score is easier to calculate than GRACE and CRUSADE scores.

Intervention: Invasive versus Conservative Management

Approach

An early invasive strategy, in the absence of contraindication, is recommended in patients with NSTE-ACS who have ST-segment changes and/or positive troponin assay on admission, or in whom these high-risk features develop over the subsequent 24 hours. Other high-risk indicators, such as recurrent ischemia or evidence of congestive heart failure, also indicate an early invasive strategy.[1,46] An early invasive strategy is also advised in patients with NSTE-ACS previously treated with CABG.[1] and in patients who have had NSTE-ACS within 6 months of a previous PCI and in whom restenosis may be the cause.[46] Indications for an initial conservative strategy include patients with life-threatening comorbid conditions or in whom the risks outweigh the potential benefits, and in low-risk patients without recurrent symptoms.[1,46]

Comparison: Invasive versus Conservative

In the meta-analysis performed by Milasinovic et al. (2015),[47] the early invasive patients received intervention between 0.5 hours and 24 hours from hospital admission and the delayed invasive patients received intervention between 20.5 hours and 86 hours from hospital admission. From the large study population used, they were able to conclude that an earlier invasive strategy was associated with lower rates of recurrent ischemia at 6 months (4.1% compared with 7.5%).

Angiographic success (TIMI epicardial grade 2 or 3 flow) can be achieved in a large majority (95%) of patients with NSTE-ACS who undergo PCI, even in those considered to be at high risk.[48] However, the development of intraprocedural complications, such as transient or sustained loss of a side branch, abrupt closure, distal embolization, or development of the no-reflow phenomenon, may entail a four- to fivefold increase in the risk for ischemic complications and death over the next 30 days.[48] Although use of drug-eluting stents (DESs) reduces the risk for restenosis, there is a risk for late stent thrombosis following DES implantation, especially when DAPT (i.e., ASA and P2Y12 inhibitor) is discontinued. This serious complication can be reduced in the long-term in

BOX 2 Risk criteria in patients with NSTE-ACS

Very-high-risk criteria
- Hemodynamic instability or cardiogenic shock
- Recurrent or ongoing chest discomfort refractory to optimal medical therapy
- Life-threatening arrhythmias or cardiac arrest
- Mechanical complications of MI
- Acute heart failure
- Recurrent dynamic ST-T wave changes, paricularly with intermittent ST-elevation

High-risk criteria
- Rise and fall in cardiac tropon in compatible with MI
- Dynamic ST-T wave changes without symptoms (silent)
- Elevated TIMI (>4) or GRACE (>140) risk score

Intermediate-risk criteria
- Diabetes mellitus
- Renal insufficiency (eGFR <60 mL/min/173 m^2)
- LVEF <40% or congestive heart failure
- Early post-MI angina
- Prior CABG
- TIMI (2–3) or GRACE (109–140) risk score

Low-risk criteria
- None of the characteristics mentioned above

CABG, coronary artery bypass graft; eGFR, estimated glomerular filtration rate; NSTE-ACS, non-ST elevation acute coronary syndrome; MI, myocardial infraction; PCI, percutaneous coronary intervention.

patients with DESs, by continuing DAPT beyond 12 months after stenting.[48]

Both North American and European guidelines recommend using a "heart team" approach to guide decisions regarding revascularization that includes input from interventional cardiologists and cardiothoracic surgeon in patients with LMA and complex CAD. Factors that favor CABG include multiple and complex coronary lesions, presence of DM, LV systolic dysfunction, and DAPT intolerance. Factors favoring PCI include high risk of operative mortality, prior thoracotomy, and advanced CKD.[1]

Table 2 and box 2 shows the management of NSTE-ACS[49] patients according to risk stratification.

Rehabilitation

Non-ST elevation-ACS is a heterogeneous syndrome, not a specific disease. Subgroups of patients who respond to specific therapies should be identified. Specifically, there is considerable variation in the responses to antiplatelet agents and anticoagulants, in terms of both efficacy and safety. Efforts should be elevated to identify predictors of responses to these agents.

The time of discharge is important to let the patient know the importance of continuance of the antiplatelet agents and to teach the patient regarding the modifiable risk factors and the impact they have on the disease process.

The management strategies often depend on risk assessment, available facilities and financial constraints. An analysis of data from Indian ACS registries[50] highlight the problems related to accessibility of health care, literacy, and economic status on management outcomes. NSTEMI patients are older, have more risk factors and present late. The utilization of evidence based medication is less.

Inadequate access to health care, difficulty in transportation and poor socioeconomic background are impediments to the care of patients in rural areas. In urban centers, out of pocket expenses remain challenging for patients.

REFERENCES

1. Amsterdam E, Wenger N, Brindis R, et al. 2014 AHA/ACC Guideline for the management of patients with non-ST-elevation acute coronary syndromes: Executive summary: A Report of the American College of Cardiology/American Heart Association Task Force on Practice Guidelines. Circulation. 2014;130(25): 2354-94.
2. Prabhakaran D, Jeemon P, Roy A. Cardiovascular diseases in India. Circulation. 2016;133(16):1605-20.
3. Braunwald E, Morrow D. Unstable Angina: Is It time for a requiem?. Circulation. 2013;127(24):2452-7.
4. Libby P. Mechanisms of acute coronary syndromes and their implications for therapy. New Eng J Med. 2013;368(21):2004-13.
5. Herren K. Emergency management of cardiac chest pain: a review. Emerg Med J. 2001;18(1):6-10.
6. Mistry N, Vesely M. Acute coronary syndromes. Cardiol Clin. 2012;30(4):617-27.
7. Fesmire F, Percy R, Bardoner J, et al. Usefulness of automated Serial 12-Lead ECG monitoring during the initial emergency department evaluation of patients with chest pain. Ann Emerg Med. 1998;31(1):3-11.
8. Thygesen K, Alpert J, Jaffe A, et al. Third universal definition of myocardial infarction. Circulation. 2012;126(16):2020-35.
9. Kraaijeveld A, de Jager S, de Jager W, et al. CC Chemokine Ligand-5 (CCL5/RANTES) and CC Chemokine Ligand-18 (CCL18/PARC) Are Specific markers of refractory unstable angina pectoris and are transiently raised during severe ischemic symptoms. Circulation. 2007;116(17):1931-41.
10. Beygui F, Silvain J, Pena A, et al. Usefulness of biomarker strategy to improve GRACE score's prediction performance in patients with non–ST-segment elevation acute coronary syndrome and low event rates. Am J Cardiol. 2010;106(5):650-8.
11. Viswanathan K, Kilcullen N, Morrell C, et al. Heart-type fatty acid-binding protein predicts long-term mortality and re-infarction in consecutive patients with suspected acute coronary syndrome who are troponin-negative. J Am Coll Cardiol. 2010;55(23):2590-8.
12. Koga S, Ikeda S, Yoshida T, et al. Elevated levels of systemic pentraxin 3 are associated with thin-cap fibroatheroma in coronary culprit lesions. JACC: Cardiovasc Interv. 2013;6(9):945-54.
13. O'Malley R, Bonaca M, Scirica B, et al. Prognostic performance of multiple biomarkers in patients with Non–ST-segment elevation acute coronary syndrome. J Am Col Cardiol. 2014;63(16):1644-53.
14. Thelin J, Borna C, Erlinge D, et al. The combination of high sensitivity troponin T and copeptin facilitates early rule-out of ACS: a prospective observational study. BMC Cardiovasc Disorders. 2013;13(1).
15. Eek C, Grenne B, Brunvand H, et al. Strain echocardiography predicts acute coronary occlusion in patients with non-ST-segment elevation acute coronary syndrome. Eur J Echocardio. 2010;11(6):501-8.
16. Hoffmann U, Truong Q, Schoenfeld D, et al. Coronary CT Angiography versus Standard Evaluation in Acute Chest Pain. New Eng J Mede. 2012;367(4): 299-308.
17. Litt H, Gatsonis C, Snyder B, et al. CT Angiography for Safe Discharge of Patients with possible acute coronary syndromes. New Eng J Med. 2012;366(15): 1393-403.

18. Goldstein J, Chinnaiyan K, Abidov A, et al. The CT-STAT (coronary computed tomographic angiography for systematic triage of acute chest pain patients to treatment) Trial. J Am Coll Cardiol. 2011;58(14):1414-22.
19. Hollander J, Than M, Mueller C. State-of-the-art evaluation of emergency department patients presenting with potential acute coronary syndromes. Circulation. 2016;134(7):547-64.
20. Raman S, Simonetti O, Winner M, et al. Cardiac magnetic resonance with edema imaging identifies myocardium at risk and predicts worse outcome in patients with non–ST-segment elevation acute coronary syndrome. J Am Coll Cardiol. 2010;55(22):2480-8.
21. Granger C. Predictors of hospital mortality in the global registry of acute coronary events. Arch Intern Med. 2003;163(19):2345.
22. Antman E, Cohen M, Bernink P, et al. The TIMI Risk score for unstable angina/ Non–ST elevation MI. JAMA. 2000;284(7):835.
23. Yan A, Jong P, Yan R, et al. Clinical trial–derived risk model may not generalize to real-world patients with acute coronary syndrome. Am Heart J. 2004;148(6):1020-7.
24. Samaha F, Kimmel S, Kizer J, et al. Usefulness of the TIMI risk score in predicting both short- and long-term outcomes in the Veterans Affairs Non–Q-Wave Myocardial Infarction Strategies In-Hospital (VANQWISH) Trial. Am Jo Cardiology. 2002;90(9):922-6.
25. Bradshaw P, Ko D, Newman A, et al. Validation of the Thrombolysis In Myocardial Infarction (TIMI) risk index for predicting early mortality in a population-based cohort of STEMI and non-STEMI patients. Can J Cardiology. 2007;23(1):51-6.
26. Bradshaw P. Validity of the GRACE (Global Registry of Acute Coronary Events) acute coronary syndrome prediction model for six month post-discharge death in an independent data set. Heart. 2006;92(7):905-9.
27. Singh M. Scores for Post-Myocardial Infarction Risk Stratification in the Community. Circulation. 2002;106(18):2309-14.
28. Yan A, Yan R, Tan M, et al. Risk scores for risk stratification in acute coronary syndromes: useful but simpler is not necessarily better. Eur Heart J. 2007;28(9): 1072-8.
29. Boersma E, Pieper K, Steyerberg E, et al. Predictors of outcome in patients with acute coronary syndromes without persistent ST-segment Elevation: Results From an International Trial of 9461 Patients. Circulation. 2000;101(22):2557-67.
30. Gale C, Manda S, Weston C, et al. Evaluation of risk scores for risk stratification of acute coronary syndromes in the Myocardial Infarction National Audit Project (MINAP) database. Heart. 2008;95(3):221-7.
31. Fox K, Dabbous O, Goldberg R, et al. Prediction of risk of death and myocardial infarction in the six months after presentation with acute coronary syndrome: prospective multinational observational study (GRACE). BMJ. 2006;333(7578):1091.
32. Tang E, Wong C, Herbison P. Global Registry of Acute Coronary Events (GRACE) hospital discharge risk score accurately predicts long-term mortality post acute coronary syndrome. American Heart Journal. 2007;153(1):29-35.
33. Kurz D, Bernstein A, Hunt K, et al. Simple point-of-care risk stratification in acute coronary syndromes: the AMIS model. Heart. 2008;95(8):662-8.
34. Piombo A, Gagliardi J, Guetta J, et al. A new scoring system to stratify risk in unstable angina. BMC Cardiovasc Disord. 2003;3(1).
35. Aragam K, Tamhane U, Kline-Rogers E, et al. Does simplicity compromise accuracy in ACs risk prediction? A Retrospective Analysis of the TIMI and GRACE Risk Scores. PLoS ONE. 2009;4(11):e7947.
36. de Araújo Gonçalves P, Ferreira J, Aguiar C, et al. TIMI, PURSUIT, and GRACE risk scores: sustained prognostic value and interaction with revascularization in NSTE-ACS. Eur Heart J. 2005;26(9):865-72.
37. Mehran R, Pocock S, Nikolsky E, et al. A risk score to predict bleeding in patients with acute coronary syndromes. J Am Coll Cardiol. 2010;55(23):2556-66.
38. Steg P, Huber K, Andreotti F, et al. Bleeding in acute coronary syndromes and percutaneous coronary interventions: position paper by the Working Group on Thrombosis of the European Society of Cardiology. Eur Heart J. 2011;32(15):1854-64.
39. Subherwal S, Bach R, Chen A, Gage B, Rao S, Newby L et al. Baseline Risk of Major Bleeding in Non-ST-Segment-Elevation Myocardial Infarction: The CRUSADE (Can Rapid risk stratification of Unstable angina patients Suppress ADverse outcomes with Early implementation of the ACC/AHA guidelines) Bleeding Score. Circulation. 2009;119(14):1873-82.
40. Abu-Assi E, Raposeiras-Roubin S, Lear P, Cabanas-Grandío P, Girondo M, Rodríguez-Cordero M et al. Comparing the predictive validity of three contemporary bleeding risk scores in acute coronary syndrome. European Heart Journal: Acute Cardiovascular Care. 2012;1(3):222-31.
41. Soukoulis V, Boden W, Smith S, O'Gara P. Nonantithrombotic Medical Options in Acute Coronary Syndromes: Old Agents and New Lines on the Horizon. Circulation Research. 2014;114(12):1944-58.
42. Mewton N, Croisille P, Gahide G, Rioufol G, Bonnefoy E, Sanchez I et al. Effect of Cyclosporine on Left Ventricle Remodeling after Reperfused Myocardial Infarction. Archives of Cardiovascular Diseases Supplements. 2010;2(1):19.
43. Hansen M, Sørensen R, Clausen M, et al. Risk of Bleeding With Single, Dual, or Triple Therapy With Warfarin, Aspirin, and Clopidogrel in Patients With Atrial Fibrillation. Archives of Inter Med. 2010;170(16).
44. Lip G, Windecker S, Huber K, et al. Management of antithrombotic therapy in atrial fibrillation patients presenting with acute coronary syndrome and/or undergoing percutaneous coronary or valve interventions: a joint consensus document of the European Society of Cardiology Working Group on Thrombosis, European Heart Rhythm Association (EHRA), European Association of Percutaneous Cardiovascular Interventions (EAPCI) and European Association of Acute Cardiac Care (ACCA) endorsed by the Heart Rhythm Society (HRS) and Asia-Pacific Heart Rhythm Society (APHRS). Eur Heart J. 2014;35(45):3155-79.
45. Hsieh M, Lee C, Chen C, et al. Predictive performance of HAS-BLED risk score for long-term survival in patients with non-ST elevated myocardial infarction without atrial fibrillation. J Cardiol. 2017;69(1):136-43.
46. Gibson C, Mehran R, Bode C, et al. Prevention of Bleeding in Patients with Atrial Fibrillation Undergoing PCI. New Eng J Med. 2016;375(25):2423-34.
47. Milasinovic D, Milosevic A, Marinkovic J, et al. Timing of invasive strategy in NSTE-ACS patients and effect on clinical outcomes: A systematic review and meta-analysis of randomized controlled trials. Atherosclerosis. 2015;241(1): 48-54.
48. Pride Y, Mohanavelu S, Zorkun C, et al. Association between angiographic complications and clinical outcomes among patients with acute coronary syndrome undergoing percutaneous coronary intervention. JACC: Cardiovasc Interv. 2012;5(9):927-35.
49. Gray H, Henderson R, de Belder M, et al. Early management of unstable angina and non-ST-segment elevation myocardial infarction: summary of NICE guidance. Heart. 2010;96(20):1662-8.
50. Negi P, Merwaha R, Panday D, et al. Multicenter HP ACS Registry. Ind Heart J. 2016;68(2):118-27.

hs-cTroponin in Acute Coronary Syndrome: Current Status

Amal K Banerjee

INTRODUCTION

Chest pain is one of the most common reasons for presentation to hospitals worldwide. Despite the majority of patients not having acute coronary syndrome (ACS), hospital admission for observation and serial cardiac troponin (cTn) testing is required in many patients to identify those with and without myocardial injury.

The field of ACS is rapidly changing. Besides new drugs, the evolution is mainly driven by the introduction of novel biomarkers in an effort to respond to the partly unmet need for better diagnosis, prognostication, and management of patients. Novel biomarkers may improve diagnostic accuracy, identify subgroups of patients who may benefit from a specific therapeutic modality in the acute phase, and reveal pathophysiological insights that need to be addressed by long-term medical treatment. In this context, the new-generation cTn assays provide considerably more sensitive and timely diagnosis of ACS.[1] The highly sensitive new-generation cTn assays modify the classification of patients with non–ST-segment elevation acute coronary syndrome (NSTE-ACS) by increasing the percentage of cases with NSTE myocardial infarction (MI) and limiting that of unstable angina (UA) (Fig. 1).[2] As a result, this reclassification[2] creates a need for novel prognostication models that would identify high-, moderate-, and low-risk patients and thus guide our treatment decisions. In particular, the long-term benefit of an invasive approach in the subgroup of patients who are reclassified from UA to NSTE myocardial infarction has not yet been proven by large randomized trials. Whether this need is addressed by novel biomarkers remains to be seen.

Despite uneasiness among clinicians about the increasing sensitivity of assays for cTn, it is rare that clinical algorithms for laboratory-based tests have as much data to guide decision making as do high-sensitivity assays for

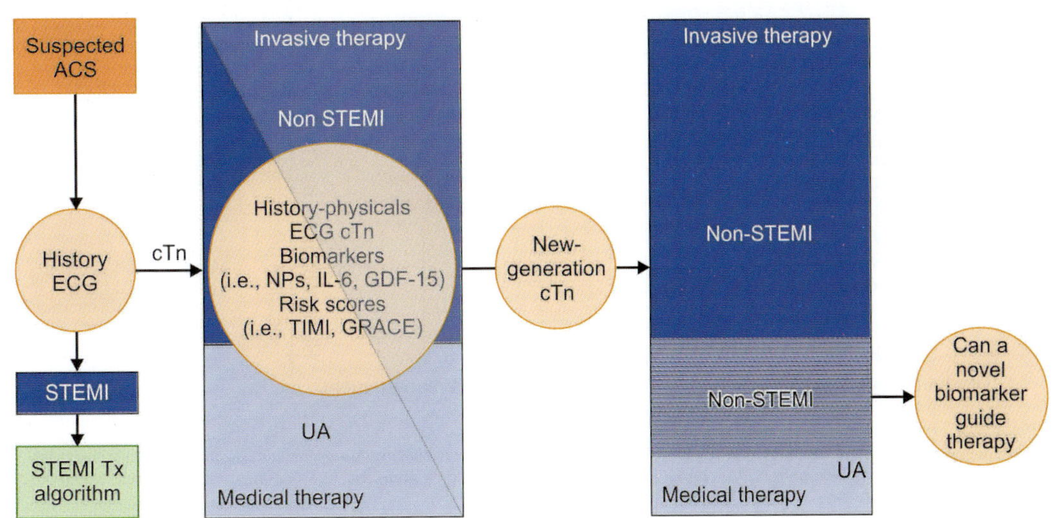

ACS, acute coronary syndrome(s); cTn, cardiac troponin; ECG, electrocardiogram; NP, natriuretic peptides; STEMI, ST-segment elevation myocardial infarction; Tx, therapy; UA, unstable angina.

FIG. 1: The role of highly sensitive new-generation cTn in the diagnosis and risk stratification of patients with ACS.

cTn for diagnosis (rule-in) or exclusion (rule-out) of MI. Rather, the proliferation of research evaluating variations in such algorithms in the emergency department (ED) has the potential to overwhelm clinicians with options. Of the emerging applications for hsTn, the rapid rule-out of MI in the ED is the application most likely to be embraced by clinicians.[3] This application most directly leverages the superior analytic and clinical sensitivity of hsTn assays as an advantage by translation into a robust negative predictive value (NPV) for MI.

CLINICAL PERSPECTIVE

Recently, high-sensitivity cardiac troponin (hs-cTn) assays have been implemented into routine clinical care in Europe, Canada, Australia, New Zealand, and other countries. These assays overcome some of the limitations of conventional cTn assays, particularly the sensitivity deficit at presentation.[4,5] hs-cTn assays provide higher early diagnostic accuracy for acute myocardial infarction (AMI) when compared with conventional cTn assays.[6,7] However, their clinical introduction has also been associated with challenges, particularly the interpretation of mild elevations.

CLINICAL PRACTICE GUIDELINES

The most recent European Society of Cardiology (ESC) guidelines for the management of ACSs in patients presenting without persistent ST-segment elevation[8] proposed a new algorithm using high-sensitivity troponin: a 1-hour rule-in and rule-out algorithm.

Rule-in and Rule-out Algorithms in ESC 2015 Guidelines on Management of ACS[8]

Due to the higher sensitivity and diagnostic accuracy for the detection of acute MI at presentation, the time interval to the second cTn assessment can be shortened with the use of high-sensitivity assays. This may reduce substantially the delay to diagnosis, translating into shorter stays in the emergency department and lower costs.[8]

It is recommended to use the 0-hour/3-hour algorithm (Flowchart 1).[8] As an alternative, 0-hour/1-hour assessments are recommended when hs-cTn assays with a validated algorithm are available (Flowchart 2).[8] The 0-hour/1-hour algorithms rely on two concepts: first, hs-cTn is a continuous variable and the probability of MI increases with increasing hs-cTn values;[9] second, early absolute changes of the levels within 1-hour can be used as surrogates for absolute changes over 3-hour or 6-hour and provide incremental diagnostic value to the cTn assessment at presentation. The cut-off levels within the 0-hour/1-hour algorithm are assay specific.[8-10]

Characteristics of 0-hour/3-hour and 0-hour/1-hour Algorithms[8]

"The negative predictive value for MI in patients assigned to rule-out exceeded 98% in several large validation cohorts.[9-13] Used in conjunction with clinical and ECG findings, the 0-hour/1-hour algorithm may allow the identification of candidates for early discharge and outpatient management. The positive predictive value for MI in those patients meeting the rule-in criteria was 75–80%.[1,9,11,13] Most of the rule-in

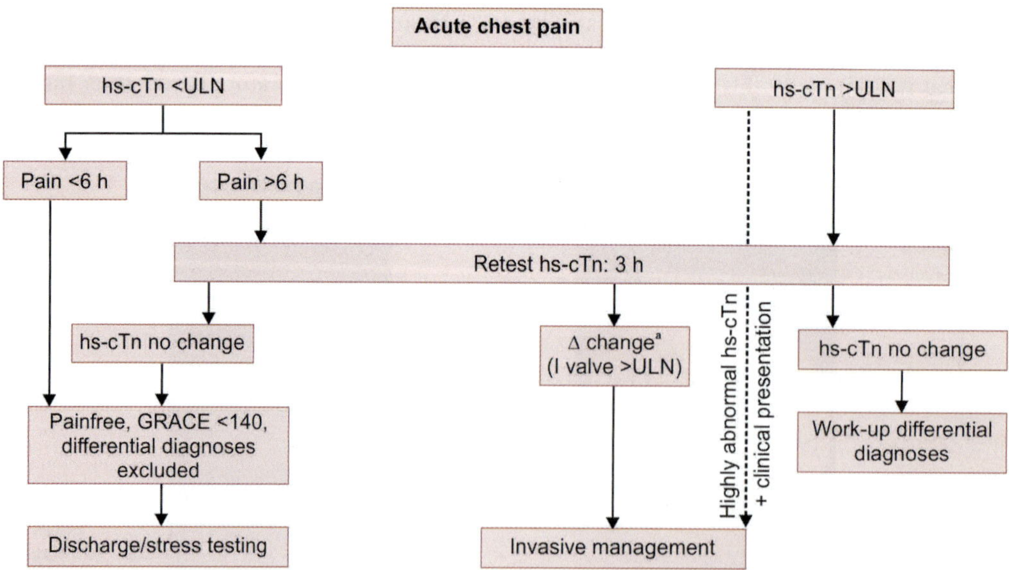

GRACE, Global Registry of Acute Coronary Events score; hs-cTn, high-sensitivity cardiac troponin; ULN, upper limit of normal, or 99th percentile of healthy controls; [a]Δ, change, dependent on assay. Highly abnormal hsTn defines values beyond 5-fold the upper limit of normal.

FLOWCHART 1: 0-hour/3-hour rule-out algorithm of non-ST-elevation acute coronary syndromes using high-sensitivity cardiac troponin assays.

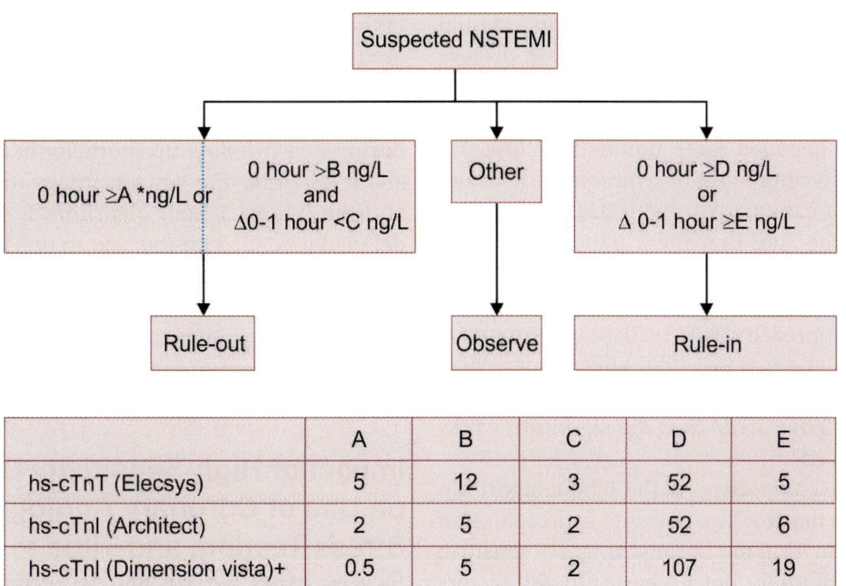

	A	B	C	D	E
hs-cTnT (Elecsys)	5	12	3	52	5
hs-cTnI (Architect)	2	5	2	52	6
hs-cTnI (Dimension vista)+	0.5	5	2	107	19

*Only applicable if chest pain onset >3 h.

hs-cTnT, high-sensitivity cardiac troponin T; hs-cTnI, high-sensitivity cardiac troponin I; NSTEMI, non-ST-elevation myocardial infarction.

FLOWCHART 2: 0-hour/1-hour rule-in and rule-out algorithms using high-sensitivity cardiac troponins (hs-cTn) assays in patients presenting with suspected non-ST-elevation myocardial infarction (NSTEMI) to the emergency department. 0-hour and 1-hour refer to the time from first blood test. NSTEMI can be ruled-out already at presentation, if the hs-cTn concentration is very low. NSTEMI can also be ruled out by the combination of low baseline levels and the lack of a relevant increase within 1-hour. Patients have a high likelihood for NSTEMI if the hs-cTn concentration at presentation is at least moderately elevated or hs-cTn concentrations show a clear rise within the 1st hour. Cut-off levels are assay-specific. Cut-off levels for other hs-cTn assays are in development.

patients with diagnoses other than MI did have conditions that usually require inpatient coronary angiography for accurate diagnosis, including takotsubo cardiomyopathy and myocarditis.[9,13,14] Patients who do not qualify for rule-out or rule-in represent a heterogeneous group that may require further investigations, if no alternative explanation for the cTn elevation is identified. A large proportion of these patients may require a further hs-cTn assessment (e.g., at 3-hour). For rapid rule-out, alternative approaches to the 0-hour/1-hour or 0-hour/3-hour algorithms have been adequately validated and may be considered. A 2-h rule-out protocol combining the Thrombolysis in Myocardial Infarction (TIMI) risk score with ECG and hs-cTn at presentation allowed a safe rule-out in up to 40% of patients."[15]

"When using any algorithm, three main caveats should be considered—(1) algorithms should only be used in conjunction with all available clinical information, including detailed assessment of chest pain characteristics and ECG; (2) in patients presenting very early (e.g., within 1 hour from chest pain onset), the second cTn level should be obtained at 3-hour, due to the time dependency of troponin release; (3) as late increases in cTn have been described in approximately 1% of patients, serial cTn testing should be pursued if the clinical suspicion remains high or whenever the patient develops recurrent chest pain.[16] High-sensitivity cTn assays also maintain high diagnostic accuracy in patients with renal dysfunction. To ensure the best possible clinical use, assay-specific optimal cut-off levels, which are higher in patients with renal dysfunction, should be used."[17]

RISK ASSESSMENT AND OUTCOMES

Beyond diagnostic utility, cTn levels add prognostic information in terms of short- and long-term mortality to clinical and ECG variables. While hs-cTn T and I seem to have comparable diagnostic accuracy, high-sensitivity cardiac troponin T (hs-cTnT) has greater prognostic accuracy.[18] The higher the high-sensitivity troponin levels at presentation, the greater the risk of death.[9]

Sometimes Earlier may not be Better

The ESC guidelines 15 algorithm opened a wide debate regarding its efficacy and safety. Allan S Jaffe et al. from the Mayo Clinic in Rochester, Minnesota, USA challenge this notion.[19] They argue that, although these algorithms may represent an advance in the early diagnosis of chest pain patients, the ESC guidelines may have overlooked some gaps in the evidence for these approaches that could inadvertently disadvantage patients.

The hs-cTn 0-hour/1-hour algorithm, they said, proposed in the ESC guidelines on the management of NSTEMI might allow a rapid rule in and rule out of a large proportion of patients with suspected NSTEMI. A critical question is: Should the 1-hour algorithm for rule-in and rule-out of AMI be used universally? This approach might substantially speed up the triage of patients with suspected NSTEMI. Yet, some concern has recently been raised on this universal application regardless of symptom duration, overall clinical risk, and sex.

Guideline mandated diagnostic assessments should be applicable to all possible patients within a given disease state. To accomplish this goal, the 1-hour algorithm would have required a more extensive database than the one used.[8] The studies relied on included large numbers of low risk patients presenting early after onset of symptoms but lacked substantial numbers of early patients with AMI. This group is critical to study to be sure that these patients manifest elevations even early after AMI so they can be distinguished from those without AMI. The largest number of AMIs in the studies evaluating the approach was 443 with only 106 patients presenting in less than or equal to 3-hour after onset.[20] How many presented in less than 2-hour is unclear. "Thus, we have insufficient knowledge about how the algorithm works in patients early after AMI".[19]

It is likely that some components of the 1-hour algorithm will work well. It may be that low hs-cTn values at presentation is a good way to exclude AMI, not because they are sensitive at detecting myocardial injury but because the risk factors associated with ischemic heart disease cause increases in hs-cTn within the normal range so baseline values are not apt to be low. Thus, low values define a low-risk group.[20] "However, we are less confident about some of the other recommendations such as utilizing a solitary fixed cut off for diagnosis of AMI and the application of this approach too all patients with possible AMI including those with renal failure, acute illness, the elderly and those who present early. Until these issues are clarified clinicians should take an extra caution in the interest of safe patient care".[19]

Marco Roffi from the Hôpitaux Universitaire in Geneva, Switzerland, contradicting Jaffe et al. mention that the 2015 ESC guidelines propose two hs-cTn-based diagnostic algorithms for patients presenting with acute chest pain and/or suspected AMI to the emergency department. By including the new hs-cTn 0-hour/1-hour algorithm, the novel ESC guidelines have tried to balance diagnostic accuracy and speed carefully and guide physicians toward the best possible clinical use of high-sensitivity cardiac troponins.

Two Large Multicenter Studies Seem to Confirm the Effectiveness and Safety of the Algorithm Proposed by ESC

In one study in 2,222 patients, Pickering et al.[21] found that the 0-hour/1-hour algorithm using hs-c TnT allowed to safely rule out about 50% of patients who had a prevalence of MI less than 0.5. Similar results were obtained using hs-cTnI.[21] This study has also shown that the sensitivity of the 0-hour/1-hour high-sensitivity troponin T and high-sensitivity troponin I algorithms was not as high as reported in the derivation studies referenced in the ESC guidelines. The study has further suggested, that the ESC guidelines 0-hour/1-hour algorithm should only be implemented with safeguards, including robust clinical risk assessment, the assessment will likely reduce the proportions of patients who will be eligible for this rapid rule-out algorithm and the use of the rule-in algorithm to rapidly transit emergency patients to the cardiology services will depend on local acceptance of moderate positive predictive values.

In the other study in 2,828 patients, Boeddinghaus et al.[22] found very similar results using hs-c TnI. Furthermore during 2-year follow-up mortality in ruled out patients was about 2% only. The key advantage of the 1-hour algorithm and the 0-hour/1-hour algorithm is that they also provide detailed guidance for the rule-in of AMI. On the other hand, the need for two measurements is a logistic disadvantage in comparison with the single-measurement strategies. Because of its stringent and robust methodology, this study also provided accurate estimates for the real sensitivity and NPV of the respective strategies.[22]

Impact of High-Sensitivity Cardiac Troponin on Use of Coronary Angiography, Cardiac Stress Testing, and Time to Discharge in Suspected Acute Myocardial Infarction

In a very important clinical study, [23] Raphael Twerenbold et al. have shown that hs-cTn assays provide higher diagnostic accuracy for AMI as compared with conventional assays. They have also concern that use of hs-cTnT may also result in an increased use of unnecessary coronary angiographies due to their ability to detect cardiomyocyte injury in conditions other than AMI. The authors therefore evaluated the impact of the clinical introduction of hs-cTnT assays on the use of coronary angiography, stress testing, and time to discharge in 2,544 patients presenting to the emergency department with symptoms suggestive of an ACS. The patients were derived from a multicenter study either before (i.e., in 1,455 patients) or after (i.e., in 1,089 patients) the introduction of hs-cTnT assays. AMI was the clinical discharge diagnosis in 14% before and in 10% after the introduction of hs-cTnT assays; while at 9%, UA was less often the clinical discharge diagnosis than with conventional assays, where it was 14%. The rate of coronary angiography was similar before and after the introduction of hs-cTnT assays, as was the percentage of coronary angiographies showing no stenosis. In contrast, the use of stress testing was substantially reduced from 29 to 19% with high-sensitivity assays. In outpatients, the median time to discharge decreased by 79 minutes with high-sensitivity assays, and total costs decreased by 20%.

The authors conclude that the introduction of hs-cTn assays does not lead to an increased or inappropriate use of coronary angiography, but is associated with an improved rule-out process and thereby reduces the need for stress testing and time to discharge.[23]

CONCLUSION

Though conventional troponin (cTn) methods are of substantial importance and have changed the landscape of modern cardiology, the relatively high imprecision of many cTn assays (especially at very low analyte concentrations) leaves them unable to resolve small differences in biomarker values. In turn, this results in lower sensitivity for detecting small amounts of myocardial necrosis, such as that seen in patients at first contact, or resolve small changes in closely spaced serial samples. In this regard, several hours must often pass before a definitive rise in cTn might occur; this troponin blind interval is a major concern with cTn methods, slowing down triage, and creating apprehension and clinical delays.

Developed in response to calls for increased assay precision at low troponin concentration,[24] hsTn assays appear to overcome many limitations of cTn. In several clinical trials such as the Advantageous Predictors of Acute Coronary Syndrome Evaluation (APACE) study,[1] it was found hsTn testing allowed for more rapid identification or exclusion of AMI when compared with cTn. Based on these and other data,[25] hsTn testing is now accepted and in use in several countries, with strategies incorporating rapid hsTn testing protocols (based on a 0–3-hour approach or a 0–1-hour approach), even incorporated in European clinical practice guidelines.[8] Finally, it is worth mentioning that this is a rapidly moving field and further research is needed to understand the clinical utility and cost-effectiveness of this approach to risk stratification.

REFERENCES

1. Reichlin T, Hochholzer W, Bassetti S, et al. Early diagnosis of myocardial infarction with sensitive cardiac troponin assays. N Engl J Med. 2009;361:858-67.
2. Filippatos G, Farmakis D, Parissis J. Novel biomarkers in acute coronary syndromes: new molecules, new concepts, but what about new treatment strategies? J Am Coll Cardiol.1914;63:1654-6
3. Morrow DA. Evidence-based algorithms using high-sensitivity cardiac troponin in the emergency department. JAMA Cardiol. 2016;1:379-81.
4. Apple FS, Smith SW, Pearce LA, et al. Use of the centaur TnI-ultra assay for detection of myocardial infarction and adverse events in patients presenting with symptoms suggestive of acute coronary syndrome. Clin Chem. 2008;54:723-8.
5. Giannitsis E, Kurz K, Hallermayer K, et al. Analytical validation of a high-sensitivity cardiac troponin T assay. Clin Chem. 2010;56:254-61.
6. Keller T, Zeller T, Peetz D, et al. Sensitive troponin I assay in early diagnosis of acute myocardial infarction. N Engl J Med. 2009;361:868-77.
7. Twerenbold R, Reiter M, Reichlin T, et al. Early diagnosis of acute myocardial infarction in patients with pre-existing coronary artery disease using more sensitive cardiac troponin assays. Eur Heart J. 2012;33:988-97.
8. Roffi M, Patrono C, Collet JP, et al. Management of Acute Coronary Syndromes in Patients Presenting without Persistent ST-Segment Elevation of the European Society of Cardiology. 2015 ESC Guidelines for the management of acute coronary syndromes in patients presenting without persistent ST-segment elevation: Task Force for the Management of Acute Coronary Syndromes in Patients Presenting without Persistent ST-Segment Elevation of the European Society of Cardiology (ESC). Eur Heart J. 2016;37:267-315.
9. Reichlin T, Schindler C, Drexler B, et al. One-hour rule-out and rule-in of acute myocardial infarction using high-sensitivity cardiac troponin T. Arch Intern Med. 2012;172:1211-8.
10. Rubini Gimenez M, Hoeller R, Reichlin T, et al. Rapid rule out of acute myocardial infarction using undetectable levels of high-sensitivity cardiac troponin. Int J Cardiol. 2013;168:3896-901.
11. Giannitsis E, Becker M, Kurz K, et al. High-sensitivity cardiac troponin T for early prediction of evolving non-ST-segment elevation myocardial infarction in patients with suspected acute coronary syndrome and negative troponin results on admission. Clin Chem. 2010;56:642-50.
12. Body R, Carley S, McDowell G, et al. Rapid exclusion of acute myocardial infarction in patients with undetectable troponin using a high-sensitivity assay. J Am Coll Cardiol. 2011;58:1332-9.
13. Rubini Gimenez M, Twerenbold R, Jaeger C, et al. One-hour rule-in and rule-out of acute myocardial infarction using high-sensitivity cardiac troponin I. Am J Med. 2015;128:861-870.e4.
14. Zhelev Z, Hyde C, Youngman E, et al. Diagnostic accuracy of single baseline measurement of Elecsys troponin T high-sensitive assay for diagnosis of acute myocardial infarction in emergency department: systematic review and meta-analysis. BMJ. 2015;350:h15.
15. Cullen L, Mueller C, Parsonage WA, et al. Validation of high-sensitivity troponin I in a 2-hour diagnostic strategy to assess 30-day outcomes in emergency department patients with possible acute coronary syndrome. J Am Coll Cardiol. 2013;62:1242-9.
16. Reichlin T, Twerenbold R, Wildi K, et al. Prospective validation of a 1-hour algorithm to rule-out and rule-in acute myocardial infarction using a high sensitivity cardiac troponin T assay. CMAJ. 2015;187:E243-52.
17. Twerenbold R, Wildi K, Jaeger C, et al. Optimal cutoff levels of more sensitive cardiac troponin assays for the early diagnosis of myocardial infarction in patients with renal dysfunction. Circulation. 2015;131:2041-50.
18. Rubini Gimenez M, Twerenbold R, Reichlin T, et al. Direct comparison of high-sensitivity-cardiac troponin I vs. T for the early diagnosis of acute myocardial infarction. Eur Heart J 2014;35:2303-11.
19. Crea F, Jaffe AS, Collinson PO, et al. Should the 1h algorithm for rule in and rule out of acute myocardial infarction be used universally? Eur Heart J. 2016;37:3316-23.
20. Hoeller R, Rubini Gimenez M, Reichlin T, et al. Normal presenting levels of high-sensitivity troponin and myocardial infarction. Heart. 2013;99: 1567 72.
21. Pickering JW, Greenslade JH, Cullen L, et al. Assessment of the European Society of Cardiology 0-hour/1-hour algorithm to rule-out and rule-in acute myocardial infarction. Circulation. 2016;134:1532-41.
22. Boeddinghaus J, Nestelberger T, Twerenbold R, et al. Direct comparison of 4 very early rule-out strategies for acute myocardial infarction using high-sensitivity cardiac troponin I. Circulation. 2017;135:1597-611.
23. Twerenbold R, Jaeger C, Rubini Gimenez M, et al. Impact of high sensitivity cardiac troponin on use of coronary angiography, cardiac stress testing, and time to discharge in suspected acute myocardial infarction. Eur Heart J. 2016;37:3324-32.
24. Thygesen K, Alpert JS, Jaffe AS, et al. Writing Group on the Joint ESC/ACCF/AHA/WHF Task Force for the Universal Definition of Myocardial Infarction. Third universal definition of myocardial infarction. Eur Heart J. 2012;33: 2551-67.
25. Mueller C, Giannitsis E, Christ M, et al. TRAPID-AMI Investigators. Multicenter evaluation of a 0-hour/1-hour algorithm in the diagnosis of myocardial infarction with high-sensitivity cardiac troponin T. Ann Emerg Med. 2016;68:76-87.

CHAPTER 40

Managing Acute Coronary Syndrome in Renal Dysfunction

Parayoru K Asokan, Kailash K Goyal

INTRODUCTION

Presence of renal dysfunction in patients with acute coronary syndrome (ACS) is common and is associated with both short- and long-term poor prognosis.[1,2] The National Cardiovascular Data Registry Acute Coronary Treatment and Intervention Outcomes Network (NCDR-ACTION) registry showed that 42.9% of patients with non-ST-elevation myocardial infarction (NSTEMI) and 30.5% of patients with STEMI have chronic kidney disease (CKD), and defined as a glomerular filtration rate (GFR) less than 60 mL/min/1.73 m^2.[3] Despite a high prevalence, patients with CKD are often excluded from ACS clinical trials,[4,5] which results in lack of data and insufficient treatment for this high-risk population. Further, the fear of complications such as bleeding and contrast-induced nephropathy (CIN) deters an interventional cardiologist from using invasive diagnostic and revascularization procedures in these patients contributing to poor outcomes. In this review, we aim to highlight the unique features and briefly summarize the available evidence associated with managing ACS in patients with renal dysfunction.

PATHOPHYSIOLOGY

Several studies have shown a higher burden of multivessel disease, longer stenoses, more severe calcification, and chronic occluded lesions compared with the general population.[6-8] Moreover, atherosclerotic plaque composition assessed with intravascular ultrasound (IVUS) demonstrated greater necrotic core and dense calcium with less fibrous tissue in CKD, suggesting that renal dysfunction not only results in greater plaque burden, but also alters coronary atherosclerotic plaque composition to a less stable phenotype.[9] This accelerated disease may be due to the presence of risk factors such as chronic inflammation, chronic oxidative stress, changes in nitric oxide availability, chronic phosphate retention, secondary hyperparathyroidism, and elevated levels of fibroblast growth factor 23.[10-12] Patients with CKD have also been shown to have an accelerated infarct expansion in association with enhanced inflammation and oxidative stress, as compared with non-CKD patients.

DIAGNOSIS OF ACUTE CORONARY SYNDROME IN PATIENTS WITH RENAL DYSFUNCTION

The clinical presentation of ACS in patients with CKD is markedly different from that of patients without CKD. Data from the SWEDEHEART Registry (Swedish Web System for Enhancement and Development of Evidence-based Care in Heart Disease Evaluated According to Recommended Therapies) showed that the incidence of chest pain and typical electrocardiogram (ECG) findings decrease with worsening renal function and presentation with heart failure increases.[13] The diagnostic value of baseline ECG is often limited by nonspecific changes due to left ventricular hypertrophy and electrolyte disturbances. To complicate things further, troponin levels may remain chronically elevated and are less specific for the diagnosis of ACS in patients with renal dysfunction. However, increase in troponin levels 2–3 times the upper limit of normal with a rise and fall pattern likely indicates myocardial infarction.

MANAGEMENT

Anticoagulant Therapy

Heparin is the standard management in patients with ACS and the two preparations available are unfractionated heparin (UFH) and low-molecular weight heparin (LMWH). Primary route of UFH elimination is via the reticuloendothelial system (RES) and hence a dose modification is not required in patients with renal dysfunction. Enoxaparin (most commonly used LMWH), on the other hand, is cleared primarily by renal mechanism. A substudy of the EXTRACT (Enoxaparin and Thrombolysis Reperfusion for Acute Myocardial Infarction Treatment)–TIMI 25 trial showed that with every 30 mL/minute decrease in creatinine clearance (CrCl), the risk of major and minor bleeding increased by 50%[14] suggesting that dosage adjustment is needed in these patients to minimize the bleeding risk. The current US Food and Drug Administration-approved dose for enoxaparin in ACS patients with CrCl less than 30 mL/minute/1.73 m^2 is 1 mg/kg subcutaneously every 24 hours. Table 1 shows the dose modification needed for various drugs used in ACS for patients with renal dysfunction.

Fondaparinux is an indirect factor Xa inhibitor and recommended as the preferred anticoagulant in UA/NSTEMI patients being managed with a conservative strategy who have an increased risk of bleeding. In a subanalysis of OASIS-5 (Fifth Organization to Assess Strategies in Acute Coronary Syndrome) trial,[15] fondaparinux was associated with low rates of bleeding compared to enoxaparin across all quartiles of renal dysfunction. Hence, it may be preferred over enoxaparin in patients with CrCl between 30 mL/minute and 59 mL/minute/1.73 m^2 but should be avoided, if CrCl less than 30 mL/minute/1.73 m^2, as it is excreted unchanged through renal mechanism.

Antiplatelets

Aspirin

McCullough et al.[16] showed that aspirin reduced in-hospital mortality by 64.3–80% across all quartiles of CrCl in patients with CKD and ACS. In a study by Yan et al.[17] aspirin was associated with improved 1-year survival to a similar extent among those with normal and impaired renal function. Similarly, in a meta-analysis of 287 randomized trials,[18] antiplatelet therapy produced a 41% proportional reduction in serious vascular events and no significant increase in extracranial bleeds in patients undergoing hemodialysis. Thus, the available data suggest that aspirin therapy is safe as well as effective in ACS patients with renal dysfunction and should be used to reduce the risk of death and vascular events.

Dual Antiplatelet Therapy

Dual antiplatelet therapy (DAPT) with aspirin and an additional agent (clopidogrel, ticagrelor, or prasugrel) are used routinely in patients with ACS. Observed rates

TABLE 1: Dose modification of various drugs in patients with acute coronary syndrome and renal dysfunction

Drug	Route of elimination	Effect of renal dysfunction on dose	Remarks
Unfractionated heparin	RES	None	Preferred over LMWH in patients with renal dysfunction
LMWH	Renal (40%)	Dose should be reduced by half in patients with CrCl <30 mL/min/1.73 m^2	Increased risk of bleeding in patients with CKD
Fondaparinux	Renal	Avoid if CrCl <30 mL/min/1.73 m^2	May be preferred over enoxaparin in patients with GFR between 30 and 59 mL/min/1.73 m^2
Aspirin	Renal	None	Should be used in patients with CKD presenting with ACS
Clopidogrel	Renal (50%), feces (50%)	None	Should be considered in CKD patients presenting with ACS
Prasugrel	Renal (60–70%)	None	Should be considered in CKD patients not requiring dialysis
Ticagrelor	Biliary	None	Should be considered in CKD patients not requiring dialysis
Abciximab	RES	None	Increased risk of bleeding in patients with CKD
Eptifibatide	Renal (50%)	Dose should be reduced by half in patients with CrCl <30 mL/min/1.73 m^2	Increased risk of bleeding in patients with CKD
Tirofiban	Renal (40–70%)	Dose should be reduced by half in patients with CrCl < 30 mL/min/1.73 m^2. Contraindicated in patients on dialysis	Increased risk of bleeding in patients with CKD
Statins	Hepatic	None	Should be considered in CKD patients presenting with ACS
Beta-blockers:			Should be used in CKD patients presenting with ACS
• Propranolol	Hepatic	None	
• Metoprolol	Hepatic	None	
• Carvedilol	Hepatic	None	
• Atenolol	Renal	Should be modified according to creatinine clearance	

ACS, acute coronary syndrome; CKD, chronic kidney disease; CrCl, creatinine clearance; LMWH, low-molecular weight heparin; RE,: reticuloendothelial system; GFR, glomerular filtration rate.

of bleeding have been higher with clopidogrel than with placebo in CKD patients, but several studies such as CURE,[19] CREDO,[20] or CLARITY-TIMI 28[21] showed that there was no significant interaction based on renal function and no significant increase in risk with the use of clopidogrel in ACS patients with CKD. Similarly, the efficacy associated with prasugrel compared with clopidogrel and the efficacy and safety associated with ticagrelor compared with clopidogrel were evident in patients with and without CKD, and the data suggest these agents should be considered in CKD patients who are not considered to be at high risk of bleeding.

Glycoprotein IIb/IIIa Inhibitors

Abciximab is cleared via the RES, and there is no current recommendation for dose adjustment for patients with CKD. Eptifibatide and tirofiban are dependent on renal clearance for elimination and hence a dose adjustment is required. Frilling et al.[22] compared the efficacy of abciximab in normal and CKD patients. Patients in either group had similar clinical outcomes. The CKD patients had more episodes of major bleeding but similar episodes of minor bleeding and thrombocytopenia. Several other studies using glycoprotein (GP) IIb/IIIa receptor antagonists in CKD patients with ACS showed a reduction in ischemic events and a variable increase in the risk of bleeding events. So, the currently available data suggest that these agents can be used cautiously with proper dose modification.

Statins

Statins have proved to be effective in preventing cardiovascular events in the general population, however, randomized trials of statin therapy in patients with CKD yielded mixed results. Studies like AURORA[23] and ALERT,[24] which mostly included dialysis-dependent patients showed no benefit of statin therapy. However, the Study of Heart and Renal Protection trial (SHARP) randomized patients with CKD (both on dialysis and not on dialysis) to 20 mg simvastatin plus 10 mg ezetimibe or placebo and showed a benefit of simvastatin plus ezetimibe therapy on the risk of the primary composite endpoint of first major atherosclerotic event.[25] Similarly, a meta-analysis of randomized trials showed that statin use for primary prevention consistently lowers the risk of death and major cardiovascular events by 20% in patients with CKD and not on dialysis.[26] So, data show a consistent benefit with regard to a reduction in cardiovascular events with statin therapy in CKD patients who present with ACS and support the routine use of statins in this population.

Beta-blocker Therapy

The β-blockers are recommended for all patients with ACS unless contraindicated. Metoprolol, propranolol, and carvedilol are all extensively hepatically metabolized and do not require dose adjustments in renal impairment. Atenolol is renally eliminated and requires dose adjustment in those with renal impairment. An observational study showed that β-blocker use was associated with a 40% relative reduction in mortality among those undergoing dialysis and a 56% relative reduction among those without end-stage renal disease (ESRD)[27] and so should be considered in all patients presenting with ACS.

Angiotensin Blockade

Angiotensin-converting enzyme (ACE) inhibitors/angiotensin receptor blockers (ARBs) are recommended by current guidelines to be initiated and continued indefinitely in all patients with ACS and a left ventricular ejection fraction (LVEF) less than 40% and also for those with hypertension, diabetes mellitus (DM), and CKD unless contraindicated. The most common concerns with ACE inhibitors or ARBs, however, include perceived worsening renal function and hyperkalemia. There is no absolute level of serum creatinine (SCr) that precludes the use of these agents; however, caution is warranted, if the SCr exceeds 2.5 mg/dL, and these can be used as long as the SCr does not increase beyond this point and the serum potassium remains less than 5.5 mEq/L.

Aldosterone Receptor Antagonists

Aldosterone antagonists such as spironolactone and eplerenone are recommended for post-myocardial infarction (MI) patients who are receiving therapeutic doses of an ACE inhibitor and a β-blocker, have a LVEF less than 40%, and have either DM or heart failure. But there are concerns regarding the increased risk of life-threatening hyperkalemia attributable to aldosterone antagonists, particularly when combined with angiotensin blockade. Therefore, the American College of Cardiology/American Heart Association guidelines recommend against using aldosterone blockade, if significant renal dysfunction (SCr >2.5 mg/dL in men and >2.0 mg/dL in women) or hyperkalemia (serum potassium >5.0 mEq/L) coexists.[28]

Fibrinolytic Therapy

The commercially available thrombolytics (alteplase, reteplase, tenecteplase, and streptokinase) do not require dose adjustment for CKD. Several observational studies have evaluated the association of CKD with outcomes and the treatment effect of fibrinolytic therapy in STEMI patients. Data from these studies showed increasing rates of intracranial hemorrhage with worsening renal function. Despite this, fibrinolytic therapy should be considered as a treatment strategy for CKD patients presenting with STEMI when primary percutaneous coronary intervention (PCI) is not available. However, given the increased rates of intracranial hemorrhage observed with worsening renal function, careful consideration of the benefits, and risk of fibrinolytic therapy in this population are required.

Percutaneous Coronary Intervention

Primary PCI, whenever available, should be the treatment of choice in patients with STEMI as the cardiovascular risk is greater than the risk of requiring renal replacement therapy (RRT) in most of the patients. Sadeghi et al.[29] evaluated the potential impact of renal insufficiency in patients undergoing primary PCI in the Controlled Abciximab and Device Investigation to Lower Late Angioplasty Complications (CADILLAC) trial. In patients with estimated glomerular filtration rate (eGFR) less than 60, procedural success rates were lower (87.2% vs. 92%, $p = 0.01$), and was associated with 9-fold greater mortality at 1 month and a fivefold increase in mortality at 1-year. Further, in a single-center retrospective study,[30] the 30-day and 6-month mortality were reduced from 22 to 3.6% ($p < 0.03$) and from 25.4 to 7.1% ($p < 0.05$) among renal dysfunction patients who underwent PCI during hospitalization. This suggests that mild-to-moderate renal insufficiency in the setting of STEMI is associated with increased mortality but an early PCI may be beneficial among such patients.

Renal dysfunction is a strong independent predictor of mortality in patients with NSTE-ACS. In a study by Keeley et al.,[31] there was a reduction in 6-month mortality in patients with CKD stage 3 and 4 and NSTE-ACS with early revascularization. The SWEDEHEART study, however, suggested that an early invasive strategy was harmful for CKD five patients with NSTE-ACS and should be tried to be managed with optimal medical therapy. A detailed algorithm regarding management of ACS in patients with renal dysfunction is shown in flowchart 1.

Contrast-induced Nephropathy

Contrast-induced nephropathy, also known as contrast-induced acute kidney injury (CI-AKI), is an iatrogenic renal injury that follows intravascular administration of radiopaque contrast media (ROCM) in susceptible individuals. The most widely used definition is the increase in SCr more than or equal to 0.5 mg/dL or 25% increase of SCr from the baseline value at 48 hours after CM administration. Serum cystatin C levels have also been evaluated as an early marker of CI-AKI. In a study by Briguori et al.[32] performed on CKD patients undergoing percutaneous transluminal coronary angioplasty (PTCA), increase of cystatin C levels more than or equal to 10% at 24 hours after the procedure was found to reliably predict the patients with high risk of CI-AKI. Pre-existent stage-3 CKD, defined as an eGFR less than 60 mL/min/1.73 m^2, is the most commonly identified risk factor for CIN and all the measures to prevent CIN should be taken meticulously in such patients. The most commonly used measures to prevent CIN are:

- Use minimum amount of CM
- Avoid concomitant use of other nephrotoxic drugs
- Hydrate the patient with isotonic saline and/or sodium bicarbonate before and after the procedure
- *N-acetylcysteine (NAC)*: Although the strength of the evidence is low, NAC is a well tolerated and inexpensive drug and it has a relatively good profile of adverse effects. Thus, in 2012, Kidney Disease: Improving Global Outcomes (KDIGO) guidelines suggested NAC for patients with high risk of CI-AKI.[33] There is no consensus on the dose of the NAC, however, it is usually used at a dose of 600–1,200 mg orally twice daily
- *Prefer isoosmolar contrast media (IOCM) or hypoosmolar contrast media (LOCM) over hyperosmolar CM*: In a meta-analysis,[34] a mild decrease in the risk of CI-AKI was found with iodixanol (IOCM) when compared to iohexol (LOCM), however, no difference was found between the groups in terms of risk of RRT, cardiovascular outcomes, or death. Therefore, KDIGO guidelines do not make a recommendation about the preference of IOCM or LOCM due to lack of reliable evidence[33]

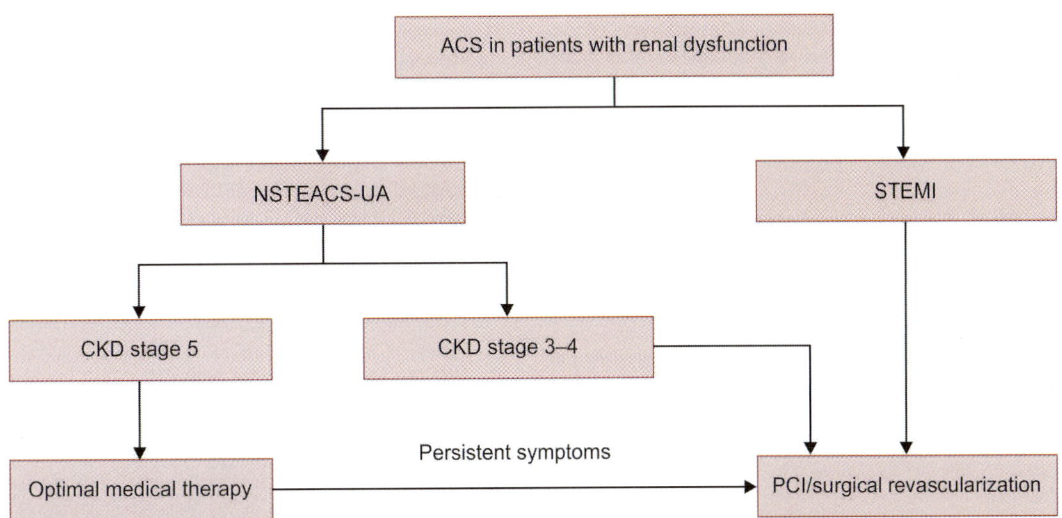

NSTEACS-UA, non-ST elevation acute coronary syndromes-unstable angina; PCI, percutaneous coronary intervention; STEMI, ST-elevation myocardial infarction.

FLOWCHART 1: Algorithm for management of acute coronary syndrome (ACS) in patients with chronic kidney disease (CKD).

- *Remote ischemic preconditioning (RIP)*: It is based on a hypothesis that a transient ischemia of an organ may protect against an ischemic injury of another distant organ. This is mostly induced by arm ischemia performed by inflation of blood pressure cuffs during or before the procedure. Few studies have shown that RIP decreases the risk of CI-AKI.[35,36] However, further randomized clinical trials are needed
- *Prophylactic hemodialysis/hemofiltration*: Prophylactic hemodialysis (HD)/hemofiltration (HF) has not been found to be protective against CI-AKI. In a meta-analysis, no beneficial effect of these treatment modalities was found against CI-AKI.[37] Furthermore, HD was found to increase the risk of CI-AKI. Thus, prophylactic renal replacement treatment is not recommended.

CONCLUSION

Presence of renal dysfunction should not prevent an ACS patient from receiving standard guideline-directed therapy. Patients with CKD can receive antithrombotic therapy, DAPT, standard medical therapy, as well as coronary revascularization therapy but with an increased risk of bleeding. These patients have poor prognosis compared to those without renal dysfunction, however, adherence to guideline-based therapy appears to be associated with improved short- and long-term mortality.

REFERENCES

1. Wright RS, Reeder GS, Herzog CA, et al. Acute myocardial infarction and renal dysfunction: a high-risk combination. Ann Intern Med. 2002;137:563-70.
2. Shlipak MG, Heidenreich PA, Noguchi H, et al. Association of renal insufficiency with treatment and outcomes after myocardial infarction in elderly patients. Ann Intern Med. 2002;137:555-62.
3. Fox CS, Muntner P, Chen AY, et al. Use of evidence-based therapies in short-term outcomes of ST-segment elevation myocardial infarction and non-ST-segment elevation myocardial infarction in patients with chronic kidney disease: a report from the National Cardiovascular Data Acute Coronary Treatment and Intervention Outcomes Network registry. Circulation. 2010;121(3):357-65.
4. Coca SG, Krumholz HM, Garg AX, et al. Underrepresentation of renal disease in randomized controlled trials of cardiovascular disease. JAMA. 2006;296:1377-84.
5. Charytan D, Kuntz RE. The exclusion of patients with chronic kidney disease from clinical trials in coronary artery disease. Kidney Int. 2006;70:2021-30.
6. Nakano T, Ninomiya T, Sumiyoshi S, et al. Association of kidney function with coronary atherosclerosis and calcification in autopsy samples from Japanese elders: the Hisayama study. Am J Kidney Dis. 2010;55(1):21-30.
7. Kawai H, Sarai M, Motoyama S, et al. Coronary plaque characteristics in patients with mild chronic kidney disease. Analysis by 320-row area detector computed tomography. Circ J. 2012;76(6):1436-41.
8. Schwarz U, Buzello M, Ritz E, et al. Morphology of coronary atherosclerotic lesions in patients with end-stage renal failure. Nephrol Dial Transplant. 2000;15(2):218-23.
9. Baber U, Stone GW, Weisz G, et al. Coronary plaque composition, morphology, and outcomes in patients with and without chronic kidney disease presenting with acute coronary syndromes. JACC Cardiovasc Imaging. 2012;5:S53-61.
10. Madore F. Uremia-related metabolic cardiac risk factors in chronic kidney disease. Semin Dial. 2003;16(2):148-56.
11. Naito K, Anzai T, Yoshikawa T, et al. Impact of chronic kidney disease on postinfarction inflammation, oxidative stress, and left ventricular remodeling. J Card Fail. 2008;14(10):831-8.
12. Gutierrez OM, Januzzi JL, Isakova T, et al. Fibroblast growth factor 23 and left ventricular hypertrophy in chronic kidney disease. Circulation. 2009;119(19):2545-52.
13. Szummer K, Lundman P, Jacobson SH, et al. SWEDEHEART. Relation between renal function, presentation, use of therapies and in-hospital complications in acute coronary syndrome: data from the SWEDEHEART register. J Intern Med. 2010;268:40-9.
14. Fox KA, Antman EM, Montalescot G, et al. The impact of renal dysfunction on outcomes in the ExTRACT-TIMI 25 trial. J Am Coll Cardiol. 2007;49:2249-55.
15. Fox KA, Bassand JP, Mehta SR, et al. OASIS 5 Investigators. Influence of renal function on the efficacy and safety of fondaparinux relative to enoxaparin in non ST-segment elevation acute coronary syndromes. Ann Intern Med. 2007;147:304-10.
16. McCullough PA, Sandberg KR, Borzak S, et al. Benefits of aspirin and beta-blockade after myocardial infarction in patients with chronic kidney disease. Am Heart J. 2002;144:226-32.
17. Yan AT, Yan RT, Tan M, et al. Canadian Acute Coronary Syndromes (ACS) Registry Investigators. Treatment and one-year outcome of patients with renal dysfunction across the broad spectrum of acute coronary syndromes. Can J Cardiol. 2006;22:115-20.
18. Antithrombotic Trialists' Collaboration. Collaborative meta-analysis of randomised trials of antiplatelet therapy for prevention of death, myocardial infarction, and stroke in high risk patients. BMJ. 2002;324:71-86.
19. Keltai M, Tonelli M, Mann JF, et al. CURE Trial Investigators. Renal function and outcomes in acute coronary syndrome: impact of clopidogrel. Eur J Cardiovasc Prev Rehabil. 2007;14:312-8.
20. Best PJ, Steinhubl SR, Berger PB, et al. CREDO Investigators. The efficacy and safety of short- and long-term dual antiplatelet therapy in patients with mild or moderate chronic kidney disease: results from the Clopidogrel for the Reduction of Events during Observation (CREDO) trial. Am Heart J. 2008;155:687-93.
21. Ahmed S, Michael Gibson C, Cannon CP, et al. Impact of reduced glomerular filtration rate on outcomes in patients with ST-segment elevation myocardial infarction undergoing fibrinolysis: a CLARITY-TIMI 28 analysis. J Thromb Thrombolysis. 2011;31:493-500.
22. Frilling B, Zahn R, Fraiture B, et al. Comparison of efficacy and complication rates after percutaneous coronary interventions in patients with and without renal insufficiency treated with abciximab. Am J Cardiol. 2002;89:450-2.
23. Fellström BC, Jardine AG, Schmieder RE, et al. AURORA Study Group. Rosuvastatin and cardiovascular events in patients undergoing hemodialysis. N Engl J Med. 2009;360:1395-407.
24. Holdaas H, Fellström B, Jardine AG, et al. Assessment of LEscol in Renal Transplantation (ALERT) Study Investigators. Effect of fluvastatin on cardiac outcomes in renal transplant recipients: a multicentre, randomised, placebo-controlled trial. Lancet. 2003;361:2024-31.
25. Baigent C, Landray MJ, Reith C, et al. SHARP Investigators. The effects of lowering LDL cholesterol with simvastatin plus ezetimibe in patients with chronic kidney disease (Study of Heart and Renal Protection): a randomised placebo-controlled trial. Lancet. 2011;377(9784):2181-92.
26. Palmer SC, Navaneethan SD, Craig JC, et al. HMG CoA reductase inhibitors (statins) for people with chronic kidney disease not requiring dialysis. Cochrane Database Syst Rev. 2014;31(5):CD007784.
27. Berger AK, Duval S, Krumholz HM. Aspirin, beta-blocker, and angiotensin-converting enzyme inhibitor therapy in patients with end-stage renal disease and an acute myocardial infarction. J Am Coll Cardiol. 2003;42:201-8.
28. Antman EM, Hand M, Armstrong PW, et al. 2007 Focused update of the ACC/AHA 2004 Guidelines for the Management of Patients with ST-Elevation Myocardial Infarction: a report of the American College of Cardiology/American Heart Association Task Force on Practice Guidelines (Writing Group to Review New Evidence and Update the ACC/AHA 2004 Guidelines for the Management of Patients With ST-Elevation Myocardial Infarction). J Am Coll Cardiol. 2008;51:210-47.

29. Sadeghi HM, Stone GW, Grines CL, et al. Impact of renal insufficiency in patients undergoing primary angioplasty for acute myocardial infarction. Circulation. 2003;108:2769-75.
30. Hobbach HP, Gibson CM, Giugliano RP, et al. The prognostic value of serum creatinine on admission in fibrinolytic-eligible patients with acute myocardial infarction. J Thromb Thrombolysis. 2003;16:167-74.
31. Keeley EC, Kadakia R, Soman S, et al. Analysis of long-term survival after revascularization in patients with chronic kidney disease presenting with acute coronary syndromes. Am J Cardiol. 2003;92:509-14.
32. Briguori C, Visconti G, Rivera NV, et al. Cystatin C and contrast-induced acute kidney injury. Circulation. 2010;121:2117-22.
33. KDIGO. Clinical Practice Guideline for Acute Kidney Injury. Kidney Int Suppl. 2012;2:8.
34. Eng J, Wilson RF, Subramaniam RM, et al. Comparative Effect of Contrast Media Type on the Incidence of Contrast-Induced Nephropathy: A Systematic Review and Meta-analysis. Ann Intern Med. 2016;164:417-24.
35. Igarashi G, Iino K, Watanabe H, et al. Remote ischemic pre-conditioning alleviates contrast-induced acute kidney injury in patients with moderate chronic kidney disease. Circ J. 2013;77:3037-44.
36. Er F, Nia AM, Dopp H, et al. Ischemic pre-conditioning for prevention of contrast medium-induced nephropathy: randomized pilot RenPro Trial (Renal Protection Trial). Circulation. 2012;126:296-303.
37. Cruz DN, Goh CY, Marenzi G, et al. Renal replacement therapies for prevention of radiocontrast-induced nephropathy: a systematic review. Am J Med. 2012;125:66-78.e3.

SECTION 7

ST-Segment Elevation Myocardial Infarction

CHAPTER 41

Burden and Outcome of STEMI in India

Santanu Guha, Avik Karak

PREAMBLE

Mr AB, a 45-year-old farmer, residing at a remote village area of Bengal, presented to a small rural hospital in a small town of Midnapore, India, at 11:30 PM with severe chest pain. The hospital was a 10-bed facility with a small emergency room. The entire staff consisted of just three nurses and a junior doctor. The duty nurse recorded an electrocardiogram (ECG) and sent it to the doctor's house through a ward boy, situated 15 minutes away. The doctor diagnosed an anterior ST-segment elevation myocardial infarction (STEMI). However, he wanted to consult with the senior doctor to confirm the diagnosis before starting streptokinase (SK). However, he decided to go to the hospital to see the patient as he was having ongoing pain. He advised the relatives to shift the patient to a higher medical center in the closest city located 120 km away—a 3-hour journey. They decided to wait until next morning to organize funds to arrange for the transfer. The patient started to deteriorate and became hypotensive from early morning before the contemplated transfer and succumbed at 6.30 AM, before the transportation to the city hospital or the senior doctor could confirm the diagnosis. This is not an isolated case history. The names may be different but progressively younger men and women are dying every day of acute myocardial infarction (AMI) without proper medical attention. With the turn of the century, cardiovascular diseases (CVDs) have become the leading cause of mortality in India.[1] Approximately, 3–4% of Indians in rural areas and 8–10% in urban areas have coronary artery disease (CAD). Indians are more likely to develop CAD at younger ages during an individual's productive years resulting in loss of potentially productive years of life in India.[2,3]

BURDEN OF CARDIOVASCULAR DISEASES IN INDIA

Cardiovascular disease is the leading cause of death in India accounting for approximately 21% of deaths in the year 2010, with 10% of deaths due to CAD. The Global Burden of Disease study estimated an age-standardized CVD death rate is 272 per 100,000 in Indian population in comparison to the global average of 235 per 100,000 population. The World Health Organization (WHO) estimated that India would lose $237 billion from the loss of productivity and spending on health care over a 10-year period (2005–2010) with the current burden of CVD.[4] There are no nationally representative surveillance data on the prevalence of CVD and the secular trends of CVD mortality in India at present. However, three large prospective studies from India recently have suggested a higher proportion of mortality attributable to CVD (30–42%) and an age-standardized CVD mortality rate of 255–525 per 100,000 population in men and 225–299 per 100,000 population in women in comparison with the Global Burden of Disease Study (2010).[5-7] Ischemic heart disease (IHD) and cerebrovascular accident (CVA) constitutes the majority of CVD mortality in India (83%), with IHD being predominant (Fig. 1).[8] The years of life lost

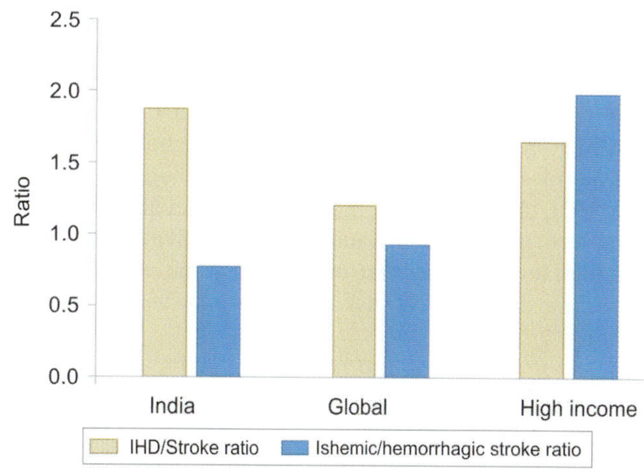

FIG. 1: Ischemic heart disease to stroke ratio and ischemic to hemorrhagic stroke ratio in India in comparision with global data.[8]

attributable to CVD in India increased by 59% from 1990 to 2010 (23.2 -37 million).[9] Several small cross-sectional studies performed in different parts of the country suggested a rapid increase in the IHD burden over the past few decades.[10-32] The prevalence of IHD has increased by almost sevenfolds to approximately 14% in 2013 from a meager 2% in 1960 with a higher margin of increase in the rural areas where the prevalence has quadrupled (1.7-7.4%).[10-22,31,32] The higher case fatality of acute coronary syndrome (ACS) could also result in the underestimation of prevalence among Indians.[33]

BURDEN OF CARDIOVASCULAR DISEASE RISK FACTORS

It is estimated that, currently approximately 275 million individuals aged more than 15 years consume tobacco in India.[34] The rate of fruit and vegetables consumption is low in India. The National Family Health Survey-3 (NFHS-3), covering 156,316 individuals in India, reported that half of the population in its survey consumed zero to one serving of fruit in a week.[35] Time-series data on nutrient intake captured from the National Sample Survey Organization surveys indicate that, Indians' fat intake increased from 24 to 36 g/day and from 36 to 50 g/day in rural and urban individuals, respectively from 1972 to 2000.[36] The Indian Council of Medical Research-India Diabetes (ICMR-INDIAB) study is a large cross-sectional survey which assessed physical activity using the global physical activity questionnaire in 14,227 individuals aged more than or equal to 20 years showed that one of every two were considered physically inactive and less than 10% of the studied population engaged in recreational physical activity.[37] The prevalence of hypertension in Indian adults is in the tune of 30% (34% in urban areas and 28% in rural areas).[38] The average blood pressure has increased in the past two decades in India whereas in most Western nations it has declined.[39] Prospective Urban and Rural Epidemiology (PURE) study (83% of the participants being from India) showed that low educational status is associated with lower rates of awareness, treatment, and control of hypertension.[40] Urban areas of India has seen a doubling in the prevalence of diabetes mellitus (DM) in the past 20 years, from 9 to 17%, whereas it has nearly quadrupled, from 2 to 9% in the rural areas.[41] There has been a rapid rise in the mean levels of total cholesterol, low-density lipoprotein (LDL) cholesterol, non-high-density lipoprotein (non-HDL) cholesterol, and triglycerides (TG) as shown in serial epidemiological studies.[42] Low-HDL cholesterol was the most common abnormality.[43] Long-term material deprivation, unhealthy living conditions, and high levels of stress are other factors that also appear to contribute to excess CVD risk among socially deprived groups in India.[44,45]

DETERMINANTS OF CARDIOVASCULAR DISEASE IN INDIANS

There are significant variations between various CVD risk factors within different regions. Southern states of India have a higher prevalence of DM whereas hypertension appears to be higher in the North-eastern states.[46] The social determinants play an important role in the heterogeneity apart from the cultural diversities and variations in the economic development. Suboptimal social characteristics such as low educational, occupational, and socioeconomic status (SES) were associated with a clustering of more than or equal to three CV risk factors and a higher Framingham risk score in a cross-sectional study of CV risk factors in Jaipur.[47,48] Social determinants play a major role in determining outcomes after a CVD event as shown in the CREATE (Clinical Trial of Reviparin and Metabolic Modulation in Acute Myocardial Infarction Treatment Evaluation) registry where the outcomes after ACS were worse in lower-SES individuals.[3]

EPIDEMIOLOGY OF STEMI IN INDIA

About 30 million individuals in India have CAD.[32] With 381.5 per 100,000 CVD deaths in India, India ranked higher than Britain, US, and China in the WHO report in 2004.[4] The fact that the mean age of occurrence of STEMI in Indians is 5–10 years lower than Western population was supported by a study done in Karnataka.[49] Abnormal lipids, smoking, hypertension, diabetes, abdominal obesity, psychosocial factors, low fruit and vegetable consumption, and lack of physical activity were the eight coronary risk factors as identified by the INTERHEART-South Asia study which accounted for 89% of the cases of all AMI in Indians. The INTERHEART study also revealed that Indians who developed STEMI had lower LDL and HDL cholesterol levels than others in the study. Apolipoprotein B/apolipoprotein A1 (ApoB/ApoA1) showed the strongest association with the risk of AMI in Indians.[50] This shows that Indians deserve a separate consensus in the management of ACS as there are many unknown factors at play. We can extrapolate data and latest trends from the few but significant registries like the CREATE registry, Kerala ACS registry, OASIS-2, DEMAT registry, North East (NE) registry and Himachal Pradesh registry for STEMI patients in India.[3,33,51-54]

Presentation of ACS Patients as STEMI

The CREATE registry showed that STEMI accounted for 60% of ACS, while in Kerala ACS registry STEMI constituted only 40% which is slightly higher than that seen in many international registries. The Kerala ACS registry of the patients presenting a similar proportion of men as with the other Indian ACS registries which was higher when compared with the National Cardiovascular Data Registry in the US, Euro Heart Survey ACS II registry in Europe and Global Registry of Acute Coronary Events (GRACE) registry.[55-57]

Case Fatality Rates in India

In-hospital mortality rate for STEMI in the Kerala ACS registry (8.2%) and CREATE registry (8.6%) were similar but were higher than GRACE (7%) and Euro Heart Survey ACS II (6%).[3,54,56,57]

Delayed Presentation Time

In India various registries have shown trends of late presentation which hampers timely intervention which influences the prognosis and outcome of the STEMI patients.

Reperfusion Strategies are Underutilized

Thrombolytic therapy and primary percutaneous coronary intervention (PCI) are two commonly used reperfusion strategies. Kerala ACS registry reported a lower rate of utilization of thrombolysis in comparison to CREATE as well as GRACE registry.[3,57] Thrombolysis was used in 41% of STEMI patients but when used, was generally prompt with less than one-third patients exceeding the door to needle times of more than 30 minutes. Approximately, half of the patients presenting with the diagnosis of STEMI received some form of reperfusion [thrombolysis, PCI or coronary artery bypass grafting (CABG)]. Primary PCI in STEMI, the gold standard of treatment, is available to a very small proportion of STEMI patients in India.

Inappropriate diagnosis and thrombolysis was one of the most worrisome factors in the management of STEMI as shown in the Kerala ACS registry[54] where 19% of non-STEMI (NSTEMI) and 10% of unstable angina (UA) patients also received thrombolysis and this was more common in the rural, non-teaching, and low volume centers. This percentage was much higher than that reported in the Western population (2.5–5%).[58]

Practice Pattern and Guideline Adherence

Secondary analysis of the Kerala ACS registry showed that optimal in-hospital and discharge medical care defined as receiving dual antiplatelet therapy (DAPT), β-blockers, statin, and parenteral anticoagulation (in-hospital only), were given in 40% and 46% of admissions, respectively. Patients receiving optimal in-hospital medical care had 21% lower rate of in-hospital major adverse cardiac events (MACE). The CREATE registry[3] reported a lower use of β-blockers and statins and a higher use of angiotensin-converting enzyme inhibitors/angiotensin II receptor blockers (ACEIs/ARBs) when compared with the Kerala ACS Registry[54] with an unfortunately even lower postdischarge rates of optimal medical care. The PURE registry reported that less than half of patients with prevalent CVD take more than or equal to one medication for secondary prevention.[40]

Gender Differences in Presentation and Management

Kerala ACS registry (5,825 women out of 25,748 ACS patients) showed that women at presentation were approximately five years older than men with moderately higher rates of previous MI. Gender differences in the outcome of death or in the composite outcome of death, reinfarction, stroke, heart failure (HF), and cardiogenic shock were not statistically significant even after adjustment for possible confounding factors. The DEMAT registry (1,565 ACS patients from ten tertiary care centers in India) also corroborated that after adjustment for age, education, history of CAD, STEMI presentation, and reperfusion of any type, there was no evidence of increased risk of death at 30 days among women, nor was there any difference between death, rehospitalization, and cardiac arrest at 30 days in comparison to men.[51]

The Economic Impact in India

Out of pocket expenditure (OOPE) amounts to up to nine times of the total household expenditures, depending on the SES and type of treatment availed, imposing a large financial burden on families. The high OOPE and catastrophic health expenditure (CHE) have been reported elsewhere due to CVD-related hospitalizations (including ACS) where India (Kerala) had the highest 15-month OOPE and more than 80% of the low- and middle-income groups and more than 60% of the high-income group experienced CHE.[59]

Onset of Cardiovascular Disease and High Fatality

The INTERHEART study (across 52 countries) reported the occurrence of MI at an early age among patients from South Asia at a median age of 52 years in comparison with 62 years in the European origin cohort.[2] Gupta et al.,[60] in their study of age-specific trends in CV risk factors among the adolescent and young demonstrated that CV risk factors increase exponentially with age after Indians reach the 30–39-year age group. More severe manifestations of CVD and higher fatality rates are an additional cause of concern.[40] In the PURE study, the incidence of major CV events and mortality among individuals of low-income countries (96% from South Asia, of whom 83% were from India) was higher than in middle- and high-income countries, despite having a lower conventional CVD risk factor burden.[40]

OUTCOME OF STEMI

Patients in India who have ACS have a higher rate of STEMI than do patients in developed countries. Various studies in the Indian subcontinent have studied the outcomes of STEMI in India. The following section focuses on the various studies with attention to the outcomes of STEMI patients in India.

Isezuo et al.[61] carried out a cross-sectional retrospective analysis of 1,468 ACS patients in Chennai. The time from onset of symptoms to presentation ranged from 5 to 120 minutes (median 5 h, mode 24 h) in patients with STEMI. The median time from onset of symptoms to hospitalization was 360 minutes, with 50 minutes from hospital to thrombolysis in the CREATE registry [which enrolled 20,937 patients, of which 12,405 (60.6%) had STEMI]. Medical therapy including antiplatelet drugs; ACEI/ARB were prescribed more in STEMI than in NSTEMI. About 58·5% of patients with STEMI received thrombolysis predominantly with SK (96.3%). Fewer patients with STEMI than those with NSTEMI or UA were given β-blockers; statins. Coronary angiography (CAG) was performed in 80.6% of patients in the study by Isezuo et al. The CAG rate was higher in the STEMI group than NSTEMI/UA group which was statistically significant. Single vessel disease was more frequent in the STEMI group than the other group. About 20.3% of patients were thrombolyzed (streptokinase in 94.0%), while 53.3% and 10.3% had primary PCI and CABG, respectively in the STEMI group. About 16.1% of STEMI patients had sole medical therapy. Importantly, the rate of utilization of some form of reperfusion therapy was higher in the current than previous reports from India.[3,62] Patients who had PCI were significantly younger than those who had only medical treatment in both the studies. Though CAG rate was higher in males than females, there were no statistically significant gender differences in the rates of PCI and CABG. Among the complications arrhythmias (3.7%), resuscitated cardiac arrest (1.8%) and intracardiac thrombus (1.5%) were the predominant ones. Seven days, 30 days, 6 months, and 1-year mortality rates were 0.4%, 0.7%, 2.0%, and 2.5%, respectively with total of 37 casualties reported in 1 year. Mortality increased with increasing age group and at higher risk stratification which was not statistically significant. At 1 year of follow up, reinfarction, resuscitated cardiac arrest and major bleeding were seen in 59/1,463 (4.0%), 26/1,468 (1.8%), 16/1,468 (1.1%), and 5/1,171 (0.4%) of the patients, respectively. Composite MACE comprising deaths, MI, stroke, cardiac arrest and bleeding at 1 year occurred in 9.7% of the study population. The deceased were predominantly the elderly and had renal dysfunction (higher serum creatinine) and severe left ventricular (LV) dysfunction. In the CREATE registry death, reinfarction, and stroke occurred in 8.6%, 2.3%, and 0.7% of STEMI patients, respectively at 30 days in comparison to NSTEMI or UA patients where death, reinfarction, and stroke occurred in 3.7%, 1.2%, and 0.3% patients, respectively. SES influenced the key treatments: more rich patients were given thrombolytics, β-blockers, statins, ACEIs/ARBs, PCI, and CABG surgery than poor patients. These differences resulted in a significant 2.7% absolute higher 30-day mortality in the poorest group when compared to the richest group, though rates of reinfarction or stroke were similar. Adjustment for treatments between the different strata of SES (but not risk factors and baseline characteristics) eliminated the differences in mortality between the rich and the poor, suggesting that better treatment of established CAD offers an opportunity to improve outcome of STEMI patients across the varied SES distribution in India. Higher number of poor patients might have died before reaching hospital resulting in under estimation of the actual mortality. It can be hypothecated that mortality can be reduced, if all patients, across all SES spectrum, had access to similar health care facilities, reached hospital rapidly, and received similar treatments.[63]

In Kerala ACS registry data from 25,748 consecutive ACS admissions were collected from 125 hospitals from May 2007 to May 2009 the unadjusted in-hospital mortality rate was 8.2% in STEMI patients, compared with substantially lower rates in NSTEMI (1.8%) and UA (0.9%) patients. STEMI patients had a higher nonfatal MACE (stroke, reinfarction, HF, or cardiogenic shock) rates. STEMI patients had a higher risk of in-hospital death and in-hospital MACE when compared to patients with UA. Delayed presentation significantly affected the outcome of the STEMI patients as demonstrated by the fact that symptom-to-door time of more than 6 hours was associated with higher in-hospital mortality, and in-hospital MACE. Door-to-needle time less than 30 minutes resulted in lower in-hospital mortality and in-hospital MACE in STEMI patients proving that early intervention significantly improved the outcomes. Patients in the Kerala ACS registry included patients slightly older than those in prior Indian ACS registries. Predischarge medical therapy with DAPT was high and similar to prior literature. Beta-blockers and statins were used more commonly than prior Indian registry data, while heparin, ACEI/ARBs, and CCBs were used less commonly. Though CAG rates were lower than prior Indian data (20% vis-a-vis 23% in the CREATE registry),[3] the PCI rates were higher (12% vs. 7.5% in the CREATE registry).[3] Both CAG and PCI rates were substantially lower than those in the ACTION[64,65] and Euro Heart Survey ACS I and II.[57,66] Thrombolysis in the setting of a STEMI diagnosis was lower in the Kerala ACS registry reported a lower rate of utilization of thrombolysis than CREATE[3] as well as GRACE.[57]

There were trends towards increasing annual rates of admission for ACS, CAG, PCI, and use of ACEIs/ARBs and β-blockers during the study period of 1 year in the study done by Isezuo et al. along with decreasing rates of mortality and CABG (Fig. 2).

Outcomes of ACS has been influenced by the hospital setting as suggested in the AMIS registry,[67] where the hospitals categorized as grade A characterized by 24 hours coronary care unit, cardiac catheterization, and cardiac surgery services had lower mortality than category B hospitals where these services were either unavailable or were not

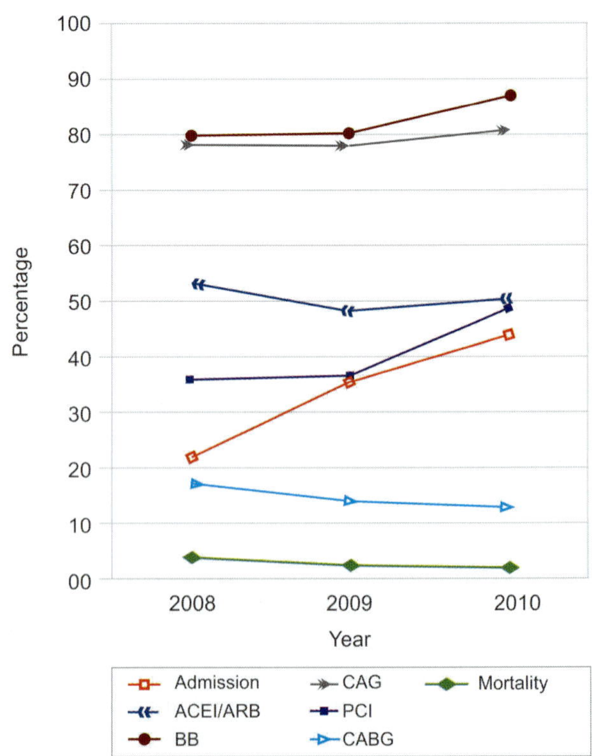

CAG, coronary angiography; ACEI/ARB, angiotensin-converting enzyme inhibitors/angiotensin II receptor blocker; BB, beta-blocker; CABG, coronary artery bypass grafting; PCI, percutaneous coronary intervention.

FIG. 2: Trends in interventions and mortality.

obtainable to the same extent (2.8% vs. 4.0%). Contrary to the belief that mortality in ACS is higher in Indians than the whites,[68,69] a recent meta-analysis (of four recently published studies) demonstrated that the prognosis of CAD in South Asian population is not worse than whites, and the increased mortality rates in the former are due to the higher incidence of fatal and non-fatal CAD. Another recent study comparing South Asian STEMI population with the Europeans showed that though the former were younger and more likely to be diabetic, the survival at discharge was comparable.[70] The low mortality rate in the study by Isezuo et al. could have been influenced by the fact that the study population belonged predominantly to low or intermediate-risk group with lower rates of fatal outcomes and the clinical determinants of mortality were largely similar to the findings in previous reports.[57,70-71] Another interesting observation recently was the higher mortality rates among young women with ACS with the difference disappearing with increasing age, with long-term prognosis similar or even better among elder women. They nonetheless probably indicate that the CAD epidemic is still on-going in India, and that there is increased awareness of the disease among the populace and improved compliance with evidence-based treatment guidelines among the physicians. Trends towards increasing admission rate for ACS, utilization of therapeutic advances, and fall in mortality were observed.

The outcome of timely fibrinolysis along with contemporary antiplatelets and antithrombotic (tenecteplase was used as the thrombolytic agent) followed by timely CAG in the pharmaco-invasive approach has been compared with the standard primary PCI in the STEPP-AMI study.[72] Two hundred STEMI patients aged less than 75 years, who underwent either primary PCI or a pharmaco-invasive strategy within 12 hours of symptom onset were followed up for 1 year. The primary end-point (composite of death, cardiogenic shock, reinfarction, repeat revascularization of the culprit artery and congestive heart failure) was similar between the two groups at 30 days, 3 months, 6 months, and 1 year, although primary PCI had a trend towards benefit during the early phase of follow-up. Relatively affluent patients underwent primary PCI, a plausible explanation for the better long-term outcomes due to lifestyle changes and better adherence to medication. The findings corroborated with the well-known STREAM study.[73] Another important finding in this study is the nonrequirement of a stent in a significant number of patients who underwent thrombolysis followed by CAG due to insignificant disease (6.7%) and a better infarct related artery (IRA) patency rate and lesser thrombus burden. Failed thrombolysis occurred in 12.1% patients which is much less than that reported in the STREAM study (36.3%). The mortality rates in the pharmaco-invasive group stabilized after the initial three months period (6.7% followed by 8.9% after 3 months) whereas it continued to increase in the primary PCI group (1.3% at 30 days, 2.6% at 3 months, 3.2% at 6 months and 4.5% at 1 year). Another interesting finding is that the bleeding risk was similar between the two groups which were contrary to the previous studies which had a higher bleeding in the thrombolysis arm. The increased utilization of the radial access for CAG in comparison to primary PCI could have been the reason for the similar rates of bleeding. The results of this study demonstrate the safety and efficacy of the pharmaco-invasive strategy in comparison to primary PCI under the age of 75 years which can alleviate the logistic and geographic barriers of primary PCI in the treatment of STEMI in India.[74]

Interesting findings have surfaced from the Tamil Nadu-STEMI (TN-STEMI) program. The implementation of the hub and spoke model of health care delivery for ACS as a system of care for the low and middle-income countries (LMICs) has proved to be beneficial. One-year mortality was lower in the postimplementation phase in the TN-STEMI program though there were no statistically significant differences between the pre- and postimplementation phases for cardiogenic shock, stroke, or in-hospital mortality. Patients presenting to the hub hospitals had a significantly lower in-hospital mortality compared to those who were initially evaluated at the spoke health care centers during the preimplementation phase, but this difference was abolished in the postimplementation phase. Postimplementation phase also saw an increase in utilization rates of medical therapy like aspirin, statins, and DAPT. Focusing on primary PCI as the exclusive mode of reperfusion is not feasible while developing a system of care for the LMICs despite its proven benefits. TN-STEMI program boasted of several of its key features like high rates of reperfusion at baseline (approximately 90%) reflecting the institution of care processes around measurement in the preimplementation phase, establishing transfer of patients with STEMI using ambulance services with paramedics,[75] use of the STEMI information technology kit for diagnosis and monitoring; the features which resulted in the findings of stable reperfusion rates and times to treatment combined with increases in primary PCI and the pharmaco-invasive approach after its implementation. The ominous finding from the TN-STEMI program was an increased utilization of primary PCI and the pharmaco-invasive approach in the spoke health care centers (by almost 10-fold from 3.5 to 31.3%) and a reduction of stand-alone fibrinolysis from 53.6% of patients in the preimplementation phase to 29.4% in the postimplementation phase.[76,77]

CONCLUSION

There is a high burden of CVD especially ACS accounting for a significant percentage of mortality among the Indian population. STEMI is a major public health problem, often impacting the most productive years of an individuals' life. STEMI affects younger population in India when compared to the Western population. Various socioeconomic factors and CVD risk factors are unique to Indians affecting the epidemiology and burden of STEMI among Indians. More resources are needed to be directed towards applying the existing knowledge base to tackle the CVD epidemic in policy, programs, capacity building, and research arenas to address the socioeconomic differentials in the burden of disease and healthcare needs of Indians. Out-of-pocket payment for medical care is the most common payment method for medical services in India, where insurance coverage is low, an issue which needs attention especially affecting the lower SES. Evidence-based pharmacotherapy and interventions as well as outcomes were favorably comparable to the data from developed nations. Trends towards increasing admission rate for ACS, utilization of therapeutic advances and fall in mortality were observed. Pharmaco-invasive therapy can be an excellent alternative to primary PCI in financially constrained situations and the age-old SK has beyond doubt proved its efficacy in saving lives. There are numerous data of ACS in India to date, and these demonstrate opportunities for improving the quality of ACS management by focusing on reducing symptom-to-door time, door-to-needle time, and inappropriate use of thrombolysis and increasing use of recommended drugs.

REFERENCES

1. Srinath RK, Shah B, Varghese C, et al. Responding to the threat of chronic diseases in India. Lancet. 2005;366:1744-9.
2. Joshi P, Islam S, Pais P, et al. Risk factors for early myocardial infarction in South Asians compared with individuals in other countries. JAMA. 2007;297:286-94.
3. Xavier D, Pais P, Devereaux PJ, et al. CREATE registry investigators. Treatment and outcomes of acute coronary syndromes in India (CREATE): a prospective analysis of registry data. Lancet. 2008;371:1435-42.
4. WHO. The top ten causes of death. WHO Fact sheet No. 310. 2011.
5. Pednekar MS, Gupta R, Gupta PC. Illiteracy, low educational status, and cardio-vascular mortality in India. BMC Public Health. 2011;11:567.
6. Soman CR, Kutty VR, Safraj S, et al. All-cause mortality and cardiovascular mortality in Kerala state of India: results from a 5-year follow-up of 161,942 rural community dwelling adults. Asia Pac J Public Health. 2011;23:896-903.
7. Joshi R, Cardona M, Iyengar S, et al. Chronic diseases now a leading cause of death in rural India–mortality data from the Andhra Pradesh Rural Health Initiative. Int J Epidemiol. 2006;35:1522-9.
8. Institute of Health Metrics and Evaluation (2016). GBD Compare 2010. [online]. Available from http:// vizhub.healthdata.org/gbd-compare/ [Accessed August 2018].
9. Institute of Health Metrics and Evaluation. (2014). GBD Profile: India. [online]. http:// www.healthdata.org/sites/default/files/files/country_profiles/GBD/ihme_gbd_country_report_india.pdf [Accessed August 2018].
10. Mathur KS. Environmental factors in coronary heart disease. An epidemiological survey at Agra (India). Circulation. 1960;21:684-9.
11. Padmavati S. Epidemiology of cardiovascular disease in India. II. Ischemic heart disease. Circulation. 1962;25:711-7.
12. Sarvotham SG, Berry JN. Prevalence of coronary heart disease in an urban population in northern India. Circulation. 1968;37:939-53.
13. Gupta SP, Malhotra KC. Urban–rural trends in the epidemiology of coronary heart disease. J Assoc Physicians India. 1975;23:885-92.
14. Chadha SL, Radhakrishnan S, Ramachandran K, et al. Epidemiological study of coronary heart disease in urban population of Delhi. Indian J Med Res. 1990;92:424-30.
15. Sinha PR, Gaur SD, Somani PN. Prevalence of coronary heart disease in an urban community of Varanasi. Indian J Comm Med. 1990;15:82-5.
16. Gupta R, Prakash H, Majumdar S, et al. Prevalence of coronary heart disease and coronary risk factors in an urban population of Rajasthan. Indian Heart J. 1995;47:331-8.
17. Begom R, Singh RB. Prevalence of coronary artery disease and its risk factors in the urban population of South and North India. Acta Cardiol. 1995;50:227-40.
18. Mohan V, Deepa R, Rani SS, et al. Prevalence of coronary artery disease and its relationship to lipids in a selected population in South India: The Chennai Urban Population Study (CUPS No. 5). J Am Coll Cardiol. 2001;38:682-7.
19. Gupta R, Gupta VP, Sarna M, et al. Prevalence of coronary heart disease and risk factors in an urban Indian population: Jaipur Heart Watch-2. Indian Heart J. 2002;54:59-66.
20. Pinto VG, Motghare DD, Ferriera AMA, et al. Prevalence of coronary heart disease in an urban community of Goa South Asian J Prev Cardiol. 2004;8:211-5.
21. Kamili M, Dar I, Ali G, et al. Prevalence of coronary heart disease in Kashmiris. Indian Heart J. 2007;59:44-9.
22. Dewan BD, Malhotra KC, Gupta SP. Epidemiological study of coronary heart disease in rural community in Haryana. Indian Heart J. 1974;26:68-78.
23. Jajoo UN, Kalantri SP, Gupta OP, et al. The prevalence of coronary heart disease in rural population from central India. J Assoc Physicians India. 1988;36:689-93.
24. Chadha SL, Gopinath N, Radhakrishnan S, et al. Prevalence of coronary heart disease and its risk factors in a rural community in Haryana. Indian J Comm Med. 1989;14:141-7.
25. Kutty VR, Balakrishnan KG, Jayasree AK, et al. Prevalence of coronary heart disease in the rural population of Thiruvananthapuram district, Kerala, India. Int J Cardiol. 1993;39:59-70.
26. Wander GS, Khurana SB, Gulati R, et al. Epidemiology of coronary heart disease in a rural Punjab population– prevalence and correlation with various risk factors. Indian Heart J. 1994;46:319-23.
27. Gupta R, Gupta VP, Ahluwalia NS. Educational status, coronary heart disease, and coronary risk factor prevalence in a rural population of India. BMJ. 1994;309:1332-6.
28. Kumar R, Singh MC, Singh MC, et al. Urbanization and coronary heart disease: a study of urban-rural differences in northern India. Indian Heart J. 2006;58: 126-30.
29. Chow C, Cardona M, Raju PK, et al. Cardiovascular disease and risk factors among 345 adults in rural India–the Andhra Pradesh Rural Health Initiative. Int J Cardiol. 2007;116:180-5.
30. Gupta R, Joshi P, Mohan V, et al. Epidemiology and causation of coronary heart disease and stroke in India. Heart. 2008;94:16-26.
31. Praveen PA, Roy A, Anand K, et al. Rising prevalence of coronary heart disease (CHD) in urban Delhi, India-results from a repeat cross-sectional study. Eur Heart J. 2013;34(suppl 1):470.
32. Gupta R. Recent trends in coronary heart disease epidemiology in India. Indian Heart J. 2008;60(2 suppl B):B4-18.
33. Prabhakaran D, Yusuf S, Mehta S, et al. Two-year outcomes in patients admitted with non-ST elevation acute coronary syndrome: results of the OASIS registry 1 and 2. Indian Heart J. 2005;57:217-25.
34. Giovino GA, Mirza SA, Samet JM, et al. Tobacco use in 3 billion individuals from 16 countries: an analysis of nationally representative cross-sectional household surveys. Lancet. 2012;380:668-79.
35. Ministry of statistics and programme implementation. (2013). SARRC Development Goals-India Country Report [online]. Available from http://mospi.nic.in/mospi_new/upload/SAARC_Development_Goals_%20India_ Country_Report_29aug13.pdf [Accessed August 2018].
36. Ramachandran P. The Double Burden of Malnutrition in India. Food and Agriculture Organization; 2006.
37. Anjana RM, Pradeepa R, Das AK, et al. Physical activity and inactivity patterns in India – results from the ICMR-INDIAB study (Phase-1) [ICMR-INDIAB-5]. Int J Behav Nutr Phys Act. 2014;11:26.
38. Anchala R, Kannuri NK, Pant H, et al. Hypertension in India: a systematic review and meta-analysis of prevalence, awareness, and control of hypertension. J Hypertens. 2014;32:1170-7.
39. Danaei G, Finucane MM, Lin JK, et al. Global Burden of Metabolic Risk Factors of Chronic Diseases Collaborating Group (Blood Pressure). National, regional, and global trends in systolic blood pressure since 1980: systematic analysis of health examination surveys and epidemiological studies with 786 country-years and 5.4 million participants. Lancet. 2011;377:568-77.
40. Chow CK, Teo KK, Rangarajan S, et al. Prevalence, awareness, treatment, and control of hypertension in rural and urban communities in high-, middle-, and low-income countries. JAMA. 2013;310:959-68.
41. Gupta R, Guptha S, Sharma KK, et al. Regional variations in cardiovascular risk factors in India: India heart watch. World J Cardiol. 2012;4:112-20.
42. Gupta R, Guptha S, Agrawal A, et al. Secular trends in cholesterol lipoproteins and triglycerides and prevalence of dyslipidemias in an urban Indian population. Lipids Health Dis. 2008;7:40.
43. Joshi SR, Anjana RM, Deepa M, et al. Prevalence of dyslipidemia in urban and rural India: the ICMR-INDIAB study. PLoS One. 2014;9:e96808.

44. Chandola T. Ethnic and class differences in health in relation to British South Asians: using the new National Statistics Socio-Economic Classification. Soc Sci Med. 2001;52:1285-96.
45. Kutty VR, Thankappan KR, Kannan KP, et al. How socioeconomic status affects birth and death rates in rural Kerala, India: results of a health study. Int J Health Serv. 1993;23:373-86.
46. Anjana RM, Ali MK, Pradeepa R, et al. The need for obtaining accurate nationwide estimates of diabetes prevalence in India – rationale for a national study on diabetes. Indian J Med Res. 2011;133:369-80.
47. Gupta R, Kaul V, Agrawal A, et al. Cardiovascular risk according to educational status in India. Prev Med. 2010;51:408-11.
48. Jeemon P. Socio-economic status and cardiovascular risk among Indians. Prev Med. 2011;52:471-2.
49. Sharma R, Bhairappa S, Prasad SR, et al. Clinical characteristics, angiographic profile and in hospital mortality in acute Coronary syndrome patients in south Indian population. Heart India. 2014;2(3).
50. Karthikeyan G, Teo KK, Islam S, et al. Lipid profile, plasma apolipoproteins, and risk of a first myocardial infarction among Asians: an analysis from the INTERHEART Study. J Am Coll Cardiol. 2009;53(3):244-53.
51. Pagidipati NJ, Huffman D, Jeemon P, et al. Association between gender, process of care measures, and outcomes in ACS in India: results from the detection and management of coronary heart disease (DEMAT) registry. PLoS One. 2013;8(4):e6206.
52. Negi PC, Merwaha R, Paday D. Multicentre HP ACS registry. Indian Heart J. 2015;07-27.
53. Iqbal F, Barkataki JC. Spectrum of acute coronary syndrome in North Eastern India: a study from a major center. Indian Heart J. 2013;68:128-31.
54. Mohanan PP, Mathew R, Harikrishnan S, et al. Presentation, management, and outcomes of 25 748 acute coronary syndrome admissions in Kerala, India: results from the Kerala ACS Registry. Eur Heart J. 2013;34(2):121-9.
55. Brindis RG, Fitzgerald G, Anderson HV, et al. The American college of cardiology-National cardiovascular data registry: building a national clinical data repository. J Am Coll Cardiol. 2001;37(8):2240–5.
56. Mandelzweig L, Battler A, Boyko V, et al. The second Euro Heart Survey on acute coronary syndromes: characteristics, treatment, and outcome of patients with ACS in Europe and the Mediterranean Basin in 2004. Eur Heart J. 2006;27(19):2285-93.
57. Fox KA, Goodman SG, Klein W, et al. Management of acute coronary syndromes. Variations in practice and outcome: findings from the global registry of acute coronary events (GRACE). Eur Heart J. 2002;23:1177-89.
58. Allen LA, O'Donnell CJ, Giugliano RP, et al. Care concordant with guidelines predicts decreased long-term mortality in patients with unstable angina pectoris and non-ST elevation myocardial infarction. Am J Cardiol. 2004;93(10):1218-22.
59. Daivadanam M, Thankappan KR, Sarma PS, et al. Catastrophic health expenditure & coping strategies associated with acute coronary syndrome in Kerala, India. Indian J Med Res. 2012;136:585-94.
60. Gupta R, Misra A, Vikram NK, et al. Younger age of escalation of cardiovascular risk factors in Asian Indian subjects. BMC Cardiovasc Disord. 2009;9:28.
61. Isezuo S, Subban V, Krishnamoorthy J, et al. Characteristics, treatment and one-year outcomes of patients with acute coronary syndrome in a tertiary hospital in India. Indian Heart J. 2014;66:156-63.
62. Misiriya KJ, Sudhayakumar N, Khadar SA, et al. The clinical spectrum of acute coronary syndromes: experience from a major center in Kerala. J Phys Assoc Physicians India. 2009;57:377-83.
63. Patel A, Vishwanathan S, Nair T, et al. Sex Differences in the Presentation, Diagnosis, and Management of Acute Coronary Syndromes findings from the Kerala (India) ACS Registry. Glob Heart. 2015;10(4):273-80.
64. Peterson ED, Roe MT, Mulgund J, et al. Association between hospital process performance and outcomes among patients with acute coronary syndromes. JAMA. 2006;295:1912-20.
65. Roe MT, Messenger JC, Weintraub WS, et al. Treatments, trends, and outcomes of acute myocardial infarction and percutaneous coronary intervention. J Am Coll Cardiol. 2010;56:254-63.
66. Hasdai D, Behar S, Wallentin L, et al. A prospective survey of the characteristics, treatments and outcomes of patients with acute coronary syndromes in Europe and the Mediterranean basin; the Euro Heart Survey of Acute Coronary Syndromes (Euro Heart survey ACS). Eur Heart J. 2002;23:1190-201.
67. Dragana R, Rene' S, Markus S, et al (for the AMIS Plus Investigators). Outcome of patients with acute coronary syndrome in hospitals of different sizes. Swiss Med Wkly. 2010;140:314 e322.
68. Huffman MD, Rao KD, Pichon-Riviere A, et al. A cross-sectional study of the microeconomic impact of cardiovascular disease hospitalization in four low- and middle-income countries. PLoS One. 2011;6:e20821.
69. Mendis S, Abegunde D, Yusuf S, et al. WHO study on prevention of recurrences of myocardial infarction and stroke (WHO-PREMISE). Bull World Health Organ. 2005;83:820-9.
70. Arshad S, Dhakam S, Awan S. Outcomes in ST Elevation Myocardial Infarction; a comparison of a tertiary care center in Pakistan with European centers. J Pak Med Assoc. 2011;61:1215.
71. Awad HH, Zubaid M, Alsheikh-Ali AA, et al. Comparison of characteristics, management practices, and outcomes of patients between the global registry and the Gulf Registry of Acute Coronary Events. Am J Cardiol. 2011;108:1252-8.
72. Constantinides SS, Gieowarsingh S, Halim M, et al. Predictors of mortality in patients with acute coronary syndrome undergoing percutaneous coronary intervention. Heart. 2003;89:1245-6.
73. Filippo O, Marcello G, Francesca AN, et al. Elevated cardiac troponin levels predict the risk of adverse outcome in patients with acute coronary syndromes. Am Heart J. 2000;140:917-27.
74. Armstrong PW, Gershlick AH, Goldstein P, et al. Fibrinolysis or Primary PCI in ST-Segment Elevation Myocardial Infarction. N Engl J Med. 2013;368:1379-87.
75. Jernberg T, Johanson P, Held C, et al. Association between adoption of evidence-based treatment and survival for patients with ST-elevation myocardial infarction. JAMA. 2011;305:1677-84.
76. Razzak JA, Kellermann AL. Emergency medical care in developing countries: is it worthwhile? Bull World Health Organ. 2002;80(11):900-5.
77. Victor SM, Subban V, Alexander T, et al. A prospective, observational, multicentre study comparing tenecteplase facilitated PCI versus primary PCI in Indian patients with STEMI (STEPP —AMI). Open Heart. 2014;1:e000133.

CHAPTER 42

Choosing Fibrinolytics in STEMI: Economics over Efficacy?

Mullasari S Ajit, Meenakshi MS

INTRODUCTION

Since the first description of angina pectoris by Herbeden in 1772[1] to our current understanding of the genetic and molecular basis of coronary artery disease, the pathways of discovery, innovation, and therapeutic advancements have been truly remarkable. The fibrinolytic property of streptokinase (SK) was established in 1933 by William Tillet and Garner,[2] but the intravenous use of SK for clot resolution began in the 1980s. The breakthrough in the management of ST-elevation myocardial infarction (STEMI) patients was in 1986 when the GISSI I (Gruppo Italiano per lo Studio della Streptochinasi nell'Infarto Miocardico) trial, the first large randomized trial, showed that intravenous thrombolytic therapy with SK improved survival. The antigenicity and less fibrin specificity of SK were undesirable properties, which prompted interest in finding other potential fibrinolytic agents such as tissue plasminogen activator (t-PA).

Choosing fibrinolytics in STEMI—economics over efficacy? The answer is definitely efficacy. But what in the Indian scenario? We have multiple tiers of healthcare systems, variable strata of population with different economical status. We do not have a common protocol of coronary care management from community to tertiary care level across the country and a universal comprehensive government insurance policy for all. Hence, we need to consider the economics in the poor and uninsured patients.

IMPORTANCE OF EARLY REVASCULARIZATION

Evidence from several randomized controlled trials (RCTs) shows that early revascularization, whether primary percutaneous coronary intervention (PPCI) or fibrinolysis, decreases the infarct size, preserves left ventricular function, and improves survival rates. PPCI has been proved to be the gold standard in achieving better thrombolysis in myocardial infarction III (TIMI III) flow and improved survival,[3] when done with a door to balloon time of less than 90 minutes.[4] But this can be achieved in only 10% of the Indian population.[5] Early reperfusion with thrombolysis is a good and feasible option in a developing country like India where PPCI is not possible for most of the patients.[6]

Data from the CREATE[5] registry, a large prospective registry of acute coronary syndrome patients across major cities of India, shows that 60% of patients had STEMI (compared to 40% in developed countries) and the median time from onset of symptoms to hospital arrival was 300 minutes (140–170 minutes in developed countries). Among them, 59% received fibrinolytic therapy with a time interval of 50 minutes to undergo fibrinolysis after reaching the hospital and 9% underwent PCI during their hospitalization. The initial delay is by the patient due to lack of awareness, lack of access, lack of transfer facilities, and lack of knowledge about PCI capable centers.

PHARMACOINVASIVE STRATEGY

The pharmacoinvasive (PI) approach is gaining momentum in recent years. The STREAM trial (strategic reperfusion early after myocardial infarction) showed that a strategy involving early fibrinolysis with bolus tenecteplase (TNK) and adjunctive pharmacotherapy followed by PCI offers similar efficacy as PPCI in patients with STEMI who presented within 3 hours of symptom onset and who could not undergo PPCI within 1 hour of first medical contact (FMC). At 1 year, the combined endpoint of death, shock, reinfarction, and stroke did not show difference in both arms. The FAST-MI (French registry of Acute ST-elevation and non-ST-elevation Myocardial Infarction) study from France also showed lower 5-year mortality in the PI arm.

The STEPP-AMI[7] trial, a prospective, observational, multi centric trial from India evaluated the efficacy of early fibrinolytic treatment with TNK followed by PCI (pharmacoinvasive) in patients presenting within 3–24 hours compared to PPCI and concluded that PI strategy was safe, with 80% patency of infarct related artery (IRA), lower thrombus burden and better TIMI III flows at the time of the procedure and the outcomes were comparable with PPCI at 1 year.

FIBRINOLYTIC DRUGS—CLASSIFICATION AND COMPARISON

The available fibrinolytics (Table 1) are classified based on fibrin specificity. The commonly used fibrinolytics are compared in table 2. Thrombolysis can be initiated by the activation of the endogenous fibrinolytic system. The plasminogen activators convert plasminogen to plasmin, which degrades fibrin, a major constituent of clots. The fibrin-specific agents such as t-PA and its derivatives act in the presence of fibrin and do not induce a systemic lytic state but the less fibrin-specific agent such as streptokinase (SK) activates plasminogen irrespective of its association with fibrin and leads to degradation of fibrinogen, plasminemia, and depletion of coagulation factors.

Although by definition fibrinolytic therapy dissolves thrombus, paradoxically, the thrombin released from clot lysis may be prothrombotic as well.[8] SK induces thromboxane (TXA2) synthesis and activates platelets, particularly in the presence of high titers of anti-SK antibodies.[9] These may be the factors associated with increased reocclusion rates and adjunctive therapy with antiplatelets, anticoagulants, and GP IIb/IIIa inhibitors helps in maintaining IRA patency rates and prevent ischemic complications during PCI.

The platelet activation and platelet aggregation inhibition varies with different lytic agents, which warrants further studies on the optimum timing of PCI after thrombolysis. The optimal time would be theoretically, one when there is less prothrombotic effect and less bleeding. The platelet activation inhibition of newer fibrinolytics persists for 2 hours and that for SK persists for almost 12 hours.[8] For practical purposes as per guideline recommendation, the optimal timing for PCI after newer fibrinolytics is 3 hours[3,8] and the radial route is preferred.

EFFICACY OF FIBRINOLYTICS—BASED ON TRIALS

Streptokinase

The GISSI 1 trial and the International Study of Infarct Survival (ISIS) trials firmly established the efficacy of intravenous SK in acute myocardial infarction (AMI). In the GISSI trial, at 21 days there was 18% reduction in mortality following SK compared to the control group. The extent of the benefit was related to the time of onset of chest pain to SK infusion [risk ratio (RR) 0.74, 0.80, 0.87, and 1.19 for the 0–3, 3–6, 6–9 and 9–12 hours subgroups]. In ISIS-2 trial, patients with AMI randomized to SK and aspirin compared with neither treatment resulted in significant reduction not only in death (8% vs. 13.2%), but also stroke (0.6% vs. 1.1%) and reinfarction (1.8% vs. 2.9%). The GISSI trial marked the beginning of early revascularization in STEMI.

Alteplase

The Global Use of Strategies to Open Occluded Coronary Arteries (GUSTO), GISSI, and ISIS investigators compared intravenous SK and t-PA in STEMI patients. Although no significant difference was observed between SK and t-PA in GISSI-2 and ISIS-3, the GUSTO trial demonstrated that an accelerated regimen of t-PA resulted in 14% reduction in mortality at 30 days and slight excess of hemorrhagic stroke. The phase-I TIMI trial demonstrated that alteplase resulted in reperfusion of twice as many occluded IRA compared with SK at 90 minutes.

Reteplase

Reteplase (r-PA) compared to accelerated alteplase infusion demonstrated no significant benefit in terms of reduction in 30-day mortality in GUSTO III trial. r-PA + abciximab did not provide significant benefit in 30 day survival in the GUSTO V trial. However a double dose r-PA (10 + 10 MU) utilized in the revitalising areas by planning, investment and development (RAPID) trial resulted in complete, rapid and sustained thrombolysis of IRA at 90 minutes and at 5–14 days (63% vs. 49%, p = 0.019; and 88% vs. 71%, p <0.001) compared with alteplase and improved regional and global left ventricular function at discharge. The RAPID II trial further confirmed the advantage of r-PA over accelerated t-PA in achieving higher rates of early reperfusion in the IRA and fewer coronary interventions. This, however, did not translate into improved clinical outcomes in the International Joint Efficacy Comparison of Thrombolytics (INJECT) trial, which demonstrated no significant difference between r-PA and SK in reducing 35-day mortality.

Tenecteplase

A single bolus TNK increased IRA patency rates (64% TIMI III flow with 50 mg bolus dose) in the TIMI 10A trial. In the TIMI 10B trial, TNK (40 mg) and alteplase produced similar rates of TIMI grade 3 flow at 90 minutes (62.8% vs. 62.7%, respectively, P = NS). Subsequently, the Assessment of the Safety and Efficacy of a New Thrombolytic (ASSENT-1) trial

TABLE 1: Available fibrinolytics

	Fibrin specific	Nonfibrin specific
First generation	–	Streptokinase* Urokinase
Second generation	Tissue plasminogen activator	Pro-urokinase (saruplase)
Third generation	• Alteplase* • Reteplase* • Tenecteplase* • Lanoteplase • Monteplase • Pamiteplase • Staphylokinase • Desmoteplase	APSAC (anistreplase)

*commonly used and clinically approved fibrinolytic agents.

TABLE 2: Comparison of frequently used fibrinolytics

	Tenecteplase (TNK)	Reteplase (r-PA)	Alteplase (t-PA)	Streptokinase (SK)
Dose	Single IV weight Based bolus$	10U+10U IV 30 minutes apart	90 minute weight based infusion¢	1.5 million units over 30–60 minutes
Plasminogen activation	Direct	Direct	Direct	Indirect
Fibrin specificity	++++	++	++	No
Fibrinogen depletion	Minimal	Moderate	Mild	Marked
Activity on platelet rich clot	+++	+	++	--
Antigenic	No	No	No	Yes
Half-life (min)	20	16	4	20
Resistance to PAI-I	Yes	No	No	No
Intracranial hemorrhage§	0.7%	0.6%	0.7%	0.4%
Cost (rupees)€	45,000	25,000–35,000	50,000	2,000–4,000
Patency at 90 minute	++++	++++	+++	+
TIMI 2 or 3 flow (%)	63%	60%	54%	32%

$Bolus of 30 mg for weight less than 60 kg, 35 mg for 60–69 kg, 40 mg for 70–79 kg, 45 mg for 80–89 kg and 50 mg for 90 kg or greater.
¢Accelerated infusion with bolus of 15 mg followed by infusion of 0.75 mg/kg for 30 minutes, then 0.5 mg/kg (maximum 35 mg) over next 60 minutes, total dose not to exceed 100 mg.
€Cost in Indian rupees. Range of cost given depending on the various brands available.
§Intracranial hemorrhage is based on the presence of multiple risk factors. Based on many studies, the common risk factors include elderly, low body weight, and hypertension.

showed that the safety profile of TNK was comparable to alteplase. Assessment of the Safety and Efficacy of a New Thrombolytic (ASSENT-2) trial compared single-bolus TNK with accelerated dose t-PA and the 30-day mortality rate was 6.17% vs. 6.15%, intracranial hemorrhage (ICH) was 0.93% and 0.94%, major bleeding occurred in 4.66% and 5.94% (p = 0.0002). There was no specific subgroup of patients for whom TNK or t-PA was significantly better, except patients treated after 4 hours of symptom onset, in whom the mortality rate was 7.0% with TNK and 9.2% with t-PA. Furthermore, the ASSENT-3 trial demonstrated that the addition of enoxaparin to TNK reduced ischemic complications at the cost of increased bleeding.

CHOICE OF FIBRINOLYTIC IN ST-ELEVATION MYOCARDIAL INFARCTION

Early revascularization and establishing flow is very important in salvaging the myocardium in AMI. The TN-STEMI project with the "hub-and-spoke" model-of-care showed the importance of "any" form of early reperfusion after symptom onset followed by early coronary intervention. In south India, this model of system of care resulted in 3.4% absolute reduction in mortality at the end of 1 year in 2,167 patients. The majority of this difference was in the spoke centers (3.3% mortality reduction compared to only 1.1% in the hub centers), mainly due to early transfer to PCI centers with or without fibrinolysis.[10]

Multiple trials showed evidence for safety and efficacy of one drug over the other. The PI trials such as STREAM, CARESS-AMI, TRANSFER-AMI, and STEPP-AMI used mainly TNK as the fibrinolytic agent and showed better patency rates of IRA and the MACCE rates in the PI group with TNK as compared to the primary PCI group. The greater convenience, simplicity in dosing, ease and speed of administration make TNK as the fibrinolytic of choice in all patients, in most situations.

But in the real world situation, cost and availability of bolus fibrinolytics is a major concern thus refocusing on SK. The circulating high titers of anti SK antibodies[11,12] in endemic tropical countries, like India, leads to increased hypotension and allergic reactions and may be the cause for more reocclusion rates with standard dose of SK. But the recent subgroup analysis of the PI arm of the TN-STEMI[13] program showed that, in the 94% of the patients in the PI arm who had thrombolysis with SK followed by a system of care, the postimplementation group of systems of care as compared to the preimplementation group, showed improved IRA patency (86% vs. 70.2%; p <0.001), better TIMI 3 flow (25.4% vs. 37.5%; p = 0.027), and less thrombus burden (49.1% vs. 73.4%; p <0.001), translating into lower target revascularization and fewer admissions in the PI arm. The mortality, reinfarction and stroke, in the postimplementation PI group with SK was comparable to that with newer fibrinolytics. The 2013 consensus statement for early reperfusion and PI approach in Indian STEMI patients, suggested that the choice of fibrinolytic is TNK (LOE Grade 1A), reteplase (LOE Grade 1B) and alteplase (LOE Grade 1C), and SK is used only when a fibrin-specific agent is not available or unaffordable (LOE Grade 2B).[14]

Reteplase and TNK are given as bolus agents making it suitable for prehospital fibrinolysis at community level or in the ambulance, whereas SK and alteplase given over 1 hour infusion, make it suitable for in-hospital use, rather than at community level. In patients, presenting within 4 hours of symptom onset, the speed of reperfusion is important and TNK is the preferred agent, which acts quickly with bolus dose and has high patency rates. In those presenting after 4 hours of symptom onset, with lower risk of death, MI involving small territory and high risk of ICH (e.g., acute hypertension), SK, accelerated t-PA, reteplase, and TNK have approximately equivalent outcomes.

Rural patients with prolonged transport time to PCI capable centers or patients in urban setting where delay in transfer is expected due to distance or heavy traffic congestion, bolus fibrinolytics are preferred at community level. Patients reaching PCI capable or noncapable centers, in whom a door to balloon time of less than 90 minutes cannot be achieved due to prolonged transfer times, nonavailability of cath laboratory or manpower or financial issues may be thrombolyzed with bolus fibrinolytic agents. Patients not affordable for bolus fibrinolytics may be thrombolyzed with SK before prompt shifting to PCI capable centers.

CONCLUSION

Tenecteplase with its ease of dosing, speed of administration, and better patency rates, is the default choice of fibrinolytic in STEMI patients. But SK, reteplase, or alteplase may be chosen according to the availability, affordability, and physician's choice and experience. The goal of early revascularization with primary PCI, or thrombolysis with any fibrinolytic drug, should be initiated within 90 minutes or 30 minutes of FMC, respectively. Thrombolysis should be followed by transfer to PCI capable center as early as possible, which would be the practical approach in managing STEMI patients in low- and middle-income countries, like India. The government should provide a universal system of care for STEMI patients, with primary PCI and bolus fibrinolytics made available for all, across the country, at affordable costs.

REFERENCES

1. Heberden W. Some account of a disorder of the breast. Medical Transactions. 1772;2:59-67.
2. Tillett WS, Garner RL. The fibrinolytic activity of hemolytic streptococci. J Exp Med. 1933;58:485-502.
3. O'Gara PT, Kushner FG, Ascheim DD, et al. ACCF/AHA guideline for the management of ST-elevation myocardial infarction: executive summary. J Am Coll Cardiol. 2013;61(4):485-510.
4. Nallamothu BK, Antman EM, Bates ER. Primary percutaneous coronary intervention versus fibrinolytic therapy in acute myocardial infarction: does the choice of fibrinolytic agent impact on the importance of time-to-treatment? Am J Cardiol. 2004;94:772-4.
5. Xavier D, Pais P, Devereaux PJ, et al. Treatment and outcomes of acute coronary syndromes in India (CREATE): a prospective analysis of registry data. Lancet. 2008;371:1435-42.
6. Alexander T, Mehta S, Mullasari A, et al. Systems of care for ST-elevation myocardial infarction in India. Heart. 2012;98(1):15-7.
7. Victor SM, Subban V, Alexander T, et al. A prospective, observational, multicentre study comparing tenecteplase facilitated PCI versus primary PCI in Indian patients with STEMI (STEPP-AMI). Open Heart. 2014;1:e000133.
8. Moser M, Nordt T, Peter K, et al. Platelet Function During and After Thrombolytic Therapy for Acute Myocardial Infarction With Reteplase, Alteplase, or Streptokinase. Circulation. 1999;100:1858-64.
9. Vaughan DE, Houtte EV, Declerck PJ, et al. Streptokinase-Induced Platelet Aggregation Prevalence and Mechanism. Circulation. 1991;84:84-91.
10. Alexander T, Mullasari AS, Joseph G, et al. A system of care for patients with ST-Segment elevation myocardial infarction in India: the Tamil Nadu-ST-Segment elevation myocardial infarction program. JAMA Cardiol. 2017;2(5):498-505.
11. Alexander T, Krishnaswami S, Kanduri S. Anti-streptokinase levels in Indian patients. Int J Cardiol. 1991;32:361-4.
12. Subhendu MS, George OK, Prakash JA. Antistreptokinase antibodies and the response to thrombolysis with streptokinase in patients with acute ST elevation myocardial infarction. Heart Asia. 2012;4(1):7-10.
13. Raja DC, Subban V, Victor SM, et al. The impact of systems-of-care on pharmacoinvasive management with streptokinase: The sub-group analysis of the TN-STEMI Programme. Indian Heart J. 2017;69:573-9.
14. Dalal JJ, Alexander T, Banerjee PS, et al.; Cardiocare STEMI experts. 2013 Consensus statement for early reperfusion and pharmaco-invasive approach in patients presenting with chest pain diagnosed as STEMI (ST elevation myocardial infarction) in an Indian Setting Developed in collaboration with STEMI India. J Assoc Phys India. 2014:62.

CHAPTER 43

Routine PCI after IV Thrombolysis—Is it Ready for Prime Time?

Lekha Pathak, Ankur Jhavar

INTRODUCTION

Currently, patients who present with ST-segment elevation myocardial infarction (STEMI), their management involves critical timed decision in every aspect of care including primary reperfusion strategy, triage and timely transfer to a percutaneous coronary intervention (PCI) capable tertiary center. At present, other ideal alternative option for STEMI patients residing in remote areas where primary PCI is not available is fibrinolytic therapy. Unlike unstable angina/non-ST-segment elevation myocardial infarction (UA/NSTEMI), STEMI is mostly characterized by total occlusion of the infarct-related artery.

Current STEMI 2017 guidelines[1] involve time slab of 120 minutes to reach to PCI capable center. If expected time delay is more, fibrinolysis (unless contraindicated) should be instituted. Complete reperfusion with reduced morbidity and mortality is desired outcome of any modality of therapy for STEMI patients. Timely reperfusion has gained superior importance than complete or near-complete reperfusion. Time has been given crucial importance when considering which reperfusion therapy approach is to be used.

Final infarct size is one of the best predictor of long-term adverse events in STEMI survivors. The introduction of a specific infarct-limiting therapy in clinical practice might have a massive clinical and socioeconomic impact. Primary angioplasty is considered gold standard, although multiple conditions attenuated superior result in India, some of them being skilled operator, economical and logistical factors, and well-equipped catheterization laboratories. If primary PCI takes more than 120 minutes from diagnosis, associated with higher mortality even in well-developed centers, they achieve mechanical reopening of infarct-related artery without much benefit. In India, 70% of patients with acute myocardial infarction (AMI) present in non-PCI centers. Instituting reperfusion therapy as early as possible is crucial. It is proposed that if fibrinolytic therapy is part of the primary reperfusion strategy, a strategy of routine or adjunctive PCI is superior to rescue or selective ischemia-guided PCI with respect to adverse events. This approach is popularly known as pharmacoinvasive strategy.[2]

STRATEGY CLOCK IN STEMI

The short- and long-term prognosis of STEMI patients depends not only on reperfusion but also with time delay for initiation of treatment. Prehospital delay has been considered as marker for increased morbidity and mortality; however, the benefit is highly dependent on the time between the onset of symptoms and start of reperfusion therapy.[3,4]

Although primary PCI is unequivocally superior to thrombolysis, the time to revascularization is still better marker of overall outcome. In meta-analysis of six randomized trials, prehospital thrombolysis has shown to shorten the time from symptom onset to treatment by 60 minutes with 17% reduction in the overall mortality.[5] Data from CAPTIM (Comparison of primary Angioplasty and Prehospital fibrinolysis In acute Myocardial infarction) and WEST (Which Early ST-elevation myocardial infarction Therapy) trials, have suggested mortality benefit with prehospital thrombolysis for early presenters. The absolute survival benefit of angioplasty compared with fibrinolysis decreased by 0.24% for every additional 10-minute delay.[6] PCI remained superior to fibrinolysis when time delay related to PCI extended to 120 minutes. Life saved by reperfusion per 1,000 treated patients is 65, 27, 25 and 8 when performed at 1 hour, 2–3 hours, 4–6 hours and 7–12 hours, respectively.[7]

TREATMENT DELAY IN STEMI

Apart from prehospital delay, other type of delay is health system-related delay, i.e., between first medical contact (FMC) to reperfusion treatment which is always a major concern. Health system-related delay directly correlates with increased mortality in STEMI patients as a rule "time is muscle" considering STEMI patients. Challenges to institution of early primary PCI include economical support, geographical area, trained cardiologist as well as other medical staff and well-equipped catheterization laboratories. Practical application of STEMI guidelines is very difficult and many times not been fulfilled by many centers.

REPERFUSION STRATEGIES

Fibrinolysis

Nine landmark trials by the Fibrinolytic Therapy Trialists' Collaborative Group[8] compared the outcomes of patients undergoing fibrinolytic therapy and those of controls and demonstrated statistically significant absolute reduction in 35-day mortality rates of approximately 30 per 1,000 for patients who arrived at the hospital within 6 hours of the onset of symptoms (Table 1). The greatest benefit was observed among patients with left bundle branch block (LBBB) or anterior STEMI.

Fibrinolytic therapy is currently indicated for patients with STEMI who have experienced symptom onset within the previous 12 hours and in whom electrocardiography (ECG) demonstrates ST-segment elevation of more than 0.1 mV in at least two contiguous precordial leads or at least two adjacent limb leads or new LBBB. The fibrinolytic agents currently approved for treating patients with STEMI include streptokinase, alteplase, reteplase, and tenecteplase. The thrombolysis in myocardial infarction (TIMI), phase 1 trial randomly assigned 290 patients with evolving AMI to alteplase or to streptokinase. Alteplase was far superior in achieving coronary reperfusion; twice as many occluded infarct-related arteries opened after 90 minutes with alteplase than with streptokinase. Assessment of the Safety of a New Thrombolytic (ASSENT)-2 trial,[9] randomly assigned 16,949 patients to weight based single-bolus tenecteplase or to accelerated alteplase infusion. The 30-day mortality rates were virtually identical. Tenecteplase has become the most widely used fibrin-specific agent because of advantage of single bolus dosing. If the reperfusion strategy is fibrinolysis, the goal is to inject the bolus of fibrinolytic within 10 minutes from STEMI diagnosis. This time is selected based on the median time from randomization to bolus recorded in the Strategic Reperfusion Early After Myocardial Infarction (STREAM) trial, which was 9 minutes.

TABLE 1: Important time targets in acute ST-segment elevation myocardial infarction (STEMI)

Intervals	Time targets
Maximum time from first medical contact (FMC) to electrocardiography (ECG) and diagnosis[a]	≤10 min
Maximum expected delay from STEMI diagnosis to primary percutaneous coronary intervention (PCI) (wire crossing) to choose primary PCI strategy over fibrinolysis (if this target time cannot be met, consider fibrinolysis)	≤120 min
Maximum time from STEMI diagnosis to wire crossing in patients presenting at primary PCI hospitals	≤60 min
Maximum time from STEMI diagnosis to wire crossing in transferred patients	≤90 min
Maximum time from STEMI diagnosis to bolus or infusion start of fibrinolysis in patients unable to meet primary PCI target times	≤10 min
Time delay from start of fibrinolysis to evaluation of its efficacy (success or failure)	60–90 min
Time delay from start of fibrinolysis to angiography (if fibrinolysis is successful)	2–24 hours

[a]ECG should be interpreted immediately.

Primary Percutaneous Coronary Intervention

Twenty-three randomized clinical trials[10] compared primary angioplasty in myocardial infarction (PAMI) with fibrinolytic therapy and demonstrated that PAMI was better than fibrinolysis in reducing the incidence of short-term and long-term adverse outcomes, including death. It was found that patients undergoing PAMI, increases in the door-to-balloon time (especially by >2 hours) were associated with higher mortality rates.

Selection of either fibrinolysis or PAMI as the appropriate reperfusion strategy should depend on the clinical scenario. Primary PCI is generally preferable if it is rapidly available because it yields better outcome than fibrinolysis. The effectiveness of both fibrinolytic therapy and PAMI diminishes with the passage of time. Thus, PCI is generally preferred for patients who arrive at the hospital late after the onset of symptoms (>3 hours). Early initiation of fibrinolytic therapy may lead to outcomes that are similar to or better than those achieved with PCI.

Routine PCI after Fibrinolytic Treatment (Facilitated PCI)

This approach involves fibrinolysis followed by early and mandatory PCI. This procedure tries to improve patency by fibrinolysis before performing PCI. Potential advantages of this approach include earlier time to reperfusion, smaller infarct size, better patient stability, lower infarct artery thrombus burden, and greater procedural success rate. However, higher mortality was seen with this approach mostly due to stent restenosis rather than bleeding complications. Firstly, the prothrombotic circumstance caused by short application of fibrinolytic agents may have limited the benefit of PCI. Secondly, fibrinolytic agent would soften the fresh thrombus and divide them into small pieces. Thirdly, the differences in time of reperfusion may affect first 2 hours after the onset of infarction, and the time interval can hardly be met in many of the included studies which enrolled patients with less than 12 hours, 6 hours or 3 hours of symptom onset. Therefore, the time-dependency of PCI-mediated salvage may be considerably attenuated.[11]

Rescue Percutaneous Coronary Intervention

In this approach, those patients who suffer failed thrombolysis are treated with emergency PCI to salvage jeopardized myocardium. Failed thrombolysis usually manifests as persistent ischemic symptoms, hemodynamic instability and failure to achieve 50–70% resolution of maximal ST-segment elevation at 90 minutes after initiation of infusion. This approach was proved to be more effective than repeat thrombolysis.

Pharmacoinvasive Strategy

Recently, a strategy of combining fibrinolysis followed by transfer for early PCI ("pharmacoinvasive PCI") has been shown to be an effective reperfusion strategy for STEMI patients presenting to non-PCI hospitals compared with fibrinolysis alone. In contrast to facilitated PCI, this approach includes PCI which follows fibrinolysis after some delay so that early prothrombotic phase would get resolved preventing the increased incidence of stent restenosis. This strategy aims at reduction of mortality seen with facilitated PCI.

Pharmacoinvasive strategy consists of administration of fibrinolysis at a non-PCI center followed by immediate transfer to a PCI-capable hospital for routine early catheterization performed within 2–24 hours of start of fibrinolytic therapy, regardless of whether thrombolysis results in successful reperfusion or not. Thus, the time to PCI is longer than with facilitated PCI.[12]

In the recent past, several clinical trials and patient registries using pharmacoinvasive strategy [GRACIA-2[13] (Grupo de Análisis de la Cardiopatía Isquémica Aguda) TRANSFER-AMI[14] (Trial of Routine Angioplasty and Stenting after Fibrinolysis to Enhance Reperfusion in Acute Myocardial Infarction), FAST-MI (French Registry of Acute ST-elevation or Non-ST-elevation Myocardial Infarction),[15] WEST[16]] have demonstrated mortality that is comparable to that documented with primary PCI. These trials reinforced that pharmacologic regimen rapidly delivered, coupled with routine coronary intervention within 24 hours of initial treatment, may not be different from timely expert PCI.

Gracia-2 Trial[13]

This trial (n = 212) compared full tenecteplase followed by stenting within 3–12 hours of randomization (early routine post-fibrinolysis angioplasty; 104 patients) with primary stenting with abciximab within 3 hours of randomization (primary angioplasty; 108 patients) compared primary versus facilitated angioplasty. All patients received clopidogrel, aspirin and enoxaparin to prevent reocclusion. The results showed that early routine post-fibrinolysis angioplasty resulted in higher frequency of complete epicardial and myocardial reperfusion following angioplasty. Thus, the pharmacoinvasive approach was equivalent to primary PCI despite performance of a delayed PCI.

Transfer-AMI Trial[14]

This study was conducted in Canada in high-risk STEMI (n = 1,059) patients transferred from community hospital to regional PCI center for urgent PCI within 6 hours of thrombolysis. It showed reduction in additional 6% death or myocardial infarction in post-tenecteplase angioplasty (30-day mortality 17.2% vs. 11.0%, p = 0. 004), when performed after 6 hours of onset of symptoms.[14]

FAST-MI Trial[15]

Data of 1,714 patients from FAST-MI also showed a pharmacoinvasive strategy that combines thrombolysis with a liberal use of PCI yields early and 1-year survival rates that are comparable to those of PAMI.

WEST Trial[16]

In this study, 304 patients were randomized to tenecteplase alone and PCI if required and compared with PAMI. The trial showed similar low mortality in both the groups. Coronary intervention was done within 24 hours of initial therapy. This reinforced that pharmacologic regimen rapidly delivered, coupled with routine coronary intervention within 24 hours of initial treatment, may not be different from timely expert PCI.

The European Society of Cardiology (ESC) 2017 STEMI guidelines recommend early routine angiography 2–24 hours after successful thrombolysis. This time window avoids PCI during the prothrombotic period in the first few hours after thrombolysis and minimizes the risk of reocclusion with PCI delay of more than 24 hours (class IIa recommendation) (Table 2, Box 1 and Flowchart 1).[1] A pharmacoinvasive strategy improved outcomes because the delay between thrombolysis and PCI was more than 2 hours, i.e., long enough to prevent bleeding complications, and because most patients randomized in these trials presented within

TABLE 2: What is new in 2017 ST-segment elevation myocardial infarction (STEMI) guidelines?

Recommendation	Trial	COR/LOE
Additional lipid lowering therapy if LDL >1.8 mmol/L (70 mg/dL)	IMPROVE-IT, FOURIER	II A
Complete revascularization during index primary PCI in STEMI patients with shock	Expert opinion	II A
Cangrelor if $P2Y_{12}$ inhibitors have not been given	CHAMPION	II B
Switch to potent $P2Y_{12}$ inhibitors 48 hours after fibrinolysis	Expert opinion	II B
Extend ticagrelor up to 36 hours in high risk patients	PEGASUS-TIMI 54	II B
Use of polypill to increase adherence	FOCUS	II B
Routine use of deferred stenting	DANAMI 3-DEFER	III

COR, class of recommendation; LDL, low-density lipoprotein; LOE, level of evidence; PCI, percutaneous coronary intervention; STEMI, ST-segment elevation myocardial infarction; DANAMI 3-DEFER, deferred versus conventional stent implantation in patients with ST-segment elevation myocardial infarction; PEGASUS-TIMI 54, Prevention of Cardiovascular Events in Patients with Prior Heart Attack Using Ticagrelor Compared to Placebo on a Background of Aspirin-Thrombolysis In Myocardial Infarction 54; IMPROVE-IT, IMProved Reduction of Outcomes–Vytorin Efficacy International Trial)

Source: STEMI 2017 European Society of Cardiology guidelines.[1]

BOX 1 2017 revised concepts

1. Time limits for routine opening of an infarct-related artery—0–12 hours (Class 1); 12–48 hours (Class IIa); more than 48 hours (Class III).
2. ECG at presentation—left bundle branch block and right bundle branch block are considered equal for recommending urgent angiography, if ischemia persists.
3. Time to angiography after fibrinolysis—timeframe is set in 2–24 hours after successful fibrinolysis.
4. Patients taking anticoagulants—acute and chronic management presented.
5. Strategy selection and time delays:
   a. Clear definition of first medical contact (FMC)
   b. Definition of "Time 0" to choose reperfusion strategy (i.e., strategy clock starts at the time of STEMI diagnosis)
   c. Selection of PCI over fibrinolysis when anticipated delay from STEMI diagnosis to wire crossing is less than 120 minutes.
   d. Maximum delay time from STEMI diagnosis to bolus of fibrinolysis agent is set in 10 minutes.
   e. "Door-to-balloon" term is eliminated from the guidelines.

Source: STEMI 2017 European Society of Cardiology guidelines.[1]

2–3 hours of symptom onset, when the time to reperfusion is critical.[17] After 3 hours, the PCI-mediated myocardial salvage is less time-dependent.[18]

Pathak Trial[19]

This study compared primary angioplasty versus post-tenecteplase angioplasty in ST elevation AMI in 200 cases and found no difference between post-tenecteplase and PAMI patients with regard to infarct size and left ventricular ejection fraction which are powerful predictors of survival after AMI. Rather post-fibrinolysis angioplasty resulted in better and higher TIMI 3 epicardial and TIMI myocardial perfusion grade (TMPG) 3 myocardial perfusion. The post-tenecteplase angioplasty provided wider window from 3 to 12 hours for coronary intervention in STEMI, from FMC.

STREAM Study[20]

This study evaluated whether a fibrinolytic-therapy approach consisting of prehospital or early fibrinolysis with contemporary antiplatelet and anticoagulant therapy, coupled with

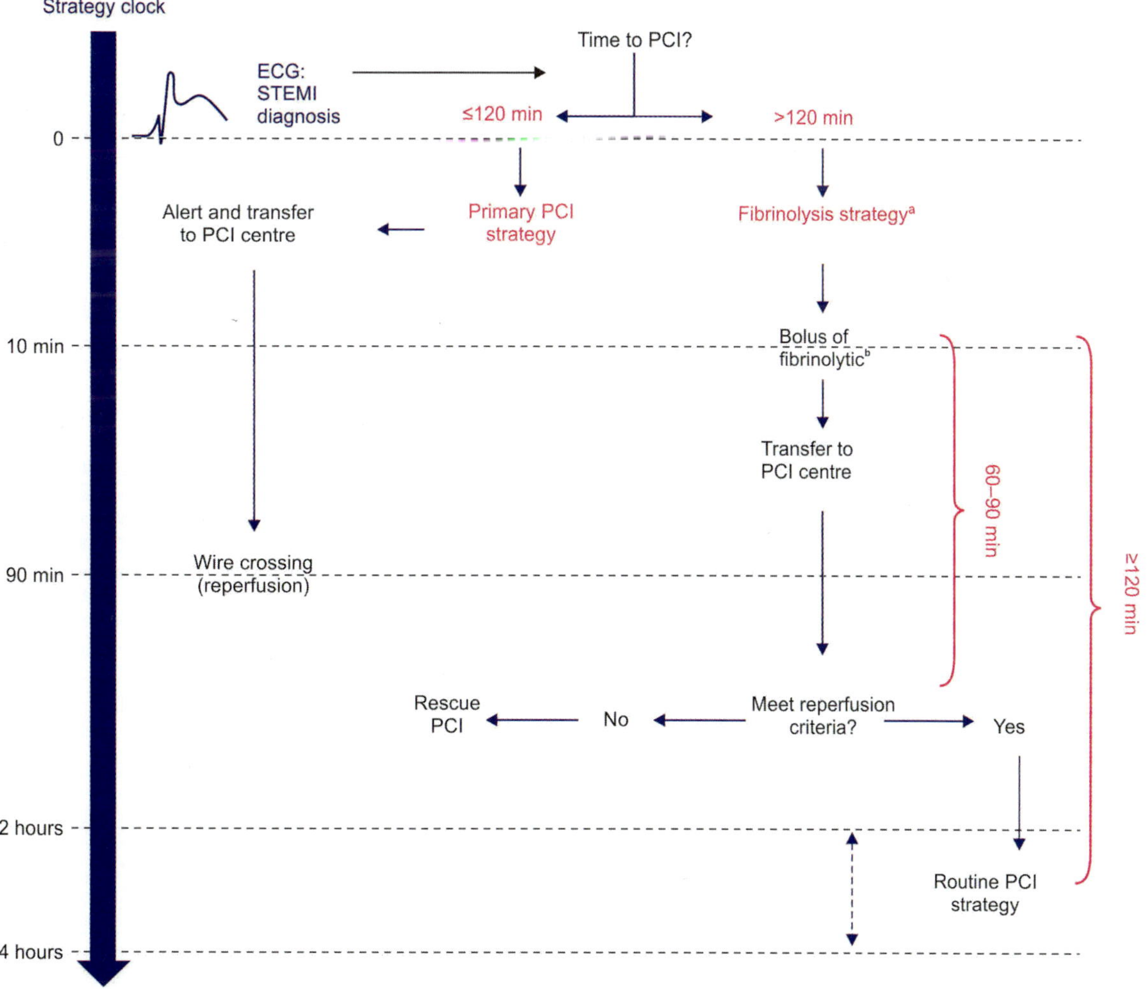

[a]If fibrinolysis is contra-indicated, direct for primary PCI strategy regardless of time to PCI.
[b]10 min is the maximum target delay time from STEMI diagnosis to fibrinolytic bolus administration, however, it should be given as soon as possible after STEMI diagnosis.
PCI, percutaneous coronary intervention; STEMI, ST-segment elevation myocardial infarction.

FLOWCHART 1: Electrocardiography in the diagnosis of STEMI.
Source: STEMI 2017 European Society of Cardiology guidelines.[1]

timely coronary angiography, provides a clinical outcome similar to that with primary PCI in patients with STEMI who present early after symptom onset. In this trial, 1,892 patients with STEMI who presented within 3 hours after symptom onset were randomly assigned to undergo either primary PCI or fibrinolytic therapy with bolus tenecteplase clopidogrel, and enoxaparin before transport to a PCI-capable hospital. If fibrinolysis failed, emergency angiography was performed otherwise; it was performed after 6–24 hours. Emergency angiography was required in 36.3% patients whereas the remainder of patients underwent angiography at a median of 17 hours after randomization. Thus, early prehospital fibrinolysis along with antithrombotics coupled with timely coronary angiography resulted in effective reperfusion in patients who presented within 3 hours after symptom onset. However, increased risk of intracranial bleeding was a concern with early fibrinolytic therapy.[20]

CONCLUSION

Primary angioplasty in myocardial infarction is most preferable reperfusion strategy at present. However, multiple reasons being logistic, timely intervention possibilities may not be possible for many STEMI patients. Most STEMI patients are getting treated with fibrinolysis as of easy availability of pharmacological treatment than still at large deficit of appropriate catheterization laboratory centers in Indian scenario. Debate continues as to whether, and when, patients treated with fibrinolysis should undergo subsequent PCI. Current data support the strategy of early routine PCI after fibrinolysis rather than the conservative standard care approach.

REFERENCES

1. Ibanez B, James S, Agewall S, et al. 2017 ESC Guidelines for the management of acute myocardial infarction in patients presenting with ST-segment elevation: The Task Force for the management of acute myocardial infarction in patients presenting with ST-segment elevation of the European Society of Cardiology (ESC). Eur Heart J. 2018;39(2):119-177.
2. Abbott JD. Pharmacoinvasive strategy for ST-segment elevation myocardial infarction: wading through the treatment options. Circ Cardivasc Interv. 2010;3: 294-6.
3. Berger PB, Ellis SG, Holmes DR Jr, et al. Relationship between delay in performing direct coronary angioplasty and early clinical outcome in patients with acute myocardial infarction: results from the global use of strategies to open occluded arteries in Acute Coronary Syndromes (GUSTO-11b) trial. Circulation. 1999;100(1):14-20.
4. Zahn R, Schiele R, Gitt AK, et al. Impact of prehospital delay on mortality in patients with acute myocardial infarction treated with primary angioplasty and intravenous thrombolysis. Am Heart J. 2001;142:105-11.
5. Morrison LI, Verbeek PR, McDonald AC, et al. Mortality and prehospital thrombolysis for acute myocardial infarction: a meta-analysis. IAMA. 2000;283: 2686-92.
6. Westerhout CM, Bonnefoy E, Welsh RC, et al. The influence of time from symptom onset and reperfusion strategy on 1-year survival in ST-elevation myocardial infarction: a pooled analysis of an early fibrinolytic strategy versus primary percutaneous coronary intervention from CAPTIM and WEST. Am Heart J. 2011;161(2):283-90.
7. Boersma E, Maas AC, Dockers IW, et al. Early thrombolytic treatment in acute myocardial infarction: reappraisal of the golden hour. Lancet. 1996;348:771.
8. Indications for fibrinolytic therapy in suspected acute myocardial infarction: collaborative overview of early mortality and major morbidity results from all randomised trials of more than 1000 patients. Fibrinolytic Therapy Trialists' (FTT) Collaborative Group. Lancet. 1994;343(8893):311-22.
9. Van De Werf F, Adgey J, Ardissino D, et al. Single-bolus tenecteplase compared with front-loaded alteplase in acute myocardial infarction: the ASSENT-2 double-blind randomised trial. Lancet. 1999;354(9180):716-22.
10. Keeley EC, Boura JA, Grines CL. Primary angioplasty versus intravenous thrombolytic therapy for acute myocardial infarction: A quantitative review of 23 randomised trials. Lancet. 2003;361:13-20.
11. Ellis SG, Tendera M, de Belder MA, et al. Facilitated PCI in patients with ST-elevation myocardial infarction. N Engl J Med. 2008;358:2205-17.
12. Hanna EB, Hennebry TA, Abu-Fadel MS. Combined reperfusion strategies in ST-segment elevation MI: Rationale and current role. Cleve Clin J Med. 2010;77(9):629-38.
13. Ferna'ndez-Avile's F, Alonso JJ, Pena A, et al. Primary angioplasty vs. early routine post fibrinolysis angioplasty for acute myocardial infarction with ST segment elevation: the GRACIA-2 non-inferiority, randomized, controlled trial. Eur Heart J. 2007;28:949-60.
14. Cantor WJ, Fitchett D, Borgundvaag B, et al. Routine Early Angioplasty after Fibrinolysis for Acute Myocardial Infarction. N Engl J Med. 2009;360:2705-18.
15. Danchin N, Coste R, Ferrières J, et al. Comparison of Thrombolysis Followed by Broad Use of Percutaneous Intervention with Primary Percutaneous Coronary Intervention for ST-Segment Elevation Acute Myocardial Infarction: Data from the French Coronary Registry on Acute ST-Elevation (FAST-MI). Circulation. 2008;118:268-76.
16. Armstrong PW. A comparison of pharmacologic therapy with/without timely coronary intervention vs. primary percutaneous intervention early after ST-elevation myocardial infarction: the WEST (Which Early ST-elevation myocardial infarction Therapy) study. Eur Heart J. 2006;2711:530-8.
17. Van de Werf F, Bax J, Betriu A, et al. Management of acute myocardial infarction in patients presenting with persistent ST-segment elevation: The Task Force on the Management of ST-Segment Elevation Acute Myocardial Infarction of the European Society of Cardiology. Eur Heart J. 2008;29:2909-45.
18. Liu F, Guo Q, Xie G, et al. Percutaneous Coronary Intervention after Fibrinolysis for ST-Segment Elevation Myocardial Infarction Patients: An Updated Systematic Review and Meta-Analysis. PLoS One. 2015;10(11):e0141855.
19. Pathak LA, Ratnaparkhi GR, Shcth S. Post Tenectplase Angioplasty vs PAMI in ST Elevation MI. Indian Heart J. 2011;63:245-9.
20. Armstrong PW, Gershlick AH, Goldstein P, et al. Fibrinolysis or primary PCI in ST-segment elevation myocardial infarction. N Engl J Med. 2013;368:1379-87.

CHAPTER 44

Revascularizing Nonculprit Artery in AMI: Uniform Strategy or Case-based Approach

Ranjit K Nath, Kewal C Goswami

INTRODUCTION

Primary angioplasty or primary percutaneous coronary intervention (PCI) has been proved to be an excellent therapy for ST-elevation myocardial infarction (STEMI) that has been shown to improve immediate and long-term outcomes. While there is ample evidence to demonstrate that immediate revascularization is required to open the infarct related artery (IRA), the clinician is faced with the dilemma of how to treat other diseased vessels which are seen in up to 50% of patients presenting with an STEMI.[1] The short-term and long-term prognosis of patients with multivessel coronary artery disease (MVCAD) is worse than the patients who have single vessel disease.[2] The worse prognosis of MVCAD is stems from clinical variables because such as older age, multiple risk factors or associated comorbid conditions, pre-existing ventricular dysfunction, additional vulnerable plaques, diffuse endothelial dysfunction, microvascular spasm, or inflammation, slow-flow or decreased contractility in noninfarct zones.[3-5]

Because of increased risk of subsequent MI and mortality in patients with MVCAD, these patient needs to be managed timely. The adverse impact of nonculprit lesions in STEMI patients raises the question as to whether revascularization will improve their outcomes. Many observational and randomized studies have shown that revascularization of nonculprit lesions will reduce the major adverse cardiac event (MACE). However, the optimal management strategy for management of MVCAD in STEMI patients is still controversial. Currently available evidence addressing the management of nonculprit coronary stenotic lesions at the time of primary PCI has yielded conflicting result.

The 2015 American College of Cardiology (ACC)/American Heart Association (AHA)/Society for Cardiovascular Angiography and Interventions (SCAI) guidelines[6] currently recommend consideration of multivessel PCI (MVPCI) either at the time of primary PCI or as a staged procedure (class IIb), modified from culprit-vessel PCI (CV-PCI) only in the absence of hemodynamic instability (class III). The 2017 European Society of Cardiology (ESC) guidelines for the management of acute myocardial infarction (AMI) in patients presenting with ST-segment elevation recommends routine revascularization of non-IRA lesions to be considered in STEMI patients with multivessel disease before hospital discharge (class IIa) or during index procedure in patients with cardiogenic shock.[7]

APPROACH TO THE MANAGEMENT OF NONCULPRIT LESIONS IN STEMI

There can be various treatment approaches to manage STEMI patients with MVCAD either at the time of primary PCI or by staged approach (Flowchart 1).

Complete Revascularization during Index Procedure versus Culprit-Vessel Only

There are some advantages and disadvantages of complete revascularization during index procedure (Table 1) in comparison to the CV only approach. In the PRAMI (Preventive Angioplasty in Acute Myocardial Infarction) trial 465 patients with acute STEMI were randomized to either CV-PCI only (231 patients) or MVPCI involving CV and preventive PCI of other angiographically significant coronary stenosis (234 patients). PCI of the nonculprit lesions had to be performed at the index procedure and staged procedures were discouraged. Lesions that were more than 50% diameter stenosis in the non-CV were considered significant. Fractional flow reserve (FFR) was not used to assess lesion severity. Patients in cardiogenic shock, chronic total occlusions (CTOs) of the non-CV or those with significant left main disease were excluded. Among the patients who underwent CV only PCI, subsequent PCI was recommended only for refractory angina with objective evidence of ischemia.[8] Although this study planned to recruit 600 patients, it had to be prematurely stopped at 23 months due to highly significant difference

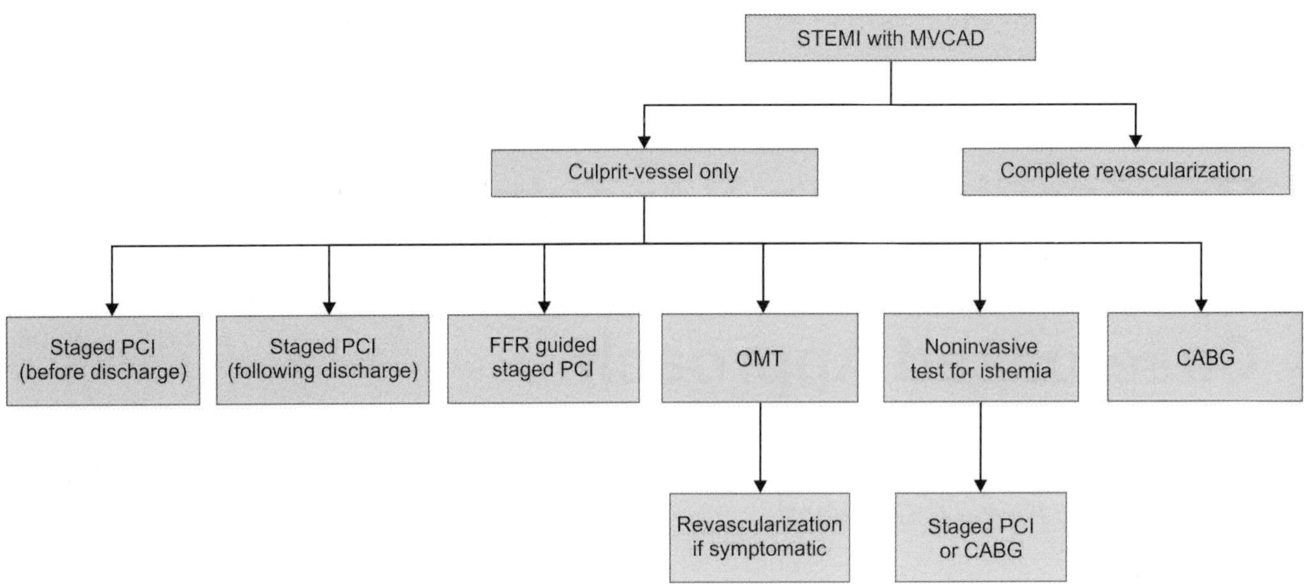

CABG, coronary artery bypass grafting; FFR, fractional flow reserve; MVCAD, multivessel coronary artery disease; OMT, optimal medical therapy; PCI, percutaneous coronary intervention; STEMI, ST-elevation myocardial infarction.

FLOWCHART 1: Various options for management of MVCAD in acute myocardial infarction.

TABLE 1: Advantages and disadvantages of multivessel percutaneous coronary intervention in acute myocardial infarction

Advantages	Disadvantages
• Decreases complications of repeated procedures • Decreases chance of in-hospital recurrent ischemia or related arrhythmias • Improves blood supply to hibernating myocardium or watershed area of infarction, hence improves ejection fraction and remodeling • Reduces subsequent urgent revascularization • Decreases duration of hospital stay, hence increases cost-effectiveness • May decrease future MI and related mortality • When access is very difficult or limited, repeat procedure may not be possible	• Procedure duration is long • More radiation exposure • Higher contrast use may cause contrast-induced nephropathy which can increase hospital morbidity and mortality • Increased risk of stent thrombosis • Increased periprocedural MI risk • Nonculprit lesion severity may be exaggerated because of more catecholamine release, producing vasoconstriction • More chance of slow-flow • Occlusion/dissection/no-flow-related complication of major noninfarct artery can be catastrophic • Operator experience becomes important factor in handling complex cases

MI, myocardial infarction; PCI, percutaneous coronary intervention.

in the primary composite outcome of cardiovascular death, nonfatal MI and refractory angina favoring preventive PCI [9% vs. 22%, hazard Ratio (HR) 0.35]. There were 21 events in the multivessel group versus 53 events in the culprit-vessel only (CVO) group, with nearly half of the events driven by refractory angina. Even when analyzed for the variables of death and nonfatal MI, the HR favored preventive PCI (HR 0.36). Thus, this trial demonstrated fewer MACE events amongst patients treated with MVPCI at the time of STEMI. However, this trial was limited by the liberal definition of lesion severity as well as the small number of events.

The CvLPRIT (Complete versus Lesion-only Primary PCI Trial) randomly assigned 296 patients to complete revascularization during the index hospitalization or IRA-only revascularization.[9] The criteria for significant nonculprit stenosis were more than 70% diameter stenosis in other coronary arteries. Around 64% of patients received complete revascularization at the time of primary PCI in complete revascularization group and in remaining one-third of patients revascularization was done before hospital discharge. FFR assessment was not used to look into the hemodynamic significance of the nonculprit lesions. The primary composite end point at 12 months occurred less often in the complete revascularization group (10.0% vs. 21.2%; HR 0.45, 95% CI 0.24–0.84). The MACE curves between the two groups separated early at approximately a month from the event and continued to do so even at one year. Most importantly there was no difference in the safety end points between the two approaches (major bleeding, contrast-induced nephropathy, or stroke). However, this trial was not powered to detect differences in the individual components of the primary composite end point of all-cause mortality, recurrent MI, heart failure, or repeat revascularization.

From CvLPRIT trial the following conclusions can be made:

- It showed 55% reduction in MACE in those patients with STEMI who underwent revascularization of nonculprit lesion in index admission with no adverse safety signal
- Those patients with immediate nonculprit lesion PCI showed a strong trend towards improved clinical outcomes compared with those undergoing a staged in-hospital procedure
- As the staging was based on clinicians' decisions and was nonrandomized, and also the number of patient in each strategy was less, it is difficult to draw a definite conclusion
- In view of the early separation of outcome measures in event curves, it can be suggested that a postdischarge late complete revascularization approach may not be a better option than in-hospital complete PCI.

The ACC guidelines presently do not clearly define whether revascularization of nonculprit lesion during performed in the index period or whether they should be performed as a staged procedure. The ESC guidelines however recommend that nonculprit revascularization during index PCI should only performed in patients presenting with cardiogenic shock.[7]

From a practical standpoint considering the possible risks and benefits of index complete revascularization, it may not be suitable to perform complete revascularization in all patients with AMI with MVCAD at the index period. Decision should be individualized based on patient condition, operator efficiency, availability of tools, and manpower, etc.

Complete revascularization at the time of index procedure is not recommended in following patients:

- Patients with less than TIMI III flow in the CV after angioplasty
- Acute hemodynamic or arrhythmic instability after CV angioplasty
- Who have risk factors for contrast induced nephropathy (like anemia, diabetes, known renal dysfunction or history of medical renal disease)
- Complex nonculprit lesions like calcified lesion, bifurcation, tortuous vessels, and anomalous origin
- Bleeding or other complications after culprit vessel PCI
- Chronic total occlusion lesions in non-CV
- If the patient has indication for valve surgery or coronary artery bypass grafting (CABG) for other vessel disease like complex left main disease or mechanical complication.

Culprit Vessel Only Primary PCI versus Staged PCI

Staged PCI of nonculprit arteries have some advantages especially in patients with advanced age, additional comorbid conditions and low left ventricular ejection fraction (LVEF). It is also associated with a lesser chance of developing contrast induced nephropathy.

The DANAMI-3-PRIMULTI (Third Danish Study of Optimal Acute Treatment of Patients with STEMI: Primary PCI in Multivessel Disease) trial randomly assigned 627 patients after culprit lesion treatment to either no further treatment (313 patients) or complete revascularization of nonculprit lesions (314 patients). Complete revascularization was usually done after 2 days of index primary PCI and unlike PRAMI or CvLPRIT trial, FFR-guided PCI of the nonculprit lesions (>50% diameter stenosis) was performed in this trial.[10] Patients in cardiogenic shock or those with indication for CABG were not included in this trial. The primary composite end point of all-cause mortality, nonfatal infarction, and ischemia-driven revascularization of lesions in non-IRAs occurred less often in the group with complete revascularization than in the CV only group (13% vs. 22%). The reduction in events was driven by a 69% reduction in the need for repeat revascularizations (5% vs. 17%). There was no difference in cardiac death or reinfarction between the two groups.

One important point observed was that approximately one-third of patients did not undergo nonculprit lesion revascularization in complete revascularization group, as FFR value was found to be above 0.80 despite the fact that initial angiogram showed significant stenosis. This supports that during AMI there is an increased chance that nonsignificant lesion may appear significant because of vasospasm and FFR will definitely play a role in such scenario and will improve the outcome.

Multivessel PCI versus Staged PCI

Observational studies by Varani et al.[11] and Jensen et al.[12] have shown increased mortality in MVPCI during index procedure group when compared to staged PCI group. They found a longer hospital stay and higher in-hospital mortality in MVPCI group than in the staged procedure group. This increased mortality could be because clinically more critical patients may have been selected for multivessel primary PCI. Also, this may be related to prolonged procedure-related complications like slow-flow in non-CV, large contrast load, hemodynamic instability like hypotension or arrhythmias, etc. Suboptimal result after angioplasty in culprit vessel before proceeding for nonculprit lesion revascularization can be another factor of poorer outcome.

Is Staged PCI Better then Multivessel PCI?

Recent meta-analysis by Li et al.[13] has shown benefit of both short and long term mortality favoring staged PCI. This may be because of:

- Procedures done in routine hours with better support and tools
- Procedures done or supervised by experienced operators
- Patient already stabilized
- Already on adequate medications like dual antiplatelet therapy (DAPT), high-dose statin, and other required medicines
- Can have a plan in managing complex cases.

Chronic Total Occlusion as Nonculprit Vessel in STEMI

The occurrence of CTO in STEMI patients is not uncommon and its reported incidence varies from 10 to 15%. Presence of CTO significantly increases mortality in these patients.[14] Randomized trial have not shown any benefit of opening CTO lesions in patients of AMI. The benefit of opening the CTO was studied in the EXPLORE (Evaluating Xience and Left Ventricular Function in Percutaneous Coronary Intervention on Occlusions after ST-Elevation Myocardial Infarction) trial.[15] About 304 patients with STEMI who underwent primary PCI and also had concurrent CTO in nonculprit vessels were included. A total of 150 patients were randomly assigned to early PCI of the CTO, and the remaining 154 patients were assigned to conservative treatment. Procedural success for CTO was 77%. This study has shown additional PCI of opening of CTO within 1 week of AMI was feasible and safe, but the primary outcomes of improvement in LVEF and left ventricular (LV) end diastolic volume at 4 months were not significant. However, in a subgroup analysis, patients who had CTO in the left anterior descending artery had a significantly higher LV function than in those who did not undergo a CTO recanalization strategy.

Thus, revascularization of CTO of nonculprit arteries in patients with AMI may not be beneficial or necessary, and if at all required it has to be done in a staged manner after testing for inducible ischemia. Factors determining need and success of CTO revascularization of nonculprit arteries will depend on (i) large area of supply by the CTO vessel; (ii) patient comorbid conditions and EF; (iii) the lesion complexity, calcification, etc., (iv) more importantly the experience and availability of CTO tools.

Meta-analysis on MVCAD in STEMI

A recent network meta-analysis by Elgendy et al. in 2017[16] included ten randomized trials with 2,285 patients from the available trials. They compared four treatment strategies in STEMI with MVCAD undergoing primary PCI in these patients:

- Complete revascularization performed at the time of index procedure
- Culprit lesion only approach
- Staged PCI of nonculprit lesion performed before hospital discharge
- Staged PCI of nonculprit lesions performed a few weeks after discharge (not dictated by presence or absence of symptoms).

After median follow up of 25 months the following observations were made:

- Patients who underwent complete revascularization, regardless of strategy (at the time of index procedure or as a staged procedure) had a lower risk of MACE [risk ratio (RR) 0.57, 95% CI 0.42–0.77] as compared with those undergoing just CV-PCI
- The composite primary end point in these patients (MACE) has been largely due to a lower rate of urgent revascularization in the MVPCI arm as compared to culprit vessel only arm
- Multivessel PCI has been associated with a lower risks of all-cause mortality and recurrent MI (RR 0.76, 95% CI 0.52–1.12 and 0.55, 95% CI 0.23–1.28, respectively).

Percutaneous Coronary Intervention in STEMI with Cardiogenic Shock

The earlier common practice was that, if patient was in shock then non-CV should be opened at the same time and recent ESC (2017) guidelines also has given this a class IIa recommendation for MVPCI at index period if patient is in cardiogenic shock. But the recent CULPRIT-SHOCK trial has included 706 patients with STEMI who had MVCAD and in cardiogenic shock has shown some different findings.[17] These patients were randomized either to culprit lesion only with options of staged PCI or complete revascularization at index period.

At 30 days the following points were noted:

- The primary end point of death from any cause or renal replacement therapy were higher in MVPCI group
- Recurrent MI or hospitalization for congestive heart failure were also higher in MVPCI group
- Staged or urgent revascularization was higher in culprit vessel only group
- Lack of benefit of MVPCI may be because of more dye use in MVPCI group causing contrast nephropathy as acute coronary syndrome (ACS) itself is a risk factor for nephropathy and also toxic effect of dye on myocardium whose function is already compromised by STEMI.

Therefore the role of nonculprit vessel angioplasty or complete revascularization in the setting of cardiogenic shock is not shown to be definitely beneficial in the only randomized trial done in this area till date. Hence the treatment needs to be strategized patient to patient. Complete revascularization may turn out to be beneficial in subgroup of young patients (age <50 years) with AMI. Result was neutral in female patients, diabetics, and anterior location of STEMI.

Technical possibility of better outcome can be expected if:

- The nonculprit lesions are critical but type A, short, proximal coronary lesions of major arteries and can be opened up easily without much additional time or contrast load
- Can be performed by experienced operators, avoiding prolonged ischemia to non-CV by complications like slow-flow, dissection, wedging by guide catheter, etc
- If required circulatory support is available and instituted in time.

Role of Fractional Flow Reserve in STEMI Patients with MVCAD

Fractional flow reserve use during ACS is controversial, and is because of important prerequisite for use of FFR of "maximal hyperemia". Patients with ACS will have blunted response to adenosine; hence the optimal hyperemia may not be achieved effectively leading to FFR value being falsely negative.

Fractional Flow Reserve in Culprit Vessel

Fractional flow reserve may be of use in cases where deferred stenting of CV is planned, which is not a commonly used strategy of managing AMI. In fact the expert consensus statement of SCAI by Lofti A et al. said that FFR should not be performed in the culprit lesions in patients with ACS.[18]

Fractional Flow Reserve in Nonculprit Lesions

The Compare-acute trial[19] included 885 patients with STEMI to undergo complete revascularization of nonculprit lesion or no revascularization after primary angioplasty in a 1:2 ratio. FFR was done in both groups and the cut-off point for PCI was FFR value of less than or equal to 0.80 in revascularization group. The primary composite end point of death from any cause, nonfatal MI, revascularization, and cerebrovascular events at 12 months occurred less frequently in the complete revascularization group than in the CVO group (7.8% vs. 20.5%). This difference was primarily driven by reduction in repeat revascularization. In most cases, revascularization took place during the index procedure as compared to DANAMI-3-PRIMULTI trial, where FFR was done in staged procedure and it also showed improved outcome at 12-month in patients who underwent FFR-guided PCI of nonculprit lesion. So, results from these two trails suggest superior outcomes of FFR-guided nonculprit vessel angioplasty in a strategy of complete revascularization in AMI compared to angiographically guided revascularization.

Post-PCI Fractional Flow Reserve

Post-PCI FFR can be improved by postdilatation and by implanting additional stents, if the value is low after stenting. Studies have shown obtaining final FFR values of more than 0.91 had a significantly lower adverse event rate compared with a final FFR of less than or equal to 0.91 (19% vs. 30%; $p = 0.03$).[20]

CONCLUSION

Patients with MVCAD in STEMI have higher risk for future morbidity and mortality mainly because of repeat MI or need for revascularization of nonculprit lesions. Evidence from randomized trials have shown that complete revascularization is better in terms of reduction in MACE than the CVO revascularization, but the difference is mainly driven by the need for repeat revascularization in non-CV, and not by death or MI. Among complete vessel revascularization groups, the staged PCI before hospital discharge seems to have better short- and long-term mortality benefit when compared to complete revascularization during index procedure. The recent culprit shock trial questioned the role of complete revascularization in cardiogenic shock during index PCI. FFR-guided complete revascularization has shown to be beneficial when strategy of complete revascularization is adopted, avoiding unwanted PCI. There are number of ongoing trials that are going to address this question in further detail. The ASSIST-MI trial be assessing infarct size by cardiac magnetic resonance imaging (MRI) to evaluate strategy of MVPCI versus culprit vessel only approach. The COMPLETE study will assess culprit only versus staged PCI with FFR in 3,900 patients. The CROSS-AMI study will be evaluating staged PCI versus ischemia-guided strategy in 400 patients.

REFERENCES

1. Park DW, Clare RM, Schulte PJ, et al. Extent, location, and clinical significance of non-infarct related coronary artery disease among patients with ST-elevation myocardial infarction. JAMA. 2014;312:2019-27.
2. Sorajja P, Gersh BJ, Cox DA, et al. Impact of multivessel disease on reperfusion success and clinical outcomes in patients undergoing primary percutaneous coronary intervention for acute myocardial infarction. Eur Heart J. 2007;28:1709-16.
3. Asakura M, Ueda Y, Yamaguchi O, et al. Extensive development of vulnerable plaques as a pan-coronary process in patients with myocardial infarction: an angioscopic study. J Am Coll Cardiol. 2001;37:1284-8.
4. Gibson CM, Ryan KA, Murphy SA, et al. TIMI Study Group. Impaired coronary blood flow in nonculprit arteries in the setting of acute myocardial infarction. J Am Coll Cardiol. 1999;34:974-82.
5. Grines CL, Topol EJ, Califf RM, et al. TAMI Study Group. Prognostic implications and predictors of enhanced regional wall motion of the noninfarct zone after thrombolysis and angioplasty therapy of acute myocardial infarction. Circulation. 1989;80:245-53.
6. Levine G, O'Gara P, Bates E, et al. 2015 ACC/AHA/SCAI focused update on primary percutaneous coronary intervention for patients with ST-elevation myocardial infarction: an update of the 2011 ACCF/AHA/SCAI guideline for percutaneous coronary intervention and the 2013 ACCF/AHA guideline for the management of ST-elevation myocardial infarction: a report of the American College of Cardiology/American Heart Association Task Force on Clinical Practice Guidelines and the Society for Cardiovascular Angiography and Interventions. J Am Coll Cardiol. 2016;87(6):1001-19.
7. Ibanez B, James S, Agewall S, et al. 2017 ESC Guidelines for the management of acute myocardial infarction in patients presenting with ST-segment elevation: The Task Force for the management of acute myocardial infarction in patients presenting with ST-segment elevation of the European Society of Cardiology (ESC). Eur Heart J. 2018;39,119-7.
8. Wald DS, Morris JK, Wald NJ, et al. PRAMI Investigators. Randomized trial of preventive angioplasty in myocardial infarction. N Engl J Med. 2013;369: 1115-23.
9. Gershlick AH, Khan JN, Kelly DJ, et al. Randomized trial of complete versus lesion-only revascularization in patients undergoing primary percutaneous coronary intervention for STEMI and multivessel disease: the CvLPRIT trial. J Am Coll Cardiol. 2015;65:963-72.
10. Engstrøm T, Kelbæk H, Helqvist S, et al. DANAMI-3-PRIMULTI Investigators. Complete revascularization versus treatment of the culprit lesion only in patients with ST-segment elevation myocardial infarction and multivessel disease: an open-label, randomised controlled trial. Lancet. 2015;386:665-71.
11. Varani E, Balducelli M, Aquilina M, et al. Single or multivessel percutaneous coronary intervention in ST-elevation myocardial infarction patients. Catheter Cardiovasc Interv. 2008;72:927-33.
12. Jensen LO, Thayssen P, Farkas DK, et al. Culprit only multivessel coronary interventions in patients with ST-segment elevation myocardial infarction and multivessel disease. Euro Intervention. 2012;8:456-64.
13. Li Z, Zhou Y, Xu Q, et al. Staged versus One-Time Complete Revascularization with Percutaneous Coronary Intervention in STEMI Patients with Multivessel Disease: A Systematic Review and Meta-Analysis. PLoS One. 2017;12:e0169406.
14. Claessen BE, Dangas GD, Weisz G, et al. Prognostic impact of a chronic total occlusion in a non-infarct-related artery in patients with ST-segment elevation myocardial infarction: 3-year results from the HORIZONS-AMI trial. Eur Heart J. 2012;33:768-5.
15. Henriques JP, Hoebers LP, Råmunddal T, et al. Percutaneous Intervention for Concurrent Chronic Total Occlusions in Patients with STEMI: The EXPLORE Trial. J Am Coll Cardiol. 2016;68:1622-32.
16. Elgendy IY, Mahmoud AN, Kumbhani DJ, Bhatt DL, Bavry AA. Complete or Culprit-Only Revascularization for Patients With Multivessel Coronary Artery

Disease Undergoing Percutaneous Coronary Intervention: A Pairwise and Network Meta- Analysis of Randomized Trials. JACC Cardiovasc Interv. 2017;10:315-24.
17. Thiele H, Akin I, Sandri M, et al. PCI strategies in patients with acute myocardial infarction and cardiogenic shock. N Engl J Med. 2017;377:2419-32.
18. Lotfi A, Jeremias A, Fearon WF, et al. Expert consensus statement on the use of fractional flow reserve, intravascular ultrasound, and optical coherence tomography: a consensus statement of the Society of Cardiovascular Angiography and Interventions. Catheter Cardiovasc Interv. 2014;83:509-18.
19. Smits PC, Abdel-Wahab M, et al. Fractional Flow Reserve-Guided Multivessel Angioplasty in Myocardial Infarction. N Engl J Med. 2017;376:1234-44.
20. Kasula S, Agarwal SK, Hacioglu Y, et al. Clinical and prognostic value of poststenting fractional flow reserve in acute coronary syndromes. Heart. 2016;102:1988-94.

CHAPTER 45

Improving Outcomes of Primary Percutaneous Coronary Intervention: Technical Aspects

Ambukeshwar Singh, Ayush Shukla, Nakul Sinha

INTRODUCTION

Coronary artery disease (CAD) is one of the most common noncommunicable diseases in our country causing significant mortality and morbidity. Acute ST-segment elevation myocardial infarction (STEMI) is a common presentation of CAD resulting in high morbidity and mortality. Timely reperfusion therapy has proven to be the best therapeutic option for the management of STEMI.[1] Primary percutaneous coronary intervention (PCI) is the most effective and predictable form of reperfusion therapy with low complication rate in comparison to thrombolysis with different agents.[2] According to the American College of Cardiology/American Heart Association (ACC/AHA) and the European Society of Cardiology (ESC) guidelines, primary PCI for management of STEMI is class IA indication within 12 hours of initiation of myocardial infarction (MI) and also highly effective between 12–24 hours if there is clinical and/or electrocardiography (ECG) evidence of ongoing ischemia. In case thrombolysis is contraindicated, it should be offered irrespective of time delay after the onset of MI.[3,4] Worldwide figures indicate a 3–5% mortality at 30 days, 2.5% reinfarction, and 1% stroke after primary PCI.[2]

PREHOSPITAL OR PATIENT PREPARATION

Early diagnosis of STEMI and early reperfusion of the culprit vessel by primary PCI is the central concept of STEMI management and the best method of achieving its benefits. For achieving this goal, certain practical points and protocols have demonstrated universal ability. Early transportation of a patient to a cath laboratory-enabled center is one of the important steps. An 8 years follow-up study found a significant mortality benefit with primary (direct) transportation of patient to a cardiac center versus secondary transportation from another hospital.[5] This should be accompanied by a prior information with (preferably) electronic transfer of relevant parameters, preparedness of the on-call team with a ready cath laboratory, quick part and patient preparation, monitoring of relevant parameters, and a screening Echo to rule out any surprises being some of the essential components. Modifications depending on local prevailing facilities and conditions are preferable keeping in view the primary goal of offering an early revascularization. It is preferable that all the team members are assigned a fixed role to not only make things more efficient but also not to miss any important step. A designated team leader should assume the overall responsibility of supervising the preparations.

We will now attempt to outline only those current technical concepts and practices which are believed or have been shown to exert a positive (either direct or indirect) impact on the short and long-term outcome of primary angioplasty. There are many other equally important ancillary measures which will have to be judiciously employed depending on the clinical condition of the patient and are directed more toward stabilizing the patient's condition so that he/she can withstand the procedure better.

LOADING DOSE

The loading doses of antiplatelets should be given as early as possible after the diagnosis of STEMI is established. According to latest ESC and ACC guidelines, ticagrelor 180 mg or prasugrel 60 mg is the preferred antiplatelet agents after ruling out absolute contraindications. In case of nonavailability of these agents, use of clopidogrel must not be delayed. If there is a possibility of delay due to any reason, parenteral anticoagulant (enoxaparin) should be given. The role of cangrelor IV is under investigation.

Many trials have indicated a positive effect of preloading with high dose statins before PCI for ACS showing some benefit in recurrent MI, angina, and mortality along with thrombolysis in myocardial infarction (TIMI) and TIMI myocardial perfusion (TMP) scores.[6]

ROLE OF COUNSELING

While the patient is being prepared, a physician may be available to converse and explain to the family members regarding the disease, present condition of patient, along with relevant information regarding primary angioplasty including risks and benefit involved in the procedure. This is likely to make the family and attendants understand and appreciate better about the procedural risks and benefits and help in endorsing the decision immediately after the findings of angiography are communicated to them. This effort may primarily be seen as a time-saving measure to speed-up the process of revascularization.

ANGIOGRAPHY

Access Site

In the RIVAL (RadIal Vs femorAL access for coronary inter vention) study STEMI subgroup and RIFLE-STEACS (RadIal versus FemoraL randomizEd investigation in ST-Elevation Acute Coronary Syndrome) trial, transradial approach was not only associated with a significant reduction of primary end point (death/MI/stroke), but also mortality in primary PCI.[7,8] The STEMI-RADIAL (ST-Elevation Myocardial Infarction treated by RADIAL or femoral approach) trial showed that transradial approach resulted in significant reduction in major bleeding compared to transfemoral approach but at the cost of significant increase in access site crossover with transradial approach.[9] If there is more than 3–5 minutes delay in getting transradial access or catheter passage due to spasm or an anomaly, it is better to crossover to transfemoral route. If there is indication of temporary pacing or one is suspecting bradyarrhythmia during procedure, transfemoral venous access should preferably be taken. Sometimes left radial artery can be easily cannulated and the intervention done smoothly with only minor positional adjustments.

Catheter Selection

In case of transradial access, tiger catheter is preferred one. Minimum but adequate numbers of angiographic view with use of lesser amount of dye or contrast is the foremost important precaution to be taken. In transfemoral access, nonculprit vessel maybe imaged first followed by culprit vessel directly with a guiding catheter. This usually avoids time delay in cath laboratory, all types and all sizes of catheters must be available, and in case of difficulty in engagement of vessel ostia, we should shift to another type of catheter instead of wasting time. A guiding catheter with good support and backup characteristics should be preferred mostly depending on the primary operator choice. Wider internal diameter catheters are usually more helpful in case thrombosuction, larger stents or a bifurcation strategy is required. Sheathless catheters having a smaller external but comparable internal diameter, can provide a viable solution in females, shorter patients or thinner radials.

Wiring

As most of the time culprit artery is totally occluded with thrombus with no antegrade flow, a soft tip wire with low tip load should be used, at least initially. After crossing the proximal portion of culprit artery, one should take an angiogram, as most of the time there is some antegrade trickling of dye which help in localizing the subsequent course of artery and negotiation of the wire.

Sex Differences

Generally all the large studies have shown a less favorable outcome for females versus males in primary PCI results. A recent pooled analysis, together with a German and European registry all bear testimony to this trend[10-12] This is probably a worldwide phenomenon, though more apparent in Indian conditions and is mostly related to low awareness, late recognition and more hesitation, indecision or inability to seek specialized treatment for acute myocardial infarction (AMI) in case of females with more subsequent delays coupled with economic factors.

Complete versus Culprit Vessel Only Revascularization

This has been a subject of much thought and debate recently specially highlighted by the PRAMI (PReventive angioplasty in Acute Myocardial Infarction) trial results,[13] though its design and conductance had been called in question. The COMPARE-ACUTE (FFR guided primary multivessel PCI to improve guideline indexed actual standard of care) trial[14] which compared a culprit only strategy with a fractional flow reserve (FFR)-guided complete revascularization, showed similar mortality but, expectedly a lower subsequent intervention rate in the latter group. A meta-analysis of six studies favored the group with staged revascularization of nonculprit lesions with a significantly decreased mortality.[15] However, the final word is still pending and possibly this aspect will still generate debate with personal and operator preferences also influencing the decision, of course influenced by the patients overall condition and tolerance of the culprit vessel revascularization which has to be done first. Another reasonable strategy advocates revascularization of nonculprit significant lesions before discharge.

Sometimes identification or recognition of the culprit vessel can be a matter of concern especially between left circumflex coronary artery (LCX) and right coronary artery (RCA). If the lesion morphology and ECG evidences are not very helpful, it is better to do both rather than spend valuable time in solving the issue.

Occasionally once the primary, proximal culprit lesion has been opened one encounters a distal chronic total occlusion (CTO) with a sizeable and good size distal vessel filling retrogradely. It is judicious to only do the culprit lesion, beyond a short attempt at probing the CTO, since otherwise the time, contrast load, and other factors may adversely affect the result of the primary PCI.

Predilatation

A strategy of "quick in-quick out" is probably the best in primary PCI as it also saves time and time is muscle. The benefits of direct stenting include reduced procedure time, quick restoration of antegrade flow, less thrombus fragmentation, and/or distal displacement and thus reduced chances of slow flow/no-reflow. Having said that it is also of utmost importance that the final result of angioplasty be at least optimal if not perfect. After wiring through the occluded artery, if antegrade flow is inadequate in even outlining the distal vessel, a strategy of uninflated (but perhaps at a neutral pressure) balloon passage can be helpful by partially displacing the thrombus distally and permitting distal assessment of the vessel health. However, this can be offset by attempt at direct stenting which if successful can perhaps contain the thrombus better between the stent struts and the vessel walls with minimal displacement. Data from the EUROTRANSFER registry suggest that when anatomically and technically feasible, the use of direct stenting techniques may result in improved long-term survival in patients with STEMI undergoing primary PCI.[16] If even after a balloon passage, the flow does not improve and the operator believes that the lesion is an acute-on-chronic one, a short predilatation with a semicompliant balloon at low-to-moderate pressures may be necessary.

Postdilatation

Observational studies indicate that stent postdilatation does not seem to have any detrimental effects on patients' final angiographic results and long-term clinical outcomes. However, the option is left on the operator if he/she feels that the stent is under expanded. Slow flow/no-reflow may be induced by postdilatation at high pressures. In a study by Tasal et al., 405 patients were retrospectively evaluated, and it was found that postdilatation did not adversely affect the final angiographic parameters, and seemed to decrease the probability of stent thrombosis and target vessel revascularization (TVR).[17] In another recent study by Soylu K et al., 124 patients were randomized to routine or no post dilatation during primary PCI with the former strategy being found to be associated with an increased risk of slow flow or no reflow in patients without angiographic stent expansion problems.[18]

Adjunctive Medications

The prehospital routine upstream use of glycoprotein (GP) IIb/IIIa inhibitors before primary PCI has not been demonstrated to offer any benefit and possibly increases the bleeding risk.[19] Using GP IIb/IIIa inhibitors as bailout therapy in the event of angiographic evidence of a large thrombus, slow- or no-reflow, and other thrombotic complications is reasonable, although this strategy has not (and can possibly never be) been tested in a randomized trial.

Overall, at the present moment, there is no evidence to recommend the routine use of GP IIb/IIIa inhibitors for primary PCI. The intracoronary administration of GP IIb/IIIa inhibitors is also not superior to its IV use.[20]

SLOW FLOW OR NO REFLOW

"Slow flow" and "no flow" represent differing degrees of the same phenomenon where a decrease in antegrade epicardial flow is there in the absence of a mechanical occlusion mostly due to distal microembolization and sludging. Certain drugs used by intracoronary route have been shown to reduce and perhaps reverse this phenomenon, but sometimes it can be extremely troublesome. Prevention is invariably a better option. Nicorandil has been used as an intravenous infusion for 24 hours after primary PCI to prevent slow flow. Adenosine has a role in prevention and treatment both. If it still happens during the procedure, the following drugs may prove to be helpful--adenosine 10–120 μg bolus, verapamil 100–200 μg bolus, or nitroprusside 50–200 μg; maximum up to 1,000 μg. However, there is no fixed protocol or sequence which has been found to be consistently helpful.

Cardiogenic Shock

Different trials have mostly indicated that in hemodynamically stable patients, complete revascularization of physiologically significant lesions may be beneficial in preventing progression of impending shock, but in unstable patients this strategy is likely to cause more harm. Thus, presently only culprit vessel revascularization, in the presence of cardiogenic shock, is the accepted strategy.[21,22]

Timing of initiation of Impella device has also evoked some interest, with a registry data favoring early pre-PCI use of Impella in such situations with demonstration of a significant early survival benefit.[23]

Thrombosuction

Since DeWoods landmark demonstration of thrombus being the primary culprit in the majority of AMIs, thrombus management has been at the core of interventional practices in AMI. A major limitation of primary PCI is the possibility of distal embolization of thrombus and failure to restore flow at the microvascular level even after creating a viable lumen in the artery. Indirect measures of microvascular tissue perfusion, such as the degree of ST-segment resolution or angiographic myocardial blush grade, have been shown to correlate with probability of death after primary PCI. Removal of thrombus by manual thrombectomy before stent deployment has the potential of reducing distal embolization and improving microvascular perfusion. The thrombus aspiration during PCI in AMI TAPAS (The Thrombus Aspiration during PCI in AMI Study) study showed improved myocardial blush grade (primary outcome) and lower mortality with thrombectomy.[24] Practice guidelines were subsequently altered to recommend routine manual thrombectomy. As a result, thrombectomy became a part of clinical practice and its use grew very rapidly. Subsequently meta-analyses[25] suggested that routine thrombosuction might increase the risk of stroke, but this finding was cautiously interpreted because it was based on a small number of events. Later, the thrombus aspiration in ST elevation myocardial infarction in Scandinavia (TASTE)[26] trial showed no reduction in mortality at 30 days up to 1 year with routine thrombectomy. Although updated meta-analyses of thrombectomy that included the TASTE trial continued to suggest that a modest but clinically important benefit is possible, the efficacy of this procedure presently remains uncertain. In TOTAL trial[27] a strategy of routine manual thrombectomy during primary PCI did not reduce the risk of the primary outcome of cardiovascular death, recurrent MI, shock or heart failure within 6 months as compared with strategy of PCI alone with thrombectomy only permitted as a bailout. Stroke rates were higher in patients who had undergone routine thrombectomy than in those who underwent PCI only. After the results of TOTAL trial, ACC/AHA focused update 2015 has classified routine manual aspiration thrombectomy during primary PCI as a class III indication and class IIb for selective and bailout procedures. A recent meta-analysis of all the three major trials (TAPAS, TASTE, TOTAL)[28] found no difference in major end points. However, in a subgroup of patients with high thrombus burden, thrombus aspiration was associated with a slight reduction in CV mortality (2.5% vs. 3.1%, CI 0.65–0.98; p = 0.03) but with an increase in stroke or transient ischemic attack (TIA). Perhaps, in the near future improved thrombus detection and characterization techniques (not all TIMI 0 flow are large thrombus—there can be significant underlying lesions also), better patient selection, and improved hardware can show us the correct way in different patients.

Choice of Stent

The central principle remains same as for conventional angioplasty—A drug-eluting stent (DES) is almost always better than a bare-metal stent (BMS). In a large-network meta-analysis of trials assessing the safety and efficacy of DES versus BMS in the setting of STEMI, Palmerini and colleagues found significantly lower rates of cardiac death or MI and stent thrombosis in cobalt-chromium-based everolimus eluting stents (CoCr-EES) compared with both BMS and first-generation DES. Nearly all DES types also carried lower 1-year TVR rates than BMS. The authors concluded that DES were superior to BMS in STEMI patients, with lower rates of MACE and improved efficacy seen at as little as 30 days from the index procedure and maintained for up to 2 years.[29]

In a pooled subgroup analysis from three randomised trials [the Intracoronary Stenting and Angiographic Results: test efficacy of 3 limus-eluting stents (ISAR TEST) 3, ISAR TEST 4 and Limus Eluted from A Durable versus ERodable Stent coating (LEADERS)] comparing outcomes in patients with acute MI between biodegradable polymer (BP) DESs (Yukon or Biomatrix) and durable polymer (DP) DESs (Cypher) at 4 years, MACE was significantly reduced with BP DES stents [hazard ratio (HR) 0.59, 95% confidence interval (CI) 0.39–0.90; p = 0.01). Trends toward reduction were also seen for cardiac death and MI, and definite or probable stent thrombosis (3.6% vs. 7.1%, HR 0.49, 95% CI 0.22–1.11; p = 0.09). Thus biodegradable polymer DESs demonstrated a reduction in clinically indicated target lesion revascularization and very late definite stent thrombosis up to 4 years in comparison to durable polymer DES, an effect which is likely to be potentially magnified in patients with STEMI.[30]

Another concept that held a brief promise, during evolution of primary PCI was use of MGuard stent—a balloon expandable BMS (stainless steel-strut width-100 µmm) along with a protection net (mesh sleeve fibres of 20 µmm polyethylene terephthalate) with a net aperture size of 150 × 180 µmm. The belief was that it would be effective in minimizing distal embolization. However, its use was associated with some limitations like deliverability related to a higher crossing profile, a possible compromise of side branches due to its double-layer design, and a higher restenosis rates.

The MGuard stent can rarely also be used in vein grafts causing AMI when conventional PCI with distal protection devices is not feasible, as well as to seal coronary perforations that persist despite prolonged balloon inflation.

DEFERRED STENTING

The concept of deferred stent implantation even after restoration of near normal epicardial flow by a minimalist immediate mechanical intervention (MIMI) for STEMI management was proposed for the first time by Isaaz et al.[31] Subsequent observational studies suggested that deferred stenting could have higher procedural success, and better 6-month ejection fraction together with lower rates of adverse events compared to immediate stenting. However, according to a recent comparative meta-analysis, a deferred-stenting strategy did not reduce the occurrence of no or slow reflow, death, MI, or repeat revascularization compared with immediate stenting in patients with STEMI but showed an improved LV function in the long term.[32] In DANAMI-3-DEFER study, deferred stenting (48 hours after the index procedure) had no effect on the primary clinical outcome. Routine deferred stenting was associated with a higher need for TVR.[33] Based on these findings, routine use of deferred stenting is not recommended at present and we suggest reserving this strategy only for those patients where there is a large residual visible thrombus and near TIMI III flow has been achieved.

CONCLUSION

The primary goal of any medical treatment in medical science is to relieve symptoms and prolong life--these are very admirably, quickly, and reliably achieved by performing a primary PCI in a patient with a STEMI, with a good end result in terms of vessel patency (both acute and chronic) and achieving TIMI 3 flow with TMP grade 3. The balance of speed, logistics, technique, and maturity is perhaps tested to the utmost during this procedure. A judicious combination of these qualities based on sound and up-to-date knowledge and current concepts defines a wise interventionalist likely to deliver the goods most of the time. Achieving a cosmetically good result may sometimes be compromised for safety and settling for a cosmetically adequate but a functionally good and safe result. Our first responsibility and endeavor should be to help the patient with minimal possibility of harm rather than satisfy our technical egos in pursuit of perfection.

REFERENCES

1. Alexander T, Mehta S, Mullasari A, et al. Systems of care for ST-elevation myocardial infarction in India. Heart. 2012;98:15e17.
2. Keeley EC, Boura JA, Grines CL. Primary angioplasty versus intravenous thrombolytic therapy for acute myocardial infarction: A quantitative review of 23 randomised trials. Lancet. 2003;361:13-20.
3. O'Gara PT, Kushner FG, Ascheim DD, et al. 2013 ACCF/AHA guideline for the management of ST–elevation myocardial infarction: A report of American College of Cardiology Foundation/American Heart Association Task Force on Practice Guideline. Circulation. 2013;127:e362.
4. Ibanez B, James S, Agewall S, et al. 2017 ESC guidelines for the management of acute myocardial infarction in patients presenting with ST- elevation. Eur Heart J. 2017;1-8.
5. Almawiri A, Jan V, Ziad A, et al. Mortality benefit of primary transportation to a PCI-capable center persists through an eight-year follow-up in patients with ST-segment elevation myocardial infarction. J Interv Cardiol. 2017;30:522-6.
6. Lampropoulos K, Megalou A, Bazoukis G, et al. Pre-loading therapy with statins in patients with angina and acute coronary syndromes undergoing PCI. J Interv Cardiol. 2017;30:507-13.
7. Jolly SS, Yusuf S, Cairns J, et al: Radial versus Femoral access for coronary angiography and intervention in patients with acute coronary syndrome (RIVAL): A randomized, parallel group multicenter trial. Lancet. 2011;377:1409-20.
8. Romagnoli E, Biondi-Zoccai G, Sciahbasi A, et al. Radial versus femoral randomized investigation in ST-segment elevation acute coronary syndrome: The RIFLE-STEACS. J Am Coll Cardiol. 2012;60:2481-9.
9. Bernat I, Horac D, Stasek J, et al. ST-segment elevation myocardial infarction treated by radial or femoral approach in a multicenter randomized clinical trial: The STEMI-RADIAL trial. J Am Coll Cardio. 2014;I63:964-72.
10. Kosmidou I, Redfors B, Selker HP, et al. Infarct size, left ventricular function, and prognosis in women compared to men after primary percutaneous coronary intervention in ST-segment elevation myocardial infarction: results from an individual patient-level pooled analysis of 10 randomized trials. Eur Heart J. 2017;38:1656-63.
11. Heer T, Hochadel M, Schmidt K, et al. Sex differences in percutaneous coronary intervention-insights from the coronary angiography and PCI registry of the German society of cardiology. J Am Heart Assoc. 2017;6:e004972.
12. Kunadian V, Qiu W, Lagerqvist B, et al. Gender differences in outcomes and predictors of all-cause mortality after percutaneous coronary intervention (data from United Kingdom and Sweden). Am J Cardiol. 2017;119:2106.
13. Wald DS, Morris JK, Wald NJ, et al. Randomized trial of preventive angioplasty in myocardial infarction. N Engl J Med. 2013;369(12):1115-23.
14. Smits PC, Abdel-Wahab M, Neumann FJ, et al. Fractional flow reserve-guided multivessel angioplasty in myocardial infarction. N Engl J Med. 2017; 376(13):123444.
15. Agarwal N, Jain A, Garg J, et al. Staged versus index procedure complete revascularization in ST-elevation myocardial infarction: a meta-analysis. J Interv Cardiol. 2017;30:397-404.
16. Dziewierz A, Siudak Z, Rakowski T, et al. Impact of direct stenting on outcome of patients with ST-elevation myocardial infarction transferred for primary percutaneous coronary intervention (from the EUROTRANSFER registry).Catheter Cardiovasc Interv. 2014;84(6):925-31.
17. Tasal A, Bacaksiz A, Vatankulu MA, et al. Is postdilatation with a noncompliant balloon necessary after coronary stent deployment during primary angioplasty? J IntervCardiol. 2013;26(4):325-31.
18. Soylu K, Ataş AE, Yenerçağ M, et al. Effect of routine postdilatation on final coronary blood flow in primary percutaneous coronary intervention patients without angiographic stent expansion problems. J Invest Med. 2018.
19. Ellis SG, Tendera M, de Belder MA, et al. Facilitated PCI in patients with ST-elevation myocardial infarction. N Engl J Med. 2008;358(21):2205-17.
20. Friedland S, Eisenberg MJ, Shimony A. Meta-analysis of randomized controlled trials of intracoronary versus intravenous administration of glycoprotein IIb/IIIa inhibitors during percutaneous coronary intervention for acute coronary syndrome. Am J Cardiol. 2011;108(9):1244-51.
21. Thiele H, Akin I, Sandri M, et al. PCI strategies in patients with acute myocardial infarction and cardiogenic shock. N Engl J Med. 2017;377:2419-32.
22. Ouweneel DM, Eriksen E, Sjauw KD, et al. Percutaneous mechanical circulatory support versus intra-aortic balloon pump in cardiogenic shock after acute myocardial infarction. J Am Coll Cardiol. 2017;69:278-87.
23. Meraj PM, Doshi R, Schreiber T, et al. Impella 2.5 initiated prior to unprotected left main PCI in acute myocardial infarction complicated by cardiogenic shock improves early survival. J Interv Cardiol. 2017;30:256-63.
24. Svilaas T, Vlaar PJ, Van der Horst IC, et al. Cardiac death and reinfarction after 1 year in the thrombus aspiration during Percutaneous coronary intervention in acute myocardial infarction Study (TAPAS): A 1 year follow-up study. Lancet. 2008;371:1915-20.
25. Lagerqvist B, Frobert O, Olivecrona GK, et al. Outcomes at 1 year after thrombus aspiration for myocardial infarction. N Engl J Med.. 2014;371:1111-20.
26. Frobert O, Lagerqvist B, Olivecrona GK, et al. thrombus aspiration during during ST-segment elevation myocardial infarction. N Engl J Med. 2014;371:786.
27. Jolly SS, Cairns JA, Yusuf S, et al. Outcomes after thrombus aspiration for ST elevation myocardial infarction: 1 year follow-up of the prospective randomized TOTAL trial. Lancet. 2016;387;127-35.
28. Jolly SS, James S, Dzavik V, et al. Thrombus aspiration in ST segment elevation myocardial infarction. An individual patient meta-analysis. Thrombectomy Trialists Collaboration. Circulation. 2017;135(2).143-52.
29. Palmerini T, Biondi-Zoccai G, Della Riva D, et al. Clinical outcomes with drug-eluting and bare-metal stents in patients with ST-segment elevation myocardial infarction: evidence from a comprehensive network meta-analysis. J Am Coll Cardiol. 2013;62(6):496-504.
30. de Waha A, King LA, Stefanini G, et al. Long-term outcomes of biodegradable polymer versus durable polymer drug eluting stents in patients with acute ST segment elevation myocardial infarction: a pooled analysis of individual patients from three randomized trials. Euro Inter. 2015;10:1425-31.
31. Isaaz K, Robin C, Cerisier A, et al. A new approach of primary angioplasty for ST elevation acute myocardial infarction based on minimalist immediate mechanical intervention. Coron Artery Dis. 2006;17:261-9.
32. Belle L, Motreff P, Mangen L, et al. Comparison of immediate with delayed stenting using the minimalist immediate mechanical intervention approach in acute ST segment elevation myocardial infarction: the MIMI study. Circ Cardiovasc Interv. 2016;9(3):e003388.
33. Kelbaek H, Hofsten DE, Kober L, et al. Deferred versus conventional stent implantation in patients with ST-segment elevation myocardial infarction (DANAMI 3-DEFER): An open-label, randomized controlled trial. Lancet. 2016; 387(10034):2199-206.

CHAPTER 46

Late Presenters with STEMI: Which is the Best Strategy?

Soumitra Kumar

INTRODUCTION

Any patient presenting 24 hours after onset of chest pain secondary to ST-elevation myocardial infarction (STEMI) represents a failure of the prevailing STEMI care system. The "total ischemic time" (symptom onset to initiation of reperfusion therapy) has two components: (1) patient delay and (2) system delay (including first medical contact to diagnosis and diagnosis to initiation of reperfusion therapy). The mean "total ischemic time" in Kerala Acute Coronary Syndrome (ACS) Registry[1] was 5 hours. When a patient presents as late as 24 hours after onset of symptoms, patient-related delay accounts for the main reason of delay and system-related delay becomes relatively insignificant. Proportion of latecomers (>12 h) is significant even in data from the west: 12% in GRACE (the Global Registry of Acute Coronary Events) study[2] and as high as 40% in the TETAMI (Treatment of Acute ST-Segment Elevation Myocardial Infarction Patients Ineligible for Reperfusion) study.[3] In an Indian study[4] done from Uttar Pradesh, India, 32.3% patients with STEMI presented after 24 hours.

Major benefit of revascularization of the infarct-related artery (IRA) is when the time from the onset of symptoms is less than 12 hours (Fig. 1). In the TETAMI Registry, 30 days mortality was only 4.4% in patients who received reperfusion therapy, but 12% in patients who did not receive it. Triple end point of death, myocardial reinfarction or recurrent angina occurred in only 11% of patients who were reperfused versus in 19.1% of patient who were not reperfused. In the ACOS registry, in-hospital mortality was 14% among nonreperfused patients compared to only 6.3% among reperfused patients.[5]

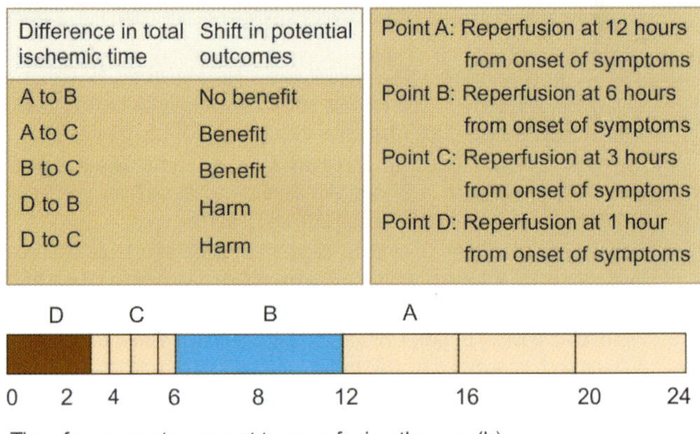

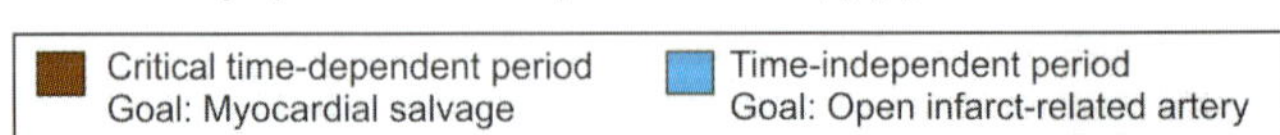

FIG. 1: Relationship of outcome and myocardial salvage as a function of total ischemic time.

RISK STRATIFICATION IN LATECOMERS AFTER STEMI

- *Clinical*: In the presence of hemodynamic or electrical instability and/or if patient continues to experience symptoms, a reperfusion-based strategy using percutaneous coronary intervention (PCI) is recommended and endorsed by the current guidelines [American College of Cardiology/American Heart Association/The Society for Cardiovascular Angiography and Interventions (ACC/AHA/SCAI) and European Society of Cardiology/European Association for Cardio-Thoracic Surgery (ESC/EACTS)][6,7]
- *Electrocardiography (ECG)*: Predictive value of negative T wave as a marker of reperfusion is strong. When T waves are positive, probability of occluded IRA is high. Negative T waves in "early" latecomers can thus push invasive strategy with the expectation to salvage the greatest amount of residual ischemic myocardium[8]
- *Angiographic*: Patency of IRA is important determinant of quantum of salvage by PCI independent of its timing. In their pivotal studies, Reimer and Jennings[9] emphasized by their work in a dog model that reperfusion must be established within the first 3 hours of onset of symptoms to achieve significant myocardial salvage. However, there exists an important yet unrecognized interplay between

time to reperfusion and presence of residual coronary flow within the area at risk. Beyond 4 hours of symptoms, significant salvage only occurred in the presence of well-developed collateral vessels or preserved antegrade flow in the IRA. The time-related transmural progression of infarction is greater in patients with no residual flow in the myocardium in jeopardy and presence of collateral flow or antegrade flow in the IRA can indeed increase the time-window for perfusion in humans[10]

- *Left ventricular (LV) systolic function*: Among patients with STEMI, adverse events are markedly increased in those with LV ejection fraction (LVEF) less than 40% even when undergoing primary PCI;[11] however, given the prospect of myocardial salvage, these high-risk patients stand to accrue substantial clinical benefits from the procedure as well
- *Stress testing*: Exercise testing is useful in assessing exercise capacity, identifying persistent ischemia, and risk stratification for future cardiac events. Submaximal testing may be done in asymptomatic patients after 3–5 days and symptom-limited testing may be done in the same subset of patients after 5 days

The DANAMI-1 (DANish trial in Acute Myocardial Infarction)[12] and SWISS (Swiss Interventional Study on Silent Ischemia)[13] trials have demonstrated beneficial effects of PCI performed late after myocardial infarction (MI) in patients with persistent ischemia on stress testing. The INSPIRE (Investigating New Standards for Prophylaxis in Reducing Exacerbations) trial[14] assessed use of myocardial perfusion imaging for defining initial patient risk and in guiding role of intensive medical therapy versus coronary revascularization for reducing the total LV perfusion defect and extent of scintigraphic ischemia on single photon emission computed tomography (SPECT) imaging. Myocardial perfusion positron emission tomography (PET) provides an option for patient groups who may be more difficult to image with SPECT myocardial perfusion imaging (MPI), including obese patients, women, patients with previous nondiagnostic tests, and patients with poor LV function attributable to coronary artery disease (CAD) considered for revascularization

- *Myocardial viability*: In the VIAMI (Viability-Guided Angioplasty After Acute Myocardial Infarction) trial,[15] patients not treated with primary or rescue PCI but otherwise in the non-high-risk category were subjected to either invasive (PCI) or a conservative (ischemia-guided) strategy if the infarct area was proven to be viable. Benefit in terms of composite end points of death, MI or unstable angina is seen at follow-up of 1 year and at long-term follow-up of median 8 years with initial in-hospital invasive strategy. The same investigators also reported in a substudy of the trial on the influence of viability and revascularization on LV remodeling. Viability early after acute myocardial infarction (AMI) is associated with improvement in LV function after revascularization. When viable myocardium is not revascularized, the LV tends to remodel with increased LV volumes, without improvement of EF. Absence of viability results in ventricular dilatation and deterioration of LVEF, irrespective of revascularization status.

Various modalities which can be utilized to assess myocardial viability are thallium-201 or technetium-99m, SPECT, fluorodeoxyglucose (FDG)-PET, dobutamine stress ECHO, dobutamine stress cardiac MRI, and contrast-enhanced MRI.

REPERFUSION PCI IN LATECOMERS WITH STEMI

Open Artery Hypothesis

This hypothesis was first proposed by Eugene Braunwald in 1989 when he noted that patients with spontaneous recanalization of the IRA had fewer adverse events during following weeks and months. These effects are not likely to be attributable to small benefits in infarct salvage and probably arise from limitation of infarct expansion, reduction of LV remodeling development, scaffolding effect of reperfused vessel, a conduit for collateral vessel, improvement of blood supply to hibernating myocardium, increased infarct wound healing, development of contraction band necrosis rather that coagulation necrosis in infarcted myocardium, reduction of myocardial apoptosis, increased baroreceptor sensitivity and vagal activity and reduced ventricular arrhythmia. These mechanisms extended the time window of ischemia to 12 hours and possibly 24 hours after onset of AMI. However, the period after 24 hours of onset of AMI is more challenging. On the basis of OAT (The Occluded Artery Trial) study,[16] routine PCI 3 days to weeks after AMI is not recommended for persistently occluded IRA in asymptomatic high-risk patients, since higher reinfarction rates were seen in the PCI group and yet, no difference were seen between PCI and conservative groups in terms of event-free survival after median follow-up of 3.2 years or LV systolic function at 1 year. Subsequently, Abbate et al.[17] performed a meta-analysis and systematic review of randomized trials (total of 3,560 patients from OAT, SWISS III and several other small studies (Table 1) comparing late PCI (defined as >12 hours from symptom onset) with medical therapy in hemodynamically stable patients with primary end point of survival. PCI was associated with an overall improvement in survival with an odds ratio of 0.49 [95% confidence interval (CI): 0.26–0.94]. In addition, a greater improvement in cardiac function was observed over time in patients assigned to PCI than medically managed patients supporting the concept that late revascularization may reverse adverse cardiac remodeling over longer-term.

Based on these trial results, it is also reasonable to expect that those with a totally occluded IRA on initial diagnostic angiogram are less likely to see a survival benefit from late revascularization than those with subtotal occlusions, unless there are other high-risk features, such as inducible ischemia or significant viability. It is likely that patients with subtotal occlusions are more likely than those with total occlusions to have ongoing ischemia, which can predispose to further cell death. Late reperfusion probably beneficially interrupts this process and reduces the extent of adverse remodeling

TABLE 1: Randomized clinical studies of late perfusion more than 24 hours after onset of acute myocardial infarction

Study	No. of patients rep.: +/-	Method for rep	Time to rep	Sustained patency rep. +/-	Overall outcome
Topol et al. TAMI-6	71, 34/37	tPA+/–PTCA	12–48 h	60%/38% at 6 months	Negative (modality, LV volume, LV systolic function at 6 months)
Dzavik et al. TOMIIS	44, 25/19	PTCA	5–42 days; mean 21 days	43%/19% at 4 months	Negative (clinical outcomes, LV size and EF at 4 months); positive in the subset (LVEF at 4 months)
Horie et al.	83, 44/39	PTCA	>24 h	96%/13% at 6 months	Positive (LV volume at 6 months; death, recurrent MI, congestive heart failure at 50 months)
Yousef et al. TOAT	66, 32/34	Stenting	3 days–6 weeks; mean, 26 days	91%/19% at 12 months	Greater LV dilation but improved exercise tolerance and QoL with reperfusion at 12 months
Steg et al. DECOPI	212, 109/103	Stenting	2–15 days	83%/34% at 6 months	Improved LVEF but no difference in clinical outcomes at 2 years
Hochman et al.	2166, 1082/1084	Stenting	3–28 days; median, 8 days	–	Negative (event-free survival at 4 years) trend toward higher reinfarction rates in reperfusion
Davik etal.	381, 150/136	Stenting	3–28 days; median,10 days	83%/25% at 1 year	Negative (LVEF at 4 years); trend toward less LV dilation in reperfusion

LVEF, left ventricular ejection fraction; MI, myocardial infarction; PTCA, percutaneous transluminal coronary angioplasty; tPA, tissue plasminogen activator; LV, left ventricular; QoL, quality of life; rep, reperfusion.

occurring in this setting. The BRAVE-2 (The Beyond 12 hours Reperfusion Alternative Evaluation) study[18] enrolled STEMI patients between 12 and 48 hours and SPECT study at a median of 7.1 days showed a statistically significant reduction in final infarct size in those assigned to the invasive strategy. Thus, "not so latecomers" (12–48 hours) may stand to gain through reperfusion of hibernating myocardium in peri-infract region. Busk et al.[19] compared infarct size and myocardial salvage after primary angioplasty in patients presenting with symptoms less than 12 h versus 12–72 hours. Final infarct size in late presents (>12 h) was larger than in early presenters (<12 h) after primary angioplasty for STEMI. However, they concluded that substantial myocardial salvage could be obtained beyond 12 hours limit, even when the infarct-related artery was totally occluded.

Challenges of Late Revascularization

- Success rates as defined by residual diameter stenosis less than 20%; epicardial TIMI-3 grade flow do not exceed 85–90%. Ongoing microvascular damage also interferes with TIMI-3 perfusion grades
- Total occlusion of an IRA is commonly associated with a significant thrombotic burden. The thrombus is at least partially organized and thus mechanically more resistant to guidewire recanalization
- However, paradoxically, periprocedural complications occur only in a minority of patients with adverse coronary lesion features (e.g., unprotected left main lesion, true bifurcation disease, and severe calcification) or heavy thrombus burden
- When thrombus is angiographically evident, aggressive antithrombotic therapy and mechanical thrombectomy prior to stent implantation may be helpful in minimizing distal embolization and recurrent MI
- Remaining interventional strategy, e.g., choice of bare-metal versus drug-eluting stents, use of debulking or imaging [intravascular ultrasound (IVUS) or optical coherence tomography (OCT)], short- versus long-term dual antiplatelet therapy, should be decided on a case-by-case basis.

Overall, rationale and current guidelines for reperfusion with PCI for latecomers with STEMI has been summarized in boxes 1 and 2.

NONREPERFUSION OPTIONS FOR LATE PRESENTERS WITH STEMI

Antithrombotic Therapy

- *Oral acetylsalicylic acid (ASA)*: Current guidelines for treatment of STEMI in patients with platelet counts in the normal range recommend that ASA (aspirin) therapy is associated with relative risk reduction (RRR) in mortality rate of 20–25% irrespective of whether patients are receiving reperfusion therapies.[19] True aspirin hypersensitivity remains an exception and use of ASA was not associated with more severe bleeding
- *Thienopyridines*: The ACOS Registry[5] reported that addition of clopidogrel to aspirin showed a reduction in major adverse cardiac and cerebrovascular events (death, nonfatal reinfarction and nonfatal stroke) in all subgroups of patients with STEMI including those who were not reperfused. The subgroup analysis of the COMMIT (ClOpidogrel and Metoprolol in Myocardial Infarction Trial)[20] showed similar reduction of primary endpoints with clopidogrel irrespective of treatment with fibrinolytic agents (11% reduction with fibrinolytic therapy vs. 7% without)[21]

BOX 1 Rationale of reperfusion with percutaneous coronary intervention for latecomers (>24 h) with STEMI

- The late open artery hypothesis is that coronary revascularization may yield clinically relevant benefit even when performed more than 12 h from symptom onset in a time-independent fashion. Proposed mechanisms for this include limitation of infarct expansion and remodeling through the influx of inflammatory cells and reduction in cellular degeneration through apoptosis
- Early support for this theory came from retrospective observation studies that found patency of the infarct-related artery (IRA) following thrombolytic therapy to be a favorable prognostic sign
- The BRAVE-2 study demonstrated that patients treated with an immediate invasive strategy within 12–48 h of acute myocardial infarction had reduced mortality at 4 years
- Patients with evidence of silent ischemia showed significant benefit from late PCI with a reduction in major adverse clinical events over a 10-year follow-up period in the Swiss Interventional Study on Silent Ischemia Type II study
- Myocardial viability may also be an important factor in determining who may benefit from late PCI based on early results from the Viability in Acute Myocardial Infarction trial
- Stable asymptomatic patients presenting more than 3 days from symptom onset who have total occlusion of the IRA and no evidence of severe silent ischemia showed no difference in overall mortality or major adverse clinical events in the Open Artery Trial
- Studies with higher event rates in the control arm have shown greater benefit from late PCI, suggesting that it is higher risk patients that have the most to gain from late revascularization
- Trials that enrolled patients with subtotal occlusion tended to show more benefit from PCI than those that only enrolled patients with total IRA occlusion, suggesting those with subtotal occlusions are more likely to have underlying viability and/or ischemia
- Busk et al. reported that substantial myocardial salvage can be obtained beyond the 12 h limit, even when the IRA is totally occluded
- A meta-analysis of randomized trials comparing late PCI to medical therapy demonstrated improved survival and greater improvement in cardiac function over time
- Late revascularization presents special challenges to the interventional cardiologist, requiring careful analysis of patient and angiographic variables to determine the most appropriate strategy
- Given the complexity and variety of possible factors in the spectrum of stable patients presenting late with acute myocardial infarction, we propose a patient-tailored approach and a management strategy based on the existing evidence

PCI, percutaneous coronary intervention.

- *Glycoprotein IIb/IIIa receptor blockers*: The TETAMI randomized trial[22] demonstrated that addition of tirofiban to either unfractionated heparin (UFH) or low-molecular-weight heparin (LMWH) did not provide additional benefit irrespective of the use of reperfusion. There are no data to support the use of intravenous glycoprotein IIb/IIIa inhibitors alone as an antiplatelet agent in the absence of reperfusion in STEMI

BOX 2 The European Society of Cardiology (ESC) 2017 STEMI guidelines[27]

- In patients with time from symptom-onset >12 h, a primary percutaneous coronary intervention (PCI) strategy is indicated in the presence of ongoing symptoms suggestive of ischemia, hemodynamic instability or life-threatening arrhythmias (class IC recommendation)
- A routine primary PCI strategy should be considered in patients presenting late (12–48 h) after symptom onset (class IIa B recommendation)
- In asymptomatic patients, routine PCI of an occluded IRA >48 h after onset of STEMI is not indicated (class IIIA recommendation)

- *Unfractionated heparin*: Systematic overview by Collins et al.[23] revealed that in absence of aspirin, heparin therapy reduced mortality; however, in presence of aspirin, adding UFH reduced mortality and reinfarction but there was a significant excess of major bleeds (1% vs. 0.7%, $p < 0.001$)
- *Low-molecular-weight heparin*: Available data-suggest that compared with UFH, LMWHs given along with aspirin provide significant benefit in STEMI patients who present late or are ineligible for reperfusion therapy. Their use in these patients is supported by both current European and North American STEMI guidelines[24]
- *Fondaparinux*: In the subgroup of OASIS-6 trial,[25] in which patients did not receive reperfusion therapy, fondaparinux as compared to usual care (UFH infusion or placebo) significantly reduced the composite of death or myocardial reinfarction without increasing severe bleedings or strokes
- *Parenteral direct thrombin inhibitor*: There are no data available on the role of direct thrombin inhibitors in STEMI with no-reperfusion therapy.

Nonantithrombotic Therapies

- *Beta-blockers*: There is significant evidence of benefit with early use of beta-blockers in wide subset of STEMI patients without any contraindications. Benefits have been demonstrated for patients with and without concomitant fibrinolytic therapy and both early and late after STEMI
- *Renin–angiotensin–aldosterone system inhibitors*: A large number of randomized clinical trials have assessed the role of angiotensin-converting enzyme inhibitors (ACEI) early in the course of acute MI. The SMILE (Survival of Myocardial Infarction Long-term Evaluation) trial[26] comprised only patients with anterior MI who had not received fibrinolytic therapy. Early use of an ACE inhibitor, zofenopril, in this trial conferred a trend of reduction in mortality in the first 6 weeks. These data support the role of ACEI with or without reperfusion therapy in STEMI
- *Nitrates*: These are useful only in patients suffering from recurrent angina and should not be used if consequent hypotension limits the administration of beta-blockers or ACEI, who have significant prognostic benefits for STEMI patients

- *Statins*: Early use of statins in ACS patients reduces both short- and long-term adverse outcomes.[20] However, recent statin trials were conducted in the setting of STEMI receiving reperfusion therapy.

CONCLUSION

- Late presenters of STEMI are well beyond the scope of conventional revascularization of IRA less than 12 hours after onset of STEMI and they have a higher incidence of death, myocardial reinfarction, and recurrent angina
- It should be remembered that delayed revascularization of IRA is fraught with lower success rate and benefits are also less certain
- Benefits of routine, i.e., nonischemia driven PCI of an angiographically significant stenosis in a patent infarct-related artery more than 24 hours after STEMI, are less well established but may have a survival benefit by virtue of improved cardiac function. Delayed PCI of a totally occluded infarct artery more than 48 hours after STEMI should not be undertaken in clinically stable patient without demonstrable evidence of ischemia or viability.

REFERENCES

1. Mohanan PP, Mathew R, Harikrishna S, et al. Presentation, management and outcomes of 25748 acute coronary syndrome admissions in Kerala. India: results from the Kerala ACS Registry. Eur Heart J. 2013;34(2):121-9.
2. Eagle KA, Nallamothu BK, Mehta RH, et al. Trends in acute reperfusion therapy for ST-segment elevation myocardial infarction from 1999 to 2006: we are getting better but we have got a long way to go. Eur Heart J. 2008;29:609-17.
3. Cohen M, Gensini GF, Maritz P, et al. on behalf of the TETAMI Investigators. Prospective evaluation of clinical outcomes after ST-segment elevation myocardial infarction in patients who are ineligible for reperfusion therapy; preliminary results from the TETAMI registry and randomized trial. Circulation. 2003;108(Suppl 3):14-21.
4. Agarwal V, Lohiya BV, Sihag BK, et al. Clinical profile with angiographic correlation in naïve acute coronary syndrome. J Clin Diagn Res. 2016;10(9):10-4.
5. Zeymer U, Gitt AK, Junger C, et al. Clopidogrel in addition to aspirin reduces in-hospital major cardiac and cerebrovascular events in unselected patients with acute ST segment elevation myocardial infarction. Thromb Haemostat. 2008;99:155-60.
6. Levine GN, Bates ER, Blankenship JC, et al. 2011 ACCF/AHA/SCAI guideline for percutaneous coronary intervention. J Am Coll Cardiol. 2011;58:e44-122.
7. Windecker S, Kolh P, Alfonso F, et al. 2014 ESC/EACTS Guidelines on myocardial revascularization. Eur Heart J. 2014;35(37):2541-619.
8. Ripa MS. The ECG as decision support in STEMI. Dan Med J. 2012;59(3):B4413.
9. Reimer KA, Jennings RB. The "Wavefront Phenomenon" of myocardial ischemic cell death II. Transmural progression of necrosis within the framework of ischemic bed size (myocardium at risk) and collateral flow. Lab Invest. 1979;40:633-44.
10. Octz-Perez JT, Lee DC, Meyers SN, et al. Determinants of myocardial salvage during acute myocardial infarction. J Am Coll Cardiol. 2010;3(5):491-500.
11. Ng VG, Lansky AJ, Stone GW, et al. Eur Heart J Acute Cardiovasc Care. 2014;3(1):67-77.
12. Madsen JK, Grande P, Saunamaki K, et al. Danish multicenter randomized study of invasive versus conservative treatment in patients with inducible ischemia after thrombolysis in acute myocardial infarction (DANAMI). DANISH trial in Acute Myocardial Infarction. Circulation. 1997;96(3):748-55.
13. Erne P, Schoenenberger AW, Burckhardt D, et al. Effects of percutaneous coronary interventions in silent ischemia after myocardial infarction the SWISS II randomized controlled trial. JAMA. 2007;297(18):1985-91.
14. Mahamarian JJ, Shaw LJ, Olszewski GH, et al. Adenosine sestamibi SPECT post-infarction evaluation (INSPIRE) trial: A randomized prospective multicenter trial evaluating the role of adenosine Tc-99m sestamibi SPECT for assessing risk and therapeutic outcomes In survivors of acute myocardial infarction. J Nucl Cardiol. 2004;11(4):458-69.
15. Van Loon RB, Veen G, Baur LH, et al. Long-term follow-up of the viability guided angioplasty after acute myocardial infarction (VIAMI) trial. Int J Cardiol. 2015;186:111-6.
16. Hochman JS, Lamas GA, Buller CE, et al. Coronary intervention for persistent occlusion after myocardial infarction. N Engl J Med. 2006;355:2395-407.
17. Abbate A, Biondi-Zoccai GG, Appleton DL, et al. Survival and cardiac remodeling benefits in patients undergoing late percutaneous coronary intervention of the infarct-related artery: evidence from a meta-analysis of randomized controlled trials. J Am Coll Cardiol. 2008;51(9):956-64.
18. Schoemig A, Mehilli J, Antoniucci D, et al. Mechanical reperfusion in patients with acute myocardial infarction presenting more than twelve hours from symptom onset. JAMA. 2005;293:2865-72.
19. Busk M, Kaltoft A, Nielsen SS, et al. Infarct size and myocardial salvage after primary angioplasty in patients presenting with symptoms for <12 h vs. 12-72 h. Eur Heart J. 2003;30:1322-30.
20. Van de Werf F, Bax J, Betriu A, et al. Management of acute myocardial infarction in patients with persistent ST-segment elevation: the Task Force on the Management of ST-Segment Elevation Acute Myocardial Infarction of the European Society of Cardiology. Eur Heart J. 2008;29:2909-45.
21. Chen ZM, Jiang LX, Chen YP, et al. Addition of clopidogrel to aspirin in 45,852 patients with acute myocardial infarction: randomized placebo-controlled trial. Lancet. 2005;366:1607-21.
22. Cohen M, Gensini GF, Maritz F, et al. The safety and efficacy of subcutaneous enoxaparin versus intravenous unfractionated heparin and tirofiban versus placebo in the treatment of acute ST-segment elevation myocardial infarction patients ineligible for reperfusion (TETAMI): a randomized trial. J Am Coll Cardiol. 2003;42:1348-56.
23. Collins R, MacMohan S, Flather M, et al. Clinical effects of anticoagulant therapy in suspected acute myocardial infarction: systematic overview of randomized trials. BMJ. 1996;313:652-9.
24. Thomas D, Gingliano RP. Management of ST-segment elevation myocardial infarction: comparison of updated guidelines from North America and Europe. Am Heart J. 2009;158:695-705.
25. Oldgren J, Wallentin L, Afzal R, et al. Effects of fondaparinux in patients with ST-segment elevation acute myocardial infarction not receiving reperfusion treatment. Eur Heart J. 2008;29:315-23.
26. Ambrosioni E, Borghi C, Magnami B. The effect of the angiotensin-converting enzyme inhibitor Zofenopril on mortality and morbidity after anterior myocardial infarction. The survival of Myocadial Infarction Long Term Evaluation (SMILE) Study Investigators. N Engl J Med. 1995;332:80-5.
27. Ibanez B, James S, Agewal S, et al. 2017 ESC Guidelines for Management of Acute Myocardial Infarction in Patients Presenting with ST-segment Elevation: The Task Force for the Management of Acute Myocardial Infarction in Patients presenting with ST-segment Elevation of the European Society of Cardiology (ESC). Eur Heart J. 2018;39:79-90.

CHAPTER 47

Acute Coronary Syndrome in Elderly

Surender Deora, Kewal C Goswami

INTRODUCTION

Aging is inevitable and irreversible demographic phenomenon. It not only affects the individual but also the whole society directly or indirectly. With the improvement in living conditions, better available healthcare facilities and declining fertility, there is demographic shift with more ageing population in the society. Cardiovascular disease (CVD) is the most common cause of morbidity and mortality in elderly and acute coronary syndrome (ACS) contributes to one-third of total deaths in United States.[1] In India also, CVD is the leading cause of death in 20.3% in men and 16.9% in women.[2] The definition of elderly varies with different countries and population. Most of the developed countries use the cutoff of 65 years for elderly but the United Nations has accepted the chronological age of 60 years as cutoff. In India, population age more than 60 years are categorized as elderly and according to population census 2011, there are 104 million elderly populations with 53 million females and 51 million males which is expected to increase three times to reach 300 million by 2050.[3] The population of elderly in India is gradually increasing with 5.6% in 1961 which increased to 8.6% in 2011 and will be 20% of the total population in 2050. Most of the elderly population lives in rural area (~71%) as compared to 29% in urban area.[4]

The clinical presentation and management of ACS in elderly is challenging and is different as compared to younger patients. Advanced age itself is the most important risk factor for coronary heart disease and is an independent predictor of poor outcome. The mortality of ACS in elderly rises exponentially with age. Also there is paucity of data of ST-elevation myocardial infarction (STEMI) in the elderly population as they are underrepresented in majority of the clinical trials. In 593 published studies of ACS from 1996–2000, elderly individuals were only 6.7%.[5] Even with newer trials like TRITON-TIMI 38 (Trial to Assess Improvement in Therapeutic Outcomes by Optimizing Platelet Inhibition with Prasugrel) and PLATO (Platelet Inhibition and Patient Outcomes) the representation of elderly population was 13% and 15%, respectively.[6,7] The morbidity and mortality is high in elderly population as compared to younger population.[8] The in hospital mortality is 2.1% in patients less than 55 years of age and it is increased to 26.3% in patients more than 85 years.[9] Even the patients more than 80 years of age have double the mortality rate as compared to patients of 70 years.[10] With the improvement in medical and invasive treatment, the mortality of ACS is declining but the burden of the disease is increasing as the elderly population is increasing because of the increased life expectancy. These elderly patients also may have the history of coronary artery disease in the young and are being treated previously either medically or by any invasive modality. Repeat ACS in these patients are more challenging because of extensive coronary artery disease and associated other organ diseases.

CHALLENGES IN ELDERLY

There are various factors which makes diagnosis and treatment in elderly population challenging. Usually the elderly patients have late presentation of STEMI because of various comorbid and socioeconomic factors. The symptoms are vague in nature and typical angina is less common.[11] The autonomic symptoms like dyspnea, nausea, vomiting, and syncope are more common.[12] Neurocognitive abnormalities are also frequently seen in this patient population which sometime makes the history taking and clinical examination difficult. The associated comorbid conditions like anemia, arthritis, hiatal hernia, abdominal discomfort, and renal dysfunction may mask the ischemic symptoms.[13] More often these patients presents with heart failure. The interpretation of electrocardiogram may also be difficult because of the pre-existing conduction defects, pacing rhythm, left ventricular hypertrophy or previous myocardial infarction.[14] Moreover, the elderly ACS patients usually present without significant

ST elevation because of more severe coronary involvement that may result in rich collateral network and ischemic preconditioning. The cardiac reserve is less and the chances of diastolic dysfunction are more. The coronaries are more diffusely diseased and calcified which makes the interventions more challenging and more prone for complications.[15,16]

MANAGEMENT

The prognosis of ACS has improved significantly in the last two decades with evidence-based therapies. The benefit of more aggressive treatment in elderly is high as they are at the greatest risk of complications. The benefit of guideline-directed therapy has been seen in elderly patients with non-ST-elevation myocardial infarction (NSTEMI) with reduced in-hospital mortality.[17] However, in real world clinical practice, the elderly are being treated more conservatively and even guideline-directed therapy not given because of fear of high risk of complications and therefore, has high mortality in spite of advancement in ACS management.[18,19] The management of elderly ACS patients depends on ischemic burden of the disease. The approach to the elderly patients with STEMI should be individualized depending on comorbid conditions, ischemic burden, estimated life expectancy and patient choice. The patients with extensive ischemia need more aggressive therapies with antithrombin, antiplatelets and early percutaneous coronary intervention (PCI) and therefore should be risk stratified before initiating any treatment. There are no separate risk stratification score for elderly but the ACS validated score systems like TIMI risk score, GRACE (Global Registry of Acute Coronary Events) score can be used in elderly because age has been included as important predictor of survival and complication. Baseline functional status and frailty are also important predictors of bleeding, longer hospital stay, increased morbidity and mortality.[20,21] The Gold Standards Framework (GSF) criteria may also help in deciding whether elderly ACS patient needs medical management or more aggressive invasive approach.[22]

MEDICAL MANAGEMENT

The standard and goal of medical care remains same as in young population and is to save the myocardium as much as possible along with the symptom relief. Oxygen support, antiplatelets, statins, beta-blockers, and angiotensin-converting enzyme (ACE) inhibitors are indicated in the pharmacotherapy as in other ACS patients except if any contra-indications are there. Thrombolytics are to be used in STEMI patients if the delay for primary PCI is more than expected time of 120 minutes. Elderly patients should not be denied fibrinolytic therapy although the risk of complications especially intracranial hemorrhage is more. But in real world scenario, the fibrinolytics are less commonly used in elderly. A study by Anderson et al. has shown that only 40% of the patients with STEMI aged between 75 and 84 years and only 20% above 85 years of age received fibrinolytic therapy.[23] The choice of fibrinolytic therapy in elderly is not well defined. In the GUSTO I (Global Utilization of Streptokinase and TPA for Occluded coronary arteries) trial, the patients above 85 years of age fared better with streptokinase and but because of limited data the relative superiority cannot be proved.[24] Fibrin-specific agents like reteplase and tenecteplase are usually preferred and have relatively lower risk of bleeding as compared to streptokinase but are costly. An observational registry by Toleva et al. has shown the in-hospital death rate in the elderly with no reperfusion therapy was 20%, with primary PCI 13%, and with fibrinolysis 9%.[25] In their study, 30% of elderly patients with STEMI received no reperfusion as compared to 13% of the younger patients. Thus in conclusion, the outcomes of fibrinolysis in elderly population are excellent with the selective use of fibrinolytic agents.

Anticoagulants have been shown to decrease the mortality in ACS patients. In EXTRACT-TIMI 25 (the Enoxaparin and Thrombolysis Reperfusion for Acute Myocardial Infarction treatment thrombolysis in myocardial infarction) study, the dose of enoxaparin in elderly more than 75 years of age was modified with no loading dose and maintenance dose of 0.75 mg/kg every 12 hourly.[26] There was no statistical difference in bleeding or hemorrhagic stroke was observed in elderly patients with age more than 75 years.

Antiplatelets should be given in all elderly patients with ACS. The loading dose of aspirin in elderly especially more than 75 years of age is 200 mg followed by 100 mg maintenance dose. Adjunctive antiplatelet like clopidogrel, prasugrel and ticagrelor should also be administered as per the indication similar to the young ACS patients but with caution especially in patients above 75 years of age. There are no specific studies in elderly patients with ACS for the antiplatelet but the data is from subgroup analysis of the other studies. The use of dual antiplatelet, i.e., adding clopidogrel to aspirin in CURE (Clopidogrel in Unstable Angina to Prevent Recurrent Events) study has shown benefit in reducing the primary end-point in NSTEMI patients. The subgroup analysis of CURE study in patients above 65 years of age has not shown any benefit in absolute or relative terms.[27] Prasugrel, a $P2Y_{12}$ receptor inhibitor is contraindicated in elderly population of more than 75 years and if weight is less than 60 kg. In TRITON-TIMI 38, there was no net benefit in elderly patients more than 75 years of age with ACS undergoing PCI and given 10 mg prasugrel because of increased risk of major bleeding and therefore suggested 5 mg in elderly patients. Similarly in PLATO trial of ticagrelor no net benefit was observed in elderly patients more than 75 years of age. Ticagrelor is an effective and more potent antiplatelet than clopidogrel but is costly which may be a limitation in old age patients especially in India and other developing countries. The American College of Cardiology (ACC)/American Heart Association (AHA) guideline is not clear on choice of second antiplatelet in elderly patients.[28] An ongoing study "POPular AGE" is an open label, multicenter trial in NSTEMI patients above 70 years of age randomized to either clopidogrel or more potent $P2Y_{12}$ inhibitor (prasugrel or ticagrelor).[29] The results

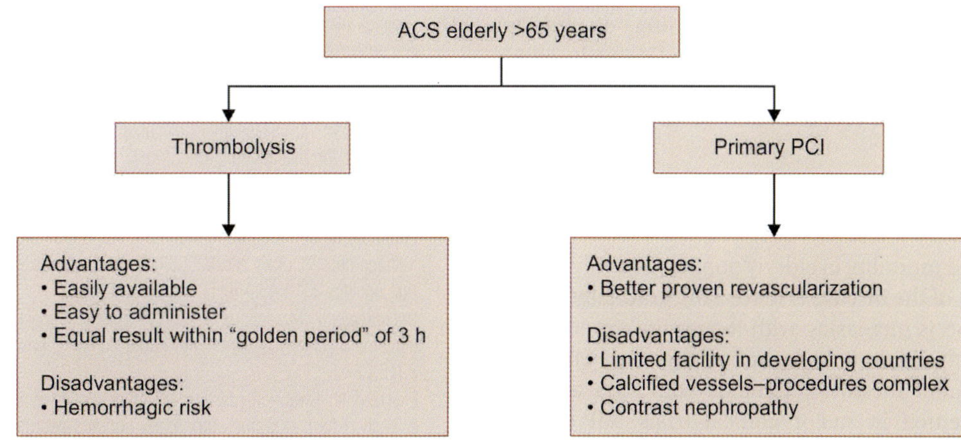

PCI, percutaneous coronary intervention; ACS, acute coronary syndrome.

FLOWCHART 1: Advantages and disadvantages of thrombolysis versus primary percutaneous coronary intervention.

of this study may give some evidence in choosing second antiplatelet agent in ACS patients.

High-dose statins in elderly has been proved as effective and safe as in younger population. A subgroup analysis from PROVE IT-TIMI 22 (the Pravastatin or Atorvastatin Evaluation and Infection Therapy–Thrombolysis in Myocardial Infarction 22) has shown a greater reduction in adverse events and similar side effect in elderly who received high-dose statin regimen as compared to younger patients.[30] Beta-blockers are also relatively less frequently used in elderly. An observational study has shown that half of the elderly patients more than 65 years of age did not receive beta-blocker therapy. Patients with early beta-blockers therapy had lower in hospital mortality rate than who did not receive it.[31] ACE inhibitors have been shown to reduce mortality at 1 year in elderly patients with STEMI.[32] The patients with age 55–74 years, anterior STEMI and heart rate more than 80/min are the most to be benefited.[33]

The side effect of polypharmacy is more in elderly. The adverse drug reaction increases with concurrent increase in the number of medication. With two medications it is 13% which increases to 38% with four medications and 82% with seven or more medications.[34] Therefore, in elderly selective medication according to guidelines should be used only and with caution.

THROMBOLYSIS VERSUS PRIMARY PERCUTANEOUS CORONARY INTERVENTION

Reperfusion therapies including fibrinolysis are indicated in elderly patients up to the age of 85 years.[35] The choice of preferred revascularization therapy by PCI or fibrinolysis does not depends on age but on many factors, e.g., time from presentation, door to balloon time, comorbid conditions, renal function and hemodynamic condition at the time of presentation (Flowchart 1).[36] The FRISC II (FRagmin and Fast Revascularization during InStability in Coronary artery disease) study was the first to show the clinical benefit of invasive strategy in NSTEMI patients and the most of the benefit was in patients above 65 years of age although patients above 75 years of age were excluded.[37] Similarly, the benefit of invasive strategy was noted in TACTICS (Treat Angina with Aggrastat and Determine Cost of Therapy with an Invasive or Conservative Strategy) study with ACS patients above 65 years of age in reducing death, nonfatal myocardial infarction and rehospitalization at 6 months.[38] The transradial approach is preferred over femoral approach in elderly patients because less access site bleeding complications but with higher crossover to femoral approach.[39] The elderly ACS patients usually more often presents with NSTEMI and have complex multivessel disease and diabetes. This subset of patients is more often benefited by coronary artery bypass surgery as compared to PCI but with more prolonged hospital stay and post-surgical recovery.[40] But due to wide heterogeneity in elderly patients in terms of chorological age and biological age, each patient should be individualized for the choice of revascularization therapy. Patient should be counseled about the disease and its associated risk and prognosis, quality of life after revascularization and side effect of the medications especially need of dual antiplatelet post-PCI.

CARDIAC REHABILITATION

Elderly patients after ACS need special attention as they are vulnerable because of frailty, comorbid conditions, multiple medications and decreased neurocognitive abilities. There is increased risk of rehospitalization and death from cardiac and noncardiac causes and the mortality increases by 50% every 10-year after the age of 65 years.[41] Patients should be discharged with clear advice for the compliance of medications and their schedule in local language, exercise and diet instructions and importance of cardiac rehabilitation. Lifestyle modifications, psychosocial support, and monitoring of risk factors are some of the components of cardiac rehabilitation.[42] Exercise training of elderly improves the sense of well-being, functional capacity, and cardiorespiratory efforts. Patients with strict compliance to medications and cardiac rehabilitation programs have less rehospitalization rates.

CONCLUSION

The morbidity and mortality in elderly population with ACS is high. The burden of the disease is increasing gradually as the elderly population is increasing with longer life expectancy. There is limited available data regarding the most effective way of management in elderly patients with ACS as they are underrepresented in major clinical trials. All elderly patients cannot be treated in the same way and treatment for each patient is to be individualized. Special attention has to be given to the associated comorbid conditions, ischemic burden and bleeding risk. Patients should be counseled for cardiac rehabilitation program to improve the quality of life post-ACS.

REFERENCES

1. Mozaffarian D, Benjamin EJ, Go AS, et al. Heart disease and stroke statistics – 2016 update: a report from the American Heart Association. Circulation. 2016;133:e38-360.
2. Registrar General of India. Causes of Deaths in India, 2001–2003. Office of the Registrar General, New Delhi, India 2009.
3. Caring for elders: Early responses. India ageing report 2017. United Nations Population Funds 2017.
4. Elderly in India: Profile and programmes in 2016. Central Statistics Office Ministry of Statistics and Programme Implementation, Government of India. 2016.
5. Lee PY, Alexander KP, Hammill BG, et al. Representation of elderly persons and women in published randomized trials of acute coronary syndromes. JAMA. 2001;286:708-13.
6. Wiviott SD, Braunwald E, McCabe CH, et al. Prasugrel versus clopidogrel in patients with acute coronary syndromes. N Engl J Med. 2007;357(20):2001-15.
7. Wallentin L, Becker RC, Budaj A, et al. Ticagrelor versus clopidogrel in patients with acute coronary syndromes. N Engl J Med. 2009;361(11):1045-57.
8. Hafiz AM, Jan MF, Mori N, et al. Contemporary clinical outcomes of primary percutaneous coronary intervention in elderly versus younger patients presenting with acute ST-segment elevation myocardial infarction. J Interv Cardiol. 2011;24:357-65.
9. Boucher JM, Racine N, Thanh TH, et al. Age-related differences in in-hospital mortality and the use of thrombolytic therapy for acute myocardial infarction. CMAJ. 2001;164:1285-90.
10. Halon DA, Adawi S, Dobrecky-Mery I, et al. Importance of increasing age on the presentation and outcome of acute coronary syndromes in elderly patients. J Am Coll Cardiol. 2004;43:346-52.
11. Mehta RH, Rathore SS, Radford MJ, et al. Acute myocardial infarction in the elderly: differences by age. J Am Coll Cardiol. 2001;38:736-41.
12. Gregoratos G. Clinical manifestations of acute myocardial infarction in older patients. Am J Geriatr Cardiol. 2001;10:345-7.
13. Grosmaitre P, Le Vavasseur O, Yachouh E, et al. Significance of atypical symptoms for the diagnosis and management of myocardial infarction in elderly patients admitted to emergency departments. Arch Cardiovasc Dis. 2013;106:586-92.
14. Boie ET. Initial evaluation of chest pain. Emerg Med Clin North Am. 2005;23:937-7.
15. Liberman A. Acute coronary syndromes in the elderly—Which is the difference? Rev Soc Cardiol Estado de São Paulo. 2002;4:497-510.
16. Wang TY, Gutierrez A, Peterson ED. Percutaneous coronary intervention in the elderly. Nat Rev Cardiol. 2011;8:79-90.
17. Skolnick AH, Alexander KP, Chen AY, et al. Characteristics, management, and outcomes of 5,557 patients age ≥90 years with acute coronary syndromes: results from the CRUSADE Initiative. J Am Coll Cardiol. 2007;49(17):1790-7.
18. Alexander KP, Newby LK, Armstrong PW, et al. Acute coronary care in the elderly, part II: ST-segment-elevation myocardial infarction: a scientific statement for healthcare professionals from the American Heart Association Council on Clinical Cardiology: in collaboration with the Society of Geriatric Cardiology. Circulation. 2007;115:2570-89.
19. Saunderson CE, Brogan RA, Simms AD, et al. Acute coronary syndrome management in older adults: Guidelines, temporal changes and challenges. Age Ageing. 2014;43:450-5.
20. Decourcelle V, Marechaux S, Pincon C, et al. Impact of functional decline on outcome in elderly patients with acute coronary syndromes. Am J Crit Care. 2013;22:e1-11.
21. Ekerstad N, Swahn E, Janzon M, et al. Frailty is independently associated with short-term outcomes for elderly patients with non-ST-segment elevation myocardial infarction. Circulation. 2011;124:2397-404.
22. Moretti C, Quadri G, D'Ascenzo F, et al. THE STORM (acute coronary Syndrome in paTients end Of life and Risk assesMent) study. Emerg Med J. 2016;33:10-6.
23. Alexander KP, Newby LK, Armstrong PW, et al. Acute coronary care in the elderly (part II), ST-segment elevation myocardial infarction: a statement for healthcare professionals from the American Heart Association Council of Clinical Cardiology, in collaboration with the Society of Geriatric Cardiology. Circulation. 2007;115:2570-89.
24. White HD, Barbash GI, Califf RM, et al. Age and outcome with contemporary thrombolytic therapy: results from the GUSTO-I trial. Global Utilization of Streptokinase and TPA for Occluded coronary arteries trial. Circulation. 1996;94:1826-33.
25. Toleva O, Ibrahim Q, Brass N, et al. Treatment choices in elderly patients with ST: Elevation myocardial infarction-insights from the Vital Heart Response registry. Open Heart. 2015;2(1):e000235.
26. Antmam EM, Morrow DA, McCabe CH, et al. Enoxaparin versus unfractionated heparin as antithrombin therapy in patients receiving fibrinolysis for ST elevation myocardial infarction. Design and rationale for the Enoxaparin and Thrombolysis Reperfusion for Acute Myocardial Infarction treatment thrombolysis in myocardial infarction study (EXTRACT-TIMI 25). Am Heart J. 2005;149:217-26.
27. Yusuf S, Zhao F, Mehta SR, et al. Effects of clopidogrel in addition to aspirin in patients with acute coronary syndromes without ST-segment elevation. N Engl J Med. 2001;345(7):494-502.
28. Amsterdam EA, Wenger NK, Brindis RG, et al. 2014 AHA/ACC guideline for the management of patients with non-ST-elevation acute coronary syndromes: executive summary: A report of the American College of Cardiology/ American Heart Association Task Force on Practice Guidelines. Circulation. 2014;130(25):2354-94.
29. Qaderdan K, Ishak M1, Heestermans AA, et al. Ticagrelor or prasugrel versus clopidogrel in elderly patients with an acute coronary syndrome: Optimization of antiplatelet treatment in patients 70 years and older—rationale and design of the POPular AGE study. Am Heart J. 2015;170(5):981-5.
30. Ray KK, Bach RG, Cannon CP, et al. Benefits of achieving the NCEP optional LDL-C goal among elderly patients with ACS. Eur Heart J. 2006;27(19):2310-6.
31. Krumholz HM, Radford MJ, Wang Y, et al. Early beta-blocker therapy for acute myocardial infarction in elderly patients. Ann Intern Med. 1999;131(9):648-54.
32. Krumholz HM, Chen YT, Wang Y, et al. Aspirin and angiotensin-converting enzyme inhibitors among elderly survivors of hospitalization for an acute myocardial infarction. Arch Intern Med. 2001;161(4):538-44.
33. ACE Inhibitor Myocardial Infarction Collaborative Group. Indications for ACE inhibitors in the early treatment of acute myocardial infarction systematic overview of individual data from 100000 patients in randomized trials. Circulation. 1998;97:2202-12.
34. Goldberg RM, Mabee J, Chan L, et al. Drug-drug and drug-disease interactions in the ED: Analysis of a high-risk population. Am J Emerg Med. 1996;14(5):447-50.
35. White HD, Barbash GI, Califf RM, et al. Age and outcome with contemporary thrombolytic therapy. Results from the GUSTO-I trial. Global Utilization of

Streptokinase and TPA for Occluded coronary arteries trial. Circulation. 1996;94(8):1826-33.

36. O'Gara PT, Kushner FG, Ascheim DD, et al. 2013 ACCF/AHA guideline for the management of ST-elevation myocardial infarction: A report of the American College of Cardiology Foundation/American Heart Association Task Force on Practice Guidelines. J Am Coll Cardiol. 2013;61(4):e78-140.
37. Invasive compared with non-invasive treatment in unstable coronary-artery disease: FRISC II prospective randomised multicentre study. FRagmin and Fast Revascularisation during InStability in Coronary artery disease Investigators. Lancet. 1999;354(9180):708-15.
38. Cannon CP, Weintraub WS, Demopoulos LA, et al. TACTICS (Treat Angina with Aggrastat and Determine Cost of Therapy with an Invasive or Conservative Strategy)–Thrombolysis in Myocardial Infarction 18 Investigators. Comparison of early invasive and conservative strategies in patients with unstable coronary syndromes treated with the glycoprotein IIb/IIIa inhibitor tirofiban. N Engl J Med. 2001;344(25):1879-87.
39. Cantor WJ, Mehta SR, Yuan F, et al. Radial versus femoral access for elderly patients with acute coronary syndrome undergoing coronary angiography and intervention: insights from the RIVAL trial. Am Heart J. 2015;170(5):880-6.
40. Amsterdam EA, Wenger NK, Brindis RG, et al. 2014 AHA/ACC guideline for the management of patients with non-ST-elevation acute coronary syndromes: A report of the American College of Cardiology/American Heart Association Task Force on Practice Guidelines. Circulation. 2014;130(25):e344-426.
41. Lopes RD, Gharacholou SM, Holmes DN, et al. Cumulative incidence of death and rehospitalization among the elderly in the first year after NSTEMI. Am J Med. 2015;128:582-90.
42. Pasquali SK, Alexander KP, Peterson ED. Cardiac rehabilitation inn the elderly. Am Heart J. 2001;142:748-55.

CHAPTER 48

Right Ventricular Myocardial Infarction: An Update

Shishu Shankar Mishra, Biswaranjan Mishra

INTRODUCTION

Worldwide coronary artery disease (CAD) is a leading cause of morbidity and mortality. It is a huge health burden to the mankind and all nations in the contemporary time. A great amount of knowledge and research has accumulated on the left ventricular myocardial infarction (LVMI). Right ventricular (RV) involvement in myocardial infarction (MI) was first described in 1974.[1] RV myocardium receives blood supply from both right and left coronary arteries. RV wall is thinner compared to LV. Therefore, right ventricular myocardial infarctions (RVMIs) are relatively small and most of the myocardium remains viable. Subsequently, high rate of in-hospital mortality was seen to be associated with RVMI.[2]

DEFINITION

With a clinical background of MI, diagnosis of RVMI is made by the presence of elevation of the ST-segment more than equal to 1 mm in leads augmented vector right, V1, and/or in the right precordial leads V3R and V4R. It is recommended to record V3R and V4R seeking ST-segment elevation, to identify concomitant RVMI. Right-sided electrocardiography (ECG) is the most sensitive and specific, as ST elevation in V4R more than 1 mm has 100% sensitivity, 87% specificity, and 92% predictive accuracy.[3]

INCIDENCE

Isolated RVMI is rare, it is commonly associated with LVMI.[4] In inferior wall MI (IWMI) and posterior MI of LV, the incidence of RVMI varies from 24 to 50%, out of which up to 50% are hemodynamically compromised. Compared to LVMI, RVMI is relatively rare. Lower incidence of RVMI is explained by its lower oxygen demand and increased supply. Relatively lower muscle mass and less workload keep the oxygen demand low, at the same time, coronary supply to RV muscles occurs in both systole and diastole along with more extensive collateralization which increases the supply. RV myocardium also receives oxygen from inside the RV cavity by diffusion because of its thin wall.[5]

PATHOPHYSIOLOGY

The right coronary artery (RCA) primarily supplies the right ventricle. The first branch of RCA, conus artery, supplies blood to the RV outflow tract whereas the second branch supplies to the sinoatrial node. Then it courses in the atrioventricular (AV) groove giving off multiple small branches to anterior RV. RCA then divides into the acute marginal branch that runs anteriorly along the diaphragm, and the posterior descending artery (PDA) that runs posteriorly. In 90% of patients the PDA supplies the AV node; in the remaining 10% it receives blood from the left circumflex artery. PDA also supplies the inferior wall of both ventricles. PDA may arise from the left coronary circulation in 15% of the population called left dominant coronary circulation.[6] Proximal RCA occlusions, occlusion of the RV branch or acute marginal branch result in RVMI. Occlusion of the left circumflex coronary artery in left dominant coronary circulation may also cause a RVMI.[7]

Right ventricular ischemia and infarction result in reduced RV systolic contraction along with RV diastolic dysfunction raising the RV filling pressure. This leads to a reduction in RV output and blood supply to the lungs and an increase in right atrial pressure. Reduced pulmonary flow decreases pulmonary venous return to left atrial (LA) and LV. In other words, it decreases LV preload or LV filling. This is expressed as reduced LV output and reduced systolic blood pressure (BP) in spite of a normally contracting LV. RV infarction leads to RV dilatation which alters the motion of the interventricular septum. Leftward shift of septum during diastole also impedes LV filling and further reduces cardiac output. LV dyssynchrony due to abnormal septal motion and loss of AV synchrony when there is AV block may also contribute to decreased cardiac output. Dilatation of RV enlarges the tricuspid annulus resulting in tricuspid regurgitation (TR) further jeopardizing forward RV output.

Increased RA pressure raises the jugular venous pressure (JVP) and increased systemic venous pressure may cause an edematous state.[8]

When RCA occlusion is proximal to right atrial branch, right atrial ischemia diminishes its contraction and increases RA pressure further increasing chance of atrial arrhythmia.[9] Increased RA pressure cause secretion of atrial natriuretic peptide which may also adversely affect the already compromised hemodynamics.

Elevated right-sided filling pressure in presence of normal pulmonary artery and left-sided filling pressure is the hallmark of RVMI. RA pressure of 10 mm Hg and with pulmonary artery wedge pressure 1–5 mm Hg, had a sensitivity of 73% and a specificity of 100% in identifying hemodynamically important RVMI.[10] RV pressure tracing may show an early diastolic dip and plateau resembling restrictive-constrictive physiology. Increased RA pressure may cause a right-to-left shunt across a stretched foramen ovale decreasing systemic saturation.[11]

CLINICAL PRESENTATION

Chest pain, diaphoresis, nausea, and vomiting are the hallmark of clinical presentation in MI including RVMI. AV block and arrhythmia can produce syncope and palpitation. Hypotension may be responsible for postural symptoms and fatigue. Signs of right heart failure such as edema and raised JVP are often seen. When RA ischemia is absent, JVP shows prominent "a" with a prominent "x" descent, but when RA contraction is compromised due to RA ischemia, "a", "x", and "y" descent are diminished. In presence of significant TR, both "v" waves and "y" descent are prominent. TR murmur may be heard in some cases. Marked sensitivity to preload reducing agents such as nitrates, morphine, and diuretics is a clue to presence of RVMI. Rarely, it may be present with RV free wall rupture causing cardiac tamponade.[12]

The classical triad of presentation of RVMI are hypotension, raised JVP and clear lung fields. Jugular venous distention on inspiration, the Kussmaul's sign in a setting of IWMI indicates presence of RVMI. Pulsus paradoxus which represents an exaggeration of the normal inspiratory decline in systemic arterial pressure may be appreciated in some cases. At times, these signs appear only after administration diuretics or nitrates.[13]

DIFFERENTIAL DIAGNOSIS

The classical triad of hypotension, raised JVP, and clear lung fields may be observed in cardiac tamponade, constrictive pericarditis, restrictive cardiomyopathy, acute pulmonary embolism, severe pulmonary hypertension, right-sided obstructive mass lesions, and acute severe TR. Careful history, ECG changes, and particularly echocardiography can easily differentiate each condition. [14]

Electrocardiography

The ST-segment elevations in leads II, III, and augmented vector foot are almost always present as RVMIs are usually associated with an IWMI. Several ECG findings arouse suspicion of associated RVMI. Disproportionately greater ST-segment elevation in lead III than in lead II is pathognomonic of RVMI.[15] An ST-segment elevation in lead V4R more than 1 mm is a reliable marker of RVMI with a sensitivity of 93% and specificity of 95%. Elevation of ST segment across the entire right precordium from V1R through V6R may also occur which is 100% sensitive, 87% specificity with 92% predictive accuracy (Fig. 1). Height of ST-segment elevation in V4R has also been found to be an independent predictor of adverse outcome.[16]

Rarely an isolated RVMI may present with ST-segment elevation in leads V1–V4 making an erroneous diagnosis of anterior wall MI. But there are some differentiating features. ST-segment vector analysis shows the mean vector in RV infarction usually is directed anteriorly and to the right (>100). But in an anteroseptal infarct, the mean ST-segment vector is directed leftward between –30° and –90°. Thus mean ST-segment vector can differentiate between MI at these two different sites.[17]

Arrhythmias are quite frequent in a setting of RVMI. There is a very high incidence of severe conduction disorders, complete AV or sinoatrial blocks which is present in nearly 50% of cases with ST elevation or a QS pattern in V3R, and/or V4R.[18] The incidence of sustained ventricular tachycardia (VT) is also high. Although anterior wall LVMI is associated with the highest mortality rates, but incidence of significant AV block and arrhythmias is higher when inferior wall LVMI is associated with RVMI.[19]

Biomarkers

Cardiac enzymes will be elevated in RVMI quite similar to LVMI. As the mass of myocardium involved is less, it does not play a significant role in diagnosis of RVMI. Similarly, biomarkers may not be of much help in differentiating between hemodynamically significant pulmonary embolism and RVMI.[20]

Echocardiography

The sensitivity and specificity of echo is 82% and 93%, respectively, for the detection of RV infarction. RV free wall hypokinesia is most specific for the diagnosis of RVMI. Wall

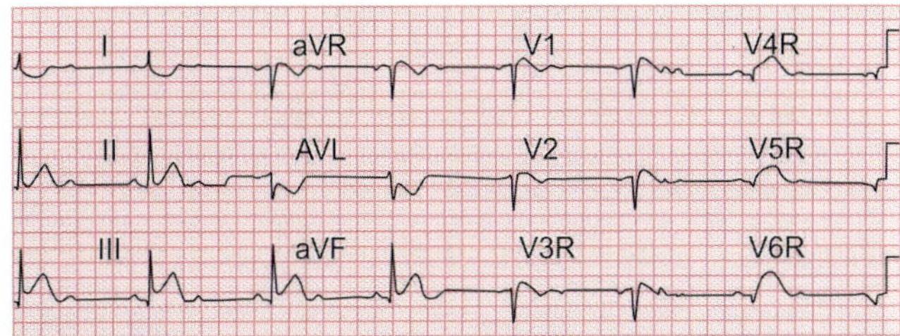

aVR, augmented vector right; aVL, augmented vector left; aVF, augmented vector foot.

FIG. 1: Electrocardiography in inferior wall myocardial infarction (MI) with right ventricular MI showing ST elevation in inferior leads, note the ST elevation in lead III is more than lead II, recording of right-sided leads V3R to V6R show ST elevation.

motion abnormality usually resolves in 3 months of time.[21] Dilation of RV is often seen with paradoxical septal motion. Systolic function is depressed as measured by tricuspid annular plane systolic excursion (TAPSE) and tissue Doppler bases tricuspid annular systolic motion. Calculation of RV ejection fraction (EF) shows lower values using two-dimensional (2D) or three-dimensional (3D) based methods. Doppler examination frequently shows presence of TR. A low-velocity TR is hallmark of RVMI (Fig. 2).[22] An abnormally elevated RV myocardial performance index (MPI) of greater than equal to 0.30 or greater is suggestive of the presence of a RV infarction. Recently, newer techniques like 2D speckle tracking is gaining importance in diagnosis of RVMI.[23]

Nuclear Imaging

Radionuclide ventriculography and 99mTc-pyrophosphate myocardial scintigraphy are sometimes used to assess RV wall motion and RV function including RV EF. RV dilatation

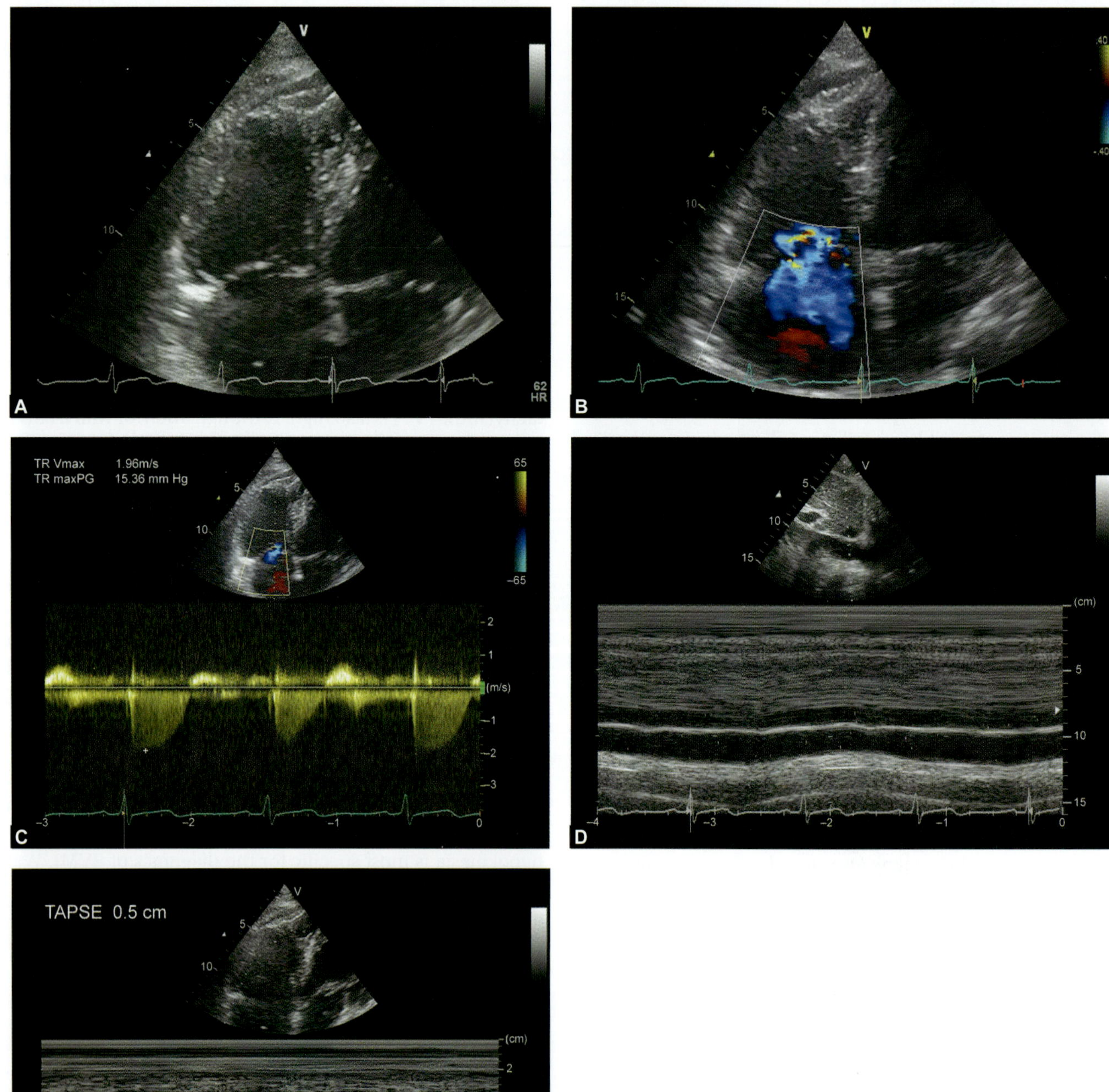

FIG. 2: A, Echocardiography in right ventricular myocardial infarction showing dilated hypokinetic right ventricular (RV); **B,** color Doppler interrogation shows presence of tricuspid regurgitation; **C,** continuous-wave Doppler shows a low-velocity tricuspid regurgitation; **D,** inferior vena cava is dilated with absent respiratory variation indicating right heart failure;. **E,** right ventricular annular plane systolic excursion (TAPSE) of 5 mm indicating RV dysfunction.

and free wall hypokinesia give a diagnosis of RVMI. The 99mTc-pyrophosphate myocardial scintigraphy is useful to detect RVMI, but clinical utility is less due to logistic issues.[24]

Cardiovascular Magnetic Resonance

Cardiovascular magnetic resonance (CMR) can accurately identify RVMI, but less availability, cost and patient discomfort in acute setting restrict its use in clinical practice.[25] RV free wall myonecrosis indicated by late gadolinium enhancement and obstruction are independent predictors of long-term outcome.[26]

Coronary Angiography

Coronary angiography (CAG) is the gold standards for definitive diagnosis. Its role in initial evaluation and workup are limited. This invasive procedure is mainly used during intervention.

MANAGEMENT

The use of statin, dual antiplatelet agents, and supplemental oxygen are similar to all MIs. The special precautions and treatment modalities are highlighted below.

Avoidance of Nitrates and Diuretics

Drugs that produce venodilatation like, nitrates and diuretics reduce RV filling further and can exacerbate the state of low cardiac output and hypotension in RVMI. Therefore, it is critically important to avoid nitrates and diuretics once the diagnosis of RVMI is made or suspected.[27]

Intravenous Fluid

The most important hemodynamic consequence of RV ischemia is significant decrease in LV preload. Mechanism of decreased LV preload is RV diastolic and systolic dysfunction that leads to decreased RV output, less blood returns to LV, reducing the filling (preload) of the LV. Therefore, the initial treatment requires the administration of IV crystalloid fluid sufficiently to increase RV filling. Generally 300–600 mL of normal saline is infused intravenously preferably through a central line over 10–15 minutes initially as fluid challenge. Clinical response depends upon the baseline intravascular volume status. In volume depleted patients cardiac output increases and BP rises, but in patients with normal volume status there will be no change in cardiac output and BP. Further volume loading of RV may be harmful as it hampers LV filling through interventricular interactions and raised intrapericardial pressure. It is pertinent to have invasive hemodynamic monitoring to see that RA pressure and pulmonary capillary wedge pressure (PCWP) does not exceed 20 mm Hg.[28]

Positive Inotropic Agent

After initial fluid challenge, if BP and cardiac output does not improve, but at the same time RA pressure and PCWP rise as seen by hemodynamic monitoring then positive inotropic agents such as dobutamine should be infused. In such cases, dobutamine infusion has shown to improve RV output, BP and RV EF. Inhaled nitric oxide when combined with dobutamine has the added benefit of reducing pulmonary vascular resistance (PVR) which decreases RV afterload. Milrinone, a phosphodiesterase III inhibitor, may also improve RV dysfunction by improving RV contractility. However, due to its nonselective action there is a risk of exacerbating systemic hypotension. The calcium sensitizer levosimendan may also improve RV function, by improving cardiac myocyte sensitivity to intracellular calcium without increasing calcium concentrations. These drugs produce increased inotropy as well as peripheral vasodilatation.[29]

Restoration of Coronary Blood Flow

Early establishment of coronary blood flow is the key to a successful treatment. Early thrombolysis improves hemodynamics, clinical course and decrease mortality.[4] Timely primary percutaneous coronary intervention (PCI) can dramatically improve clinical, hemodynamic, and survival parameters (Fig. 3). Early reperfusion also helps in stabilizing electrically and reduces chances of ventricular arrhythmias.[30]

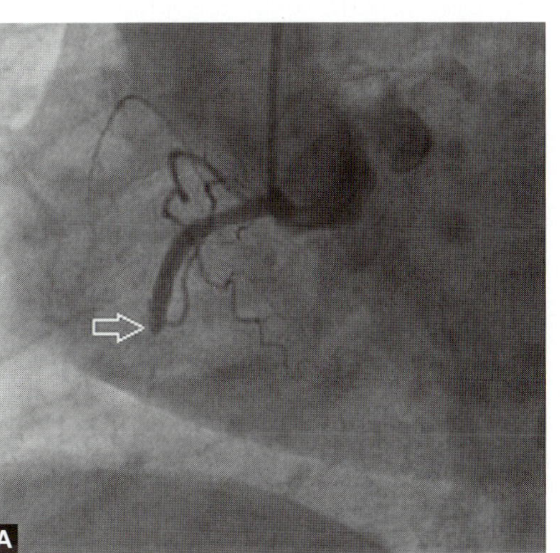

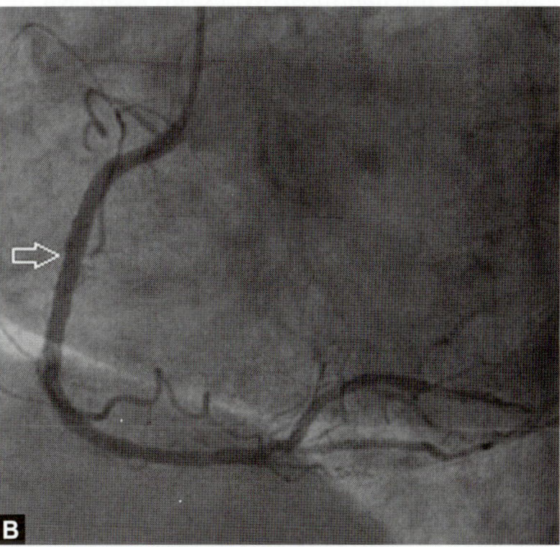

FIG. 3: **A,** Complete occlusion of proximal right coronary artery in a patient presenting with inferior and right ventricular MI (arrow); **B,** Post primary PCI establishment of flow (arrow) resulting in marked improvement in clinical and hemodynamic parameters.

Intra-Aortic Balloon Counterpulsation and Right Ventricular Assist Devices

Intra-aortic balloon counterpulsation (IABP) and RV assist devices are reserved for medically refractory cases despite successful reperfusion. IABP not only increases RV perfusion pressure, but also helps in improving septal contraction in an otherwise poorly contracting RV. RV assist device such as Tandem-Heart Percutaneous Ventricular Assist Device (Cardiac Assist Inc, USA) is able to bypass the dysfunctional RV allowing it to recover. Both surgical and percutaneous devices have shown to improve survival, venoarterial extracorporeal membrane oxygenation systems can bypass the pulmonary circulation too to further reduce RV load particularly in presence of pulmonary hypertension and pulmonary embolism.[31]

Correction of Arterial Ventricular Dyssynchrony

Restoration of sinus rhythm when there is atrial fibrillation (AF) and AV sequential pacing when there is AV block improves hemodynamics.[32]

Inhaled Nitric Oxide

When there is refractory hypotension due to RVMI, inhaled nitric oxide has been tried successfully. It acts by decreasing PVR but without any effect on systemic vascular resistance. LV filling improves leading to improvement of cardiac output and BP.[33]

Valve Replacement or Repair

Severe TR acts as a deterrent on improvement of forward RV cardiac output. In the setting of RVMI, both valve replacement and repair with annuloplasty rings can be used with good outcomes.

Patent Foramen Ovale Occluder Device

When hypoxemia occur secondary to right-to-left shunt across the atrial septum, occluding device closure of the same should be considered. Inhaled nitric oxide can decrease the right-to-left shunting till a device is placed.

PROGNOSIS

Short-term prognosis of patients presenting with RVMI is worse than those with isolated LVMI. In a study of 200 consecutive cases of acute inferior wall LVMI Zehender et al. found ST elevation in lead V4R has a highly negative predictive factor of both in-hospital mortality (31% vs. 6%) and all major in-hospital complications (64% vs. 28%).[34] In another study, Jacobs et al. did not find significant difference of mortality in acute MI presenting with cardiogenic shock due to either predominant RV or LV failure.[35] Foussas et al. found no significant difference in long-term mortality between patients with and without a RVMI, the poor in-hospital prognosis for patients with RVMIs was attributed to life-threatening arrhythmias.[36]

CONCLUSION

Up to half of patients presenting with inferior LVMI has RVMI. Associated RVMI makes IWMI a special subclass having unique clinical, ECG, echocardiography, and hemodynamic findings. Routine recording of right-sided chest leads in IWMI is able to identify most cases. Presentation with high-grade AV block, sustained arrhythmias, low cardiac output, hypotension and right heart failure despite an adequate LV function and clear lung fields make RVMI a special category for prompt identification and management. Imaging techniques particularly echocardiography plays a crucial role in the diagnosis. Judicious management particularly avoidance of preload reducing agents, IV fluid, and inotropes should be considered. Early primary PCI, IABP, and RV assist devices and in selected cases tricuspid valve surgery, nitric oxide inhalation and device occlusion of PFO are lifesaving procedures, with positive outcome often saves life.

REFERENCES

1. Cohn JN, Guiha NH, Broder MI, et al. Right ventricular infarction. Clinical and hemodynamic features. Am J Cardiol. 1974;33(2):209-14.
2. Goldstein JA. Pathophysiology and management of right heart ischemia. J Am Coll Cardiol. 2002;40(5):841-53.
3. Thygesen K, Alpert JS, Jaffe AS, et al. Writing Group on the Joint ESC/ACCF/AHA/WHF Task Force. Third universal definition of myocardial infarction. Eur Heart J. 2012;33(20):2551-67.
4. Berger PB, Ryan TJ. Inferior myocardial infarction. High-risk subgroups. Circulation. 1990;81(2):401-11.
5. Andersen HR, Falk E, Nielsen D. Right ventricular infarction: frequency, size and topography in coronary heart disease: A prospective study comprising 107 consecutive autopsies from a coronary care unit. J Am Coll Cardiol. 1987;10(6):1223-32.
6. Cohn JN, Guiha NH, Broder MI, et al. Right ventricular infarction. Clinical and hemodynamic features. Am J Cardiol. 1974;33(2):209-14.
7. Ondrus T, Kanovsky J, Novotny T, et al. Right ventricular myocardial infarction: From pathophysiology to prognosis. Exp Clin Cardiol. 2013;18(1):27-30.
8. Haji SA, Movahed A. Right ventricular infarction—diagnosis and treatment. Clin Cardiol. 2000;23(7):473-82.
9. Lopez-Sendon J, Coma-Canella I, Gamallo C. Sensitivity and specificity of hemodynamic criteria in the diagnosis of acute right ventricular infarction. Circulation. 1981;64(3):515-25.
10. Goldstein AJ. Acute right ventricular infarction. Cardiol Clin. 2012;30(2):219-32.
11. Laham RJ, Ho KKL, Douglas PS, et al. Right ventricular infarction complicated by acute right-to-left shunting. Am J Cardiol. 1994;74:824-6.
12. Elkayam U, Halprin SL, Frishman W, et al. Echocardiographic findings in cardiogenic shock due to right ventricular myocardial infarction. Cathet Cardiovasc Diagn. 1979;5(3):289-94.
13. Sharpe DN, Botvinick EH, Shames DM, et al. The noninvasive diagnosis of right ventricular infarction. Circulation. 1978;57(3):483-90.
14. Tomala M, Miszalski-Jamka T, Zajdel W, et al. Angiographic result of index PCI determines the presence of right ventricular infarction in patients with acute inferior myocardial infarction. Int J Cardiovasc Imaging. 2015;31 (8):1591-601.
15. Moye S, Carney MF, Holstege C, et al. The electrocardiogram in right ventricular myocardial infarction. Am J Emerg Med. 2005;23(6):793-9.
16. Robalino BD, Whitlow PL, Underwood DA, et al. Electrocardiographic manifestations of right ventricular infarction. Am Heart J. 1989;118(1):138-44.
17. Sharpe DN, Botvinick EH, Shames DM, et al. The noninvasive diagnosis of right ventricular infarction. Circulation. 1978;57(3):483-90.
18. Barrillon A, Chaignon M, Guize L, et al. Premonitory sign of heart block in acute posterior myocardial infarction. Br Heart J. 1975;37(1):2-8.
19. Zehender M, Kasper W, Kauder E, et al. Right ventricular infarction as an independent predictor of prognosis after acute inferior myocardial infarction. N Engl J Med. 1993;328(14):981-8.

20. Andersen HR, Nielsen D, Falk E. Right ventricular infarction: larger enzyme release with posterior than with anterior involvement. Int J Cardiol. 1989;22(3):347-55.
21. Strauss HD, Sobel BE, Roberts R. The influence of occult right ventricular infarction on enzymatically estimated infarct size, hemodynamics and prognosis. Circulation. 1980;62(3):503-8.
22. Chockalingam A, Gnanavelu G, Alagesan R, et al. Myocardial performance index in evaluation of acute right ventricular myocardial infarction. Echocardiography. 2004;21(6):487-94.
23. Nourian S, Hosseinsabet A, Jalali A, et al. Evaluation of right atrial function by two-dimensional speckle-tracking echocardiography in patients with right ventricular myocardial infarction. Int J Cardiovasc Imaging. 2016;33(1).
24. O'Rourke RA, Dell'Italia LJ. Diagnosis and management of right ventricular myocardial infarction. Curr Probl Cardiol. 2004;29(1):6-47.
25. Masci PG, Francone M, Desmet W, et al. Right ventricular ischemic injury in patients with acute ST-segment elevation myocardial infarction: characterization with cardiovascular magnetic resonance. Circulation. 2010;122(14):1405-12.
26. Miszalski-Jamka T, Klimeczek P, Tomala M, et al. Extent of RV dysfunction and myocardial infarction assessed by CMR are independent outcome predictors early after STEMI treated with primary angioplasty. JACC Cardiovasc Imaging. 2010;3(12):1237-46.
27. Goldstein JA, Vlahakes GJ, Verrier ED, et al. The role of right ventricular systolic dysfunction and elevated intrapericardial pressure in the genesis of low output in experimental right ventricular infarction. Circulation. 1982;65(3):513-22.
28. Goldstein JA, Vlahakes GJ, Verrier ED, et al. Volume loading improves low cardiac output in experimental right ventricular infarction. J Am Coll Cardiol. 1983;2(2):270-8.
29. Dell'Italia LJ, Starling MR, Blumhardt R, et al. Comparative effects of volume loading, dobutamine, and nitroprusside in patients with predominant right ventricular infarction. Circulation. 1985;72(6):1327-35.
30. Bowers TR, O'Neill WW, Grines C, et al. Effect of reperfusion on biventricular function and survival after right ventricular infarction. N Engl J Med. 1998; 338(14):933-40.
31. Berman M, Tsui S, Vuylsteke A, et al. Life-threatening right ventricular failure in pulmonary hypertension: RVAD or ECMO? J Heart Lung Transplant. 2008;27(10):1188-9.
32. Mavric Z, Zaputovic L, Matana A, et al. Prognostic significance of complete atrioventricular block in patients with acute inferior myocardial infarction with and without right ventricular involvement. Am Heart J. 1990;119(4): 823-8.
33. Inglessis I, Shin JT, Lepore JJ, et al. Hemodynamic effects of inhaled nitric oxide in right ventricular myocardial infarction and cardiogenic shock. J Am Coll Cardiol. 2004;44(4):793-8.
34. Zehender M, Kasper W, Kauder E, et al. Right ventricular infarction as an independent predictor of prognosis after acute inferior myocardial infarction. N Engl J Med. 1993;328(14):981-8.
35. Jacobs AK, Leopold JA, Bates E, et al. Cardiogenic shock caused by right ventricular infarction: A report from the SHOCK registry. J Am Coll Cardiol. 2003;41(8):1273-9.
36. Foussas SG, Zairis MN, Tsiaousis GZ, et al. The impact of right ventricular involvement on the postdischarge long-term mortality in patients with acute inferior ST-segment elevation myocardial infarction. Angiology. 2010;61(2):179-83.

CHAPTER 49

Cardiogenic Shock in Myocardial Infarction: Optimal Approach

Siddharthan Deepti, Sandeep Singh

INTRODUCTION

Cardiogenic shock is a devastating complication of acute myocardial infarction (MI). It is associated with a dismal prognosis despite recent advances in the care of patients with acute MI and the benefits associated with early use of reperfusion strategies. This chapter will review the definitions, incidence, outcomes, and optimal management of cardiogenic shock complicating MI.

DEFINITIONS

Cardiogenic shock is defined clinically as persistent hypotension [systolic blood pressure (SBP) <90 mm Hg for ≥30 minutes, or requirement of vasopressors and/or mechanical support to achieve SBP ≥90 mm Hg] despite adequate filling status with signs of impaired end-organ perfusion and pulmonary congestion.[1] Signs of hypoperfusion include cold/clammy skin and extremities, altered mental status, dizziness, loss of consciousness, oliguria (urine output <30 mL/hour), resting tachycardia, narrow pulse pressure, and increased arterial lactate levels (>2 mmol/L). In hemodynamic terms, it is characterized by a decrease in cardiac index (CI) associated with pulmonary capillary wedge pressure more than or equal to 15 mm Hg. Thus, pragmatically speaking, cardiogenic shock is a clinical diagnosis and may be defined as state of ineffective cardiac output resulting from a primary cardiac disorder leading to inadequate tissue perfusion.[2]

INCIDENCE, TEMPORAL TRENDS, AND ETIOLOGIES

The most common cause of cardiogenic shock is acute MI. Other than acute MI, cardiogenic shock may also be caused by decompensated valvular heart disease, acute myocarditis, and certain arrhythmias. For the purpose of this chapter, the focus will be on the management of cardiogenic shock caused by acute MI.

The incidence of cardiogenic shock complicating MI has been reported as ranging from 5 to 10%.[3] There are conflicting reports on the temporal trends of cardiogenic shock in MI with some studies reporting a decrease in incidence over time while others showing a slight but statistically significant upward trend.[4,5] The wide variability in the overall incidence rates and the differences in temporal trends have been attributed to the variations in the definitions of acute MI and cardiogenic shock, the characteristics of the population studied, and the rates of use of therapeutic options that may reduce the risk of cardiogenic shock. The incidence of cardiogenic shock in MI is greater in women and Asian and Pacific Islanders compared to whites, African Americans, and Hispanics.

The majority of patients with MI develop cardiogenic shock during the first 24 hours; only a minority develop this complication before hospital admission or late (>24 hours) after hospital admission. The median time of onset of cardiogenic shock after MI is around 6 hours. The most common cause of cardiogenic shock in acute MI is left ventricular (LV) dysfunction accounting for approximately 80% of cases, followed by severe mitral regurgitation (6.9%), ventricular septal rupture (VSR) (3.9%), right ventricular (RV) failure (2.8%), and cardiac tamponade (1.4%).

OUTCOMES

Cardiogenic shock remains the leading cause of death in patients with MI, though in-hospital mortality rates have reduced from formerly 80% to 35–50%. Mortality is highest (~80%) in cardiogenic shock resulting from VSR. The post-hospital outcomes in survivors of cardiogenic shock show a higher risk of death and/or hospitalization during the first year after discharge. The risk is time-dependent and is clustered mainly in the first 60 days after discharge.

MANAGEMENT

Flowchart 1 provides an overview of the management of acute MI complicated by cardiogenic shock.

Reperfusion Therapy

Reperfusion is the mainstay of management of cases of MI complicated by cardiogenic shock. The preferred modality for reperfusion is percutaneous coronary intervention (PCI). As a result of its limited efficacy, thrombolysis followed by transfer to a PCI-capable center should only be reserved for cases in which PCI-mediated reperfusion is estimated to occur in more than 120 minutes.[6]

The efficacy of early revascularization in this subset was first demonstrated by the landmark randomized trial, "SHOCK"' (Should We Emergently Revascularize Occluded Coronaries for Cardiogenic Shock) published nearly two decades ago.[7] This trial randomized patients with shock due to LV failure complicating MI to emergency revascularization or initial medical stabilization. Although the primary endpoint, 30-day mortality was not significantly different in the two groups [46.7% vs. 56.0%; difference, –9.3%; 95% confidence interval (CI) for the difference, –20.5 to 1.9%; p = 0.11], there was a survival benefit in the long-term, with significantly lower mortality at 6 months, 12 months, and through long-term follow-up (6 years). Accordingly, a class IB recommendation has been given to immediate PCI in patients with cardiogenic shock, if coronary anatomy is suitable. The rates of revascularization in this subset in the real world range from 27 to 54% in the USA, 47% in the GRACE registry, and 50% in a French registry to as high as 70% in a Swiss registry.

Culprit-only Percutaneous Coronary Intervention

The majority of patients with cardiogenic shock have multivessel or left main coronary artery disease. For example, in the SHOCK trial registry, of all the patients who underwent angiography, 16% had significant left main disease and 53% had three vessel disease. Based on pathophysiologic considerations, the guidelines gave a class II-C recommendation for consideration for complete revascularization during the index procedure in patients presenting with cardiogenic shock. This recommendation has however been challenged by the recently published "CULPRIT-SHOCK" trial.[8,9] This trial compared culprit-vessel-only PCI with immediate PCI of all obstructive lesions (i.e., those with >70% stenosis of the diameter) in patients who had MI with cardiogenic shock. The study showed a significant clinical benefit of a culprit-lesion-only strategy with a reduction in the primary endpoint of 30-day mortality (an absolute 8.2% reduction) or severe renal failure requiring renal replacement therapy.[8] At 1-year follow up, there was no significant difference in mortality between the two groups. The rates of rehospitalization for heart failure and repeat revascularization were, however, higher in the culprit-lesion-only PCI group at 1 year. This has been attributed to better survival of patients at extreme risk of death in the culprit-lesion-only PCI arm, who would have otherwise not survived long enough to develop heart failure.[9] Thus, as of now, the evidence is in favor of employing a strategy of culprit-lesion-only PCI over initial multivessel PCI for patients with cardiogenic shock. However, it should be noted that the decision needs to individualized depending on the patient's characteristics. For example, intuitive revascularization of a

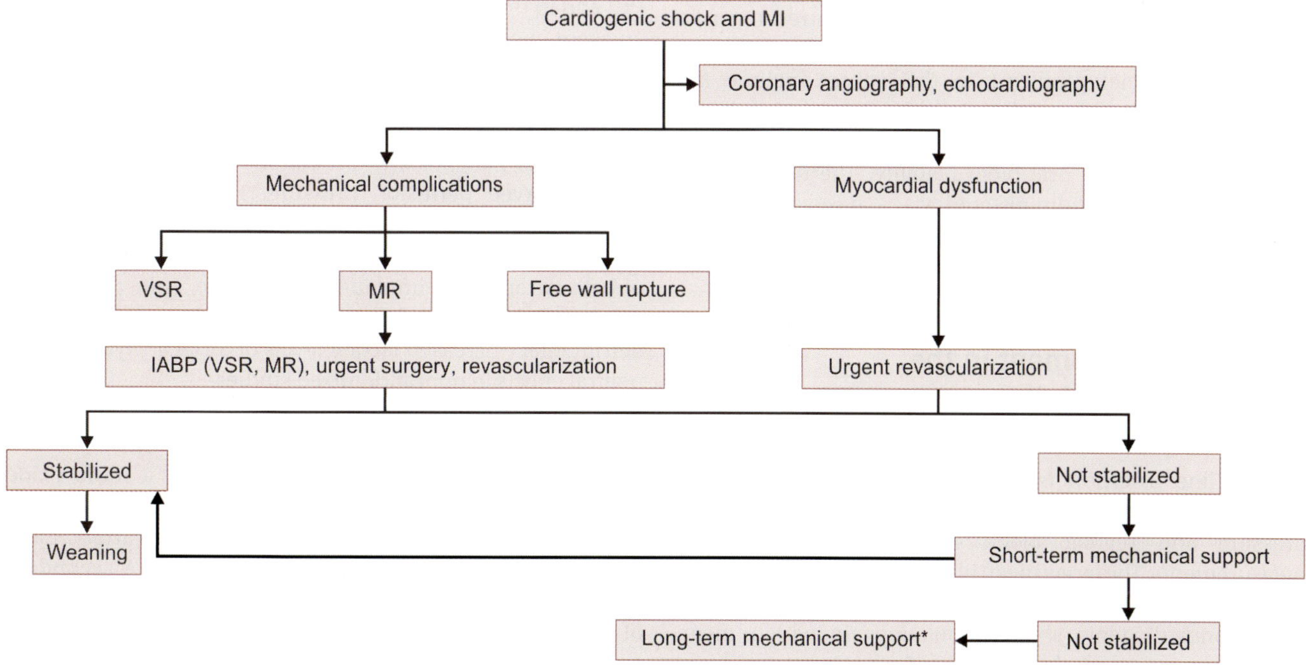

FLOWCHART 1: Algorithm for management of acute myocardial infarction complicated by cardiogenic shock.

concomitant high-grade proximal left anterior descending coronary artery with less than TIMI 3 flow after dealing with an occluded right coronary artery culprit lesion may not be entirely inappropriate in a properly selected patient.

Access-Radial versus Femoral

The preferential use of radial arterial access for PCI in cardiogenic shock has been favored by the guidelines, if performed by an experienced radial operator, although, the benefit is less well established in this subset compared to patients presenting without shock. Radial access has been shown to be associated with a reduction in all-cause mortality as well as major adverse cardiac and cerebral events at 30-day follow-up in survivors of cardiogenic shock in a meta-analysis of registry patients. However, it should be kept in mind that obtaining a radial artery access may be challenging in hypotensive patients.

Role of Immediate Coronary Artery Bypass Graft (CABG) Surgery

No clear evidence exists to guide CABG vs. PCI in patients with MI complicated by cardiogenic shock, who are found to have multivessel or left main disease. Observational reports have shown no difference in the outcomes between the two. In the real world, the rates of immediate coronary artery bypass graft (CABG) in this subset have remained around 5–6% compared to PCI which have improved from 26–54%.

Antithrombotic Therapies as Adjuncts to Percutaneous Coronary Intervention

There are no separate randomized trials for patients with cardiogenic shock with regard to antiplatelet and anticoagulant drugs. The data from the trials performed in stable patients undergoing primary PCI is inferred to make similar recommendations for patients having cardiogenic shock. The special problems in this subset include the inability to swallow the oral antiplatelet drugs in intubated patients and the impaired enteral perfusion in the state of shock decreasing the oral bioavailability. The tablets need to be crushed and administered via a nasogastric tube. More liberal use of glycoprotein IIb/IIIa inhibitors or the parenteral antiplatelet cangrelor may be considered, though the evidence for the same is lacking.

Medical Management in the Coronary Care Unit

Monitoring

Arterial line insertion is recommended based on expert consensus for continuous monitoring of arterial blood pressure and regular blood gas analysis and lactate measurements. The target mean blood pressure in cardiogenic shock has not been established and has been extrapolated from noncardiogenic shock populations in which mean arterial pressure more than or equal 65 mm Hg is considered a reasonable target. Insertion of a central venous catheter should be considered; it aids in monitoring of central venous pressure and provide a preferential route for administration of vasoactive substances. Lastly, monitoring with a pulmonary artery catheter has not been found to be of any clinical benefit in randomized studies and meta-analyses. However, pulmonary artery catheter has still been afforded a place in the major guidelines as a tool to provide hemodynamic data that can confirm the presence and severity of cardiogenic shock, RV involvement, and measurements of pulmonary artery pressures, transpulmonary gradient, and vascular resistance of the pulmonary or systemic arterial beds. It can also help in monitoring responses to therapeutic interventions. A class IIb recommendation has been given to use of pulmonary artery catheter in diagnosis and guiding therapy, especially in cases of diagnostic or management uncertainty or in patients with moderate to severe cardiogenic shock who are unresponsive to initial therapy.

Echocardiography

Serial transthoracic echocardiographic examinations are recommended at diagnosis and during coronary care unit (CCU) stay to evaluate changes in biventricular function, valve dysfunction, and exclusion or diagnosis of mechanical complications. LV ejection fraction and severity of mitral regurgitation have been identified as independent echocardiographic predictors of outcomes in a substudy from the SHOCK trial. Echocardiography may also aid in hemodynamic monitoring by providing estimates of cardiac output and filling pressures; though use in this area is not firmly established yet and can prove challenging.

Vasoactive Drugs

Vasopressors and/or inotropes may be required in the prehospital setting, in the catheterization laboratory during PCI and in the CCU. There is limited evidence for selection of an agent in cardiogenic shock. Norepinephrine is considered to be the agent of choice as first-line therapy as it has been shown to be safer than dopamine, vasopressin, or epinephrine and has a lower risk of arrhythmias. Dobutamine should be preferred in patients with predominant low cardiac output and preserved perfusion pressure. Regarding inodilators, levosimendan finds a place in patients on chronic beta-blocker therapy because its inotropic effect being independent of beta-adrenergic stimulation. Dopamine, epinephrine and vasopressin are not preferred as these have been found to have detrimental (increased lactate levels or atrial arrhythmias) or neutral effects in nonrandomized studies.

Nonvasoactive Pharmacologic Therapy

The "TRIUMPH" trial evaluated tilarginine, a nitric oxide synthase inhibitor, in patients with refractory cardiogenic shock complicating MI despite an open infarct artery. Early mortality rates were high in the therapy arm. A secondary analysis of the data from this trial showed administration of β-blockers or renin-angiotensin-aldosterone system antagonists in 25% of patients within the first 24 hours after cardiogenic shock diagnosis. Higher 30-day mortality was observed in the recipients of these agents.

Early statin use has been associated with a favorable outcome in an analysis from the Korean Acute Myocardial Infarction Registry. Critical care bundles of best-practice prevention strategies should be implemented to prevent hospital-acquired infections, stress ulcers, delirium, critical illness neuropathy, and venous thromboembolism.

Mechanical Circulatory Support

Intra-aortic Balloon Pump

The role of routine use of intra-aortic balloon pump (IABP) has been downgraded to class IIIB recommendation based on the results of the "IABP-SHOCK II" trial.[10] This study compared standard therapy (early revascularization with best available medical care) with and without IABP in 600 patients with cardiogenic shock secondary to MI. No difference was observed in 30-day mortality (39.7% vs. 41.3%; relative risk 0.96, 95% CI 0.79–1.17) or in any key secondary endpoints such as length of ICU stay, renal function, or the rates of major bleeding, peripheral ischemic complications, sepsis, or stroke. There were no significant differences in these endpoints on follow-up at 12 months. However, crossover rate was high in the control group. There is a possibility that the trial enrolled patients without rapid deterioration and the sample is more representative of patients stabilized on vasopressor or inotropic support. The role of IABP in patients with severe shock with rapid deterioration requires further study. Currently, IABP is to be considered only in patients with cardiogenic shock secondary to mechanical complications.

Percutaneous Active Mechanical Circulatory Support Devices

There is lack of high-quality evidence to support the use of percutaneous active mechanical circulatory support (MCS) devices like TandemHeart and Impella as therapeutic adjuncts in the cardiogenic shock population. Temporary MCS devices can be used as a bridge to recovery, whereby the MCS is removed after correction of shock; a bridge to a bridge, whereby the MCS provides time for a provisional plan to transition to durable MCS after clinical stabilization; or a bridge to decision, in cases where hemodynamic instability, neurological uncertainty or multisystem organ failure may preclude a comprehensive assessment for durable MCS or transplantation.

The Impella CP, 5.0 unloads the LV completely with simple percutaneous insertion unlike the TandemHeart which requires an atrial septal puncture. Recently, a small study, the IMPRESS-in-Severe-SHOCK trial, compared Impella CP and IABP in patients with ST-elevation myocardial infarction (STEMI)-associated cardiogenic shock requiring MCS.[11] The trial was markedly underpowered for the assessment of the primary endpoint of all-cause 30-day mortality and failed to show any difference in the two groups. However, there was no benefit with respect to the other nonclinical endpoints as well including arterial lactate levels. This raises concerns about the efficacy of the device. On the other hand, registry data suggests improved outcomes using early active hemodynamic support with Impella CP in cardiogenic shock in patients with isolated left ventricle failure. An adequately powered trial is needed before routine use of this device can be recommended.

A pilot feasibility study (the Detroit cardiogenic shock initiative) examined the effect of early MCS before PCI in patients who present with acute MI complicated by cardiogenic shock and observed favorable trends in survival.[12] The protocol of PCI following MCS needs to be validated in larger national studies before its widespread application.

Venoarterial Extracorporeal Membrane Oxygenation

Venoarterial extracorporeal membrane oxygenation (VA-ECMO) provides both respiratory and cardiac support and is appealing as a potential first-line MCS device in cardiogenic shock in view of possibility of its rapid deployment, applicability in case of malignant arrhythmias, and rapid improvement in oxygenation. The drawbacks include requirement of a specialist team for insertion and running and a relevant risk of thromboembolic events and limb ischemia. The increasing use of ECMO in patients with cardiogenic shock is promising; however, there is paucity of evidence to support its routine use. A recent observational study found increased mortality and higher cost of care without significant increase in length of stay with use of ECMO in cardiogenic shock. Future research including randomized studies is needed to clarify the role of this modality in this population.

Currently, percutaneous MCS devices have been given a class IIb-C recommendation for use in refractory cardiogenic shock.

Cardiogenic Shock Secondary to Mechanical Complications

Cardiogenic shock secondary to a mechanical complication of MI carries worse prognosis, especially with VSR where the early mortality is as high as 80%. The incidence of VSR previously ranged from 1 to 2% with a decrease to 0.2% in the current era of primary PCI. Immediate surgical closure is recommended in current guidelines in patients with cardiogenic shock not responding to medical therapy. IABP may be considered for initial stabilization before coronary angiography and surgery. Immediate percutaneous extracorporeal life support might be required in cases of refractory cardiogenic shock. However, surgery has been found to be futile with mortality approaching 100% in a subset of patients with VSR including the very elderly and patients with poor RV function. A possible alternative is percutaneous device closure of the VSR. There is paucity of hard evidence in favor of device closure of VSR. A meta-analysis of all published reports has shown similar mortality data with percutaneous VSR closure and surgery.

Papillary muscle rupture leading to acute mitral regurgitation and cardiogenic shock may complicate a minority (~0.25%) of cases of MI. Emergency surgery (valve repair/replacement) is recommended in this situation. Afterload reduction and IABP may help in stabilizing the patient in preparation for angiography and surgery. Operative mortality is high (20–25%).

Ventricular free wall rupture is known to complicate 2–3% of cases of MI. Emergent surgery is vital. Pericardiocentesis can be a life-saving temporizing measure in manifest tamponade and circulatory collapse.

Cardiogenic Shock with Right Ventricular Infarction

Acute RV infarction leading to cardiogenic shock is a special situation in which, in addition to reperfusion, volume support is indicated to maintain increased filling pressures and maximize flow to the left ventricle. Since, the viability of RV remains preserved longer after MI unlike its left counterpart, late reperfusion is an option in patients with inferior wall MI and RV dysfunction. Right ventricular assist device (RVAD) like the Impella RP system may be considered in patients with refractory RV shock. The prognosis of patients with cardiogenic shock secondary to RV infarction is no different than those without it.

Multiorgan Dysfunction in Cardiogenic Shock

Pulmonary edema usually accompanies cardiogenic shock and may necessitate mechanical ventilation in 60–80% of cases to improve gas exchange and to relieve the work of breathing. Acute kidney injury is seen in roughly one-third of patients with cardiogenic shock. Management is supportive with correction of hypoperfusion and avoidance or minimal use of nephrotoxic agents. Significant elevation of hepatic transaminases is observed with severe hypoperfusion and portends worse prognosis. As in renal dysfunction, restoration of hepatic perfusion is the key to management.

Cardiac arrest has been reported in 29–41% of patients with cardiogenic shock complicating MI. The management of brain injury in resuscitated patients is not clear. General postresuscitation measures include monitoring of hemodynamics, oxygenation, and ventilation to avoid secondary brain injury. Hypothermia is known to provide profound neuroprotection after resuscitation from cardiac arrest. Moderate hypothermia was evaluated in a small, nonrandomized study in 14 patients with severe cardiogenic shock with or without cardiac arrest (COOL Shock Study I & II). It was found to be safe and feasible in this setting with improvement in parameters of cardiac function for the duration of therapy. The role of hypothermia in patients on ECMO support is being investigated in an ongoing multicenter randomized controlled trial (HYPO-ECMO: NCT02754193).

Assessment of Prognosis

Multiple scoring systems have been developed to predict clinical outcomes in patients with cardiogenic shock. Some of the models are derived for the general ICU patients and include the APACHE (Acute Physiology and Chronic Health Evaluation)-II score and SAPS (Simplified Acute Physiology Score)-II scoring systems. Specific to cardiogenic shock, three scoring systems are available, the Sleeper score (derived from the SHOCK trial), the CardShock risk score, and the IABP-SHOCK II risk score.

Independent predictors of mortality in the Sleeper score include anoxic brain injury, shock at admission, noninferior wall MI, increasing age, end-organ hypoperfusion, renal dysfunction (serum creatinine ≥1.9 mg/dL), prior CABG and SBP at admission. The CardShock risk score includes seven prognostic variables that were found to be independently associated with increased mortality: ACS etiology, age, previous MI, prior CABG, confusion, low LV ejection fraction, and blood lactate levels. Lastly, the IABP-SHOCK II risk score recognizes six variables as independent predictors for 30-day mortality: age more than 73 years, prior stroke, glucose at admission above 191 mg/dL, creatinine at admission above 1.5 mg/dL, thrombolysis in MI flow grade less than 3 after PCI, and arterial blood lactate at admission above 5 mmol/L.

These scoring systems find utility in counseling patients and families, in healthcare policy resource utilization decisions, in quality improvement systems, and design of trials to test novel therapies.

CONCLUSION

Cardiogenic shock is a life-threatening complication of acute MI that continues to have extremely high mortality in spite of advances in the care of patients with MI over the last two decades. As of now, reperfusion with PCI is the mainstay of management of these patients. Key aspects have been explored in randomised trials, the most important of which have been summarized in table 1. However, there are several issues that await clarification in future studies including the role of MCS, immediate CABG and optimal monitoring techniques.

TABLE 1: Important trials in management of cardiogenic shock complicating myocardial infarction

Trial	Findings
SHOCK (1991)[7]	• N = 302 • Survival benefit in the long-term with emergency revascularization
IABP-SHOCK II (2012)[10]	• N = 600 • No improvement in mortality at 30 days with IABP use
CULPRIT-SHOCK (2017, 2018)[8,9]	• N = 706 • Lower 30-day risk of death or severe renal failure with culprit lesion only PCI compared to immediate multivessel PCI*
IMPRESS-in-Severe Shock (2017)[11]	• N = 48 • No difference in 30-day mortality between Impella and IABP

*No significant difference in 1-year mortality between the two groups. Higher rates of rehospitalization for heart failure and repeat revascularization in the culprit lesion only PCI group at 1 year.

IABP, intra-aortic balloon pump; PCI, percutaneous coronary intervention.

REFERENCES

1. Mebazaa A, Combes A, van Diepen S, et al. Management of cardiogenic shock complicating myocardial infarction. Intensive Care Med. 2018 [Epub ahead of print].
2. van Diepen S, Katz JN, Albert NM, et al. Contemporary Management of Cardiogenic Shock: A Scientific Statement From the American Heart Association. Circulation. 2017;136(16):e232-68.
3. Kolte D, Khera S, Aronow WS, et al. Trends in incidence, management, and outcomes of cardiogenic shock complicating ST-elevation myocardial infarction in the United States. J Am Heart Assoc. 2014;3(1):e000590.
4. Jeger RV, Radovanovic D, Hunziker PR, et al. Ten-year incidence and treatment of cardiogenic shock. Ann Intern Med. 2008;149(9):618-26.
5. Goldberg RJ, Spencer FA, Gore JM, et al. Thirty-year trends (1975 to 2005) in the magnitude of, management of, and hospital death rates associated with cardiogenic shock in patients with acute myocardial infarction: a population-based perspective. Circulation. 2009;119:1211-9.
6. Ibanez B, James S, Agewall S, et al. 2017 ESC Guidelines for the management of acute myocardial infarction in patients presenting with ST-segment elevation: The Task Force for the management of acute myocardial infarction in patients presenting with ST-segment elevation of the European Society of Cardiology (ESC). Eur Heart J. 2018;39(2):119-77.
7. Hochman JS, Sleeper LA, Webb JG, et al. Early revascularization in acute myocardial infarction complicated by cardiogenic shock: SHOCK Investigators: Should We Emergently Revascularize Occluded Coronaries for Cardiogenic Shock. N Engl J Med. 1999;341:625-34.
8. Thiele H, Akin I, Sandri M, et al for the CULPRIT-SHOCK Investigators. PCI strategies in patients with acute myocardial infarction and cardiogenic shock. N Engl J Med. 2017;377:2419-32.
9. Thiele H, Akin I, Sandri M, et al. One-Year Outcomes after PCI Strategies in Cardiogenic Shock. N Engl J Med. Published online 25 Aug 2018. doi: 10.1056/NEJMoa1808788
10. Thiele H, Zeymer U, Neumann F-J, et al for the IABP-SHOCK II Trial Investigators. Intra-aortic balloon support for myocardial infarction with cardiogenic shock. N Engl J Med. 2012;367(14):1287-96.
11. Ouweneel DM, Eriksen E, Sjauw KD, et al. Percutaneous Mechanical Circulatory Support Versus Intra-Aortic Balloon Pump in Cardiogenic Shock After Acute Myocardial Infarction. J Am Coll Cardiol. 2017;69(3):278-87.
12. Basir MB, Schreiber T, Dixon S, et al. Feasibility of early mechanical circulatory support in acute myocardial infarction complicated by cardiogenic shock: The Detroit cardiogenic shock initiative. Catheter Cardiovasc Interv. 2018;91(3):454-61.

CHAPTER 50

Optimizing STEMI Care—Developing Regional Networks

Sabarirajan Sokkaiyan, Thomas Alexander

INTRODUCTION

The development and use of reperfusion therapy in ST-elevation myocardial infarction (STEMI) has been one of the great achievements of modern medicine in the United States of America and Western Europe. In the 1960s, 1-year mortality rates after STEMI approached 30% in these countries. However, their numbers are dramatically different today: under ideal circumstances, reperfusion therapy—in combination with cardiac care units and other evidence-based treatments—has now lowered 1-year mortality rates after STEMI to well under 10% in clinical trials. The goal of the last two decades in these countries has been to translate these outcomes under "ideal circumstances" into "real-world" practice.[1]

Cardiovascular disease (CVD) is a major cause of morbidity and mortality in India. The recent nationwide survey published in Lancet has shown that the epidemiologic transition toward lifestyle diseases has been completed in all states in India.[2] CVD is now the dominant cause of death in India and therefore must be an area of priority in both planning and resource allocation. While public education to improve preventive strategies and to educate people on early recognition and management of coronary risk factors is important, there remains an urgent need to plan and improve acute cardiac care especially in managing patients with acute coronary syndrome (ACS).

Experience from the developed countries clearly show that developing regional STEMI networks significantly reduces morbidity and mortality of ACS. However, these systems require a high level of trained manpower, emergency medical services (EMS), and finance to implement. Low- and middle-income countries (LMIC) such as India will find replicating similar systems difficult and impractical. Therefore, it is imperative that STEMI networks developed for LMIC are not only practical but also accessible and equitable to the large number of patients who are from the below poverty level (BPL) strata of the society.[3]

MAGNITUDE OF THE PROBLEM

There are no accurate estimates of STEMI in India. Expert estimates indicate there could be between 1,500 and 2,000 STEMI per million per year. If this were to be accurate, then there could be upward of 2.0 million STEMI cases every year. This is a huge burden that requires urgent attention.

Data from the CREATE registry, published over a decade ago, looked at hospital data from 89 centers from 50 cities across India. There were 20,468 patients of which 12,405 had STEMI. Total 58.5% had thrombolysis and 8% had primary percutaneous coronary intervention (PCI).[4] The Kerala ACS Registry showed that 41.4% had thrombolysis and 12.9% had primary PCI. Thus, these registry data, acquired over a decade ago, show a 55–65% reperfusion rate.[5] Over the last decade these rates could have improved. However, these are mostly urban data and Kerala has been the best state in terms of healthcare delivery and social and health indices, and so may reflect a "best case scenario" and may not reflect the ground realities in the other parts of the country.

Data presented at the Interventional Council of India, showed that approximately 64,000 primary PCI were performed in 2016. Data collected from the pharmaceutical industry has shown that approximately 430,000 doses of thrombolytic doses were dispensed in 2016. Thus approximately 500,000 reperfusions were instituted in 2016 and would indicate only 25% of STEMI patients had reperfusion therapy.

It is therefore imperative to improve access to reperfusion therapy across the country.

Barriers to Access of Appropriate Care

- *Patient factors*:
  - Nonrecognition of symptoms
  - Gender disparity
  - Cost of medical care.
- *Transportation factors*:
  - Lack of ambulance services
  - Clear delineation of "STEMI hospital"

- *Hospital factors*:
    - Absence of clear protocol
    - Absence of trained "STEMI teams".

Some of the nonsystem delays can be overcome by public education, using prehospital electrocardiography (ECG) as in the STEMI INDIA project, and accrediting and publicizing "STEMI hospitals". This will ensure that patients do not lose time when they are admitted to "non-STEMI" hospitals and then must be transferred to another hospital for STEMI management. Thus, critical delays associated with "door-in-door-out" can be avoided.

Access to ambulance services and availability of universal insurance coverage for STEMI patients will ensure that all patients with STEMI can access appropriate care. For this it is important that governments, both at the Centre and the States, work together with the scientific societies to understand and help to implement these programs.

STEMI—Acute Care at First Point of Contact

In the absence of a clear-cut and well-developed STEMI network in India, patients present to a variety of medical facilities with complaints of chest pain. It is imperative to develop clear guidelines to assist these facilities in the appropriate management of STEMI patients.

These could include:

- Physician clinic or primary health centers (PHCs)
- Community health centers (CHCs) or hospitals with no coronary care unit (CCU) facility
- Thrombolytic center with CCU but without a cardiac catheterization facility
- Center with cardiac catheterization laboratory and primary PCI facility.

There have been recent attempts to develop guidelines to help PHCs and CHCs to manage patients with chest pain, as also to improve facilities and develop protocols to help manage patients with ACS. However, these initiatives will take time and require significant government funding.

DEVELOPING REGIONAL STEMI NETWORKS—THE STEMI INDIA EXPERIENCE

Regional STEMI networks to manage patients with STEMI have been developed in the United States and Europe and have played a critical role in reducing mortality in patients with STEMI. These systems have critically combined a well-developed EMS system with a strategy of primary PCI as the mode for reperfusion. This system is critically dependent on a high quality of infrastructure and medical capability. Countries such as India and other LMIC can seldom replicate these models.

The STEMI India model combines the two proven reperfusion strategies of primary PCI with the pharmaco-invasive strategy to build a hub-and-spoke model.[6] The hub centers, located mostly in urban areas, have cath laboratories and STEMI patients self-presenting or transported to these centers have primary PCI here. These hospitals also catheterize and do PCI for patients transferred from the spokes after thrombolysis—the pharmaco-invasive strategy of reperfusion. The hubs are connected to multiple spoke hospitals that are in the peripheral and rural areas. Patients presenting here are thrombolyzed and then shifted to the hub for catheterization (Fig. 1).

The TN-STEMI Project

The initial pilot study was the Kovai Erode Pilot study involving 84 patients over a 6-month period. The study tested the feasibility of the hub-and-spoke model and could show remarkable improvement in access to STEMI care. This was published in the Heart Journal.[7]

Based on this a larger study was planned and conducted in Tamil Nadu—The TN-STEMI Programme.[8] This study was partly funded by the Indian Council of Medical Research (ICMR) and partly by STEMI India. The study had the active participation of the Tamil Nadu State Government through the Tamil Nadu Health Systems Project (TNHSP), the State ambulance network through GVK-EMRI (Emergency Management and Research Institute), and the State CM Health Insurance Scheme for BPL patients. The study was conducted in four clusters in Tamil Nadu.

The program resulted in the creation of an integrated, regional quality improvement program that linked the 35 spoke healthcare centers to the four large PCI hub hospitals and leveraged recent developments in public health insurance schemes, EMS, and health information technology.

This multicenter, prospective, observational program studied 2,420 patients 20 years or older with confirmed ECG and symptoms or signs consistent with STEMI at primary care clinics, small hospitals, and PCI hospitals in the southern state of Tamil Nadu in India. Data were collected from the four clusters before implementation of the program (pre-implementation data). There was a 12-week period for the pre-implementation data acquisition with the period extending from August 7, 2012, through January 5, 2013. The program was then implemented in a sequential manner across the four clusters, and data were collected in the same manner (post-implementation data) from June 12, 2013, through June 24, 2014, for a mean 32-week period.

Primary outcomes focused on the proportion of patients undergoing reperfusion, timely reperfusion, and post-fibrinolysis angiography and PCI. Secondary outcomes were in-hospital and 1-year mortality.

A total of 2,420 patient with STEMI [2,034 men (84.0%) and 386 women (16.0%); mean (SD) age, 54.7 (12.2) years] (898 in the preimplementation phase and 1,522 in the postimplementation phase) were enrolled, with 1,053 patients (43.5%) from the spoke healthcare centers. Missing data were common for systolic blood pressure [213 (8.8%)], heart rate [223 (9.2%)], and anterior myocardial infarction location [279 (11.5%)]. Overall reperfusion use and times to reperfusion were similar [795 (88.5%) vs. 1372 (90.1%);

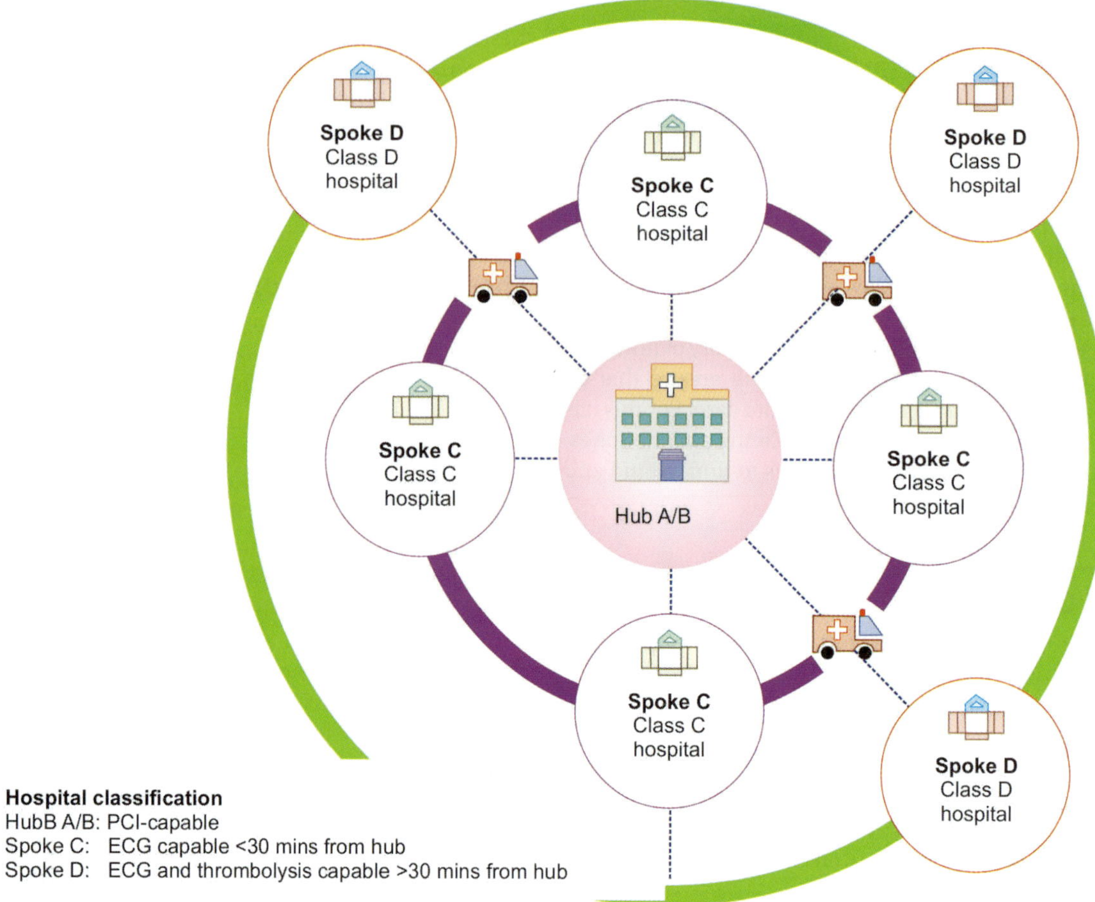

ECG, electrocardiography; PCI, percutaneous coronary intervention.

FIG. 1: The hub-and-spoke model for STEMI care model. This example from the STEMI India program is a well-tested formulation shown to work well in resource-challenged locations.

Source: Alexander T, Mullasari AS, Kaifoszova Z, et al. Framework for a National STEMI Program: Consensus document developed by STEMI INDIA, Cardiological Society of India and Association Physicians of India. Indian Heart J. 2015;67(5):497-502.

p = 0.21]. Coronary angiography [314 (35.0%) vs. 925 (60.8%); p <0.001] and PCI [265 (29.5%) vs. 707 (46.5%); p <0.001] were more commonly performed during the postimplementation phase. In-hospital mortality was not different [52 (5.8%) vs. 85 (5.6%); p = 0.83], but 1-year mortality was lower in the postimplementation phase [134 (17.6%) vs. 179 (14.2%); p = 0.04], and this difference remained consistent after multivariable adjustment (adjusted odds ratio, 0.76; 95% confidence interval, 0.58–0.98; p = 0.04).

The Way Forward

Based on the success of the TN-STEMI Programme, the ICMR invited the health secretaries of 18 states and held a dissemination workshop to highlight the benefits of the TN-STEMI Programme and the modalities for a successful implementation. The Union Health Ministry has resolved to provide states with 60% of the cost of running a similar program. This should give a fillip to the program with many states implementing a similar program.

CONCLUSION

A hub-and-spoke model in South India improved STEMI care through greater use of PCI and has been shown to improve 1-year mortality. This model may serve as an example for developing STEMI systems of care in India and other low- to middle-income countries.

Working together with the government, utilizing technological innovation and working together with Cardiological Society of India (CSI) and STEMI India, it is possible to develop these regional STEMI networks. In an environment of resource constraints with a burgeoning population with coronary artery disease and STEMI, a comprehensive national STEMI program is critical to deliver reperfusion for all.

REFERENCES

1. O'Gara P, Kushner FG, Ascheim DD, et al. 2013 ACCF/AHA guideline for the management of ST-elevation myocardial infarction: executive summary: a report of the American College of Cardiology Foundation/American Heart Association Task Force on Practice Guidelines. Circulation. 2013;127:529-55.

2. India State-Level Disease Burden Initiative Collaborators. Nations within a nation: variations in epidemiological transition across the states of India, 1990–2016 in the Global Burden of Disease Study. The Lancet. 2017;390(10111): 2437-60.
3. Kaifoszova Z, Kala P, Alexander T, et al. Stent for Life Initiative: leading example in building STEMI systems of care in emerging countries. EuroIntervention. 2014;10 Suppl T:T87-95.
4. Xavier D, Pais P, Devereaux PJ, et al. Treatment and outcomes of acute coronary syndromes in India (CREATE): a prospective analysis of registry data. Lancet. 2008;371:1435-42.
5. Mohanan PP, Mathew R, Harikrishnan S, et al. Presentation, management, and outcomes of 25 748 acute coronary syndrome admissions in Kerala, India: Results from the Kerala ACS Registry. Euro Heart J. 2013;34(2): 121-9.
6. Alexander T, Victor SM, Mullasari AS, et al. Protocol for a prospective, controlled study of assertive and timely reperfusion for patients with ST-segment elevation myocardial infarction in Tamil Nadu: the TN-STEMI program. BMJ Open. 2013;3:e003850.
7. Alexander T, Mehta S, Mullasari A, et al. Systems of care for ST-elevation myocardial infarction in India. Heart. 2012;98:15-7.
8. Alexander T, Mullasari AS, Joseph G, et al. A System of Care for Patients With ST-Segment Elevation Myocardial Infarction in India: The Tamil Nadu–ST-Segment Elevation Myocardial Infarction Program. JAMA Cardiol. 2017;2(5):498-505.

SECTION 8

Dual Antiplatelet Therapy

CHAPTER 51

Choice of Dual Antiplatelet Therapy in Acute Coronary Syndrome: Is There a Consensus?

Hiremath MS, Deore RA

INTRODUCTION

As per National Informatics Center (NIC) data in 2015,[1] 30 lacs patients suffered from acute coronary syndrome (ACS). Of these 12 lacs received medical management, 67,000 received primary percutaneous intervention (PCI), and rest did not get the appropriate treatment.

Central to ACS is the vulnerable plaque rupture with formation of arterial thrombus triggering the positive feedback mechanism. This leads to platelet activation and fibrin formation leading to platelet aggregation. So, antiplatelets and anticoagulants are the mainstay of therapy for ACS (Fig. 1).

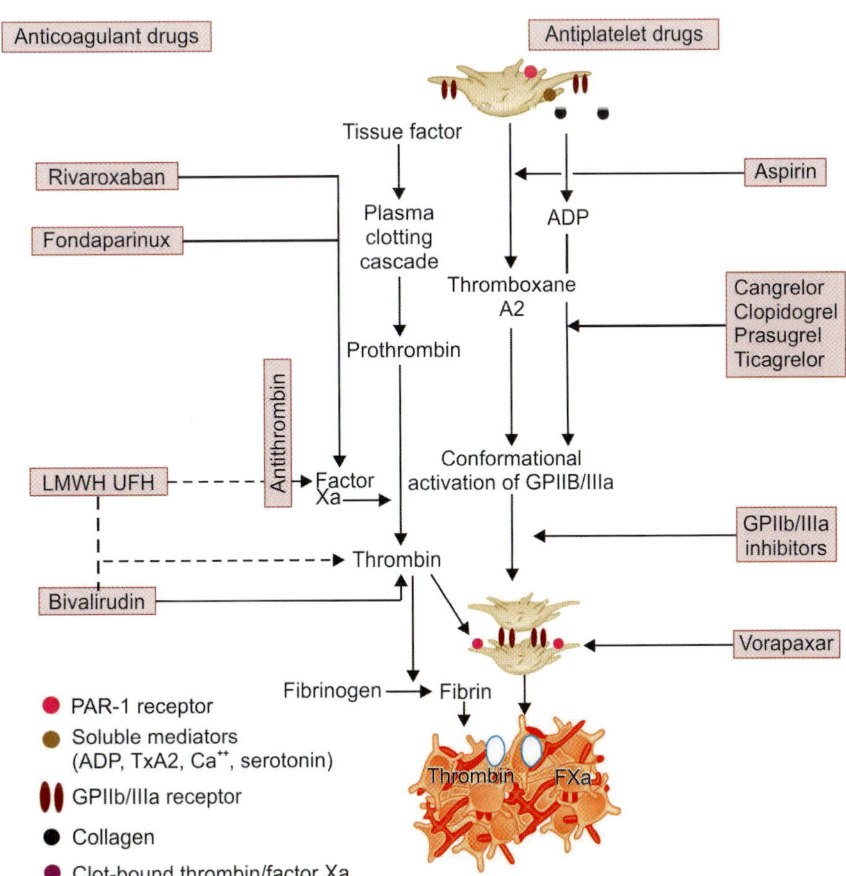

ADP, adenosine diphosphate; LMWH, low molecular-weight heparin; UFH, unfractionated heparin.

FIG.1: Antithrombotic and antiplatelet drugs for acute coronary syndromes. Figure depicts the targets available that can be used to inhibit coagulation and platelet aggregation.

In 1996, Schwomig et al.[2] first described the role of dual antiplatelet therapy (DAPT; aspirin with ticlopidine) over anticoagulation (aspirin with heparin followed by phenprocoumon) in patients undergoing intracoronary stent placement. Compared to anticoagulation group, DAPT group experienced 82% less myocardial infarctions (MIs) and 78% lesser repeat revascularization. In DAPT group, 1.6% patients reached primary cardiac end points and 1.2% reached primary noncardiac end points compared to 6.2% and 12.3% in anticoagulation group, respectively. This started the era of DAPT therapy in post-PCI population.

ASPIRIN

Aspirin is an inhibitor of cyclooxygenase I (COX-I) inhibitor leading of irreversible functional platelet inhibition, which lasts for the approximate 8–9 days life span of a circulating platelet. ISIS-2 (Second International Study of Infarct Survival) trial aspirin when used in post-thrombolysis patients significantly reduced early vascular mortality and this beneficial effect was maintained event at 10 years postevent.[3,4] The antiplatelet effect of aspirin is at the dose range of 50–325 mg/day, with optimal effect at the dose of 75 mg/day, as proven in CURRENT OASIS-7 (Clopidogrel and Aspirin Optimal Dose Usage to Reduce Recurrent Events—Seventh Organization to Assess Strategies in Ischemic Syndromes) trial.[5] There is no incremental benefit with higher doses of aspirin above 100 mg/day, above which bleeding risk increases incrementally. Most of the bleeding events with aspirin are gastrointestinal, at the incidence rate of ≈2% per year.

Aspirin remains the backbone of anti-thrombotic therapy over which other antiplatelets are added.

TICLOPIDINE

Addition of second antiplatelet agent, adenosine diphosphate (ADP) receptor antagonist was shown to be superior by Schwomig et al.,[2] but hematological side effects (gastrointestinal problems—diarrhea, abdominal pain, nausea, and vomiting, neutropenia in approximately 2.4% of patients, severe neutropenia in 0.8% of patients, and, rarely, thrombotic thrombocytopenia purpura) and availability of superior molecule (clopidogrel) have rendered ticlopidine obsolete.

CLOPIDOGREL

Clopidogrel remains the most extensively studied and the most commonly used second antiplatelet in the DAPT-regimen. Clopidogrel, thienopyridine class, is a prodrug which irreversibly inhibits $P2Y_{12}$-receptor. The first randomized controlled trial (RCT) of clopidogrel in ACS patients was CURE (Clopidogrel in Unstable Angina to Prevent Recurrent Ischemic Events)[6] trial. In this trial of the 12,562 patients with non-ST elevation acute myocardial infarction (AMI), 6,259 were given clopidogrel (300 mg immediately, followed by 75 mg once daily) and placebo arm was given only aspirin for 3–12 months. About 9.3% patients in the clopidogrel arm achieved primary end points (a composite of death from cardiovascular (CV) causes, nonfatal MI, or stroke) compared to 11.4% patients in the placebo arm [relative risk with clopidogrel as compared with placebo, 0.80; 95% confidence interval (CI) 0.72 to 0.90; p <0.001]. Similar benefit was also seen in secondary outcome of refractory ischemia (16.5% in study group vs. 18.8% in placebo group; relative risk, 0.86, p <0.001). In the angioplasty subgroup of the same study (PCI-CURE[7]) the benefit was even greater with 30% relative risk reduction in the primary end points. But this was at the expense of higher major bleeding in the clopidogrel-arm compared to the placebo arm (3.7% vs. 2.7%; relative risk, 1.38; p = 0.001), though life-threatening bleeds (2.1% vs. 1.8%, p = 0.13) and the hemorrhagic strokes were not significant.

Further clopidogrel was studied in ST-elevation myocardial infarction (STEMI) in CLARITY TIMI-28 trial [The Clopidogrel as Adjunctive Reperfusion Therapy (CLARITY)-Thrombolysis in Myocardial Infarction (TIMI)].[8] In this trial, 3,491 STEMI patients were randomized to clopidogrel plus aspirin or aspirin only arm. The primary efficacy end point was the composite of an occluded infarct-related artery (defined by TIMI flow grade of 0 or 1) on angiography, death from any cause before angiography could be performed, or recurrent MI before angiography. There was 6.7% absolute reduction in the primary efficacy end points in the study group (15% in clopidogrel arm vs. 21.7% in placebo-arm). Similar to CURE study, there was an angioplasty subgroup of this trial (CLARITY-PCI)[9] which showed 46% relative risk reduction in the, the 30-day composite of CV death, MI, or stroke (6.2% vs. 3.6%; p = 0.008) without any significant difference in major or minor bleeding between the two groups.

Medically managed STEMI patients were studied in COMMIT trial (The Clopidogrel and Metoprolol in Myocardial Infarction Trial).[10] There was 9% relative risk reduction in the DAPT arm (aspirin plus clopidogrel) compared to placebo arm (aspirin alone), corresponding to nine fewer events per 1,000 patients treated for about 2 weeks. There was also a significant 7% proportional reduction in any death (7.5% DAPT arm vs. 8.1% aspirin only arm; p = 0.03). This effect is of independent of the other treatments used without significant increase in the risk of any bleeding either overall [134 (0.58%) vs. 125 (0.55%); p = 0.59], or in patients aged older than 70 years or in those given fibrinolytic therapy.

The Clopidogrel for High Atherothrombotic Risk and Ischemic Stabilization, Management, and Avoidance (CHARISMA)[11] trial studied role of clopidogrel in patients with either clinically evident cardiovascular disease (CVD) (secondary prevention) or multiple risk factors (primary prevention). A total of 15,603 patients were randomized to aspirin plus clopidogrel or aspirin plus placebo and followed for a median of 28 months. There was no difference in the primary end point of CV death, MI, or stroke, although the secondary end point, which included hospitalizations for ischemia, was significantly reduced. In this trial, there was a suggestion of benefit with clopidogrel treatment in patients with symptomatic atherothrombosis (secondary prevention group) and a suggestion of harm in patients with multiple risk factors (primary prevention group).

Interindividual variability in responsiveness to clopidogrel: Clopidogrel being a prodrug requires 2-step conversion to its active metabolite, R-130964 in liver mediated by several CYP450 isoenzymes. Major genetic polymorphism in isoenzymes of CYP2C19 leads to loss of function, which is responsible variable response to clopidogrel, incidence being 20%. *CYP2C19**2 and *3 variants account for 99% of the loss-of-function alleles in Asians. Genetic analysis of CURE and CHARISMA study showed no impact of reduced function alleles on potential benefits of clopidogrel plus aspirin in the study population. More minor degrees of bleeding did seem to be associated with CYP2C19 polymorphisms. So these studies did not find any role of clopidogrel genotyping in stable coronary artery disease patients.[12] The Food and Drug Administration (FDA) announced a "Boxed Warning" on March 12, 2010, about the diminished effectiveness of clopidogrel in patients with an impaired ability to convert the drug into its active form. The FDA label revision does not mandate testing for *CYP2C19* genotypes or overall platelet function.[13]

Besides genetics, drug–drug interaction is an important cause for clopidogrel variability. Pharmacokinetic and pharmacodynamic data show proton-pump inhibitors (PPI) attenuate antiplatelet efficacy of clopidogrel, supplemented by various observational studies.[14] Based on populations from two randomized trials, the PRINCIPLE (Prasugrel In Comparison to Clopidogrel for Inhibition of Platelet Activation and Aggregation) TIMI-44 trial[15] and the TRITON (Trial to Assess Improvement in Therapeutic Outcomes by Optimizing Platelet Inhibition with Prasugrel)–TIMI-38 trial,[16] PPI treatment attenuated the pharmacodynamic effects of clopidogrel and, to a lesser extent, those of prasugrel; but PPI treatment did not affect the clinical outcome of patients given clopidogrel or prasugrel. The US-FDA notifies that for patients taking clopidogrel the need for starting or continuing treatment with PPI should be re-evaluated and if required, other drugs to reduce gastric acidity to be preferred like H2-blockers or antacids.[13]

Higher loading doses (600–900 mg) have been evaluated.[17,18] They appear to be safe and more rapidly acting; however, it must be recognized that the database for such higher loading doses is not sufficiently robust to formulate definitive recommendation (Table 1).

TABLE 1: Oral antiplatelet agents for acute coronary syndrome

	Aspirin	Clopidogrel	Prasugrel	Ticagrelor
Molecule chemical class	Acetysalicylic acid	Thienopyridine	Thienopyridine	Cyclopentyl-triazolo-pyrimidine
Route of administration	Oral	Oral	Oral	Oral
Mechanism of action	Cyclo-oxygenase-1 inhibition	$P2Y_{12}$ receptor inhibition	$P2Y_{12}$ receptor inhibition	$P2Y_{12}$ receptor inhibition
Loading dose	150–300 mg (80–150 mg intravenously)	300–600 mg	60 mg	180 mg
Maintenance dose	75–150 daily	75 mg daily	10 (5) mg daily	90 mg twice daily
Activation	Prodrug, hydrolysis by an esterase	Prodrug, variable hepatic metabolism	Prodrug, predictable hepatic metabolism	Active drug with additional active metabolite
Action	Irreversible	Irreversible	Irreversible	Reversible
Action onset	30–40 min	2–6 hours	30 min	30 min
Action duration	5 days	3–10 days	7–10 days	3–5 days
Interruption before surgery	No interruption when possible (5 days if high bleeding risk surgery)	5 days	7 days	5 days
Plasmatic half-life of prodrug	2–3 hours	30–60 min	30–60 min	6–12 hours
Inhibition of adenosine reuptake	No	No	No	Yes
Indications	• Stable CAD • ACS	• Stable CAD • ACS	• ACS scheduled for PCI	• ACS • Stable CAD after MI
Contraindications	• Active bleeding • Hypersensibility to aspirin • Severe hepatic failure	• Active bleeding • Severe hepatic failure	• Active bleeding • History of stroke or TIA • Severe hepatic failure (Child-Pugh C)	• Active bleeding • History of intracranial bleeding • Moderate to severe hepatic failure • Coadministration with potent cytochrome CYP3A4 inhibitors

ACS, acute coronary syndrome; CAD, coronary artery disease; MI, myocardial infraction; PCI, percutaneous intervention; TIA, transient ischemic attack.

PRASUGREL

Prasugrel—a novel thienopyridine—is a prodrug, inhibits adenosine diphosphate-induced platelet aggregation more rapidly, more consistently, and to a greater extent than do standard and higher doses of clopidogrel. Prasugrel was first studied in 10,074 moderate- to high-risk ACS patients (74% were NSTEMI) in TRITON-TIMI-38[16] trial. Patients were randomly assigned 13,608 patients with moderate-to high-risk ACS, of whom 10,074 (74%) had unstable angina (UA)/non-ST-segment elevation myocardial infarction (NSTEMI), to receive prasugrel (a 60-mg loading dose and a 10-mg daily maintenance dose) or clopidogrel (a 300-mg loading dose and a 75-mg daily maintenance dose) after coronary anatomy was defined, for a median follow-up of 14.5 months. Total 12.1% patients in the prasugrel arm experienced the primary efficacy end point [a composite of the rate of death due to CV causes (including arrhythmia, congestive heart failure, shock, and sudden or unwitnessed death), nonfatal MI, or nonfatal stroke] compared to 9.9% in clopidogrel arm [hazard ratio (HR) for prasugrel vs. clopidogrel, 0.81; 95% CI, 0.73–0.90; $p < 0.001$]; conferring significant 2.2% absolute reduction and a 19% relative reduction with prasugrel. There was significant reductions in secondary end points of MI (9.7% for clopidogrel vs. 7.4% for prasugrel; $p < 0.001$), urgent target-vessel revascularization (3.7% vs. 2.5%; $p < 0.001$), and stent thrombosis (2.4% vs. 1.1%; $p < 0.001$). This was at the expense of statistically insignificant increase in major bleeding (2.4% in prasugrel arm and 1.8% in clopidogrel arm; HR, 1.32; 95% CI, 1.03–1.68; $p = 0.03$), life-threatening bleeding (1.4% vs. 0.9%; $p = 0.01$), including nonfatal bleeding (1.1% vs. 0.9%; HR, 1.25; $p = 0.23$) and fatal bleeding (0.4% vs. 0.1%; $p = 0.002$). In the few patients who underwent coronary artery bypass graft (CABG), TIMI major bleeding through 15 months was also greater with prasugrel than with clopidogrel (13.4% vs. 3.2%, respectively; HR for prasugrel: 4.73; 95% CI: 1.90–11.82; $p < 0.001$). The net clinical benefit in the TRITON-TIMI-38 study demonstrated a primary efficacy and safety end point rate of 13.9% in the clopidogrel group versus 12.2% in the prasugrel group (HR: 0.87; 95% CI: 0.79–0.95; $p = 0.004$). The US-FDA labeling information, derived from *post hoc* analysis of the trial patients suggested that there were three subgroups of ACS patients who did not have favorable clinical benefit from prasugrel because of higher risk of fatal or intracranial bleed. These subgroups were patients with a history of stroke or transient ischemic attack before enrolment, patients with a body weight of less than 60 kg had no net benefit, patients age more than 75 years.

Two double blind, placebo-controlled RCTs have addressed the question of DAPT timing in ACS. The Targeted Platelet Inhibition to Clarify the Optimal Strategy to Medically Manage Acute Coronary Syndromes (TRILOGY ACS) trial[19] randomized patients with ACS who were initially medically managed with prasugrel or clopidogrel, in comparison to TRITON-TIMI-38 trial which prasugrel was given to ACS patients only after coronary anatomy is defined and patients are destined for PCI. For medically managed CS patients prasugrel did not offered any benefit over clopidogrel and similar risk of bleeding observed.

In a NSTE-ACS (non-ST-segment elevation acute coronary syndromes) cohort, the ACCOAST study[20] compared prasugrel pretreatment (30 mg preangiography, followed by 30 mg postangiography), with 60 mg prasugrel loading postangiography and pre-PCI. There was no difference in the primary end point of CV death, stroke, MI, and urgent revascularization; although bleeding was nearly twice as high in the pre-treatment arm. This led to guideline recommendation guideline to recommend of avoiding pretreatment with prasugrel in patients diagnosed with NSTE-ACS.

TICAGRELOR

Ticagrelor is the first nonthienopyridine, direct ADP blocker and reversibly inhibits the $P2Y_{12}$ platelet receptor leading to more rapid and consistent platelet inhibition. Adenosine reuptake is also inhibited by ticagrelor, this causes symptoms of dyspnea (≈5%) and bradycardia with occasional sinus pauses.

The Platelet Inhibition and Patient Outcomes (PLATO) study[21] was a large, global, randomized clinical trial comparing ticagrelor (180 mg loading dose, followed by 90 mg twice daily) and clopidogrel (300–600 mg loading dose at investigator discretion, followed by 75 mg daily), and enrolled 18,624 patients with ACS. At 12 months, the primary end point—a composite of death from vascular causes, MI, or stroke—had occurred in 9.8% of patients receiving ticagrelor as compared with 11.7% of those receiving clopidogrel (HR, 0.84; 95% CI, 0.77–0.92; $p < 0.001$). The rate of death from any cause was also reduced with ticagrelor (4.5%, vs. 5.9% with clopidogrel; $p < 0.001$). PLATO major bleeding (the primary safety end point) was not different between the study arms. This was attributed to the rapidly reversible mechanism of action of ticagrelor. There was more non-CABG-related major bleeding observed in the ticagrelor group compared with clopidogrel (4.5% vs. 3.8%; HR, 1.19; $p = 0.03$), whereas CABG-related major bleeding was similar between the treatments (Table 2).

A phenomenon of "North American Paradox" was noted, in which patients enrolled in the United States had outcomes favoring clopidogrel and qualitatively different from the overall results of the trial. Extensive analyses suggested that a different dose of aspirin used in the United States compared with the rest of the world (325 mg vs. ≤100 mg) explained much of this difference. The hypothesis for this phenomenon was—higher doses of aspirin given with ticagrelor are associated with increased bleeding risks with the possibility of reduced efficacy as well. Ticagrelor in Patients With ST-Elevation Myocardial Infarction Treated With Pharmacological Thrombolysis—TREAT trial[22] is a multicenter, randomized, open-label with blinded end point adjudication trial that enrolled 3,799 patients (younger than 75 years) with STEMI receiving fibrinolytic therapy in 152 sites from ten countries. The primary outcome of TIMI major

TABLE 2: Summary of outcomes from PLATO and TRITON-TIMI 38 trials in patients with non-ST-segment elevation acute coronary syndromes (NSTE-ACS) or ST-segment elevation myocardial infarction (STEMI)

	PLATO		TRITON-TIMI-38	
Outcome	NSTE-ACS	STEMI	NSTE-ACS	STEMI
No. of patients	11080	7544	10074	3534
Median age, years	64	59	61.2–62.1	58–59
Prior myocardial infarction, no. (%) of patients	2810 (25)	1014 (13)	2075 (21)	359 (10)
Prior PCI, no. (%) of patients	1862 (17)	630 (8)	1597 (16)	N/A
PCI on study, no. (%) of patients	5710 (52)	6158 (82)	99.1	3425 (97)
Primary end point (cardio-vascular death, myocardial infarction, stroke)	10.0% T vs. 12.3% C p = 0.001	9.4% T vs. 10.8%C p = 0.07	9.30% T vs. 11.23% C p = 0.002	10.0% P vs. 12.4% C p = 0.02
All-cause mortality	4.3% T vs. 5.8% C p = 0.002	5.0% T vs. 6.1%c p = 0.05	N/A	3.3% P vs. 4.3% C p = 0.11
Cardiovascluar death	3.7% T vs. 4.9% C p = 0.007	4.5% T vs. 5.5% C p = 0.07	1.78% P vs. 1.83% C p = 0.88	2.4% P vs. 3.4% C p = 0.13
Myocardial infarction	6.6% T vs. 7.7% C p = 0.04	4.7% T vs. 5.8% C p = 0.03	7.26% P vs. 9.46% C p <0.001	6.8% P vs. 9.0% C p = 0.02
Stroke	1.3% T vs. 1.4% C p = 0.79	1.7% T vs. 1.0% C p = 0.02	0.97% P vs. 0.91% C p = 0.75	1.6% P vs. 1.5% C p = 0.91
Major bleeding	13.4% T vs. 12.6% C p = 0.26	9.0%T vs. 9.2% C p = 0.76	N/A	N/A
CABG-related major bleeding	N/A	5 .1%T vs. 5.8%C p = 0.30	N/A	18.8% P vs. 2.7% C p = 0.003
Non-CABG-related major bleeding	4.8% T vs. 3.8% p = 0.01 TIMI: 2.9% T vs. 2.2% C p = 0.01	4.1%T vs. 3.7% C p = 0.61 TIMI: 2.5% T vs. 2.2% C p = 0.60	2.16%P vs. 1.55% C p = 0.02	2.4% P vs. 2.1% C p = 0.65
Life-threatening bleeding	6.6% T vs. 6.5% C p = 0.56	4.7% T vs. 4.9% C p = 0.86	N/A	1.3% P vs. 1.1% C p = 0.75
Fatal bleeding	0.3% T vs. 0.4% C p = 0.37	0.2% T vs. 0.1% c N/A	0.28% P vs. 0.06% C p = 0.008	0.45% P vs. 0.13% C p = 0.10

CABG, coronary artery bypass graft; PCI, percutaneous intervention coronary; PLATO, The Platelet Inhibition and Patient Outcomes; TRITON-TIMI, Trial to Assess Improvement in Therapeutic Outcomes by Optimizing Platelet Inhibition with Prasugrel-Thrombolysis in Myocardial Infarction; T, test/study population; C, control population.

bleeding occurred in 0.73% of the ticagrelor group versus 0.69% of the clopidogrel group (p <0.001 for noninferiority). Although the trial was not powered for efficacy, there was no apparent ischemic benefit with ticagrelor. Among patients less than 75 years of age who were treated with fibrinolysis for STEMI, delayed administration of ticagrelor was noninferior to clopidogrel. Ticagrelor represents a treatment option in such patients (i.e., clopidogrel allergy); however, unless future trials show otherwise, ticagrelor is not preferential to clopidogrel after fibrinolysis for STEMI.

As per both European and American guidelines for management of ACS, aspirin forms the backbone DAPT-regimen. For second antiplatelet therapy, ticagrelor (regardless of initial treatment strategy) or prasugrel (only for patients undergoing invasive management) should be preferred over clopidogrel. But clopidogrel is the still the most commonly used second antiplatelet because of wide availability and low cost (Flowchart 1).

CONCLUSION

For patients with ACS, aspirin forms the backbone of DAPT. For second antiplatelet, amongst the three available $P2Y_{12}$ inhibitors, ticagrelor has the most rapid-onset of action, most potent and having least side effects, also it can be used for medically managed patients and patients undergoing intervention. So, ticagrelor is the preferred second antiplatelet agent in the DAPT regimen. Clopidogrel being the most extensively studied drug, it is preferred in the patients with multiple risk factors and comorbities. Prasugrel, though highly potent, has very limited utility because of risk of bleeding.

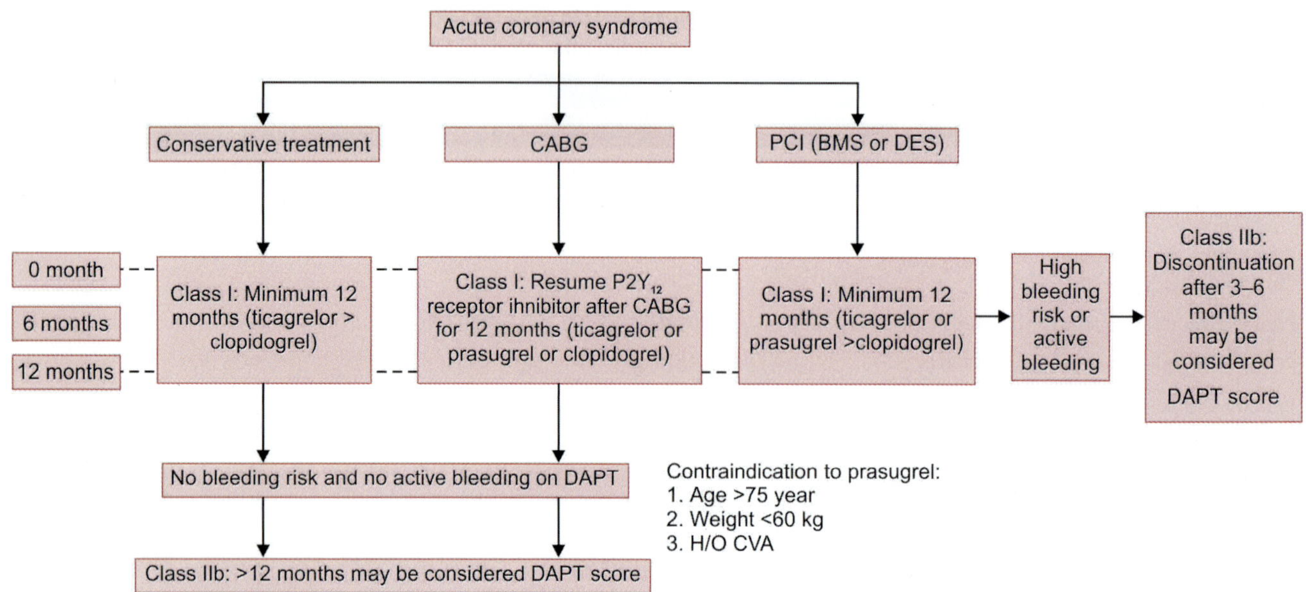

ACS, acute coronary syndrome; BMS, bare-metal stent; CABG, coronary artery bypass graft; CVA, cerebral vascular accident; H/o, history of; DAPT, dual antiplatelet therapy; DES, drug-eluting stent; PCI, percutaneous coronary intervention.

FLOWCHART 1: Proposed algorithm for "Choice of DAPT in ACS".

REFERENCES

1. Growth of Interventional Cardiology in India: NIC data; 2016-17.
2. Schwomig A, Neumann FJ, Kastrati A, et al. A randomized comparison of antiplatelet and anticoagulant therapy after the placement of coronary-artery stents. N Engl J Med. 1996;334:1084-9.
3. ISIS-2 (Second International Study of Infarct Survival) Collaborative Group. Randomised trial of intravenous streptokinase, oral aspirin, both, or neither among 17,187 cases of suspected acute myocardial infarction: ISIS-2. Lancet. 1988;2:349-60.
4. Baigent, C, Collins R, Appleby P, et al. ISIS-2: 10-year survival among patients with suspected acute myocardial infarction in randomised comparison of intravenous streptokinase, oral aspirin, both, or neither. The ISIS-2 (Second International Study of Infarct Survival) Collaborative Group. BMJ. 1998;316:1337-43.
5. Mehta SR, Bassand JP, Chrolavicius S, et al. Dose comparisons of clopidogrel and aspirin in acute coronary syndromes. N Engl J Med. 2010;363:930-42.
6. Yusuf S, Zhao F, Mehta SR, et al. Effects of clopidogrel in addition to aspirin in patients with acute coronary syndromes without ST-segment elevation. N Engl J Med. 2001;345:494-502.
7. Mehta SR, Yusuf S, Peters RJ, et al. Effects of pretreatment with clopidogrel and aspirin followed by long-term therapy in patients undergoing percutaneous coronary intervention: The PCI-CURE study. Lancet. 2001;358:527-33.
8. Sabatine MS, Cannon CP, Gibson CM, et al. Addition of clopidogrel to aspirin and fibrinolytic therapy for myocardial infarction with ST-segment elevation. N Engl J Med. 2005;352:1179-89.
9. Sabatine MS, Cannon CP, Gibson CM, et al. Effect of clopidogrel pretreatment before percutaneous coronary intervention in patients with ST-elevation myocardial infarction treated with fibrinolytics: The PCI-CLARITY study. JAMA. 2005;294:1224-32.
10. Chen ZM, Jiang LX, Chen YP, et al. Addition of clopidogrel to aspirin in 45,852 patients with acute myocardial infarction: randomised placebo-controlled trial. Lancet. 2005;366:1607-21.
11. Bhatt DL, Fox KA, Hacke W, et al. Clopidogrel and aspirin versus aspirin alone for the prevention of atherothrombotic events. N Engl J Med. 2006;354:1706-17.
12. Paré G, Mehta SR, Yusuf S, et al. Effects of CYP2C19 genotype on outcomes of clopidogrel treatment. N Engl J Med. 2010;363:1704-14.
13. Holmes DR Jr, Dehmer GJ, Kaul S, et al. ACCF/AHA clopidogrel clinical alert: Approaches to the FDA "boxed warning": A report of the American College of Cardiology Foundation Task Force on clinical expert consensus documents and the American Heart Association. J Am Coll Cardiol. 2010;56:321-41.
14. Simon T, Verstuyft C, Mary-Krause M, et al. Genetic determinants of response to clopidogrel and cardiovascular events. N Engl J Med. 2009;360:363-75.
15. Wiviott SD, Trenk D, Frelinger AL, et al. Prasugrel compared with high loading- and maintenance-dose clopidogrel in patients with planned percutaneous coronary intervention: The Prasugrel in Comparison to Clopidogrel for Inhibition of Platelet Activation and Aggregation-Thrombolysis in Myocardial Infarction 44 trial. Circulation. 2007;116:2923-32.
16. Wiviott SD, Braunwald E, McCabe CH, et al. Prasugrel versus clopidogrel in patients with acute coronary syndromes. N Engl J Med. 2007;357:2001-15.
17. von Beckerath N, Taubert D, Pogatsa-Murray G, et al. Absorption, metabolization, and antiplatelet effects of 300-, 600-, and 900-mg loading doses of clopidogrel: results of the ISAR-CHOICE (Intracoronary Stenting and Antithrombotic Regimen: Choose Between 3 High Oral Doses for Immediate Clopidogrel Effect) Trial. Circulation. 2005;112:2946.
18. Mehta SR, Yusuf S, Granger CB, et al. Design and rationale of the MICHELANGELO Organization to Assess Strategies in Acute Ischemic Syndromes (OASIS)-5 trial program evaluating fondaparinux, a synthetic factor Xa inhibitor, in patients with non-ST-segment elevation acute coronary syndromes. Am Heart J. 2005;150:1107.
19. Roe MT, Armstrong PW, Fox KA, et al. Prasugrel versus clopidogrel for acute coronary syndromes without revascularization. N Engl J Med. 2012;367:1297-1309.
20. Montalescot, G, Bolognese L, Dudek D, et al. Pretreatment with prasugrel in non-ST-segment elevation acute coronary syndromes. N Engl J Med. 2013;369:999-1010.
21. Wallentin L, Becker RC, Budaj A, et al. Ticagrelor versus clopidogrel in patients with acute coronary syndromes. N Engl J Med. 2009;361:1045-57.
22. Berwanger O, Nicolau JC, Carvalho AC, et al. Ticagrelor vs clopidogrel after fibrinolytic therapy in patients with ST-elevation myocardial infarction: A randomized clinical trial. JAMA Cardiol. 2018;3(5):391-9.

CHAPTER 52

Optimal Duration of Dual Antiplatelet Therapy after Acute Coronary Syndrome: Current Status

Dhiman Kahali, Vivek Singh Rathore

INTRODUCTION

Acute coronary syndrome (ACS) is a disease spectrum that comprises of unstable angina, ST-segment elevation myocardial infarction (STEMI) and non-STEMI (NSTEMI). It is the main cause of mortality in coronary artery disease (CAD) and represents a principle form of its clinical presentation.

Antiplatelet therapy is the treatment where platelet activation and aggregation are reduced, which are the primary steps toward the formation of a thrombus after the disruption of plaque.

Although there are several potential combinations of antiplatelet therapy, the term and acronym dual antiplatelet therapy (DAPT) is used to specifically refer to combination antiplatelet therapy with the drugs aspirin along with a $P2Y_{12}$ receptor inhibitor (clopidogrel, prasugrel, or ticagrelor).

Dual antiplatelet therapy which includes acetylsalicylic acid (ASA) in addition to a $P2Y_{12}$ inhibitor is the principle treatment after an ACS or after patients undergoing a percutaneous coronary intervention (PCI), toward preventing recurrent ischemic events such as stent thrombosis.

Ever since the dawn of drug-eluting stents (DESs) era the rates of restenosis have dramatically decreased. Though the first-generation DESs have been associated with a slighter increased rates of stent thrombosis, which is the complication most feared in coronary stenting as it has higher mortality. Ever since the introduction of the new, second-generation DES, along with the usage of stronger $P2Y_{12}$ inhibiting drugs, the stent thrombosis rates have halved. The second-generation DES are indeed superior in all aspects.

Due to the improved status of the stents available to us today, the focus is now shifting toward the flipside of DAPT, such as the bleeding. The most important risk factor of stent thrombosis is due to discontinuation of clopidogrel prematurely. The quest to strike the right balance between lower complications of coronary stents and increased awareness of bleeding from DAPT leads to the probing question—What is the optimal duration of DAPT?

Dual antiplatelet therapy is mandatory in the first months after stent implantation until endothelialization has been completed. As the risk of late stent thrombosis is less of a concern with second-generation DES, prolonged DAPT is now more aimed at preventing (recurrent) myocardial infarction (MI) not related to the implanted stent. Thus, rather than focusing on the stent or the angiogram alone, the key to success is to treat the patient's overall thrombotic risk.[1]

RISK STRATIFICATION TOOLS FOR ISCHEMIA AND BLEEDING RISKS

The probing decision for a DAPT duration depends largely on the ischemic versus bleeding risks, and with the help of scoring systems it helps to tailor the DAPT duration maximizing ischemic protection and reduce the bleeding risks in a patient (Table 1).

The Dual Antiplatelet Therapy Score

The DAPT score was initially validated in patients who were enrolled in PROTECT (Patient-Related Outcomes with Endeavor vs. Cypher Stenting) trial.[2] This prediction rule identified nine factors [age, congestive heart failure/low left ventricular ejection fraction (LVEF), vein graft stenting, MI at presentation, prior MI or PCI, diabetes, stent diameter <3 mm, smoking, and paclitaxel-eluting stent] resulting in a score ranging from –2 to +10].[3]

Within the DAPT trial,[4] a high-risk score (i.e., a score ≥2) showed a reduction in MI or stent thrombosis and cardiovascular (CV) or cerebrovascular events risk after a prolonged, 30-month DAPT, with only a modest increase in bleeding risk. And a low-risk score (<2) selected patients recruited in the DAPT trial who did not derive any reduction of ischemic events from prolonging DAPT, with a significant increase in moderate or major bleeding.[4]

PRECISE-DAPT Score

The PRECISE-DAPT[5] (Predicting Bleeding Complications in Patients Undergoing Stent Implantation and Subsequent

TABLE 1: DAPT score and PRECISE-DAPT score systems

	PRECISE-DAPT score	DAPT score
Time of use	At the time of coronary stenting	After 12-month of uneventful DAPT
DAPT duration strategies assessed	Short DAPT (3–6 months) vs. Standard/long DAPT (12–24 months)	Standard DAPT (12 months) vs. Long DAPT (30 months)
Score calculating	HB: ≥12, 11-5, 11, 10-5, ≤10 WBC: ≤5, 8, 10, 12, 14, 16, 18, ≥20 Age: ≤50, 60, 70, 80, ≥90 CrCl: ≥100, 80, 60, 40, 20, 0 Prior bleeding: No, Yes Score Points: 0, 2, 4, 6, 8, 10, 12, 14, 16, 18, 20, 22, 24, 26, 28, 30	Age ≥75 −2 pt 65 to <75 −1 pt 65 0 pt Cigarette smoking +1 pt Diabetes mellitus +1 pt MI at presentation +1 pt Prior PCI or prior MI +1 pt Paclitaxel-eluting stent +1 pt Stent diameter <3 mm +1 pt CHF or LVEF <30% +2 pt Vein graft stent +2 pt
Score range	0 to 100 points	−2 to 10 points
Decision making cut-off suggested	Score ≥25 → Short DAPT Score <25 → Standart/long DAPT	Score ≥2 → Long DAPT Score <2 → Standart DAPT

CHF, congestive heart failure; CrCl, creatinine clearance; DAPT, dual antiplatelet therapy; LVEF, left ventricular ejection fraction; MI, myocardial infarction; PCI, percutaneous coronary intervention; WBC, white blood cells.

Dual Antiplatelet Therapy) study had patients with CAD who underwent PCI either elective, urgent, or emergent. It generated a five-item [age, creatinine clearance (CrCl), hemoglobin, white blood cell count, and prior spontaneous bleeding] prediction algorithm in patients being treated with DAPT for out-of-hospital bleeding.[5]

This score was assessed in the PLATO (Platelet Inhibition and Patient Outcomes) trial[6] and the Bern PCI registry. It was seen that a high-bleeding risk according to PRECISE-DAPT (PRECISE-DAPT score ≥25) a prolonged DAPT was not associated with ischemic benefit but a high-bleeding burden.[5]

Though, these risk prediction systems have not been tested as prospective randomized studies hence their value remains unclear.

TYPE OF P2Y$_{12}$ INHIBITOR AND TIMING OF INITIATION

Clopidogrel

Clopidogrel is the safer drug, especially in terms of skin and gastrointestinal disorders, neutropenia, and allergy though they have a similar degree of P2Y$_{12}$ inhibition and bleeding risk.

Prasugrel

Prasugrel's P2Y$_{12}$ inhibition is faster and greater having a more consistent degree of activity compared to clopidogrel. Prasugrel needs two metabolic steps in forming the active metabolite that is similar to clopidogrel active metabolite.

Ticagrelor

Ticagrelor comes from a newer chemical class, cyclopentyl-triazolopyrimidine, which is a direct oral, reversibly binding P2Y$_{12}$ inhibitor with nearly 12 hours of plasma half-life.

P2Y$_{12}$ Inhibitors in Patients of STEMI Treated with Lysis

The P2Y$_{12}$ inhibitor which has been extensively studied in patients with STEMI undergoing initial treatment with thrombolysis is clopidogrel. The STREAM study (Strategic Reperfusion Early after Myocardial Infarction)[7] took patients below 75 years with clopidogrel 300 mg loading dose and to those above 75 years of age 75 mg once daily without loading dose.

While prasugrel or ticagrelor were allowed as per protocol in patients with prior treatment with lysis in P2Y$_{12}$ inhibitor-naïve patients or those with prior clopidogrel administration, respectively, there are insufficient safety data to recommend their concomitant use during or soon after thrombolysis.[3]

The TREAT (Ticagrelor in Patients with ST-Elevation Myocardial Infarction Treated with Pharmacological Thrombolysis) trial[8] infers that among patients below 75 years treated with fibrinolysis after STEMI, late administration of ticagrelor was noninferior to clopidogrel. There was no excess of major bleeding, fatal bleeding, or intracranial bleeding with ticagrelor versus clopidogrel. Ticagrelor represents a treatment option in such patients (i.e., clopidogrel allergy); however, unless future trials show otherwise, ticagrelor is not preferential to clopidogrel after fibrinolysis for STEMI.[9]

TABLE 2: Recommendations on $P2Y_{12}$ inhibitor selection and timing (ESC, 2017)[3]

Recommendation	Class
In ACS, ticagrelor (180 mg loading dose, 90 mg twice daily) on top of aspirin is recommended, regardless of initial treatment strategy, including patients pretreated with clopidogrel (which should be discontinued when ticagrelor is commenced)	I B
In patients with ACS undergoing PCI, prasugrel (60 mg loading dose, 10 mg daily dose) on top of aspirin is recommended for $P2Y_{12}$ inhibitor-naïve patients with NSTE-ACS or initially conservatively managed STEMI if indication for PCI is established, or in STEMI patients undergoing immediate coronary catheterization	I B
Pretreatment with a $P2Y_{12}$ inhibitor is generally recommended in patients in whom coronary anatomy is known and the decision to proceed to PCI is made and in patients with STEMI	I A
In patients with NSTE-ACS undergoing invasive management, ticagrelor administration (180 mg loading dose, 90 mg twice daily), or clopidogrel (600 mg loading dose, 75 mg daily dose) if ticagrelor is not an option, should be considered as soon as the diagnosis is established	IIa C
In patients with stable CAD, pretreatment with clopidogrel may be considered if the probability of PCI is high	–
Clopidogrel (600 mg loading dose, 75 mg daily dose) with aspirin is recommended in stable CAD patients undergoing coronary stent implantation and in ACS patients who cannot receive ticagrelor or prasugrel, including those with prior intracranial bleeding or indication for OAC	–
Clopidogrel (300 mg loading dose in patients aged <75 years, 75 mg daily dose) is recommended on top of aspirin in STEMI patients receiving thrombolysis	–

ACS, acute coronary syndrome; CAD, coronary artery disease; ESC, European Society of Cardiology; NSTE, non-ST-segment elevation myocardial infarction; OAC, oral anticoagulant; PCI, percutaneous coronary intervention; STEMI, ST-segment elevation myocardial infarction.

TABLE 3: Measures to minimize bleeding while on dual antiplatelet therapy[3]

Recommendations	Class
Radial over femoral access is recommended for coronary angiography and PCI if performed by an expert radial operator	I A
In patients treated with DAPT, a daily aspirin dose of 75–100 mg is recommended	I A
A PPI in combination with DAPT is recommended	I B
Routine platelet function testing to adjust antiplatelet therapy before or after elective stenting is not recommended	III A

DAPT, dual antiplatelet therapy; PCI, percutaneous coronary intervention; PPI, proton pump inhibitor.

Timing of Initiation of $P2Y_{12}$ Inhibitor

A reasonable approach to start $P2Y_{12}$ inhibitor according to their approval studies is to start clopidogrel and ticagrelor as soon as possible whereas for prasugrel, it must be started only after decision for PCI based on coronary anatomy is established (Table 2).

Aspirin in Patients Treated with DAPT

Low-dose aspirin (<100 mg daily) is associated with less major and total bleeding while being compared with high doses, as because daily doses of 30–50 mg is usually adequate to inactivate the platelet cyclooxygenase-1 enzyme and inhibit thromboxane production completely.

Also, it must be noted that the efficacy of ticagrelor is reduced with higher doses of aspirin (>300 mg daily) compared to lower doses (<100 mg daily). To balance between the bleeding risks and ischemic events 75–100 mg of aspirin apparently is the optimal range.

Type, Dose of $P2Y_{12}$ Inhibitor and Duration of Treatment

According to the varying stages of CAD, the type and dose of $P2Y_{12}$ inhibitor are well established. Ongoing bleeds or previous intracranial hemorrhage are common contraindications for prasugrel and ticagrelor. And in patients below 75 years, weighing under 60 kg or with history of cerebrovascular accident; prasugrel should not be used.

It is very common to switch between the $P2Y_{12}$ inhibitors mainly in episodes of minor bleeding or in those patients who have a low platelet reactivity which acts as a marker for risk for major bleeding (Table 3).

There are no properly powered randomized data on the long-term safety or efficacy of "switching" patients treated for weeks or months with a $P2Y_{12}$ inhibitor to a different $P2Y_{12}$ inhibitor. Therefore, this practice is generally discouraged.[3]

According to the 2017 European Society of Cardiology (ESC) guidelines,[3] in patients with ACS who were previously exposed to clopidogrel, switching from clopidogrel to ticagrelor is recommended early after hospital admission at a loading dose of 180 mg irrespective of timing and loading dose of clopidogrel, unless contraindications to ticagrelor exist is a class I A indication (Fig. 1).

DAPT AFTER PERCUTANEOUS CORONARY INTERVENTION FOR ACS

DAPT with Novel $P2Y_{12}$ Inhibitors for 1 Year after PCI for ACS

Though both prasugrel and ticagrelor significantly increase risk of thrombolysis in myocardial infarction (TIMI) major noncoronary artery bypass grafting (non-CABG) related

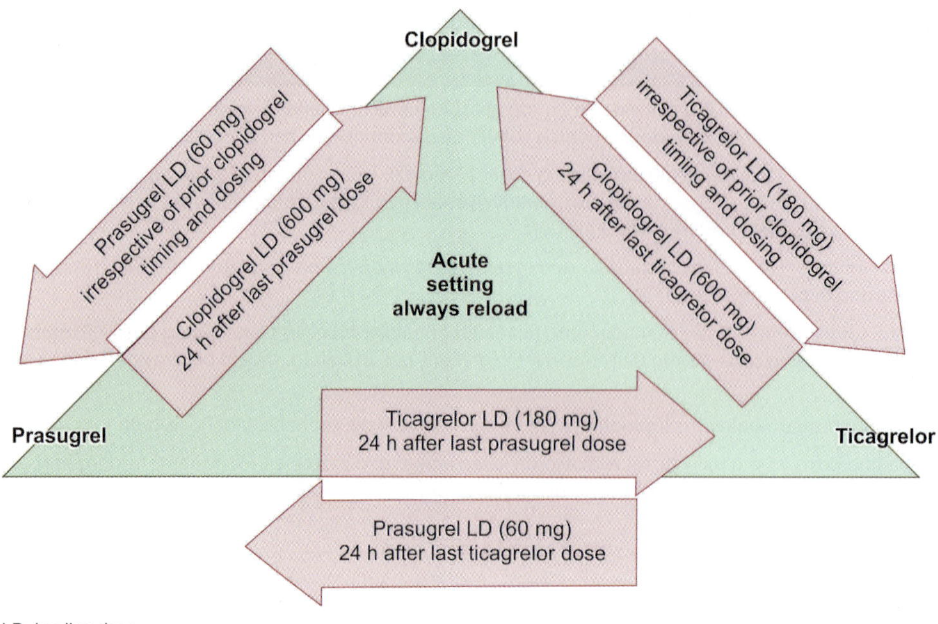

LD, loading dose

FIG. 1: Switching between oral P2Y$_{12}$ inhibitors.

bleeds but the risk-benefit ratios are favorable. Data has established the 1-year course of DAPT, preferably with prasugrel or ticagrelor, for patients undergoing PCI for ACS, unless contraindicated.[3]

DAPT with Ticagrelor for Secondary Prevention after Myocardial Infarction

In the PEGASUS (Prevention of Cardiovascular Events in Patients with Prior Heart Attack Using Ticagrelor Compared to Placebo on a Background of Aspirin) trial,[10] all the primary endpoints were consistently reduced with ticagrelor versus placebo, which was statistically significant for both 60 mg and 90 mg after MI and with 60 mg for stroke. There was an overall trend in reduction of CV mortality.

Those patients who had continued their treatment without (a major) interruption (≤30 days) derived more benefit from extended ticagrelor intake than those who interrupted their thienopyridine treatment for longer periods of time.[3] Study result suggests that the patients who could continue the initial thienopyridine treatment were getting relatively greater benefit with DAPT continuation with ticagrelor.[3]

Patients having lower-extremity artery disease (LEAD), who are at greater ischemic risk, benefit hugely from extended ticagrelor. In this group of patients with ticagreolor versus placebo showed better primary efficacy endpoints and fewer ischemic and revascularization procedures were needed.

DAPT with Thienopyridines (Clopidogrel or Prasugrel) for Secondary Prevention after Myocardial Infarction

In the DAPT trial, trialists investigated the risks and benefits of extended versus standard duration of DAPT in patients with or without MI. Prasugrel was given to one-third of the patients with MI and two-thirds received clopidogrel. In post-MI patient, extended DAPT when compared to aspirin alone showed reduction in stent thrombosis and major adverse cardiac events (MACE) significantly.

A meta-analysis study on DAPT effect (extended duration) in those patients who had MI including the PEGASUS and the subgroups of MI of studies—CHARISMA[11] (Clopidogrel for High Atherothrombotic Risk and Ischemic Stabilization, Management, and Avoidance), PRODIGY[12] (Prolonging Dual Antiplatelet Treatment After Grading Stent-Induced Intimal Hyperplasia), and DES-LATE[13] (Drug-Eluting Stent-Late Coronary Arterial Thrombotic Event) with clopidogrel as well as ARCTIC-Interruption[14] (dual-antiplatelet treatment beyond 1 year after DES implantation) and DAPT with clopidogrel or prasugrel interprets that there is a decrease in MACE when compared to giving aspirin alone. This benefit is attained at the cost of increased bleeding risk. Though the CV mortality reduction with DAPT was significant, but the absolute risk reduction was small (0.3%) with no difference seen in the all-cause mortality. This suggests a consistent effect amongst the three classes of P2Y$_{12}$ inhibitors (ticagrelor, clopidogrel, or prasugrel).

Beyond 1 year duration, it is reasonable to consider ticagrelor 60 mg twice a day as the drug of choice in prolonged DAPT in stable post-MI patients who have a lower bleeding risk, and to have clopidogrel as the reserved alternative if ticagrelor cannot be used (Table 4).

Shortening of DAPT Duration in Patients at High-bleeding Risk

After an ACS, the status of high-risk for bleeding is more challenging with regards to the duration and choice of DAPT (Fig. 2).

TABLE 4: Dual antiplatelet therapy duration in patients with acute coronary syndrome treated with percutaneous coronary intevention[3]

Recommendations	Class
In patients with ACS treated with coronary stent implantation, DAPT with a $P2Y_{12}$ inhibitor on top of aspirin is recommended for 12 months unless contraindicated (e.g., PRECISE-DAPT >25)	I A
In patients with ACS and stent implantation, who are at high-risk of bleeding, discontinuation of $P2Y_{12}$ inhibitor therapy after 6 months should be considered.	IIa B
In patients with ACS treated with bioresorbable vascular scaffolds, DAPT for at least 12 months should be considered	IIa C
In patients with ACS who have tolerated DAPT without a bleeding complication, continuation of DAPT for longer than 12 months may be considered	IIb A
In patients with MI and high ischemic risk, who have tolerated DAPT without a bleeding complication, ticagrelor 60 mg twice a day (bid) for longer than 12 months on top of aspirin may be preferred over clopidogrel or prasugrel	IIb B

ACS, acute coronary syndrome; DAPT, dual antiplatelet therapy; MI, myocardial infarction.

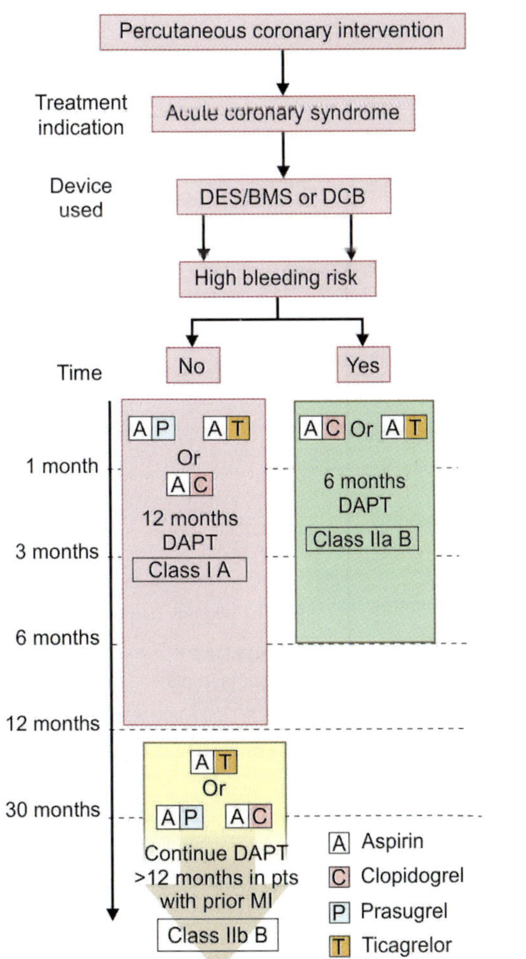

BMS, bare metal stent; DAPT, dual antiplatelet therapy; DCB, drug-coated balloon; DES, drug-eluting stents; MI, myocardial infarction.

FIG. 2: Duration of DAPT in patients undergoing percutaneous coronary intervention.

A meta-analysis that includes six trials which compare the DAPT for 3 and 6 months duration to the 12-month duration suggested to consider to discontinue $P2Y_{12}$ inhibitor after a period of 6 months when the bleeding risk is high (Table 4).

DAPT IN PATIENTS TREATED WITH CABG SURGERY FOR ACS

Background

In ACS patients, the advantages of DAPT over aspirin alone is adequately proven to reduce the ischemic risks, but due to lack of dedicated studies in patients who will undergo CABG the evidence of DAPT benefits is limited.

There is an increase in the risk of perioperative bleed, increased need for transfusions and re-exploration when DAPT is continued till CABG, therefore it is recommended that $P2Y_{12}$ inhibitor should be stopped prior to an elective CABG whenever possible. An alternative is to defer elective surgeries until the DAPT treatment is completed.

In cases that are urgent, mostly the ACS group of patients, the thrombotic risk must be evaluated against the perioperative bleeding risk, while one waits for the effect of the drug $P2Y_{12}$ inhibitor to wear off (Table 5).

$P2Y_{12}$ Inhibitors

These drugs have different pharmacokinctic and pharmacodynamics properties and different inhibitory effects on platelets, thus the safe period for discontinuation of these agents also vary. In the CURE (Clopidogrel in Unstable Angina to Prevent Recurrent Events) trial,[15] the substudy of the CABG group showed that discontinuation more than 5 days before CABG does not increase the bleeding risk. For prasugrel, a 7-day interval is recommended from the TRITON-TIMI 38 (Trial to Assess Improvement in Therapeutic Outcomes by Optimizing Platelet Inhibition with Prasugrel-TIMI)[16] and a 5-day period for ticagrelor.

However, newer data from the studies such as Swedish study and PLATO trial incline more toward a discontinuation period of 3 days.

Acetylsalicylic Acid

A meta-analysis which included 13 trials showed that ASA decreases the risk of perioperative MI while increasing postoperative bleeding, red cell transfusions, and increased surgical re-exploration.

The ASA of 100 mg was compared to placebo in the ATACAS (Aspirin and Tranexamic Acid for Coronary Artery Surgery)[17] trial, where ASA was given on the day of the surgery in CABG patients. The ASA did not have any significant effect on the perioperative bleeding and neither did it reduce the incidence of thrombotic events.

Considering in to, the available evidence suggests that ASA given until the day of cardiac surgery has been associated with slight increase in risk of bleeding complications and significant decreased risk of perioperative MI. Platelet transfusions can be used if bleeding occurs during surgery. ASA can also be considered to be given throughout the perioperative period.

TABLE 5: Dual antiplatelet therapy in patients treated with cardiac surgery[3]

Recommendations	Class
In patients on aspirin who need to undergo nonemergent cardiac surgery, it is recommended to continue aspirin at a low daily regimen throughout the perioperative period	I C
In patients treated with DAPT after coronary stent implantation who subsequently undergo cardiac surgery, it is recommended to resume $P2Y_{12}$ inhibitor therapy postoperatively as soon as is deemed safe so that DAPT continues until the recommended duration of therapy is completed	I C
In patients on $P2Y_{12}$ inhibitors who need to undergo nonemergent cardiac surgery, postponing surgery for at least 3 days after discontinuation of ticagrelor, at least 5 days after clopidogrel, and at least 7 days after prasugrel should be considered	IIa B
In CABG patients with prior MI who are at high risk of severe bleeding (e.g., PRECISE-DAPT ≥25), discontinuation of $P2Y_{12}$ inhibitor therapy after 6 months should be considered	IIa C
Platelet function testing may be considered to guide decisions on timing of cardiac surgery in patients who have recently received $P2Y_{12}$ inhibitors	IIb B
In patients perceived to be at high ischemic risk with prior MI and CABG, who have tolerated DAPT without a bleeding complication, treatment with DAPT for longer than 12 months and up to 36 months may be considered	IIb C

CABG, coronary artery bypass grafting; DAPT, dual antiplatelet therapy; MI:,myocardial infarction.

Testing of Platelet Function

There is a wide variability amongst the different drugs of $P2Y_{12}$ inhibitor group in terms of platelet inhibitory effect, duration, and magnitude of antiplatelet effect. The platelet function test may help in deciding the timing of surgery and also guide to gauge the antiplatelet effect where the duration of drug discontinuation is not clear.

The assessment of platelet aggregation capacity in the preoperative period can predict bleeding complications that is CABG-related in clopidogrel and ticagrelor-treated patients of ACS (Fig. 3).

The results suggest that in patients with ACS who are referred for CABG, the platelet function test is helpful in guiding the timing of CABG in patients taking $P2Y_{12}$ inhibitors.

DAPT FOR PATIENTS WITH MEDICALLY MANAGED ACS

In ACS patients who are being managed medically, the studies from which the evidence is derived are the CHARISMA and CURE trials for clopidogrel, TRILOGY ACS (The Targeted Platelet Inhibition to Clarify the Optimal Strategy to Medically Manage Acute Coronary Syndromes) trial[18] for prasugrel, and the PLATO and PEGASUS trials for ticagrelor (Fig. 4).

The CURE study shows evidence that a DAPT treatment of 9-month duration is beneficial when compared to a 1 month treatment in the NSTE-ACS patient group, irrespective of the management strategy.

Although the overall result of the CHARISMA trial do not show benefit of DAPT over aspirin alone, but the patients of post-MI subset in the CHARISMA trial shows benefit of DAPT in terms that antiplatelet drugs beyond 1 year reduce long-term ischemic recurrences, even if it is at the cost of higher bleeding episodes.

The results of TRILOGY study were negative for prasugrel in medically managed ACS.

In the medically managed subset of patients of the PLATO trial there was benefit from ticagrelor 90 mg given twice daily when compared to clopidogrel with overall mortality reduction.

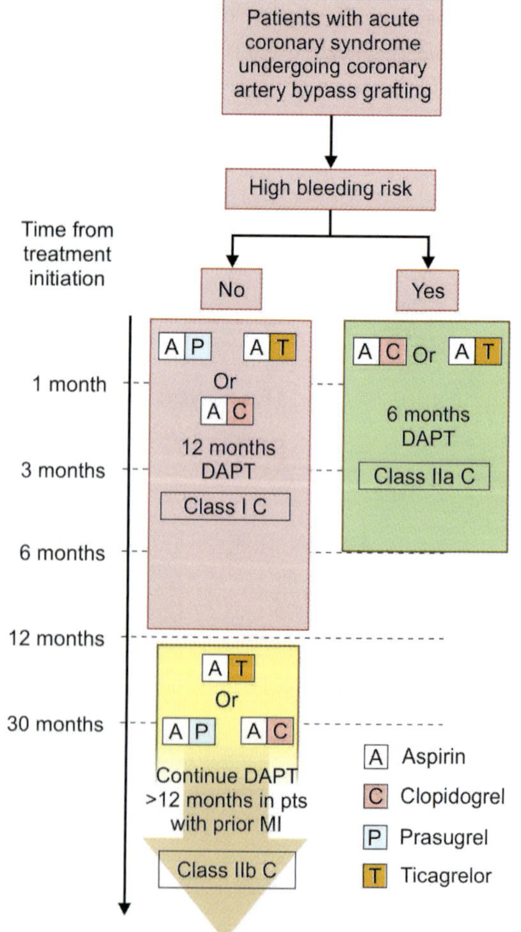

DAPT, dual antiplatelet therapy; MI, myocardial infarction.

FIG. 3: DAPT duration in patients with acute coronary syndrome undergoing coronary artery bypass grafting.

The PEGASUS trial draws evidence that consistent benefits and risks are drawn from ticagrelor.

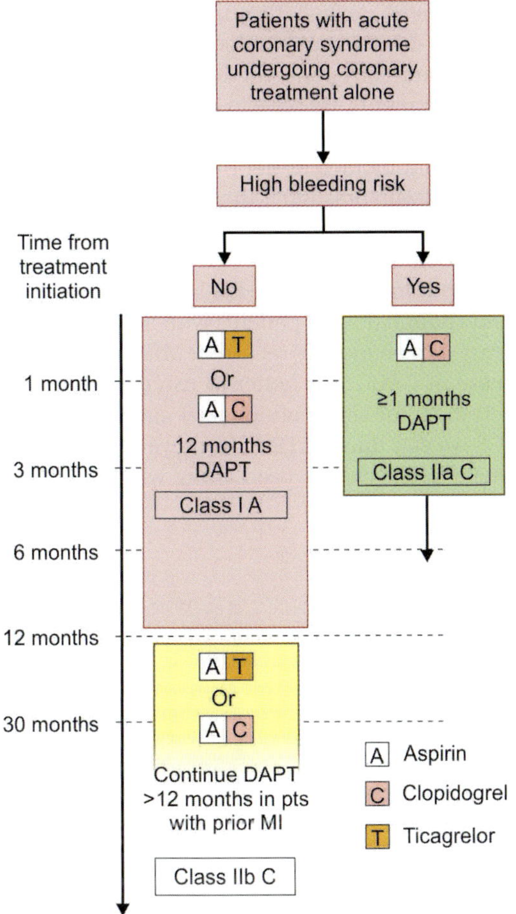

DAPT, dual antiplatelet therapy; MI, myocardial infarction.

FIG. 4: Duration of DAPT in patients with acute coronary syndrome undergoing medical treatment alone.

TABLE 6: Dual antiplatelet therapy duration in patients with ACS undergoing medical therapy management[3]

Recommendations	Class
In patients with ACS who are managed with medical therapy alone and treated with DAPT, it is recommended to continue $P2Y_{12}$ inhibitor therapy (either ticagrelor or clopidogrel) for 12 months	I A
Ticagrelor is recommended over clopidogrel, unless the bleeding risk outweighs the potential ischemic benefit	I B
In medically managed ACS at high-risk of bleeding (e.g., PRECISE-DAPT >25), DAPT for at least 1 month should be considered	IIa C
In patients with prior MI at high ischemic risk who are managed with medical therapy alone and have tolerated DAPT without a bleeding complication, treatment with DAPT in the form of ticagrelor 60 mg bid with aspirin for longer than 12 months and up to 36 months may be considered	IIb B
In patients with prior MI not treated with coronary stent implantation, who have tolerated DAPT without a bleeding complication and who are not eligible for treatment with ticagrelor, continuation of clopidogrel with aspirin for longer than12 months may be considered	IIb C
Prasugrel is not recommended in medically managed ACS patients	III B

ACS, acute coronary syndrome; DAPT, dual antiplatelet therapy; MI, myocardial infarction; PRECISE-DAPT, Predicting Bleeding Complications in Patients Undergoing Stent Implantation and Subsequent Dual Antiplatelet Therapy.

Multiple sources reveal that the patients of ACS being medically managed receive the DAPT treatment less frequently comparing to the group of patients who undergo PCI (Table 6).

RESISTANCE TO DRUGS

It must be noted that resistance with both aspirin and clopidogrel is prevalent and can be deduced from the fact that a large number of patients despite being on these antiplatelets in adequate dosage and complete compliance may still have ischemic events.

Aspirin resistance has been estimated to exist, anywhere from 5 to 45% of the population. This prevalence of aspirin resistance is very important and of great alarming clinical concern. Aspirin resistance generally describes the failure of aspirin to produce an expected biological response (i.e., inhibition of platelet aggregation) or preventing the atherothrombotic events.[19]

Clopidogrel resistance is said to be clopidogrel fails to achieve the platelet inhibition effect. The initial results indicate that clopidogrel's low antiplatelet effect may lead to have more risk of having CV events. The interpatient variability in clopidogrel response is multifactorial. It can be due to extrinsic or intrinsic mechanisms such as drug-drug interactions involving cytochrome P450 3A4 (CYP3A4), or genetic polymorphisms of the $P2Y_{12}$ receptor and CYP3As.[19]

In more advanced countries the practice of genetic testing to determine the susceptibility or resistance to the antiplatelet drugs is on the rise, however given the factors of cost and availability it still remains to be in use in India.

DURATION OF DAPT AFTER PCI IN PATIENTS WITH PERIPHERAL ARTERY DISEASE

Every third patient affected by CAD also has a coexisting peripheral artery disease (PAD). Considering in totality, antiplatelet therapy should be used for patients who are having a high-risk for ischemia such as the patients who are having polyvascular atherosclerosis in multiple vascular beds.

When considered in totality, antiplatelet therapy in patients who are at a higher ischemic burden (i.e., patients with atherosclerosis of multiple vascular beds). Overall ischemic burden (polyvascular atherosclerosis), clinical risk factors for disease progression, DAPT tolerance in the 1st year, and bleeding risk affect the risk-benefit ratio of prolonged DAPT in patients with MI and PAD.[20] So all high ischemic burden patients must be evaluated individually to determine the risks and the benefits of a prolonged regime of DAPT. With the data that is available to us, a prolonged regime (>12 month) of DAPT should be considered strongly in patients post PCI with evidence of PAD and with absence of any excessive risk of bleeding.

Recommendations in Peripheral Artery Disease

At present, there is no evidence of use of aspirin in asymptomatic patients. The AHA/ACC (American Heart Association/American College of Cardiology) guidelines[21] for ankle-brachial index less than 0.90 recommend use of antiplatelets as reasonable, whereas the ESC does not recommend its use in asymptomatic patients.

Patients with symptomatic PAD should be treated with antithrombotic therapy to reduce CV risk.[21] Single antiplatelet therapy with either aspirin or clopidogrel is recommended.[21] For those undergoing surgical revascularization, aspirin, clopidogrel, and rivaroxaban plus aspirin are all reasonable recommendations.

CONCLUSION

It will be fair to say that the optimal duration of DAPT after ACS is still debatable. To summarize, with the present stage of our knowledge DAPT should be continued till 1 year in a patient of ACS after PCI or even if on medical treatment following ACS. As SMART DATE (Safety of 6-month Duration of Dual Antiplatelet Therapy After Acute Coronary Syndromes) trial[22] has clearly shown that discontinuing DAPT after 6 months results in increased incidents of MI and recurrent ischemic events, but if the chance of bleeding is very high, in those population or in the elderly patients DAPT can be stopped at 6 months. After stenting with a newer DES it is now somewhat acceptable, but as a routine we should continue DAPT till 1 year after the procedure and then we can think of discontinuing it. However, if the patient has got high chances of thrombosis such as in diabetics, patients with excessive thrombus load, recurrent angina then we may continue DAPT. And here a better choice would be low dose of ticagrelor 60 mg bid along with small dose of aspirin 75 mg daily till 3 years following the MI and the incidents of bleeding is not high, but the reduction of events is much lower because we know at 1–3 years after ACS, 1 in 8 patients tend to have recurrent ischemic event. It is relatively recent and important evidence that to prevent recurrent ischemic events in high-risk patients, it is fair enough to continue DAPT up to 3 years. And in our practice also we find that the incidents of bleeding are not so high in routine population even if we continue to use DAPT for longer durations. In an ongoing study on ticagrelor in the Indian population, we have seen that the incidents of bleeding are not high even if we continue it for another 2–3 years, but there is reduction of events in the trial, but due to confidentially agreement we cannot tell details of the trial data as it is not yet submitted.

So to conclude we should continue DAPT for 1 year after stenting in a patient of ACS or even with medical treatment and after 1 year in high thrombotic risk patient we can continue low-dose ticagrelor along with aspirin for another 2–3 years without any concern. Regarding the medical treatment of ACS patients, we have to give low-dose aspirin along with clopidogrel or ticagrelor 90 mg bid, but prasugrel has not been recommended as per the negative results found in TRILOGY trial with prasugrel. There are recommendations by the different international societies stating that ticagrelor and prasugrel should be used more frequently in patients with high thrombus load and where the blood is procoagulant like in diabetic population, in patients with STEMI or NSTEMI or in patients with chances of recurrent MI or recurrent ACS.

In case of CABG it is better to use the DAPT for a year and then to go for single antiplatelet agent. For PAD, along with ACS we can think of DAPT for a year and then a single antiplatelet agent can be used along with other drugs and trained exercise program.

REFERENCES

1. Navarese EP, Andreotti F, Schulze V, et al. Optimal duration of dual antiplatelet therapy after percutaneous coronary intervention with drug eluting stents: meta-analysis of randomised controlled trials. BMJ. 2015;350:h1618.
2. Camenzind E, Wijns W, Mauri L, et al. Rationale and design of the Patient Related Outcomes with Endeavor versus Cypher stenting trial (PROTECT): randomized controlled trial comparing the incidence of stent thrombosis and clinical events after sirolimus or zotarolimus drug-eluting stent implantation. Am Heart J. 2009;158(6):902-9.
3. Valgimigli M, Bueno H, Byrne RA, et al. 2017 ESC focused update on dual antiplatelet therapy in coronary artery disease developed in collaboration with EACTS. Eur J Cardiothorac Surg. 2018;53(1):34-78.
4. Mauri L, Kereiakes DJ, Yeh RW, et al. Twelve or 30 months of dual antiplatelet therapy after drug-eluting stents. New Engl J Med. 2014;371(23):2155-66.
5. Costa F, van Klaveren D, James S, et al. Derivation and validation of the predicting bleeding complications in patients undergoing stent implantation and subsequent dual antiplatelet therapy (PRECISE-DAPT) score: a pooled analysis of individual-patient datasets from clinical trials. Lancet. 2017;389(10073): 1025-34.
6. Wallentin L, Becker RC, Budaj A, et al. Ticagrelor versus clopidogrel in patients with acute coronary syndromes. N Engl J Med. 2009;361(11):1045-57.
7. Armstrong PW, Gershlick AH, Goldstein P, et al. Fibrinolysis or primary PCI in ST-segment elevation myocardial infarction. N Engl J Med. 2013;368(15): 1379-87.
8. Berwanger O, Nicolau JC, Carvalho AC, et al. Ticagrelor versus clopidogrel after fibrinolytic therapy in patients with ST-elevation myocardial infarction: rationale and design of the ticagrelor in patients with ST-elevation myocardial infarction treated with thrombolysis (TREAT) trial. Am Heart J. 2018;202:89-96.
9. O'gara PT, Kushner FG, Ascheim DD, et al. 2013 ACCF/AHA guideline for the management of ST-elevation myocardial infarction: executive summary: a report of the American College of Cardiology Foundation/American Heart Association Task Force on Practice Guidelines. J Am Coll Cardiol. 2013;61(4):485-510.
10. Bonaca MP, Bhatt DL, Cohen M, et al. Long-term use of ticagrelor in patients with prior myocardial infarction. N Engl J Med. 2015;372(19):1791-800.
11. Bhatt DL, Flather MD, Hacke W, et al. Patients with prior myocardial infarction, stroke, or symptomatic peripheral arterial disease in the CHARISMA trial. J Am Coll Cardiol. 2007;49(19):1982-8.
12. Valgimigli M, Borghesi M, Tebaldi M, et al. Should duration of dual antiplatelet therapy depend on the type and/or potency of implanted stent? A pre-specified analysis from the prolonging dual antiplatelet treatment after grading stent-induced intimal hyperplasia study (PRODIGY). Eur Heart J. 2013;34(12): 909-19.
13. Lee CW, Ahn JM, Park DW, et al. Optimal duration of dual antiplatelet therapy after drug-eluting stent implantation: a randomized, controlled trial. Circulation. 2014;129(3):304-12.

14. Collet JP, Silvain J, Barthélémy O, et al. Dual-antiplatelet treatment beyond 1year after drug-eluting stent implantation (ARCTIC-Interruption): a randomised trial. Lancet. 2014;384(9954):1577-85.
15. Peters RJ, Mehta SR, Fox KA, et al. Effects of aspirin dose when used alone or in combination with clopidogrel in patients with acute coronary syndromes: observations from the clopidogrel in unstable angina to prevent recurrent events (CURE) study. Circulation. 2003;108(14):1682-7.
16. Wiviott SD, Braunwald E, McCabe CH, et al. Prasugrel versus clopidogrel in patients with acute coronary syndromes. N Engl J Med. 2007;357(20):2001-15.
17. Myles PS, Smith JA, Forbes A, et al. Stopping vs. continuing aspirin before coronary artery surgery. N Engl J Med. 2016;374(8):728-37.
18. Wiviott SD, White HD, Ohman EM, et al. Prasugrel versus clopidogrel for patients with unstable angina or non-ST-segment elevation myocardial infarction with or without angiography: a secondary, prespecified analysis of the TRILOGY ACS trial. Lancet. 2013;382(9892):605-13.
19. Nguyen TA, Diodati JG, Pharand C. Resistance to clopidogrel: a review of the evidence. J Am Coll Cardiol. 2005;45(8):1157-64.
20. Bonaca MP, Sabatine MS. Antiplatelet therapy for long-term secondary prevention after myocardial infarction. JAMA Cardiol. 2016;1(6):627-8.
21. Hussain MA, Al-Omran M, Creager MA, et al. Antithrombotic therapy for peripheral artery disease: recent advances. J Am Coll Cardiol. 2018;71(21):2450-67.
22. Hahn JY, Song YB, Oh JH, et al. 6-month versus 12-month or longer dual antiplatelet therapy after percutaneous coronary intervention in patients with acute coronary syndrome (SMART-DATE): a randomised, open-label, non-inferiority trial. The Lancet. 2018;391(10127):1274-84.

Switching Between DAPT Agents: The Right Strategy

Harinder K Bali, Hiteshi KC Chauhan

DUAL ANTIPLATELET THERAPY CLINICAL CONUNDRUM UNRAVELED

Dual antiplatelet therapy (DAPT), comprising of aspirin given in conjunction with a P2Y12 receptor antagonist, is the backbone of treatment strategy in patients presenting with acute coronary syndromes (ACS) with the aim of preventing atherothrombotic events.[1-5]

With a research timeline spanning 22 years[6] and with over 35 randomized clinical trials, DAPT is one of the most meticulously and extensively researched treatment strategies in the annals of cardiovascular medicine (Fig. 1).[2] Over the last two decades, DAPT has undergone rapid evolution from being merely a "local" stent-related treatment strategy to a wider "systemic" one capable of preventing thrombotic arterial occlusions.[2]

Despite intense clinical research leading to updated guidelines and focused updates on DAPT, practicing clinicians, across the world, often find it difficult to incorporate these into practice, especially considering different patient subsets, varied clinical settings, cost constraints, and drug availability issues in different geographical locations.[1-5]

Availability of multiple oral P2Y12 inhibitors and a novel intravenous (IV) P2Y12 inhibitor has given physicians

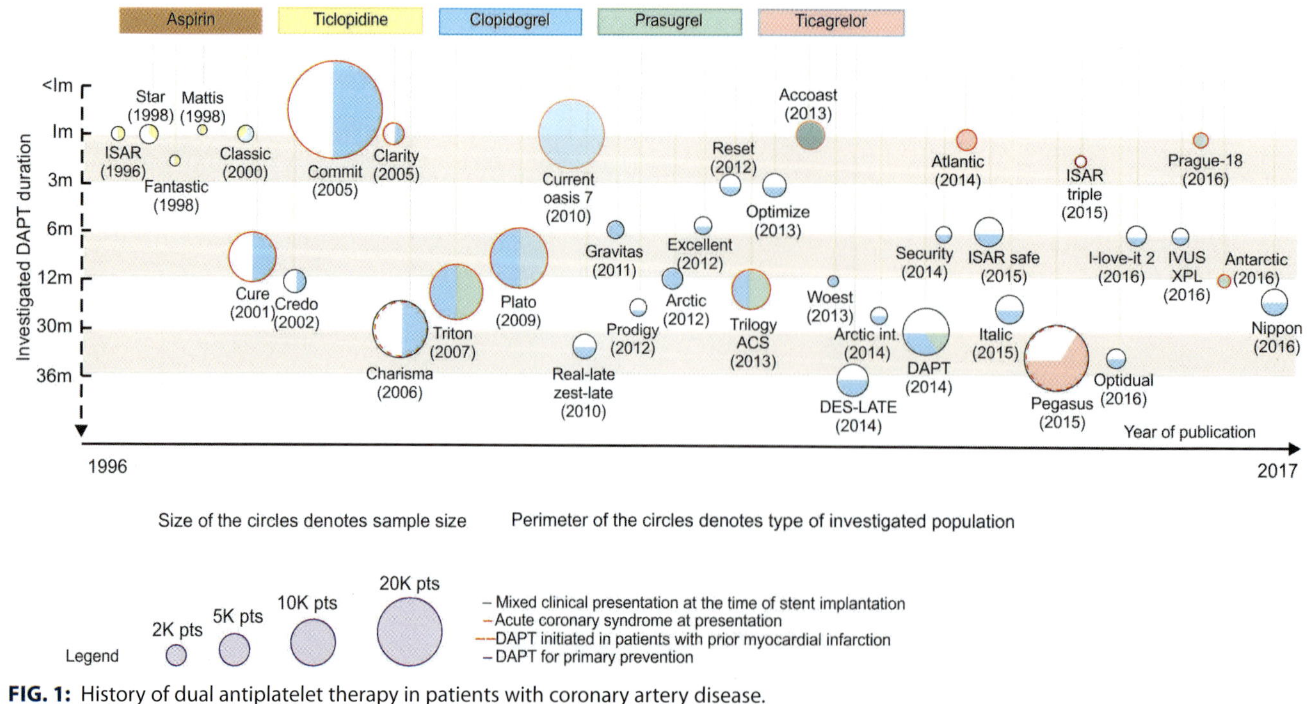

FIG. 1: History of dual antiplatelet therapy in patients with coronary artery disease.

Source: Reprinted with permission from: 2017 ESC focused update on dual antiplatelet therapy in coronary artery disease developed in collaboration with EACTS: The Task Force for dual antiplatelet therapy in coronary artery disease of the European Society of Cardiology (ESC) and of the European Association for Cardio-Thoracic Surgery (EACTS). Eur Heart J. 2017;39(3):213-60.

the apparently attractive option of switching antiplatelet therapy to address a multitude of factors: patient-specific characteristics, drug compliance issues, adverse effects, drug-drug interactions (DDIs) and cost considerations.[7,8] Therefore, in spite of lingering concerns fueled by paucity of scientifically reliable data on safety and efficacy of switching between DAPT agents, it is undertaken quite frequently in clinical practice.[2]

All the aforementioned factors deepen the recurrent clinical dilemma physicians' face regarding personalization of DAPT therapy, including optimal type, duration, and ideal timing of switching of DAPT agents, while treating patients with different clinical manifestations of coronary artery disease (CAD).

It is, therefore, extremely important for physicians to be well versed with drug pharmacology, different switching modalities, available literature[1-8] and latest consensus recommendations to decide upon the right timing and strategy of switching antiplatelet therapies.[9]

The treating physician must tailor DAPT therapy for each individual patient after meticulously evaluating the trade-off between ischemic and bleeding risk: at initiation, during follow-up, and at completion.[7]

P2Y12 Receptor Antagonists

Pharmacological Profile

The unique pharmacological properties of P2Y12 receptor antagonists are of utmost clinical significance (Table 1).[8,9] While switching P2Y12 inhibitors, these differences in their pharmacological profile, including drug half-life, site and mechanism of binding of P2Y12 receptors, and rate of onset and offset of drug effect, may enhance the potential for DDIs due to either inadequate or excessive platelet reactivity. This may lead to adverse clinical outcomes (thrombotic or bleeding complications, respectively).[9-11]

Oral P2Y12 Receptor Antagonists

- *Ticlopidine*: The first available platelet P2Y12 inhibitor, ticlopidine, is no longer used due to safety concerns[12]
- *Clopidogrel*: This "staple" quintessential second-generation thienopyridine retains its position of being the most prescribed P2Y12 inhibitor, worldwide.[1,13] This prodrug is ~85% hydrolyzed by human carboxylesterase-1 into an inactive metabolite after intestinal absorption.[14] Thereafter, cytochrome P-450 isoenzymes oxidize the remaining 15% to create an active metabolite, which binds the adenosine diphosphate (ADP) site irreversibly. The variable pharmacodynamic response to this drug attributable to myriad of factors, ranging from pharmacological properties to genotype polymorphism, lessens its stability and potency.[15]

  In patients with stable CAD[1,2] and in those presenting with ST-elevation myocardial infarction (STEMI) after thrombolysis,[16,17] clopidogrel is strongly recommended as compared to its newer counterparts
- *Prasugrel*: It is also a prodrug-like clopidogrel. However, its active metabolite is generated faster and in higher plasma concentration via a single-step hepatic cytochrome [CYP] oxidation. Therefore, this third-generation thienopyridine achieves higher, consistent and more potent platelet inhibitory effect, as compared to clopidogrel.[14] Due to irreversible binding of active metabolite and enhanced platelet inhibition achieved by prasugrel, platelet recovery time is longer at 7–10 days after treatment discontinuation, as compared to clopidogrel (5–7 days)[18,19]

TABLE 1: Pharmacological profile of P2Y12—receptor inhibitors

	Clopidogrel	Prasugrel	Ticagrelor	Cangrelor
Drug class	**Thienopyridine**	**Thienopyridine**	**Cyclopentyl triazolopyrimidine**	**ATP analogue**
Administrative route	Oral	Oral	Oral	Intravenous
Dosing frequency	Once daily	Once daily	Twice daily	Bolus, infusion
Onset of action	2–8 h	30 min–4 h	30 min–4 h	2 min
Offset of action	5–7 days	7–10 days	3–5 days	30–60 min
P2Y12—receptor blockade	Irreversible	Irreversible	Reversible	Reversible
Prodrug	Yes	Yes	No	No
Half-life:				
A. Parent drug	~6 h	<5 min	6–12 h	3–6 min
B. Active metabolite	30 min	• Distribution half-life—30–60 min • Elimination half-life—2–15 h	8–12 h	Not applicable
Binding site	ADP	ADP	Allosteric	Undetermined
Type of binding	Competitive	Competitive	Noncompetitive	Undetermined

ADP, adenosine diphosphate; ATP, adenosine triphosphate.

- *Ticagrelor*: This oral cyclopentyl-triazolopyrimidine is a direct-acting compound, which does not require hepatic metabolism. However, an active metabolite produced by the CYP3A4/5 enzymes is responsible for one-third of its effect.[20] This drug reversibly binds the P2Y12 receptors at a unique site through a noncompetitive, allosteric mechanism.[20]

  Ticagrelor rates higher on both potency and predictability, as compared to the older P2Y12 receptor antagonists.[20] However, this drug has two limitations: a quicker offset of action due to its reversible binding and a relatively short half-life of 6–12 hours, which necessitates a twice daily dosing and may compromise long-term compliance.[21]

  The newer, more potent kids on the P2Y12-inhibitor block—prasugrel and ticagrelor—are recommended as first-line agents in ACS and in patients undergoing percutaneous coronary intervention (PCI), as they remarkably decrease the incidence of ischemic events, particularly the risk of stent thrombosis (ST).[22,23]

Intravenous P2Y12 Receptor Inhibitor

Cangrelor: The only intravenous P2Y12 receptor inhibitor currently available is an ATP analogue, which directly and reversibly binds to the P2Y12 receptor at an undetermined site. Its effect is dose-dependent and is distinguished by a high level of receptor occupancy.[24,25] Cangrelor is rapidly inactivated by ectonucleotidase via dephosphorylation. Therefore, platelet function is recovered within ~60 minutes of stopping its infusion.[24,25]

Optimal Aspirin Dosing with P2Y12 Receptor Inhibitors

The optimal aspirin dose in patients on DAPT, which imparts maximal ischemic protection and minimal bleeding risk, is 75–100 mg.[26-32] In patients on ticagrelor, a lower dose of aspirin is recommended as higher aspirin doses are known to compromise the efficacy of this potent P2Y12 inhibitor.[33]

SWITCHING MODALITIES

Translation of Evidence from Randomized Trials, Registries, and Pharmacodynamic Studies into Clinical Practice

Switching DAPT agents should be approached with caution—as per latest guidelines[2] and expert consensus statement[9]—due to valid safety concerns. However, as already discussed, in clinical practice, certain scenarios may necessitate switching of DAPT agents[2] (Table 2).

As there is paucity of dedicated large scale clinical studies, current recommendations on switching modalities mostly rely on results of pharmacodynamic studies, sometimes exclusively so (Fig. 2).[2] Obviously, these pharmacodynamic studies do not have as compelling a scientific rationale as multicentric randomized clinical trials.

We would discuss each switching modality, taking into account the evidence from randomized trials, registries, and pharmacodynamic studies, to finally converge into latest expert recommendations on switching DAPT agents in clinical practice.

Switching modalities are categorized into:

- Switching between various oral P2Y12 receptor antagonists
- Switching between different oral P2Y12 receptor inhibitors and the novel IV P2Y12 antagonist.

SWITCHING BETWEEN VARIOUS ORAL P2Y12 INHIBITORS

In concordance with Academic Research Consortium (ARC) definition for ST time is established as per index event leading to initiation of P2Y12 receptor antagonist.[34] Switching between oral agents may, therefore, be categorized into acute (<24 h), early (1 day to <30 days), late (30 days to 1-year), and very late (beyond 1 year).[9]

Switching is subdivided into escalation, de-escalation, and change.[2,8,9]

TABLE 2: Common clinical scenarios leading to P2Y12 inhibitor switching

Escalation from clopidogrel to prasugrel or ticagrelor	De-escalation from prasugrel or ticagrelor to clopidogrel	Changes between prasugrel and ticagrelor
A. Patients with ACS on clopidogrel	A. Patients with major bleeding (resolved) with high-risk features (clinical or angiographic) for ST or ACS	A. Patients with intolerance or side effects to a drug having high-risk features (clinical or angiographic) for thrombotic events
B. Patients with ST or ACS on clopidogrel	B. Patients with minor bleeding on either drug likely to affect compliance to it	B. Patients with ST or ACS on either drug
C. Poor metabolizers of clopidogrel	C. Intolerance or side effects to either drug in patients without high-risk features (clinical or angiographic) for ACS/ST	C. Patients on concomitant CYP3A inducers affecting ticagrelor metabolism
–	D. Patients having clinical indication for concurrent oral anticoagulation	–
–	E. Affordability issues, inadequate insurance, nonavailability of newer DAPT agents in a geographic region	–

ACS, acute coronary syndrome; DAPT, dual antiplatelet therapy; ST, stent thrombosis.

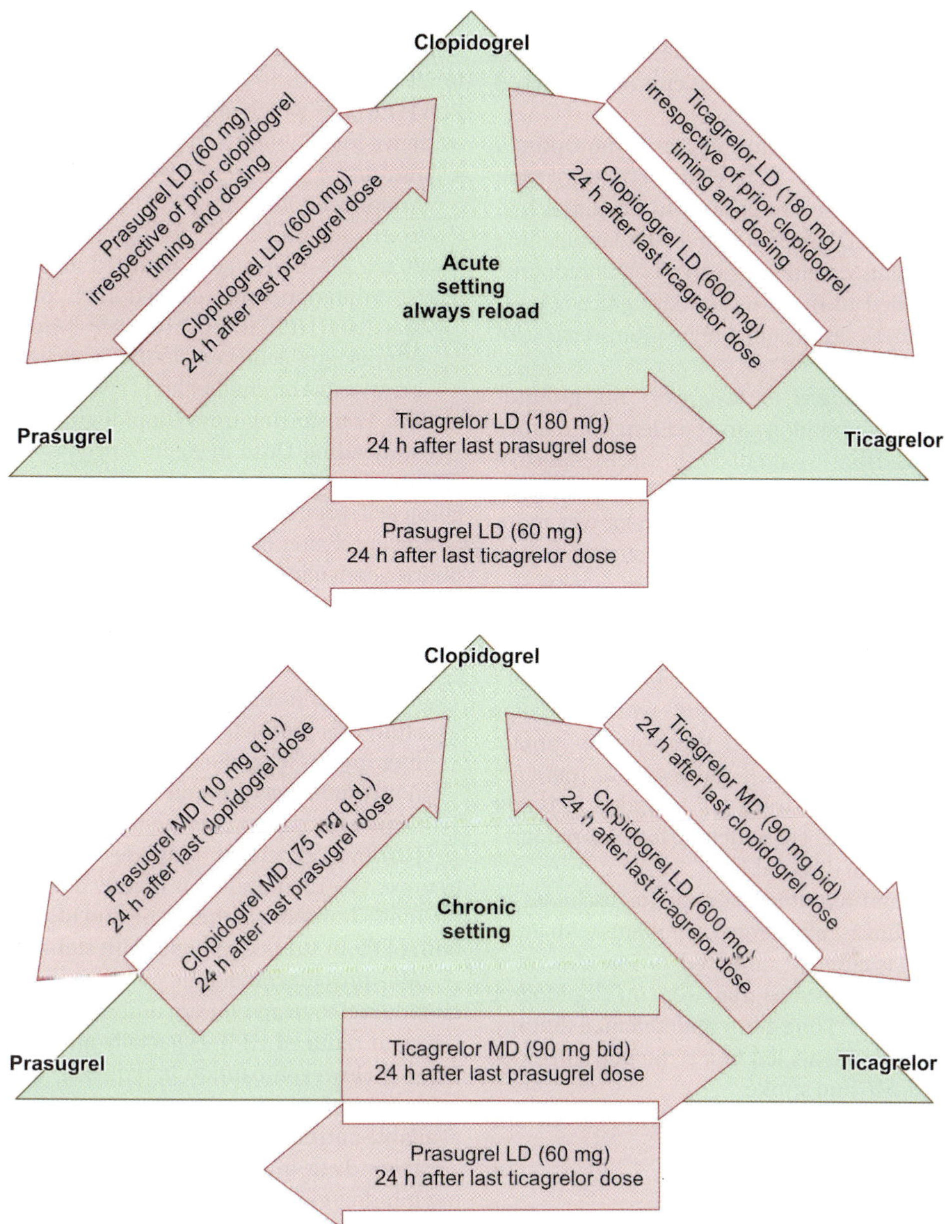

FIG. 2: Algorithm for switching between oral P2Y12 inhibitors in the acute and chronic setting.

Source: Reprinted with permission from: 2017 ESC focused update on dual antiplatelet therapy in coronary artery disease developed in collaboration with EACTS: The Task Force for dual antiplatelet therapy in coronary artery disease of the European Society of Cardiology (ESC) and of the European Association for Cardio-Thoracic Surgery (EACTS). Eur Heart J. 2017;39(3):213-60.

Escalation

Change from a less efficacious, oral P2Y12 antagonist with lower potency to a more efficacious and more potent oral P2Y12 receptor inhibitor is termed as escalation.

Evidence from Clinical Trials, Registries, and Pharmacodynamic Studies

Evidence from Clinical Trials

- *Escalation from clopidogrel to prasugrel*: In the pivotal Therapeutic Outcomes by Optimizing Platelet Inhibition with Prasugrel - Thrombolysis in Myocardial Infarction 38 (TRITON-TIMI 38) trial, prasugrel was proven superior to clopidogrel in reducing ischemic endpoints, highlighted by a marked risk reduction for myocardial infarction (MI).[23] The obvious caveat was higher rates of both non-coronary artery bypass grafting (CABG) and CABG-related major bleeding events in patients on prasugrel. However, this trial included only P2Y12-receptor-antagonist-naïve patients. Therefore, despite the compelling evidence it generated for the use of prasugrel; it, unfortunately, was unable to address the clinical consequences of this switching modality.[23]

In contradiction, patients on a maintenance dose (MD) of clopidogrel at time of randomization were included in A Comparison of Prasugrel at the Time of Percutaneous Coronary Intervention or as Pretreatment at the Time of Diagnosis in Patients with Non-ST Elevation Myocardial

Infarction (ACCOAST) trial.[35] However, irrespective of clopidogrel pretreatment, there was no ischemic benefit and more major bleeding complications in patients administered prasugrel at time of diagnosis.[35]

In the Targeted Platelet Inhibition to Clarify the Optimal Strategy to Medically Manage ACS (TRILOGY-ACS) trial, almost two-thirds of patients randomized to prasugrel had received a loading dose (LD) of clopidogrel. Similar bleeding risk was found in patients on either prasugrel or clopidogrel. However, this trial failed to reach its primary efficacy endpoint and therefore, these results need to be interpreted with caution[36]

- *Escalation from clopidogrel to ticagrelor:* The groundbreaking PLATElet inhibition and patient Outcomes (PLATO) trial proved that in patients with ACS, irrespective of prior exposure to clopidogrel and treatment strategy (medical vs. invasive management), ticagrelor was more efficacious than clopidogrel in reducing ischemic events and as safe with no increase in major bleeding events.[22]

However, as proven by the Administration of Ticagrelor in the Cath Laboratory or in the Ambulance for New ST Elevation Myocardial Infarction to Open the Coronary Artery (ATLANTIC) trial, prehospital treatment with ticagrelor in patients with acute STEMI failed to positively impact coronary reperfusion before PCI.[37] However, as patients on clopidogrel at presentation were not included, it is not possible to comment on impact of switching from clopidogrel to ticagrelor from results of this trial.[37]

Au contraire, around one-third of patients, included in the Prevention of Cardiovascular Events in Patients with Prior Heart Attack Using Ticagrelor Compared to Placebo on a Background of Aspirin (PEGASUS) trial, were on clopidogrel at time of randomization.[38] Long-term maintenance therapy with ticagrelor in these patients led to a reduction in risk of cardiovascular death, MI, and stroke.

However, this superiority was partially offset by an increase in major bleeding rates.[38]

Evidence from Registries

Numerous registries have documented prevalence of escalation from clopidogrel to the novel P2Y12 inhibitors from 5 to 50%.[39-50] This "upgrade" switch occurs mostly in the catheterization laboratory during, or immediately after PCI.[9] There are myriad of reasons necessitating this switch, including patient-specific factors, presentation with STEMI, in-hospital reinfarction, and socioeconomic characteristics.[8,9] Although, these registries have documented no major safety concerns associated with switching, the fact that none of them were designed or powered for clinical outcomes dilutes the significance of these results, compelling one to view them with skepticism.[2,8,9,39-50]

Evidence from Pharmacodynamic Studies

The failure of the TRITON-TIMI 38 trial to define an optimal strategy regarding escalation from clopidogrel to prasugrel has fueled a large number of pharmacodynamic studies being conducted on this switching strategy.[8,23,51-66]

Au contraire, the paucity of pharmacodynamic studies on switching from clopidogrel to ticagrelor[64-69] is attributable, in all likelihood, to indisputable clinical evidence from the PLATO trial,[22] which abbreviates requirement of any further evidence for all intent and purpose.[9]

- *Escalation from clopidogrel to prasugrel:* The Switching Antiplatelet Therapy (SWAP) study evaluated the switch from clopidogrel to prasugrel in patients with ACS.[52] 60 mg LD of prasugrel achieved increased levels of platelet inhibition and reduced high on-treatment platelet reactivity (HPR) within 2 hours.[52,70] After 1-week, 10 mg MD of prasugrel achieved similar levels of platelet inhibition, irrespective of whether an LD was administered.[52]

The Transferring from Clopidogrel Loading Dose to Prasugrel Loading Dose in Acute Coronary Syndrome Patients (TRIPLET) trial concluded that in patients with ACS undergoing PCI, pretreatment with clopidogrel (adding a 60 mg LD of prasugrel after 600 mg LD of clopidogrel) had no additive pharmacodynamic benefit, as compared to administering 60 mg LD of prasugrel alone[57]

- *Escalation from clopidogrel to ticagrelor:* The Response to Ticagrelor in Clopidogrel Non-responders and Responders and the Effect of Switching Therapies (RESPOND) study was conducted in patients with stable CAD on aspirin therapy.[67] Ticagrelor therapy was efficacious in patients nonresponsive to clopidogrel.[67] Its antiplatelet effect was same in clopidogrel responders and nonresponders.[67]

However, given that "upgrade" switching from clopidogrel to novel P2Y12 inhibitors is mainly done in the acute setting, the main limitation of the SWAP and RESPOND trials was that both of them studied patients with stable CAD only.[52,67]

All pharmacodynamic studies on escalation from clopidogrel to ticagrelor document enhanced platelet inhibition and reduced HPR, especially after administration of an LD.[51-74] However, caution is required, while translating this evidence into practice, as clinical outcomes study data is not available currently.

Drug-drug interactions in patients previously exposed to clopidogrel (irrespective of whether they were given LDs or are on long-term maintenance therapy) are rare, while switching over to prasugrel or ticagrelor. This is because substantial numbers of P2Y12 receptors are still uninhibited in patients treated with clopidogrel, which are then subsequently blocked by LD of either prasugrel or ticagrelor.[8]

Translation of Evidence into Clinical Practice

- *Escalation during early, especially acute, phase of treatment:* Inadequate platelet inhibition may lead to ST in these patients, given high thrombotic milieu of coronary vasculature in first few weeks after an ACS or PCI.[10,11] In the acute phase, escalation from clopidogrel to prasugrel or ticagrelor should occur with 60 mg or 180 mg LD, respectively.[9] An LD is administered independent of timing of last dose of clopidogrel. Thereafter, it is reasonable to transit to long-term maintenance therapy with either prasugrel 10 mg in a once daily dosing regimen or ticagrelor 90 mg twice a day[2,9]

- *Escalation during chronic or late phase of treatment:* In chronic or late phase of treatment, an LD regimen is not required. The patient may be started on a MD regimen of 10 mg once daily prasugrel or 90 mg twice daily ticagrelor approximately 24 hours after last dose of clopidogrel.[2,8,9]

De-escalation

Stepping down from novel P2Y12 inhibitors to clopidogrel is defined as de-escalation.[9]

The prevalence of "downgrade" switching is 5–14% in in-patients. Patients at higher risk for bleeding—"elderly patients, patients having low-body weight, those with history of cerebrovascular accident, patients recuperating from CABG, those diagnosed with atrial fibrillation or flutter, or while starting oral anticoagulation"—are usually de-escalated to clopidogrel while in-hospital.[9]

Switching between P2Y12 receptor inhibitors, mostly de-escalation is done in 5–8% of patients' postdischarge.[9,39-44] De-escalation in outside hospital scenario is usually attributable to cost issues, increased risk of bleeding with prasugrel or ticagrelor or significant nonbleeding side effects such as dyspnea with ticagrelor.[22,38,75,76]

Evidence from Clinical Trials, Registries, and Pharmacodynamic Studies

Evidence from Clinical Trials and Registries

In the Timing of Optimal Platelet Inhibition After Acute Coronary Syndrome (TOPIC) study, in patients with ACS at 1-month post-PCI, switching from ticagrelor or prasugrel directly to clopidogrel was found to reduce bleeding rates with no documented increase in ischemic occurrences.[77] The caveat was that this study was inadequately powered to assess ischemic outcomes.[78]

In patients diagnosed as ACS undergoing percutaneous coronary revascularization, a "guided de-escalation strategy", comprising of prasugrel administration in acute phase, followed by de-escalation to clopidogrel in maintenance phase, was compared to the standardized protocol of long-term treatment with prasugrel in the Testing Responsiveness to Platelet Inhibition on Chronic Antiplatelet Treatment for ACS (TROPICAL-ACS) trial.[79]

At 1-year, net clinical benefit was similar in both groups with no increase in ischemic events and statistically insignificant reduction in bleeding.[79]

However, the Switching from Clopidogrel to New Oral Antiplatelet Agents During Percutaneous Coronary Intervention (SCOPE) registry results infuse a note of caution into considering an early de-escalation of P2Y12 inhibitors in patients with ACS. This switch makes them vulnerable to increase in platelet reactivity and HPR in acute phase.[50] Therefore, early de-escalation of P2Y12 inhibitors in these patients may increase risk of ischemic events without a reduction in bleeding rates.[50] However, upgrade switching from old to novel P2Y12 inhibitors led to no ischemic or bleeding risk during the entire study period and was deemed safe.[50]

Evidence from Pharmacodynamic Studies

Pharmacodynamic studies associated with de-escalation to clopidogrel therapy are few in number and show high platelet reactivity and HPR rates.[54,55,64,67,80-82]

Speed of offset of drug action has important therapeutic implications during de-escalation therapy. Important considerations are delineating the optimal time to administer clopidogrel dose and to determine whether clopidogrel should be given as an LD or just a MD of clopidogrel is adequate, especially in patients at high bleeding risk.[8,80]

In the Optimising crossover from ticagrelor to clopidogrel in patients with acute coronary syndrome (CAPITAL OPTI-CROSS) study, the "downgrade" switch to clopidogrel was made at next scheduled dose of ticagrelor.[78,80] However, based on pharmacodynamics data from the RESPOND study, clopidogrel dose may be administered up to 24 hours after last ticagrelor dose.[67]

These pharmacodynamic studies report lower bleeding events. Despite a higher number of patients with HPR, there is no report of increase in the incidence of thrombotic events.[9,54,55,64,67,80-82]

De-escalation therapy carries a risk of DDI, particularly when crossing over from ticagrelor to clopidogrel, as highlighted by the Switching Antiplatelet Therapy - 4 (SWAP - 4) study results.[8,80,83]

It is not sure whether an LD of clopidogrel would mitigate the high levels of platelet reactivity in entirety.[83]

Considering the paucity of data, potential for DDIs during de-escalation therapy related to high HPR and most importantly, the fact that all aforementioned studies were inadequately powered for clinical outcomes; the optimal strategy to de-escalate from novel P2Y12 inhibitors to clopidogrel is undefined, as of now.[2,9] Large scale studies are definitely the need of the hour to evaluate the safety and efficacy of de-escalation strategy, especially in the acute setting.

Translation of Evidence into Clinical Practice

De-escalation from Ticagrelor to Clopidogrel

Considering the rapid offset of action of ticagrelor, de-escalation should be done with a 600 mg LD of clopidogrel, regardless of timing of switching (acute, early, or late).[9] This confers a short-term 48 hours pharmacodynamic advantage and potentially obliterates the time gap in platelet inhibition.[8] However, in patients at high bleeding risk, it is reasonable to de-escalate to clopidogrel with a MD only.[8,9]

De-escalation from prasugrel to clopidogrel:

- *During early, especially acute, phase of treatment:* It may be reasonable to de-escalate with 600 mg LD of clopidogrel
- *During chronic or late phase of treatment:* In stable patients or in chronic setting, clopidogrel in a MD of 75 mg may be administered approximately 24 hours from last dose of prasugrel.[2,8,9]

Changes

"Parallel" switching between novel P2Y12 inhibitors—prasugrel and ticagrelor—are called changes.[9]

Prevalence of this switch in registries ranges from 2 to 4%.[8,39-42]

With its once daily dosing, switching over to prasugrel from ticagrelor may improve long-term patient compliance to therapy.[8] In patients at high-risk for ischemic events, ticagrelor-associated dyspnea is another important reason to switch over to prasugrel.[9] Patients with ACS pretreated with prasugrel prior to a coronary angiogram and those, who are not scheduled to undergo coronary revascularization, may be switched to ticagrelor.[39,42,44]

Evidence from Clinical Trials, Registries, and Pharmacodynamic Studies

There is scant evidence to endorse a switch between prasugrel and ticagrelor.[39-42,84,85]

- *Switch from ticagrelor to prasugrel*: In the Switching Antiplatelet Therapy [SWAP-2] study, there was a documented increase in platelet reactivity in patients crossed over to prasugrel therapy measured 12 hours after last MD of ticagrelor. In addition, at 24 hours and 48 hours, platelet reactivity increased in the prasugrel group, as compared to preswitch levels.[84] An LD of prasugrel partially offset this increased reactivity, but did not bring it down to preswitch levels.[84]

  Switching to prasugrel may be extended to approximately 24 hours after last dose of ticagrelor. This may provide extra time for P2Y12 receptor blockade to decline and thereby, limit increases in platelet reactivity[9,84]
- *Switch from prasugrel to ticagrelor*: The Switching Antiplatelet Therapy [SWAP-3] study documented that crossover from prasugrel to ticagrelor was associated with transiently higher levels of platelet inhibition, regardless of administration of LD.[85] However, no DDIs or increase in HPR rates were noted during the study.[85]

Translation of Evidence into Clinical Practice

- *Switching from ticagrelor to prasugrel*: 60 mg LD of prasugrel is preferred, regardless of timing (early or late). It is best to avoid switching with a 10 mg MD, as pharmacodynamic data suggests a potential DDI[2,8,9]
- *Switching from prasugrel to ticagrelor*: A standard 90 mg twice daily MD regimen may be used, as pharmacodynamic studies do not suggest any DDI related to this change.[9,85]

Summation of evidence from clinical trials and registries on switching between oral P2Y12 receptor inhibitors[9,39-48,77,79] is highlighted in table 3.

Recommendations on switching between oral P2Y12 inhibitors in clinical practice[2,8,9] are highlighted in table 4.

TABLE 3: Switching oral P2Y12 receptor inhibitors: Evidence from major randomized clinical trials and registries

Study Acronym	Study authors	Clinical presentation	Switching modality (prevalence)	Clinical outcomes
GRAPE	Alexopoulos et al.[39]	ACS undergoing PCI	**Escalation** C →P: 40.1% C →T: 50.3% **De-escalation** P →C: 1% T →C: 4.3% **Change** Between P and T: 4.3%	1-month outcome: Higher risk of bleeding and less MACE in patients switched from C to P or T compared with those treated with C only
MULTIPRAC	Clemmensen et al.[40]	STEMI	**Escalation** C →P: 48.7% C →T: 11.6% **De-escalation** P →C: 8.3% **Change** P →T: 2.8%	In-hospital outcomes: No differences in MACE and non-CABG related bleeding in patients switched from C to P vs. patients on P only
TRANSLATE-ACS	Bagai et al.[41]	NSTEMI, STEMI	**Escalation** C →P: 10.4% C →T: 1% **De-escalation** P →C: 11.5% T →C: 2.1% **Change** Between P and T: P →T: 0.3% T →P: 3.4%	6-month outcome: No significant differences in MACE and bleeding in between groups

Continued

Continued

Study Acronym	Study authors	Clinical presentation	Switching modality (prevalence)	Clinical outcomes
FAST-MI	Schiele et al.[42]	NSTEMI, STEMI	**Escalation** C →P: 16.5% **De-escalation** P →C: 4.6%	N/A
EYESHOT	De Luca et al.[43]	NSTE-ACS, STEMI	**Escalation** Cath-lab switch: C →P/T: 3% At discharge switch: C →P/T: 9.6% Switch in medically managed patients: C →P/T: 2% **De-escalation** In cath-lab switch: P/T →C: 0.3% At discharge switch: P/T →C: 3.2% Switch in medically managed patients: P/T→C: 3.4% **Change** Cath-lab switch: C →P/T: 3% At discharge switch: C →P/T: 9.6%	N/A
ACTION Registry GWTG and Cath PCI	Bagai et al.[44]	NSTEMI and STEMI undergoing PCI	**Escalation** C →P: 5.2% C →T: n/a **De-escalation** P →C: 11.5%	N/A
–	De Luca et al.[45]	STEMI, UA undergoing PCI	150 patients switched from C to P matched with 300 C only treated patients	30 days outcome: No differences in MACE, NACE and bleeding between groups.
–	Loh et al.[46]	ACS undergoing PCI	**Escalation** C →P: 14.8%	In-hospital outcomes: Mace greater, but no differences in bleeding between patients switched to P compared to those on P only
–	Almendro-Delia et al.[47]	ACS	**Escalation** C →P: 25% **Change** P →T: 0.3%	In-hospital outcomes: No difference in bleeding and MACE between patients who switched to P compared with those on C only
TRANSLATE-ACS	Zettler et al.[48]	NSTEMI, STEMI	**Escalation** C → P: 91.7% C →T: 8.3% **De-escalation** P →C: 97.4% T →C: 87.5% **Change** Between P and T: P →T: 2.6% T →P: 12.5%	In the 7 days preceding the switch from clopidogrel, 18.5% had a MACE and 5.6% had a definite stent thrombosis event. GUSTO moderate or severe bleeding event occurred in 0.3% in those switched from P; postdischarge switching was uncommonly associated with MACEs or bleeding events

Continued

Continued

Study Acronym	Study authors	Clinical presentation	Switching modality (prevalence)	Clinical outcomes
TRANSLATE-ACS	Bagai et al.[49]	NSTEMI,STEMI undergoing PCI with HPR on clopidogrel	**Escalation** C →P: 30.7% (HPR) C →P: 4.4% (w/o HPR)	1-year outcomes: ADP receptor switching not significant associated with increased hazard of MACE/ bleeding
SPACE	De Luca et al.[50]	ACS undergoing PCI	**Escalation** In cath-lab switch: C →P: 2.1% C →T: 0.2% At discharge switch: C →P: 0.4% C →T: 0.6% After discharge switch: C→P: 0.3% C→T: 0.3% From admission to follow-up switch: C →P: 1.2% C →T: 1.4% **De-escalation** At discharge switch: P →C: 0.8% T →C: 1% After discharge switch: P →C: 0.7% T →C: 0.8% From admission to follow-up switch: P →C: 1.3% T→C: 1.8% **Change** At discharge switch: P →T: 0.3% T →P: 0.2% After discharge switch: P→T: 1.6% T →P: 1.4% From admission to follow-up switch: P →T: 1.9% T →P: 1.6%	Cumulative incidence of MACE—1.6% and NACE—5.6% Patients receiving an upgrade switching: No ischemic or bleeding events during study period Patients with downgrade switching: Independent predictor of NACE
TOPIC	Cuisset et al.[77]	–	**De-escalation** P/T →C: 50%	Outcomes at 1 year: Net clinical benefit: 13.4% in patients who switched, 26.3% in patients who did not switch
TROPICAL-ACS	Sibbing et al.[79]	Biomarker positive ACS with a successful PCI	**Escalation** C →P: 39% **De-escalation** P →C: 50%	Outcomes at 1-year: Net clinical benefit: 7% in patients who switched (guided de-escalation group), 9% in patients who did not switch (control group, 12 months on P)

ACS, acute coronary syndrome; ADP, adenosine diphosphate; CABG, coronary artery bypass grafting; MACE, major adverse cardiovascular events; NACE, net adverse clinical event; NSTEMI, non-ST elevation myocardial infarction; PCI, percutaneous coronary intervention; STEMI, ST elevation myocardial infarction; UA, unstable angina.

TABLE 4: Recommendations on switching between oral P2Y12 inhibitors

P2Y12 inhibitor stopped	P2Y12 inhibitor started	Recommendation
	Acute or early phase	
Escalation:		
Clopidogrel	Prasugrel	• 60 mg LD, irrespective of last clopidogrel dose • Start MD ~24 h after last clopidogrel dose
Clopidogrel	Ticagrelor	• 180 mg LD, irrespective of last clopidogrel dose • Start MD ~24 h after last clopidogrel dose
De-escalation:		
Prasugrel	Clopidogrel	600 mg LD 24 h after last prasugrel dose
Ticagrelor	Clopidogrel	600 mg LD 24 h after last ticagrelor dose
Change:		
Prasugrel	Ticagrelor	180 mg LD 24 h after last prasugrel dose
Ticagrelor	Prasugrel	60 mg LD 24 h after last ticagrelor dose
	Late or very late phase	
Escalation:		
Clopidogrel	Prasugrel	10 mg MD 24 h after last clopidogrel dose
Clopidogrel	Ticagrelor	• 90 mg twice daily • Start MD 24 h after last clopidogrel dose
De-escalation:		
Prasugrel	Clopidogrel	75 mg MD 24 h after last prasugrel dose
Ticagrelor	Clopidogrel	600 mg LD, 75 mg MD 24 h after last ticagrelor dose
Change:		
Prasugrel	Ticagrelor	90 mg MD 24 h after last prasugrel dose
Ticagrelor	Prasugrel	60 mg LD 24 h after last ticagrelor dose

LD, loading dose; MD, maintenance dose.

SWITCHING BETWEEN ORAL AND INTRAVENOUS P2Y12 INHIBITORS

Bridging

Switching from an oral P2Y12 inhibitor to cangrelor is termed as bridging.[9]

Patients scheduled for surgical procedures require discontinuation of oral P2Y12 inhibitor therapy to mitigate their bleeding risk and should be "bridged" over to cangrelor.[2,8,9]

Evidence from Clinical Trials, Registries, and Pharmacodynamic Studies

The Bridging Antiplatelet Therapy with Cangrelor in Patients Undergoing Cardiac Surgery (BRIDGE) trial[86] and various *in vitro* and *ex vivo* investigations[87-92] highlighted that cangrelor resulted in high levels of platelet inhibition and no DDI in patients discontinuing thienopyridine therapy before cardiac surgery.[86-92] The reason for no DDI is probably that patients on oral P2Y12 inhibitors have unbound receptors that are occupied and inhibited by cangrelor.[9]

However, there is extremely scarce data to endorse safety and efficacy of cangrelor as a bridging modality in real-world clinical practice.[9,93]

Translation of Evidence into Clinical Practice

Effects of oral P2Y12 inhibitors persist with significant levels of P2Y12 inhibition after drug discontinuation.[93] Therefore, bridging with cangrelor should be initiated according to timing of discontinuation of the specific drug: earlier in patients on clopidogrel or ticagrelor (2–3 days) and later in patients on prasugrel (3–4 days).[9]

Transition

When a switch occurs from IV cangrelor to oral P2Y12 inhibitors, mostly after PCI, it is termed as transition.[9]

Evidence from Clinical Trials, Registries, and Pharmacodynamic Studies

In the Cangrelor versus Standard Therapy to Achieve Optimal Management of Platelet Inhibition (CHAMPION-PHOENIX) trial, cangrelor infusion during PCI led to a significant decrease in ischemic events, including ST, with no increase in severe bleeding.[94]

However, in absence of any clinical outcomes study, single-center observational data[95,96] are grossly inadequate to prove either safety or efficacy of this novel IV P2Y12 inhibitor in patients, subsequently transited to oral P2Y12 receptor inhibitors.

A multitude of pharmacodynamic studies have investigated the potential for DDI during concomitant administration of these drugs.[86-91,97-99] These DDIs are a potential nightmare for interventional cardiologists as reduced platelet inhibition may lead to thrombotic events in the peri-PCI period.

- *Transition from cangrelor to clopidogrel*: Administration of clopidogrel during cangrelor infusion was associated with a diminished antiplatelet effect, as active metabolites of thienopyridines are unable to bind to P2Y12 receptors, as the latter are still blocked by cangrelor.[99,100]

By the time receptors become free for binding by thienopyridines after stopping cangrelor infusion, majority of active metabolites are eliminated from the system, thus compromising maintenance of platelet inhibition levels.[9,100]

However, when clopidogrel is administered after cangrelor infusion, its antiplatelet effect is retained as cangrelor has a rapid offset of action and subsequently, P2Y12 receptor site become free to bind to active metabolite of clopidogrel[8,9,90,91,97]

- *Transition from cangrelor to prasugrel*: As already discussed, prasugrel has a higher concentration and longer half-life, as compared to that of clopidogrel.[14] Therefore, an LD of prasugrel given at time of initiation of cangrelor infusion led to a faster and stronger platelet inhibition in stable patients undergoing an elective PCI in the Impact of Extent of Clopidogrel-Induced Platelet Inhibition During Elective Stent Implantation on Clinical Event Rate-Advanced Loading Strategies (ExcelsiorLOAD2)[101]
- *Transition from cangrelor to ticagrelor*: In contradiction to thienopyridines, no interaction was observed for transition from cangrelor to ticagrelor. This is probably attributable to its unique pharmacodynamic properties—it is direct acting, binds the P2Y12 receptor at a distinct site, and has a half-life of 6–12 hours. The latter is of utmost clinical significance as it implies that postdiscontinuation of cangrelor infusion, it is still systemically present to bind with P2Y12 receptors.[9,89] Therefore, ticagrelor can be administered prior to initiation of, during, or after discontinuation of, cangrelor infusion without any DDIs.

Translation of Evidence into Clinical Practice

- *After noncardiac surgery:* Clopidogrel in LD should be resumed after noncardiac surgery as soon as possible. It is not advisable to administer potent P2Y12 inhibitors—prasugrel or ticagrelor—after major noncardiac surgery, considering their potency may heighten the risk of serious bleeding in these patients[2,8,9]
- *At time of PCI:*[8,9] In patients on cangrelor infusion during PCI, timing of transition to oral P2Y12 inhibitors is drug-specific.
  - *Cangrelor to clopidogrel:* Loading dose of 600 mg of clopidogrel may be given at time of stopping cangrelor infusion
  - *Cangrelor to prasugrel:* Loading dose of 60 mg of prasugrel may be given either at time of discontinuing cangrelor infusion or up to 30 minutes before end of infusion
  - *Cangrelor to ticagrelor:* Ticagrelor can be administered at any time prior to, during or at end of cangrelor infusion.

Summation of evidence from pharmacodynamic studies on switching between IV or oral P2Y12 receptor inhibitors[9,51-57,59-69,80-82,86,89,90,91,97,98,101] is highlighted in table 5.

TABLE 5: Switching Oral or intravenous P2Y12 receptor inhibitors: evidence from pharmacodynamic studies

Study acronym	Authors	Clinical presentation	Switching modality	Clinical outcomes
–	Rollini et al.[51]	CAD	Escalation: C → P	Outcomes at 1 week: Two minor bleeding
SWAP	Angiolillo et al.[52]	Prior ACS	Escalation: C → P	Outcomes at 15 days: Bleeding by TIMI criteria was reported in 12.5% of the C 75 mg MD group, 8.5% of the P 10 mg MD group, and 13.6% of the P LD + MD group
–	Payne et al.[53]	Healthy subjects	Escalation: C → P	Outcomes at 22 days: No differences in bleeding episodes or other adverse events
PRINCIPLE-TIMI44	Wiviott et al.[54]	Planned PCI	Escalation: C → P	Outcomes at 29 days: Bleeding occurred in four subjects switching from C to P
			De-escalation: P → C	Outcomes at 29 days: No bleeding events in subject switching from P to C
ACAPULCO	Montalescot et al.[55]	UA/NSTEMI	Escalation: C → P De-escalation: P → C	Outcomes at 60 days: There were no differences in any non-CABG-related TIMI major or GUSTO severe/life-threatening bleeding events
TRIGGER-PCI	Trenk et al.[56]	Stable CAD with HPR undergoing PCI	Escalation: C → P	Outcomes at 6 months: TIMI major non-coronary artery bypass graft bleeding occurred in three patients on P and one patient on C
TRIPLET	Diodati et al.[57]	ACS undergoing planned PCI	Escalation: C → P	Outcomes at 72 hours: Treatment-emergent adverse events were three in the placebo LD/P 60 mg group; four in the C 600 mg LD/P 60 mg LD group; and seven in the C 600 mg LD/P 30 mg
			Escalation: C → T	Outcomes at 1 week: One minor bleeding, 26 patients with dyspnea
–	Nührenberg et al.[59]	STEMI undergoing PCI	Escalation: C → P	N/A

Continued

Continued

Study acronym	Authors	Clinical presentation	Switching modality	Clinical outcomes
–	Parodi et al.[60]	CAD undergoing PCI	Escalation: C → P	Outcomes in hospital and at 6 months: There were no differences in major or minor TIMI bleeding rates or in BARC bleeding rates or ischemic events between the patients switching and naïve
–	Aradi et al.[61]	ACS undergoing PCI	Escalation: C → P	Outcomes at 1 year: Rates of thrombotic complications in HPR group were similar to those in the no HPR group without any difference in MACE. No excess of major bleeding after switching to P in HPR group compared to those without HPR
–	Mayer et al.[62]	ACS with HPR undergoing PCI	Escalation: C → P	Outcomes at 30 days: 1.7% combined death/stent thrombosis and 8.7% TIMI major bleeding
–	Lhermusier et al.[63]	ACS with planned invasive strategy	Escalation: C → P	Outcomes at discharge: No differences in bleeding between groups
–	Lhermusier et al.[64]	ACS	Escalation: C → P	N/A
			Escalation : C → T	Outcomes at 24 hours: One bleeding event following switch to T 90 mg
–	Alexopoulos et al.[65]	ACS with HPR	Escalation: C → P	Outcomes at 30 days: No patient exhibited a major adverse cardiovascular event or a major bleeding event
			Escalation: C → T	Outcomes at 30 days: No major adverse cardiovascular event or a major bleeding event
–	Koul et al.[66]	STEMI undergoing PCI	Escalation: C → P	Outcomes in-hospital: 1.1% major bleeding
			Escalation: C → T	Outcomes in-hospital: 3.3 % major bleeding
RESPOND	Gurbel et al.[67]	Stable CAD	Escalation: C → T	Outcomes at 30 days: Four patients (two nonresponders and two responders) experienced the five serious adverse events, and all events occurred during or after T therapy. One major and three minor bleeding events occurred during T treatment, and no bleeding events occurred during C treatment
SHIFT-OVER	Caiazzo et al.[68]	ACS	Escalation: C → T	Outcomes at 30 days: No deaths nor strokes were reported after switch
CAPITAL RELOAD	Hibbert et al.[69]	STEMI	Escalation: C → T	N/A
CAPITAL OPTI-CROSS	Pourdjabbar et al.[80]	ACS	De-escalation: T → C	Outcomes at 30 days: No differences in MACE, TIMI major bleeding or stent thrombosis between groups
–	Kerneis et al.[81]	ACS	De-escalation: P → C	Outcomes at 30 days: No major bleedings
POBA	Deharo et al.[82]	ACS with LPR	De-escalation : P → C	Outcomes at 30 days: No bleeding events after switching to C
–	Angiolillo et al.[86]	ACS	Thienopyridine → Cangrelor	Study-defined excessive CABG—surgery-related bleeding not significantly different between Cang (11.8%) or placebo (10.4%). Ischemic end points prior to surgery were low: 2.8% with Cang, 4.0% with placebo
–	Schneider et al.[89]	Stable CAD	Cangrelor → Ticagrelor	No adverse events during study duration

Continued

Continued

Study acronym	Authors	Clinical presentation	Switching modality	Clinical outcomes
–	Schneider et al.[90]	Stable CAD	Cangrelor → Prasugrel	No adverse events during study duration
–	Schneider et al.[91]	Stable CAD	Cangrelor → Clopidogrel	N/A
Predefined substudy of CHAMPION-PCI and CHAMPION-PLATFORM randomized trials	Angiolillo et al.[97]	CAD undergoing PCI	Cangrelor → Clopidogrel	Not Reported
–	Steinhubl et al.[98]	Healthy subjects	Cangrelor → Clopidogrel	N/A
ExcelsiorLOAD2 Trial	Hochholzer et al.[101]	CAD without MI	Cangrelor → Oral P2Y12 Inhibitors	The incidence of 30-day ischemic and bleeding events similar between groups

CAD, coronary artery disease; ACS, acute coronary syndromes; PCI, percutaneous coronary intervention; TIMI, thrombolysis in myocardial infarction; MD, maintenance dose; LD, loading dose;CABG, coronary artery bypass surgery; NTEMI, non—ST-segment elevation myocardial infarction; STEMI, ST-segment elevation myocardial infarction; UA, unstable angina; HPR, high on-treatment platelet reactivity; MI, myocardial infarction; N/A, not applicable.

TABLE 6: Recommendations on bridging or transitioning between intravenous and oral P2Y12 inhibitors

Bridging: From oral to IV P2Y12 inhibitor			
Oral P2Y12 inhibitor	**IV P2Y12 inhibitor**	**Days to withhold P2Y12 inhibitor prior to procedure**	**Recommendation**
Clopidogrel	Cangrelor	5	Initiate cangrelor 0.75 mcg/kg/min without bolus 2–3 days after stopping clopidogrel
Prasugrel	Cangrelor	7	Initiate cangrelor 0.75 mcg/kg/min without bolus 3–4 days after stopping prasugrel
Ticagrelor	Cangrelor	5	Initiate cangrelor 0.75 mcg/kg/min without bolus 2–3 days after stopping ticagrelor
Transitioning: From IV to oral P2Y12 inhibitor			
IV P2Y12 inhibitor	**Oral P2Y12 inhibitor**	**Days to withhold P2Y12 inhibitor prior to procedure**	**Recommendation**
Cangrelor	Clopidogrel	N/A	600 mg LD to be given immediately after cangrelor infusion is discontinued
Cangrelor	Prasugrel	N/A	60 mg LD to be given immediately after cangrelor infusion is discontinued
Cangrelor	Ticagrelor	N/A	180 mg LD to be given at start of cangrelor infusion (ideal) or up to infusion discontinuation

LD, loading dose; N/A, not applicable; IV, intravenous.

Recommendations on switching between IV and oral P2Y12 inhibitors in clinical practice[2,8,9] are provided in table 6.

PLATELET FUNCTION TESTING AND SWITCHING OF P2Y12 INHIBITORS

In patients on P2Y12 receptor antagonists, high and low platelet reactivity is a strong indicator of ischemic and bleeding risk, respectively.[2,11] Therefore, scientifically speaking, individualized antiplatelet therapy based on platelet function monitoring should be advocated to adjust or switch antiplatelet therapy.[2,102] However, randomized trials demonstrate no significant clinical impact of using platelet function tests to either modify or switch therapy.[56,103-106]

THE WAY FORWARD: WHAT IS THE RIGHT STRATEGY TO SWITCH DAPT?

Switching between DAPT agents remains a clinical conundrum. As current recommendations are derived largely from pharmacodynamic studies and registry data, dedicated prospective studies are needed to provide important insights into optimal and clinically safe switching strategies.

Until new clinical or pharmacokinetic/pharmacodynamics data become available, one has no option, but to adhere to current evidence. However, as practicing physicians, it is imperative that one tailors switching of DAPT, if required, on an individualized basis; keeping in view pharmacological properties of P2Y12 inhibitor therapies and timing of disease presentation (acute or chronic).

REFERENCES

1. Levine GN, Bates ER, Blankenship JC, et al. 2011 ACCF/AHA/SCAI guideline for percutaneous coronary intervention: a report of the American College of Cardiology Foundation/American Heart Association Task Force on Practice Guidelines and the Society for Cardiovascular Angiography and Interventions. Circulation. 2011;124:e574-651.
2. Valgimigli M, Bueno H, Byrne RA, et al. 2017 ESC focused update on dual antiplatelet therapy in coronary artery disease developed in collaboration with EACTS: the Task Force for dual antiplatelet therapy in coronary artery disease of the European Society of Cardiology (ESC) and of the European Association for Cardio-Thoracic Surgery (EACTS). Eur Heart J. 2017;39(3):213-60.
3. O'Gara PT, Kushner FG, Ascheim DD, et al. 2013 ACCF/AHA guideline for the management of ST-elevation myocardial infarction: a report of the American College of Cardiology Foundation/American Heart Association Task Force on Practice Guidelines. Circulation. 2013;127(4):e362-425.
4. Amsterdam EA, Wenger NK, Brindis RG, et al. 2014 AHA/ACC guideline for the management of patients with non-ST- elevation acute coronary syndromes: a report of the American College of Cardiology/American Heart Association Task Force on Practice Guidelines. J Am Coll Cardiol. 2014;64(24):e139-228.
5. Windecker S, Kolh P, Alfonso F, et al. 2014 ESC/EACTS guidelines on myocardial revascularization: the Task Force on Myocardial Revascularization of the European Society of Cardiology (ESC) and the European Association for Cardio-Thoracic Surgery (EACTS). Developed with the special contribution of the European Association of Percutaneous Cardiovascular Interventions (EAPCI). Eur Heart J. 2014;35:2541-619.
6. Schomig A, Neumann FJ, Kastrati A, et al.A randomized comparison of antiplatelet and anticoagulant therapy after the placement of coronary artery stents. N Engl J Med. 1996;334:1084-9.
7. Valgimigli M, Costa F, Byrne R, et al. Dual antiplatelet therapy duration after coronary stenting in clinical practice: results of an EAPCI survey. Euro Intervention. 2015;11:68-74.
8. Rollini F, Franchi F, Angiolillo DJ. Switching P2Y12-receptor inhibitors in patients with coronary artery disease. Nat Rev Cardiol. 2016;13:11-27.
9. Angiolillo DJ, Rollini F, Storey RF, et al. International expert consensus on switching platelet $P2Y_{12}$ receptor-inhibiting therapies. Circulation. 2017;136(20):1955-75.
10. Tantry US, Bonello L, Aradi D, et al; Working Group on On-Treatment Platelet Reactivity. Consensus and update on the definition of on-treatment platelet reactivity to adenosine diphosphate associated with ischemia and bleeding. J Am Coll Cardiol. 2013;62:2261-73.
11. Aradi D, Kirtane A, Bonello L, et al. Bleeding and stent thrombosis on P2Y12-inhibitors: collaborative analysis on the role of platelet reactivity for risk stratification after percutaneous coronary intervention. Eur Heart J. 2015;36:1762-71.
12. Angiolillo DJ. The evolution of antiplatelet therapy in the treatment of acute coronary syndromes: from aspirin to the present day. Drugs. 2012;72:2087-116.
13. Sherwood MW, Wiviott SD, Peng SA, et al. Early clopidogrel versus prasugrel use among contemporary STEMI and NSTEMI patients in the US: insights from the National Cardiovascular Data Registry. J Am Heart Assoc. 2014;3:e000849.
14. Farid NA, Kurihara A, Wrighton SA. Metabolism and disposition of the thienopyridine antiplatelet drugs ticlopidine, clopidogrel, and prasugrel in humans. J Clin Pharmacol. 2010;50:126-42.
15. Campo G, Valgimigli M, Gemmati D, et al. Poor responsiveness to clopidogrel: drug-specific or class-effect mechanism? Evidence from a clopidogrel-to-ticlopidine crossover study. J Am Coll Cardiol. 2007;50:1132-7.
16. Sabatine MS, Cannon CP, Gibson CM, et al. CLARITY-TIMI 28 Investigators. Addition of clopidogrel to aspirin and fibrinolytic therapy for myocardial infarction with ST-segment elevation. N Engl J Med. 2005;352:1179-89.
17. Chen ZM, Jiang LX, Chen YP, et al. Addition of clopidogrel to aspirin in 45,852 patients with acute myocardial infarction: randomised placebo-controlled trial. Lancet. 2005;366:1607-21.
18. Bernlochner I, Morath T, Brown PB, et al. A prospective randomized trial comparing the recovery of platelet function after loading dose administration of prasugrel or clopidogrel. Platelets. 2013;24:15-25.
19. Price MJ, Walder JS, Baker BA, et al. Recovery of platelet function after discontinuation of prasugrel or clopidogrel maintenance dosing in aspirin-treated patients with stable coronary disease: the recovery trial. J Am Coll Cardiol. 2012;59:2338-43.
20. Husted S, vanGiezen JJ. Ticagrelor: the first reversibly binding oral P2Y12 receptor antagonist. Cardiovasc Ther. 2009;27:259-74.
21. Gurbel PA, Bliden KP, Butler K, et al. Randomized double-blind assessment of the ONSET and OFFSET of the antiplatelet effects of ticagrelor versus clopidogrel in patients with stable coronary artery disease: the ONSET/OFFSET study. Circulation. 2009;120:2577-85.
22. Wallentin L, Becker RC, Budaj A, et al; PLATO Investigators. Ticagrelor versus clopidogrel in patients with acute coronary syndromes. N Engl J Med. 2009;361:1045-57.
23. Wiviott SD, Braunwald E, McCabe CH, et al; TRITON-TIMI 38 Investigators. Prasugrel versus clopidogrel in patients with acute coronary syndromes. N Engl J Med. 2007;357:2001-15.
24. Franchi F, Angiolillo DJ. Novel antiplatelet agents in acute coronary syndrome. Nat Rev Cardiol. 2015;12:30-47.
25. Franchi F, Rollini F, Muñiz-Lozano A, et al. Cangrelor: a review on pharmacology and clinical trial development. Expert Rev Cardiovasc Ther. 2013;11:1279-91.
26. Antithrombotic Trialists' Collaboration. Collaborative meta-analysis of randomised trials of antiplatelet therapy for prevention of death, myocardial infarction, and stroke in high-risk patients. BMJ. 2002;324(7329):71-86.
27. Peters RJ, Mehta SR, Fox KA, et al. Effects of aspirin dose when used alone or in combination with clopidogrel in patients with acute coronary syndromes: observations from the Clopidogrel in Unstable angina to prevent Recurrent Events (CURE) study. Circulation. 2003;108:1682-7.
28. Serebruany VL, Steinhubl SR, Berger PB, et al. Analysis of risk of bleeding complications after different doses of aspirin in 192,036 patients enrolled in 31 randomized controlled trials. Am J Cardiol. 2005;95:1218-22.
29. Jolly SS, Pogue J, Haladyn K, et al. Effects of aspirin dose on ischaemic events and bleeding after percutaneous coronary intervention: insights from the PCI-CURE study. Eur Heart J. 2009;30:900-7.
30. Xian Y, Wang TY, McCoy LA, et al. Association of discharge aspirin dose with outcomes after acute myocardial infarction: insights from the Treatment with ADP Receptor Inhibitors: Longitudinal Assessment of Treatment Patterns and Events after Acute Coronary Syndrome (TRANSLATE-ACS) Study. Circulation. 2015;132:174-81.
31. Steinhubl SR, Bhatt DL, Brennan DM, et al; CHARISMA Investigators. Aspirin to prevent cardiovascular disease: the association of aspirin dose and clopidogrel with thrombosis and bleeding. Ann Intern Med. 2009;150:379-86.
32. Mehta SR, Tanguay JF, Eikelboom JW, et al. Double-dose versus standard-dose clopidogrel and high-dose versus low-dose aspirin in individuals undergoing percutaneous coronary intervention for acute coronary syndromes (CURRENT-OASIS 7): a randomised factorial trial. Lancet. 2010;376:1233-43.
33. Mahaffey KW, Wojdyla DM, Carroll K, et al. Ticagrelor compared with clopidogrel by geographic region in the Platelet Inhibition and Patient outcomes trial. Circulation. 2011;124:544-54.
34. Cutlip DE, Windecker S, Mehran R, et al. Clinical end points in coronary stent trials: a case for standardized definitions. Circulation. 2007;115(17):2344-51.
35. Montalescot G, Bolognese L, Dudek D, et al; ACCOAST Investigators. Pre-treatment with prasugrel in non-ST-segment elevation acute coronary syndromes. N Engl J Med. 2013;369:999-1010.
36. Roe MT, Armstrong PW, Fox KA, et al; TRILOGY ACS Investigators. Prasugrel versus clopidogrel for acute coronary syndromes without revascularization. N Engl J Med. 2012;367:1297-309.
37. Montalescot G, van 't Hof AW, Lapostolle F, et al.; ATLANTIC Investigators. Prehospital ticagrelor in ST-segment elevation myocardial infarction. N Engl J Med. 2014;371:1016-27.
38. Bonaca MP, Bhatt DL, Cohen M, et al.; PEGASUS-TIMI54 Steering Committee and Investigators. Long-term use of ticagrelor inpatients with prior myocardial infarction. N Engl J Med. 2015;372:1791-800.
39. Alexopoulos D, Xanthopoulou I, Deftereos S, et al. In-hospital switching of oral P2Y12 inhibitor treatment in patients with acute coronary syndrome undergoing percutaneous coronary intervention: prevalence, predictors and short-term outcome. Am Heart J. 2014;167:68-76.e2.
40. Clemmensen P, Grieco N, Ince H, et al.; MULTIPRAC study investigators. MULTInational non-interventional study of patients with ST-segment elevation myocardial infarction treated with PRimary Angioplasty and Concomitant use of upstream antiplatelet therapy with prasugrel or clopidogrel: the European MULTIPRAC Registry. Eur Heart J Acute Cardiovasc Care. 2015;4:220-9.

41. Bagai A, Peterson ED, Honeycutt E, et al. In-hospital switching between adenosine diphosphate receptor inhibitors in patients with acute myocardial infarction treated with percutaneous coronary intervention: insights into contemporary practice from the TRANSLATE-ACS study. Eur Heart J Acute Cardiovasc Care. 2015;4: 499-508.
42. Schiele F, Puymirat E, Bonello L, et al. Switching between thienopyridines in patients with acute myocardial infarction and quality of care. Open Heart. 2016;3:e000384.
43. De Luca L, Leonardi S, Cavallini C, et al.; EYE- SHOT Investigators. Contemporary antithrombotic strategies in patients with acute coronary syndrome admitted to cardiac care units in Italy: the EYESHOT study. Eur Heart J Acute Cardiovasc Care. 2015;4:441-52.
44. Bagai A, Wang Y, Wang TY, et al. In-hospital switching between clopidogrel and prasugrel among patients with acute myocardial infarction treated with percutaneous coronary intervention: insights into contemporary practice from the National Cardiovascular Data Registry. Circ Cardiovasc Interv. 2014;7:585-93.
45. De Luca G, Verdoia M, Schaffer A, et al. Switching from high-dose clopidogrel to prasugrel in ACS patients undergoing PCI: a single-center experience. J Thromb Thrombolysis. 2014;38:388-94.
46. Loh JP, Pendyala LK, Kitabata H, et al. Safety of reloading prasugrel in addition to clopidogrel loading in patients with acute coronary syndrome undergoing percutaneous coronary intervention. Am J Cardiol. 2013;111:841-5.
47. Almendro-Delia M, Blanco Ponce E, Gomez-Domínguez R, et al. Safety and efficacy of in-hospital clopidogrel-to-prasugrel switching in patients with acute coronary syndrome: an analysis from the "real world." J Thromb Thrombolysis. 2015;39:499-507.
48. Zettler ME, Peterson ED, McCoy LA, et al.; TRANSLATE-ACS Investigators. Switching of adenosine diphosphate receptor inhibitor after hospital discharge among myocardial infarction patients: insights from the Treatment with Adenosine Diphosphate Receptor Inhibitors: Longitudinal Assessment of Treatment Patterns and Events after Acute Coronary Syndrome (TRANSLATE-ACS) observational study. Am Heart J. 2017;183:62-8.
49. Bagai A, Peterson ED, McCoy LA, et al. Association of measured platelet reactivity with changes in P2Y12 receptor inhibitor therapy and outcomes after myocardial infarction: Insights into routine clinical practice from the TReatment with ADP receptor iNhibitorS: Longitudinal Assessment of Treatment Patterns and Events after Acute Coronary Syndrome (TRANSLATE-ACS) study. Am Heart J. 2017;187:19-28.
50. De Luca L, D'Ascenzo F, Musumeci G, et al. Incidence and outcome of switching of oral platelet P2Y12 receptor inhibitors in patients with acute coronary syndromes undergoing percutaneous coronary intervention: the SCOPE registry. Euro Intervention. 2017;13:459-66.
51. Rollini F, Franchi F, Cho JR, et al. A head-to-head pharmacodynamic comparison of prasugrel vs. ticagrelor after switching from clopidogrel in patients with coronary artery disease: results of a prospective randomized study. Eur Heart J. 2016;37:2722-30.
52. Angiolillo DJ, Saucedo JF, Deraad R, et al.; SWAP Investigators. Increased platelet inhibition after switching from maintenance clopidogrel to prasugrel in patients with acute coronary syndromes: results of the SWAP (SWitching Anti Platelet) study. J Am Coll Cardiol. 2010;56:1017-23.
53. Payne CD, Li YG, Brandt JT, et al. Switching directly to prasugrel from clopidogrel results in greater inhibition of platelet aggregation in aspirin-treated subjects. Platelets. 2008;19:275-81.
54. Wiviott SD, Trenk D, Frelinger AL, et al.; PRINCIPLE TIMI 44 Investigators. Prasugrel compared with high loading- and maintenance-dose clopidogrel in patients with planned percutaneous coronary intervention: the Prasugrel in Comparison to Clopidogrel for Inhibition of Platelet Activation and Aggregation-Thrombolysis in Myocardial Infarction 44 trial. Circulation. 2007;116:2923-32.
55. Montalescot G, Sideris G, Cohen R, et al. Prasugrel compared with high-dose clopidogrel in acute coronary syndrome: the randomised, double-blind ACAPULCO study. Thromb Haemost. 2010;103:213-23.
56. Trenk D, Stone GW, Gawaz M, et al. A randomized trial of prasugrel versus clopidogrel in patients with high platelet reactivity on clopidogrel after elective percutaneous coronary intervention with implantation of drug eluting stents: results of the TRIGGER-PCI (Testing Platelet Reactivity In Patients Undergoing Elective Stent Placement on Clopidogrel to Guide Alternative Therapy With Prasugrel) study. J Am Coll Cardiol. 2012;59:2159-64.
57. Diodati JG, Saucedo JF, French JK, et al. Effect on platelet reactivity from a prasugrel loading dose after a clopidogrel loading dose compared with a prasugrel loading dose alone: Transferring From Clopidogrel Loading Dose to Prasugrel Loading Dose in Acute Coronary Syndrome Patients (TRIPLET): a randomized controlled trial. Circ Cardiovasc Interv. 2013;6:567-74.
58. Cuisset T, Gaborit B, Dubois N, et al. Platelet reactivity in diabetic patients undergoing coronary stenting for acute coronary syndrome treated with clopidogrel loading dose followed by prasugrel maintenance therapy. Int J Cardiol. 2013;168:523-8.
59. Nührenberg TG, Trenk D, Leggewie S, et al. Clopidogrel pre-treatment of patients with ST-elevation myocardial infarction does not affect platelet reactivity after subsequent prasugrel-loading: platelet reactivity in an observational study. Platelets. 2013;24:549-53.
60. Parodi G, De Luca G, Bellandi B, et al. Switching from clopidogrel to prasugrel in patients having coronary stent implantation. J Thromb Thrombolysis. 2014;38:395–401.
61. Aradi D, Tornyos A, Pintér T, et al. Optimizing P2Y12 receptor inhibition in patients with acute coronary syndrome on the basis of platelet function testing: impact of prasugrel and high-dose clopidogrel. J Am Coll Cardiol. 2014;63:1061-70.
62. Mayer K, Schulz S, Bernlochner I, et al. A comparative cohort study on personalised antiplatelet therapy in PCI-treated patients with high on-clopidogrel platelet reactivity: results of the ISAR-HPR registry. Thromb Haemost. 2014;112:342-51.
63. Lhermusier T, Lipinski MJ, Drenning D, et al. Switching patients from clopidogrel to prasugrel in acute coronary syndrome: impact of the clopidogrel loading dose on platelet reactivity. J Interv Cardiol. 2014;27:365-72.
64. Lhermusier T, Voisin S, Murat G, et al. Switching patients from clopidogrel to novel P2Y12 receptor inhibitors in acute coronary syndrome: comparative effects of prasugrel and ticagrelor on platelet reactivity. Int J Cardiol. 2014;174:874-6.
65. Alexopoulos D, Galati A, Xanthopoulou I, et al. Ticagrelor versus prasugrel in acute coronary syndrome patients with high on-clopidogrel platelet reactivity following percutaneous coronary intervention: a pharmacodynamic study. J Am Coll Cardiol. 2012;60:193-9.
66. Koul S, Andell P, Martinsson A, et al. A pharmacodynamic comparison of 5 anti-platelet protocols in patients with ST-elevation myocardial infarction undergoing primary PCI. BMC Cardiovasc Disord. 2014;14:189.
67. Gurbel PA, Bliden KP, Butler K, et al. Response to ticagrelor in clopidogrel non-responders and responders and effect of switching therapies: the RESPOND study. Circulation. 2010;121:1188-99.
68. Caiazzo G, De Rosa S, Torella D, et al. Administration of a loading dose has no additive effect on platelet aggregation during the switch from ongoing clopidogrel treatment to ticagrelor in patients with acute coronary syndrome. Circ Cardiovasc Interv. 2014;7:104-12.
69. Hibbert B, Maze R, Pourdjabbar A, et al. A comparative pharmacodynamic study of ticagrelor versus clopidogrel and ticagrelor in patients undergoing primary percutaneous coronary intervention: the CAPITAL RELOAD study. PLoS One. 2014;9:e92078.
70. Saucedo JF, Angiolillo DJ, DeRaad R, et al. SWAP Investigators. Decrease in high on-treatment platelet reactivity (HPR) prevalence on switching from clopidogrel to prasugrel: insights from the Switching Anti-Platelet (SWAP) study. Thromb Haemost. 2013;109:347-55.
71. Michelson AD, Frelinger AL 3rd, Braunwald E, et al; TRITON-TIMI 38 Investigators. Pharmacodynamic assessment of platelet inhibition by prasugrel vs. clopidogrel in the TRITON-TIMI 38 trial. Eur Heart J. 2009;30:1753-63.
72. Bliden KP, Tantry US, Storey RF, et al. The effect of ticagrelor versus clopidogrel on high on-treatment platelet reactivity: combined analysis of the ONSET/OFFSET and RESPOND studies. Am Heart J. 2011;162:160-5.
73. Storey RF, Angiolillo DJ, Patil SB, et al. Inhibitory effects of ticagrelor compared with clopidogrel on platelet function in patients with acute coronary syndromes: the PLATO (PLATelet inhibition and patient Outcomes) PLATELET sub-study. J Am Coll Cardiol. 2010;56:1456-62.
74. Cannon CP, Harrington RA, James S, et al. PLATelet inhibition and patient Outcomes Investigators. Comparison of ticagrelor with clopidogrel in patients with a planned invasive strategy for acute coronary syndromes (PLATO): a randomised double-blind study. Lancet 2010;375:283-93.

75. Alexopoulos D, Xanthopoulou I, Perperis A, et al. Dyspnea in patients treated with P2Y12 receptor antagonists: insights from the GReek Anti PlatElet (GRAPE) registry. Platelets. 2017;2:1-7.
76. Bonaca MP, Bhatt DL, Oude Ophuis T, et al. Long-term tolerability of ticagrelor for the secondary prevention of major adverse cardiovascular events: a secondary analysis of the PEGASUS-TIMI 54 Trial. JAMA Cardiol. 2016;1:425–32.
77. Cuisset T, Deharo P, Quilici J, et al. Benefit of switching dual antiplatelet therapy after acute coronary syndrome: the TOPIC (Timing of Platelet Inhibition After Acute Coronary Syndrome) randomized study. Eur Heart J. 2017;38(41):3070-8.
78. Mehta SR, Armstrong PW, Cantor WJ, et al. 2018 Canadian Cardiovascular Society/Canadian Association of Interventional Cardiology Focused Update of the Guidelines for the Use of Antiplatelet Therapy. Can J Cardiol. 2018;34(3):214-33.
79. Sibbing D, Aradi D, Jacobshagen C, et al.; TROPICAL-ACS Investigators. Guided de-escalation of antiplatelet treatment in patients with acute coronary syndrome undergoing percutaneous coronary intervention (TROPICAL-ACS): a randomised, open-label, multicentre trial. Lancet. 2017;390(10104):1747-57.
80. Pourdjabbar A, Hibbert B, Chong AY, et al. A randomised study for optimising crossover from ticagrelor to clopidogrel in patients with acute coronary syndrome: The CAPITAL OPTI-CROSS Study. Thromb Haemost. 2017;117(02):303-10.
81. Kerneis M, Silvain J, Abtan J, et al. Switching acute coronary syndrome patients from prasugrel to clopidogrel. JACC Cardiovasc Interv. 2013;6:158-65.
82. Deharo P, Pons C, Pankert M, et al. Effectiveness of switching "hyper responders" from prasugrel to clopidogrel after acute coronary syndrome: the POBA (Predictor of Bleeding with Antiplatelet drugs) SWITCH study. Int J Cardiol. 2013;168: 5004-5.
83. Franchi F, Rollini F, Rios JR, et al. Pharmacodynamic Effects of Switching From Ticagrelor to Clopidogrelin Patients With Coronary Artery Disease: Results of the SWAP (Switching Antiplatelet Therapy)-4 Study. Circulation. 2018;137(23): 2450-62.
84. Angiolillo DJ, Curzen N, Gurbel P, et al. Pharmacodynamic evaluation of switching from ticagrelor to prasugrel in patients with stable coronary artery disease: results of the SWAP-2 Study (Switching Anti Platelet-2). J Am Coll Cardiol. 2014;63:1500-9.
85. Franchi F, Faz GT, Rollini F, et al. Pharmacodynamic effects of switching from prasugrel to ticagrelor: results of the prospective, randomized SWAP-3 study. JACC Cardiovasc Interv. 2016;9:1089-98.
86. Angiolillo DJ, Firstenberg MS, Price MJ, et al. BRIDGE Investigators. Bridging antiplatelet therapy with cangrelor in patients undergoing cardiac surgery: a randomized controlled trial. JAMA. 2012;307:265-74.
87. Rollini F, Franchi F, Tello-Montoliu A, et al. Pharmacodynamic effects of cangrelor on platelet P2Y12 receptor- mediated signaling in prasugrel-treated patients. JACC Cardiovasc Interv. 2014;7:426-34.
88. Rollini F, Franchi F, Thano E, et al. In vitro pharmacodynamic effects of cangrelor on platelet P2Y12 receptor-mediated signaling in ticagrelor-treated patients. JACC Cardiovasc Interv. 2017;10:1374-5.
89. Schneider DJ, Agarwal Z, Seecheran N, et al. Pharmacodynamic effects during the transition between cangrelor and ticagrelor. JACC Cardiovasc Interv. 2014;7:435-42.
90. Schneider DJ, Seecheran N, Raza SS, et al. Pharmacodynamic effects during the transition between cangrelor and prasugrel. Coron Artery Dis. 2015;26: 42-8.
91. Schneider DJ, Agarwal Z, Seecheran N, et al. Pharmacodynamic effects when clopidogrel is given before cangrelor discontinuation. J Interv Cardiol. 2015;28:415-9.
92. Dovlatova NL, Jakubowski JA, Sugidachi A, et al. The reversible P2Y antagonist cangrelor influences the ability of the active metabolites of clopidogrel and prasugrel to produce irreversible inhibition of platelet function. J Thromb Haemost. 2008;6:1153-9.
93. Vaduganathan M, Qamar A, Singh A, et al. Cangrelor use since FDA approval: a single-center, real-world experience at a tertiary care hospital. J Am Coll Cardiol. 2017;69:463-4.
94. Bhatt DL, Stone GW, Mahaffey KW, et al; CHAMPION PHOENIX Investigators. Effect of platelet inhibition with cangrelor during PCI on ischemic events. N Engl J Med. 2013;368:1303-13.
95. Badreldin HA, Carter D, Cook BM, et al. Safety and tolerability of transitioning from cangrelor to ticagrelor in patients who underwent percutaneous coronary intervention. Am J Cardiol. 2017;120:359-61.
96. Franchi F, Rollini F, Park Y, et al. A safety evaluation of cangrelor in patients undergoing PCI. Expert Opin Drug Saf. 2016;15:275-85.
97. Angiolillo DJ, Schneider DJ, Bhatt DL, et al. Pharmacodynamic effects of cangrelor and clopidogrel: the platelet function sub-study from the Cangrelor Versus Standard Therapy to Achieve Optimal Management of Platelet Inhibition (CHAMPION) trials. J Thromb Thrombolysis. 2012;34:44-55.
98. Steinhubl SR, Oh JJ, Oestreich JH, et al. Transitioning patients from cangrelor to clopidogrel: pharmacodynamic evidence of a competitive effect. Thromb Res. 2008;121:527-34.
99. Schneider DJ. Transition strategies from cangrelor to oral platelet P2Y12 receptor antagonists. Coron Artery Dis. 2016;27:65-9.
100. Judge HM, Buckland RJ, Jakubowski JA, et al. Cangrelor inhibits the binding of the active metabolites of clopidogrel and prasugrel to P2Y12 receptors in vitro. Platelets. 2016;27:191-5.
101. Hochholzer W, Kleiner P, Younas I, et al. Randomized Comparison of oral P2Y12-receptor inhibitor loading strategies for transitioning from cangrelor: the ExcelsiorLOAD2 Trial. JACC Cardiovasc Interv. 2017;10:121-9.
102. Bonello L, Tantry US, Marcucci R, et al; the Working Group on High On-Treatment Platelet Reactivity. Consensus and future directions on the definition of high on-treatment platelet reactivity to adenosine diphosphate. J Am Coll Cardiol. 2010;56:919-33.
103. Price MJ, Berger PB, Teirstein PS, et al.; GRAVITAS Investigators. Standard- vs high-dose clopidogrel based on platelet function testing after percutaneous coronary intervention: the GRAVITAS randomized trial. JAMA. 2011;305:1097-105.
104. Collet JP, Cuisset T, Range G, et al. Bedside monitoring to adjust antiplatelet therapy for coronary stenting. N Engl J Med. 2012;367:2100-9.
105. Collet JP, Cuisset T, Rangé G, et al.; ARCTIC Investigators. Bedside monitoring to adjust antiplatelet therapy for coronary stenting. N Engl J Med. 2012;367: 2100-9.
106. Cayla G, Cuisset T, Silvain J, et al; ANTARCTIC Investigators. Platelet function monitoring to adjust antiplatelet therapy in elderly patients stented for an acute coronary syndrome (ANTARCTIC): an open-label, blinded-endpoint, randomised controlled superiority trial. Lancet. 2016;388:2015-22.

CHAPTER 54

Management of Bleeding in Planned or Unplanned Surgery in a Patient on Dual Antiplatelet Therapy

Sameer Dani

INTRODUCTION

In this industrialized world, patients suffering from cardiovascular diseases are increasing day by day and a number of them are treated with percutaneous coronary intervention (PCI) with stent implantation for major coronary events. Platelets play a major role in the pathogenesis of these events.

Platelet aggregation and rupture of unstable plaque lead to thrombus which underlies the pathogenesis for acute coronary syndrome (ACS).[1,2] In medical practice, dual antiplatelet therapy (DAPT) is routinely used as a mainstay therapy for ACS.[3] In cases of ACS where PCI was done with the use of ballooning or stent implantation, risk of stent thrombosis and during the phase of re-endothelialization the use of DAPT is unavoidable.[4]

Dual antiplatelet therapy itself carries a risk of bleeding in patients who are taking it regularly for ACS and who are not even exposed to any surgical procedures.[5] In early postoperative period in addition to bleeding risk there are higher chances of risk of thrombosis due to hypercoagulable state as a result of systemic inflammation.[6,7] Out of all the patients undergoing PCI, approximately 6–20% are posted for noncardiac surgery within the first 2 years after PCI.[8] Out of these, 45–50% who received a drug-eluting stent (DES) undergo surgery in less than 12 months, in which, the use of DAPT is compulsory.[9] Patient on perioperative DAPT should be individualized with the combined decision of anesthesiologist, cardiologist, and surgeon to lower the risk of both ischemia and bleeding.

DUAL ANTIPLATELET THERAPY AND PHARMACOLOGY

Aspirin and a P2Y12 inhibitors are together considered as DAPT, but the available antiplatelets can be generally classified into five types based on their mechanism of action: cyclooxygenase (COX)-1 inhibitor (aspirin), P2Y12 inhibitors (clopidogrel, prasugrel, ticagrelor, cangrelor), glycoprotein (GP) IIb/IIIa inhibitors (abciximab, eptifibatide, tirofiban), phosphodiesterase-III inhibitors (dipyridamole, cilostazol), and protease-activated receptor-1 inhibitor (vorapaxar). Cilostazol is mostly used in patients with peripheral arterial disease. Similarly, there is not much evidence regarding the use of vorapaxar in addition with DAPT in patients of coronary artery disease (Table 1).

Timing of platelet transfusion or discontinuation of DAPT will be decided after having the knowledge of pharmacokinetics and pharmacodynamics about various antiplatelets.

TABLE 1: Antiplatelets

	Administration route/mode of action	Onset/elimination half-life	% inhibition of platelet function	Recovery after discontinuation
Aspirin	Oral/irreversible cyclooxgenase-1 inhibitor	20–45 min/2–4 h	60–70%	5 days
Clopidogrel	Oral/irreversible P2Y12 inhibitor	12–24 hr/4–6 h	60–70%	5–7 days
Prasugrel	Oral/irreversible P2Y12 inhibitor	0.5–4 hr/7 h	90%	7–10 days
Ticagrelor	Oral/reversible P2Y12 inhibitor	0.5–4 hr/7 h	90%	3–5 days
Cangrelor	Intravenous/reversible P2Y12 inhibitor	Immediate/3–5 min	>90%	30–60 min
Abciximab	Intravenous/reversible glycoprotein IIb/IIIa inhibitor	Immediate/10–30 min	~100%	12 h
Tirofiban	Intravenous/reversible glycoprotein IIb/IIIa inhibitor	Immediate/2–2.5 h	~100%	4 h
Eptifibatide	Intravenous/reversible glycoprotein IIb/IIIa inhibitor	Immediate/2–2.5 h	~100%	4 h

PREVENTION OF BLEEDING

Assessment of Bleeding Risk

"DAPT score" may be useful for decisions about whether to continue DAPT in postangioplasty patients. In patients treated for 1 year with DAPT without significant bleeding or ischemic events, the patients with high DAPT score (≥2) have a favorable benefit-risk ratio with prolonged DAPT because prolonged DAPT reduces both ischemic and bleeding complications when compared with nonprolonged DAPT.[10]

The 2017 Focused Update on DAPT provides a comprehensive set of recommendations for the routine use of DAPT after coronary artery stenting, with perhaps the underlying message being that an individual assessment of high bleeding [e.g., predicting bleeding complication in patients undergoing stent implantation and subsequent dual antiplatelet therapy (PRECISE-DAPT) score ≥25] or ischemic risk (e.g., DAPT score ≥2 and/or complex PCI) may justify a shorter or longer DAPT duration, respectively, than the hitherto accepted standard of 6 months (clopidogrel) in stable or 12 months (ticagrelor or prasugrel) in ACS patients (Table 2).

Bleeding Risk According to Types of Surgery

Surgery can be divided into low, intermediate, and high-risk categories, with estimated 30-day cardiac event rates for major adverse cardiac events of less than 1%, 1–5%, and more than or equal to 5%, respectively (Table 3).[20,21]

In surgeries with low bleeding risk, the patient need not discontinue DAPT perioperatively while during surgeries with intermediate bleeding risk, continuing aspirin throughout the procedure and P2Y12 inhibitor therapy should be stopped whenever possible and can be started as early as possible in postoperative period. Those who undergo noncardiac surgeries with high-risk bleeding may face more challenges in decision making whether to stop or continue DAPT.[22-24] In these cases, particular consideration should be given to discontinue P2Y12 inhibitor therapy timely to decrease off-therapy period before surgery.

Timing of Discontinuation of Dual Antiplatelet Therapy in Elective Noncardiac Surgery

In patients who have undergone DES implantation recently, timing of elective noncardiac surgery depends upon:

- Major risk of stent thrombosis if there is definite need of stopping DAPT
- It also carries risk of complication by delaying required surgery
- Risk of bleeding during and prior to procedure will be there with continued use of DAPT.

Also as we have described above, surgery is related to systemic proinflammatory and prothrombotic effect mainly during early postoperative period with higher risk of stent thrombosis (Fig. 1).

TABLE 2: Risk scores validated for dual antiplatelet therapy duration decision making[11-19]

	PRECISE-DAPT score[18]	DAPT score[15]
Time of use	At the time of coronary stenting	After 12-month of universal DAPT
DAPT duration strategies assessed	Short DAPT (3–6 months) vs. Standard/long DAPT (12–24 months)	Standard DAPT (12 months) vs. Long DAPT (30 months)
Score calculating[a]	Hb: ≥12 11-5 11 10-5 ≤10 WBC: ≤5 8 10 12 14 16 18 ≥20 Age: ≤50 60 70 80 ≥90 CrCl: ≥100 80 60 40 20 0 Prior bleeding: No Yes Score Points: 0 2 4 6 8 10 12 14 16 18 20 22 24 26 28 30	Age ≥75 −2 pt 65 to <75 −1 pt 65 0 pt Cigarette smoking +1 pt Diabetes mellitus +1 pt MI at presentation +1 pt Prior PCI or prior MI +1 pt Paclitaxel-eluting stent +1 pt Stent diameter <3 mm +1 pt CHF or LVEF <30% +2 pt Vein graft stent +2 pt
Score range	0 to 100 points	−2 to 10 points
Decision making cut-off suggested	Score ≥25 → Short DAPT Score <25 → Standard/long DAPT	Score ≥2 → Long DAPT Score <2 → Standard DAPT
Calculator	www.precisedaptscore.com	www.daptstudy.org

[a]For the PRECISE-DAPT score, use the score nomogram: mark patient's value for each of the five clinical varibles of the score and draw a vertical line to the 'point' axis to determine the number of points obtained for each clinical variable. Then summate the points obtained for each clinical variable to the total score.

For the DAPT score, summate positive points for each value and subtract values for age to the total score

CHF, congestive heart failure; CrCl, creatinine clearance; DAPT, dual antiplatelet therapy; LVEF, left ventricular ejection fraction; MI, myocardial infarction; PCI, percutaneous coronary intervention; WBC, white blood cells.

TABLE 3: Types of surgery

Low risk (<1%)	Intermediate risk (1–5%)	High risk (>5%)
Superficial surgery Breast Dental Endocrine: Thyroid Eye Reconstruction Carotid asymptomatic (CEA or CAS) Gynecology: Minor Orthopedic: Minor Urological: Minor (Transurethral resection of the prostate)	Intraperitoneal: Splenectomy, hiatal hernia repair, cholecystectomy Carotid symptomatic (CEA or CAS) Peripheral arterial angioplasty Endovascular aneurysm repair Head and neck surgery Neurological or orthopedic: Major (hip and spine surgery) Urological and gynecological: Major Renal transplant Intrathoracic: Nonmajor	Aortic and major vascular surgery Open lower limb revascularization or amputation or thromboembolectomy Duodenopancreatic surgery Liver resection, bile duct surgery Esophagectomy Repair of perforated bowel Adrenal resection Total cystectomy Pneumonectomy Liver or pulmonary transplant

CEA, carotid endarterectomy; CAS, carotid artery stenting.

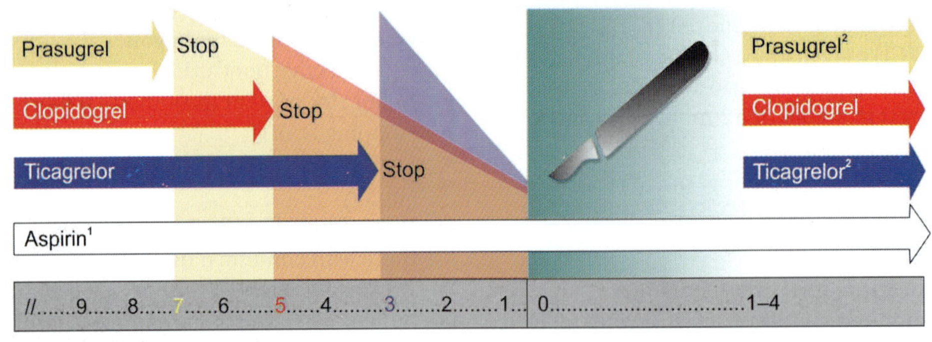

= Expected average platelet function recovery.

¹Decision to stop aspirin throughout surgery should be made on a single case basis taking into account the surgical bleeding risk.

²In patients not requiring oral anticoagulant.

FIG. 1: Time frames of minimal discontinuation and reimplementation of dual antiplatelet therapy for patients undergoing elective noncardiac surgery.[25,26]

Guidelines for the Timing of Noncardiac Surgery in Relation to Newer Generation Drug-eluting Stent

In the era of new antiplatelet agents, there has also been continuous development in the efficacy of DES. The previous guidelines were mostly based on first-generation sirolimus- or paclitaxel-eluting stents. But, now the ACC/AHA (American College of Cardiology/American Heart Association), 2016, guidelines give data regarding the use of newer generation DES (with elution of everolimus or zotarolimus). Clearly, newer generation DES shows less thrombogenicity and better ischemic protection, thus requiring a shorter period for re-endothelialization.[27] Hence, the necessary duration of DAPT after DES placement has been shortened in the new guidelines. Compared with prolonged DAPT, short-term DAPT is associated with similar rates of MACE but lower rates of bleeding after DES placement.[28] The updated 2016 ACC/AHA guidelines recommended elective noncardiac surgery to be performed 6 months after newer generation DES placement, and if the risk-benefit ratio of delaying the required surgery versus risk of stent thrombosis is more, then surgery could be considered at least 3 months after DES placement[29] in contrast to a year with first-generation stents as some of studies also hypothesized that myocardial ischemia is the leading cause of postoperative mortality and morbidity in patients undergoing major vascular surgery as platelets have been implicated in the pathogenesis of acute thrombotic events (Flowchart 1).[30]

However, if emergency or urgent noncardiac surgery is required, then a decision to continue aspirin or DAPT should be individualized with consensus of the cardiologist, anesthesiologist, and surgeon, with the risk weighed against the benefits of continuing DAPT.[31]

Dual Antiplatelet Therapy versus Single Antiplatelet Therapy

According to the European Society of Cardiology (ESC), 2017, guidelines, DAPT discontinuation is recommended in the form of stopping P2Y12 inhibitors at least 3 days before surgery for ticagrelor, at least 5 days for clopidogrel and at least 7 days for prasugrel.

Single antiplatelet therapy (SAPT)—if the bleeding risk is not very high, then it is recommended to continue aspirin and DAPT is to be started as early as possible postoperatively. This is primarily based on expert opinions.

However, patients undergoing elective noncardiac surgery within first month of treatment with PCI should not discontinue DAPT.

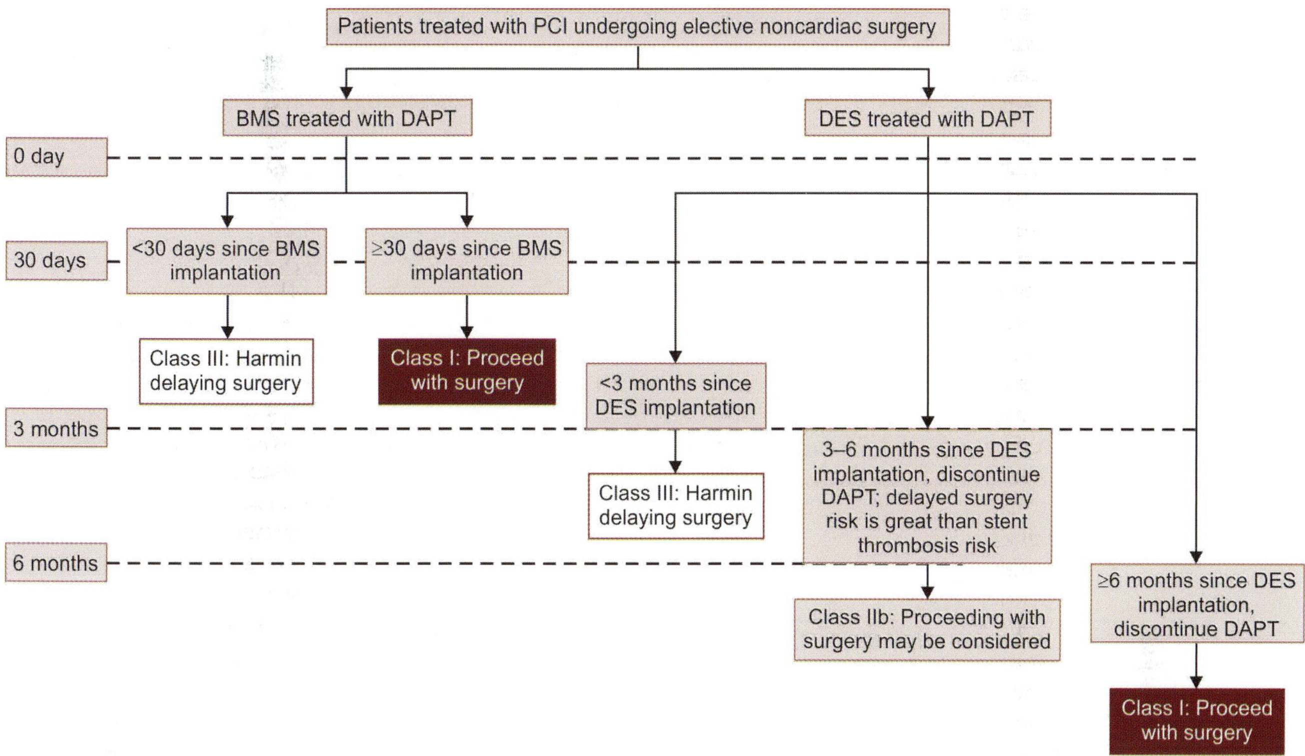

BMS, bare-metal stent; PCI, percutaneous coronary intervention; DAPT, dual antiplatelet therapy; DES, drug-eluting stent.

FLOWCHART 1: Recommendations for the timing of elective noncardiac surgery in patients with coronary stents.

TREATMENT OF BLEEDING

Bleeding complications such as major hemorrhages do not occur very frequently with the use of DAPT; however, minor bleeding complications can occur which can be managed with various pharmacological and nonpharmacological measures described below. In case of minor bleeding in which hemostatic agents were used, once hemostasis is achieved, consider the starting of antiplatelets as early as possible.[32-34]

In case of emergent surgery, reversal of the antiplatelet effect by platelet transfusion may be considered which carries the risk of significant arterial thrombosis.

General Measures to Stop Bleeding

Nonpharmacological Measures

In cases where bleeding is not significant, general nonpharmacological measures and discontinuation of DAPT are sufficient to treat the bleeding (Box 1). Some techniques like plasmapheresis or hemofiltration can reduce plasma concentration of antiplatelets in some cases and these are also not easily accessible in all emergency settings.

BOX 1 General nonpharmacological measures

- Stop DAPT
- Timing and dose of drug
- Presence of associated comorbidities
- Look for bleeding site
- Send complete blood count, prothrombin time, activated partial thromboplastin time, thrombin time, fibrinogen concentration, creatinine concentration
- Intravenous fluids and red cell transfusion to make patient hemodynamically stable and also apply mechanical pressure, if possible
- Use endoscopic, radiological, or surgical measures wherever applicable

DAPT, dual antiplatelet therapy.

General Hemostatic Agents

There is no specific antidote available to reverse DAPT. However, few prohemostatic agents are available which can be useful for reversal of the effect of antithrombotic drugs in some situations. For example, recombinant activated factor VII (rFVIIa), prothrombin complex concentrates (PCC), and activated PCC [APCC; e.g., factor VIII inhibitor bypass activity (FEIBA)] are often considered. Antithrombotic effect reversal with rFVIIa is not approved,[35] but it is still considered as a last option when all other attempts have failed and when the risks and benefits are carefully explained.

PCC and fresh frozen plasma (FFP) are used to reverse vitamin K antagonists (VKAs), but their role as a reversal agent for DAPT is doubtful (Box 2).[36]

Practical Recommendations for Management of Bleeding

Flowchart 2 shows practical recommendations for management of bleeding.

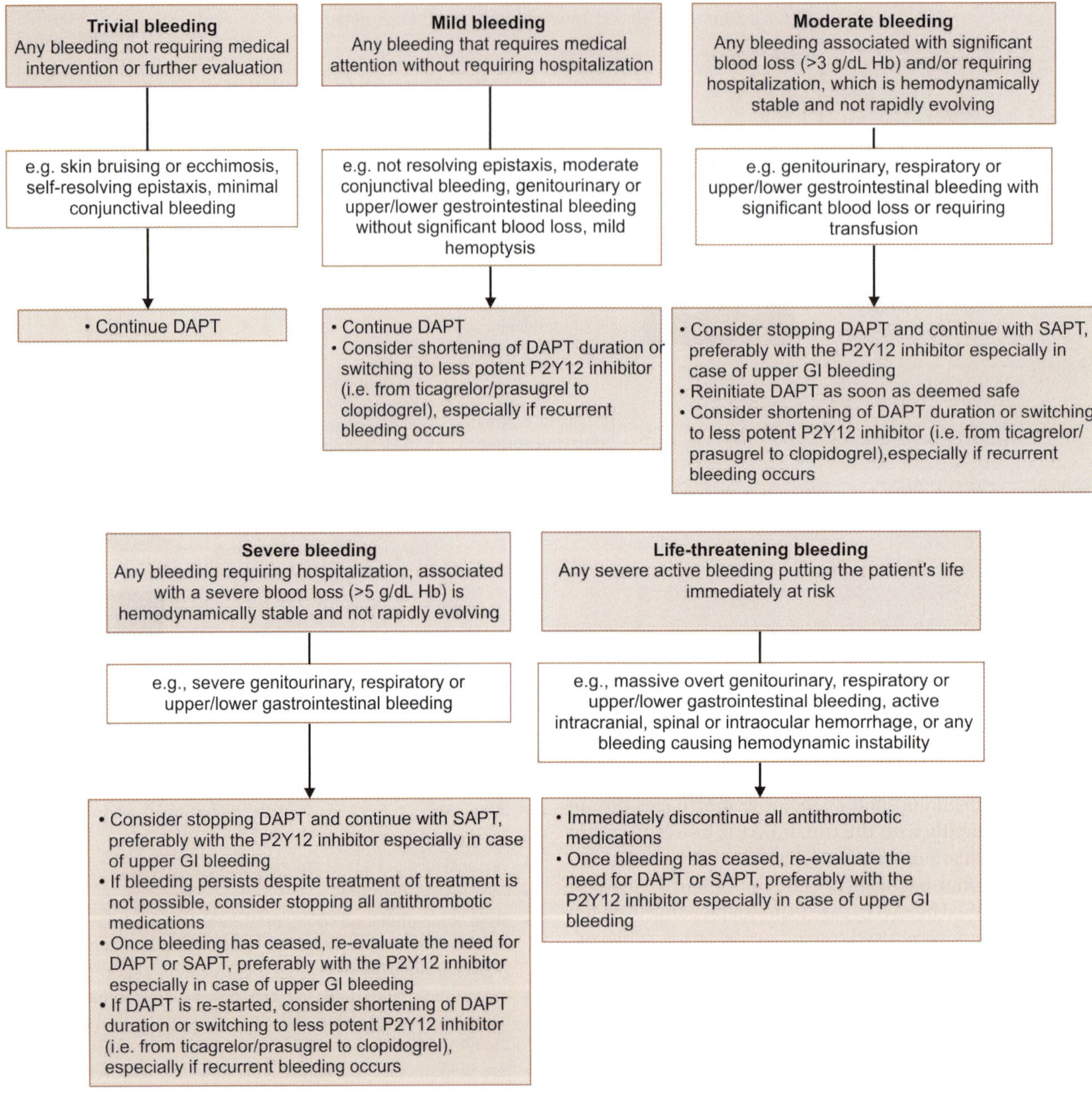

DAPT, dual antiplatelet therapy; GI, gastrointestinal; SAPT, single antiplatelet therapy.

FLOWCHART 2: Management of bleeding.

BOX 2 Pharmacological and blood component prohemostatic measures

- Tranexamic acid
- Desmopressin
- Fresh frozen plasma
- Cryoprecipitate
- Platelet transfusion
- Fibrinogen concentrate
- Prothrombin complex concentrate
- Activated prothrombin complex concentrate
- Recombinant factor VIIa

CONCLUSION

While balancing risks of bleeding versus thrombotic events, the relative adverse events must be considered. Rarely, the bleeding is life-threatening in comparison with the potential consequences of stent thrombosis.

Sudden discontinuation of DAPT can lead to a rebound effect marked by an excessive thromboxane A2 activity and inflammatory prothrombotic state, increased platelet adhesion, and aggregation.

Surgery further increases the prothrombotic and inflammatory state, which, combined with incompletely endothelialized DES, can lead to stent thrombosis and, consequently, myocardial infarction and/or death.[37]

In a patient treated with DAPT after coronary stent implantation, who must undergo surgical procedures that mandate the discontinuation of P2Y12 inhibitor therapy, it is recommended that aspirin be continued if possible and P2Y12 platelet receptor inhibitor be started as soon as possible after the surgery. There are no clinical evidence-based trials or studies that have shown benefits of IV antiplatelet agents used as bridging therapy in patients who require to stop DAPT temporarily before noncardiac surgery—class 1 recommendation of ACC guidelines.

An elective noncardiac surgery should not be performed within at least 1 month after bare-metal stent (BMS) implantation or within 3 months after DES implantation in patients in whom DAPT will need to be discontinued perioperatively—class 3 recommendation of ACC guidelines.

After coronary stent implantation, elective surgery requiring discontinuation of P2Y12 inhibitor should be considered after 1 month irrespective of the stent type if aspirin can be maintained throughout the perioperative period—*Class 2a recommendation of ESC guidelines.*

Discontinuation of P2Y12 inhibitors should be considered at least 3 days before for ticagrelor, at least 5 days for clopidogrel and at least 7 days for prasugrel—class 2a recommendation of ESC guidelines.

It is not recommended to discontinue DAPT within the first month of treatment in patients undergoing elective noncardiac surgery—class 3 recommendation of ESC guidelines.

If emergency or urgent noncardiac surgery is required, then a decision to continue aspirin or DAPT should be individualized with consensus of the cardiologist, anesthesiologist, and surgeon, with the risk weighed against the benefits of continuing DAPT.

REFERENCES

1. Falk E, Nakano M, Bentzon JF, et al. Update on acute coronary syndromes: The pathologists' view. Eur Heart J. 2013;34:719-28.
2. Gidron Y, Gilutz H, Berger R, et al. Molecular and cellular interface between behavior and acute coronary syndromes. Cardiovasc Res. 2002;56:15-21.
3. Amsterdam EA, Wenger NK, Brindis RG, et al. 2014 AHA/ACC guidelines for the management of patients with non-ST-elevation acute coronary syndromes: A report of the American College of Cardiology/American Heart Association Task Force on Practice Guidelines. Circulation. 2014;130:e344-426.
4. Mehran R, Baber U, Steg PG, et al. Cessation of dual antiplatelet treatment and cardiac events after percutaneous coronary intervention (PARIS): 2-year results from a prospective observational study. Lancet. 2013;382:1714-22.
5. Doyle BJ, Rihal CS, Gastineau DA, et al. Bleeding, blood transfusion, and increased mortality after percutaneous coronary intervention: implications for contemporary practice. J Am Coll Cardiol. 2009;53:2019-27.
6. Priebe HJ. Triggers of perioperative myocardial ischaemia and infarction. Br J Anaesth. 2004;93:9-20.
7. Kim NY, Shim JK, Bang SO, et al. Effects of ulinastatin on coagulation in high-risk patients undergoing off-pump coronary artery bypass graft surgery. Korean J Anesthesiol. 2013;64:105-11.
8. Hawn MT, Graham LA, Richman JR, et al. The incidence and timing of noncardiac surgery after cardiac stent implantation. J Am Coll Surg. 2012;214:658-66.
9. Fleisher LA, Fleischmann KE, Auerbach AD, et al. 2014 ACC/AHA guidelines on perioperative cardiovascular evaluation and management of patients undergoing noncardiac surgery: a report of the American College of Cardiology/American Heart Association Task Force on Practice Guidelines. Circulation. 2014;130:e278-333.
10. Yeh RW, Secemsky E, Kereiakes DJ, et al. Development and validation of a prediction rule for benefit and harm of dual antiplatelet therapy beyond one year after percutaneous coronary intervention: An analysis from the randomized Dual Antiplatelet Therapy Study. JAMA. 2016;315(16):1735-49.
11. Bueno H, Fernandez-Aviles F. Use of risk scores in acute coronary syndromes. Heart. 2012;98:162-8.
12. Antman EM, Cohen M, Bernink PJ, et al. The TIMI risk score for unstable angina/non-ST elevation MI: A method for prognostication and therapeutic decision making. JAMA. 2000;284:835-42.
13. Boersma E, Pieper KS, Steyerberg EW, et al. Predictors of outcome in patients with acute coronary syndromes without persistent ST-segment elevation. Results from an international trial of 9461 patients. The PURSUIT Investigators. Circulation. 2000;101:2557-67.
14. Fox KA, Dabbous OH, Goldberg RJ, et al. Prediction of risk of death and myocardial infarction in the six months after presentation with acute coronary syndrome: Prospective multinational observational study (GRACE). BMJ. 2006;333:1091.
15. Subherwal S, Bach RG, Chen AY, et al. Baseline risk of major bleeding in non-ST-segment-elevation myocardial infarction: The CRUSADE (Can Rapid risk stratification of Unstable angina patients Suppress ADverse outcomes with Early implementation of the ACC/AHA Guidelines) bleeding score. Circulation. 2009;119:1873-82.
16. Mehran R, Pocock SJ, Nikolsky E, et al. A risk score to predict bleeding in patients with acute coronary syndromes. J Am Coll Cardiol. 2010;55:2556-66.
17. Mathews R, Peterson ED, Chen AY, et al. In-hospital major bleeding during ST-elevation and non-ST-elevation myocardial infarction care: Derivation and validation of a model from the ACTION Registry(R)-GWTG. Am J Cardiol. 2011;107:1136-43.
18. Costa F, Tijssen JG, Ariotti S, et al. Incremental value of the CRUSADE, ACUITY, and HAS-BLED risk scores for the prediction of hemorrhagic events after coronary stent implantation in patients undergoing long or short duration of dual antiplatelet therapy. J Am Heart Assoc. 2015;4:e002524.
19. Mahaffey KW, Yang Q, Pieper KS, et al. Prediction of one-year survival in high-risk patients with acute coronary syndromes: Results from the SYNERGY trial. J Gen Intern Med. 2008;23:310-6.
20. Kristensen SD, Knuuti J, Saraste A, et al. 2014 ESC/ESA Guidelines on non-cardiac surgery: Cardiovascular assessment and management: The Joint Task Force on non-cardiac surgery: Cardiovascular assessment and management of the European Society of Cardiology (ESC) and the European Society of Anaesthesiology (ESA). Eur Heart J. 2014;35:2383-431.
21. Glance LG, Lustik SJ, Hannan EL, et al. The Surgical Mortality Probability Model: Derivation and validation of a simple risk prediction rule for noncardiac surgery. Ann Surg. 2012;255:696-702.
22. Chapman TW, Bowley DM, Lambert AW, et al. Haemorrhage associated with combined clopidogrel and aspirin therapy. Eur J Vasc Endovasc Surg. 2001;22:478-9.
23. Ernst A, Eberhardt R, Wahidi M, et al. Effect of routine clopidogrel use on bleeding complications after transbronchial biopsy in humans. Chest. 2006;129:734-7.
24. Moore M, Power M. Perioperative hemorrhage and combined clopidogrel and aspirin therapy. Anesthesiology. 2004;101:792-4.
25. Abualsaud AO, Eisenberg MJ. Perioperative management of patients with drug-eluting stents. JACC Cardiovasc Interv. 2010;3:131-42.
26. Dimitrova G, Tulman DB, Bergese SD. Perioperative management of antiplatelet therapy in patients with drug-eluting stents. HSR Proc Intensive Care Cardiovasc Anesth. 2012;4:153-67.
27. Fleisher LA, Fleischmann KE, Auerbach AD, et al. 2014 ACC/AHA guidelines on perioperative cardiovascular evaluation and management of patients undergoing noncardiac surgery: A report of the American College of Cardiology/American Heart Association Task Force on Practice Guidelines. J Am Coll Cardiol. 2014;64:e77-137.

28. Palmerini T, Sangiorgi D, Valgimigli M, et al. Short- versus long-term dual antiplatelet therapy after drug-eluting stent implantation: an individual patient data pairwise and network meta-analysis. J Am Coll Cardiol. 2015;65:1092-1102.
29. Levine GN, Bates ER, Bittl JA, et al. 2016 ACC/AHA guidelines focused update on duration of dual antiplatelet therapy in patients with coronary artery disease: A report of the American College of Cardiology/American Heart Association Task Force on clinical practice guidelines: An Update of the 2011 ACCF/AHA/SCAI guidelines for percutaneous coronary intervention, 2011 ACCF/AHA guidelines for coronary artery bypass graft surgery, 2012 ACC/AHA/ACP/AATS/PCNA/SCAI/STS guidelines for the diagnosis and management of patients with stable ischemic heart disease, 2013 ACCF/AHA guidelines for the management of ST-elevation myocardial infarction, 2014 AHA/ACC guidelines for the management of patients with non-ST-elevation acute coronary syndromes, and 2014 ACC/AHA guidelines on perioperative cardiovascular evaluation and management of patients undergoing noncardiac surgery. Circulation. 2016;134:e123-55.
30. Rajagopalan S, Ford I, Bachoo P, et al. Platelet activation, myocardial ischemic events and postoperative non-response to aspirin in patients undergoing major vascular surgery. J Thromb Haemost. 2007;5:2028-35.
31. Diamantis T, Tsiminikakis N, Skordylaki A, et al. Alterations of hemostasis after laparoscopic and open surgery. Hematology. 2007;12:561-70.
32. Howard-Alpe GM, de Bono J, Hudsmith L, et al. Coronary artery stents and non-cardiac surgery. Br J Anaesth. 2007;98:560-74.
33. Bhala N, Taggar JS, Rajasekhar P, et al. Anticipating and managing bleeding complications in patients with coronary stents who are receiving dual antiplatelet treatment. Br Med J. 2011;343:d4264.
34. Korte W, Cattaneo M, Chassot PG, et al. Peri-operative management of antiplatelet therapy in patients with coronary artery disease: joint position paper by members of the working group on Perioperative Haemostasis of the Society on Thrombosis and Haemostasis Research (GTH), the working group on Perioperative Coagulation of the Austrian Society for Anesthesiology, Resuscitation and Intensive Care (ÖGARI) and the Working Group Thrombosis of the European Society for Cardiology (ESC). Thromb Haemost. 2011;105(5): 743-9.
35. Sorour Y, Van Veen JJ, Makris M. Recombinant factor VIIa for unlicensed indications—A definite No or a cautious maybe in selected patients. Int J Clin Pract. 2010;64:1468-71.
36. Crowther MA, Warkentin TE. Bleeding risk and the management of bleeding complications in patients undergoing anticoagulant therapy: Focus on new anticoagulant agents. Blood 2008;111:4871-9.
37. Newsome LT, Weller RS, Gerancher JC, et al. Coronary artery stents: II. Perioperative considerations and management. Anesth Analg. 2008;107:570-90.

SECTION 9

Coronary Intervention

CHAPTER 55

History and Evolution of Coronary Intervention

Dev B Pahlajani, Akshay Mehta

INTRODUCTION

Coronary angiography and intervention are the most common invasive and interventional procedures performed all over the world. It is estimated that more than 3 million coronary interventional procedures are performed annually across various countries with India contributing half a million of them.

Evolution of coronary intervention is the result of curiosity to know the physiology and anatomy of the cardiovascular system, ingenuity of the earlier researchers, with the aim to provide relief to the victims of cardiac ailments. While to the contemporary practitioner of intervention cardiology, the procedure may appear very simple with a comment "after all what is so big about it?", one must not forget the challenges of unknown, ethics, primitive technological, and engineering material at disposal to these scientists of the earlier era. The evolution to the present state should be credited to the courage and daring with coordination among physicians, physicists, engineers, technologists and in the modern era with the pharmaceutical and device industry.

History of coronary intervention is incomplete without acknowledging the early work performed in animals, and cardiac catheterization and coronary angiography in humans that ultimately laid the firm foundation of coronary intervention as we perform today.

Phases of evolution: One could divide the evolution of coronary intervention in four phases:

1. Early animal experiments to understand the physiology of cardiovascular system
2. Development of X-ray systems
3. Cardiac catheterization and coronary angiography in humans
4. Coronary intervention.

Early animal experiments: While Greeks and Romans used to perform "medical procedures" by introducing needles and tubes during early era, the subsequent experiments in humans were performed only in cadavers by introducing needles and pipes in vascular system.

Credit for understanding the cardiac physiology can be attributed to Claude Bernard, a French physiologist (1813–1878). He performed several invasive experiments in dogs. He introduced a small glass tube in the jugular vein of a dog and measured intracardiac pressures by connecting it to "cardiodynamometer" and showed that the right ventricular pressure was lower than the arterial pressure. He can be given the credit for detailed description of cardiac catheterization in animals.

Auguste Chauveau (1827–1917) a veterinary physician and Étienne Marey (1830–1904) an engineer, technologist and physician, again a French physiologist, described the simultaneous pressure tracings in left ventricle and aorta in awake horse and gave account of intracardiac pressure recordings in various cardiac chambers. They commented that "one can be reassured of the innocuity of this method by examining the horse who is scarcely disturbed with the procedure!!"

In late 19th century, cardiac catheterization became routine in physiology laboratories. However, its application in humans remained elusive for few decades.

X-rays: The soul of cardiovascular invasive and interventional procedures:

One wonders what would have been the face of diagnostic and therapeutic cardiovascular intervention had there been no discovery of X-rays !

Credit for the development of coronary angiography and cardiovascular intervention squarely rests on the serendipitous discovery of X-rays by German physicist, Wilhelm Röntgen in 1895. On November 8, 1895 while experimenting, he observed that certain rays were emitted during passing of current through discharge tube. Not knowing the significance of these rays he called them X-rays. He recorded the first X-ray pictures of the hand of his wife with wedding ring. On January 18, 1896 an X-ray machine was

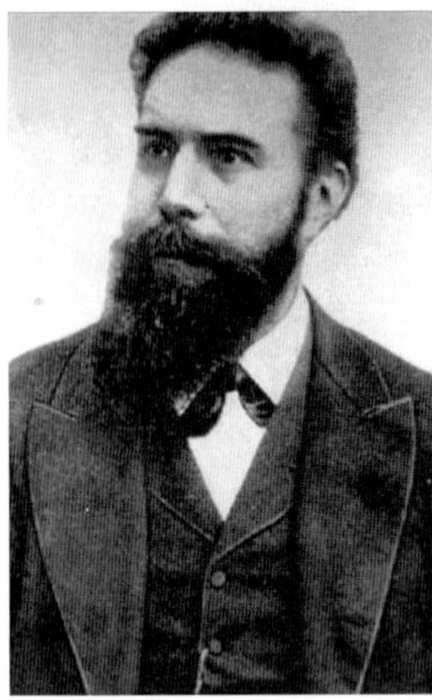

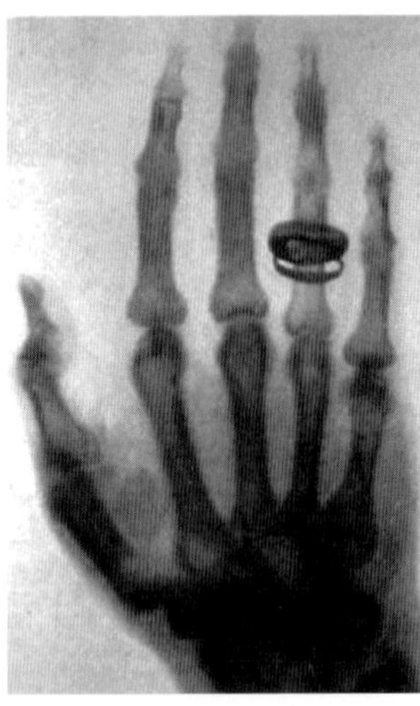

FIG. 1: Wilhelm Röntgen with the first X-ray of his wife's hand with the wedding ring.

formally displayed by Henry Louis Smith and fully functional unit was introduced at the World Fair by Clarence Daily in 1904 (Fig. 1).

Subsequently several refinements, like live fluoroscopy, cine angiography have made it possible to perform the invasive procedures.

Cardiac catheterization in humans: Werner Forssmann, a German Urologist, can be given the credit for performing the first cardiac catheterization in human. No doubt there were some earlier attempts to perform human catheterization which either failed or did not provide the desired outcome. Born on August 29, 1904, it is reported that he performed several experiments on himself. Fascinated by the work of Claude Bernard, Chauveau, and Marey who had performed cardiac catheterization in animals, he desired to perform the cardiac catheterization through the cubital vein. He discussed the plans with his chief, Dr Schneider, and his colleagues. There was strong resistance from academic community. However, with the chief's encouragement he performed the initial animal experiment to assess the safety of the procedure. In his first attempt, he opened his left cubital vein and inserted the lubricated catheter with help of his colleague Peter Romeis and pushed the catheter for about 35 cm. However, the catheter could not be pushed further and had to be abandoned since Romeis thought that the experiment was dangerous. Later, Forssmann with the help of his surgical nurse Gerda Deisen, could open his left arm vein and introduced the catheter for 30 cm. Initially, the nurse thought that the experiment was supposed to be performed on her. With her help he went to the X-ray department, one floor below and advanced the catheter upto 60 cm in the region of the right atrium. He was criticized intensely. However, the chief Snuger authorized the second catheterization to be performed in a woman dying of puerperal sepsis with shock. The aim was to administer intracardiac adrenaline and strophanthin. It may appear ironical that this case could indeed, might have been the first "therapeutic cardiac catheterization". In November 1929 paper entitled "DIE SONDIERUNG DES RECHTEN HERZENS" (Catheterization of the right heart) was published. Forssmann moved to Berlin to work in Charite hospital in Berlin. However, was fired from his work which was not considered to be ethical by chief Ferdinand Sauerbruch proclaiming "he could lecture in a circus but never in a respectable German University". He joined Eberswalde and carried out at least 6 additional safe catheterizations. In October 1956, he was awarded Nobel Prize in medicine, physiology which he shared with Andre Cournand and Dickinson Richards. At the awarding ceremony Professor Lil Hestrand commented that Forssmann was working in a milieu that did not clearly grasp the great value of his idea. Subsequently, the procedure was adapted in various institutions with variously designed catheters and material (Fig. 2).

Andre Cournand and Dickinson W Richards worked together in New York and performed various studies on the hemodynamics and relationship between the heart and the lungs. They also reported on the cardiac output measurements and published several papers on the techniques and

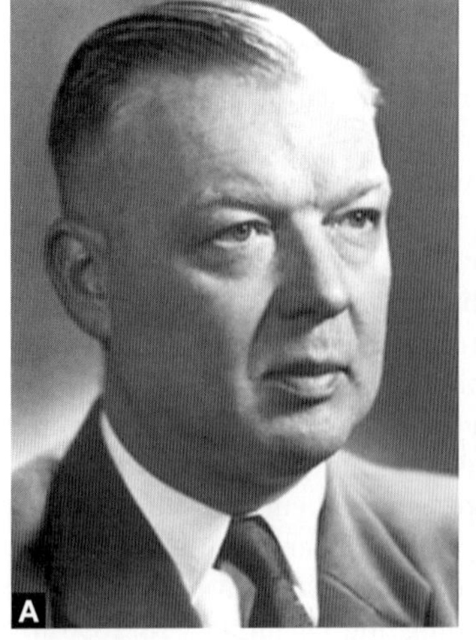

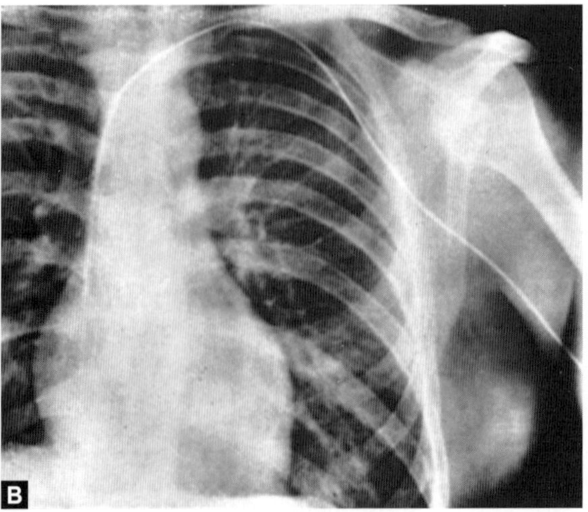

FIG. 2: A, Dr Werner Forssmann; **B,** Catheter through left cubital vein in right atrium.

advances like new catheters, new pressure recorders which resulted in better and safer intravascular recordings. In 1942 they dared to advance the catheter in right ventricle and pulmonary artery. They also studied hemodynamics in shock with measurement of arterial blood pressure, cardiac output, blood gases, and other biochemical parameters.

ARRIVAL OF CORONARY ANGIOGRAPHY

While indirect visualizations of the coronary arteries by injecting into the ascending aorta had been practiced by Charles Dotter who suggested that one could occlude the ascending aorta with a balloon and then dye could be injected into the ascending aorta to temporarily arrest the heart so as to visualize the coronary arteries; however, it was left to the keen observation of Mason Sones in Cleveland clinic who observed that 40 cc of contrast which got injected into the right coronary artery could be tolerated without any untoward side effects except bradycardia. This particular case could be considered as the path breaking case for the futuristic treatment of coronary artery disease. This first selective coronary arteriogram performed by Dr Mason Sones in Cleveland Clinic on October 30, 1958 could be considered as serendipitous discovery. A young man of 26 years of age, was undergoing cardiac catheterization for evaluation of his rheumatic disease of mitral and aortic valve. After completing left ventricular angiogram, Dr Sones intended to perform aortic root shoot. Dr Sones was observing 11 inch image intensifier while sitting underneath in the pit to monitor the injection. A 50 cc of contrast was inadvertently delivered directly into the right coronary artery. Fearing the worst, Dr Sones as he described, grabbed the scalpel to open the chest and perform open cardiac massage. However, he was astonished to find the patient had brief period of bradycardia which recovered after coughing and injection of atropine. This was indeed a serendipitous event which heralded the beginning of new era in cardiology to selectively opacify coronary arteries (Fig. 3). This will open up the flood gates for the accurate diagnosis of coronary arteries, to judge its prognosis and appropriately tailored scientific treatment.

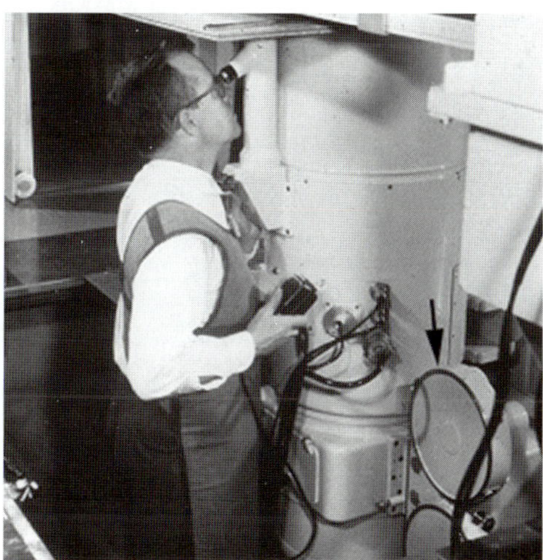

FIG. 3: Dr Mason Sones in his cardiac catheterization laboratory.

Needless to say that without selective visualization of coronary arteries subsequent coronary artery bypass graft surgery and percutaneous transluminal coronary angioplasty (PTCA) would not have been light of the day. As a matter of fact before Sones's work, attempts were made to image coronary arteries by Radner in 1945, to use trans-sternal puncture to inject contrast. However, this was associated with too many complications and therefore the procedure had to be abandoned. The selective opacification by contrast medium was fraught with fear and some of the skeptics felt that introducing oxygen-free medium into the coronary circulation which is already compromised by atherosclerosis could be dangerous and lead to sudden death.

Subsequently, Sones designed the catheters which had a relatively thick shaft (8F) which tapered to soft and flexible tip of small diameter (5F). He was also instrumental in coordinating with Philips North America to develop 5 inch image intensifier which was better suited for coronary artery visualization than earlier larger intensifiers. It was only 4 years later in 1962 that Sones published his paper on 1,000 coronary angiography cases since Sones wanted to acquire complete knowledge and experience before publishing. It may appear news to many practitioners of cardiology that Sones was dyslexic (and reluctant to write and read). Sones also advocated the importance of visualization of coronary arteries in multiple views. It is surprising that as late as 1996, a leading article which appeared in Lancet wrote "as an aid to ischemic heart disease it seems at present to offer little that cannot be more easily obtained by methods such as good history taking and electrocardiography." However, clinicians all over the world realized that there was no equivalent test to coronary arteriography.

While Sones technique was performed through the brachial cutdown route an important path changing modification occurred when Dr Melwyn Judkins designed his preshaped catheters which could be introduced through transfemoral approach. Because of the simplicity of the procedure and no cutdown the Judkins catheter technique became widely popular.

Development of Coronary Balloon Angioplasty

Dr Andreas Roland Gruentzig could rightfully be called as the father of coronary angioplasty (Fig. 4). Born in Dresden, Germany on June 25, 1939 and having obtained his training in Zurich in the University Hospital of Zurich, Switzerland, he was fascinated with the work of balloon angioplasty in the peripheral arteries by Dotter. He performed the dilatation of the superficial femoral artery with the help of Eberhard Zietler and started following the technique of Dotter on his own, together with Meira Schlumpf his personal assistant and was instrumental in designing several balloon catheters for dilating peripheral arteries. While designing various catheters he had to approach several plastic experts to get the appropriate shape of the balloon. This involved trying various forms of polyvinyl chloride (PVC) or rubber so as to form the appropriate and safe pressure resistant cylindrical balloons.

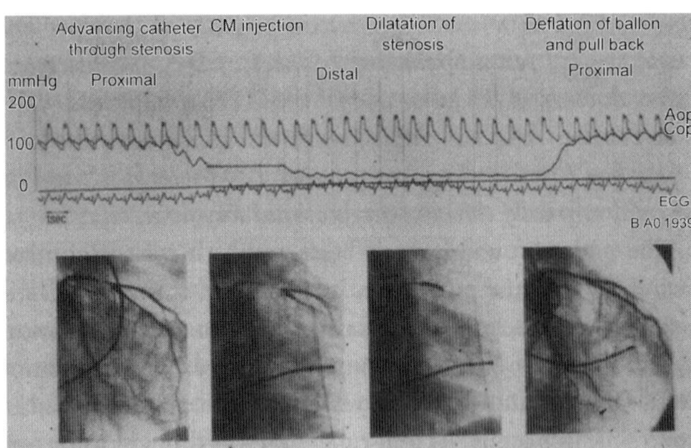

FIG. 4: First coronary angioplasty by Dr Andreas Gruentzig.

In the beginning, the entire designing and the construction was conceived on his kitchen table in his apartment. He even assumed that silk stocking would be required to prevent PVC balloon from turning in the spherical shape with increasing pressure. In his own recounts he mentions the developments of the balloon catheter by writing "I spent the next two years contacting manufacturing plants in an attempt to solve this problem. Especially fruitful was the cooperation of a factory that produced shoe laces and which provided me with silk meshes which I planned to wrap around the balloon, thus limiting its outer diameter. I then needed a very thin balloon to insert within the mesh. It was at that time that I met a retired chemist, Dr Hopff, a Professor emeritus of chemistry of the Technical University of Zurich. He introduced me to PVC compounds. I started to experiment with this material and studied his book on organic chemistry. I acquired some small thin PVC material used as insulation for electrical wires. Following the description in his book, I heated a localized segment of the tubing and applied compressed air pressure resulting in a localized aneurysm of the tubing. I used a second outer tubing measuring 4 mm in diameter to confine the diameter of the segment. After hundreds of experiments most of which were performed in my own kitchen I was able to form a sausage-shaped distensible segment which I tried to reinforce with the silk mesh. When I mounted the material on normal catheter tubing and applied pressure to distend the aneurysmal segment, I suddenly realized that the strength of this material was so great that the silk mesh was not necessary. This was a great breakthrough and enabled me to reduce the size of the catheter."

There were severe criticisms especially by the surgeons and particularly by the internists as regards to the safety of his procedure. However, Dr Ake Senning, a well-known cardiovascular surgeon, in his institute supported him to further develop the methods to remove the blocks in the occluded arteries. The earlier designs were of single lumen catheters. However, he was in search of technique to produce double lumen catheters and ultimately could get help from Schneider Medintag Company. On October 22, 1975, he performed the first canine coronary angioplasty after cardiac surgeon Marko Turina had produced coronary stenosis with silk ligature and in about years "time several dogs" angioplasty was performed and he was ready to perform coronary angioplasty in the clinical use, since the double lumen catheter had been produced by Schneider Medintag. However, he found it difficult to get the first patient. Though according to the historical records it is mentioned that the first angioplasty was performed intraoperatively, actually attempt to perform angioplasty in Catheterization Laboratory was attempted earlier to intraoperative procedure. On March 22, 1976, a 63-year-old man was referred to Gruentzig with several myocardial infarctions, unstable angina, severe triple vessel disease, left main stenosis, and peripheral vascular disease and was turned down by cardiac surgeons. After some initial hesitations he attempted to perform the procedure from left brachial artery. However, he could not engage coronary ostium due to bulky 10F guiding catheter. The procedure was abandoned. The patient expired after few days. However, Dr Richard K Myler from San Francisco, USA was impressed by Dr Gruentzig's presentation of dog experiments during the annual convention of the American Heart Association in Miami in November 1976 (Fig. 5). He invited him to perform the procedure intraoperatively during open heart surgery by a team of Elias Hanna. The team consisted of Hanna, Myler, and Gruentzig.

However, Dr Gruentzig was keen to perform the procedure in the cardiac catheterization laboratory. He had to wait until September 1977 when Dr Bernhard Meire referred 38 years old patient who had unstable angina pains of several weeks duration and the angiography had shown discrete left anterior descending (LAD) lesion. As a matter of fact patient was advised CABG surgery and to the good luck of Dr Gruentzig and the future interventional cardiology community, patient agreed to undergo the LAD dilatation procedure. The procedure was performed in the University Hospital of Zurich. Postprocedure angiography has been performed which revealed patent LAD. The first patient became friend of Andrea Gruentzig and used to participate as a popular delegate in live teaching course of angioplasty.

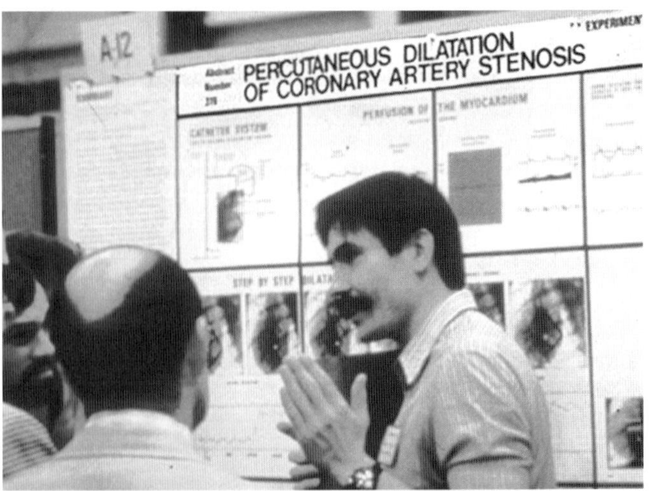

FIG. 5: Dr Andreas Gruentzig at American Heart Association meeting with his presentation.

In addition to developing balloon angioplasty technique, it was to the credit of Dr Gruentzig that he started live demonstration courses. Four such courses were held in Zurich before he moved to USA. During these courses some of the stalwarts and who is who of cardiovascular specialty would be the ones who would be attending these courses. One could meet Dotter, Gruentzig, Mason Sones and Judkins under one roof. Unfortunately all of them died in 1985. Angioplasty thus proved to be a small step for Gruentzig, but a huge leap for percutaneous treatment of coronary artery disease. The numbers slowly tended to grow and it was not surprising that angioplasty numbers have now outnumbered the surgical numbers.

In the beginning, the procedure was recommended for some selective cases. However, the next major step was by John Simpsons who proposed removable of guide wire which would allow the torque control. He named it "steerable guide wire". He designed the wire which had solid core which was tapered toward the distal end to increase flexibility. The guide wire could be moved independently and facilitate the negotiation of the vessel by the balloon. However, these were over the wire systems and maneuvering was little more cumbersome. The next was monorail system developed by Bonzel. The term monorail was coined by Bernhard Meire.

NEW DEVICES

Subsequent to balloon angioplasty acceptance as a definite procedure for treating obstructive coronary artery disease, several problems were encountered by the angioplasters. Some of them were (A) calcified and bulky lesions, (B) small diameter vessels, (C) restenosis, and (D) of course the greatest challenge that would jeopardize the life of the patient, was the acute reclosure after balloon angioplasty due to dissection of the artery and impending acute myocardial infarction. In the early era of angioplasty, it was mandatory to have stood by surgical back up. The interventional cardiologists, engineers, technologists worked together to address some of these problems so as to make the procedure accepted by the patients easily and match the results of coronary artery bypass graft surgery. The result was development of several new adjunctive devices.

Directional Atherectomy

This was one of the first new devices and John Simpson in 1985 was instrumental in developing this device with Flexicut Device Company. The technique could cut huge bulky or calcified plaques giving a larger lumen diameter. However, the procedure later became unpopular since the device was bulky needing large guide catheter, with risk of dissection and arterial closure and myocardial infarction. Moreover, it failed to show reduction in rates of restenosis.

Transluminal extraction catheter (TEC) was designed by Starr. It was over the wire conical system with two stainless steel cutters which cut and aspirated the atheromatous material. Its use was largely defined in the saphenous vein grafts.

Rotational Atherectomy

This high-speed rotational atherectomy device was developed by Auth, a Biomed Engineer who started to investigate the rotational atherectomy as an alternative to debulking with directional coronary atherectomy (DCA) or TEC. The burr spins at 160,000–200,000 p/m pulverizing plaque and calcium in tiny particles. After several experiments the first case of rotational atherectomy in humans was performed by Zaka in Houston and the first coronary rotational atherectomy on January 06, 1988 by Fourrer Bernard in a 68-year-old woman with stable angina. Apart from stents, rotational atherectomy has withstood the test of time. The frequency of its use varies from operator to operator and probably its use is in the range of 5–10% .However, its use is limited to severely calcified lesion.

Laser Angioplasty

It was introduced in interventional cardiology during the beginning years of 1980s and was used in patients with total occlusion and became popular procedure in early 80s. However, the earlier data indicated higher restenosis rate and failed to show benefit of laser and comparable techniques.

Brachytherapy

Several autopsy specimens and animal experiment showed that restenosis occurred due to neointimal proliferation. To reduce the risk of neointimal proliferation, brachytherapy with gamma and beta radiation obtained through different sources and devices was explored. Several post-brachytherapy patients developed stent thrombosis. With the advent of drug-eluting stents, brachytherapy was removed from the market.

Coronary Stents

Stents have been the most important innovation in the field of coronary angioplasty after balloon angioplasty. Stents were able to address two major challenges of balloon angioplasty: (1) acute closure during the angioplasty procedure could be handled affectively since, it provided scaffold to the dissected intima and (2) reduced the risk of restenosis.

The word stent is named after Charles Stenting, an English dentist, who used the dental impression in 1856. The history of first coronary artery stenting started with meeting of two Swedish individuals at a gathering. Wallsten was a designer of a revolutionary machine intended to manufacture paper and Senning one of the most popular surgeon from Switzerland. Dr Senning explained to Wallsten the difficulties of treating aortic dissection. Wallsten agreed to design endovascular prosthesis and created the Wallstent. Subsequently, Puel implanted the first coronary stent on March 28, 1986 and subsequently Sigwart and Puel continued to carry on with their work on stents. Subsequently, new designs like Palmas Schatz, Wiktor, Gianturco-Roubin, NIR, and Multilink flooded the market. These stents tackled the issue of acute reclosure and reduced the incidence of restenosis, but not to a large numbers. There was need to reduce neointimal proliferation. In 1999, Cordis introduced rapamycin-coated stent called CYPHER. Rapamycin and its analogs decrease neointimal proliferation and thus would reduce the chances of restenosis. First implantation and data was published in First In Man (FIM) trial by Patrick Serruys and Eduardo Sousa from Rotterdam and Sao Paulo. Subsequently, several large scale trials have shown favorable results of drug-eluting stents. Currently, several analogs of rapamycin have been used on cobalt-chromium platform. The field is ever expanding with newer metallic bioabsorbable stents under trial.

HISTORY OF FRACTIONAL FLOW RESERVE, INTRAVASCULAR ULTRASOUND, AND OPTICAL COHERENCE TOMOGRAPHY

Fractional Flow Reserve

Like present times, the quandary faced by clinicians at the beginning of invasive coronary angiography in the seventies was to determine which lesions were important, and which were not. There were very few techniques for measuring human coronary blood flow. In 1974, Dr K. Lance Gould demonstrated that coronary flow reserve (CFR) or hyperemic maximal to basal flow ratio could be related to stenosis severity, and perhaps overcome the limitations and ambiguity of the coronary angiogram for detection of ischemia.

In animal experiments, he showed that CFR began to decline when stenoses were more than 60% narrow and resting flow decreased when stenoses were more than 90% narrowed. Hence, it was thought that coronary physiology could predict anatomy and vice versa. However, it was realized that in human patients, unlike in the experimental dogs, CFR was poorly related to the angiographic percentage narrowing, because of two factors: (1) the inability of the angiogram to precisely determine the stenosis area and length, and (2) the fact that some patients had microvascular disease and an impaired coronary flow reserve, even with normal coronary arteries.

However, Dr Andreas Gruentzig's coronary angioplasty balloon catheter changed cardiology history on July 12, 1979, when it used a small pressure lumen to measure translesional gradients.

He reported the first "nonoperative dilatation of the coronary artery stenosis"; that is, percutaneous coronary balloon angioplasty, in the New England Journal of Medicine. This paper showed the method and results of the dilating Grüntzig catheter inflating in a stenosis. The measurement of the pressure gradient before and after the balloon inflation and deflation was used to guide the procedure, and overcome the very poor angiographic image quality at that time. However, pressure measurements during PTCA were questioned, because of the technical difficulty of measuring pressure through a large 4.5F catheter with a small, fluid-filled pressure lumen.

Over the next few years, coronary angiography improved dramatically and many like Dr Jeff Hartzler, did not feel the need for measurement of pressure to do angioplasty.

Nico Pijls from Eindhoven, the Netherlands, and Bernard De Bruyne in Aalst, Belgium, were the first to begin using a 0.014-inch hollow sensor angioplasty guide wire to measure pressure across a stenosis. With this invention, the evolution of the pressure-only flow reserve theory could be tested, which culminated in the derivation and application of the fractional flow reserve (FFR) concept. FFR is the percent of stenotic flow to normal flow across a stenosis. The flow ratio is computed from the distal or aortic pressure measurements at maximal hyperemia. One important aspect in the development of the FFR was the incorporation of venous pressure to account for collateral flow, making the validation successful in both the animal lab as well as in clinical outcome studies.

In 1996 the validation of FFR, published in the New England Journal of Medicine by Nico, Bernard, and others, demonstrated a strong relationship of myocardial ischemia to an FFR value of 0.75. The sensitivity of FFR in the identification of reversible ischemia was 88%, the specificity 100%, the positive predictive value 100%, the negative predictive value 88%, and the accuracy 93%.

The rest, as they say, is history!

The future of coronary physiology over the next decade is the validation and application of noninvasive imaging-based FFR such as FFRCT (computed tomography-derived FFR), using 3D reconstruction of the arterial imaging scan and applying computational fluid dynamics.

Another development is the resting pressure ratio of the instantaneous wave-free ratio which obviates the use of vasodilator injection for hyperemia.

Quantitative flow ratio (QFR) does away with both pressure wires and induction of hyperemia. It is based on computation of standard invasive coronary angiographic imaging and is derived from fluid dynamic equations incorporating vessel geometry, assumptions on flow through a stenosis, and vessel tapering.

Thus, these are exciting times for coronary physiology and interventional cardiology.

Intravascular Ultrasound

Tremendous advances have occurred during the last 40 years in the field of medical imaging of the heart and the coronary vasculature, triggered by the increasing need to reduce or prevent coronary artery disease.

Although in 1960s and early 1970s, noninvasive method was the most preferred method for the clinical use of heart and great arteries, with increased understanding of coronary artery diseases, noninvasive method alone could not have sufficient resolution and penetration depth to give a direct image of smaller size vessel like coronary arteries.

Due to these limitations of noninvasive method, intravascular imaging route led to the development of X-ray angiography in the 1960s, balloon angioplasty and related techniques in the late 1970s and early 1980s. Meanwhile, in the early 1970s, academic research programs focused on developing two-dimensional real-time ultrasound imaging of the heart, transferring in particular knowledge from underwater acoustics to medicine. This noninvasive route led to echocardiography, an imaging modality acclaimed for its radiation-free nature but lacking the resolution to image the coronary vasculature.

The first trial of using ultrasound invasively to make image of mammalian lumen was done by Cieszynski in 1956, where a single-element echo catheter was used to measure a dog's cardiac chamber dimensions. In 1969, the cross-section image of an animal's cardiac chamber was first reconstructed and reported with ultrasound by Eggleton et al. In the same year, the first design of cylindrical transducer was first designed by Carelton et al.

From the time of the first implantation of coronary stent in human in 1986, cardiologists were trying to find ways how to investigate coronary vessels *in vivo* from inside. The first method used for this purpose was angioscopy, a method that allows only surface assessment of the vessel.

A need was felt in the early 1990s to provide high-resolution images of diseased coronary artery wall structures, referred to as vulnerable plaques and primarily responsible for myocardial infarctions, when false-negative coronary angiography cases became evident. Intravascular ultrasound (IVUS) is a catheter-based echocardiography modality that was patented by Bom in 1972 and further developed to investigate the status of the coronary artery wall.

Twenty years after its introduction in the clinic in the early 1990s, IVUS technology continues to bring scientific insight into the pathophysiology of the coronary artery disease and not only helps guiding percutaneous coronary interventions, but also research into plaque growth and regression.

Optical Coherence Tomography

Predicting the risk for future acute cardiovascular events requires knowledge of plaque composition, which is not yet provided by conventional IVUS, although several IVUS signal processing techniques have been developed at research level to augment IVUS capabilities in detecting and characterizing coronary artery plaques at risk.

Optical coherence tomography (OCT) was first described more than two decades ago when it was used to image the peripapillary area of the human retina *in vitro*. Eleven years later, OCT was used to image atherosclerotic plaques in human coronary arteries. The image resolution achievable with OCT (axial: 10 μm, lateral: 20–40 μm) far surpasses that of IVUS (100–200 μm). Histological studies have shown that certain adverse plaque phenotypes are associated with the onset of an acute coronary syndrome (ACS). With its excellent spatial resolution, OCT is ideally placed to identify vulnerable plaque that could result in ACS.

While IVUS offers an improved imaging depth for the assessment of lipid or necrotic plaques, intravascular OCT offers better penetration and enhanced imaging of calcific tissue. Intravascular OCT requires a short injection of contrast (e.g., 2–3 seconds) in a similar way to obtain an angiographic image. IVUS does not require a contrast injection as ultrasounds can penetrate through blood.

Since, its first clinical application reported by Huang and coworkers in 1991, suggesting the principle of its use both in ophthalmology and interventional cardiology, the method has developed rapidly and is now used in increasing number of cases, both in routine clinical situations and research projects. Its detailed intravascular imaging ability, providing real-time information of the intracoronary pathology has benefited interventional cardiology tremendously.

Future of Optical Coherence Tomography in Interventional Cardiology

Optical coherence tomography imaging technique is constantly developing and opening new horizons in the coronary interventions. One is development of the software for the 3D reconstruction of the OCT image. In the near future, introduction of the micro-OCT system is expected which should provide extreme image resolution (up to 1 μm). With this level of resolution cellular structure of endothelial tissue should be assessable. One can only imagine its application not only in the evaluation of disease process but also in its prevention.

REFERENCES

1. Forssmann W. Die Sondierung des rechten Herzens. Klin Wschr. 1929;8:2085.
2. Cournand A, Ranges H. Catheterization of the right auricle in man. Proc Soc Exp Biol Med. 1941;46:462-6.
3. Cournand A. Cardiac catheterization; development of the technique, its contributions to experimental medicine, and its initial applications in man. Acta Med Scand Suppl. 1975;579:3-32.
4. Radner S. An attempt at the roentgenologic visualization of coronary blood vessels in man. Acta Radiol (Old Series). 1945;26:497-502.
5. Dotter C, Judkins M. Transluminal treatment of arteriosclerotic obstruction: Description of a new technic and a preliminary report of its application. Circulation. 1964;3:654-70.
6. Dotter CT, Frische LH, Hoskinson WS, et al. Coronary arteriography during induced cardiac arrest and aortic occlusion. Arch Intern Med. 1959;104:720-9.
7. Bertrand ME, Meier B. A history of cardiac catheterization. Percutaneous Interventional Cardiovascular Medicine. The PCR-EAPCI Textbook. 2012. pp. 3-40.
8. Sones FM, Shirey EK. Cine coronary arteriography. Mod Concepts Cardiovasc Dis. 1962;31:735-8.
9. Sheldon WC. Pathfinders of the Heart: The History of Cardiology at the Cleveland Clinic. Bloomington, IN: Xlibris Corporation, 2008:26-7.
10. Judkins MP. Selective coronary arteriography. Part 1. A percutaneous transfemoral technic. Radiology. 1967;89:815-24.
11. Gruentzig A, Turina M, Schneider J. Experimental percutaneous dilatation of coronary artery stenosis (abstract). Circulation. 1976;53:II-81.
12. Gruentzig A. Transluminal dilatation of coronary-artery stenosis. Lancet. 1978; 1:263.
13. Meier B. The first patient to undergo coronary angioplasty: 23-year follow-up. N Engl J Med. 2001;344:144-5.
14. Hurst J. The first coronary angioplasty as described by Andreas Gruentzig. Am J Cardiol. 1986;57:185-6.
15. Gruentzig AR, Senning A, Siegenthaleer WE. Nonoperative dilatation of coronary-artery stenosis: Percutaneous transluminal coronary angioplasty. N Engl J Med. 1979;301:61-8.
16. Simpson JB, Baim DS, Robert EW, et al. A new catheter system for coronary angioplasty. Am J cardiol. 1982;49:1216-22.
17. Bonzel T, Wollschlager H, Just H. A new catheter system for the mechanical dilatation of coronary stenoses with exchangeable intracoronary catheters, fast flow of the contrast agent and improved control. Biomed Tech (Berl). 1986;31:195-200.
18. Simpson J, Johnson D, Thapliyal HV. Transluminal atherectomy: A new approach to the treatment of atherosclerotic vascular disease. Circulation. 1985;72:111.

19. Sigwart U, Puel J, Mirkovitch V, et al. Intravascular stents to prevent occlusion and restenosis after transluminal angioplasty. N Engl J Med. 1987;316:701-6.
20. Serruys PW, de Jaegere P, Kiemeneij F, et al. A comparison of balloon-expandable-stent implantation with balloon angioplasty in patients with coronary artery disease. Benestent Study Group. N Engl J Med. 1994;331:489-95.
21. Morice MC, Serruys PW, Sousa JE, et al. Randomized study with the Sirolimus-Coated Bx Velocity Balloon-Expandable Stent in the treatment of patients with de Novo Native Coronary Artery Lesions. A randomized comparison of a sirolimus-eluting stent with a standard stent for coronary revascularization. N Engl J Med. 2002;346:1773-80.
22. Tahara N, Imaizumi T, Virmani R, et al. Clinical feasibility of molecular imaging of plaque inflammation in atherosclerosis. J Nucl Med. 2009;50:331-4.
23. Gould KL, Lipscomb K, Hamilton GW. Physiologic basis for assessing critical coronary stenosis. Instantaneous flow response and regional distribution during coronary hyperemia as measures of coronary flow reserve. Am J Cardiol. 1974;33(1):87-94.
24. Pijls NH, van Son JA, Kirkeeide RL, et al. Experimental basis of determining maximum coronary, myocardial, and collateral blood flow by pressure measurements for assessing functional stenosis severity before and after percutaneous transluminal coronary angioplasty. Circulation. 1993;87:1354-67.
25. Yoxen E. Seeing with sound: a study of the development of medical images. The Social Construction of Technological Systems: New Directions in the Sociology and History of Technology. Boston: MIT Press. 1987;281.
26. Huang D., Swanson EA, Lin CP, et al. Optical coherence tomography. Science. 1991;254:1178-81.

CHAPTER 56

Bifurcation Stenting: Optimal Strategy in 2018

Ashwin B Mehta, Nihar Mehta

INTRODUCTION

Coronary artery bifurcations are prone to develop atherosclerotic plaques due to turbulent blood flow and high-shear stress. Bifurcation lesions are commonly accounting for approximately 15–20% of all percutaneous coronary interventions (PCIs).[1,2] Bifurcation stenting in 2018 is still complex, since it is associated with a high risk of stent thrombosis and significant restenosis. With the use of drug-eluting stents (DESs) there has been reduction in the rate of restenosis and reintervention as compared to bare-metal stents (BMSs).[3] This subset of coronary artery disease intervention poses unique challenge of obtaining optimal result in the main vessel (MV) while maintaining the side branch (SB) patency. Understanding the anatomy and physiology of the coronary bifurcation lesions is essential to achieve this goal. While stenting of the MV and stenting of the SB to salvage it if flow is impaired (provisional strategy) is preferred, there are instances where upfront elective two-stent strategy needs to be used. The carina and SB ostium are central to the bifurcation anatomy and several strategies can be used to ensure the optimal results.

DEFINITIONS AND CLASSIFICATIONS

A coronary bifurcation lesion is defined as a coronary artery narrowing occurring adjacent to, and/or involving, the origin of a significant SB (Fig. 1). A significant SB is a branch, closure of which could lead to important adverse sequelae to the patient. Usually these are SBs more than 2.0 mm in diameter.

A bifurcation lesion involves three distinct anatomical segments; the proximal MV, the distal MV, and the SB. The bifurcation carina is the transition zone between the MV and the SB and is the core of the bifurcation anatomy.

In an attempt to simplify classifications, Medina et al. proposed a classification which is easier to remember in comparison to older ones. However, the Medina classification has shortcomings. It does not relate to angulation of the distal main branch (MB) and SB, length of the SB, plaque distribution, and the size of the proximal healthy segment which all affects the strategy and decision making (Fig. 2).[4]

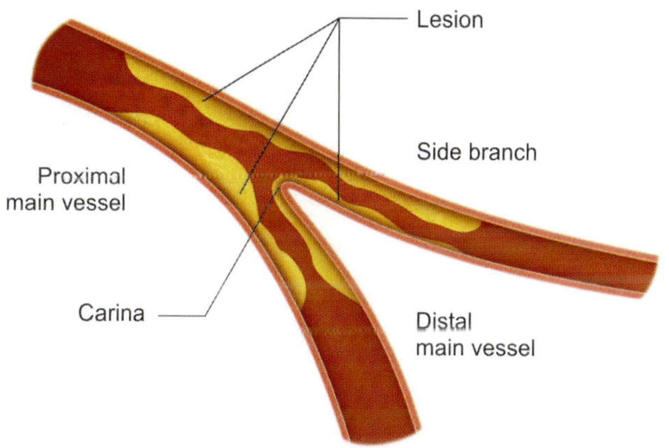

FIG. 1: Anatomy of a coronary bifurcation.

A "true bifurcation lesion" is one in which both the MV and the SB have more than 50% stenosis (Medina types 1,1,1 or 1,0,1 or 0,1,1). A "pseudo bifurcation lesion" is one which does not have significant disease at the ostium of the SB (Medina types 1,1,0 or 1,0,0 or 0,1,0).

ANATOMICAL CONSIDERATIONS

Angle assessment in bifurcation lesions is used to measure two angles: (i) The "Take-off Angle" or proximal angle or angle A (*Access* angle) between the proximal MV and the SB and (ii) The "Carina angle" or angle B (*Between*) between the distal MV and the SB (Fig. 3). The angle A gives a measure of difficulty in accessing the SB. The acuteness of Angle B increases the risk of carina displacement and SB occlusion (SBO) after stent placement. The angles between the distal MV and SB (angle B) affect the outcome of PCI pertaining to ease of wire access and stent deliverability, plaque shift or "snow-ploughing" effect and complete coverage of ostium of SB.[4]

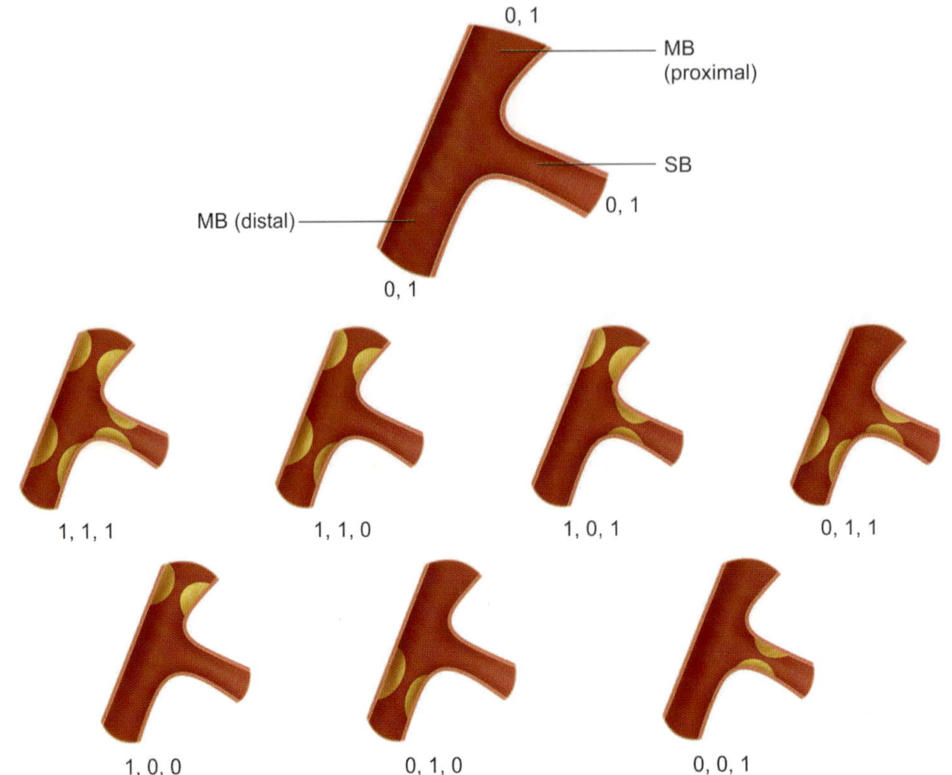

MB, main branch; SB, side branch.

FIG. 2: Medina classification of bifurcation lesions.[5]

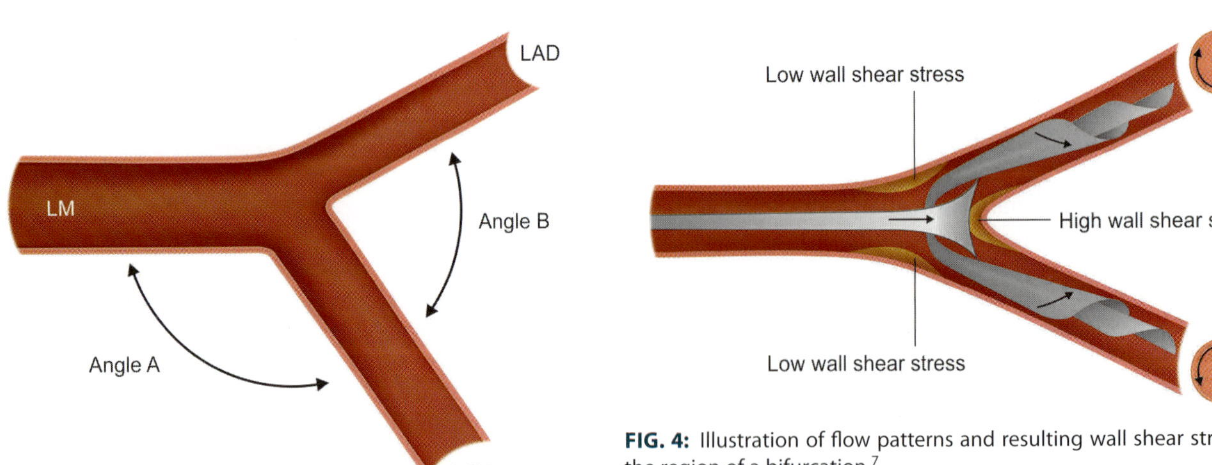

LAD, left anterior descending artery; LCX, left circumflex artery; LM, left main.

FIG. 3: Anatomy of the bifurcation angle.

FIG. 4: Illustration of flow patterns and resulting wall shear stress in the region of a bifurcation.[7]

- Angle B when less than 70°, it is called a "Y-angulation" and allows easy wire access to the SB, but plaque shifting is potentially more pronounced and precise stent placement with complete ostial coverage is often difficult or geometrically impossible.
- Angle B when more than 70°, it is called a "T-angulation" and wire access to the SB is usually more difficult. However, plaque shifting is less frequent and precise stent placement with complete ostial coverage is technically easier and more likely.

Plaque distribution in bifurcation lesions is localized exclusively to the outer wall of one or both daughter vessels where the wall shear stress (WSS) is low. The term "WSS" refers to the stress on the arterial wall due to the friction associated with the viscous fluid flowing past the arterial wall (Fig. 4). Atherosclerosis occurs early in areas of nonuniform and low WSS. On the other hand, areas of uniform, high WSS are protected. Thus, the carina is usually protected and the plaques develop in both branches opposite to the carina.[6,7] In studies done using intravascular ultrasound (IVUS), this theory has been supported showing sparing of the carina.[8]

RELATION BETWEEN SIZES OF VESSELS: MURRAY'S LAW[9] AND FINET'S LAW[10]

In the bifurcation anatomy, it is important to understand the relationship between the sizes of the vessels. The fact that the MV is larger than the MB is frequently forgotten during procedures.

There is an important mother daughter mathematical relationship first described by Murray, based on the principle of minimum work.[9] Murray's law states that the size of the proximal MV (D_{MV}) and the size of the daughter vessels (D_{MB} and D_{SB}) are represented by the following formula:

$$D_{MV}^3 = D_{MB}^3 + D_{SB}^3$$

This formula has been proven in normal and diseased vessels by IVUS study.[11] It, however, was incorrect in calcified vessels and in the culprit lesions of acute coronary syndrome. The following implications can be derived from this formula.

- The difference in the diameter (size discrepancy) between the proximal MV and distal main branch (MB) is dependent on the size of the SB. The larger the SB, the more is the size discrepancy. Therefore, it is imperative to perform the proximal optimization technique (POT) in bifurcation lesions with a large SB (details of POT are described later)
- When kissing balloon inflation is performed with balloons sized according to the two branches—MB and SB, the balloons would always be oversized for the proximal MV. According to Murray's law, the sum of the cross-sectional areas of the balloons of the two branches would be larger than the cross-sectional area of the proximal MV. Therefore, it would be advisable to be conservative in balloon inflation pressures, going up to only moderate pressures during kissing balloon inflation (kissing balloon inflation is described later).

Finet et al. modified this to derive the simple formula:[10]

$$D_{MV} = 0.678\ (D_{MB} + D_{SB})$$

This formula can be used to calculate the size of one vessel if the sizes of the other two vessels in the bifurcation are known. However, this relationship can be quite variable according to the vessel size. For example, if the SB is small, the calculated value of the MV is smaller than the MB, which cannot be true![12]

To summarize, the relationship between the size of the MV, MB, and SB are the key to select the optimal strategy of POT and kissing balloon inflation. Considering the variation in the size of the branches and the inadequacy of the Murray's and Finet's laws, IVUS should be used for optimal sizing and improved cardiovascular outcomes.[13]

PLAQUE SHIFT VERSUS CARINA SHIFT

The most common complication of bifurcation stenting is the closure of the SB. The major mechanism for SBO was assumed to be plaque shift from the MV to the SB. However, the carina was found to be spared of atherosclerotic plaque burden due to high WSS (Fig. 4).[7] Scanty plaque at the carina could not be the cause for major plaque shift. Carina shift is a major contributor to anatomical SBO, which has been proven by IVUS study of the MV and SB (Fig. 5).[14]

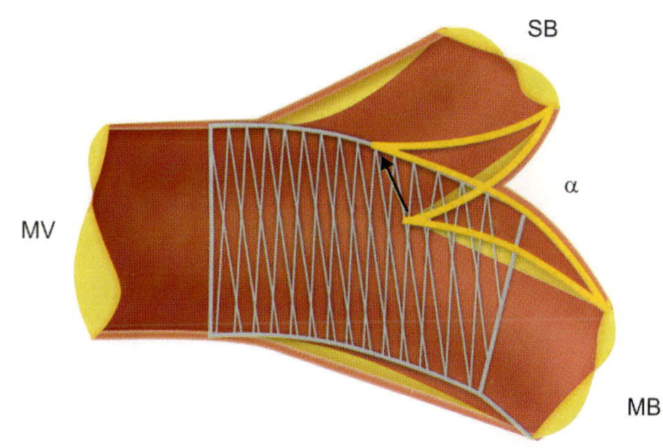

MB, main branch; MV, main vessel; SB, side branch.

FIG. 5: Carina shift during stenting according to size of MV.[14]

Conversely, functional studies using fractional flow reserve (FFR) showed opposite results. Kang et al. evaluated the MV and SB using FFR and IVUS in a study of 40 patients and showed that carina shift was mostly not associated with a significant drop in FFR. Abnormal FFR in the SB was almost always associated with plaque shift.[15] Angiographically, carina shift can look exaggerated but is often functionally insignificant.

The main causes of SBO due to plaque shift were identified as proximal MV disease, SB ostial disease, and acute coronary syndrome.[16] An IVUS study showed that plaque shift mainly comes from proximal MV disease.[14] The bifurcation angle was not a major predictor of SBO which suggested that carina shift was not the main reason for SB compromise.

To summarize, the compromise of the SB after provisional MV stenting is usually due to carina shift and is functionally not significant. Significant SBO usually results from plaque shift, for which the main predictor is proximal MV disease burden.

THREATENED SIDE BRANCH MORPHOLOGIES: PREVENTING SIDE BRANCH OCCLUSION

The major cause of complexity during bifurcation stenting is the occlusion of the SB. The main goal is identifying the SB at risk and preserving it.

The concept of "threatened SB morphologies" needs special consideration as regards to the incidence of SBO. In studies done comparing the incidence of SBO based on threatened versus nonthreatened SB morphologies, the incidence of SBO was significantly higher in threatened morphologies (80%) as compared to nonthreatened morphologies (7.9%) (Fig. 6).[4]

The COBIS (Coronary BIfurcation Stenting) II registry of 2,227 patients who were treated with provisional stenting identified the following predictors of SBO:[16]

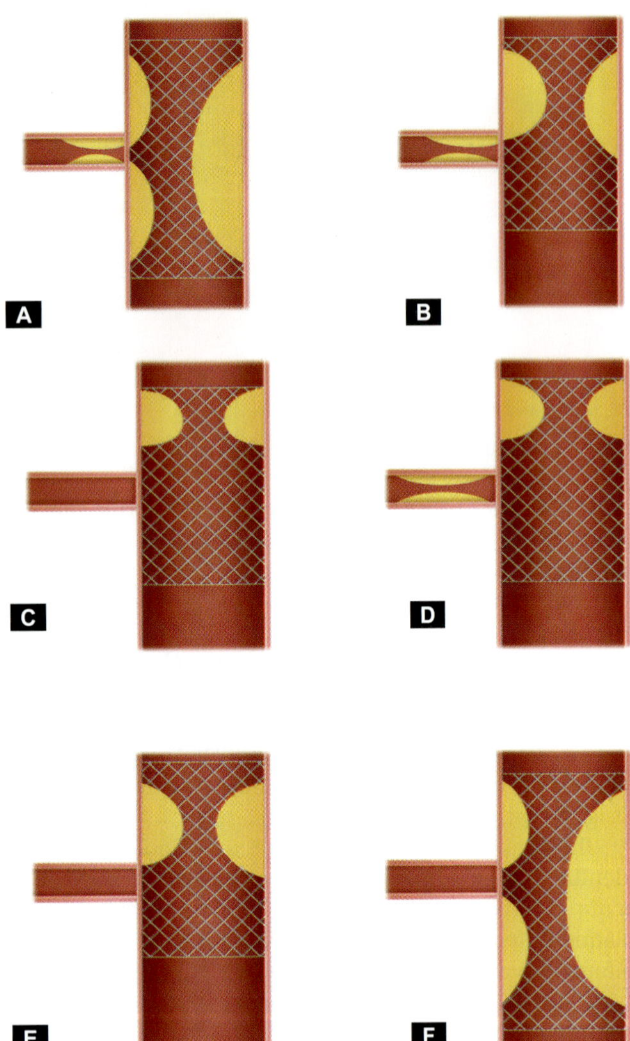

FIG. 6: Threatened side branch morphologies:[4] **A,** Side branch (SB) with more than 50% ostial narrowing where the origin is completely spanned by either the diseased segment or the index lesion; **B,** SB arises adjacent to or is partially contiguous with the diseased index lesion. Nonthreatened SB morphologies includes: **C,** SB without ostial narrowing; **D,** SB with ostial involvement; **E,** Disease-free SB arising adjacent to diseased segment of the parent vessel; **F,** SB without ostial disease arising from parent vessel lesion spanning the entire origin of the SB.

- Side branch ostial disease
- Side branch lesion length
- Diseased MB
- Non-left main bifurcations
- Acute coronary syndrome.

On the other hand, SB predilatation, jailed wire technique, and IVUS guidance were not predictors of SBO.

STENTING STRATEGY IN BIFURCATION LESIONS—ONE OR TWO STENTS?

The strategy to use one stent (in the MV) or two stents (one in the MV and one in the SB) for the treatment of bifurcation lesions has been long debated.[14-16] The most important initial questions are whether the SB is large enough (>2.25 mm diameter) and whether the SB supplies a large enough territory to justify its intervention. In the provisional SB stenting strategy, the MV is stented first and the SB is stented through the MV stent, only if necessary. Thus, the use of the second stent is provisional.

The primary reason why the PCI of bifurcation lesions has been a challenge is the risk of SBO or compromise after treating the MV. Hence, understanding the anatomic attributes characterizing the lesion including the bifurcation angle, the size of SB, myocardial territory supplied by the SB, lesion length in SB, and distribution of MV disease are essential. Thus the approach of "one for all" is not practical in all bifurcations. Hence, provisional stenting should not be used as a default strategy in "high-risk bifurcations" that involve a large SB. In some patients, elective double stenting (EDS) strategy is opted for to reduce the risk of large SB compromise.[4]

Provisional Side Branch Stenting Strategy

This strategy involves stenting the MV first. If necessary, a second stent is delivered to the SB through the MV stent in a classic T, T-stenting and protrusion (TAP) (T and small protrusion), inverted culotte or internal crush technique. Use of the second stent is only provisional.

Steps

- *Wiring both the branches*: Wiring starts with the most difficult branch. The second wire is inserted into the easier branch by limited rotation manoeuvres to avoid wire wrap. The wire inserted in the SB should be without hydrophilic or polymer coating because the coating may get peeled off during removal of the jailed wire. The advantage of securing the SB with a wire is that it serves as a marker to find the SB lumen, if an occlusion occurs
- *Predilatation*: Predilatation of the MB is left to the operator's discretion. Predilatation of the SB does reduce the risk of SB compromise after MV stenting and also relieves ischemia in the SB territory. It can, however, produce a dissection in the SB. The subsequent step of rewiring the SB through the distal strut of the MB stent may be difficult in presence of dissection. Therefore, predilatation of the SB is reasonable to reduce SB compromise in a high-risk lesion, but the operator should avoid dissections in the SB[12]
- *Stenting the MV across the SB*: The selection of the stent is important. The cell area should allow access to the SB ostium. The diameter of the stent should be selected according to the distal MB (not the proximal MB) in order to avoid excess carina shifting (Fig. 5). Ideally, the stent size should be selected using IVUS. The proximal part of the stent prior to the bifurcation may be dilated with a short 0.5 mm bigger balloon. This is called "POT technique". This results in optimal diameter of the proximal part of the stent and allows the struts of the stent to face the SB which allows subsequent rewiring of the SB (Fig. 7).[17] The POT technique has been shown to reduce

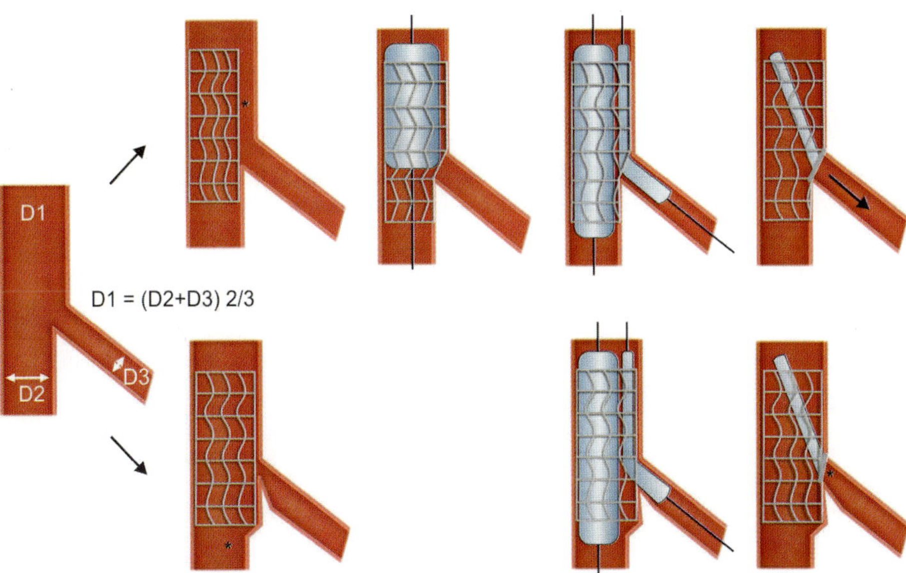

FIG. 7: Consequence of choice of diameter of main vessel (MV) stent. Up—selection according to the diameter of the distal MV followed by proximal optimization technique technique. Down—selection according to the diameter of the proximal MV.

the restenosis rates in the MV when the size of the SB is more than 2.5 mm.[16] An interesting finding was that there was no benefit of POT if final kissing inflation (FKI) was performed, probably due to the effect of two balloons expanded in the proximal MV[16]

- *Side branch rewiring or guide wire exchange*: This step starts with removal of the wire in the MB and inserting it into the SB. Alternatively, a third wire can be used to go through the struts of the MB stent into the SB so that MB position of the initial wire is not disturbed. The SB jailed wire is then removed or passed into the MB if MB wire was removed. The maneuvering of the wire through the MB stent strut should be done carefully, such that the wire enters the distal most strut of the stent. Final kissing balloon inflation performed after this "distal cross" of the guide wire allows correction of the MV stent deformation, allows better scaffolding to the SB ostium, and facilitates better future access to the SB. On the other hand, FKI performed after "proximal cross" of the guide wire results in MV stent deformation and poor SB ostium scaffolding (Fig. 8)[18]
- *Final kissing balloon inflation*: Two short balloons are selected based on the diameter of the distal vessels. They are inflated simultaneously to perform the FKI. For the optimal result of FKI, distal crossing of the wire is preferable.

A subanalysis of the CACTUS trial showed that FKI was associated with a lower major adverse cardiac event (MACE) rate and better angiographic result.[19] However, the Nordic-Baltic Bifurcation III Study randomized 477 patients to FKI versus no FKI in patients treated with MV stenting. This study showed no difference in the MACE rate or event free survival at 6 months. FKI resulted in better angiographic results, especially in true bifurcation lesions. FKI resulted in longer contrast use, angiography, and procedure times.[18] Koo et al. advocated the use of FFR guided jailed SB intervention. Their study of 110 patients showed no difference in the clinical outcomes at 9 months between the groups with or without FFR guided SB angioplasty.[20,21]

The conclusion drawn from these studies does not support routine balloon dilatation of the SB, but advocates use of FFR to guide intervention in a jailed SB. However, after SB ballooning, FKI is mandatory since SB ballooning deforms the MV stent.

- *POT-side-POT (re-POT)*:[12,22] The main goal in coronary bifurcation stenting is optimal expansion of the MV and MB stent. Although, the key issue is preserving the SB patency, but clinical outcomes are highly dependent on the MV stent expansion, particularly in the provisional stenting strategy.[12] Therefore, FKI can be replaced by a second POT. In case the SB needs to be treated, it is rewired and ballooned. This will lead to MV stent deformation which can be corrected by a second POT or a re-POT instead of a FKI. This simplifies the procedure.

The most challenging part of re-POT is precise location of POT balloon. It should cover the proximal edge of stent carina, which can be done by aligning the proximal edge of distal balloon marker with the tip of stent carina (Fig. 9).[12,22] The impact of this technique needs to be evaluated in clinical trails.

- *Provisional SB stenting*: In about 70–80% of cases, the procedure ends at the previous step. In about 20% results in the SB were unsatisfactory after FKI:[20]
    - More than 75% residual stenosis
    - Dissection in SB
    - Thrombolysis in myocardial infarction (TIMI) flow grade less than 3 in a SB more than 2.5 mm diameter
    - Fractional flow reserve less than 0.75
    - Persistent intraprocedural angina or electrocardiogram (ECG) changes.

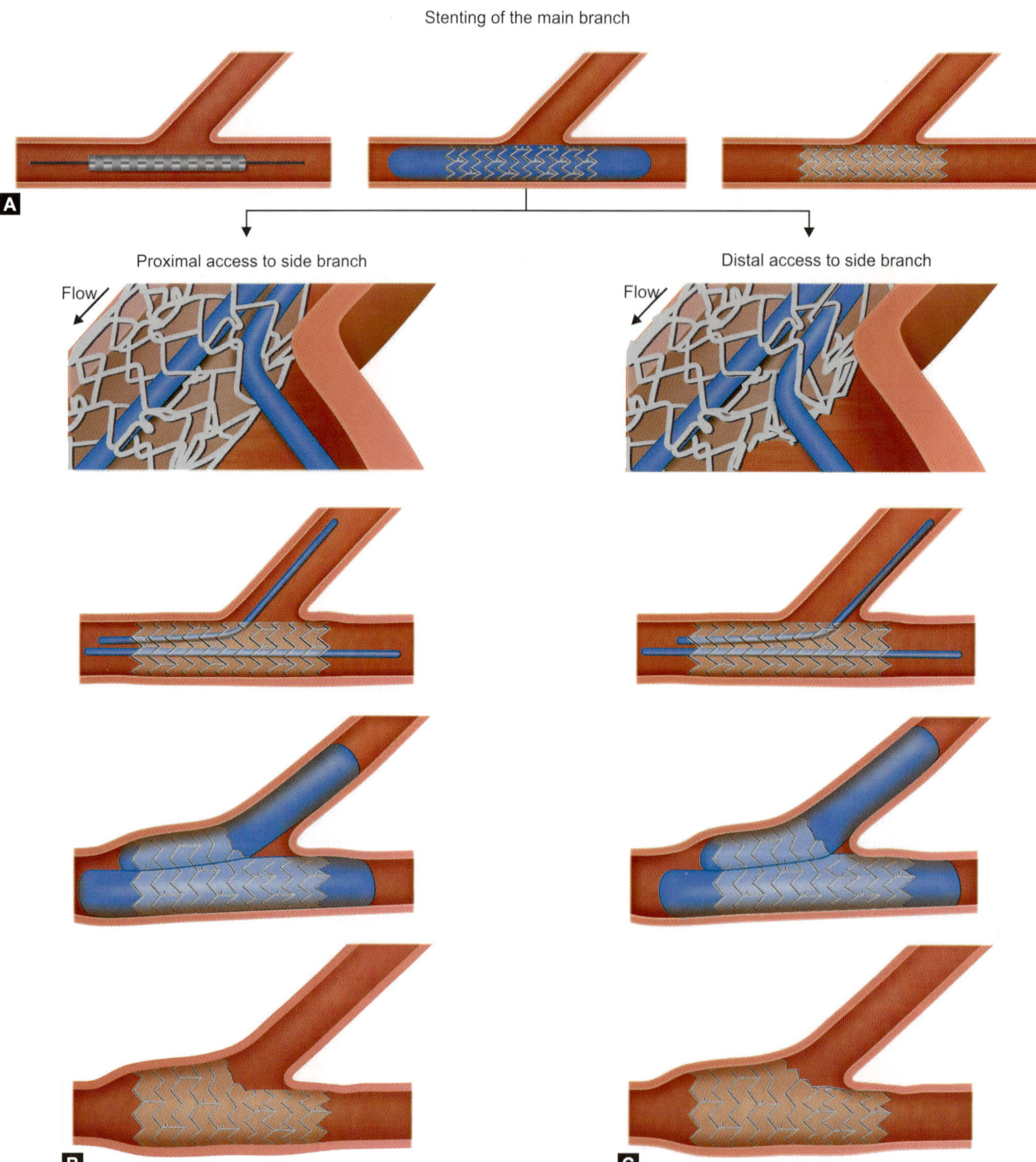

FIG. 8: Proximal versus distal cross during guidewire recrossing and result after final kissing balloon inflation.[18]

In these situations, stenting of the SB is done using reverse T technique, TAP technique, reverse crush or inverted culotte technique.

Evidence for Provisional Stenting Strategy and Indications for Side Branch Stenting

The current evidences favor the provisional stenting strategy as the preferred strategy for bifurcation stenting. The results of several randomized studies and prospective registries were pooled into meta-analyses.[23-26] Overall, the meta-analyses did not reveal any differences at 6–7 month follow-up in terms of mortality, MACE, and target lesion revascularization (TLR), although there was a significant difference in favor of the single-stent group in the Bifurcation Coronary Study (BBC) One study.[27]

The Nordic Baltic Bifurcation Study IV randomized 450 patients to compare provisional SB stenting versus two-stent strategy in treatment of true bifurcation lesions with a

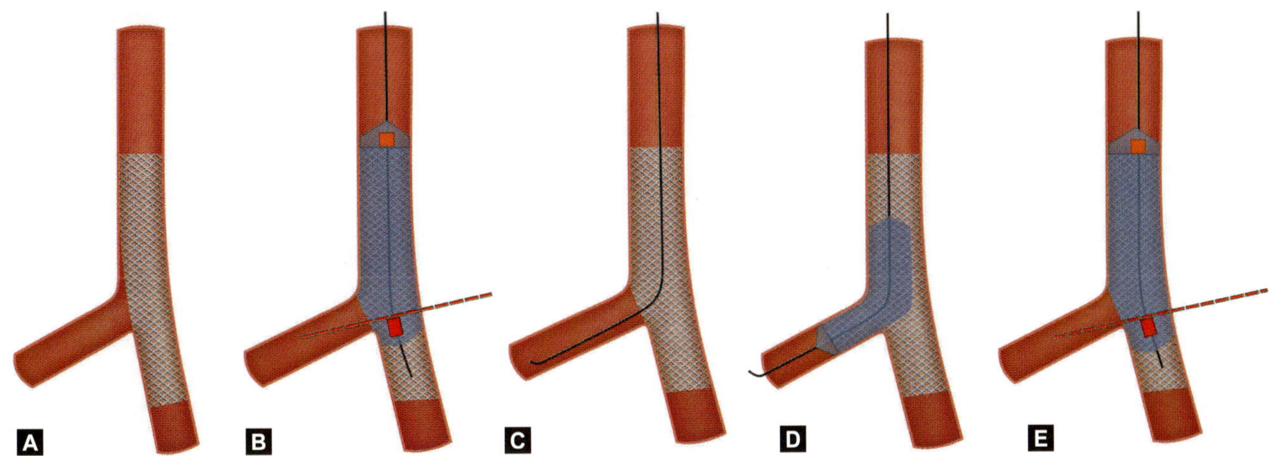

FIG. 9: The POT-side-POT technique. **A,** Stenting the main vessel and main branch (MB) according to the distal MB size; **B,** Proximal optimization therapy (POT); **C,** Re-wiring the side branch; **D,** Side branch balloon dilatation; **E,** Re-POT (second POT).[22]

large SB. After 2 years, two-stent techniques for treatment of true bifurcation lesions with a large SB showed no significant difference in MACE rate compared to provisional SB stenting.[28]

To determine the indication for SB stenting in a provisional stenting strategy, the SMART-STRATEGY (Smart Angioplasty Research Team-Optimal Strategy for Side Branch Intervention in Coronary Bifurcation Lesions) trial divided patients into a conservative group and a aggressive group. In the conservative group, SB stenting was indicated if TIMI flow less than 3 in non-left main bifurcation or if the diameter stenosis was more than 50% or dissection occurred in left main bifurcation. In the aggressive group, SB stenting was indicated if diameter stenosis more than 50% or dissection in non-left main or if the diameter stenosis was more than 30% or dissection occurred in left main bifurcation. Target vessel failure (TVF), the primary endpoint was similar between two groups (9.4% vs. 9.2%, p = 0.97). The mortality was numerically lower (0.8% vs. 2.3%, p = 0.62) in conservative group, although not statistically significant. Periprocedural myocardial infarction (MI) was significantly lower in consevative group (5.5% vs. 17.7%, p = 0.002).[29]

The European Bifurcation Coronary TWO (EBC TWO) trial compared provisional one-stent technique with elective two-stenting in the large caliber true bifurcation lesions (SB diameter ≥2.5 mm) and significant ostial disease length (≥5 mm), but MACE was not different between two groups.[30]

Based on these data, current opinion favors provisional SB stenting with placement of DES in the MV. One should be conservative in stenting of the SB.

Elective Double Stent Strategy

Although provisional stenting has been a preferred option according to many randomized controlled trial, in situations where the SB is large or severely diseased, or supplies a large area of myocardium, the two-stent strategy is still often preferred because of its superior acute angiographic result and lower risk of SB compromise.

Indications

- True bifurcation lesions—MV and SB have more than 50% stenosis (Medina classification 1,1,1 or 1,0,1 or 0,1,1)
- Side branch supplies a large area of myocardium
- Side branch has a diameter appropriate for stenting; more than 2.25 mm
- Side branch lesion is severe and/or long
- Wide angle between the MV and SB that would lead to difficulty in recrossing the SB after MV stenting.

Amongst the various two-stent strategies, the operator should select the strategy which is most familiar to him. Several trials have evaluated the best two-stent strategy, but the results are quite variable. The BBK II trial[31] found culotte technique had a reduced restenosis rate compared to T stenting, whereas the NORDIC II trial[32] showed culotte technique has similar results compared with crush technique. Conversely, the double kissing (DK) Crush III trial[33] showed that culotte was inferior to the DK Crush technique in the left main bifurcation lesions.

The DKCRUSH I bifurcation study by Chen et al. showed that the DK Crush technique reduced the incidence of stent thrombosis, TLR, and cumulative MACE rate at 8 months when compared to classical crush technique.[34] The DKCRUSH II study showed that the DK Crush technique reduced the restenosis rate and thus the TLR and target vessel revascularization at 12 months as compared to provisional stenting.[35] DKCRUSH-V study[36] showed that DK Crush technique showed a lower rate of target lesion failure at 12 months when compared to provisional stenting in the left main bifurcation lesions.

In the light of these trials with varying results, the optimal result in terms of stent apposition and expansion are more important than the stenting strategy. Currently, popular techniques are the T stenting, TAP technique, mini-crush, DK Crush, and mini-culotte techniques.

TIPS AND TRICKS[30]

- *Guide catheter*: The 7F or 8F guide catheters are preferred to reduce friction among the hardware and allow easy

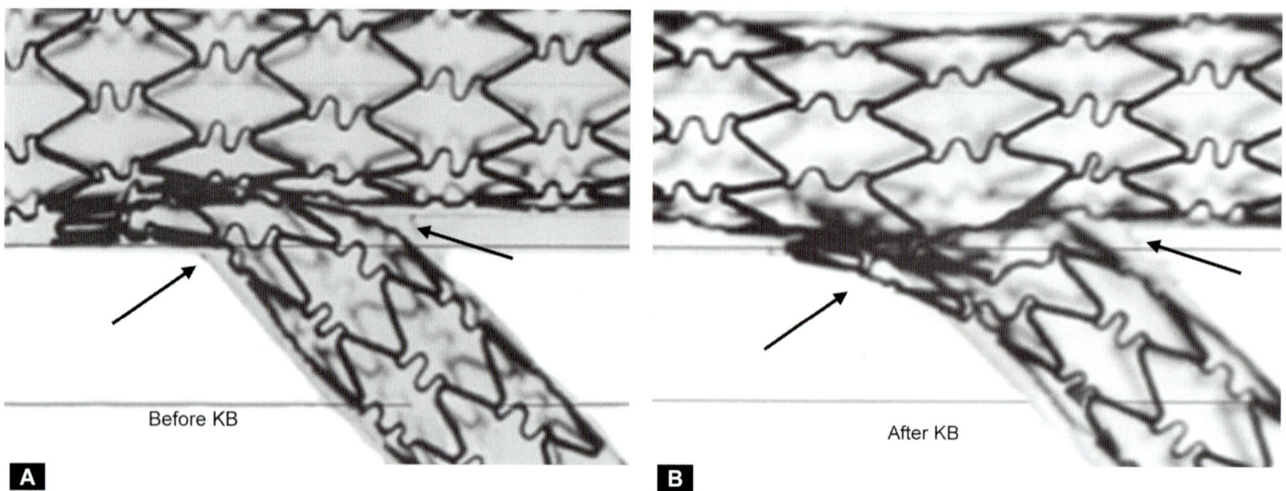

FIG. 10: DK crush technique: The distal cross may lead to a gap in stent coverage at the carina after kinal kissing balloon inflation. In this technique, proximal or mid cross is preferred.[37]

manipulation. They also provide better support for stent delivery

- *Wiring the vessel*: Wire the branch which seems more difficult first, where manipulation and rotation are expected. This will minimize wire crisscrossing. During insertion of the second wire, minimal rotation should be done. Both wires should be kept separate on the table
- *Lesion preparation*: Lesions in proximal MV, distal MV, or SB should be adequately prepared before stent deployment. In case of severely calcified lesions, rotational atherectomy may be used. Cutting balloons may be used in fibrotic lesions. The main problem with aggressive balloon dilatation is dissection
- *Stent selection and deployment*: When using EDS strategy, drug eluting stents have proven to be more effective than BMSs.[18,19] Sizing of the stent is also essential for optimal results. IVUS should be used to choose the optimal stent size and to assess the adequate stent deployment or requirement for post dilatation of the stents.
- *Jailed guide wire*:
  - When a stenting strategy involves jailing the guide wire, a nonhydrophilic guide wire should be used. This is because the coating on the hydrophilic guidewires may get peeled off when pulling it back
  - During deployment of the stent which jails the guide wire (jailing stent), nominal pressure should be used so that retrieval of the jailed wire is easier
  - During forceful removal of the jailed wire, the guide catheter may get deep throated. To avoid this, the guide catheter should be pulled back into the aorta before removing the jailed wire. In case the "jailed wire" cannot be pulled back easily, a balloon can be advanced over the jailed wire
- Stents used should have ideal stent strut expansion for optimal SB crossing. Hence, stents with "open cell" design are preferred
- *Side branch re-crossing*: Distal crossing close to the carina is preferred to ensure adequate geometry of the carina, correction of the MV stent deformation, and scaffolding of the SB ostium (Fig. 8). An exception to this rule is in case of the DK Crush technique where proximal or mid-cross is preferred to distal cross. This is based on bench testing which shows that after crushing, a trough is created between the MV and SB stent struts on the side opposite to the crushed part. If the wire recrosses distally, it may cross this trough, before entering the SB stent. After kissing balloon inflation in this case, there could be a potential gap in the coverage of the stents at the level of the carina (Fig. 10)[37]
- *Final kissing balloon inflation*: Using noncompliant balloon is an essential step to optimize results. Balloon pressures during FKI should be nominal
- *Hemodynamic support*: May be necessary, especially with left main PCI. Intra-aortic balloon pump may be need urgently or may be used electively in some cases
- *Dual antiplatelet therapy*: should continue for 12 months after the procedure at least, to reduce the risk of stent thrombosis.

CONCLUSION

In the current era of PCI, coronary bifurcations still remain a complex subset. Despite the favorable results shown by multiple trials on coronary bifurcations, achieving success of these interventions requires a learning curve. Understanding of the anatomy of the coronary bifurcation with regards to MV and SB involvement, the carina, angulations, and myocardial territory supplied are of crucial importance. IVUS is extremely useful to determine the sizes of the vessels and selection of the stent sizes in bifurcation anatomy.

As SBO is a serious complication, anatomical risk stratification of threatened SBs is useful to preserve the SB.

However, the most important predictor of clinical outcomes is the MV stent expansion. Using techniques like proximal optimization therapy, FKI or re-POT are important steps to ensure that the geometry of the stent and carina are preserved.

As per the current evidence, provisional strategy using one stent is the strategy of choice where the risk of the loss of SB by SBO is small or not consequential. In case of a SB narrowing during provisional stenting, FFR guided angioplasty may be performed. In most instances, angiographic SB pinching is due to carina shift rather than plaque shift and does not show any functional significance.

It is sensible to resort to the strategy of EDS when the loss of SB is undesirable like in presence of a large SB (>2.25 mm), severe ostial and/or long segment involvement and wide angle (angle B) with anticipated difficulty in recrossing into SB. Out of all the available techniques for elective double vessel stenting, a choice has to be made on the basis of anatomy, feasibility, operator preference, and experience to deliver a good short-term and long-term results.

REFERENCES

1. Dauerman H, Higgins P, Sparano A, et al. Mechanical debulking versus balloon angioplasty for the treatment of true bifurcation lesions. J Am Coll Cardiol. 1998;32:1845-52.
2. Lefevre T, Louvard Y, Morice MC, et al. Stenting of bifurcation lesions: classification, treatments, and results. Cathet Cardiovasc Intervent. 2000;49: 274-83.
3. Colombo F, Biondi-Zoccai G, Infantino V, et al. A long-term comparison of drug-eluting versus bare metal stents for the percutaneous treatment of coronary bifurcation lesions, Acta Cardiol. 2009;64(5):583-8.
4. Moussa I, Colombo A. Coronary artery bifurcation interventions; bridging the gap between research and practice; Tips and Tricks in Interventional Therapy of Coronary Bifurcation Lesions. Abingdon, United Kingdom: Taylor & Francis; 2010. pp. 1-13.
5. Medina A, Suárez de Lezo J, Pan M. A new classification of coronary bifurcation lesions. Rev Esp Cardiol. 2006;59(2):183.
6. Louvard Y, Sashikand G, Lefevre T, et al. Angiographic predictors of side branch occlusion during treatment of bifurcation lesions. Cath Cardiovasc Interv. 2005 (Abstr Supp).
7. Moore JE Jr, Timmins LH, LaDisa JF. Coronary artery bifurcation biomechanics and implications for interventional strategies. Catheter Cardiovasc Interv. 2010;76:836-43.
8. Oviedo C, Maehara A, Mintz G, et al. A critical intravascular ultrasound appraisal of the angiographic classification of bifurcation lesions: where is the plaque really located? J Am Coll Cardiol. 2008;51 (Poster 2902-2916):B23-98.
9. Murray CD. The physiological principle of minimum work: I. The vascular system and the cost of blood volume. Proc Natl Acad Sci USA. 1926;12(3):207-14.
10. Finet G, Gilard M, Perrenot B, et al. Fractal geometry of arterial coronary bifurcations, a quantitative coronary angiography and intravascular ultrasound analysis. EuroIntervention. 2008;3:490-8.
11. Hahn JY, Gwon HC, Kwon SU, et al. Comparison of vessel geometry in bifurcation between normal and diseased segments: intravascular ultrasound analysis. Atherosclerosis. 2008;201:326-31.
12. Gwon HC. Understanding Coronary Bifurcation Stenting. Korean Circ J. 2018; 48(6):481-91.
13. Kim JS, Hong MK, Ko YG, et al. Impact of intravascular ultrasound guidance on long-term clinical outcomes in patients treated with drug-eluting stent for bifurcation lesions: data from a Korean multicenter bifurcation registry. Am Heart J 2011;161:180-7.
14. Xu J, Hahn JY, Song YB, et al. Carina shift versus plaque shift for aggravation of side branch ostial stenosis in bifurcation lesions: volumetric intravascular ultrasound analysis of both branches. Circ Cardiovasc Interv. 2012;5:657-62.
15. Kang SJ, Kim WJ, Lee JY, et al. Hemodynamic impact of changes in bifurcation geometry after single-stent cross-over technique assessed by intravascular ultrasound and fractional flow reserve. Catheter Cardiovasc Interv. 2013;82:1075-82.
16. Hahn JY, Chun WJ, Kim JH, et al. Predictors and outcomes of side branch occlusion after main vessel stenting in coronary bifurcation lesions: results from the COBIS II Registry (COronary BIfurcation Stenting). J Am Coll Cardiol. 2013;62:1654-9.
17. Darremont O. The POT Technique. Valencia: European Bifurcation club; 2007.
18. Niemela M, Kervinen K, Erglis A, et al. Randomized comparison of final kissing balloon dilatation versus no final kissing balloon dilatation in patients with coronary bifurcation lesions treated with main vessel stenting. The Nordic Baltic Bifurcation Study III. Circulation. 2011;123:79-86.
19. Colombo A, Bramucci E, Saccà S, et al. Randomized study of the crush technique versus provisional side-branch stenting in true coronary bifurcations: the CACTUS (Coronary Bifurcations: Application of the Crushing Technique Using Sirolimus-Eluting Stents) Study. Circulation. 2009;119(1):71-8.
20. Koo BK, Park KW, Kang HJ, et al. Physiological evaluation of the provisional side branch intervention strategy for bifurcation lesions using fractional flow reserve. Eur Heart J. 2008;29(6):726-32.
21. Albiero R, Boldi E. Provisional stenting technique of non-left main coronary bifurcation lesions: Patient selection and technique. In: Moussa I, Colombo A (Eds). Tips and Tricks in Interventional Therapy of Coronary Bifurcation Lesions. Abingdon, United Kingdom: Taylor & Francis; 2010. pp. 49-66.
22. Derimay F, Souteyrand G, Motreff P, et al. Sequential proximal optimizing technique in provisional bifurcation stenting with everolimus-eluting bioresorbable vascular scaffold fractal coronary bifurcation bench for comparative test between absorb and XIENCE Xpedition. JACC Cardiovasc Interv. 2016; 9(13);1397-406.
23. Brar SS, Gray WA, Dangas G, et al. Bifurcation stenting with drug-eluting stents: a systematic review and meta-analysis of randomised trials. EuroIntervention. 2009;5(4):475-84.
24. Katritsis DG, Siontis GC, Ioannidis JP. Double versus single stenting for coronary bifurcation lesions: a meta-analysis. Circ Cardiovasc Interv. 2009;2(5):409-15.
25. Hakeem A, Khan FM, Bhatti S, et al. Provisional vs. complex stenting strategy for coronary bifurcation lesions: meta-analysis of randomized trials. J Invasive Cardiol. 2009;21(11):589-95.
26. Niccoli G, Ferrante G, Porto I, et al. Coronary bifurcation lesions: to stent one branch or both? A meta-analysis of patients treated with drug eluting stents. Int J Cardiol. 2010;139(1):80-91.
27. Hildick-Smith D, de Belder AJ, Cooter N, et al. Randomized trial of simple versus complex drug-eluting stenting for bifurcation lesions: the British Bifurcation Coronary Study: old, new, and evolving strategies, Circulation. 2010;121(10):1235-43.
28. Maeng M, Holm NR, Erglis A, et al. Long-term results after simple versus complex stenting of coronary artery bifurcation lesions: Nordic Bifurcation Study 5-year follow-up results. J Am Coll Cardiol. 2013;62(1):30-4.
29. Song YB, Hahn JY, Song PS, et al. Randomized comparison of conservative versus aggressive strategy for provisional side branch intervention in coronary bifurcation lesions: results from the SMART-STRATEGY (Smart Angioplasty Research Team-Optimal Strategy for Side Branch Intervention in Coronary Bifurcation Lesions) randomized trial. JACC Cardiovasc Interv. 2012;5:1133-40.
30. Lassen JF, Burzotta F, Banning AP, et al. Percutaneous coronary intervention for the left main stem and other bifurcation lesions: 12th consensus document from the European Bifurcation Club. EuroIntervention. 2018;13:1540-53.
31. Ferenc M, Gick M, Comberg T, et al. Culotte stenting vs. TAP stenting for treatment of de-novo coronary bifurcation lesions with the need for side-branch stenting: the Bifurcations Bad Krozingen (BBK) II angiographic trial. Eur Heart J. 2016;37:3399-405.

32. Erglis A, Kumsars I, Niemelä M, et al. Randomized comparison of coronary bifurcation stenting with the crush versus the culotte technique using sirolimus eluting stents: the Nordic stent technique study. Circ Cardiovasc Interv. 2009;2:27-34.
33. Chen SL, Xu B, Han YL, et al. Comparison of double kissing crush versus Culotte stenting for unprotected distal left main bifurcation lesions: results from a multicenter, randomized, prospective DKCRUSH-III study. J Am Coll Cardiol. 2013;61:1482-8.
34. Chen SL, Zhang JJ, Ye F, et al. Study comparing the double kissing (DK) crush with classical crush for the treatment of coronary bifurcation lesions: the DKCRUSH-1 Bifurcation Study with drug-eluting stents. Eur J Clin Invest. 2008;38:361-71.
35. Chen SL, Santoso T, Zhang JJ, et al. A randomized clinical study comparing Double Kissing Crush with Provisional Stenting for treatment of Coronary Bifurcation Lesions: Results from the DKCRUSH-II (Double Kissing Crush versus Provisional Stenting Technique for Treatment of Coronary Bifurcation Lesions) trial. J Am Coll Cardiol. 2011;57:914-20.
36. Chen SL, Zhang JJ, Han Y, et al. Double kissing crush versus provisional stenting for left main distal bifurcation lesions: DKCRUSH-V randomized trial. J Am Coll Cardiol. 2017;70:2605-17.
37. Ormiston JA, Webster MW, Webber B, et al. The "crush" technique for coronary artery bifurcation stenting: insights from micro-computed tomographic imaging of bench deployments. JACC Cardiovasc Interv. 2008;1(4):351-7.

CHAPTER 57

Left Main Coronary Artery Stenting in 2018

DS Gambhir

INTRODUCTION

Significant left main coronary artery (LMCA) disease, defined as 50% diameter stenosis, corresponding to 75% of area stenosis is observed in approximately 5–10% of patients who undergo coronary angiography for symptomatic coronary artery disease (CAD).[1,2] When treated medically, significant LMCA disease carries a mortality of 50% within 3 years after diagnosis.[3,4] With the advent of coronary artery bypass surgery (CABG) and availability of its long-term follow-up results[5,6] which established its superiority over medical therapy, CABG was accepted as the gold standard for the treatment of significant LMCA stenosis. In its initial publication on the results of balloon angioplasty by Gruntzig et al.,[7] this procedure was considered unsuitable, and in fact contraindicated, in patients with LMCA disease. However, after the introduction of drug-eluting stents (DESs) resulting in significant reduction in need for repeat revascularization, there was resurgence of enthusiasm in the role of stenting for LMCA disease.

This chapter will focus on the results of comparison between stenting using DES with CABG, very long-term results of stenting, strategies for left main (LM) bifurcation stenting, and the role of adjunct modalities in the treatment of unprotected LMCA disease.

STENTING VERSUS BYPASS SURGERY FOR LEFT MAIN CORONARY ARTERY DISEASE

Both US and European guidelines have recommended CABG in most patients with LMCA disease.[8,9] However, the widespread availability of DES associated with improvement in techniques of coronary stenting has lowered the threshold for performing percutaneous coronary intervention (PCI) instead of CABG for LMCA disease. Also, several large registries and randomized controlled trials have demonstrated that results of LMCA stenting are comparable to CABG.[10-12] This chapter will focus on the results of four recent prospective, randomized trials, comparing long-term results of PCI using DES with CABG (Table 1).

SYNTAX trial.[13] Subgroup analysis of patients with unprotected LMCA stenosis comparing PCI using DES with CABG on 705 patients and publication of 5-year follow-up results, there was no difference in major adverse cardiac and cerebrovascular events (MACCEs) between the two modalities of treatment (36.9% vs. 31.0%; p = 0.12). On further analysis, stratified according to the SYNTAX score, MACCE was significantly higher with PCI (46.5% vs. 29.7%; p = 0.003) in the high-risk group (SYNTAX score ≥33). Repeat revascularization rate were found to be higher in the PCI-treated patients regardless of SYNTAX score (26.7% vs. 15.5%; p <0.01). There was, however, no difference in the mortality between two groups, while the lower incidence of stroke rate after PCI persisted at 5 years (1.5% vs. 4.3%; p = 0.003). These findings were confirmed by the smaller LE MANS study[14] and PRECOMBAT trial.[15]

The MAIN COMPARE registry[10] enrolled 2240 patients undergoing CABG or PCI with stents [bare-metal stents (BMSs) in early phase and DES in the subsequent period]. There was no difference between the two groups with regard to composite end point of death, Q-wave myocardial infarction (MI), or stroke at minimum follow-up of 3 years. However, target vessel revascularization (TVR) was significantly higher in the PCI group as compared to CABG (p <0.001).

The greatest limitation of these studies[10-15] was the use of either BMS or first generation of DES leading to higher rate of TVR. Recent meta-analysis[16,17] have shown progressive decline in TVR, after the introduction of newer generation of DES. More recently, two large randomized trials using relatively current generation of DES and contemporary surgical techniques have been reported with somewhat conflicting results.[18,19]

The NOBLE trial[18] is a prospective, non-inferiority trial which randomized 1201 patients to PCI of LMCA stenosis with BIOLIMUS-eluting stent (n = 598) or CABG (n = 603).

TABLE 1: Major trials comparing percutaneous coronary intervention (PCI) versus coronary artery bypass grafting (CABG) for left main coronary artery disease, depicting the results of end points at long-term follow-up (values indicate hazard ratio, PCI vs. CABG; p value in brackets)

Trial (year)	No. of patients		Maximum FU (Years)	End points			References
	PCI	CABG		All-cause mortality	Repeat revascularization	MI	
SYNTAX (LM subgroup) (2013)	351	348	5	0.88 (NS)	1.82 (p = 0.001)	1.67 (NS)	11
PRECOMBAT (2015)	300	300	5	0.73 (NS)	1.86 (p = 0.020)	1.20 (NS)	29
NOBLE (2016)	598	603	5	1,07 (NS)	1.50 (p = 0.03)	2.88 (p = 0.004)	18
EXCEL (2016)	948	957	3	1.34 (NS)	1.72 (p <0.001)	0.93 (NS)	19

CABG, coronary artery bypass grafting; FU, follow-up; LMCA, left main coronary artery; MI, myocardial infarction; PCI, percutaneous coronary intervention; NS, not significant.

LM bifurcation stenting was performed in 88% of patients with two-stent techniques in 35% of these patients. The primary endpoint—composite of MACCE (death from any cause, nonprocedural MI, repeated revascularization or stroke) occurred in 28% of patients after PCI and 15% in the CABG group which exceeded the prespecified noninferiority margin. At 5-years, there was no significant difference between the two groups in all-cause mortality or stroke. Repeat revascularization rates were higher in PCI versus CABG group (15% vs. 10%; p = 0.03), as were nonprocedural MI (6% vs. 2%; p = 0.004). Treatment with BMS in 8% patients, along with higher strut thickness of BIOLIMUS-eluting stent compared to new generation everolimus-eluting stent could have adversely influenced the incidence of TVR, non-procedural MI and stent thrombosis in the PCI group.

The EXCEL trial.[19] This trial was designed to assess the previous observations that patients with low or intermediate (≤32) SYNTAX score had similar outcomes after PCI or CABG. In this randomized trial, 1,905 patients with unprotected LMCA disease were randomized to PCI (n = 948) treated with XIENCE stent versus CABG (n = 957). The primary end point—composite of death, stroke or MI at 3 years, occurred in 15.4% of patients in the PCI group and 14.7% in the CABG group (p = 0.02, for noninferiority). However, ischemia-driven revascularization remained higher in the PCI group (12.6% vs. 7.5%; p <0.001). This trial, therefore, confirmed that PCI using new generation stents and CABG have similar outcomes with regard to mortality, stroke, and MI at 3 years follow-up in patients with low-to-intermediate risk coronary anatomy and SYNTAX score of less than or equal to 32.

The conflicting outcomes between NOBLE and EXCEL trials could be explained by: (1) use of different generation of stents, (2) inclusion of repeat revascularization in the composite primary endpoint in the NOBLE trial, and (3) inclusion of patients with low or intermediate SYNTAX score in the EXCEL trial.

Meta-analysis

Several meta-analysis have been performed to compare the long-term efficacy and safety of PCI using DES versus CABG in patients with LMCA disease.[20-23] However, these included, both observational and randomized studies, different types of stents including BMSs and did not incorporate the results of two recent randomized trials—NOBLE[18] and EXCEL.[19] These meta-analysis were further limited by assessment of short- and midterm outcomes.[20-25] To overcome the limitations of previously published meta-analysis, Giacoppo et al.[26] published the results of meta-analysis of four randomized clinical trials, which included 4,394 patients,[11,15,18,19,27-29] all of whom were treated with DES and were followed up for three or more years with an objective to compare the long-term safety and efficacy of PCI with DES versus CABG in patients with significance LMCA disease. The primary endpoint was a composite of all-cause death, MI or stroke at the longest available follow-up. Secondary end points included repeat revascularization and composite of all-cause death, MI, stroke or repeat revascularization. Among 4,394 patients included in the primary analysis, 2,197 patients underwent PCI with DES and 2,197 were treated by CABG. All studies except EXCEL[19] reported a follow-up of 5 years. Both modalities of treatment showed comparable outcomes with regard to all-cause death, MI or stroke at long-term follow-up. Kaplan–Meir analysis did not show significant differences between two treatments over time with a cumulative incidence of 18.3% in the PCI group and 16.7% in the CABG group at 5 years follow-up. PCI had numerical advantage over CABG during the first 2 years, which, however, reversed over the next 3–5 years, with nonsignificant benefit of CABG over PCI. Overall, MACCEs were similar for the two modalities [hazard ratio (HR) 1.05, 95% confidence interval (CI) 0.90–1.23; p = 0.53].

Influence analysis in this meta-analysis revealed that heterogeneity was mainly due to the NOBLE trial[18]—the only study which showed superiority of CABG over PCI. The results remained consistent after including patients with low to intermediate SYNTAX scores (1–32) (HR 1.02; 95% CI 0.74–1.41; p = 0.89). The grouping of trials according to generation of DES used for PCI did not show any significant differences in the primary endpoint between patients who underwent PCI with first-generation or second-generation DES.

In another recently published meta-analysis[30] of six randomized trials including 4,686 patients with a median follow-up of 39 months, there were no significant differences between PCI versus CABG in the risk of all-cause mortality or cardiac mortality. However, the relative risk of mortality tended to be lower with PCI compared to CABG among patients in the lower SYNTAX score tertile, similar in the intermediate tertile, and higher in the upper-SYNTAX score tertile. The long-term composite risk of death, MI or stroke was similar between PCI and CABG. However, PCI was associated with greater rates of unplanned revascularization compared with CABG (HR 1.74; 95% CI 1.47–2.07). The authors concluded that both procedures resulted in similar long-term outcomes. While PCI offers an early safety advantage, CABG demonstrates greater durability for treatment of LMCA stenosis.

All the meta-analyses[20-23] have consistently shown that need for repeat revascularization was significantly higher after PCI compared to CABG. There was no significant influence of DES generation on the incidence of repeat revascularization.[26] The second-generation DES and first-generation DES groups showed a similar risk of repeat revascularization.[26].

VERY LONG-TERM FOLLOW-UP AFTER LEFT MAIN CORONARY ARTERY STENTING

While comparing LMCA stenting with CABG, one of the most important limitations is the nonavailability of very long-term (10 years or more) follow-up results after LMCA intervention. In the ASAN-MAIN registry,[31] 10-year results after implantation of BMS for unprotected LMCA stenosis highlighted the safety of procedure with cardiac mortality similar to CABG (6.9% vs. 11.0%; p = 0.1). However, repeat revascularization (43.1% vs.6.7%; p <0.001) and TLR (24.9% vs. 4.9%; p <0.001) were higher in BMS group compared to CABG. LE MANS RCT[32] was the first study which reported 10-year results of LMCA intervention, compared to CABG. Although the number of patients included was very small in both groups: PCI (n = 52) and CABG (n = 53), the survival rate was close to 70% in the PCI group and MACCE-free survival was numerically better for PCI. The rate of repeat revascularization was comparable between PCI and CABG groups (p = 0.46), mainly due to an increase in repeat revascularization in the CABG group 2 years after the operation. The study thus demonstrated durability of PCI for LMCA stenosis in the short-, long- and very long-term follow-up.[32]

These preliminary findings of LE MANS study should be regarded as mere observations rather than definitive and conclusive in the absence of large-randomized controlled trials such as SYNTAX[13] or PRECOMBAT.[15] Moreover, the analysis of SYNTAX score revealed that all patients included in this study had SYNTAX score less than 32 (low and middle groups). Therefore, excellent results observed in LE MANS study[32] may not be applicable to patients with more complex lesions. More data from large, prospective and randomized studies should be available before any definite conclusions can be drawn with regard to long-term durability of PCI for LMCA disease.-

CURRENT GUIDELINES FOR LEFT MAIN CORONARY ARTERY STENTING

The current PCI guideline for the treatment of LMCA stenosis was recently updated to a class IIb indication with a B level of evidence from the American College of Cardiology/American Heart Association and European Society of Cardiology.[33] In addition, the European Society of Cardiology and European Association for Cardio-Thoracic Surgery reported the following indications of LMCA stenting relative to CABG:[34] (1) isolated or single vessel disease, ostium/shaft, class IIa B; (2) isolated or single vessel disease, distal bifurcation, class IIb B; (3) LM plus two- or three-vessel disease, SYNTAX score 32 or less, class IIb B; (4) LM plus two- or three-vessel disease, SYNTAX score 33 or more class III B. Therefore, DES implantation is currently considered as an alternative option for selected patients with unprotected LMCA disease.

SELECTION OF LEFT MAIN BIFURCATION STENTING STRATEGY

There is no consensus with regard to optimal strategy for LM bifurcation stenting. Although several techniques have been described, the provisional one-stent approach has been considered as the most preferred strategy in comparison to elective two-stent strategy for PCI of LM bifurcation stenosis.

Provisional One-stent Technique

This consists of deploying a single stent from LM to left anterior descending (LAD) across the ostium of left circumflex (LCx). It is preferred in patients with insignificant focal stenosis at the ostium of LCx or nondominant left coronary system. In contrast, a large dominant LCx (≥2.5 mm in diameter) with significant long stenosis at the origin of LCx which has a narrow angle of origin with LAD, often requires elective two-stent strategy. Evaluation by fractional flow reserve (FFR) for LCx stenosis provides valuable information for need to intervene.

Several studies have reported that, compared to two-stent strategy, this approach is associated with more favorable outcome including lower risk of major adverse cardiac events (MACE),[35-37] death,[37] MI,[36,37] and TVR.[36-38] The incidence of stent thrombosis is also lower with one-stent approach.[37,38] Based upon several observational studies, the provisional one-stent approach is preferred for the treatment of LM bifurcation stenosis[39] and more than 60% of patients in the real world get treated by this approach.[36] However, this strategy remains to be evaluated in randomized controlled studies.

Final Kissing Balloon Inflation (FKI) in Provisional Stenting

Although, this step is frequently performed in patients undergoing provisional one-stent approach, its role is unclear and controversial. Out of 413 patients who underwent provisional single-stent treatment, 96 received FKI after main vessel stenting.[40] During a 2-year follow-up, the rate of composite death, MI and TLR did not differ significantly between groups with or without FKI (12.5% vs. 8.5%; p = 0.82), regardless of angiographic side branch (SB) stenosis. Although statistically insignificant, there was a trend toward more frequent TVR in the FKI group (8.1% vs. 4.8%; p = 0.83). Another small study showed similar results.[41] It seems, therefore, that FKI may not provide improvement in long-term clinical outcomes after main vessel stenting in provisional one-stent approach for LM bifurcation stenosis.

Side Branch Stenting in Provisional Stenting

Stenting of LCx after main vessel stenting in provisional stenting approach is often required in patients who develop compromise in LCx flow leading to ischemic symptoms or signs. It is also indicated in patients who develop flow-limiting dissection of LCx origin following FKI. Two small pilot studies evaluated the benefit of FFR in decision-making for LCx stenting after main vessel stenting in LM bifurcation treatment.[42,43] These studies observed that only one-third of angiographically significant LCx ostial stentoses were found to have FFR less than 0.80. It is, therefore, suggested that FFR provides useful information in guiding treatment of LCx ostial stenosis. An FFR of more than or equal to 0.80 is a strong predictor of favorable survival and low event rates in patients with intermediate disease.[44,45]

Stenting of LCx in provisional stenting can be performed by using one of the following techniques: (1) provisional T stenting, (2) the T-and-protrusion (TAP) technique, (3) reverse crush, and (4) provisional culotte. Each of these techniques have their advantages and limitations.

Elective Two-stent Approach

A planned two-stent strategy is used if there is significant stenosis of distal LMCA extending into both LAD and LCx branches, and possibility of acute hemodynamic collapse or periprocedural MI in the event of abrupt occlusion of LCx. A large number of elective two-stent techniques and their modifications have been proposed for LM bifurcation stenting. These include: TAP technique, crush and its variants—mini crush and double kissing and crush (DK crush), culotte, and simultaneous kissing stent (SKS technique). Since all LM bifurcations are not the same, selection of an appropriate technique depends upon consideration of several variables such as relative size of LM and its main branches (MBs), the bifurcation angle and the severity and length of stenosis at LCx origin. Equally important criteria are the experience and expertise of the operator in performing a particular technique.

Crush Techniques

The classical crush technique provides complete lesion coverage for SB ostium and generally used in patients with LM bifurcation angle of less than 70°. However, covering the SB ostium with three layers of stents can make the FKI technically difficult and even failure in approximately 15–20% of cases. The Mini-Crush technique avoids a large area with three layers of stent struts, and thereby improves the success of FKI, and minimizes residual metallic stenosis at the SB ostium.[46] Another modification called DK crush technique comprises additional kissing balloon inflation between SB crushing and MB stenting. It has been reported to facilitate FKI and enhances stent apposition.[47]

Culotte Technique

It consists of sequential implantation of two stents in both the branches, with the MB stent implanted through the SB stent, and thus forming a double layer of stents in the main vessel. This technique is suitable for all angles of bifurcation and provides near-perfect coverage of SB ostium.

Simultaneous Kissing Stent Technique

In this technique, both the stents—LM to LAD and LM to LCx are delivered and implanted together, thereby forming a double-barrel, metallic carina in LMCA. SKS is preferred in emergency situations of LMCA occlusion with a narrow angle of bifurcation and diameter of LMCA much bigger (at least two-thirds) compared to the combined sizes of LAD and LCx. This technique, though simple and easy to perform, is rarely used because of difficulty in placing a stent proximal to the double barrel, if required to seal a dissection, the formation of a new diaphragmatic metal membrane, difficulty in wiring for PCI of restenosis, and treatment of distal vessel stenosis.

Need for Proximal Optimization Technique

Since the LMCA diameter is often much larger than the distal MB diameter, proximal optimization of stent deployment is very important for adequate stent apposition in the LM bifurcation intervention.[48] This facilitates recrossing the SB through a distal stent cell and avoid abluminal rewiring by a second wire. The choice of stent diameter should be based upon the distal MB reference diameter to minimize carina shifting.[49] The stent selected for LM to LAD should be such that it should be expandable to the reference diameter of LMCA.

ROLE OF ADJUST DEVICES

Intravascular Ultrasound

It is a useful adjunct imaging modality which can provide valuable information including lesion morphology and dimensions during LMCA stenting.[50] It enables interventionist to provide adequate information on stent apposition and adequate coverage of lesions, after implantation.[51,52] Recent meta-analyses have demonstrated that intravascular ultrasound (IVUS)-guided PCI is associated with lower risk of death, MI, TVR, and stent thrombosis after DES implantation.[53,54] In patients with unprotected LMCA stenosis, the beneficial effects of IVUS-guided stenting on clinical outcomes were reported by the MAIN COMPARE multicenter registry which enrolled 975 patients with LMCA stenosis who underwent PCI under IVUS guidance or angiography alone.[55] In the propensity score matched comparison, IVUS guidance showed a trend toward lower rates of mortality at 3 years (6% with IVUS vs. 13.6% in angiography group; $p = 0.063$). Andell et al.[56] investigated the clinical outcomes of IVUS guidance on composite end point of all-cause mortality, restenosis or definite stent thrombosis in patients undergoing unprotected LMCA-PCI in a nationwide population-based observational study using SCAAR registry. After adjusting for potential

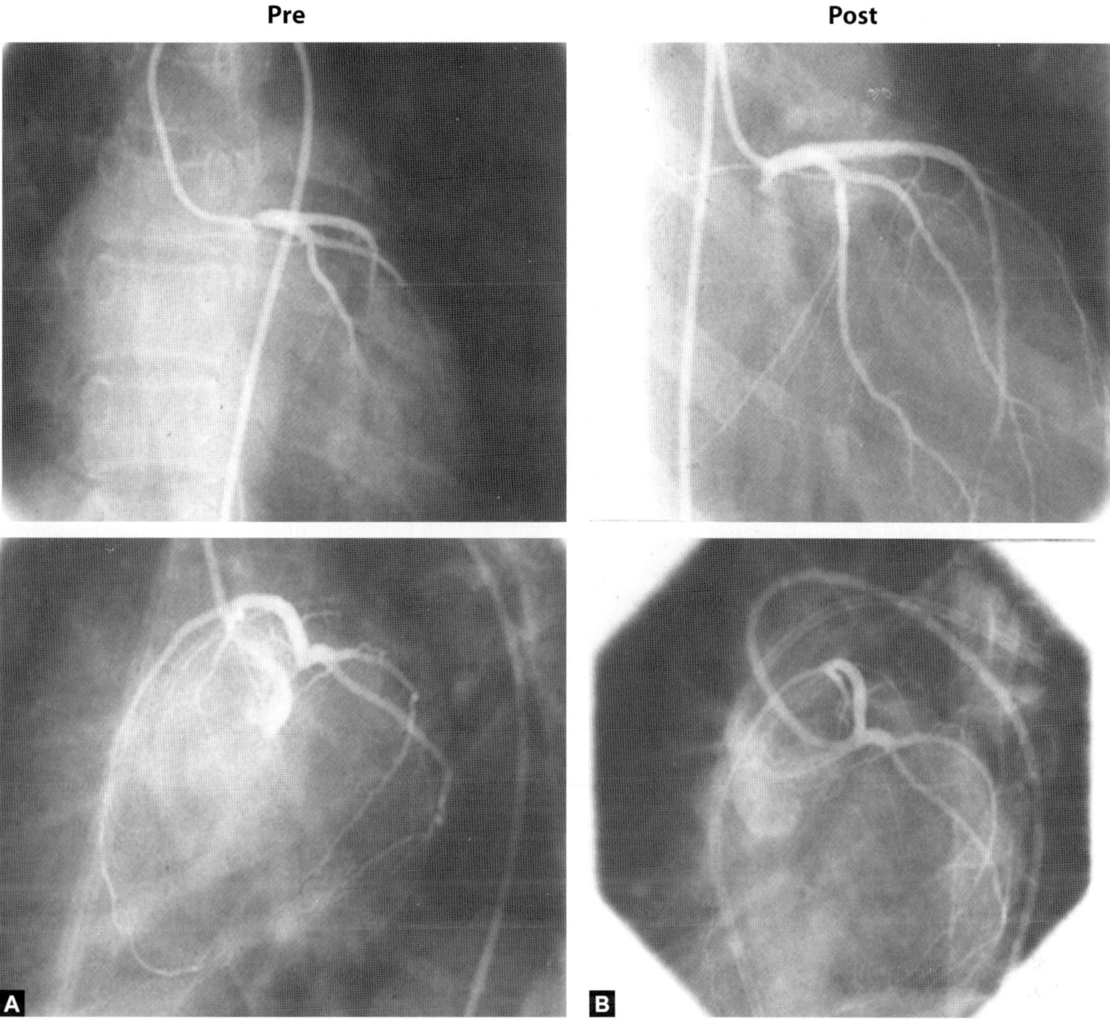

FIG. 1: Left main ostial stenting using Palmaz Schatz coronary stent under cardiopulmonary support (the first case performed by the author).

cofounder, IVUS-guided approach was associated with significantly lower incidence of primary composite endpoint of all-cause mortality, restenosis or definite stent thrombosis (p = 0.003).

Although large, prospective studies and registry data suggest improved outcomes with IVUS-guided DES implantation for LMCA stenosis, randomized trials are underpowered to assess the clinical utility of this approach.

Malapposition with underdeployment of stent increases the risk of stent thrombosis and restenosis. Kang et al.[57] studied the optimal IVUS-derived minimal stent cross-sectional area (MSA) for prevention of in-stent restenosis (ISR) in 403 patients undergoing DES implantation for LMCA stenosis. The best IVUS-derived MSA which predicted angiographic ISR on segmental basis were: 5.0 mm^2 for LCx ostium, 6.3 mm^2 for the LAD ostium, 7.2 mm^2 for the polygon of confluence (POC), and 8.2 mm^2 for the proximal LMCA above the POC. The operator should, therefore, attempt to achieve these values by using high pressure post-stent balloon dilatation.

Role of Optimal Coherence Tomography

Optimal coherence tomography (OCT) can provide accurate information of the arterial wall, including LMCA disease. Preprocedure OCT can be used to assess the lesion morphology-fatty, fibrofatty, calcific, or thrombotic. It can assess the thickness of calcium in the vessel wall, and thereby helps to decide the strategy for lesion modification before stenting. It enables precise online measurement of length and diameter of LMCA for selection of appropriate size of stent. Dissection resulting from predilatation can be easily detected, and taken into consideration while deciding the stent length. After deployment of stents, OCT can be used to verify that the guidewire recrosses into SB through the distal stent cell to ensure optimal scaffolding and minimal metal carina.[58] Post-stent deployment, OCT helps to assess the stent expansion, and occurrence of edge dissection. Three-dimensional evaluation with OCT ensures evaluation of LCx ostium and carina, and enables to detect any strut protruding at the ostium of LCx.

Hemodynamic Support

Although intra-aortic balloon pump is not routinely required during LMCA stenting, it should be used selectively to prevent hemodynamic collapse in patients with severely depressed LV function.

PERSONAL EXPERIENCE

The author performed the first case of LM stenting 20 years ago in a young pregnant patient who presented with recurrent episodes of syncope and found to have 90% ostial stenosis of LMCA (Fig. 1).[59] From 2004 to 2017, I have performed LMCA stenting in 463 patients of whom 310 (67%) were distal LM bifurcation stenosis. Single-stent approach was used in 130 (28%), two-stent strategy in 322 (69%), and LM-triple stenting in 11 (2.5%) of cases.

The various two-stent techniques for LM bifurcation stenting used were: SKS (30%), V-stenting (20%), DK crush (20%), TAP (16%), Mini-Crush (9%), T-stenting (4.6%), and culotte (1%). Use of adjunct devices included rotablation in 58%, IVUS in 28%, IABP in 21%, and OCT in 2.2% patients. Angiographic success was achieved in 460 (99%) and clinical success in 452 (97.5%). Major in-hospital complications included death (1%) and reintervention (0.6%). No patient required emergency CABG. Our experience highlights the safety of LM bifurcation stenting using DES.

CONCLUSION

Considering all the data available in the literature, the optimal management of unprotected LMCA disease is still a subject of debate. Most studies have suggested that, whereas there is no difference in mortality between the two treatment strategies, a recent meta-analysis[25] shows no difference in safety end points. In patients with LM associated with complex multi-vessel disease, CABG is superior to stenting with better long-term results. For patients with low or intermediate risk (SYNTAX score ≤32), both therapies are comparable but PCI is associated with less morbidity, shorter hospital stay and lower incidence of stroke when compared to CABG. However, repeat revascularization rates are higher despite using the latest generation of DES. Given the lack of mortality difference between the two treatment modalities, the focus should shift at improving the outcomes for both PCI and CABG in the treatment of LMCA stenosis.

REFERENCES

1. Proudfit WL, Shirey EK, Sones FM Jr. Distribution of arterial lesions demonstrated by selective cinecoronary arteriography. Circulation. 1967;36:54-62.
2. Stone P, Goldschlager N. Left main coronary artery disease: Review and appraisal. Cardiovasc Med. 1979;4:165-77.
3. Cohen MV, Gorlin R. Main left coronary artery disease. Clinical experience from 1964-1974. Circulation. 1975;52:275-85.
4. Taylor HA, Deumite NJ, Chaitman BR, et al. Asymptomatic left main coronary artery disease in the Coronary Artery Surgery Study (CASS) registry. Circulation. 1989;79:1171-79.
5. Taggart DP, Kaul S, Boden WE, et al. Revascularization for unprotected left main stem coronary artery stenosis: stenting or surgery. J Am Coll Cardiol. 2008;51:885-92.
6. Chaitman BR, Fisher LD, Bourassa MG, et al. Effect of coronary bypass surgery on survival patterns in subsets of patients with left main coronary artery disease. Report of the Collaborative Study in Coronary Artery Surgery (CASS). Am J Cardiol. 1981;48:765-77.
7. Grüntzig AR, Senning A, Siegenthaler WE. Nonoperative dilatation of coronary-artery stenosis: percutaneous transluminal coronary angioplasty. N Engl J Med. 1979;301:61-8.
8. Fihn SD, Blankenship JC, Alexander KP, et al. 2014 ACC/AHA/AATS/PCNA/SCAI/STS focused update of the guideline for the diagnosis and management of patients with stable ischemic heart disease: a report of the American College of Cardiology/American Heart Association Task Force on Practice Guidelines, and the American Association for Thoracic Surgery, Preventive Cardiovascular Nurses Association, Society for Cardiovascular Angiography and Interventions, and Society of Thoracic Surgeons. J Am Coll Cardiol. 2014;64:1929-49.
9. Windecker S, Kolh P, Alfonso F, et al. 2014 ESC/EACTS Guidelines on myocardial revascularization: The Task Force on Myocardial Revascularization of the European Society of Cardiology (ESC) and the European Association for Cardio-Thoracic Surgery (EACTS) developed with the special contribution of the European Association of Percutaneous Cardiovascular Interventions (EAPCI). Eur Heart J. 2014;35:2541-619.
10. Seung KB, Park DW, Kim YH, et al. Stents versus Coronary-artery bypass grafting for left main coronary artery disease. N Engl J Med. 2008;358:1781-92.
11. Mohr FW, Morice MC, Kappetein AP, et al. Coronary artery bypass graft surgery versus percutaneous coronary intervention in patients with three-vessel disease and left main coronary disease: 5-year follow-up of the randomised, clinical SYNTAX trial. Lancet. 2013;381:629-38.
12. Boudriot E, Thiele H, Walther T, et al. Randomized comparison of percutaneous coronary intervention with sirolimus-eluting stent versus coronary artery bypass grafting in unprotected left main stem stenosis. J Am Coll Cardiol. 2011;57:538-45.
13. Morice MC, Serruys PW, Kappetein AP, et al. Five-year outcomes in patients with left main disease treated with either percutaneous coronary intervention or coronary artery bypass grafting in the Synergy Between Percutaneous Coronary Intervention With TAXUS and Cardiac Surgery trial. Circulation. 2014;129:2388-94.
14. Buszman PE, Kiesz SR, Bochenek, et al. Acute and late outcomes of unprotected left main stenting in comparison with surgical revascularization. J Am Coll Cardiol. 2008;51:538-45.
15. Ahn JM, Roh JH, Kim YH, et al. Randomized trial of stents versus bypass surgery for left main coronary artery disease: 5-year outcomes of the PRECOMBAT study. J Am Coll Cardiol. 2015;65:2198-06.
16. Palmerini T, Biondi-Zoccai G, Della Riva D, et al. Clinical outcome with bioabsorbable polymer versus durable polymer-based drug-eluting and bare metal stents: evidence from a comprehensive network meta-analysis J Am Coll Cardiol. 2014;63:299-07.
17. Bangalore S, Kumar S, Fusaro M, et al. Short-and long-term outcomes with drug-eluting and bare-metal coronary stents: a mixed treatment comparison analysis of 117762 patient-years of followup from randomized trials: Circulation. 2012;125;2873-91.
18. Mäkikallio T, Holm NR, Lindsay M, et al. NOBLE Study Investigators. Percutaneous coronary angioplasty versus coronary artery bypass grafting in treatment of unprotected left main stenosis (NOBLE): a prospective, randomised, open-label, non-inferiority trial. Lancet. 2016;388:2743-52.
19. Stone GW, Sabik JF, Serruys PW, et al. EXCEL Trial Investigators. Everolimus-eluting stents or bypass surgery for left main coronary artery disease. N Engl J Med. 2016;375:2223-35.
20. Capodanno D, Stone GW, Morice MC, et al. Percutaneous coronary intervention versus coronary artery bypass graft surgery in left main coronary artery disease: a meta-analysis of randomized clinical data. J Am Coll Cardiol. 2011;58:1426-32.
21. Gargiulo G, Tamburino C, Capodanno D. Five-year outcomes of percutaneous coronary intervention versus coronary artery bypass graft surgery in patients with left main coronary artery disease: an updated meta-analysis of randomized trials and adjusted observational studies. Int J Cardiol. 2015;195:79-81.
22. Athappan G, Patvardhan E, Tuzcu ME, et al. Left main coronary artery stenosis: a meta-analysis of drug-eluting stents versus coronary artery bypass grafting. JACC Cardiovasc Interv. 2013;6:1219-30.

23. Nerlekar N, Ha FJ, Verma KP, et al. Percutaneous coronary intervention using drug-eluting stents versus coronary artery bypass grafting for unprotected left main coronary artery stenosis: a meta-analysis of randomized trials. Circ Cardiovasc Interv. 2016;9:e004729.
24. Liberati A, Altman DG, Tetzlaff J, et al. The PRISMA statement for reporting systematic reviews and meta-analyses of studies that evaluate healthcare interventions: explanation and elaboration. BMJ. 2009;339:b2700.
25. Kappetein AP, Feldman TE, Mack MJ, et al. Comparison of coronary bypass surgery with drug-eluting stenting for the treatment of left main and/or three-vessel disease: 3 year follow-up of the SYNTAX trial. Eur Heart J. 2011;32:2145-34.
26. Giacoppo D, Colleran R, Cassese S, et al. Percutaneous coronary intervention vs coronary artery bypass grafting in patients with left main coronary artery stenosis a systematic review and meta-analysis. JAMA Cardiol. 2017;2:1079-88.
27. Serruys PW, Morice MC, Kappetein AP, et al. SYNTAX Investigators. Percutaneous coronary intervention versus coronary-artery bypass grafting for severe coronary artery disease. N Engl J Med. 2009;360:961-72.
28. Morice MC, Serruys PW, Kappetein AP, et al. Outcomes in patients with de novo left main disease treated with either percutaneous coronary intervention using paclitaxel-eluting stents or coronary artery bypass graft treatment in the Synergy Between Percutaneous Coronary Intervention With TAXUS and Cardiac Surgery (SYNTAX) trial. Circulation. 2010;121:2645-53.
29. Park SJ, Kim YH, Park DW, et al. Randomized trials of stents versus bypass surgery for left main coronary artery disease. N Engl J Med. 2011;364:1718-27.
30. Tullio P, Serruys P, Kappetein AP, et al. Clinical outcome with percutaneous coronary revascularization vs coronary artery bypass grafting surgery in patients with unprotected left main coronary artery disease: A meta-analysis of 6 randomized trials and 4686 patients. Am Heart J. 2017;190:54-63.
31. Park DW, Kim YH, Yun SC, et al. Long-term outcomes after stenting versus coronary artery bypass grafting for unprotected left main coronary artery disease: 10-year results of bare-metal stents and 5-year results of drug-eluting stents from the ASAN-MAIN (ASAN Medical Center-Left MAIN Revascularization) Registry. J Am Coll Cardiol. 2010;56:1366-75.
32. Buszman PE, Buszman PP, Banasiewicz-Szkróbka I, et al. Left main stenting in comparison with surgical revascularization: 10-year outcomes of the (Left Main Coronary Artery Stenting) LE MANS Trial. JACC Cardiovasc Interv. 2016;9:318-27.
33. American College of Cardiology Foundation/American Heart Foundation Task Force: 2012 ACCF/AHA/ACP/AATS/PCNA/SCAI/STS guideline for the diagnosis and management of patients with stable ischemic heart disease: a report of the American College of Cardiology Foundation/American Heart Association Task Force on practice guidelines, and the American College of Physicians, American College of Thoracic Surgery, Preventive Cardiovascular Nurses Association, Society for Cardiovascular Angiography and Interventions, and Society of Thoracic Surgeons. Circulation. 2012;126:e354-471.
34. Task Force on Myocardial Revascularization of the European Society of Cardiology (ESC) and the European Association for Cardio Thoracic Surgery (EACTS): European Association for Percutaneous Cardiovascular Interventions (EAPCI) et al. Guidelines on myocardial revascularization. Eur Heart J. 2010;31:2501-55.
35. Palmerini T, Marzocchi A, Tamburino C, et al. Impact of bifurcation technique on 2-year clinical outcomes in 773 patients with distal unprotected left main coronary artery stenosis treated with drug-eluting stents. Circ Cardiovasc Interv. 2008:185-92.
36. Kim WJ, Kim YH, Park DW, et al. Comparison of single-versus two-stent techniques in treatment of unprotected left main coronary bifurcation disease. Catheter Cardiovasc Interv. 2011;77:775-82.
37. Song YB, Hahn JY, Yang JH, et al. Differential prognostic impact of treatment strategy among patients with left main versus non-left main bifurcation lesions undergoing percutaneous coronary intervention: results from the COBIS (Coronary Bifurcation Stenting) Registry II. JACC Cardiovasc Interv. 2014;7:255-63.
38. Toyofuku M, Kimura T, Morimoto T, et al. Three-year outcomes after sirolimus-eluting stent implantation for unprotected left main coronary artery disease: insights from the j-Cypher registry. Circulation. 2009;120:1866-74.
39. Lassen JF, Holm NR, Stankovic G, et al. Percutaneous coronary intervention for coronary bifurcation disease: consensus from the first 10 years of the European Bifurcation Club meetings. EuroIntervention. 2014;10:545-60.
40. Park SJ, Park HS, Kang SH, et al. TCT-234 Is final kissing ballooning mandatory in the treatment of distal left main disease treated by simple cross over stenting? J Am Coll Cardiol. 2014;64:11S.
41. Rha SW, Elnagar A, Choi BG, et al. As-174 Role of final kissing balloon for unprotected distal left main bifurcation intervention with single stent strategy. Am J Cardiol. 2012;109:S86-7.
42. Kang SJ, Ahn JM, Kim WJ, et al. Functional and morphological assessment of side branch after left main coronary artery bifurcation stenting with cross-over technique. Catheter Cardiovasc Interv. 2014;83:545-52.
43. Nam CW, Hur SH, Koo BK, et al. Fractional flow reserve versus angiography in left circumflex ostial intervention after left main crossover stenting. Korean Circ J. 2011;41:304-7.
44. Hamilos M, Muller O, Cuisset T, et al. Long-term clinical outcome after fractional flow reserve-guided treatment in patients with angiographically equivocal left main coronary artery stenosis. Circulation. 2009;120:1505-12.
45. Courtis J, Rodes-Cabau J, Larose E, et al. Usefulness of coronary fractional flow reserve measurements in guiding clinical decisions in intermediate or equivocal left main coronary stenoses. Am J Cardiol. 2009;103:943-9.
46. Ormiston JA, Webster MW, Webber B, et al. The "Crush" technique for coronary artery bifurcation stenting: insights from micro-computed tomographic imaging of bench deployments. JACC Cardiovasc Interv. 2008;1:351-57.
47. Chen SL, Xu B, Han YL, et al. Comparison of double kissing crush versus culotte stenting for unprotected distal left main bifurcation lesions: results from a multicenter, randomized, prospective DKCRUSH-III Study. J Am Coll Cardiol. 2013;61:1482-88.
48. Hildick-Smith D, Lassen JF, Albiero R, et al. Consensus from the 5th European Bifurcation Club meeting. EuroIntervention. 2010;6:34-8.
49. Kang SJ, Mintz GS, Kim WJ, et al. Changes in left main bifurcation geometry after a single-stent crossover technique: an intravascular ultrasound study using direct imaging of both the left anterior descending and the left circumflex coronary arteries before and after intervention. Circ Cardiovasc Interv. 2011;4: 355-61.
50. Nissen SE, Yock P. Intravascular ultrasound: novel pathophysiological insights and current clinical applications. Circulation. 2001;103:604-16.
51. Witzenbichler B, Maehara A, Weisz G, et al. Relationship between intravascular ultrasound guidance and clinical outcomes after drug-eluting stents: the assessment of dual antiplatelet therapy with drug-eluting stents (ADAPT-DES) study. Circulation. 2014;129:463-70.
52. Fitzgerald PJ, Oshima A, Hayase M, et al. Final results of the Can Routine Ultrasound Influence Stent Expansion (CRUISE) Study. Circulation. 2000;102: 523-30.
53. Ahn JM, Kang SJ, Yoon SH, et al. Meta-analysis of outcomes after intravascular ultrasound-guided versus angiography-guided drug-eluting stent implantation in 26,503 patients enrolled in three randomized trials and 14 observational studies. Am J Cardiol. 2014;113:1338-47.
54. Jang JS, Song YJ, Kang W, et al. Intravascular ultrasound-guided implantation of drug-eluting stents to improve outcome: a meta-analysis. JACC Cardiovasc Interv. 2014;7:233-43.
55. Park SJ, Kim YH, Park DW, et al. Impact of intravascular ultrasound guidance on long-term mortality in stenting for unprotected left main coronary artery stenosis. Circ Cardiovasc Interv. 2009;2:167-77.
56. Andell P, Karlsson S, Mohammad MA, et al. Intravascular ultrasound guidance is associated with better outcome in patients undergoing unprotected left main coronary artery stenting compared with angiography guidance alone. Circ Cardiovascular Interv. 2017;10:e004813.
57. Kang SJ, Ahn JM, Song H, et al. Comprehensive intravascular ultrasound assessment of stent area and its impact on restenosis and adverse cardiac events in 403 patients with unprotected left main disease. Cir Cardiovasc Interv. 2011;4:562-79.
58. Alegria-Barrero E, Foin N, Chan PH, et al. Optical coherence tomography for guidance of distal cell recrossing in bifurcation stenting: Choosing the right cell matters. EuroIntervention. 2012;8:205-13.
59. Gambhir DS, Singh S, Trehan V, et al. Elective stenting of unprotected left main coronary artery ostial stenosis: short-and midterm results. Ind Heart J. 1998;50:183-6.

CHAPTER 58

Current Update in the Treatment of Calcified Lesions

Matthew I Tomey, Samin Sharma

INTRODUCTION

Calcification is a defining feature of advanced coronary atherosclerotic plaque[1] and remains a challenge to optimal percutaneous coronary intervention (PCI). Calcified lesions are more difficult to cross and dilate. They are also more likely to be associated with suboptimal stent deployment, angiographic complications, and adverse clinical outcomes. Severe calcification often accompanies other complex lesion features such as chronic total occlusion, tortuosity, diffuse disease, or lesion location at a bifurcations or arterial ostium. With aging of the population and, in particular, management of coronary artery disease (CAD) in older adults undergoing transcatheter aortic valve replacement, the challenges of managing calcified coronary plaque have grown only more common in the contemporary cardiac catheterization laboratory. At one time, moderate or severe calcification conferred a 60–85% likelihood of success and a moderate risk of procedural complications.[2,3] Today, calcified lesions can be treated with an extremely high likelihood of success, with rates of angiographic and procedural success exceeding 99% in the drug-eluting stent era.[4] In this updated review, we provide our perspective on the present landscape of options for managing calcified plaque in 2018.

IDENTIFICATION AND CLASSIFICATION OF CALCIFICATION

A key principle in the successful interventional management of calcified CAD is that calcification should be recognized and characterized before the start of intervention. Anticipation of challenges posed by calcification permits appropriate preparation, device selection, and strategic planning and may help to avoid complications.

The primary method for recognition and qualification of lesion calcification continues to be fluoroscopy. In addition to being ubiquitous, fluoroscopy is highly specific for coronary calcification. As mineral content within coronary plaque accumulates, coronary artery calcium becomes progressively radiopaque (like bone) and visible by fluoroscopy. Current angiographic criteria for calcification of coronary plaque define moderate calcification as densities evident during the cardiac cycle before injection of contrast medium and severe calcification as radiopacities evident without cardiac motion before injection of contrast medium, typically involving both sides of the arterial wall (similar to "tram tracks").[5]

Yet as interventional cardiologists have long appreciated, fluoroscopy can be insensitive for detection of fibrocalcific plaque and inaccurate in discrimination of calcification as severe versus not severe and superficial versus deep. Growth in experience with advanced intravascular imaging modalities including intravascular ultrasound (IVUS) and optical coherence tomography (OCT) has confirmed this and today offers interventional cardiologists with additional options to refine diagnosis of coronary calcification in preparation for PCI. Using IVUS, plaque calcification appears as shadowing of deeper arterial structures with an acoustic signature that is brighter than the reference adventitia.[6] IVUS permits description of the arc, length, distribution, and depth of coronary calcium. On IVUS examination, calcification graded as severe by fluoroscopy is typically associated with a large arc of superficial calcium involving at least three quadrants.[6] Using time domain[7] and frequency domain[8] OCT examination, plaque calcification appears as a well-delineated signal-poor region with sharply defined borders. Variable attenuation of light by plaque lipid content can interfere with accurate measurement of calcium on OCT examination.

In our practice, we do not routinely use IVUS or OCT for the purpose of grading lesion calcification. These tools can be useful, however, in equivocal cases. In our experience, findings on intravascular imaging in such cases have underscored the need for a high-index of suspicion for fibrocalcific plaque in patients with high-risk clinical features such as advanced age, chronic kidney disease, and prior history of coronary artery bypass graft surgery (CABG).

PATIENT AND LESION SELECTION

Prerequisite to lesion-specific interventional management of calcified CAD is global assessment of the patient and appropriateness of PCI. Updated appropriate use criteria for coronary revascularization in stable ischemic heart disease provide guidance on the recommended role of PCI in different clinical and anatomic scenarios.[9] Calcification can influence this calculus in several ways. Lesion calcium can confound angiographic estimation of obstruction, leading to either over- or underestimation of diameter stenosis.[10] Both in isolation and in conjunction with other complex lesion features, calcification contributes to the SYNTAX score, influencing consideration of PCI versus CABG.

In our clinical experience caring for patients with calcified CAD, scenarios arise not infrequently in which coronary revascularization is indicated and coronary anatomy is favorable for CABG, but overall assessment of the patient by a heart team leads to recommendation against surgery. Examples include patients requiring reoperative heart surgery; older patients with severe aortic stenosis assigned to transcatheter aortic valve replacement; patients with severe left ventricular dysfunction; and patients with multiple comorbidities conferring high surgical risk. As a consequence of this selection process, patients undergoing PCI for calcified CAD often have multiple high-risk features and limited reserve to tolerate complications.

WIRE SELECTION

Standard "workhorse" guidewires are usually sufficient for PCI of calcified lesions. When severe calcification is accompanied by significant angulation or arterial tortuosity, the properties of a chosen guidewire may have greater impact on the performance of PCI. In such cases, guidewires with hydrophilic coating may help to facilitate wire manipulation and delivery of interventional devices. If device delivery across calcified segments is impossible despite use of a hydrophilic guidewire, other options may include addition of a second "buddy" wire or deep coronary intubation with a child-in-mother catheter.

When an atheroablative strategy is planned, a specialty guidewire is required for compatibility with the chosen atheroablative device. Manipulation and lesion crossing with these finer wires are possible but can be more challenging, with risks of wire kinking and dissection. In most cases, we primarily wire with a hydrophilic guidewire within a microcatheter, such as the FineCross® MG (Terumo Interventional Systems, Tokyo; Japan) or Threader™ (Boston Scientific, Natick; MA). In addition to supporting wire manipulation and permitting subsequent exchange for an 0.009" RotaWire™ (for rotational atherectomy; Boston Scientific, Natick; MA) or 0.012" ViperWire™ (for orbital atherectomy; Cardiovascular Systems, Inc., St Paul; MN), the use of a microcatheter provides an additional gauge of stenosis severity and likelihood of crossing with an atheroablative device. As a rule of thumb, if our microcatheter does not cross, we will instead primarily wire with and proceed directly to atheroablation using a smallest size burr or crown.

MODIFICATION OF CALCIFIED LESIONS

Whereas emphasis in an earlier era of PCI was placed on "debulking" of calcified plaque, focus today is instead placed on modification of lesion properties to facilitate subsequent balloon angioplasty and stenting. Multiple devices for this purpose are available today (Table 1),[11] which can be loosely divided into techniques based on balloon inflation and techniques based on atheroablation: rotational atherectomy, orbital atherectomy, and excimer laser coronary angioplasty (ELCA). In our practice, we favor an up-front strategy of atheroablation for target lesions associated with moderate or severe calcification (Flowchart 1). Although the largest randomized trial of an atheroablative strategy in the drug-eluting stent era (the Rotational Atherectomy Prior to Taxus Stent Treatment for Complex Native Coronary Artery Disease study, ROTAXUS) did not show reduction in major adverse cardiac events (MACEs),[12] strategic success was indeed superior with rotational atherectomy as compared with traditional balloon angioplasty for moderately or severely calcified lesions, as has been our experience.

Both rotational and orbital atherectomy can be highly effective for facilitating PCI of calcified lesions and we continue to incorporate both tools in our practice. For many calcified lesions, either device can be used effectively and safely and device selection is influenced predominantly by operator and laboratory preference and comfort. In some cases, however, details of coronary anatomy can favor preferential use of one device or the other. Here, we will compare and contrast the two techniques (Table 2).

Rotational and orbital atherectomy share common principles. Both exploit the material properties of calcium to selectively ablate calcified plaque and to facilitate device

TABLE 1: Interventional adjuncts to balloon angioplasty for modification of calcified lesions

Approach	Example
Scoring balloon angioplasty	AngioSculpt® (AngioScore, Inc., Fremont; CA)
Cutting balloon angioplasty	Wolverine™ (Boston Scientific, Natick; MA)
Constrained semicompliant balloon angioplasty	Chocolate® (TriReme Medical, Pleasanton; CA)
Rotational atherectomy	Rotablator™ (Boston Scientific, Natick; MA)
Orbital atherectomy	Diamondback 360® (Cardiovascular Systems, Inc., St Paul; MN)
Excimer laser coronary angioplasty	CVX-300® (Spectranetics, Colorado Springs; CO)

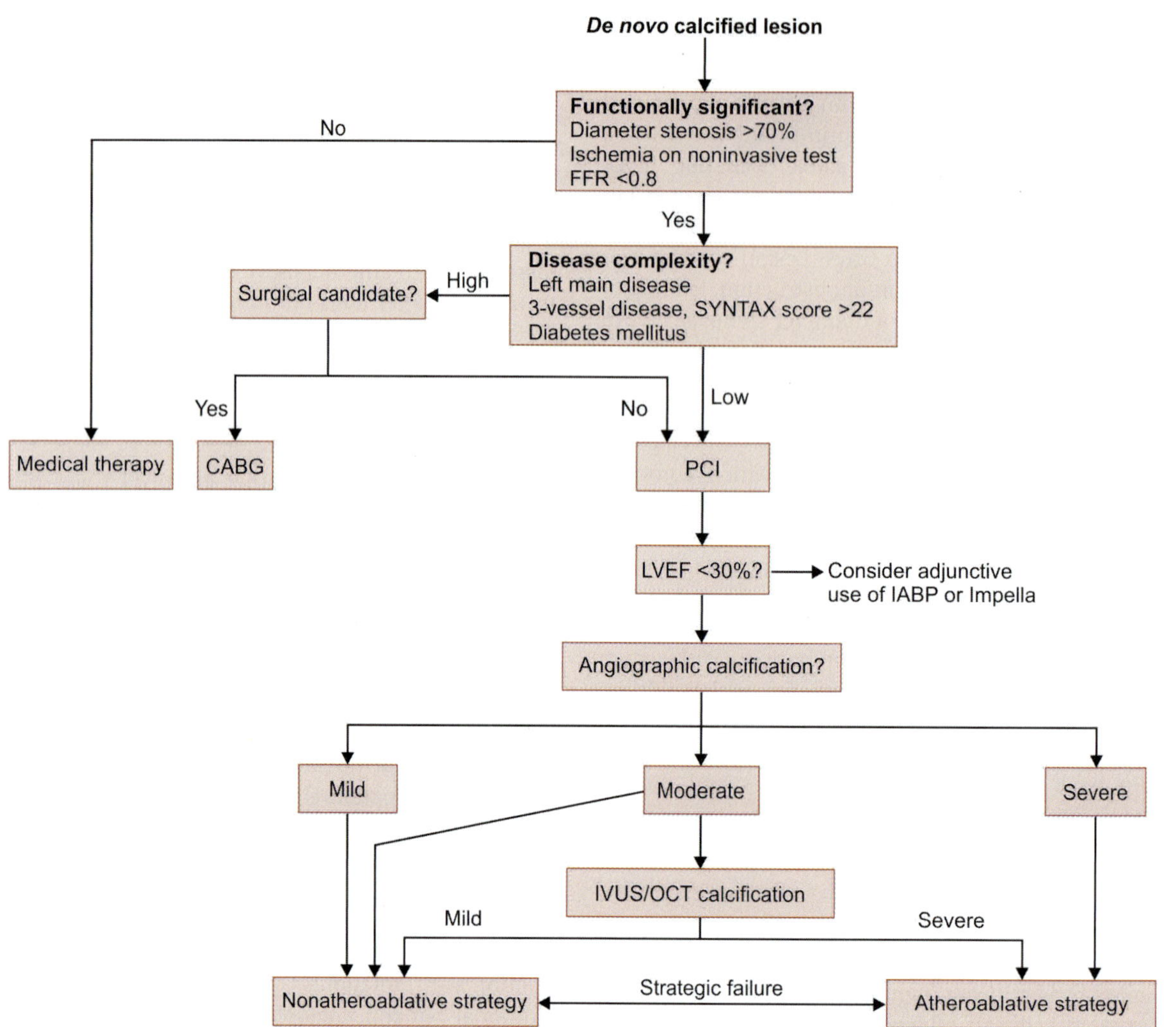

CABG, coronary artery bypass graft surgery; FFR, fractional flow reserve; IABP, intra-aortic balloon pump; IVUS, intravascular ultrasound; LVEF, left ventricular ejection fraction; OCT, optical coherence tomography; PCI, percutaneous coronary intervention.

FLOWCHART 1: In patients with *de novo* calcified lesions for whom PCI is indicated clinically, lesion modification via atheroablation is appropriate in order to facilitate procedural success when calcification is severe. If calcification severity is intermediate or indeterminate by angiography, intravascular imaging with IVUS or OCT may be useful for reclassification.

Source: Adapted from Tomey et al.[13] with permission from the author and Publisher.

advancement through jagged calcified segments.[13]. Rapid rotation of the rotational atherectomy burr (differential cutting) and rapid orbiting of the orbital atherectomy crown (differential sanding) preferentially ablates hard, inelastic tissue which, unlikely healthy arterial wall, cannot stretch away from the ablative device. High speed of device rotation or orbit displaces friction orthogonally and facilitates forward motion of the device across plaque. Diamond chips on the surface of the burr or crown ablate calcified plaque into microscopic particles which traverse the coronary microvasculature and eventually undergo phagocytosis within the reticuloendothelial system.[14]

Shared complications of rotational and orbital atherectomy include clinical complications common to PCI, including bleeding, vascular complications, stroke, myocardial infarction, urgent CABG and death and angiographic complications, including dissection, perforation, acute closure, side branch loss, and slow-flow/no-reflow.[15] Incidence of slow-flow/no-reflow during atheroablation is significantly lower today, down from as high as 15% in early series of rotational atherectomy[16] to as low as 0.0–2.6% in more recent series.[13] It is our belief that this reduction derives from iterative improvements in operator technique, optimal antiplatelet therapy, incorporation of a continuously infusing flush cocktail, and careful attention to maintaining adequate coronary perfusion pressure.[13] Very low observed rates of slow-flow/no-reflow using the orbital atherectomy may relate to design features that provide for higher flow of flush cocktail (18 mL/min) and an orbiting crown less likely to obstruct the lumen,[17] promoting clearance of debris and reducing microvascular obstruction.[18]

TABLE 2: Comparison of rotational atherectomy and orbital atherectomy

	Rotational atherectomy	Orbital atherectomy
Wire	0.009" RotaWire™	0.012" ViperWire™
Lubricant	RotaGlide™	ViperSlide™
Ablative device	"Burr"	"Crown"
Diamond chips	Anterior only	Anterior and posterior
Sizes	Multiple (1.25, 1.5, 1.75, 2.0, 2.25, 2.38, 2.5 mm), interchangeable	Single (1.25 mm), with larger path carved by higher speed
Guide catheter size	6 Fr: for 1.25, 1.5, 1.75 mm burrs 7 Fr: for 2.0 mm burr 8 Fr: for 2.25, 2.38, 2.5 mm burrs	6 Fr
Axial motion	Rotational	Elliptical
Longitudinal motion	Pecking, intermittent	Gradual, continuous
Direction of ablation	Forward only	Forward and backward
Maximum run	20 s	25 s
Difficulty of setup	Higher	Lower
Learning curve	Longer	Shorter
Body of experience	Decades	Years
Effect on plaque	Shallower dissections	Deeper dissections

PERFORMANCE OF ATHEROABLATION

Vascular Access and Guide Catheter Selection

Selection of vascular access approach, sheath, and guide catheter for a given patient should balance simultaneous goals of reducing bleeding and vascular complications and providing adequate support for atheroablation. For most patients, a 6 French system is adequate to support atheroablation, accommodating the orbital atherectomy crown and rotational atherectomy burr sizes up to 1.75 mm, and readily permitting either a transfemoral or transradial approach. Indeed, it is important to note that atheroablation is feasible from the radial approach with comparable procedural success.[19,20] Support can be further enhanced by use of a long sheath; selection of a guide catheter shape associated with extra back-up; and use of a child-in-mother catheter. The 7 French or larger systems may be desired or needed for cases in which complex bifurcation PCI is anticipated or requirement for a 2.0 mm or larger rotational atherectomy burr. In such cases, transfemoral access may be preferred, although some patients may be eligible for transradial access using sheathless guide catheters with internal diameters up to 7.5 French or 7 French glide sheaths with a 6 French profile. Coaxial guide placement is essential to facilitate burr or crown passage and avoid dissections.

Wiring

Prior to beginning atheroablation, it is necessary to position a device-specific wire (RotaWire™ or ViperWire™) across the target lesion with its radiopaque tip positioned as far distally as possible within the target vessel, avoiding small branches and eliminating any distal loops, bends, or kinks. This will reduce risk of wire fracture and coronary perforation. Although this can be accomplished by wiring primarily with the RotaWire™ or ViperWire™, the properties of lesions selected for atherectomy can make this challenging and predispose to wire kinking. Instead, it can be easier to first wire with a workhorse or specialty 0.014" coronary guide wire and then exchange for the RotaWire™ or ViperWire™ using a microexchange catheter or over-the-wire balloon.

Properties of a chosen wire influence its tendency to wire bias, with stiffer wires conferring greater wire bias and preferential ablation at the lesser curvatures of angulated segments. This is particularly relevant to rotational atherectomy as the path of atheroablation tracks coaxially with the path of the central guidewire. This property of stiffer wires (e.g., the extra support RotaWire™) can be exploited deliberately to enhance modification of plaques predominantly localized to the lesser curvature, although significant care is required in treatment of highly angulated segments to avoid dissection and perforation. The stiffer extra support RotaWire™ is also preferred for treatment of ostial lesions. Otherwise, in our practice, the floppy RotaWire™ remains suitable for most lesions treated with rotational atherectomy, and the ViperWire™ is used for all cases of orbital atherectomy.

Both as preparation for subsequent angioplasty and stenting and as a safety precaution in case device delivery is required urgently, as in cases of dissection and perforation, we recommend preparing a standard workhorse wire with an appropriate curve in advance of beginning atheroablation.

Burr and Crown Selection

In rotational atherectomy, the ultimate cross-sectional area of atheroablation approximates that of the largest burr size used.

Although larger burrs (with a burr:artery ratio >0.7) effect greater plaque debulking, smaller burrs (with burr:artery ratio <0.7) permit equivalent angiographic and procedural success with fewer angiographic complications, reduced periprocedural creatine kinase (CK)-MB release, smaller sheaths and guide catheters and, in turn, lower vascular and bleeding complications.[21,22] Accordingly, as procedural goals have shifted from plaque debulking to lesion modification, the optimal final burr:artery ratio is 0.5–0.6. In many cases, this can be accomplished with a single appropriately sized burr (Table 1). For epicardial vessels less than 3 mm in diameter, a 1.5 mm burr is usually appropriate. For epicardial vessels larger than 3 mm in diameter, a 1.75 mm burr is generally sufficient. In some cases, a stepped burr strategy may be preferable; factors favoring this approach include inability to cross the target lesion with a microexchange catheter or balloon and severe angulation, tortuosity or eccentricity. In such cases, initial rotational atherectomy using a 1.25 mm burr is preferred. Analogously, in cases in which an initially selected 1.5 mm or larger burr fails to crack a lesion or encounters excessive decelerations, downsizing the burr can be useful to facilitate lesion modification and reduce risk of procedural complications. Conversely, if attempted balloon dilatation is not successful after initial ablation with a 1.25 mm burr, upsizing to a 1.5 mm or 1.75 mm burr may be required to effect sufficient lesion modification.

The Diamondback 360® Coronary Orbital Atherectomy System currently uses a single 1.25 mm "classic crown." Unlike rotational atherectomy, with orbital atherectomy, the ultimate cross-sectional area of atheroablation is larger than the crown and dependent upon the speed of lesion crossing, the rotational speed, and the number of passes. Larger luminal areas are associated with slower lesion crossing, faster rotational speed, and increased numbers of passes. In a carbon block model, using a 1.25 mm crown and 20 forward and backward passes over approximately 5 minutes of treatment time, a rotational speed of 80,000 rpm was associated with a maximum luminal diameter of 1.64 mm and a rotational speed of 120,000 rpm was associated with a maximum luminal diameter of 1.84 mm. Of note, whereas rotational atherectomy tends to generate a mostly cylindrical lumen in treated areas after atheroablation, in clinical practice, orbital atherectomy can produce lumina of irregular shapes with variable degrees of guttering. In our practice, we have found that the slower rotational speed of 80,000 rpm is safe and effective for the vast majority of treated lesions.

Flush Solution

A pressurized, continuous flush solution is essential with both rotational and orbital atherectomy to lubricate the atheroablative device, to minimize thermal injury and to promote microvascular clearance of debris.

For rotational atherectomy, the traditional composition of the flush solution included heparinized saline, vasodilators, and RotaGlide™ lubricant, a especially designed solution comprised of olive oil, egg yolk, phospholipids, sodium deoxycholate, L-histidine, disodium ethylenediamine-tetraacetic acid (EDTA), sodium hydroxide, and water. In comparison with heparinized saline alone, addition of RotaGlide™ lubricant is associated with reduced heat generation. Due to its composition, RotaGlide™ is contraindicated in patients with allergies to egg or olive oil; use of flush solutions omitting RotaGlide™ have been reported with comparable procedural success.[23] Vasodilators incorporated in flush solutions, included for the purpose of preventing slow-flow/no-reflow, have included nitroglycerin, verapamil, nicardipine, adenosine, and nicorandil, in varied combinations.[16,24-28] As rotational atherectomy technique has improved, many users have found it possible to diminish or eliminate inclusion of vasodilators in the flush solution,[29] maintaining low rates of slow-flow/no-reflow while avoiding hypotension and bradycardia. Today, we recommend a standard rotational atherectomy flush solution composed of heparinized saline and RotaGlide™ only, reserving vasodilators for provisional use.

In the case of orbital atherectomy, flush solution is comprised of normal saline and ViperSlide™, a proprietary lubricant especially designed for the orbital atherectomy system. No additional vasodilators are required to be added to this cocktail and we again favor only provisional use of intracoronary vasodilators during performance of orbital atherectomy. Of note, a safety mechanism in the orbital atherectomy system prohibits device activation in the absence of continuous pressurized flush solution.

Adjunctive Pharmacology

Patients undergoing atheroablation should receive optimal anticoagulation and antiplatelet therapy for PCI in accordance with standard practices. Glycoprotein IIb/IIIa inhibitors (GPI) were associated with reduction in periprocedural CK-MB release and slow-flow/no-reflow phenomenon in earlier series of rotational atherectomy, reflecting the integral role of thrombosis to these complications.[30] With advances in anticoagulant and antiplatelet therapies and recognition of bleeding complications associated with routine GPI use, however, GPI should today be reserved for only provisional use.

Temporary Pacing

Transient microvascular ischemia of the cardiac conduction system and associated atrioventricular block can occur during atheroablation of the right coronary artery, dominant left circumflex artery, or, in the setting of chronic total occlusion of the dominant vessel, atheroablation of a vessel providing major collateral circulation.[31] In anticipation of that possibility, insertion of a transvenous pacemaker historically was considered prerequisite to atheroablation for such a vessel.

More recently, preemptive insertion of a transvenous pacemaker in this situation has become less uniform, with some operators preferring provisional use and initial management with atropine, aminophylline or antivagal maneuvers. Reasons for this transition include recognition of risk of ventricular perforation and cardiac tamponade; reduced severity of distal microembolization and microvascular ischemia with optimal technique; and recognition of the usually transient and remediable nature of atrioventricular block during atheroablation.

Mechanical Circulatory Support

Atheroablation in and of itself is not an indication for mechanical cardiac support. When temporary mechanical circulatory support is otherwise indicated for high-risk PCI, however, such support may permit more complete revascularization and greater operator comfort and possibly safety using atheroablative devices. In a randomized study comparing the Impella Recover LP 2.5 versus intra-aortic balloon counterpulsation for support of elective high-risk PCI, rotational atherectomy was employed more extensively at operator discretion in subjects assigned to Impella support with higher periprocedural CK-MB release but no increase in death or large (clinically-relevant) myocardial infarction and, in fact, a significant reduction in major adverse events at 3-month follow-up.[32]

Preparatory Steps

Once optimal anticoagulation and antiplatelet therapy have been confirmed, and the RotaWire™ or ViperWire™ is positioned appropriately across the lesion, key steps are taken to ensure readiness for atheroablation and swift response to potential complications. We recommend preemptively opening and preparing a noncompliant balloon sized 1:1 to the reference vessel diameter. Once the chosen device has been opened and assembled, outside of the body, the operator must verify free flow of flush solution through the distal end of the device; free movement of the advancer knob, and, once loaded on the back end of the wire, device rotation at the appropriate speed. For the great majority of lesions, we favor a set rotational speed of 140,000–160,000 rpm for rotational atherectomy and 80,000 rpm for orbital atherectomy.[33] The device is then advanced over the wire through and just beyond the tip of the guide catheter. It is not necessary to activate rotation of the device during advance through the guide. As the device advances, an assistant withdraws the wire at an equal pace in order to maintain stable wire position within the vessel. We favor active use of fluoroscopy at low magnification during this process to verify stability of wire position. Finally, before beginning atheroablation, three steps are taken to remove tension from the system in order to prevent the device from jumping forward and, potentially, causing dissection, perforation or entrapment. First, unlock and gently advance and retract the device. Second, disengage the hemostatic valve on the guide catheter and gently advance and retract the drive shaft. Third, transiently activate the device at a low rotational speed. In the case of rotational atherectomy, this is accomplished by tapping on the foot pedal while in Dynaglide mode. In the case of orbital atherectomy, this is performed by briefly toggling the device on and then off.

Device Motion and Ablation Speed

Proper technique in device motion plays an important role in the efficacy and safety of rotational and orbital atherectomy, and it is important to recognize that optimal motion differs for the two devices.

For rotational atherectomy, technique has improved iteratively over decades of use with less excessive deceleration and stalling, less distal thromboembolization, and less thermal injury.[34] In addition to appropriate burr sizing, fundamental elements of optimal rotational atherectomy technique today include (1) a rotational speed of 140,000–160,000 rpm, (2) gradual burr advancement with a slow, pecking to-and-fro motion, (3) short ablation runs lasting no more than 15–20 seconds, pausing between runs, and (4) avoidance of decelerations greater than 5,000 rpm. Visual, tactile, and auditory feedback provides additional signals concerning resistance to burr advancement. Once the lesion has been fully crossed, rotational atherectomy is completed with a final polishing run, which should be smooth and without resistance. For lesions that cannot be crossed despite optimal technique, options to be considered include higher speeds, downsizing the burr, upgrading support using a more supportive guide catheter or adding a child-in-mother catheter. Of note, whereas early literature associated higher rotational speeds with risk of slow flow due to increased platelet aggregation, higher speed ablation may today be safe when combined with other elements of optimal technique. In recent randomized comparison of low-speed (140,000 rpm) versus high-speed (190,000 rpm) rotational atherectomy, there was no difference detected in incidence of slow flow.[35]

For orbital atherectomy, in contrast, the optimal device motion[17] entails not pecking but rather slow and steady advance. The crown should be brought to approximately 5 mm proximal to the target lesion and then advanced, initially with low rotational speed (80,000 rpm), at a rate of approximately 1 mm/second, monitoring on fluoroscopy to ensure 1:1 movement of the crown and advancer knob. A run of orbital atherectomy, not to exceed 30 seconds in duration, consists of multiple passes at this speed forward and backward through a target lesion, maintaining continuous movement and finally returning to a proximal resting point outside the lesion. Multiple runs may be required to completely treat a lesion, with a total treatment time not to exceed 5 minutes. As with rotational atherectomy, we advocate concluding orbital atherectomy with a final polishing run.

Procedure Completion and Device Removal

At the conclusion of atheroablation, the rotational atherectomy burr is removed by activating Dynaglide™ mode, pressing the brake defeat button, and manually withdrawing the burr while stepping on the foot pedal at low-rotational speed. As the burr is withdrawn, an assistant advances the RotaWire™ at an equal pace in order to maintain stable wire position within the vessel. Mechanics of device removal are similar for orbital atherectomy, noting that a new GlideAssist™ mode (akin to Dynaglide™) has recently been added to permit activation of the device at slow rotational speed (5,000 rpm) to facilitate device tracking and removal.

Once the device is out of the body, cineangiography is indicated to assess the effects of atheroablation and to exclude incident complications. Safe performance of atheroablation without use of contrast has been described, but pending additional data, this approach remains exploratory and should be limited to highly experienced operators skilled with both atheroablative devices and intravascular imaging.[36]

POSTATHEROABLATION ANGIOPLASTY AND STENTING

In the absence of complications, the prepared workhorse guide wire is advanced across the lesion and balloon angioplasty and stent implantation proceed in standard fashion. Due to the calcific nature of lesions treated, noncompliant balloons are the standard of care for postatheroablation balloon angioplasty. In the current era, noting high rates of restenosis and repeat revascularization in calcified lesions with or without adjunctive use of atheroablation,[37] contemporary drug-eluting stents should be considered the treatment of choice, sized 1:1 to the reference vessel diameter. In a series of 1,176 *de novo* coronary lesions treated with rotational atherectomy from 2002 to 2013, drug eluting stents were associated with a more than 50% reduction in MACEs [hazard ratio 0.42, 95% confidence interval (CI) 0.26–0.67, p <0.001].[38] In target vessels for which reference vessel size is angiographically ambiguous, postatherectomy IVUS or OCT may be a useful guide for optimal stent sizing.

COMPARATIVE EFFICACY

To date, no trial has compared orbital and rotational atherectomy with respect to efficacy endpoints. Early insights from plaque imaging after atheroablation suggest that there are differences between the two techniques in their effects on plaque. In a series of 20 patients with OCT imaging before and after orbital atherectomy (n = 10) or rotational atherectomy (n = 10), orbital atherectomy was associated with deeper dissections, especially in plaques with comparatively less calcium and more lipid content.[39] Orbital atherectomy was associated in this small series with improved stent expansion and lower incidence of stent strut malposition (4% vs. 8%, p = 0.038). Additional comparative data on procedural outcomes, 30-day and 1-year clinical outcomes after rotational and orbital atherectomy are anticipated from the Multicenter Prospective Study to Evaluate Outcomes of the Moderate to Severely Calcified Coronary Lesions (MACE; ClinicalTrials.gov Identifier: NCT01930214), which was completed in June 2017.

OTHER DEVICES

An effective alternative to rotational or orbital atherectomy for modification of calcified or fibrocalcific plaque is photoablation with ELCA.[40-45] ELCA works by directing pulses of ultraviolet light to coronary plaque via optical fibers. These pulses cause vaporization of water, dissociation of carbon-carbon bonds, and molecular vibration leading to plaque destruction. Appropriate eye protection is required with use of ELCA. Unlike rotational and orbital atherectomy, which require placement of a RotaWire™ or ViperWire™, ELCA is compatible with a standard coronary guidewire. This feature can be quite useful for severe lesions and chronic total occlusions through which an exchange catheter cannot cross and exchange to or primary writing with a RotaWire™ or ViperWire™ is not possible. In our practice, ELCA serves a specialty role for such lesions, as well as selected recalcitrant undilatable lesions and in-stent restenosis within calcified lesions.

Atheroablation is not required for treatment of all calcified lesions, and in particular those with less than severe calcification. Indeed—with some effort—comparable results can be achieved with "plain old balloon angioplasty",[46] cutting and scoring balloon angioplasty.[47] No significant difference in clinical outcomes was observed in the randomized ROTAXUS trial with a primary strategy of rotational atherectomy,[37] and additional data are awaited from the randomized ECLIPSE trial comparing orbital atherectomy versus conventional balloon angioplasty, currently enrolling (ClinicalTrials.gov Identifier: NCT03108456). Should these approaches fail to effectively prepare a lesion, however, secondary conversion to an atheroablative strategy may be required. Should complications of balloon angioplasty occur, such as dissection, secondary application of atheroablation may be relatively contraindicated. Operators should practice within the scope of their training and comfort. We strongly advocate that operators who treat calcified and complex lesions should gain proper training in and comfort with use of atheroablative devices so that patients can be offered the benefit of atheroablation as an up front strategy when appropriate.

CONCLUSION

The availability and maturation of multiple techniques for atheroablation today makes effective interventional management of calcified CAD possible and safe in the overwhelming majority of cases. Comfort in diagnosis and management of calcified coronary plaque has become ever more important as our population ages. The subset of older adults undergoing evaluation for transcatheter aortic valve replacement constitutes an important and growing population of patients who benefit from optimal interventional management of calcified CAD. In 2018, it is incumbent upon interventional cardiologists who treat these patients to develop proficiency in a full spectrum of tools for interventional management, including atheroablative devices. We strongly advocate the establishment of centers of excellence for interventional management of calcified CAD that will serve both as leaders in patient care and education.

REFERENCES

1. Stary HC, Chandler AB, Dinsmore RE, et al. A definition of advanced types of atherosclerotic lesions and a histological classification of atherosclerosis. A report from the Committee on Vascular Lesions of the Council on Arteriosclerosis, American Heart Association. Circulation. 1995;92:1355-74.
2. Ryan TJ, Faxon DP, Gunnar RM, et al. Guidelines for percutaneous transluminal coronary angioplasty. A report of the American College of Cardiology/American Heart Association Task Force on Assessment of Diagnostic and Therapeutic Cardiovascular Procedures (Subcommittee on Percutaneous Transluminal Coronary Angioplasty). Circulation, 1988;78:486-502.
3. Bredlau CE, Roubin GS, Leimgruber PP, et al. In-hospital morbidity and mortality in patients undergoing elective coronary angioplasty. Circulation. 1985;72:1044-52.
4. Bangalore S, Vlachos HA, Selzer F, et al. Percutaneous coronary intervention of moderate to severe calcified coronary lesions: insights from the National Heart, Lung, and Blood Institute Dynamic Registry. Catheter Cardiovasc Interv. 2011;77:22-8.
5. Moussa I, Ellis SG, Jones M, et al. Impact of coronary culprit lesion calcium in patients undergoing paclitaxel-eluting stent implantation (a TAXUS-IV sub study). Am J Cardiol. 2005;96:1242-7.
6. Mintz GS, Popma JJ, Pichard AD, et al. Patterns of Calcification in Coronary Artery Disease: A Statistical Analysis of Intravascular Ultrasound and Coronary Angiography in 1155 Lesions. Circulation. 1995;91:1959-65.
7. Yabushita H, Bouma BE, Houser SL, et al. Characterization of human atherosclerosis by optical coherence tomography. Circulation. 2002;106:1640-5.
8. Mehanna E, Bezerra HG, Prabhu D, et al. Volumetric characterization of human coronary calcification by frequency-domain optical coherence tomography. Circ J. 2013;77:2334-40.
9. Patel MR, Calhoon JH, Dehmer GJ, et al. ACC/AATS/AHA/ASE/ASNC/SCAI/SCCT/STS 2017 Appropriate Use Criteria for Coronary Revascularization in Patients With Stable Ischemic Heart Disease: A Report of the American College of Cardiology Appropriate Use Criteria Task Force, American Association for Thoracic Surgery, American Heart Association, American Society of Echocardiography, American Society of Nuclear Cardiology, Society for Cardiovascular Angiography and Interventions, Society of Cardiovascular Computed Tomography, and Society of Thoracic Surgeons. J Am Coll Cardiol. 2017;69:2212-41.
10. Topol EJ, Nissen SE. Our preoccupation with coronary luminology. The dissociation between clinical and angiographic findings in ischemic heart disease. Circulation. 1995;92:2333-42.
11. Waller BF. "Crackers, breakers, stretchers, drillers, scrapers, shavers, burners, welders and melters"—the future treatment of atherosclerotic coronary artery disease? A clinical-morphologic assessment. J Am Coll Cardiol. 1989;13:969-87.
12. Abdel-Wahab M, Richardt G, Joachim Buttner H, et al. High-speed rotational atherectomy before paclitaxel-eluting stent implantation in complex calcified coronary lesions: the randomized ROTAXUS (Rotational Atherectomy Prior to Taxus Stent Treatment for Complex Native Coronary Artery Disease) trial. JACC Cardiovasc Interv. 2013;6:10-9.
13. Tomey MI, Kini AS, Sharma SK. Current status of rotational atherectomy. JACC Cardiovasc Interv. 2014;7:345-53.
14. Hansen DD, Auth DC, Vracko R, et al. Rotational atherectomy in atherosclerotic rabbit iliac arteries. Am Heart J. 1988;115:160-5.
15. Cavusoglu E, Kini AS, Marmur JD, et al. Current status of rotational atherectomy. Catheter Cardiovasc Interv. 2004;62:485-98.
16. Hanna GP, Yhip P, Fujise K, et al. Intracoronary adenosine administered during rotational atherectomy of complex lesions in native coronary arteries reduces the incidence of no-reflow phenomenon. Catheter Cardiovasc Interv. 1999;48:275-8.
17. Shlofmitz E, Martinsen BJ, Lee M, et al. Orbital atherectomy for the treatment of severely calcified coronary lesions: evidence, technique, and best practices. Expert Rev Med Devices. 2017;14:867-79.
18. Galougahi KK, Bhatti N, Shlofmitz R, et al. TCT-236 Effects of Orbital Versus Rotational Atherectomy Facilitated PCI on the Coronary Microcirculation. J Amn Coll Cardiol. 2016;68:B96.
19. Kotowycz MA, Khan SQ, Freixa X, et al. Rotational atherectomy through the radial artery is associated with similar procedural success when compared with the transfemoral route. Coron Artery Dis. 2015;26:254-8.
20. Watt J, Oldroyd KG. Radial versus femoral approach for high-speed rotational atherectomy. Catheter Cardiovasc Interv. 2009;74:550-4.
21. Whitlow PL, Bass TA, Kipperman RM, et al. Results of the study to determine rotablator and transluminal angioplasty strategy (STRATAS). Am J Cardiol. 2001;87:699-705.
22. Safian RD, Feldman T, Muller DW, et al. Coronary angioplasty and Rotablator atherectomy trial (CARAT): immediate and late results of a prospective multicenter randomized trial. Catheter Cardiovasc Interv. 2001;53:213-20.
23. Whiteside HL, Ratanapo S, Sey A, et al. Efficacy of a heparin based rota-flush solution in patients undergoing rotational atherectomy. Cardiovasc Revasc Med. 2017;19(3 Pt B):333-7.
24. Tsubokawa A, Ueda K, Sakamoto H, et al. Effect of intracoronary nicorandil administration on preventing no-reflow/slow flow phenomenon during rotational atherectomy. Circ J. 2002;66:1119-23.
25. Matsuo H, Watanabe S, Watanabe T, et al. Prevention of no-reflow/slow-flow phenomenon during rotational atherectomy—a prospective randomized study comparing intracoronary continuous infusion of verapamil and nicorandil. Am Heart J. 2007;154:994.e1-6.
26. Iwasaki K, Samukawa M, Furukawa H. Comparison of the effects of nicorandil versus verapamil on the incidence of slow flow/no reflow during rotational atherectomy. Am J Cardiol. 2006;98:1354-6.
27. Cohen BM, Weber VJ, Blum RR, et al. Cocktail attenuation of rotational ablation flow effects (CARAFE) study: pilot. Cathet Cardiovasc Diagn. 1996;Suppl 3:69-72.
28. Tsao TP, Cheng SM, Cheng CC, et al. Comparison of intracoronary adenosine and isosorbide dinitrate on no-reflow/slow flow during rotational atherectomy. Acta Cardiol. 2009;64:225-30.
29. Lee MS, Kim MH, Rha SW. Alternative Rota-Flush Solution for Patients With Severe Coronary Artery Calcification who Undergo Rotational Atherectomy. J Invasive Cardiol. 2017;29:25-8.
30. Kini A, Reich D, Marmur JD, et al. Reduction in periprocedural enzyme elevation by abciximab after rotational atherectomy of type B2 lesions: Results of the Rota ReoPro randomized trial. Am Heart J. 2001;142:965-9.
31. Mitar MD, Ratner S, Lavi S. Heart block and temporary pacing during rotational atherectomy. Can J Cardiol. 2015;31:335-40.
32. Dangas GD, Kini AS, Sharma SK, et al. Impact of hemodynamic support with Impella 2.5 versus intra-aortic balloon pump on prognostically important clinical outcomes in patients undergoing high-risk percutaneous coronary intervention (from the PROTECT II randomized trial). Am J Cardiol. 2014;113:222-8.
33. Reisman M, Shuman BJ, Dillard D, et al. Analysis of low-speed rotational atherectomy for the reduction of platelet aggregation. Cathet Cardiovasc Diagn. 1998;45:208-14.
34. Reisman M, Shuman BJ, Harms V. Analysis of heat generation during rotational atherectomy using different operational techniques. Cathet Cardiovasc Diagn. 1998;44:453-5.
35. Sakakura K, Funayama H, Taniguchi Y, et al. The incidence of slow flow after rotational atherectomy of calcified coronary arteries: A randomized study of low speed versus high speed. Catheter Cardiovasc Interv. 2017;89:832-40.
36. Karimi Galougahi K, Mintz GS, Karmpaliotis D, et al. Zero-contrast percutaneous coronary intervention on calcified lesions facilitated by rotational atherectomy. Catheter Cardiovasc Interv. 2017;90(4):E85-9.
37. de Waha S, Allali A, Buttner HJ, et al. Rotational atherectomy before paclitaxel-eluting stent implantation in complex calcified coronary lesions: Two-year clinical outcome of the randomized ROTAXUS trial. Catheter Cardiovasc Interv. 2016;87:691-700.
38. Kawamoto H, Latib A, Ruparelia N, et al. In-hospital and midterm clinical outcomes of rotational atherectomy followed by stent implantation: the ROTATE multicentre registry. EuroIntervention. 2016;12:1448-56.
39. Kini AS, Vengrenyuk Y, Pena J, et al. Optical coherence tomography assessment of the mechanistic effects of rotational and orbital atherectomy in severely calcified coronary lesions. Catheter Cardiovasc Interv. 2015;86(6):1024-32.
40. Bilodeau L, Fretz EB, Taeymans Y, et al. Novel use of a high-energy excimer laser catheter for calcified and complex coronary artery lesions. Catheter Cardiovasc Interv. 2004;62:155-61.
41. Ahmed WH, al-Anazi MM, Bittl JA. Excimer laser-facilitated angioplasty for undilatable coronary narrowings. Am J Cardiol. 1996;78:1045-6.

42. Henson KD, Leon MB, Popma JJ, et al. Treatment of refractory coronary occlusions with a new excimer laser catheter: preliminary clinical observations. Coron Artery Dis. 1993;4:1001-6.
43. Wolfe CL, Landin RJ, Linnemeier TJ, et al. Successful excimer laser angioplasty following unsuccessful primary balloon angioplasty. Cathet Cardiovasc Diagn. 1993;28:273-8.
44. Fretz EB, Smith P, Hilton JD. Initial experience with a low profile, high energy excimer laser catheter for heavily calcified coronary lesion debulking: parameters and results of first seven human case experiences. J Interv Cardiol. 2001;14:433-7.
45. Ben-Dor I, Maluenda G, Pichard AD, et al. The use of excimer laser for complex coronary artery lesions. Cardiovasc Revasc Med. 2011;12:69.e1-8.
46. Tian W, Mahmoudi M, Lhermusier T, et al. Comparison of Rotational Atherectomy, Plain Old Balloon Angioplasty, and Cutting-Balloon Angioplasty Prior to Drug-Eluting Stent Implantation for the Treatment of Heavily Calcified Coronary Lesions. J Invasive Cardiol. 2015;27:387-91.
47. Karvouni E, Stankovic G, Albiero R, et al. Cutting balloon angioplasty for treatment of calcified coronary lesions. Catheter Cardiovasc Interv. 2001;54:473-81.

CHAPTER 59

Protected Percutaneous Coronary Interventions: Treating the Complex Higher-risk Indicated Patients

Mathew Samuel Kalarickal, Ramachandran Paramasivam

INTRODUCTION

Treatment of complex and high-risk procedure is not a new invention or technology. High risk patients were treated even in the 80s and 90s with balloons even when the stents were not available. Those days even dual antiplatelet treatment was not in practice. Aspirin alone was the main stay.

Coronary artery disease (CAD) is the leading cause of mortality not only in the developed world and also in the developing countries. The enormous disease burden underscores the importance of prompt identification and appropriate treatment of these patients to improve outcomes. In patients with CAD, extent and severity of coronary ischemia remains the major determinant of mortality and hence, medical treatment alone may not be adequate in those subset of patients with large ischemic burden. The benefit of revascularization is directionally proportional to the extent of ischemia and the completeness of revascularization.

With increasing life-expectancy and extensive prevalence of coronary risk factors, the number of patients with CAD presenting at an advanced age and with high-risk clinical presentation in on the rise. At the same time, better understanding of the disease, accumulating experience, and availability of better hardwares have led to increasing competence among interventional cardiologist dealing complex lesion subsets. This resulted in the birth of a new subspecialty in interventional cardiology called "Complex High-risk Indicated Patients (CHIP)—interventions".[1]

COMPLEX HIGH-RISK INDICATED PATIENTS

There is no universal definition for CHIP (Table 1). Current risk assessment incorporates the following three important areas: (1) patient comorbidities (advanced age, frailty, chronic obstructive pulmonary disease, etc.) decides patient's physical ability to withstand the procedure; (2) adverse coronary anatomical features (calcification, chronic total occlusion, last surviving vessel, degenerated vein graft, etc.) determines the complexity of the intervention; and (3) unfavorable

TABLE 1: Complex High Risk Indicated Patients

Patient comorbidities	Clinical presentation	Complexity of coronary anatomy	Adverse hemodynamics
• Age >70 years • Frailty • History of cerebrovascular accident • Diabetes mellitus • Chronic kidney disease • Peripheral vascular disease • Chronic lung disease • Severe aortic stenosis	• STEMI • ACS with unstable hemodynamics, dysrhythmia, or refractory angina • Mechanical complications of AMI • Cardiogenic shock • Congestive cardiac failure • Coronary intervention after resuscitated cardiac arrest • Severe left ventricular dysfunction	• Intervention to unprotected left main vessel or left main equivalent • Distal left main bifurcation intervention • Multivessel disease • Degenerated vein graft intervention • Last remaining coronary conduit vessel • Chronic total occlusion with J-CTO score >2 • SYNTAX score >33	• Low cardiac output (Cardiac Index <2.2 L/min/m^2) • Elevated LV filling pressure (PCWP >15 mm Hg) • Elevated pulmonary artery pressure (mean >50 mm Hg)

ACS, acute coronary syndrome; AMI, acute myocardial infarction; STEMI, ST-elevation myocardial infarction; J-CTO, Multicenter Chronic Total Occlusion Registry of Japan; LV, left-ventricular; PCWP, pulmonary capillary wedge pressure.

hemodynamics, poor left-ventricular (LV) function, and associated valve disease determines hemodynamic stability during procedure.

During the procedure, contrast injections, balloon dilatations, atherectomy device passes, and stent manipulations transiently disturb the blood flow to the target coronary vessel which results in negative inotropic effect.[2] High-risk patients have limited ability to withstand the adverse hemodynamic effects of dysrhythmia, ischemia-reperfusion injury, or no-reflow associated with percutaneous coronary interventions (PCI) and these type of patients may have significantly low cardiovascular reserve and are increasingly susceptible to postischemic stunning.

CHIP PCI HOSPITAL

For running a successful CHIP program, the hospital must possess following basic facilities:

- At least two CHIP qualified physicians and a team of interventionists, trained nurses, and technical staff offering 24 × 7 emergency PCI services
- Catheterization laboratory with capabilities of atherectomy, intravascular imaging, and physiology, and hemodynamic support devices
- Cardiothoracic surgery facilities with 24 × 7 availability
- Intensive care physician and nurses trained in handing high-risk cardiac patients
- Administrative and economic support from the management for the program.

CHIP PHYSICIAN

Complex high-risk indicated patients' interventions are different from routine coronary interventions. Physician performing CHIP interventions should have specific skill sets to handle complex anatomical subsets and complications during procedure. CHIP operator should be a high volume operator with significant proportion of them being complex interventions involving left main coronary artery and bifurcation lesions requiring double stent strategy, chronic total occlusion recanalization—both antegrade and retrograde techniques and calcified lesion intervention involving atherectomy devices. They should also possess good knowledge of intravascular imaging and physiology. In addition, he should be competent to handle procedure complications such as coronary perforation, access site complications and device embolization and entrapment.

PATIENT EVALUATION AND PROCEDURE PLANNING

Preprocedure evaluation and planning are the cornerstones of the CHIP interventions. Maximum possible information regarding the patient's past medical and surgical history has to be obtained from the case records and treating primary care physician. Reviewing all previous procedure records is essential. For example, number of bypass grafts implanted during previous coronary artery bypass graft surgery, type of stents implanted and complications happened during previous procedure. During the assessment, it is also important to decide on the requirement of pulmonary artery pressure monitoring and hemodynamic support at the time procedure.

Once evaluation is completed, the whole information regarding the patient has to be discussed in the heart team meeting and appropriate consensus to be arrived.

In addition, it is prudent to involve experts from specialties such as heart failure, electrophysiology, and cardiac intensive care in the management of patients with other associated cardiac illnesses.[3]

The pros and cons of the procedure have to be explained in detail to the patient and the relatives and informed consent to be obtained.

HEMODYNAMIC SUPPORT DEVICES

Hemodynamic support devices are the cornerstone of CHIP procedures. They stabilize patient's hemodynamics during procedure to facilitate the procedure. There are various types support devices with different levels of back up support available for clinical use.

Intra-aortic Balloon Pump

Inflation of the balloon in early diastole augments diastolic pressure that leads to increased coronary perfusion pressure whereas deflation of balloon at end diastole decreases the aortic systolic pressure which decreases the LV afterload. Intra-aortic balloon pump (IABP) support provides up to 0.5 L/min of cardiac output.

In BCIS-1 trial, patients undergoing high-risk PCI [left ventricular ejection fraction (LVEF) <30% and extensive CAD] were randomized to either routine IABP or no planned IABP prior to PCI. There was no difference in the primary endpoint of major adverse cardiac and cerebrovascular events (MACCEs) at 28 days although there was a marked reduction in procedural complications. Bleeding and access-site complications trended higher toward routine IABP use. Although, there was no difference in 6-month mortality, it was significantly reduced at 51 months follow up. The IABP-SHOCK II study randomized 600 patients presented with acute myocardial infarction (AMI) complicated by cardiogenic shock (CS) to routine IABP versus no IABP.[4] By 30 days, the primary endpoint of all-cause mortality (39.7% vs. 41.3%, p value 0.69), and secondary endpoints of bleeding, sepsis, and stroke were similar between the groups.

The CRISP AMI trial[5] evaluated the role of prophylactic IABP insertion in patients undergoing primary PCI (PPCI) for anterior wall STEMI without CS in reducing the mean infarct size measured by cardiac MRI imaging between 3 days and 5 days of post-procedure. The primary endpoints were not statistically significant between the two groups. Secondary cardiac MRI imaging measures of mean LVEF and LV systolic volume were also similar.

Advantages

- Readily available in catheterization laboratories
- Small access size comparing to other devices (8F)
- Ease of percutaneous implantation.

Disadvantages

- Increase cardiac output only by 0.5 L/min
- Not reliable in patients with dysrhythmia
- Increase risk of access site complications, hemolysis, aortic dissection, atheroembolism, stroke, and infection.

Although the vast experience exists with the use of IABP, it provides minimal hemodynamic support, which may not be adequate for severe forms of CS. IABP has been studied extensively and has not reduced mortality in patients with CS or high-risk-PCI except in the setting of STEMI patients treated with fibrinolysis.

Impella

Impella recover LP 2.5 (Abiomed) is a microaxial rotatory blood pump that expels the blood directly from LV to the aorta which in turn decreases end-diastolic pressure, end-diastolic volume and end-systolic volume. In this way, Impella directly unloads the left ventricle, increase cardiac output and coronary perfusion[6]. Impella LP 2.5 delivers an output up to 2.5 L/min. Impella CP device provides an output up to 4 L/min and Impella 5.0 device up to 5 L/min. The first two devices are implanted percutaneously and last through surgical cut down.

In PROTECT I study,[7] enrolling patients with LMCA or sole remaining conduit and severe LV dysfunction, the device was technically successful in all cases with a low complication rate. In PROTECT II trial, 452 patients undergoing elective high-risk PCI were randomized to IABP or Impella 2.5. The primary endpoint of 30-day major adverse events (a composite of 11 end points) in intention-to-treat analysis was not different between the devices, however, it showed a trend favoring Impella in the per-protocol population analysis. At 90 days per-protocol defined major adverse events were significantly lower in the Impella group.

Currently, FDA approves Impella device for patients with CS after AMI or CABG.

Advantages

- Easy to use
- Augment cardiac output by 2.5–5 L/min
- Does not require stable cardiac rhythm.

Disadvantages

- Not universally available
- Requires 12–14 Fr access/surgical access for Impella 5
- Nonpulsatile flow
- Risk of displacement
- Access site complications, increase risk of atheroembolisation, stroke, and infection.

Extracorporeal Life Support

Extracorporeal life support (ECLS), formerly known as extracorporeal membrane oxygenation (ECMO), is a modified heart lung machine that can be implanted percutaneously. It has a venous cannula (18–21 Fr) that is placed in the right atrium via the femoral vein and an arterial cannula (16–19 Fr) placed either in the iliac artery or descending aorta. The blood drawn from the right atrium is accelerated through a centrifugal pump and oxygenated in a membrane oxygenator before delivered to the arterial system. Depending on the size of the cannula, ECLS delivers an output up to 7 L/min.[8-10]

Although ECMO provides considerable hemodynamic support, it imposes significant increase in afterload that in turn intensifies LV wall stress and oxygen demand. This may be deleterious to an already compromised left ventricle.

Advantages

- Augment cardiac output by more than 4.5 L/min
- Does not require stable cardiac rhythm
- Can be used to support the circulation up to several weeks.

Disadvantages

- Not widely available
- Nonpulsatile flow
- Possible poor perfusion of coronaries and cerebral circulation
- May require concomitant use of IABP
- Access site complications, limb ischemia, systemic inflammatory response, renal failure, systemic embolization, stroke, and infection
- Need for perfusionist.

Although there are few single center studies that evaluated ECMO in the setting of CHIP PCI, there are no major randomized studies.

TandemHeart

TandemHeart is a percutaneous ventricular assist device which works without the need of external oxygenator or a heat exchanger. In TandemHeart, the inflow cannula (21 Fr) placed in the left atrium via transseptal puncture from the right femoral vein, outflow cannula (15–17 Fr) is implanted at the level of aortic bifurcation via right femoral artery. The device pump cycles the oxygenated blood from left atrium into femoral artery. TandemHeart device provides up to 4 L/min of cardiac output.

This device indirectly unload the left ventricle, reduces the cardiac filling pressures and myocardial oxygen demand. However may paradoxically increase the myocardial demand due to rise in afterload in patients with CS with severe LV dysfunction. In such case scenario additional LV unloading devices like IABP or Impella may be necessary.

In Thiele H et al. study randomized AMI patients complicated by CS to IABP (n = 20) and TandemHeart (n = 21) before revascularization.[10] Although TandemHeart device enhanced hemodynamic and metabolic parameters more effectively, this did not result in a survival benefits.[11]

Advantages

- Can augment cardiac output by up to 4–5 L/min

- Support the circulation up to 14 days
- Does not require stable cardiac rhythm.

Disadvantages

- Requires transseptal puncture and difficult to use in emergencies
- Right atrial displacement of cannula from left atrium leads to profound desaturation.
- Access site complications, atheroembolism, stroke, infection and hemolysis.

POST-PROCEDURE CARE

Postprocedural care following implantation of support devices consists of transfer of the patient to ICU, continuous monitoring in ICU, weaning, and removal. Qualified staff and own hospital protocol is important. Care should be exercised in transferring the patients to ICU to prevent device displacement and loss of hemodynamic support. Patients should be periodically monitored for anticoagulation levels and hemolysis. It is also important to watch for device migration, bleeding, and limb ischemia.[12].

Hemodynamic support devices weaning may start in catheterization laboratory after the procedure. If an IABP is used, assistance is reduced from 1:1 to 1:2 for 10 minutes, followed by 1:3 for 10 minutes. If hemodynamic parameters are good for 10 minutes, then the device can be removed. For Impella device, the level of support is reduced by two levels every 10 minutes until P-2. If the patient continues to hemodynamically stable on level P-2 for 10 minutes, then the device can be removed. At the time of device removal, the device is turned down to P-1 level and pulled back into the descending thoracic aorta. Once in the descending thoracic aorta, the device can be turned off completely to P-0 and removed.[13-15]

If weaning done in ICU, it should be started immediately in patients who demonstrate hemodynamic improvement with good end organ perfusion and can be carried out over few hours. IABP should be weaned with a stepwise decrease in assisted beats from 1:1 to 1:2 to 1:3 over several hours. If hemodynamics remained stable on 1:3 for 3 hours, then the device is set back at 1:1, heparin infusion is stopped and once the aPTT is less than 50 seconds the device can be removed. Impella should be weaned over hours with reduction in level of support by two levels every 2–3 hours until the level P-2. Once patient is remained stable at level P-2 for 2–3 hours the device can be removed. Arterial access site can be closed with the preclose technique, surgical closure, or manual pressure.

Mechanical support devices are compared in table 2 and recommendations for use during CHIP PCI provided in table 3.

CURRENT EVIDENCE

Complex high-risk indicated patients form a specific subgroup of patients who need an advanced level of care compared to the routine patients undergoing revascularization. The randomized trials evaluating effectiveness of different treatment strategies for patients with CAD hardly represent this subset of patients. Although revascularization appears to be beneficial in CHIP population, it has to born in mind that the procedure involves a higher level of risk to the patient and also has economic implications for the health care system. So, this approach needs to be evaluated in major randomized trials before its wide spread adaptation in clinical practice.[16,17]

CONCLUSION

Patients undergoing elective high-risk PCI should be transferred to high-volume centers with operators specialized

TABLE 2: Comparison of various mechanical support devices

	IABP	IMPELLA	TANDEMHEART	VA- ECMO
Cardiac output	0.3 - 0.5 L/min	1-5 L/min	2.5 to 5 L/min	3 to 7 L/min
Maximum implant days	Weeks	7 days	14 days	Weeks
Mechanism of action	Aorta	LV to aorta	LA to aorta	RA to aorta
Sheath size	7 to 8 Fr	13 to 14 Fr	15 to 17 Fr arterial 21 Fr venous	14 to 16 Fr Arterial 18 to 21 Fr venous
Femoral artery size	> 4 mm	Impella 2.5 and CP 5.5 mm Impella 5.0–8 mm	8 mm	8 mm
Cardiac synchrony	Yes	No	No	No
Coronary perfusion	↑	↑	–	–
LVEDP	↓	↓↓	↓↓	–
Myocardial O_2 demand	↓	↓↓	–↓	–
Cardiac flow	↑	↑↑	↑↑	↑↑
Afterload	↓	↓	↑	↑↑↑
MAP	↑	↑↑	↑↑	↑↑
Vascular complications	+	++	+++	++++

IABP, intra-aortic balloon pump; LA, left atrium; LV, left-ventricular; LVEDP, left ventricular end-diastolic pressure; RA, right atrium; VA-ECMO, venoarterial extracorporeal membrane oxygenation.

TABLE 3: Guidelines on use of hemodynamic support devices in high-risk percutaneous coronary intervention (PCI)

2013 ACCF/AHA Guideline for the Management of ST-Elevation Myocardial Infarction (STEMI)
Class IIa: • The use of intra-aortic balloon pump (IABP) counterpulsation can be useful for patients with cardiogenic shock after STEMI who do not quickly stabilize with pharmacological therapy (455–459). (Level of evidence: B) Class IIb: • Alternative LV assist devices for circulatory support may be considered in patients with refractory cardiogenic shock. (Level of evidence: C)
PCI, 2011[16]
• A hemodynamic support device is recommended for patients with cardiogenic shock after STEMI who do not quickly stabilize with pharmacological therapy (Class I, Level of Evidence: B). • Elective insertion of an appropriate hemodynamic support device as an adjunct to PCI may be reasonable in carefully selected high-risk patients (Class IIb, Level of Evidence: C) High-risk patients include: • Unprotected left main or last remaining conduit PCI • Cardiogenic shock • PCI of a vessel subtending a large territory on a background of severely depressed left ventricular function
UA/NSTEMI, 2013[17]
• IABP is reasonable in UA/NSTEMI patients for continuing or frequently recurring severe ischemia despite intensive medical therapy, hemodynamic instability pre- or postangiography, and for mechanical complications of MI Class IIa, Level of Evidence: C

ACCF, American College of Cardiology Foundation; AHA, American Heart Association; LV, left-ventricular; MI, myocardial infarction; UA/NSTEMI, unstable angina/non–ST-segment elevation myocardial infarction.

in treatment of complex higher-risk indicated patients. Collective team based approach is needed for appropriate patient selection, treatment, and subsequent care of these patients. Each institution should familiar with at least two support devices including IABP and Impella or TandemHeart in order to provide safe and efficient delivery of care in patients with high-risk-PCI. Finally CHIP PCI shows great promise in advancing the interventional cardiology but it is not without risk.

Complex high-risk indicated patients terminology is a new but the technology is old. Most of the devices IABP, femorofemoral bypass was in use even in the 1990s itself. ECMO is a modification of femorofemoral bypass. Impella is an addition which is very useful in high-risk patients.

REFERENCES

1. Hachamovitch R, Hayes SW, Friedman JD, et al. Comparison of the short-term survival benefit associated with revascularization compared with medical therapy in patients with no prior coronary artery disease undergoing stress myocardial perfusion single photon emission computed tomography. Circulation. 2003;107:2900-7.
2. Smith SC Jr, Feldman TE, Hirshfeld JW Jr, et al. American College of Cardiology/ American Heart Association Task Force on Practice Guidelines; ACC/AHA/SCAI Writing Committee to Update the 2001 Guidelines for Percutaneous Coronary Intervention. ACC/AHA/SCAI 2005 guideline update for percutaneous coronary intervention: a report of the American College of Cardiology/American Heart Association Task Force on Practice Guidelines (ACC/AHA/SCAI Writing Committee to Update the 2001 Guidelines for Percutaneous Coronary Intervention) J Am Coll Cardiol. 2006;47;e1-121.
3. Kirtane AJ, Doshi D, Leon MB, et al. Treatment of Higher-Risk Patients with an Indication for Revascularization Evolution within the Field of Contemporary Percutaneous Coronary Intervention Circulation. 2016;134:422-31.
4. Thiele H, Zeymer U, Neumann FJ, et al. Intraaortic balloon support for myocardial infarction with cardiogenic shock. N Engl J Med. 2012;367:1287-96.
5. Patel MR, Smalling RW, Thiele H, et al. Intraaortic balloon counterpulsation and infarct size in patients with acute anterior myocardial infarction without shock: the CRISP AMI randomized trial. JAMA. 2011;306:1329-37.
6. Naidu SS. Novel percutaneous cardiac assist devices—the science of and indications for hemodynamic support. Circulation. 2011;123:533-43.
7. Dixon SR, Henriques JP, Mauri L, et al. A prospective feasibility trial investigating the use of the Impella 2.5 system in patients undergoing high-risk percutaneous coronary intervention (The PROTECT I Trial): initial U.S. experience. JACC Cardiovasc Interv. 2009;2:91-6.
8. Kenneth LA. Extracorporeal cardiopulmonary bypass support: a historical and current perspective. In: Shawl F (Ed). Supported Complex and High Risk Coronary Angioplasty. Boston, MA: Kluwer Academic Publishers; 1991.
9. Shawl F. Percutaneous cardiopulmonary bypass support: technique, indications, and complications. In: Shawl F (Ed). Supported Complex and High Risk Coronary Angioplasty. Boston, MA: Kluwer Academic Publishers; 1991.
10. Jones H, Kalisetti D, Gaba M, et al. Left ventricular assist for high-risk percutaneous coronary intervention. J Invasive Cardiol 2012;24:544–50.
11. Thiele H, Sick P, Boudriot E, et al. Randomized comparison of intra-aortic balloon support with a percutaneous left ventricular assist device in patients with revascularized acute myocardial infarction complicated by cardiogenic shock. Eur Heart J. 2005;360:1276-83.
12. Rihal CS, Naidu SS, Givertz MM, et al. 2015 SCAI/ACC/HFSA/STS Clinical Expert Consensus Statement on the Use of Percutaneous Mechanical Circulatory Support Devices in Cardiovascular Care: Endorsed by the American Heart Association, the Cardiological Society of India, and Sociedad Latino Americana de Cardiologia Intervencion; Affirmation of Value by the Canadian Association of Interventional Cardiology—Association Canadienne de Cardiologie d'intervention. J Am Coll Cardiol. 2015;65:e7-26.
13. Impella 2.5 with the Automated Impella Controller, Circulatory Support System: Instructions for Use and Clinical Reference Manual. Danvers, MA: Abiomed; 2015.
14. Impella CP. Circulatory Support System. Instructions for Use and Clinical Reference Manual. Danvers, MA: Abiomed; 2015.
15. Cohen HA, Henriques JPS. Percutaneous ventricular support. Interv Cardiol Clin. 2013;2:397-498.
16. Levine GN, Bates ER, Blankenship JC, et al. 2011 ACCF/AHA/SCAI guideline for percutaneous coronary intervention. A report of the American recovery after myocardial infarction. Circ Cardiovasc Interv. 2013;6:166-75.
17. Anderson JL, Adams CD, Antman EM, et al. 2012 ACCF/AHA focused update incorporated into the ACCF/AHA 2007 guidelines for the management of patients with unstable angina/non-ST-elevation myocardial infarction: a report of the American College of Cardiology Foundation/ American Heart Association Task Force. J Am Coll Cardiol. 2013;61:e179-347.

CHAPTER 60

Ostial Coronary Lesions: Tips and Tricks for the Interventionist

Pravesh Vishwakarma, Rishi Sethi

INTRODUCTION

By definition, ostial lesions are the lesions within 3 mm of origin of the vessel from aorta or parent vessel. Ostial lesions continue to challenge the skills of an interventionist despite several advancements in percutaneous coronary intervention (PCI) techniques in last 40 years. Due to unique anatomic and histologic characteristics, these lesions tend to have poor outcomes (short-term as well as long-term) as compared to lesions in nonostial location. And also, for all practical purposes, lesions very close to ostium (up to 5–6 mm) should be considered as ostial due to similar challenges posed by them during PCI.

Depending on the origin, ostial lesions can be categorized into aorto-ostial lesions [e.g., right coronary artery (RCA), left main coronary artery (LMCA), and saphenous grafts arising from aorta] and branch ostial lesions [e.g., left anterior descending artery (LAD) and left circumflex (LCx) ostial lesions; diagonal, obtuse marginal, posterior descending artery (PDA), and posterolateral branch (PLV) ostial lesions].

This chapter will focus mainly on challenges encountered and their solutions for aorto-ostial interventions. Many of these technical considerations apply to branch ostial lesions as well but these lesions are in essence bifurcation lesions (median class—0, 1, 0 or 0, 0, 1) with the plaque often extending to main branch. Hence, intervention at branch ostial junctions should be planned according to bifurcation characteristics with an individualistic approach.

MORPHOLOGY AND HISTOLOGY

Aorto-ostial lesions have a unique three-dimensional funnel-shaped morphology with variable take off angles from aorta. These may be associated with diffuse or focal coronary artery disease at other locations and are usually atheromatous in origin. Isolated aorto-ostial lesions are usually seen in females more commonly involve RCA[1,2] and are due to nonatherosclerotic causes such as inflammatory aortic disease (e.g., syphilitic, Takayasu arteritis), prior radiotherapy or aortic valve surgery, congenital arterial hypoplasia or extrinsic compression by a dilated pulmonary artery.[3]

Ostial lesions tend to have higher fibrous tissue and calcium content and minimal atheromatous plaque.[4] They have high rigidity and increased recoil tendency causing suboptimal acute luminal gain. There is also increased intimal hyperplasia after stenting leading to increased rates of target lesion revascularization (TLR). Introduction of drug-eluting stents (DES) has led to reduced restenosis and other complication rates as compared to balloon angioplasty and bare metal stents, but results at ostial location still remain inferior to those at nonostial lesions.[5] Hence, optimal PCI with a well deployed DES remains the only guarantee to best possible long-term outcome. Knowing the tips and tricks to tackle an ostial lesion comes handy in these situations. Various challenges expected and their solutions are discussed in the following text.

DIAGNOSTIC CHALLENGES

- Appropriate evaluation of ostial disease is often challenging. Catheter-induced coronary vasospasm is a close mimic, especially in RCA and should be ruled out before proceeding with PCI. Intracoronary nitroglycerine can help differentiate between spasm and true lesion
- Deep intubation beyond lesion may miss ostial disease. This usually happens with small sized (4 or 5 Fr) diagnostic catheters. Absence of contrast backflow into aortic sinus and pressure damping or ventricularization may be the clues. But pressure damping effect may not be seen in catheters with side holes and also if the catheter is noncoaxial. Stagnant dye (nonclearance or nonwashout of contrast) in coronary should prompt the operator to look for a catheter deep throated into significant ostial-proximal lesion. Failure to recognize it may lead to prolonged coronary ischemia and arrhythmic complications. Catheter needs to be disengaged before next injection to allow the artery to "breath" in between injections. Nonselective

root injections close to ostium may be helpful but are not sufficient to opacify and characterize coronary lesions. Deep intubation of coronaries can also be prevented by slight clockwise or anticlockwise rotation of catheter, keeping the catheter tip nonaligned to coronary ostial axis. Repeated need to engage and disengage catheter can increase the risk of ostial damage and dissection. Forceful contrast injections should be avoided as it may also cause intimal disruption and coronary dissection

- Accurate assessment of lesion severity by quantitative coronary analysis is not possible because of absence of proximal reference segment. Fractional flow reserve (FFR) can be help in estimating physiological significant of lesion. Of note, for aorto-ostial lesions, pressure equalization needs to be done in aorta with guiding disengaged away from ostium. Continuous intravenous infusion of adenosine is more reliable for inducing hyperemia as compared to intracoronary bolus because of need to engage to inject adenosine and rapidly disengage to do measurements
- Among imaging modalities, intravascular ultrasound (IVUS) is of particular help. Detailed plaque morphology (plaque burden, lipid core, fibrotic plaque, and calcification) as well as lesion severity [minimum luminal area (MLA)] can be assessed, helps plan adjunctive strategy like cutting balloon for fibrotic plaque and rotablation for calcified lesion. However, noncoaxial course of IVUS catheter with a disengaged guide catheter may lead to overestimated MLA and failure to recognize the severity. Optical coherence tomography (OCT) has limited utility because effective clearance of blood from lumen requires guide catheter to be engaged selectively and this would prevent ostial plaque visualization behind the catheter. Computed tomography coronary angiography (CTCA) may be extremely helpful in cases where a critically narrowed and/or anomalously placed ostium does not allow selective engagement and coronary artery visualization.

SELECTION OF HARDWARES

Radial versus Femoral Access

Considering the unequivocal advantage in terms of bleeding complications and survival benefits, it is impractical to advise against radial access over femoral. Moreover, it is a matter of operator's experience and personal preference. In some cases with challenging anatomy, femoral access can provide better guiding catheter stability and more control over catheter manipulations.

Guiding Catheter Selection

The best guiding catheter for ostial lesion would be a less aggressive one without active support or a tendency to wedge in the diseased ostium occluding the coronary blood flow. An aggressive catheter may repeatedly get deep throated into lesion compromising the blood flow, and need to repeatedly engage and disengage can increase the risk of coronary dissection. For RCA and saphenous venous grafts, Judkins right, multipurpose, Amplatz right curves are preferred. For ostial LMCA lesions, Judkins left curve with or without short tip can be used (Fig. 1).

Guiding catheters with side holes may be used for ostial chronic total occlusions, but for nonocclusive stenosis, we advise guiding catheters without side holes. Presence of side holes may fail to show warning sign of pressure damping or ventricularization in case of deep wedging, and are never sufficient to maintain blood supply of coronaries. Another drawback is contrast wastage and inadequate opacification of arteries, hence increased contrast burden during the procedure.

Another very relevant option in those situations where the risk of deep engagement is causing problems is to upsize the guiding catheter. A larger size guide would abut against the outer side of the ostial funnel and thus would have less chances of engaging deep.

Guiding Catheter Maneuvers

The purpose of catheter manipulations is to avoid impeding coronary blood flow due to catheter wedging in lesion, to avoid ostial dissection by catheter due to repeated trauma at diseased segment and to efficiently engage or disengage the catheter for precise stent placement without losing complete access to artery.

As soon as the catheter engages the ostium, pressure waveform changes (damping or ventricularization) are seen. These changes may be used throughout the procedure as a surrogate marker of engagement thus avoiding unnecessary contrast injections. For LMCA, guiding catheter may be gently withdrawn to disengage till the pressure waveform is normalized. For RCA, the guiding catheter is disengaged by giving a gentle counterclockwise torque with a purpose to creating a malalignment between guide and coronary axis. This prevents accidental deep intubation into RCA at the cost of reduced guiding support. Hence, while giving counterclockwise rotation, guide catheter is gently pushed down by a couple of millimeters so that guiding does not flip back completely into ascending aorta. Alternatively, after wiring and guiding, wire may be gently pulled out together as one unit; or wire may be pushed into distal coronary tree thereby pushing the guiding back. During these maneuvers, guidewire must be parked distal enough in coronary bed to support disengaged guiding catheter.

By doing the reverse maneuvers, catheter may be engaged again to increase the guide support while delivering a hardware like percutaneous transluminal coronary angioplasty (PTCA) balloons or stent. Guiding catheter stability may also be improved by using a second guidewire into distal coronary bed as "buddy wire" or into conus or acute marginal branch as "anchoring wire" or with a PTCA balloon over it as "anchoring balloon" technique. Sometimes, guiding catheter's tendency to deep intubation may be controlled by a "floating wire" in aortic sinus where second guidewire, placed free floating into aortic sinus, acts as a barrier between catheter tip and ostium.

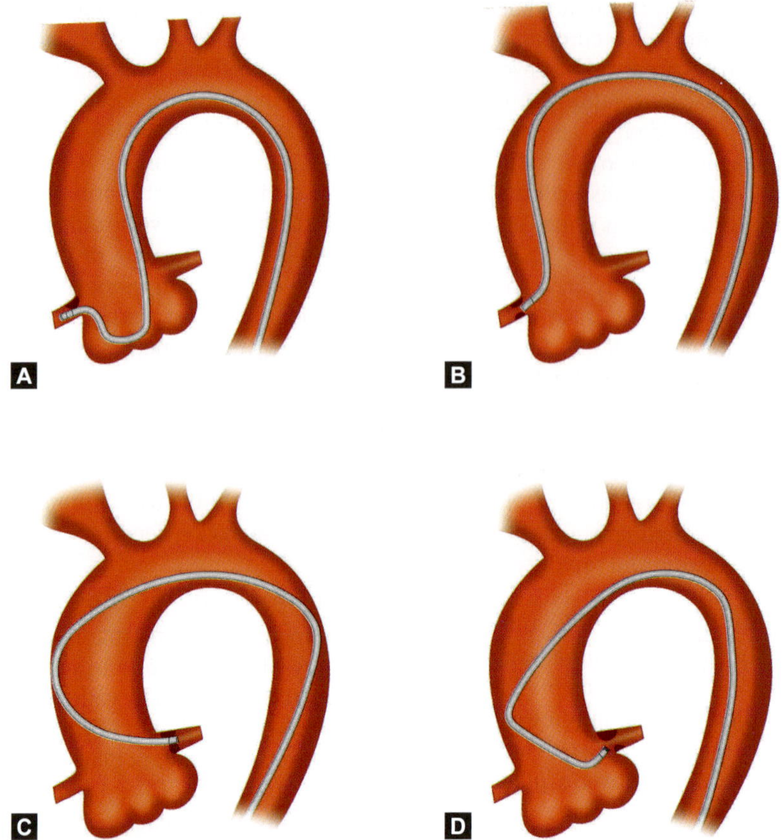

EBU, extra back up; LMS, left main stem; RCA, right coronary artery.

FIG. 1: Selecting a guiding catheter shape for aorto-ostial lesion. Choosing a less aggressive catheter avoids deep seating, thereby reducing the risk of flow impediment as well as ostial dissection. **A,** Amplatz catheter—deep engagement of RCA; **B,** Judkins catheter—minimal engagement of RCA; **C,** EBU catheter—deep engagement of LMS; **D,** Judkins catheter—minimal engagement of LMS.

Wire Selection

Standard workhorse wires are usually sufficient for ostial lesions. Even intermediate or extra support wires may be preferred. In general, hydrophilic or light support wires should be avoided for lack of adequate support to guiding catheter and heightened risk of coronary perforations. Additional wires may be used (as buddy wire or anchoring wire) to increase the guide support as described earlier in the text.

In critically stenosed ostial disease where ischemia burden is huge, e.g., in ostial LMCA lesions, it is preferable to preload the guidewire inside the guiding catheter. As soon as the catheter tip engages the ostium, wire is quickly advanced into distal coronary artery and catheter is disengaged promptly, thus significantly reducing ischemia duration.

Lesion Preparation

Optimal lesion preparation is essential not only for adequate stent expansion but also to avoid stent migration. It relieves ischemia and increases time window for catheter and stent manipulation. As the aorto-ostial lesions are rigid and fibrotic, one should have low threshold to predilate. We advise an aggressive predilatation in almost all cases of aorto-ostial lesions. Predilatation is done with compliant PTCA balloon preferably 0.5 mm smaller than distal normal reference segment (balloon to artery ratio 0.7:0.9), partially hanging in aorta and partially inside coronary artery beyond the ostium and guiding catheter disengaged to avoid balloon damaging the catheter. Satisfactory endpoint is disappearance of balloon waist during inflation and without elastic recoil after the balloon is deflated. Resistant lesions may cause watermelon seeding of the balloon, i.e., balloon slips proximally or distally before it achieves full inflation. This problem can be circumvented by using longer balloons and a very slow inflation (at rate of 1 atm at a time or even less) while simultaneously maintaining a push or pull on balloon catheter shaft. Some of nonyielding lesions can be successfully dilated by using noncompliant balloons at high pressures close to rated burst pressure (RBP). But, very high-pressure predilatation can cause undesirable complications such as intramural hematoma and/or coronary dissection leading to luminal compromise. Forceful injections should be avoided as it can cause dissection at ostium to extend antegradely down the coronaries as well as retrogradely causing aortic root dissections. These problems can be avoided by using scoring balloon or cutting balloon, which create controlled dissections as compared to noncompliant balloons. If cutting balloon or scoring balloon is not available, a noncompliant balloon over primary wire along with a second wire as buddy wire between balloon and plaque can lead to focused force dilatation of lesion. Intracoronary imaging modalities like IVUS can help plan these adjunctive devices from the outset by characterizing the plaque morphology, e.g., cutting balloon or scoring balloon for fibrotic plaques and rotablation for heavily calcified plaques, especially superficial ring calcium. If rotablation is chosen, maintaining a stable coaxial guide position is a challenge with ostial lesions and burring should start from within the guiding catheter so as not to miss the ostial lesion.

Stent Selection

There is no doubt that DES have an advantage over bare metal stents with respect to lower TLR rates and ostial lesions are no exception. Elasticity and rigidity at aorto-ostial location necessitates a stent with good radial strength to avoid excessive recoil. Slotted tube stents may be preferable over single coil stents. In case of ambiguous ostium, it may be difficult to predict the stent length with certainty so it is better to choose a little longer stent so as to cover the whole lesion up to distal edge.

Stent Positioning

Optimal stent positioning requires entire circumference of the proximal stent edge to be within the aorto-ostial landing zone (AOLZ) which is circumferential area within 1 mm of true ostium (i.e., aorto-ostial plane). Variable ostial location as well as angles of takeoff and suboptimal visualization from a disengaged guiding catheter make the identification of true ostium or AOLZ one of the trickiest jobs by a two-dimensional coronary angiography. IVUS studies have shown geographic miss in 10% of cases[6] while a CTCA study showed it in 87% of cases.[7] This is why it is recommended to cover the whole ostium while keeping one or two struts hanging into aorta rather than struggling to visualize AOLZ. Proximal protrusion more than recommended (positive geographic miss) can make the coronary artery "nonengageable" for future interventions, while missing the ostium (negative geographic miss) can lead to increased risk of stent thrombosis as well as stent restenosis.

Optimal Angiographic Views

For an ostial lesion, optimal angiographic view is the one, which demarcates aorto-ostial plane that is to say the view which separates aortic sinus from coronary ostium without any overlap. Owing to variable anatomy, there is no one angulation which suites all. It should be tailored according to individual anatomy. Multiple orthogonal angiographic views should be used to minimize overlap or foreshortening. Flecks of calcium in aortic root close to ostium may also help identify the ostium. For RCA, optimal view is obtained with a left anterior oblique view with or without slight caudal angulation.

TABLE 1: Optimal angiographic views to best delineate ostia of various coronaries

Coronary vessel ostium	Optimal view
Left main coronary artery	AP cranial, LAO cranial, and RAO cranial
Right coronary artery (RCA)	LAO, LAO caudal, lateral view
Aortocoronary grafts	• LAO for RCA grafts • RAO for LAD, LCx saphenous grafts
Left anterior descending (LAD) artery	LAO caudal, AP caudal, and RAO caudal
Left circumflex artery (LCx)	LAO caudal, AP caudal, and LAO cranial
Diagonal branches	LAO cranial, LAO caudal
Obtuse marginal branches	LAO caudal, LAO cranial
PDA and PLV	AP cranial, LAO cranial

AP, anteroposterior; LAO, left anterior oblique; RAO, right anterior oblique; PDA, posterior descending artery; PLV, posterolateral branch.

Sometimes, lateral view may give the best demarcation of true ostium. For LMCA ostium, cranial views are best with slight left or right anterior oblique angulation. Caudal (left anterior oblique—caudal, right anterior oblique—caudal) views may supplement and help give better estimate of aorto-ostial plane (Table 1).

Stent Deployment

Stent is loaded in guiding catheter just proximal to the tip. Now, guiding catheter is made coaxial with coronary artery. This allows ostial engagement causing some pressure damping. Stent is quickly delivered into the vessel with proximal stent marker just distal to catheter tip. Guidewire is pushed in distal circulation to provide maximum support. Now all three (guiding catheter, stent, and guidewire) move as one unit. Tightening the Y-connector may help making the assembly act as one. The whole system is gently retracted (in case of RCA, anticlockwise torque on guiding may be used) to bring the proximal stent marker just proximal to true ostium. This in turn automatically disengages the ostium and pressure comes back to normal waveform. Now system layout is like guiding catheter disengaged and just proximal stent balloon freely floating in aortic sinus supported by wire and stent shaft, and proximal stent marker just outside the ostium and proximal stent edge at the ostium. Magnification and StentBoost[8] can assist in confirming the same. It should be noted that proximal stent marker is not at the stent edge but 0.5–1 mm proximal to stent edge (depending on stent manufacturer). This is important so that proximal stent edge is covering the circumference of ostium. For added safety, stent edge may be kept 1–2 mm hanging into aortic root. As the catheter tip is just proximal to stent marker, contrast injections are able to delineate margins of aortic sinus while partly filling the ostium. Before the stent is deployed, final position must be confirmed in multiple views. If satisfied, stent can be deployed at nominal pressure. After first inflation, balloon is deflated, retracted a few millimeters into aorta and reinflated to high pressures to ensure complete expansion as well as stent apposition. Pulling on an incompletely deflated balloon can also suck the guiding catheter in and lead to stent deformation, another unrecognized cause of geographic miss. It is very important to allow enough time for balloon to deflate completely before attempting pull back.

Before stent balloon is taken out completely, guiding catheter should be made coaxial and railed-in over the deflated balloon to engage stented ostium. This step is important in case postdilatation is needed and one may not be able to deliver noncompliant balloon in noncoaxial and disengaged guiding catheter. Caution should be taken not to use force as it can cause longitudinal compression and deformation of stent. It may be the reason behind classical teaching of guiding catheter to avoid touching the stent and many of operators advising against this step. High pressure postdilatation should be done at ostial lesions to correct any recoil, underexpansion or malapposition. Higher sized noncompliant balloon can be used at proximal edge of stent to achieve the "funneling" of ostium.

Excessive respiratory or cardiac movement can be hindrance in achieving stable stent position. Respiratory motions can be minimized by asking the patient to hold breath. Some patients may not be able to tolerate it for a long time resulting in deep inspiration at the least desired time. It is better to ask patients to take gentle shallow breaths. Cardiac motions can be difficult to overcome. Beta-blockers, intracoronary adenosine or rapid ventricular pacing may be helpful in reducing stent excursions. Partially inflating the stent at 2–3 atm (partial preinflation technique)[9] increases the stent weight as well as profile, thus limit stent oscillations and stent can be fully deployed after final position adjustment. This technique can be disastrous if lesion is not prepared well, can result in stent getting stuck at wrong place or stripped off the balloon.

SPECIAL TECHNIQUES FOR OSTIAL STENT PLACEMENT

Floating Wire Technique

Guiding tip is retracted back and a second steerable soft-tipped guidewire is placed into aortic sinus between guiding tip and ostium. Guiding catheter is advanced over primary wire till its forward movement is stopped by second floating wire (Fig. 2). This technique also described as "sepal wire technique" for ostial LMCA stenting[10] works 2-fold—prevents guiding from jumping into ostium and simultaneously marks the junction of ostium to aortic sinus. It can really help when true ostium is ambiguous and cannot be defined by traditional angiographic views.

Tail Wire Technique (Szabo's Technique)

This technique[11] utilizes a second guidewire to anchor the stent exactly at the ostium. Primary guidewire goes in the target vessel and the second guidewire (i.e., anchor wire) is placed in aorta (for aorto-ostial lesion) (Fig. 3) or the side branch (for branch ostial lesions) (Fig. 4). The stent is loaded on primary wire and the proximal end (tail) of anchor wire is threaded through the proximal most stent strut cell. Threading can be facilitated by inflating the stent at 2–4 atm while most of stent is still inside the stent cap or sleeve except for proximal 2–3 struts which flare; balloon is deflated, anchor wire tail is threaded through flared proximal most stent strut and then stent is manually recrimped over balloon (modified Szabo's technique). Stent is advanced over both the wire until anchor wire stops its forward motion declaring that proximal edge has reached ostium. Stent is deployed first at low pressures; anchor wire is removed followed by stent balloon inflation at high pressures. Tail wire technique ensures high angiographic success but perfect ostial placement could not be documented in bench testing and IVUS and also is not without complications. Intertwined wires may restrict

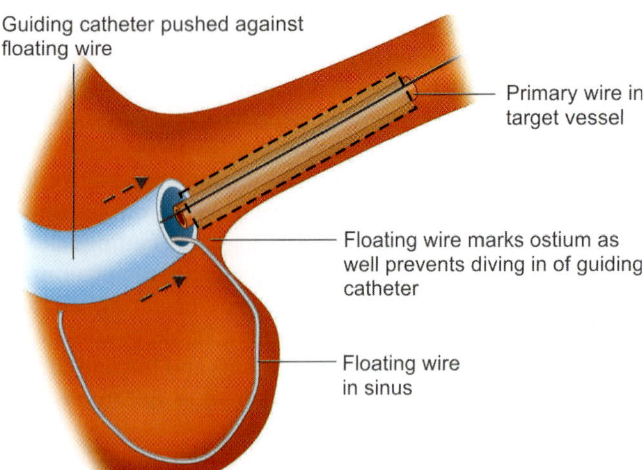

FIG. 2: Floating wire technique. This technique, primarily intended to prevent repeated deep engagement of guiding into ostium, utilizes a secondary wire left floating into aortic sinus between the guiding catheter and coronary ostium. Guiding catheter is advanced over primary wire against the floating wire, which prevents guiding from entering the ostium.

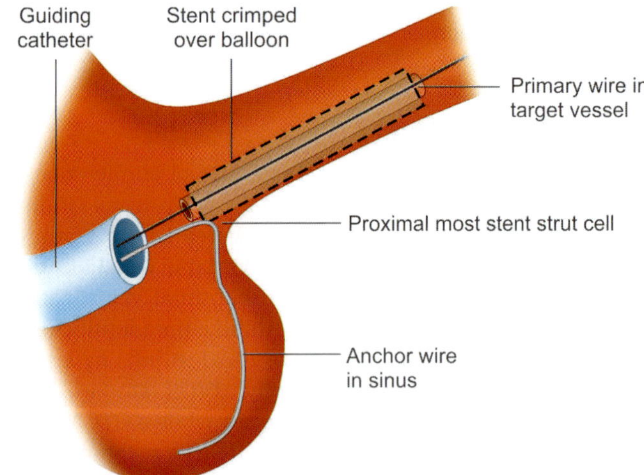

FIG. 3: Szabo's (tail wire) technique for aorto-ostial lesion. The anchor wire goes through the proximal-most struts of stent and lies free into aortic sinus. It anchors the stent at the ostium, thus, avoiding geographic miss.

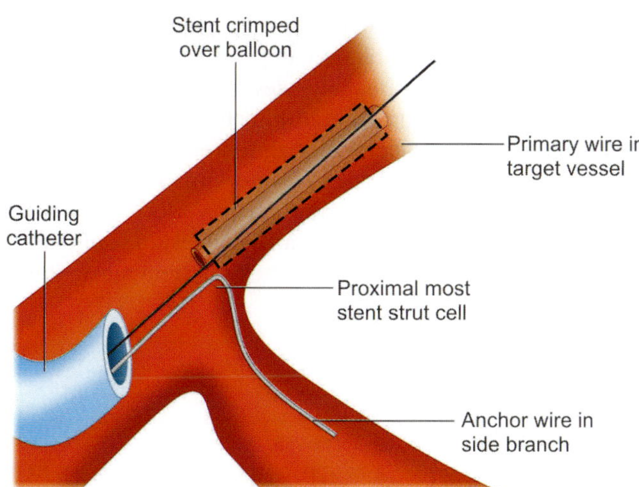

FIG. 4: Szabo's (tail wire) technique for branch-ostial lesion. The anchor wire goes through the proximal-most struts of stent and lies into side branch. It anchors the stent at the ostium, thus avoiding geographic miss.

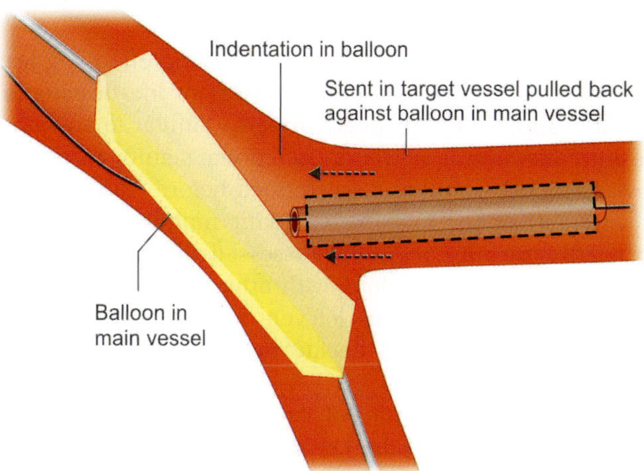

FIG. 6: Stent pull back technique. An inflated balloon is placed in main vessel and the stent in side branch is pulled back till slight indentation appears at the balloon (also known as balloon indentation technique). This prevents overhanging of stent struts in main lumen while ensuring adequate ostial coverage.

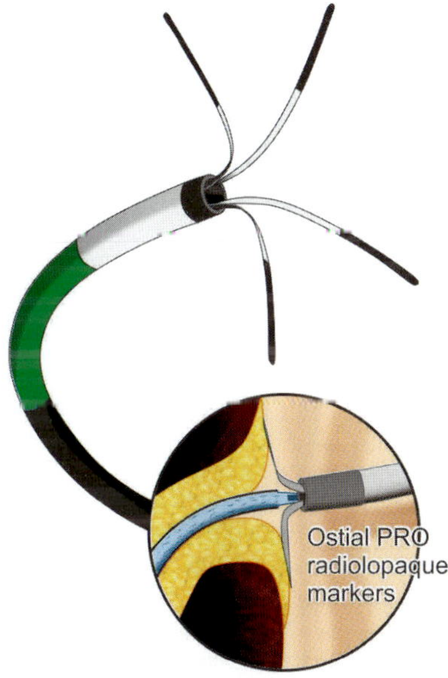

FIG. 5: Ostial Pro™ stent system. Ostial Pro™ device has four self-expanding nitinol legs protruding from distal catheter end which prevents deep engagement of ostium and also marks the aorto-ostial plane for correct stent placement.

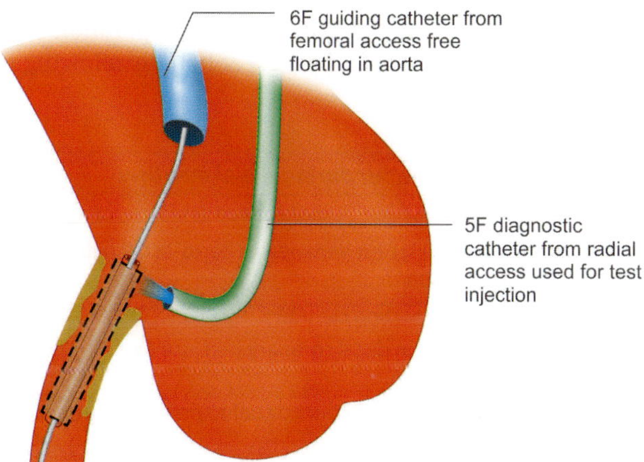

FIG. 7: Two-catheter technique. One guiding catheter and one diagnostic catheter are used simultaneously from different access sites. Guiding catheter is used to deliver stent and is kept disengaged away from ostium while diagnostic catheter placed close to ostium is used to give test injections to visualize stent placement.

forward movement of stent, inadequate crimping may result in stent getting stripped off balloon during delivery or stent positioning, forcing the stent can create bend in anchor wire at ostial location causing wire to stuck and avulsion of stent during forceful withdrawal of wire.

Ostial Pro™ Stent System

Self-expanding nitinol feet at the tip of guiding catheter assist in stable positioning (Fig. 5), prevent diving of catheter into ostial lesion and provide a visual aid to align the stent at the aorto-ostial plane.[12]

Stent Pull Back Technique

In branch ostial lesions, a small balloon is inflated at low pressure in main vessel while stent in branch ostium is pulled back till slight indentation is seen on the balloon in main vessel (Fig. 6). This ensures fewer ostial misses and need for additional stents.[13]

Two-catheter Technique

Sometimes, stent position and ostium cannot be visualized adequately once the guiding is backed out in aorta. Simultaneous use of a second 4 or 5 Fr diagnostic catheter (Fig. 7) placed close to ostium from different access site allows optimal visualization through diagnostic catheter, while maintaining the stable position of guiding catheter away from ostium.[14]

CONCLUSION

Ostial lesions are notorious and even simple-looking lesions may end up in suboptimal results or life-threatening complications if not planned properly. Similar to any other lesion, anatomical as well as functional significance of an ostial stenosis should be ascertained before embarking on revascularization. In a patient with multivessel disease, ostial disease must be carefully assessed not as an individual lesion, but in totality along with other prognostic lesions. Factors like diabetic status, left ventricular ejection fraction, syntax score may help decide between coronary artery bypass surgery and PCI.

Thorough evaluation of angiographic findings and detailed planning are the key to achieve the best possible PCI outcome. Anticipation of difficulties and possible complications during a procedure is the sixth sense of an interventionist and help him develop a plan well ahead of time. Choosing a less aggressive guiding catheter, keeping the guide out of ostium or keeping it malaligned to avoid deep engagement and avoiding forceful test injections can help in minimizing ostial trauma and hence ostial and aortic root dissections. Adequate lesion preparation is the most crucial step. IVUS can be a great help by allowing the interventionist to choose between simple balloon dilatation, cutting balloon or rotablation depending on the plaque morphology. Optimal imaging views and various special techniques like floating wire and anchor wire can help in precise ostial stent placement. Aggressive postdilatation to attain optimal stent expansion is important for best possible long-term outcomes. Box 1 summarizes various steps to be taken care of while dealing with an ostial lesion. Familiarity to challenges and various techniques can help tackle these lesions successfully.

BOX 1 Tips to remember during ostial stenting

- Rule out ostial spasm
- Define the view which best demarcates aorto-ostial plane during diagnostic angiogram
- Use less aggressive guiding catheters
- Keep guidewire park in distal coronary bed, use extra support or buddy wire if needed
- Keep guiding disengaged or noncoaxial to preserve coronary blood flow
- Avoid forceful contrast injections
- Adequate lesion preparation using proper sized balloon; consider cutting balloon or rotablation if intravascular ultrasound suggests so
- Keep proximal stent marker well (2–3 mm) inside the aorta (stent edge is 0.5–1 mm inside markers)
- Utilize multiple views
- Ask the patient to breath slow and shallow
- High pressure stent deployment to ensure stent is well expanded
- High pressure postdilatation

REFERENCES

1. Stewart JT, Ward DE, Davies MJ, et al. Isolated coronary ostial stenosis: observations on the pathology. Eur Heart J. 1987;8:917-20.
2. Rissanen V. Occurrence of coronary ostial stenosis in a necropsy series of myocardial infarction, sudden death, and violent death. Br Heart J. 1975;37:182-91.
3. Jaffe R, Halon DA, Shiran A, et al. Percutaneous treatment of aorto-ostial coronary lesions: Current challenges and future directions. Int J Cardiol. 2015;186:61-6.
4. Popma JJ, Dick RJ, Haudenschild CC, et al. Atherectomy of right coronary ostial stenoses: initial and long-term results, technical features and histologic findings. Am J Cardiol. 1991;67:431-3.
5. Hsieh IC, Chen CC, Chang SH, et al. Acute and long-term outcomes of drug-eluting stent implantations in aorto-ostial, left anterior descending artery-ostial, and nonostial lesions. Catheter Cardiovasc Interv. 2013;82:727-34.
6. Patel Y, Depta JP, Patel JS, et al. Impact of intravascular ultrasound on the long-termclinical outcomes in the treatment of coronary ostial lesions. Catheter Cardiovasc Interv. 2016;87(2):232-40.
7. Rubinshtein R, Ben-Dov N, Halon DA, et al. Geographic miss with aorto-ostial coronary stent implantation: insights from high-resolution coronary computed tomography angiography. Euro Intervention. 2015;11(3):301-7.
8. Vuurmans T, Patterson MS, Laarman GJ. StentBoost used to guide management of a critical ostial right coronary artery lesion. J Invasive Cardiol. 2009;21:19-21.
9. Hildick-Smith DJ, Shapiro LM. Ostial left anterior descending coronary artery stent positioning: partial preinflation prevents stent oscillation and facilitates accurate deployment. J Interv Cardiol. 2001;14:439-42.
10. Chan CK, Fung RC. "Sepal wire technique"--a novel technique for aorto-ostial left main stenting. J Invasive Cardiol. 2011;23(5):211-2.
11. Szabo S, Abramowitz B, Vaitkus PT. New Technique of Aorto-Ostial Stent Placement. Am J Cardiol. 2005;96:212H.
12. Fischell TA, Saltiel FS, Foster MT, et al. Initial clinical experience using an ostial stent positioning system (Ostial Pro) for the accurate placement of stents in the treatment of coronary aorto-ostial lesions. J Invasive Cardiol. 2009;21:53-9.
13. Kini AS, Moreno PR, Steinheimer AM, et al. Effectiveness of the stent pull back technique for non-aorto ostial lesions of native coronary arteries. Am J Cardiol. 2005;96:1123-8.
14. Lambros J, Fairshid A, Pitney MR. Simultaneous use of a diagnostic catheter to facilitate stent deployment in aorto-ostial lesions: A case report. Catheter cardiovasc Diagn. 1997;40:210-1.

CHAPTER 61

Approach to Management of Chronic Total Occlusion

Pravin K Goel, Roopali Khanna

INTRODUCTION

Chronic total occlusion (CTO) is observed in 16–52% of cases undergoing coronary angiography but constitute only 10–15% of cases undergoing percutaneous coronary intervention (PCI).[1] PCI of CTO lesions is not performed by many interventionists due to fear of procedural failure and complications such as vessel perforation, contrast nephropathy, higher interventional costs, prolonged procedure time, a longer radiation exposure than routine angioplasty, skepticism of benefit and most importantly paucity of widespread expertise and specifically skilled operators. With improving techniques and hardware for PCI and the increasing role of PCI in the management of obstructive coronary artery disease (CAD), CTO, being the most challenging subset, remain the last or unconquered frontier.[2-4] The purpose of a PCI in CAD is to reduce symptoms and possible future events. These benefits however have not been established at length and study outcomes vary from one study to another. The anticipated benefits of CTO-PCI should exceed the procedural risk. Benefits of CTO-PCI assumed are:

- Improvement in angina
- Improvement in quality of life
- Improved exercise capacity
- Improved left ventricular ejection fraction (LVEF)
- Improvement in cardiac mortality.

Risk associated with CTO-PCI can be categorized into acute and chronic:

- *Acute risk include*:
  - Renal injury
  - Emergency coronary artery bypass graft
  - Periprocedural myocardial infarction (MI)
  - Pericardial tamponade
  - Vascular access complication.
- *Chronic risk include*:
  - *Stent related complication*: Stent thrombosis and stent restenosis
  - Radiation injury.

The CTO interventions as a whole have their benefit, even less well established and available literature shows conflicting results.[5-7] Moreover, technical challenges involved in CTO procedures, and the unpredictability of the result, along with limited operator expertise has precluded prospective trials. Till date only three prospective trials have been conducted in patients undergoing CTO-PCI but only one is published till date.

The EXPLORE (Evaluating Xience and Left Ventricular Function in Percutaneous Coronary Intervention on Occlusions After ST-Elevation Myocardial Infarction) trial evaluated whether patients with STEMI and concurrent CTO in a non-infarct-related artery benefit from additional PCI of CTO shortly after primary PCI with primary outcome of improvement in LVEF and left ventricular end-diastolic volume (LVEDV) as assessed by cardiac magnetic resonance imaging after 4 months.[8] A total of 150 patients were enrolled in CTO-PCI group and 154 patients were kept on medical treatment with no CTO-PCI. There was no significant difference in LVEF and LVEDV at end of 4 months but subgroup analysis revealed significant improvement in LVEF in patient with left anterior descending (LAD) artery, CTO emphasizing the importance of extent of myocardial supply of the CTO artery.

The DECISION-CTO (Drug-Eluting Stent Implantation versus Optimal Medical Treatment in Patients with Chronic Total Occlusion) trial (NCT01078051) was presented at the 2017 American College of Cardiology meeting. It randomized 834 CTO patients between optimized medical treatment (OMT) alone and CTO-PCI with OMT. At median follow-up of 3.1 years there was no significant difference with respect to the primary endpoint of the composite of death, MI, stroke, or any revascularization. There were various limitations in the trial, being a underpowered trial, large number of crossover between the two arms, including periprocedural MI as the primary endpoint and early termination of study because of slow enrollment.

The EuroCTO (A Randomized Multicenter Trial to Evaluate the Utilization of Revascularization or Optimal Medical Therapy for the Treatment of Chronic Total Coronary Occlusions) trial (NCT01760083) was presented at the 2017 EuroPCR meeting. It randomized 407 CTO patients into CTO-PCI group and OMT only group. The primary endpoint was improvement in angina as assessed by Seattle Angina Questionnaire. There was significant improvement in angina in patient undergoing CTO-PCI as compared to OMT.

Several observation and retrospective studies have assessed long-term outcome of CTO-PCI compared with medical therapy and have shown lower major adverse cardiac events in CTO-PCI group.[9-11] A study from our institute assessed long-term follow-up in 549 patients undergoing CTO-PCI with median follow-up of 2.9 years.[12] Primary endpoint was defined as event free survival of major adverse cardiac event including death, MI, repeat revascularization [PCI, or coronary artery bypass grafting (CABG)] and recurrent or continued angina. Each individual adverse event was considered as a secondary endpoint. Kaplan-Meier survival analysis showed a better event-free survival in CTO success versus failure ($p = 0.03$). Our study showed successful CTO-PCI was associated with a higher total event free survival but a nonsignificant all-cause mortality difference on long-term follow-up. Complete revascularization was also associated with a better total event-free survival but a significantly lower all-cause mortality in addition at long-term follow-up. There was no significant difference in repeat revascularization rates (repeat PCI and or CABG) in either groups.

When to do Chronic Total Occlusion-Percutaneous Coronary Intervention ?

Evidence of ischemia in the territory supplied by the occluded vessel is a must to treat CTO. This can be confirmed by either clinically evident angina or reversible ischemia documented in a noninvasive study preprocedure in absence of evident angina. Further, territory supplied by the vessel being intervened must have a myocardial supply weightage of at least 10% of the entire myocardium or more, else the risk benefit ratio does not favor intervention.[13] This will be indirectly equal to a vessel with myocardial value of at least 1.5 as per Green lane scoring system.[14]

IMAGING OF CHRONIC TOTAL OCCLUSION LESIONS

Apart from new materials and techniques, the constant devezlopment of cardiovascular imaging modalities has helped to improve success and safety of CTO-PCI. Noninvasive imaging technique of coronary computed tomography angiography (coronary CTA) and imaging with intravascular ultrasonography (IVUS) have emerged as a reliable tool to help in CTO intervention. However coronary angiography still forms the basis of a CTO intervention.

Coronary angiography: Several of CTO lesions histopathologically are less than complete with tiny microchannels connecting proximal to distal stump. These microchannels could be evident on delayed frames on a proper frame by frame analysis of the angiogram in two orthogonal views. The filling pattern of the distal vessel needs to be analyzed frame by frame to differentiate a very slow antegrade filling through microchannels or bridging collaterals or filling retrograde through ipsilateral or contralateral collaterals. Simultaneous injection of feeder vessel and recipient vessel with feeder vessel injection preceding the recipient gives a very good assessment of the length of occlusion almost as good as coronary CTA and should be done in all cases with contralateral collaterals.

Coronary computed tomography angiography: Computed tomography angiography provide good detailed information on lesion length, vessel course, tortuosity, calcification grade, stump morphology, distal vessel opacity, presence of side branches, and presence of bridging collaterals. The only negative side of asking for coronary CTA in all CTO cases is the contrast used (at least additional 50–100 mL) and extra radiation dose in a patient who is due for a long procedure.[15]

Intravascular ultrasonography: IVUS provides an axial spatial resolution of 80–150 μm and therefore precise visualization of lumen and vessel wall is possible. IVUS (unlike conventional angiography) can visualize the position of a guidewire within an occluded segment. Thus, intimal and subintimal guidewire tracking can be distinguished, which is crucial for antegrade as well as retrograde wiring techniques. Furthermore, IVUS can be helpful in identifying an ostially located entrance, especially in the unfavorable situation of a stumpless CTO with a side branch at occlusion site. Finally, the usual IVUS information on the target lesion, such as lesion length, lumen area, plaque composition and distribution plays an important role in optimizing stent implantation and reducing in-stent restenosis.[16,17]

PREDICTORS OF CHRONIC TOTAL OCCLUSION-PERCUTANEOUS CORONARY INTERVENTION SUCCESS

Various scores have been postulated regarding predictors of success of CTO-PCI based on lesion specific and patient profile (Table 1). The J-CTO score is a commonly used scoring model and was derived from a study on 479 CTO cases, to estimate the likelihood of successful guidewire crossing within 30 minutes based on five criteria (intralesion >45° bend, length ≥20 mm, calcification, blunt stump, and previously failed attempt).[18] The PROGRESS-CTO (PROspective Global REgiStry for the Study of Chronic Total Occlusion Intervention) score includes ambiguous proximal cap, left circumflex target artery, moderate/severe proximal tortuosity and lack of interventional collaterals giving equal score to each characteristics. The ORA score (ostial location, Rentrop filling of distal target vessel <2 and age ≥75 years) giving Rentrop filling score 2 and rest of the predictors 1 score.[19,20] A weighted score (W-CTO) was developed by us for predicting success of antegrade wire crossing in CTO-PCI.[21] The presence of blunt stump, length of occlusion,

TABLE 1: Various scoring system for predictors of CTO-PCI success

	J-CTO	PROGRESS-CTO	ORA	W-CTO
Stump morphology	Blunt stump (1)	Ambiguous cap (1)	–	Blunt stump (2)
Length of occlusion	≥20 (1)	–	–	≥20 (1.5)
Tortuosity	>45 (1)	Moderate to severe proximal tortuosity (1)	–	>45 (1)
Previous attempt	Yes (1)	–	–	–
Calcification	Mild to moderate (1)	–	–	Yes (1)
Ostial location	–	–	Yes (1)	–
Target vessel	–	Left circumflex artery (1)	Rentrop filling <2 (2)	Rentrop filling <2 (1)
Distal target vessel	–	Poor interventional collaterals (1)	–	–
Age	–	–	>75 years (1)	–
Total score	5	4	4	6.5

CTO, chronic total occlusion; PCI, percutaneous coronary intervention.

presence of calcification, presence of tortuosity and Rentrop filling <2 were given respective score of +2, +1.5, +1, +1, and +1 with total score of 6.5. Score values of 0–2, >2–4, and >4 were classified as low, intermediate and high levels of difficulty for CTO-PCI success and were associated with 98%, 74.2%, and 42.5% ($p < 0.0001$) success rate. The predictability of antegrade wire crossing success was demonstrated to be marginally better with the W-CTO score as compared to the J-CTO score [ROCAUC of 0.82 (J-CTO) versus 0.86 (W CTO), $p = 0.009$). These CTO score helps in assessing the success rate and should be applied by operators especially less experienced operators for selecting the case which to perform and which to refer to be performed by more experienced operator.

HYBRID ALGORITHM FOR CHRONIC TOTAL OCCLUSION-PERCUTANEOUS CORONARY INTERVENTION

There are three major techniques for crossing CTO lesion: (1) antegrade wire escalation, (2) antegrade dissection re-entry, and (3) retrograde approach. According to the angiographic characteristics of occlusion the type of approach can be selected (Flowchart 1).

CHRONIC TOTAL OCCLUSION-PERCUTANEOUS CORONARY INTERVENTION TECHNIQUES

Antegrade Wiring

Antegrade approach using a single wire escalation technique and/or parallel wire technique is attempted before changing to a more complex antegrade dissection re-entry approach. For an antegrade procedure intimal plaque tracking is crucial as success rates decrease substantially once the wire enters the subintimal space. Intimal plaque tracking can either be achieved by loose tissue tracking or by intentional intimal plaque tracking. The concept of loose tissue tracking is based on the histopathological finding that angiographic determined occlusions frequently show residual lumen patency with microchannels and loose connective tissue around them.[22,23] It is therefore recommend starting the wiring procedure with a soft tapered tip wire like Fielder XT/XTR and changing to an intermediate-stiffness guidewire like Fielder XTA or Gia 1 or Gia 2 depending upon the tactile feedback of the resistance being witnessed in the tissue and the penetrating power of the wire. A tapered tip wire is more likely to enter loose connective tissue and once entered an intermediate wire will automatically track the tissue with low resistance rather than penetrating into the hard atherosclerotic plaque. This concept is supported by the PIKACHU trial (Prospective Multicenter Registry of IKAzuchi-X for Chronic Total OcclUsion) where approximately 70% of CTOs could be crossed with an intermediate-stiffness 0.010 inch hydrocoated wire.[25] In the parallel wire method, a wire which enters the subintimal space is left there, and a second wire is inserted alongside to find a new channel. When this technique is successful, the following findings are often noted: (1) the second wire crosses over the first inside the CTO; (2) the second wire shows more acute curve than the first wire; (3) the second wire penetrates the lesion from the outer curvature of the coronary artery and then is advanced along the same curvature of the vessel. Indeed, the second wire should be operated intentionally to achieve these findings so that the probability of success increases and the duration of the procedure is shortened. A crusade catheter could be used to bring in the second wire.

The "CrossBoss and Stingray Re-Entry System" (Boston Scientific, Natick, MA, USA) has recently been developed to antegrade dissection re-entry technique.[26,27]

Retrograde Approach

The retrograde approach requires more operator expertise and has high risk for periprocedural complications like cardiac tamponade due to collateral perforation, donor vessel ischemia, ostial dissection. Choosing the interventional

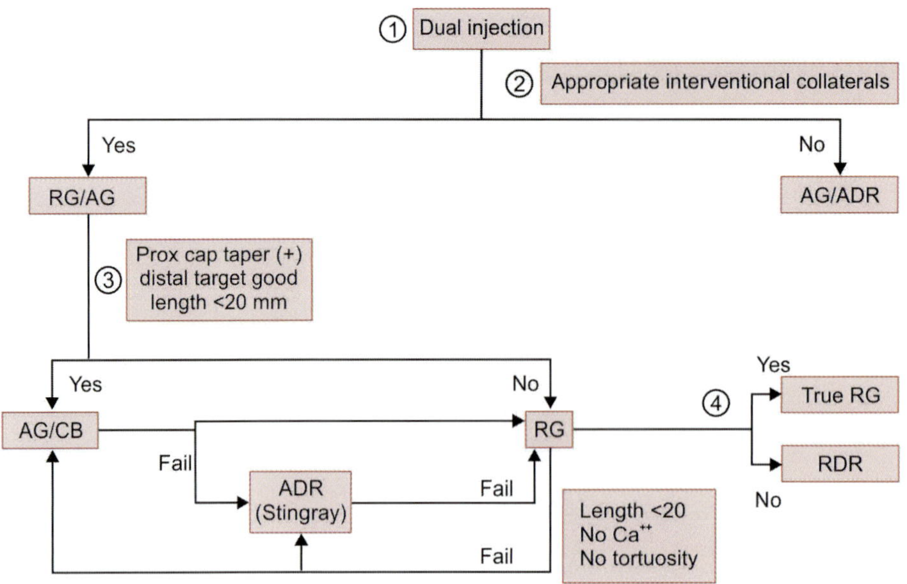

FLOWCHART 1: Hybrid algorithm: an approach to chronic total occlusion-percutaneous coronary intervention (CTO-PCI).

collateral is the first key step. Unfortunately such channels are usually of small caliber (100–200 µm) and often present a tortuous course making them fairly vulnerable. As injury to an epicardial channel can easily cause cardiac tamponade and therefore selection of a septal channel is preferred septal collaterals.[28]

"Wire Crossed Balloon Not Crossed"—What Next?

Balloon uncrossable CTOs are rarely found that cannot be crossed with a balloon after successful guidewire crossing. This is often observed in chronic calcific CTOs. These lesions are usually approached with a combination of lesion modification techniques (such as use of microcatheters and multiple balloons) and improving guide support, use of anchoring techniques and use of guide catheter extensions. Other techniques described to cross the balloons in such cases. This includes advancing a microcatheter or Tornus antegradely which creates a small channel over which a small size (1.2 mm × 6 mm) balloon could then advance. If this fails one could use other techniques like the anchor balloon technique or a guideliner as described by others. One could also experience in these chronic lesions at times a situation that balloon has crossed but fails to inflate because of calcium or otherwise. In this situation one may need plaque modification using score balloon, cutting balloon or rotablator.[29-32]

COMPLICATIONS OF CHRONIC TOTAL OCCLUSION-PERCUTANEOUS CORONARY INTERVENTION

We need to be well aware that CTO-PCI are complex procedures and are not free from complications. Pooled analysis of complications include death 0.2%, emergent CABG surgery 0.1%, stroke less than 0.01%, MI 2.5%, Q-wave MI 0.2%, coronary perforation 2.9%, tamponade 0.3%, and contrast nephropathy 3.8% in a series by Patel et al. compared with successful procedures, unsuccessful procedures had higher rates of death (0.42% vs. 1.54%; p <0.001), perforation (3.65% vs. 10.70%; p <0.001), and tamponade (0% vs. 1.65%; p <0.001).[24]

When Not to do Chronic Total Occlusion?

Although techniques have improved with great success and impervious safety, we would still advocate to avoid CTO interventions in a few select settings as follows: (1) if two or more major vessels have a CTO; (2) CTOs are present in sequence in same vessel; (3) a small vessel with CTO is not worth the effort; (4) a very long CTO with heavy calcification; (5) very tortuous CTO anatomy with heavy calcification of vessel; (6) a CTO from ostium of artery; and (7) CTOs distal to complex proximal vessel lesions, e.g., CTO of LAD beyond a severe/moderate LM bifurcation stenosis or CTO of CX/OM beyond an ostial CX calcific stenosis. Retrograde approach to do CTO-PCI should not be used if donor artery is heavily calcified or with mild or moderate long segment disease which otherwise would not need anything to be done or would risk donor artery closure.

CONCLUSION

With improvement in techniques and hardware the success of CTO-PCI has significantly increased. Appropriate selection of case and CTO technique can make it a safe procedure. PCI for CTO is an approachable goal with good skills and an experienced operator, a good understanding of the disease, availability of required hardware and wisdom of when to do and when not to do or when to stop.

REFERENCES

1. Grantham JA, Marso SP, Spertus J, et al. Chronic total occlusion angioplasty in the United States. J Am Coll Cardiol Intv. 2009;2:479-86.
2. Fefer P, Knudtson ML, Cheema AN, et al. Current perspectives on coronary chronic total occlusions: the Canadian Multicenter Chronic Total Occlusions Registry. J Am Coll Cardiol. 2012;59:991-7.
3. Joyal D, Afilalo J, Rinfret S. Effectiveness of recanalization of chronic total occlusions: a systematic review and meta-analysis. Am Heart J. 2010;160: 179-87.
4. Tajti P, Nicholas MB, Karmpaliotis D, et al. Update in the Percutaneous Management of Coronary Chronic Total Occlusions. JACC: Cardiovasc Interv. 2018;11:615-25;(7):615-25.
5. Jones DA, Weerackody R, Rathod K. Successful recanalization of chronic total occlusions is associated with improved long-term survival. JACC Cardiovasc Interv. 2012;5:380-8.
6. George S, Cockburn J, Clayton TC, et al. Long-term follow-up of elective chronic total coronary occlusion angioplasty: analysis from the U.K. Central Cardiac Audit Database. J Am Coll Cardiol. 2014; 64:235-43.
7. Suero JA, Marso SP, Jones PJ, et al. Procedural outcomes and long-term survival among patients undergoing percutaneous coronary intervention of chronic total occlusion in native coronary arteries: a 20-year experience. J Am Coll Cardiol. 2001;38:409-14.
8. Henriques JP, Hoebers LP, Ramunddal T, et al. Percutaneous intervention for concurrent chronic total occlusions in patients with STEMI: the EXPLORE trial. J Am Coll Cardiol. 2016;68:1622-32.
9. Jones DA, Weerackody R, Rathod K. Successful recanalization of chronic total occlusions is associated with improved long-term survival. JACC Cardiovasc Interv. 2012;5:380-8.
10. George S, Cockburn J, Clayton TC, et al. Long-term follow-up of elective chronic total coronary occlusion angioplasty: analysis from the U.K. Central Cardiac Audit Database. J Am Coll Cardiol. 2014;64:235-43.
11. Mehran R, Claessen BE, Godino C, et al. Long-Term outcome of percutaneous Coronary intervention for chronic total occlusions. JACC Cardiovasc Interv. 2011;4:952-61.
12. Goel PK, Khanna R, Pandey CM, et al. Long-term outcomes post chronic total occlusion intervention-implications of completeness of revascularization. J Interv Cardiol. 2018;31:293-301.
13. Hachamovitch R, Hayes SW, Friedman JD, et al. Comparison of the short-term survival benefit associated with revascularization compared with medical therapy in patients with no prior coronary artery disease undergoing stress myocardial perfusion single photon emission computed tomography. Circulation. 2003;107:2900-7.
14. Brandt PW, Patridge JB, Wattie WJ. Coronary arteriography; method of the arteriogram report and a scoring system. Clin Radiol.1977;28:361-5.
15. Yokoyama N, Yamamoto Y, Suzuki S, et al. Impact of 16-slice computed tomography in percutaneous coronary intervention of chronic total occlusions. Cathete Cardiovasc Interv. 2006;68:1-7.
16. Matsubara T, Murata A, Kanyama H, et al. IVUS-guided wiring technique: promising approach for the chronic total occlusion. Catheter Cardiovasc Interv. 2004;61:381-6.
17. Park Y, Park HS, Jang GL, et al. Intravascular ultrasound guided recanalization of stump less chronic total occlusion. Int J Cardiol. 2011;148:174-8.
18. Morino Y, Abe M, Morimoto T, et al. Predicting successful guidewire crossing through chronic total occlusion of native coronary lesions within30 minutes: the J-CTO (Multicenter CTO Registry in Japan) score as a difficulty grading and time assessment tool. JACC Cardiovasc Interv. 2011;4:213-21.
19. Christopoulos G, Kandzari DE, Yeh RW, et al. Development and validation of a novel scoring system for predicting technical success of chronic total occlusion percutaneous coronary interventions: the PROGRESS CTO (Prospective Global Registry for the Study of Chronic Total Occlusion Intervention) score. J Am Coll Cardiol Intv. 2016;9:1-9.
20. Galassi AR, Boukhris M, Azzarelli S, et al. Percutaneous coronary revascularization for chronic total occlusions: a novel predictive score of technical failure using advanced technologies. J Am Coll Cardiol Intv. 2016;9:911-22.
21. 21.Khanna R, Pandey CM, Bedi S, et al. A weighted angiographic scoring model (W-CTOscore) to predict success of antegrade wire crossing in chronic total occlusion: analysis from a single centre. Asia Interv. 2018;4:18-25.
22. Srivatsa SS, Edwards WD, Boos CM, et al. Histologic correlates of angiographic chronic total coronary artery occlusions: influence of occlusion duration on neovascular channel patterns and intimal plaque composition. J Am Coll Cardiol. 1997;29:955-63.
23. Munce NR, Strauss BH, Qi X, et al. Intravascular and extravascular microvessel formation in chronic total occlusions a micro-CT imaging study. JACC Cardiovasc Imaging. 2010;3:797-805.
24. Patel Y, Depta JP, DeMartini TJ. Complications of chronic total occlusion percutaneous coronary intervention. Interv. Cardiol. 2013;5(5):567-75.
25. Matsukage T, Masutani M, Yoshimachi F, et al. A prospective multicenter registry of 0.010-inch guidewire and compatible system for chronic total occlusion: the PIKACHU registry. Catheter Cardiovasc Interv. 2010;75:1006-12.
26. Ochiai M, Ashida K, Araki H, et al. The latest wire technique for chronic total occlusion. Ital Heart J. 2005;6:489-93.
27. Werner GS. The BridgePoint devices to facilitate recanalization of chronic total coronary occlusions through controlled subintimal reentry. Expert Rev Med Devices. 2011;8:23-9.
28. Surmely JF, Katoh O, Tsuchikane E, et al. Coronary septal collaterals as an access for the retrograde approach in the percutaneous treatment of coronary chronic total occlusions. Catheter Cardiovasc Interv. 2007;69:826-32.
29. Hu XQ, Tang L, Zhou SH, et al. A novel approach to facilitating balloon crossing chronic total occlusions: the "wire-cutting" technique. J Interv Cardiol. 2012;25:297-303.
30. Michael TT, Banerjee S, Brilakis ES. Subintimal distal anchor technique for "balloon-uncrossable" chronic total occlusions. J Invasive Cardiol. 2013;25:552-4.
31. Kovacic JC, Sharma AB, Roy S, et al. Guide Liner mother-and-child guide catheter extension: a simple adjunctive tool in PCI for balloon uncrossable chronic total occlusions. J Interv Cardiol. 2013;26:343-50.
32. Fernandez JP, Hobson AR, McKenzie D, et al. Beyond the balloon: excimer coronary laser atherectomy used alone or in combination with rotational atherectomy in the treatment of chronic total occlusions, non-crossable and non-expansible coronary lesions. EuroIntervention. 2013;9:243-50.

CHAPTER 62

Hybrid Coronary Revascularization

C Raghu

INTRODUCTION

Over the past six decades the gold standard for myocardial revascularization has been coronary artery bypass grafting (CABG). Balloon angioplasty was first performed in 1977 as an alternative to bypass,[1] and has evolved to implantation of stents into the coronary arteries, known as percutaneous coronary intervention (PCI). Revascularization by CABG and PCI is different approaches each with its own strengths and weaknesses. Of late, attempts are being made to combine these two approaches together to maximize patient outcomes and recovery.

BENEFITS OF CORONARY ARTERY BYPASS GRAFTING OVER PERCUTANEOUS CORONARY INTERVENTION

As per latest guidelines, CABG is proven to be superior to medical therapy for the treatment of advanced coronary artery disease (CAD).[2] Major reason for the success of CABG is revascularization of the left anterior descending artery (LAD), which supplies a majority of the myocardium performed by anastomozing the left internal mammary artery (LIMA) to the LAD. Freedom from atherosclerosis contributes the long-term patency rates of LIMA to LAD up to 95% at 10 years.[3] These results could be replicated both with open and minimally invasive approaches to CABG.[4] Repeat revascularization were more common after PCI of the LAD compared to CABG.

In the past two decades many studies comparing CABG to PCI showed that major adverse cardiac or cerebrovascular events (MACCE) were more common in the PCI group.[5,6] Despite large prospective trials and many observational studies supporting the benefits of CABG over PCI, in practice PCI is performed much more frequently.

WHY PERCUTANEOUS CORONARY INTERVENTION IS PREFERRED IN PRACTICE?

Percutaneous coronary intervention is preferred over CABG because of the minimally invasive nature of the approach. Patients are typically return back home within 48 hours after PCI, especially after elective cases, and periprocedure complications are often lower. Neurological complications such as stroke and neurocognitive dysfunction are lower with PCI compared to CABG.[5,6] CABG needs sternotomy so there is risk of deep sternal wound infection. In addition, CABG has higher rates of blood transfusion, atrial fibrillation, and overall morbidity and short-term mortality.

Mid-term and long-term rates of MACCE following PCI are higher than CABG, which is attributable to higher rates of repeat interventions. Even though repeat interventions are an important outcome measure, they are not viewed as seriously as CABG related morbidity. 5-year mortality rates are not different between PCI and CABG in both the SYNTAX (Synergy between PCI with Taxus and Cardiac Surgery)[7] and BEST (randomized Comparison of Coronary Artery Bypass Surgery and Everolimus-Eluting Stent Implantation in the Treatment of Patients with Multivessel Coronary Artery Disease trial).[6] Current generation drug-eluting stents (DESs) have improved rates of stent thrombosis and mortality over bare-metal stents (BMS) and early DES.[8] Owing to these advantages, lesions that were previously treated only with CABG are now being approached by PCI. For example, patients with unprotected left main disease have historically been referred for CABG, but recent trials have shown similar MACCE rates with PCI.[9]

Beyond stents numerous other advances such as radial access decreasing major bleeding,[10] optical coherence tomography, and intravascular ultrasound have improved outcomes in chronic total occlusions PCI[11] and fractional flow reserve (FFR) betters the necessity for PCI.[12]

IN CORONARY ARTERY BYPASS GRAFTING, WHICH IS THE PREFERRED SURGICAL CONDUIT?

Saphenous vein grafts (SVGs) are routinely used as additional conduits for vessels other than LAD. Compared to LIMA, SVGs are associated with inferior longevity.[13] Alternately, use of multiple arterial grafts is shown to be superior to SVGs. Common arterial conduits include the right internal mammary or radial arteries. Despite lack of strong evidence, current Society of Thoracic Surgeons guidelines recommend considering the use of multiple arterial grafts when possible.[14] But in practice, only about 7% of CABG operations are performed with more than one arterial graft.[14]

WHICH IS BETTER ON-PUMP VERSUS OFF-PUMP SURGERY?

Off-pump coronary artery bypass (OPCAB) was originally developed in the 1970s to decrease the risks of CABG associated with cardiopulmonary bypass (CPB), including stroke, inflammation, blood usage, kidney injury, etc. Currently the initial enthusiasm seen with OPCAB during 1990–2000s has slightly decreased. Evidence in the form of ROOBY (Randomized On/Off Bypass) and GOPCABE (German Off Pump CABG Trial in Elderly Patients) trials contributed to this. ROOBY trial showed higher MACCE at 1 year, lower graft patency, and lower rates of complete revascularization with OPCAB.[15] The GOPCABE trial studied a higher-risk group than ROOBY and did not find any superiority of OPCAB.

MINIMALLY INVASIVE DIRECT CORONARY ARTERY BYPASS SURGERY

Minimally invasive direct coronary artery bypass (MIDCAB) is a technique designed to reduce the invasiveness of CABG by avoiding a median sternotomy. MIDCAB, introduced in 1995, is commonly performed via an inframammary left anterior thoracotomy in the fourth or fifth interspace. Comparing MIDCAB and OPCAB, there was no difference in graft patency[16] but with additional advantages of quicker recovery, decreased ventilator times, and hospital length of stay. Limitation with the MIDCAB approach is the significant learning curve and related technical difficulty of the procedure.

ROBOTIC-ASSISTED CORONARY ARTERY BYPASS GRAFTING

A novel approach to surgery using robots was approved for use in 2000 (Intuitive Surgical, Sunnyvale, CA, USA). Surgeons sit at a console rather than standing at the bedside, controlling robotic arms that are performing surgery. Robotic surgery is a shot in the arm for minimally invasive surgery. Instead of long instruments that can only be manipulated outside the body in endoscopic surgery, robotic instruments maintain full range of motion inside the body cavity. This allows unprecedented operative precision. The use of a three-dimensional high-definition camera greatly improves visualization of the operative field creating a clarity that was never seen in endoscopic surgery.

With the robotic arm, superior degrees of freedom to operate and improved visualization, the LIMA can be dissected from the chest wall using the robotic console. Using a robotic approach sternotomy can easily be avoided along with its attendant sternal wound infection, prolonged recovery, and poor cosmesis.

ENDOSCOPIC BYPASS GRAFTING

Total endoscopic coronary artery bypass grafting (TECAB) is the extension of utilizing robotics into coronary anastomosis. Some centers have used this exclusively with the LIMA-to-LAD, while others have demonstrated the feasibility of complete revascularization with TECAB. While TECAB is commonly performed off-pump, CPB may be used in cases where the patient's hemodynamics does not tolerate positioning.

The major advantage of robotic-assisted CABG and TECAB are shorter hospital stays and quicker return to work compared to single-vessel OPCAB. Long-term MACCE rates have been reported with this approach. During the learning curve with TECAB conversion to sternotomy and longer operating hours are common, especially if multiple grafting is needed. The rate of these challenges seems to decline with experience.

HYBRID CORONARY REVASCULARIZATION

From the discussion above, one can easily understand that multiple strategies exist for performing myocardial revascularization. The spectrum of approaches ranging from PCI to ONCAB represents escalating degrees of invasiveness. Patients perceive that PCI is quick and easy while CABG is a painful operation after which patients spend a considerable time in intensive care and require prolonged recovery. At the same time, they may be unwilling to trade an early short-term risk or death, stroke, or infection for a potentially long-term, prolonged, and better quality of life.

To assuage patients' fears about open surgery, various minimally invasive techniques have been developed including OPCAB, MIDCAB, and robotic approaches. The major limitation with these novel approaches is many centers have not adopted them. This is due in part due to the potentially steep learning curves and during this learning curve even in the best hands; outcomes and graft occlusion rates may not be as good as traditional open surgery. LIMA-to-LAD anastomosis is most easily performed with minimally invasive techniques since the LAD courses on the anterior

BOX 1 Goals of hybrid revascularization

- Achieve similar or better postoperative morbidity and mortality than open CABG
- Maintain equivalent patency of LIMA-to-LAD to open techniques
- Improve recovery from surgery (length of stay, return to work and activity)
- Improve rates of repeat interventions and long-term outcomes over PCI
- Achieve excellent patient satisfaction
- Ensure cost effectiveness in the short and long term

CABG, coronary artery bypass grafting; LAD, left anterior descending artery; LIMA, left internal mammary artery; PCI, percutaneous coronary intervention.

TABLE 1: Which is the first procedure in hybrid interventions?

Positives	Negatives
PCI first	
• Ability to treat culprit lesion first • Bail-out to conventional CABG if procedure unsuccessful	• Need for antiplatelet agent to protect stent during surgery • No LIMA-to-LAD protection during PCI
CABG and PCI same time	
• Convenient for patient • Potentially reduced length of stay	• Logistically challenging, requires a hybrid operating room • Bleeding risk due to antiplatelet load for PCI
CABG first – most common approach	
• Have LIMA-to-LAD protection for PCI • Can initiate antiplatelet agents without fear of surgical bleeding	• Second surgery required if PCI unsuccessful

CABG, coronary artery bypass grafting; LAD, left anterior descending artery; LIMA, left internal mammary artery; PCI, percutaneous coronary intervention.

surface of the heart and can be readily accessed through minimally invasive incisions.

Hybrid coronary revascularization (HCR) has been developed to address these various issues. HCR in principle is to perform the LIMA-to-LAD anastomosis using a minimally invasive surgical technique and revascularize the rest of the coronary lesions with PCI.[17] This represents a "best of both worlds" approach.

Goals of HCR are summarized in box 1.

Hybrid coronary revascularization first reported in 1996,[18] till date has more than 3,000 cases reported in the literature.[19] But HCR is currently applicable to a minority of patients with CAD. In a multicenter observational study, 12% of patients presenting with significant CAD were found eligible for HCR by both a surgeon and cardiologist.[20] MIDCAB, robotic-assisted CABG, and TECAB are all used frequently as the surgical approach. PCI and CABG can be performed in the same operative setting, but more commonly the procedures are performed separately (often several days apart). The optimal timing for HCR has not yet been studied. Theoretical strengths and weaknesses of each approach are summarized in table 1. The preferred timing of HCR is best tailored to the individual patient and center.

HYBRID OUTCOMES

With improved technical expertise and technological advances results with PCI continue to get better, in the form of reduced rates of reintervention. With LIMA-to-LAD using minimally invasive surgical approaches recent series demonstrated excellent rates of LIMA patency (96–100%). There were few conversions to sternotomy, length of stay was low, and mid- and long-term rates of MACCE were not concerning. These data support the safety and efficacy of minimally invasive coronary revascularization (one of the main goals of HCR).

A number of large series of HCR have recently been performed, summarized in table 2. Postoperative survival (99–100%) and LIMA patency rates (95–100%) were excellent. Conversions to sternotomy were uncommon, consistent across different minimally invasive strategies. Reinterventions when required, were most commonly for

TABLE 2: Recent series of HCR

Year	Surgical technique	n	Survival (%)	LIMA patency (%)	Survival	LOS days	CTS (%)
2011[21]	Mid CAB	104	100	100	1 (18 months)	8.2	1
2013[22]	Mid CAB	166	98.8	100	17 (5 years)	6.5	2.4
2014[23]	Robotic	96	100	94	21 (5 years)	4	2.1
2014[24]	TECAB	180	100	NR	20 (5 years)	6	2.2
2014[25]	Mid CAB	98	100	99	10.2 (1 year)	8.8	6
2014[26]	Robotic	300	98.7	97.6	NR	5	2
2015[27]	Mid CAB	100	100	95	20 (1 year)	8	0

CAB, coronary artery bypass; CTS, conversion to sternotomy; HCR, hybrid coronary revascularization; LIMA, left internal mammary artery; LOS, length of stay; MACCE, major adverse cardiac or cerebrovascular events; n, no. of patients; TECAB, total endoscopic coronary artery bypass grafting.

previous PCI targets or coronaries not previously intervened on; there did not appear to be any significant issues with the LIMA-to-LAD anastomosis at the intermediate term (up to 5 years).

CONCLUSION

Compared to traditional open CABG, minimally invasive techniques to CABG provide an excellent alternative in carefully selected patients. Over the past two decades, the MIDCAB technique has been well established, with many groups showing excellent results. Another exciting novel vista robotic surgery showed excellent results. A substantial learning curve to all these minimally invasive techniques limits their acceptance across many centers. Results from both MIDCAB and robotic approaches, especially patency of the LIMA-to-LAD anastomosis, are excellent and appear to be equivalent to one performed via a sternotomy.

Hybrid coronary revascularization takes advantage of the excellent durability of the LIMA-to-LAD anastomosis and combines with latest PCI technologies to provide an excellent alternative to open CABG. The key for the success in developing HCR at a center is a dedicated surgeon and interventional cardiologist. HCR by nature is multidisciplinary and a heart team approach for patients with coronary disease is essential; this will ensure ideal patient selection and optimize results. HCR has developed to combine the superior results obtained with both approaches. Though in near future practice of HCR may not radically change the way how CABG is performed. But as surgeons acquire the necessary skill set with minimally invasive CABG techniques, HCR is a therapy for niche centers.

REFERENCES

1. Hurst JW. The first coronary angioplasty as described by Andreas Gruentzig. Am J Cardiol. 1986;57:185-6.
2. Patel MR, Dehmer GJ, Hirshfeld JW, et al. ACCF/SCAI/STS/AATS/AHA/ASNC/HFSA/SCCT 2012 appropriate use criteria for coronary revascularization focused update: a report of the American College of Cardiology Foundation Appropriate Use Criteria Task Force, Society for Cardiovascular Angiography and Interventions, Society of Thoracic Surgeons, American Association for Thoracic Surgery, American Heart Association, American Society of Nuclear Cardiology, and the Society of Cardiovascular Computed Tomography. J Thorac Cardiovasc Surg. 2012;143:780-803.
3. Loop FD, Lytle BW, Cosgrove DM, et al. Influence of the internal-mammary-artery graft on 10-year survival and other cardiac events. N Engl J Med. 1986;314:1-6.
4. Thiele H, Neumann-Schniedewind P, Jacobs S, et al. Randomized comparison of minimally invasive direct coronary artery bypass surgery versus sirolimus-eluting stenting in isolated proximal left anterior descending coronary artery stenosis. J Am Coll Cardiol. 2009;53:2324-31.
5. Park SJ, Ahn JM, Kim YH, et al. Trial of everolimus-eluting stents or bypass surgery for coronary disease. N Engl J Med. 2015;372:1204-12.
6. Farkouh ME, Domanski M, Sleeper LA, et al. Strategies for multi-vessel revascularization in patients with diabetes. N Engl J Med. 2012;367:2375-84.
7. Serruys PW, Morice MC, Kappetein AP, et al. Percutaneous coronary intervention versus coronary artery bypass grafting for severe coronary artery disease. N Engl J Med. 2009;360:961-72.
8. Palmerini T, Benedetto U, Biondi-Zoccai G, et al. Long-term safety of drug-eluting and bare-metal stents: Evidence from a comprehensive network meta-analysis. J Am Coll Cardiol. 2015;65:2496-507.
9. Ahn JM, Roh JH, Kim YH, et al. Randomized trial of stents versus bypass surgery for left main coronary artery disease: 5-year outcomes of the PRECOMBAT study. J Am Coll Cardiol. 2015;65:2198-2206.
10. Valgimigli M, Gagnor A, Calabro P, et al. Radial versus femoral access in patients with acute coronary syndromes undergoing invasive management: A randomized multi-center trial. Lancet. 2015;385:2465-76.
11. Kim BK, Shin DH, Hong MK, et al. Clinical impact of intravascular ultrasound-guided chronic total occlusion intervention with zotarolimus-eluting versus biolimus-eluting stent implantation: Randomized study. Circ Cardiovasc Interv. 2015;8:e002592.
12. van Nunen LX, Zimmermann FM, Tonino PA, et al. Fractional flow reserve versus angiography for guidance of PCI in patients with multi-vessel coronary artery disease (FAME): 5-year follow-up of a randomized controlled trial. Lancet. 2015;386:1853-60.
13. Mehta RH, Ferguson TB, Lopes RD, et al. Saphenous vein grafts with multiple versus single distal targets in patients undergoing coronary artery bypass surgery: One-year graft failure and five-year outcomes from the Project of Ex-Vivo Vein Graft Engineering via Transfection (PREVENT) IV trial. Circulation. 2011;124:280-8.
14. Aldea GS, Bakaeen FG, Pal J, et al. The society of thoracic surgeons clinical practice guidelines on arterial conduits for coronary artery bypass grafting. Ann Thorac Surg. 2016;101:801-9.
15. Shroyer AL, Grover FL, Hattler B, et al. On-pump versus off-pump coronary-artery bypass surgery. N Engl J Med. 2009;361:1827-37.
16. Diegeler A, Borgermann J, Kappert U, et al. Off-pump versus on-pump coronary-artery bypass grafting in elderly patients. N Engl J Med. 2013;368:1189-98.
17. Detter C, Reichenspurner H, Boehm DH, et al. Minimally invasive direct coronary artery bypass grafting (MIDCAB) and off-pump coronary artery bypass grafting (OPCAB): Two techniques for beating heart surgery. Heart Surg Forum. 2002;5:157-62.
18. Popma JJ, Nathan S, Hagberg RC, et al. Hybrid myocardial revascularization: An integrated approach to coronary revascularization. Catheter Cardiovasc Interv. 2010;75(Suppl 1):S28-34.
19. Angelini GD, Wilde P, Salerno TA, et al. Integrated left small thoracotomy and angioplasty for multi-vessel coronary artery revascularization. Lancet. 1996;347:757-8.
20. Panoulas VF, Colombo A, Margonato A, et al. Hybrid coronary revascularization: Promising, but yet to take off. J Am Coll Cardiol. 2015;65:85-97.
21. Puskas JD, Ascheim D, Halkos M, et al. Hybrid coronary revascularization for the treatment of coronary artery disease: A multicenter observational study. J Am Coll Cardiol. 2013;61:E1741.
22. Hu S, Li Q, Gao P, et al. Simultaneous hybrid revascularization versus off-pump coronary artery bypass for multi-vessel coronary artery disease. Ann Thorac Surg. 2011;91:432-8.
23. Repossini A, Tespili M, Saino A, et al. Hybrid revascularization in multi-vessel coronary artery disease. Eur J Cardiothorac Surg. 2013;44:288-93.
24. Adams C, Burns DJ, Chu MW, et al. Single-stage hybrid coronary revascularization with long-term follow-up. Eur J Cardiothorac Surg. 2014;45:438-42.
25. Bonaros N, Schachner T, Kofler M, et al. Advanced hybrid closed chest revascularization: An innovative strategy for the treatment of multi-vessel coronary artery disease. Eur J Cardiothorac Surg. 2014;6:e94-102.
26. Gąsior M, Zembala MO, Tajstra M, et al. Hybrid revascularization for multi-vessel coronary artery disease. JACC Cardiovasc Interv. 2014;7:1277-83.
27. Yang M, Wu Y, Wang G, et al. Robotic total arterial off-pump coronary artery bypass grafting: seven-year single-center experience and long-term follow-up of graft patency. Ann Thorac Surg. 2015;100:1367-73.

CHAPTER 63

Should all Percutaneous Coronary Interventions be Radial Only?

Tejas Patel, Surender Deora, Sanjay Shah

BACKGROUND

Before reaching the final phase of optimization, any new technique or technology goes through various phases of observations. The overall experience, supported by data demonstrates the exceptional quality of a particular technology or technique, which eventually leads to natural devolution and extinction of an outmoded method. Cardiac catheterization and coronary angiography are glaring examples. In a span of less than a decade the Mason Sones' brachial artery cut-down is long gone, having given way to Judkin's transfemoral approach (TFA). Kiemeneij demonstrated the safety of percutaneous coronary interventions (PCI) through the transradial approach (TRA), without major bleeding risks engendered by TFA in heavily anticoagulated patients. The evolving data supporting TRA over TFA has generated strong opinions amongst interventional cardiologists aligned with one technique over the other.[1] Which technique is quicker, safer, cost-effective, more comfortable, and easily reproducible? It took about two decades for the interventional cardiologists to be convinced regarding the overall superiority of TRA over TFA.[4-15]

Transradial approach was largely guided by case reports, case series and small randomized studies, during the first decade of its inception.[4-6] Subsequently, many studies examined the different technical aspects, outcomes, advantages and disadvantages of TRA.[4-15] Over 1,500 positive papers have been published on transradial interventions (TRI), forming a robust evidence base to drive its practice. In spite of being a globally accepted technique, the recognition of TRA in some parts seems to be slower as compared to many other parts of the world.[2,3] Young cardiologists are particularly more enthusiastic to adopt TRA. However, many senior interventional cardiologists who have practiced TFA for several decades are not very keen for change. The major cause of their reluctance is an occasional negative experience with a complex PCI in a patient on whom they are forced to use TRA. It is important to understand that there is a definite "new learning curve" for TRA, even for the most experienced interventional cardiologist.[4-6] During this phase, the operator has to deal with some cases of failure and change-overs, lengthier procedural time and higher radiation exposure, which induces negative feelings for TRA. However, once the learning curve is over the operator will have the confidence to overcome all of the aforementioned barriers. Exponential growth in the number of interventional cardiologists has led to a reduction of individual procedural volume creating a challenge for a new cardiologist to overcome the learning curve. A practical solution for this problem is to work in groups of two, three or four preferably having one reasonably experienced radial operator available. Regardless of the superiority of the TRA, the transformation of a femoral operator into an accomplished radial operator will not be possible without an organized and concerted effort. The perpetuation of a femoral operator's prior negative experience becomes his "Achilles heel" and prevents him from being able to accept a slightly more complex technique despite its superior safety record. Nonetheless, the operator can overcome most of the technical problems related to TRI with increasing experience and persistence, much like that required to conquer the occasional problems encountered in TFA. In order to achieve overall acceptability of any procedure, it is important to engender confidence of a high success rate even for low volume operators and beginners. In order to demonstrate the clinical advantage of TRA over TFA, dedicated radial operators took almost two decades to complete clinical trials due to the lack of industry resources and general ignorance of many interventional cardiologists.

Primary Percutaneous Coronary Interventions and Transradial Approach

Patients presenting with ST-elevation myocardial infarction (STEMI) not only benefit from the utilization of aggressive anticoagulant and antiplatelet therapy, but also demonstrate higher rates of bleeding complications compared to low-risk patients. TRA is therefore an effective approach for primary PCI.[7-15] The large multicenter studies have demonstrated reduction in bleeding and improvement in patient outcomes using TRA.[7-10] Although most studies report no delay in door-to-balloon times with TRA versus TFA, some do report delay up to 11 minutes. In the absence of data from large randomized studies, the clinical impact of any small delay in reperfusion should not be measured against the benefit of decrease in bleeding. It is recommended that primary PCI via TRA be attempted only once the operator is fully facile with complex PCI using this technique, because delays appear to be more common with less experienced radial operators. Simultaneous preparation of groin is generally recommended for primary PCI procedures planned through TRA, so that delay can be minimized if cross-over becomes necessary and the groin is ready to receive large caliber hemodynamic support system (i.e., intra-aortic balloon pump or Impella device), should they become necessary.[4,5] Although, it is not a routine practice, we recommend that beginners inject contrast through the puncture cannula to define the vascular anatomy before introducing the radial sheath. If anatomy in unfavorable, immediate switch-over to TFA will save important initial time. As experience increases, the number of cross-over reduces remarkably. It is important to avoid working through extreme subclavian tortuosities and arteria lusoria during the initial phase of the TRI program.[4-6]

Chronic Total Occlusions and Transradial Approach

Chronic total occlusions (CTOs) intervention is a difficult and challenging procedure. The success rate has increased from 60% to almost 90% amongst accomplished operators. While TFA is traditionally preferred, in last decade a good number of studies have shown feasibility, efficacy and equivalent success rates using TRA.[4-6,17] Although, an experienced radial operator should be able to treat almost any CTO, a beginner should avoid long segment CTOs with flat stumps and presence of intra-arterial collaterals.

Left Main Coronary Artery Lesions and Transradial Approach

In last several years several trials have documented the feasibility, safety and results of left main coronary artery (LMCA) stenting.[6-8,33,34] Although most studies have been performed through TFA, a few have demonstrated success of TRA for LMCA stenting.[4-6,16] Right atrium (RA) having diameter more than 2 mm can accommodate a 7 F introducer sheath. If a 7 F guide catheter is necessary and RA diameter is small, sheathless guide system, modified sheathless guide catheter (Combo) technique, slender technique or balloon-assisted tracking (BAT) technique can help successful passage of a 7 F guide catheter.[4-6]

Transradial Approach—Impact on Bleeding Incidence and Outcomes

Periprocedural bleeding remains an important complication of PCI.[4-15] Many studies have demonstrated that the most common site of bleeding in patients of PCI is related to the vascular access site and that bleeding is associated with worse short- and long-term outcomes.[3-15] TRA has not only shown reduction in bleeding and improvement in clinical outcomes, but also mortality benefit.[4-15] Rao et al., retrospectively analyzed data from 593,094 procedures in the National Cardiovascular Data Registry (606 sites; 2004 to 2007).[12] They evaluated trends in use and outcomes of TRA for PCI. TRA was associated with a procedural success rate similar to TFA, and with significantly lower rates of bleeding and vascular complications, even amongst high-risk groups including elderly patients, women, and patients with acute coronary syndrome (ACS). In the (Mortality benefit of Reduced Transfusion after PCI via the Arm or Leg) MORTAL study reported on reductions in mortality, likely mediated through reduced transfusions after PCIs performed through TRA when compared with TFA.[11] This study evaluated 38,872 PCI procedures in 32,822 patients in British Columbia and Canada. TFA was used in 79.5% of PCIs and TRA in 20.5%. In the TFA group, 2.8% of procedures were associated with the need for periprocedural transfusions, while in the TRA group and only 1.4% of the procedures required a transfusion. Thus, the transfusion rate was associated with a significant reduction in mortality at 1 month and 1 year. The death rates at 1 month of the transfused group versus the non-transfused group were 12.6% and 1.3%, respectively. At the end of 1 year, the death rates were 22.9% and 3.2%. In Radial verus Femoral access for coronary intervention (RIVAL) study,[17] out of 7,021 patients with ACS from 158 hospitals in 32 countries, 3,507 patients were randomly assigned in TRA group and 3,514 to TFA group.[7] Although, the study concluded that both TRA and TFA are safe and effective for PCI, the local vascular complication rate was significantly lower in TRA group (n = 42 for TRA group versus n = 106 for TFA group, $p < 0.001$). Investigators also observed statistically significant (40%) relative reduction in the risk of death, myocardial infarction (MI), stroke or non-coronary artery bypass graft (CABG)-related major bleeding and a significant (61%) relative reduction in the risk of death among STEMI patients treated via radial route. They also showed a significant reduction in the risk of the primary outcome (51%) amongst PCI centers that performed the highest volume of radial procedures. RIFLE-STEACS (Radial versus Femoral Randomized Investigation in ST-segment Elevation Acute Coronary Syndrome) was a prospective randomized parallel group multicenter study for evaluation of TRA versus TFA for primary PCI.[8] A total of 1,001 patients were randomized between these two groups. The investigators found that at 1 month, the rate of net adverse clinical events (NACE) was significantly lower in the radial group versus the femoral group (13.6% vs. 21%). This difference was determined by a reduction of both the major adverse cardiac and cerebrovascular events (7.2% vs. 11.4%) and of bleeding (7.8% vs. 12.2%). In particular, the rate of cardiac death at 1 month was 9.2% in the femoral group and 5.2% in the radial group.

Radiation Exposure and Transradial Approach

Increased operator radiation exposure with TRA has been a concern. This results primarily from a more proximity to the radiation source.[4,5] Medial positioning of the arm following access and attention to radiation shielding helps to mitigate this concern. Radiation exposure decreases as the operator experience increases. Absolute increase in fluoroscopy time and dose area product (DAP) with TRA compared to TFA is small, likely representing minimal risk to the patient (0.002% increase in lifetime cancer risk), and must be balanced against the significant benefits of decreased access site complications and bleeding.[4,5] The REVERE (Randomized Evaluation of Vascular Entry Site and Radiation Exposure) study randomized patients to TFA, right TRA and left TRA in 1:1:1 fashion, and has shown patient's exposure being similar for all groups.[18] Similarly, the FERARI study showed that the mean fluoroscopy time, median DAP, procedural duration and the amount of contrast agent used were not significantly different in TRA versus TFA groups.[19]

Transradial Approach: Quality of Life and Economic Benefits

Early ambulation provides potential cost reduction through various avenues, including expedited room turnover or increased throughput (both through cath lab and recovery unit); reduced intensity of care required by nursing and support staff; shorter length of stay; enhanced ability to perform same day PCI; and a more rapid return to productivity for working patients.[4-6,20-22] Large groin hematoma and retroperitoneal hematoma can lead to need for several additional investigations, (i.e., femoral vascular ultrasound, computed tomography (CT) of abdomen or pelvis and lab investigations), blood transfusions and longer hospital stay.[4-6] This additional cost of treating the complications and prolonged hospital stay can be reduced using TRA. Cooper et al., compared quality of life parameters of patients undergoing TFA and TRA.[20] Of patients, who have had both TFA and TRA, 80% had strong preference for TRA, 18% were undecided and only 2% had strong preference for TFA. Amoroso et al., quantified the workload for both cath lab and recovery area nurses following 260 consecutive TRI (n = 208) and transfemoral intervention (TFI) (n = 52) procedures. The workload was significantly reduced for TRI procedures (TRI = 86 min vs. TFI = 174 min, $p < 0.001$) and for TRI recovery time (TRI = 386 min vs. TFI = 720 min).[21] The workload and time savings were related to less time spent for sheath removal, early patient mobility, shorter recovery time and shorter time to ambulation. It is also rational to expect that those patients experiencing access site complications, significantly more frequent with TFA, would be delayed in returning to work by an extended recovery. Although early ambulation is possible with use of femoral vascular closure devices, there is no reduction in bleeding and vascular complication rates and approximately 5 times the closure cost of a radial hemostasis device.[4-6] So, improved quality of life for the patients, relatively shorter and relaxed periprocedural care for the nursing and supportive staff and significant cost savings for the hospital management are good reasons to use TRA.

CONCLUSION

In a nutshell, everyday practice is now driven by "evidence-based medicine" instead of "personal experience" or "anecdotal" medicine. International guidelines are regularly published and periodically updated to provide busy professionals guidance on how their practice should evolve over the time. As the superiority of TRA over TFA is well documented, it is high time to change the mindset.

REFERENCES

1. Kiemeneij F, Laarman GJ, Odekerken D, et al. A randomized comparison of percutaneous transluminal coronary angioplasty by the radial, brachial and femoral approaches: the access study. J Am Coll Cardiol. 1997;29(6):1269-75.
2. Bertrand OF, Rao SV, Pancholy S, et al. Transradial approach for coronary angiography and interventions: Results of the first international transradial practice survey. JACC Cardiovasc Interv. 2010;3(10):1022-31.
3. Feldman DN, Swaminathan RV, Kaltenbach LA, et al. Adoption of radial access and comparison of outcomes to femoral access in percutaneous coronary intervention: An updated report from the national cardiovascular data registry (2007-2012). Circulation. 2013;127(23):2295-306.
4. Caputo RP, Tremmel JA, Rao S, et al. Transradial arterial access for coronary and peripheral procedures: Executive summary by the Transradial Committee of the SCAI. Catheter Cardiovasc Interv. 2011;78(6):823-39.
5. Rao S, Tremmel J, Gilchrist I, et al. Best Practices for Transradial Angiography and Intervention: A Consensus Statement From the Society for Cardiovascular Angiography and Intervention's Transradial Working Group. Catheter Cardiovasc Interv. 2014;83(2):228-36.
6. Hamon M, Pristipino C, Di Mario C, et al. Consensus document on the radial approach in percutaneous cardiovascular interventions: Position paper by the European Association of Percutaneous Cardiovascular Interventions and Working Groups on Acute Cardiac Care and Thrombosis of the European Society of Cardiology. EuroIntervention. 2013;8(11):1242-51.
7. Mehta SR, Jolly SS, Cairns J, et al. Effects of radial versus femoral artery access in patients with acute coronary syndromes with or without ST-segment elevation. J Am Coll Cardiol. 2012;60(24):2490-9.
8. Romagnoli E, Biondi-Zoccai G, Sciahbasi A, et al. Radial versus femoral randomized investigation in ST-segment elevation acute coronary syndrome: the RIFLE-STEACS (Radial Versus Femoral Randomized Investigation in ST-Elevation Acute Coronary Syndrome) study. J Am Coll Cardiol. 2012;60(24):2481-9.
9. Bernat I, Horak D, Stasek J, et al. ST-segment elevation myocardial infarction treated by radial or femoral approach in a multicenter randomized clinical trial: the STEMI-RADIAL trial. J Am Coll Cardiol. 2014;63(10):964-72.
10. Valgimigli M, Gagnor A, Calabró P, et al. Radial versus femoral access in patients with acute coronary syndromes undergoing invasive management: a randomized multicenter trial. Lancet. 2015;385(9986):2465-76.
11. Ferrante G, Rao SV, Jüni P, et al. Radial Versus Femoral Access for Coronary Interventions Across the Entire Spectrum of Patients With Coronary Artery Disease: A Meta-Analysis of Randomized Trials. JACC Cardiovasc Interv. 2016;9(14):1419-34.
12. Rao SV, Ou FS, Wang TY, et al. Trends in the prevalence and outcomes of radial and femoral approaches to percutaneous coronary intervention: a report from the national cardiovascular data registry. JACC Cardiovasc Interv. 2008;1(4):379-86.
13. Yatskar L, Selzer F, Feit F, et al. Access site hematoma requiring blood transfusion predicts mortality in patients undergoing percutaneous coronary intervention: Data from the National Heart, Lung and Blood Institute Dynamic Registry. Catheter Cardiovasc Interv. 2007;69(7):961-6.
14. Manoukian SV, Feit F, Mehran R, et al. Impact of major bleeding on 30-day mortality and clinical outcomes in patients with acute coronary syndromes, an analysis from the ACUITY Trial. J Am Coll Cardiol. 2007;49(12):1362-8.
15. Chase AJ, Fretz EB, Warbutton WP, et al. Association of the arterial access site at angioplasty with transfusion and mortality, the M.O.R.T.A.L. study (Mortality benefit Of Reduced Transfusion after percutaneous coronary intervention via the Arm or Leg). Heart. 2008;94(8):1019-25.

16. Gili S, D'Ascenzo F, Di Summa R, et al. Radial versus Femoral Access for the Treatment of Left Main Lesion in the Era of Second-Generation Drug Eluting Stents. Am J Cardiol. 2017;120(1):33-9.
17. Tanaka Y, Moriyama N, Ochiai T, et al. Transradial coronary interventions for complex chronic total occlusions. J Am Coll Cardiol Intv. 2017;10(3):235-43.
18. Pancholy SB, Joshi P, Shah S, et al. Effect of vascular access site choice on radiation exposure during coronary angiography: The REVERE Trial (randomized evaluation of vascular entry site and radiation exposure). JACC Cardivasc Interv. 2015;8(9):1189-96.
19. Bechera T, Behnesa M, Unsala M, et al. Radiation exposure and contrast agent use related to radial versus femoral arterial access during percutaneous coronary intervention (PCI)—results of the FERARI study. Cardiovasc Revasc Med. 2016;17:505-50.
20. Cooper CJ. El-Shiekh RA, Cohen DJ, et al. Effect of transradial access on quality of life and cost of cardiac catheterization: A randomized comparison. Am Heart J. 1999;138(3 Pt 1):430-6.
21. Amoroso G, Sarti M, Bellucci R, et al. Clinical and procedural predictors of nurse workload during and after invasive coronary procedures: The potential benefit of a systematic radial access. Eur J Cardiovasc Nurs. 2005;4(3):234-41.
22. Bradley SM, Rao SV, Curtis JP, et al. Change in hospital-level use of transradial percutaneous coronary intervention and periprocedural outcomes: insights from the national cardiovascular data registry. Circ Cardiovasc Qual Outcomes. 2014;7(4):550-9.

CHAPTER 64

Contemporary Coronary Stents: Implications for My Practice

Neha Maddali, Kevin Marzo, Ramesh Daggubati

INTRODUCTION

Since Andreas Gruentzig's invention of the first balloon angioplasty in 1977,[1] percutaneous coronary intervention (PCI) has become one of the most commonly performed therapeutic procedures in the United States and around the world.[2] Preliminary attempts to utilize balloon angioplasty were restricted by the occurrence of restenosis in approximately 30–50% of patients[2] and enormously high rates of sudden vessel closure, dissection, and arterial recoil. These limitations prompted the innovation of the bare-metal stent (BMS) in the mid 1980s as a framework for vessels with the objective of maintaining luminal integrity.[2] In 1986, Ulrich Sigwart, and Jacques Puel initiated the second revolution in interventional cardiology with the first implantation of a self-expanding Wallstent in human coronary arteries (Fig. 1).[3] Julio Palmaz and Richard Schatz manufactured the widely used Food and Drug Administration (FDA) approved stent in the USA in 1994 (Fig. 2). The Palmaz-Schatz (Johnson and Johnson) is a balloon expandable slotted tube stent design that was well studied and most used in 1990s.[4] Around the same time, Cesare Gianturco and Gary Roubin developed a balloon expandable coil stent with wrapped stainless steel which was FDA approved in 1993 for acute vessel closure as a bail out therapy (Fig. 3).[2]

However, since its creation and first implantation, although BMS has been shown to reduce clinical and angiographic restenosis by 20–30%,[5] vessel response to stent-mediated injury and endothelial cell denudation induces neointimal hyperplasia.[6,7] This proliferation and migration of vascular muscle cells ultimately results in vessel shrinkage,

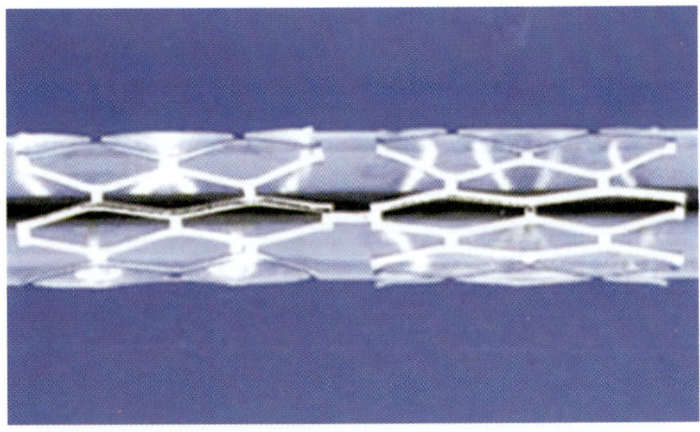

FIG. 2: The Palmaz-Schatz stent.

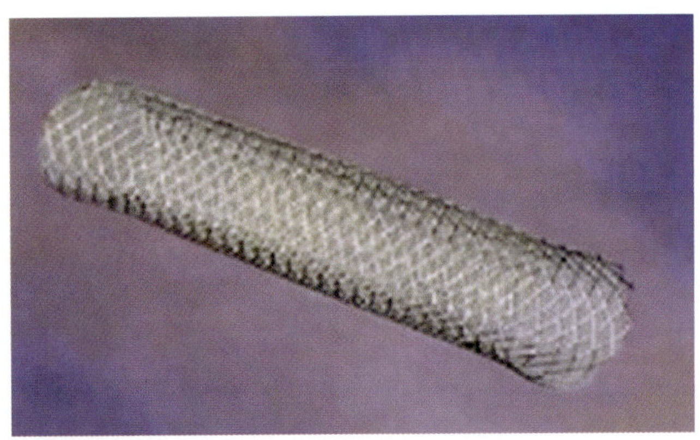

FIG. 1: The Wallstent, this was the first self-expanding stent ever used in humans.

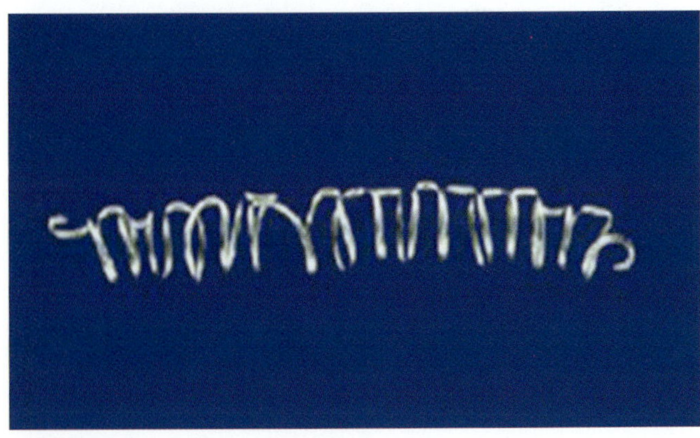

FIG. 3: The Gianturco-Roubin stent.

decreased arterial lumen space, and a necessity for revascularization.[2]

Hence, the first generation drug-eluting stent (DES) was designed to minimalize the prospect of in-stent restenosis (ISR). The DES consists of a BMS structure coated in a polymer and controlled release antiproliferative drugs. The drugs, i.e., paclitaxel and zotarolimus, disrupt the central molecular processes linked to ISR.

In comparison to BMSs, first-generation and improved second-generation DESs demonstrate the declining need for revascularization. This usage parallels itself in clinical medicine, in 2006, approximately 76% of all stents inserted in patients were DESs,[8] and in the United States, DESs are now implanted in over 500,000 patients annually.[9] Yet although practitioners are cognizant of its potential benefits in treating coronary disease, the New England Journal of Medicine issued evidence of an increased risk in stent thrombosis (ST), in addition to comparable risks of myocardial infarction (MI) and death to BMSs, after insertion of DESs releasing sirolimus and paclitaxel. This report, along with other papers displayed at the European Society of Cardiology Congress in 2006, questioned the stent's clinical efficacy and long-term safety.[10] Since the report's publication, substantial improvements have been made to DES technology to increase public safety; these new developments, particularly ultra-thin DESs, promote its revitalization in the clinical field. The ultra-thin DESs have thinner struts and new biocompatible polymers with the objective of diminishing vascular damage. This chapter focuses on the improved design, safety, and efficiency of the next generation ultra-thin DES and bioresorbable stent systems against first generation DESs and its implications for prospective clinical practice.

DESIGN

The stent platform is comprised of three significant components: (1) metallic stent, (2) antiproliferative drug, and (3) polymer coating for steady drug release (Fig. 4).[5] There are three basic stent designs which are coil, tubular mesh, and slotted tube stents.

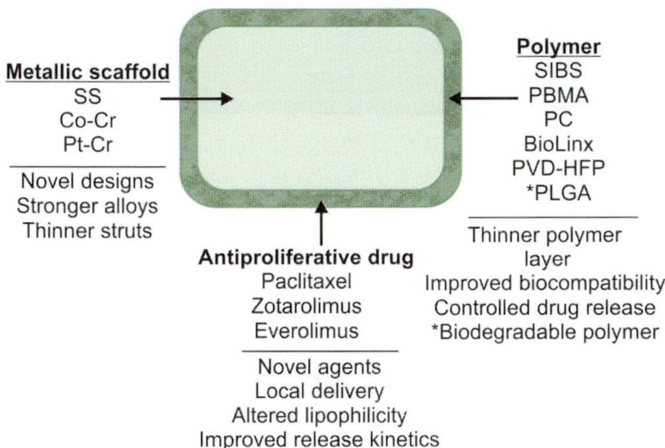

PBMA, poly(n-butyl methacrylate); PC, phosphorylcholine; PLGA, poly(lactic-co-glycolic acid); PVD-HFP, poly(vinylidene fluoride-co-hexafluoropropylene); SIBS, poly(styrene-b-isobutylene-b-styrene; Co-Cr, cobalt-chromium; Pt-Cr, platinum-chromium.

FIG. 4: Cross-section of drug-eluting stent platform.

Metallic Stent Scaffold

Drug-eluting stent metallic platforms must possess a low-crimped profile and elevated flexibility to withstand transportation from the femoral or radial arteries to throughout the vigorous cardiovascular system. Furthermore, the platform should retain high radial strength to maintain a constant vessel diameter and homogeneously distribute the drug throughout the stent to the surrounding vessel. To ensure these prerequisites, scholars utilized biologically inert metals with high radial strength. First-generation DESs were primarily composed of stainless steel and had a large stent strut thickness of 135 μm.[11] However, due to incipient parallels between strut thickness and ISR rates, metallic alloys such as cobalt-chromium and platinum-chromium have antiquated steel stents. These alloys contribute to the slenderness of second generation DESs, while maintaining corrosion resistance and simultaneously increasing yield strength, radiopacity, and flexibility. In addition to material substance, geometric configuration is vital to determining stent thickness. Scaffolds with fewer hoop connectors sanction vessel conformability and increased elasticity, reducing the risk of restenosis, arterial injury, and thrombogenicity after implantation.[2] Table 1 portrays FDA approved DES and their relative metals and thicknesses.[2,5]

Antiproliferative Drug

A drug-eluting stent implantation can often induce mechanical injury to the proximate vessel. This injury activates an automatic healing reaction: platelet stimulation, thrombus formation, and monocyte and neutrophil collection all occur at the implantation site.[7] As smooth muscle cells activate, proliferate, and migrate to the stent, the responses eventually lead to neointimal hyperplasia and ISR. Thus, to combat neointimal growth but maintain vascular healing, antiproliferative or antirestenosis drugs are embedded within the stent polymer to reduce restenosis and ISR rates. The main antiproliferative drugs in clinical use include paclitaxel, sirolimus, zotarolimus, everolimus, and ridaforolimus.[5] Paclitaxel and sirolimus were particularly utilized in first-generation DESs. Paclitaxel stabilizes microtubules and averts smooth muscle cell proliferation by halting the cell cycle in the G0-G1 and G2-M phase. Sirolimus binds to the cytosolic FK binding protein 12 (FKBP12) to interrupt and suspend the cell cycle in the G1-S phase.[7] This disrupts the cytostatic proliferation of vascular smooth muscle cells.[12] Both zotarolimus, the first treatment created for ISR, and everolimus, which are used in second generation DESs, are analogs of sirolimus.

Polymer Coating

Polymer coatings that encase the abluminal surface of the metallic stent function as drug carriers by enabling controlled and confined drug release. When the coatings amalgamate with antiproliferative or antirestenotic drugs, a drug-polymer matrix forms and diffuses. The diffusion rate is dependent on the material, structure, and quantity of polymers utilized in the drug-polymer matrix.

TABLE 1: Drug-eluting stents approved by the Food and Drug Administration

Variable	Paclitaxel-eluting stents		Sirolimus-eluting stent	Everolimus-eluting stents			Zotarolimus-eluting stents	
	Type 1	Type 2		Type 1	Type 2	Type 3	Type 1	Type 2
Commercial name	Taxus Express	Taxus Liberté	Cypher	Xience	Promus	Promus Element	Endeavor	Resolute Integrity, Onyx
Manufacturer	Boston Scientific	Boston Scientific	Cordis, Johnson and Johnson	Abbott Vascular	Boston Scientific	Boston Scientific	Medtronic	Medtronic
Scaffold material	Stainless steel	Stainless steel	Stainless steel	Cobalt-chrome	Cobalt-chrome	Platinum-chrome	Cobalt-chrome	Cobalt-chrome
Strut thickness (μm)	132	97	140	81	81	81	91	91

First Generation			Newer second Generation			Third Gen
Cypher™	TAXUS Express™	TAXUS Liberte™	Resolute Onyx™	Xience Sierra™	PROMUS Premier™	SYNERGY™
Drug type						
Sirolimus	Paclitaxel	Paclitaxel	Zotarolimus	Everolimus	Everolimus	Everolimus
Drug concentration						
1.4 μg/mm²	1 μg/mm²	1 μg/mm²	1.6 μg/mm²	1 μg/mm²	1 μg/mm²	~1 μg/mm²
Average coating thickness						
7 μm/side	16 μm/side	14 μm/side	6 μm/side	8 μm/side	8 μm/side	4 μm
Strut thickness						
140 μm (0.0055")	132 μm (0.0052")	96 μm (0.0038")	81 μm (0.0035")	81 μm (0.0032")	81 μm (0.0032")	74 μm (0.0029")
BMS platform						
Bx Velocity™	Express™	Liberte™	Integrity™	Vision™ and Multi Link 8™	Element™	SYNERGY™
Material						
Stainless steel	Stainless steel	Stainless steel	Cobalt platinum iridium	Cobalt chromium	Platinum chromium	Platinum chromium

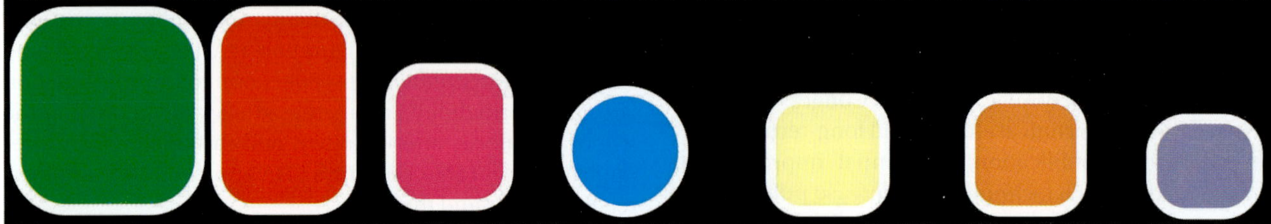

BMS, bare-metal stent.

FIG. 5: Strut profiles for contemporary stent platforms.

Currently, in first- and second-generation DESs, permanent synthetic polymer coats, i.e., poly(ethylene-co-vinyl acetate) (PEVA), poly(n-butyl methacrylate) (PBMA), and tri-block copolymer, poly(styrene-b-isobutylene-b-styrene) (SIBS), have proven most efficacious in local drug delivery from the stent to the surrounding vessel.[7] However, clinical evidence correlates permanent DES polymer coats to probable hypersensitivity, late ST, and insufficient reendothelialization. These critical issues led to the development of highly biocompatible permanent polymers such as phosphorylcholine (PC) and copolymer, poly(vinylidene fluoride-co-hexafluoropropylene) (PVDF-HFP) in ultra-thin DESs. The polymers imitate the phospholipids on erythrocyte surfaces; this action induces marginal thrombogenicity and lowers vessel injury.[7] Furthermore, the advanced polymers decrease complete strut thickness by reducing polymer thickness by 40–70%.[5] The new EluNIR Medinol stents have an elastic polymer coating.

Recent research has fixated on contemporary biodegradable polymers and their potential in reducing restenosis rates (Fig. 5). These polymers permit an even smaller effective strut thickness as the polymers resorb after a period of drug elution. The 74 µm SYNERGY bioabsorbable polymer (BP)-DES contains a platinum-chromium metallic stent and biodegradable poly(lactic-co-glycolic acid) (PGLA) polymer; demonstrated in the randomized EVOLVE (Evaluation of Cinacalcet Hydrochloride Therapy to Lower Cardiovascular Events) trials, the platform has exhibited clinical efficacy and safety.[7] At a 2-year review, patients with SYNERGY have not witnessed any augmentation in the 1.1% target lesion revascularization (TLR) and 0% ST rates from their 1st year examination.[13] Platforms such as SYNERGY have pioneered the development of ultra-thin struts and have sparked early clinical research to develop even thinner and more effective struts by replacing the polymer coating with "microfabricated and nanofabricated reservoirs" on the metallic scaffold.[14]

IMPLICATIONS ON CLINICAL PRACTICE

As technology has evolved, it has become more and more difficult to show superiority between stents of the same generation. In the next few segments, we will highlight on few features that may help one choose a particular type of stent.

Significance of Strut Thickness in Drug-eluting Stents

Stent strut thickness is crucial to determining a platform's safety and clinical efficacy. Thinner stents have a plethora of advantages over antiquated BMSs and first- and second-generation DESs, including a reduced risk of side branch occlusion, simplicity in tracking the stent inside the vessel, and improved flexibility.[15] Strut fractures were more common with the first-generation DES.

In a trial investigating the correlation between ST and *ex vivo* flow loop stent design, results indicated thick-strut stents of 162 µm were 1.5-fold more thrombogenic than thinner stents of 81 µm with an identical composition, structure, polymer coating, and antiproliferative drug (Fig. 6).[7] Additionally, after a 3 days of implantation in porcine coronary arteries, thick struts indicated an 60% increase in thrombosis and an overall accumulation in fibrin deposition than thin struts.[16]

A thinner strut thickness moreover accelerates stent endothelialization than its thinner counterparts. Due to a smaller area, the thinner stent does not require as much neo-intimal tissue coverage. In a preclinical study examining strut thickness effect on strut tissue coverage in rabbit models,

		Durable polymer coated		Biosorbable polymer coated					
	EluNIR Modinol	Xience CoCr EES	Resolute Onyx	Biomatrix	Nobori	SYNERGY	BioMime	MiStent	Orsiro
	CoCr-RES	Promus PtCr-EES	CoPi-ZES	316L-BES	316L-BES	PtCr-EES	CoCr-SES	CoCr-SES	CoCr-SES
Strut thickness	74 µm 0.0029"	81 µm 0.0032"	81 µm 0.0032"	120 µm 0.0046"	125 µm 0.0047"	74 µm 0.0029"	65 µm 0.0026"	64 µm 0.0025"	61 µm 0.0025"
Polymer	Elasto-meric	PVDF	BioLinx	PLA	PLA	PLGA	PLLA + PLGA	PLGA	PLLA Probio
Distribution/ thickness	Conformal 6 µm/side	Conformal 7–8 µm/side	Conformal 6 µm/side	Abluminal 10 µm	Abluminal 20 µm	Abluminal 4 µm	Conformal 2 µ/2 µ	Conformal 5 µm/side	Conformal 3.5 µm/side

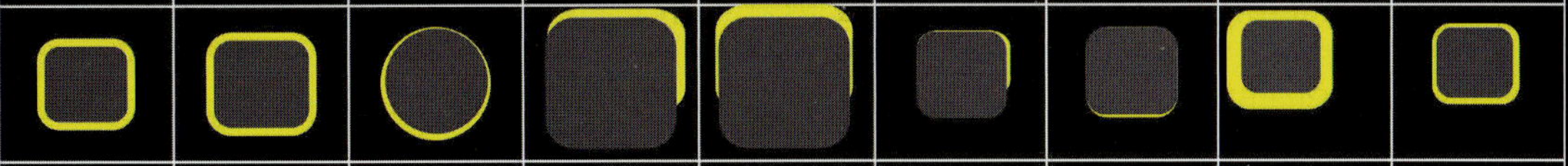

BES, biolimus-eluting stent; DES: drug-eluting stent; EES, everolimus-eluting stent; PLA, polylactic acid; PLGA, poly(lactic-co-glycolic acid); PLLA, poly(L-lactide); PVDF, poly(vinylidene fluoride); RES, ridaforolimus-eluting stent; SES, sirolimus-eluting stent; ZES, zotarolimus-eluting stent.

FIG. 6: Strut and coating thickness in new stent platforms.

after a 14-day period, strut tissue coverage was highest (95%) in thinner struts (81 μm) in comparison to the 97 μm (88%) and 132 μm (77%) thicker struts. The study concluded strut thickness modulated blood flow. Thus, as a result, stagnation and recirculation are more probable to transpire in thicker struts.[17]

Furthermore, clinical evidence suggests strut thickness determines the efficacy review of certain coronary devices. For instance, in the ISAR-STEREO (Intracoronary Stenting and Angiographic Results: Strut Thickness Effect on Restenosis Outcome) trial, a thin-strut of 50 μm displayed over a 10% reduction of binary restenosis (BR) at a 6-month angiogram follow-up from a 140 μm thick strut BMS. Therefore, the reduction of BR lead to a decrease (13.8–8.6%; $p = 0.03$) in repeat intervention and revascularization at the target vessel.[18] Results indicate that thicker struts trigger greater on-site coronary inflammation, vessel damage, and disturb the internal elastic lamina than thinner-strut platforms. The resulting inflammation induces in-stent neointimal hyperplasia, ultimately promoting restenosis.[15]

Clinical Efficacy of Biodegradable and Bioresorbable Drug-eluting Stents

Although once thought to be effective and promising, recent research has questioned biodegradable and bioresorbable DES clinical efficacy. Many of the stents, specifically the Abbott Vascular Absorb Bioresorbable Vascular Scaffold (BVS) system, have been recalled in response to meta-analyses from recent studies.[19] The ABSORB III trial 2 years results were presented at the American College of Cardiology assembly in 2017 and dampened hope for bioresorbable stents use in the future. In the ABSORB trials, the rate of ischemia-driven TLR (ID-TLR) and target vessel MI was higher with BVSs in comparison to DESs.[20] In addition, Absorb BVS had slightly higher rates of target lesion failure (TLF), scarce cases of late ST, and a generally greater percentage of poor outcomes compared to Xience, a DES. However, although the technology has had several impediments, companies are still optimistically insisting to improve the BVS platforms to eventually improve patient outcomes.

Clinical Efficacy of Ultra-thin Drug-eluting Stents

Since the release of ultra-thin strut DESs, only few clinical trials have been performed for three ultra-thin strut stents. The stents include the BioMime sirolimus-eluting stent (SES) (65 μm strut thickness), the MiStent SES (64 μm strut thickness), and the Orsiro SES (60 μm strut thickness). One such study, the BIOTRONIK (A Prospective Randomized Multicenter Study to Assess the Safety and Effectiveness of the Orsiro Sirolimus Eluting Coronary Stent System in the Treatment of Subjects with up to Three *De Novo* or Restenotic Coronary Artery Lesions), or the BIOFLOW V trial, has showcased the ultra-thin DES's superiority to fluropolyer-based everolimus-eluting stent (EES) and potential safety. In the trial, both the Orsiro SES and the Xience EES were evaluated. Results indicated that the Orsiro SES was more effective in reducing TLF and were inferior to fluoropolymer EESs.[21]

Additionally, the Merit V trial indicated a lower risk of MI in the BioMime SES in comparison to the Xience EES (0.6% vs. 4.8%; $p = 0.03$). While the results do not precisely determine an explanation for the lower MI rate in ultra-thin DESs, the rates are feasibly accredited to the reduced rate of ST due to a reduction in stent strut thickness.

DRUG-ELUTING STENT SAFETY AND EFFICACY IN SPECIFIC PATIENT POPULATIONS

Acute Myocardial Infarction

Drug-eluting stent implantation is a very common therapeutic procedure in acute coronary syndromes.[5] Acute coronary syndrome can initiate future stent malapposition and potential delayed arterial vessel healing. Thus, many patients with these syndromes are denied potentially helpful clinical treatment. However, new DES platforms, such as ultra-thin struts, have been found to be safe and effective in patients suffering from this disease. The EXAMINATION trial revealed patients with ST-elevation MI (STEMI) had lower rates of TLR in EES to BMS.[5]

Chronic Kidney Disease

Chronic kidney disease (CKD) is a common comorbidity with many cardiovascular diseases, and in conjunction, CKD can increase mortality and morbidity rates. Additionally, after BMS or first-generation DES implantation, CKD is concomitant with restenosis and ST. Unlike previous DES, second- and current-generation DES have showed a high-efficacious rate among clinical trials in patients with CKD.[5,22]

Diabetes Mellitus

Patients with diabetes mellitus (DM) are at an extremely high risk for restenosis, MI, repeat revascularization, and mortality after stent implantation.[23] Previous research has approximated DES and BMS platforms to be equally as successful if dual antiplatelet therapy (DAPT) is used for a minimum of 6 months. However, in certain aspects, DESs have proven to be superior in lowering restenosis rates in diabetics. A 42-trial mixed treatment comparison meta-analysis concluded that DES were noninferior to BMS and additionally decreased TVR rates in DES platforms.[24] Although DESs are more commonly utilized, the preeminent DES platform for diabetic treatment remains uncertain. In an effort to specialize a DES for diabetic patients, the Medtronic stent resolute zotarolimus-eluting stent was manufactured, becoming the first FDA approved stent for patients with DM.[25,26]

High-bleeding Risk Patients

The SYNERGY bioabsorbable polymer everolimus DES is commonly used in patients with high-bleeding risk presumably due to the need of shorter DAPT duration in such patients. However, similar results were seen with durable

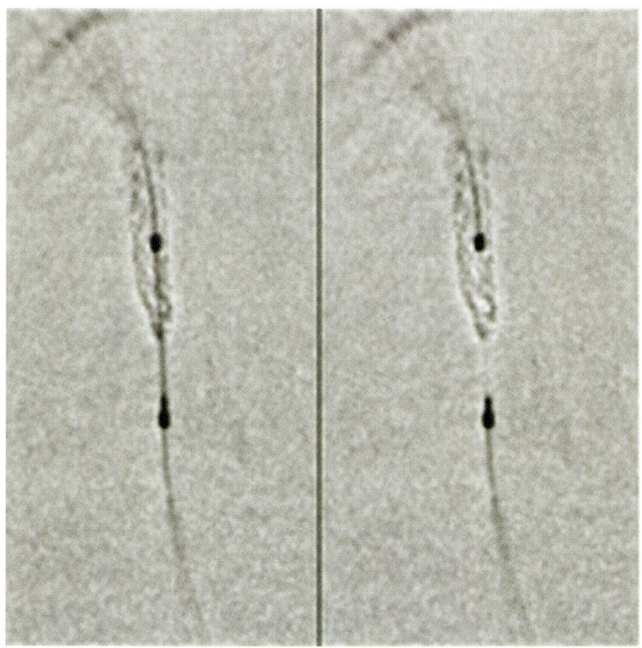

FIG. 7: Incidence of longitudinal deformation in vessel after stent implantation.

polymer thin or ultrathin stents in smaller clinical trials. US FDA has not made any recommendations to shorten the DAPT with any currently approved stents though guidelines recommend to shorten DAPT in low ischemic risk and high-bleeding risk patients.

Bioresorbable Vascular Scaffolds

Though currently BVS are not used except in clinical trials, one has to marvel at the idea of nonmetallic scaffold. Strut thickness of the first-generation BVS was larger than the first-generation DES. Second-generation BVS with 100–125 μm strut thickness are being evaluated in large clinical trials by Meril Lifesciences and REVA Medical.[27,28]

Safety Outcomes and Complications of Newer DES: Longitudinal Deformation

Although there are many strengths to DES, it is equally as important to discuss the stents' weaknesses in clinical practice and trial. Some modifications introduced in novel stent platforms may result in a reduction in their longitudinal strength as a derivative of attempting to increase flexibility (Fig. 7).[29] Longitudinal stent deformation is outlined as the reduction of a platform in the longitudinal axis after a successful stent implantation.[5] This deformation can lead to the protrusion of struts into the vessel lumen. This malposition may eventually result in disruption of blood flow and increased ST.[30] Longitudinal stent deformation occurs in 0.1–1.0% of total DES platform insertions. The rates of stent deformation are lower in older generation stiffer DES struts.[5] Recent research is concentrated on stents focused on specific lesions to avoid longitudinal compression.

CONCLUSION

Drug-eluting stents were developed to reduce the risk of ISR seen with BMS. Concerns for high-risk of late and very late adverse events seen with first-generation DESs have significantly decreased with the use of contemporary platforms, owing to advances in technology including scaffold design, novel metallic alloys leading to thinner struts, polymer biocompatibility, and antiproliferative drug development and delivery. Several randomized controlled trials and meta-analyses, have consistently shown the efficacy and safety of contemporary DES platforms in both short-term and long-term follow-up. Given their proven efficacy and safety profile, the use of contemporary DESs has become standard in most clinical scenarios, including high-risk settings such as CKD, acute MI, and diabetic population.

REFERENCES

1. Barton M, Grüntzig J, Husmann M, et al. Balloon angioplasty–the legacy of Andreas Grüntzig, M.D. (1939–1985). Front Cardiovasc Med. 2014;1:15.
2. Stefanini GG, Holmes DR Jr. Drug-eluting coronary-artery stents. N Eng J Med. 2013;368(3):254-65.
3. Iqbal J, Gunn J, Serruys PW. Coronary stents: historical development, current status and future directions. Br Med Bull. 2013;106:193-211.
4. Serruys PW, Emanuelsson H, van der Giessen W, et al. Heparin-coated Palmaz-Schatz stents in human coronary arteries: Early outcome of the Benestent-II Pilot Study. Circulation. 1996;93(3):412-22.
5. Partida RA, Yeh RW. Contemporary drug-eluting stent platforms: design, safety, and clinical efficacy. Cardiol Clin. 2017,35(2).281-90.
6. Van der Heiden K, Gijsen FJ, Narracott A, et al. The effects of stenting on shear stress: relevance to endothelial injury and repair. Cardiovasc Res. 2013;99(2):269-75.
7. Martin DM, Boyle FJ. Drug-eluting stents for coronary artery disease: a review. Med Eng Phys. 2011;33(2):148-63.
8. US Food and Drug Administration. Circulatory System Devices Panel. Washington, DC: Meeting minutes; 2006.
9. Roger VL, Go AS, Lloyd-Jones DM, et al. Heart disease and stroke statistics—2012 update: a report from the American Heart Association. Circulation. 2012;125(1):e2-220.
10. Lagerqvist B, James SK, Stenestrand U, et al. Long-term outcomes with drug-eluting stents versus bare-metal stents in Sweden. N Eng J Med. 2007;356(10):1009-19.
11. Ho MY, Chen CC, Wang CY, et al. The development of coronary artery stents: from bare-metal to bio-resorbable types. Metals. 2016;6(7):168.
12. Serruys P, Gershlick AH. Handbook of Drug-Eluting Stents. United Kingdom: Taylor & Francis; 2005.
13. Boston Scientific. (2013). Boston Scientific Promus PREMIER™ and SYNERGY™ Drug-Eluting Stent Systems Provide Exceptional Safety and Efficacy Data. [online] Available from: http://news.bostonscientific.com/2013-05-22-Boston-Scientific-Promus-PREMIER-And-SYNERGY-Drug-Eluting-Stent-Systems-Provide-Exceptional-Safety-And-Efficacy-Data.
14. Huang Y, Ng HC, Ng WX, et al. Drug-eluting biostable and erodible stents. J Control Release. 2014;193:188-201.
15. Piccolo R, Thomas P. Cardiac Interventions Today - The Impact of Thin-Strut, Biodegradable Polymer Stent Designs. Available from: https://citoday.com/2017/02/the-impact-of-thin-strut-biodegradable-polymer-stent-designs?center=18.
16. Kolandaivelu K, Swaminathan R, Gibson WJ, et al. Stent thrombogenicity early in high-risk interventional settings is driven by stent design and deployment and protected by polymer-drug coatings. Circulation. 2011;123:1400-9.
17. Soucy NV, Feygin JM, Tunstall R, et al. Strut tissue coverage and endothelial cell coverage: a comparison between bare metal stent platforms and platinum

chromium stents with and without everolimus-eluting coating. EuroIntervention. 2010;6(5):6307.
18. Kastrati A, Mehilli J, Dirschinger J, et al. Intracoronary stenting and angiographic results: strut thickness effect on restenosis outcome (ISAR-STEREO) trial. Circulation. 2001;103(23):2816-21.
19. Australian Government Department of Health Therapeutic Goods Administration. (2017). Absorb Bioresorbable Vascular Scaffold System. [online] Available from https://www.tga.gov.au/alert/absorb-bioresorbable-vascular-scaffold-system [Accessed September 2018].
20. Pavasini R, Serenell M, Gallo F, et al. Effectiveness and safety of the ABSORB bioresorbable vascular scaffold for the treatment of coronary artery disease: systematic review and meta-analysis of randomized clinical trials. J Thorac Dis. 2017;9(Suppl 9):S887-97.
21. Bangalore S, Toklu B, Patel N, et al. Newer generation ultra-thin strut drug-eluting stents versus older second-generation thicker strut drug-eluting stents for coronary artery disease: a meta-analysis of randomized trials. Circulation. 2018.
22. Lee JM, Kang J, Lee E, et al. Chronic kidney disease in the second-generation drug-eluting stent era: pooled analysis of the Korean multicenter drug-eluting stent registry. JACC Cardiovasc Interv. 2016;9(20):2097-109.
23. Garg P, Normand SL, Silbaugh TS, et al. Drug-eluting or bare-metal stenting in patients with diabetes mellitus: results from the Massachusetts Data Analysis Center Registry. Circulation. 2008;118(22):2277-85.
24. Bangalore S, Kumar S, Fusaro M, et al. Outcomes with various drug-eluting or bare metal stents in patients with diabetes mellitus: mixed treatment comparison analysis of 22 844 patient years of follow-up from randomised trials. BMJ. 2012;345:e5170.
25. ICH GCP. (2015). Efficacy and Safety of RESOLUTE Zotarolimus-Eluting Stent in Treatment of Chinese Diabetic Coronary Lesions. [online] Available from https://ichgcp.net/clinical-trials-registry/NCT01747356 [Accessed September 2018].
26. Vardi M, Burke DA, Bangalore S, et al. Long-term efficacy and safety of Zotarolimus-eluting stent in patients with diabetes mellitus: pooled 5-year results from the ENDEAVOR III and IV Trials. Cathet Cardiovasc Interv. 2013;82(7):1031-8.
27. Nebeker JR, Virmani R, Bennett CL, et al. Hypersensitivity cases associated with drug-eluting coronary stents: a review of available cases from the research on adverse drug events and reports (RADAR) project. J Am Coll Cardiol. 2006;47(1):175-81.
28. Schwartz RS, Chronos NA, Virmani R. Preclinical restenosis models and drug-eluting stents: still important, still much to learn. J Am Coll Cardiol. 2004;44(7):1373-85.
29. Romaguera R, Roura G, Gomez-Lara J, et al. Longitudinal deformation of drug-eluting stents: evaluation by multislice computed tomography. J Invasive Cardiol. 2014;26(4):161-6.
30. Panoulas VF, Demir OM, Ruparelia N, et al. Longitudinal deformation of a third generation zotarolimus eluting stent: "The Concertina Returns!" World J Cardiol. 2017;9(1):60-4.

CHAPTER 65

Fractional Flow Reserve and Instantaneous Wave-free Ratio—Which Should Be the Gold Standard?

Nagendra Boopathy Senguttuvan, Nitish Naik, Kewal C Goswami

INTRODUCTION

Clinical improvement after percutaneous coronary intervention (PCI) is based on intervening on lesions that are hemodynamically significant. Assessing hemodynamic significance of coronary lesions, it is not a new entity for interventional community. Andreas Gruntzig did his first angioplasty after assessing the pressure gradient across the lesion in proximal left anterior descending artery (LAD).[1] Until a decade ago, angiography was considered the gold standard before any form of coronary intervention. However with its inherent limitations,[2] it often misses eccentric lesions especially in the ostium or in a highly tortuous anatomy or in a calcified spot. Physiological assessment of coronary stenosis has revealed that nearly one-third of intermediate severity lesions (diameter stenosis from 50% to 70%) are in fact functionally significant. About 20% of the lesions that have a diameter stenosis of 70–90% are not functionally significant. Imaging tools such as intravascular ultrasound (IVUS) and optical coherence topography (OCT) are being used since many years to assess the significance of lesions and to assess the result of PCI. However, both these techniques still serve only anatomical and morphological analysis of coronary lesions rather than their functional significance.

Different physiological modalities have been used to assess the significance of coronary lesions before interventions including coronary flow reserve (CFR), fractional flow reserve (FFR), and relative flow reserve (RFR). CFR is the ratio of maximal hyperemic blood flow to the baseline coronary blood flow. It is dynamic and hence is often affected by variables such as heart rate, blood pressure, and microvascular resistance. With increasing coronary stenosis, CFR is reduced though the baseline flow remains largely unchanged to a coronary stenosis severity of up to 90% or more. FFR is the ratio of maximal hyperemic blood flow in a coronary with a stenosis to the maximal hyperemic blood flow in the same vessel without a stenosis. Thus in an artery without any stenosis, FFR should be 1.0. The use of FFR to guide clinical management is now well established and its use have been proved in many trials.[3-6] Recently, even resting indices of coronary blood flow have been studied in patients with coronary artery disease (CAD) to assess the significance of lesions that include Pd/Pa (ratio of distal pressure to proximal pressure) and instantaneous wave-free ratio (iFR).[7] A lot of evidence has now accumulated comparing the efficacy of resting indices, especially iFR to FFR. In this review, we intend to discuss currently available evidence on FFR and iFR to help clinicians in identifying the modality that will be relevant in decision-making in clinical practice.

FRACTIONAL FLOW RESERVE

Fractional flow reserve was first described *in vivo* by Pijls et al.[3] in 1993. It is defined as the ratio of maximal flow in the coronary artery with stenosis to the maximal flow that happens in the same vessel in a hypothetical situation without stenosis. By following work of Gould[8] who proposed that coronary arterial circulation with lesion behaved as electrical circuit with a serial connections, Pijls proposed that flow was directly proportional to pressure given the resistance was kept stable and minimum using Ohm's law.[3] When resistance is constant, pressure is directly proportional to the flow.[3] FFR measures the flow across a lesion by quantifying the pressure across the lesion, when resistance is constant and at its lowest level. Coronary arterioles play the primary role in increasing the coronary circulation resistance. By achieving vasodilation of arterioles (maximal hyperemia), pressure measured across a lesion helps to assess the flow across lesions. Hence, it represents the amount of blood flow limitation attributable due to the presence of an epicardial stenosis. Hence, FFR can be defined as the ratio of distal pressure to the proximal pressure across a stenosis at maximal hyperemia (see Fig. 1).

$FFR = Pd–Pv/Pa–Pv$

where Pd is the distal pressure; Pa the proximal pressure (aortic pressure); Pv the coronary venous pressure

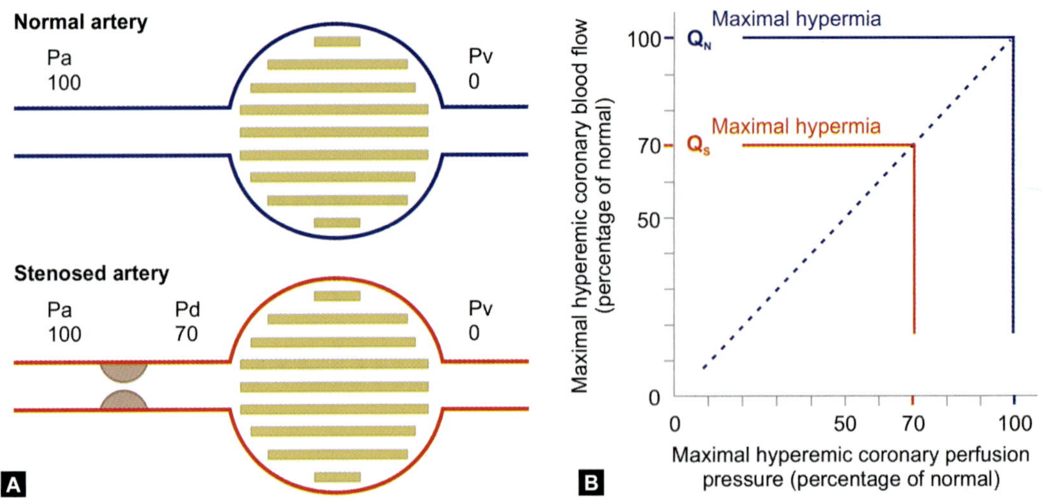

FIG. 1: **A,** Schematic representation of FFR physiology (Pa, aortic pressure; Pd, pressure distal to stenosis; Pv, central venous pressure); **B,** Linear relationship of coronary blood flow at maximal hyperemia to coronary pressure. Q_N and Qs are coronary blood flow during maximal hyperemia is normal and stenosed arteries respectively.

TABLE 1: Pharmacological agents used to achieve maximal hyperemia during FFR

Agent	Route	Dose	Peak effect	Duration
Adenosine	Intravenous	Infusion: 140 µg/kg/min	30–45 s	2 min infusion
	Intracoronary	LCA: 200 µg	<10 s	<20 s
		RCA: 100 µg		
Papaverine	Intracoronary	LCA: 16–20 µg	10–30 s	45–60 s
		RCA: 12–16 µg		
Regadenoson	Intravenous	400 µg bolus	30 s	2.5 min

LCA, left coronary artery; RCA, right coronary artery.

As coronary venous pressure is low, it can be removed from the equation making:

FFR = Pd/Pa

Maximal hyperemia is achieved by intracoronary nitroglycerine (NTG) along with intracoronary or intravenous (IV) adenosine.[9] Other agents such as papaverine, regadenoson, and sodium nitroprusside have also been used to produce maximal vasodilatation (Table 1). Initial studies recommended a value of ≤0.75 as definitely significant and values between 0.76 and 0.8 to be considered in the gray zone; however, current guidelines suggest that values ≤0.80 be considered as abnormal and values >0.80 be considered as insignificant.

ADVANTAGES OF FRACTIONAL FLOW RESERVE

Fractional flow reserve is easy to perform in the catheterization laboratory and easy to interpret with less intra- and interobserver variations. There are a number of companies that are now providing FFR commercially (Table 2). FFR accounts not only for the vessel stenosis but also for collateral flow and the size of the distal myocardial bed. It is independent of heart rate, blood pressure, and left ventricular (LV) function. However, care needs to be taken in performing FFR during maximal hyperemia and making sure that all precautions are taken to ensure accurate pressure measurements (Box 1). FFR values may be false negative if there is inadequate hyperemia due to inappropriate dose, damping from the guide catheter (preventing increase in blood flow), or in an acute coronary syndrome (ACS) due to microvascular dysfunction. These values may be false positive due to incorrect calibration or signal drift in the guide catheter or guidewire. Recently, it was postulated that FFR may vary in patients with arterial

TABLE 2: Available FFR technologies

Manufacturer	Name of product	Method	Advantages
Abbott St. Jude	Certus	Piezoelectric pressure wire	Wireless connection of wire with machine
	Aeris		Thermodilution blood flow measurement
Philips Volcano	Verrata	Piezoelectric pressure wire	FFR; iFR
			Doppler-tipped pressure and flowire
Boston Scientific	COMET	Optical sensor wire	Less likely to be affected by signal drift, better wire performance
Opsens Medical	OptoWire	Optical sensor wire	Less likely to be affected by signal drift, better wire performance
Acist Medical	Navvus	Optical sensor monorail microcatheter	Improved steerability;
			any guidewire may be used

FFR, fractional flow reserve; iFR, instantaneous wave-free ratio.

BOX 1 Steps of FFR

- Anticoagulation to achieve therapeutic levels as in PCI
- Place the wire flat and flush FFR wire in its delivery spiral package with 10–20 mL of saline
- Connect the FFR wire with the machine; in wireless systems, the wire will communicate with the machine
- Remove FFR wire and introduce into the guide catheter gently after making the standard tip-shaping technique on the wire as required for the lesion
- Advance the wire such that the junction of the radio-opaque and radiolucent region of the wire (where the pressure transducer is located) is just beyond the tip of the guiding catheter. Nitroglycerine can be administered to prevent coronary vasospasm
- Ensure that the guide catheter is properly hooked without damping or ventricularization. If there is an ostial lesion, then guide catheter should be unhooked and the radiopaque–radiolucent junction of wire should be in the aortic root
- Remove the introducer needle, flush the guide, and then equalize the readings of the pressure from the guide catheter and the pressure wire. Ensure there is no contrast in the guide to prevent spurious readings. The Y connector should be closed tightly to prevent leakage and fall in pressure. The Pd and Pa reading ratio should be 1.0. If the difference between the two pressures exceeds 15 mm Hg then FFR readings are not valid
- Ensure that the pressure transducers are at mid-chest level. If the transducers are positioned above the mid-chest level, then the pressure will be underestimated (pressure is too low). If the pressure transducer is located too high, then the pressure will be overestimated (pressure too high)
- Once equalized, the pressure wire should be advanced to beyond the lesion under evaluation such that the pressure transducer is beyond the lesion. The introducer may be reinserted if needed to facilitate smooth handling of the wire. However, after parking the wire beyond the lesion being tested, the introducer should be removed before making any measurements
- The wire should be positioned such that the pressure transducer is at least three vessel diameter lengths beyond the lesion to prevent overestimation just beyond the lesion due to turbulence
- Check FFR value once the wire is beyond the lesion being evaluated. Wait for pressures to stabilize. If baseline resting Pd/Pa is <0.80, then the lesion is significant at rest and pharmacological hyperemia is not required
- If resting Pd/Pa is >0.80, then administer coronary vasodilator as per protocol. Ensure appropriate dose is administered
- Measure FFR reading at maximal hyperemia; document and store reading
- Once FFR reading is taken gently, withdraw wire and recheck that both pressures are equal to ensure that there is no drift
- If there are multiple lesions/tandem lesions, then assess FFR of the entire vessel. FFR wire may be withdrawn during maximal hyperemia to assess individual lesions if clinically necessary
- Take a final angiogram after removal of the wire to check for any wire-related complications
- If FFR is significant then PCI can be performed on the FFR wire by disconnecting the wire from the analyzer. Post-PCI measurements can be taken by reconnecting the pressure wire and with maximal hyperemia

FFR, fractional flow reserve; PCI, percutaneous coronary intervention.

hypotension[10] findings which need to be confirmed in larger studies. At present, it is considered to be the gold standard for assessing a lesion's functional significance.[11]

CLINICAL UTILITY OF FRACTIONAL FLOW RESERVE

Clinical use of FFR is now well established in assessing intermediate-grade lesions during coronary intervention. The deferral of percutaneous intervention (DEFER) study[4] where CAD patients with FFR >0.75 and FFR <0.75 underwent revascularization or medical therapy. Patients with FFR <0.75 who did not get revascularized had more major adverse coronary events (MACE). On the contrary, patients with FFR >0.75 who did not undergo revascularization did equally good as compared to those with FFR <0.75 who underwent revascularization. In the landmark FAME-1 (FFR vs. angiography for multivessel evaluation 1) study,[5,12] it was observed that FFR-guided PCI is better than angiography-guided PCI. In FAME substudy,[13] it was found that 20% of lesion which had been classified as significant by angiogram (70–90%) was found to be physiologically insignificant. A total of 497 patients were studied who were stratified into tertiles based on their syntax score.[14] After determining the functional syntax score (FSS) for each patient (calculating syntax score only for lesions that are functionally significant), they observed that 32% changed to a low-risk category from intermediate- or high-risk group that would have resulted in change in their treatment modality. It was noticed that FSS and procedure time were the only factors that were associated independently with 1 year MACE. It was also found that FSS had a better predictive accuracy for MACE as compared with conventional syntax score. It was also observed that the presence of angiographically significant, but functionally insignificant, lesion that led to residual syntax score did not affect the prognosis of the patients.[15] This study emphasizes that almost one in three patients landed up in appropriate change in treatment modality after FSS assessment. FFR was found to be equally good in female patients,[16] in patients with unstable angina, and non-ST elevation myocardial infarction (NSTEMI).[17] FFR was also shown to be useful in patients with severe LV dysfunction, unless their lesion is very tight which may lead to clinically irrelevant overestimation of FFR.[18] It was also found that the chance to have a MACE due to FFR insignificant lesion is 0.02% over a year, which is very minimal. FFR-guided PCI was found to be superior to medical therapy alone in patients with CAD.[19] A 5-year follow-up of FAME-2 study showed an initial FFR-guided PCI in patients with stable CAD with a significantly fewer rate of composite end point that included death, myocardial infarction (MI), and urgent revascularization.[20] It also showed that those who had FFR >0.8 had a favorable outcome with medical therapy alone.[20]

Grafting vessels with a stenosis >50% is standard practice in patients scheduled for surgery, though it is known that rates of graft failure are higher in patients with insignificant stenosis. In a small study, patients who had 50–70% stenosis and were scheduled for bypass surgery underwent FFR at the time of angiography. These patients were reevaluated a year later to assess graft patency. There was a higher rate of graft failure when these were done in FFR negative lesions though angiographic stenosis was 50–70%.

Fractional flow reserve also helps in assessing long lesions to assess their hemodynamic significance. FFR wire pullback during sustained maximal hyperemia can help decide significance of long lesions guiding therapy. In assessing serial lesions/long lesions the total FFR across all lesions should be measured with IV adenosine as per standard protocol. If the summed FFR of the entire segment is <0.80, then a pressure pullback during IV adenosine hyperemia should be performed to assess individual lesions. Decision for PCI of the most severely narrowed lesion is then determined by the lesion that produces the biggest pressure gradient. After stenting the lesion with the largest ΔP, the remaining lesion/s FFR should be reassessed.

Fractional flow reserve is also a useful strategy for bifurcation lesions. It has been shown that though jailed side branches often have angiographically significant disease, most of these vessels have FFR values >0.75.

Assessing equivocal ostial or body lesions in the left main is as per standard protocols except that care needs to be taken that the guide catheter does not wedge as well as that the equalization of pressures is done in the aortic root. For intermediate severity distal lesions of the left main involving the bifurcation, FFR has to be assessed in both the LAD and left circumflex arteries. It is generally useful to first assess FFR in the less diseased of the two vessels, preferably the LAD using a manual slow pullback—if the FFR is <0.80 then it needs revascularization. If it is >0.85 then it does not merit any intervention. If the value is between 0.8 and 0.85 and there is significant distal disease in the other vessel, the decision should be based on additional imaging (IVUS). The presence of significant coexistent disease in the LAD and/or circumflex artery will increase FFR across the left main if these lesions supply a large area of jeopardized myocardium; if these lesions are in distal branches their effect on FFR of the left main will be minimal.

Assessment of vein grafts using FFR varies according to the presence or absence of antegrade flow in the graft. In grafts that have no antegrade flow, FFR accurately depicts blood flow in the distal myocardial bed. However, in grafts that have residual flow as well as collateral flow, FFR may be normal.

CASE STUDY

A 75-year-old elderly man presented with NSTEMI. Coronary angiogram done elsewhere was reported to have a critical diagonal disease with borderline LAD disease (Fig. 2A) and was advised to have a PCI to diagonal and was put on maximal medical treatment. However, he was having recurrent unstable angina. Hence, he was taken up for FFR-guided PCI-to-LAD. Even without adenosine, Pd/Pa was significant (0.73). He underwent PCI-to-LAD and diagonal using V-stenting strategy (Fig. 2B) and is doing fine. But for FFR, the decision would have been to perform PCI of the diagonal branch alone which would have risked leaving him with an unstable significant plaque in LAD.

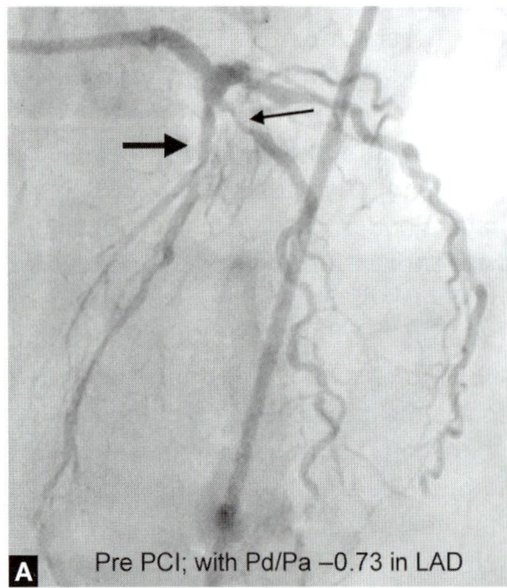

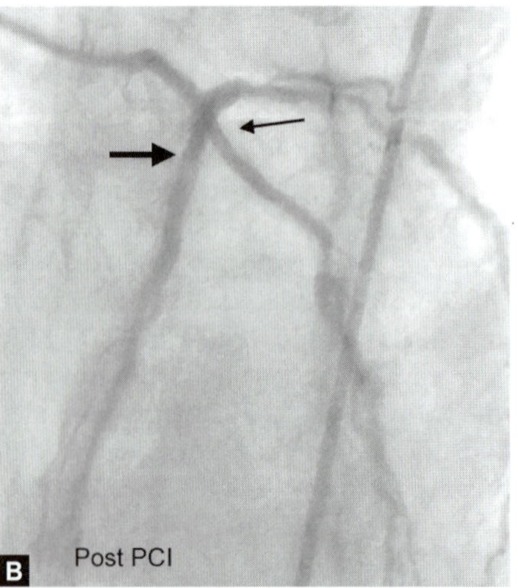

AP, anteroposterior; FFR, fractional flow reserve; LAD, left anterior descending artery; PCI, percutaneous coronary intervention.

FIG. 2: A, AP Cranial projection showing an angiographically mild proximal LAD lesion (bold black arrow) and a tight diagonal lesion (small black arrow). FFR was 0.73 across the proximal LAD lesion (significant); **B,** PCI was done using a V stent strategy.

Reproduced with permission from Evangel Publishers.

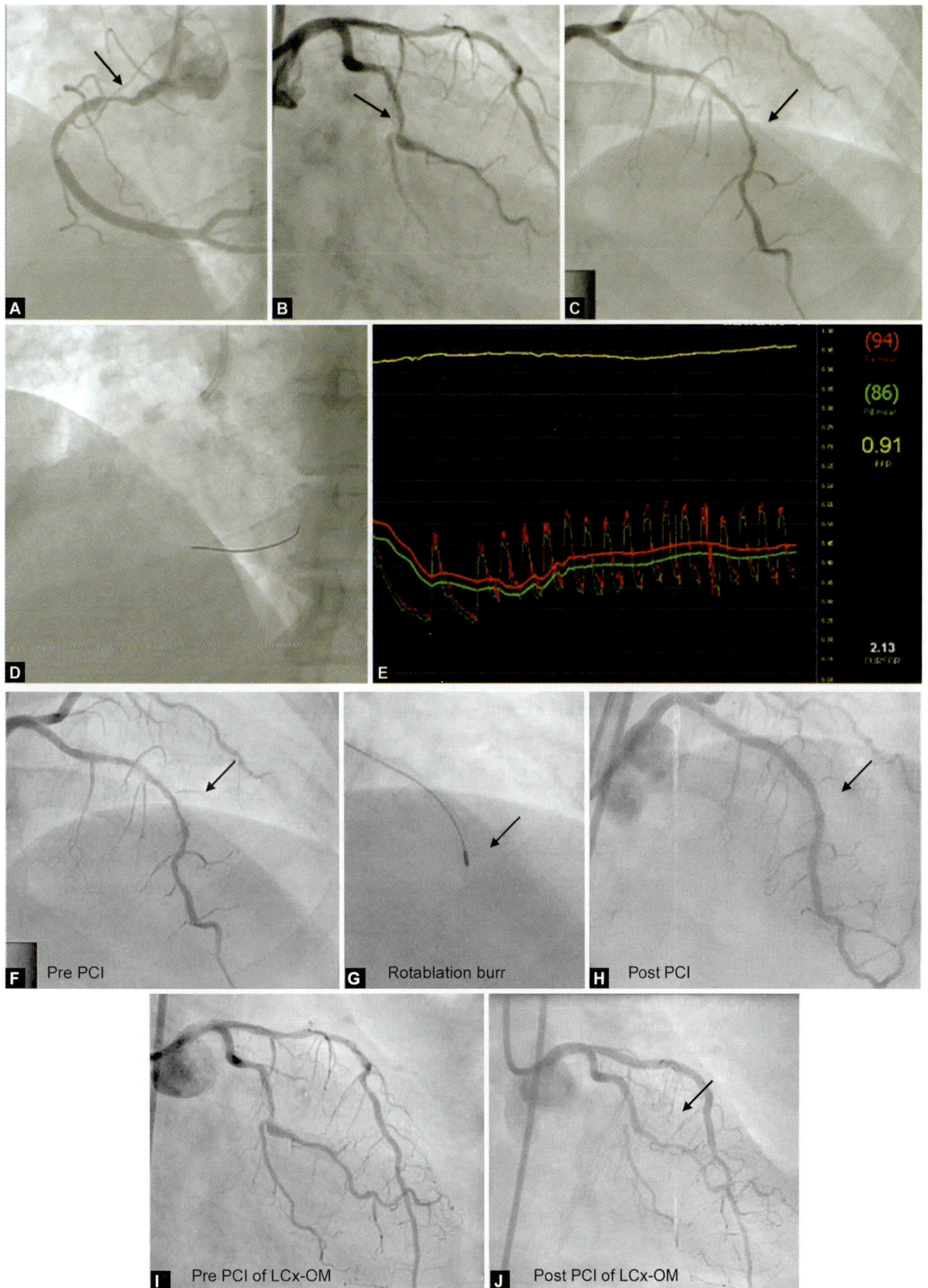

LAD, left anterior descending artery; LCx, left circumflex artery; PCI, percutaneous coronary intervention; PTCA, percutaneous transluminal coronary angioplasty; RCA, right coronary artery.

FIG. 3: There is an angiographically significant long RCA disease and borderline calcific LAD and LCx disease. FFR of the RCA was 0.91 (insignificant) while FFR of LAD and LCx was significant. LAD was intervened using rotablation followed by stenting (Panels F, G, H) while LCx underwent PTCA followed by stenting (Panels I, J).

Reproduced with permission from Evangel Publishers.

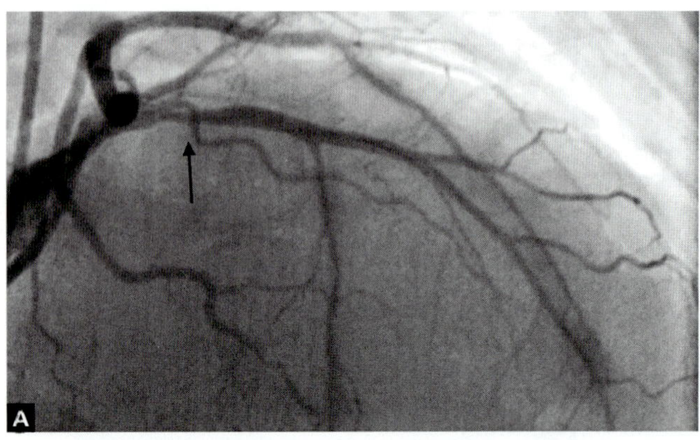

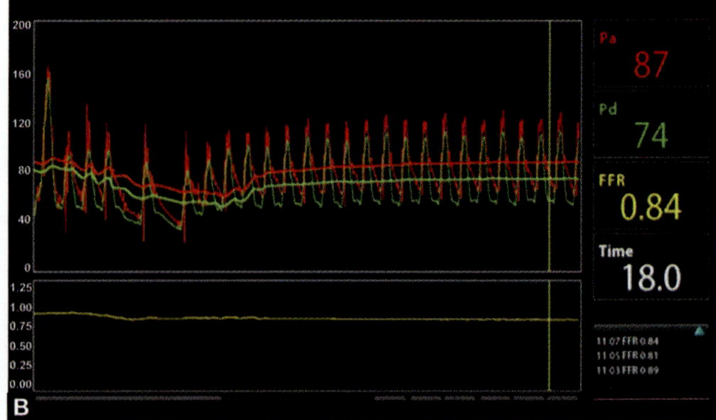

FFR, fractional flow reserve; RAO, right anterior oblique.

FIG. 4: RAO cranial projection showing an angiographically borderline to significant appearing lesion (black arrow). FFR was 0.84 across this lesion (insignificant).

Reproduced with permission from Evangel Publishers.

Additional case examples where FFR significantly changed management strategy in patients are provided in figures 3 and 4.

INSTANTANEOUS WAVE-FREE PRESSURE RATIO

In spite of the established value of FFR-guided revascularization, it is not commonly used in routine clinical practice due to various reasons including operator's preference, increased time with FFR, side effects of adenosine, and added cost of these procedures. Recently, resting indices of coronary blood flow have been proposed to assess the significance of lesions. Among them, Pd/Pa and iFR are the most well studied. Using coronary wave intensity analysis there is a period in diastole during which there are no waves from the aortic pressure head or from the reflected pressure waves from the coronary microcirculation. This wave-free period can be used for assessing FFR as there is minimal coronary resistance though coronary blood flow is at its peak. Pd/Pa during this phase is called iFR. This method is emerging as a potent competitor of FFR as the gold standard modality to assess the significance of lesions (Fig. 5). Mamas et al.[21] observed significant linear correlation between Pd/Pa and FFR. Sen et al. found that intracoronary resistance is constant and minimum during a particular wave-free period during diastole. They compared the intracoronary resistance at rest measured during the wave-free period with that of postvasodilatation (during FFR). It was concluded that iFR (ratio of distal to proximal pressure measured during this wave-free period) correlated very closely with FFR.[7] Jeremias et al.[22] studied the relation between Pd/Pa, iFR, and FFR. They found that the appropriate cut-off point of iFR and Pd/Pa for FFR ≤0.80 were 0.90 and 0.92 respectively with no significant difference between these resting measures. They found that iFR and Pd/Pa can predict positive or negative FFR with an accuracy of 90% in two-thirds and half of the patients respectively. There are several assumptions in the measurement of iFR. Foremost important assumption in iFR measurement is wave-free interval where the coronary

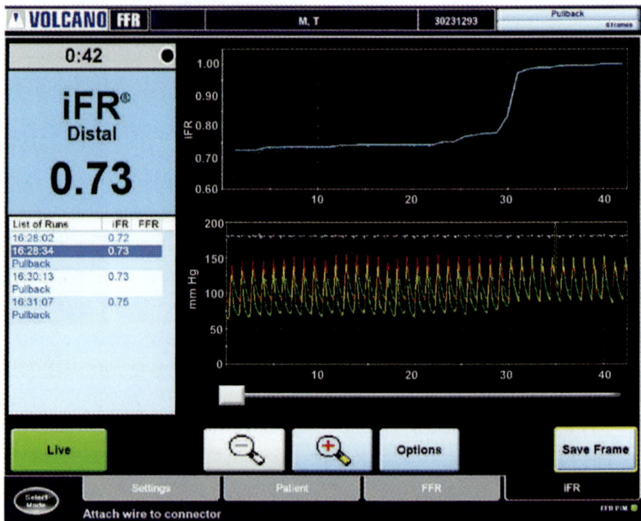

iFR, instantaneous wave-free ratio.

FIG. 5: IFR pullback using the Phillips Volcano system.

Image courtesy: Phillips India, reproduced with permission.

resistance is not only minimal but is also near equivalent to the coronary resistance measured with maximal hyperemia. It is also presumed that the pressure coronary flow relationship is proportional during this period. Though assumptions have not been perfect, that is the microvascular resistance measured in wave-free period is higher than that of maximal hyperemia-related microresistance, landmark studies have been published recently that compared the efficacy of FFR with iFR-guided revascularization.

COMPARISON OF INVASIVE PHYSIOLOGICAL INDICES TO NONINVASIVE PHYSIOLOGY MEASURED BY POSITRON EMISSION TOMOGRAPHY

There is always a debate whether CFR is better or FFR is better. Hwang et al. studied the relation between invasive physiological indices such as FFR, iFR, and Pd/Pa to noninvasively measured parameters such as CFR and RFR by ammonia-based positron emission tomography (PET). They found significant correlation between invasive physiological indices and PET-derived CFR and RFR.

HYBRID APPROACH

A hybrid approach of combining iFR with FFR was proposed to increase the identification of physiologically significant lesions. Rivero et al.[23] suggested a hybrid approach of doing iFR for all and doing intracoronary adenosine fractional flow reserve (IC-FFR) for individuals with iFR between 0.85 and 0.92 increased the sensitivity, positive predictive value, and specificity of this strategy.

STANDALONE INSTANTANEOUS WAVE-FREE RATIO APPROACH

Two large randomized studies compared the efficacy of iFR-based revascularization versus FFR-guided revascularization. They have taken 0.89 as the cut-off point for iFR and 0.8 as cut-off point for FFR.

DEFINE-FLAIR[24] was a randomized, noninferiority trial that enrolled 2,492 patients with CAD. They were randomized in 1:1 fashion to undergo either iFR- or FFR-guided coronary revascularization. The primary end point was the 1 year risk of MACE, which were a composite of death, nonfatal MI, or unplanned revascularization. No difference in primary end point was observed between the groups at 1 year [6.8% in the iFR group vs. 7.0% in the FFR group ($p < 0.001$ for noninferiority)]. There was also no difference in the secondary end points that included individual components of primary end points separately. The number of patients who had adverse procedural symptoms and clinical signs was significantly lower in the iFR group (3.1% vs. 30.8%, $p \leq 0.001$). It was also noticed that the median procedural time was significantly shorter in iFR arm (40.5 min vs. 45.0 min, $p = 0.001$). One important point, that needs to be emphasized, is the increased use of revascularization in FFR arm. In other words, functionally significant lesions were lower with iFR as compared to FFR [iFR (28.6% vs. 34.6%, $p = 0.004$)], and hence led to fewer revascularization procedures (47.5% vs. 53.4%, $p = 0.003$) with similar 1 year clinical outcome.

Instantaneous wave-free ratio-SWEDE-HEART study[25] was a multicentric, open-labeled, noninferiority, randomized controlled trial. This trial enrolled 2,037 patients with stable angina or ACS with indication of physiological assessment and randomized them to iFR- versus FFR-guided revascularization. Primary end point was the composite of death from any cause/nonfatal MI or unplanned revascularization within 12 months of the procedure. The primary end point was observed in 6.7% in iFR group versus 6.1% in FFR-guided group ($p = 0.007$ for noninferiority). A significant higher proportion of patients in FFR group developed chest discomfort as compared to iFR group (related to adenosine). This study concluded that coronary revascularization guided by iFR was noninferior to revascularization guided by FFR at 12 months with lower adverse procedural reactions and shorter procedural time. A meta-analysis studying death and MI combining both DEFINE-FLAIR and iFR-SWEDE-HEART trials has been conducted.[26] Though numerically higher death rates were observed in iFR arm, these were not statistically significant.

There are some limitations of both these trials. It is well known that iFR and FFR were concordant in 80% of cases.[27] Hence, both these trials could affect the outcomes of 20% individuals only. This will decrease the power of the study drastically. Though the vessel involved were reported, location of disease in particular vessel were not reported in both these trials. Previously Kobayashi et al.[28] reported that resting indices including contrast FFR, iFR, and Pd/Pa are less accurate in identifying the significance of lesions in LM/pLAD as compared with non-LM/pLAD. This is likely due to the huge amount of myocardial mass supplied by LM/pLAD.

MERITS AND DEMERITS

One major advantage of iFR is virtual PCI, that is effect of virtual PCI (Fig. 3) on tandem lesions. It was shown to be accurate and was helpful in changing the treatment strategy in one-third of patients.[29] Another point that was shown in the patient level analysis of the above two studies showed that patients with ACS had more MACE as compared to stable CAD in FFR arm unlike iFR arm where there was no significant difference. In difficult to wire lesions, microcatheter-based FFR could be used.[30]

CONCLUSION

Using physiology-based revascularization strategy either by FFR or iFR seems to be the best method to assess intermediate-grade lesions. Though FFR-based revascularization strategy is considered the gold standard modality until recently, a simpler, less time-consuming and more patient-friendly product; iFR, which has been found to be noninferior to FFR is now available. We believe using iFR technology may allow us to use the benefit of the physiology in many of our patients routinely. It does not imply that centers/operators using FFR routinely for intermediate lesions should change to iFR. It is rather time that interventional cardiologists start incorporating functional PCI using iFR or FFR to improve patient outcomes when clinically indicated. The emergence of even newer technologies such as quantitative flow ratio (QFR) which is computed as a 3D reconstruction of the diseased coronary artery from angiographic views may simplify functional assessment even further.

REFERENCES

1. History of Coronary Angioplasty [online]. Available from: www.pcronline.com/About-PCR/40-years-angioplasty/The-History-of-Coronary-Angioplasty-the-book [accessed August 2018].
2. Mintz GS, Popma JJ, Pichard AD, et al. Limitations of angiography in the assessment of plaque distribution in coronary artery disease: a systematic study of target lesion eccentricity in 1446 lesions. Circulation. 1996;93(5):924-31.

3. Pijls NH, van Son JA, Kirkeeide RL, et al. Experimental basis of determining maximum coronary, myocardial, and collateral blood flow by pressure measurements for assessing functional stenosis severity before and after percutaneous transluminal coronary angioplasty. Circulation. 1993;87(4):1354-67.
4. Zimmermann FM, Ferrara A, Johnson NP, et al. Deferral vs. performance of percutaneous coronary intervention of functionally non-significant coronary stenosis: 15-year follow-up of the DEFER trial. Eur Heart J. 2015;36(45):3182-8.
5. Tonino PAL, De Bruyne B, Pijls NHJ, et al. Fractional flow reserve versus angiography for guiding percutaneous coronary intervention. N Engl J Med. 2009;360(3):213-24.
6. Pijls NH, De Bruyne B, Bech GJ, et al. Coronary pressure measurement to assess the hemodynamic significance of serial stenoses within one coronary artery: validation in humans. Circulation. 2000;102(19):2371-7.
7. Sen S, Escaned J, Malik IS, et al. Development and validation of a new adenosine-independent index of stenosis severity from coronary wave-intensity analysis: results of the ADVISE (ADenosine Vasodilator Independent Stenosis Evaluation) study. J Am Coll Cardiol. 2012;59(15):1392-402.
8. Gould KL. Coronary artery stenosis and reversing atherosclerosis, 2nd edition. London and New York: Hodder Education Publishers; 1999. p 704.
9. Vranckx P, Cutlip DE, McFadden EP, et al. Coronary pressure-derived fractional flow reserve measurements: recommendations for standardization, recording, and reporting as a core laboratory technique. Proposals for integration in clinical trials. Circ Cardiovasc Interv. 2012;5(2):312-7.
10. Verdier-Watts F, Rioufol G, Mewton N, et al. Influence of arterial hypotension on fractional flow reserve measurements. EuroIntervention. 2015;11(4):416-20.
11. Toth GG, Johnson NP, Jeremias A, et al. Standardization of fractional flow reserve measurements. J Am Coll Cardiol. 2016;68(7):742-53.
12. van Nunen LX, Zimmermann FM, Tonino PAL, et al. Fractional flow reserve versus angiography for guidance of PCI in patients with multivessel coronary artery disease (FAME): 5-year follow-up of a randomised controlled trial. Lancet Lond Engl. 2015;386(10006):1853-60.
13. Nam CW, Mangiacapra F, Entjes R, et al. Functional SYNTAX score for risk assessment in multivessel coronary artery disease. J Am Coll Cardiol. 2011;58(12):1211-8.
14. Serruys PW, Morice MC, Kappetein AP, et al. Percutaneous coronary intervention versus coronary-artery bypass grafting for severe coronary artery disease. N Engl J Med. 2009;360(10):961-72.
15. Kobayashi Y, Nam CW, Tonino PAL, et al. The prognostic value of residual coronary stenoses after functionally complete revascularization. J Am Coll Cardiol. 2016;67(14):1701-11.
16. Kim HS, Tonino PAL, De Bruyne B, et al. The impact of sex differences on fractional flow reserve-guided percutaneous coronary intervention: a FAME (fractional flow reserve versus angiography for multivessel evaluation) substudy. JACC Cardiovasc Interv. 2012;5(10):1037-42.
17. Layland J, Oldroyd KG, Curzen N, et al. Fractional flow reserve vs. angiography in guiding management to optimize outcomes in non-ST-segment elevation myocardial infarction: the British Heart Foundation FAMOUS-NSTEMI randomized trial. Eur Heart J. 2015;36(2):100-11.
18. Kobayashi Y, Tonino PAL, De Bruyne B, et al. The impact of left ventricular ejection fraction on fractional flow reserve: Insights from the FAME (fractional flow reserve versus angiography for multivessel evaluation) trial. Int J Cardiol. 2016;204:206-10.
19. De Bruyne B, Fearon WF, Pijls NHJ, et al. Fractional flow reserve-guided PCI for stable coronary artery disease. N Engl J Med. 2014;371(13):1208-17.
20. Xaplanteris P, Fournier S, Pijls NHJ, et al. Five-year outcomes with PCI guided by fractional flow reserve. N Engl J Med. 2018 19;379(3):250-9.
21. Mamas MA, Horner S, Welch E, et al. Resting Pd/Pa measured with intracoronary pressure wire strongly predicts fractional flow reserve. J Invasive Cardiol. 2010;22(6):260-5.
22. Jeremias A, Maehara A, Généreux P, et al. Multicenter core laboratory comparison of the instantaneous wave-free ratio and resting Pd/Pa with fractional flow reserve: the RESOLVE study. J Am Coll Cardiol. 2014;63(13):1253-61.
23. Rivero F, Cuesta J, Bastante T, et al. Diagnostic accuracy of a hybrid approach of instantaneous wave-free ratio and fractional flow reserve using high-dose intracoronary adenosine to characterize intermediate coronary lesions: Results of the PALS (practical assessment of lesion severity) prospective study. Catheter Cardiovasc Interv Off J Soc Card Angiogr Interv. 2017;90(7):1070-6.
24. Davies JE, Sen S, Dehbi HM, et al. Use of the instantaneous wave-free ratio or fractional flow reserve in PCI. N Engl J Med. 2017;376(19):1824-34.
25. Götberg M, Christiansen EH, Gudmundsdottir IJ, et al. Instantaneous wave-free ratio versus fractional flow reserve to guide PCI. N Engl J Med. 2017;376(19):1813-23.
26. Berry C, McClure JD, Oldroyd KG. Meta-analysis of death and myocardial infarction in the DEFINE-FLAIR and iFR-SWEDEHEART trials. Circulation. 2017;136(24):2389-91.
27. Hennigan B, Oldroyd KG, Berry C, et al. Discordance between resting and hyperemic indices of coronary stenosis severity: the VERIFY 2 study (a comparative study of resting coronary pressure gradient, instantaneous wave-free ratio and fractional flow reserve in an unselected population referred for invasive angiography). Circ Cardiovasc Interv. 2016;9(11): e004016.
28. Kobayashi Y, Johnson NP, Berry C, et al. The influence of lesion location on the diagnostic accuracy of adenosine-free coronary pressure wire measurements. JACC Cardiovasc Interv. 2016;9(23):2390-9.
29. Kikuta Y, Cook CM, Sharp ASP, et al. Pre-angioplasty instantaneous wave-free ratio pullback predicts hemodynamic outcome in humans with coronary artery disease: primary results of the international multicenter iFR GRADIENT registry. JACC Cardiovasc Interv. 2018;11(8):757-67.
30. Menon M, Jaffe W, Watson T, et al. Assessment of coronary fractional flow reserve using a monorail pressure catheter: the first-in-human ACCESS-NZ trial. EuroIntervention. 2015;11(3):257-63.

CHAPTER 66

Optical Coherence Tomography in Coronary Artery Disease: A Review

Ashwat S Dhillon, Leah Raj, Anil Kumar Mehra

INTRODUCTION

Coronary angiography is the most easily accessible and universally used current method to assess coronary anatomy and as a guide to therapy including percutaneous coronary intervention (PCI), but it only provides a luminogram. In order to study arterial lumen as well as arterial wall structure, intravascular ultrasound (IVUS) and intracoronary optical coherence tomography (OCT) are currently available modalities of invasive imaging. IVUS has been in use for over 30 years with limited routine clinical penetration despite proven improvement in major adverse cardiac event (MACE) with IVUS-guided PCI use compared to angiography-guided PCI.[1] OCT is a recently developed new tool available for clinical use in its current form since 2007. Although, there are no large scale clinical data with OCT in comparison to angiography-guided PCI, it has distinct technological advantages as an imaging modality compared to IVUS. It is important as an interventional cardiologist to understand the advantages and disadvantages of both imaging modalities for clinical use. Adequate training in the acquisition of images and especially image interpretation may be an important factor in addition to cost and time, in the variable utilization of these important technologies for guidance during PCI and follow-up.

PRINCIPLES OF OPTICAL COHERENCE TOMOGRAPHY

Optical coherence tomography is a light interference-based imaging technique that uses near-infrared (NIR) light with a central wavelength range of 1250–1350 nm to generate cross-sectional (tomographic) view of the vasculature.[2] The key features of the three-dimensional (3D) cross-sectional images are: a very high spatial resolution (10 µm or less vs. 100 µm by IVUS) and high tissue contrast.[3] OCT is based on the principle of light interference, i.e., backscattered (reflected) from the analyzed tissue. Current commercially available system of intracoronary OCT (Ilumien Optis PCI Optimization System, Light Lab Imaging Inc., St Jude Medical, MA) employ a technique known as frequency domain (FD) OCT that enables imaging at 180 frames/sec with imaging length of 75 mm in survey mode and 54 mm in high-resolution images.

Introduction of FD-OCT with rapid automatic analysis and display of the 3D data of the coronary artery imaging has made possible for it to be used as a routine intravascular imaging tool for guidance during PCI. In FD-OCT, NIR light generated from fast tunable laser with variable narrow frequency sweep travels through an optical fiber and is projected after splitting on to a fixed reference mirror as well as outwards and perpendicular to the catheter on to the vasculature at variable depth. The backscattered (reflected) interference signals of different wavelengths and amplitude from both the mirror and the tissue are detected and amplified. The Fourier transformation converts it into an amplitude versus depth for display as an axial image (A-line image). As the catheter rotates, there are 500 A-line scan images generated per frame to combine and display as a B-mode cross-sectional tomographic view of the structure. The motor drive unit of the current system rotates the probe and automatically pulls back spirally at a speed of 30 mm/sec generating 180 frames/sec and this is displayed as the longitudinal view (L-view). The rapid scan and pullback allows the imaging to be done without the need for the occlusion of the blood vessel being imaged with no effect of the rapid motion of the heart during the cardiac cycle on the images.[1] OCT has a 10 times higher axial (≈10 µm) and lateral resolution (≈30 µm), but lower penetration depth compared with IVUS (1–3 mm vs. 8–10 mm). Another limitation is scattering of NIR light and its high-signal attenuation by the blood cells in the lumen. Therefore, it requires catheter to be flushed with high viscosity solution (iso-osmolar contrast) and temporary complete removal of the blood from the lumen during imaging by the contrast injection. This ensures a very high contrast between lumen and the intimal interface.

PREPARATION OF IMAGING SYSTEM AND IMAGE ACQUISITION

The OCT system consists of the Dragonfly Imaging Catheter, Drive-motor and Optical Coupler (DOC), and Ilumien Optis Integrated computer system (Light-Lab Imaging Inc., St Jude Medical, MA) to acquire images and analyze as well as perform automatic or manual measurements after completion of image acquisition.

The Dragonfly Imaging Catheter is a 0.014 inch wire compatible 2.7 F rapid exchange intravascular catheter with an external sheath and an internal rotating fiber optic imaging core, which emits the infrared light as well as captures the reflected backscattered light waves. The imaging core is driven by a stainless steel torque wire connected to the DOC and pulled back automatically after activation along the length of the imaging window of the external sheath.

At present, in order to provide adequate and rapid injection of contrast during image acquisition, a guide catheter with at least a 6 F size without side holes and coaxially alignment in the coronary artery is recommended. The outer sheath is flushed with 3–5 cc of contrast medium so no blood elements can enter between the optical probe and the sheath. The OCT catheter is connected to the DOC. The catheter is advanced over the wire. The Dragonfly Duo Intravascular Imaging Catheter has three radiopaque markers at the distal tip, imaging lens and 50 mm proximal to the lens (Fig. 1).The lens marker is placed just distal to the intended segment to be studied. If blood is detected inside the sheath of the imaging catheter, purge it with 3 cc attached syringe with contrast, then enable live view. Autocalibrate the catheter by making sure the calibration markers are at the outer edge of the sheath. Enable pullback recording while injecting contrast medium (12–20 cc at rate of 4 cc/sec manually or automatically). Catheter pullback is activated automatically by detection of contrast medium at the lens and the probe is rapidly pulled back by the DOC inside the sheath in 2.5 seconds. When the pullback is finished, the OCT probe returns to its initial position and if needed, a new imaging run can be initiated. The acquired images are available for immediate review and analysis in short axis, long axis, and 3D view. The current generation imaging display system can coregister the angiography and OCT images for better understanding of coronary anatomy and lesion characteristics.

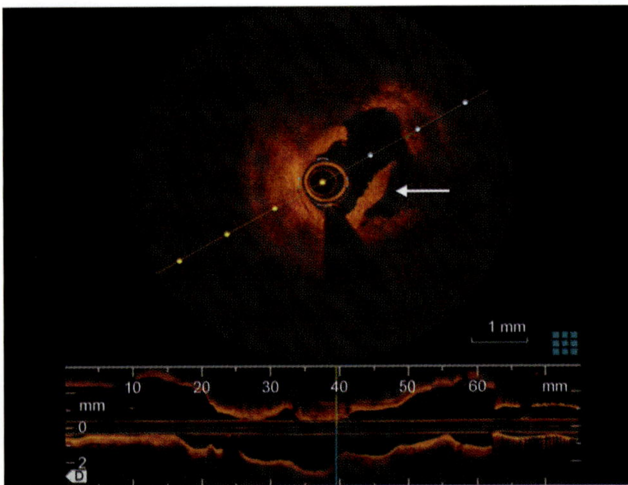

FIG. 1: Ruptured plaque.

OPTICAL COHERENCE TOMOGRAPHY INTERPRETATION IN INTRACORONARY IMAGING

Optical coherence tomography images have been validated against histology for accurate analysis of normal vessels as well as plaque composition, including fibrous cap thickness, lip core assessment, macrophage accumulation, calcification, and neovascularization.[4] OCT has been found to have a 10 times higher axial (≈10 μm) and lateral resolution (≈30 μm), but lower penetration depth (1–3 mm) compared with IVUS.[5] Therefore, visualization of the complete depth of a lesion is difficult especially in the presence of lipid-rich tissue.

The different vascular tissue layers have variable backscattering and attenuation properties as they interact with infrared light. High backscattering by a tissue gives it a high-pixel intensity [bright picture, Internal and external elastic lamina (EEL), fibrous tissue] whereas low backscattering will be seen as a darker, low pixel intensity region (media layer and calcium). The second interaction that defines tissue is attenuation. A high attenuation means the light cannot penetrate to deeper tissue (lipids and red thrombus) whereas low attenuation means light passes through the tissue to deeper layers that can be seen in images (calcium, fibrous tissue). Other features used in image interpretation are homogeneous versus heterogeneous composition (fibrous plaque and lipid versus calcium respectively), sharp versus diffuse edges (calcium versus lipids). Further, due to high axial and longitudinal resolution, OCT allows for measurement of thickness and arc of tissues. OCT has also been used to identify atherosclerotic plaque with high-risk features such as thin fibrous cap, cholesterol clefts and increased macrophage infiltration (irregular bright structures in intima).[6] The ability of OCT to detect the composition of tissue is based on the certain characteristic light interaction patterns.[7] Normal coronary arterial segments in OCT images appear as a three-layer structure with bright internal and EEL with a thin layer of low-intensity media in between. The adventitia is identified with the tissue beyond EEL and vasa vasorum within it. Abnormal segments can be classified as:

- *Fibrous plaque*: Finely textured homogeneous, high backscattered (signal-rich bright image) with low attenuation, (bright image with visualization of intima, media, and adventitia in the entire vessel thickness)
- *Calcific plaque*: Sharply bordered region with heterogeneous low backscatter and low attenuation (heterogeneously darker region with sharp borders and visible deeper layers)
- *Lipid-rich plaque*: High attenuating, signal poor region with poorly defined borders. High backscatter on the surface and poor backscatter under it. The intima

media may not be visible beyond the lipid content of plaque (bright fibrous cap with diffuse homogeneous darker image underneath and indistinct edges and no visualization of deeper structures)

- *White thrombus*: Low attenuating, poorly defined mass "floating" with high backscatter, in the vessel (bright tissue with irregular edges seen on the surface with complete visualization of deeper structures). The white thrombus consists of platelets and white blood cells
- *Red thrombus*: High backscatter on the surface with high attenuating irregular mass attached to vessel wall that casts a shadow on wall behind mass (a bright surface structure with darker deeper nonvisible tissue). The red thrombus is rich in fibrin and red blood cells.

Artifacts seen with OCT can include residual blood in the vessel lumen or swirl; blood inside the probe; non-uniform distortion; fold over, saturation or sew-up artifact; and Z-offset drift. All of these artifacts are relatively uncommon with the exception of residual blood in the lumen and blood inside the probe. The first one is easily remedied with better contrast injection, and the second one by simply flushing the OCT catheter. Some of the artifacts in OCT are due to guidewire, stent struts (ghost reflection artifacts) or due to catheter and/or arterial rapid movement [stitching artifact/ image malalignment (Fig. 2)].[7]

Vulnerable Plaque Assessment

Optical coherence tomography has an advantage over IVUS for identification of vulnerable plaque. High-resolution images of bright fibrous tissue obtained by OCT make it possible to accurately measure the thickness of the fibrous cap in μm. Further, easy identification of a lipid core with thin fibrous cap (<65 μm) defines a thin-cap fibroatheroma (TCFA) as vulnerable plaque (Figs. 3 and 4). In addition, OCT may be able to identify the mechanism of acute coronary syndrome (ACS) by identification of plaque erosion (intact intima with white thrombus) versus plaque rupture (loss of integrity of intimal layer with white or red thrombus in the lumen).

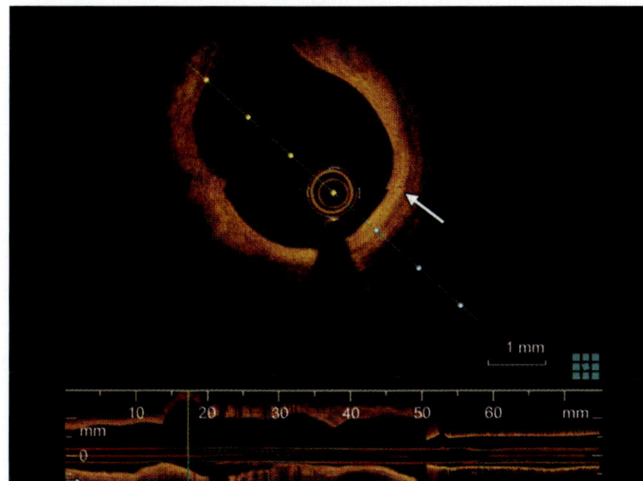

FIG. 2: Stitching artifact.

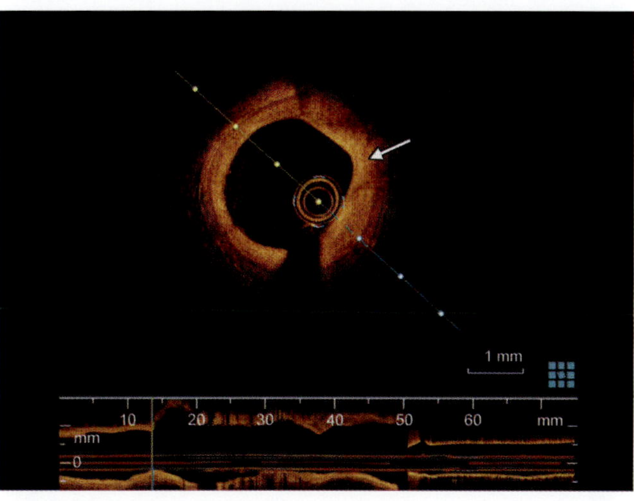

FIG. 3: Fibrotic plaque with thick fibrous cap.

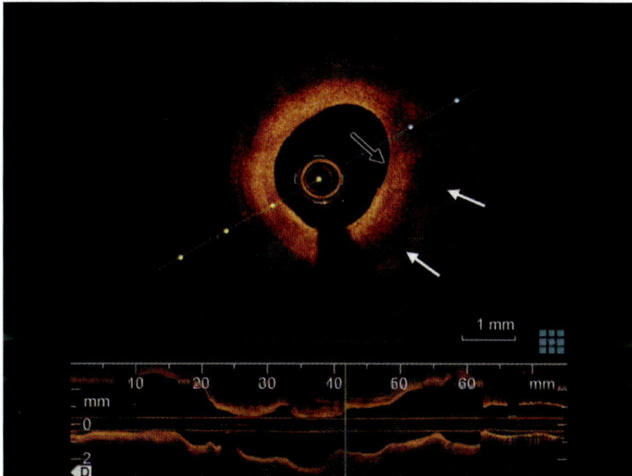

FIG. 4: Fibrotic plaque with lipid core (white arrows) and thin fibrous cap (black arrow).

OPTICAL COHERENCE TOMOGRAPHY VERSUS INTRAVASCULAR ULTRASOUND

Optical coherence tomography as an imaging modality has certain distinct advantages and disadvantages compared to IVUS, which may be useful in evaluation of specific clinical settings.

Advantages

- Optical coherence tomography images are easy to interpret and system interface is superior due to very rapid automatic analysis and display of stents with lumen profile
- Near-field spatial resolution is 10 times higher compared with IVUS, which allows for more accurate assessment of vulnerable plaque, coronary dissection, stent edge dissections, tissue coverage of stent struts, and stent malapposition (Fig. 5)
- Determination of calcium thickness (which is not possible with IVUS); total calcium arc more than 180°

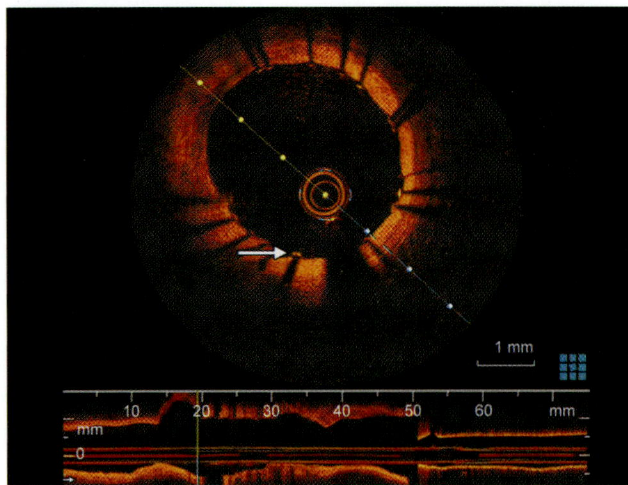

FIG. 5: Stent strut malapposition.

and increased calcium thickness more than 0.5 mm are all associated with greater risk of stent under-expansion. Therefore, one may need to aggressively predilatate after rotational atherectomy, prior to stent placement

- Accuracy of identification of white and red thrombus (identification of mechanisms of ACS), stent failure (stent thrombosis and restenosis)
- Guidance of bioresorbable scaffold implantation
- Optical coherence tomography offers better accuracy for stent apposition and edge dissection during PCI
- Optical coherence tomography offers the ability to measure full volumetric lumen analysis due to high resolution of longitudinal view compared with IVUS, resulting in greater accuracy for selection of stent size.[8]

Disadvantages of Optical Coherence Tomography

- Additional contrast load in patients with renal insufficiency increases the risk of contrast-induced nephropathy
- Swirling artifacts created by inadequate clearance of blood from the arterial lumen by inadequate injection, larger arterial lumen size or rapid blood flow
- Since contrast detection at the optical probe is necessary to initiate pullback, predilation of the lesion may be necessary preintervention in cases with obstruction by the catheter
- Inability to assess aorto-ostial lesions (left main or right coronary artery) as proper catheter engagement is needed for adequate contrast flush
- Depth penetration is limited, so the recommended size of the vessels is less than 3.5 mm
- Optical coherence tomography cannot identify EEL area accurately in lipid-rich plaques or larger arteries. IVUS enables better EEL visibility compared to OCT, and therefore leads to "more aggressive" stent sizing with larger minimum stent area (MSA) during PCI compared to OCT[9,10]
- There is limited clinical outcome data for OCT-guided versus angiography-guided PCI. The only major study looking at this is a recently published observational trial.[11]

CORRELATION OF OPTICAL COHERENCE TOMOGRAPHY WITH FRACTIONAL FLOW RESERVE

Although OCT is an excellent tool to assess atherosclerosis, it is limited in its inability to assess the functional significance of moderate coronary atherosclerotic lesions. Although, minimal luminal area (MLA) or minimal luminal diameter (MLD) by OCT has limited correlation with fractional flow reserve (FFR), except in the case of the left main coronary artery.[12-14] OCT-derived MLA thresholds have reasonably high-positive predictive value (80–92%) but lower negative predictive value for physiological significance of coronary artery stenosis (66–89%).[15-20] Therefore, PCI based on OCT-derived MLA alone is not routinely recommended.

CLINICAL UTILITY OF OPTICAL COHERENCE TOMOGRAPHY IMAGING

Clinical utility of OCT in diagnosis of coronary artery disease is limited to:

- Angiographically ambiguous lesions (e.g., dissection, thrombus, calcified nodule)
- Assessment of left main stenosis (except ostial) especially with distal lesions in the left anterior descending (LAD) or left circumflex (LCX) arteries, which may make FFR assessment difficult or uncertain.
- Suspected culprit lesion of ACS to identify plaque erosion versus rupture, which may identify some erosion in patients, who can be treated medically without stent implantation.
- Rate of periprocedural complications with stent implantation (malapposition, stent thrombosis, no reflow).
- Complex bifurcation lesion for preprocedure planning.

Utility of Optical Coherence Tomography in Procedural Planning of Percutaneous Coronary Intervention

The use of OCT or IVUS should be considered for PCI planning and optimization in patients undergoing interventions for chronic total occlusion, long lesions, left main lesions, bifurcation stenting with two stents, and in calcified lesions. If OCT is used in such scenarios, the guidelines recommend a set of parameters for stent selection and optimization.

Lesion Preparation

As stated earlier, OCT has higher tissue penetration into calcium compared to IVUS.[21,22] Accurate assessment of thickness and length of calcified plaque can guide decision making about lesion preparation. Regular or scoring balloons can fracture thin, concentric calcium. On the other hand, for concentric and thicker calcified plaque, atherectomy versus aggressive predilatation with noncompliant balloons may be considered. For lipid-rich plaque, predilation with an undersized balloon or a direct stenting strategy may be employed.

STENT SELECTION (DIAMETER AND LENGTH)

Stent Diameter

Stent underexpansion is an important predictor of early stent thrombosis and restenosis after drug-eluting stent (DES) implantation. Based on the currently available data from the ILUMIEN III trial and OPINION (the OPtical frequency domain imaging vs. INtravascular ultrasound in percutaneous coronary InterventiON) study, the best approach for stent size selection by OCT is to use distal lumen reference (less aggressive to more aggressive: mean distal lumen diameter, mean distal EEL diameter if two orthogonal measurements feasible or a single distal EEL diameter).[23,24] The stent size can be chosen as 0.25 mm up if one uses lumen diameter versus rounded down if one uses EEM diameter (3.30 mm mean lumen diameter will need 3.5 mm stent vs. 3.30 mm EEL will need 3.0 m stent). Subsequent dilatation of the mid and proximal part of the stent can be done to optimize stent expansion in these segments. Intravascular imaging results in implantation of larger diameter and length of stent, and larger final in-lesion minimum lumen diameter compared with angiographic guidance.[25,26] When comparing IVUS versus OCT guidance, if you size by distal lumen diameter, OCT guidance leads to around 10% lower diameter; a small but significant difference in the average stent size (OCT 2.92 ± 0.39 mm versus IVUS 2.99 ± 0.39 mm, $p = 0.005$) with no effect on long-term angiographic follow-up. If one uses EEM diameter then there is no difference in stent size when using OCT vs. IVUS guidance.[24] It has also been shown that luminal volumetric dimensions measured by OCT resulted in smaller MSA and lower stent expansion with OCT compared to IVUS.[9] Other studies have shown that OCT guided PCI resulted in smaller MSA, smaller stent diameters, and smaller maximum balloon diameters compared to IVUS guided PCI.[10,24,27] One strategy that has been suggested for OCT-guided PCI is to measure reference diameters pre-PCI to guide stent sizing, deploy the stent, assess angiographic success (postdilate if needed), and then repeat OCT prior to completion of procedure.[23]

Stent Length Selection

Optical coherence tomography can aid in stent length selection by showing regions of the coronary artery with eccentric calcification or lipid-rich plaque (>50%) at the proximal or distal edge of the proposed stent implantation. As such defining the normal coronary segment helps avoid edge dissection and stent complications. The coregistration of angiography and OCT can be used as a clinical tool can optimize stent implantation by selecting appropriate landing zone and length of the stents, thereby resulting in a trend toward reduced major stent edge dissection.

OPTIMIZATION AFTER STENT DEPLOYMENT

Stent Expansion

Whether adequate stent expansion should be defined by imaging modalities as absolute area or relative area (relative to reference segments) remains controversial. In general, greater achievable absolute stent expansion by OCT or IVUS results in improved long-term stent patency and better clinical outcomes. Based on the available data, large percentage of patients (~50%) do not achieve strict predefined relative reference criteria for stent expansion in randomized controlled trials with both IVUS and OCT. These did not translate proportionally into worse clinical outcomes. Therefore available evidence would suggest that an absolute MSA of more than 4.5 mm^2 by OCT and more than 5.5 mm^2 by IVUS and relative MSA more than 80% of the mean reference segment area should be considered adequate stent expansion in non-LM lesions. This cutoff may not be achievable in small vessels or may result in stent under-expansion in large vessels. In left main coronary artery (LM), based on IVUS studies the MSA should be more than 7 mm^2 for distal LM and more than 8 mm^2 for proximal left main. OCT with lumen profile in longitudinal view allows easy detection of stent under-expansion with rapid automatic calculation of the luminal stent area at the potential under-expanded stent site in reference to distal and proximal reference segment. OCT-angiography coregistration can help in identification of the under-expanded stent segments, which can then be postdilated appropriately. Accurate postdilation of only the under-expanded stent segment helps to avoid unnecessary postdilatation, especially near stent edges, thereby lowering the risk of edge dissection.[28]

Stent Malapposition

Acute stent malapposition (the lack of contact of stent struts with the vessel wall) is common as detected by OCT, with studies showing an incidence of 39–84% compared to IVUS (~15%).[29-32] OCT has a better resolution than IVUS to measure accurately the axial distance of stent strut from the vessel wall [incomplete stent apposition (ISA) distance] and its longitudinal extent. It is more common when stent is placed in a tortuous segment of the artery. Acute stent malapposition may resolve by neointimal tissue growth if the ISA distance is less than 0.4 mm and the length of malapposition is less than 1 mm.[33] However, the findings of three large OCT registries of stent thrombosis have shown higher incidence of malapposition in acute, subacute as well as late stent thrombosis.[34] Therefore, it may be prudent to avoid extreme malapposition and correct it safely at the time of stent implantation when anatomically feasible. Late acquired malapposition (due to positive remodeling) is difficult to diagnose unless intravascular imaging was done at the time of initial stent placement; but has been identified as a cause of late and very late stent thrombosis.

Tissue Prolapse

Optical coherence tomography is superior in detection and identification of tissue characteristics of the material found protruding through stent struts into lumen (tissue prolapse). It is more common in patients undergoing PCI for ACS with plaque rupture than chronic stable plaques or ACS with plaque erosion. Although, large tissue prolapse (definition unclear) is related to acute stent thrombosis and periprocedural complications but there are no guidelines for the management of small tissue prolapse.[35]

Edge Dissection

Optical coherence tomography due to its high resolution is ideal in identifying edge dissections as well as in-stent dissections. Based on the randomized and observational studies of routine OCT imaging post stent implantation, minor edge dissections are very common (20–40%), do not portray adverse clinical outcomes and do not require routine additional intervention. In contrast large edge dissections with more than 60° arc, more than 2 mm length, involving the medial or at the distal edge should be treated with additional stenting.[36,37] Identification of intramural or extramural hematoma at the stent edge by OCT should also be treated to reduce acute stent thrombosis.

Bioabsorbable Stent Implantation

Due to currently available technology of bioabsorbable stent (thick stent struts and low radiopacity), proper identification of lesion morphology by OCT is very important in stent selection. OCT also provides the poststent implantation optimization to avoid stent underexpansion and malapposition.

CONCLUSION

In comparison to IVUS, OCT imaging clearly has an advantage in assessment of plaque morphology; is as good as IVUS in guiding the optimization of PCI procedure; is better in evaluation of stent-related complications but has limited clinical data to date. However, the coronary images obtained are simple to acquire and can be learned to interpret. Familiarity with image interpretation and advancement in technology such as coregistration of angiography, 3D OCT and FFR as well as 3D reconstruction of implanted stent will only further enhance our comfort for its use in routine clinical practice because it clearly has a role in improvement in short- and long-term clinical outcomes in patients with coronary artery disease.

REFERENCES

1. Ahn JM, Kang SJ, Yoon SH, et al. Meta-analysis of outcomes after intravascular ultrasound-guided versus angiography-guided drug-eluting stent implantation in 26,503 patients enrolled in three randomized trials and 14 observational studies. Am J Cardiol. 2014;113:1338-47.
2. Roleder T, Jakala J, Kaluza GL, et al. The basics of intravascular optical coherence tomography. Postepy w kardiologii interwencyjnej = Adv Interventional Cardiol. 2015;11:74-83.
3. Popescu DP, Choo-Smith LP, Flueraru C, et al. Optical coherence tomography: Fundamental principles, instrumental designs and biomedical applications. Biophy Revi. 2011;3:155.
4. Yabushita H, Bouma BE, Houser SL, et al. Characterization of human atherosclerosis by optical coherence tomography. Circulation. 2002;106:1640-5.
5. Koskinas KC, Ughi GJ, Windecker S, et al. Intracoronary imaging of coronary atherosclerosis: Validation for diagnosis, prognosis and treatment. Eur Heart J. 2016;37:524-35a-c.
6. Sinclair H, Bourantas C, Bagnall A, et al. Oct for the identification of vulnerable plaque in acute coronary syndrome. JACC Cardiovasc Imaging. 2015;8:198-209.
7. Tearney GJ, Regar E, Akasaka T, et al. Consensus standards for acquisition, measurement, and reporting of intravascular optical coherence tomography studies: A report from the international working group for intravascular optical coherence tomography standardization and validation. J Am Coll Cardiol. 2012;59:1058-72.
8. Guagliumi G, Sirbu V, Petroff C, et al. Volumetric assessment of lesion severity with optical coherence tomography: Relationship with fractional flow. EuroIntervention. 2013;8:1172-81.
9. Habara M, Nasu K, Terashima M, et al. Impact of frequency-domain optical coherence tomography guidance for optimal coronary stent implantation in comparison with intravascular ultrasound guidance. Circ Cardiovasc Interv. 2012;5:193-201.
10. Maehara A, Ben-Yehuda O, Ali Z, et al. Comparison of stent expansion guided by optical coherence tomography versus intravascular ultrasound: The ILUMIEN II study (observational study of optical coherence tomography [oct] in patients undergoing fractional flow reserve [ffr] and percutaneous coronary intervention). JACC Cardiovasc Interv. 2015;8:1704-14.
11. Prati F, Di Vito L, Biondi-Zoccai G, et al. Angiography alone versus angiography plus optical coherence tomography to guide decision-making during percutaneous coronary intervention: The centro per la lotta contro l'infarto-optimisation of percutaneous coronary intervention (CLI-OPCI) study. EuroIntervention. 2012;8:823-9.
12. Nascimento BR, de Sousa MR, Koo BK, et al. Diagnostic accuracy of intravascular ultrasound-derived minimal lumen area compared with fractional flow reserve--meta-analysis: Pooled accuracy of ivus luminal area versus ffr. Catheter Cardiovasc Interv. 2014;84:377-85.
13. Stefano GT, Bezerra HG, Attizzani G, et al. Utilization of frequency domain optical coherence tomography and fractional flow reserve to assess intermediate coronary artery stenoses: Conciliating anatomic and physiologic information. Int J Cardiovasc Imaging. 2011;27:299-308.
14. D'Ascenzo F, Barbero U, Cerrato E, et al. Accuracy of intravascular ultrasound and optical coherence tomography in identifying functionally significant coronary stenosis according to vessel diameter: A meta-analysis of 2,581 patients and 2,807 lesions. Am Heart J. 2015;169:663-73.
15. Shiono Y, Kitabata H, Kubo T, et al. Optical coherence tomography-derived anatomical criteria for functionally significant coronary stenosis assessed by fractional flow reserve. Circ J. 2012;76:2218-25.
16. Gonzalo N, Escaned J, Alfonso F, et al. Morphometric assessment of coronary stenosis relevance with optical coherence tomography: A comparison with fractional flow reserve and intravascular ultrasound. J Am Coll Cardiol. 2012; 59:1080-9.
17. Pawlowski T, Prati F, Kulawik T, et al. Optical coherence tomography criteria for defining functional severity of intermediate lesions: A comparative study with FFR. Int J Cardiovasc Imaging. 2013;29:1685-91.
18. Reith S, Battermann S, Jaskolka A, et al. Relationship between optical coherence tomography derived intraluminal and intramural criteria and haemodynamic relevance as determined by fractional flow reserve in intermediate coronary stenoses of patients with type 2 diabetes. Heart. 2013;99:700-7.
19. Pyxaras SA, Tu S, Barbato E, et al. Quantitative angiography and optical coherence tomography for the functional assessment of nonobstructive coronary stenoses: Comparison with fractional flow reserve. Am Heart J. 2013;166:1010-18.
20. Zafar H, Ullah I, Dinneen K, et al. Evaluation of hemodynamically severe coronary stenosis as determined by fractional flow reserve with frequency domain optical coherence tomography measured anatomical parameters. J Cardiol. 2014;64:19-24.

21. Kobayashi Y, Okura H, Kume T, et al. Impact of target lesion coronary calcification on stent expansion. Circ J. 2014;78:2209-14.
22. Karimi Galougahi K, Shlofmitz RA, Ben-Yehuda O, et al. Guiding light: Insights into atherectomy by optical coherence tomography. JACC Cardiovasc Interv. 2016;9:2362-3.
23. Ali ZA, Maehara A, Genereux P, et al. Optical coherence tomography compared with intravascular ultrasound and with angiography to guide coronary stent implantation (ILUMIEN III: Optimize PCI): A randomised controlled trial. Lancet. 2016;388:2618-28.
24. Kubo T, Shinke T, Okamura T, et al. Optical frequency domain imaging vs. Intravascular ultrasound in percutaneous coronary intervention (opinion trial): One-year angiographic and clinical results. Eur Heart J. 2017;38:3139-47.
25. Chieffo A, Latib A, Caussin C, et al. A prospective, randomized trial of intravascular-ultrasound guided compared to angiography guided stent implantation in complex coronary lesions: The AVIO trial. Am Heart J. 2013;165:65-72.
26. Hong SJ, Kim BK, Shin DH, et al. Effect of intravascular ultrasound-guided vs angiography-guided everolimus-eluting stent implantation: The IVUS-XPL randomized clinical trial. JAMA. 2015;314:2155-63.
27. Otake H, Kubo T, Takahashi H, et al. Optical frequency domain imaging versus intravascular ultrasound in percutaneous coronary intervention (OPINION trial): Results from the opinion imaging study. JACC Cardiovasc Imaging. 2018;11:111-23.
28. Romagnoli E, Sangiorgi GM, Cosgrave J, et al. Drug-eluting stenting: The case for post-dilation. JACC. Cardiovascular Interv. 2008;1:22-31
29. Prati F, Romagnoli E, Burzotta F, et al. Clinical impact of OCT findings during PCI: The CLI-OPCI II study. JACC Cardiovasc Imaging. 2015;8:1297-305.
30. Gutierrez-Chico JL, Wykrzykowska J, Nuesch E, et al. Vascular tissue reaction to acute malapposition in human coronary arteries: Sequential assessment with optical coherence tomography. Circ Cardiovasc Interv. 2012;5:20-29, S21-8.
31. Im E, Kim BK, Ko YG, et al. Incidences, predictors, and clinical outcomes of acute and late stent malapposition detected by optical coherence tomography after drug-eluting stent implantation. Circ Cardiovasc interv. 2014;7:88-96.
32. Soeda T, Uemura S, Park SJ, et al. Incidence and clinical significance of poststent optical coherence tomography findings: One-year follow-up study from a multicenter registry. Circulation. 2015;132:1020-9.
33. Gonzalo N, Barlis P, Serruys PW, et al. Incomplete stent apposition and delayed tissue coverage are more frequent in drug-eluting stents implanted during primary percutaneous coronary intervention for st-segment elevation myocardial infarction than in drug-eluting stents implanted for stable/unstable angina: Insights from optical coherence tomography. JACC Cardiovasc interv. 2009;2:445-52.
34. Adriaenssens T, Joner M, Godschalk TC, et al. Prevention of Late Stent Thrombosis by an Interdisciplinary Global European Effort I. Optical coherence tomography findings in patients with coronary stent thrombosis: A report of the prestige consortium (prevention of late stent thrombosis by an interdisciplinary global european effort). Circulation. 2017;136:1007-21.
35. Sohn J, Hur SH, Kim IC, et al. A comparison of tissue prolapse with optical coherence tomography and intravascular ultrasound after drug-eluting stent implantation. Int J Cardiovasc Imaging. 2015;31:21-9.
36. Guo J, Chen YD, Tian F, et al. Optical coherence tomography assessment of edge dissections after drug-eluting stent implantation in coronary artery. Chin Med J. 2012;125:1047-50.
37. Chamie D, Bezerra HG, Attizzani GF, et al. Incidence, predictors, morphological characteristics, and clinical outcomes of stent edge dissections detected by optical coherence tomography. JACC Cardiovasc Interv. 2013;6:800-13.

CHAPTER 67

Stem Cells in Cardiovascular Disease: Is there an indication?

Vijay Iyer

INTRODUCTION

Cardiovascular disease remains the leading cause of death worldwide, getting 17 million people each year.[1] The World Health Organization estimates that by 2020 this number reached 24 million.[2,3] With complex multifactorial pathologies, including both genetic and environmental factors, cardiac disease continues to be difficult to prevent. Current strategies against cardiac vessel disease into prevention, i.e., the effectiveness of drug strategies, vary among individuals, and surgical intervention is not be applicable to all patients. New approaches need to be established to better understand the mechanism for coronary vessel disease and improved diagnostic and therapeutic 70s, particularly in the context of heart failure (HF), lifestyle changes, and pharmacological and/or surgical intervention.

Over the last 20 years, there has been interest in harnessing and promoting the innate and regenerative ability of injured organs to treat disease. The exciting preclinical findings in stem cell biology and the growing expertise and cell isolation and handling has increased interest in cell-based therapy for cardiovascular disease.[4] In more than 200 clinical trials and 50 meta-analysis we have improved our understanding off the potential use of stem cells for improving cardiac function. Despite the lack of a trial that conclusively demonstrates clinical efficacy, this safety and feasibility of several different cell types are now established. This field is now placed to anchor the next phase of trials that most likely will pave the pathway for a cell-based therapy with efficacy.

There is a dire need for therapies for cardiovascular disease due to the increasing number of patients worldwide. HF continues to be a major problem worldwide and despite the use of evidence-based therapies, such as angiotensin-converting enzyme inhibitors, beta-blockers, and mineralocorticoid receptor antagonist and angiotensin receptor neprilysin inhibitors mortality continues to be unacceptably high. Furthermore, drug therapy for HF is efficacious only in a subset of patients with no appropriate therapy for preserved ejection fraction or for worsening chronic HF.

The traditionally held opinion was that the heart is a terminally differentiated organ with little to no regenerative capacity. This changed after the identification of a small resident population of multipotent cardiac stem cells (CSCs) reframing the heart has an organ that the capacity for self-renewal. It is now understood that although they are terminally differentiated cells, there is a 1–2% cardiomyocyte turnover per year in childhood.[5,6] However, the heart is unable to adequately compensate in the face of overwhelming cardio myocyte loss seen in acute myocardial infarction (AMI) and HF. Stem cells, defined by the inability to self-renew and differentiated into at least one of the cell type were investigated as a means to directly replace lost myocardium and stimulate endogenous repair. This review will focus on the clinical data available from trials in stem-cell therapy.

CHALLENGES IN CELL THERAPY

The field of stem-cell therapy applied to clinical cardiovascular problems as some significant challenges. The challenges are listed in box 1.[7]

The potency of injected cells is often poor diminishing their inability to be effective in larger animal studies and in humans. Current approaches have attempted to precondition these cells by culturing them in hypoxic medium, by the addition of several growth factors like transforming growth factor (TGF), vascular endothelial growth factor (VEGF), and fibroblast growth factor (FGF) as well as the proto-oncogene Pim-1. Additional approaches have been combined two different types of cell types to improve the potency.

A second major problem with cardiac regeneration therapy has been the poor engraftment under tension-off the administered cells. The approaches being used to overcome these include repeated injections of cell types in therapy, the administration of cells by electro anatomic directed trans-endocardial injection instead of coronary artery infusion, the use of a bio-matrix to enhance cell engraftment.

BOX 1 Challenges in cell therapy for cardiovascular disease

- Selection of cell recipient
- Selection of cell donors
- Selection of appropriate cells
- Route and method of delivery
- Retention of stem cells
- Optimizing cell potency
- Determining the optimal dose and number of doses of cells
- Creating bio scaffolds to help delivery of cells
- Standardization of preclinical studies to help measure the appropriate end points in clinical trials
- Determining the optimum timing of cell administration.

CELL TYPES AND MECHANISMS

The early studies of therapy hypothesized that transplanted cells could differentiate into myocytes and therefore regenerate the myocardium. This however appears to be a rare event in larger animal studies and in humans.[8,9] Even in the studies that have shown improvement in myocardial function, i.e., little evidence that cells have engrafted.[9] This has shifted the focus to paracrine mechanisms as the main mode of benefit from stem cells.[10] The multitude of mechanisms proposed include secretion of growth hormones, cytokines, metalloproteinase, exosomes, and mitochondrial transfer. A number of adverse cardiac remodeling events occur in damaged myocardium that include imbalanced extracellular matrix turnover and fibrosis, acute and chronic inflammation, oxidative stress, abnormal energy metabolism, and oxygen consumption, increased apoptosis, endothelial dysfunction and reduced vasculogenesis, all of which are targets for stem-cell therapies. It is very likely that different cell types have different mechanisms by which the may have a positive benefit. Preclinical studies to investigate these are continuing.

The paracrine mechanism of stem cell benefit was derived from early studies that showed that bone marrow-conditioned medium, i.e., cell-free medium in which bone marrow cells had been cultured, acquired VEGF and monocyte chemoattractant protein from the cultured cells.[11] Additionally, the transendocardial injection of autologous bone marrow into place with induced myocardial ischemia increased collateral perfusion and improved function in the ischemic myocardium presumably because of the above-mentioned growth factors.[12] Additional studies, both in small and larger animals with coronary occlusion suggested that cell-free mesenchymal cell culture medium alone was able to provide the same benefit as the stem cells themselves. All of these together have supported the paracrine mechanism of action of stem cells.

It is now believed that the transfer of cytokines, chemotherapy cries, and growth factors from stem cells is mediated by small extracellular vesicles called exosomes.[13] These are of endosomal origin within a lipid bilayer and are between 30 and 120 nm in diameter. Some current approaches are targeting exosomes as possible drug delivery vehicles that can be produced in robust quantities *in vitro* by immortalized stem cells.

Early studies are stem cells in clinical trials were primarily derived from adult sources such as bone marrow and adipose tissue. There were often delivered as unfractionated populations of cells or as purified unmodified single cell types. The early trials of unfractionated bone marrow mononuclear cells which is a heterogeneous population comprising mesenchymal stem cells, endothelial progenitor cells and hematopoietic stem cells were largely neutral but safe.[14]

The next generation of cell therapies included progenitor cells isolated from cardiac tissue, allogeneic cell products, human pluripotent stem cells, and stem cells that have been lineage directed via chemical or genetic treatments to take on a specific cell phenotype. This group includes c-Kit+ (CD 117+) CSCs and cardiosphere-derived cells (CDC). CSCs are derived from adult hearts and displays strong paracrine signaling and demonstrate multi-lineage trans-differentiation *in vitro*.[15] CDCs are a heterogeneous population of cells derived from myocardial tissue that form self-adherent clusters *in vitro* and include both CSCs and supporting cells among others. Lineage-directed cells are those that have been treated to express a specific phenotype. These bone marrow-derived mesenchymal stem cells were treated with a cocktail of trophic factors to elicit a cardiac phenotype. The cells are typically isolated from young healthy donors and can be saved for later delivery and delivered as an off-the-shelf product, eliminating the need for long waiting periods required to expand autologous cell populations.[16] More recent approaches have included pluripotent cells such as embryonic stem cells (ESCs) and induced pluripotent stem cells (iPSCs).

CLINICAL TRIALS WITH STEM CELLS

There have been a number of clinical trials utilizing stem cells in AMI, ischemic cardiomyopathy, and nonischemic dilated cardiomyopathy. These trials are summarized in Tables 1–3.[17]

Clinical trials in stem-cell therapy in cardiovascular medicine often preceded a clear understanding of the mechanism of actions of the cell types being utilized. The consequence of this was that the endpoints chosen in these trials were probably inadequate or inappropriate. A number of these trials utilized surrogate endpoints. A surrogate endpoint is a functional or biochemical marker that substitutes for a clinical endpoint but is expected to predict clinical benefit based on evidence. The benefit of a surrogate endpoint is that it can overcome some of the financial burden associated with large sample size needed for clinical endpoints.

In HF trials a number of endpoints having utilized that include left ventricular ejection fraction (LVEF), left ventricular end-systolic, and end-diastolic volume. These surrogate endpoints often predict mortality in HF trials.[18] In addition patient functional status and quality of life (QoL) or important markers and HF trials and often reflect the symptomatic burden of the HF syndrome. A number of tools having utilized to assess QoL among HF patient's and include

TABLE 1: Stem cell trials in acute myocardial infarction

Trial	Follow-up (months)	n	Timing of cell delivery (post-MI)	Cell type and dose	LV assessment	LVEF	Volumes	Scar size
TOPCARE-AMI	12	59	5 days	CPCs; BMMNCs 7.3×10^6	LVG	↑	↓ESV	↓
BOOST	6	60	5 days	2.4×10^9 BMMNCs vs. placebo	cMRI	↑	NS	NA
REPAIR-AMI	4	204	3–5 days	190×10^6 BMMNCs vs. placebo	LVG	↑	NS	NA
TIME	6	120	3 vs. 7 days	150×10^6 BMMNCs vs. placebo	cMRI	NS	NS	NS
LateTime	6	87	2–3 weeks	150×10^6 BMMNCs vs. placebo	cMRI	NS	NS	NS
SWISS-AMI	12	192	5–7 days vs. 3–4 weeks	153×10^6 BMMNCs vs. control	cMRI	NS	NS	NS
BOOST-2	6	188	7 days	20.6×10^6 vs. 7.0×10^6 BMMNCs vs. placebo	cMRI	NS	NS	NS
PreSERVE-AMI	12	161	4–11 days	14.9×10^6 CD34+ vs. placebo	cMRI	NS	NS	NS

↑ indicates increase; ↓ indicates decrease.

AMI, acute myocardial infarction; BMMNCs, bone marrow mononuclear cells; CD34+, hematopoietic stem cells; cMRI, cardiac magnetic resonance imaging; CPCS, circulating progenitor cells; LVEF, left ventricular ejection fraction; LVG, left ventriculogram; n, number of patients; NA, not available; NS: not assessed.

TABLE 2: Stem cell trails in ischemic cardiomyopathy

Trial	Follow-up	n	Cell type, dose, and treatment groups	Delivery method	End point evaluation	LVEF	LV volumes	Scar size	NYHA class	Functional capacity	QoL
TOPCARE-CHD	3 months	75	22×10^6 CPCs vs. 205×10^6 BMMNCs vs. control	IC	LVG	BMMNC ↑LVEF	NS	NS	↑	NA	NA
FOCUS	6 months	92	100×10^6 BMMNCs vs. placebo	TESI	Echo SPECT	NS	NS	NS	NS	NS	NA
MSC-HF	6 months	55	77×10^6 BM-MSC vs. placebo	TESI	cMRI or CT	↑	↓ESV	↓	NS	NS	NS
SCIPIO	4 months	23	1×10^6 CSCs vs. control	IC	Echo/cMRI	↑	NA	↓	↓	NA	↓
POSEIDON	13 months	30	$20,100,200 \times 10^6$ BM-MSCs (allo vs. auto)	TESI	cMRI	NS	Allo:↓EDV	↓	NS	Auto:↑	Auto:↑
CADUCEUS	6 months	31	$12.5–25 \times 10^6$ CDCs vs. control	IC	cMRI	NS	NS	↓	NS	NS	NS
CHART-1	39 weeks	351	$9.7 \times 10^6 – 1.2 \times 10^6$ cardiopoietic cells vs. sham	TESI	Echo	NS	NS	NA	NA	NS	NS
TAC-HFT	12 months	65	100×10^6 BM-MSCs vs. 100×10^6 BMMNCs vs. placebo	TESI	cMRI/CT	NS	NS	MSC:↓	NS	MSC:↑	↑
RIMECARD	12 months	30	1×10^6/kg UC-MSC vs. placebo	IV	Echo/cMRI	↑	↑	EDV	NA	↑	↑
ATHENA	12 months	31	80×10^6 vs. 40×10^6 ARDCs vs. placebo	TESI	Echo	NS	NA	NA	↑	↑	↑
Perin et al.[31]	4 months	21	25.5×10^6 BCMMNCs vs. control	TESI	Echo	↑	↓ESV	NA	NA	↑	NA

↑ indicates increase; ↓ indicates decrease.

allo, allogeneic; ADRCs, adipose derived regenerative cells; auto, autologous; BMMNCs, bone marrow mononuclear cells; BM-MSCs, bone marrow derived mesenchymal cells; CDCs, cardiosphere derived cells; cMRI, cardiac magnetic resonance imaging; CPCs, circulating progenitor cells; CT, computed tomography; echo, echocardiography; EDV, end diastolic volume; EF, ejection fraction; ESV, end systolic volume; IC, intracoronary; IV, intravenous; LV, left ventricle; LVEF, left ventricular ejection fraction; n, number of patients; NA, not assessed; NS, not significant; NYHA, New York heart association, QoL, quality of life; SPECT, single-photon emission tomography; TESI, transendocardial stem cell injection; UC-MSCs, umbilical cord derived mesenchymal stem cells.

TABLE 3: Stem cell trials in nonischemic cardiomyopathy

Trial	Follow-up	n	Cell type and dose	Delivery method	End point evaluation	LVEF	LV volumes	NYHA	Functional capacity	QoL
TOPCARE-DCM	1 year	33	BMMNC 259 ± 135 × 10^6	IC	LVG	↑	NS	NA	NA	NA
ABCD	3 year	85	BMMNC 168 ± 96 × 10^6	IC	Echo	↑	↓ ESV	NA	NA	↑
MiHeart	12 months	160	BMMNC vs. placebo	IC	Echo	NS	NS	NS	NS	NS
Vrtovec et al.[40]	12 months, 5 years	110	CD34+ 113 ± 26 × 10^6 vs. control	IC	Echo	↑	NS	NA	↑	NA
POSEIDON-DCM	12 months	37	1 × 10^6 Allo-BM-MSC 1 × 10^6 auto BM-MSC	TESI	cMRI/CT	↑	NS	NS	↑ Allo	↑ Allo
Butler et al.[42]	3 months	22	Ischemia tolerant MSC 1.5 × 10^6/kg vs. placebo	IV	Echo/cMRI	↑	↑ EDV	↑	↑	↑
Xian et al.[43]	12 months	53	5.1 × 10^8 BMMNC vs. 4.9 × 10^8 BM-MSC vs. placebo	IC	Echo	↑	↓ BMMNC	↑	NA	NA

↑ indicates increase; ↓ indicates decrease.

allo, allogeneic; ADRCs, adipose derived regenerative cells; auto, autologous; BMMNCs, bone marrow mononuclear cells; BM-MSCs, bone marrow derived mesenchymal cells; CDCs, cardiosphere derived cells; cMRI, cardiac magnetic resonance imaging; CPCs, circulating progenitor cells; CT, computed tomography; echo, echocardiography; EDV, end diastolic volume; EF, ejection fraction; ESV, end systolic volume; IC, intracoronary; IV, intravenous; LV, left ventricle; LVEF, left ventricular ejection fraction; n, number of patients; NA, not assessed; NS, not significant; NYHA, New York heart association; QoL, quality of life; SPECT, single-photon emission tomography; TESI, transendocardial stem cell injection.

the Minnesota living with HF questionnaire and the Kansas City cardiomyopathy questionnaire. Markers of symptoms and functionality such as the New York Heart Association class and the Canadian cardiovascular society score for angina are also important endpoints especially in refractory angina trials. The measurement of infarct size has been an important endpoint in some AMI trials. The assessment of this is typically done with echocardiography or magnetic resonance imaging. The use of serum markers like B-type natriuretic peptide and N-terminal pro B-type natriuretic peptide is also being utilized in the HF trials.

Most trials that have been recently designed have measured a multitude of endpoints that will allow us to understand how best to designed the next phase of clinical trials. The utilization of surrogate endpoints in early face trials is reasonable but the next phase of trials will need to measure heart endpoints such as mortality, cardiovascular events and hospitalizations. These will obviously require adequately powered longitudinal placebo control studies.

Trials in Acute Myocardial Infarction

Early trials in cell-based therapy were in the clinical area of AMI. Most trials were designed around the concept of cardioprotection with the intent of using intracoronary infusion of stem cells in addition to percutaneous intervention in the setting of AMI. The early trials used bone marrow derives mononuclear cells which were harvested from patient's 1–12 days after percutaneous intervention and delivered the same day. TOPCARE-AMI and BOOST evaluated bone marrow to mononucleosis is delivered an average of 5 days after AMI.[19,20] Trials reported improvement in LVEF in the treatment during a short follow-up period. REPAIR-AMI was the largest trial for AMI and was designed to assess the efficacy of bone marrow mononuclear cells. This study randomized patients receiving cells or placebo 3–7 days after AMI. At 4 months, LVEF was significantly improved with an average 5.5% in the cell therapy group compared with only 3% in the placebo group. At 1 year the composite of death, myocardial infarction and need for repeat revascularization, was lower in the cell therapy group. This effect on mortality, but not improvement in LVEF was maintained at 5 years.

A number of subsequent trials including TIME, Late TIME, SWISS-AMI, BOOST-2 and MiHeart/AMI have not been able to demonstrate improvement severe left ventricle systolic function and response to cell therapy.[21-25] Most of these trials used different populations of bone marrow-derived cells. Significantly these trials utilized cardiac magnetic resonance imaging (MRI) as the standard for assessing left ventricular systolic function. Subsequent treatment analysis have shown that trials of utilized echocardiography as a marker of LVEF of demonstrated improvement in left ventricular systolic function one that have utilized cardiac MRI (disease which is considered medical center for evaluating left ventricular function) have not demonstrated a benefit of several therapy in improvement in left ventricle systolic function in the setting of AMI. These findings suggest that the trials to follow should utilize cardiac MRI as the preferred modality of assessing left ventricular systolic function both for regional and global function.

Bone marrow mononuclear cells have not shown much efficacy and recent trials suggesting that mesenchymal stem cells may be more appropriate candidates. A number of smaller phase II studies have shown promise in the utilization of mesenchymal stem cells in the setting of AMI.

Trials in Refractory Angina

With improvements in percutaneous revascularization as well as coronary artery bypass grafting the persistent problem of a large number of people who cannot be adequately revascularized and have refractory angina is growing. Stem cells at an attractive option for these patients since therapy shown to stimulate neoangiogenesis and improve perfusion. This population of cells studied with a CD34 positive circulating progenitor cells that showed a reduction in angina frequency compared to the placebo group after 12 months. The RENEW trial utilizing autologous CD34 positive cells isolated from peripheral blood enrolled 112 patients and demonstrated improvement in total exercise time at 3 months and an reduction in angina frequency at 6 months compared to patients treated with placebo only.[26-28]

There has been subsequent treatment and allergies all 6 trials using stem cells refractory angina utilizing CD34 positive cells suggesting a reduction in number of angina episodes and improved exercise tolerance as well as myocardial perfusion. Therefore, despite the fact that no single trial has shown an improvement in mortality this may be a therapeutic option for some patients for refractory angina.

Trials in Ischemic Cardiomyopathy

Ischemic cardiomyopathy offers the most promising area of therapeutic benefit with cell-based therapy. Most of these patients have a chronic syndrome secondary to loss of myocyte function and the cellular renewal of degenerated myocytes in this setting is most likely to offer both a mortality and symptomatic benefit.

Clinical trials and ischemic cardiomyopathy of utilized a number of different kinds of cell types that include bone marrow-derived mononuclear cells and second-generation cells. Early trials also utilized skeletal myoblasts that were injected into the myocardium at the time of coronary artery bypass surgery. However, the cells were shown to be extremely arrhythmogenic and this approach has since been abandoned.[29]

The earliest trial of bone marrow-derived mononuclear cells in congestive HF patient's utilized direct injections after electromechanical mapping into areas of infarct. These trials suggested an improvement in left ventral systolic function by 9% and reduction in left ventricle and systolic volume and scar sites.[29,30] The endpoint of exercise capacity was also significantly improved at 6 months and 12 months. A number of the other trials have been summarized in table 1. Meta-analysis of trials utilizing bone marrow-derived mononuclear cells in ischemic cardiomyopathy does reveal an improvement in left ventricle systolic function. The cells however may not have significant efficacy in older patients as a consequence more recent trials are investigating more purified cell types, allogeneic transplants and combination of cells.

Mesenchymal some cells from the bone marrow are also excellent candidates for regenerative therapy since the exhibit a fourfold constellation of phenotypic activity that includes immunomodulation, antipyretic effects, stimulation of new angiogenesis, and activation of endogenous cardiac repair pathways. Most of these effects are thought to be because of paracrine mechanisms. The early trials involving autologous mesenchymal stem cells are summarized in table 2.[31-33] Subsequently, allogeneic stem cells were also tested these trials collectively showed improvements in left ventricular remodeling, improvements in QoL, functional status, and in some cases also improvement in left systolic function. Stem cells derived from umbilical cord who also been tested in trials with variable results.

Adipose-derived regenerative cells were tested in a number of trials that were essentially neutral or negative.

Cardiac stem cells similar to mesenchymal stem cells secrete cytokines and growth factors. Incomplete clinical models there appeared to be beneficial and was subsequently tested in phase I trials in humans. In small numbers of patients improvements in left ventricle systolic function were seen. These trials were early and did utilize cardiac MRI for evaluation of left ventricular function and the newer trials utilizing CSCs will be testing these effects more rigorously.[34,35]

Cardiosphere-derived cells are a promising mixture of cells that are rich in the CD-105 cell surfaces marker and demonstrate a paracrine effect, i.e., probably more potent than the CSCs. The CADUCEUS trial was a proof of clots of trial and 33 patient's vancomycin received autologous CDCs or standard of care. In no myocardial biopsies were performed to obtain samples and CDCs were grown. The cells were delivered within intracoronary infusion one and a half to 3 months after myocardial infarction. Cardiac MRI showed reductions in myocardial scar size in the treatment arm. A subsequent trial, ALLSTAR, utilized a similar strategy in patients with left ventricular dysfunction secondary to a myocardial infarction within the last 12 months. However, this trial was halted early due to lack of benefit.

Cardiopoietic stem cells are second-generation therapeutic cells that include mesenchymal stem cells that have been treated to optimize to cardioprotective functions. The cells were tested in patients with ischemic cardiomyopathy and ejection fraction of less than 35%. The composite endpoint that included mortality, worsening HF, 6 minute walk distance, left ventricular end-systolic volume and LVEF measured by echocardiography did not show any difference between the sham and the cell therapy groups. However, in those patients who had a baseline larger than left ventricular end diastolic volume there appeared to be a positive reduction in both end-diastolic and end-systolic volume in the cell treated. This further highlights that selective populations of patient's might benefit even within these clinical trials that have shown to be overall negative.[16]

A number of preclinical studies have shown that combinations of stem cell types especially mesenchymal stem cells and cardiopoietic stem cells have a synergistic effect in the cardiac repair process.[4] These combinations are being tested in randomized controlled trials in patients with ischemic cardiomyopathy.

The interpretation of trials and ischemic cardiomyopathy is fraught with confusion because of the different endpoints being utilized. It is important to assess just mortality and LVEF improvements but also recurrent cardiovascular events, QoL, and functional status improvements since they're equally meaningful.

NONISCHEMIC DILATED CARDIOMYOPATHY

Nonischemic cardiomyopathy is marked by a significant immunological component, a lower scar burden and a larger proportion of dysfunctional viable myocardium. This makes it a potential therapeutic target for cell-based therapy. Cardiac MRI studies that have measured scar volume and the extent of dysfunctional viable myocardium have shown that dysfunctional viable myocardium is an independent predictive improvement in LVEF, wall motion score and end-systolic volume index. Stem-cell therapies are known to work in part because of immunomodulatory signaling and reversal of myocardial dysfunction. Theoretically, this would suggest that nonischemic cardiomyopathy would be a good therapeutic target for cell-based therapies. The number of trials in nonischemic cardiomyopathy is relatively smaller compared to those an AMI and ischemic cardiomyopathy and summarized in table 3.[36-42]

These trials included the use of bone marrow-derived mononuclear cells, CD34 positive cells from peripheral blood, allogeneic, and autologous bone marrow denied mesenchymal stem cells. Many of these trials of shown improvements in LVEF. The changes and left ventricular volumes have been more variable as have changes in functional status and functional capacity.

FUTURE DIRECTIONS IN CELL THERAPY AND LESSONS LEARNED

It is important to recognize that cell-based therapy has only been investigated over the last 20 years. This is a relatively small period of time and the field is still very young. The early irrational exuberance has been tempered by some of the neutral and negative outcomes of trials. However, it is extremely promising that in most of these trials so therapy has been shown to be extremely safe. In many of these trials that are somebody positive outcomes that give us hope for future trials. Preclinical work on understanding the mechanism of action continues to grow and will help us decide better trials with more specific endpoints that can be measured. The different kinds of stem cells being studied is also increasing. The iPSCs are specifically of great interest since they alleviate a number of ethical and availability concerns. The preclinical work with the cells is progressing rapidly and clinical trials with the cells are very close.

The experience with the trial so far has enhance on understanding of the paracrine mechanism of benefit from the cells as well as the possible need for repeated dosing like drug therapy. In conclusion stem-cell-based therapy for cardiovascular disease continues to remain an exciting area of research and in combination with advances in bioengineering scaffolds and the understanding from preclinical work, will most likely provide exciting results in the near future that will add to the armamentarium off therapies available for patients with cardiovascular disease.

It is important that there are no current guidelines which approve the stem cells for use routinely in cardiovascular disease. Therefore, patients should only be treated within the confines of appropriate randomized control trials.

REFERENCES

1. Joseph P, Leong D, McKee M, et al. Reducing the global burden of cardiovascular disease, part 1: the epidemiology and risk factors. Circ Res. 2017;121:677-94.
2. Benjamin EJ, Blaha MJ, Chiuve SE, et al. American Heart Association Statistics Committee and Stroke Statistics Subcommittee. Heart disease and stroke statistics-2017 update: a report from the American Heart Association. Circulation. 2017;135:e146-603.
3. Heidenreich PA, Albert NM, Allen LA, et al. American Heart Association Advocacy Coordinating Committee; Council on Arteriosclerosis, Thrombosis and Vascular Biology; Council on Cardiovascular Radiology and Intervention; Council on Clinical Cardiology; Council on Epidemiology and Prevention; Stroke Council. Forecasting the impact of heart failure in the United States: a policy statement from the American Heart Association. Circ Heart Fail. 2013;6:606-19.
4. Wysoczynski M, Khan A, Bolli R. New Paradigms in cell therapy: repeated dosing, intravenous delivery, Immunomodulatory actions and new cell types. Circ Res. 2018;123:138-58.
5. Beltrami AP, Barlucchi L, Torella D, et al. Adult cardiac stem cells are multipotent and support myocardial regeneration. Cell. 2003;114:763-76.
6. Bergmann O, Zdunek S, Felker A, et al. Dynamics of cell generation and turnover in the human heart. Cell. 2015;161:1566-75.
7. Braunwald E. Cell-Based therapy in cardiac regeneration: An overview. Circ Res2018;123:132-7.
8. Hatzistergos KE, Quevedo H, Oskouei BN, et al. Bone marrow mesenchymal stem cells stimulate cardiac stem cell proliferation and differentiation. Circ Res. 2010;107:91-22.
9. Wu T, Cieply K, Nalesnik MA et al. Minimal evidence of transdifferentiation from recipient bone marrow to parenchymal cells in regenerating and long-surviving human allografts. Am J Transplant. 2003;3:1173-81.
10. Gnecchi M, He H, Liang OD, et al. Paracrine action accounts for marked protection of ischemic heart by Akt-modified mesenchymal stem cells. Nat Med. 2005;11:367-8.
11. Kinnaird T, Stabile E, Burnett MS, et al. Local delivery of marrow-derived stromal cells augments collateral perfusion through paracrine mechanisms. Circulation. 2004:109:1543-9.
12. Yoshioka T, Ageyama N, Shibata H et al. Repair of infarcted myocardium mediated by transplanted bone marrow derived Cd34+ stem cells in a nonhuman primate model. Stem Cells. 2005:23:355-64.
13. Garikipati V, Shoja-taheri F, Davis M, et al. Extracellular vesicles for cardiac repair. Circ Res. 2018;123:188-204.
14. Sanganalmath SK, Bolli R. Cell therapy for heart failure: a comprehensive overview of experimental and clinical studies, current challenges, and future directions. Circ Res. 2013;113:810-34.
15. Bearzi C, Rota M, Hosoda T, et al Human cardiac stem cells. Proc Natl Acad Sci USA. 2007;104:14068-73.
16. Bartunek J, Terzic A, Davison BA, et al. CHART Program. Cardiopoietic cell therapy for advanced ischaemic heart failure: results at 39 weeks of the

prospective, randomized, double blind, sham-controlled CHART-1 clinical trial. Eur Heart J. 2017;38:648-60.
17. Bannerjee M, Bolli R, Hare JM. Clinical studies in Cell therapy in Cardiovascular Medicine. Recent developments and Future Directions. Circ res. 2018;123: 266-87.
18. Biomarkers Definitions Working Group. . Biomarkers and surrogate endpoints: preferred definitions and conceptual framework. Clin Pharmacol Ther. 2001;69:89-95.
19. Assmus B, Schächinger V, Teupe C, et al. Transplantation of progenitor cells and regeneration enhancement in acute myocardial infarction (TOPCARE-AMI). Circulation. 2002;106:3009-17.
20. Wollert KC, Meyer GP, Lotz J, et al. Intracoronary autologous bone-marrow cell transfer after myocardial infarction: the BOOST randomised controlled clinical trial. Lancet. 2004;364:141-8.
21. Traverse JH, Henry TD, Pepine CJ, et al. Cardiovascular Cell Therapy Research Network (CCTRN). Effect of the use and timing of bone marrow mononuclear cell delivery on left ventricular function after acute myocardial infarction: the TIME randomized trial. JAMA. 2012;308:2380-9.
22. Traverse JH, Henry TD, Ellis SG, et al. Cardiovascular Cell Therapy Research Network. Effect of intracoronary delivery of autologous bone marrow mononuclear cells 2 to 3 weeks following acute myocardial infarction on left ventricular function: the LateTIME randomized trial. JAMA. 2011;306:2110-9.
23. Wollert KC, Meyer GP, Müller-Ehmsen J, et al. Intracoronary autologous bone marrow cell transfer after myocardial infarction: the BOOST-2 randomised placebo-controlled clinical trial. Eur Heart J. 2017;38:2936-43.
24. Quyyumi AA, Vasquez A, Kereiakes DJ, et al. PreSERVE-AMI: a randomized, double-blind, placebo-controlled clinical trial of intracoronary administration of autologous CD34+ cells in patients with left ventricular dysfunction post STEMI. Circ Res. 2017;120:324-31.
25. Nicolau JC, Furtado RHM, Silva SA, et al. ACCMiHeart/AMI Investigators. . Stem-cell therapy in ST-segment elevation myocardial infarction with reduced ejection fraction: a multicenter, double-blind randomized trial. Clin Cardiol. 2018;41:392-9.
26. Hare JM, Traverse JH, Henry TD, et al. A randomized, double-blind, placebo-controlled, dose-escalation study of intravenous adult human mesenchymal stem cells (prochymal) after acute myocardial infarction. J Am Coll Cardiol. 2009;54:2277-86.
27. Sanz-Ruiz R, Casado Plasencia A, Borlado LR, et al. Rationale and design of a clinical trial to evaluate the safety and efficacy of intracoronary infusion of allogeneic human cardiac stem cells in patients with acute myocardial infarction and left ventricular dysfunction: the randomized multicenter double-blind controlled CAREMI trial (Cardiac Stem Cells in Patients With Acute Myocardial Infarction). Circ Res. 2017;121:71-80.
28. Povsic TJ, Henry TD, Traverse JH, et al. RENEW Investigators. The RENEW trial: efficacy and safety of intramyocardial autologous CD34(+) cell administration in patients with refractory angina. JACC Cardiovasc Interv. 2016;9:1576-85.
29. Menasché P, Hagège AA, Scorsin M, et al. Myoblast transplantation for heart failure. Lancet. 2001;357:279-80.
30. Perin EC, Dohmann HF, Borojevic R, et al. Transendocardial, autologous bone marrow cell transplantation for severe, chronic ischemic heart failure. Circulation. 2003;107:2294-302.
31. Perin EC, Willerson JT, Pepine CJ, et al. Cardiovascular Cell Therapy Research Network (CCTRN). Effect of transendocardial delivery of autologous bone marrow mononuclear cells on functional capacity, left ventricular function, and perfusion in chronic heart failure: the FOCUS-CCTRN trial. JAMA. 2012;307:1717-26.
32. Heldman AW, DiFede DL, Fishman JE, et al. Transendocardial mesenchymal stem cells and mononuclear bone marrow cells for ischemic cardiomyopathy: the TAC-HFT randomized trial. JAMA. 2014;311:62-73.
33. Florea V, Rieger AC, DiFede DL, et al. Dose comparison study of allogeneic mesenchymal stem cells in patients with ischemic cardiomyopathy (The TRIDENT study). Circ Res. 2017;121:1279-90.
34. Chugh AR, Beache GM, Loughran JH, et al. Administration of cardiac stem cells in patients with ischemic cardiomyopathy: the SCIPIO trial: surgical aspects and interim analysis of myocardial function and viability by magnetic resonance. Circulation. 2012;126:S54-64.
35. Kapelios CJ, Nanas JN, Malliaras K. Allogeneic cardiosphere-derived cells for myocardial regeneration: current progress and recent results. Future Cardiol. 2016;12:87-100.
36. Fischer-Rasokat U, Assmus B, Seeger FH, et al. A pilot trial to assess potential effects of selective intracoronary bone marrow-derived progenitor cell infusion in patients with nonischemic dilated cardiomyopathy: final 1-year results of the transplantation of progenitor cells and functional regeneration enhancement pilot trial in patients with nonischemic dilated cardiomyopathy. Circ Heart Fail. 2009;2:417-23.
37. Seth S, Bhargava B, Narang R et al. AIIMS Stem Cell Study Group. The ABCD (Autologous Bone Marrow Cells in Dilated Cardiomyopathy) trial a long-term follow-up study. J Am Coll Cardiol. 2010;55:1643-44.
38. Martino H, Brofman P, Greco O, et al. Dilated Cardiomyopathy Arm of the MiHeart Study Investigators. Multicentre, randomized, double-blind trial of intracoronary autologous mononuclear bone marrow cell injection in non-ischemic dilated cardiomyopathy (the dilated cardiomyopathy arm of the MiHeart study). Eur Heart J. 2015;36:2898-04.
39. Vrtovec B, Poglajen G, Lezaic L, et al. Effects of intracoronary CD34+ stem cell transplantation in nonischemic dilated cardiomyopathy patients: 5-year follow-up. Circ Res. 2013;112:165-73.
40. Hare JM, DiFede DL, Rieger AC, et al. Randomized comparison of allogeneic versus autologous mesenchymal stem cells for nonischemic dilated cardiomyopathy: POSEIDON-DCM Trial. J Am Coll Cardiol. 2017;69:526-37.
41. Butler J, Epstein SE, Greene SJ, et al. Intravenous allogeneic mesenchymal stem cells for nonischemic cardiomyopathy: safety and efficacy results of a phase II-A randomized trial. Circ Res. 2017;120:332-40.
42. Xiao W, Guo S, Gao C, et al. D. A randomized comparative study on the efficacy of intracoronary infusion of autologous bone marrow mononuclear cells and mesenchymal stem cells in patients with dilated cardiomyopathy. Int Heart J. 2017;58:238-44.

CHAPTER 68

Future of Interventional Cardiology

VK Bahl, Dinkar Bhasin

INTRODUCTION

It has been over 40 years since the first percutaneous coronary intervention (PCI) was done and 15 years since transcatheter aortic valve replacement was developed. These procedures have evolved considerably and have likely reached peak levels of safety and efficacy. The focus of interventional cardiology has now shifted to novel therapies for other forms of structural heart disease. Herein, we review the new interventional technologies on the horizon.

PERCUTANEOUS MITRAL VALVE THERAPIES

Surgical repair of mitral valve (MV) is often successful but, in contemporary practice, patients with severe mitral regurgitation (MR) have several comorbid conditions which increase the risk of surgical therapy. Hence, arises the need for safe and efficacious percutaneous therapies for MV. Technologies have been developed for both primary and secondary MR and these device systems target the various components of MV apparatus including the valve leaflets, annulus, chordae, and ventricular attachments. The most widely studied device is MitraClip (Abbott Vascular) which has been compared in a randomized control trial (RCT) to surgical therapy, while evidence for other devices is either preclinical or preliminary.

MitraClip involves implantation of 1–4 mm V-shaped clips across anterior and posterior mitral leaflets, approximating them and converting a single large regurgitant orifice into two small orifices. The procedure is done under transesophageal echo and fluoroscopic guidance. A 24Fr delivery sheath is introduced into left atrium (LA) via trans-septal puncture. A single clip is generally sufficient for functional MR while degenerative MV disease often requires at least two clips for additional stability. The EVEREST II trial compared MitraClip with surgical therapy and showed that with MitraClip there were increased rates 3+ to 4+ MR (12.3% vs. 1.8%; $p = 0.02$), higher rates of surgery (27.9% vs. 8.9%; $p = 0.003$) but similar 5-year mortality rates (20.8% and 26.8%; $p = 0.4$).[1] Currently, MitraClip is considered a class IIb recommendation in patients who are not operable or at high risk with surgery.[2,3] The PASCAL device (Edwards Lifesciences, California, USA) is a similar device that allows each MV leaflet to be grasped independently followed by apposition. It has been used on compassionate grounds in patients with severe MR which is not suited for repair with MitraClip.[4]

Devices targeting the chordal apparatus include the NeoChord DS1000 (Neochord, Inc.) and Harpoon TSD-5 devices (Harpoon Medical). Both are polytetrafluoroethylene (PTFE) sutures implanted on a beating heart using minimally invasive transapical approach and are tethered to the apical myocardium, thereby, preventing leaflet prolapse. Initial experience with the NeoChord device showed a reduction in MR severity to grade ≤ +2 in over 85% of the patients and the device was CE approved in 2012.[5]

A wide range of percutaneous mitral annuloplasty devices have also been developed. The Cardioband (Valtech Cardio, or Yehuda) device is a polyester band with multiple 6 mm stainless steel anchors and is implanted via 25Fr trans-septal access system into the atrial aspect of the mitral annulus posteriorly. The band is tightened after implantation resulting in annular shortening.[6] The Carillon device (Cardiac Dimensions) is another option for percutaneous annuloplasty that is delivered into the coronary sinus. It consists of a curvilinear nitinol wire with two self-expanding nitinol anchors at either end which are implanted in the coronary sinus and great cardiac vein, along the posterior atrioventricular groove resulting in the approximation of the posterior mitral annulus.[7] Mitraign (Mitralign, Inc., Tewksbury, MA) is a suture-based annuloplasty technology. It involves delivery of a suture and pledgets along the posterior margins of the annulus (P1 and P3 scallops) from the left ventricle (LV) aspect using a deflectable catheter. The suture and pledgets are tightened resulting in narrowing of the anteroposterior dimension of MV annulus.

Percutaneous ventriculoplasty devices have been developed to improve LV geometry and decrease MR.[8] VenTouch (Mardil Medical) consists of an inflatable chamber positioned along the external posterolateral aspect of LV by a left thoracotomy. Inflation of the device reduces LV and annular dimensions and improves leaflet coaptation. The Accucinch system (Ancora Heart) consists of multiple nitinol anchors connected by a nitinol wire and is delivered via retrograde access across the aortic valve into the base of the LV. Tightening of the nitinol wire cinches the basal LV and hence, the mitral annulus, thereby improving leaflet apposition.

Transcatheter MV replacement is a feasible option when percutaneous repair is not possible or has failed. However, unlike aortic valve replacement, MV interventions are more complex. The annulus is saddle-shaped increasing risk of paravalvular leak and annular calcification is rare, making anchorage of the valve difficult. Critical nearby structures such as the left ventricular outflow tract, conduction system, and the circumflex artery are at risk of iatrogenic damage. The use of trancatheter aortic valves such as the Sapient XT valve via transapical approach was associated with poor results, necessitating the development of special valves for the mitral position. The currently available valves include CardiAQ (CardiAQ Valve Technologies), Tiara (Neovasc Inc., British Columbia, Canada), Tendyne (Tendyne Inc.), and Medtronic-Intrepid (Medtronic Inc.). All valves are trileaflet bioprosthetic valves with self-expanding nitinol frame. Valve anchoring is either axial to the LV apex (Tendyne) or radial to the annulus with most devices having addition design features to reduce paravalvular leak. Delivery approaches vary among the devices being apical or trans-septal with delivery systems ranging in size from 26 to 42 Fr.[9]

Percutaneous Tricuspid Valve Therapies

The significance of functional tricuspid regurgitation (TR) has been highlighted in recent studies showing that it is associated with decreased long-term survival independent of left ventricular function, right ventricular function, or pulmonary hypertension.[10] Surgery for severe TR is associated with a high mortality and medical management alone is often suboptimal. There is a growing unmet need for effective percutaneous tricuspid valve (TV) interventions for patients with functional TR. The major mechanisms of functional TR are annular dilation and leaflet tethering because of structural changes in the right ventricle. Several devices targeting these pathophysiologic mechanisms have been developed but the clinical experience is limited. Preoperative evaluation involves the use of multimodality imaging including transthoracic echocardiography (TTE), transesophageal echocardiography (TEE), and computed tomography (CT) for delineation of the anatomy of the valve and neighboring structures such as coronary sinus ostium and the right coronary artery. The procedures are done using TEE and fluoroscopic guidance.

Annuloplasty devices reduce the tricuspid annulus by percutaneous or minimally invasive procedures. The Trialign device (Mitralign, Inc., Tewksbury, USA) is similar to the Mitralign device used for percutaneous MV annuloplasty. It percutaneously delivers pledgets and sutures the anteroposterior and septoposterior commissures of the TV reducing the annulus size. A recent study with this device showed a 30-day success rate of 80% with a significant reduction in severity of TR and improvement in New York Heart Association (NYHA) functional class.[11] Tricinch (4Tech Cardio, Galway, Ireland) is another percutaneous device being studied for TV annuloplasty and consists of a stainless-steel cork-screw implant that is delivered transcavally into the anterior TV annulus, and is connected by an adjustable Dacron band to a self-expanding nitinol stent implanted in the inferior vena cava (IVC). The implant tenses the TV annulus, decreases its dimensions, and decreases TR. The stent in the IVC maintains the tension. The Cardioband, used for percutaneous MV annuloplasty, has also been implanted for the TV annuloplasty.

The FORMA repair system (Edwards Lifesciences, California, USA) is a novel coaptation device which aims to reduce the effective regurgitant orifice area by providing a structure on which the TV leaflets can coapt. It consists of a rail which is screwed to the RV apex and a spacer anchored to this rail, which facilitates coaptation. The spacer consists of foam-filled polymer balloon with holes in its shaft and undergoes passive expansion after deployment. A recent study of 18 patients reported a success rate of 89% with no major peri-procedural complications and reduction in severity of TR in 46% at 1-year. Significant improvement in NYHA class and 6-minute walk distance (6MWD) were reported.[12]

MitraClip has been used in the tricuspid position for clipping the anterior and posterior tricuspid leaflets and reducing the regurgitant orifice. Observational data from 64 patients showed that the procedure was successful in 97% and reduction of TR severity by at least 1 grade occurred in 91% of the patients. There was a significant improvement in the NYHA class and 6MWD.[13]

Caval valve implantation involves heterotopic valve implantation in the IVC and the superior vena cava (SVC) in contrast to orthotropic valve implantation which is done at the site of normal TV. The valves do not prevent TR but decrease the hemodynamic consequences and right-sided congestive symptoms. However, they are only useful for patients with pulsatile blood flow in the vena cava and evidence of systolic flow reversal. The Tric Valve (P&F Products & Features Vertriebs GmbH, Austria, and Braile Biomedica, Brazil) consists of two self-expanding bioprosthetic valves made of bovine pericardium on a nitinol frame. One valve is implanted in the SVC-right atrium (RA) junction and other at the IVC-RA junction above the diaphragm to avoid hepatic vein compromise. The procedure is straightforward but the valve has only been used on a compassionate basis in severely ill patients, often with multiple comorbidities, and systematic data are lacking. Commercially available balloon-expandable valves used to treat aortic stenosis, such as Edwards Sapien XT or Sapien 3 (Edwards Lifesciences, California, USA) valve, have also been implanted in the vena cava to decrease regurgitant flow. This procedure requires presenting of large-sized vena cava to stabilize the valves and is generally done only for the IVC. These valves have also been used for valve-in-valve and valve-in-ring procedures for patients who have previously undergone TV replacement and TV repair, respectively.[14]

Left Atrial Appendage Occlusion

Warfarin therapy decreases the risk of stroke in patients with atrial fibrillation (AF) by over 60% compared to placebo.[15] Over 90% of the thrombi in nonvalvular AF form in the left atrial appendage (LAA) and the majority of the AF-related strokes occur from embolism of LAA thrombi.[16] Percutaneous LAA occlusion was developed as a treatment option for stroke prevention in patients who have AF but cannot tolerate long-term oral anticoagulation. Eligible candidates include patients with prior severe bleeding (intracranial bleed or severe gastrointestinal bleed), patients requiring combined use of dual antiplatelet therapy and anticoagulation, patients with labile international normalized ratio (INR) values, patients with thrombocytopenia or other coagulation defects, poor compliance with anticoagulant therapy, and patients with recurrence of stroke on oral anticoagulation. The procedure is contraindicated in patients with absolute contraindications to anticoagulation as postprocedure anticoagulation is necessary. The Watchman device (Boston Scientific, Minnesota, USA) is the only device tested in RCTs and approved by FDA for percutaneous LAA occlusion.

The Watchman device is a self-expanding nitinol cage covered with a PTFE membrane and has ten fixation anchors for holding the device in the LAA. The device is available in 5 sizes from 21 to 33 mm (in 3 mm increments); the size corresponds to the width of the expanded device at its shoulders. Preprocedural evaluation requires baseline TEE and CT imaging to assess LAA anatomy and rule out pre-existing thrombi. The device is selected based on the maximum width of LAA ostium; 8–20% compression of the original device size is acceptable. Implantation is done via antegrade access across the atrial septum using a 14 Fr delivery sheath. Aspirin (81–100 mg) is started one day before the procedure and warfarin is added postprocedure to maintain an INR between 2–3 for at least 45 days or longer depending upon TEE assessment after that interval. After stopping warfarin, clopidogrel is added to aspirin and continued until 6 months after implantation, and thereafter aspirin (300–325 mg) is continued indefinitely.[17,18]

Two RCTs (PROTECT-AF and PREVAIL) have evaluated the Watchman device in comparison to oral anticoagulation.[19,20] Meta-analysis of these trials demonstrated that the Watchman device was noninferior to warfarin therapy for postprocedure ischemic stroke or systemic embolism.[21] Significantly lower rates of nonprocedure related [hazard ratio (HR) = 0.48; p = 0.0003] major bleeding, hemorrhagic stroke (HR: 0.20; p = 0.0022), and all-cause mortality (HR: 0.73; p = 0.035) were observed in the device group. Recent observational studies have reported procedural success rates of more than 98% and rates of major periprocedural complications being less than 2% (pericardial tamponade in ~1% patients).[22] The Amplatzer Amulet LAA occlusion device (Abbott Vascular, Illinois, USA) is currently being studied in a noninferiority trial comparing it with the Watchman device.

Patent Foramen Oval Occlusion

Cryptogenic ischemic stroke is diagnosed when the recognizable causes of stroke have been excluded including atheroembolism, cardioembolic stroke, small vessel disease, coagulation disorders, and arterial dissection. The prevalence of patent foramen ovale (PFO) in cryptogenic stroke is 40–50%.[23] The reference standard for noninvasive detection of PFO is TEE with a bubble contrast study. Transcranial Doppler has a sensitivity of 97% and specificity of 93%.[24] The sensitivity and specificity of TTE with harmonic imaging and using bubble contrast is 91% and 93%, respectively.[25] Percutaneous PFO occlusion has emerged as a treatment option for patients with cryptogenic stroke and PFO.

The most widely used device is the Amplatzer PFO occluder (Abbott Vascular, Illinois, USA). The device is made of nitinol and consists of two disks with a 3-mm long connecting waist. Each disk has polyester mesh to prevent flow across the device. The device is available in 3 sizes: 18 mm, 25 mm, and 35 mm. The size is based on the RA disk size and decided based on the distance of the PFO from the aortic root and SVC orifice. The procedure is done under intracardiac echocardiography or TEE guidance. The device is delivered across the PFO using dedicated 8–9F delivery sheaths. NobleStitch EL device (HeartStitch, Inc., California, USA) uses a percutaneously delivered prolene sutures to appose the ostium primum and secundum and is in investigational stages.

Evidence from initial studies was conflicting. However, three recent trials that compared PFO closure to medical therapy for cryptogenic stroke (one trial each for Amplatzer device and Gore device, while the third allowed the physician to choose from a variety of devices) showed lower rates of recurrent stroke with device closure, although, rates of AF in patients undergoing device closure were higher.[26-28] A meta-analysis of all available RCTs showed that device closure decreases the risk of recurrent stroke by nearly two-thirds. However, the absolute annual risk of recurrent stroke with medical therapy alone was low (1.17%) and the number needed to treat (NNT) with device closure to prevent one stroke was 176. The benefit depends upon the size of the shunt with greater risk reduction in patients who have a large shunt (presence of >30 microbubbles in LA within three cycles after right atrial opacification) with a NNT of 96 but no benefit in patients with a small shunt. Device therapy resulted in a four-times higher annual risk of AF [risk ratio = 4.68, 95% confidence interval (CI) 2.19–10.00, $p < 0.001$, heterogeneity $I^2 = 27.5\%$] with a number needed to harm of 85.[29] However, other studies have shown that such AF generally occurs early (<45 days) as a single episode of paroxysmal AF and less than 4% of the patients with AF progress to permanent AF.[30] There was no difference in the rates of major bleeding and procedure-related complications in various trials ranged from 2.4 to 5.9%. Other meta-analyses have reported higher rates of absolute risk reduction ranging from 1.8 to 2.2%.[31,32] Further, the risk of AF may depend upon the device used with one trial using a particular device showing no increase in rates of AF.[27] Another small trial compared PFO device closure with antiplatelet therapy in patients with high-risk PFO defined as PFO with an atrial septal aneurysm, hypermobility (phasic septal excursion into either atrium ≥10 mm), or PFO size (maximum separation of the septum primum from the secundum) more than or equal to 2 mm. There was no recurrence of stroke at the end of 2 years in the device group compared with a rate of 12.9% in patients on medication alone.[33]

Interatrial Shunt Device

Heart failure with a preserved ejection fraction (HFpEF) comprises nearly 50% of all patients with heart failure. The pathophysiologic basis is abnormal left ventricular relaxation resulting in elevation of LA pressure, pulmonary congestion, and leading to symptoms. The interatrial shunt device (Corvia Medical) was designed to percutaneously create an iatrogenic defect in interatrial septum with the objective of decompressing LA and reducing LA pressure. Eligible candidates are patient with NYHA class II–IV symptoms, LV ejection fraction more than or equal to 40% and elevated pulmonary capillary wedge pressure (PCWP ≥15 mmHg resting or ≥ during 25 supine bicycle exercise). The device is made of nitinol with an outer diameter of 18 mm and creates an 8 mm atrial septal defect. It is deployed by a standard interatrial septal puncture using a preloaded 16 Fr delivery system.

Limited evidence is available for the use of this device. A phase I study showed a success rate of 94% (64 out of 68 patients) and no major device-related complications during 6 months follow-up with reduction in resting PCWP in over 50% of the patients.[34] A phase II sham-controlled RCT with 44 patients showed a significant reduction in PCWP during exercise and no major adverse cardiac, cerebrovascular, and renal events at 1 month.[35]

Another device which has been developed is the V-Wave shunt device (V-Wave, Caesarea, Israel). It is an hourglass-shaped implant with a nitinol frame, PTFE encapsulation and a one-way bioprosthetic valve (porcine pericardium) to prevent paradoxical embolism. A proof-of-concept cohort study in patients with heart failure with reduced ejection fraction (EF <40%; n = 10 patients) showed improvement in NYHA class in eight patients and reduction in PCWP by 6 mmHg at 3 months.[36]

Robotic Percutaneous Coronary Intervention

Robotic PCI was developed to reduce the risk of radiation exposure and orthopedic injuries to PCI operator. The robotic system consists of a bedside robotic arm and a radiation shielded physician workstation located in the cath lab. The robotic arm has a disposable cassette in which the angioplasty equipment including wires, balloons, and stents are loaded. Vascular access is obtained manually, the coronary artery is engaged with the guide catheter by the operator, and the guide catheter is connected to the Y-connector of the robotic arm. The guidewire is advanced through the opposite end of the robotic arm into the guide catheter. Thereafter, the guidewire is advanced under robotic control. Angioplasty catheters are loaded manually and are then advanced by robotic assistance. The workstation has a console with three joysticks for manipulating the wire, balloon catheter, and guide catheter. It also displays hemodynamic data, vital parameters, and fluoroscopic image with the facility of computerized angiographic analysis. Corindus CorPath 200 (Corindus Vascular Robotics, Massachusetts, USA) was approved by the FDA in 2012 and the second-generation system CorPath GRX has been recently approved.

The PRECISE (Percutaneous Robotically Enhanced Coronary Intervention) trial was a multicenter registry study of 164 patients which showed that robotic PCI is feasible and safe in simple lesions without an increase in patient radiation or contrast use.[37] The CORA-PCI (Complex Robotically Assisted Percutaneous Coronary Intervention) study evaluated CorPath 200 in a real-world cohort of 315 patients. Technical success with robotic PCI was 91.7%, manual assistance was required in 11.1% of cases, and manual conversion in 7.4%. Clinical success, stent use, and fluoroscopy time were similar between robotic and conventional PCI. However, procedure time was longer in the robotic group (44:30 ± 26:04 mins vs. 36:34 ± 23:03 mins; p = 0.002).[38] There is also some evidence to suggest a trend toward decreased geographic miss with robotic PCI, as the robotic system allows sub-millimeter movements of angioplasty equipment.

The greatest drawback of this system is the absence of tactile feedback. It also does not allow the use of over the wire equipment such as over the wire balloons, microcatheters, and rota-ablation catheters and hence, has limited utility for complex lesions. Further, simultaneous balloon inflation as needed in dedicated bifurcation lesions is also not possible. While the angioplasty equipment can be advanced using the robotic arm, balloon and stent inflation is done by the operator. Lastly, the robotic PCI increases the operator learning curve, procedure time, and cost. Robotic systems have also been studied for electrophysiologic radiofrequency ablation procedures.

Quantitative Flow Ratio

Fractional flow reserve (FFR) is considered the reference standard for evaluation of intermediate coronary stenosis but requires expensive pressure wires, use of intravenous adenosine, and increases the procedure time. Quantitative flow ratio (QFR) is a computer-derived FFR calculated from three-dimensional quantitative angiography (3D-QCA) without the use of adenosine. A diagnostic angiogram is performed in two projections which are at least 25° apart and 3D-QCA reconstruction done. The contrast flow velocity is estimated by frame count during baseline conditions. The QFR is then calculated using complex computerized equations that derive the pressure drop across a lesion based on the geometry of the stenosis as assessed by 3D-QCA.[39] A prospective study of 308 patients showed that QFR had a higher sensitivity and specificity for detecting hemodynamically-significant stenosis when compared with QCA considering FFR as gold standard (sensitivity: 94.6% vs. 62.5%, difference: 32.0%, p <0.001; specificity: 91.7% vs. 58.1%, difference: 36.1%, p <0.001). The overall patient-level diagnostic accuracy of QFR was 92.4%.[40]

Coronary Lithoplasty

Coronary lithoplasty is a novel technique to tackle calcified coronary lesions. The lithoplasty system consists of a 6F compatible balloon angioplasty catheter that is introduced on a standard guidewire to the target lesion. The catheter contains electrohydraulic lithotripsy emitters which convert electrical energy into acoustic pressure pulses that disrupt coronary calcium. The balloon is connected to the generator, inflated at a pressure of 4 atmosphere and prespecified lithotripsy pulses delivered. Optical coherence tomography studies have shown that lithoplasty results in circumferential fractures in superficial and deep calcium increasing the minimum luminal area.[41] Limited observational data (DISRUPT-CAD study, n = 60 patients) available for the device shows good procedural success rates, with rates of stent delivery being 100% and with no flow-limiting dissections, abrupt closure or perforation being reported. The device is approved by FDA for peripheral interventions and has received the CE approval for coronary interventions.[42]

Coronary Sinus Reducer for Refractory Angina

Coronary sinus reducer (CSR) is a novel treatment option for patients with refractory angina who are not candidates for revascularization. Data from animal studies has shown that obstruction of the coronary sinus increases the coronary venous pressure, redistributes the blood from ischemic to nonischemic zones, and reduces myocardial ischemia. Surgical narrowing of the coronary sinus improves myocardial perfusion. Percutaneous implantation of CSR is based on the same principle by creating a focal narrowing in the coronary sinus by utilizing an implantable device.

The CSR (Neovasc Medical, Inc., Or Yehuda, Israel) is a balloon-mounted, bare metal, stainless steel stent which on expansion is shaped like an hourglass (the balloon has the same shape). The device is available in a single size and is suitable for variable anatomies. The procedure is performed under fluoroscopic guidance via right jugular venous approach. The coronary sinus is cannulated using a diagnostic 6F multipurpose or Amplatz catheter, a selective angiogram is done to assess anatomy and a 9F-guiding catheter is advanced over the diagnostic catheter. The device is advanced over a coronary guidewire and balloon inflated at 2–6 atmospheres. The procedure is done on an outpatient basis, and dual antiplatelet therapy is advised for 6 months after the procedure.[43] The device received CE approval in November 2011 but is not currently approved by the FDA.

The best available evidence for CSR comes from a small RCT comparing CSR to placebo. There was a significantly greater number of patients who experienced a reduction in Canadian Cardiovascular Society angina scale by 2 classes (35% vs. 15%; p = 0.02%) and improvement in the quality of life as assessed by Seattle Angina Questionnaire after CSR implantation. However, the trial did not show any difference between the two groups in exercise time or provocable ischemia as assessed by dobutamine echocardiography, and cardiovascular outcomes were not assessed.[44] Compassionate use of the CSR for patients with microvascular angina has also been reported, with limited data available on the same.

Percutaneous Ventricular Restoration

Percutaneous ventricular restoration (PVR) involves delivery of a ventricular partition device to isolate the aneurysmal LV apex from the remaining cavity, thereby, decreasing LV volume, restoring geometry and improving ventricular mechanics. The Parachute device (CardioKinetix Inc., California, USA) consists of an occlusive PTFE membrane bonded to a self-expanding nitinol frame in the shape of an inverted umbrella. It has 16 metallic struts with 2 mm anchors at the wide end which engage the myocardium and a collapsible foot which rests on the LV apex. The device is available in eight sizes. It is delivered by retrograde transaortic access with a 14–16F guide catheter by using a screwing delivery system which has an inflatable balloon for expanding the device and engaging the myocardium. Preprocedure screening is done by TTE and all eligible patients should undergo contrast-enhanced CT for evaluating cardiac anatomy. Anatomic criteria for device therapy are ejection fraction less than 40% with akinetic or aneurysmal apex, LV end-diastolic diameter greater than 55 mm, LV wall thickness greater than 3.5 mm, apical dimensions 4 × 5 cm, and normal trabeculations and papillary muscles.[45]

Evidence for the use of parachute device is available from observational studies. The largest study, PARACHUTE III (n = 100 patients) demonstrated procedural success rate of 97% with major periprocedural adverse events at 7% with one death. At the end of 1 year, there was significant LV volume reduction, improvement in 6MWD and mean NYHA class.[46] A large pivotal RCT to test the efficacy of PVR is currently underway.

Endogenous Tissue Restoration

Percutaneous valve implantation has revolutionized the management of valvular disorders. However, the implanted prostheses are xenografts made from native animal valves or pericardium that incite a chronic inflammatory reaction and undergo structural degeneration requiring repeat interventions. Endogenous tissue restoration (Xeltis BV, Eindhoven, Netherlands) is a novel technology for valve replacement that aims to provide a synthetic bioresorbable scaffold which allows the endogenous host tissue to regenerate. Unlike standard bioresorbable polymers, such as polyglycolic acid, these scaffolds are made of a special supramolecular polymer which is electrospun into matrices allowing space for native tissue to regrow. The technology has been used to develop extracardiac Fontan conduits, valved pulmonary conduits for right ventricular outflow tract reconstruction, and aortic valves.[47] The Fontan conduit has been studied in five children and 2-year follow-up results showed good hemodynamic and structural performance. The pulmonary valved conduit has undergone a successful preclinical study and has been successfully implanted in 12 children with good periprocedural outcomes and long-term results are awaited. A preclinical animal study of the aortic valve has shown good hemodynamic results with only mild AR being reported.[48] These valves may usher in a new frontier in valve replacement therapy in the coming years.

Pulmonary Artery Denervation

An imbalance between the local vasoconstrictor and vasodilator tone, and an exaggerated local baroreflex has been implicated in increasing the pulmonary artery pressures (PAP) in patients with idiopathic pulmonary artery hypertension. Pulmonary artery denervation (PADN) was initially studied in animals where it was successful in abolishing the elevation of PAP that occurs after occlusion of an interlobar artery.[49] Animal studies also showed that there is an immediate decrease in mean PAP and pulmonary vascular resistance and this is associated with histologic changes in the adventitial nerves.[50] Ablation is done using a dedicated 7Fr PADN radiofrequency catheter with 10 ablation electrodes arranged in a circular fashion. The catheter is introduced into the main pulmonary artery (MPA) in an 8 Fr sheath and ablation is given at three levels: proximal to the bifurcation in the MPA, distal to the bifurcation in the right pulmonary artery, and distal to the bifurcation in left pulmonary artery.

The first-in-man study of PADN in 13 patients with idiopathic pulmonary arterial hypertension not responding to medical therapy showed a significant reduction in mean PAP (55.5–36.5 mmHg, p <0.01) and improvement in 6MWD (324 ± 21 m to 491 ± 38 m, p <0.006) over a period of 3-months.[51] The phase II results of PADN study showed that there was a hemodynamic success (defined as a reduction in mean PAP by at least 10% of baseline) in 94% patients. There was an absolute decrease in mean systolic PAP and mean PAP of –10 mmHg and –7 mmHg, respectively, within 24 hours with no major periprocedural complications. At 6 months there was a significant decrease in mean PAP (44.8 ± 16.4 vs. 53.1 ± 19.1) and PVR (8.4 ±5.4 Woods units vs. 13.2 ± 6.9 Woods units), increase in 6MWD by a mean of 94 ± 73 m, and WHO functional class improved in 63.6% patients.[52] A small study in 16 patients with chronic thromboembolic pulmonary hypertension with residual hypertension after pulmonary endarterectomy also showed a reduction in mean PAP (37.3–24.6 mmHg; p = 0.01) and decrease in PVR (672 dyn·s·cm^{-5} to 386 dyn·s·cm^{-5}; p = 0.02).[53]

Renal Denervation

Renal denervation targets the renal sympathetic nervous system supply by percutaneous radiofrequency ablation in the renal arteries. The procedure was developed as a treatment option for resistant hypertension. Initial studies showed a significant reduction in systolic blood pressure (SBP) and excellent procedural safety, but the sham-controlled SYMPLICITY HTN-3 trial showed no significant difference in mean office SBP or mean ambulatory blood pressure after 6 months.[54] The SYMPLICITY HTN-3 trial, however, had several limitations confounding the interpretation and generalization of results. The enrolled patients had treatment-resistant hypertension and underwent frequent drug changes during the study period. The ablation catheter (Simplicity Flex Catheter, Medtronic, Inc., California, USA) used was unipolar, required precise positioning and multiple ablations from distal to proximal, such that the complexity of the procedure may have resulted in incomplete denervation.[55]

The SPYRAL HTN-OFF MED was a sham-controlled proof-of-concept RCT designed to assess the effects of renal denervation on SBP in treatment naïve patients. The trial used an advanced, easy-to-use, self-positioning catheter (Symplicity Spyral Catheter, Medtronic, Inc., California, USA) with multiple electrodes, giving simultaneous four-quadrant ablations which were done in the main and side branches. The 3 month results of the trial showed significant decrease in office and 24-hour ambulatory blood pressure in the renal denervation group: 24-hour SBP –5.5 mmHg (95% CI –9.1 to –2.0; p = 0.0031); 24-hour diastolic blood pressure (DBP) –4.8 mmHg (–7.0 to –2.6; p <0.0001); office SBP –10.0 mmHg (–15.1 to –4.9; p = 0.0004); and office DBP –5.3 mmHg (–7.8 to –2.7; p = 0.0002). No significant changes were seen in the sham-control group. No major adverse events were observed in either group.[56] The SPYRAL HTN-ON MED trial was a similarly designed study (sham-controlled proof-of-concept RCT; n = 80) but evaluated renal denervation in patients with uncontrolled hypertension on antihypertensive therapy. At 6 months, the change in blood pressure was significantly greater in the renal denervation group than the sham-control group: office SBP (difference –6.8 mmHg, 95% CI –12.5 to –1.1; p = 0.0205) and 24-hour SBP (difference –7.4 mmHg, –12.5 to –2.3; p = 0.0051). No major adverse events were observed.[57]

A recently developed technology utilizes endovascular ultrasound energy for thermal ablation of renal sympathetic nerves (Paradise renal denervation system, ReCor Medical, California, USA). The catheter is placed percutaneously in the renal arteries, centered with a water-filled cooling balloon and achieves a circumferential ring of ablation. The RADIANCE-HTN SOLO study was a single-blinded sham controlled RCT (n = 146) evaluating this technology which showed significantly greater reduction in daytime ambulatory SBP with renal denervation [–8.5 mmHg, standard deviations (SD) 9.3] than with the sham procedure (–2.2 mmHg, SD 10.0; baseline-adjusted difference between groups: –6.3 mmHg, 95% CI –9.4 to –3.1, p = 0.0001). There were no major adverse events in either group.[58]

CONCLUSION

Several upcoming technologies are set to revolutionize interventional cardiology. Foremost among them are devices for percutaneous mitral and tricuspid valve repair. PFO occlusion has shown benefit in the management of cryptogenic stroke. Interatrial shunt device offers a novel treatment strategy for patients with HFpEF. QFR allows physiologic assessment during routine coronary angiogram using special software. Renal artery denervation has witnessed renewed interest with encouraging results from recent trials. Pulmonary artery denervation offers a new therapeutic option for patients with pulmonary hypertension. Finally, in the future, prosthetic implants may be replaced by the endogenous tissue restoration which allows regeneration of native tissue over bioresorbable scaffolds.

REFERENCES

1. Feldman T, Kar S, Elmariah S, et al. (2015). Randomized Comparison of Percutaneous Repair and Surgery for Mitral Regurgitation. [online] Available from http://www.onlinejacc.org/content/66/25/2844 [Accessed July 2018].
2. Nishimura RA, Otto CM, Bonow RO, et al. 2017 AHA/ACC Focused Update of the 2014 AHA/ACC Guideline for the Management of Patients With Valvular Heart Disease: A Report of the American College of Cardiology/American Heart Association Task Force on Clinical Practice Guidelines. Circulation. 20171;135(25):e1159-95.
3. Baumgartner H, Falk V, Bax JJ, et al. 2017 ESC/EACTS Guidelines for the management of valvular heart disease. [online] Available from https://academic.oup.com/eurheartj/article/38/36/2739/4095039#supplementary-data [Accessed July 2018].
4. Praz F, Spargias K, Chrissoheris M, et al. Compassionate use of the PASCAL transcatheter mitral valve repair system for patients with severe mitral regurgitation: a multicentre, prospective, observational, first-in-man study. Lancet Lond Engl. 2017;390:773-80.
5. Seeburger J, Rinaldi M, Nielsen SL, et al. Off-pump transapical implantation of artificial neo-chordae to correct mitral regurgitation: the TACT Trial (Transapical Artificial Chordae Tendinae) proof of concept. J Am Coll Cardiol. 2014;63:914-9.
6. Maisano F, Taramasso M, Nickenig G, et al. Cardioband, a transcatheter surgical-like direct mitral valve annuloplasty system: early results of the feasibility trial. Eur Heart J. 2016;37:817-25.
7. Schofer J, Siminiak T, Haude M, et al. Percutaneous Mitral Annuloplasty for Functional Mitral Regurgitation: Results of the CARILLON Mitral Annuloplasty Device European Union Study. Circulation. 2009;120:326-33.
8. Sorajja P, Leon MB, Adams DH, et al. Transcatheter Therapy for Mitral Regurgitation Clinical Challenges and Potential Solutions. Circulation. 2017;136: 404-17.
9. Al-Lawati A, Cheung A. Transcatheter Mitral Valve Replacement. Interv Cardiol Clin. 2016;5:109-15.
10. Nath J, Foster E, Heidenreich PA. Impact of tricuspid regurgitation on long-term survival. J Am Coll Cardiol. 2004;43:405-9.
11. Hahn RT, Meduri CU, Davidson CJ, et al. Early Feasibility Study of a Transcatheter Tricuspid Valve Annuloplasty: SCOUT Trial 30-Day Results. J Am Coll Cardiol. 2017;69:1795-806.
12. Perlman G, Praz F, Puri R, et al. Transcatheter Tricuspid Valve Repair With a New Transcatheter Coaptation System for the Treatment of Severe Tricuspid Regurgitation. JACC Cardiovasc Interv. 2017;10:1994-2003.
13. Nickenig G, Kowalski M, Hausleiter J, et al. Transcatheter Treatment of Severe Tricuspid Regurgitation With the Edge-to-Edge MitraClip Technique. Circulation. 2017;135:1802-14.
14. Lauten A, Dreger H, Laule M, et al. Caval Valve Implantation. Interv Cardiol Clin. 2018;7:57-63.
15. Stroke Prevention in Atrial Fibrillation Study. Final results. Circulation. 1991; 84:527-39.
16. Blackshear JL, Odell JA. Appendage obliteration to reduce stroke in cardiac surgical patients with atrial fibrillation. Ann Thorac Surg. 1996;61:755-9.
17. Price MJ. The WATCHMAN Left Atrial Appendage Closure Device. Interv Cardiol Clin. 2018;7:201-12.
18. Piccini JP, Sievert H, Patel MR. Left atrial appendage occlusion: rationale, evidence, devices, and patient selection. Eur Heart J. 2016;38(12):869-76.
19. Reddy VY, Doshi SK, Sievert H, et al. Percutaneous left atrial appendage closure for stroke prophylaxis in patients with atrial fibrillation: 2.3-Year Follow-up of the PROTECT AF (Watchman Left Atrial Appendage System for Embolic Protection in Patients with Atrial Fibrillation) Trial. Circulation. 2013;127:720-9.
20. Holmes DR, Kar S, Price MJ, et al. Prospective randomized evaluation of the Watchman Left Atrial Appendage Closure device in patients with atrial fibrillation versus long-term warfarin therapy: the PREVAIL trial. J Am Coll Cardiol. 2014;64:1-12.
21. Reddy VY, Doshi SK, Kar S, et al. 5-Year Outcomes After Left Atrial Appendage Closure. J Am Coll Cardiol. 2017;70:2964-75.
22. Boersma LVA, Schmidt B, Betts TR, et al. Implant success and safety of left atrial appendage closure with the WATCHMAN device: peri-procedural outcomes from the EWOLUTION registry. Eur Heart J. 2016;37:2465-74.
23. Mojadidi MK, Zaman MO, Elgendy IY, et al. Cryptogenic Stroke and Patent Foramen Ovale. J Am Coll Cardiol. 2018;71:1035-43.
24. Mojadidi MK, Roberts SC, Winoker JS, et al. Accuracy of Transcranial Doppler for the Diagnosis of Intracardiac Right-to-Left Shunt: A Bivariate Meta-Analysis of Prospective Studies. JACC Cardiovasc Imaging. 2014;7:236-50.
25. Mojadidi MK, Winoker JS, Roberts SC, et al. Two-dimensional echocardiography using second harmonic imaging for the diagnosis of intracardiac right-to-left shunt: a meta-analysis of prospective studies. Int J Cardiovasc Imaging. 2014;30:911-23.
26. Mas JL, Derumeaux G, Guillon B, et al. Patent Foramen Ovale Closure or Anticoagulation vs. Antiplatelets after Stroke. N Engl J Med. 2017;377:1011-21.
27. Saver JL, Carroll JD, Thaler DE, et al. Long-Term Outcomes of Patent Foramen Ovale Closure or Medical Therapy after Stroke. N Engl J Med. 2017;377:1022-32.
28. Søndergaard L, Kasner SE, Rhodes JF, et al. Patent Foramen Ovale Closure or Antiplatelet Therapy for Cryptogenic Stroke. N Engl J Med. 2017;377:1033-42.
29. Ahmad Y, Howard JP, Arnold A, et al. Patent foramen ovale closure vs. medical therapy for cryptogenic stroke: a meta-analysis of randomized controlled trials. Eur Heart J. 2018;39:1638-49.
30. Staubach S, Steinberg DH, Zimmermann W, et al. New onset atrial fibrillation after patent foramen ovale closure. Catheter Cardiovasc Interv. 2009;74(6):889-95.
31. Abo-salem E, Chaitman B, Helmy T, et al. Patent foramen ovale closure versus medical therapy in cases with cryptogenic stroke, meta-analysis of randomized controlled trials. J Neurol. 2018;265:578-85.
32. Mojadidi MK, Elgendy AY, Elgendy IY, et al. Transcatheter Patent Foramen Ovale Closure After Cryptogenic Stroke. JACC Cardiovasc Interv. 2017;10:2228-30.
33. Lee PH, Song J-K, Kim JS, et al. Cryptogenic Stroke and High-Risk Patent Foramen Ovale. J Am Coll Cardiol. 2018;71:2335-42.
34. Hasenfuß G, Hayward C, Burkhoff D, et al. A transcatheter intracardiac shunt device for heart failure with preserved ejection fraction (REDUCE LAP-HF): a multicentre, open-label, single-arm, phase 1 trial. The Lancet. 2016;387:1298-304.
35. Feldman T, Mauri L, Kahwash R, et al. Transcatheter Interatrial Shunt Device for the Treatment of Heart Failure With Preserved Ejection Fraction (REDUCE LAP-HF I [Reduce Elevated Left Atrial Pressure in Patients With Heart Failure]): A Phase 2, Randomized, Sham-Controlled Trial. Circulation. 2018;137:364-75.
36. Trigo MD, Bergeron S, Bernier M, et al. Unidirectional left-to-right interatrial shunting for treatment of patients with heart failure with reduced ejection fraction: a safety and proof-of-principle cohort study. The Lancet. 2016;387:1290-7.
37. Weisz G, Metzger DC, Caputo RP, et al. Safety and feasibility of robotic percutaneous coronary intervention: PRECISE (Percutaneous Robotically-Enhanced Coronary Intervention) Study. J Am Coll Cardiol. 2013;61:1596-600.
38. Mahmud E, Naghi J, Ang L, et al. Demonstration of the Safety and Feasibility of Robotically Assisted Percutaneous Coronary Intervention in Complex Coronary Lesions. JACC Cardiovasc Interv. 2017;10:1320-7.
39. Tu S, Barbato E, Köszegi Z, et al. Fractional Flow Reserve Calculation From 3-Dimensional Quantitative Coronary Angiography and TIMI Frame Count. JACC Cardiovasc Interv. 2014;7:768-77.
40. Xu B, Tu S, Qiao S, et al. Diagnostic Accuracy of Angiography-Based Quantitative Flow Ratio Measurements for Online Assessment of Coronary Stenosis. J Am Coll Cardiol. 2017;70:3077-87.
41. Ali ZA, Brinton TJ, Hill JM, et al. Optical Coherence Tomography Characterization of Coronary Lithoplasty for Treatment of Calcified Lesions. JACC Cardiovasc Imaging. 2017;10:897-906.

42. Brinton TJ. (2016). DISRUPT CAD: A multicenter, prospective, single-arm study of percutaneous lithoplasty prior to stent implantation in heavily calcified coronary lesions. [online] Available from https://www.tctmd.com/slide/disrupt-cad-multicenter-prospective-single-arm-study-percutaneous-lithoplasty-prior-stent [Accessed July 2018].
43. Benedetto D, Abawi M, Stella PR, et al. (2016). Percutaneous Device to Narrow the Coronary Sinus: Shifting Paradigm in the Treatment of Refractory Angina? A Review of the Literature. [online] Available from http://journal.frontiersin.org/article/10.3389/fcvm.2016.00042/full [Accessed July 2018].
44. Verheye S, Jolicœur EM, Behan MW, et al. Efficacy of a Device to Narrow the Coronary Sinus in Refractory Angina. N Engl J Med. 2015;372:519-27.
45. Dhakal BP, Oliveira GH. Percutaneous Ventricular Restoration with a Partitioning Device for Ischemic Heart Failure Treatment. Curr Heart Fail Rep. 2017;14:87-99.
46. Thomas M, Nienaber CA, Ince H, et al. Percutaneous ventricular restoration (PVR) therapy using the Parachute device in 100 subjects with ischaemic dilated heart failure: one-year primary endpoint results of PARACHUTE III, a European trial. EuroIntervention 2015;11(6):710-7.
47. Serruys P, Miyazaki Y, Katsikis A, et al. Restorative valve therapy by endogenous tissue restoration: tomorrow's world? Reflection on the EuroPCR 2017 session on endogenous tissue restoration. EuroIntervention. 2017;13:AA68-77.
48. Yosuke M, Soliman OI, Mohammad A, et al. (2017). Acute performance of a novel restorative transcatheter aortic valve: preclinical results. [online] Available from: https://www.pcronline.com/eurointervention/127th_issue/volume-13/number-12/225/acute-performance-of-a-novel-restorative-transcatheter-aortic-valve-preclinical-results.html [Accessed July 2018].
49. Shao-Liang C, Yao-Jun Z, Lin Z, et al. (2013). Percutaneous pulmonary artery denervation completely abolishes experimental pulmonary arterial hypertension in vivo. [online] Available from https://www.pcronline.com/eurointervention/61st_issue/volume-9/number-2/43/percutaneous-pulmonary-artery-denervation-completely-abolishes-experimental-pulmonary-arterial-hypertension-in-vivo.html [Accessed July 2018].
50. Rothman AMK, Arnold ND, Chang W, et al. Pulmonary Artery Denervation Reduces Pulmonary Artery Pressure and Induces Histological Changes in an Acute Porcine Model of Pulmonary Hypertension. Circ Cardiovasc Interv. 2015;8(11):e002569.
51. Chen SL, Zhang FF, Xu J, et al. Pulmonary artery denervation to treat pulmonary arterial hypertension: the single-center, prospective, first-in-man PADN-1 study (first-in-man pulmonary artery denervation for treatment of pulmonary artery hypertension). J Am Coll Cardiol. 2013;62(12):1092-100.
52. Chen SL, Zhang H, Xie DJ, et al. Hemodynamic, functional, and clinical responses to pulmonary artery denervation in patients with pulmonary arterial hypertension of different causes: phase II results from the Pulmonary Artery Denervation-1 study. Circ Cardiovasc Interv. 2016;9(1):e003463.
53. CHernyavskiy AM, Edemskiy AG, Novikova NV, et al. [Radiofrequency Pulmonary Artery Ablation for Treatment of Residual Pulmonary Hypertension After Pulmonary Endarterectomy]. Kardiologiia. 2018;(4):15-21.
54. Bhatt DL, Kandzari DE, O'Neill WW, et al. A Controlled Trial of Renal Denervation for Resistant Hypertension. N Engl J Med. 2014;370:1393-401.
55. Kandzari DE, Bhatt DL, Brar S, et al. Predictors of blood pressure response in the SYMPLICITY HTN-3 trial. Eur Heart J. 2015;36:219-27.
56. Townsend RR, Mahfoud F, Kandzari DE, et al. Catheter-based renal denervation in patients with uncontrolled hypertension in the absence of antihypertensive medications (SPYRAL HTN-OFF MED): a randomised, sham-controlled, proof-of-concept trial. The Lancet. 2017;390:2160-70.
57. Kandzari DE, Böhm M, Mahfoud F, et al. Effect of renal denervation on blood pressure in the presence of antihypertensive drugs: 6-month efficacy and safety results from the SPYRAL HTN-ON MED proof-of-concept randomised trial. The Lancet. 2018;391:2346-55.
58. Azizi M, Schmieder RE, Mahfoud F, et al. Endovascular ultrasound renal denervation to treat hypertension (RADIANCE-HTN SOLO): a multicentre, international, single-blind, randomised, sham-controlled trial. The Lancet. 2018;391:2335-45.

SECTION 10

Intervention in Structural Heart Disease

CHAPTER 69

TAVR: Indications and Limitations in Clinical Practice

Tarun Chakravarty, Matthias Raschpichler, Chinar Patel, Raj Makkar

INTRODUCTION

Transcatheter aortic valve replacement (TAVR) is a minimally invasive treatment option for severe aortic stenosis (AS). The first case of TAVR in a human was performed in 2002 by Professor Alain Cribier.[1] With improved TAVR device technology, increasing operator experience, refinement in procedural techniques and patient selection, the field of TAVR has rapidly evolved. TAVR is now routinely performed for the treatment of severe symptomatic AS. A total of 54,782 TAVR procedures with commercially approved devices were performed in the United States from 2012 through December 2015.[2] In this chapter, we review the clinical evidence supporting the current indications for TAVR;[3-9] as well as limitations of this technology.

ELIGIBILITY FOR TRANSCATHETER AORTIC VALVE REPLACEMENT

The clinical trials evaluating the safety and efficacy of TAVR have enrolled patients, based on their surgical risk profile. The surgical risk in patients with severe symptomatic AS was assessed based on the Society of Thoracic Surgery (STS) risk score as well as presence of comorbidities that may not be captured in the STS score, for instance, extensively calcified (porcelain) aorta, cirrhosis, chest wall deformity or deleterious effects of chest wall irradiation, oxygen-dependent respiratory insufficiency, and/or frailty. Based on the surgical risk, the patients in clinical trials were stratified, according to surgical risk, into extreme risk/inoperable (STS score ≥15%; or risk of morbidity and mortality ≥50%),[3,8] high risk but operable (STS ≥10%; or 30-day mortality/morbidity ≥ 50%),[4,7] intermediate risk [STS 4–8% in PARTNER (Placement of Aortic Transcatheter Valves) 2A or STS 3–15% in SURTAVI (Surgical Replacement and Transcatheter Aortic Valve Implantation) trial][9,10] and low risk (STS <2% in PARTNER 3 or STS <3% in Evolut low-risk trial). The risk adjudication in all randomized controlled trials (RCTs) was performed by two cardiothoracic surgeons.

Randomized Clinical Trials (Table 1)

Extreme Risk to Inoperable Patients

The PARTNER 1B trial randomized 358 extreme risk to inoperable patients to transfemoral TAVR with Edwards SAPIEN valve (n = 179) (Edwards Lifesciences Inc., Irvine; CA) or standard therapy (including balloon aortic valvuloplasty) (n = 179).[3] The primary end point was rate of death from any cause. At 1 year, the rate of death from any cause was 30.7% with TAVR, as compared with 50.7% with standard therapy ($p < 0.001$). TAVR, compared with standard therapy, was also associated with a significant reduction in the composite rate of death/rehospitalization as well as significant improvement in quality of life. At 5 years, all-cause mortality was 71.8% in the TAVR group versus 93.6% in the standard treatment group ($p < 0.0001$).[5]

Following the results of the PARTNER 1B trial, a prospective nonrandomized registry of self-expanding CoreValve (Medtronic Inc., Minneapolis; MN) was initiated to evaluate the effectiveness of CoreValve for the treatment of extreme/prohibitive risk patients with severe AS.[8] To estimate the rate of death or major stroke in patients with AS at prohibitive risk for surgery treated with standard therapy, an objective performance goal (OPG) of 43% was determined from a meta-analysis of seven balloon aortic valvuloplasty studies as well as the results of the PARTNER 1B trial. The rate of all-cause mortality or stroke at 1 year observed during the study was 26.0% versus 43.0% with the OPG ($p < 0.0001$).

High Risk but Operable Patients

The PARTNER 1A trial randomized 699 high-risk patients with symptomatic severe AS to TAVR with Edwards SAPIEN valve (n = 348) or surgical aortic valve replacement (SAVR) (n = 351).[4] The primary end point was death from any cause at 1 year. The rate of death from any cause after at 1 year was not different after TAVR and SAVR, 1 year death rate being 24.2% and 26.8%, respectively ($p = 0.44$). At 5 years, the rate of death was 67.8% in the TAVR group compared with 62.4% in

TABLE 1: Summary of randomized clinical trials and prospective registries of transcatheter aortic valve replacement

	30-day outcomes					1-year outcomes		2-year outcomes		5-year outcomes	
	Mortality	Stroke	Moderate to severe PVL	Pacemaker	Major vascular complication	Mortality	Stroke	Mortality	Stroke	Mortality	Stroke
Extreme risk studies											
PARTNER 1B	5.0%	6.7%	11.8%	3.4%	16.2%	30.7%	10.6%			71.8%	16.0%
CoreValve extreme-risk study	8.4%	4.0%	11.4%	21.6%	8.2%	24.3%	7.0%				
High-risk studies											
PARTNER 1A	3.4%	4.7%	12.2%	3.8%	11.0%	24.2%	6.0%			67.8%	10.4%
CoreValve high-risk study	3.3%	4.9%	9.0%	19.8%	5.9%	14.2%	8.8%				
Intermediate risk studies											
PARTNER 2A	3.9%	5.5%	3.7%	8.5%	7.9%	12.3%	8.0%	16.7%	10%		
SURTAVI trial	2.2%	3.4%	10.0%	25.9%	6.0%	6.7%	5.4%	11.4%	6.2%		
Sapien 3 study	1.1%	2.7%	1.2%	10.2%	6.1%	7.4%	4.6%				

PVL, paravalvular leak.

the SAVR group (p = 0.76). There were no cases of structural valve deterioration requiring surgical valve replacement in either group. Moderate or severe aortic regurgitation was more frequent in the TAVR group, noted in 40 (14%) of 280 patients in the TAVR group and two (1%) of 228 in the SAVR group (p <0.0001), and was associated with increased 5-year risk of mortality in the TAVR group (72·4% for moderate or severe aortic regurgitation versus 56·6% for those with mild aortic regurgitation or less; p = 0.003).[6]

A similar randomized trial of 795 high risk but operable patients with symptomatic severe AS randomized patients to TAVR with CoreValve (n = 394) or SAVR (n = 401), primary end point of the study being rate of death at 1 year.[7] In the as-treated population, the rate of death at 1 year was significantly lower in the TAVR group than in the surgical group (14.2% vs. 19.1%) (p <0.001 for noninferiority; p = 0.04 for superiority). The results were similar in the intention-to-treat analysis.

Intermediate-risk Patients

The PARTNER 2 trial randomized 2,032 intermediate-risk patients with symptomatic severe AS to TAVR with SAPIEN XT valve (Edwards Lifesciences Inc., Irvine; CA) or SAVR.[10] The primary end point was all-cause mortality or disabling stroke at 2 years. There was no significant difference in the rates of death or nondisabling stroke at 2 years between TAVR and SAVR groups (19.2% vs. 21.1%, p = 0.25). Patients undergoing TAVR had large aortic valve areas and lower rates of acute kidney injury, severe bleeding, and new-onset atrial fibrillation; surgery resulted in fewer major vascular complications and less paravalvular aortic regurgitation. In conclusion, TAVR was noninferior to SAVR for the treatment of symptomatic severe AS in intermediate surgical-risk patients.

Like PARTNER 2 trial, SURTAVI trial randomized intermediate-risk patients to TAVR with self-expanding CoreValve/Evolut-R (n = 879) or SAVR (n = 867).[9] The primary end point was death or disabling stroke at 2 years. At 2 years, there was no difference in the incidence of primary end point between TAVR and SAVR groups (12.6% vs. 14%, p >0.999). TAVR was associated with lower aortic valve mean gradients, lower incidence of acute kidney injury, atrial fibrillation and higher incidence of permanent pacemaker (PPM) and residual aortic regurgitation.

Low-risk Patients

The PARTNER 3 trial (NCT02675114) randomized low-risk patients to TAVR with SAPIEN 3 valve or SAVR. The Medtronic Evolut low-risk study (NCT02701283) randomized low-risk patients with symptomatic severe AS to TAVR with Evolut valve or SAVR. Both the trials have completed enrollment; results are pending.

TRANSCATHETER AORTIC VALVE REPLACEMENT FOR DEGENERATIVE BIOPROSTHETIC AORTIC VALVES

Transcatheter aortic valve-in-valve (ViV) implantation has become the preferred treatment for degenerated bioprosthetic aortic valves, especially in patients at intermediate to high risk for redo surgery. The largest body of evidence supporting ViV as a treatment alternative for these patients comes from the Valve-in-Valve International Data (VIVID) registry.[11] In a VIVID registry report of 459 patients with degenerated bioprosthetic valves undergoing ViV implantation, 30-day mortality and major stroke rate was 7.6% and 1.7%, respectively. Survival at 1 year was 83.2%. Patients in the stenosis group had worse 1-year survival [76.6%; 95% confidence interval (CI), 68.9–83.1%) in comparison with the regurgitation group (91.2%; 95% CI, 85.7–96.7%) (p = 0.01). Patients with small valves had worse 1-year survival (74.8%,

95% CI, 66.2–83.4%) versus with intermediate-sized valves (81.8%; 95% CI, 75.3–88.3%) and with large valves (93.3%; 95% CI, 85.7–96.7%) (p = 0.001). These outcomes are comparable to the outcomes of TAVR for the treatment of native AS. The PARTNER 2 ViV trial and continued access registries enrolled 365 high-risk patients with symptomatic degeneration of surgical aortic bioprostheses.[12] At 30 days, all-cause mortality was 2.7%, stroke was 2.7%, major vascular complication was 4.1%, conversion to surgery was 0.6%, coronary occlusion was 0.8%, and new pacemaker insertion was 1.9%. 1-year all-cause mortality was 12.4%. At 1 year, mean gradient was 17.6 mm Hg and effective orifice area was 1.16 cm^2.

CURRENT GENERATION COMMERCIALLY AVAILABLE TRANSCATHETER AORTIC VALVE

The randomized TAVR trials were performed with the early generation TAVR valves. The current generation TAVs used in contemporary clinical practice, including balloon-expandable SAPIEN 3 and self-expanding Evolut PRO valves, have only been studied in prospective registries. Nevertheless, these registries have demonstrated excellent procedural outcomes with the SAPIEN 3 and Evolut valves.

SAPIEN 3 Valve

In the SAPIEN 3 study, 1,077 intermediate-risk patients with severe symptomatic AS underwent TAVR with SAPIEN 3 valve.[13] Compared to the previous generations of balloon-expandable valves, the SAPIEN 3 valve system (Edwards Lifesciences Inc., Irvine; CA) has improved geometry of the trileaflet bovine pericardial valve; different cobalt alloy frame, which is longer than the early version of the balloon-expandable valve system (SAPIEN XT valve) with more open outlet cells and denser inlet cells; a polyethylene terephthalate fabric skirt sewn to the bottom portion of the interior and exterior of the frame [providing an external circumferential seal to reduce paravalvular leak (PVL)]; four valve sizes (20 mm, 23 mm, 26 mm, and 29 mm diameters); and lower profile delivery catheters with more precise valve positioning inserted through 14 or 16 French expandable sheaths for transfemoral access. At 1 year, mortality was rate 7.4%, disabling stroke rate was 2.0%, moderate-severe PVL rate was 2.0% and aortic valve reintervention rate was 1%. Following propensity score matching with intermediate-risk patients who underwent SAVR in the PARTNER 2 clinical trials, TAVR with SAPIEN 3 valve was both noninferior (pooled weighted proportion difference of –9·2%; 90% CI –12·4 to –6; p <0.0001) and superior (–9.2%, 95% CI –13.0 to –5.4; p <0.0001), compared to SAVR.

Evolut PRO Valve

Medtronic Evolut PRO valve (Medtronic Inc., Minneapolis; MN) was designed with an external pericardial wrap with the intent to reduce PVL while maintaining the benefits of a low profile, self-expanding, and repositionable supra-annular valve. In the Medtronic Evolut PRO study, 60 patients with severe symptomatic AS underwent TAVR with Evolut PRO valve.[14] At 30 days, mortality rate was 1.7%, disabling stroke rate was 1.7% and more than and equal to moderate PVL rate was 0%.

INDICATIONS FOR TRANSCATHETER AORTIC VALVE REPLACEMENT

Based on the available evidence from RCTs as well as large multicenter registries, TAVR is recommended for symptomatic patients with severe AS and a prohibitive risk for SAVR who have a predicted post-TAVR survival greater than 12 months. TAVR is a reasonable alternative to SAVR for symptomatic patients with severe AS and an intermediate surgical risk, depending on patient-specific procedural risks, values, and preferences. For severely symptomatic patients with bioprosthetic aortic valve stenosis judged by the heart team to be at high or prohibitive risk of reoperation, and in whom improvement in hemodynamics is anticipated, a transcatheter ViV procedure is reasonable. Although guidelines do not recommend for or against TAVR for the treatment of specific anatomic subsets, for instance, bicuspid AS or pure native aortic regurgitation, it may be reasonable to perform TAVR in experienced centers for these indications in carefully screened high-risk patients.

LIMITATIONS OF TRANSCATHETER AORTIC VALVE REPLACEMENT

With contemporary device technology and improved procedural techniques, TAVR is successfully performed by transfemoral approach in most patients with excellent procedural outcomes. The main limitations of TAVR include need for PPMs, strokes, valve thrombosis, and lack of data on long-term durability. The need for alternate access, PVL, vascular complications, and bleeding complications has become less frequent with the newer generation TAVR devices.

Permanent Pacemaker Implantation

The incidence of PPM implantation varies according to the transcatheter valve type, rates being higher with self-expanding valves compared to balloon-expandable valves. The rate of PPM implantation was 3.5% with the first generation Edwards SAPIEN valve,[3,4] 8.5% with the second generation Sapien XT valve[10] and 13% with the current generation SAPIEN 3 valve.[13] The rates of PPM implantation were higher with the self-expanding CoreValve/Evolut valve; rates being 19.6% in the CoreValve high-risk study[7] and 26% in the SURTAVI intermediate-risk study.[9] The highest PPM rates are associated with implantation of a mechanically expanding Lotus valve, rates being 35.5% in the randomized controlled REPRISE trial.[15] With improved implantation techniques, especially high deployment of the valves, the PPM rates have come down with all valve types. While pacemaker implantation does not impact mortality after TAVR, it is not benign. The need for PPM implantation after TAVR is associated with prolonged hospitalization; increased risk of rehospitalization; less improvement in ejection fraction in patients with depressed ejection fraction at baseline; and increased procedural costs.[16,17]

Stroke

Stroke after TAVR is associated with increased mortality, worse quality of life and increased healthcare costs. In the PARTNER 1 TAVR trials using first generation Edwards SAPIEN valve, stroke rates were higher with TAVR compared to SAVR (5.4% vs. 2.4% at 30 days). With improved TAVR technology, better patient screening and improved procedural understanding, stroke rates after TAVR have decreased significantly. The Medtronic high-risk CoreValve study that was initiated after the PARTNER 1 trial demonstrated a lower stroke rate with TAVR, compared to SAVR; although the differences were not significantly different (4.9% vs. 6.2%). PARTNER 2A trial comparing TAVR with Sapien XT valve with SAVR demonstrated similar stroke rates between TAVR and SAVR. The SURTAVI trial comparing TAVR with CoreValve versus SAVR in intermediate-risk patients demonstrated lower strokes rates with TAVR (3.4% vs. 5.3%). Strokes continue to be a devastating complication of TAVR. The SAPIEN 3 registry of intermediate and high-risk patients demonstrated a stroke rate of 2.7% at 30 days after TAVR, disabling stroke rates being 1.0%.[13] The use of cerebral embolic protection devices to decrease periprocedural strokes after TAVR is an area of ongoing research. The SENTINEL trial compared cerebral embolic protection with the Sentinel device, randomizing patients in a 1:1:1 manner to Sentinel device with magnetic resonance imaging (MRI), Sentinel device with no MRI imaging or TAVR without the use of Sentinel device.[18] The use of Sentinel device during TAVR was associated with a significant reduction in stroke rates at 72 hours post-TAVR. Based on these data, the Sentinel device was approved by the Food and Drug Administration (FDA) for use during TAVR. A significant proportion of patients develop new onset atrial fibrillation after TAVR, which is also a significant predictor of strokes after TAVR. In conclusion, the stroke rates have decreased with contemporary valve types and procedural techniques, being comparable, if not lower than the stroke rates after SAVR. These stroke rates can potentially be reduced further with the use of cerebral protection devices, detection and treatment of new onset atrial fibrillation and optimization of postprocedural antiplatelet and antithrombotic therapy.

Valve Thrombosis

Subclinical leaflet thrombosis was recently reported in 10–15% of patients undergoing TAVR. Subclinical leaflet thrombosis is missed routinely on transthoracic echocardiography (TTE); is readily detected with contrast computed tomography (CT) of the valve; is less common in patients on anticoagulation; resolves with the initiation of anticoagulation; and is associated with increased aortic valve gradients compared to patients with no subclinical leaflet thrombosis (although the gradients are still within the expected range after TAVR) (Fig. 1).[19-22] In a registry of 931 patients undergoing contrast CT after bioprosthetic aortic valve replacement, subclinical leaflet thrombosis was more frequent in transcatheter valves, compared to surgical valves.[20] Most of the small studies did not notice a relationship between valve thrombosis and stroke rates; however, the two largest studies reported

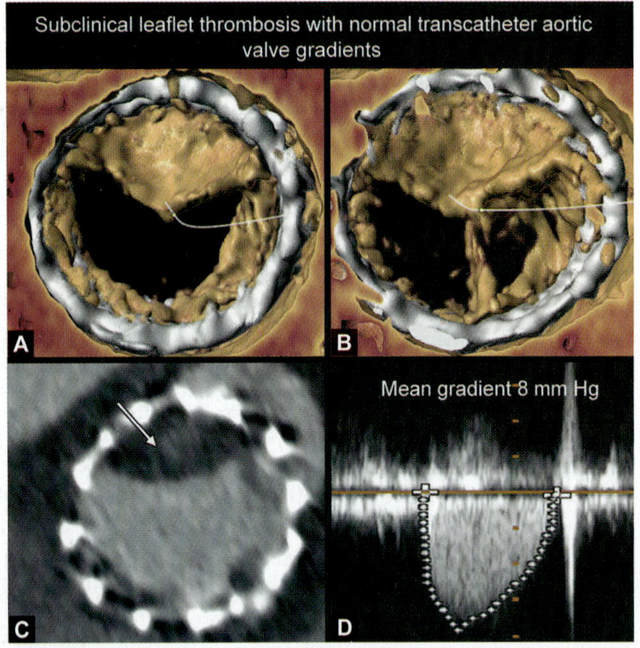

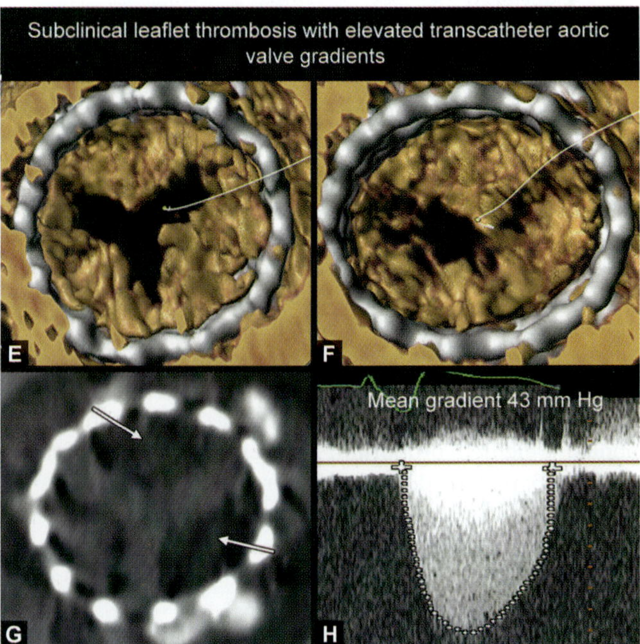

FIG. 1: Subclinical leaflet thrombosis, associated with normal gradients and elevated aortic valve gradients. (A–D) Reduced leaflet motion during systole (A) and diastole (B); in the presence of hypoattenuation associated leaflet thickening (C) and normal aortic valve gradients (D). (E–H) Reduced leaflet motion during systole (E) and diastole (F); in the presence of hypoattenuation associated leaflet thickening (G) and normal aortic valve gradients (H).

an increased incidence of transient ischemic attacks with subclinical leaflet thrombosis (although the stroke rates were not different). While subclinical leaflet thrombosis is frequent, clinically significant valve thrombosis of TAVs resulting in heart failure or thromboembolic complications is rare, occurring in only up to 0.5% of the patients after TAVR.[23] Whether subclinical leaflet thrombosis is an innocent imaging finding; or if it really impacts valve hemodynamics, clinical outcomes and valve durability needs to be determined with prospective randomized trials with long-term follow-up. The role of routine anticoagulation after TAVR for the prevention of subclinical leaflet thrombosis and its impact on clinical outcomes is being evaluated in the GALILEO trial (NCT02556203) and ATLANTIS trial (NCT02664649).

Valve Durability

Transcatheter aortic valve replacement was initially performed in high-risk patients, who had limited life expectancy due to the presence of comorbidities. In the PARTNER 1 trial of inoperable patients with severe AS, only 1 out of 169 patients who did not undergo TAVR was alive at 5 years. In the PARTNER 1 trial of high-risk patients, 67.8% of the patients undergoing TAVR had died by 5 years. Given the high mortality in the high-risk patients undergoing TAVR in the early TAVR era, there is paucity of evidence on the long-term durability of TAVs. Nevertheless, the limited datasets available on valve durability of TAVR valves are reassuring, within the limitations of poor long-term survival in majority of patients. A report from the 5-year follow-up from the PARTNER 1 trial (with 5-year follow-up echocardiograms available in 424 patients undergoing TAVR) demonstrated valve durability of Edwards SAPIEN valve, without structural valve degeneration at 5 years. Long-term durability of TAVs will be available from the low-risk and intermediate-risk study, with longer life-expectancy.

Other Limitations

The rates of vascular complications, bleeding complications, need for alternate access, and paravalvular regurgitation have become less common with improved device design; smaller caliber delivery systems; improved patient screening; and improved operator experience. The newer TAVs (SAPIEN 3, Evolut PRO, and Lotus) have moderate-severe PVL rates of less than 2–3%. The incidence of vascular complications and bleeding complications; as well as the need for alternate access, continues to decline with the availability of 14 French delivery systems.

CONCLUSION

In summary, TAVR is a breakthrough technology and is the standard of care for the treatment of severe symptomatic AS in high-risk patients; an alternative to SAVR for intermediate-risk patients or for the treatment of high-risk patients with degenerative bioprosthetic aortic valves. With device iterations, accumulating clinical experience, and better patient screening, the incidence of complications after TAVR continues to decline.

REFERENCES

1. Cribier A, Eltchaninoff H, Bash A, et al. Percutaneous transcatheter implantation of an aortic valve prosthesis for calcific aortic stenosis: first human case description. Circulation. 2002;106(24):3006-8.
2. Grover FL, Vemulapalli S, Carroll JD, et al. 2016 Annual Report of The Society of Thoracic Surgeons/American College of Cardiology Transcatheter Valve Therapy Registry. J Am Coll Cardiol. 2017;69(10):1215-30.
3. Leon MB, Smith CR, Mack M, et al. Transcatheter aortic-valve implantation for aortic stenosis in patients who cannot undergo surgery. N Engl J Med. 2010;363(17):1597-607.
4. Smith CR, Leon MB, Mack MJ, et al. Transcatheter versus surgical aortic-valve replacement in high-risk patients. N Engl J Med. 2011;364(23):2187-98.
5. Kapadia SR, Leon MB, Makkar RR, et al. 5-year outcomes of transcatheter aortic valve replacement compared with standard treatment for patients with inoperable aortic stenosis (PARTNER 1): a randomised controlled trial. Lancet. 2015;385(9986):2485-91.
6. Mack MJ, Leon MB, Smith CR, et al. 5-year outcomes of transcatheter aortic valve replacement or surgical aortic valve replacement for high surgical risk patients with aortic stenosis (PARTNER 1): a randomised controlled trial. Lancet. 2015;385(9986):2477-84.
7. Adams DH, Popma JJ, Reardon MJ. Transcatheter aortic-valve replacement with a self-expanding prosthesis. N Engl J Med. 2014;371(10):967-8.
8. Popma JJ, Adams DH, Reardon MJ, et al. Transcatheter aortic valve replacement using a self-expanding bioprosthesis in patients with severe aortic stenosis at extreme risk for surgery. J Am Coll Cardiol. 2014;63(19):1972-81.
9. Reardon MJ, Van Mieghem NM, Popma JJ, et al. Surgical or transcatheter aortic-valve replacement in intermediate-risk patients. N Engl J Med. 2017;376(14):1321-31.
10. Leon MB, Smith CR, Mack MJ, et al. Transcatheter or surgical aortic-valve replacement in intermediate-risk patients. N Engl J Med. 2016;374(17):1609-20.
11. Dvir D, Webb JG, Bleiziffer S, et al. Transcatheter aortic valve implantation in failed bioprosthetic surgical valves. JAMA. 2014;312(2):162-70.
12. Webb JG, Mack MJ, White JM, et al. Transcatheter aortic valve implantation within degenerated aortic surgical bioprostheses: PARTNER 2 Valve-in-valve registry. J Am Coll Cardiol. 2017;69(18):2253-62.
13. Thourani VH, Kodali S, Makkar RR, et al. Transcatheter aortic valve replacement versus surgical valve replacement in intermediate-risk patients: a propensity score analysis. Lancet. 2016;387(10034):2218-25.
14. Forrest JK, Mangi AA, Popma JJ, et al. Early outcomes with the Evolut PRO repositionable self-expanding transcatheter aortic valve with pericardial wrap. JACC Cardiovasc Interv. 2018;11(2):160-8.
15. Feldman TE, Reardon MJ, Rajagopal V, et al. Effect of mechanically expanded vs self-expanding transcatheter aortic valve replacement on mortality and major adverse clinical events in high-risk patients with aortic stenosis: The REPRISE III randomized clinical trial. JAMA. 2018;319(1):27-37.
16. Chamandi C, Barbanti M, Munoz-Garcia A, et al. Long-Term outcomes in patients with new permanent pacemaker implantation following transcatheter aortic valve replacement. JACC Cardiovasc Interv. 2018;11(3):301-10.
17. Nazif TM, Dizon JM, Hahn RT, et al. Predictors and clinical outcomes of permanent pacemaker implantation after transcatheter aortic valve replacement: the PARTNER (Placement of AoRtic TraNscathetER Valves) trial and registry. JACC Cardiovasc Interv. 2015;8(1 Pt A):60-9.
18. Kapadia SR, Kodali S, Makkar R, et al. Protection against cerebral embolism during transcatheter aortic valve replacement. J Am Coll Cardiol. 2017;69(4):367-77.
19. Makkar RR, Fontana G, Jilaihawi H, et al. Possible subclinical leaflet thrombosis in bioprosthetic aortic valves. N Engl J Med. 2015;373(21):2015-24.
20. Chakravarty T, Sondergaard L, Friedman J, et al. Subclinical leaflet thrombosis in surgical and transcatheter bioprosthetic aortic valves: an observational study. Lancet. 2017;389(10087):2383-92.
21. Pache G, Schoechlin S, Blanke P, et al. Early hypo-attenuated leaflet thickening in balloon-expandable transcatheter aortic heart valves. Eur Heart J. 2015;37(28):2263-71.
22. Hansson NC, Grove EL, Andersen HR, et al. Transcatheter aortic valve thrombosis: incidence, predisposing factors, and clinical implications. J Am Coll Cardiol. 2016;68(19):2059-69.
23. Latib A, Naganuma T, Abdel-Wahab M, et al. Treatment and clinical outcomes of transcatheter heart valve thrombosis. Circ Cardiovasc Interv. 2015;8(4):e001779.

CHAPTER 70

Imaging for Transcatheter Aortic Valve Implantation: Practical Aspects

Kinjal Banerjee, Nyal Borges, Parth Parikh, Samir Kapadia

INTRODUCTION

Transcatheter aortic valve implantation (TAVI) has dramatically changed management of patient with severe aortic stenosis (AS). Patients previously considered inoperable are often excellent candidates for TAVI. The indications for transcatheter aortic valve replacement (TAVR) have now been expanded to patients with high- and intermediate-surgical risk for surgical aortic valve replacement (SAVR) as well. Without direct visualization and access to the valve, multimodality imaging plays an immense role in accurate planning and successful execution of the procedure.

PLANNING PHASE

The process begins with the evaluation of a patient with severe AS as a candidate for TAVR. Broad objectives in the planning phase include the following described here.

Patient Selection

While the indications for TAVI are expanding, appropriate patient selection is an essential part of a successful procedure. The first goal is to establish severe AS and indications for a valve replacement. Ruling out other severe valvular lesions is also an important part of establishing suitability for TAVI. Patient with concomitant severe mitral pathology may benefit more from a combined open surgical procedure.

Elderly patients with significant calcific AS often have concomitant multi-vessel coronary artery disease. A patient who may need coronary artery bypass graft (CABG) now or in the near future may benefit from a combined open surgical procedure.

Transthoracic Echocardiography

By the time a patient is seen by a Heart Team, the patient usually has had a transthoracic echocardiography (TTE) (Fig. 1). A two-dimensional TTE provides an initial assessment of severity of AS, morphology of the aortic valve, and coexisting valve lesions like mitral regurgitation (MR). It also provides an estimation of left ventricular (LV) and right ventricular (RV) function, among other parameters. This is a good starting point, and is enough to give a rough idea of patient suitability for TAVI. It is best to consider the TTE as a firewall to exclude patients who are not candidates for TAVI and thus to avoid further, potentially unnecessary, testing. The most important information that TTE provides is with regards to severity of AS. Aortic valve area and peak and mean gradients are important measurements. In patients with low-gradient AS careful measurement of flow should be undertaken. Patients with low flow (35 mL/m^2) are defined as low-flow AS patients. Some elderly patients, particularly men above 80 years of age with low-flow low-gradient AS should be screened for TTR amyloid using pyrophosphate scan or cardiac magnetic resonance imaging (MRI). Patients with amyloidosis have worse prognosis with or without TAVI. In some patients with advanced amyloidosis, TAVI may not help to improve symptoms particularly if AS is not critical.

Cardiac Catheterization

Most centers routinely obtain a diagnostic cardiac catheterization prior to TAVI. This serves several purposes. First, a diagnostic coronary angiogram assesses coronary pathology and helps decide the need for intervention. The optimal timing of intervention for coronary lesions is a matter of debate. However, for patients with multi-vessel disease, a combined CABG and aortic valve replacement (AVR) may be a more suitable procedure. Further, a combined TAVR and percutaneous coronary intervention (PCI) has been shown to be feasible and safe. However, patients with a low ejection fraction less than 30% and high STS score more than or equal to 10 have been shown to have higher risk of 30-day mortality after PCI. Second, it serves as a secondary modality to evaluate LV hemodynamics. Invasive pressure measurements are not routinely necessary with high quality echocardiographic Doppler estimation, but may serve to provide additional assessment.

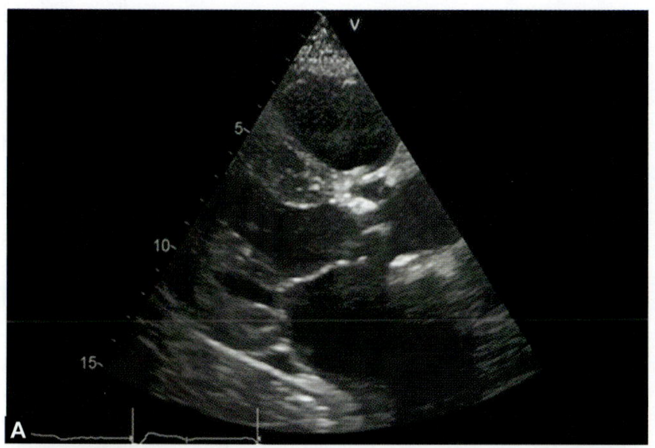

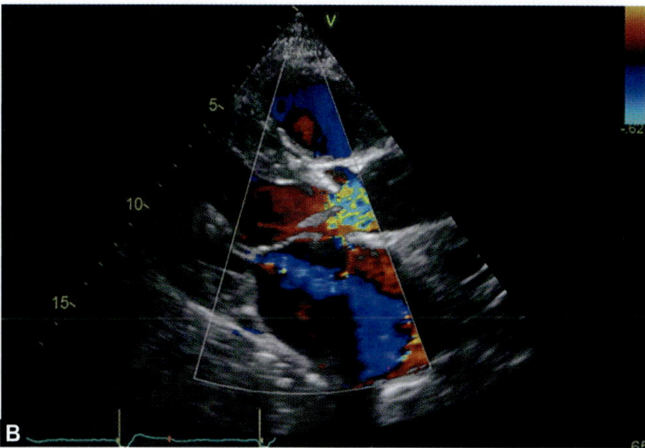

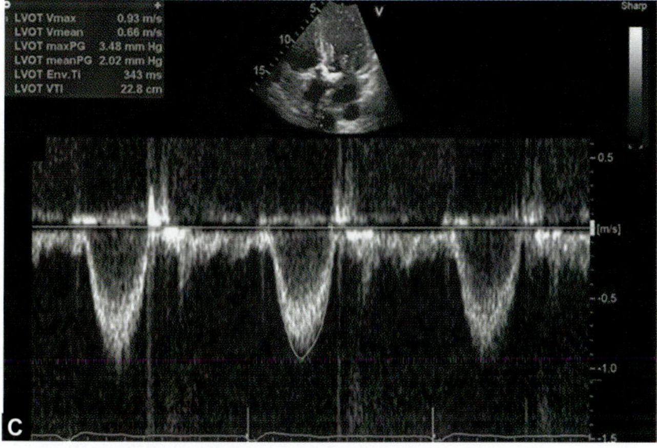

FIG. 1: Transthoracic echocardiography showing severe aortic stenosis.

Transesophageal Echocardiography

Preprocedural transesophageal echocardiography (TEE) with three-dimensional imaging may be used to further assess the aortic root, especially in the setting of morphological anomalies of the aortic valve. It may serve to help annular sizing in patients unable to undergo a contrast-enhanced computed tomography (CT) scan due to renal impairment. However, in many centers cardiac MRI can be performed to evaluate the aortic annulus. Therefore, TEE is sparingly used for preprocedural planning at this time.

PLANNING PHASE: PROCEDURAL PLANNING

Once indications for AVR have been firmly established, and TAVR is considered, more concrete anatomical information is needed to plan the procedure. Special emphasis is placed on detailed aortic root anatomy (Fig. 2), to aid in valve sizing, coronary anatomy in relation to aortic valve and annular calcification. Evaluation of access for TAVI is another important goal for preprocedural planning.

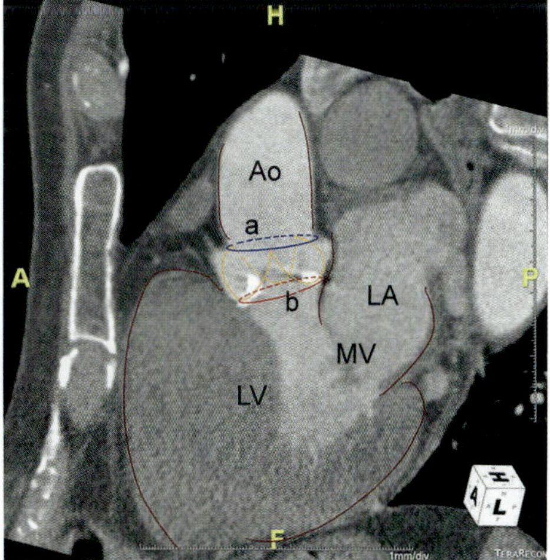

LA, left atrium; LV, left ventricle; MV, mitral valve; Ao, aorta.

FIG. 2: Basic anatomy of the aortic root. **A,** Sinotubular junction; **B,** Aortic annular plane defined by lowest point of three cusps.

Computed Tomography Imaging Protocol: Basics and Objectives

To obtain optimal images of the aorta, several conditions should be met. Firstly, iodinated contrast provides good delineation of the aorta and blood vessels. Imaging must be obtained in the arterial phase to allow acquisition of the aorta, down to the iliac and femoral arteries. In patients with a contraindication to iodinated contrast, e.g., renal disease, noncontrast CT images may suffice for access evaluation in many patients but root assessment is not possible with noncontrast CT alone. As indicated above, TEE or cardiac MRI may be considered. Second, electrocardiographic (ECG) gating is necessary to eliminate motion artifacts, and also allows measurement of the aortic annulus in specific phases of the cardiac cycle. Some centers prefer prospective ECG gating, where the patient is exposed to X-rays only during a specific phase of the cardiac cycle. While this generates similar image quality and reduces radiation exposure, images are often restricted to a single phase of the cardiac cycle and lacks the flexibility of retrospectively gated images. Images are reconstructed using multiplanar views for accurate measurement of annulus (Fig. 3) Images are obtained in 0.5 mm thickness for the annulus but 3 mm thickness may be adequate for access evaluation in abdomen and pelvis. Annular measurements are usually taken in systolic phase of the cardiac cycle. Centerline reconstructions allow imaging of the aorta, iliac, and femoral arteries in planes perpendicular to blood flow irrespective of curvature of these arteries.

The following measurements are necessary for the aortic root:

- *Aortic annulus*: The aortic annular is defined as the plane that passes through the lowest point of all three aortic cusps. The area of the aortic annulus is measured as a polygon, and then converted to a diameter. Similarly, the diameter is also estimated by measuring the perimeter of the aortic annulus. This measurement is extremely critical as it provides vital information for sizing of the prosthetic transcatheter heart valve (THV). Incorrect sizing can have devastating consequences, with undersized valves at risk for paravalvular leakage (PVL) and embolization, while oversized valves may cause conduction anomalies or even an annular rupture. Area-based sizing is considered standard and reproducible, and tend to yield more conservative estimates of annular size for balloon expandable valves. For self-expanding valves, where valves conform to annulus, perimeter-based sizing is used more commonly. The degree of oversizing is an important parameter in procedure planning, and is associated with procedural success and complications. Recommended oversizing ratios vary by valve models and technologies
- *Height of coronary ostium*: The distance from the aortic annulus plane to the opening of the left main coronary artery is an important measurement. Ensuring adequate clearance of the coronary ostium allows the valve to be implanted without impinging on coronary blood flow, and allows the coronary arteries to be accessed in the future. Other measurements used to assess ostial clearance are mean sinus of Valsalva diameter and sinus or annulus diameter ratio. Effaced sinuses with low coronary arteries and bulky calcification of leaflets have been associated with higher risk of coronary occlusion with TAVR
- *Valve morphology*: A gross assessment of the valvular morphology is essential to a successful procedure. Calcification of the aortic root may put the patient at risk for PVL, conduction abnormalities or even annular rupture. Specific measures can be taken in patients with bicuspid valves to appropriately select and place the valve
- *Sinotubular junction (STJ) and ascending aorta*: The STJ diameters are a sizing parameter for self-expanding valves which extend proximally beyond the STJ. Severe calcification of the STJ and ascending thoracic aorta puts the patient at risk of multiple complications, including aortic wall dissection, rupture, and embolic complications
- *Concomitant cardiac pathology*: Pathology involving the mitral valve, left ventricular outflow tract (LVOT), or interventricular septum may complicate, or exclude the option of, TAVI for a patient. Similarly, the presence of an intraventricular thrombus is also a contraindication for TAVI
- *Access feasibility*: Transfemoral TAVR requires a sheath of 14F–18F sheath dependent on specific TAVR device. The arterial phase of the CT scan is used to assess the descending aorta and the iliac and femoral arteries. Excessive tortuosity, significant calcifications, atherosclerotic occlusive disease or aneurysmal changes put the patient at some risk of access-related complications like bleeding, hematoma or pseudoaneurysms, as well as embolic complications including stroke. If transfemoral

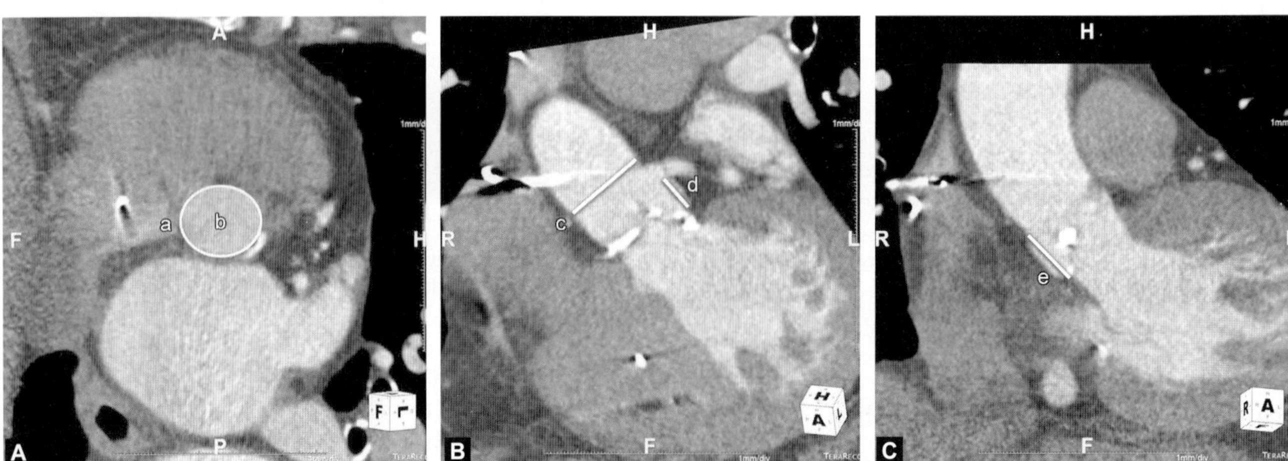

FIG. 3: Multidetector computed tomography imaging for procedural planning. **A,** Perimeter-derived area of annulus; **B,** Estimated area of annulus; **C,** Diameter at sinotubular junction; **D,** Height of coronary ostia from aortic annulus; **E,** Sinus height, measured from aortic annulus.

access is unsuitable, the patient may be a candidate for an alternative access route, the most common of which is trans-subclavian followed by transaortic access. Transapical access is also used sometimes but it is rare these days with availability of TAVI devices requiring smaller access
- Estimation of aortic valve plane for device implantation using fluoroscopy. Identification of a plane perpendicular to the native annulus (coplanar angulation) may reduce the need for multiple dye injections during the procedure to align fluoroscopic imaging to the valve.

PROCEDURE PHASE

Being a minimally invasive transcatheter procedure, intra-procedural imaging plays an essential part of the entire procedure. The main aims of intraprocedural imaging are:

- Procedural guidance, appropriate positioning of THV across the valve and deployment
- Identification of complications intraoperatively, with the potential to intervene immediately.

Fluoroscopy

Fluoroscopy is the primary imaging modality used for guidance during the procedure. Identification of a coplanar angle during procedural planning can reduce both dye injection and radiation exposure during aligning the fluoroscope to an optimal angle perpendicular to the native valve. Biplane fluoroscopy can provide an additional dimension to imaging, and allow guidance in two separate orthogonal planes. Dye injections allow visualization of aorta and aortic valve (Fig. 4), and allow positioning of the THV across the native aortic valve (Fig. 5A). The depth of implantation is estimated as the depth of the distal edge of the valve from the noncoronary sinus. The valve is expanded (for balloon-expandable valves) or deployed (for self-expanding valves) under real-time fluoroscopic guidance (Figs. 5B and C). Once the valve is deployed, further dye injections allow visualization of the positioned valve in relation to the aortic root (Fig. 6). Retrievable valves can be repositioned before they are released from the deployment catheter. Further, aortic regurgitation (AR) can be assessed by regurgitation of dye from the aorta into the LV cavity. A final dye injection is usually recorded at the end of valve deployment to document procedure success, lack of significant AR, and final implantation depth. As the catheter is withdrawn, dye is injected into the iliofemoral system to ensure there are no vascular complications.

Role of Transesophageal Echocardiography during Transcatheter Aortic Valve Implantation

Transesophageal echocardiography may be used to provide an additional layer of real-time guidance during the procedure. It allows high-resolution imaging of the aortic valve, and can aid with positioning of the valve prior to deployment. Three-dimensional reconstruction provides an anatomically correct image of the aortic valve and aortic root both before and after deployment of the valve. In the event of PVL, TEE can precisely localize the regurgitant jet and allow assessment of severity. Mild PVL is common after TAVI, but moderate or severe PVL need intervention, typically a balloon postdilation. Rarer complications like a valve embolization, new wall motion abnormality, pericardial effusion, severe valvular regurgitation, rupture of the annulus or dissection of the aorta can be rapidly identified by intraprocedural TEE.

There is a growing trend of performing TAVI under conscious sedation without general anesthesia. This serves to reduce anesthesia-related complications and to shorten hospital stay after the procedure. Therefore, in the current era TEE is not performed at the time of procedure. In this situation TTE is a must. Just after valve deployment TTE is performed to rule out pericardial effusion, PVL and new wall motion abnormalities. TAVI should not be performed without availability of echocardiographic machine in the cath laboratory.

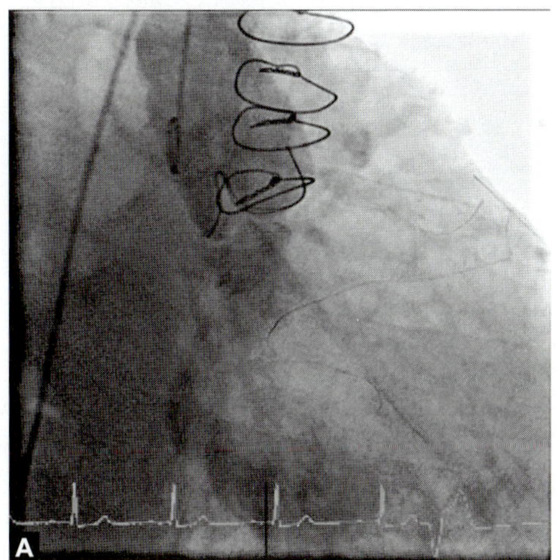

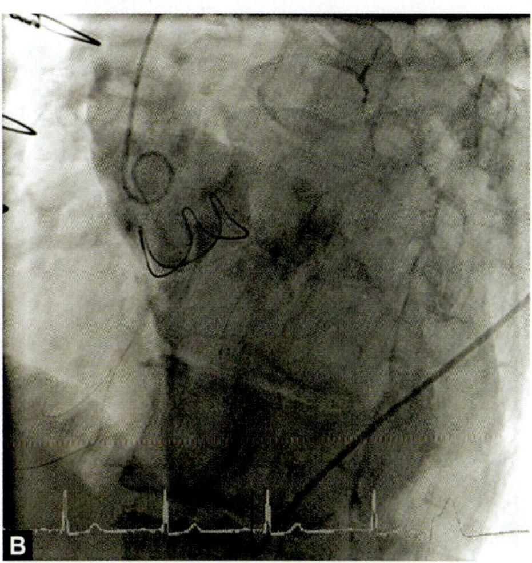

FIG. 4: Aortogram showing aorta and aortic root in a patient with a prior surgically implanted bioprosthetic valve.

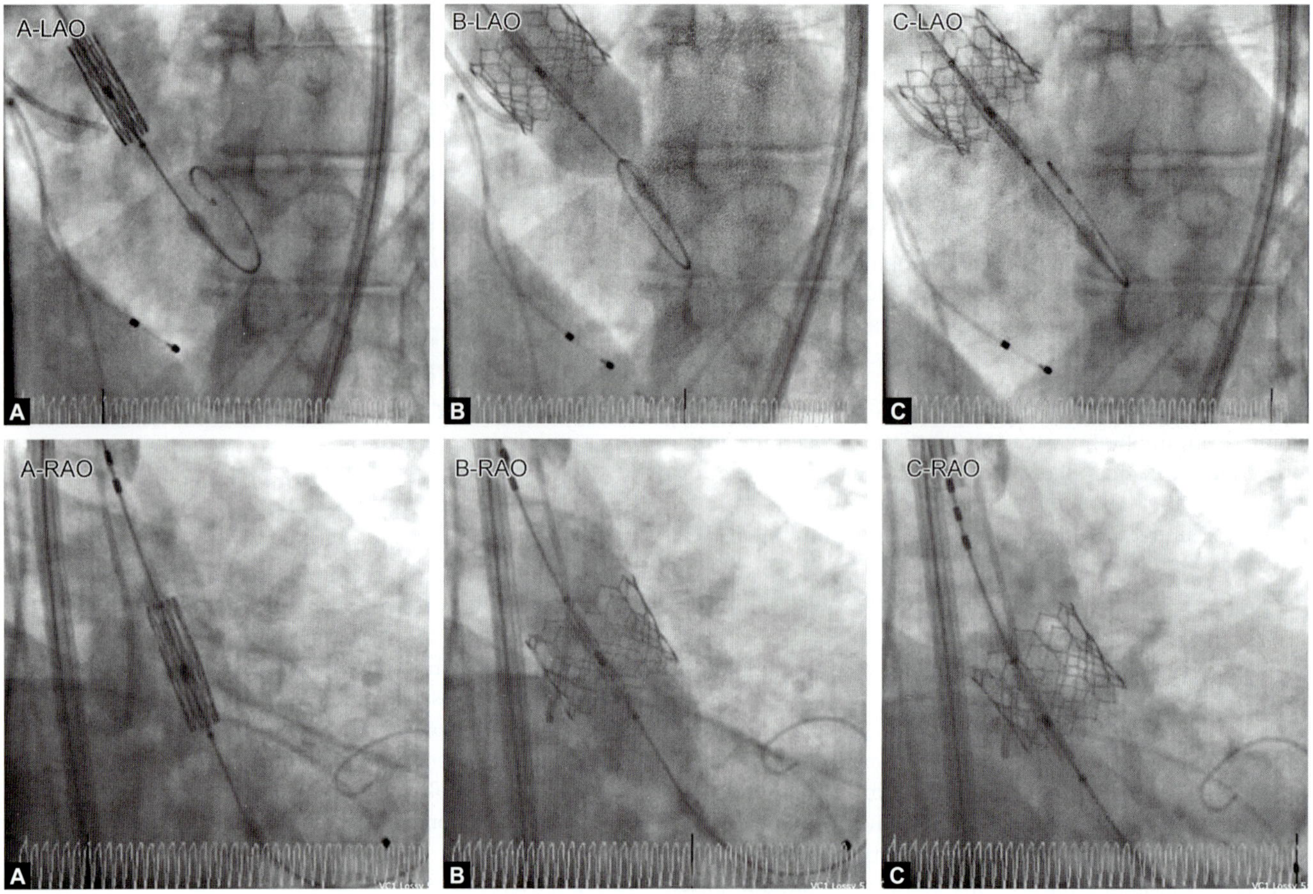

FIG. 5: Fluoroscopy images showing deployment of Edwards SAPIEN 3 valve. **A,** Valve positioned across the aortic annulus prior to deployment; **B,** Balloon at maximal expansion to deploy valve; **C,** Valve remains expanded as the balloon is collapsed. Note rapid pacing via temporary wire placed in right ventricle.

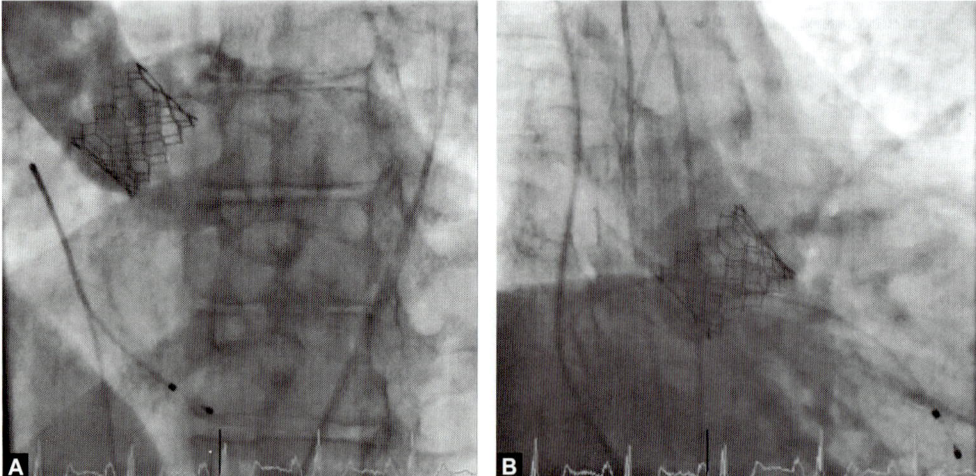

FIG. 6: Aortogram after valve deployment to check positioning of the valve, implantation depth, and aortic regurgitation. The coronary ostia may be engaged and separate images obtained if there is suspicion for coronary obstruction.

POSTPROCEDURE FOLLOW-UP

Patients undergoing TAVI need follow-up after the procedure. Parameters to monitor include:

- Valve gradient and effective orifice area for baseline assessment and for future diagnosis of worsening valve function
- *Aortic regurgitation*: Central and paravalvular
- *Other complications*: Leaflet thrombosis, device migration, and endocarditis
- *Changes in cardiac structure and function*: Effect of valve replacement on LV hypertrophy, mitral valve function, and other cardiac pathology.

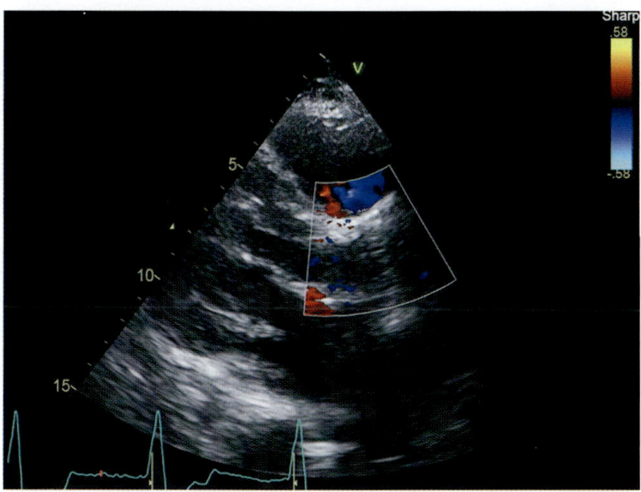

FIG. 7: Transthoracic echocardiogram obtained postprocedure, showing valve *in situ* and no aortic regurgitation.

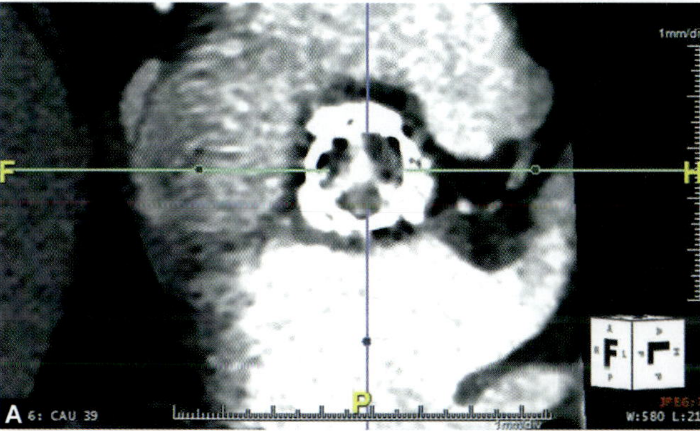

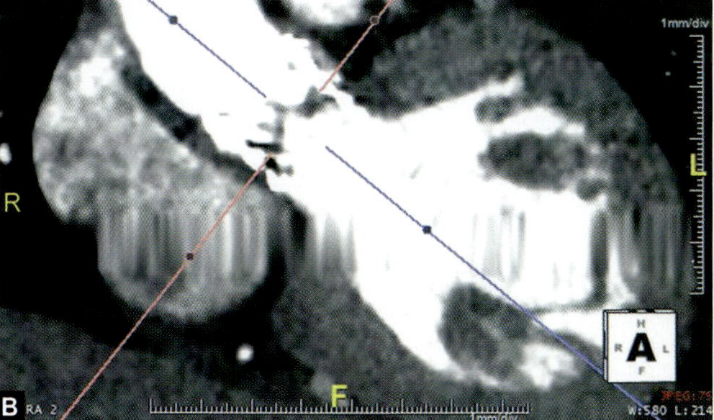

FIG. 8: Post-transcatheter aortic valve replacement CT imaging with contrast showing hypoattenuated leaflet thickening.

Transthoracic echocardiography is adequate for follow-up in most patients (Fig. 7). If valve gradient is increasing or there is valvular AR, hypoattenuated leaflet thickening (HALT) is suspected. HALT is properly diagnosed with contrast gated CT scan imaging in all cardiac cycles (Fig. 8). TEE is not as sensitive as CT but can be used in patients with severe renal insufficiency.

CONCLUSION

Successful TAVI is dependent on appropriate patient selection, thorough procedure planning, and real-time guidance during the procedure. At each of these stages, imaging plays an important role. TTE provides a basic starting in point in confirming the indications of AVR. CT scanning plays a vital role in access planning and valve sizing. Fluoroscopy forms the mainstay of intraprocedure real-time guidance, and for assessment of immediate postprocedure complications. TEE and MRI serve as backup imaging modalities when standard imaging is not possible, or further detail is necessary.

REFERENCES

1. Otto CM, Kumbhani DJ, Alexander KP, et al. 2017 ACC expert consensus decision pathway for transcatheter aortic valve replacement in the management of adults with aortic stenosis: A Report of the American College of Cardiology Task Force on Clinical Expert Consensus Documents. J Am Coll Cardiol. 2017;69(10):1313-46.
2. Nishimura RA, Otto CM, Bonow RO, et al. 2014 AHA/ACC guideline for the management of patients with valvular heart disease: A report of the American College of Cardiology/American Heart Association Task Force on Practice Guidelines. J Am Coll Cardiol. 2014;63:e57.
3. Nishimura RA, Otto CM, Bonow RO, et al. 2017 AHA/ACC focused update of the 2014 AHA/ACC guideline for the management of patients with valvular heart disease: A report of the American College of Cardiology/American Heart Association task force on clinical practice guidelines. J Am Coll Cardiol. 2017;17:36019.
4. Bonow RO, Brown AS, Gillam LD, et al. ACC/AATS/AHA/ASE/EACTS/HVS/SCA/SCAI/SCCT/SCMR/STS 2017 appropriate use criteria for the treatment of patients with severe aortic stenosis: A report of the American College of Cardiology Appropriate Use Criteria Task Force, American Association for Thoracic Surgery, American Heart Association, American Society of Echocardiography, European Association for Cardio-Thoracic Surgery, Heart Valve Society, Society of Cardiovascular Anesthesiologists, Society for Cardiovascular Angiography and Interventions, Society of Cardiovascular Computed Tomography, Society for Cardiovascular Magnetic Resonance, and Society of Thoracic Surgeons. J Am Coll Cardiol. 2017;70:2566.
5. Baumgartner H, Falk V, Bax JJ, et al. 2017 ESC/EACTS Guidelines for the management of valvular heart disease. Eur Heart J. 2017;38:2739.
6. Bloomfield GS, Gillam LD, Hahn RT, et al. A practical guide to multimodality imaging of transcatheter aortic valve replacement. JACC Cardiovasc Imaging. 2012;5:441.
7. Leon MB, Smith CR, Mack MJ, et al. Transcatheter or surgical aortic-valve replacement in intermediate-risk patients. N Engl J Med. 2016;374:1609.
8. Leon MB, Smith CR, Mack M, et al. Transcatheter aortic-valve implantation for aortic stenosis in patients who cannot undergo surgery. N Engl J Med. 2010;363:1597.
9. Binder RK, Webb JG, Willson AB, et al. The impact of integration of a multidetector computed tomography annulus area sizing algorithm on outcomes of transcatheter aortic valve replacement: a prospective, multicenter, controlled trial. J Am Coll Cardiol. 2013;62:431.
10. Jilaihawi H, Kashif M, Fontana G, et al. Cross-sectional computed tomographic assessment improves accuracy of aortic annular sizing for transcatheter aortic valve replacement and reduces the incidence of paravalvular aortic regurgitation. J Am Coll Cardiol. 2012;59:1275.
11. Kurra V, Schoenhagen P, Roselli EE, et al. Prevalence of significant peripheral artery disease in patients evaluated for percutaneous aortic valve insertion: Preprocedural assessment with multidetector computed tomography. J Thorac Cardiovasc Surg. 2009;137:1258.

12. Joshi SB, Mendoza DD, Steinberg DH, et al. Ultra-low-dose intra-arterial contrast injection for iliofemoral computed tomographic angiography. JACC Cardiovasc Imaging. 2009;2:1404.
13. Piazza N, de Jaegere P, Schultz C, et al. Anatomy of the aortic valvar complex and its implications for transcatheter implantation of the aortic valve. Circ Cardiovasc Interv. 2008;1:74.
14. Willson AB, Webb JG, Labounty TM, et al. 3-dimensional aortic annular assessment by multidetector computed tomography predicts moderate or severe paravalvular regurgitation after transcatheter aortic valve replacement: A multicenter retrospective analysis. J Am Coll Cardiol. 2012;59:1287.
15. Plank F, Friedrich G, Bartel T, et al. Benefits of high-pitch 128-slice dual-source computed tomography for planning of transcatheter aortic valve implantation. Ann Thorac Surg. 2012;94:1961.
16. Tsang W, Bateman MG, Weinert L, et al. Accuracy of aortic annular measurements obtained from three-dimensional echocardiography, CT and MRI: Human in vitro and in vivo studies. Heart. 2012;98:1146.
17. Rogers T, Waksman R. Role of CMR in TAVR. JACC Cardiovasc Imaging. 2016; 9:593.
18. Tuzcu EM, Kapadia SR, Schoenhagen P. Multimodality quantitative imaging of aortic root for transcatheter aortic valve implantation: more complex than it appears. J Am Coll Cardiol. 2010;55:195.
19. Hahn RT, Nioara A, Kapadia S, et al. Echocardiographic imaging for transcatheter aortic valve replacement. J Am Soc Echocardiogr. 2018;31:405.
20. Kapadia S, Tuzccu EM, Svensson LG. Anatomy and flow characteristics of neosinus: Important consideration for thrombosis of transcatheter aortic valves. Circulation. 2017;136:1610.

CHAPTER 71

Alcohol Ablation for HOCM: Progress over the Past Two Decades

Hubert Seggewiss, Angelika Koljaja-Batzner

INTRODUCTION

Hypertrophic cardiomyopathy (HCM) is the most common genetic heart disease with an estimated incidence between 0.2 and 0.6%.[1,2] The most important pathophysiologic finding is left ventricular obstruction with significant impact on symptoms and prognosis of the patients.[3] In 1995, alcohol septal ablation was introduced as new treatment option and alternative to surgical myectomy in symptomatic patients with hypertrophic obstructive cardiomyopathy (HOCM).[4] In this chapter, we describe the developments of the treatment within the last two decades.

HISTORICAL DEVELOPMENT OF PERCUTANEOUS SEPTAL ABLATION

After introduction of percutaneous treatment of coronary artery disease in the late 1970s advances in interventional techniques widened the therapeutic options into the field of valvular and structural heart diseases. Three observations were important for the development of percutaneous septal reduction therapy in HOCM.

Sigwart et al. reported on impaired systolic wall motion by temporary balloon occlusion of coronary arteries.[5] Come et al. observed disappearance of left ventricular obstruction in patients with HOCM following myocardial infarction.[6] Finally, Brugada et al. successfully treated malignant ventricular tachycardia by septal artery occlusion with alcohol injection into septal branches.[7] Simultaneously, performed animal studies showed that use of absolute alcohol resulted in more homogeneous scars.

All these observations led to the primary idea of percutaneous treatment of septal hypertrophy in HOCM patients by G Berghoefer (personal communication).[8] He developed the hypothesis that occlusion of a septal coronary branch supplying the hypertrophied septal area with consecutive therapeutic infarction may result in gradient reduction. Identification of the target septal branch should be done by echo contrast study during temporary balloon occlusion of the target branch. Berghoefer discussed that the definitive septal branch occlusion should be performed either chemically by alcohol injection or mechanically by deployment of coils. Unfortunately, Berghoefer could not transfer his idea into clinical practice.

It took some years until Kuhn et al. published their studies of the effect of temporary balloon occlusion in patients with HOCM in the early 1990s.[9] In the meantime Sigwart has treated patients with the alcohol ablation. He published the results of the first three patients in 1995.[4] The first publication of the new treatment option for symptomatic patients with HOCM opened the discussion about the long-term effect of the induced myocardial scar.[10] Despite the discussion septal ablation became popular worldwide.[8,11-13] Introduction of myocardial contrast echo guidance in 1996 by Faber et al. was the major step for this acceptance as first choice treatment in most patients.[11]

INDICATION FOR SEPTAL ABLATION

Symptomatic (dyspnea, angina, exercise-related syncope) patients with significant obstruction (>30 mm Hg at rest and >50 mm Hg at provocation) despite optimal medical therapy (beta-blocker or verapamil without vasodilating drugs) should be considered for septal reduction treatment. From the morphologic standpoint patients isolated non-systolic anterior motion (non-SAM)-related mitral valve disease should primarily undergo myectomy. But, clearly SAM-related outflow tract gradient with consecutive mitral regurgitation and patients with mid-cavitary obstruction can be successfully treated by percutaneous transluminal septal myocardial ablation (PTSMA).[14] Patients with additional cardiac diseases are primarily candidates for combined surgical therapy although combined interventional treatment can be performed, especially in patients with coronary artery disease.[15] Patients with prior myectomy and insufficient result had been successfully treated.[16] In summary, indication for septal ablation is an individual decision taking into account clinical and morphologic aspects as well as the patient's choice after detailed information about the different treatment options.

TECHNIQUE OF SEPTAL ABLATION

First of all, it has to be stated that treatment of symptomatic patients with HOCM is an elective procedure in order to improve the quality of life. Therefore, achievement of a satisfactory result and avoidance of complications are equivalent therapeutic aims. An indispensible requirement is that alcohol septal ablation should be performed only by an experienced multidisciplinary team in the treatment of HCM including an experienced interventional cardiologist who is familiar in the management of all potential interventional complications and an experienced echocardiographer. Due to the large number of anatomic variations a certain number of procedures are necessary in order to maintain the interventional skills.[17]

After introduction of percutaneous septal alcohol septal ablation for treatment of symptomatic patients with HOCM a large number of technical variants have been used and described.[18] As in most centers we use echocardiographic guided ablation which was introduced as PTSMA.[19]

A diagnostic catheterization is required to exclude coronary artery disease in symptomatic patients, define a potential target septal branch, and measure left ventricular outflow tract gradient (LVOTG). Simultaneous pressure recording of aortic and left ventricular pressures (Fig. 1) is necessary in order to measure accurate LVOTG at rest, during Valsalva maneuver, and postextrasystolic beat (Brockenbrough phenomenon), especially in patients with atrial fibrillation.

To perform PTSMA, we prefer two arterial accesses. A coronary angioplasty guide catheter is inserted via the right femoral artery and a special pigtail catheter via the left femoral artery. Simultaneous recording of the aortic pressure through the guide catheter and the left ventricular pressure through the pigtail catheter enables earliest diagnosis of hemodynamic changes during ablation, especially potential complications like pericardial tamponade.

Up to 50% of the treated patients develop temporary complete heart block at any time of the procedure. Therefore, placement of a temporary pacemaker lead is mandatory in patients without pacemaker or implantable cardioverter defibrillator (ICD). To avoid rarely observed loss of capture after alcohol injection, especially in high risk patients [previous myectomy, baseline left bundle branch block (LBBB), septal pacing], output increase of permanent

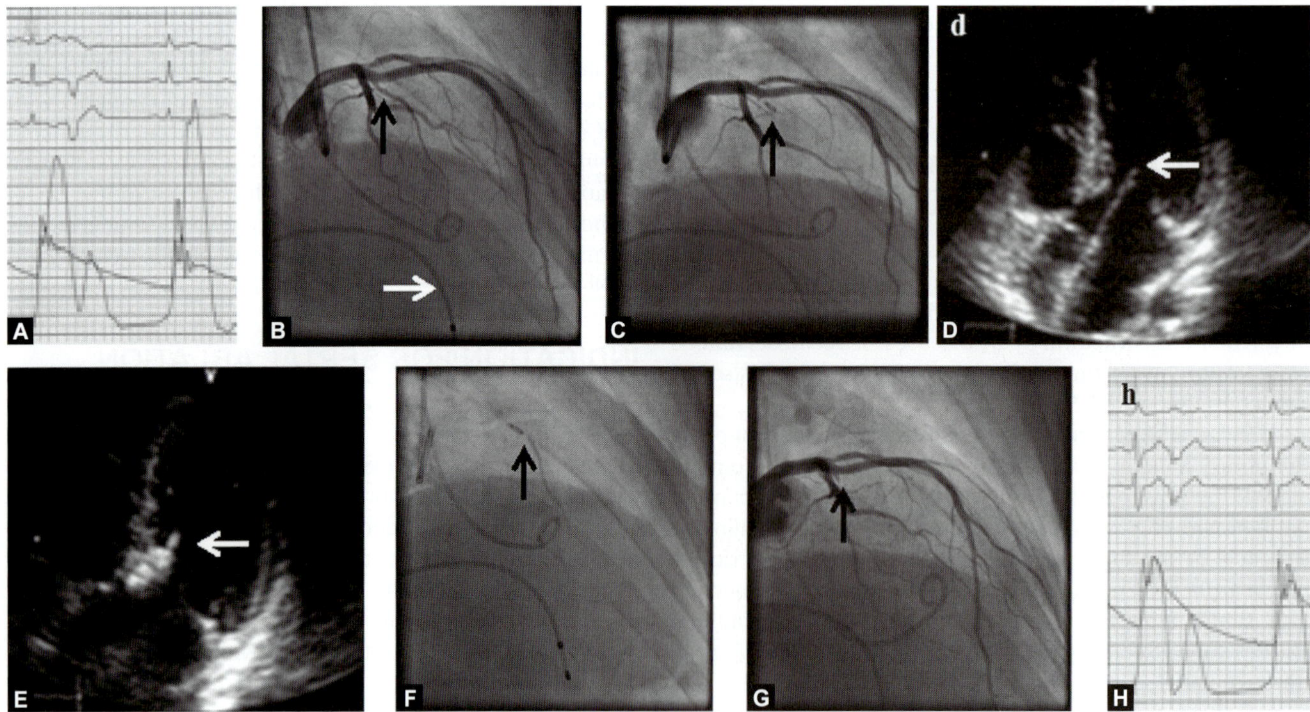

FIG. 1: Echo-guided septal ablation (percutaneous transluminal septal myocardial ablation); **A,** Simultaneous pressure recording of left ventricular outflow tract and aorta at rest and post extrasystole; **B,** Baseline coronary angiography of the left coronary artery with estimated target branch (black arrow) and temporary pacemaker lead (white arrow); **C,** Placement of the "over-the-wire" balloon into the target septal branch (black arrow); **D,** Modified baseline four-chamber view in transthoracic echocardiogram with systolic anterior motion (SAM) septal contact (arrow); **E,** Echo contrast depot in the basal septum at SAM septal contact (arrow); **F,** Injection of contrast dye through the central lumen of the "over-the-wire" balloon (arrow); **G,** Occluded septal branch (branch) after balloon withdraw 10 minutes after last alcohol injection; **H,** final hemodynamic measurement with gradient at rest and post extrasystole.

pacemaker or ICD is recommended. Weight adjusted heparin at the beginning of the procedure as well as opiate analgesia before alcohol injection are administered intravenously as a routine.

Left coronary angiography [usually in right anterior oblique (RAO) cranial view] permits the identification of possible target septal branches. In patients with left ventricular outflow tract obstruction commonly the first large septal branch or one of its side branches is considered as target vessel. Nevertheless, the diagonal and intermediate branches and rarely, the right coronary artery should also be carefully inspected for the existence of atypically originating septal branches.

An angioplasty floppy guidewire with standard length is advanced in the supposed target septal branch. Sometimes, it may be necessary to try differently shaped wires due to the enormous variety of septal branches anatomy. A mildly oversized short (6–10 mm) over-the-wire (OTW) balloon is advanced into the septal branch and inflated. Inflation pressures above the nominal pressure should be avoided as they result in compression of the central lumen of the catheter. Usually, balloon sizes are 1.5–2.5 (rarely 3.0) mm. The occluded balloon should avoid alcohol spilling to the left anterior descending (LAD), thus avoiding infarction of non-target myocardial areas. Avoidance of the parent vessel dissection can be achieved by positioning the balloon distally the origin of the target branch.

Identification of the target septal branch is the most critical part as alcohol misplacement could lead to necrosis in unwanted left and right ventricular areas like free-walls or papillary muscles with potential mitral or tricuspid valve regurgitation. Furthermore, an excessive anatomic variation with potential collateralization in the septal artery system has been described.[20] Postmortem studies have shown that, the first septal branch supplies the right ventricular free wall in 2 out of 10 patients and led to incomplete supply of the basal septum in 4 out of 10 patients.[21] In 1996, Faber et al. had detected alcohol misplacements in the septal area during the early series. Therefore, they invented echocardiographic guidance of the procedure in August 1996 which was presented at the American Heart Association (AHA) annual scientific meeting in 1996. (Fig. 2) Each predicted target septal branch should be tested with myocardial contrast echocardiography.[11,22,23]

After balloon placement and before inflation, multiple transthoracic echocardiographic views (parasternal, apical, and subcostal) are taken and recorded. Thereafter, the balloon catheter is inflated and the guidewire withdrawn. About

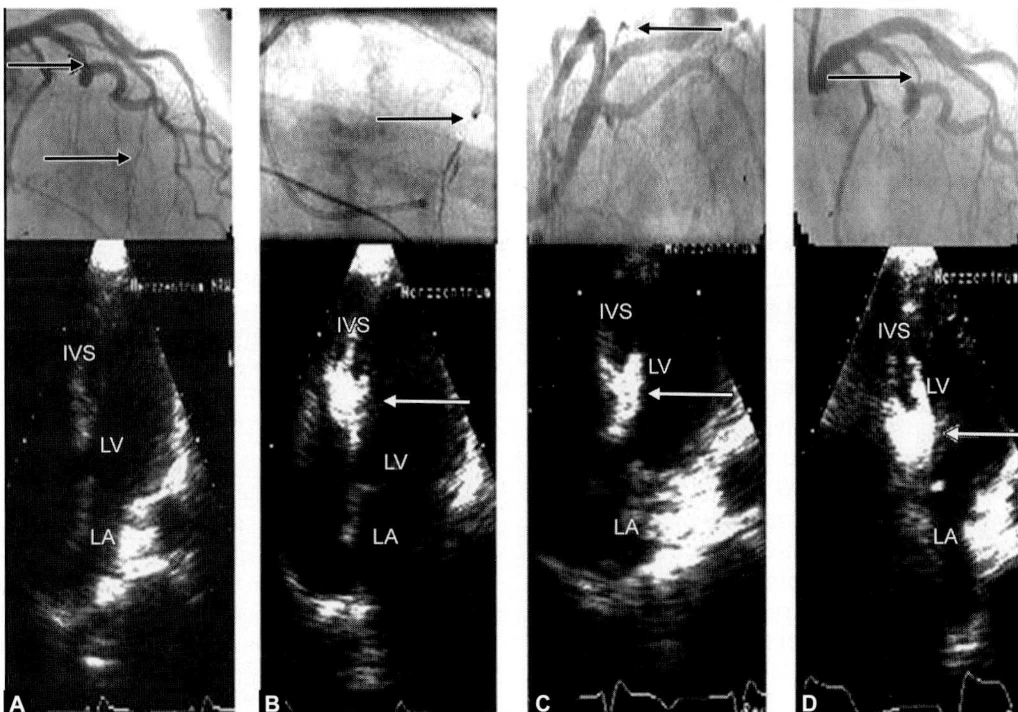

IVS, intraventricular septum; LV, left ventricle; LA, left atrium.

FIG. 2: First ever echo-guided septal ablation (upper line angiography, lower line transthoracic echocardiography); **A,** Angiographic documentation of atypical (upper arrow) and typical (lower arrow) septal branches. Echocardiographic four-chamber view [intraventricular septum (IVS), left ventricle, left atrium]; **B,** Contrast injection through "over-the-wire" balloon in the typical branch (black arrow) with echo contrast depot in the mid-septal intraventricular septum (IVS) (white arrow); **C,** Contrast injection through "over-the-wire" balloon in the atypical branch (black arrow) with echo contrast depot in the subaortic IVS (white arrow); **D,** Final angiography with occlusion of the atypical septal branch (black arrow) and perfect located alcohol depot (white arrow).

1-2 mL of echocardiographic contrast agent is injected through the balloon catheter with simultaneous transthoracic echocardiography repeating the previous recorded views in order to exclude misplacements which may lead to complications in case of alcohol injection. After withdraw of the mostly used contrast agent Levovist® (Bayer, Germany) from the market, we compared different echocardiographic contrast agents in vitro and during septal ablation. Finally, cooled (4°C) agitated gelatine polysuccinate (Gelafundin®, B Braun, Melsungen, Germany), a colloid plasma volume substitute, offers the best contrasting properties and stability.[23] The use of Gelafundin® gives reliable information regarding contrast opacification of any other cardiac structure (right ventricle, papillary muscle, and other areas of left ventricle). After confirmation with myocardial contrast echocardiography, selective angiography of the target septal branch through the inflated balloon catheter should document the adequate sealing of the septal branch and exclude filling of any other coronary artery through septal collaterals.[24,25] Diagnostic accuracy of this important step will be improved by increasing the frame rate during contrast injection. In case of retrograde filling of the LAD or any other vessel the collateralizing septal branch can be occluded by a monorail balloon.[24] After identification of the ideal septal branch up to 2–3 cc of absolute alcohol is slowly injected through the central lumen of the OTW balloon under continuous fluoroscopic—to exclude instability and dislocation of the balloon, hemodynamic, and electrocardiographic control. Injection rate is 1 cc/min followed by angiographic control of the left coronary artery after each cc of alcohol. Injected alcohol amount should be 1 cc/1 cm septal thickness.[26]

Any catheter dislocation or resistance during injection should lead to immediate cessation of injection to avoid alcohol spilling. The balloon is left in place for 10 minutes after final alcohol injection. Shorter time have been associated with higher complication risk due to alcohol backflow.[27]

After balloon retraction, a final angiogram documents occlusion of the septal branch without complications of any other vessel. Thereafter, final measurement of LVOTG at rest and provocation are repeated. As we are aware of hemodynamic remodeling and scar formation with further gradient reduction up to 12 months after alcohol injection we plan ablation of further septal branches only in patients with combined subaortic and mid-cavitary obstruction in one session to reduce the risk of complications and keep to therapeutic scar as small as necessary.

After removal of the right femoral artery sheath and arterial closure with a closure device, the patient will subsequently stay in the coronary care unit for at least 48 hours under constant hemodynamic and rhythm control. Cardiac enzyme measurements every 6–8 hours allow documentation of peak creatine kinase (CK) value. In absence of third-degree atrioventricular (AV) block, the temporary pacemaker will be removed the morning after the procedure. In case an ongoing heart block requiring temporary pacing the jugular or subclavian venous access is preferable in order to reduce the risk of lower limb venous thrombosis. After 48 hours we decide on implantation of a permanent pacemaker or ICD in case of increased risk of sudden cardiac death according to the clinical risk stratification models.[28-30] Hospital discharge usually takes place after 1 week of permanent electrocardiographic monitoring being aware of the risk of late heart block.

The described actual technique is the result of permanent steps to reduce complications and improve hemodynamic and clinical results. Main steps of this improvement were the introduction of echo contrast guidance and reduction of the amount of alcohol. Other discussed technical aspects like, intracardiac echocardiography or preinterventional computed tomography (CT) coronarography for choosing the target septal branch did not gain widespread acceptance.

ACUTE RESULTS AND COMPLICATIONS

Since, the first report of percutaneous treatment of symptomatic patients with HOCM by Sigwart a large number of consistent reports have shown acute hemodynamic success in more than or equal to 90% of the patients mainly treated with the echocardiography-guided technique.[4,8,11-13,26,30-37]

Faber et al. reported in the first series of 61 patients with echo-guided septal ablation compared to the initial 30 patients with nonecho-guided ablation a superiority with respect to acute gradient reduction (>50% gradient reduction 92% vs. 70%) and need for permanent pacemaker implantation (7% vs. 17%). Reduction of LVOT obstruction resulted in symptomatic improvement and in increased of exercise capacity.[19]

From the very beginning of percutaneous septal ablation concerns about the risk of procedure-related acute and late complications had been discussed. Despite the reduction of reported complication rates due to increased experience of the interventional cardiologists it should be addressed that avoidance of complications should be the main goal of this elective procedure beside the achievement of a good hemodynamic and clinical success. Up to now there is an open discussion about the numbers of required procedures to achieve and maintain large enough experience to perform safe procedures.

The most common complication after alcohol septal ablation is complete heart block requiring permanent pacing. Despite the reduction of heart block after introduction of echo-guided ablation up to 50% of patients may develop conduction problems in the first hours after alcohol injection, which resolves spontaneously in most cases (either in the cath laboratory or in the coronary care unit). This is due to the close proximity of the first septal branch with the His bundle or the right bundle branch.[38,39] As pointed out before placement of a temporary pacemaker before alcohol injection is an absolute requirement of the procedure because the development of heart block is not predictable.

Faber et al. developed a scoring system based on ECG parameters, hemodynamic variables and myocardial enzyme release for the prediction of pacemaker dependency after alcohol septal ablation which turned out to be a sufficient help in clinical routine.[40] Patients with pre-existing left bundle branch block are at higher risk to develop complete heart block as nearly 50% of the patients develop complete right bundle branch block. In such patients implantation of a permanent pacemaker before alcohol septal ablation can be discussed. As pointed out before preprocedural ICD implantation is certainly reasonable in case of an increased risk of sudden cardiac death according to the commonly used risk stratification models.

Advances of the initial technique of alcohol septal ablation with the addition of myocardial contrast echocardiography and use of lower alcohol volumes resulted in a reduced need for permanent pacing after the intervention. Finally, about 10% of the patients will require a permanent pacemaker.[11,41-43]

Like any interventional procedure alcohol septal ablation may be complicated by technical problems. Reported complications include coronary dissection, coronary spasm, ventricular fibrillation, cardiac tamponade mainly due to temporary pacemaker lead, pulmonary embolism, cardiogenic shock, stroke, and problems with the puncture site.[33] As in our personal experience in about 2,000 ablations without coronary spasm and ventricular fibrillation we would postulate that leakage and misplacement of alcohol are the main reasons for these reported complications. Therefore, special care should be taken to avoid alcohol leakage to the LAD due to retrograde flow through an incompletely sealed septal branch or through collateral flow to other septal branches that could lead to an unwanted infarction.[24,25] Dislocation or rupture of the balloon during alcohol injection as well as too early deflation and retraction of the balloon after alcohol injection are also possible causes of alcohol spilling.[27,44] These complications can be avoided by careful intervention following a strict interventional protocol (use of slightly oversized balloon, careful angiographic exploration of the septal branch, thorough observation of the balloon during slow alcohol injection, well-timed deflation 10 minutes after alcohol injection).[22] The described complications associated with the technical part of the procedure are influenced by the considerable learning curve and are rare in high-volume centers.[36,45] In addition, it should be mentioned that the procedure can and should be abandoned if the operator has the impression of a potential complication.

FOLLOW-UP RESULTS

From the very beginning of PTSMA follow-up studies have shown ongoing hemodynamic and clinical improvement with further reduction of the left ventricular outflow tract obstruction during the first year due to postprocedural remodeling.[31]

The mean residual LVOTG decreased from 60–70 mm Hg to 15–20 mm Hg. Patients with higher residual gradients have an increased all-cause mortality at follow-up.[35,43,46] Mainly due to the anatomic variation of the septal artery system[21] 14% of patients may require a second ablation to get an adequate result.[47]

Successful ablation results in reduction of SAM-related mitral regurgitation and pulmonary artery pressure.[11,31] Hemodynamic improvement after ASA is associated with symptomatic improvement and increased exercise capacity. The subjective improvement has been verified by objective measurements of exercise performance on cardiopulmonary exercise testing.[26,48]

With introduction of septal ablation for symptomatic patients with HOCM, concern was raised on the potential negative effect of creating a myocardial scar in patients who were already at risk for ventricular arrhythmias.[10] This presumption was supported by initial case reports of ventricular arrhythmias occurring after septal ablation.[49]

We reported on an up to 8 years follow-up in the first 100 consecutive symptomatic patients treated with echocardiography-guided technique. Only one sudden cardiac death was observed, and event-free survival at 5 years was 82%.[31] A more recent study on 178 consecutive patients treated with septal ablation provided similar results. Survivals after 1, 5, and 10 years were 97%, 92%, and 82%, respectively, and did not differ from survival in an age- and sex-matched general population. The only independent predictor of all-cause mortality was age at the time of ablation.[50]

A study on 470 consecutive patients treated with echo-guided ablation between 1996 and 2010 in Germany and Denmark addressed the question of sudden cardiac death during follow-up. Before ablation, 25% of the patients had more than or equal to 2 risk factors for sudden death with a significant reduction to 8% after ablation. The observed 10-year survival was 88%, and survival free of sudden death was 95%, which was similar to that of a matched general population.[43]

Veselka et al. reported on the results of the Euro-ASA registry in which 1,275 patients underwent the procedure in 10 European tertiary referral centers in 7 countries. The 10-year overall survival was 77%, whereas sudden death-free survival was 90%. Follow-up in this study exceeded 7,000 patient-years with a sudden death rate of 0.6% per year. The combined rate of sudden and cardiovascular mortality was relatively low at 1.2% per patient-year.[35] In summary, an expected increase of cardiac mortality after septal ablation has not been observed.

CONCLUSION

In patients with symptomatic HOCM despite optimal medical therapy PTSMA has been established as effective alternative to the previous gold standard surgical myectomy. The optimal therapy of an individual HOCM patient should be found in the context of a HCM team, consisting of experts of both treatment methods and the disease itself. Decisive criteria are anatomical findings as well as cardiac and noncardiac comorbidities. Both methods should not be regarded as competing, but complementary treatment methods. Procedural success is related to the experience of the surgeon or interventionalist.

REFERENCES

1. Maron BJ, Gardin JM, Flack JM, et al. Prevalence of hypertrophic cardiomyopathy in a general population of young adults. Echocardiographic analysis of 4111 subjects in the CARDIA Study. Coronary Artery Risk Development in (Young) Adults. Circulation. 1995;92(4):785-9.
2. Semsarian C, Ingles J, Maron MS, et al. New perspectives on the prevalence of hypertrophic cardiomyopathy. J Am Coll Cardiol. 2015;65(12):1249-54.
3. Maron MS, Olivotto I, Betocchi S, et al. Effect of left ventricular outflow tract obstruction on clinical outcome in hypertrophic cardiomyopathy. N Engl J Med 2003;348(4): 295-303.
4. Sigwart U. Non-surgical myocardial reduction for hypertrophic obstructive cardiomyopathy. Lancet 1995;346(8969):211-4.
5. Sigwart U, Grbic M, Essinger A, et al. Improvement of left ventricular function after percutaneous transluminal coronary angioplasty. Am J Cardiol. 1982;49(4):651-7.
6. Come PC, Riley MF. Hypertrophic cardiomyopathy. Disappearance of auscultatory, carotid pulse, and echocardiographic manifestations of obstruction following myocardial infarction. Chest. 1982;82(4):451-4.
7. Brugada P, de Swart H, Smeets JL, et al. Transcoronary chemical ablation of ventricular tachycardia. Circulation. 1989;79(3):475-82.
8. Seggewiss H, Gleichmann U, Faber L, et al. Percutaneous transluminal septal myocardial ablation in hypertrophic obstructive cardiomyopathy: acute results and 3-month follow-up in 25 patients. J Am Coll Cardiol. 1998;31(2):252-8.
9. Kuhn H, Gietzen F, Leuner C, et al. Induction of subaortic septal ischaemia to reduce obstruction in hypertrophic obstructive cardiomyopathy. Studies to develop a new catheter-based concept of treatment. Eur Heart J. 1997;18(5):846-51.
10. Goodwin JF, Oakley CM. Non-surgical myocardial reduction for hypertrophic obstructive cardiomyopathy. Lancet. 1995;346(8990):1624.
11. Faber L, Seggewiss H, Fassbender D, et al. Percutaneous transluminal septal myocardial ablation in hypertrophic obstructive cardiomyopathy: acute results in 66 patients with reference to myocardial contrast echocardiography. Z Kardiol. 1998;87(3):191-201.
12. Nagueh SF, Groves BM, Schwartz L, et al. Alcohol septal ablation for the treatment of hypertrophic obstructive cardiomyopathy. A multicenter North American registry. J Am Coll Cardiol. 2011;58(22):2322-8.
13. Gietzen FH, Leuner CJ, Raute-Kreinsen U, et al. Acute and long-term results after transcoronary ablation of septal hypertrophy (TASH). Catheter interventional treatment for hypertrophic obstructive cardiomyopathy. Eur Heart J. 1999;20(18):1342-54.
14. Seggewiss H, Faber L. Percutaneous septal ablation for hypertrophic cardiomyopathy and mid-ventricular obstruction. Eur J Echocardiogr. 2000;1(4):277-80.
15. Seggewiss H, Faber L, Meyners W, et al. Simultaneous percutaneous treatment in hypertrophic obstructive cardiomyopathy and coronary artery disease: a case report. Cathet Cardiovasc Diagn. 1998;44(1):65-9.
16. Rigopoulos AG, Seggewiss H. Twenty years of alcohol septal ablation in hypertrophic obstructive cardiomyopathy. Curr Cardiol Rev. 2016;12(4):285-96.
17. Harold JG, Bass TA, Bashore TM, et al. ACCF/AHA/SCAI 2013 update of the clinical competence statement on coronary artery interventional procedures: a report of the American College of Cardiology Foundation/American Heart Association/American College of Physicians Task Force on Clinical Competence and Training (Writing Committee to Revise the 2007 Clinical Competence Statement on Cardiac Interventional Procedures). J Am Coll Cardiol. 2013;62(4): 357-96.
18. Nishimura RA, Seggewiss H, Schaff HV. Hypertrophic obstructive cardiomyopathy: surgical myectomy and septal ablation. Circ Res. 2017;121(7):771-83.
19. Faber L, Seggewiss H, Gleichmann U. Percutaneous transluminal septal myocardial ablation in hypertrophic obstructive cardiomyopathy: results with respect to intraprocedural myocardial contrast echocardiography. Circulation. 1998;98(22):2415-21.
20. Angelini P. The "1st septal unit" in hypertrophic obstructive cardiomyopathy: a newly recognized anatomo-functional entity, identified during recent alcohol septal ablation experience. Tex Heart Inst J. 2007;34(3):336-46.
21. Singh M, Edwards WD, Holmes DR Jr, et al. Anatomy of the first septal perforating artery: a study with implications for ablation therapy for hypertrophic cardiomyopathy. Mayo Clin Proc. 2001;76(8):799-802.
22. Seggewiss H. Current status of alcohol septal ablation for patients with hypertrophic cardiomyopathy. Curr Cardiol Rep. 2001;3(2):160-6.
23. Pfeiffer B, Rigopoulos A, Seggewiss H. Myocardial contrast echocardiography guided alcohol septal ablation in hypertrophic obstructive cardiomyopathy with a new echocardiographic contrast agent. Dtsch Med Wochenschr. 2012;137(41):2093-6.
24. Koljaja-Batzner A, Pfeiffer BHS. Septal Collateralization to Right Coronary Artery in Alcohol Septal Ablation. Solution to a Dangerous Pitfall. JACC-Card Intervent. [In Press].
25. Rigopoulos A, Sepp R, Palinkas A, et al. Alcohol septal ablation for hypertrophic obstructive cardiomyopathy: collateral vessel communication between septal branches. Int J Cardiol. 2006;113(2):e67-9.
26. Faber L, Seggewiss H, Welge D, et al. Echo-guided percutaneous septal ablation for symptomatic hypertrophic obstructive cardiomyopathy: 7 years of experience. Eur J Echocardiogr. 2004;5(5):347-55.
27. Ruzyllo W, Chojnowska L, Demkow M, et al. Left ventricular outflow tract gradient decrease with non-surgical myocardial reduction improves exercise capacity in patients with hypertrophic obstructive cardiomyopathy. Eur Heart J. 2000;21(9):770-7.
28. Elliott PM, Anastasakis A, Borger MA, et al. 2014 ESC Guidelines on diagnosis and management of hypertrophic cardiomyopathy: the Task Force for the Diagnosis and Management of Hypertrophic Cardiomyopathy of the European Society of Cardiology (ESC). Eur Heart J. 2014;35(39):2733-79.
29. O'Mahony C, Jichi F, Pavlou M, et al. A novel clinical risk prediction model for sudden cardiac death in hypertrophic cardiomyopathy (HCM risk-SCD). Eur Heart J. 2014;35(30):2010-20.
30. Faber L, Seggewiss H, Welge D, et al. Predicting the risk of atrioventricular conduction lesions after percutaneous septal ablation for obstructive hypertrophic cardiomyopathy. Z Kardiol. 2003;92(1): 39-47.
31. Seggewiss H, Rigopoulos A, Welge D, et al. Long-term follow-up after percutaneous septal ablation in hypertrophic obstructive cardiomyopathy. Clin Res Cardiol. 2007;96(12):856-63.
32. Sorajja P, Valeti U, Nishimura RA, et al. Outcome of alcohol septal ablation for obstructive hypertrophic cardiomyopathy. Circulation. 2008;118(2):131-9.
33. Alam M, Dokainish H, Lakkis N. Alcohol septal ablation for hypertrophic obstructive cardiomyopathy: a systematic review of published studies. J Interv Cardiol. 2006;19(4):319-27.
34. Liebregts M, Faber L, Jensen MK, et al. Outcomes of Alcohol Septal Ablation in Younger Patients With Obstructive Hypertrophic Cardiomyopathy. JACC Cardiovasc Interv. 2017;10(11):1134-43.
35. Veselka J, Jensen MK, Liebregts M, et al. Long-term clinical outcome after alcohol septal ablation for obstructive hypertrophic cardiomyopathy: results from the Euro-ASA registry. Eur Heart J. 2016;37(19):1517-23.
36. Veselka J, Faber L, Jensen MK, et al. Effect of Institutional Experience on Outcomes of Alcohol Septal Ablation for Hypertrophic Obstructive Cardiomyopathy. Can J Cardiol. 2018;34(1):16-22.
37. Veselka J, Faber L, Liebregts M, et al. Outcome of alcohol septal ablation in mildly symptomatic patients with hypertrophic obstructive cardiomyopathy: A Long-Term Follow-Up Study Based on the Euro-Alcohol Septal Ablation Registry. J Am Heart Assoc. 2017;6(5).
38. Talreja DR, Nishimura RA, Edwards WD, et al. Alcohol septal ablation versus surgical septal myectomy: comparison of effects on atrioventricular conduction tissue. J Am Coll Cardiol. 2004;44(12):2329-32.
39. Seggewiss H, Rigopoulos A. Alcohol septal ablation for hypertrophic obstructive cardiomyopathy. Percutaneous Interventional Cardiovascular Medicine: The PCR-EAPCI Textbook. 2012. pp. 461-76.
40. Faber L, Welge D, Fassbender D, et al. Percutaneous septal ablation for symptomatic hypertrophic obstructive cardiomyopathy: managing the risk of procedure-related AV conduction disturbances. Int J Cardiol. 2007;119(2):163-7.
41. Fifer MA. Controversies in cardiovascular medicine. Most fully informed patients choose septal ablation over septal myectomy. Circulation. 2007;116(2):207-16; discussion 16.

42. Veselka J, Zemanek D, Tomasov P, et al. Complications of low-dose, echo-guided alcohol septal ablation. Catheter Cardiovasc Interv. 2010;75(4):546-50.
43. Jensen MK, Prinz C, Horstkotte D, et al. Alcohol septal ablation in patients with hypertrophic obstructive cardiomyopathy: low incidence of sudden cardiac death and reduced risk profile. Heart. 2013;99(14):1012-7.
44. Antolinos Pérez MJ dlMVG, Gimeno Blanes JR, Cerdán Sánchez Mdel C, et al. Balloon rupture and alcohol leakage into the left anterior descending coronary artery during percutaneous septal ablation for hypertrophic obstructive cardiomyopathy. Rev Esp Cardiol. 2005;58(7):872-4.
45. Sorajja P, Binder J, Nishimura RA, et al. Predictors of an optimal clinical outcome with alcohol septal ablation for obstructive hypertrophic cardiomyopathy. Catheter Cardiovasc Interv. 2013;81(1):E58-67.
46. Sorajja P, Ommen SR, Holmes DR Jr, et al. Survival after alcohol septal ablation for obstructive hypertrophic cardiomyopathy. Circulation. 2012;126(20):2374-80.
47. Fernandes VL, Nielsen C, Nagueh SF, et al. Follow-up of alcohol septal ablation for symptomatic hypertrophic obstructive cardiomyopathy the Baylor and Medical University of South Carolina experience 1996 to 2007. JACC Cardiovasc Interv. 2008;1(5):561-70.
48. Faber L, Welge D, Fassbender D, et al. One-year follow-up of percutaneous septal ablation for symptomatic hypertrophic obstructive cardiomyopathy in 312 patients: predictors of hemodynamic and clinical response. Clin Res Cardiol. 2007;96(12):864-73.
49. Nishimura RA, Ommen SR. Septal reduction therapy for obstructive hypertrophic cardiomyopathy and sudden death: what statistics cannot tell you. Circ Cardiovasc Interv. 2010;3(2):91-3.
50. Veselka J, Krejci J, Tomasov P, et al. Long-term survival after alcohol septal ablation for hypertrophic obstructive cardiomyopathy: a comparison with general population. Eur Heart J. 2014;35(30):2040-5.

CHAPTER 72

Percutaneous Management of Paravalvular Leak: Patient Selection and Outcomes

A Sreenivas Kumar, Ramakrishna Janapati

INTRODUCTION

Paravalvular leak (PVL) is defined as an abnormal retrograde flow between the implanted prosthetic valve and annulus of the native valve. The prosthetic valve regurgitation includes regurgitation through the valve (transvalvular) as well as paravalvular regurgitation (also known as paravalvular leak). PVL can occur after (1) surgical valve replacement; (2) surgical valve repair; or (3) after percutaneous valve implantation. PVL is a rare complication associated with surgical or percutaneous valve implantations. Previous studies reported an incidence of PVL around 2–10% in aortic valve replacements and 7–17% in the mitral valve (MV) implantation.[1,2] Only 1–5% of patients with PVLs can had serious clinical manifestations[3,4] and majority of the PVL had benign clinical course. Definitive treatment of significant PVL requires redo surgical repair or replacement, but it is associated with significant morbidity and mortality. Percutaneous treatment of PVL has been rapidly evolving therapy for significant PVL. With increasing operator experience and better availability of percutaneous closure devices, the transcatheter treatment of PVL was associated with lower morbidity, mortality, shorter duration of procedure time and hospitalization.[5]

ETIOLOGY OF PARAVALVULAR LEAK

Paravalvular leak results from the incompetent seal between the native annulus and prosthetic sewing ring. Several factors increase the risk of PVL that includes abnormal pressure or traction forces on implanted prosthesis, slow resorption of annular calcium, postoperative infections, continuous suturing of mitral prosthesis, smaller size prosthetic valve, and location of valve implant. PVL can occur early after surgery or it may be delayed complication and early occurrence usually associated with technical aspects. Delayed PVLs can result from infective endocarditis with suture dehiscence and slow resorption of annular calcium.[6,7]

CLINICAL DIAGNOSIS

The most common presenting symptoms and signs of significant PVL includes that of congestive heart failure (CHF) from fluid overload in 90% of cases and hemolytic anemia in 30–40% cases. Anemia may be the presenting sign due to intravascular hemolysis. Majority of patients had New York Heart Association (NYHA) class III or more symptoms. Clinical examination had a limited sensitivity and specificity in detecting significant PVL. Mitral PVLs may present with a pansystolic murmur heard over the left sternal border, with radiation of murmur depending on the direction of regurgitant jet. In aortic PVLs, a high-pitched decrescendo early diastolic murmur heard at the neoaortic area. Hemolytic anemia is more commonly observed in patients with smaller size leaks with high-velocity jets, pre-existing anemia, and with increased red blood cells (RBCs) fragility due to folate or iron deficiency. Hemolysis can be diagnosed by a serum lactate dehydrogenase (LDH) level more than 450 U/L and any two of the four following criteria: blood hemoglobin less than 13.8 g/dL for men or less than 12.4 g/dL for women, serum haptoglobin less than 50 mg/dL, and reticulocyte count more than 2%.[8] In addition, plasma free hemoglobin levels more than 40 mg/dL are suggestive of intravascular hemolysis. Plasma N-terminal pro-brain natriuretic peptide (NT-proBNP) is usually elevated (>400 pg/mL) in patients with CHF and increases as the severity of aortic or mitral regurgitation increases.[9,10]

IMAGING

Imaging provides a pivotal role in diagnosis of PVL, and to detect the size, extent location, number of leaks. Imaging also plays an essential role during and after procedure to assess the success of the procedure and residual leaks. Imaging is useful to assess the left ventricular (LV) function, to detect any active infective endocarditis, excessive rocking motion of the prosthetic valve and severity of regurgitation. In most cases echocardiography is useful for definitive diagnosis of PVL. Other imaging modalities that are increasingly used for evaluation of PVL are cardiac computed tomography (CT) and magnetic resonance imaging (MRI).

Echocardiography

Echocardiogram is the mainstay of imaging modality for diagnosis of PVL and both transthoracic and transesophageal echocardiography (TEE) are utilized for evaluation of prosthetic valves. TTE provides both functional and anatomic information of prosthetic valve. TTE is routinely used for assessment of prosthetic valve mobility, chamber size, and function and transvalvular gradients. However, TTE is limited by acoustic shadowing, metallic artifacts, and with limited imaging windows in postoperative patients. TEE provides better spatial resolution of prosthetic valve function and evaluation of prosthetic valve leaks, and is superior to TTE especially for imaging of mitral prosthesis. For aortic PVL the acoustic shadowing prevents the assessment of posteriorly located PVL by TTE parasternal long-axis view and anteriorly located PVL by TEE midesophageal views. Three-dimensional (3D) TEE provides better assessment of PVL size and shape when compared to two-dimensional (2D) TEE.[11] 3D TEE is most useful for intraprocedural guidance and it provides superior assessment over 2D TEE during procedure. Several studies had used different grading schemes for assessment of severity of PVL and most commonly used in the previous studies was a 3-class grading system (mild, moderate, and severe) and some other studies had used a 4-class grading scheme (grades 1, 2, 3, 4) similar to native valve regurgitation. More recently a unified 5-class grading system was proposed which classifies PVL as trace, mild, mild-to-moderate, moderate, moderate-to-severe, and severe. The PVL severity was classified based on several qualitative and quantitative parameters such as vena contracta width, jet density, jet deceleration time, diastolic flow reversal in the descending aorta regurgitant volume, and regurgitant fraction (Table 1).

TABLE 1: Parameters to define the severity of mitral and aortic PVL

Mild mitral PVL	Severe mitral PVL
Normal sewing ring motion	Sewing ring motion usually abnormal
Jet features: Narrow jet width, infrequent multiple, no proximal flow convergence	Jet features: Wide jet width, frequently multiple, proximal flow convergence visible
% LVOT diameter <30%	% LVOT diameter ≥60%
Circumferential extent <10%	Circumferential extent ≥30%
Normal LV size	Moderately or severely dilated LV size
Vena contracta width <4 mm	Vena contracta width >6 mm
Incomplete or faint spectral Doppler	Dense spectral Doppler
Quantitative criteria for mild MVR PVL	**Quantitative criteria for severe MVR PVL**
RVol <30 mL	RVol ≥60 mL
RF <30%	RF ≥50%
EROA <0.1 cm^2	EROA ≥0.3 cm^2
Mild aortic PVL	**Severe aortic PVL**
Normal sewing ring motion	Sewing ring motion usually abnormal
Jet features: Narrow jet width, infrequent multiple, no proximal flow convergence	Jet features: Wide jet width, frequently multiple, proximal flow convergence visible
% LVOT diameter <30%	% LVOT diameter ≥60%
Circumferential extent <10%	Circumferential extent ≥30%
Normal LV size	Moderately or severely dilated LV size
Vena contracta width <4 mm	Vena contracta width ≥6 mm
Incomplete or faint spectral Doppler	Dense spectral Doppler
PHT >500 ms	PHT <200 ms
Diastolic flow reversal absent or brief	Holodiastolic flow reversal (end-diastolic velocity >20–30 cm/s)
Quantitative criteria for mild AVR PVL	**Quantitative criteria for severe AVR PVL**
RVol <30 mL	RVol ≥60 mL
RF <30%	RF ≥50%
EROA <0.1 cm	EROA ≥0.3 cm

AVR, aortic valve replacement; EROA, effective regurgitant orifice area; LVOT, left ventricular outflow tract; MVR, mitral valve replacement; PVL, paravalvular leak; PHT, pressure half-time; RF, regurgitant fraction; RVol, regurgitant volume.

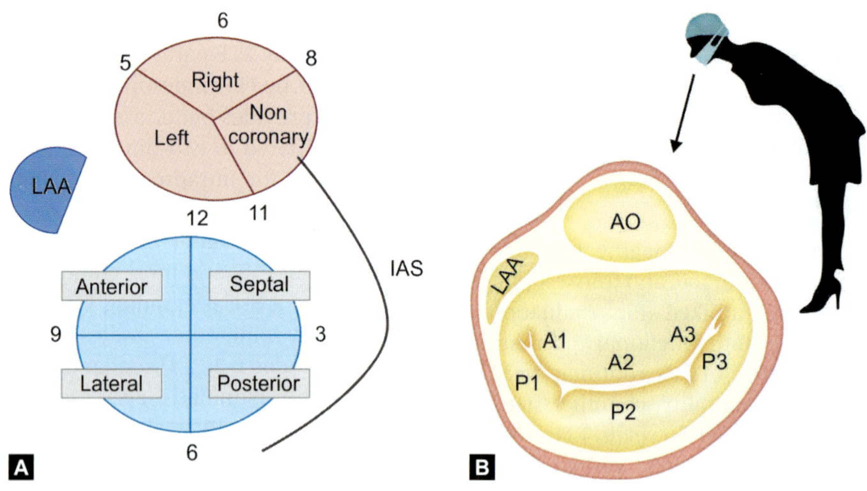

LAA, left atrial appendage; IAS, interatrial septum; AO, aorta.

FIG. 1: Mitral and aortic valves from a surgeon's view.

For mitral PVL pulmonary venous flow reversal in systole was considered as a specific sign of severe mitral PVL.[12] Precise quantification of PVL can be difficult in majority of cases due to various artifacts.

To provide uniformity in reporting and for better communication between the interventionalist and echocardiographer, the leak location should be reported in a clockwise fashion from a surgical view of mitral and aortic valves (Fig. 1). For aortic valve the commissure between left and right coronary cusp was assigned at 5 o'clock position, between right and noncoronary at 8 o'clock and 11 o'clock position was assigned to the commissure between left and noncoronary sinuses. Most of aortic PVLs are located between right and noncoronary cusps.[13] Similarly, for mitral PVL by rotating the TEE probe and echocardiographic image, the MV and aortic valve are oriented in a fashion that aortic valve is at the top of MV when viewed from atrium. The junction between aortic valve and anterior mitral annulus was assigned as 12 o'clock position and 6 o'clock was assigned to midpoint of posterior annulus. The interatrial septum and posteromedial commissure are at 3 o'clock and left atrial appendage and anterolateral commissure at 9 o'clock location. The aortomitral curtain at the 11 o'clock position is the most common location for mitral PVL followed by at 5 and 6 o'clock, representing the posterior wall of mitral ring.[14]

Computed Tomography

With advances in cardiac CT it is possible to assess the PVL in a greater detail. Retrospective electrocardiogram (ECG)-gated image acquisition with 3D or 4D-reconstruction utilizing volume rendering techniques has been used in PVL assessment.[15,16] Better quality images were obtain when patient heart rates were slower, longer diastolic frames and in closed leaflet position. Even with CT imaging of PVL can produce hyperdense or hypodense image artifacts.

Cardiac Magnetic Resonance Imaging

Cardiac magnetic resonance imaging (CMR) is utilized for accurate quantification of regurgitation, quantification of antegrade and retrograde flow and for assessment of cardiac chamber size and function. Velocity-encoded phase-contrast magnetic resonance (MR) is utilized for reproducible assessment of regurgitant fraction and regurgitant volumes. CMR is especially useful for assessment of bioprosthetic valves, annuloplasty rings and metallic artifacts may impair mechanical valve assessment. With advances in MR technology it is now possible for 3D reconstruction of PVL with complex anatomy.[17]

Fluoroscopy

Prosthetic valves needs to be profiled in multiple angulated views to document the valve leaflet motion and for assessment of paravalvular regurgitations. Biplane imaging provides two orthogonal views simultaneously and useful for oblique and angulated projections. Left anterior oblique caudal fluoroscopic imaging differentiates medial versus lateral paravalvular defects, and right anterior oblique view differentiates anterior versus posterior location of PVL. Fluoroscopy is also useful to detect any impingement of PVL closure device on the prosthetic valves before releasing the closure device. Coronary angiogram should be done to locate the distal left anterior descending (LAD) near apex during Transapical access for PVL closure.

Multimodality Imaging

All the imaging modalities will complement each other whereas 2D or 3D TEE provides real time image guidance during PVL closure, and fluoroscopy will detect the prosthetic valve movement and impingement of device on prosthetic valve movement during procedure. For anteriorly located aortic PVLs intracardiac echocardiography (ICE) may be

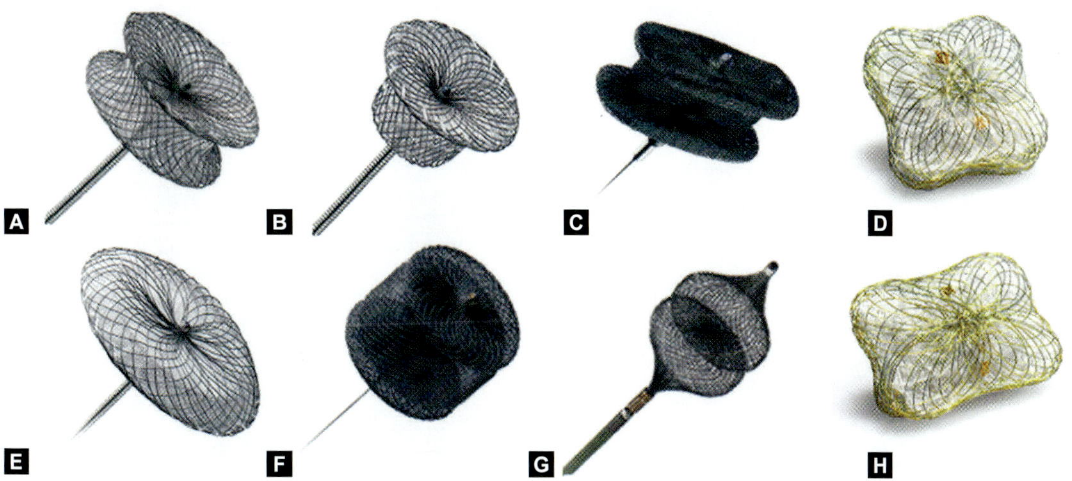

FIG. 2: Paravalvular leak closure devices: **A,** Amplatzer muscular ventricular septal defect occluder; **B,** Amplatzer duct occluder; **C,** Amplatzer vascular plug III; **D,** Occlutech paravalvular leak device (square-shaped design); **E,** Amplatzer septal occluder; **F,** Amplatzer vascular plug II; **G,** Amplatzer vascular plug IV; **H,** Occlutech paravalvular leak device (rectangular-shaped design).

helpful. Fusion imaging techniques may enable the real time display of 4D reconstructed CT images adjacent to or on over laid on live fluoroscopy image there by reducing the duration of procedure.

INDICATIONS FOR PARAVALVULAR LEAK CLOSURE

The percutaneous treatment of PVL is a Class IIa [American College of Cardiology/American Heart Association (ACC/AHA) 2014 guidelines] indication for high-risk surgical patients who had an indication for PVL closure.[18]

Absolute Indications[19]

- Symptoms of heart failure due to PVL
- Significant hemolysis due to PVL
- Moderate PVL with declining left ventricular ejection fraction (LVEF)
- Moderate PVL with progressive LV enlargement.

Relative Indications[19]

- Risk of endocarditis
- Asymptomatic mild or moderate PVL
- Mild or moderate PVL after transcatheter aortic valve implantation (TAVI).

Contraindications

- Active endocarditis
- Regurgitation involving one-third of prosthetic valve annulus
- Rocking motion of prosthetic valve.

DEVICES FOR PERCUTANEOUS PARAVALVULAR LEAK CLOSURE

The currently used PVL closure devices are made-up of woven nitinol mesh that can be retrievable and repositionable. Only very few purpose-specific devices exist. The AMPLATZER^{TM} vascular plug III (AVP III; St Jude Medical) and the Occlutech PVL device (PLD; Occlutech, Germany) are the only two devices designed specifically for PVL closure. The other devices that are currently used off-label for PVL closure, have been designed for closure other congenital cardiovascular defects like atrial septal defect, ventricular septal defect, and patent ducts arteriosus (Fig. 2). The Amplatzer devices are the most commonly used for PVL closure worldwide. The AVP II device is most commonly used in the USA and while in Europe the most frequently used device is the AVP III;, however, only Occlutech device is approved by the European commission for PVL closure.

TECHNIQUE OF TRANSCATHETER PARAVALVULAR LEAK CLOSURE

Generally procedure is performed under general anesthesia with 3D TEE as it takes long time for percutaneous PVL closure. In case of aortic PVL procedure can be completed under conscious sedation.

Mitral Transcatheter Paravalvular Leak Closure

The various approaches that had been used for mitral PVL closure includes antegrade-transseptal approach, retrograde transaortic approach, and transapical approach. Under fluoroscopic guidance in the most commonly used antegrade approach once successful transseptal puncture is made, a diagnostic catheter usually multipurpose or Judkins right catheter was advanced over the wire into left atrium (LA) (Fig. 3A). The mitral prosthetic valve is profiled in multiple angulated views usually in RAO (tangential view) and LAO caudal view (enface view for MV) to have a clear idea about the prosthetic valve motion. Systemic heparinization administered to prevent thrombus formation in catheters or

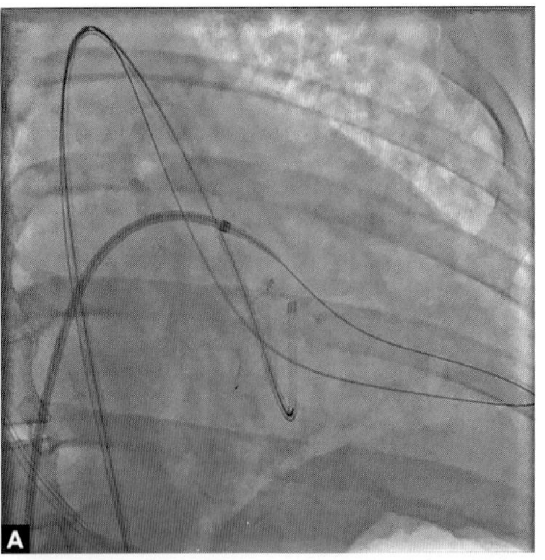

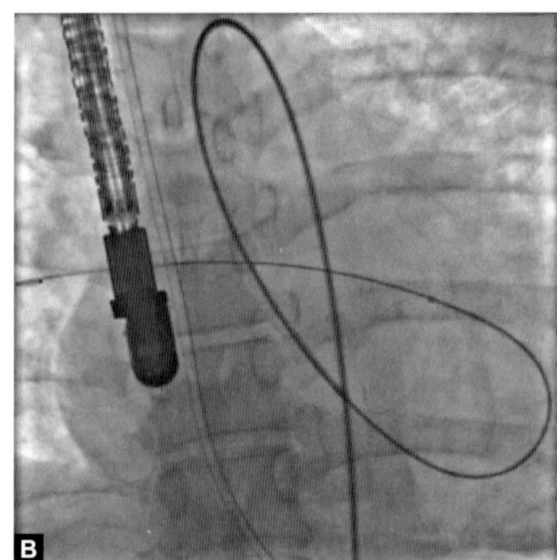

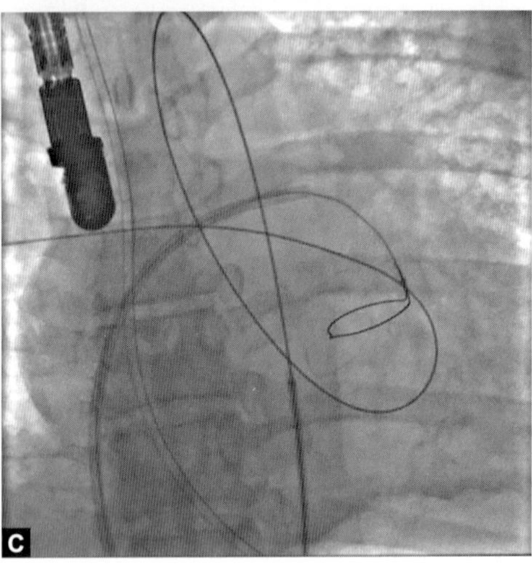

FIG. 3: A, Antegrade crossing of the paravalvular leak with septal puncture; **B,** Crossing the bioprosthetic mitral PVL in a retrograde route; **C,** Creating the arteriovenous loop with snaring of the retrograde wire in left atrium through a septal puncture.

over the valves. The PVL was crossed with a hydrophilic guide wire (Terumo wire) under TEE guidance. Sometimes it may be helpful to use a deflectable catheter (Agilis catheter, St Jude Medical) for crossing the PVL especially in septal PVL. The hydrophilic guide wire is exchanged for a stiffer (Amplatz Extra-Stiff) wire with forming a loop in LV. Sometimes the formation of a venoarterial loop may be required for additional support by snaring the wire in aorta or in LA. After this a 6F guide catheter (usually 6F multipurpose guide) was advanced over the wire into LV. An AVP device up to size 12 mm can fit in a 6F coronary guide catheter without excessive resistance. Based on the size of the defect single or multiple devices can be deployed sequentially through the same guide catheter. It is important to confirm the normal movement of mechanical leaflets before releasing the device. If the leaflet motion is impaired, the device needs to be repositioned or to choose a smaller device.

In retrograde transaortic approach the PVL is crossed from LV to LA with a hydrophilic guide wire over a diagnostic catheter usually a Judkins right catheter (Fig. 3B) or a flexible tip catheter. After crossing MV the wire is snared in LA through a transseptal puncture and an arteriovenous loop is created (Fig. 3C). Finally the device is deployed over the venous access catheter through the transseptal puncture.

For difficult cases like posterior, medially located defects and in patients with double-mechanical valve placement the alternative approach is through the LV apex. The advantage with transapical access is easy to cross the PVL and less difficulty in deploying the PVL devices. However, this approach is associated with higher procedural complications like coronary perforation, pericardial effusion, and the need for a separate device for apical access closure.

Aortic Paravalvular Leak Closure

Most of aortic PVLs are smaller than mitral PVL and are usually closed with a single-closure device. The most commonly used approach for aortic PVL closure is retrograde approach through the transfemoral access. In retrograde approach the coaxial system consisting of a 6F coronary guide catheter (multipurpose catheter) with 5F diagnostic catheter [Amplatz left (AL1) or Judkins right (JR)] and a 0.035 inch Terumo wire or flexible tip stiff wire is commonly used. After crossing the defect the coaxial system can be advanced into LV and device can be deployed. Alternatively, for difficult cases the guide wire can be exchanged for a stiffer wire (Amplatz Extra-Stiff) with a stable loop in LV or an arteriovenous loop may need to be created for additional support as described for mitral PVL. The other approach is transapical access as described earlier.

Paravalvular Leak Closure after Transcatheter Aortic Valve Replacement

With increasing use of transcatheter aortic valve replacement (TAVR) for aortic valve replacement, PVLs can occur due to undersized prosthetic valve, malapposition of valve due to heavy calcification. The malapposition can be treated by balloon postdilation, whereas moderate-to-severe PVL can be treated by vascular plug or AVP IV device. The AVP IV device is smaller in size (4–8 mm) and is easier to deliver through a 4F catheter. With improved design of prosthetic valves with adequate sealing skirts the incidence of PVL had decreased considerably.

OUTCOMES AND COMPLICATIONS OF PARAVALVULAR LEAK CLOSURE PROCEDURES

Technical success of PVL closure was defined as correct placement of the device across PVL without any residual leak and without any prosthetic valve dysfunction. Clinical success was defined according to the clinical indication for PVL closure such that improvement in hemolysis and more than equal to 1-stage improvement in NYHA functional state. With increasing operator experience the technical success of PVL closure ranges between 77 and 90% across various studies and clinical success ranges between 67 and 77% depending on the indication of PVL closure.[20,21] Successful device closure is associated with improved quality of life and reduction in overall mortality and morbidity.[22] The reported major complications with tanscatheter PVL closure include emergency cardiac surgery for failed device closures, mechanical valve interference, embolization of prosthetic device, stroke, worsening of hemolysis, and death during or immediately after the procedure.[23]

MEDICAL THERAPY

For patients who were using anticoagulation prior to PVL closure to be continued after the procedure with metallic valves and patients with atrial arrhythmias. At least 3 months of dual antiplatelet therapy is recommended for bioprosthetic valve patients.

CONCLUSION

Transcatheter closure of symptomatic PVL is associated with less procedural morbidity and mortality rate than surgical closure of PVL. Successful percutaneous closure of PVL is associated with long-term morality benefit in symptomatic patients. With improved design of newer devices, availability of exclusive devices for PVL and with increasing operator experience the technical and clinical success of percutaneous closure PVL is improving.

REFERENCES

1. Ionescu A, Fraser AG, Butchart EG. Prevalence and clinical significance of incidental paraprosthetic valvar regurgitation: a prospective study using transesophageal echocardiography. Heart. 2003;89(11):1316-21.
2. Kliger C, Eiros R, Isasti G, et al. Review of surgical prosthetic paravalvular leaks: diagnosis and catheter-based closure. Eur Heart J. 2013;34(9):638-48.
3. Pate GE, Al Zubaidi A, Chandavimol M, et al. Percutaneous closure of prosthetic paravalvular leaks: case series and review. Catheter Cardiovasc Interv. 2006;68(4):528-33.
4. Rallidis LS, Moyssakis IE, Ikonomidis I, et al. Natural history of early aortic paraprosthetic regurgitation: a five-year follow-up. Am Heart J. 1999;138(2 Pt 1):351-7.
5. Yang C, Liu Y, Tang J, et al. Prognosis of transcatheter closure compared with surgical repair of paravalvular leak after prosthetic valve replacement: a retrospective comparison. Thorac Cardiovasc Surg. 2018.
6. De Cicco G, Lorusso R, Colli A, et al. Aortic valve periprosthetic leakage: anatomic observations and surgical results. Ann Thorac Surg. 2005;79(5):1480-5.
7. De Cicco G, Russo C, Moreo A, et al. Mitral valve periprosthetic leakage: anatomical observations in 135 patients from a multicentre study. Eur J Cardiothorac Surg. 2006;30(6):887-91.
8. Skoularigis J, Essop MR, Skudicky D, et al. Frequency and severity of intravascular hemolysis after left-sided cardiac valve replacement with medtronic hall and St Jude medical prostheses, and influence of prosthetic type, position, size and number. Am J Cardiol. 1993;71(7):587-91.
9. Gerber IL, Stewart RA, French JK, et al. Associations between plasma natriuretic peptide levels, symptoms, and left ventricular function in patients with chronic aortic regurgitation. Am J Cardiol. 2003;92(6):755-8.
10. Sutton TM, Stewart RA, Gerber IL, et al. Plasma natriuretic peptide levels increase with symptoms and severity of mitral regurgitation. J Am Coll Cardiol. 2003;41(12):2280-7.
11. Garcia-Fernandez MA, Cortes M, Garcia-Robles JA, et al. Utility of real-time three-dimensional transesophageal echocardiography in evaluating the success of percutaneous transcatheter closure of mitral paravalvular leaks. J Am Soc Echocardiogr. 2010;23(1):26-32.
12. Zoghbi WA, Chambers JB, Dumesnil JG, et al. Recommendations for evaluation of prosthetic valves with echocardiography and doppler ultrasound: a report from the American Society Of Echocardiography's Guidelines And Standards Committee And The Task Force On Prosthetic Valves. J Am Soc Echocardiogr. 2009;22(9):975-1014.
13. De Cicco G, Lorusso R, Colli A, et al. Aortic valve periprosthetic leakage: anatomic observations and surgical results. Ann Thorac Surg. 2005;79(5):1480-5.
14. De Cicco G, Russo C, Moreo A, et al. Mitral valve periprosthetic leakage: Anatomical observations in 135 patients from a multicentre study. Eur J Cardiothorac Surg. 2006;30(6):887-91.
15. Suh YJ, Hong GR, Han K, et al. Assessment of mitral paravalvular leakage after mitral valve replacement using cardiac computed tomography: comparison with surgical findings. Circ Cardiovasc Imaging. 2016;9(6):e004153.
16. Suchá D, Symersky P, Tanis W, et al. Multimodality imaging assessment of prosthetic heart valves. Circ Cardiovasc Imaging. 2015;8(9):e003703.
17. Ruiz CE, Hahn RT, Berrebi A, et al. Clinical trial principles and endpoint definitions for paravalvular leaks in surgical prosthesis: an expert statement. J Am Coll Cardiol. 2017;69(16):2067-87.
18. Nishimura RA, Otto CM, Bonow RO, et al. 2014 AHA/ACC Guideline for the Management of Patients With Valvular Heart Disease: executive summary: a report of the American College of Cardiology/American Heart Association Task Force on Practice Guidelines. Circulation. 2014;129(23):2440-92.
19. Nietlispach F, Maisano F, Sorajja P, et al. Percutaneous paravalvular leak closure: chasing the chameleon. Eur Heart J. 2016;37(47):3495-502.
20. Ruiz CE, Jelnin V, Kronzon I, et al. Clinical outcomes in patients undergoing percutaneous closure of periprosthetic paravalvular leaks. J Am Coll Cardiol. 2011;58(21):2210-7.
21. Sorajja P, Cabalka AK, Hagler DJ, et al. Long-term follow-up of percutaneous repair of paravalvular prosthetic regurgitation. J Am Coll Cardiol. 2011;58(21):2218-24.
22. Millán X, Skaf S, Joseph L, et al. Transcatheter reduction of paravalvular leaks: a systematic review and meta-analysis. Can J Cardiol. 2015;31(3):260-9.
23. Cruz-Gonzalez I, Rama-Merchan JC, Rodríguez-Collado J, et al. Transcatheter closure of paravalvular leaks: state of the art. Neth Heart J. 2017;25(2):116-24.

CHAPTER 73

Left Atrial Appendage Closure Device for Stroke Prevention in Atrial Fibrillation

Balbir Singh

INTRODUCTION

Atrial fibrillation (AF) is the most common arrhythmia seen in clinical practice, and the incidence increases with age. It is associated with significant mortality and morbidity, mainly due to stroke and heart failure. AF is associated with five times higher stroke rates as compared to those without AF.[1] For prevention of this complication, treatment options have been either with warfarin or with the newer anticoagulant agents. This anticoagulant therapy has been proven to effectively prevent thromboembolic strokes, but the increased risk of serious bleeding prevents many patients from taking this therapy. Therefore, there is always a need for alternative therapies with lower bleeding risk.[2]

Percutaneous left atrial appendage (LAA) occlusion is an evolving therapy, which should be taken into consideration in those patients with AF with a high stroke risk and contraindications for oral anticoagulant (OAC).

This chapter aims at discussing the scope for LAA closure, the available LAA occlusion devices, and their clinical evidence until now.

EXISTING OPTIONS OF STROKE PREVENTION IN ATRIAL FIBRILLATION

Several randomized controlled trials have proved the efficacy of OACs in preventing strokes and reducing mortality, these trials have also shown that antiplatelets are not useful for this purpose.

However, OACs are associated with increased bleeding to the tune of incidence of 2–4% per year which is substantial and also with some life-threatening bleeds like intracranial hemorrhage (ICH). There was a hope that the advent of new oral anticoagulants (NOACs) such as dabigatran, apixaban, or rivaroxaban would overcome these disadvantages; however, this has not been fulfilled entirely.[3] Table 1 depicts the incidence of bleeds and compliance with these drugs.

RATIONALE FOR LEFT ATRIAL APPENDAGE OCCLUSION

The logic behind LAA occlusion is that the LAA is the primary site of thrombus formation in patients with nonvalvular atrial fibrillation (NVAF) as has been demonstrated on postmortem studies and transesophageal data. In 90% of patients with NVAF, the site of clot formation is the LAA.[4] In view of this data, it appears LAA closure will provide protection against thromboembolic episodes in patients with NVAF. As a result, the European Society of Cardiology (ESC) guidelines for the management of AF (2012) recommend that LAA closure may be considered in patients with a high stroke risk and contraindications for long-term OAC administration (Class IIb, level of evidence B). The USA

TABLE 1: Incidence of bleeds and compliance with oral anticoagulants

Parameters	Warfarin (PROTECT AF)	Dabigatran (RELY)	Apixaban (ARISTOTLE)	Rivaroxaban (ROCKET AF)
Age	71.7	71.5	70	70
Major/minor bleed	N/A	16.4	18.1	14.9
Major bleed (%)	4.1	3.1	2.1	3.6
Stroke (%)	2.7	1.1	1.3	1.7
Drug discontinuation	16–34	21	N/A	24

Food and Drug Administration (FDA) has also approved LAA closure device in recent past.

However, one must remember that many patients with NVAF have several comorbidities and could have atheromatous changes in aorta or carotids which could lead to stroke mitigating the benefit of LAA closure.

IDENTIFYING THE RIGHT PATIENT FOR DEVICE CLOSURE

Left atrial appendage closure offers an alternative to patients of NVAF who are at risk of thromboembolism and are also at high risk for bleeds or contraindications to OACs. The patients who could be considered as high risk for bleeding are:

- Coagulopathies, low platelet counts, or other disorders
- Severe hepatic or renal dysfunction
- Known vascular malformations in intestine, brain, or retina which could potentially bleed.

Other groups of patients apart from those with high bleeding risk are those who develop ischemic stroke despite well-controlled OAC or NOAC therapy and high chance of therapeutic noncompliance to OAC or NOACs (Box 1).

BOX 1 Potential indications of left atrial appendage closure

- Serious bleed with oral anticoagulants like ICH, etc.
- Contraindications to OAC-like underlying coagulopathies
- Development of stroke or SE despite controlled anticoagulation
- Intolerant to oral anticoagulants
- Not compliant on drugs

ICH, intracranial hemorrhage; OAC, oral anticoagulant; SE, status epilepticus.

INTOLERANCE OR CONTRAINDICATIONS TO ORAL ANTICOAGULANT OR NEW ORAL ANTICOAGULANTS

Transesophageal echocardiography (TEE) helps to identify the anatomy of LAA and is essential preprocedure and also during the procedure; preprocedural TEE is used to screen suitable candidates and to define LAA morphology and dimensions and exclude LAA thrombus.[2] TEE has a major role in guiding proper placement of the device and for assessing procedural complications (Fig. 1).

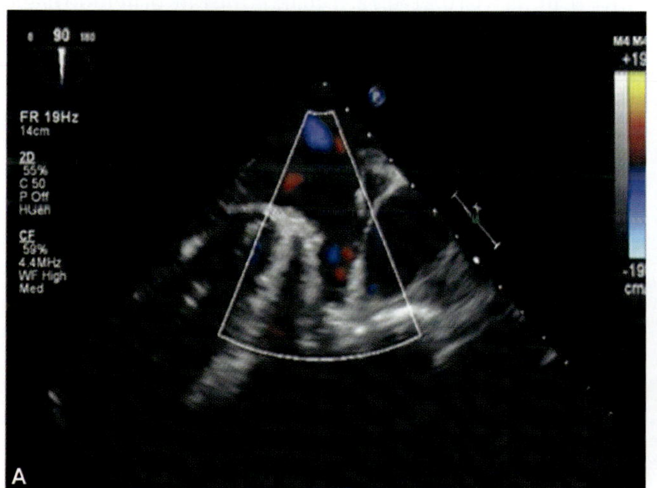

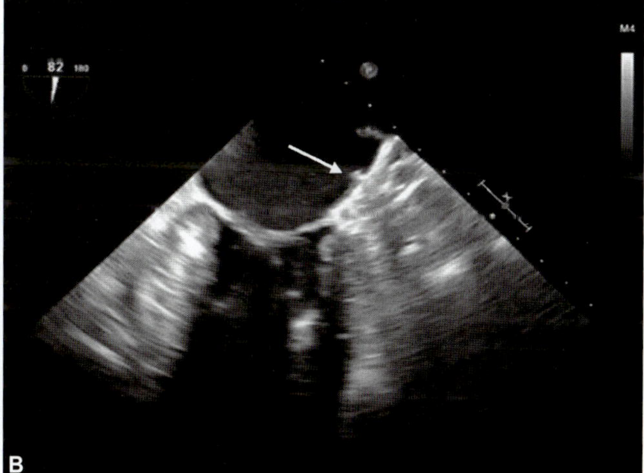

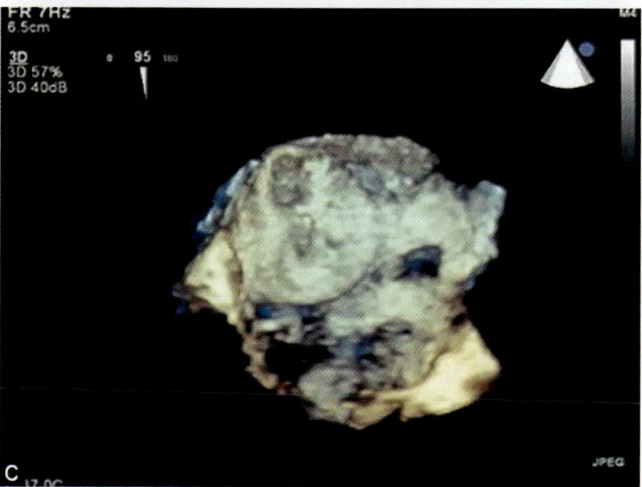

FIG. 1: **A,** and **B,** Transesophageal images during the procedure in one of our patient showing the left left atrial appendage (LAA) clearly. Dimensions are made from the neck and it also help to calculate the length of LAA; **C,** 3D image of LAA.

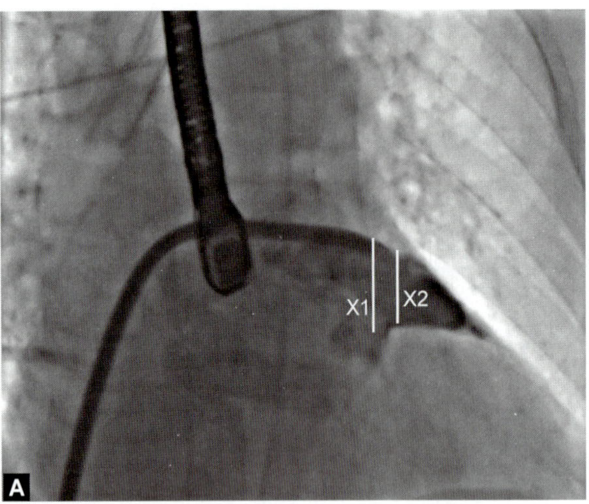

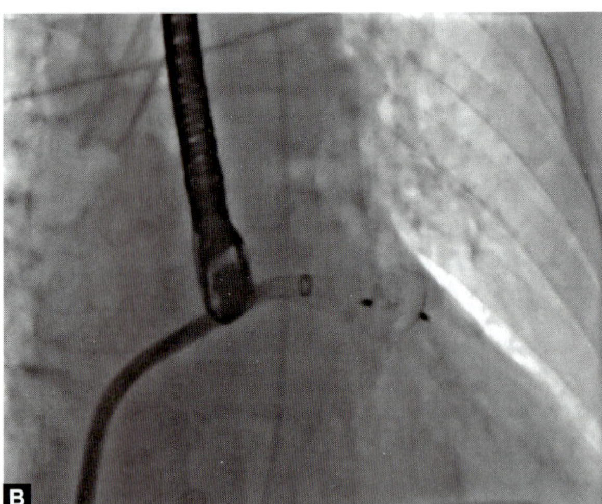

FIG. 2: The fluoroscopy images showing the deployment of the device.

DEVICE IMPLANTATION

Percutaneous LAA occlusion is usually performed under general anesthesia and with TEE and fluoroscopic guidance. The standard transseptal puncture techniques are used to position the delivery sheath and place the device in the LAA. Once in position, the device stability is confirmed by a fluoroscopy and TEE imaging. Finally, the device is released from the delivery cable by counterclockwise rotation at the shaft [these are steps for Amplatzer Cardiac Plug (ACP), St Jude Medical—Figure 2]. Until now, the WATCHMAN and ACP devices are widely used in clinical practice and WATCHMAN device is now FDA approved.

POSTPROCEDURAL TREATMENT

Dual antiplatelet therapy (DAPT) (aspirin and clopidogrel) is prescribed for the first 45 days after LAA closure and clopidogrel can then be stopped, antiplatelet therapy exists. In patients with a very high bleeding risk, it may be considered to low-dose NOAC may be needed if the device indication was for recurrent strokes despite NOACs.

CLINICAL TRIAL RESULTS[4-9]

The only prospective, randomized trial is the PROTECT AF trial in which 707 patients with NVAF were randomly assigned in a 2:1 ratio to either percutaneous LAA occlusion with the WATCHMAN device or to warfarin therapy. Patients with paroxysmal, persistent, or permanent NVAF were enrolled if they had a CHADS2 risk score more than or equal to 1. The trial demonstrated the noninferiority of WATCHMAN LAA occlusion compared with OAC therapy regarding the primary efficacy endpoint—a composite of stroke, systemic embolism, and cardiovascular death [relative risk (RR) = 0.62, 95% confidence interval (CI) 0.35–1.25]. The primary efficacy endpoint occurred in 2.3% of the device group versus 3.8% of the warfarin group (RR = 0.60, 95% CI 0.41–1.05), demonstrating a 40% RR reduction in primary efficacy in the WATCHMAN group. Cardiovascular death occurred in 1.0% of the device group versus 2.4% of the warfarin group (RR = 0.40, 95% CI 0.21–0.72, $p < 0.05$). The rate of hemorrhagic stroke was 0.2% in the device group versus 1% in the warfarin group (RR = 0.18, 95% CI 0.04–0.60, $p < 0.05$).

More recent data, from the CAP registry (n = 566, WATCHMAN), the PREVAIL study (n = 269, WATCHMAN) and a large multicenter study involving the ACP device (n = 969) show improved procedural safety, the complication rates within 7 days were 4.1%, 4.4%, and 4.1%, respectively. These lower rates of complications are due to better operator experience of device implantation.

The PREVAIL study added information to the first PROTECT AF. The major findings of this trial were:

- Left atrial appendage occlusion with the WATCHMAN device was not noninferior to warfarin for the primary efficacy composite endpoint
- The WATCHMAN device was noninferior to warfarin for the occurrence of late ischemic events, such as ischemic stroke or status epilepticus.
- The WATCHMAN procedure met the prespecified success criterion for safety events.

A recent meta-analysis with the long-term 5-year outcomes of the PREVAIL trial, combined with the 5-year outcomes of the PROTECT AF trial, demonstrate that LAAC with the WATCHMAN device provides stroke prevention in NVAF patients to a similar degree as OAC with warfarin. It also reduces mortality and risk of hemorrhagic stroke.

DISCUSSION

Left atrial appendage closure has emerged in the last decade as a useful therapy in stroke prevention in NVAF. Since the initial publications, the complication rates have significantly reduced making the procedure more attractive.

The current guidelines only justify the use of this in patients with contraindications to OAC therapy or those with poor compliance or inability to take drugs.

The future studies will shed more light on the group which will benefit the most with these drugs.

CONCLUSION

Percutaneous LAA occlusion has been shown to be a safe, efficacious, and cost-effective strategy for stroke prevention in patients with NVAF with increased stroke and bleeding risk. It is now a commonly performed procedure in many centers in Europe and US, in our experience success was obtained in all eight patients where it was attempted, however, operator experience and technique are of paramount importance.

REFERENCES

1. Wolf PA, Abbott RD, Kannel WB. Atrial fibrillation as an independent risk factor for stroke: the Framingham Study. Stroke. 1991;22:983-8.
2. Camm AJ, Lip GY, De Caterina R, et al. 2012 focused update of the ESC Guidelines for the management of atrial fibrillation: an update of the 2010 ESC Guidelines for the management of atrial fibrillation—developed with the special contribution of the European Heart Rhythm Association. Europace. 2012;14:1385-413.
3. Holmes DR, Reddy VY, Turi ZG, et al. Percutaneous closure of the left atrial appendage versus warfarin therapy for prevention of stroke in patients with atrial fibrillation: a randomised non-inferiority trial. Lancet. 2009;374:534-42.
4. Reddy VY, Möbius-Winkler S, Miller MA, et al. Left atrial appendage closure with the Watchman device in patients with a contraindication for oral anticoagulation: the ASAP study (ASA Plavix Feasibility Study with Watchman Left Atrial Appendage Closure Technology). J Am Coll Cardiol. 2013;61:2551-6.
5. Plicht B, Konorza TF, Kahlert P, et al. Risk factors for thrombus formation on the Amplatzer Cardiac Plug after left atrial appendage occlusion. JACC Cardiovasc Interv. 2013;6:606-13.
6. Reddy VY, Holmes D, Doshi SK, et al. Safety of percutaneous left atrial appendage closure: results from the Watchman Left Atrial Appendage System for Embolic Protection in Patients with AF (PROTECT AF) clinical trial and the Continued Access Registry. Circulation. 2011;23:417-24.
7. Holmes D. Preliminary results of the randomized trial of LAA closure vs warfarin for stroke/thromboembolic prevention in patients with non-valvular atrial fibrillation (PREVAIL)-late breaking clinical trial. San Francisco: American College of Cardiology; 2013.
8. Reddy V. Long term results of PROTECT AF: the mortality effects of left atrial appendage closure versus warfarin for stroke prophylaxis in AF-late breaking clinical trial. United States: Heart Rhythm Society; 2013.
9. Reddy VY, Doshi SK, Kar S. 5-Year Outcomes After Left Atrial Appendage Closure: From the PREVAIL and PROTECT AF Trials. J Am Coll Cardiol. 2017;70:2964-75.

SECTION 11

Cardiac Imaging

CHAPTER 74

Utility of Echo in Assessment and Management of Functional Mitral Regurgitation

Gonzalo Luis Alonso Salinas, Marina Pascual Izco, José Luis Zamorano

INTRODUCTION

Despite the decrease of rheumatic disease, mitral regurgitation (MR) is becoming more prevalent in parallel with population aging and the improvement and increased survival of patients with dilated cardiomyopathy (DCM) of any etiology. Approximately, 10% of the population over 75 years of age have significant MR.[1] This condition has a negative impact on prognosis, regardless of the etiology and comorbidity.

Surgical or percutaneous treatment would be performed only in patients with severe MR. Thus, a precise and accurate evaluation is required.

MECHANISM AND ETIOLOGY OF MITRAL REGURGITATION

According to MR mechanism, Carpentier classification[2] for mitral leaflets motion:

- *Type I*: Normal motion. MR is due to annular dilatation or leaflet perforation or tear
- *Type II*: Excess leaflet motion. The free edge of one or more leaflets overrides the plane of the annulus during systole (leaflet prolapse)
- *Type III*: Restricted leaflet motion.
    - Restricted in both systole and diastole
    - Restricted only in systole.

According to its etiology, if the disease is intrinsic to the valve and its structure is called primary MR; if there are no structural anomalies in the valvular apparatus is called secondary or functional MR. In this chapter, the focus will be the secondary or functional MR.

The etiologies of secondary or functional MR are mainly the ischemic heart disease and DCM. Secondary MR appears because, despite a normal and undamaged valvular apparatus, myocardial ischemia, DCM or severe left atrial (LA) dilation decreases the forces that help the mitral valve (MV) closure during the systole of the left ventricle (LV).[3] Within these pathologies, ventricular remodeling produces an altered LV geometry with an altered subvalvular apparatus, there is an apical and posterior displacement of the papillary muscles and their corresponding chordae tendineae, which pulls the mitral leaflets and progressively decreases and cancels its coaptation surface.[4] This traction or tethering that usually occurs during LV systole, can be asymmetric, caused by involvement of the posterior papillary muscle, which is visualized with the "Seagull Sign" (Fig. 1) or symmetric if it affects both papillary muscles equally.

ULTRASOUND ASSESSMENT OF FUNCTIONAL MITRAL REGURGITATION

Echocardiography (ECG) is, despite the development of other imaging techniques, the cornerstone of the study of MR. It helps us to describe the morphology of the valve, which can guide us about the etiology of MR, as well as the possibility of repair. In addition, it is a very reliable tool to quantify the severity of the regurgitation.

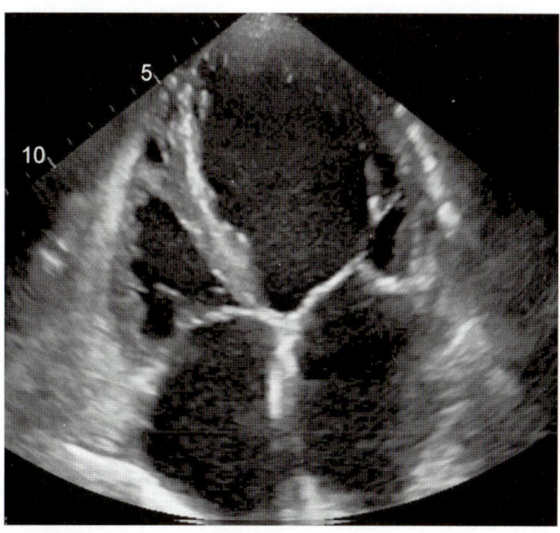

FIG. 1: Seagull's sign.

Morphological Evaluation of the Mitral Valve

Transthoracic Echocardiogram

Two-dimensional transthoracic echocardiogram (TTE) allows an accurate observation of the morphology of the MV. The location of the affected segments and the origin of the regurgitant jet, the description of the presence and extension of calcifications, as well as the anatomical changes within the valve or its annulus are fundamental parameters that we must describe to guide the management of the valve disease. Moreover, the presence of a damaged leaflet, the rupture of a papillary muscle and a large coaptation defect are specific findings of significant MR.

Recognize and identify the leaflet segments showed in each cardiac view seems fundamental. Parasternal short-axis view allows observation of the six segments of both mitral leaflets and using color Doppler technique, locates the origin of the regurgitant jet and/or the prolapsing segment. Parasternal long-axis view shows the segments A2 and P2, apical four-chambers the segments A3, A2, and P1 (from internal to external), and apical two-chambers P3, A2, and P1 in the same order.[5]

Transoesophageal Echocardiogram

Transesophageal echocardiogram (TEE) allows us to visualize the MV with higher resolution, being especially useful in those patients with a suboptimal acoustic window. MV is fully visualized in the transgastric view at 0° with the posterior leaflet in the upper part of the image and the anterior leaflet in the lower one. This view shows us the six segments, similarly to parasternal short-axis view in TTE. In sagittal view at 120° long-axis four-chambers we can visualize segments A2 and P2. From this plane, if we angulate the probe toward the aortic valve we can see A1 and P1, and if we do it toward the tricuspid valve, A3 and P3 segments. In sagittal view, from 60° to 90°, we can obtain a bicommissure vision and identify P3, A2, and P1 segments from left to right.[5]

Mitral Annulus

To describe the dilatation of the mitral annulus (MA), we use the MA/anterior leaflet ratio in parasternal long-axis view, considering the MA dilated if this ratio is greater than 1.3 in diastole. In addition, we should also measure the diameter of the ring, considering it dilated if it is greater than 35 mm. MA decreases its area in systole approximately 25% of its area in diastole.

Three-dimensional Image Assessment

When available, 3D images give us more information than a 2D assessment. Three-dimensional images can show the mitral apparatus from the LA or from the LV. The view of the MV from the LA is called the "surgeon's vision" or "*en face* view" (Fig. 2) and it has a proven value in the description of leaflet prolapse, other defects of mitral leaflets or the rupture of the chordae tendineae.[6] This is especially useful in TEE.

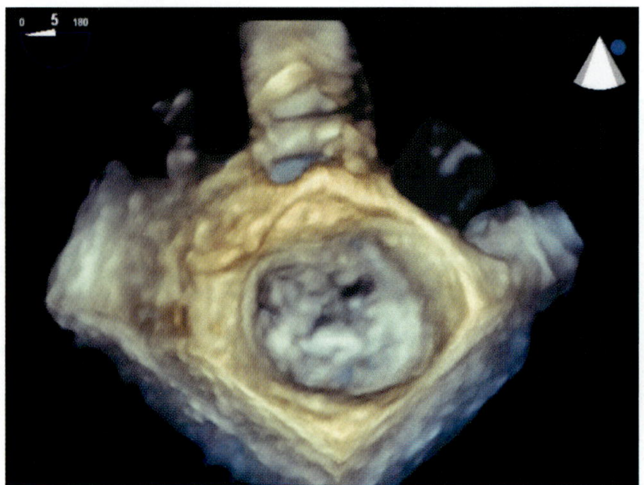

FIG. 2: Surgeon's vision or *en face* view using three-dimentional transesophageal echocardiogram.

There are three basic modes of acquiring 3D images: Real-time 3D, 3D zoom, and full volume acquisition. Each of them has a different sector width, frame rate, and spatial resolution.

- *Real-time 3D*: Uses a narrow sector for a simple image. It is useful for an initial quick approach
- *Three-dimensional zoom*: We can see the entire MV in one heartbeat. Very useful in case of atrial fibrillation, supraventricular extrasystole or frequent ventricular extrasystole, or artifact electrocardiogram (ECG)
- *Full volume acquisition*: This technique acquires several volumes in several beats: Improves temporal and spatial resolution. The higher the number of heartbeats acquired, the higher the resolution, but the quantity of artifacts produced in the image increases. It is usually combined with color Doppler technique.

Morphological description of the MV, preferably performed by TEE, can also provide information that predicts unsuccessful MV repair (Box 1).

Quantification of the Mitral Regurgitation

The quantification of MR is based on different qualitative, semiquantitative and quantitative parameters. Despite the number of different methods that can be found in the literature, no unique method is good enough to study by itself the MR, so actual recommendations integrate different methods that will be explained below.

Color Doppler

Jet area by color Doppler: It is the most widespread method. It assumes that the greater the severity of the MR, the greater the area of the jet and its extension in the LA. The main limitation of this method is that the relationship between the MR jet and its severity can present significant variability since it also depends on technical and hemodynamic factors, especially on functional MR.

BOX 1 Predictors of unsuccessful mitral valve repair

Mitral valve deformation:
- Coaptation length ≥1 cm
- Tenting area[1] >2.5–3 cm^2
- Central or posterior-medial significant regurgitant jet
- Extensae calcification
- More than or equals to 3 compromised MV segments, especially if anterior leaflet is compromised
- Mitral valve tissue lacking (uncommon in secondary MR, common in rheumatic MR or infective endocarditis)

Damaged left ventricle:
- Distance between papillary muscles >20 mm
- Distance between posterior papillary muscle and MV annulus >40 mm
- Lateral akinesia or hypokinesia

Remodeled left ventricle:
- LVEDD >65 mm
- LVESD >51 mm or LVESV> 140 mL
- Sphericity index >0.7
- Annular dilation >50 mm

Up to 50% MR recurrence after repair if:
- Diastolic annulus length ≥37 mm
- Tenting area[1] ≥1.6 cm^2
- Severe MR with central or multiple jet
- Coaptation length ≥1 cm
- LVEDD ≥65 mm or LVESD ≥51 mm
- Lateral akinesia

1, Tenting area (area between annulus plane and leaflets when coapting).
LVEDD, left ventricular end-diastolic diameter; LVESD, left ventricular end-systolic diameter; LVESV, left ventricular end-systolic volume; MR, mitral regurgitation; MV, mitral valve.

This method alone is not recommended to assess the severity of MR, but it could help us to screen it. A central jet, with an area smaller than 4 cm^2 or smaller than the 10% of LA area without associated valve anomalies, is highly suggestive of mild MR. A central jet that reaches the LA roof and pulmonary veins suggests significant MR, and a large, eccentric jet that adheres and travels around the atrial wall toward the atrial roof (Coanda effect) suggests it in the same way.[7]

Measurement of the Width of the "Vena Contracta"

The vena contracta (VC) is the narrowest segment and the fastest regurgitant flow at the level of the regurgitant orifice or immediately above it. Its width reflects the area of the regurgitant orifice thus it can be used to quantify severity.

For VC measurement, we used the parasternal long-axis and apical four-chambers views, obtaining clear vision of the regurgitant jet through the MV. The measurement of the VC in the apical two-chambers view, parallel to the coaptation line, could overestimate its severity. If possible, zooming in on the flow can help us to identify the frame where the width of the jet is smaller. The cut-offs to identify a mild MR would be those less than 0.3 cm. Those greater than 0.7 cm suggest a severe MR. Intermediate values require other quantification methods to determine severity.

The measurement of the VC assumes that the regurgitant orifice of the MR is circular. When this situation happens, it presents a good correlation with regurgitant orifice area. The problem arises when MR orifice is not circular. In these cases, the measurement of VC may underestimate the MR severity. This limitation can be solved using 3D ECG, which has been shown to be more accurate when finding a measurement completely perpendicular to the MR jet.

Another limitation appears in the cases in which the MR includes several jets, which in this case are not additive, so we should look for another measurement method. Finally, the measurement is made only on one frame, disregarding the rest of the ventricular systole period, which can cause the measurement not to be performed on the narrowest segment of the regurgitant flow.

With the ECG in two dimensions we can only approximate the width of the contracted vein, there being no such limitation within 3D ECG, which does not assume the premise of a circular regurgitant orifice. It can be used to calculate the true area of the VC.

The "surgeon's vision" or "*en face* view" provided by 3D ECG allows us to calculate the area of the VC measuring it by planimetry. It is considered that a VC area greater than 0.41 cm^2 indicates a severe MR with an 82% of sensitivity and a 97% of specificity.[8] Moreover, using 3D TTE planimetry can obtain the area of the anatomical regurgitant orifice (ARO) with high precision.

The main limitation of 3D ECG is its low spatial resolution, so in the case of a small orifice, or in the case of several small orifices, the measurement could be mistaken. Another important limitation is the time and experience necessary for its performance, which limits its diffusion together with its high interobserver variability for the selection of the measurement frame.

Proximal Isovelocity Surface Area Method

The proximal isovelocity surface area (PISA) method is based on the hemodynamic principle by which all fluid passing through an orifice undergoes an acceleration, creating hemispheres of increasing velocity and decreasing area.[9,10] With the use of color Doppler technique, this convergence zone can be identified and its radius (r) measured. This measurement allows the calculation of the effective regurgitant orifice (ERO).

The recommended view for the visualization of the hemispheres of velocity is the apical four-chambers view, nevertheless the parasternal short and long views are frequently useful in case of prolapse of the anterior mitral leaflet. In the selected view for the measurement it is recommended to enlarge the MV and use the color Doppler, reducing the Nyquist limit [aliasing velocity (AV)] to values between 15 and 40 cm/s for the best visualization of the hemisphere, which constitutes the PISA. The PISA r is measured in mesosystolic phase from the MV plane to the point at which the color changes. To complete the calculation, the maximum jet velocity (Vmax) of the MR must also be obtained. The ERO is calculated as follows:

$$ERO = 2\pi r^2 \times aV/Vmax$$

ERO, effective regurgitant orifice (cm^2); *r*, PISA radius (cm); AV, aliasing velocity (cm/s); Vmax, maximum MR jet velocity (cm/s).

The cut-offs for functional MR vary respect primary MR. An ERO smaller than 0.1 cm^2 would correspond to a mild MR, from 0.1 to 0.14 cm^2 to a mild-to-moderate MR, 0.15–0.19 cm^2 to a moderate-to-severe MR and it would be catalogued as severe MR for an ERO above 0.2 cm^2.

A simple approximation, derived from this formula, would be just to measure the r with an AV of 40 cm/s. The functional MR would be severe if the radius is greater than 0.5 cm and mild if it is less than 0.2 cm. In addition, the presence of hemispheres of velocity at AV greater than 50 cm/s indicate the presence of significant MR.

If the ERO is assumed to be a uniform, fixed hole during systole, the regurgitant volume (RVol) could be calculated by multiplying the ERO by the velocity-time integral (VTI) of the MR jet:

$$RVol = ERO \times VTI$$

RVol, regurgitant volume (mL); ERO, effective regurgitant orifice (cm^2); VTI, velocity-time integral (cm).

The cut-offs for severity in the RVol are greater than or equals to 30 mL.

The PISA method has proved to be one of the most accurate for quantifying MR severity and it is widespread in numerous cardiac imaging units, but it has several limitations. One of its limitations is to assume that the ERO is circular and the PISA is a hemisphere. Several studies have shown that in most cases this is not the case, and that in addition, correcting by changing the hemisphere for a hemiellipse translates significant differences in the calculation of the ERO.[11] This is especially relevant in functional MR where the PISA is ellipsoidal because there are two MR jets, medial and lateral to the coaptation line of both mitral leaflets. By assuming the spherical shape of the PISA, the degree of MR is significantly underestimated in functional MRs in which the long axis to short axis ratio of the ellipse is greater than 1.5. These findings explain the differences in the cut-offs for quantification.

Another limitation of PISA method consists of the dynamic nature of the MR itself. The PISA r is only measured in the frame in which it is greater, rejecting the rest of the ventricular systole. This fact could overestimate its measurement, equaling holosystolic MR to proto or telesystolic MR.

The quantification by PISA method of the MR using the 3D ECG could mitigate these limitations. On the one hand, with 3D ECG we can identify either spheroidal or ellipsoid PISA, improving calculation of its area; on the other hand, with the new advances in this technique we can achieve a high spatial and temporal resolution that allows us to visualize the entire heart cycle.

Pulsed Doppler Wave: Volumetric Method

This method can be used in addition to those already mentioned to increase the precision of the quantification, or as an alternative method when the previous ones are not feasible. It consists of calculating the RVol and the regurgitant fraction thereof by means of the difference between the mitral stroke volume (MSV) and the systemic stroke volume (SV).

For the measurement of MSV, we choose the apical four-chambers view, using apical five-chambers view for SV. Here we follow the rule that the flow that passes through an orifice can be estimated by calculating the area of that orifice and multiplying it by the VTI.

$$RVol = MSV - SV$$

$$\text{Mitral regurgitant fraction (MRF)} = (RVol/MSV) \times 100$$

$$MSV = (\text{MV length})^2 \times 0.785 \times \text{TVI mitral filling}$$

$$SV = (\text{LV outflow tract diameter})^2 \times 0.785 \times \text{TVI LV outflow tract}$$

Its main strength is that it considers the dynamic component of the MR, unlike PISA method is not a measurement of an isolated frame. If the RVol is greater than or equal to 60 mL or 50% of the SV the MR would be classified as severe, while for values lower than 30 mL or 30% we classify the MR as mild.

It has several important limitations, on the one hand it assumes that the orifice of the MR is circular, on the other it needs a precise VTI tracing. Furthermore, since the formula includes the values of the annular diameter and the outflow tract squared, small errors in these measurements could be magnified. Another important limitation is that it is not an accurate measurement in case of significant aortic valve regurgitation (AoR), due to the variations in flow that this entails.

The measurement of the LV outflow tract and the MA by 3D ECG is more accurate since it does not assume the circular geometry of these elements.

Mitral Filling Assessment: Mitral Velocity-Time Integral/Aortic Velocity-Time Integral Ratio

In the absence of mitral stenosis (MS), the increase in the velocity of mitral protodiastolic filling flow is greater as the severity of MR increases. This can be assessed by pulsed Doppler wave (PW), identifying high filling velocities of the E-wave. In the absence of MS, an E-wave peak velocity greater than 1.5 m/sec suggests severe MR. However, a dominant A-wave practically excludes it.

In addition, mitral VTI/aortic VTI ratio can be assessed to quantify the MR. A ratio greater than 1.4 suggests severe MR, while a smaller than 1 ratio suggests mild MR.

Flow Assessment in Pulmonary Veins

The normal flow in PV shows a higher velocity during ventricular systole than during diastole. As MR severity increases the velocity curve, measured by PW decreases. Moreover, in some cases, reversal flow can be documented. This fact is considered a specific marker of MR severity.

In the case of an eccentric MR jet, it may happen that this flow is reversed only in one PV, therefore the study of the four PV is recommended, especially during a transesophageal study. This evaluation is performed with PW located 1 cm deeper from the entrance of the PV from the LA.

One limitation of this method is that any situation that increases LA pressure can decrease PV flow velocity, so whenever a muffled wave appears, this increase in LA pressure should be studied by other techniques.

Continuous Doppler Wave

The evaluation of MR by CW can be used as a qualitative marker of severity. A high-density holosystolic signal, with a similar density than the antegrade flow, is suggestive of significant MR. However, a protosystolic flow or a low-density flow suggests a mild MR.

Similarly, continuous Doppler wave (CW) can inform about MR chronicity. A triangular wave is highly suggestive of severe an acute MR, while a rounded wave is consistent with chronic MR.

Therefore, table 1 summarizes the methods of quantification of MR.

Echocardiographic Impact of Mitral Regurgitation

The increase of LA filling and the LV overload that produces chronic MR leads to a dilation and progressive dysfunction of theses heart chambers. This LV dilation and dysfunction plays a fundamental role in the management of chronic MR. Three-dimensional ECG allows a more accurate assessment of it, so it should be used if available.

Left atrial dilation is part of the natural history of MR. As MR increases, LA dilates due to volume and pressure overload. We also consider LA volume within the indications for surgery management.

Another measurement that should be done in patients with significant MR is the pulmonary systolic pressure (PSP), which increases due to the increase in retrograde pressure on the LA, and the tricuspid valve annulus, since if it is dilated it may require annuloplasty during mitral repair or replacement.

Stress Transthoracic Echocardiogram

Stress TTE is useful in patients with severe asymptomatic MR, or in those with confusing symptoms, to define their functional capacity. In addition, it can inform about the left ventricular ejection fraction (LVEF), the severity of the MR and the PSP increase during exercise. An increase in PSP greater than 60 mm Hg is an indication for repair or replacement and is associated with a poor prognosis. Moreover, the inability to increase LVEF or the increase in MR measured by PISA method is associated with a poor prognosis.

In the case of functional MR quantified as moderate, an increase in ERO greater than 13 mm^2 during exercise leads to an unfavorable prognosis and it would be an indicator of repair or replacement needs.

MANAGEMENT OF FUNCTIONAL MITRAL REGURGITATION

Natural history and symptomatic course of patients with MR is related to its quantification, its chronicity and subsequent cardiac anatomy abnormalities. Patients with an insidious onset and a steadily progression of MR have a prolonged asymptomatic course due to gradual cardiac remodeling with dilation of LA and LV, which adapt heart function to this situation and a delay the increase of pulmonary pressure. This is similar in cases in which MR is acute and severe. These patients present with an acute pulmonary edema, endangering patient's life.

In functional or secondary MR, the pathology that causes it marks the natural history of the MR. Current approach consists of optimize the medical treatment including cardiac resynchronization therapy if indicated. After achieving an optimized medical treatment, if the patient is still asymptomatic, the recommendation is surgery repair or

TABLE 1: Quantification of functional mitral regurgitation

Parameter	Mild	Moderate	Severe
Qualitative			
Color Doppler jet area	Small, central, does not occupy all the systole	Intermediate	Large amplitude, Coanda effect, reaches LA ceiling
CW Doppler	Intermittent, weak	Dense	Very dense, triangular morphology
Semi quantitative			
Vena contracta	<3 mm	3–6 mm	≥7 mm
Mitral TVI/aortic TVI	<1	1–1.3	≥1.4
Mitral filling	Dominant A-wave	Variable	Dominant E-wave (>1.5 m/s)
PV flow		Systolic flow damped	Systolic flow reversed
Quantitative			
ERO	<10 mm^2	10–20 mm^2	≥20 mm^2
RVol	<15 mL	15–30 mL	≥30 mL
Volumetric method	<30 mL or <30%	Intermediate	≥60 mL or ≥50%

CW, continuous Doppler wave; ERO, effective regurgitant orifice; PV, pulmonary veins; RVol, regurgitant volume; TVI, time-velocity integral.

TABLE 2: Surgical repair or replacement in secondary mitral regurgitation[12]

Recommendations	Class	Evidence
Surgery is indicated in patients with severe secondary mitral regurgitation undergoing CABG and LVEF >30%	I	C
Surgery should be considered in symptomatic patients with severe secondary mitral regurgitation, LVEF <30% but with an option for revascularization and evidence of myocardial viability	IIa	C
When revascularization is not indicated, surgery may be considered in patients with severe secondary mitral regurgitation and LVEF <30% who remain symptomatic despite optimal medical management (including CRT if indicated) and have low surgical risk	IIb	C
When revascularization is not indicated and surgical risk is low, a percutaneous edge-to-edge procedure may be considered in patients with severe secondary mitral regurgitation and LVEF <30% who remain symptomatic despite optimal medical management (including CRT if indicated) and who have suitable valve morphology by echocardiography, avoiding futility.	IIb	C
In patients with severe secondary mitral regurgitation and LVEF <30% who remain symptomatic despite optimal medical management (including CRT if indicated) and who have no option for revascularization, the Heart Team may consider a percutaneous edge-to-edge procedure or valve surgery after careful evaluation for a ventricular assist device or heart transplant according to individual patient characteristics.	IIb	C

CABG, cardiac artery bypass grafting; CRT, cardiac resynchronization therapy; LVEF, left ventricular ejection fraction.

TABLE 3: Study of MitraClip® and Not MitraClip® feasible

	MitraClip® feasible	Not MitraClip® feasible
MV area	> 4 cm^2	Significant stenosis
MR Jet	Central	Eccentric or multiple
Calcification	Not calcified or mildly	Severe
Specific measurements	Regurgitant orifice width <15 mm Regurgitant orifice height <10 mm Coaptation depth <11 mm Coaptation length >2 mm	Height >2 mm between the leaflets

MR, mitral regurgitation; MV,mitral valve.

replacement if the LVEF is greater than 30% and the patient is candidate for revascularization. If LVEF is less than 30%, the patient is deeply symptomatic and comorbidity is low, repair or replacement may be considered even if patient is not candidate for surgical revascularization.

Table 2 summarizes the recommendations for surgical repair or replacement based on European Society of Cardiology Clinical Practice Guidelines.[12]

A recent approach in these cases is the use of MitraClip® (Abbott Vascular). This percutaneous technique, similar to Alfieri technique, is an alternative therapy that may be considered in patients in class III or IV of the New York Heart Association (NYHA) functional class classification, with severe MR and favorable anatomy (Table 3) for its implantation, but with a prohibitive surgical risk.

REFERENCES

1. Monteagudo Ruiz JM, Galderisi M, Buonauro A, et al. Overview of mitral regurgitation in Europe: Results from the European Registry of mitral regurgitation (EuMiClip). Eur Heart J Cardiovasc Imaging. 2018 [in press].
2. Carpentier A, Chauvaud S, Fabiani JN, et al. Reconstructive surgery of mitral valve incompetence: Ten-year appraisal. J Thorac Cardiovasc Surg. 1980;79(3):338-48.
3. Zamorano JL, Manuel Monteagudo J, Mesa D, et al. Frequency, mechanism and severity of mitral regurgitation: Are there any differences between primary and secondary mitral regurgitation? J Heart Valve Dis. 2016;25(6):724-9.
4. Moñivas V, Mingo S, Cobo M, et al. Papel del ecocardiogramaen la reparación mitral. Cir Cardiov. 2010;17(4):315-30.
5. Alonso Salinas GL, Pascual Izco M, Zamorano JL. Implicacionescuantificación y pronóstico de la insuficiencia mitral con técnicas de imagen. In: Cardio Imagen en la insuficienciacardiaca, García Fernández MA, Lang RM, Perez de Isla L, Gómez de Diego JJ (Eds.) CTO Editorial SL, Madrid, Spain. 2017; pp. 385-416.
6. Zamorano JL, Gonçalves A. Three-dimensional echocardiography for quantification valvular heart disease. Heart. 2013;99:811-8.
7. Gayburn PA, Weissman NJ, Zamorano JL. Quantification of mitral regurgitation. Circulation. 2012;126:2005-17.
8. Thavendiranathan P, Phelan D, Thomas JD, et al. Quantitative assessment of mitral regurgitation. Validation of new methods. J Am Coll Cardiol. 2012;60(16): 1470-83.
9. Vandervoort P, Rivera JM, Thoreau D, et al. Application of color Doppler flow imaging to calculate effective regurgitant orifice area: An assessment of valvular incompetence independent of hemodynamics. Circulation. 1993;88:1150-6.
10. Moya JL, Darriba-Pollán J, García-Lledó A, et al. Evaluation of mitral regurgitation severity using a simplified method based on proximal flow convergence. Rev Esp Cardiol. 2006;59(10):1019-25.
11. Yosefy C, Levine RA, Solis J, et al. Proximal flow convergence region as assessed by real-time 3-dimensional echocardiography: challenging the hemispheric assumption. J Am Soc Echocardiogr. 2007;20:389-96.
12. Baumgartner H, Falk V, Bax JJ, et al. 2017 ESC/EACTS Guidelines for the management of valvular heart disease. Eur Heart J. 2017;38(36):2739-91.

CHAPTER 75

Diastology Demystified

Jagdish C Mohan, Vishwas Mohan, Madhu Shukla

INTRODUCTION

Human beings engage in varying physical activity in daily life; physical exercise capacity is a manifestation of diastolic function. The heart chambers contract, eject, relax, fill, and then contract in a sequential manner (Fig. 1). The phase of relaxation and filling is called diastole (Figs. 2 to 4). Diastole fills the ventricles with adequate blood at very low pressures. There is atrioventricular (AV) coupling which maintains the relationship between peak and nadir of filling. Atrial diastole is during ventricular systole and vice versa. Relaxation aids in filling during early diastole in an active manner while there is passive gradient-dependent filling also in significant part of diastole. The phenomena of relaxation and contraction are interlinked and energy-dependent. Diastole precedes systole because no ejection is possible unless there is filling first. The processes of relaxation and filling constitute diastolic function. Increased resistance to filling is the simplest way of defining diastolic dysfunction. Increased resistance leads to elevated filling pressures. Diastolic dysfunction is the first manifestation of a disease process and explains the symptoms better. Abnormalities of diastolic function are common to virtually all forms of cardiac disease. Noninvasive evaluation of diastolic ventricular function is based on Doppler echocardiographic visualization of inflow pattern and ventricular tissue stretching, although many more parameters are described.

Left ventricular (LV) diastolic pressure becomes elevated as a compensatory mechanism to maintain cardiac output. Therefore, demonstration of elevated LV filling pressure is an important diagnostic target when using echocardiography (ECG) to evaluate diastolic function. The study of pressure-volume loop during diastole is the ideal way to understand and assess diastolic function. However, there are several surrogate methods and parameters in echo-Doppler techniques which provide reasonable, reliable, and actionable information about diastolic function. In general, diastolic dysfunction may be characterized by enlargement of upstream chamber (atrium), alteration in various phases of diastole, and raised

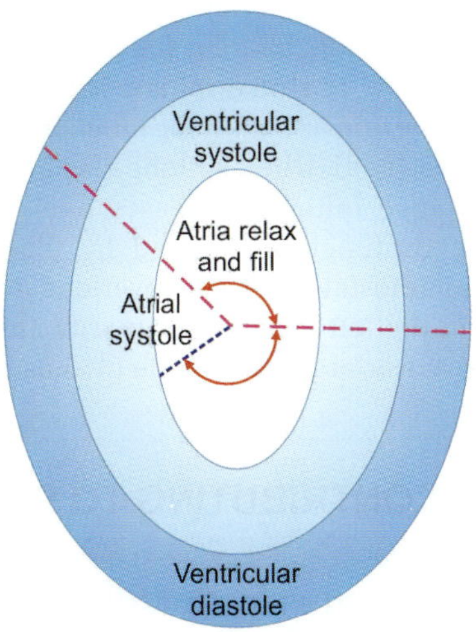

FIG. 1: Temporal components of atrial and ventricular contraction and filling.

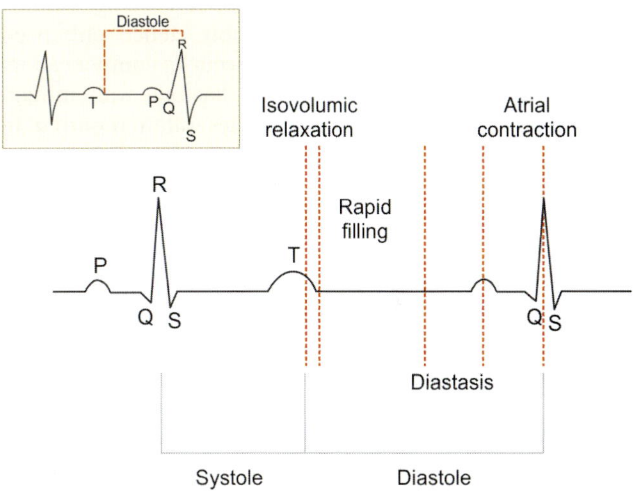

FIG. 2: Relationship of electrocardiogram to four phases of ventricular diastole.

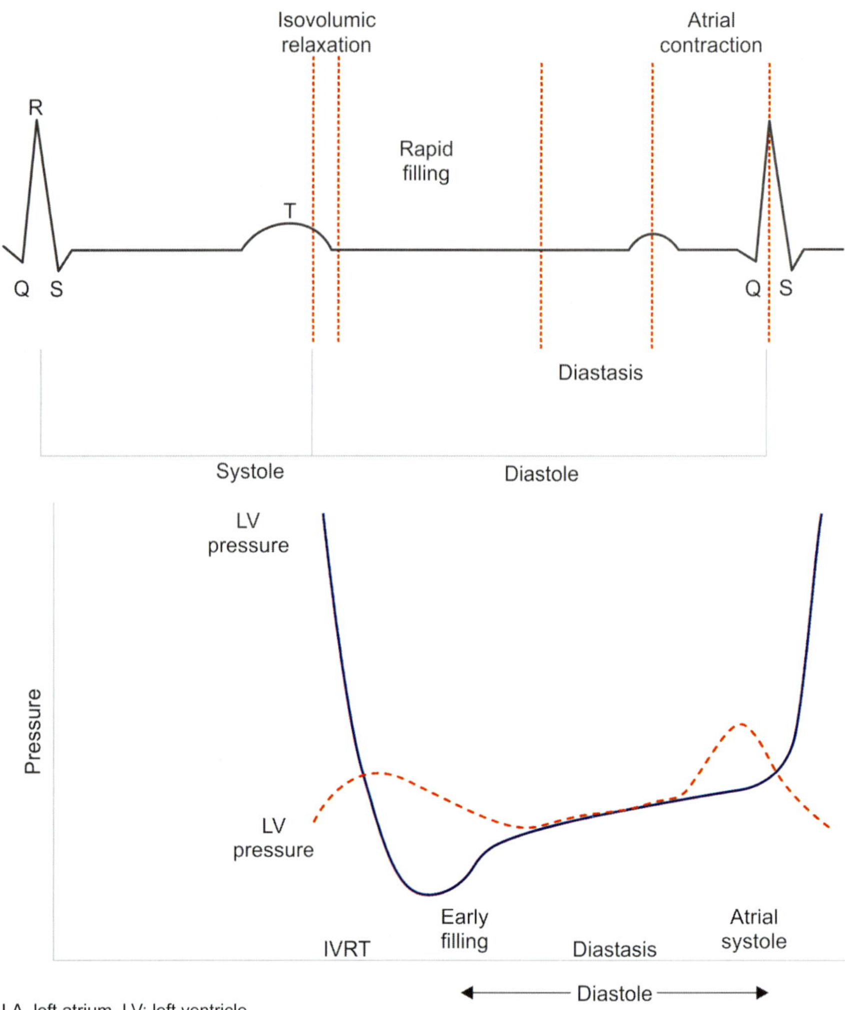

FIG. 3: Relationship of electrocardiogram, phases of diastole, and atrioventricular pressure gradients.

filling pressures. Diastolic dysfunction is dynamic and in early phases, filling pressures are not increased. Assessment of diastolic function in simulated physiological situation like exercise, may provide enhanced information. Diastolic compensatory mechanisms that maintain filling volume are the earliest evidence of dysfunction. Hence, enhanced atrial contraction is the first thing to occur in compensation. There is also evidence of regional diastolic wall motion nonuniformity. Noninvasive surrogates often reported in clinical studies reflect integrative properties of the entire chamber and lack specificity.

PHYSIOLOGY OF DIASTOLE

Form follows function. Diastolic dysfunction is a physiological expression of morphological cardiovascular disease (CVD). The healthy myocardium is an active, nonlinear, nonhomogeneous, and anisotropic viscoelastic material. During diastolic lengthening, normal cardiac muscle behaves like a spring. When the spring is more forcefully compressed during systole, diastolic lengthening is higher and vice versa (Fig. 5).

There is a certain degree of systolic elastance (slope between end-systolic pressure and end-systolic volume) and also a definite diastolic elastance in the ventricles.[1] In several disease states like hypertension, diabetes, and LV hypertrophy as also with aging, systolic elastance remains unaffected or may actually increase and diastolic elastance decreases which can be studied and assessed by echo-Doppler parameters of diastolic function (Figs. 6 and 7). A ratio of mitral E/e' to stroke volume is a good estimate of diastolic elastance and also diastolic function reserve.

On the other hand, when systolic elastance is reduced, diastolic elastance initially increases due to remodeling and diastolic dysfunction denoted by filling pressures, therein, is a manifestation of fluid overload. Most systemic diseases affect the left ventricle primarily and hence, it is pertinent to discuss largely about the LV diastolic function/dysfunction.

FACTORS CONTRIBUTING TO DIASTOLE

- Decline of the myocardial active state following systole
- Passive effects of expanded extracellular volume
- Rapid changes in atrial and ventricular pressures
- Transmitral flow

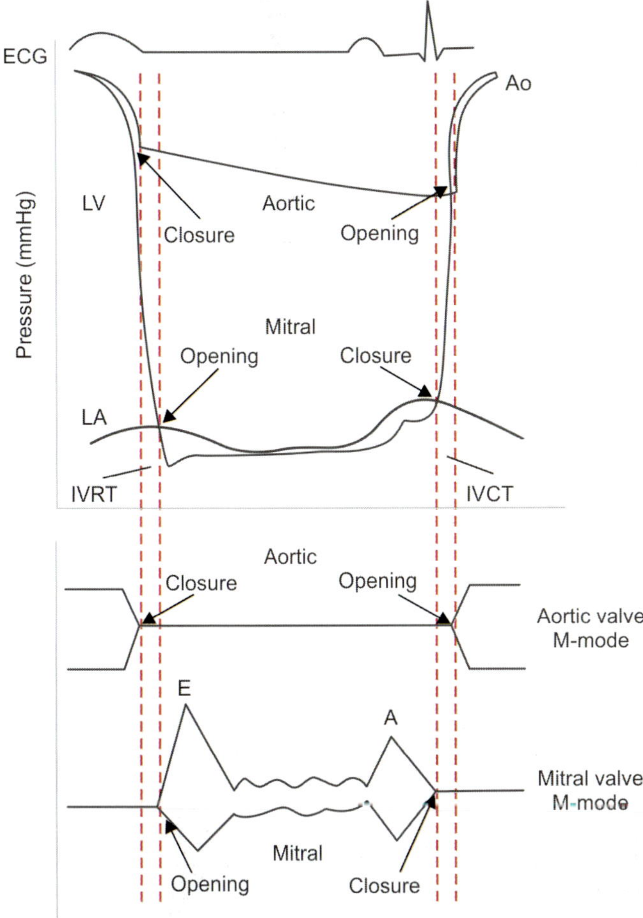

ECG, electrocardiogram; IVCT, isovolumic contraction time; IVRT, isovolumic relaxation time; LA, left atrium; LV, left ventricle.

FIG. 4: Description of the left ventricular diastole with relation to ECG, intracardiac pressures, and valvular mechanics.

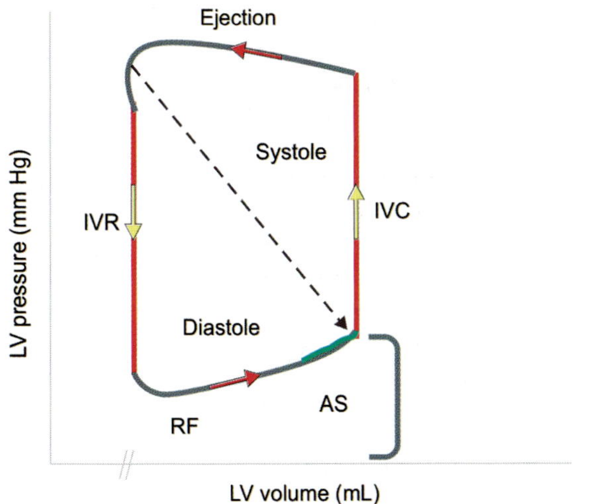

AS, atrial systole; IVC, isovolumic contraction; IVR, isovolumic relaxation; LV, left ventricle; RF, rapid filling.

FIG. 5: Left ventricular pressure-volume loop. Note that the diastole is a mirror image of systole.

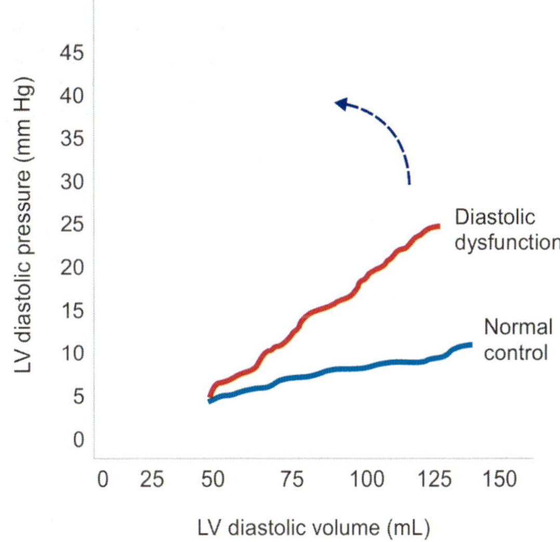

LV: left ventricle.

FIG. 6: Diastolic pressure-volume relationship (elastance) of a normal subject (blue color) and that of a subject with diastolic dysfunction (red color).

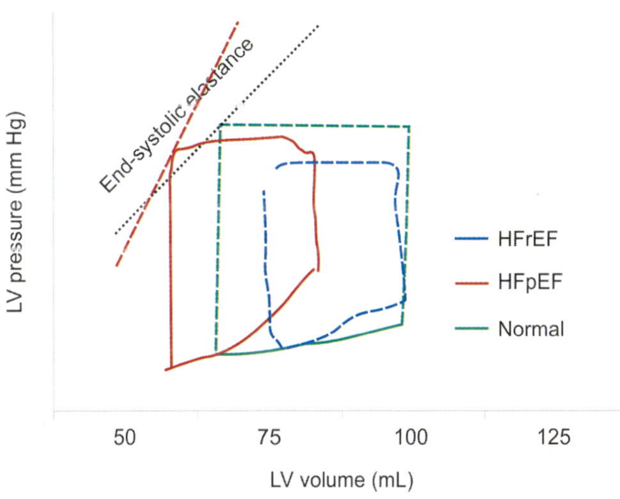

HFpEF, heart failure with preserved ejection fraction; HFrEF, heart failure with reduced ejection fraction; LV, left ventricle.

FIG. 7: Depiction of pressure-volume loop in pure diastolic heart failure (HFpEF) compared to that of normal control and systolic heart failure (HFrEF).

- Interactions with the right ventricle and pericardium
- Atrial systole.

SIGNIFICANCE OF DIASTOLIC FUNCTION

- Identification of preclinical diseases in probands
- Diagnosis and subtyping of clinical syndrome of heart failure (HF)
- Marker of incremental prognosis in diverse cardiac disorders
- Monitoring therapy and follow-up
- Understanding exercise physiology

- Cardiac versus noncardiac dyspnea
- Physiological versus pathological remodeling
- Optimizing devices and drugs response
- Evaluation of intraventricular dyssynchrony
- Study of pericardial diseases.

There is no single definition for diastolic dysfunction. Many features can get altered, and any one change or their combination is typically called diastolic dysfunction, although the pathophysiology and functional significance varies greatly.[2-4] Clinically, the most common manifestation is an elevated mean diastolic pressure and altered filling patterns, but neither of these are specific features of diastolic dysfunction (Fig. 8).

When diastolic dysfunction is detected, it has some morphological, cellular, and proteomic connotations. These are:

- A change in the extracellular matrix of the myocardium, with the formation of excess collagen tissue[5]
- At the cellular level, there is reduced phosphorylation of sarcomeric proteins
- At the proteomic level, an isoform change in important structural macromolecular proteins such as titin.[6]

Diastole starts with closure of the aortic valve and ends with onset of ventricular contraction (Fig. 9). It has an initial period of ventricular relaxation without filling [isovolumic relaxation time (IVRT)] and then three phases of ventricular filling [diastolic filling period (DFP)]. The four phases of diastole are:[7]

1. Isovolumic relaxation (IVR) phase
2. Rapid filling phase
3. Diastasis
4. Late diastolic filling due to atrial contraction.

Diastolic LV function can be assessed in each of the four phases: (1) IVR, (2) rapid filling, (3) slow filling, and (4) atrial contraction by studying the inflow Doppler pattern either in pulmonary veins or at the level of mitral orifice (Fig. 10). These four phases uniquely reflect LV physiology and are invariably accessible to noninvasive evaluation.

In brief, diastolic dysfunction is presumed when there is impaired relaxation (and decreased ventricular suction), poor filling, or loss of atrial contraction.[7]

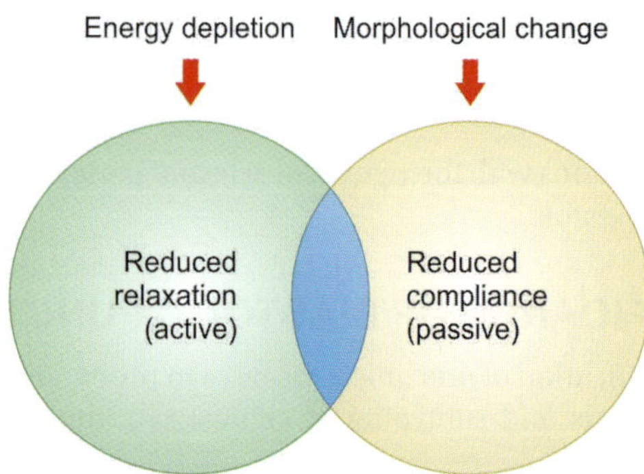

FIG. 8: Diastolic dysfunction in clinical sense is raised diastolic pressures which means reduced compliance or increased diastolic stiffness.

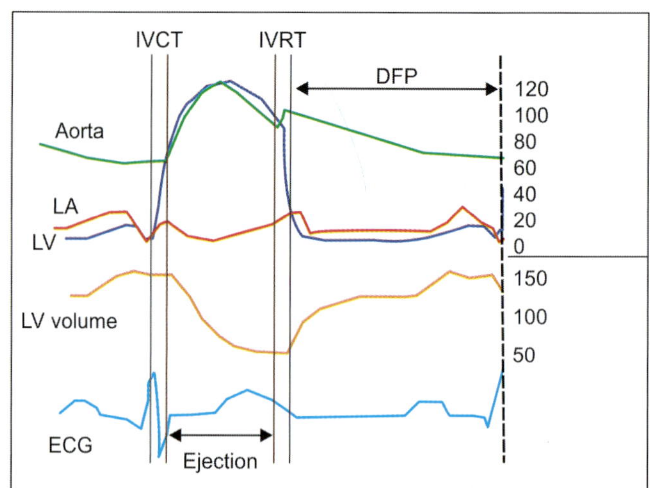

DFP, diastolic filling period; ECG, electrocardiogram; IVCT, isovolumic contraction time; IVRT, isovolumic relaxation time; LA, left atrium; LV, left ventricle.

FIG. 9: Graphic representation of various phases of the cardiac cycle of the left heart.

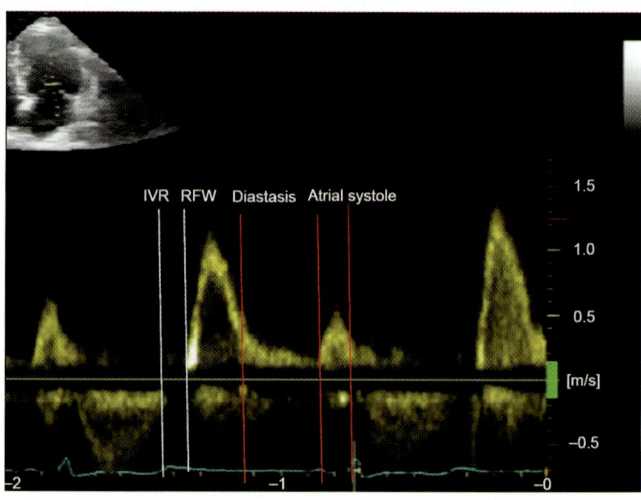

FIG. 10: Doppler interrogation with sample volume placed between the left ventricular outflow and the inflow showing all four phases of diastole: (1) IVR—isovolumic relaxation, (2) RF—rapid filling, (3) diastasis—slow filling, and (4) AC—late filling due to atrial systole.

There are two phases in systole:

1. Isovolumic contraction (IVC) phase
2. Ejection phase (ET).

Combined systolic and diastolic function can be assessed by the ratio of IVR time + IVC time/ejection time. This ratio has been called myocardial performance index.[8] Although used for prognosis in various diseased states, it has not found practical utility for daily use in most echocardiography laboratories.

Isovolumic Relaxation Time

Isovolumic relaxation time, which corresponds to the time interval from aortic valve closure to mitral valve opening, is difficult to appreciate from simultaneous LV pressure, aortic pressure, and wedge pressure recordings but is easily measured by pulsed or continuous-wave (CV) Doppler from the simultaneous display of the end of aortic ejection and the onset of mitral inflow (Fig. 11).

Isovolumic relaxation time has a predictable quantitative relationship to constant of IVR and to left atrial (LA) and aortic pressures.[8]

- Prolonged IVRT indicates impaired myocardial relaxation
- A normal IVRT is about 70 ± 12 ms, and approximately 10 ms longer in people over 40 years
- In abnormal relaxation, IVRT is usually in excess of 110 ms
- With restrictive filling, it is usually under 60 ms

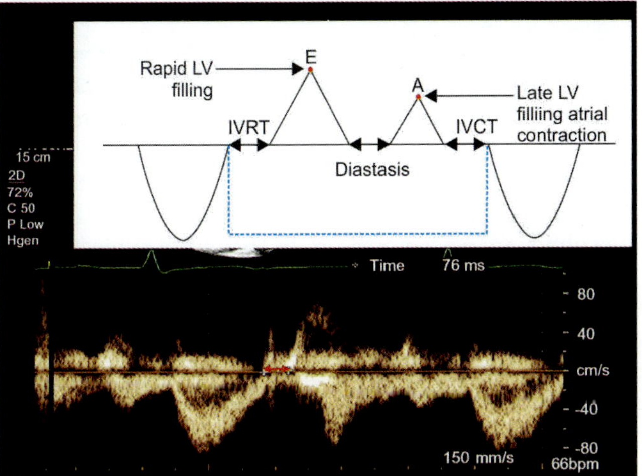

BPM, beats per minute; IVCT, isovolumic contraction time; LV, left ventricular.

FIG. 11: Doppler interrogation between LV outflow and inflow showing measurement of isovolumic relaxation time. At heart rate of 66 BPM, IVRT is 76 ms in this normal subject.

- If IVRT is prolonged (>110 ms), LA pressure is not elevated because the delay in mitral valve opening is related to lower pressure crossover between LV and LA in the setting of delayed relaxation
- It is safe to conclude that LA pressure is elevated if the IVRT is short (<60 ms) in the presence of cardiac disease and normal heart rate range.

Clinical value of IVRT as an index of diastolic LV function is limited because it depends on mitral valve opening pressures and, therefore, is not uniquely related to LV dysfunction.

Rapid Filling Phase

In early diastole, chamber wall relaxation unmasks stored elastic strain, allowing the LV to recoil and act as a suction pump by aspirating blood into the ventricle. Normal LV filling occurs rapidly early in diastole caused by a progressive pressure gradient within the ventricle and with a low LA pressure.

Rapid filling phase accounts for 70% of LV filling. It gets shorter in duration with raised filling pressures and is prolonged in subjects with impaired relaxation alone.[9] When both impaired relaxation and raised LA pressure coexist, it has variable duration like in normal subjects. Rapid filling phase is denoted by early diastolic (E) mitral flow wave and antegrade diastolic (D) flow wave of the pulmonary veins. Variables affecting rapid filling phase are shown in figure 12.

Deceleration Time of Early Filling Wave (Mitral E and Pulmonary D Waves)

Deceleration time (DT) is the duration between the peak of early filling wave and where its linear descending slope reaches zero (Fig. 13). Nonlinear slopes are not measured.

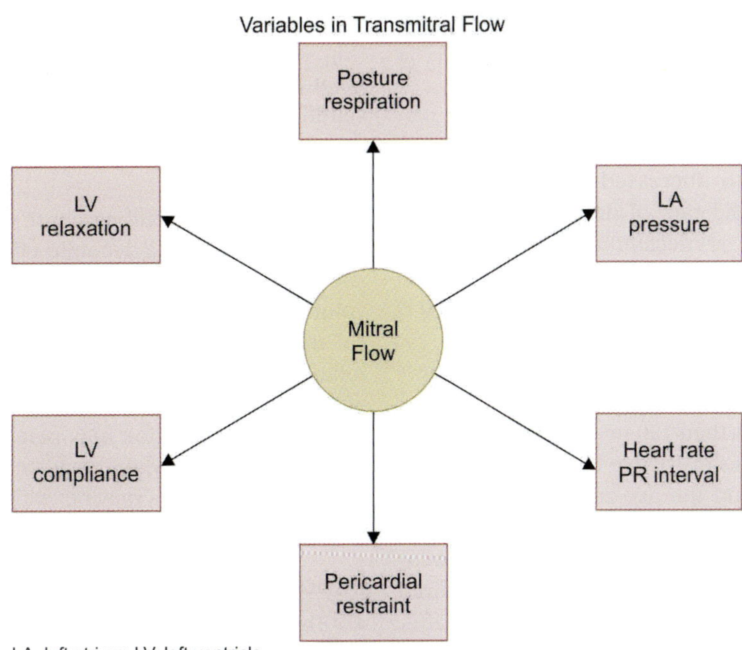

LA, left atrium; LV, left ventricle.

FIG. 12: Variables affecting rapid filling phase in diastole.

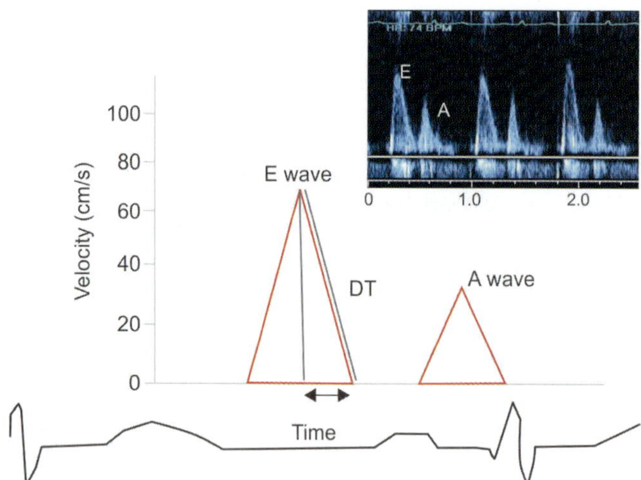

FIG. 13: Graphic display of deceleration time (DT) of mitral early filling wave.

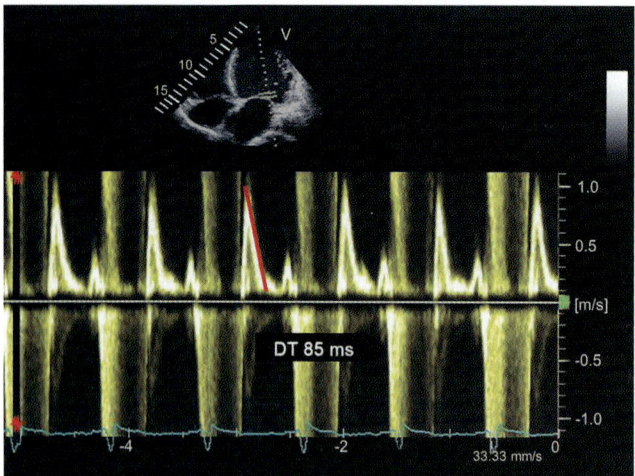

FIG. 14: Restrictive filling pattern with deceleration time (DT) of 85 ms in a 50-year-old male patient with dilated cardiomyopathy.

Conditions associated with increased LV stiffness are associated with a more rapid rate of deceleration of early filling and a shorter time for this deceleration.[10]

- It is an index of resistance to early filling with normal values in range of 150–250 ms (up to 200 ms by some). It is shorter in young subjects
- Deceleration time denotes chamber stiffness regardless of heart rate, afterload, and contractility
- Deceleration time of less than 150 ms (range 130–160 ms in some studies) indicates restrictive filling and relatively noncompliant LV beyond the age more than 45 years (Fig. 14)
- Deceleration time more than 200 ms indicates compensatory mechanism is in place to overcome impaired relaxation. Prolonging of DT during therapy after recording a very short DT initially is a positive sign of recovery when heart rates do not change significantly

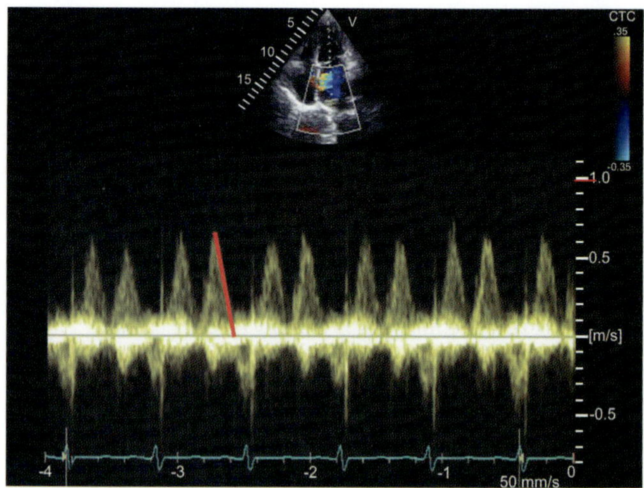

FIG. 15: Right upper pulmonary vein flow in a patient with restrictive cardiomyopathy measuring deceleration time (DT) of D wave.

- There is a close inverse relationship between DT and pulmonary wedge pressure in HF and in subjects more than 45 years of age
- Deceleration time is affected by age as well as pericardial restraint. As myocardial relaxation becomes less active with aging or abnormally delayed due to a disease process, the rate of LV pressure decline during the early diastole is reduced, and it takes a longer time to reach the minimal LV diastolic pressure
- Longer DT indicates impaired diastolic reserve. In this situation with abnormal myocardial relaxation, a reduced DFP and a lack of atrial contraction compromise LV filling further and produce clinically syndrome of effort intolerance.

During the time of early flow deceleration, there is rapid flow into the LA from the pulmonary veins. DT of pulmonary vein diastolic wave has same significance as that of mitral DT (Fig. 15). A pulmonary vein DT of less than 150 ms has much greater specificity for predicting elevated filling pressures and significant diastolic dysfunction.[11]

Diastasis

During the slow LV filling phase or diastasis, residual effects of LV relaxation and dynamic effects of fast LV inflow have subsided. This phase is used to construct diastolic LV pressure-volume relations from a single cardiac cycle and allows LV stiffness, the slope of the diastolic LV pressure-volume relation, to be derived under static conditions. In subjects with impaired relaxation and longer cardiac cycle, residual effects of LV relaxation may persist and positive filling wave during diastasis (L-wave) may be observed (Figs. 16 and 17). Mitral valve L-waves may be evident in healthy patients with relatively low heart rates.[12]

Importance of L-wave

- The L-wave (between E and A waves) may be seen in relatively bradycardic patients with normal hearts. It is usually less than 20 cm/s in velocity

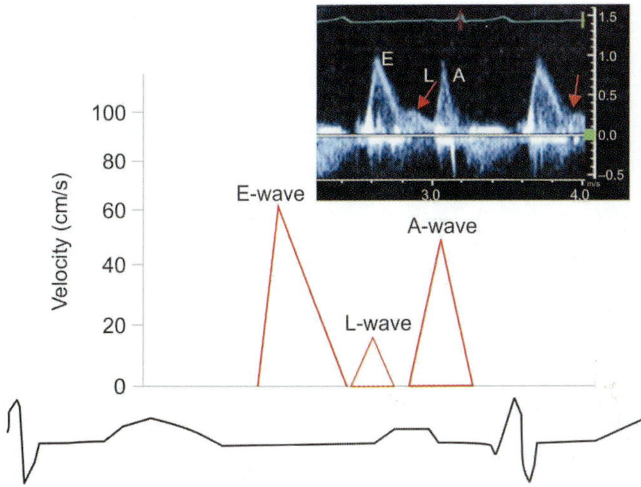

FIG. 16: Pulsed-wave Doppler mitral flow showing positive wave (L-wave) during diastasis.

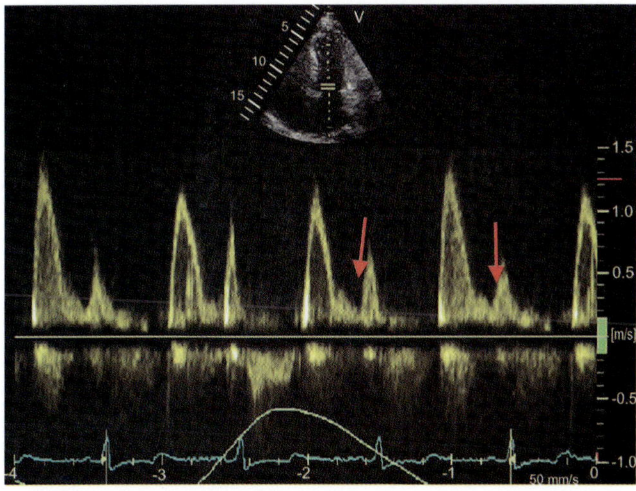

FIG. 18: Transmitral L-wave (red arrows).

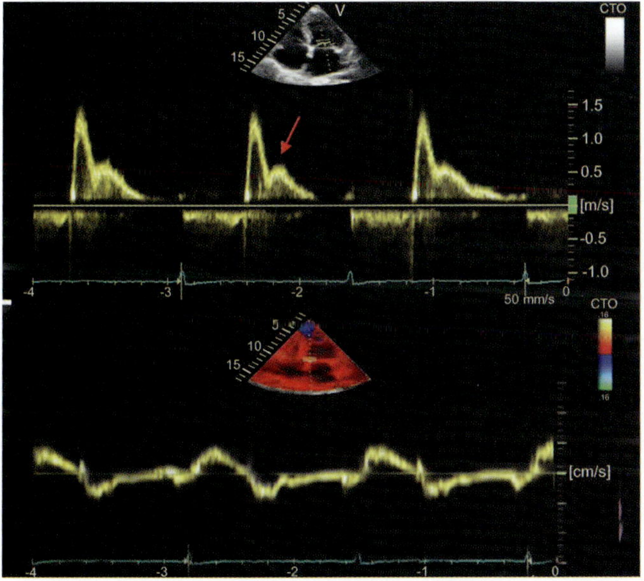

FIG. 17: Pulsed-wave Doppler mitral flow in upper panel showing prominent L-wave (red arrow), no A-wave, and bradycardia.

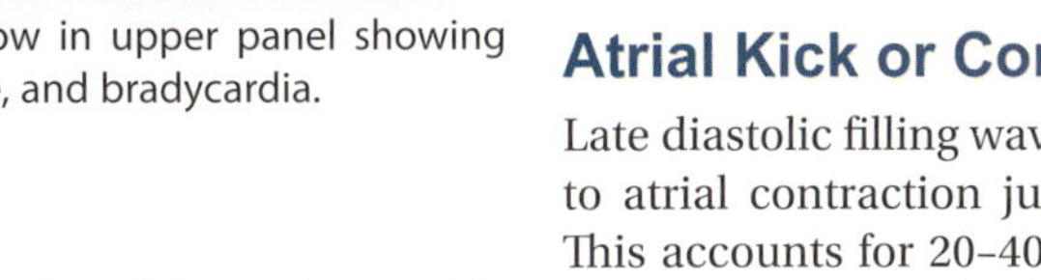

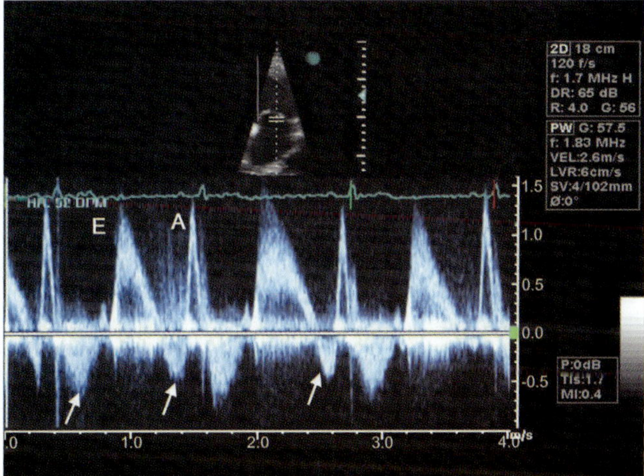

FIG. 19: Mid-diastolic negative L-wave in a patient with left ventricular (LV) diastolic dysfunction.

- A pathologic L-wave typically is found in patients with delayed active relaxation with increased LV stiffness. Its velocity is more than 20 cm/s
- In the echo laboratory, patients who exhibit transmitral L-wave, will often have clinical HF, LV hypertrophy with normal systolic function, or LV systolic dysfunction
- A pathologic L-wave is suggestive of elevated LV preload (pseudonormalization)
- A pathologic L-wave has prognostic value, in that it is predictive of future hospitalizations with HF (Fig. 18).

Occasionally, there can be negative L-wave or mid-diastolic mitral regurgitation due to rapid rise in LV diastolic pressure as a consequence of early filling (Fig. 19). Its exact significance is not clear.

Atrial Kick or Contribution

Late diastolic filling wave is of short duration and occurs due to atrial contraction just before ventricular systole begins. This accounts for 20–40% of ventricular filling and is absent in atrial fibrillation (AF) and fragmented during atrial flutter. This gets partly or completely obliterated in first-degree heart block and markedly raised ventricular stiffness. Atrial kick is reflected by late diastolic (A) mitral flow wave and atrial flow reversal (Ar) in pulmonary veins. In markedly elevated LV diastolic pressure, atrial contraction may not produce any antegrade flow wave and may be seen to send flow retrogradely in pulmonary veins due to resistance gradient (Fig. 20).

Tissue Motion and Diastolic Function

As transmitral flow commences in diastole, the mitral annulus moves upward the atrium along the long axis. Due to tissue and blood incompressibility, as the annulus rises, the

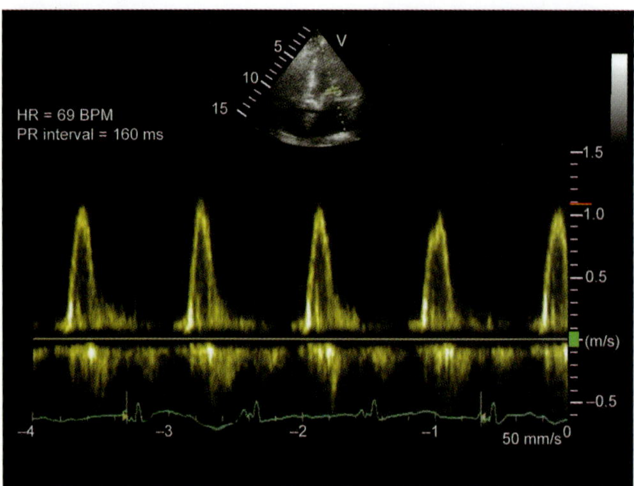

BPM, beats per minute; HR, heart rate.

FIG. 20: Monophasic mitral flow with normal PR interval and HR of 69 BPM in a 90-year-old subject.

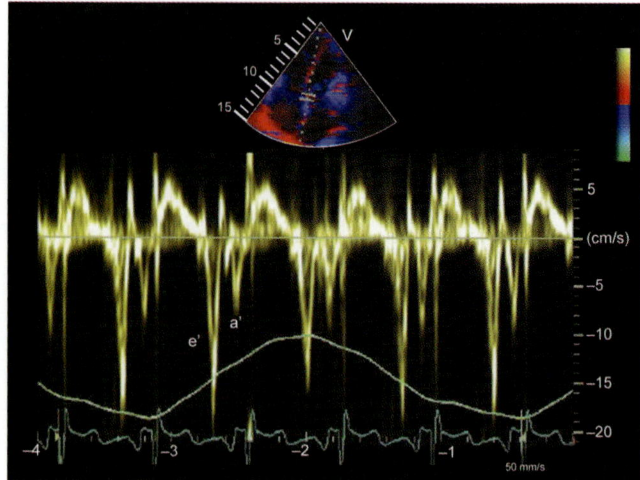

FIG. 22: Biphasic longitudinal expansion of the left ventricle during diastole. e'—early diastolic and a'—late diastolic longitudinal tissue velocity waves.

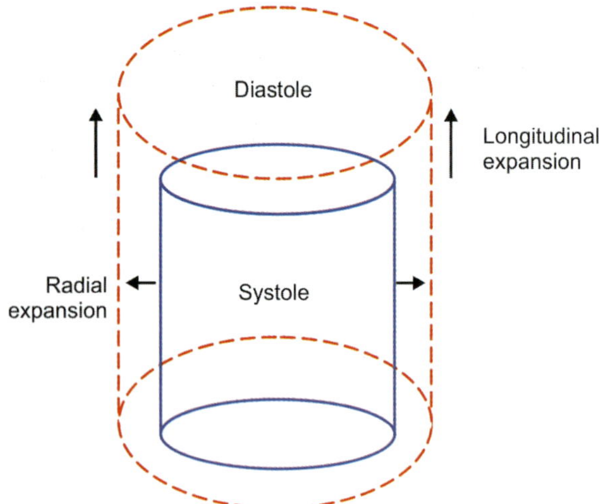

FIG. 21: Graphic display of longitudinal and radial expansion of the left ventricle during diastole (arrows).

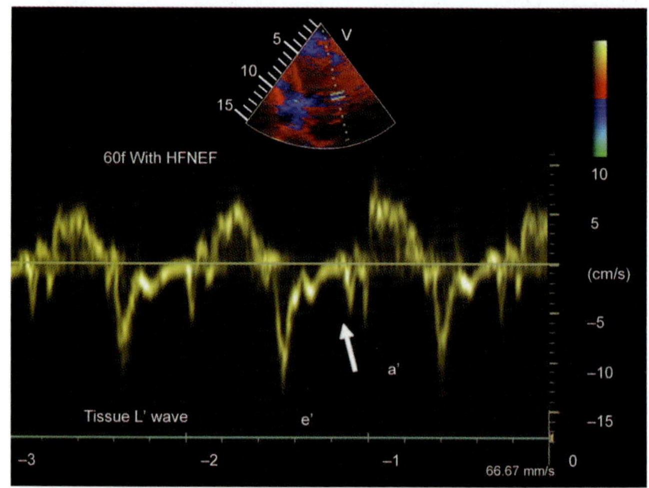

FIG. 23: Tissue L' wave in diastasis (arrow).

wall thins, and the endocardium is simultaneously displaced radially outward toward the epicardium. During filling, the short and long axes change simultaneously (Fig. 21). Hence, rate of longitudinal displacement and radial endocardial displacement are good indicators of diastolic function.[13] Early diastolic longitudinal excursion rate can be easily obtained from tissue Doppler studies (Fig. 22).

Left ventricular wall motion generates the AV pressure gradient resulting in the early transmitral flow (Doppler E-wave) and associated vortex formation.

Substantial residual LV relaxation pressures in mid-diastole present in some patients with stiff LV can result in a positive wave called tissue L' wave (Fig. 23).[14]

LEFT ATRIAL VOLUME AND DIASTOLIC FUNCTION/DYSFUNCTION

The measurement of maximum LA volume is an essential component of the comprehensive assessment of LV diastolic function.[15,16] This is based upon the premise that the form follows the function. Resistance to filling due to diastolic dysfunction causes blood stasis and stretches the chamber. More recently, LA volumes have been obtained by three-dimensional (3D) echocardiography. However, normative data in clinical practice is validated from two-dimensional (2D) echocardiography only.

The LA volume is usually measured by biplane area-length method (Fig. 24). In current guidelines, assessment of diastolic function mandates measurement of LA volume index in every subject. Although, it has limited role in assessing diastolic function or dysfunction in acute situations, it has great relevance in chronic stable CV conditions.[15]

- The LA volume can be viewed as a morphologic expression of LV diastolic dysfunction[15]
- Left atrial volume is regarded as a barometer of the chronicity of diastolic dysfunction[15]
- This simple measure of LA volume provides significant insight into an individual's risk for the development

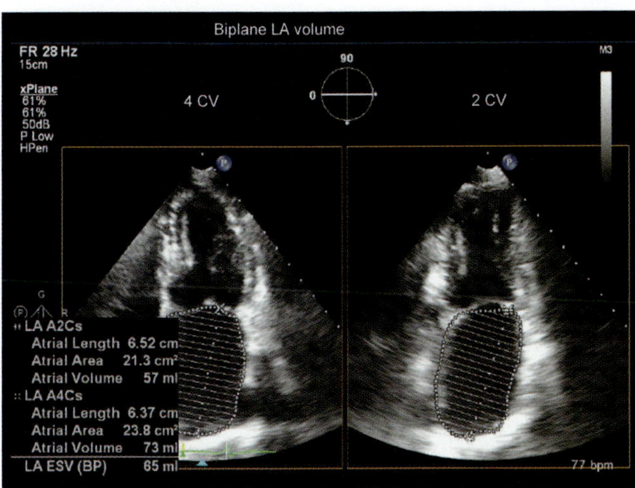

FIG. 24: Estimation of biplane end-systolic left atrial (LA) volume by area-length method.

of adverse CV events including, myocardial infarction, stroke, AF, and HF

- Normal values for LA volume are 22 ± 6 mL/m^2.[15]
- Left atrial volume is graded relative to risk, 28–33 mL/m^2 = mild; 34–39 mL/m^2 = moderate; and more than or equal to 40 mL/m^2 = high or severe.
    - *Normal subjects*: 22 ± 6 mL/m^2
    - *Mild LA enlargement*: 28–33 mL/m^2
    - *Moderate LA enlargement*: 34–39 mL/m^2.
    - *Severe LA enlargement*: More than or equal to 40 mL/m^2
- Diastolic dysfunction is more likely if the LA volume index exceeds 34 mL/m^2
- However, LA volume can increase in mitral regurgitation, athletes, and in presence of sinus bradycardia without concomitant diastolic dysfunction
- There is a fairly good positive correlation between LA volume index and grade of diastolic dysfunction
- Maximum LA systolic lengthening and its rate have also been found to correlate with diastolic dysfunction (Figs. 25 and 26)
- It is possible to use LA strain during ventricular systole along with LA pressure or its Doppler echocardiographic surrogate (E/e') to calculate LA chamber stiffness.[17] E/e; divided by LA reservoir longitudinal strain is a measure of chamber stiffness
- Left atrial stiffness has good accuracy in identifying patients in diastolic HF
- Change in volume-pressure relationships in left atrium also indicates change in material properties (ischemia, fibrosis, etc.) and physiological or pathological remodeling in the LV.

Factors extrinsic to the LV myocardium may influence the end-diastolic pressure-volume relationship. Changes in intrathoracic pressure (as with spontaneous or assisted ventilation), pericardial constraints, and interventricular interactions may each affects ventricular diastolic pressure (when referenced to atmospheric pressure), which, therefore, influences this relationship. In absence of these, intrinsic diastolic function governs this relationship. Various equations have been derived from mitral flow and tissue expansion rate to predict end-diastolic pressure. E/e' ratio has the strongest relation to pulmonary capillary wedge pressure (PCWP) [r = 0.86, PCWP = 1.55 + 1.47 (E/E$_a$)], irrespective of the pattern and ejection fraction (EF).[18]

How to perform a study focusing on diastolic function?

- After estimation of biplane LA volume, one proceeds to interrogate by pulsed-wave (PW) Doppler, four different sites as shown in figure 27
- With the patient supine, apical four-chamber views (4-CVs) using a 2.5-MHz transducer are obtained with the sample volume gated at 1.5–5 mm directed between the tips of the mitral valve leaflets and orthogonal to the mitral valve plane
- Continuous-wave Doppler is used to record aortic outflow and mitral inflow from the apical view for determination of the IVRT using a sweep speed of 100 mm/s
- In apical 4-CV, ostium of the right upper pulmonary vein is interrogated by pulsed-wave Doppler
- M-mode of the color flow propagation velocity across the mitral valve up to 4 cm into the cavity is obtained

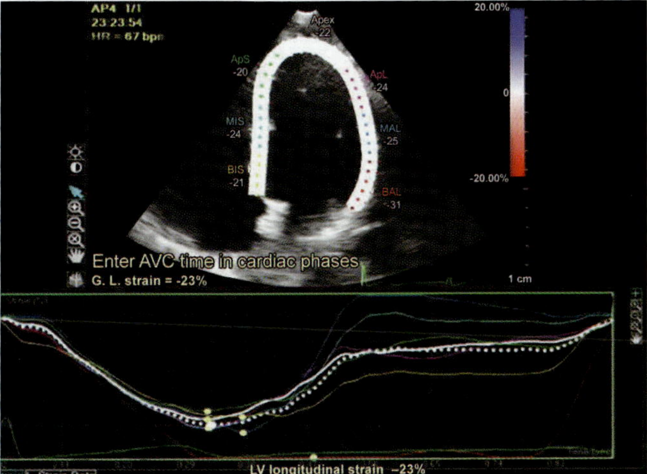

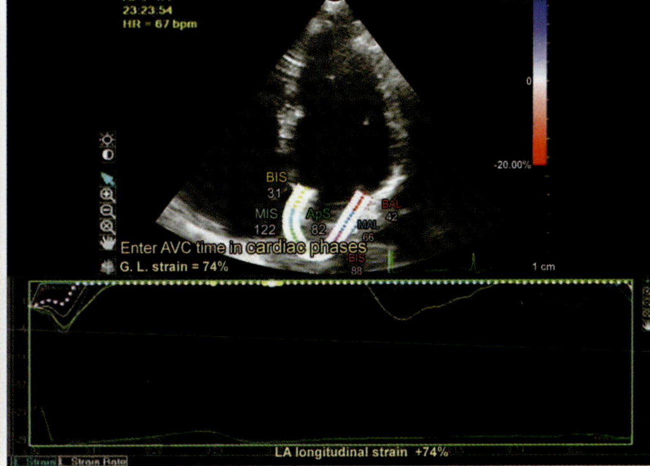

FIG. 25: Left atrial (LA) longitudinal lengthening in a normal subject compared to that of the left ventricular (LV) shortening. Typically, LA lengthening is twice or more of the LV shortening.

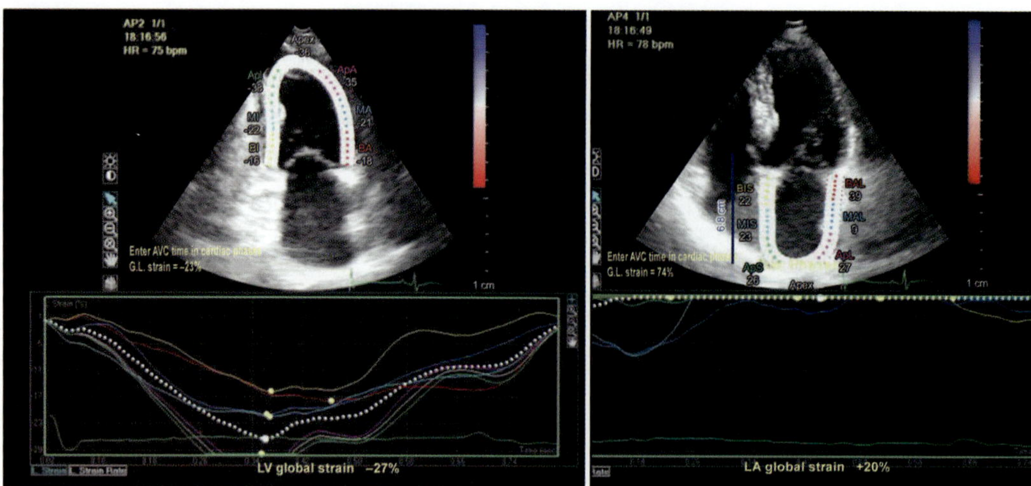

FIG. 26: Significantly reduced left atrial (LA) global strain in presence of diastolic dysfunction.

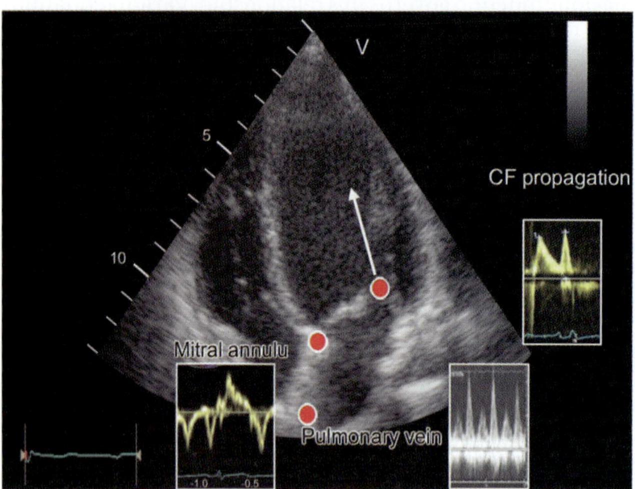

FIG. 27: Sites for assessing diastolic function in an apical four-chamber view (4-CV).

- Doppler tissue imaging (DTI) of the medial and the lateral mitral annulus and M-mode images are also recorded. DTI is performed at a sample size gated at 2.5 mm
- Effect of Valsalva maneuver is also observed for the mitral and pulmonary vein flow
- Sometimes, supine exercise is used to study diastolic function parameters. Postexercise E/A ratio as an independent determinant of severity of exercise-induced dyspnea and impaired exercise tolerance
- Longitudinal strain and untwisting rate of the LV are also recorded by acoustic speckle tracking
- After obtaining all the measurements, the diastolic dysfunction, if present, is graded and occasionally it may be noted as indeterminate if multiparameters give conflicting results and less than 50% parameters are positive for dysfunction.

MITRAL INFLOW VELOCITIES

The mitral inflow velocity profile is initially used to characterize LV filling dynamics (Fig. 28).

- E velocity (E) represents the early mitral inflow velocity and is influenced by the relative pressures between the LA and LV, which, in turn, are dependent on multiple variables including LA pressure, LV compliance, and the rate of LV relaxation[19]
- A velocity (A) represents the atrial contractile component of mitral filling and is primarily influenced by LV compliance and LA contractility. It would be absent in AF
- The DT of the E velocity is the interval from peak E to a point of intersection of the deceleration of flow with the baseline and it correlates with time of pressure equalization between the LA and LV. Incomplete or delayed relaxation causes a delay in the transfer of blood from atria to ventricle
- As the early LA and LV filling pressures either move toward or away from equilibrium, so will the DT either shorten or lengthen, respectively
- Diastolic dysfunction can be categorized into three stages based upon transmitral filling patterns:[2-4]
  1. *Grade I*: Impaired relaxation denoted by DT more than 250 ms and E/A velocity ratio less than 0.8 (Figs. 29 and 30). The American Society of Echocardiography (ASE) and European Association of Echocardiography (EAE) guidelines suggest DT more than 200 ms in grade I
     Early in the evolution of diastolic dysfunction and the delay in emptying (DT >250 ms) partially compensated by a more vigorous end-diastolic atria contraction, and, hence, the E/A ratio is reduced (<0.8)
  2. *Grade II*: Pseudonormal pattern with DT 150–250 ms and E/A ratio between 0.8 and 1.5. ASE-EAE guidelines put DT in range of 160–200 ms
     Pseudonormal pattern needs confirmation by increased LA volume (>34 mL/m^2) or mitral E wave velocity/annular tissue early diastolic velocity more than 15 (medial) or more than 13 (lateral) or pulmonary vein flow increased duration of atrial flow reversal wave or Valsalva maneuver to unearth impaired relaxation in mitral flow

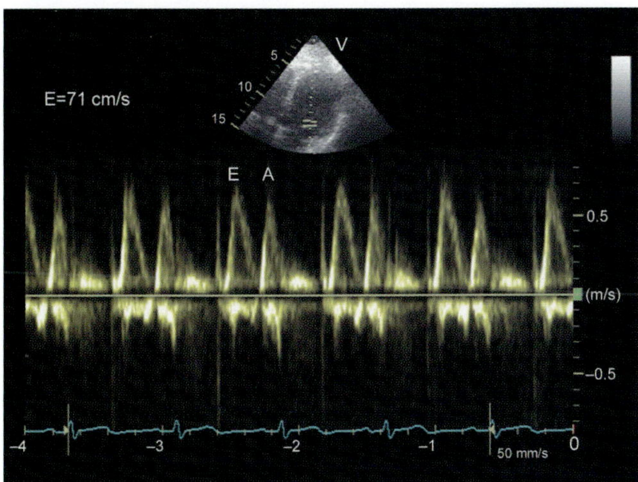

FIG. 28: Biphasic mitral flow with sample volume at the tips of the mitral leaflets.

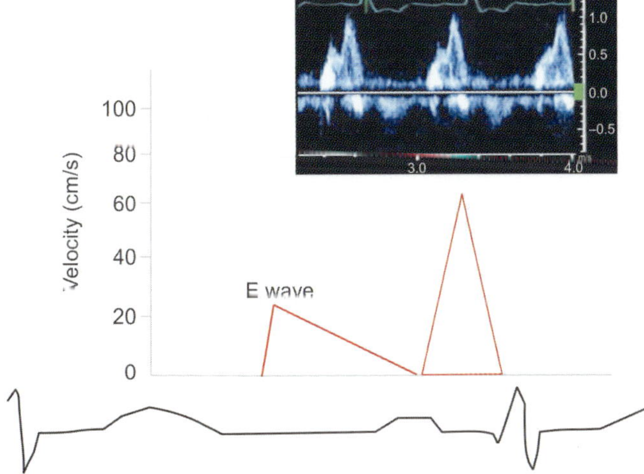

FIG. 29: Grade I diastolic dysfunction in transmitral flow with prolonged deceleration time (DT).

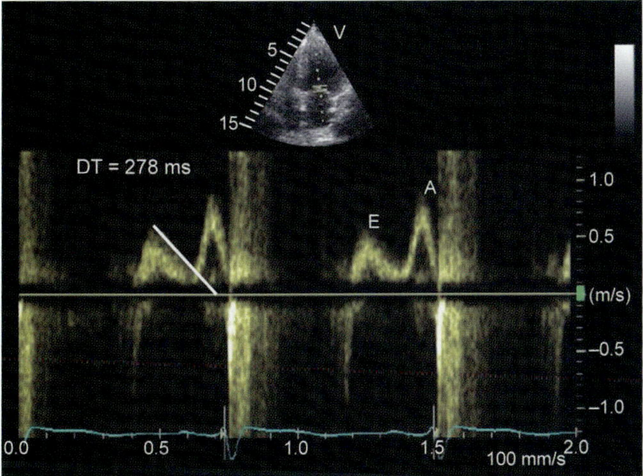

FIG. 30: Grade I diastolic dysfunction denoted by deceleration time (DT) of 278 ms and E/A 0.7.

Presence of L-wave or DT less than 150 ms could also provide clue to pseudonormal pattern if E/A velocity ratio is 0.8–1.5

3. *Grade III*: Restrictive flow or reduced compliance pattern with DT less than 160 ms and E/A ratio more than or equal to 2.0. Others have used DT cutoff limits of less than 150 ms and less than 130 ms as well.

MITRAL INFLOW MEASUREMENTS

Following measurements should be made in each examination:

- Peak early filling velocity (E-wave)
- Late diastolic filling velocity (A-wave)
- E/A ratio
- Deceleration time of early filling velocity
- Isovolumic relaxation time (ms)
- Mitral A-wave duration (obtained at the level of the mitral annulus)
- Diastolic filling time (ms)
- A-wave velocity-time integral (cm)
- Total mitral inflow velocity-time integral (and thus, the atrial filling fraction) with the sample volume at the level of the mitral annulus
- Mid-diastolic flow is an important signal to recognize. Low velocities can occur in normal subjects, but when increased (≥20 cm/s), they often represent markedly delayed LV relaxation and elevated filling pressures.

Most confusions arise in so-called pseudonormal pattern wherein one or the other parameter can be discordant (Fig. 31). Help can be obtained from using multiple parameters and any of the other abnormality could be construed as abnormal diastolic function especially if the early diastolic annular tissue velocity is significantly reduced.[3,4]

Restrictive flow is relatively easy to detect and is unambiguous in adult patients with heart disease (Fig. 32).[20] These criteria cannot be used in children and young adults who normally have large E-waves and short DT due to very active suction of the LV.

Although not supported by the ASE, others have used grade IV diastolic dysfunction as the one in which either the restrictive pattern is irreversible[21] or has monophasic flow pattern with absent A-wave despite sinus rhythm, normal PR interval, and usual heart rates (Fig. 33).

MITRAL INFLOW: ACQUISITION AND FEASIBILITY

- Pulsed-wave Doppler apical 4-CV is performed in order to obtain mitral inflow velocities to assess LV filling
- Color flow imaging can be helpful for optimal alignment of the Doppler beam, especially in the presence of a dilated left ventricle
- Continuous-wave Doppler to assess peak E (early diastolic) and A (late diastolic) velocities should be performed before applying the PW technique to ensure that maximal velocities are obtained
- A 1–3 mm sample volume is then placed between the mitral leaflet tips during diastole to record a crisp velocity profile

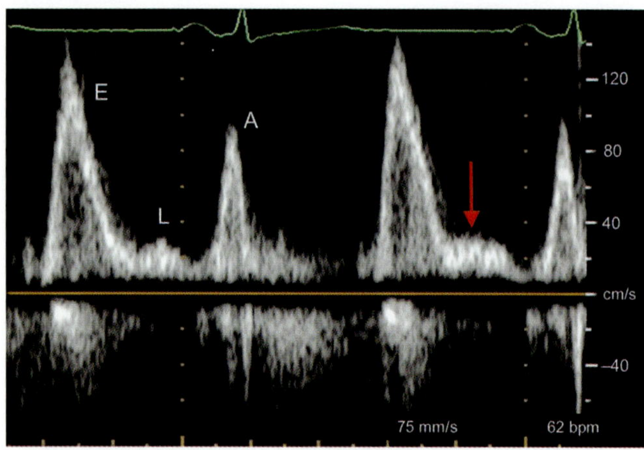

FIG. 31: Pseudonormal or grade II diastolic dysfunction denoted by presence of L-wave (arrow).

Note: E/A ratio of 1.5 and deceleration time (DT) of 180 ms.

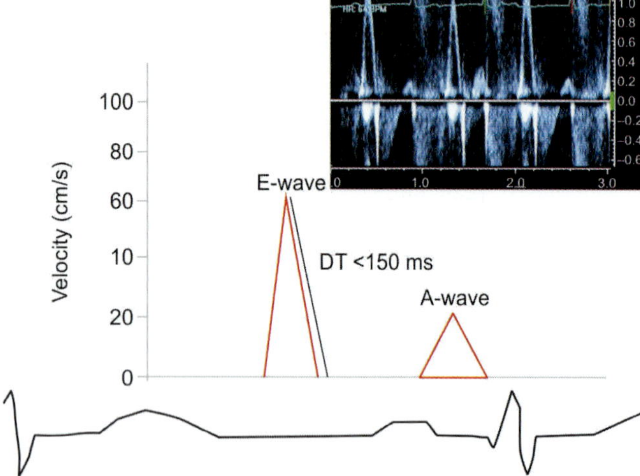

FIG. 32: Restrictive (grade III) flow pattern with short deceleration time (DT) and E/A ratio more than or equal to 2.

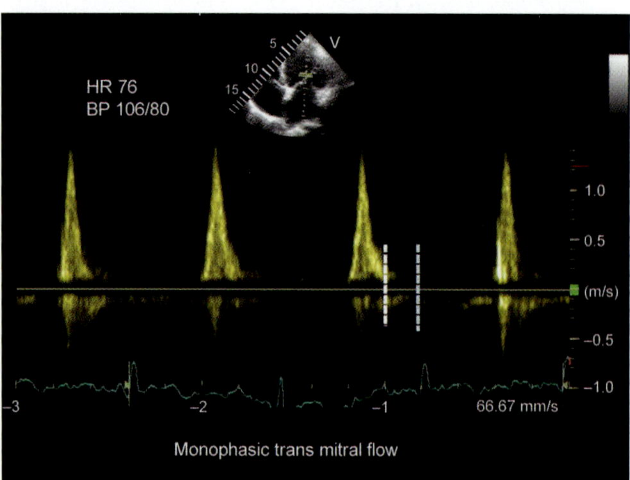

FIG. 33: Monophasic transmitral flow pattern in a patient with advanced diastolic dysfunction and heart failure due to previous anterior wall myocardial infarction.

- Optimizing spectral gain and wall filter settings is important to clearly display the onset and cessation of LV inflow
- Spectral mitral velocity recordings should be initially obtained at sweep speeds of 25–50 mm/s for the evaluation of respiratory variation of flow velocities, as seen in patients with pulmonary or pericardial disease
- If variation is not present, the sweep speed is increased to 100 mm/s, at end-expiration, and averaged over three consecutive cardiac cycles
- The Valsalva maneuver is performed by forceful expiration (about 40 mm Hg) against a closed nose and mouth, producing a complex hemodynamic process involving four phases. It helps to identify pseudonormal mitral inflow and irreversible restrictive flow. A decrease in E/A ratio more than or equal to 0.5 is the criterion (Figs. 34 and 35).

In cardiac patients, a decrease of more than or equal to 50% in the E/A ratio during Valsalva maneuver is highly specific for increased LV filling pressures, but a smaller magnitude of change does not always indicate normal diastolic function.

No change in restrictive flow is an ominous sign.[21]

MITRAL ANNULAR VELOCITIES

Diastolic tissue velocities measured at the mitral annulus show low-velocity deflections during early filling (e') and with atrial contraction (a') with great clarity.[22,23] These indicate biphasic longitudinal expansion rate of the LV (Fig. 36).

- *e'* is presumed to correlate closely with LV relaxation indexes and to be relatively preload insensitive
- Similar to mitral E flow, *e'* appears to be age dependent
- Mitral flow E depends on LA pressure, residual LV relaxation pressure, and age and because *e'* is presumed to depend only on LV relaxation pressure, dividing E by e' eliminates LV relaxation pressure and age, so the E/e' ratio becomes a noninvasive estimate of LA pressure (Fig. 37)
- Septal and lateral mitral annular *e'* velocities differ. Recent guidelines for the detection of diastolic dysfunction recommend use of an E/e' value that is the average of septal and lateral mitral annular e' and more than or equal to 14 being abnormal
- A value of medial E/e' more than or equal to 15 is usually proposed as evidence for elevated LV filling pressure and a value of E/e' less than 10 as evidence for normal LV filling pressure
- There is a wide range of E/e' values[10-14] for which additional investigations are required to obtain a LV filling pressure estimate (Fig. 38)
- Technical limitations include angle dependency, signal noise, signal drifting, spatial resolution, sample volume, and tethering artifacts
- *e'* can be decreased erroneously by mitral annular calcification, surgical rings, or prosthetic valves
- An average of septal and lateral E/e' more than or equal to 14 is suggestive of elevated filling pressures

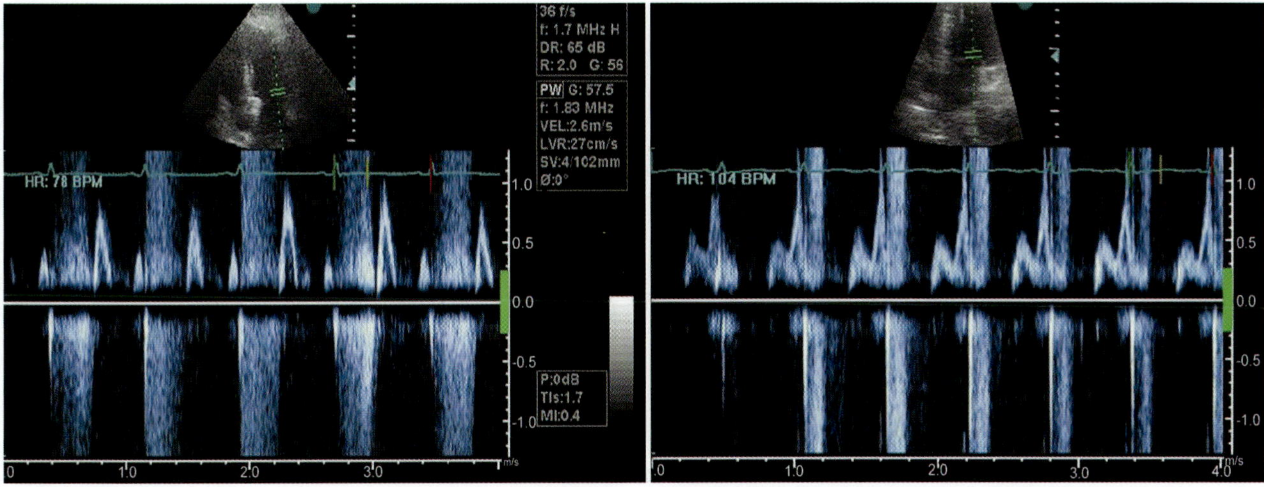

FIG. 34: Valsalva maneuver changing restrictive flow pattern (left panel) to pattern of impaired relaxation (right panel).

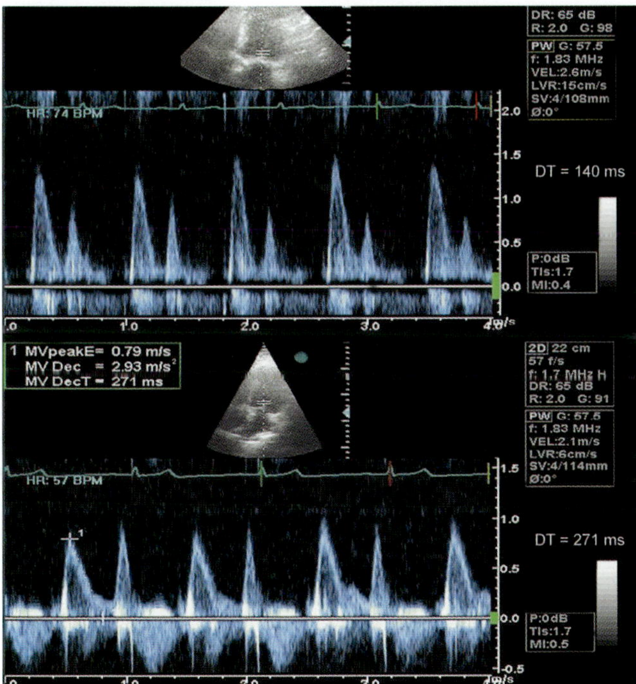

FIG. 35: Effect of Valsalva. Upper panel shows restrictive flow pattern which changes to pseudonormal pattern with an L-wave at the end of Valsalva maneuver.

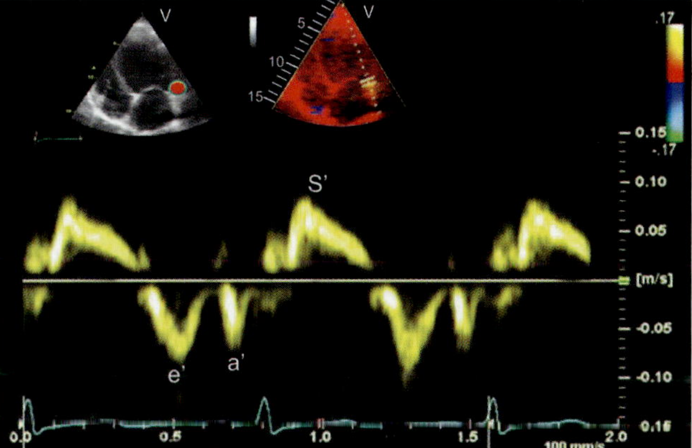

FIG. 36: Annular tissue velocities from lateral edge of the mitral annulus. See text for description.

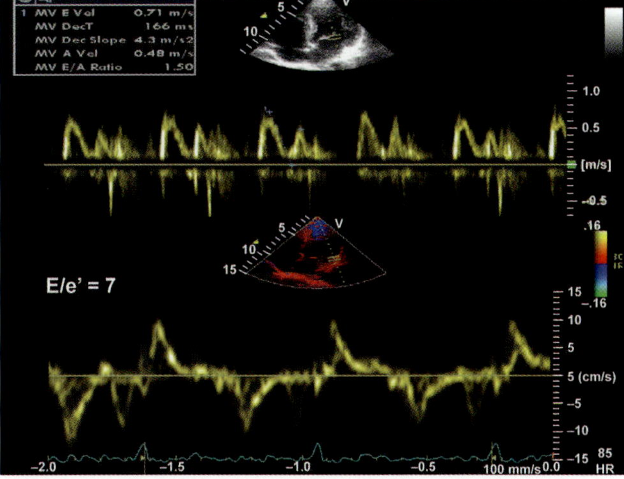

FIG. 37: Upper panel shows mitral inflow pattern and the lower panel depicts annular velocities from the lateral edge of the mitral annulus. An E/e' of 7 indicates normal diastolic function as the e' is 10 cm/s.

- A reduced s' velocity is an indirect index of diastolic dysfunction because there is a close correlation between longitudinal systolic function and early diastolic function. However, discordance is quite common
- In healthy young individuals, septal e' is more than or equal to 10 cm/s and lateral e' more than or equal to 15 cm/s at rest. But there are vendor-dependent variations
- *e'* less than 5 cm/s in cardiac disease is reflection of advanced diastolic dysfunction
- E/e' may not work well in patients with severe mitral regurgitation, intraventricular conduction delay, or pacemaker.

How to obtain annular tissue velocities?

- Pulsed-wave DTI is performed in the apical views to acquire mitral annular velocities

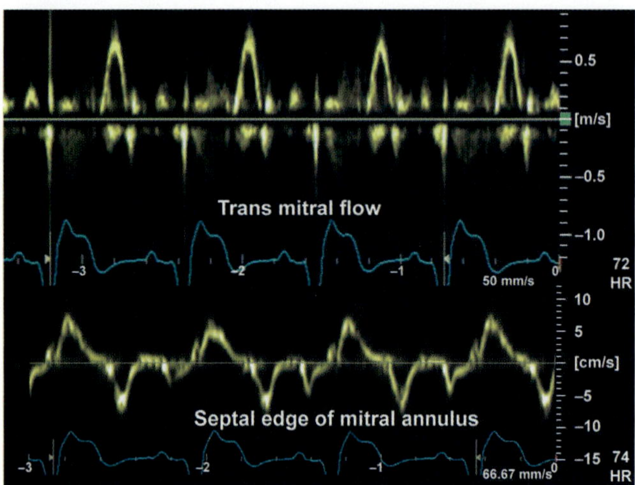

FIG. 38: Upper panel shows restrictive transmitral flow and the lower panel shows annular velocities of septal edge of the mitral annulus. An E/e′ ratio of 10 falls in indeterminate zone.

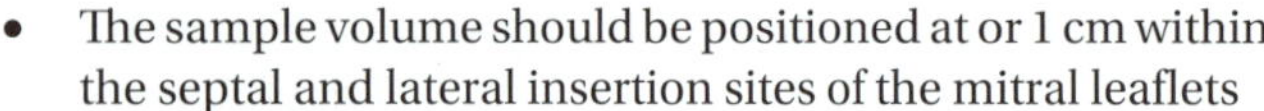

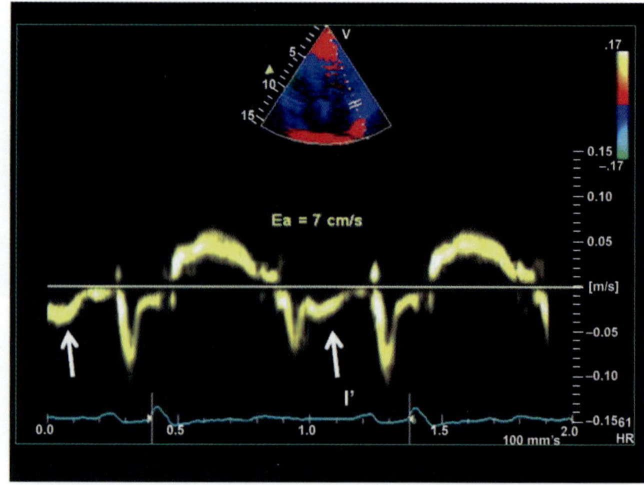

FIG. 39: Lateral edge mitral annular velocities showing l′ (arrow). Diastolic dysfunction is also suggested by e′ less than a′.

- The sample volume should be positioned at or 1 cm within the septal and lateral insertion sites of the mitral leaflets
- It is recommended that spectral recordings be obtained at a sweep speed of 50–100 mm/s at end-expiration and that measurements should reflect the average of more than or equal to three consecutive cardiac cycles
- Primary measurements include the systolic (s), early (e′), and late (a′) diastolic velocities
- For the assessment of global LV diastolic function, it is recommended to acquire and measure tissue Doppler signals at least at the septal and lateral sides of the mitral annulus and their average
- In patients with cardiac disease, e′ can be used to correct for the effect of LV relaxation on mitral E velocity, and the E/e′ ratio can be applied for the prediction of LV filling pressures
- The E/e′ ratio is not accurate as an index of filling pressures in normal subjects or in patients with heavy annular calcification, mitral valve disease, and constrictive pericarditis
- Presence of tissue Doppler wave during diastasis (*l′*) is suggestive of diastolic dysfunction (Fig. 39)
- Higher accuracy of a single-cycle E/e′ ratio in predicting mean wedge pressure in patients with AF using a dual Doppler echocardiographic probe has been shown
- Strain rate during IVRT has good correlations with the time constant of LV relaxation and –dP/dt and is not affected by changes in preload. Strain rate can be obtained by tissue velocity imaging.[24]

PRACTICAL TIPS

- In presence of normal or pseudonormal mitral flow pattern, an E/e′ ratio more than or equal to 15 obtained from either edge of the mitral annulus suggests diastolic dysfunction and possibly elevated filling pressures (Fig. 40)
- In long-standing disease, An E/e′ ratio may not accurately reflect the magnitude of filling pressures but may be indicative of stiff LV (Fig. 41)
- Greater utility of E/e′ lies in patients with systolic dysfunction as compared to those with pure diastolic dysfunction
- In relatively younger patients, this ratio has greater predictive value for filling pressure and symptoms (Fig. 42). However, it is not wise to predict filling pressures from E/e′ although one may get into the right ball-park (Fig. 43)
- If E/e′ does not clearly indicate presence of diastolic dysfunction, an e′/a′ ratio less than 1 can be used along with other data (Fig. 44)
- In elderly people, all normal-appearing mitral flow patterns cannot be regarded as pseudonormal. An E/e′ may help define the degree of normalcy (Fig. 45)
- Fusion of mitral E- and A-waves may make E/e′ calculation difficult (Fig. 46). Fusion occurs in several conditions listed here:
  - Sinus tachycardia
  - Prolonged PR interval
  - Intraventricular dyssynchrony
  - Advanced diastolic dysfunction.
- In many disease states, postsystolic tissue waves may mask tissue e′, making it difficult to estimate E/e′ ratio (Fig. 47)
- Annular postsystolic positive waves may convert severe diastolic dysfunction to mild by virtue of changing transmitral flow pattern (Fig. 48)
- An E/e′ ratio may not be reliable in presence of AF, sinus bradycardia, and first-degree AV block (Fig. 49)
- Left ventricular diastolic function can be deciphered through the evaluation not only of the relationship of the amplitude of E to e′ but also by evaluating the relationship of the timing of the onset of E to the onset of e′. Normally, mitral inflow is initiated with rapid LV relaxation and suction of blood into the LV. When this occurs, the onset of e′ will be slightly before or simultaneous with the onset of E.[25] If, however, LA pressure is elevated and LV relaxation reduced, E velocity onset may precede the onset of e′ (Fig. 50). These timing relationships have been correlated with LV filling pressure.

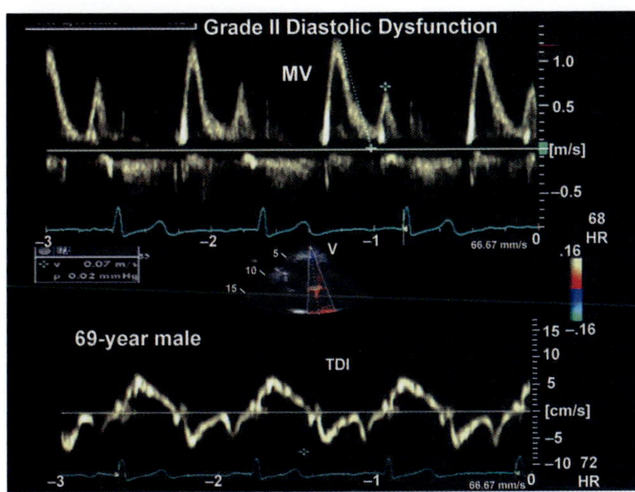

FIG. 40: Upper panel shows mitral E of 130 cm/s and the lower panel shows septal edge e' of 7 cm/s. An E/e' ratio is 19, indicating grade II diastolic dysfunction.

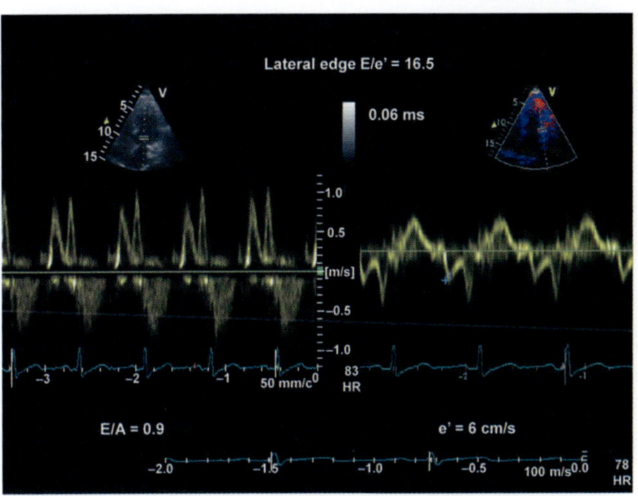

FIG. 43: Same patient as in figure 36. E/e' at lateral margin of the mitral annulus (16.5) is lower than that at the septal margin but is still way above normal. A lateral E/e' more than or equal to 13 is indicating of diastolic dysfunction.

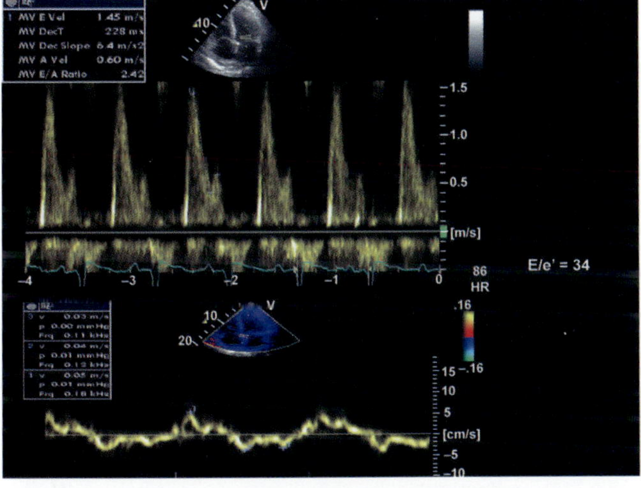

FIG. 41: Upper panel shows transmitral flow while the lower panel shows annular velocities at the septal edge in a patient on maintenance hemodialysis. An E/e' ratio of 34 does not necessarily imply very high filling pressures in this otherwise stable patient.

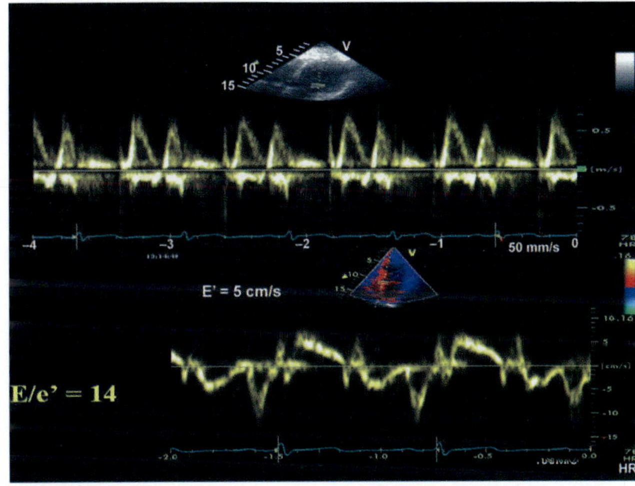

FIG. 44: An indeterminate E/e' ratio from the septal edge is complimented by absolute e' of 5 cm/s and e'/a' ratio less than 1 in suggesting diastolic dysfunction.

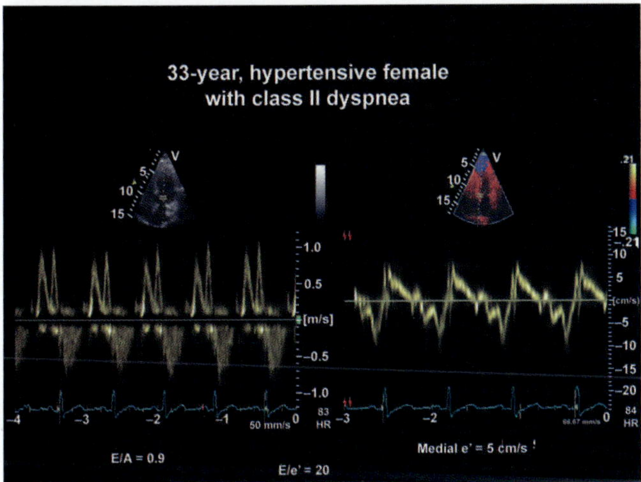

FIG. 42: Left panel shows normal transmitral flow while mitral annular velocity at septal margin is 5 cm/s and E/e' ratio of 20 is indicative of elevated filling pressures and most likely cause of dyspnea.

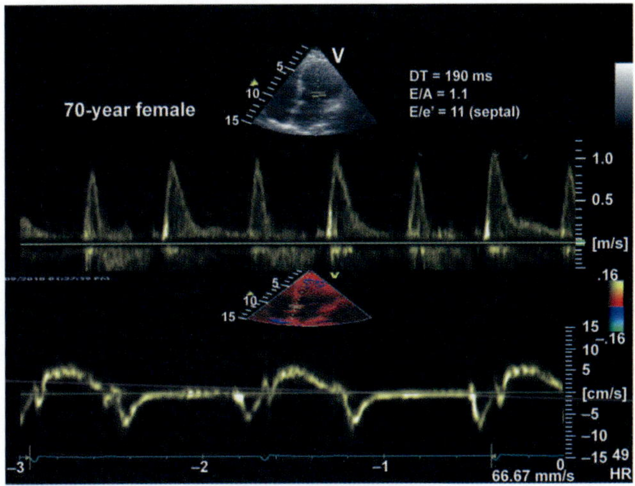

FIG. 45: A 70-year-old healthy woman with normal mitral flow and a septal edge E/e' of 11.

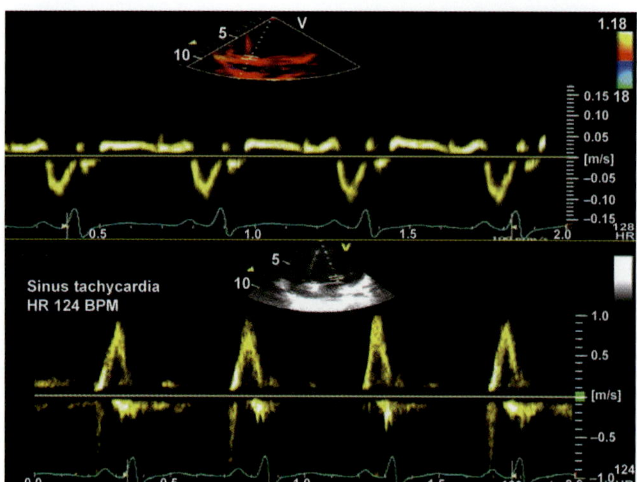

FIG. 46: Improbability of estimating E/e′ ratio due to fusion of mitral E- and A-waves in presence of sinus tachycardia and absence of annular e′ wave (upper panel).

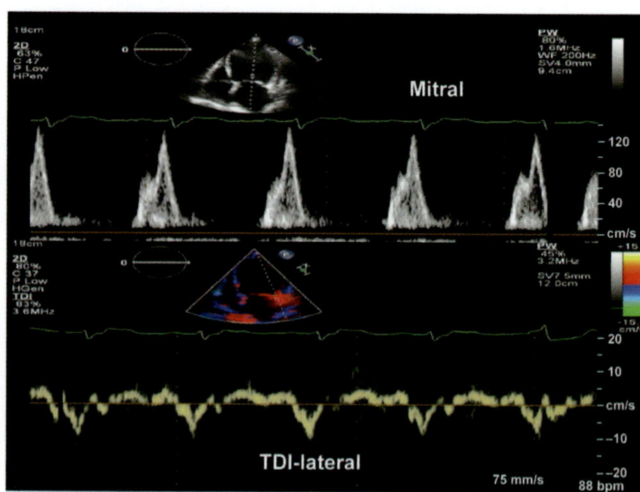

FIG. 48: Impaired relaxation pattern of mitral flow (upper panel) in a patient with advanced heart failure. Postsystolic annular waves extending into mid-diastole (lower panel).

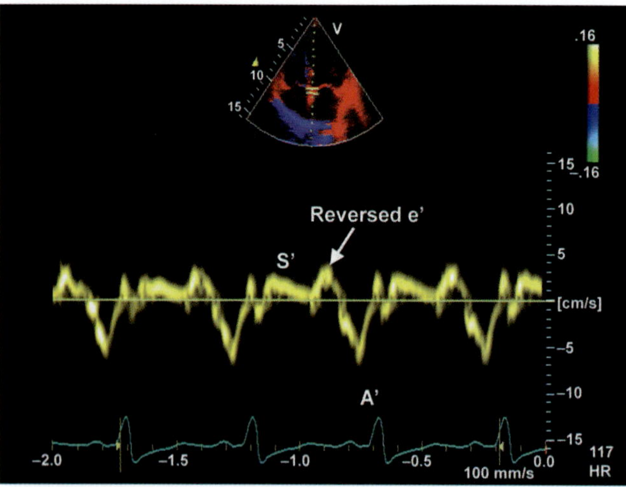

FIG. 47: Postsystolic annular tissue wave masking e′. This could be called reversed e′.

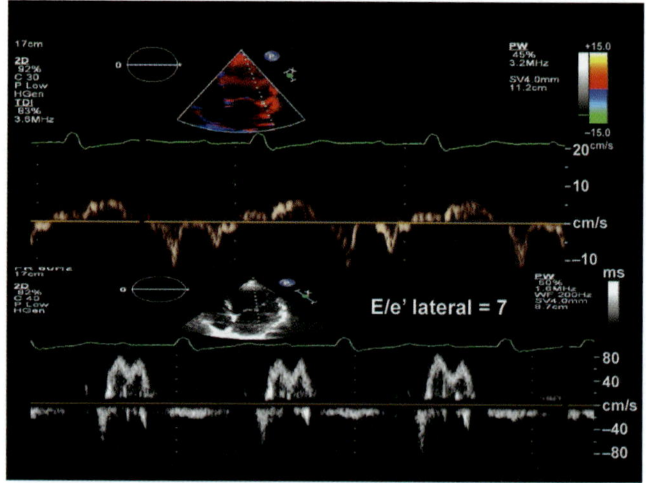

FIG. 49: E/e′ ratio of 7 (lateral) in an 84-year-old person with sinus bradycardia, first-degree atrioventricular (AV) block with, and heart failure.

PULMONARY VEIN FLOW AND DIASTOLIC FUNCTION

Pulsed-wave Doppler flow pattern of pulmonary veins shows two over-riding antegrade systolic waves (mostly seen as one, S wave), one antegrade diastolic wave (D), and a retrograde wave during atrial contraction, Ar (Figs. 51 to 53). First S wave is due to atrial relaxation and the second one (S2) due to descent of the mitral annulus during systole.

D wave occurs during opened mitral valve. Ar wave occurs following atrial contraction when blood has option of flowing antegradely into the LV as well as back in pulmonary veins depending upon the relative resistance.[26]

- The pattern of pulmonary venous flow (systolic vs. diastolic predominance) has been proposed as a predictor of diastolic dysfunction (Figs. 54 and 55). However, diastolic preponderance is invariable in children and young adults
- Ar velocity more than 35 cm/s also indicates raised filling pressures (Fig. 55)

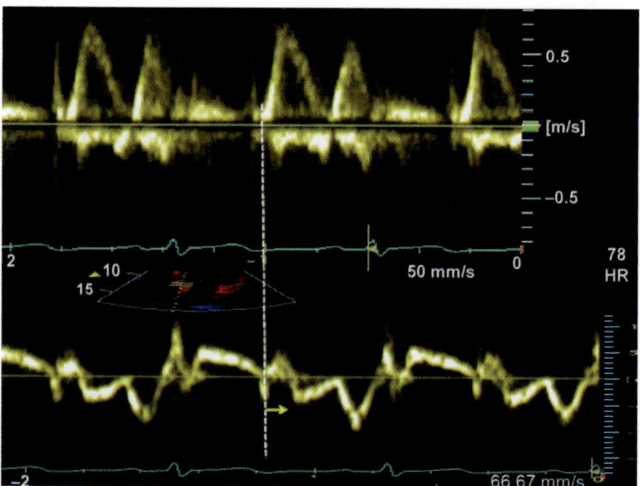

FIG. 50: Mitral E preceding tissue e′ in a patient with grade II diastolic dysfunction.

- Comparison of the duration of flow at atrial contraction across the mitral valve (on the mitral inflow velocity curve) and the duration of reversal flow back into the pulmonary veins (on the pulmonary venous velocity curves) has been repeatedly demonstrated to reflect the LV end-diastolic pressure (Fig. 56)
- If the duration of atrial reversal flow in the pulmonary vein exceeds by more than or equal to 30 ms, the duration of flow across the mitral valve, raised LV end-diastolic pressure can be diagnosed with high specificity
- The major limitations to the use of the pulmonary venous signals are that these signals are difficult to obtain and interpret. The technical feasibility of obtaining adequate signals is perhaps less than 80% of unselected patients
- Pulmonary vein flow when interpretable, is used to refining the grades of diastolic dysfunction (Figs. 57 to 60).
- Longer duration of mitral atrial flow compare to that of pulmonary vein atrial flow reversal velocity may be found in grade I diastolic dysfunction besides in normal subjects.

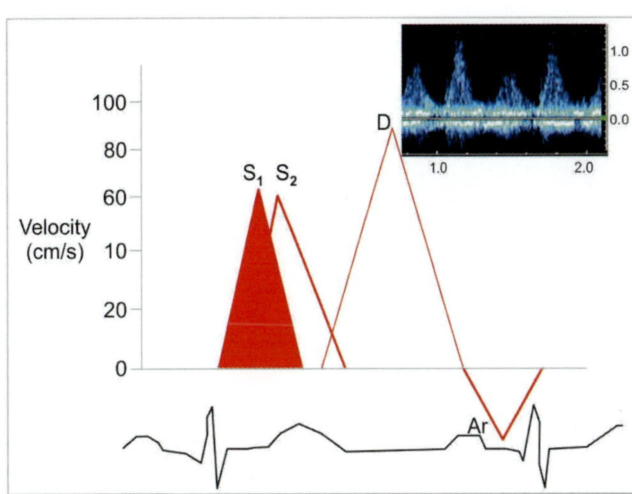

FIG. 53: Graphic representation of pulmonary vein flow in a subject with raised left ventricular (LV) filling pressure. The inset shows the real Doppler spectrum.

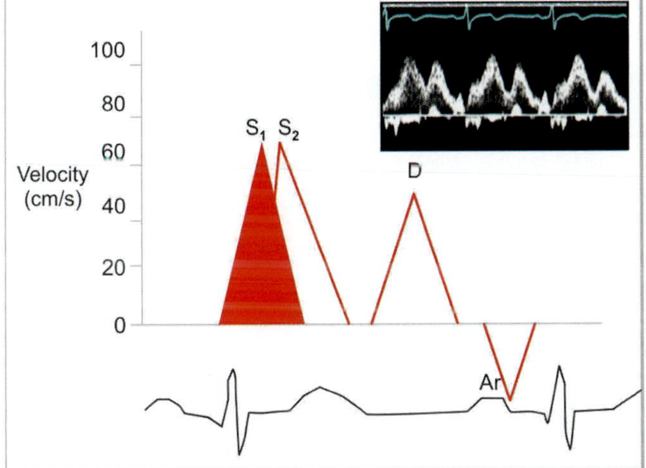

FIG. 51: Pulmonary vein flow pattern in a normal subject. Patients with grade I diastolic dysfunction have similar pattern.

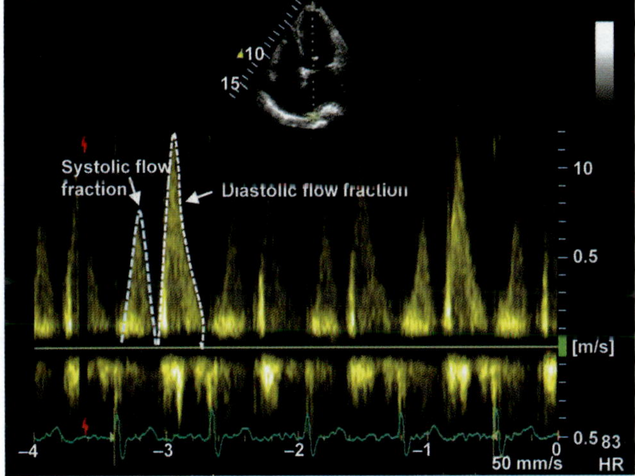

FIG. 54: Right upper pulmonary vein diastolic flow velocity and velocity-time integral is greater than systolic filling fraction in a patient with significant diastolic dysfunction.

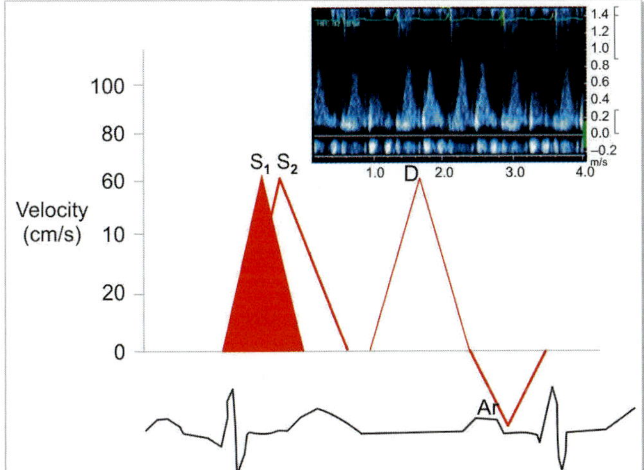

FIG. 52: Equivalent pulmonary systolic and diastolic wave but with prolonged Ar suggestive of diastolic dysfunction.

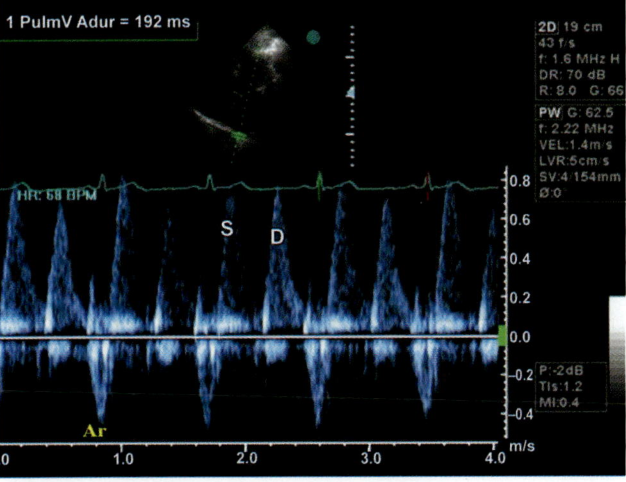

FIG. 55: Right upper pulmonary vein Ar velocity of 50 cm/s indicative of diastolic dysfunction.

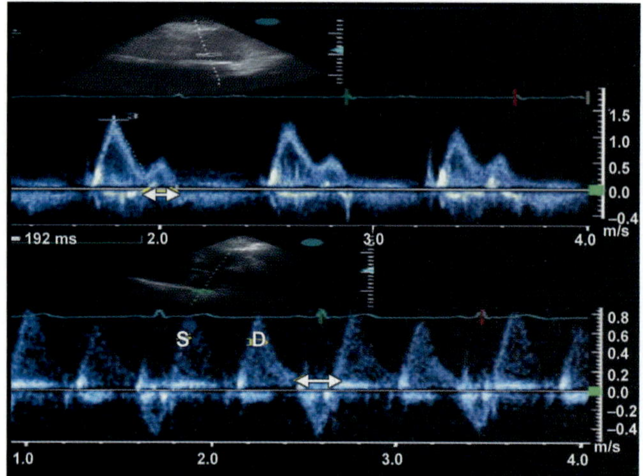

FIG. 56: Ar duration of mitral A more than 30 ms suggestive of elevated end-diastolic pressure.

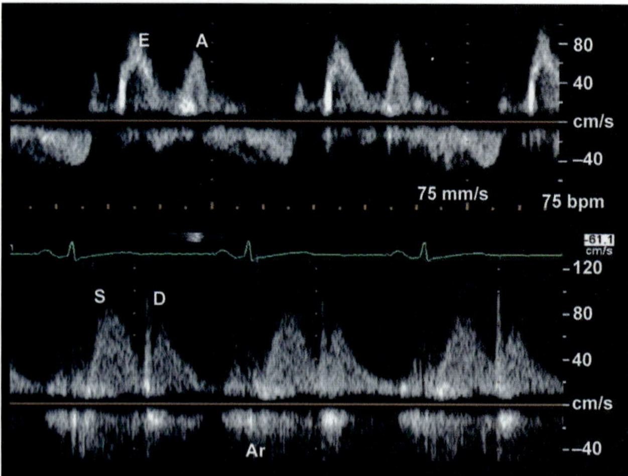

FIG. 57: Upper panel shows mitral flow pattern and the lower panel shows right upper pulmonary flow pattern. In presence of normal-appearing mitral flow, predominant systolic fraction and short Ar indicate that the above pattern is of a normal adult.

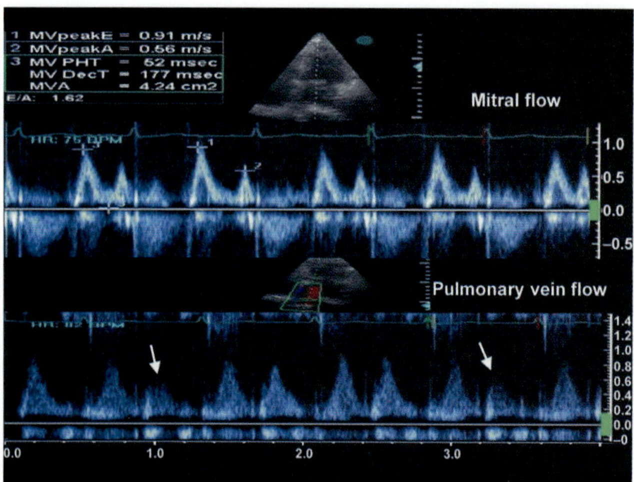

FIG. 58: Equivalent pulmonary venous systolic and diastolic flow fraction (lower panel) but with inspiratory decrease in D-wave (arrow) is suggestive of normal filling pattern.

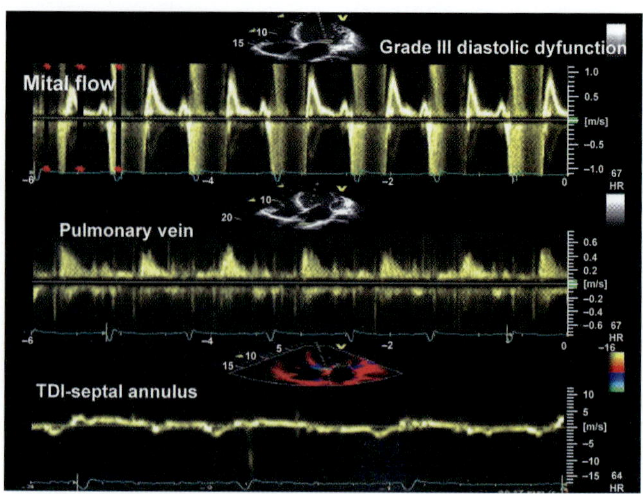

SHS, systolic heart failure; VT, ventricular tachycardia.

FIG. 59: Upper panel—mitral flow, middle panel—pulmonary flow, and lower panel—septal annular velocities. There is hardly any S-wave in pulmonary vein flow and E/e′ of 30 indicating of advanced or grade 3 diastolic dysfunction.

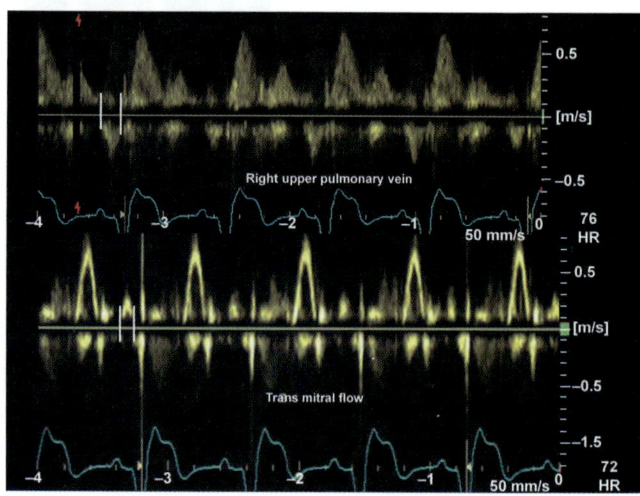

FIG. 60: Upper panel: pulmonary vein flow. Lower panel—transmitral flow. Restrictive transmitral flow is negated by normal pulmonary venous flow although Ar is 20 ms longer.

ACQUISITION OF PULMONARY VEIN FLOW SIGNALS

- Color flow imaging is useful for the proper location of the sample volume in the right upper pulmonary vein
- In a majority of the patients, the best Doppler recordings are obtained by angulating the transducer superiorly in such a manner that the aortic valve is visualized
- A 2–3 mm sample volume is placed more than 0.5 cm into the pulmonary vein for optimal recording of the spectral waveforms
- Wall filter settings must be low enough to display the onset and cessation of the atrial reversal (Ar) velocity waveform
- Pulmonary venous flow can be obtained in about 80% of ambulatory patients with an effort though the feasibility is much lower in the intensive care unit setting

- The major technical problem is LA wall motion artifacts, caused by atrial contraction, which interferes with the accurate display of Ar velocity
- Spectral recordings should be obtained at a sweep speed of 50–100 mm/s at end-expiration and measurements include the average of more than or equal to three consecutive cardiac cycles.

PULMONARY VEIN FLOW PARAMETERS

- Measurements of pulmonary venous waveforms include peak systolic (S) velocity, peak anterograde diastolic (D) velocity, the S/D ratio, systolic and diastolic filling fractions , and the peak Ar velocity in late diastole
- Other measurements are the duration of the Ar velocity, the time difference between it and mitral A-wave duration (Ar – A)
- D-wave velocity DT
- There are two systolic velocities (S1 and S2), mostly noticeable when there is a prolonged PR interval, because S1 is related to atrial relaxation. S2 should be used to compute the ratio of peak systolic to peak diastolic velocity
- S1 velocity is primarily influenced by changes in LA pressure and LA contraction and relaxation whereas S2 is related to stroke volume and pulse-wave propagation in the pulmonary arterial tree
- D-wave velocity is influenced by changes in LV filling and compliance and changes in parallel with mitral E velocity.
- Pulmonary venous Ar velocity and duration are influenced by LV late diastolic pressures, atrial preload, and LA contractility
- A decrease in LA compliance and an increase in LA pressure decrease the S velocity and increase the D velocity, resulting in an S/D ratio less than 1, systolic filling fraction less than 40%, and shortening of the DT of D velocity, usually less than 150 ms (Fig. 61).
- However, DT of mitral E and pulmonary vein D may not always be concordant as DT of D-wave tends to be nonlinear more often (Fig. 62).

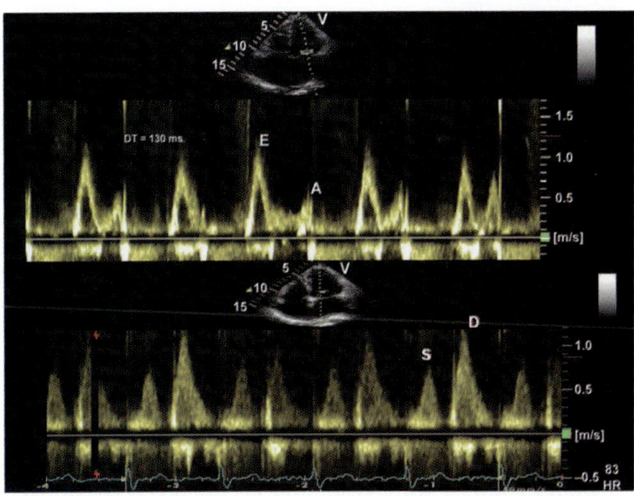

FIG. 62: Upper panel shows short deceleration time (DT) of mitral E while DT of pulmonary vein D is longer (170 ms) and nonlinear.

MITRAL FLOW PROPAGATION BY COLOR M-MODE

Assessment of flow propagation into the left ventricle is another technique that provides better ability to predict filling pressures.[27-29]

In the normal state, flow rapidly propagates into the LV cavity (Fig. 63). Early-stage relaxation abnormalities show a blunting of flow propagation.

The propagation velocity (Vp) does not show a pseudonormalization and, therefore, can be used in all levels of diastolic dysfunction.

Similar to the tissue Doppler velocities, color M-mode flow propagation has been combined in a ratio with the mitral E velocity to provide an adjusted parameter (E/Vp) with strong correlation to filling pressures and prognosis.

The chief limitations of this tool are lack of consensus on technique and theoretical concerns that this will be invalid in small LV cavities.

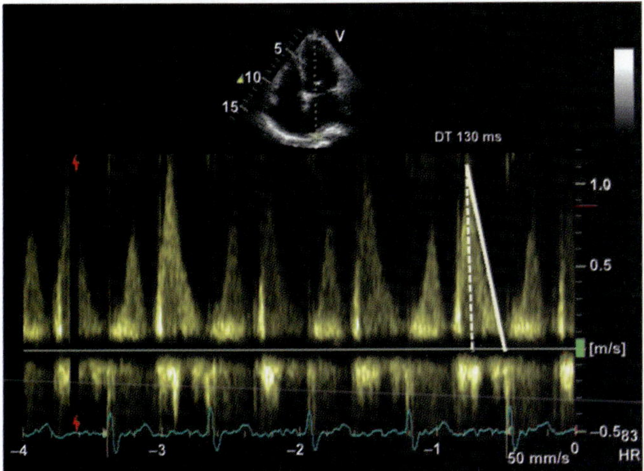

FIG. 61: Pulmonary vein D-wave more than S-wave with deceleration time (DT) of 130 ms indicating elevated left ventricular (LV) filling pressure.

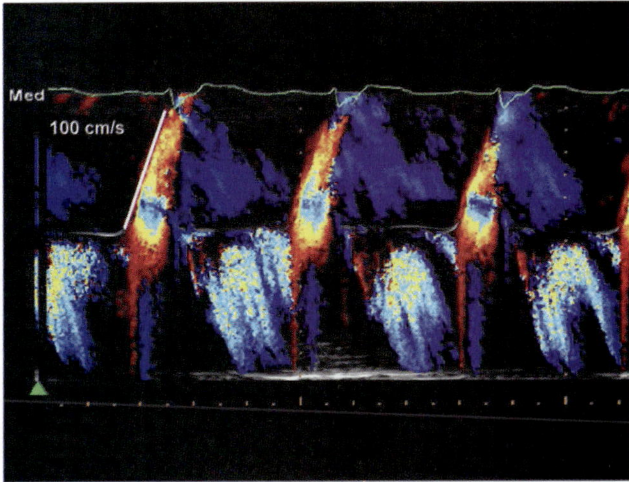

FIG. 63: Mitral flow propagation velocity by M-mode.

Practical Tips

- Acquisition is performed in the apical 4-CV, using color flow imaging
- M-mode scan line is placed through the center of the LV inflow blood column from the mitral valve to the apex, with baseline shift to lower the Nyquist limit so that the central highest velocity jet is blue
- Propagation velocity is measured as the slope of the first aliasing velocity during early filling, measured from the mitral valve plane to 4 cm distally into the LV cavity, or the slope of the transition from no color to color
- Propagation velocity more than 45–50 cm/s is considered normal
- Should other Doppler indices appear inconclusive, an E/Vp ratio more than or equal to 2.5 predicts PCWP more than 15 mm Hg with reasonable accuracy (Figs 64 and 65)
- Patients with normal LV volumes and EFs but elevated filling pressures can have misleadingly normal Vp.

Peak velocity of early-diastolic mitral flow Vp has been used as an approximation for ventricular suction.

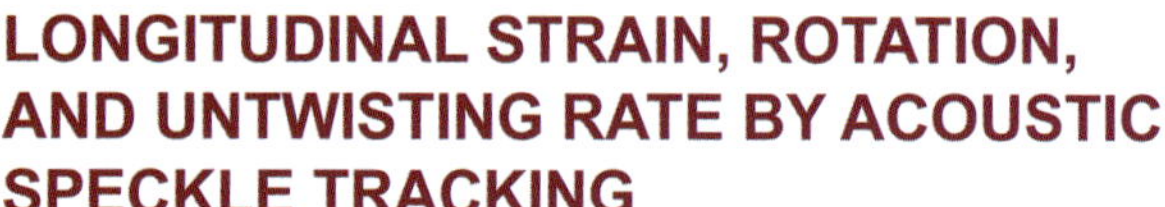

LONGITUDINAL STRAIN, ROTATION, AND UNTWISTING RATE BY ACOUSTIC SPECKLE TRACKING

- Most patients with diastolic dysfunction have impaired longitudinal strain by acoustic speckle tracking. Impaired longitudinal strain (>15%) is first indication of impaired diastolic function[30]
- Torsion and circumferential strain are normal in patients with isolated diastolic dysfunction (Fig. 66)
- Assessment of LV torsion has shown that untwisting begins before aortic valve closure and might be an important component of normal diastolic filling[29]
- Studies in human subjects using indirect indexes derived from right heart catheterization have suggested a relationship between constant of IVR and measures of untwisting
- But the relationship between directly measured diastolic function indexes with micromanometer catheters and untwisting parameters has not been established in human subjects
- Untwisting parameters are related to invasive indexes of LV relaxation and suction but not to LV stiffness. These data suggest that untwisting is an important component of early diastolic LV filling but not later diastolic events.

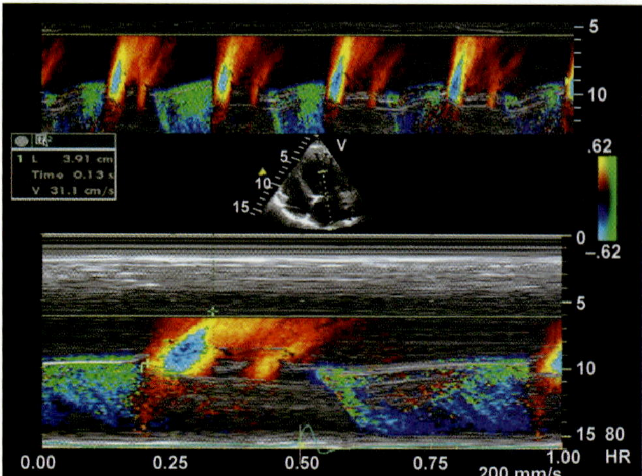

FIG. 64: Propagation velocity (Vp) of 31 cm/s in a patient with heart failure.

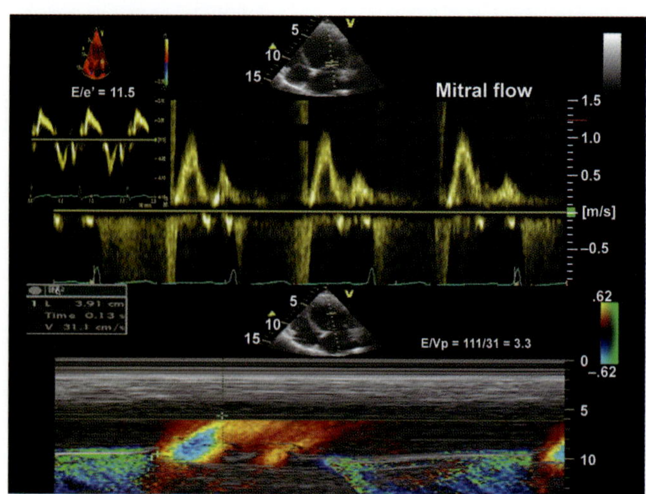

FIG. 65: A 43-year-old female with recurrent pulmonary edema. E/e' of 11.5 (lateral) is inconclusive but E/Vp of 3.3 suggests raised filling pressures.

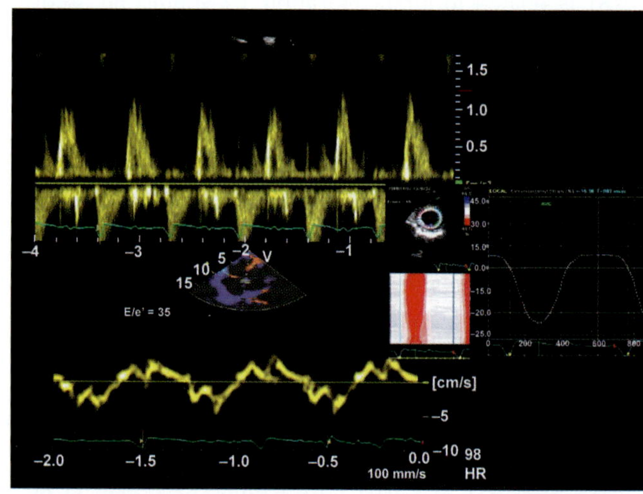

FIG. 66: Normal circumferential strain (right panel) in presence of advanced diastolic dysfunction.

DIASTOLIC STRESS TEST

Many patients present with exertional dyspnea but have normal LV filling pressures at rest. In these patients, it is important to evaluate filling pressure with exercise.[31,32]

Exercise can be performed using a supine bicycle or treadmill protocol. Because most patients have limited functional capacity, the workload starts at 25 W and increases in increments of 25 W every 3 minutes.

We need to record mitral inflow by pulsed Doppler echocardiography at the level of the mitral tips, mitral annular velocities by spectral Doppler echocardiography, and tricuspid regurgitation jet by CW Doppler (Fig. 67).

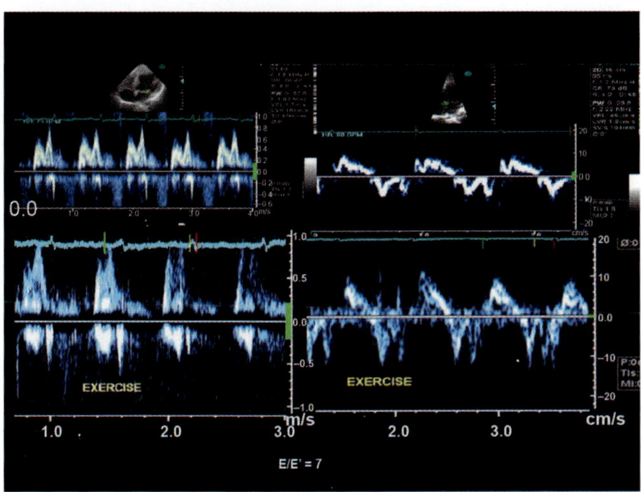

FIG. 67: Diastolic stress test in a normal person. There is proportionate increase in mitral E and e'.

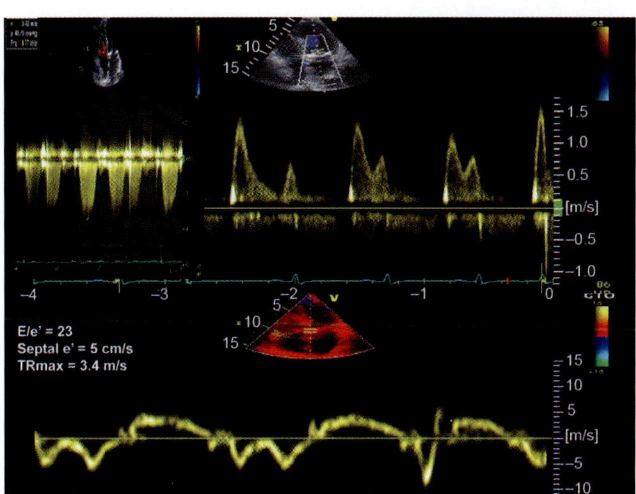

FIG. 68: An 80-year-old male with dyspnea on exertion. Three out of four parameters are abnormal suggesting diastolic dysfunction.

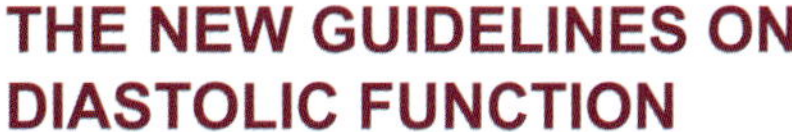

THE NEW GUIDELINES ON DIASTOLIC FUNCTION

The recent guidelines on diastolic function enunciated by the ASE and European Association of Cardiovascular Imaging focus upon four (five) parameters to decide whether diastolic function is normal or abnormal:[33]

1. Left atrial volume index (>34 mL/m^2 being abnormal)
2. Tricuspid regurgitation maximum velocity (abnormal >2.8 m/s)
3. Average E/e' >14
4. Septal *e'* (<7 cm/s being labeled abnormal)
5. Lateral *e'* (abnormal if <10 cm/s).

If less than 50% parameters are abnormal, diastolic function is presumed to be normal. If more than 50% parameters are abnormal, it is considered diastolic dysfunction (Fig. 68). As septal and lateral e' are clubbed as one parameter, then there is possibility of indeterminate diastolic function if only two out of four parameters are present.

Following is the grading of diastolic dysfunction proposed that is given in table 1.

These recommendations have significant advantages, including increased flexibility, with recognition that not all parameters are abnormal in a given case of diastolic dysfunction. These have been validated in some database.[34,35] Preload dependence, the effects of positive pressure ventilation on mitral inflow velocity, and the angle dependence of tissue Doppler are some of the technical challenges. The relationship between systolic function and myocardial relaxation is such that patients with abnormal systolic function or structural abnormalities must automatically have a degree of impaired diastolic function. Those with normal systolic function need to have impairment of diastolic function detected before subsequent grading of severity, whereas those with abnormal systolic function or structural issues must have impaired relaxation and subsequently can proceed to grading of their diastolic dysfunction.

TABLE 1: Grading of diastolic dysfunction

Parameters	Grade 1	Grade 2	Grade 3
Relaxation	Impaired	Impaired	Impaired
Left atrial (LA) pressure	Normal	Elevated	Elevated
Mitral E/A	<0.8	0.8 – <2.0	>2.0
E/e'	<10	10–14	>14
Trmax (m/s)	<2.8	>2.8	>2.8

CONCLUSION

Doppler echocardiography provides major insights into the pathophysiology of diastolic LV dysfunction. So far, however, no single Doppler echocardiographic index of diastolic LV dysfunction has been shown as a robust criterion for elevated LV filling pressures. A stepwise strategy with sequential use of multiple Doppler echocardiographic indexes reduces diagnostic sensitivity because it frequently leads to an indeterminate outcome. A multiparametric approach with age, LA volume, and clinical situation in mind are the best way of using echocardiography in detection of diastolic dysfunction because it is so complex and dependent upon multitude of variables (Fig. 69). Because of these persistent shortcomings, clinicians should continue to make critical use of current Doppler echocardiographic estimates of LV filling pressures and should not hesitate to implement invasive investigations to confirm their clinical suspicions.[34,35] Guidelines for assessing diastolic function by echocardiography are continually being updated. There is reasonable agreement in estimating diastolic function grade and LA pressure using current guidelines but accuracy is not guaranteed. Further refinements in the definition of mild and moderate dysfunction may improve agreement. There are a number of limitations to these measurements, including the need for high-quality signals, adequate flow visualization in the apical views, experience in acquisition and analysis, impact of PR interval, and heart rate, etc.

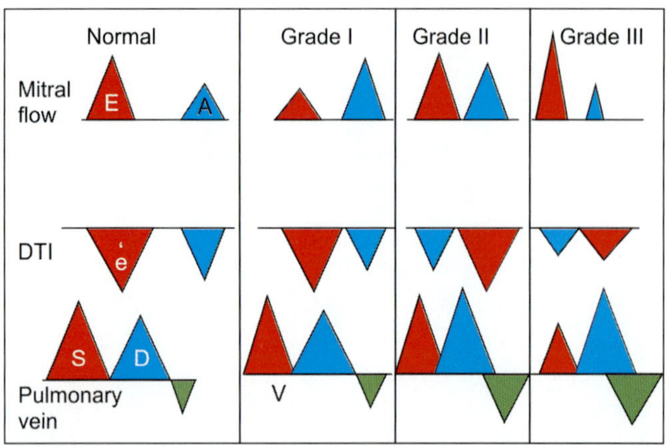

FIG. 69: A simplified schema to report diastolic function based upon pulsed-wave Doppler mitral flow, annular velocities, and pulmonary vein flow.

REFERENCES

1. Spevack DM, Karl J, Yedlapati N, et al. Echocardiographic left ventricular end-diastolic pressure volume loop estimate predicts survival in congestive heart failure. J Card Fail. 2013;19:251-9.
2. Nagueh SF, Appleton CP, Gillebert TC, et al. Recommendations for the evaluation of left ventricular diastolic function by echocardiography. Eur J Echocardiogr. 2009;10:165-93.
3. Chapman CB, Ewer SM, Kelly AF, et al. Classification of Left Ventricular Diastolic Function Using American Society of Echocardiography Guidelines: Agreement among Echocardiographers. Echocardiography. 2013,30:1022-31.
4. Dokainish H, Nguyen JS, Bobek J, et al. Assessment of the American Society of Echocardiography-European Association of Echocardiography guidelines for diastolic function in patients with depressed ejection fraction: an echocardiographic and invasive haemodynamic study. Eur J Echocardiogr. 2011;12:857-64.
5. Martos R, Baugh J, Ledwidge M. Diastolic heart failure: evidence of increased myocardial collagen turnover linked to diastolic dysfunction. Circulation. 2007;115:888-95.
6. Granzier HL, Labeit S. The giant protein titin: a major player in myocardial mechanics, signaling, and disease. Circ Res. 2004;94:284-95.
7. Gillebert TC, De Pauw M, Timmermans F. Echo-Doppler assessment of diastole: flow, function and haemodynamics. Heart. 2013;99:55-64.
8. Oh JK, Tajik J. The return of cardiac time intervals: the Phoenix is rising. J Am Coll Cardiol. 2003;42:1471-4.
9. Nishimura RA, Appleton CP, Redfield MM, et al. Noninvasive Doppler echocardiographic evaluation of left ventricular filling pressures in patients with cardiomyopathies: a simultaneous Doppler echocardiographic and cardiac catheterization study. J Am Coll Cardiol. 1996;28:1226-33.
10. Little WC, Ohno M, Kitzman DW, et al. Determination of left ventricular chamber stiffness from the time for deceleration of early left ventricular filling. Circulation. 1995;92:1933-6.
11. Rossvoll O, Hatle LK. Pulmonary venous flow velocities recorded by transthoracic Doppler ultrasound: relation to left ventricular diastolic pressures. J Am Coll Cardiol. 1993;21:1687-96.
12. Lam CS, Han L, Ha JW, et al. The mitral L wave: A marker of pseudonormal filling and predictor of heart failure in patients with left ventricular hypertrophy. J Am Soc Echocardiogr. 2005;18:336-41.
13. Dini FL, Galderisi M, Nistri S, et al. Abnormal left ventricular longitudinal function assessed by echocardiographic and tissue Doppler imaging is a powerful predictor of diastolic dysfunction in hypertensive patients: The SPHERE study. Int J Cardiol. 2013;168:3351-8.
14. Lam CS, Han L, Oh JK, et al. The mitral annular mid-diastolic velocity curve: Functional correlates and clinical significance in patients with left ventricular hypertrophy. J Am Soc Echocardiogr. 2007;21:165-70.
15. Tsang TS, Barnes ME, Gersh BJ, et al. Left atrial volume as a morphophysiologic expression of left ventricular diastolic dysfunction and relation to cardiovascular risk burden. Am J Cardiol. 2002;90:1284-9.
16. Aljaroudi W, Alraies MC, Halley C, et al. Effect of age, gender, and left ventricular diastolic function on left atrial volume index in adults without known cardiovascular disease or risk factors. Am J Cardiol. 2013;111:1517-22.
17. Khan UA, de Simone G, Hill J, et al. Depressed atrial function in diastolic dysfunction: a speckle tracking imaging study. Echocardiography. 2013;30:309-16.
18. Nagueh SF, Middleton KJ, Kopelen HA, et al. Doppler tissue imaging: a noninvasive technique for evaluation of left ventricular relaxation and estimation of filling pressures. J Am Coll Cardiol. 1997;30:1527-153.
19. Nishimura RA, Tajik AJ. Evaluation of diastolic filling of left ventricle in health and disease: Doppler echocardiography is the clinician's Rosetta Stone. J Am Coll Cardiol. 1997;30:8-18.
20. Kitabatake A, Inoue M, Asao M. Transmitral blood flow reflecting diastolic behavior of the left ventricle in health and disease–a study by pulsed Doppler technique. Jpn Circ J. 1982;46:92-102.
21. Pinamonti B, Zecchin M, Di Lenarda A, et al. Persistence of restrictive left ventricular filling pattern in dilated cardiomyopathy: an ominous prognostic sign. J Am Coll Cardiol. 1997;29:604-12.
22. Ommen SR, Nishimura RA, Appleton CP, et al. Clinical utility of Doppler echocardiography and tissue Doppler imaging in the estimation of left ventricular filling pressures: a comparative simultaneous Doppler-catheterization study. Circulation. 2000;102:1788-94.
23. Oki T, Tabata T, Yamada H, et al. Clinical application of pulsed Doppler tissue imaging for assessing abnormal left ventricular relaxation. Am J Cardiol. 1997;79:921-8.
24. Wang J, Khoury DS, Thohan V, et al. Global diastolic strain rate for the assessment of left ventricular relaxation and filling pressures. Circulation. 2007;115:1376-83.
25. Rivas-Gotz C, Khoury DS, Manolios M, et al. Time interval between onset of mitral inflow and onset of early diastolic velocity by tissue Doppler: a novel index of left ventricular relaxation: experimental studies and clinical application. J Am Coll Cardiol. 2003;42:1463-70.
26. Smiseth OA, Thompson CR, Lohavanichbutr K. The pulmonary venous systolic flow pulse—its origin and relationship to left atrial pressure. J Am Coll Cardiol. 1999;34:802-9.
27. Rivas-Gotz C, Manolios M, Thohan V, et al. Impact of left ventricular ejection fraction on estimation of left ventricular filling pressures using tissue Doppler and flow propagation velocity. Am J Cardiol. 2003;91:780-4.
28. Rivas-Gotz C, Khoury DS, Manolios M, et al. Impact of left ventricular ejection fraction on estimation of left ventricular filling pressures using tissue Doppler and flow propagation velocity. Am J Cardiol. 2002;91:780-4.
29. Brun P, Tribouilloy C, Duval AM. Left ventricular flow propagation during early filling is related to wall relaxation: a color M-mode Doppler analysis. J Am Coll Cardiol. 1992;20:420-32.
30. van Heerebeek L, Borbely A, Niessen HW. Myocardial structure and function differ in systolic and diastolic heart failure. Circulation. 2006;113:1966-73.
31. Ha JW, Oh J, Pellikka P, et al. Diastolic stress echocardiography: a novel noninvasive diagnostic test for diastolic dysfunction using supine bicycle exercise Doppler echocardiography. J Am Soc Echocardiogr. 2005;18:63-8.
32. Nasim S, Nadeem N, Zahidie A, et al. Relationship between exercise induced dyspnea and functional capacity with Doppler-derived diastolic function. BMC Res Notes. 2013;6:150.
33. Nagueh SF, Smiseth OA, Appleton CP. Recommendations for the Evaluation of Left Ventricular Diastolic Function by Echocardiography: An Update from the American Society of Echocardiography and European Association of Cardiovascular Imaging. J Am Soc Echocardiogr. 2016;29:277-314.
34. Andersen OS, Smiseth OA, Do Kanish H. Estimating Left Ventricular Filling Pressures by Echocardiography. J Am Coll Cardiol. 2017;69:1937-48.
35. Mitter SS, Shah SJ, Thomas JD. A Test in Content: E/A and E/e' to Assess Diastolic Dysfunction and LV Filling Pressures. J Am Coll Cardiol. 2017;69:1451-64.

CHAPTER 76

Echocardiographic Assessment of Right Ventricular Function

K Tamilselvan, R Alagesan

INTRODUCTION

Echocardiography is an important tool to evaluate heart chambers. Lack of well-established data coupled with excessive focus on left ventricle (LV) had resulted in lack of interest in detailed right ventricular (RV) echocardiographic study for quite some time. However, for the past two decades, evaluation of RV function is being increasingly recognized, as RV dysfunction is linked to prognosis of many conditions like coronary artery disease, pulmonary hypertension, and congenital heart disease. It is also a very powerful independent predictor of morbidity and mortality in patients with advanced heart failure requiring implanted LV assist devices and heart transplantation.

ANATOMICAL AND PHYSIOLOGICAL BASIS FOR RIGHT VENTRICULAR ECHOCARDIOGRAPHY

Right ventricular differs from LV structurally, as LV has no infundibulum and fewer trabeculation. Ventricular wall thickness and mass is lower in RV in comparison to LV. Orientation of myofibers is different as RV has only two layers, middle layer being absent. Subendocardial fibers orientation is similar in both ventricles but subepicardial fibers course obliquely in LV but circumferentially in RV. Thinner walls and prominent trabeculations due to distinct embryologic origin and hemodynamic environment (high-volume, low-pressure system), makes it difficult to characterize the walls.[1] While LV adapts better to pressure overload states, RV is suited for better adaptation to volume overload state. Both anatomical and physiological differences between the two ventricles play key roles in technical differences observed during echocardiography.

Right ventricular is triangular in the transverse plane and crescentic in the coronal plane and inflow portion of RV is perpendicular to outflow tract so that both segments are not situated in the same plane. This complex geometry prevents direct imaging of the entire RV in a single view, requiring as many views as possible for accurate assessment.[2-4] In addition to this complex three-dimensional (3D) geometry, accurate RV assessment by echocardiography is often a difficult job for the sonographers due to paucity of well-defined anatomical landmarks.

Other factors which interfere in RV assessment include the marked load dependence of RV function indices, complex contraction-relaxation pattern among the different segments of the RV, ill-defined endocardial borders due to markedly trabeculated RV and the unfavorable retrosternal location of the RV, which limits optimal imaging views.

According to the American Society of Echocardiography (ASE) guidelines, a comprehensive 2DE evaluation of the RV needs the six standardized views: parasternal long-axis (PLAX), parasternal RV inflow, parasternal short-axis (PSAX), apical four-chamber (A4C), RV-focused A4C, and subcostal views (Fig. 1). A systematic RV assessment involves evaluation of shape, thickness, area, volume, tissue characterization, and its systolic and diastolic function.

RIGHT VENTRICULAR CHAMBER DIMENSIONS ASSESSMENT

The RV consists of inflow region, RV apex and outflow tract. In the usual A4C view the LV is in the center and RV inflow tract is visualized, and the RV apex is not visualized. From this view the transducer is moved little laterally to visualize the entire RV and this view is called the RV focused A4C view. The inflow tract measurements and fractional area change are measured from this view. In addition, in this view the RV free wall is parallel to the ultrasound beam making it the best view for measuring tricuspid annular plane systolic excursion (TAPSE), tissue Doppler imaging (TDI), and tricuspid regurgitation (TR) velocity.

The diameters measured are RV basal diameter close to the tricuspid annular plane from inner border of RV free wall to the inner border of interventricular septum (IVS), mid-RV

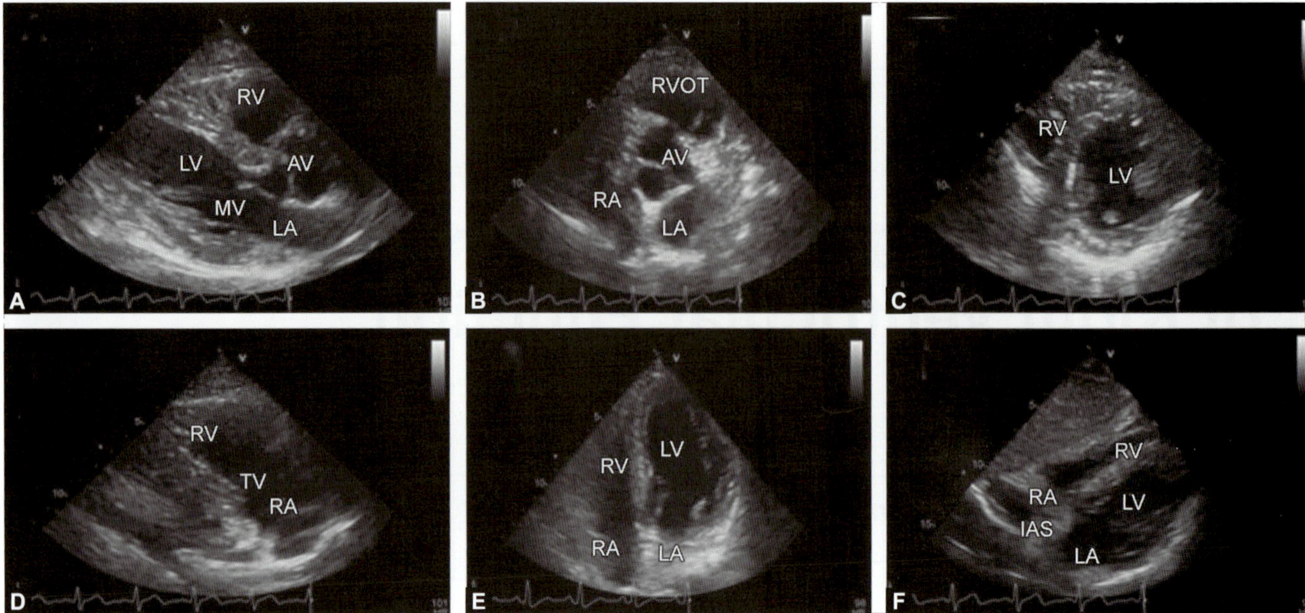

AV, atrioventricular; IAS, interatrial septum; LA, left atrium; LV, left ventricular; MV, mitral valve; RV, right ventricular; RVOT, right ventricular outflow tract; TV, tricuspid valve.

FIG. 1: Views for assessment of right ventricular (RV) function. **A,** Parasternal long-axis view; **B,** Parasternal short-axis view atrioventricular level; **C,** Parasternal short-axis view papillary muscle level; **D,** Parasternal RV inflow tract view; **E,** Apical four-chamber view; **F,** Subcostal four-chamber view.

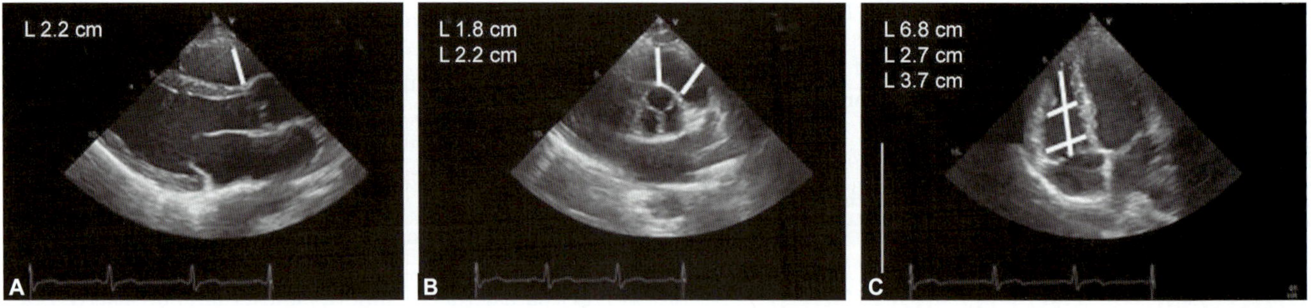

FIG. 2 : **A,** Proximal right ventricular (RV) outflow tract; **B,** Proximal and distal RV outflow tract; **C,** RV inflow tract major and minor axis.

diameter at the middle of RV at the level of papillary muscles and RV long-axis diameter from the tricuspid annulus to the RV apex. The diameters of proximal right ventricular outflow tract (RVOT) can be measured in PLAX view from anterior RV wall to septal-aortic junction. In PSAX view, distal RVOT at the level of pulmonary annulus can be measured (Fig. 2). All these measurements are taken at end diastole without oblique cuts.

While RV linear diameters are measured in end diastole, area measurements should be measured in end diastole and end systole. While trabeculations and papillary muscles are included in RV volume measurement, they should be ignored during RV thickness measurement. Normal reference values are summarized in table1.

RIGHT VENTRICULAR ANTERIOR WALL THICKNESS ASSESSMENT

Guidelines recommend that RV thickness should be measured in the subcostal four-chamber view at the level of the chordae tendineae usually opposite to the tip of the anterior tricuspid valve (TV) leaflet when fully open, at end diastole during apnea, avoiding echo dense epicardial fat and trabecula. Subcostal four-chamber view does not have the problem of near field artifacts.

ASSESSMENT OF RIGHT VENTRICULAR HEMODYNAMICS

Evaluation of right ventricle hemodynamic data involves both afterload and preload assessment which include measurement of systolic pulmonary artery pressure (SPAP), mean pulmonary artery pressure (MPAP), diastolic pulmonary artery pressure (DPAP), pulmonary vascular resistance (PVR), and assessment of filling profiles. Both volume loading and pressure loading effects on right ventricle can be assessed by looking at the IVS. In pressure overload the IVS is flat during systole and diastole making the ventricle D shaped whereas the IVS is flat only during diastole in volume overload. Right atrial pressure is estimated from measuring the size of the IVC during inspiration and expiration and calculating percentage change in IVC dimension during respiration. When the respiration is shallow the patient is asked to sniff and the change in IVC dimension is assessed (Table 2). Other secondary indices include restrictive filling pattern, e/e' >6 and systolic filling fraction >55% in hepatic venous flow Doppler spectrum.

Estimation of systolic and diastolic and MPAP is derived from peak TR and pulmonary regurgitation velocities (Table 3).

Estimation of PVR adds prognostic information on top of the diagnostic information gained from MPAP. Various methods had been suggested to estimate PVR noninvasively, especially by echocardiography. Peak TR velocity/RVOT velocity time integral (VTI) >38 provided a specificity of 100% for a PVR of >8 Wood units. In children, the ratio isovolumetric relaxation time (IVRT) to RV ejection time (RVET) correlated well with PVR, with IVRT/ET <0.3 being 97% specific for a PVR <3 Wood units. PVR calculated by cardiac catheterization is far superior than echocardiographic estimation of PVR.

TABLE 1: Normal values for right ventricular chamber dimensions and volumes

Linear dimensions	Normal range (mm)	
RV basal diameter	25–41	
RV mid diameter	19–35	
RV longitudinal diameter	59–83	
RVOT PLAX diameter	20–30	
RVOT distal diameter	17–27	
RV wall thickness	1–5	
Volumetric data	Normal range(area in cm^2/m^2, volume in mL/m^2)	
	Men	Women
RV end-diastolic area indexed to BSA*	5–12.6	4.5–11.5
RV end-systolic area indexed to BSA	2.0–7.4	1.6–6.4
RV end-diastolic volume indexed to BSA	35–87	32–74
RV end-systolic volume indexed to BSA	10–44	8–36

*Indicates body surface area.
PLAX, parasternal long-axis; RV, right ventricular; RVOT, right ventricular outflow tract.
Source: Adapted from ASE guidelines 2015.[12]

TABLE 2: Estimation of right atrial pressure

Parameters	Estimated RA pressure
IVC diameter <2.1 cm that collapses >50% with a sniff	RA pressure of 3 mm Hg (range, 0–5 mm Hg)
IVC diameter >2.1 cm that collapses <50% with a sniff	RA pressure 15 mm Hg (range, 10–20 mm Hg)
IVC size and IVC collapse does not fit into the above categories	RA pressure 8 mm Hg (range, 10–15 mm Hg)

IVC, inferior vena cava; RA, right atrial.

TABLE 3: Estimation of hemodynamic indices by echo*

Parameters	Formula
Systolic pulmonary artery pressure	$4\,(\text{TR Vmax})^2$ + right atrial pressure
Systolic pulmonary artery pressure in ventricular septal defect (VSD)	SBP – 4VSD Vmax^2
Systolic pulmonary artery pressure in patent ductus arteriosus (PDA)	SBP – 4PDA Vmax^2
Diastolic pulmonary artery pressure	4 (end-diastolic pulmonary regurgitation velocity)^2 + RA pressure
Mean pulmonary artery pressure	4 (early peak pulmonary regurgitation velocity)^2 + RA pressure
Mean pulmonary artery pressure	$79 - (0.45 \times \text{pulmonary acceleration time})$
Pulmonary vascular resistance	IVRT to RV ET ratio
	TR Vmax/VTI [(RVOT) × 10] + 0.16

*In the absence of RVOT obstruction. RA pressure to be calculated as per guidelines
ET, ejection time; IVRT, isovolumetric relaxation time; RA, right atrial; RVOT, right ventricular outflow tract; SBP, systolic blood pressure; TR, tricuspid regurgitation; VTI, velocity time integral.

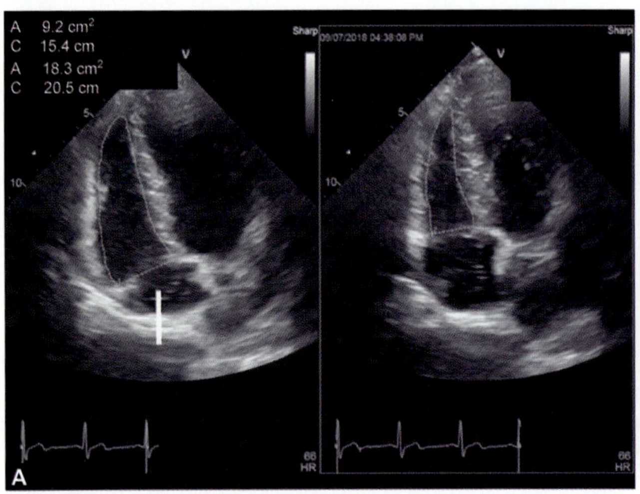

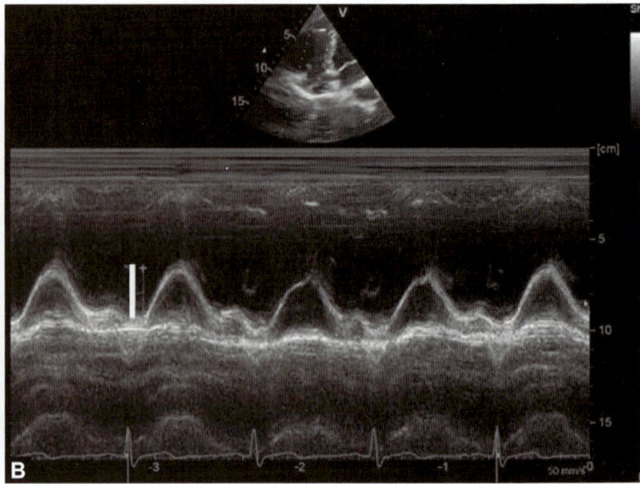

FIG. 3: **A,** Fractional area change measurement; **B,** Tricuspid annular planar systolic excursion.

ASSESSMENT OF RIGHT VENTRICULAR SYSTOLIC FUNCTION

Right Ventricular Fractional Area Change

Right ventricular fractional area change was calculated by doing planimetry involving endocardial borders from end-diastolic to end-systolic frames in RV focused A4C view (Fig. 3A). Among other parameters of RV systolic indices, RVFAC correlates well with RV ejection fraction (RVEF) measured by cardiovascular magnetic resonance (CMR).[5] Though it is not an accurate estimate of RVEF and global RV function, it serves as an independent predictor for mortality after heart failure, MI, and pulmonary embolism. The normal value is 40–56% abnormal cutoff point to predict RV dysfunction, is less than 35% (Table 4).

TABLE 4: Normal values for parameters of right ventricular function

Parameters	Cutoff values for abnormality	
	Cutoff	Range
RV fractional area change (%)	<35%	49 ± 7
TAPSE (mm)	<17	24 ± 3.5
Pulse Doppler MPI	>0.41	0.26 ± 0.085
Tissue Doppler MPI	>0.54	0.38 ± 008
Pulse Doppler S′ (cm/s)	<9.5	14.1 ± 2.3
Color Doppler S′ (cm/s)	<6	9.7 ±1.85
E-wave deceleration time (m/s)	<119 or >242	180 ± 31
E/A	<0.8 or >2.0	1.4 ± 0.43
e′/a′	0.52	1.18 ± 0.33
e′	<7.8	14 ± 3.1
E/e′	>6.0	4.0 ± 1.0
RV free wall 2D strain (%)	>–20	–29 ± 4.5
3D EF	<44%	58 ± 6.5

EF, ejection fraction; MPI, myocardial performance index; RV, right ventricular; TAPSE, tricuspid annular planar systolic excursion.

Source: Adapted from ASE guidelines 2015

Tricuspid Annular Planar Systolic Excursion

Tricuspid annular planar systolic excursion is the distance travelled by anterior tricuspid annulus from end-diastole to end-systole. It is measured by recording the M-mode by placing the cursor through the anterior tricuspid annulus as parallel as possible to the RV free wall using the zoom with low gain setting at a sweep speed of 75–100 mm/s during apnea (Fig. 3B). The amplitude of movement from end diastole to peak systole is measured in mm TAPSE is angle and load dependent.[6] It has reasonable correlation with ejection fraction (EF) measured by radionuclide angiography and CMR. Guideline recommends the use of less than 17 mm of TAPSE as abnormal. TAPSE is dependent on the longitudinal contraction of RV and so reflects only partially the status of global RV function, nevertheless TAPSE is an easily obtainable measurement with prognostic value for routine clinical use.[7]

RIGHT VENTRICULAR MYOCARDIAL PERFORMANCE INDEX

The right ventricular myocardial performance index (RVMPI) is load independent unlike majority of other RV systolic function indices, therefore found to be useful in many clinical settings especially volume loading conditions.

Tricuspid valve inflow and pulmonary valve (PV) outflow Doppler tracings are acquired in RV modified A4C view and PSAX view, with low wall filters and 75–100 mm/s sweep speed.[8] Time duration from the end of A-wave to onset of next E-wave from the tricuspid inflow Doppler tracing that is TV closure to opening time. RVET from the pulmonary Doppler tracing are measured. Isovolumic time is calculated by subtracting the RVET from TV A-wave to E-wave time duration (Fig. 4). And this isovolumetric time is divided by the RVET to get the RVMPI.[9] Whenever TR jet is holosystolic, the TV A to E time duration can be replaced by measuring the duration of TR jet. Normal reference value for RVMPI is 0.18–0.35 and cutoff value of more than 0.44 indicates RV dysfunction.

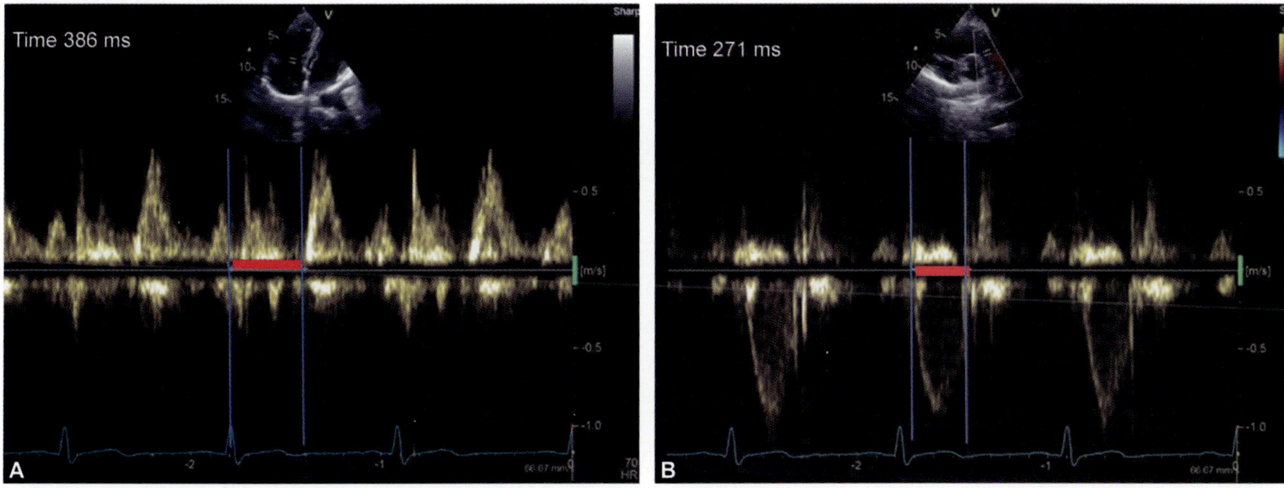

FIG. 4: **A,** Tricuspid valve closure to opening time; **B,** Pulmonary ejection time.

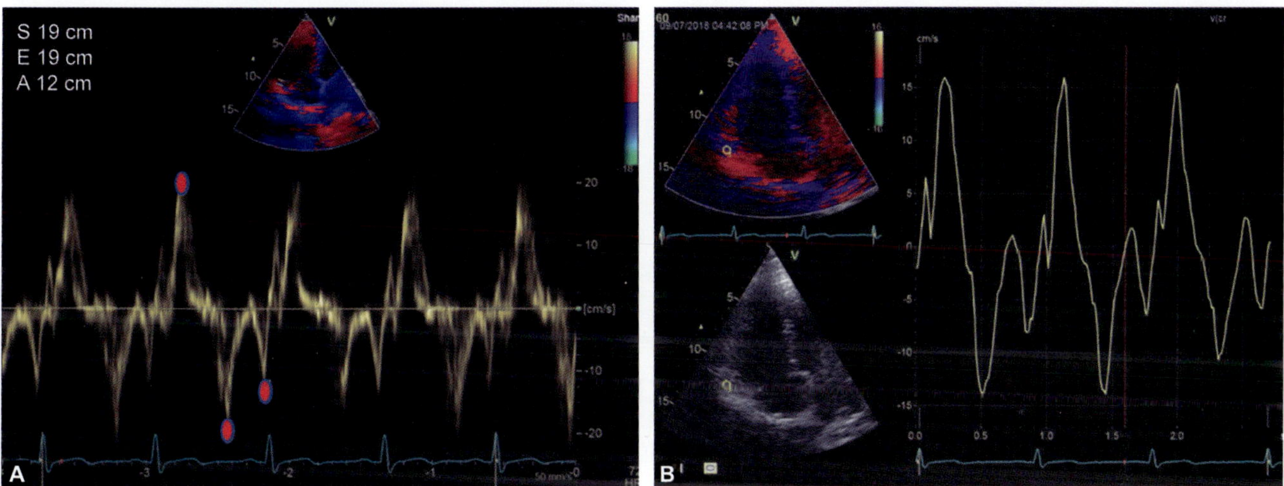

FIG. 5: **A,** Pulsed tissue Doppler from anterior tricuspid annulus; **B,** Tricuspid tissue Doppler velocity from color two-dimensional tissue Doppler.

To avoid the variation in RR interval affecting the RVMPI, it can be calculated from pulsed tissue Doppler velocity from anterior tricuspid annulus. The normal value is 0.34–0.46 with a cutoff value of more than 0.54. The RVMPI cannot be relied upon when the right atrial pressure is elevated.

TISSUE DOPPLER IMAGING OF RIGHT VENTRICULAR

Pulsed tissue Doppler velocity of tricuspid annulus is obtained by keeping the Doppler sampling volume over anterior tricuspid annulus. Proper placement of sampling volume, aligning the cursor parallel to the movement of TV annulus, increasing the frame rate by narrowing the sector, and recording during apnea will aid in getting a good tracing. The peak systolic velocity S′, early diastolic velocity E′ and atrial systolic velocity A′ can be measured (Fig. 5). The normal S′ velocity is 12–16 cm/s and the cutoff value is less than 9.5 cm/s for RV dysfunction. The RVMPI also can be calculated from the tricuspid annulus velocity.

The tissue Doppler velocity from tricuspid annulus can be measured offline from two-dimensional (2D) color tissue Doppler recording. The velocities are lower, the normal S′ velocity is 8–10.5 cm/s and abnormal cutoff point to predict RV dysfunction, is <6 cm/s by color tissue Doppler imaging and <9.5 cm/s by pulsed TDI (Table 4).[10]

Right ventricular structural and functional changes can reduce the peak systolic and diastolic tissue velocities. S′ correlated well with mildly reduced RVEF (<50%) but less with markedly reduced RVEF (<30%) by CMR.[11]

RIGHT VENTRICULAR STRAIN IMAGING

Strain and strain rate imaging are the newer and useful markers to assess RV systolic function. Strain imaging can be performed either with Doppler (TDI) or speckled tracking imaging (STI) method. Measurement of RV strain needs optimal visualization of right ventricle. Higher frame rates (above 50–100 frames/s for STI and 100–150 frames/s for TDI) achieved by narrowing the sector size and decreasing the

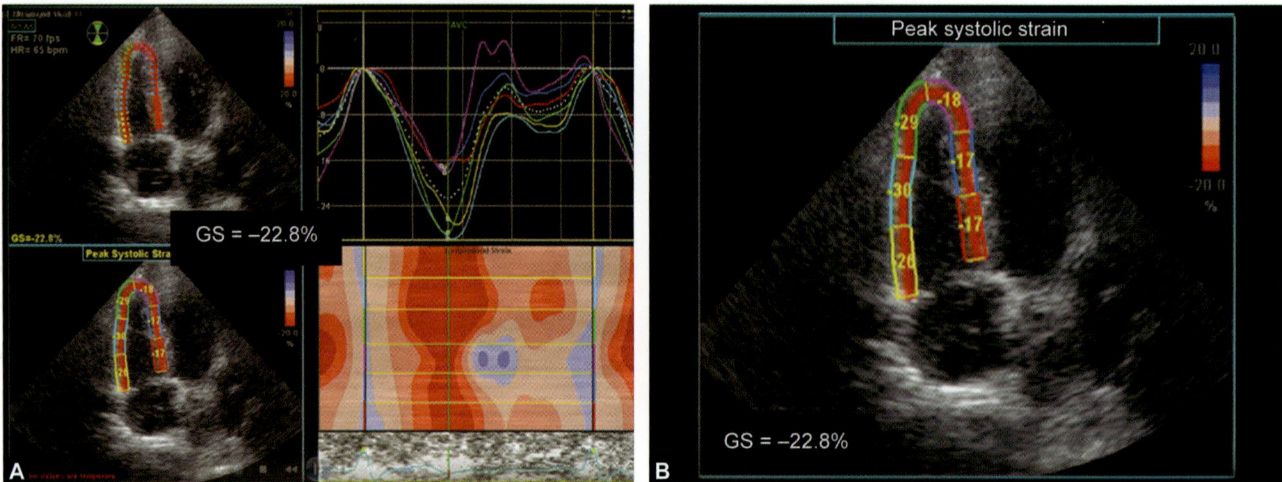

FIG. 6: Speckle tracking derived right ventricular strain. Average of the strain of three segments of free wall.

depth, images are acquired in the RV focused A4C view. Onset of QRS to PV opening is either fed manually or automated. The anterior tricuspid annulus, septal tricuspid annulus and RV apex are marked, the region of interest is reduced to fit the RV wall, the alignment with RV endocardium is checked and the process button is clicked. Peak velocity measured at the end of the T-wave, most often correlates with the peak longitudinal strain. Utilizing six segment methods on the RV-focused A4C view with high frame rates, RV free wall longitudinal strain was computed by averaging segmental peak values. Some authors prefer that the strain from IVS are discarded and only the three values from RV free wall are taken. Averaging the three gives the peak systolic RV strain (Fig. 6).

When compared to tissue Doppler strain imaging, 2D STI has low temporal resolution and dependency on image quality. In addition to the paucity of normative data and insufficient clinical validation, inter-vendor variability, the loss of speckles due to excessive motion of RV lateral wall, and the non-availability of uniform reporting of test parameters are the major limitations of 2D RV speckled tracking. 3D speckled tracking has the potential to overcome the limitations of 2D speckled tracking. However, need for separate software for RV and lower spatial resolution limits its clinical use.

The 2015 ASE/EACVI guidelines state normal values of RV free wall strain, as –29.0 ± 4.5% and the cutoff for RV dysfunction is less than –20% (the value in less negative values mean more dysfunction).[12] The RV strain varies from vendor to vendor and has not been standardized.

Right ventricular free wall longitudinal strain showed better correlation with CMR derived RVEF than other systolic function indices.[13] In patients with pulmonary arterial hypertension it was found that RV longitudinal strain and strain rate correlate well with invasive hemodynamic data and 6-minute walk distance. Moreover, significant gain in RVLS was noted when there was fall in MPAP and PVR after therapy. Kjaergaard J et al. reported the prognostic value of RV strain by Doppler tissue echocardiography in pulmonary embolism.[14] Rajagopalan et al. showed that TDI strain imaging derived RV dyssynchrony, correlated with SPAP and RV function in heart failure.[15]

Three-dimensional echocardiography of right ventricle: Three-dimensional echocardiography (3DE) mitigates the inherent limitations of 2D echocardiography (2DE) in the assessment of RV volumes and function. Live 3DE or multiple beats ECG gated 3DE are used to acquire the right ventricle images. A focused examination or a complete full volume set data are the strategies used depending upon clinical need. Complete 3D transthoracic echocardiogram (3DTTE) examination involves the parasternal, apical, and subcostal views. A complete full volume data collection can be postprocessed and displayed by four methods. They are (1) volume rendering, (2) surface rendering, (3) wireframe, and (4) 2D tomographic slicing.

A full-volume data set consists of standard 2D images in multiple cut planes of the RV sagittal, four-chamber, and coronal views (Fig. 7). These are useful in RV volume calculations and segmental wall motion assessment. Volume rendering provides a 3D visualization of structural abnormalities within the right ventricle like thrombi, masses and septal defects. Surface rendering is useful for measurement of RV volume and EF.

Using the apical long axis of the LV, multiple cuts at various levels of RV can be acquired. The basal, middle, and apical parts of RV are evaluated by these cuts. Anatomical details of right ventricle are evaluated in three axial planes, the A4C view (for RV free wall, septum and apex), the coronal view (for the RV inflow and outflow,) and the RV inflow view (for the right atrium and TV).

A dedicated software guides in identifying the center of the TV and RV apex, and then in dividing the RV into systolic and diastolic planes. Next, RV endocardial borders are traced in the coronal, sagittal, and transverse planes, performing analysis of wall motion during all phases of cardiac cycle. While the apical portion of moderator band is excluded, trabeculations are included in the endocardial border

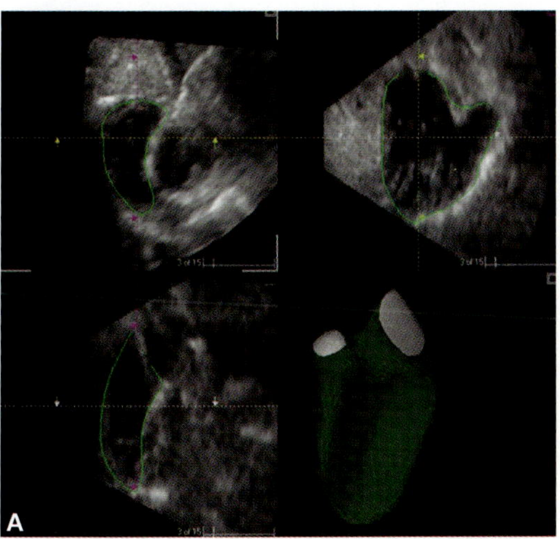
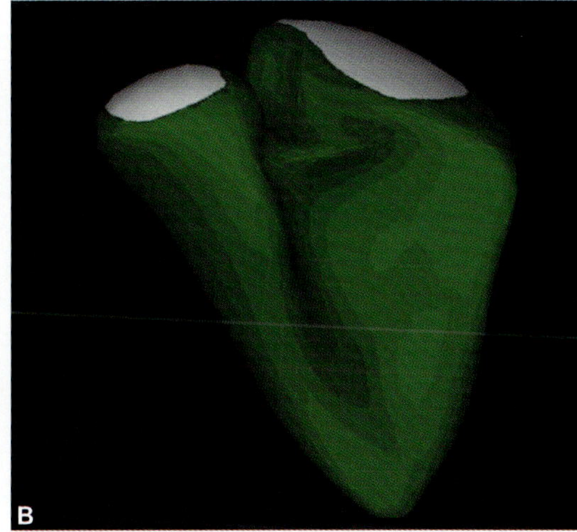

FIG. 7: Three-dimensional reconstruction of right ventricular (RV) inflow tract, RV apex and RV outflow tract from full volume data set.

tracing RV end-diastolic volume, end-systolic volume, stroke volume, and EF are derived. RVOT volume is added by this 3D volumetric method unlike the traditional 2D echo which omits it. This adds accuracy to the 3D volumetric data.[6,16] The method of disks and volumetric semiautomated border detection approach are used to quantify RV geometry and functions.[17]

A good 2DE image quality is must for a better 3DE image quality. Though varying heart rates and breath holding difficulties are some of the limitations, 3DE RV evaluation is increasingly utilized in clinical conditions like congenital heart disease and heart failure. A cutoff value less than 44% of RV EF derived by 3DE indicates RV dysfunction.

ASSESSMENT OF RIGHT VENTRICULAR DIASTOLIC FUNCTION

For right ventricle, pressure and volume are not linearly related. Therefore, correlations between RV filling profiles and chamber dimensions are not well established. RV end-diastolic or right atrial pressures serves as an indirect marker of diastolic properties. Though mean right atrial pressure is calculated in many ways by echocardiography, the tricuspid annular E/e' ratio is useful to estimate right atrial pressure.[18] ASE guidelines suggested grading of RV diastolic dysfunction based on transtricuspid flow velocity and early diastolic tricuspid annulus tissue velocity.

- Grade 1 dysfunction or impaired relaxation (tricuspid E/A ratio <0.8)
- Grade 2 dysfunction (tricuspid E/A ratio of 0.8–2.1) with tricuspid E/e' ratio >6 and
- Grade 3 dysfunction or restrictive filling (tricuspid E/A ratio >2.1 with a deceleration time <120 ms).

Though diastolic function grading of right ventricle lacks clinical data, the role of diastolic dysfunction as a prognostic factor and its importance in diagnosing early RV systolic dysfunction has been validated in clinical studies.

RIGHT VENTRICULAR WALL MOTION ASSESSMENT

Regional wall motion can be assessed by visualizing all the four segments which include anterior, inferior, and lateral walls, with infundibulum as separate entity. Apical four-chamber views allow the visualization of the lateral wall. Other useful views include parasternal RV inflow views for anterior and inferior walls and parasternal short axis view for infundibulum.

In RV myocardial infarction, the wall motion abnormality depends on the culprit vessel. Lateral and inferior wall hypokinesia is seen in proximal right coronary artery disease while isolated anterior wall hypokinesia seen in left anterior descending coronary artery involvement and isolated inferior wall hypokinesia seen in the posterior descending artery.

Regional mid- basal RV free wall hypokinesis with normal contraction of the apical segment (McConnell sign) can be sometimes seen in RV myocardial infarction, it is also very useful in pulmonary embolism. Regional RV akinesia or frank aneurysm in the "triangle of dysplasia" formed by the RV apex, the inferior wall below TV, and infundibulum is specific for arrhythmogenic RV dysplasia.[1]

TRANSESOPHAGEAL ECHOCARDIOGRAPHY

Evaluation of RV by transesophageal echocardiography (TEE) is less rewarding due to fewer additional information when compared to TTE. However, TEE can be useful in patients with acute pulmonary embolism, during cardiac surgery, patients with poor TTE windows, and in intensive care units.

CONCLUSION

Echocardiography is a very useful tool in RV functional assessment. Traditional methods are less accurate, leading to the evolving applications of RV echocardiography like speckle tracking and 3DE. Even though the surrogate parameters like fractional area change, TAPSE, RVMPI, and tissue Doppler have issues like angle and load dependency they have been documented to be useful in number of clinical studies. Speckle tracking echocardiography is angle independent, hence it is useful to assess the longitudinal contraction and intraventricular synchrony. For assessment of RV volumes and EF, 3DE is superior.

Right ventricular loading conditions impact heavily on its size, geometry and function. High load dependency of most of the echo parameters is a huge handicap in routine clinical use. Future research should address this serious issue which is increasingly noticed in device therapy in advanced heart failure. A load independent but easy to perform bedside echocardiographic method to accurately estimate RV function, is need of the hour.

REFERENCES

1. Kurtz CE. Right ventricular anatomy, function, and echocardiography evaluation. In: Otto C (Eds). The Practice Clinical of Echocardiography, 4th edition. Philadelphia: Saunders; 2012. pp. 615-28
2. Haddad F, Hunt SA, Rosenthal DN, et al. Anatomy, physiology, aging and functional assessment right ventricle. Circulation. 2008;114:1436-48.
3. Jurcut R, Giusca S, La Gerche A, et al. The echocardiographic assessment of the right ventricle: what to do in 2010. Eur J Echocardiogr. 2010;11:81-96.
4. Sanz J, Conroy J, Narula J. Imaging of the Right Ventricle. Cardiol Clin. 2012;30:189-203.
5. Anavekar NS, Gerson D, Skali H, et al. Two-dimensional assessment of right ventricular function: an echocardiographic-MRI correlative study. Echocardiography. 2007;24:452-6.
6. Kaul S, Tei C, Hopkins JM, et al. Assessment of right ventricular function using two-dimensional echocardiography. Am Heart J. 1984;107:526-31.
7. Samad BA, Alam M, Jensen-Urstad K. Prognostic impact of right ventricular involvement as assessed by tricuspid annular motion in patients with acute myocardial infarction. Am J Cardiol. 2002;90:778-81.
8. Karnati PK, El-Hajjar M, Torosoff M, et al. Myocardial performance index correlates with right ventricular ejection fraction measured by nuclear ventriculography. Echocardiography. 2008;25:381-5.
9. Tei C, Dujardin KS, Hodge DO, et al. Doppler echocardiographic index for assessment of global right ventricular function. J Am Soc Echocardiogr. 1996;9:838-47.
10. Kjaergaard J, Sogaard P, Hassager C. Right ventricular strain in pulmonary embolism by Doppler tissue echocardiography. J Am Soc Echocardiogr. 2004;17:1210-2.
11. Pavlicek M, Wahl A, Rutz T, et al. Right ventricular systolic function assessment: rank of echocardiographic methods vs. cardiac magnetic resonance imaging. Eur J Echocardiogr. 2011;12:871-80.
12. Lang RM, Badano LP, Mor-Avi V, et al. Recommendations for cardiac chamber quantification by echocardiography in adults: an update from the American Society of Echocardiography and the European Association of Cardiovascular Imaging. J Am Soc Echocardiogr. 2015;28:1-39.e14.
13. Nageh MF, Kopelen HA, Zoghbi WA, et al. Estimation of mean right atrial pressure using tissue Doppler imaging. Am J Cardiol. 1999;84:1448-51.
14. Horton KD, Meece RW, Hill JC. Assessment of the right ventricle by echocardiography: a primer for cardiac sonographers. J Am Soc Echocardiogr. 2009;22:776-92.
15. Lu X, Nadvoretskiy V, Bu L, et al. Accuracy and reproducibility of real-time three-dimensional echocardiography for assessment of right ventricular volumes and ejection fraction in children. J Am Soc Echocardiogr. 2008;21:84-9.
16. Teske AJ, De Boeck BW, Olimulder M, et al. Echocardiographic assessment of regional right ventricular function: a head-to-head comparison between 2-dimensional and tissue Doppler-derived strain analysis. J Am Soc Echocardiogr. 2008;21:275-83.
17. Chien-Chia Wu V, Takeuchi M. Echocardiographic assessment of right ventricular systolic function. Cardiovasc Diagn Ther. 2018;8:70-9.
18. Rajagopalan N, Dohi K, Simon MA, et al. Right ventricular dyssynchrony in heart failure: a tissue Doppler imaging study. J Card Fail. 2006;12:263-7.

CHAPTER 77

Longitudinal Strain Imaging: Is it a Clinical Tool? An Echocardiographic Appreciation

G Vijayaraghavan, S Sivasankaran

INTRODUCTION

Systolic function of the left ventricle (LV) is assessed by the m-mode echocardiography as end-systolic and end-diastolic diameters from which the ejection fraction is calculated.[1] End-systolic dimension has important diagnostic and prognostic value in subjects with ventricular systolic dysfunction.[2] Ejection fraction calculated from the m-mode is on a presumption that the LV is globular, which is far from the truth.[3] American Society of Echocardiography (ASE) no longer recommends measuring the LV ejection fraction from m-mode and advised all echocardiographers to use the two-dimensional (2D) echo biplane Simpson's method or use three-dimensional (3D) echo for LV ejection fraction calculation.[4] While assessing the regional myocardial function we assess the wall motion, and the terminologies advocated by the ASE are normal, hypokinetic, akinetic, dyskinetic, aneurysmal, or hyperkinetic. Wall motions are assessed by eye balling and require expertise and are purely subjective. We need a more precise measurement of the systolic parameters of LV function.[5]

DEFINITION

As the LV contracts in systole, it shortens in the longitudinal and circumferential direction (negative strain) and thickens in the radial direction (positive strain).[6] The change in length or thickness could be measured and expressed as a percentage of its diastolic length or thickness which is called the strain or deformation.[7] Longitudinal shortening is responsible for 60% of the LV ejection and is the most important component of systolic function. This longitudinal shortening varies from –15% to –30% from base to apex.[8] The circumference of the LV becomes small with systole. This systolic shortening of circumference of LV is circumferential strain which measures to –20% to –30% of its diastolic circumference. LV contraction causes radial thickening in systole. The thickening is measured as a positive strain of +30% to +60%.[9] In the short-axis view during LV systole basal segments of the LV rotates in an overall clockwise direction and apex rotates in a counter-clockwise direction when viewed from apex to base.[10] This squeezing movement of the LV is essential for the systolic ejection and is termed as twist and measures to counter-clockwise movement of about 65°and clockwise movement of about 5° in a normal individual.[11] This LV torsion is followed by rapid untwisting, which contributes to ventricular filling because LV torsion is directly related to fiber orientation in the LV wall.

LONGITUDINAL STRAIN

When you place a sample volume at the LV free wall in the apical views and record the tissue Doppler, you can demonstrate the longitudinal strain curve of that segment of the LV muscle.

Strain or deformation represents the systolic shortening of a segment of the myocardium and is expressed as a percentage of the diastolic length. This is like the ejection fraction, where it is expressed as a percentage of the diastolic volume ejected out in systole. Along with the beginning of the QRS complex of the electrocardiogram, the strain curve shows a small positive wave indicating lengthening of the myocardium lasting a few milliseconds and then a gradual negative wave. The negative wave represents the systolic shortening percentage of the myocardium in each segment. The maximal shortening occurs at the end systole or peak systole and is more than 15%.[12] This occurs toward the end of aortic systolic velocity curve at the peak of the T-wave of the electrocardiogram. The shortening percentage or strain increases as you move from base to apex.[6] From the end systole, the curve gradually goes back to the resting level of 0% at end diastole to begin the next cardiac cycle. After the peak systole, the curve may show a small wave in early diastole called the postsystolic wave. This wave normally is less in magnitude than the peak systolic strain. Normal ranges for these values are now available on publications.[13]

SPECKLE TRACKING FOR STRAIN IMAGING[14]

Strain curves were recorded using tissue Doppler echocardiography from various segments of the myocardium.[15] For accurate measurements the incident ultrasound beam should be perpendicular to the myocardium interrogated. When you look at the anatomy of the LV this is not a practical proposition while using the tissue Doppler. Strain analysis of the myocardial segments is done by the new method of speckle tracking.[16] This is a post-processing computer algorithm that uses the routine grayscale digital images. Movement of the speckle patterns in the myocardium is utilized to image the shortening of every segment during the cardiac cycle. Within each regions of interest in the myocardium, the image-processing algorithm automatically subdivides regions into blocks of pixels tracking stable patterns of speckles. Subsequent frames are then automatically analyzed by searching for the new location of the speckle patterns within each of the blocks using correlation criteria and the sum of absolute differences.[17] The location shift of these acoustic markers from frame to frame representing tissue movement provides the spatial and temporal data used to calculate velocity vectors.[18] Temporal alterations in these stable speckle patterns are identified as moving farther apart or closer together and create a series of regional strain vectors and the sum of it as strain curves.[14] The strain measurements are done by different software by various vendors. This paper describes the automatic functional imaging protocol used by GE.[19]

LONGITUDINAL STRAIN IMAGING PROTOCOL[20]

Good-quality strain imaging requires excellent apical views, four-chamber, long-axis and the two-chamber views images with a good frame rate (Fig. 1).[21] Reduce the depth of the image and the width of the sector to get good quality image without any drop outs. Increase the frame rate to more than 60 frames per sec (fps). Breath held in expiration, minimizes the motion artifacts. Apical four-chamber, long-axis and two-chamber images are to be archived for three cardiac cycles. Aortic closure marked at the peak of the electrocardiographic T-wave. Start the strain measurement with apical long-axis view and follow the machine instructions. The region of interest is marked by placing the points at the base of the LV near the atrioventricular posterior and anterior annulus and finally, the apex. The LV walls will be highlighted in colors depicting the anterior basal septum, mid-septum and apical septum, inferolateral basal wall, mid basal and apical basal wall. Strain of each segment will be inscribed in each of these segments of the LV. The strain curve will be available for each segment and an anatomical m-mode of these segments from medial base to apex and back to lateral basal wall will also be depicted. This is repeated for six segments of the apical four-chamber view and apical two-chamber views. Once all the three apical images have been interrogated and strain measured by automatic functional imaging technique, the bull's eye picture of 17 segments of the LV with measured longitudinal strain will appear on the screen. You can also get the strain curves of all the 17 segments with the bull's eye and you can highlight any segment with abnormal strain curve to analyze the curve. The color of each segment also represents the strain. Normal strain will be depicted in red and reduction of strain will be seen as light strain and if the segments lengthen instead of shortening, it will be seen as blue.

One can select bull's eye view of postsystolic index or see bull's eye view of the time to peak velocity format, which will demonstrate the timing of the peak strain from the onset of QRS complex. This, along with postsystolic strain index will identify areas where the contraction continued on to

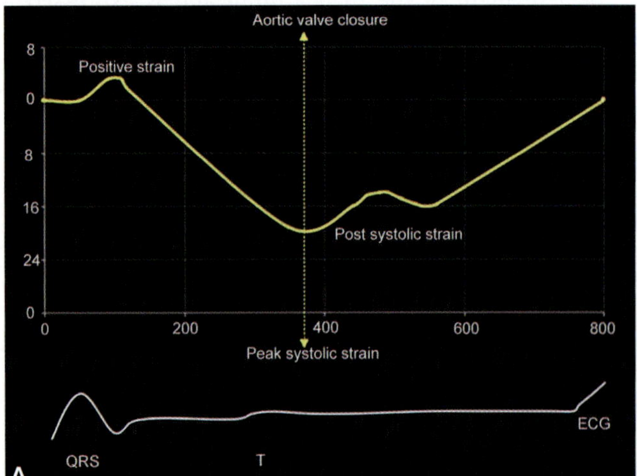

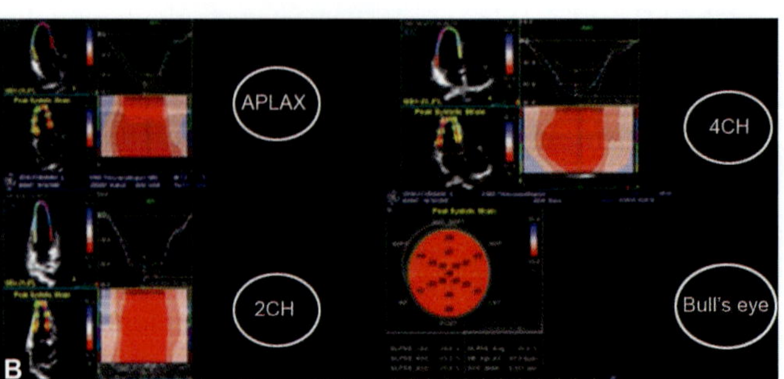

FIG. 1: Strain imaging and Bull's eye map of global myocardial strain. **A**, the myocardial strain of a myocardial segment, correlated with the electrocardiogram. P represents the small positive wave at the beginning of myocardial contraction, and S wave denotes the peak systolic strain, end systole is marked by the closure of the aortic valve. PSS denotes the post systolic wave; **B**, The Bull's eye map of all the 17 segments of the myocardium acquired by the long-axis (APLAX), two-chamber (2CH) and four-chamber (4CH) views at peak systole. Color panels show the curved or anatomical M-mode of the various segments.

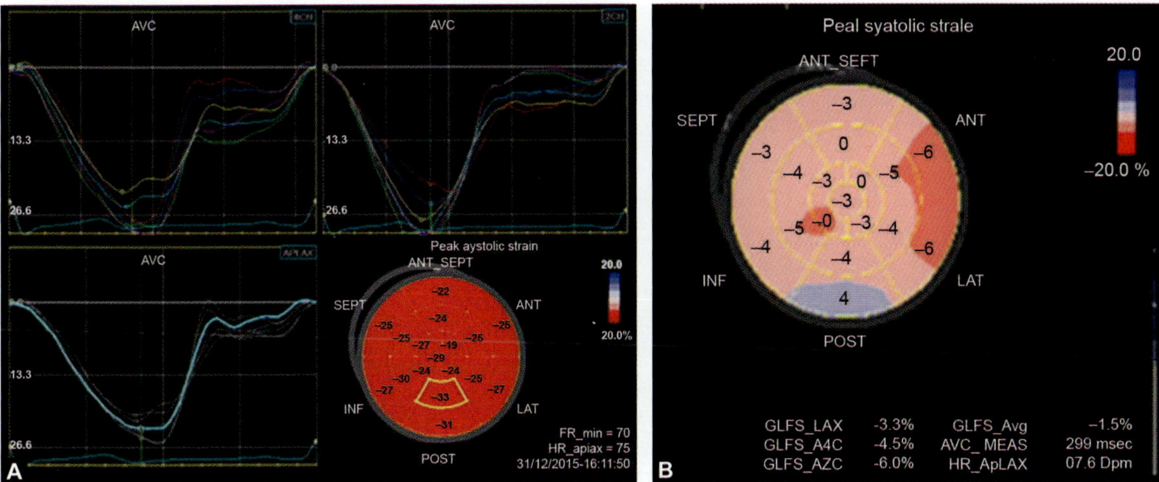

ANT, anterior; SEPT, septum; INF, inferior; LAT, lateral; POST: posterior.

FIG. 2: Bull's eye picture of segmental strain of all 17 segments of the left ventricle. **A,** Normal left ventricle, with peak systolic strain rate more than –14 in all segments; **B,** left ventricle in dilated cardiomyopathy where the peak systolic strain is less than –5 in most segments except apical septal and basal lateral walls. Inferobasal segment is dyskinetic and hence, blue with +4 strain rates.

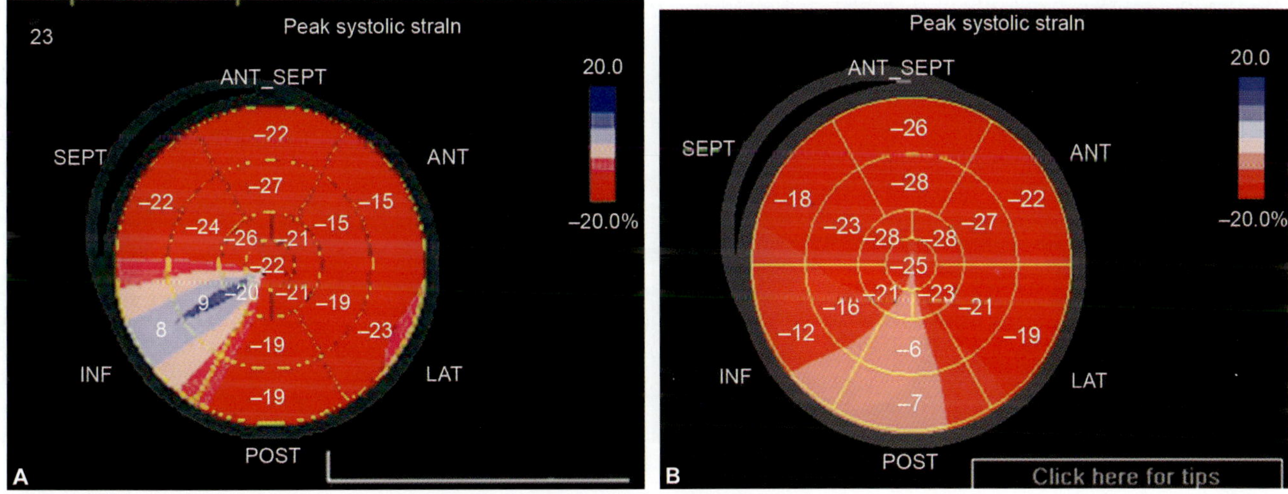

ANT, anterior; SEPT, septum; INF, inferior; LAT, lateral; POST, posterior.

FIG. 3: Bull's eye map of 17-segment global longitudinal strain before **A,** and after **B,** right coronary angioplasty in a subject with coronary artery disease. Note the positive blue strain parameters in the inferior segments which show red (negative/recovering) parameters postangioplasty.

diastole in certain myocardial segments as a pathological phenomenon.

EJECTION FRACTION AND GLOBAL LONGITUDINAL STRAIN

There is wide criticism in the method of assessment of LV function by ejection fraction. M-mode echocardiographic calculation of ejection fraction is not used now and is replaced with 2D Simson's biplane method.[4] Foreshortening is a major problem for apical imaging and may underestimate ejection fraction. Three-dimensional method is ideal but not universally available in every echo laboratory. It is in this place the global longitudinal strain (GLS) is found to be more reliable in assessing the prognosis of patients with acute heart failure.[20] The strain is labeled as mildly reduced when it is more than –12.5%, moderately reduced when it is between –8.1% and –12.5% and severely when it is less than –8.0%. This assessment of prognosis was found to be statistically more reliable than the use of ejection fraction. Figure 2 represent a patient with dilated cardiomyopathy with markedly reduced GLS of –4.5%, of course with a poor prognosis.

ISCHEMIC HEART DISEASE AND REGIONAL STRAIN[22]

Ischemic heart disease produces reduction in strain percentage in the vascular territory involved.[23] An example

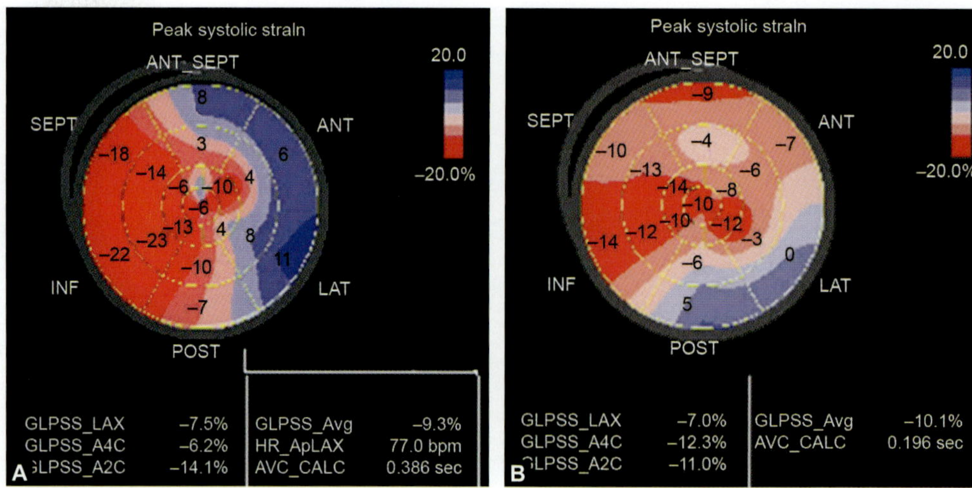

ANT, anterior; SEPT, septum; INF, inferior; LAT, lateral; POST, posterior.

FIG. 4: Bull's eye map of global longitudinal strain in coronary artery disease. **A,** in a subject with dominant left anterior descending artery infarction, where there is impaired strain in the anteroseptal anterior and lateral wall with blue regions representing dyskinesia (positive strain); **B,** Global involvement of all myocardial segments with triple vessel disease and ischemic cardiomyopathy.

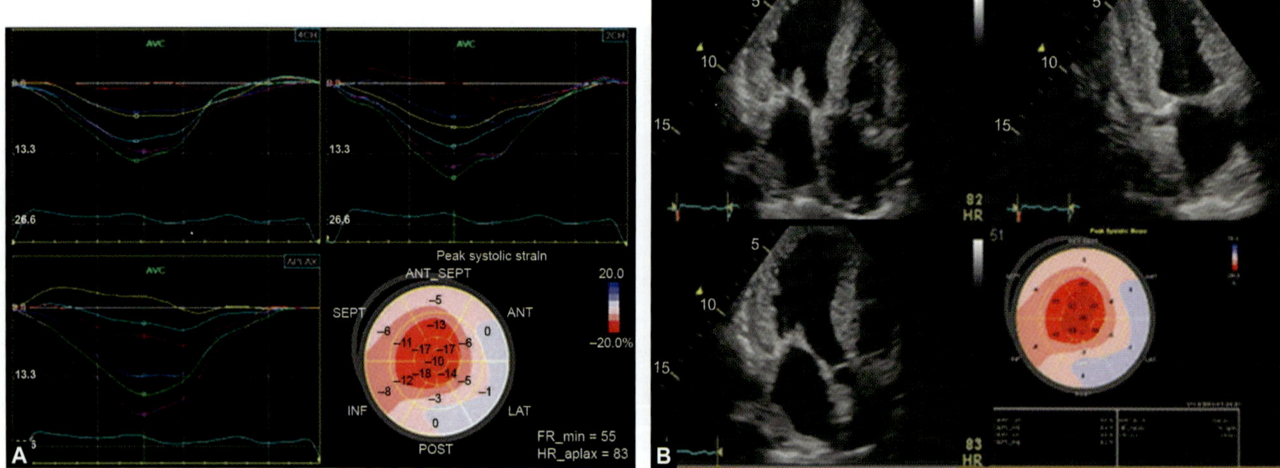

ANT, anterior; SEPT, septum; INF, inferior; LAT, lateral; POST, posterior.

FIG. 5: Typical cherry red plot of global longitudinal strain bull's eye map in cardiac amyloidosis. **A,** The velocities of the strain curves; **B,** The thickened hyperechogenic myocardium in the respective views.

of inferior wall myocardial infarction before and after angioplasty is given in figure 3. You can appreciate that before angioplasty the strain in the inferior wall segments were positive in the basal and mid segments, which completely disappeared following right coronary angioplasty. However, we can see that basal and mid segments still have low strain even though the systolic lengthening as shown by the blue color is replaced by relatively reduced strain. Global strain rate imaging can be used to assess the infarct size,[24] during exercise echocardiography[25] and for prognosticating a subject with coronary artery disease.[26]

Two examples of anterior wall infarction and ischemic cardiomyopathy are given in figures 4 and 5. In figure 4, you can see that the inferior wall strain is normal while that of the anterior septum, anterior wall and lateral wall have reduced strain with the basal and mid segments showing positive strain. This patient had a dominant left anterior descending artery. The loss of strain has resulted in the global average peak systolic strain which was only −9.3%. Figure 5 were from a patient with triple-vessel disease where the reduction of strain is present in all the territories and the patient was in congestive cardiac failure (ischemic cardiomyopathy).

INFILTRATIVE DISEASES: AMYLOIDOSIS[27]

The amyloid deposits are predominantly in the basal segments, less so in the mid segments and the apical segments are spared giving the appearance of a cherry on top of the ice-cream on strain imaging. Whether the increase torsional movements at the apex compared to base prevent the interstitial deposition is conjunctural. The strain curves

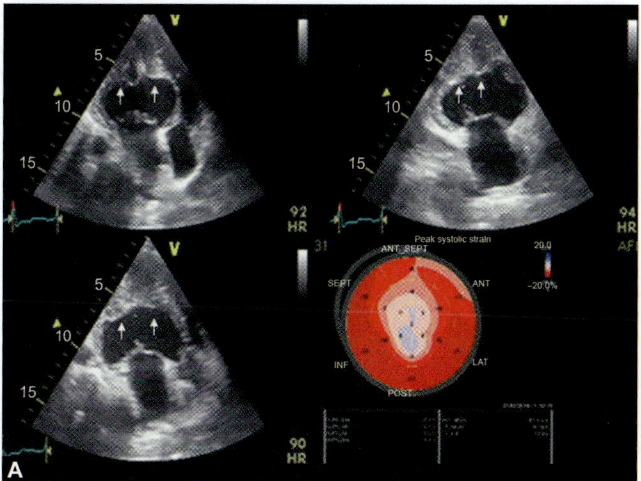

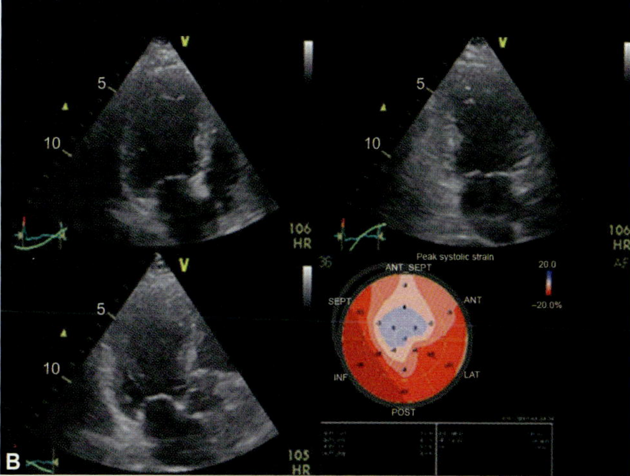

FIG. 6: Global longitudinal strain of the left ventricle represented by bull's eye map in figure **A,** Left ventricular endomyocardial fibrosis. Short arrows show the thickened calcific endocardium with ventricular apical obliteration. Corresponding myocardial segment shows reduced strain in the bull's eye plot; **B,** Apical ballooning (Takotsubo) syndrome with good strain rates at the basal segments.

depict the systolic lengthening of the basal lateral and anterior walls. The pathology of amyloidosis can be appreciated from the bright thick ventricular walls. This pattern could be seen in most of the patients with ventricular hypertrophy as the disease progresses to heart failure. Hypertensive heart disease, aortic stenosis, are clear examples.[28]

LEFT VENTRICULAR ENDOMYOCARDIAL FIBROSIS

The fibrosis and calcification of the LV apex as is seen in the 2D echo is well represented by the reduction of strain in the apical and mid segments.[29] Similar picture will be seen temporarily in patients with apical ballooning syndrome where the basal segments of the LV contracts normally and the apical segments balloon out, as figure 6.[30] In pictures of strain imaging from a patient with apical ballooning syndrome, as in figure 7, you can appreciate the positive strain in the apical segments and lengthening of segments as is depicted in the strain curves. Some of the segments peak in diastole and this postsystolic strain is classically described for ischemia.

HYPERTROPHIC CARDIOMYOPATHY

Hypertrophied muscles with myofiber disarray have no coordinated contraction and systolic shortening. In fact, it produces disordered contraction and minimal systolic shortening of many segments as shown in the strain curves from a patient, hypertrophy of anterior wall and apical inferior wall (Fig. 8).[31]

It is interesting to note that in apical hypertrophic cardiomyopathy the loss of strain is limited to the apical segments as is shown in figure 9, and the differences in the longitudinal strain helps to differentiate people with physiologic hypertrophy.[32] The regions of reduced strain correlates with pathological fibrosis on evaluation with magnetic resonance and hence is useful in prognostication.[33]

LEFT BUNDLE BRANCH, CARDIAC FAILURE, AND CARDIAC RESYNCHRONIZATION THERAPY[34]

Left bundle branch with lateral walls of the LV contracting in a delayed manner results in loss of myocardial efficiency.[35] The segments contracting after the aortic valve closure do not contribute to LV ejection but contractions occurring in early diastole hampers LV filling and adds to afterload dependant dysfunction.[36] If cardiac resynchronization therapy can make these segments contract before aortic valve closure, the problem will be solved to a large extent.[37] If strain imaging can identify the segments with delayed contraction and place the LV leads over those segments to resynchronize their contractions, one can get significant benefit in patients with cardiac failure and left bundle branch block, which has major prognostic implications.[38,39] Notice the segments with peak contractions occurring in diastole after the aortic valve closure in a patient with left bundle branch block in figure 10 and the postsystolic index being significantly abnormal over the entire inferior and lateral walls.

MYOCARDITIS

Acute ventricular dysfunction can occur in viral myocarditis as well as in allergic myocardial dysfunction, the Kounis syndrome, and near normal GLS differentiates the latter from acute myocarditis. Similarly, clinical disorders with chronic myocarditis like sarcoidosis can be picked up by strain imaging.[40] Serial longitudinal studies add additional information on prognosis.[41]

Illustrative Case Study on Myocarditis

Figure 11 depict the GLS images of the LV in a 26-year-old engineer who was admitted following an episode of acute viral fever. His dyspnea was originally being treated by the pulmonologist. Once the high-sensitive troponin T was found to be high, he was transferred to cardiology

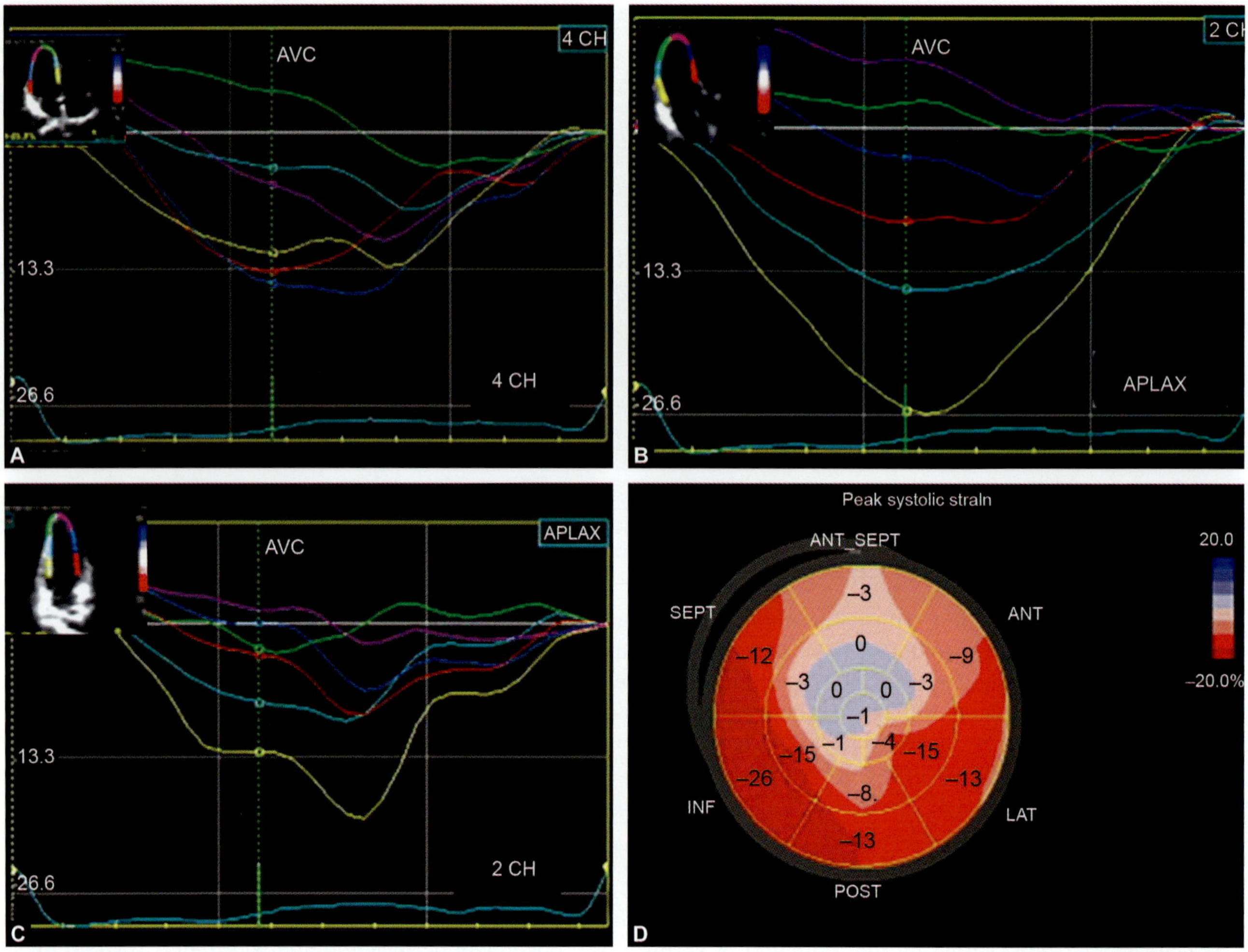

ANT, anterior; SEPT, septum; INF, inferior; LAT, lateral; POST, posterior.

FIG. 7: Global longitudinal strain depicted with the bull's eye plot, typical of apical ballooning syndrome. **A,** Apical four-chamber view; **B,** Apical long-axis view; **C,** Apical two-chamber view; **D,** The bull's eye plot. Note the basal segments shown by red and yellow lines have normal strain pattern whereas the apical segments show lengthening instead of shortening in systole. Moreover, in apical four-chamber and two-chamber views, few segments show significant post systolic strain, beyond aortic valve closure, typical of myocardial ischemia.

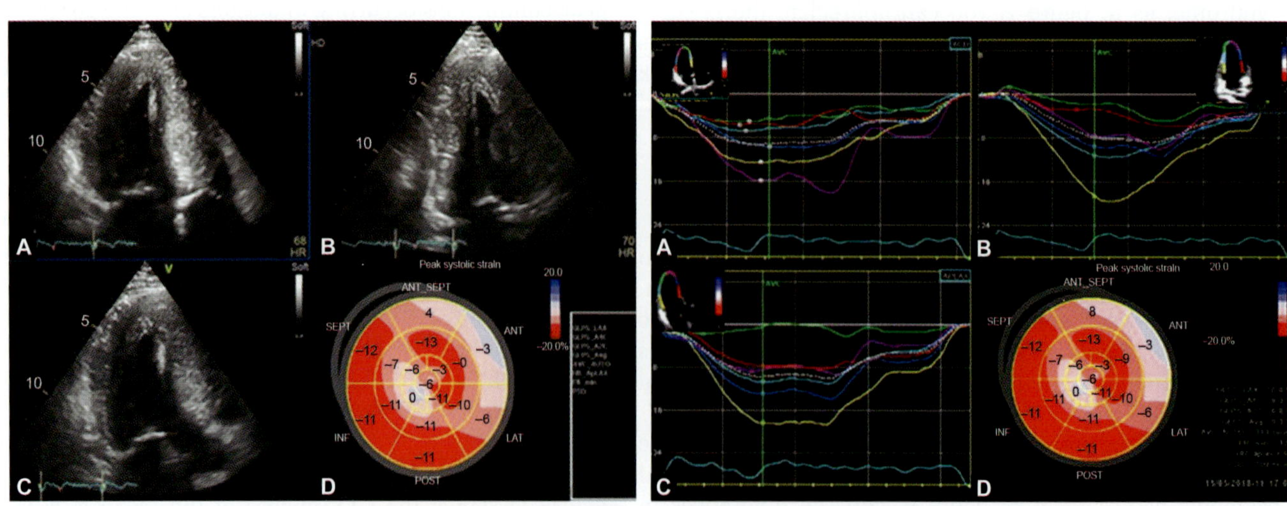

ANT, anterior; SEPT, septum; INF, inferior; LAT, lateral; POST, posterior.

FIG. 8: Global longitudinal strain imaging in hypertrophic cardiomyopathy; left panel shows the two-dimensional images and the right panel the corresponding strain velocities of the various segments. **A,** The four-chamber; **B,** Two-chamber; **C,** The apical long axis; **D,** The bull's eye map. The septal basal and mid segments shown in red and green lines show reduced strain rates consistent with the regional pathology.

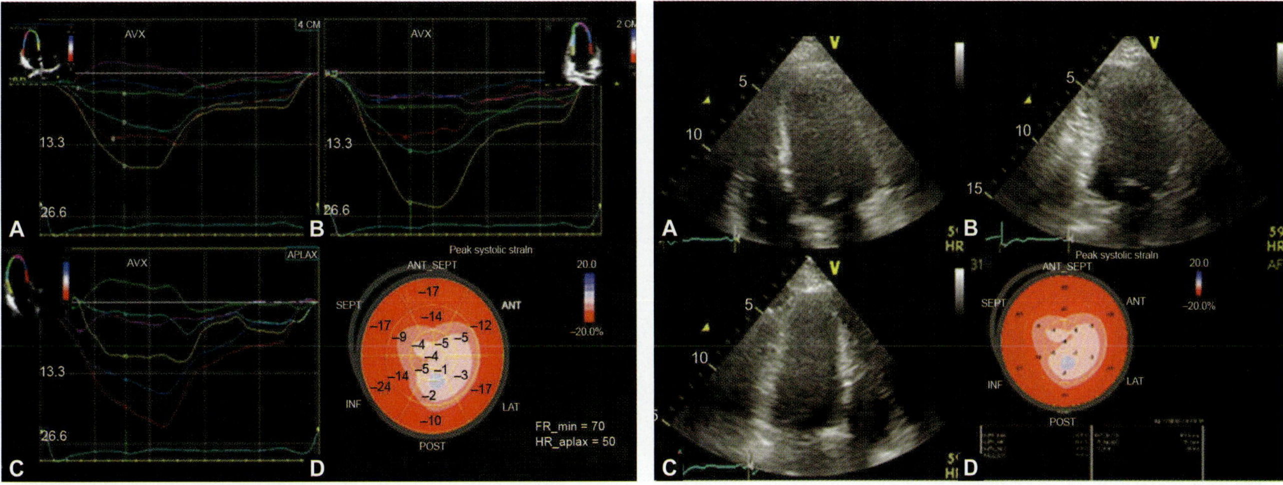

ANT, anterior; SEPT, septum; INF, inferior; LAT, lateral; POST, posterior.

FIG. 9: Global longitudinal strain imaging in apical hypertrophic cardiomyopathy; left panel shows the two-dimensional echo images and the right panel, the corresponding strain velocities of the various segments. **A,** The four-chamber; **B,** two-chamber; **C,** The apical long axis; **D,** The bull's eye map. Note the reduced strain rate along the apical segments, whereas the basal segments have normal pattern.

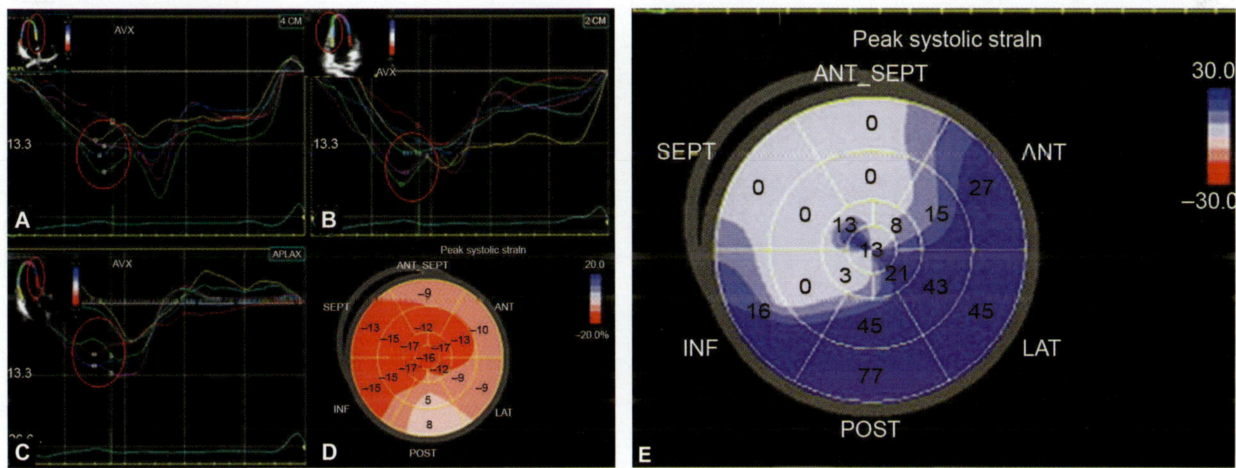

ANT, anterior; SEPT, septum; INF, inferior; LAT, lateral; POST, posterior.

FIG. 10: Global longitudinal strain in a subject with left bundle branch block. The segments contracting earlier are identified by the earlier peaking of strain as shown by the red ovals, which correspond to electrical systole. **A,** the apical 4-chamber view, shows the septal segments contracting earlier than the lateral; **B,** Apical 2-chamber view, the inferior segments contract earlier than the anterior wall; **C,** the long-axis view, the anteroseptal segments are earlier than the inferolateral wall; **D,** and **E,** shows the bull's eye map of the peak systolic strain and the post-systolic strain in the same subject.

and subsequently initiated on beta-blockers, angiotensin-converting enzyme inhibitors, and diuretics. His initial strain imaging showed marked reduction of basal and mid-wall strain with many segments showing positive strain. His average GLS was only –6.5%. His edema and dyspnea improved with treatment and he could be discharged on medications. Strain imaging done after 1 month showed remarkable improvement from –6.5% to –10.5% as shown in figure 12.

STRAIN IMAGING IN RARE SITUATIONS[42]

There are many other areas in cardiology where strain imaging has been of great use in evaluating significant pathology before any other investigations could pick up early abnormalities like myocardial ischemia,[33] LV diastolic dysfunction, subclinical myocardial dysfunction before, during and after cancer chemotherapy,[43,44] fetal echocardiography[45] and the list will increase as the experience with this new clinical modality increases.[46] Figure 13

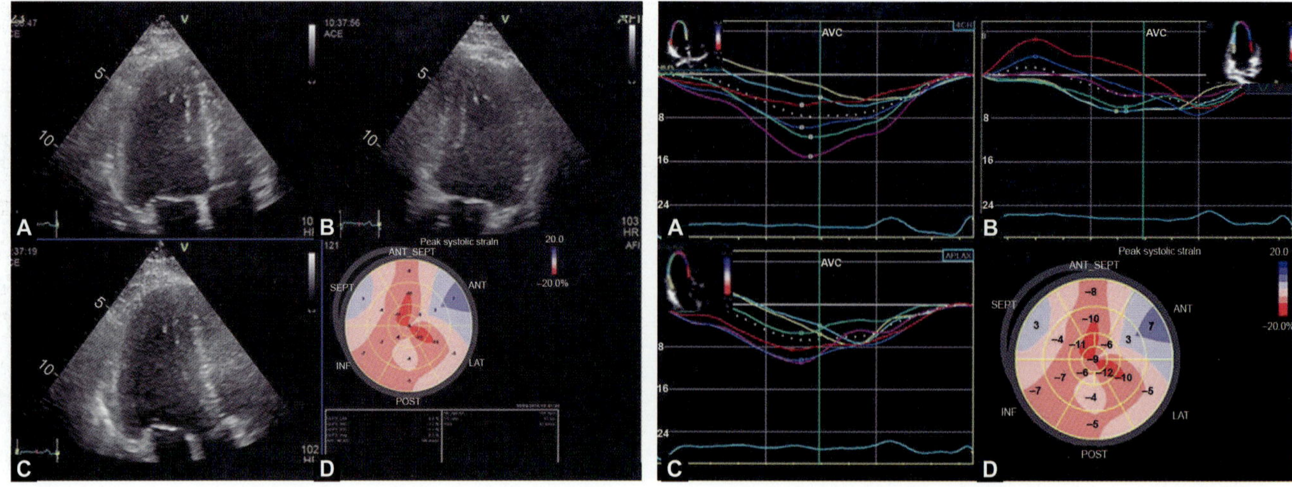

ANT, anterior; SEPT, septum; INF, inferior; LAT, lateral; POST, posterior.

FIG. 11: Global longitudinal strain in a 26-year-old gentleman who had viral myocarditis. The left panel shows the two-dimensional echo images and the right panel the strain velocities. **A,** The four-chamber view; **B,** The two-chamber view; **C,** The long-axis view; **D,** The bull's eye map. The decreased strain velocities are global and are not restricted to any coronary vascular territory.

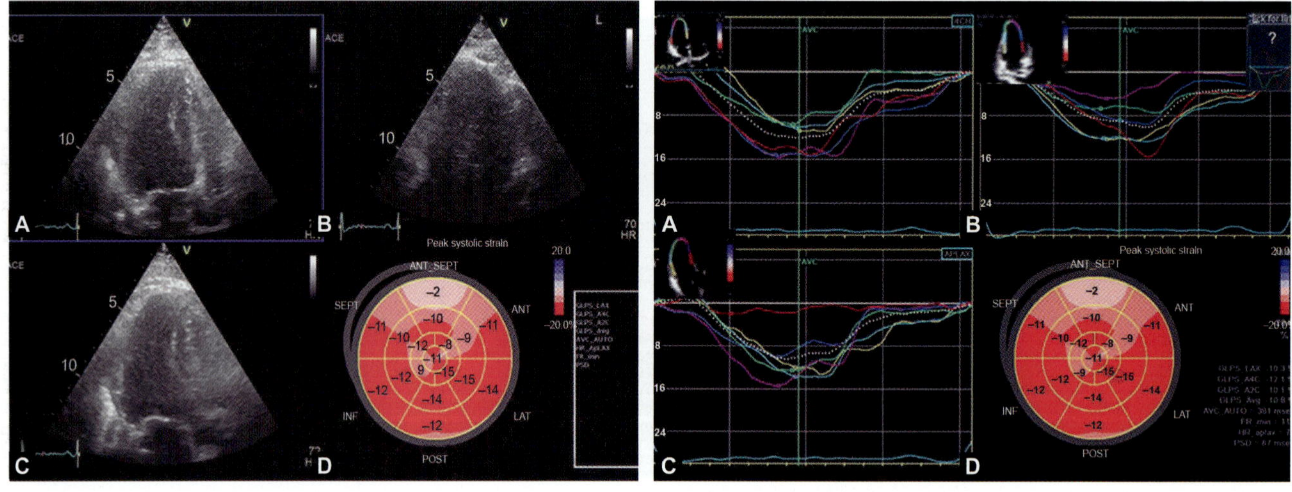

ANT, anterior; SEPT, septum; INF, inferior; LAT, lateral; POST, posterior.

FIG. 12: Global longitudinal strain in a 26-year-old gentleman who had viral myocarditis at one month follow-up. The left panel shows the two-dimensional echo images and the right panel the strain velocities. **A,** The 4-chamber view; **B,** The two-chamber view; **C,** The long-axis view; **D,** The bull's eye map. The global left ventricular function shows improvement to –10.5% from the initial value of –6% to 5% in figure 11.

illustrate the utility of GLS imaging in the diagnosis of constrictive pericarditis, compared with circumferential strain imaging.[47] Circumferential strain imaging cannot image the true apex. In constrictive pericarditis, lateral and peripheral segments are immobilized by the visceral pericardial fibrosis, in a patchy manner, whereas the septum, which is intracardiac maintains its mobility.

LIMITATIONS OF STRAIN IMAGING[48]

We have to overcome many limitations in strain imaging. In-plane deformation or displacement in a 2D sequence of images during speckle tracking, could produce artifacts in short-axis images (but less so in apical views). The 3D images could overcome this but it has low temporal and spatial resolution.[49] Ultrasound noise could reduce the frame by frame tracking of local speckle patterns. Acquiring optimized image quality is essential to reduce inter and intra-observer variation.[28] Speckle patterns may not be stable due to changes in interrogation angle, between moving tissue and ultrasonic beam. The accumulation of small random errors in detection of speckled pattern along the tracking process leads to inaccurate tracking results. As the technology develops, we may overcome some of these limitations. Two main vendors supplying the equipment for strain imaging are the QLab with cardiac motion quantification (CMQ) software of the Philips IE33 and the EchoPAC 11 of automated function imaging (AFI) from GE. The global average peak strain values

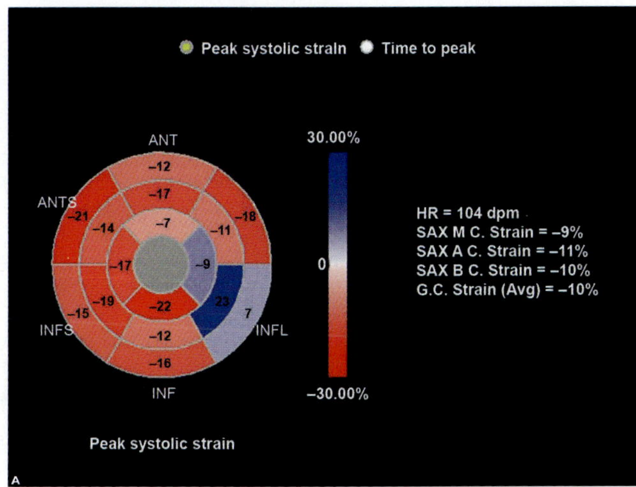

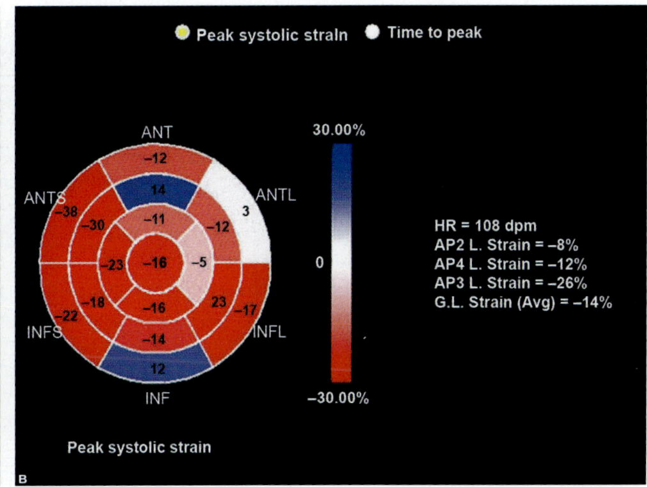

AP, anteroposterior; ANT, anterior; INF, inferior.

FIG. 13: Global strain imaging in constrictive pericarditis. **A,** The circumferential strain imaging where the left ventricular apex cannot be imaged; **B,** The global longitudinal strain imaging. Note that the circumferential strain is more affected than the longitudinal strain and the septal regions are spared. Segmental involvement is patchy and is not restricted to any vascular territory.

may show correlation, but we may find regional variation in strain values from the available vendors.[6] CMQ is more time-consuming than AFI. There was a comparative study regarding the time needed to complete the measurements using AFI with EchoPAC or CMQ with QLab in 15 subjects.[50] The time required with EchoPAC compared with QLab was 117 ± 17s versus 477 ± 43s, $p < 0.001$.

CONCLUSION

Longitudinal strain has become a clinical tool. Bull's eye pictures on the GLS along with the 2D echo images and the strain curves give important diagnostic information in a host of diseases. In ischemic heart disease the changes may appear before the wall motion and electrocardiogram changes. In congestive cardiac failure, it has important prognostic value. It can detect impending ventricular dysfunction in subjects undergoing chemotherapy with cardiotoxic drugs and help to modulate the dose. With increasing experience and vendors using comparable software of it will soon become a standard imaging format in all echocardiographic laboratories.

REFERENCES

1. Picard MH, Popp RL, Weyman AE. Assessment of left ventricular function by echocardiography: a technique in evolution. J Am Soc Echocardiogr. 2008;21(1):14-21.
2. Bhat PK, Ashwath ML, Rosenbaum DS, et al. Usefulness of left ventricular end-systolic dimension by echocardiography to predict reverse remodeling in patients with newly diagnosed severe left ventricular systolic dysfunction. Am J Cardiol. 2012;110(1):83-7.
3. Dittoe N, Stultz D, Schwartz BP, et al. Quantitative left ventricular systolic function: from chamber to myocardium. Crit Care Med. 2007;35(8 Suppl):S330-9.
4. Lang RM, Badano LP, Mor-Avi V, et al. Recommendations for cardiac chamber quantification by echocardiography in adults: an update from the American Society of Echocardiography and the European Association of Cardiovascular Imaging. J Am Soc Echocardiogr. 2015;28(1):1-39.
5. Cameli M, Mondillo S, Solari M, et al. Echocardiographic assessment of left ventricular systolic function: from ejection fraction to torsion. Heart Fail Rev. 2016;21(1):77-94.
6. Smiseth OA, Torp H, Opdahl A, et al. Myocardial strain imaging: how useful is it in clinical decision making? Eur Heart J. 2016;37(15):1196-207.
7. Claus P, Omar AMS, Pedrizzetti G, et al. Tissue tracking technology for assessing cardiac mechanics: principles, normal values, and clinical applications. JACC Cardiovasc Imaging. 2015;8(12):1444-60.
8. Lin FC, Hsieh IC, Lee CH, et al. Introduction of tissue Doppler imaging echocardiography—based on pulsed-wave mode. J Med Ultrasound. 2008; 16(3):202-9.
9. Acosta-Martínez J, López-Haldón JE, Gutiérrez-Carretero E, et al. Radial and circumferential strain as markers of fibrosis in an experimental model of myocardial infarction. Rev Esp Cardiol. 2013;66(6):508-9.
10. Opdahl A, Helle-Valle T, Remme EW, et al. Apical rotation by speckle tracking echocardiography: a simplified bedside index of left ventricular twist. J Am Soc Echocardiogr. 2008;21(10):1121-8.
11. Omar AMS, Vallabhajosyula S, Sengupta PP. Left ventricular twist and torsion: research observations and clinical applications. Circ Cardiovasc Imaging. 2015;8(6):e003029.
12. Mada RO, Lysyansky P, Daraban AM, et al. How to define end-diastole and end-systole?: Impact of timing on strain measurements. JACC Cardiovasc Imaging. 2015;8(2):148-57.
13. Yingchoncharoen T, Agarwal S, Popovic ZB, et al. Normal ranges of left ventricular strain: a meta-analysis. J Am Soc Echocardiogr. 2013;26(2):185-91.
14. Voigt JU, Pedrizzetti G, Lysyansky P, et al. Definitions for a common standard for 2D speckle tracking echocardiography: consensus document of the EACVI/ASE/ Industry Task Force to standardize deformation imaging. Eur Heart J Cardiovasc Imaging. 2015;16(1):1-11.
15. Tee M, Noble JA, Bluemke DA. Imaging techniques for cardiac strain and deformation: comparison of echocardiography, cardiac magnetic resonance and cardiac computed tomography. Expert Rev Cardiovasc Ther. 2013;11(2):221-31.
16. Choudhury A, Magoon R, Malik V, et al. Studying diastology with speckle tracking echocardiography: The essentials. Ann Card Anaesth. 2017;20(5):57-60.
17. Collier P, Phelan D, Klein A. A test in context: myocardial strain measured by speckle-tracking echocardiography. J Am Coll Cardiol. 2017;69(8):1043-56.
18. Li P, Meng H, Liu S-Z, et al. Quantification of left ventricular mechanics using vector-velocity imaging, a novel feature tracking algorithm, applied to echocardiography and cardiac magnetic resonance imaging. Chin Med J. 2012;125(15):2719-27.
19. Gorcsan J, Tanaka H. Echocardiographic assessment of myocardial strain. J Am Coll Cardiol. 2011;58(14):1401-13.

20. Negishi K, Negishi T, Kurosawa K, et al. Practical guidance in echocardiographic assessment of global longitudinal strain. JACC Cardiovasc Imaging. 2015;8(4): 489-92.
21. Marwick TH. Measurement of strain and strain rate by echocardiography: ready for prime time? J Am Coll Cardiol. 2006;47(7):1313-27.
22. Radwan H, Hussein E. Value of global longitudinal strain by two dimensional speckle tracking echocardiography in predicting coronary artery disease severity. Egypt Heart J. 2017;69(2):95-101.
23. Mada RO, Duchenne J, Voigt JU. Tissue Doppler, strain and strain rate in ischemic heart disease "How I do it". Cardiovasc Ultrasound. 2014;12:38.
24. Diao K, Yang Z, Ma M, et al. The diagnostic value of global longitudinal strain (GLS) on myocardial infarction size by echocardiography: a systematic review and meta-analysis. Sci Rep. 2017;7(1):10082.
25. Wierzbowska-Drabik K, Plewka M, Kasprzak JD. Variability of longitudinal strain in left ventricular segments supplied by non-stenosed coronary artery: insights from speckle tracking analysis of dobutamine stress echocardiograms in patients with high coronary risk profile. Arch Med Sci. 2017;13(1):82-92.
26. Yadlapati A, Maher TR, Thomas JD, et al. Global longitudinal strain from resting echocardiogram is associated with long-term adverse cardiac outcomes in patients with suspected coronary artery disease. Perfusion. 2017;32(7):529-37.
27. Liu D, Hu K, Nordbeck P, et al. Longitudinal strain bull's eye plot patterns in patients with cardiomyopathy and concentric left ventricular hypertrophy. Eur J Med Res. 2016;21(1):21.
28. Maceira AM, Tuset-Sanchis L, López-Garrido M, et al. Feasibility and reproducibility of feature-tracking-based strain and strain rate measures of the left ventricle in different diseases and genders. J Magn Reson Imaging. 2018;47(5):1415-25.
29. Vijayaraghavan G, Sivasankaran S. Tropical endomyocardial fibrosis in India: A vanishing disease! Indian J Med Res. 2012;136(5):729-8.
30. Briasoulis A, Marinescu K, Mocanu M, et al. Comparison of left ventricular contractile abnormalities in stress-induced cardiomyopathy versus obstructive coronary artery disease using two-dimensional strain imaging. Echocardiography. 2016;33(6):863-70.
31. Reant P, Mirabel M, Lloyd G, et al. Global longitudinal strain is associated with heart failure outcomes in hypertrophic cardiomyopathy. Heart. 2016;102(10): 741-7.
32. Afonso L, Kondur A, Simegn M, et al. Two-dimensional strain profiles in patients with physiological and pathological hypertrophy and preserved left ventricular systolic function: a comparative analyses. BMJ Open. 2012;2(4):e001390.
33. Saito M, Okayama H, Yoshii T, et al. Clinical significance of global two-dimensional strain as a surrogate parameter of myocardial fibrosis and cardiac events in patients with hypertrophic cardiomyopathy. Eur Heart J Cardiovasc Imaging. 2012;13(7):617-23.
34. Oyenuga OA, Onishi T, Gorcsan J. A practical approach to imaging dyssynchrony for cardiac resynchronization therapy. Heart Fail Rev. 2011;16(4):397-410.
35. Klein MR, Sundh F, Simlund J, et al. Immediate mechanical effects of acute left bundle branch block by speckle tracked strain. J Electrocardiol. 2015;48(4):643-51.
36. Aalen J, Storsten P, Remme EW, et al. Afterload hypersensitivity in patients with left bundle branch block. JACC Cardiovasc Imaging. 2018.
37. Witt CT, Kronborg MB, Nohr EA, et al. Left ventricular performance during triggered left ventricular pacing in patients with cardiac resynchronization therapy and left bundle branch block. J Interv Card Electrophysiol. 2016;46(3):345-51.
38. Hwang IC, Cho GY, Yoon YE, et al. Association between global longitudinal strain and cardiovascular events in patients with left bundle branch block assessed using two-dimensional speckle-tracking echocardiography. J Am Soc Echocardiogr. 2018;31(1):52-63.
39. Kydd AC, McCormick LM, Dutka DP. Optimizing benefit from CRT: role of speckle tracking echocardiography, the importance of LV lead position and scar. Expert Rev Med Devices. 2012;9(5):521-36.
40. Schouver ED, Moceri P, Doyen D, et al. Early detection of cardiac involvement in sarcoidosis with 2-dimensional speckle-tracking echocardiography. Int J Cardiol. 2017;227:711-6.
41. Caspar T, Fichot M, Ohana M, et al. Late detection of left ventricular dysfunction using two-dimensional and three-dimensional speckle-tracking echocardiography in patients with history of nonsevere acute myocarditis. J Am Soc Echocardiogr. 2017;30(8):756-62.
42. Govind SC, Kiotsekoglou A, Gopal AS, et al. Principles and clinical applications of strain imaging. Indian Heart J. 2011;63(2):151-64.
43. Plana JC, Galderisi M, Barac A, et al. Expert consensus for multimodality imaging evaluation of adult patients during and after cancer therapy: a report from the American Society of Echocardiography and the European Association of Cardiovascular Imaging. Eur Heart J Cardiovasc Imaging. 2014;15(10):1063-93.
44. Thavendiranathan P, Poulin F, Lim KD, et al. Use of myocardial strain imaging by echocardiography for the early detection of cardiotoxicity in patients during and after cancer chemotherapy: a systematic review. J Am Coll Cardiol. 2014;63(25 Pt A):2751-68.
45. Saini AP, Ural S, Pauliks LB. Quantitation of fetal heart function with tissue Doppler velocity imaging-reference values for color tissue Doppler velocities and comparison with pulsed wave tissue Doppler velocities. Artif Organs. 2014;38(1):87-91.
46. Joyce E, Ninaber MK, Katsanos S, et al. Subclinical left ventricular dysfunction by echocardiographic speckle-tracking strain analysis relates to outcome in sarcoidosis. Eur J Heart Fail. 2015;17(1):51-62.
47. Madeira M, Teixeira R, Costa M, et al. Two-dimensional speckle tracking cardiac mechanics and constrictive pericarditis: systematic review. Echocardiography. 2016;33(10):1589-99.
48. Kadappu KK, Thomas L. Tissue Doppler imaging in echocardiography: value and limitations. Heart Lung Circ. 2015;24(3):224-33.
49. Seo Y, Ishizu T, Aonuma K. Current status of 3-dimensional speckle tracking echocardiography: a review from our experiences. J Cardiovasc Ultrasound. 2014;22(2):49-57.
50. Patrianakos AP, Zacharaki AA, Kalogerakis A, et al. Two-dimensional global and segmental longitudinal strain: are the results from software in different high-end ultrasound systems comparable? Echo Res Pract. 2015;2(1):29-39.

CHAPTER 78

Three-Dimensional Echocardiography—Current Indications

Hardeep K Grewal, Ravi R Kasliwal

INTRODUCTION

Echocardiography, since its inception about five decades ago, has evolved to a great extent and has become the most important diagnostic tool in cardiology practice for noninvasive assessment of cardiac structure, function, and hemodynamics. The field of echocardiography has progressed from the earliest M-mode examination to two-dimensional (2D) imaging along with the development of various forms of Doppler and strain imaging. Because this modality is noninvasive, widely available, cost and time efficient and is radiation free, therefore has become the investigation of choice for various cardiac pathologies. However, 2D echocardiography (2DE) has some important limitations. Firstly, for quantification of cardiac chamber size and function, 2DE has to rely on geometric assumptions about the shape of cardiac chambers which can affect the accuracy and reproducibility of various quantitative parameters especially in patients with dilated and aneurysmal ventricles. Secondly, 2DE is a tomographic technique which provides flat views of heart and great vessels; therefore echocardiographer has to take many views and then has to mentally reconstruct the complex cardiac anatomy. These limitations have been overcome by the introduction of 3D echocardiography (3DE). Initially, this technique suffered from limitations like poor image quality as well as labor-intensive and time-consuming offline analysis. But the advancements in the ultrasound and computer processing technology have helped overcome these limitations, enabling online display of 3D images in real time (RT) with accurate, precise, and detailed assessment of cardiac structures from any spatial orientation. Although, considerable improvements are still needed before 3DE can become a truly indispensable part of echocardiographic imaging, there are several clinical conditions in which it offers definite incremental benefit.

In this review, we describe the current indications of 3DE, its incremental value over 2DE, and its limitations.

LEFT VENTRICLE ASSESSMENT

Assessment of left ventricle (LV) function and size is the most essential component of echocardiographic evaluation. There are several parameters for LV assessment like LV volumes, LV mass, LV ejection fraction (LVEF), LV regional wall motion abnormalities (LV RWMA), LV geometry and assessment of regional and global longitudinal strain.

Left Ventricle Volume and Left Ventricle Ejection Fraction

The most common assessments made using echocardiography are the LV size and LVEF calculation, and LV volumes provide estimation of both these parameters. Therefore, accurate assessment of LV volumes is essential during any echocardiographic examination. LV chamber does not have a fixed geometric shape. A healthy heart may resemble an elongated ellipse with a conical apex whereas a diseased heart may have distorted geometry. Traditionally, LV volumes are assessed by M-mode and 2DE-based methods, but all these methods suffer from technical limitations. M-mode-based formulae are based on the assumption that LV is a prolate ellipsoid and therefore, minor LV dimension is cubed to obtain LV volume. However, this assumption does not hold true in distorted ventricles as the linear measurements give information along single plane only and because one dimension is cubed so any error in the measurement also becomes very large. Therefore, the Teichholz and Quinones methods for calculating LV volumes are no longer recommended now.

Currently, recommended 2D method to assess LV volumes and LVEF is biplane method of disks (modified Simpson's method). This method is based on the principle that the total LV volume is calculated from the summation of stack of elliptical disks. In this method, LV volumes are measured by tracing the LV endocardial border from the apical four and apical two chamber views. This method has the advantage over the linear dimension method that it corrects for shape distortions and is less dependent on geometrical assumptions compared with linear dimension method. But the assumption that the ventricle can be represented by a series of stacked discs with varying diameters does not hold true in ventricles with RWMA and aneurysms. Moreover, foreshortened or off-axis views and endocardial dropout also significantly compromise the accuracy of this method. An alternative method to calculate LV volumes is area-length method especially when apical endocardial borders are not well visualized. This method is based on the assumption that LV is bullet-shaped, which again does not hold true always.

Accurate information about LV size and LVEF is important for any cardiovascular pathology from diagnostic as well as prognostic point of view. Cardiac magnetic resonance (CMR) imaging is the gold standard technique for LV quantification. But it is costly, not widely available, and requires iodinated contrast use. Moreover, CMR cannot be used in patients with implanted pacemakers and defibrillators. Adding third dimension to 2DE can overcome the limitations of both 2DE as well as of CMR imaging.

Three-dimensional echocardiography makes no geometrical assumptions about LV shape and also eliminates problems related to foreshortening and off-axis imaging because the entire LV is included in the acquired pyramidal dataset permitting proper alignment of the LV cavity (Fig. 1). The data thus acquired can be analyzed using computerized automated or semi-automated endocardial surface detection software requiring minimal manual intervention, thereby improving measurement reproducibility. The software creates a cast of LV. Within 3D dataset LV volume is calculated for each frame and plotted in the form of graph with volume against time, as shown in figure 1. LV volumes (end-diastolic and end-systolic) and EF are automatically derived from this graph and displayed. The calculation of LV volume by 3DE is found to be more accurate and reproducible when compared with conventional 2DE methods because endocardial position is measured at considerably large number of points over LV surface. Studies have shown that 3DE-based LV volumes are larger than 2DE-based values, and corresponding upper limits of the normal range are end-diastolic volumes (EDVs) of 79 mL/m^2 for men and 71 mL/m^2 for women and end-systolic volumes (ESVs) of 32 mL/m^2 for men and 28 mL/m^2 for women.[1-3]

High degree of correlation has been found between CMR-derived and 3DE-derived volume measurements.[4-8] However, several studies have shown notable underestimation of LV volumes with 3DE when compared with CMR.[2,5,8-19] Though, there are several potential reasons for such underestimation, the most likely reason seems to be the inability of 3DE to differentiate consistently between the myocardium and the trabeculae.[20] To reduce the inter-technique differences, trabeculae in the LV cavity should be included while tracing the endocardium. Another limitation of 3DE is its low temporal resolution. As a result, true end-systolic frame may not be successfully captured in single beat acquisitions. This may result in erroneous ESV calculations and EF measurements.

American Society of Echocardiography (ASE) recommends that in laboratories with experience in 3DE, 3D measurement of LV volumes and LVEF should be done, when feasible depending on the image quality.

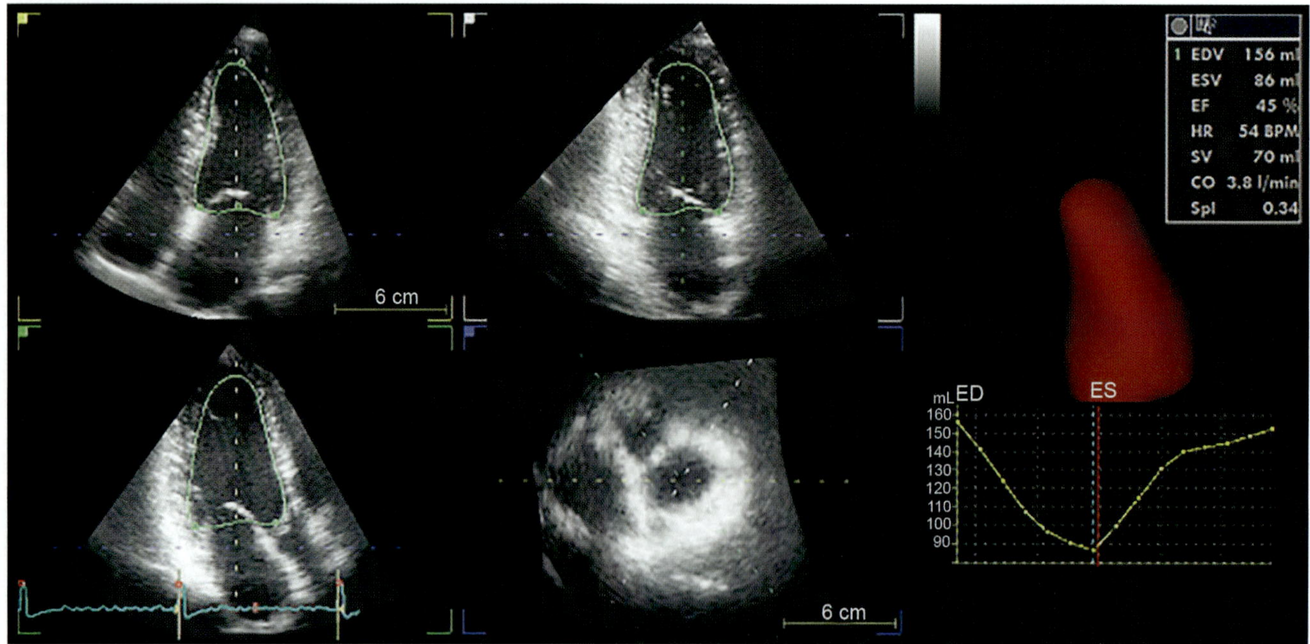

EDV, end-diastolic volumes; EF, ejection fraction; ESV, end-systolic volumes; HR, heart rate; SV: systolic volume.

FIG. 1: Estimation of left ventricular (LV) volume and ejection fraction by three-dimensional echocardiography. Single volume dataset is used. LV endocardial contour is defined in both end-diastolic and end-systolic frames and confirmed in different orthogonal planes. The analysis software then generates LV cavity cast and calculates LV volumes and ejection fraction.

Left Ventricle Mass

Left ventricle mass is a well-established prognostic marker which can independently predict adverse cardiovascular events and premature death. Because of the clinical value of LV mass, it is important to have a reliable method of its measurement. Echocardiographically, LV mass is derived from LV volume by multiplying the volume of myocardium by the myocardial density (approximately 1.05 g/mL). Therefore, all limitations of LV volume assessment are applicable to LV mass assessment also. Three-dimensional echocardiography can overcome these limitations as this is the only echocardiographic method that directly measures LV myocardial volume without any geometric assumptions regarding LV shape, therefore it is likely to provide more precise measurements of LV mass (Fig. 2).

Three-dimensional echocardiography has been found to have better interobserver agreement than 2DE.[21-23] Studies have shown that LV mass measured by 3DE has better correlation with CMR results.[4,21-30] Several studies have demonstrated the accuracy of 3DE-based measurement of LV mass, when compared to CMR, and it has been shown that the accuracy is maintained even in diseases with abnormal LV geometry as seen in hypertrophic cardiomyopathy or congenital heart diseases and in the presence of abnormal wall motion abnormalities.[25,26,31] However, one meta-analysis has suggested that LV mass measurements are more likely to be underestimated in patients with cardiac pathology than in healthy individuals.[27]

Several studies have validated the precision of 3DE-derived LV mass, however, there have been few studies determining the practicality or prognostic value of 3DE-derived LV mass estimation in large-scale clinical environments.[32] American Society of Echocardiography recommends that 3DE is preferable to 2DE, wherever feasible, for LV mass assessment, particularly in patients with asymmetric or localized hypertrophy or in distorted ventricles. However, 3DE-based LV mass data available so far in normal subjects is not enough to recommend normal reference values.

Left Ventricle Regional Wall Motion Abnormalities

The 17-segment model as suggested by ASE divides the LV into six segments (inferoseptal, anteroseptal, anterior, anterolateral, inferolateral, and inferior) at the basal and mid-ventricular level and into four segments (septal, anterior, lateral, and inferior) at the apex, with apical cap as 17th segment.[33] In 2DE, the LV needs to be scanned through different acoustic windows to image all the LV walls. Whereas in 3DE, all walls of LV can be imaged in a single volume acquisition and the entire LV can also be divided into multiple short-axis slices which can then be rotated and re-oriented at any time after acquisition and can be visualized simultaneously. These advantages, thus, allows comprehensive assessment of LV endocardial motion and myocardial thickening. The LV cast generated can be rotated on computer screen to visualize the regional contractile function of all myocardial segments. Using 3DE, a time-volume curve for each of the LV segments is displayed showing minimum and maximum volumes of that specific segment during the cardiac cycle. Hypokinetic or akinetic segments can be easily recognized by the pattern of the curve. Diseased segments have a flattened curve. This approach has been validated using CMR imaging as the standard.[17]

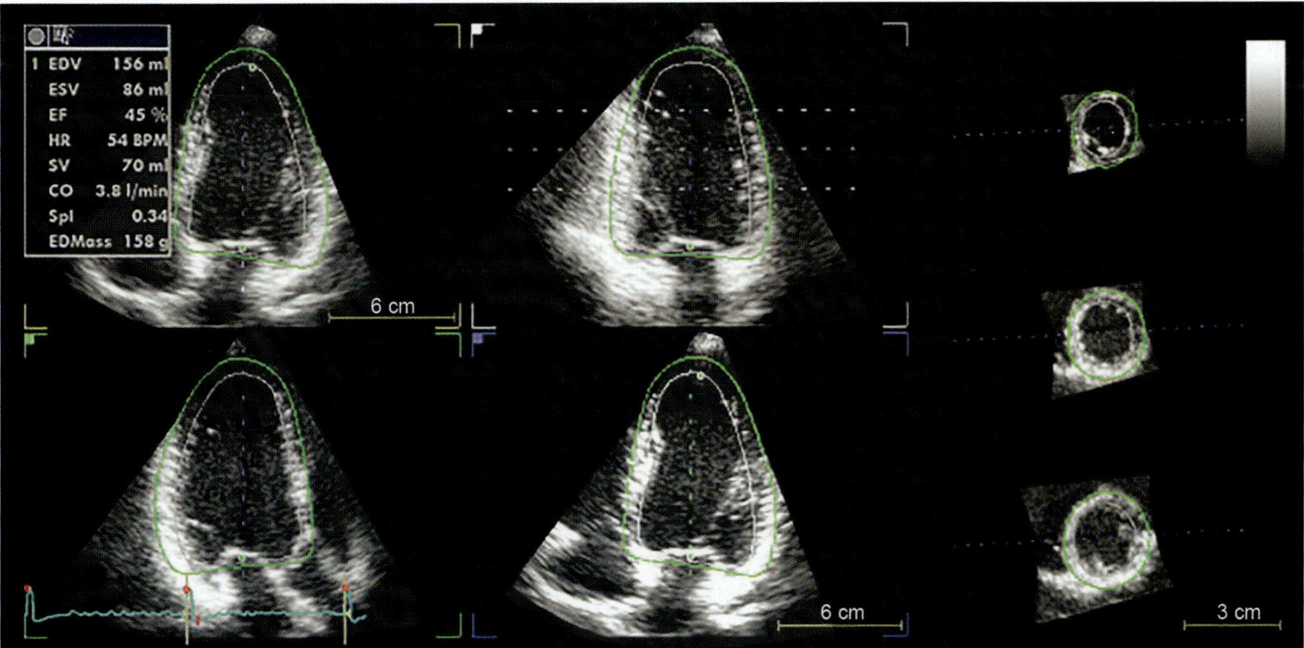

EDV, end-diastolic volumes; EF, ejection fraction; ESV, end-systolic volumes; HR, heart rate; SV, systolic volume.

FIG. 2: Estimation of left ventricular (LV) mass by three-dimensional echocardiography. Both epicardial and endocardial borders are defined, and the software automatically calculates the difference between the two volume measurements to derive LV myocardial volume and mass.

A recent observational prospective study, identified a good agreement between RT-3DE (RT3DE) and conventional 2DE in the assessment of RWMA of most segments and 3DE is found to be noninferior when compared to visual assessment by conventional 2DE. A reasonable correlation (r = 0.74) between the extent of delayed gadolinium enhancement by CMR[34] and wall motion score index by 3D-transesophageal echocardiography (3D TEE) has been reported in patients with recent myocardial infarction. It has been shown that in patients with suboptimal 3D transthoracic echocardiography (3D TTE) image quality, the use of echocardiographic contrast improves concordance of wall motion assessment with CMR.[35] Three-dimensional TTE is also useful in stress echocardiography (SE). Two-dimensional stress echocardiography (2D-SE) has its limitations because several views of the LV have to be acquired within 90 seconds of peak stress to completely visualize all LV segments. Whereas, 3DE requires only a single apical acquisition at peak stress and also avoids foreshortening, which is a frequently encountered problem in 2D-SE. This would be particularly useful in patients with rapid recovery of heart rate post-exercise. Moreover, post-processing analysis allows the assessment of images in large number of planes to ascertain the actual amount of wall motion abnormalities. Several studies have shown the feasibility of exercise and pharmacologic stress testing, with more rapid image acquisition and greater interobserver concordance in wall motion interpretation as compared to 2D TTE.[36-40] Some studies have also demonstrated that the sensitivity of 3D TTE to detect significant coronary artery disease, based on an invasive angiography as the reference standard, is equal to or better than that of 2D TTE.[36,38] Although some studies have not shown any superiority over 2D TTE.[41]

RIGHT VENTRICLE ASSESSMENT

Right ventricle (RV) has a crescent shape which wraps around the LV and can be divided into three different parts—(1) inlet, (2) apical trabecular, and (3) outlet. Because of the complex geometry, all three parts of RV cannot be visualized at the same time in 2DE and has to be imaged through multiple echocardiographic windows for complete assessment. Therefore, the conventional Simpson's method used to assess LV volumes cannot be used for RV volume assessment.

Functional assessment of RV is also difficult as the myocardial fiber orientation is different for RV when compared with LV. The RV has a poorly developed circumferential mid-layer and a longitudinal arrangement of endocardial fibers. Due to this fiber orientation, RV contracts in a peristaltic manner from inflow to outflow area. Furthermore, RV is situated anteriorly in the chest resulting in suboptimal image quality. Because of these reasons the cardiac magnetic resonance imaging (MRI) has become the gold standard as it allows RV quantification (volumes and EF) without any geometric assumptions. However, echocardiography still remains the first line imaging modality as it is widely available and time and cost efficient unlike cardiac MRI.

Two-dimensional echocardiography can assess different RV function parameters which have been found to be useful diagnostically and prognostically. However, all these parameters address RV function in an indirect manner and do not provide precise RVEF and RV volumes.[42-44] Recently, 3DE has gained acceptance for the evaluation of RV volumes and EF. Many studies, though mostly single center studies and studies conducted at centers with high level of expertise, have shown that RV assessment by 3DE is feasible, accurate, and reproducible.[2,5] A study comparing 2DE and 3DE for RV assessment showed RV volumes are significantly overestimated by 2DE by a factor of 45% and are also less reproducible than 3DE.[45] In another study of 25 patients,[46] it was demonstrated that RVEF derived from 3DE was associated with a 39% decrease in interobserver variability when compared 2DE-derived RVEF.

Several studies have shown good correlation between CMR and 3DE-derived RV volumes and EF in various clinical settings.[47-53] In one such study involving healthy individuals as well as patients with congenital heart disease and complex anatomy, RV size and function were assessed by both CMR and 3DE.[47] Both imaging modalities showed close correlation with each other for RV assessment with correlation coefficients being 0.91 for RVEF, 0.99 for RV EDV and 0.98 for ESV. The utility of 3DE-based assessment has also been demonstrated for guidance of RV endomyocardial biopsies.[54] However, data assessing the prognostic value of RV volume and RVEF is scarce. A recent study by Nagata et al.[55] has assessed the correlation between RV function and prognosis in 446 patients and the study demonstrated that RVEF assessed with 3D TTE is independently associated with cardiac outcomes and provides additional prognostic information. This study also provided the 3D RVEF cut off values to stratify prognosis of patients with different cardiac diseases: 35% for cardiac death and 41% for major adverse cardiac events.

Though studies have shown good feasibility but, in these studies, only patients with optimal image quality were included and therefore, it is difficult to extrapolate the data presented in terms of feasibility and reproducibility to everyday clinical practice. Imaging acquisition may also be difficult in patients who have dilated RV. Patients with RV pathology usually have irregular rhythm which may be source of artifacts. We need more studies to test the feasibility and reproducibility of 3DE-derived RV parameters in different clinical settings and patients. New 3D software for RV analysis is under evaluation[56] to improve accuracy and reproducibility. We hope that with newer developments in the technology RV 3D echo evaluation will become possible in everyday clinical practice.

As per recommendation by 2015 ASE guidelines for chamber quantification,[33] RV size should be routinely evaluated during echocardiography and conventional 2DE using several acoustic windows should be used as the primary approach for this purpose. However, in laboratories with experience in 3DE and when information of RV volumes may be clinically important, 3DE-based RV assessment is recommended.

LEFT ATRIAL ASSESSMENT

Left atrial (LA) size is an important prognostic factor in variety of cardiovascular diseases. Increased LA size is associated with development of atrial fibrillation (AF), stroke, and cardiovascular death.[57-59] LA size is also known as glycosylated hemoglobin of LV diastolic dysfunction as it provides information about the duration of LV diastolic dysfunction and is also a determinant of success of therapeutic procedures available for the management of AF.

Most commonly used measure of LA size is LA antero-posterior dimension obtained in parasternal long axis. However, LA volume assessment is superior over LA linear dimension, especially in patients with an enlarged left atrium.[60-63] In 2DE, LA volume is calculated by using the ellipsoidal formula or the modified Simpson method.[64,65] These formulae are also based on geometric assumptions as in LV assessment. Recent studies have shown superiority of 3DE over 2DE for estimation of LA volumes (Fig. 3).[66,67]

Recently in a study, RT3DE-derived LA volumes were compared with 64-slice computed tomography (CT) and it was found that LA volumes provided by 3DE are more precise and reproducible as compared to 2DE.[68] Similarly, in another study, 34 patients undergoing pulmonary vein isolation were enrolled and both echocardiography and CT was done to determine LA maximum and minimum volumes and LA emptying fraction. It was found that 3DE-derived measurements are more robust in terms of intra and interobserver variability[69] and also had very high degree of correlation with CT. Mor-Avi et al. performed a multicentric study and compared RT3DE LA volume against 2DE biplane volume and CMR in 92 patients.[70] It was found that CMR-derived volumes had much better correlation with 3DE for both maximum and minimum LA volumes and the biases were minimal in comparison to 2DE. Additionally, using a threshold of 34 mL/m^2, overall concordance with CMR was higher for 3DE than 2DE. In a study of 127 patients undergoing radiofrequency catheter ablation of AF, LA volumes with 3DE have also been compared with angiography and electroanatomic mapping.[68,71,72] The measurements obtained using 3DE were generally smaller than the same obtained using invasive methods. These results suggest that LA volumes assessed by angiography or electro-anatomic mapping should not be used as baseline values for noninvasive follow-up.

Although, several studies have convincingly shown that 3DE provides more accurate LA volumes than biplane 2DE,[70] it is not yet clear whether there is an additional clinical benefit of 3DE-derived LA volumes. Studies are required to determine whether the incremental precision offered by 3DE for LA size measurement really adds to the clinical decision-making.

Unlike left atrium, there is very limited data for estimation of right atrial (RA) volumes using 3DE. In a study by Keller et al.,[73] it was shown that 3DE-derived RA volume measurement is superior to 2DE-based techniques and is also comparable with CMR. A study, involving large number of healthy individuals with a wide age range,[74] provided the 3DE and 2D-speckle tracking echocardiography (STE) derived normative reference values for RA size and function. It was found that 2DE-derived RA volumes were significantly smaller than those assessed using 3DE. The 3DE-based RA volumes have shown better interobserver reproducibility than that of 2DE RA volumes.

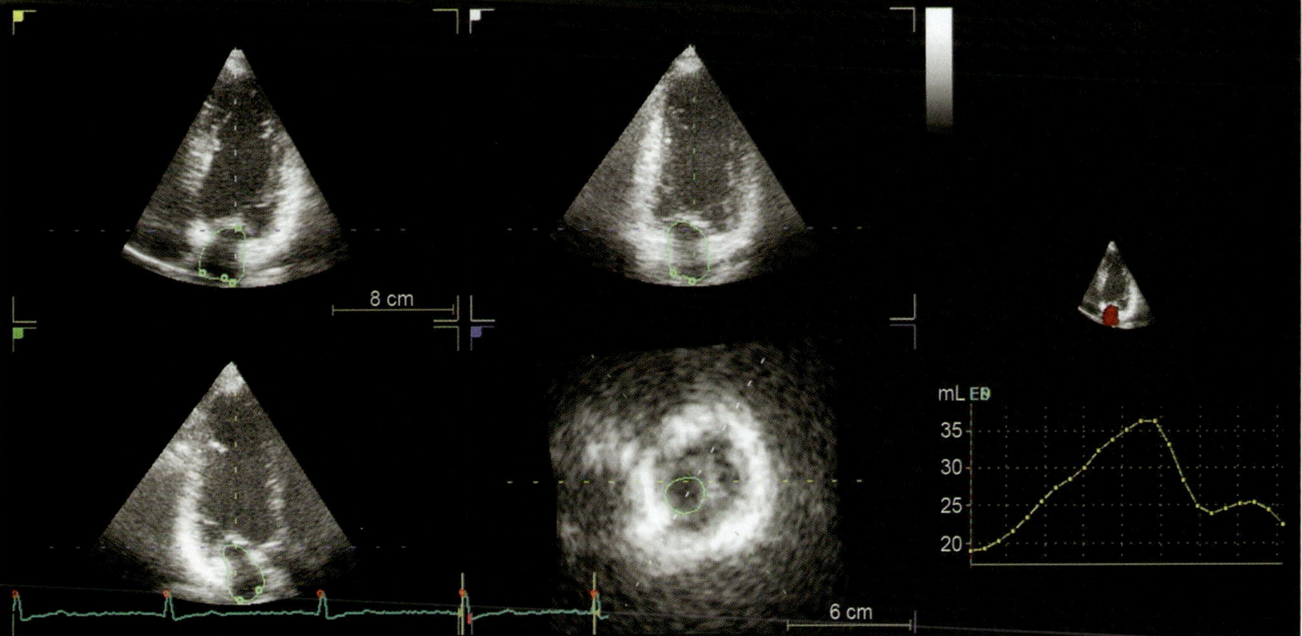

FIG. 3: Use of three-dimensional echocardiography for estimation of left atrial volume. Same principle is used as for left ventricular volume.

THREE-DIMENSIONAL STRAIN OF LEFT VENTRICLE

Two-dimensional speckle tracking strain measurement has been validated as a robust method for quantification of LV systolic function. For 2D strain, multiple views must be obtained to assess all three components of myocardial deformation (longitudinal, radial, and circumferential), but this can affect the strain measurements because of beat-to-beat variability of LV contraction. Moreover, the information collected from limited planes of LV is extrapolated for the whole LV myocardium. In 2D analysis, the out-of-plane motion of speckles due to the rotation and shortening motion of the LV cannot be quantified.[75]

Three-dimensional strain is a new technology aimed for the assessment of LV myocardial deformation and seems promising as it has the capacity to analyze all three components of strain in the same dataset.[76-80] Additionally, 3DE also provides area strain which combines the longitudinal and circumferential strain vectors, thus quantifying the deformation of the myocardial segment more comprehensively (Fig. 4). More precise LV torsion values can be obtained by simultaneous measurement of rotation in every short-axis plane and the distance between the planes. It was shown in a study of post-cardiac transplant patients with preserved LVEF that 3D speckle-tracking global longitudinal and circumferential strain, but not 2D strain, is predictive of New York Heart Association functional class.[81] These findings suggest that 3D speckle-tracking strain could be useful in predicting clinical outcomes and in various cardiac and systemic diseases. Two factors which can affect the results of 3D strain are the image quality and temporal resolution. However, we need more multicenter studies to validate this technique over the well-established 2D strain. Therefore, more data is needed to assess the reliability, feasibility, and reproducibility of this novel technique.

LEFT VENTRICLE DYSSYNCHRONY ANALYSIS

Various echocardiographic techniques have been used to diagnose intraventricular dyssynchrony in order to select patients for cardiac resynchronization therapy (CRT). Most commonly used technique for dyssynchrony evaluation is tissue Doppler method. This method has limitation that it allows simultaneous comparison of only those LV segments which are included in the scan plane which implies that all LV segments cannot be analyzed within the same cardiac cycle. LV dyssynchrony is a 3D process.[82] In this context, RT3DE can be a promising technique as it allows simultaneous dyssynchrony assessment of all myocardial segments in the same cardiac cycle.[83] The 3DE-based LV dyssynchrony assessment can be done by volumetric analysis or by tri-plane tissue synchronization imaging.[32,84] For volumetric analysis in 3DE, LV cast is divided into ASE defined 16 or 17 segments. Volume of each myocardial segment is then calculated and plotted for each cast. If all the segments of ventricle are contracting synchronously, then each segment is expected to reach its minimum volume at almost the same time during the cardiac cycle. Conversely, in a dyssynchronous LV there will be dispersion in the timing of achievement of minimum volume for each myocardial segment (Fig. 5). Systolic dyssynchrony index (SDI) can be calculated from the degree of dispersion by measuring the standard deviation of the time to achieve minimum volume. SDI can be expressed as a percentage of cardiac cycle enabling comparison between patients who have different heart rates.[83] Higher levels of dyssynchrony indicate high degree of dispersion. The

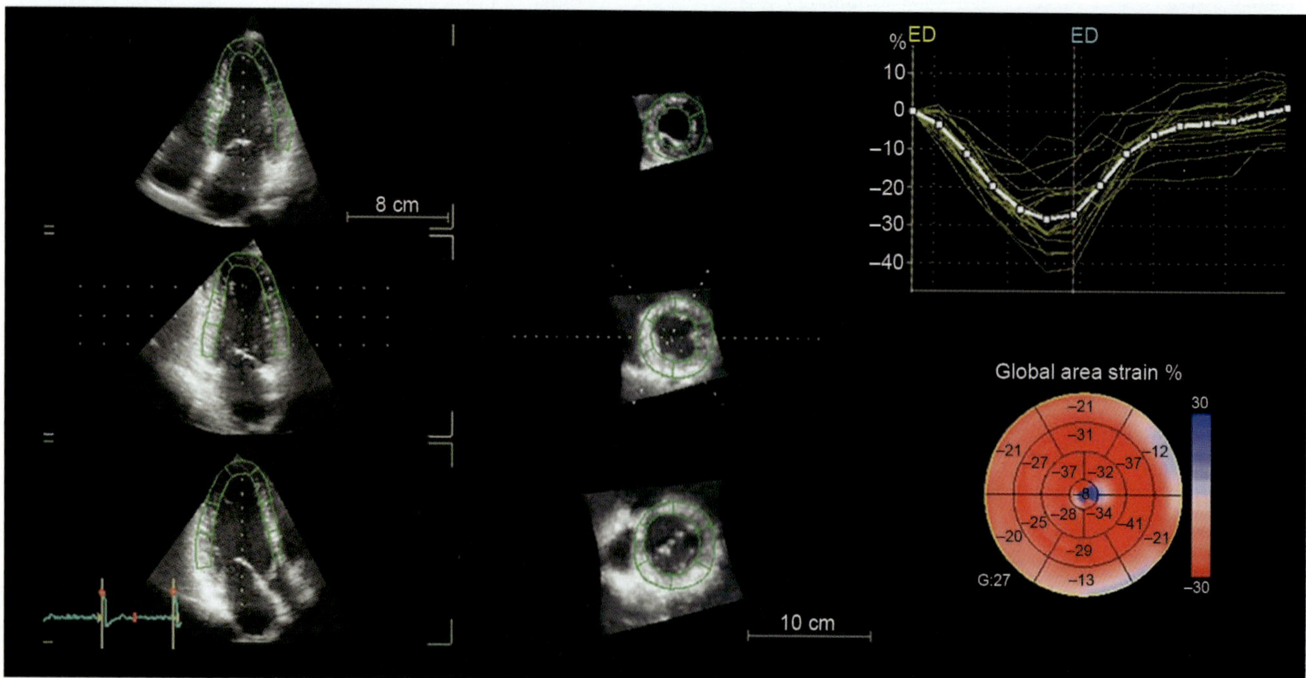

FIG. 4: Three-dimensional speckle-tracking echocardiography. From a single volume dataset, all different components of left ventricular (LV) regional and global strain are derived. Shown in this example is LV global and segmental area strain.

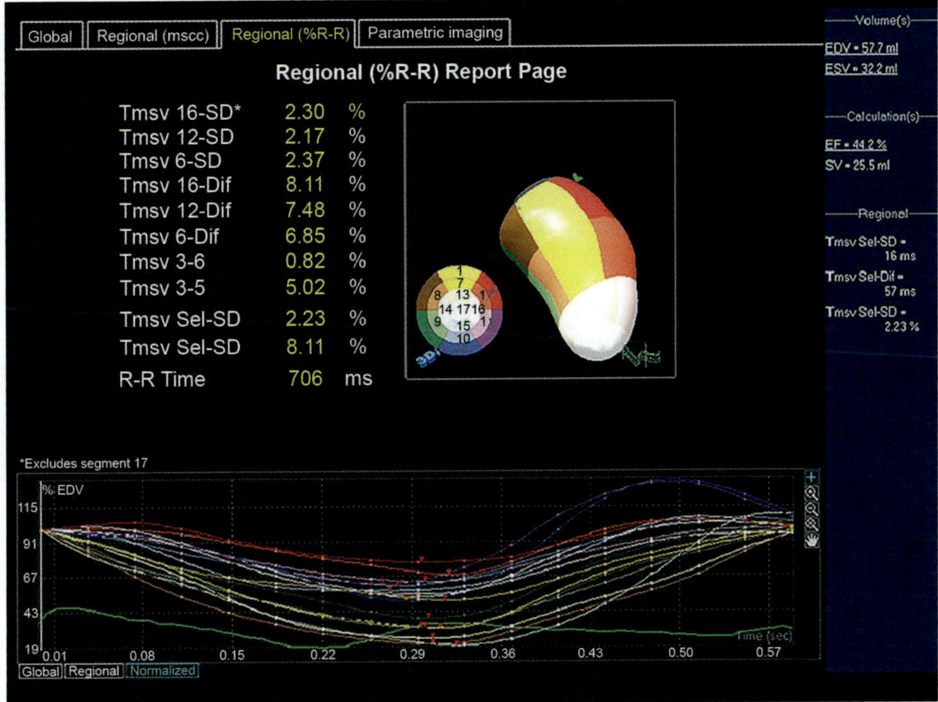

FIG. 5: Left ventricular dyssynchrony analysis by three-dimensional echocardiography. Segmental volume waveforms are created to quantify regional mechanical dispersion.

timing of contraction of different segments of LV can also be displayed in the form of parametric bull's eye. In this method, LV contraction is examined at approximately 700–800 points over the endocardial surface. Different regions of LV are color-coded according to the time of contraction and thus help in identifying the last contracting regions. This approach can be used by electrophysiologists for optimal positioning of LV electrode.

With the introduction of four-dimensional matrix phased-array transducer, triplane imaging is possible and with tissue Doppler imaging all 12-basal and mid-LV segments can be compared simultaneously from the apical window.

Real-time three-dimensional echocardiography seems promising in detecting and quantifying LV intraventricular dyssynchrony and is also useful in predicting patients who will show response to CRT and will show reverse remodeling post CRT.[85] Studies have demonstrated feasibility of RT3DE in the assessment of intraventricular LV dyssynchrony.[86] However, inter- and intra-observer reproducibility of the 3D dyssynchrony is hampered by suboptimal image quality[87] and is less robust than that of tissue Doppler imaging.[88,89] The inferior temporal resolution of 3DTTE when compared to tissue Doppler imaging is another important limitation.[90] Though with the introduction of second generation 3DE scanners, the low temporal resolution does not seem to be a major drawback for LV dyssynchrony assessment.[2] Since, 3DE measures regional volume changes and not regional velocities (as tissue Doppler imaging, which requires a high frame rate), it seems likely that echo systems using a temporal resolution of 20–30 volume/s are adequate to sample the usual frequency of regional volume curves which is less than 10Hz.[91]

Tissue Doppler methods are still considered to be the "gold standard" method for establishing dyssynchrony and it is yet to be ascertained, if 3D-based methods are superior. There is need of more data to know the accuracy, feasibility, and reproducibility of RT3DE based intraventricular dyssynchrony analysis. A reliable, clinically meaningful cut off value for the 3D dyssynchrony index remains to be established.[90] Larger, multicenter studies are required to evaluate the role of 3DE-based dyssynchrony assessment in the evaluation of patients prior to CRT.

VALVE ASSESSMENT

Three-dimensional echocardiography plays an important role in the diagnosis of valvular heart disease especially for mitral valve (MV) assessment. Image resolution, a factor of concern for transthoracic 3D imaging, has become less of an issue with the introduction of 3D TEE.

Mitral Valve

Among the four heart valves, 3DE, especially RT3D TEE, is most helpful in the diagnosis and management of MV pathologies.

Mitral Regurgitation

There are variety of mechanisms which can result in mitral regurgitation (MR). MV malcoaptation and MR can occur due to dysfunction of LV, papillary muscles, chordae tendineae, mitral annulus (MA), and the MV leaflets. Carpentier's functional classification describes the mechanism of MV dysfunction based on leaflet motion (normal motion, prolapse or restriction of a leaflet opening or closure). The rationale for treatment depends on the mechanism of MR. Therefore, it is important to identify the type and extent of leaflet motion abnormality. The 3DE provides better overall perspective in the assessment of MV pathology and severity of mitral regurgitation.

Assessment of Mitral Valve Morphology

To assess MV by 2DE, multiple views are required to scan all the segments of the two leaflets and then the operator has to mentally reconstruct the MV image. 3DE can overcome this limitation by providing the *en face* or "surgical" view of MV from the left atrium which cannot be obtained by 2DE. The image can be optimized to bring the entire leaflets and annulus into view (Fig. 6). With the help of established landmarks, the entire coaptation line can be defined from the anterolateral commissure to the posteromedial commissure, passing through the valve segments. This allows accurate assessment of each segment in relation to the MA along with evaluation of segmental prolapse or tenting in relation to the annulus. By using 3D color full volume imaging, additional smaller jets along the coaptation line and commissures can also be detected in addition to the primary jet which can result in residual regurgitation post-repair and may help the surgeon to reassess the sites of the mitral leaflet coaptation requiring attention.

Three-dimensional TEE is found to be superior to 2D TEE and 3D TTE in terms of diagnostic accuracy of localization of leaflet prolapse (96.5, 87, and 90%, respectively; $p < 0.001$)[92] and other structural defects of MV (Figs. 6 to 8). The 3D TEE is more accurate than 2D TEE at defining the extent of leaflet prolapse when compared against the surgical findings[93] (Fig. 6) and superiority is maintained even in complex cases where multiple MV segments are involved.[94] With the help of 3D TEE it was demonstrated that in MV disease, early systolic changes in MA, i.e., size reduction and deepening of MA, are less marked despite a similar amount of ventricular contraction. This ventricular-annular decoupling plays an

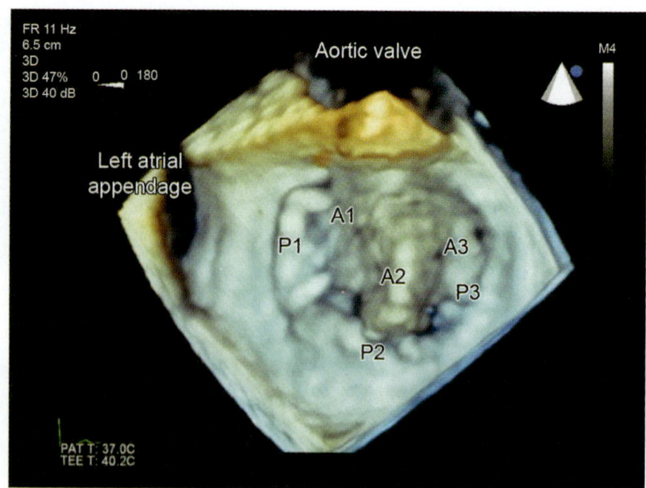

FIG. 6: *En face* view of the mitral valve as visualized from the atrial aspect. As per convention, the aortic valve is on top of the image and the left atrial appendage is towards the left side. All different scallops of anterior and posterior mitral leaflets are clearly visualized. A2 scallop prolapse can also be appreciated.

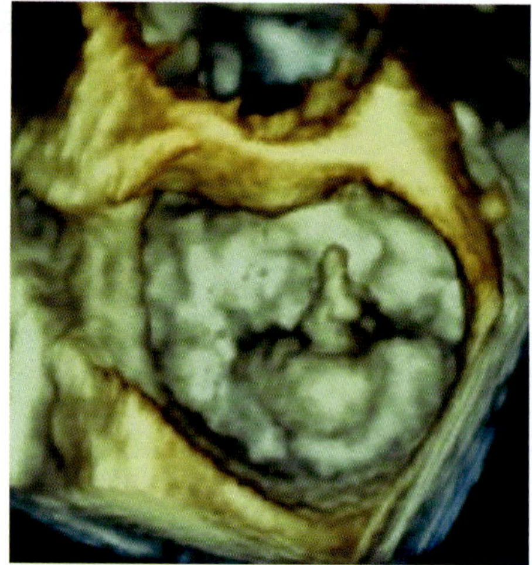

FIG. 7: Flail P2 segment of the posterior mitral leaflet. Ruptured chordae attached to the flail segment is also seen.

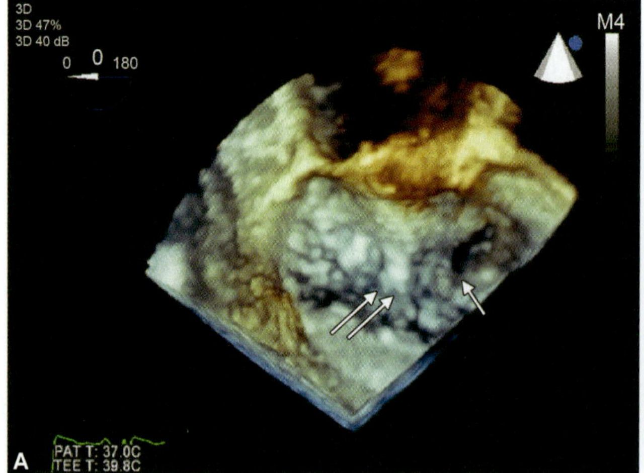

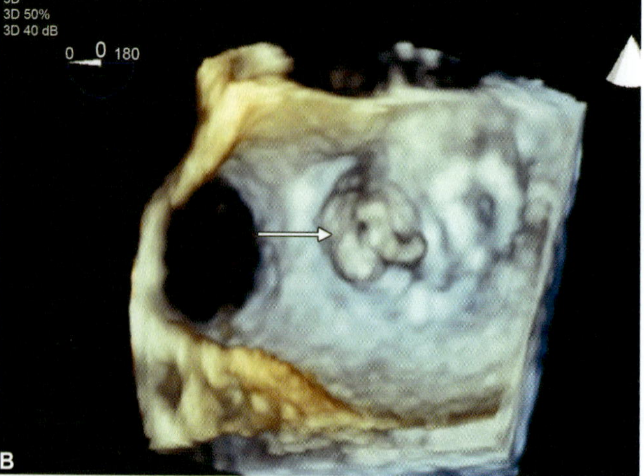

FIG. 8: Two examples highlighting utility of three-dimensional transesophageal echocardiography in the assessment of mitral valve pathologies. **A,** There is perforation in the A3 segment (single arrow) and prolapse of the A2 segment; **B,** A1 P1 segments are flail with perforation in A1 (arrow).

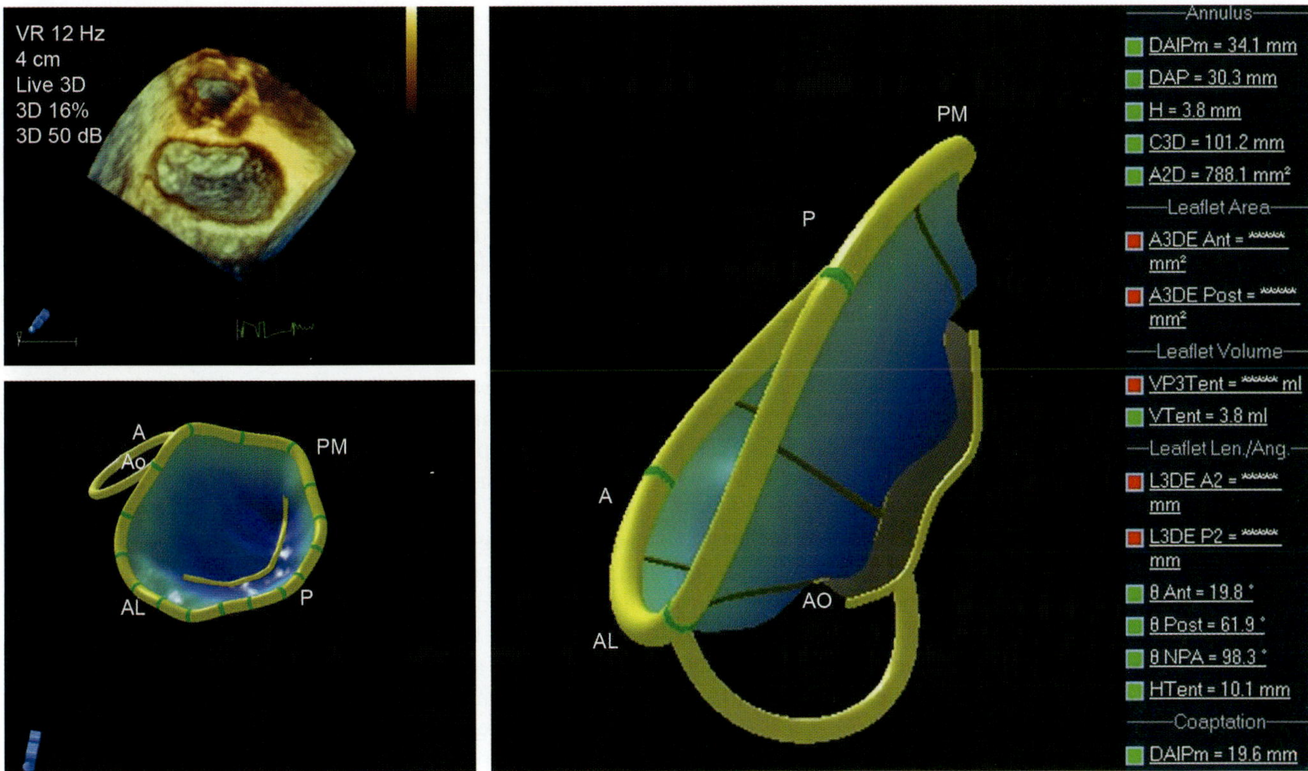

FIG. 9: Mitral valve analysis software for detailed characterization of the mitral apparatus anatomy in patients with functional mitral regurgitation.

important role in causing mitral incompetency. There is MV quantification software which enables comprehensive evaluation with precise measurements of the annulus and leaflets, aortic-mitral angles and papillary muscle position (Fig. 9) and is likely to play an important role in preoperative planning of MV repair in the future. However, there is limited published data on its clinical use.

Assessment of Mitral Regurgitation Severity

Methods used to quantify MR severity are vena contracta (VC) and proximal isovelocity surface area (PISA) assessment. PISA allows the calculation of effective regurgitant orifice area and regurgitant volume.[95] The conventional PISA method assumes a hemispheric shape of the isovelocity surface, which is usually not the case. Assessment of the severity of MR by 2DE can be challenging, particularly with eccentric jets. Three-dimensional color Doppler enables better assessment of the origin, shape, and size of jets.[96,97] The novel 3D techniques allow evaluation of the correct shape of proximal flow convergence region resulting in more precise measurement of the VC and PISA (Fig. 10).[98,99] The 3D-derived data has provided better insight in understanding the shape of the regurgitant orifice.[100] PISA is more spherical in degenerative MV disease and more elongated and elliptical in functional MR and this partly explains the discrepancies in regurgitation severity by 2D PISA methods. Underestimation of MR can be reduced from 49 to 26% with application of hemi-ellipsoid formula.[101] The VC area determined by color Doppler 3DE has also been found to be useful for quantification of MR.[99,102-105] Studies have shown that there are variety of VC shapes in functional MR patients.[103] The idea of 3D VC seems promising as it is free from geometric assumptions. Despite these advances, the routine clinical use is limited as the analysis by these methods is time-consuming. Moreover, factors like image resolution, dependence on multiple cardiac cycles (7-14 cycles) and narrow sector acquisitions increase the chances of artifacts.

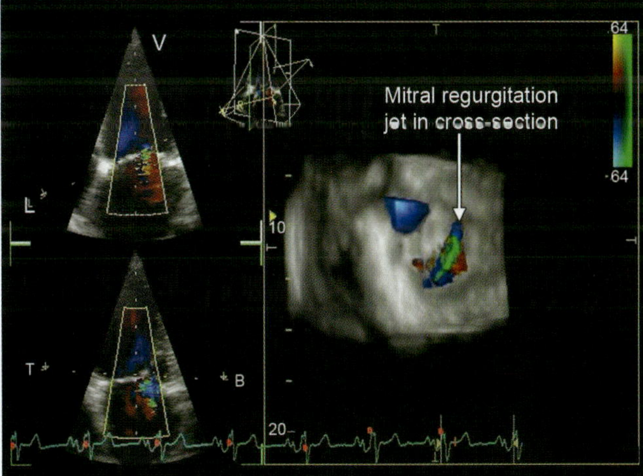

FIG. 10: Use of three-dimensional echocardiography for visualization and quantification of the shape and the size of the mitral regurgitation vena contracta.

Mitral Stenosis

Transthoracic echocardiography is usually sufficient to assess mitral stenosis (MS) severity. TEE is usually done to exclude intracardiac thrombi before a percutaneous or surgical intervention. Quantification of MS severity is usually described in terms of mean transmitral gradient and mitral orifice area.[106] The "effective" mitral orifice area can be calculated by Doppler-derived methods like pressure half-time measurement (PHT), continuity equation, and PISA method. However, these methods are influenced by many factors like heart rhythm, tachycardia, nonlinear Doppler velocity curves and associated valvular disease, and are also not reliable in the immediate post-balloon valvuloplasty period. Therefore, direct planimetry is favored to measure the true MV orifice area. This is considered to be the reference method in clinical practice. It has also been shown that this method is more closely related with the anatomic MV area (MVA) when compared with explanted valves.[107] However, obtaining the narrowest mitral orifice opening with 2D planimetry requires considerable experience and may be specifically difficult when the stenotic MV forms a funnel shape and the orifice is placed obliquely. Moreover, there is no definitive anatomical landmark to make sure that the short-axis view used to trace the MV orifice is the narrowest one, which can lead to underestimation of MS severity.[108]

Three-dimensional echocardiography can overcome the limitations of 2D MV planimetry as it allows cropping of the 3D data set and defines the true MV anatomic area. Multiplanar 3D imaging can also be used to display the orifice in both the long and the short axis. MVA planimetry by 2DE was compared with MVA by 3D TEE in 87 patients. It was demonstrated that 2D planimetry tends to overestimate MV orifice area when compared with 3D TEE measurements especially in patients with a large left atrium.[109] 3DE-based MVA is more accurate and reproducible with superior interobserver and intraobserver concordance when compared with MVA by 2D planimetry and PHT (Fig. 11).[109-111] Sugeng et al.[111] demonstrated that direct 3D planimetry of MV from ventricular aspect is the most accurate method for MVA estimation. Studies have also shown that 3DE derived MVA is highly correlated with those obtained from invasive catheter measurements using Gorlin's formula[112] in both rheumatic and calcific mitral stenosis.[113,114] Additionally, 3DE is also useful in detailed morphological assessment of mitral valvular and subvalvular apparatus which is particularly important in candidates undergoing balloon mitral valvotomy. Reliable 2D planimetry is difficult when the MV leaflets have significantly calcification. This limitation can be overcome by 3D TEE by imaging the mitral orifice from the LA *en face* view because calcific shadowing is on the ventricular side.

Percutaneous balloon mitral valvuloplasty (PBMV) is an effective therapeutic modality in selected patients with MS. Main predictor of a successful PBMV is MV morphology. Wilkins' score, based on valve structure, is most commonly used 2DE-based scoring system to predict the procedural success for mitral valvuloplasty. Anwar et al.[115] introduced a new 3DE-based score for evaluating patients with MS before valvuloplasty. This score involves the assessment of both mitral valvular and subvalvular apparatus. This score is found to be feasible and reproducible with good interobserver and intra-observer agreement in the evaluation of MV morphology in MS and can provide incremental prognostic information in addition to Wilkins' score.

The 3DE is also better in detecting complication as it can determine clearly if the increase in valve area is due to commissural splitting or leaflet tearing

Aortic Valve

Aortic valve (AV) has oblique orientation and is more complex than just its three semilunar cusps. AV with aortic root is called as AV complex and can be evaluated by TTE and TEE but for complete assessment of its complex geometry, it has to be imaged through multiple echo windows. With 3DE we can image AV from different prospective with no erroneous geometric assumptions.

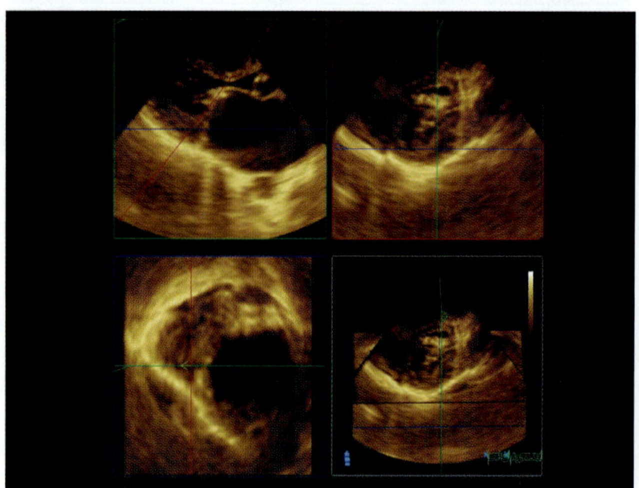

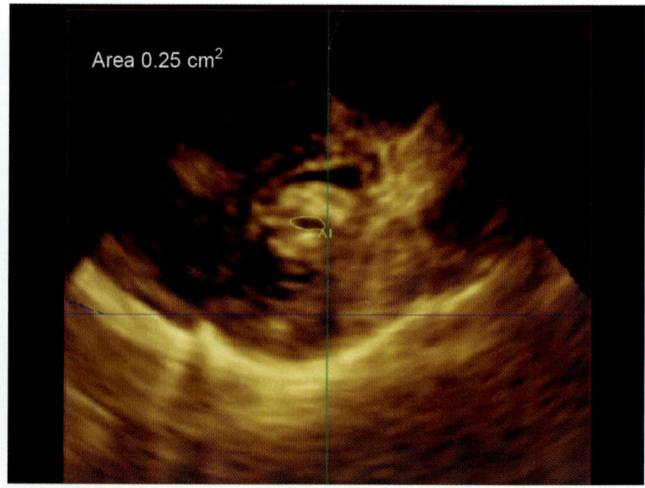

FIG. 11: Mitral valve area planimetry using three-dimensional echocardiography in a patient with rheumatic mitral stenosis. Three-dimensional echocardiography allows accurate alignment of the imaging plane at the leaflet tips so that correct measurement of mitral valve area can be performed.

Aortic Stenosis

Quantification of aortic stenosis (AS) by echocardiography is based on the measurement of gradients derived from transaortic velocities and valve area derived from continuity equation.[106] The 2DE-based calculation of the AV area (AVA) by continuity equation is based on various assumptions: firstly, left ventricular outflow tract (LVOT) is circular and can be described by its anteroposterior diameter in parasternal long-axis view; secondly, the cut plane is exactly parallel to LVOT; thirdly, pulse wave Doppler of LVOT flow is obtained at the same site where the LVOT diameter is measured. Because the LVOT area calculation involves the squaring of LVOT diameter, the LVOT diameter is a potential source of error in the AVA calculated by continuity equation.[106] Accurate measurement of LVOT geometry and size is an essential component in the quantitation of AS severity. Correct size is also important for calculating stroke volume and during interventions like transcatheter aortic valve implantation (TAVI) or for guiding the muscle reduction therapeutic procedures in hypertrophic obstructive cardiomyopathy. It has been shown by both multi-slice cardiac tomography (MSCT) and 3DE studies that LVOT has an elliptical configuration rather than a circular one.[116,117] Therefore, LVOT and aortic annulus calculation by 2DE may not give correct values. Three-dimensional TEE has the potential to overcome this limitation of 2DE by direct planimetry of aortic annulus and LVOT areas. LVOT or aortic annulus area by 3D TEE (Fig. 12) has shown good correlation with gold standard MSCT. Even the LVOT area derived from 3D TTE biplane imaging has shown improved accuracy in the stroke-volume measurement[118] and AS severity quantification, when compared with direct planimetry.[119] Studies have demonstrated that LVOT diameter-based calculations by either 2DE or 3DE result in significant underestimation of AVA (by 16.4% and 12.9%, respectively).[120] Quantification of AV complex geometry by 3D TEE has also shown good correlation with the measurements obtained by MSCT.[121] Since, 3DE-derived LV volumes has good accuracy and reproducibility, LV stroke volume can also be calculated by subtracting the end-systolic from the end-diastolic 3D LV volume. This can overcome the limitation of conventional continuity equation.[4] This approach has also been found to have better correlation with the invasive AV area calculation by Gorlin's equation than by using conventional continuity equation.[122]

In certain cases of AS, Doppler methods are not reliable to assess AS severity, as in patients with small aorta, subaortic

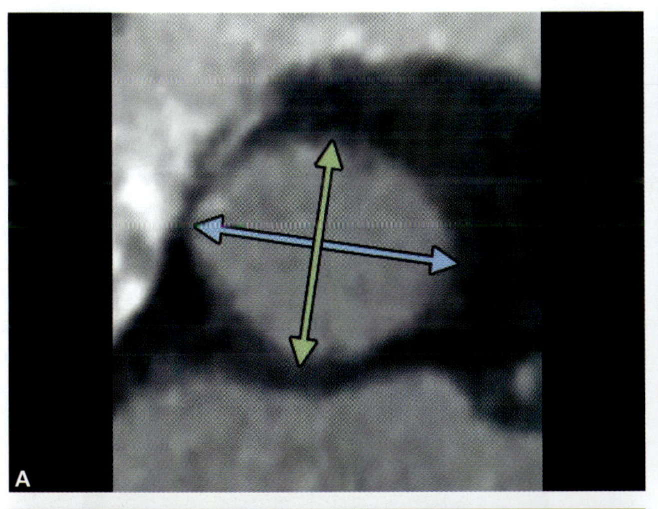

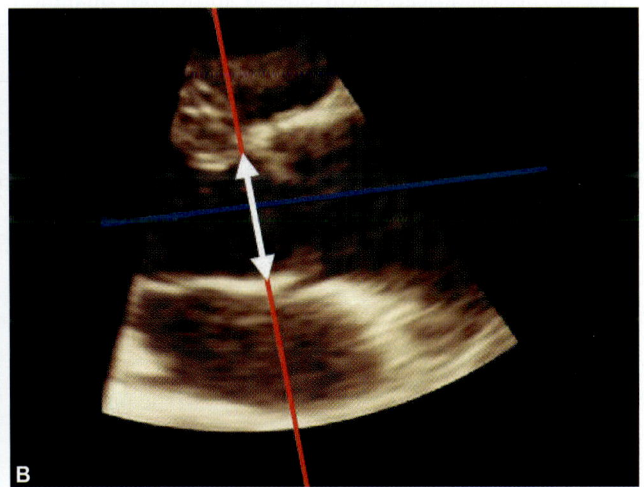

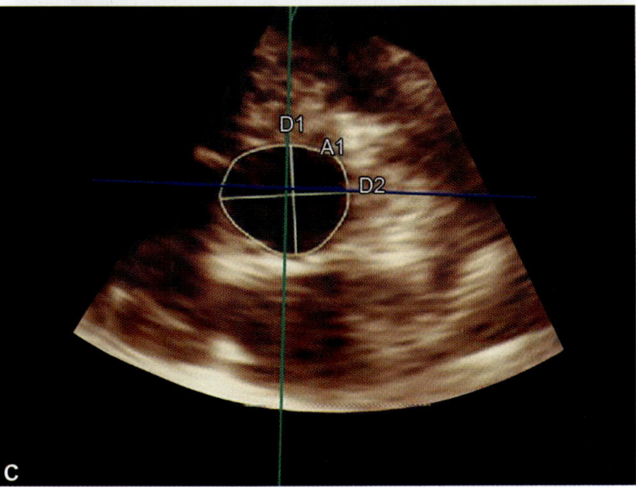

FIG. 12: Advantage of three-dimensional echocardiography for measurement of left ventricular outflow tract (LVOT) area. **A,** Computed tomography reveals oval shape of the LVO; **B,** Single measurement in two-dimensional imaging is likely to underestimate LVOT area; C, Three-dimensional echocardiography permits measurement of true LVOT area.

stenosis, significant aortic regurgitation (AR) and LV dysfunction. In these cases, direct AV planimetry becomes important for diagnosis. AVA by 2DE planimetry is prone to errors as there are high chances of off-axis imaging of the AV orifice which is a nonplanar 3D structure, especially in diseases like bicuspid or degenerative valve disease when the orifice is distorted. In addition, aortic annulus shows movement during cardiac cycle with more caudal position during isovolumic relaxation and cranial movement during early systole.[123] Therefore, fixed 2D cut plane frequently shows larger AV orifice area rather than true narrowest opening leading to overestimation of AVA.[124] The 3D TEE planimetry has shown better accuracy than 2D TEE.[125] Moreover, 3DE also provides information about valvular as well as subvalvular stenosis.

However, AVA planimetry by both 3DE and 2DE is not reliable when there is significant valvular calcification, as orifice tracing will be difficult due to artifacts like shadowing or reverberations, and also in low cardiac output states, as the anatomic area of AV opening is reduced. Another limitation of 3DE is its lower frame rate which hampers its ability to precisely capture the maximum systolic opening of the aortic cusps.

Aortic Regurgitation

Aortic regurgitation can occur due to aortic root dilatation or due to valvular abnormalities such as a bicuspid AV, rheumatic heart disease and degenerative valvular disease. RT-3D TEE can reveal important anatomical differences in various AV diseases causing AR.[126] AR severity is assessed by various qualitative and quantitative 2DE-based Doppler techniques. Most commonly used method is the ratio of AR jet width immediately below the AV to the inner LVOT width taken in the same frame. Another parameter is VC, which is the size of the jet within the leaflets and extending for a small extent into the LVOT. The assessment of exact size and shape of the VC is important in the quantification of regurgitant lesions. Generally, VCA is considered circular or elliptical, but this assumption is usually incorrect.[127] In the parasternal long-axis or apical views, only one dimension of the AR jet is visualized. Therefore, the measured size or area is based on an assumption regarding its shape. A parasternal short-axis view at the level of the AV leaflets on 2DE with color Doppler would probably define the VCA in 3D, but because of cardiac motion, it is difficult to ensure that the measured jet size is within the leaflets and not further downstream where it tends to be larger. For reliable VCA measurements short axis echo plane should be exactly parallel to the VC, which is difficult to ensure on 2DE. Whereas, a pyramidal dataset, acquired by RT3D echo, can be cropped in multiple transverse planes at any desired angle and this allows the alignment of the plane exactly parallel to the VC in a short-axis or perpendicular to the direction of AR jet in long axis, at or just below the AV level. This approach has good accuracy, when compared with magnetic resonance, angiography or comprehensive conventional Doppler evaluation.[128-130] The 3DE-derived regurgitant volume was found to have high correlation to the velocity encoded-MRI-derived regurgitant volume (r = 0.94 and –13.6 to 15.6 mL/beat, respectively). The 3DE has the potential to obviate the limitations of 2DE color Doppler and is a useful supplement to 2D TTE.

Tricuspid Valve

Tricuspid valve (TV) assessment is very important in many cardiovascular diseases. The valve has three leaflets—septal, anterior, and posterior, but all three leaflets cannot be well visualized in one view using either TTE or TEE. Whereas, 3DE provides *en face* views of TV and thus enables visualization of the entire TV from any perspective. "*En face*" views (Fig. 13) may be particularly useful in localizing leaflet pathology such as prolapse, vegetations, or perforation and are also helpful in localizing the origin of regurgitant jets and performing planimetry of the tricuspid orifice area. In patients with optimal transthoracic acoustic window, evaluation of TV anatomy and function with 3D TTE is often feasible, though its evaluation requires more experience compared with MV 3D evaluation.[131]

Tricuspid Regurgitation

Tricuspid regurgitation (TR) can be classified into two main categories—primary TR and secondary TR. Primary TR occurs when there is leaflet abnormality as seen in Ebstein's anomaly, carcinoid heart disease, and TV prolapse. In secondary TR, valve leaflets are normal and TR is caused by abnormalities of the structures supporting the valves, such as dilatation of tricuspid annulus (TA) and/or RV dilatation and dysfunction or pulmonary hypertension. The 3DE has been found to be advantageous over 2DE for assessment of TV pathologies and the location of the TR orifice.[132-134] This modality is also useful in patients with intracardiac devices to detect the location of lead and its relationship to valve leaflets and significant TR.[135-137] One of the studies revealed that 45 out of 100 patients had TV leaflet interference due to device lead and most commonly affected is septal leaflet. Device lead

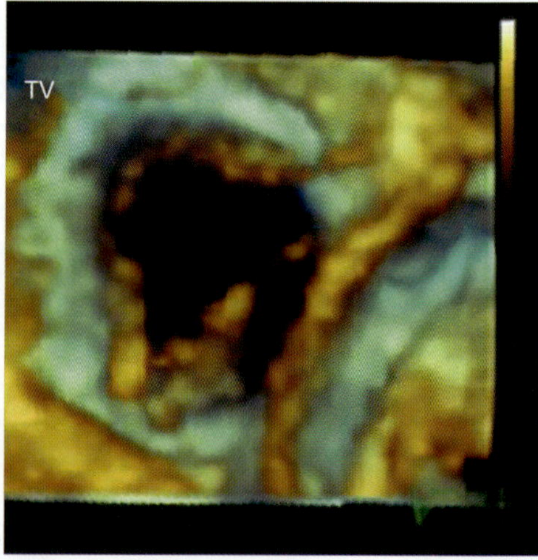

FIG. 13: *En face* view of the tricuspid valve as visualized from the ventricular aspect. All three tricuspid valve leaflets are visualized simultaneously.

interference increases the likelihood of developing significant TR by more than 10-fold.[136] TR is less commonly seen when the lead is placed in a commissural position.[135] Therefore, it was suggested that 3DE should also be done to assess lead interference in patients with significant TR.[136] Three-dimensional echocardiography also allows us to locate the anatomical regurgitant orifice of TR and to measure the VC, which was found to be more often ellipsoid than circular.[138]

Tricuspid Annulus

Tricuspid annulus (TA) size and function plays vital role in the genesis of secondary TR. The accurate analysis of the TA is also required to assess the need for a combined procedure on the TV in patients undergoing cardiac surgery for left-sided valve diseases. Significant TA dilatation is defined by a diastolic diameter more than 21 mm/m^2 or more than or equal to 40 mm in the four-chamber transthoracic view, and is considered as a criterion for concomitant tricuspid procedure in case of left-sided valve surgery.[139]

The TA is a complex nonplanar oval structure. Dilatation of the TA occurs mainly in the septolateral direction, resulting in more circular shape.[140] The recommended 2D transthoracic view for measurement of TA diameter is the apical four-chamber view[139,141] as this view has better inter-observer agreement compared with other views.[142] The TA diameter varies according to the site of measurement, with reference values ranging between 25 mm and 39 mm.[143,144] It's a dynamic structure and shows variability in size during the cardiac cycle, with an approximately 20% reduction in annular circumference with atrial systole.[145] Studies have shown that the diameter of TA is consistently underestimated by 2DE whereas 3D TTE obtained diameters has shown better correlation with those obtained from MRI.[146] Various studies have revealed that 3DE-based analysis of TA geometry and size has shown good feasibility.[139,143,144,147-151] Various measurements can be obtained from 3DE, including major and minor TA diameters, TA fractional shortening, TA area, and TA fractional area change. The 3DE has determined that not only dilatation, but structural modifications of TA also contribute in the genesis of functional TR. The extent of TV tethering can also be quantified with 3D echocardiography in terms of the tenting volume and tenting angle of the three leaflets.[152,153] All these parameters such as quantification of TA enlargement, the mode of leaflet coaptation and the degree of tenting are significantly important in making a surgical decision about TV repair or replacement. Normative data about TA diameter and function are limited. In fact, the 2D view and in which phase of cardiac cycle TA should be measured is still a matter of debate.[145] Because TA diameter is usually underestimated by 2DE, it seems necessary to redefine normal TA values with 3D imaging. Furthermore, more complicated analysis of the nonplanarity of TA can also be performed from 3D acquisitions, which have potentially important mechanistic and therapeutic implications for TV repair.[143,147]

Tricuspid Stenosis

Most common cause of tricuspid stenosis (TS) is rheumatic heart disease, affecting up to 8% of patients.[154] The 2DE estimates the severity of TS by detecting the thickening of TV leaflets, restricted valve opening and by estimation of the tricuspid transvalvular pressure gradient by continuous wave Doppler.[155] However, on 2DE it is not possible to visualize all three leaflets simultaneously and therefore, planimetry of TV area is not possible with 2DE. RT3D-TEE provides short-axis views of the valve with simultaneous viewing of the three leaflets and their junction with the annulus, enabling planimetry of TV with high accuracy. As of now we have limited data on the use of 3DE in patients with TS and we need more studies to assess its feasibility and accuracy. However, the additional knowledge obtained by 3DE can still be useful in the diagnostic and therapeutic decision making in patients with TV involvement.

Infective Endocarditis

Transesophageal echocardiography plays a pivotal role in the diagnosis and management of infective endocarditis (IE). Therefore, TEE is done in almost all suspected cases of IE.[156] The 2D TEE has sensitivity of 85–90%, with a specificity of approximately 90–100% in the detection of vegetation[157] and is also useful in evaluating complications of IE like abscess (sensitivity 90% and specificity 90%)[158] fistulae, pseudoaneurysms, and perforated leaflets. 3DE can provide better visualization about the entire cardiac structure so, it may have an incremental value over 2DE, especially when large vegetation are present. Hansalia et al.[159] compared 3D TEE and 2D TEE in 13 patients with valvular vegetation and concluded that during surgery 3D TEE was superior in determining the overall presence and exact site of valvular vegetation. These authors also suggested the possibility that 3D TEE can measure the volume of vegetation, and they showed low interobserver variability between measurements performed by means of 3DE. The improved spatial orientation of 3D TEE can provide better information regarding the relationship between vegetation, prosthesis, and adjacent structures. These advantages of 3DE might enable better risk stratification, surgical decision-making, and operative planning. In one study, it was found that[160] only 48% of abscesses detected intraoperatively correlated with preoperative 2D TEE findings. Because abscesses are not limited to specific tissue planes and can extend in directions beyond the planes, 2D TEE may not provide complete information. Moreover, 3D TEE has been found to be superior in identifying the sequelae of IE in prosthetic heart valves, especially in locating and evaluating prosthetic dehiscence, perivalvular abscesses, and valvular perforation.[159,161-164] At present 3D TEE should be used as a supplement to standard 2D and its major limitation, i.e. low frame rate should always be kept in mind as it may impair detection of smaller vegetation.

Prosthetic Valves

Transesophageal echocardiography provides better images of prosthetic valves than TTE. However, 2D TEE can fail to identify important findings as the entire prosthetic valve cannot be seen in single image. RT3D TEE allows comprehensive imaging of prosthetic valve components and is also useful in detecting associated complications (Fig. 14). This is extremely helpful in the evaluation of mechanical prosthetic valves where 2D image quality is usually suboptimal due to acoustic shadowing. Because 3D images can be cropped into multiple planes, deeper cardiac structures can be visualized more clearly when compared to 2D TEE. The 3D TEE has been found to be particularly helpful in the assessment of prosthetic valve endocarditis[165] as the "*en face*" view of prosthetic valves allows the identification of valve dehiscence, para-prosthetic leaks and involvement of adjacent cardiac structures. It has been shown that 3D imaging identifies additional vegetations which are not seen on 2D TEE[165] and can also help in distinguishing vegetation from loose suture material.

These advantages of 3D TEE can help in complete assessment of the prosthetic AV and MV and associated complications (Fig. 15).[166] Although, the visualization scores for AV are lower than for MV prostheses.[166]

TRANSCATHETER INTERVENTIONS FOR VALVULAR HEART DISEASE

Recently transcatheter valve implantation and repair have emerged as promising therapeutic procedures for patients with valvular heart disease. Procedures like TAVI and mitraclip have been found to be noninferior when compared to surgery in high-risk patients. Echocardiography plays a central role in selecting suitable patients for these interventions and for monitoring of patients during and after the procedure. The 3DE is particularly useful in intra-procedural guidance as it allows visualization of cardiac structures in RT and therefore, facilitates safe manipulation of catheters, guide wires and device deployment. The 3DE helps in achieving high success rates in these procedures while avoiding potential complications.

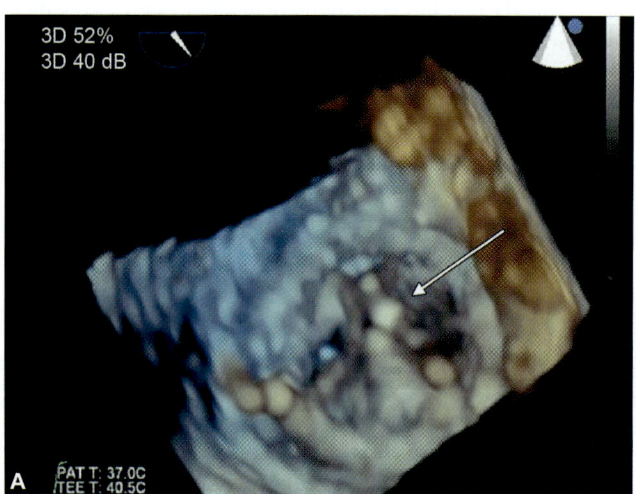

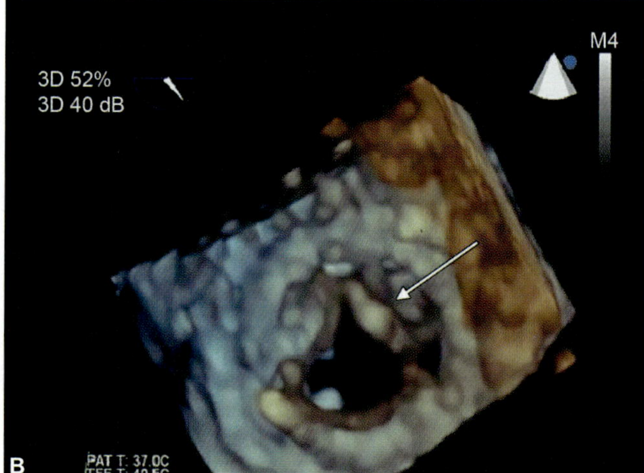

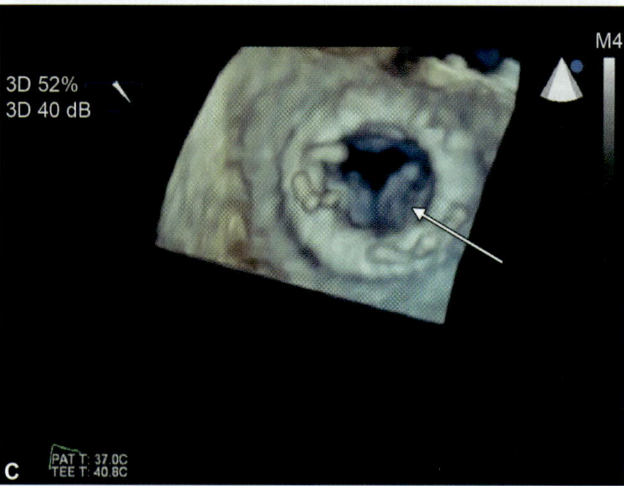

FIG. 14: Three-dimensional transesophageal echocardiography for the assessment of prosthetic mitral valve dysfunction. **A** and **B,** One of the leaflets (arrow) of the bioprosthetic valve is thickened and completely immobile; **C,** The same valve visualized from the atrial side. Diastolic frame is shown. One of the leaflets is not open (arrow), whereas the other leaflet is only partially open.

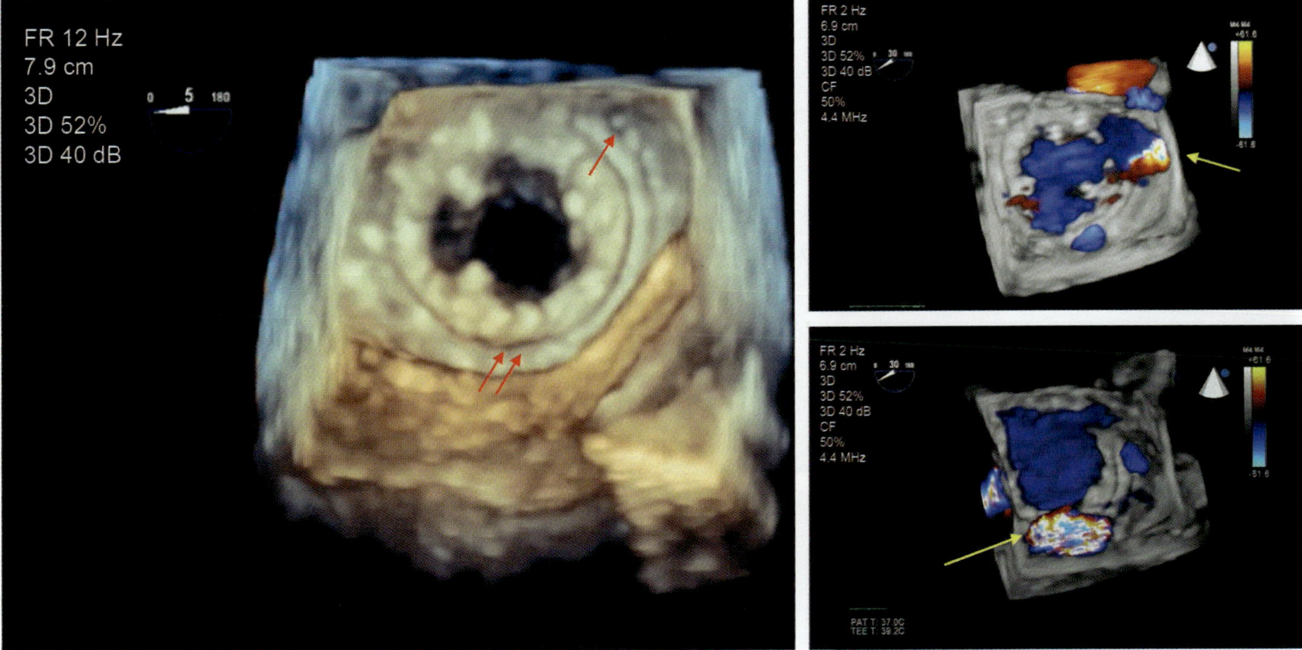

FIG. 15: Paravalvular defects around a bioprosthetic mitral valve. Left—gray scale image showing the location of the defects (arrows); Right—color Doppler confirming the presence of mitral regurgitation through these defects.

Paravalvular Leak (PVL) Closure

Transcatheter closure of PVL requires accurate assessment of the number, site and size of each defect and its relationship to the prosthesis and suture ring (Fig. 15). RT3D TEE, when compared with 2D TEE, is found to be superior in assessing these parameters as 3DE provides *en face* views of the prosthesis from both ventricular and atrial prospective. As a result, it helps in deciding if the procedure is feasible in a patient and it also shortens the procedure time because it facilitates catheter manipulation, device sizing and positioning. RT3D TEE has been found to be especially helpful during atrial trans-septal puncture and in guide wire and catheter manipulation through the defect (Fig. 16). 3D imaging is particularly advantageous as it allows visualization of the whole length of the intracardiac catheters and the attached devices and their position in relation to surrounding structures.[167,168] 3D TEE plays an important role in choice of closure device, as well as the adequacy and success of the procedure.[169] Currently, for occlusion of small paravalvular leaks Amplatzer patent ductus arteriosus (PDA) device are used and Amplatzer ventricular septal defect devices are used to occlude larger paravalvular leaks (Figs. 16 and 17).

Transcatheter Aortic Valve Replacement (TAVR)

One of the most important component affecting the procedural success of transcatheter aortic valve replacement (TAVR) is the precise measurement of AV annulus and the aortic root for appropriate selection of the prosthesis type and valve size.[170] The 3DE-based techniques have shown that the aortic annulus is oval in shape and not circular as assumed in 2DE-based calculations. The 2DE under-estimates maximum aortic annulus dimension due to off-axis imaging.[171] Accurate assessment of aortic annulus has been done by 3D TEE-guided direct planimetry and has been shown to have good correlation with results from multidetector CT (MDCT).[120] Another important measurement for the feasibility of TAVR is the distance of the annulus to the coronary artery ostia. This is usually measured by MDCT. The 2D TEE can measure the distance of aortic annulus to right coronary ostia but the annular ostial distance for left main coronary sinus cannot be measured as it lies in a plane which is not possible to image by 2D TEE. However, this distance can be measured by 3D TEE. Therefore, 3D TEE is an alternative option for these measurements especially in patients who are at higher risk of contrast-induced nephropathy. Compared to 2D, 3D TEE provides better guidance during the procedure like in guide wire manipulation while it passes through the LV, for adequate positioning of the prosthesis in relation to the native valve annulus and surrounding structures.

Mitraclip

Transesophageal echocardiography is an important imaging modality used at all stages of mitraclip procedure. Use of 3D TEE is required for adequate guidance of the clip delivery system towards the MV as 3D TEE provides better understanding of spatial relationship of clip delivery system with the surrounding structures like LA wall and MV. Three-dimensional views are useful in maneuvering the catheters in the LA cavity without touching the wall of LA and also helpful in ensuring that mitraclip device remains perpendicular to the commissure. The 3DE provides *en face* views of the repaired MV which are helpful in confirming the adequacy

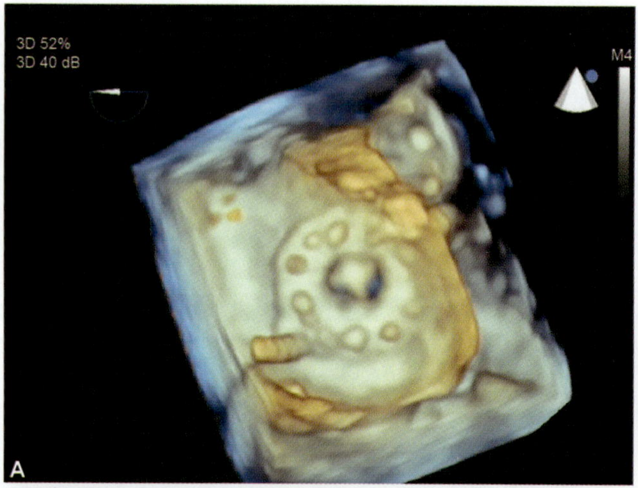

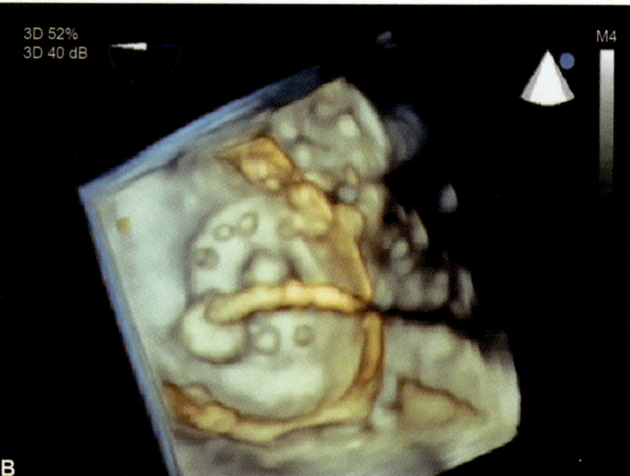

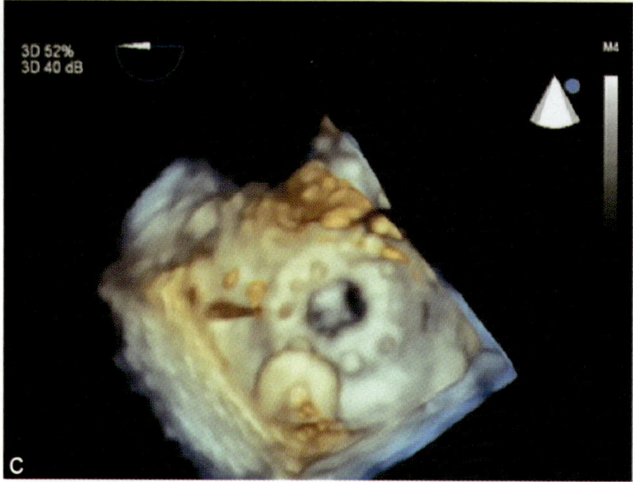

FIG. 16: Three-dimensional transesophageal echocardiography guided device closure of the paravalvular leak. **A,** Guiding sheath is traversing the defect, outside the valve; **B,** The device is being deployed; **C,** Fully deployed closure device.

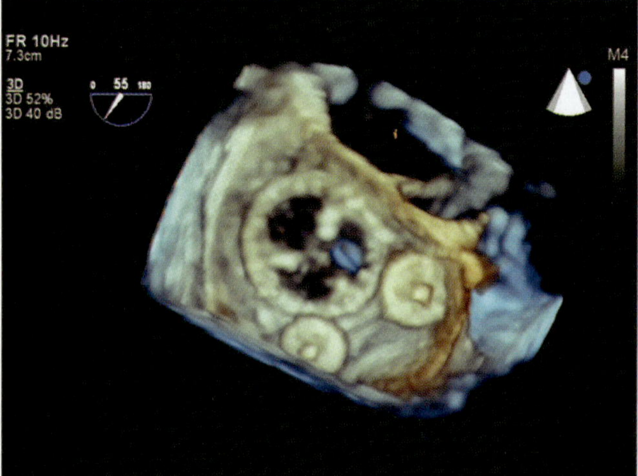

FIG. 17: Same patient as in Figure 15. Both the leaks have been closed.

of the procedure, any eccentricity of the dual orifices created by the device and location and extent of any residual regurgitation. Altiok et al.[172] compared procedural effects of percutaneous MV repair by using RT3D TEE and 2D TEE and 3D TEE was shown to be advantageous in most of the steps of percutaneous mitral repair procedure.

Transcatheter Mitral Valve Replacement

In transcatheter mitral valve replacement (TMVR), 3D TEE is extremely useful in the pre-, post-, and intra-procedural guidance. Measurement of MA is important for correct sizing of the prosthesis and for TMVR planning. Although with 2D TEE the commissural and long-axis views provide the major and minor MA diameter, respectively. However, 2D measurements do not completely describe the complex 3D MA geometry, and produced values are strongly dependent on their exact orientation. Therefore, optimal visualization of the annular plane cannot be guaranteed with 2D TEE. The 3DE has the potential to overcome these limitations as the wide angle 3D mode (zoom 3D) enables complete visualization of the entire mitral apparatus from the MA to tip of papillary muscles. However, the broader sector mode is inferior to the "live" 3D mode in terms of temporal and spatial resolution. The narrow-angle "live" 3D mode is very useful in guiding deployment of device as it has higher temporal and spatial resolution but is not sufficient to visualize the complete MV apparatus.

Although, 3D TEE is advantageous over 2D TEE in SHD interventions, but it is still not recommended as the sole imaging technique, because of the limitations with 3D TEE-like low frame rate and spatial resolution. Additionally, thin structures like interatrial septum and thin valves may show dropout artifacts resembling real holes and may result in wrong interpretation of 3D images. Ongoing advancements and understanding in 3D technology will further increase the use of this technique for guiding transcatheter interventions in SHD.

CONCLUSION

Over the past two decades, 3DE has evolved in to a useful imaging modality for the assessment of cardiac anatomy and function in a variety of clinical settings. The major advantage of 3DE is that it allows comprehensive, spatial depiction of cardiac structures without any geographical assumptions or the need for mental reconstruction. Currently, 3DE has definite incremental utility over 2DE for estimation of LV volumes, assessment of MV pathologies and for guiding certain percutaneous interventions, whereas it has potential role in several other disease conditions. Further, improvements in temporal and spatial resolution of 3DE are needed to fully realize its true potential.

REFERENCES

1. Fukuda S, Watanabe H, Daimon M, et al. Normal values of real-time 3 dimensional echocardiographic parameters in a healthy Japanese population: the JAMP-3D Study. Circ. J. 2012;76:1177-81.
2. Muraru D, Badano LP, Piccoli G, et al. Validation of a novel automated border-detection algorithm for rapid and accurate quantitation of left ventricular volumes based on three-dimensional echocardiography. Euro J Echocardio. 2010;11:359-68.
3. Aune E, Baekkevar M, Rodevand O, et al. Reference values for left ventricular volumes with real-time 3-dimensional echocardiography. Scandinavian Cardiovascular J. 2010;44:24-30.
4. Jenkins C, Bricknell K, Hanekom L, et al. Reproducibility and accuracy of echocardiographic measurements of left ventricular parameters using real-time three-dimensional echocardiography. J Am Col Cardiol. 2004;44:878-86.
5. Zeidan Z, Erbel R, Barkhausen J, et al. Analysis of global systolic and diastolic left ventricular performance using volume-time curves by real-time three-dimensional echocardiography. J Am Soc Echocardio. 2003;16:29-37.
6. Kuhl HP, Schreckenberg M, Rulands D, et al. High-resolution transthoracic real-time three-dimensional echocardiography: quantitation of cardiac volumes and function using semi-automatic border detection and comparison with cardiac magnetic resonance imaging. J Am Coll Cardiol. 2004;43:2083-90.
7. Bu L, Munns S, Zhang H, et al. Rapid full volume data acquisition by real-time 3-dimensional echocardiography for assessment of left ventricular indexes in children: a validation study compared with magnetic resonance imaging. J Am Soc Echocardio. 2005;18:299-305.
8. Gutierrez-Chico JL, Zamorano JL, Perez de Isla L, et al. Comparison of left ventricular volumes and ejection fractions measured by three-dimensional echocardiography versus by two-dimensional echocardiography and cardiac magnetic resonance in patients with various cardiomyopathies. Am J Cardiol. 2005;95:809-13.
9. Bicudo LS, Tsutsui JM, Shiozaki A, et al. Value of real time three-dimensional echocardiography in patients with hypertrophic cardiomyopathy: comparison with two-dimensional echocardiography and magnetic resonance imaging. Echocardiography (Mount Kisco, NY). 2008;25:717-26.
10. Jenkins C, Moir S, Chan J, et al. Left ventricular volume measurement with echocardiography: a comparison of left ventricular opacification, three-dimensional echocardiography, or both with magnetic resonance imaging. Euro Heart J. 2009;30:98-106.
11. Shiota T, McCarthy PM, White RD, et al. Initial clinical experience of real-time three-dimensional echocardiography in patients with ischemic and idiopathic dilated cardiomyopathy. Am J Cardiol. 1999;84:1068-73.
12. Sugeng L, Mor-Avi V, Weinert L, et al. Quantitative assessment of left ventricular size and function: side-by-side comparison of real-time three-dimensional echocardiography and computed tomography with magnetic resonance reference. Circ. 2006;114:654-61.
13. van den Bosch AE, Robbers-Visser D, Krenning BJ, et al. Real-time transthoracic three-dimensional echocardiographic assessment of left ventricular volume and ejection fraction in congenital heart disease. J Am Soc Echocardio. 2006;19:1-6.
14. Caiani EG, Corsi C, Zamorano J, et al. Improved semiautomated quantification of left ventricular volumes and ejection fraction using 3-dimensional echocardiography with a full matrix-array transducer: comparison with magnetic resonance imaging. J Am Soc Echocardio. 2005;18:779-88.
15. Lee D, Fuisz AR, Fan PH, et al. Real-time 3-dimensional echocardiographic evaluation of left ventricular volume: correlation with magnetic resonance imaging--a validation study. J Am Soc Echocardio. 2001;14:1001-9.
16. Jacobs LD, Salgo IS, Goonewardena S, et al. Rapid online quantification of left ventricular volume from real-time three-dimensional echocardiographic data. Euro Heart J. 2006;27:460-8.
17. Corsi C, Lang RM, Veronesi F, et al. Volumetric quantification of global and regional left ventricular function from real-time three-dimensional echocardiographic images. Circ. 2005;112:1161-70.
18. Nikitin NP, Constantin C, Loh PH, et al. New generation 3-dimensional echocardiography for left ventricular volumetric and functional measurements: comparison with cardiac magnetic resonance. Euro J Echocardio. 2006;7:365-72.
19. Chan J, Jenkins C, Khafagi F, et al. What is the optimal clinical technique for measurement of left ventricular volume after myocardial infarction? A comparative study of 3-dimensional echocardiography, single photon emission computed tomography, and cardiac magnetic resonance imaging. J Am Soc Echocardio. 2006;19:192-201.
20. Mor-Avi V, Jenkins C, Kuhl HP, et al. Real-time 3-dimensional echocardiographic quantification of left ventricular volumes: multicenter study for validation with magnetic resonance imaging and investigation of sources of error. JACC Cardiovasc Imaging. 2008;1:413-23.
21. Mor-Avi V, Sugeng L, Weinert L, et al. Fast measurement of left ventricular mass with real time three-dimensional echocardiography: comparison with magnetic resonance imaging. Circ. 2004;110:1814-8.
22. Yap SC, van Geuns RJ, Nemes A, et al. Rapid and accurate measurement of LV mass by biplane real-time 3D echocardiography in patients with concentric LV hypertrophy: comparison to CMR. Euro J Echocardio. 2008;9:255-60.
23. Pacileo G, Castaldi B, Di Salvo G, et al. Assessment of left-ventricular mass and remodeling in obese adolescents: M-mode, 2D or 3D echocardiography? J Cardiovas Med (Hagerstown, Md). 2013;14:144-9.
24. Caiani EG, Corsi C, Sugeng L, et al. Improved quantification of left ventricular mass based on endocardial and epicardial surface detection with real time three dimensional echocardiography. Heart (British Cardiac Society). 2006;92:213-9.
25. Chang SA, Kim HK, Lee SC, et al. Assessment of left ventricular mass in hypertrophic cardiomyopathy by real-time three-dimensional echocardiography using single-beat capture image. J Am Soc Echocard. 2013;26:436-42.
26. van den Bosch AE, Robbers-Visser D, Krenning BJ, et al. Comparison of real-time three-dimensional echocardiography to magnetic resonance imaging for assessment of left ventricular mass. Am J Cardiol. 2006;97:113-7.
27. Shimada YJ, Shiota T. A meta-analysis and investigation for the source of bias of left ventricular volumes and function by three-dimensional echocardiography in comparison with magnetic resonance imaging. Am J Cardiol. 2011;107:126-38.
28. Qin JX, Jones M, Travaglini A, et al. The accuracy of left ventricular mass determined by real-time three-dimensional echocardiography in chronic animal and clinical studies: a comparison with postmortem examination and magnetic resonance imaging. J Am Soc Echocardio. 2005;18:1037-43.
29. Lenstrup M, Kjaergaard J, Petersen CL, et al. Evaluation of left ventricular mass measured by 3D echocardiography using magnetic resonance imaging as gold standard. Scand J Clin Lab Invest. 2006;66:647-57.
30. Oe H, Hozumi T, Arai K, et al. Comparison of accurate measurement of left ventricular mass in patients with hypertrophied hearts by real-time three-

dimensional echocardiography versus magnetic resonance imaging. Am J Cardiol. 2005;95:1263-7.
31. Pouleur AC, le Polain de Waroux JB, Pasquet A, et al. Assessment of left ventricular mass and volumes by three-dimensional echocardiography in patients with or without wall motion abnormalities: comparison against cine magnetic resonance imaging. Heart. 2008;94:1050-7.
32. Marsan NA, Bleeker GB, Ypenburg C, et al. Real-time three-dimensional echocardiography as a novel approach to assess left ventricular and left atrium reverse remodeling and to predict response to cardiac resynchronization therapy. Heart rhythm. 2008;5:1257-64.
33. Lang RM, Badano LP, Mor-Avi V, et al. Recommendations for cardiac chamber quantification by echocardiography in adults: an update from the American Society of Echocardiography and the European Association of Cardiovascular Imaging. European Heart J Cardiovasc Imag. 2015;16:233-70.
34. Thorstensen A, Dalen H, Hala P, et al. Three-dimensional echocardiography in the evaluation of global and regional function in patients with recent myocardial infarction: a comparison with magnetic resonance imaging. Echocardio (Mount Kisco, NY). 2013;30:682-92.
35. Corsi C, Coon P, Goonewardena S, et al. Quantification of regional left ventricular wall motion from real-time 3-dimensional echocardiography in patients with poor acoustic windows: effects of contrast enhancement tested against cardiac magnetic resonance. J Am Soc Echocardio. 2006;19:886-93.
36. Aggeli C, Giannopoulos G, Misovoulos P, et al. Real-time three-dimensional dobutamine stress echocardiography for coronary artery disease diagnosis: validation with coronary angiography. Heart (British Cardiac Society). 2007;93:672-5.
37. Matsumura Y, Hozumi T, Arai K, et al. Non-invasive assessment of myocardial ischaemia using new real-time three-dimensional dobutamine stress echocardiography: comparison with conventional two-dimensional methods. European Heart J. 2005;26:1625-32.
38. Badano LP, Muraru D, Rigo F, et al. High volume-rate three-dimensional stress echocardiography to assess inducible myocardial ischemia: a feasibility study. J Am Soc Echocardio. 2010;23:628-35.
39. Takeuchi M, Otani S, Weinert L, et al. Comparison of contrast-enhanced real-time live 3-dimensional dobutamine stress echocardiography with contrast 2-dimensional echocardiography for detecting stress-induced wall-motion abnormalities. J Am Soc Echocardio. 2006;19:294-9.
40. Walimbe V, Garcia M, Lalude O, et al. Quantitative real-time 3-dimensional stress echocardiography: a preliminary investigation of feasibility and effectiveness. J Am Soc Echocardio. 2007;20:13-22.
41. Jenkins C, Haluska B, Marwick TH. Assessment of temporal heterogeneity and regional motion to identify wall motion abnormalities using treadmill exercise stress three-dimensional echocardiography. J Am Soc Echocardio. 2009;22:268-75.
42. Portnoy SG, Rudski LG. Echocardiographic evaluation of the right ventricle: a 2014 perspective. Current Cardiol Reports. 2015;17:21.
43. Dandel M, Hetzer R. Echocardiographic assessment of the right ventricle: Impact of the distinctly load dependency of its size, geometry and performance. Int J Cardiol. 2016;221:1132-42.
44. Rudski LG, Lai WW, Afilalo J, et al. Guidelines for the echocardiographic assessment of the right heart in adults: a report from the American Society of Echocardiography endorsed by the European Association of Echocardiography, a registered branch of the European Society of Cardiology, and the Canadian Society of Echocardiography. J Am Soc Echocardio. 2010;23:685-713; quiz 786-8.
45. Schindera ST, Mehwald PS, Sahn DJ, et al. Accuracy of real-time three-dimensional echocardiography for quantifying right ventricular volume: static and pulsatile flow studies in an anatomic in vitro model. J Ultrasound Med. 2002;21:1069-75.
46. Chua S, Levine RA, Yosefy C, et al. Assessment of right ventricular function by real-time three-dimensional echocardiography improves accuracy and decreases interobserver variability compared with conventional two-dimensional views. European J Echocardio. 2009;10:619-24.
47. Niemann PS, Pinho L, Balbach T, et al. Anatomically oriented right ventricular volume measurements with dynamic three-dimensional echocardiography validated by 3-Tesla magnetic resonance imaging. J Am Coll Cardiol. 2007;50: 1668-76.
48. Acar P, Abadir S, Roux D, et al. Ebstein's anomaly assessed by real-time 3-D echocardiography. The Annals Thoracic Surg. 2006;82:731-3.
49. Kjaergaard J, Hastrup SJ, Sogaard P, et al. Advanced quantitative echocardiography in arrhythmogenic right ventricular cardiomyopathy. J Am Soc Echocardio. 2007;20:27-35.
50. Sugeng L, Mor-Avi V, Weinert L, et al. Multimodality comparison of quantitative volumetric analysis of the right ventricle. JACC Cardiovasc Imag. 2010;3:10-8.
51. Kjaergaard J, Petersen CL, Kjaer A, et al. Evaluation of right ventricular volume and function by 2D and 3D echocardiography compared to MRI. European J Echocardio. 2006;7:430-8.
52. Gopal AS, Chukwu EO, Iwuchukwu CJ, et al. Normal values of right ventricular size and function by real-time 3-dimensional echocardiography: comparison with cardiac magnetic resonance imaging. J Am Soc Echocardio. 2007;20:445-55.
53. Grewal J, Majdalany D, Syed I, et al. Three-dimensional echocardiographic assessment of right ventricular volume and function in adult patients with congenital heart disease: comparison with magnetic resonance imaging. J Am Soc Echocardio. 2010;23:127-33.
54. Scheurer M, Bandisode V, Ruff P, et al. Early experience with real-time three-dimensional echocardiographic guidance of right ventricular biopsy in children. Echocardio (Mount Kisco, NY). 2006;23:45-9.
55. Nagata Y, Wu VC, Kado Y, et al. Prognostic Value of Right Ventricular Ejection Fraction Assessed by Transthoracic 3D Echocardiography. Circ Cardiovas Imag. 2017;10.
56. Muraru D, Spadotto V, Cecchetto A, et al. New speckle-tracking algorithm for right ventricular volume analysis from three-dimensional echocardiographic data sets: validation with cardiac magnetic resonance and comparison with the previous analysis tool. European Heart J Cardiovas Imag. 2016;17:1279-1289.
57. Vaziri SM, Larson MG, Benjamin EJ, et al. Echocardiographic predictors of nonrheumatic atrial fibrillation. The Framingham Heart Study. Circ. 1994;89:724-30.
58. Benjamin EJ, D'Agostino RB, Belanger AJ, et al. Left atrial size and the risk of stroke and death. The Framingham Heart Study. Circ. 1995;92:835-41.
59. Laukkanen JA, Kurl S, Eranen J, et al. Left atrium size and the risk of cardiovascular death in middle-aged men. Arch Intern Med. 2005;165:1788-93.
60. Pritchett AM, Jacobsen SJ, Mahoney DW, et al. Left atrial volume as an index of left atrial size: a population-based study. J Am Coll Cardiol. 2003;41:1036-43.
61. Tani T, Tanabe K, Ono M, et al. Left atrial volume and the risk of paroxysmal atrial fibrillation in patients with hypertrophic cardiomyopathy. J Am Soc Echocardio. 2004;17:644-8.
62. Tsang TS, Abhayaratna WP, Barnes ME, et al. Prediction of cardiovascular outcomes with left atrial size: is volume superior to area or diameter? J Am Coll Cardiol. 2006;47:1018-23.
63. Lester SJ, Ryan EW, Schiller NB, et al. Best method in clinical practice and in research studies to determine left atrial size. Am J Cardiol. 1999;84:829-32.
64. Khankirawatana B, Khankirawatana S, Porter T. How should left atrial size be reported? Comparative assessment with use of multiple echocardiographic methods. Am Heart J. 2004;147:369-74.
65. Aurigemma GP, Gottdiener JS, Arnold AM, et al. Left atrial volume and geometry in healthy aging: the Cardiovascular Health Study. Circ Cardiovas Imag. 2009;2:282-9.
66. Muller H, Burri H, Shah D, et al. Evaluation of left atrial size in patients with atrial arrhythmias: comparison of standard 2D versus real time 3D echocardiography. Echocardio (Mount Kisco, NY). 2007;24:960-6.
67. Anwar AM, Soliman OI, Geleijnse ML, et al. Assessment of left atrial volume and function by real-time three-dimensional echocardiography. Int J Cardiol. 2008;123:155-61.
68. Miyasaka Y, Tsujimoto S, Maeba H et al. Left atrial volume by real-time three-dimensional echocardiography: validation by 64-slice multidetector computed tomography. J Am Soc Echocardio. 2011;24:680-6.
69. Rohner A, Brinkert M, Kawel N et al. Functional assessment of the left atrium by real-time three-dimensional echocardiography using a novel dedicated analysis tool: initial validation studies in comparison with computed tomography. European J Echocardio. 2011;12:497-505.
70. Mor-Avi V, Yodwut C, Jenkins C, et al. Real-time 3D echocardiographic quantification of left atrial volume: multicenter study for validation with CMR. JACC Cardiovascular Imag. 2012;5:769-77.

71. Marsan NA, Tops LF, Holman ER, et al. Comparison of left atrial volumes and function by real-time three-dimensional echocardiography in patients having catheter ablation for atrial fibrillation with persistence of sinus rhythm versus recurrent atrial fibrillation three months later. Am J Cardiol. 2008;102:847-53.
72. Delgado V, Vidal B, Sitges M, et al. Fate of left atrial function as determined by real-time three-dimensional echocardiography study after radiofrequency catheter ablation for the treatment of atrial fibrillation. Am J Cardiol. 2008;101:1285-90.
73. Keller AM, Gopal AS, King DL. Left and right atrial volume by freehand three-dimensional echocardiography: in vivo validation using magnetic resonance imaging. European J Echocardio. 2000;1:55-65.
74. Spencer KT, Mor-Avi V, Gorcsan J, 3rd, et al. Effects of aging on left atrial reservoir, conduit, and booster pump function: a multi-institution acoustic quantification study. Heart (British Cardiac Society). 2001;85:272-7.
75. Maffessanti F, Nesser HJ, Weinert L, et al. Quantitative evaluation of regional left ventricular function using three-dimensional speckle tracking echocardiography in patients with and without heart disease. Am J Cardiol. 2009;104:1755-62.
76. Kleijn SA, Brouwer WP, Aly MF, et al. Comparison between three-dimensional speckle-tracking echocardiography and cardiac magnetic resonance imaging for quantification of left ventricular volumes and function. European Heart J Cardiovas Imag. 2012;13:834-9.
77. Reant P, Barbot L, Touche C, et al. Evaluation of global left ventricular systolic function using three-dimensional echocardiography speckle-tracking strain parameters. J Am Soc Echocardio. 2012;25:68-79.
78. Nesser HJ, Winter S. Speckle tracking in the evaluation of left ventricular dyssynchrony. Echocardiography (Mount Kisco, NY) 2009;26:324-36.
79. Kleijn SA, Aly MF, Terwee CB, et al. Reliability of left ventricular volumes and function measurements using three-dimensional speckle tracking echocardiography. European Heart J Cardiovas Imag. 2012;13:159-68.
80. Duan F, Xie M, Wang X, et al. Preliminary clinical study of left ventricular myocardial strain in patients with non-ischemic dilated cardiomyopathy by three-dimensional speckle tracking imaging. Cardiovascular Ultrasound, 2012;10:8.
81. Elefteriades JA, Farkas EA. Thoracic aortic aneurysm clinically pertinent controversies and uncertainties. J Am Coll Cardiol. 2010;55:841-57.
82. Sugeng L, Weinert L, Lang RM. Left ventricular assessment using real time three dimensional echocardiography. Heart (British Cardiac Society) 2003;89:29-36.
83. Horstman JA, Monaghan MJ, Gill EA. Intraventricular dyssynchrony assessment by real-time three-dimensional echocardiography. Cardiol Clin. 2007;25:253-60.
84. Van de Veire NR, Yu CM, Ajmone-Marsan N, et al. Triplane tissue Doppler imaging: a novel three-dimensional imaging modality that predicts reverse left ventricular remodelling after cardiac resynchronisation therapy. Heart (British Cardiac Society). 2008;94:e9.
85. Kapetanakis S, Kearney MT, Siva A, et al. Real-time three-dimensional echocardiography: a novel technique to quantify global left ventricular mechanical dyssynchrony. Circ. 2005;112:992-1000.
86. Zhang Q, Yu CM, Fung JW et al. Assessment of the effect of cardiac resynchronization therapy on intraventricular mechanical synchronicity by regional volumetric changes. Am J Cardiol. 2005;95:126-9.
87. Soliman OI, van Dalen BM, Nemes A, et al. Quantification of left ventricular systolic dyssynchrony by real-time three-dimensional echocardiography. J Am Soc Echocardio. 2009;22:232-9.
88. Takeuchi M, Jacobs A, Sugeng L, et al. Assessment of left ventricular dyssynchrony with real-time 3-dimensional echocardiography: comparison with Doppler tissue imaging. J Am Soc Echocardio. 2007;20:1321-9.
89. Russo C, Jaubert MP, Jin Z, Homma S, Di Tullio MR. Intra- and interobserver reproducibility of left ventricular mechanical dyssynchrony assessment by real time three-dimensional echocardiography. Echocardio (Mount Kisco, NY). 2012;29:598-607.
90. Gorcsan J, 3rd, Abraham T, Agler DA, et al. Echocardiography for cardiac resynchronization therapy: recommendations for performance and reporting--a report from the American Society of Echocardiography Dyssynchrony Writing Group endorsed by the Heart Rhythm Society. J Am Soc Echocardio. 2008;21:191-213.
91. Bacha EA, Zimmerman FJ, Mor-Avi V, et al. Ventricular resynchronization by multisite pacing improves myocardial performance in the postoperative single-ventricle patient. Ann Thorac Surg. 2004;78:1678-83.
92. Grewal J, Mankad S, Freeman WK, et al. Real-time three-dimensional transesophageal echocardiography in the intraoperative assessment of mitral valve disease. J Am Soc Echocardio. 2009;22:34-41.
93. Macnab A, Jenkins NP, Bridgewater BJ, et al. Three-dimensional echocardiography is superior to multiplane transoesophageal echo in the assessment of regurgitant mitral valve morphology. European J Echocardio. 2004;5:212-22.
94. Grewal J, Suri R, Mankad S, et al. Mitral annular dynamics in myxomatous valve disease: new insights with real-time 3-dimensional echocardiography. Circ. 2010;121:1423-31.
95. Zoghbi WA, Enriquez-Sarano M, Foster E, et al. Recommendations for evaluation of the severity of native valvular regurgitation with two-dimensional and Doppler echocardiography. J Am Soc Echocardio. 2003;16:777-802.
96. Belohlavek M, Foley DA, Gerber TC, et al. Three-dimensional reconstruction of color Doppler jets in the human heart. J Am Soc Echocardio. 1994;7:553-60.
97. Irvine T, Derrick G, Morris D, et al. Three-dimensional echocardiographic reconstruction of mitral valve color Doppler flow events. Am J Cardiol. 1999;84:1103-6, A10.
98. Yosefy C, Levine RA, Solis J, et al. Proximal flow convergence region as assessed by real-time 3-dimensional echocardiography: challenging the hemispheric assumption. J Am Soc Echocardio. 2007;20:389-96.
99. Yosefy C, Hung J, Chua S, et al. Direct measurement of vena contracta area by real-time 3-dimensional echocardiography for assessing severity of mitral regurgitation. Am J Cardiol. 2009;104:978-83.
100. Matsumura Y, Saracino G, Sugioka K, et al. Determination of regurgitant orifice area with the use of a new three-dimensional flow convergence geometric assumption in functional mitral regurgitation. J Am Soc Echocardio. 2008;21:1251-6.
101. Matsumura Y, Fukuda S, Tran H, et al. Geometry of the proximal isovelocity surface area in mitral regurgitation by 3-dimensional color Doppler echocardiography: difference between functional mitral regurgitation and prolapse regurgitation. Am Heart J. 2008;155:231-8.
102. Kahlert P, Plicht B, Schenk IM, et al. Direct assessment of size and shape of noncircular vena contracta area in functional versus organic mitral regurgitation using real-time three-dimensional echocardiography. J Am Soc Echocardio. 2008;21:912-21.
103. Zeng X, Levine RA, Hua L, et al. Diagnostic value of vena contracta area in the quantification of mitral regurgitation severity by color Doppler 3D echocardiography. Circ Cardiovas Imag. 2011;4:506-13.
104. Hyodo E, Iwata S, Tugcu A, et al. Direct measurement of multiple vena contracta areas for assessing the severity of mitral regurgitation using 3D TEE. JACC Cardiovas Imag. 2012;5:669-76.
105. Maragiannis D, Little SH. Quantification of mitral valve regurgitation: new solutions provided by 3D echocardiography. Current Cardiol Reports. 2013;15:384.
106. Baumgartner H, Hung J, Bermejo J, et al. Echocardiographic assessment of valve stenosis: EAE/ASE recommendations for clinical practice. J Am Soc Echocardio. 2009;22:1-23; quiz 101-2.
107. Faletra F, Pezzano A, Jr., Fusco R, et al. Measurement of mitral valve area in mitral stenosis: four echocardiographic methods compared with direct measurement of anatomic orifices. J Am Coll Cardiol. 1996;28:1190-7.
108. Vahanian A, Baumgartner H, Bax J, et al. Guidelines on the management of valvular heart disease: The Task Force on the Management of Valvular Heart Disease of the European Society of Cardiology. Euro Heart J. 2007;28:230-68.
109. Min SY, Song JM, Kim YJ, et al. Discrepancy between mitral valve areas measured by two-dimensional planimetry and three-dimensional transoesophageal echocardiography in patients with mitral stenosis. Heart (British Cardiac Society). 2013;99:253-8.
110. Schlosshan D, Aggarwal G, Mathur G, et al. Real-time 3D transesophageal echocardiography for the evaluation of rheumatic mitral stenosis. JACC Cardiovas Imag. 2011;4:580-8.
111. Sugeng L, Weinert L, Lammertin G, et al. Accuracy of mitral valve area measurements using transthoracic rapid freehand 3-dimensional scanning: comparison with noninvasive and invasive methods. J Am Soc Echocardio. 2003;16:1292-300.
112. Perez de Isla L, Casanova C, Almeria C, et al. Which method should be the reference method to evaluate the severity of rheumatic mitral stenosis? Gorlin's method versus 3D-echo. European J Echocardio. 2007;8:470-3.

113. Zamorano J, Cordeiro P, Sugeng L, et al. Real-time three-dimensional echocardiography for rheumatic mitral valve stenosis evaluation: an accurate and novel approach. J Am Coll Cardiol. 2004;43:2091-6.
114. Chu JW, Levine RA, Chua S, et al. Assessing mitral valve area and orifice geometry in calcific mitral stenosis: a new solution by real-time three-dimensional echocardiography. J Am Soc Echocardio. 2008;21:1006-9.
115. Anwar AM, Attia WM, Nosir YF, et al. Validation of a new score for the assessment of mitral stenosis using real-time three-dimensional echocardiography. J Am Soc Echocardio. 2010;23:13-22.
116. Hamdan A, Guetta V, Konen E, et al. Deformation dynamics and mechanical properties of the aortic annulus by 4-dimensional computed tomography: insights into the functional anatomy of the aortic valve complex and implications for transcatheter aortic valve therapy. J Am Coll Cardiol. 2012;59:119-27.
117. Doddamani S, Bello R, Friedman MA, et al. Demonstration of left ventricular outflow tract eccentricity by real time 3D echocardiography: implications for the determination of aortic valve area. Echocardio (Mount Kisco, NY). 2007;24:860-6.
118. Shahgaldi K, Manouras A, Brodin LA, et al. Direct measurement of left ventricular outflow tract area using three-dimensional echocardiography in biplane mode improves accuracy of stroke volume assessment. Echocardio (Mount Kisco, NY). 2010;27:1078-85.
119. Khaw AV, von Bardeleben RS, Strasser C, et al. Direct measurement of left ventricular outflow tract by transthoracic real-time 3D-echocardiography increases accuracy in assessment of aortic valve stenosis. Int J Cardiol. 2009;136:64-71.
120. Ng AC, Delgado V, van der Kley F, et al. Comparison of aortic root dimensions and geometries before and after transcatheter aortic valve implantation by 2- and 3-dimensional transesophageal echocardiography and multislice computed tomography. Circ. Cardiovascular Imag. 2010;3:94-102.
121. Otani K, Takeuchi M, Kaku K, et al. Assessment of the aortic root using real-time 3D transesophageal echocardiography. Circ J. 2010;74:2649-57.
122. Gutierrez-Chico JL, Zamorano JL, Prieto-Moriche E, et al. Real-time three-dimensional echocardiography in aortic stenosis: a novel, simple, and reliable method to improve accuracy in area calculation. Euro Heart J. 2008;29:1296-306.
123. Nakai H, Takeuchi M, Yoshitani H, et al. Pitfalls of anatomical aortic valve area measurements using two-dimensional transoesophageal echocardiography and the potential of three-dimensional transoesophageal echocardiography. European J Echocardio. 2010;11:369-76.
124. Goland S, Trento A, Iida K, et al. Assessment of aortic stenosis by three-dimensional echocardiography: an accurate and novel approach. Heart (British Cardiac Society). 2007;93:801-7.
125. Ge S, Warner JG, Jr., Abraham TP, et al. Three-dimensional surface area of the aortic valve orifice by three-dimensional echocardiography: clinical validation of a novel index for assessment of aortic stenosis. Am Heart J. 1998;136: 1042-50.
126. Shibayama K, Watanabe H, Sasaki S,, et al. Impact of regurgitant orifice height for mechanism of aortic regurgitation. JACC Cardiovas Imag. 2013;6:1347-9.
127. Shiota T, Jones M, Delabays A et al. Direct measurement of three-dimensionally reconstructed flow convergence surface area and regurgitant flow in aortic regurgitation: in vitro and chronic animal model studies. Circ. 1997;96: 3687-95.
128. Fang L, Hsiung MC, Miller AP et al. Assessment of aortic regurgitation by live three-dimensional transthoracic echocardiographic measurements of vena contracta area: usefulness and validation. Echocardiography (Mount Kisco, NY) 2005;22:775-81.
129. Perez de Isla L, Zamorano J, Fernandez-Golfin C, et al. 3D color-Doppler echocardiography and chronic aortic regurgitation: a novel approach for severity assessment. Int J Cardiol. 2013;166:640-5.
130. Chin CH, Chen CH, Lo HS. The correlation between three-dimensional vena contracta area and aortic regurgitation index in patients with aortic regurgitation. Echocardiography (Mount Kisco, NY). 2010;27:161-6.
131. Stankovic I, Daraban AM, Jasaityte R, et al. Incremental value of the en face view of the tricuspid valve by two-dimensional and three-dimensional echocardiography for accurate identification of tricuspid valve leaflets. J Am Soc Echocardio. 2014;27:376-84.
132. Patel V, Nanda NC, Rajdev S, et al. Live/real time three-dimensional transthoracic echocardiographic assessment of Ebstein's anomaly. Echocardiography (Mount Kisco, NY). 2005;22:847-54.
133. van Noord PT, Scohy TV, McGhie J, et al. Three-dimensional transesophageal echocardiography in Ebstein's anomaly. Interactive Cardiovas Thoracic Surg. 2010;10:836-7.
134. Bhattacharyya S, Toumpanakis C, Burke M, et al. Features of carcinoid heart disease identified by 2- and 3-dimensional echocardiography and cardiac MRI. Circ. Cardiovas Imag. 2010;3:103-11.
135. Mediratta A, Addetia K, Yamat M, et al. 3D echocardiographic location of implantable device leads and mechanism of associated tricuspid regurgitation. JACC Cardiovas Imag. 2014;7:337-47.
136. Addetia K, Maffessanti F, Mediratta A, et al. Impact of implantable transvenous device lead location on severity of tricuspid regurgitation. J Am Soc Echocardio. 2014;27:1164-75.
137. Klein AL, Jellis CL. 3D imaging of device leads: "taking the lead with 3D". JACC Cardiovas Imag. 2014;7:348-50.
138. Song JM, Jang MK, Choi YS, et al. The vena contracta in functional tricuspid regurgitation: a real-time three-dimensional color Doppler echocardiography study. J Am Soc Echocardio. 2011;24:663-70.
139. Vahanian A, Alfieri O, Andreotti F, et al. Guidelines on the management of valvular heart disease (version 2012): the Joint Task Force on the Management of Valvular Heart Disease of the European Society of Cardiology (ESC) and the European Association for Cardio-Thoracic Surgery (EACTS). Euro J Surg. 2012;42:S1-44.
140. Ring L, Rana BS, Kydd A, et al. Dynamics of the tricuspid valve annulus in normal and dilated right hearts: a three-dimensional transoesophageal echocardiography study. Euro Heart J Cardiovas Imag. 2012;13:756-62.
141. Nishimura RA, Otto CM, Bonow RO, et al. 2014 AHA/ACC Guideline for the Management of Patients With Valvular Heart Disease: a report of the American College of Cardiology/American Heart Association Task Force on Practice Guidelines. Circ. 2014;129:e521-643.
142. Anwar AM, Geleijnse ML, Ten Cate FJ, et al. Assessment of tricuspid valve annulus size, shape and function using real-time three-dimensional echocardiography. Interact Cardiovasc Thorac Surg. 2006;5:683-7.
143. Ton-Nu TT, Levine RA, Handschumacher MD, et al. Geometric determinants of functional tricuspid regurgitation: insights from 3-dimensional echocardiography. Circ. 2006;114:143-9.
144. Fukuda S, Saracino G, Matsumura Y, et al. Three-dimensional geometry of the tricuspid annulus in healthy subjects and in patients with functional tricuspid regurgitation: a real-time, 3-dimensional echocardiographic study. Circ. 2006;114:I492-8.
145. Miglioranza MH, Mihaila S, Muraru D, et al. Dynamic changes in tricuspid annular diameter measurement in relation to the echocardiographic view and timing during the cardiac cycle. J Am Soc Echocardio. 2015;28:226-35.
146. Anwar AM, Soliman OI, Nemes A, et al. Value of assessment of tricuspid annulus: real-time three-dimensional echocardiography and magnetic resonance imaging. Int J Cardiovasc Imaging. 2007;23:701-5.
147. Fukuda S, Gillinov AM, McCarthy PM, et al. Determinants of recurrent or residual functional tricuspid regurgitation after tricuspid annuloplasty. Circ. 2006;114:I582-7.
148. Kwan J, Kim GC, Jeon MJ, et al. 3D geometry of a normal tricuspid annulus during systole: a comparison study with the mitral annulus using real-time 3D echocardiography. European J Echocardio. 2007;8:375-83.
149. Mahmood F, Kim H, Chaudary B, et al. Tricuspid annular geometry: a three-dimensional transesophageal echocardiographic study. J Cardiothorac Vasc Anes. 2013;27:639-46.
150. Owais K, Taylor CE, Jiang L, et al. Tricuspid annulus: a three-dimensional deconstruction and reconstruction. Ann Thorac Surg. 2014;98:1536-42.
151. Park YH, Song JM, Lee EY, et al. Geometric and hemodynamic determinants of functional tricuspid regurgitation: a real-time three-dimensional echocardiography study. Int J Cardiol. 2008;124:160-5.
152. Min SY, Song JM, Kim JH, et al. Geometric changes after tricuspid annuloplasty and predictors of residual tricuspid regurgitation: a real-time three-dimensional echocardiography study. Euro Heart J. 2010;31:2871-80.

153. Schnabel R, Khaw AV, von Bardeleben RS, et al. Assessment of the tricuspid valve morphology by transthoracic real-time-3D-echocardiography. Echocardiography (Mount Kisco, NY). 2005;22:15-23.
154. Hauck AJ, Freeman DP, Ackermann DM, et al. Surgical pathology of the tricuspid valve: a study of 363 cases spanning 25 years. Mayo Clinic Proc. 1988;63:851-63.
155. Pearlman AS. Role of echocardiography in the diagnosis and evaluation of severity of mitral and tricuspid stenosis. Circ. 1991;84:I193-7.
156. Habib G, Badano L, Tribouilloy C, et al. Recommendations for the practice of echocardiography in infective endocarditis. European J Echocardio. 2010;11:202-19.
157. Evangelista A, Gonzalez-Alujas MT. Echocardiography in infective endocarditis. Heart (British Cardiac Society). 2004;90:614-7.
158. Daniel WG, Mugge A, Martin RP, et al. Improvement in the diagnosis of abscesses associated with endocarditis by transesophageal echocardiography. N Engl J Med. 1991;324:795-800.
159. Hansalia S, Biswas M, Dutta R, et al. The value of live/real time three-dimensional transesophageal echocardiography in the assessment of valvular vegetations. Echocardiography (Mount Kisco, NY). 2009;26:1264-73.
160. Hill EE, Herijgers P, Claus P, et al. Abscess in infective endocarditis: the value of transesophageal echocardiography and outcome: a 5-year study. Am Heart J. 2007;154:923-8.
161. Walker N, Bhan A, Desai J, et al. Myocardial abscess: a rare complication of valvular endocarditis demonstrated by 3D contrast echocardiography. European J Echocardio. 2010;11:E37.
162. Mukhtari O, Horton CJ, Jr., Nanda NC, et al. Transesophageal color Doppler three-dimensional echocardiographic detection of prosthetic aortic valve dehiscence: correlation with surgical findings. Echocardiography (Mount Kisco, NY). 2001;18:393-7.
163. Thompson KA, Shiota T, Tolstrup K, et al. Utility of three-dimensional transesophageal echocardiography in the diagnosis of valvular perforations. Am J Cardiol. 2011;107:100-2.
164. Chandra S, Vijay SK, Dwivedi SK, et al. Delineation of anatomy of the ruptured sinus of Valsalva with three-dimensional echocardiography: the advantage of the added dimension. Echocardiography (Mount Kisco, NY). 2012;29:E148-51.
165. Kort S. Real-time 3-dimensional echocardiography for prosthetic valve endocarditis: initial experience. J Am Soc Echocardio. 2006;19:130-9.
166. Sugeng L, Shernan SK, Weinert L, et al. Real-time three-dimensional transesophageal echocardiography in valve disease: comparison with surgical findings and evaluation of prosthetic valves. J Am Soc Echocardio. 2008;21:1347-54.
167. Perk G, Lang RM, Garcia-Fernandez MA, et al. Use of real time three-dimensional transesophageal echocardiography in intracardiac catheter based interventions. J Am Soc Echocardio. 2009;22:865-82.
168. Lee AP, Lam YY, Yip GW, et al. Role of real time three-dimensional transesophageal echocardiography in guidance of interventional procedures in cardiology. Heart (British Cardiac Society). 2010;96:1485-93.
169. Kronzon I, Sugeng L, Perk G, et al. Real-time 3-dimensional transesophageal echocardiography in the evaluation of post-operative mitral annuloplasty ring and prosthetic valve dehiscence. J Am Coll Cardiol. 2009;53:1543-7.
170. Zamorano JL, Goncalves A, Lang R. Imaging to select and guide transcatheter aortic valve implantation. Euro Heart J. 2014;35:1578-87.
171. Piazza N, de Jaegere P, Schultz C, et al. Anatomy of the aortic valvar complex and its implications for transcatheter implantation of the aortic valve. Circ Cardiovasc Interv 2008;1:74-81.
172. Altiok E, Becker M, Hamada S, et al. Optimized guidance of percutaneous edge-to edge repair of the mitral valve using real-time 3-D transesophageal echocardiography. Clin Res Cardiol German Cardiac Soc. 2011;100:675-81.

CHAPTER 79

Intervention and Fusion Echocardiography

Shantanu P Sengupta

INTRODUCTION

Structural heart disease (SHD) in elderly is associated with significant valvular heart lesions which demands surgical therapy. But advancing age is associated with higher perioperative mortality and morbidity.[1,2] Recent times has seen advances in less invasive therapies such as percutaneous or transcatheter interventions for treatment of SHD. Studies have shown that transcatheter aortic valve replacement (TAVR) is equal or better than surgical aortic valve replacement in high-risk surgical group of patients.[3] Also the effective closure of the left atrial appendage (LAA) by few recent devices has helped in the reduction of thromboembolic complications in atrial fibrillation.[4] Also many patients of severe mitral regurgitation have been benefited by percutaneous mitral valve repair using the MitraClip device.[5,6] The future is also for the use of percutaneous mitral annuloplasty ring implantation or transcatheter mitral valve replacement for mitral valve pathologies.[7,8]

Advances in cardiac imaging with its clinical implementation has helped in SHD interventions.[9] SHD interventions demand clear visualization of the important structures in a beating heart. Real-time three-dimensional (3D) transesophageal echocardiography (TEE) and multislice computed tomography (MSCT) have advanced the visualization of complex valvular morphology and helped in performing necessary precise measurements for planning and tailoring of percutaneous therapies.[9] During SHD intervention, multiple images are simultaneously shown in multiple screens which thus help in coordination of the imager and the interventionist.

Fusing echocardiography onto the fluoroscopy screen enhances workflow and improves procedural outcomes. This article is an effort to understand the concept, knowledge, and current use of fusion echocardiography for various SHD interventions in the present era of cardiology.

PROBLEMS DURING STRUCTURAL HEART DISEASE INTERVENTIONS

Structural heart disease interventions are generally performed with specialized catheters, wires, guides, sheaths, and implantation devices. This procedure is highly demanding and requires precision. SHD interventions involve a multidisciplinary approach with a strong coordination between cardiac interventionists, imagers, trained nurses, and catheterization laboratory technicians. The imaging specialist guides the interventionists in every step of the procedure with the use TEE probe limited to a narrow (although not fixed) view through the esophagus.[10,11] This needs to synchronize with the C-arm of the fluoroscopy rotation to allow multiple views of the same cardiac structure (Fig. 1).[12] A successful procedure demands a good communication between interventional cardiologist who works on the catheters and the imager who operates on the 3D echo images. Such an approach requires real-time image coregistration with a sufficient overlay visualization of both imaging modalities.[13] For this, real-time echocardiography with fusion of fluoroscopy—fusion echocardiography has recently been introduced.[14,15]

UNDERSTANDING FUSION IMAGING

Fusion of Static Images

Last one decade has seen advances in fusion of static imaging in various forms. Fusion of cardiac computed tomography (CT) images with single-photon emission computed tomography (SPECT) has helped in understanding the relationship of coronary artery anatomy to corresponding ischemic area.[16] Similar results have also been obtained with the fusion of images of MSCT and echocardiography for the identification of ischemic area.[17] For diagnosis of prosthetic valve endocarditis, fusion of cardiac CT with

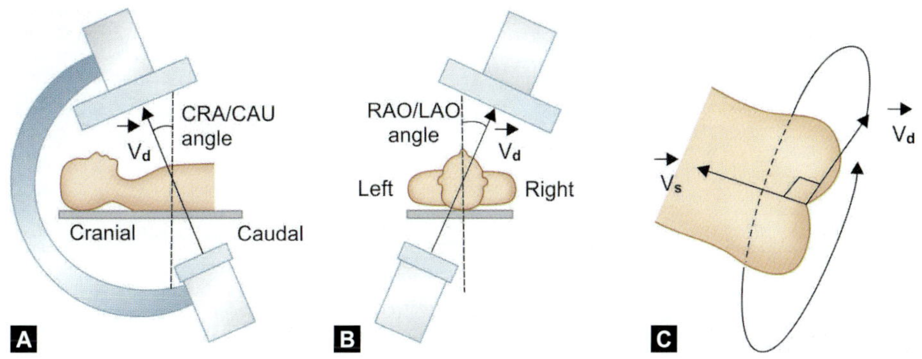

CAU, caudal; CRA, cranial; LAO, left anterior oblique; RAO, right anterior oblique.

FIG. 1: The angles in fluoroscopy. Vectors V_d and V_s are perpendicular and are optimal angles.

positron emission tomography scan imaging is rewarding.[18] And for the selection of the correct size and type of prosthetic heart valve for TAVR, fusion of MSCT data with models of prosthetic implants has been used recently.[19,20] However, these fusion imaging uses static images, which are not useful for SHD interventions, which require more dynamic imaging correlation due to presence of beating heart.

Fusion of Dynamic Images

For SHD interventions in beating heart, real-time images are acquired in a hybrid catheterization laboratory. The live images from fluoroscopy and 3D echocardiography get superimposed (Fig. 2).[21,22] The latest software called EchoNavigator (Philips Medical Systems, Best, The Netherlands) overlaps the real-time (live) images from TEE over the fluoroscopy and is one such example being extensively used for SHD interventions.

Fusion imaging enables the amalgamation of image angle acquired from echocardiographic probe and the fluoroscopic angle. Once the fusion occurs, both the images move cohesively in all angulation simultaneously. The software also uses markers or dots to identify important structures which can be used as landmarks during SHD.

Use of Real-time 3D Fusion Imaging

One of the first steps of many SHD interventions is to make an accurate and safe puncture of the inter-atrial septum (Fig. 3). The procedure type demands the site of the puncture, as in inferoposterior (i.e., for percutaneous closure of the LAA) or anterosuperior at a level of 4 cm above the mitral annulus (MitraClip implantation). Real-time TEE helps in identifying the actual puncture site.

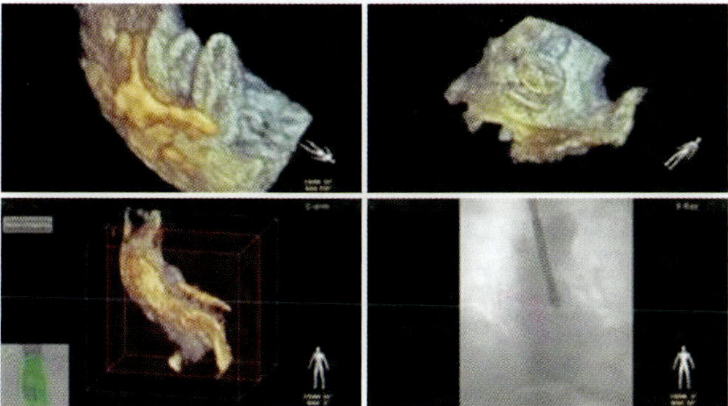

FIG 2: Integration of live images of echo and fluoroscopy.

INTERATRIAL SEPTAL DEFECT CLOSURE

Nonsurgical interventional closures of patent foramen ovale (PFO) and interatrial septal defect are being mostly done in children and adults. Usage of TEE during this procedure makes it safer. Sometimes the passage across PFO is long, narrow, and negotiating the wire can be time consuming and a marker on the fused fluoro-echo image helps in this passage. Also, many times a PFO and small atrial septal defects (ASDs) can coexist. Negotiating the septum without echocardiographic image is not advisable. To achieve complete closure, however, anatomical knowledge is mandatory. Fusion imaging with the use of a marker prevents perforation of cardiac structures and helps in complete ASD or PFO closure with safe deployment of umbrella (Fig. 4).

Closure of Paravalvular Leaks

Paravalvular leaks (PVLs) have been diagnosed and are known complications of surgical and transcatheter valve replacement procedures. These can be targeted and closed by interventional procedures. It requires precise details of the defect for the selection of the appropriate type, size, and number of device.[23] Fusion imaging has been helpful during managing PVL closure as it provides ease in diagnosis and procedural guidance.[24] A direct visualization of the defect by real-time TEE improves spatial resolution of the defect, during placement of the guide wire after transseptal puncture.[23]

Fusion imaging with EchoNavigator software has been helpful in PVL closure procedures by reducing procedural time, facilitating location of the lesion and evaluating the surrounding structures.[25] Also this software is helpful in multiple PVL and avoids the use of contrast agents in patients with renal insufficiency.

Occlusion of Left Atrial Appendage

In nonvalvular atrial fibrillation, systemic anticoagulation is needed. However, in patients where anticoagulation is

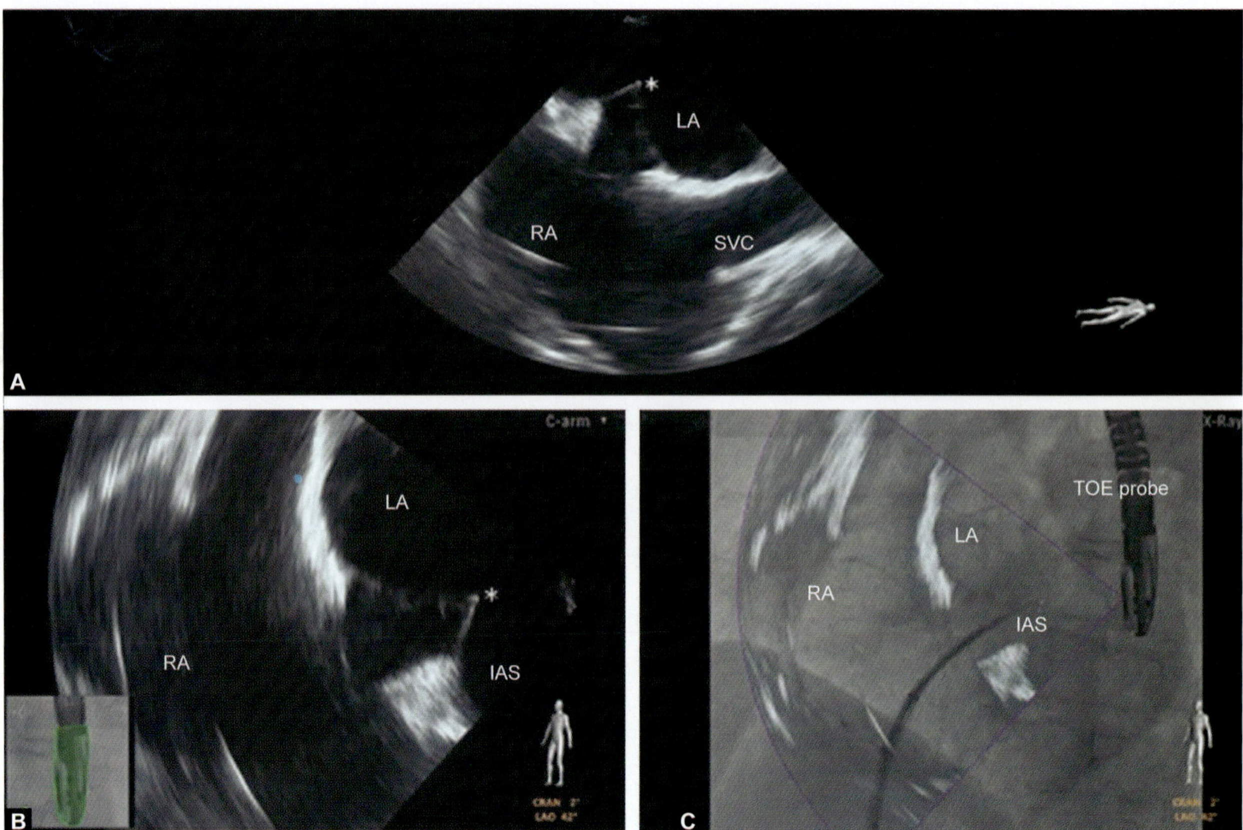

IAS, interatrial septum; RA, right atrium; SVC, superior vena cava; LA, left atrium.

FIG. 3: Septal puncture being shown during left atrial appendage closure by fusion imaging.

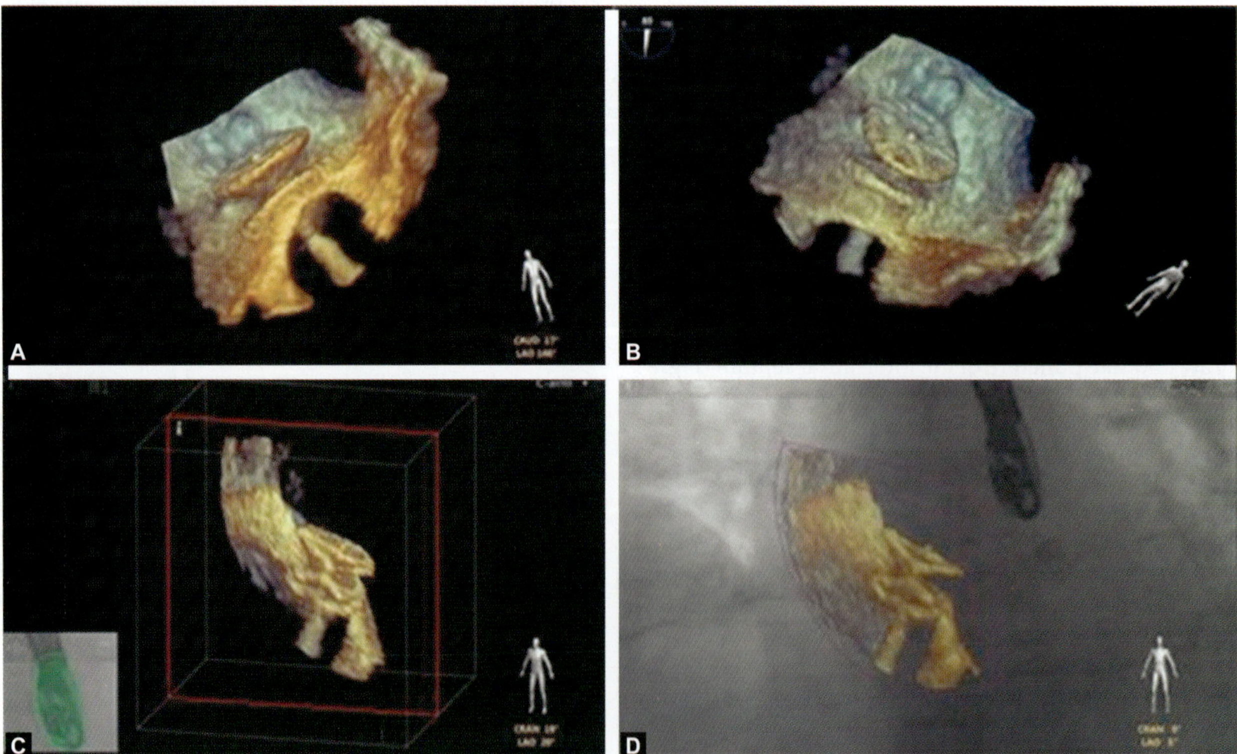

FIG. 4: Atrial septal defect closure being shown by fusion imaging.

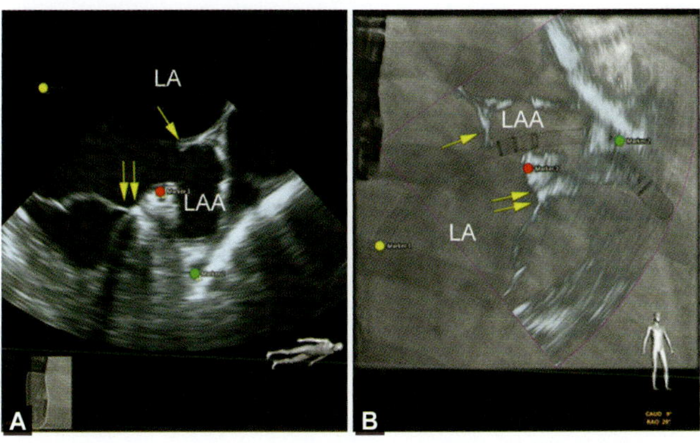

LA, left atrium; LAA, left atrial appendage.

FIG. 5: Fusion imaging showing left atrial appendage closure.

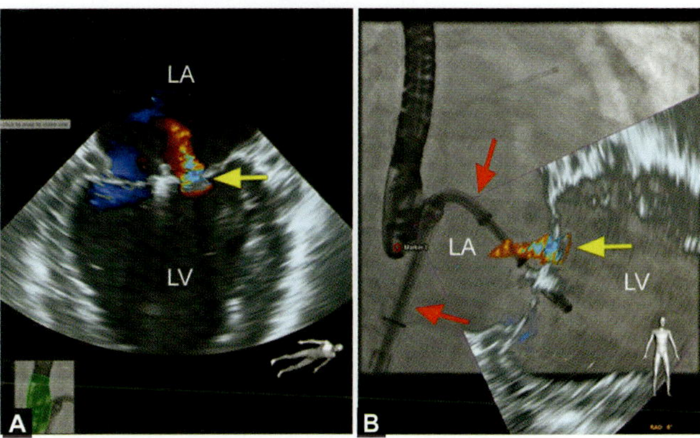

LA, left atrium; LV, left ventricle.

FIG. 6: Fusion imaging during MitraClip procedure.

contraindicated, device closure of LAA has been shown to be safe and effective.[26] During this procedure, guiding wire is crossed through the interatrial septum into the left atrium and the occluder is placed into the LAA. The complication which is expected is perforation of the LAA wall and laceration of the pulmonary artery which can cause pericardial tamponade and immediate death. Fusion echocardiography helps in preventing this complication.

The markers available in EchoNavigator localize the echocardiographic images which appear in the coregistered X-ray images. This allows positioning and alignment of the catheter in the LAA and facilitates the placement of the closure device.[27] These markers can be placed at any level like at the LAA orifice at the level of the circumflex artery or the orifice of the left upper pulmonary vein or at the tip of the LAA.[28] Many times it has been seen that 3D orientation of the LAA can be challenging because of the complex structure.[29] The direct overlay of the real-time 3D TEE echocardiographic information before, during, and after the procedure is helpful to understand the complex relationship between the device and the anatomy of the LAA (Fig. 5).

MITRAL VALVE INTERVENTIONS

Percutaneous Mitral Valve Repair Using MitraClip

Precision is the key during maneuvering the MitraClip device during mitral valve repair. This prevents complications like perforation of the aortic root or left atrial wall. The best way is to direct visualize the mitral valve apparatus by 3D TEE with offline reconstruction techniques. Fluoroscopy also helps in localizing the orientation of guiding system with respect to the structures of the MitraClip and its grippers. Fusion imaging helps in combining these two modalities and compliments the understanding of the orientation of changes during the procedure. During this procedure, localization of the exact site of transseptal puncture in the fossa ovalis is crucial for successful device delivery. The EchoNavigator system helps in localizing the exact location for the transseptal puncture on the TEE images. The same marker simultaneously appears on fluoroscopy together with the echocardiographic image. This augments the localization of precise puncture site and assures the crossing of the device through the interatrial septum.

Fusion imaging is helpful for the safety of the MitraClip procedure. It helps the interventional cardiologist to locate three echocardiographic orientation points (interatrial septum at puncture site, crista terminalis between pulmonary vein and the LAA and the center of the mitral valve) into the fluoroscopic image (Fig. 6). The main complication during this procedure is perforation of the atrial septal wall by the MitraClip leading to cardiac tamponade.

Transcatheter Mitral Valve Replacement

There has been an increase interest and usage of transcatheter mitral valve replacement in last couple of years. This includes valve-in-ring by either transseptal or transapical approach and transapical valve-in-valve options.[30,31] During this procedure, the annuloplasty ring or valve prosthesis can be used as markers. Fusion imaging is however be used for choosing the proper access site. The correct position and function of the implanted prosthetic valve is usually controlled by TEE and is seen on fusion imaging.

Fusion imaging is a mandate for the recently introduced mitral valve prostheses that will be used as percutaneous valve-in-native-valve procedure.[30] If fluoroscopy is used alone, important landmarks are not seen; e.g., during transcatheter mitral valve replacement interventions, mitral annulus or the aortomitral connection are not visible on fluoroscopy alone. For this simultaneous use of 3D TEE is mandatory. In addition, the orientation of the prosthesis is of crucial importance, and proper alignment can be achieved by fused imaging. With the more usage of interventional cardiology for SHD management, there is a great future for real-time fused imaging in this field of managing mitral valve pathologies.

AORTIC VALVE INTERVENTIONS

Transcatheter aortic valve implantation (TAVI) has now been accepted as the treatment of choice for patients with severe

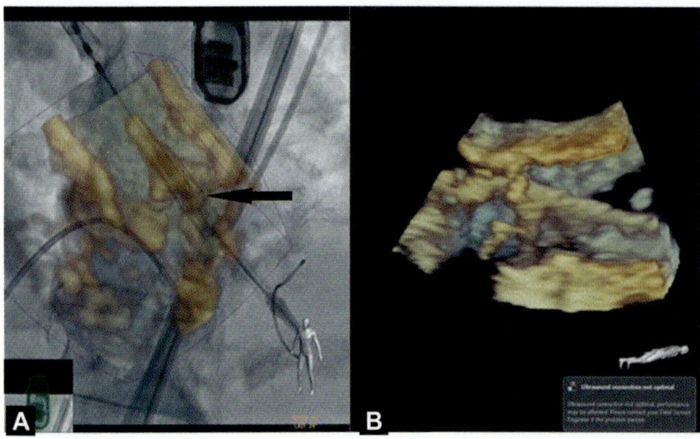

FIG. 7: Fusion imaging during transcatheter aortic valve replacement procedure.

aortic stenosis patients who are in high risk for surgery.[4] Three-dimensional TEE is very useful before, during and after aortic valve implantation as it facilitates precise aortic annular sizing and exact delineation of the hinge points during valve deployment.[32]

In order to optimize TAVI procedural safety and effectiveness, fusion imaging enables a precise knowledge of the anatomy of the aortic root and its surrounding structures.[17] During TAVI interventions, important landmarks of the aortic root such as the leaflets, the coronary cusps, the sinotubular junction, the anatomic ventriculo-arterial junction, the aortic-mitral curtain and the virtual ring formed by the hinge points of the aortic valvar leaflets are not visible on fluoroscopy but on echocardiography. In addition, the orientation of the prosthesis is crucial for procedural success. The EchoNavigator system allows the transfer of specific echocardiographic markers onto the fluoroscopic image (Fig. 7). This enables marking of the level of the annulus and correction of the position of the gantry to the point where all three hinge point markers derived from echocardiography create one orthogonal plane, and thus facilitating catheter guidance and prosthesis placement.[18] It is important to generate a straight line of perpendicularity in order to reach the correct image plain for implantation of the valve.[19] Fusion imaging helps in this.

CONCLUSION

The need of fusion imaging is going to increase due to an increase in aging population going for SHD interventions. The EchoNavigator system from Philips has been an advancement which has helped in fusion of echo and fluoroscopic data in real-time during percutaneous cardiac interventions. It has also helped in better communication between interventional cardiologist and cardiac imager. In conclusion, fusion imaging using the EchoNavigator system has now become a robust tool for SHD intervention and has the advantage of being safe, accurate, and effective. The system is now being used in many in procedures where real-time 3D TEE information is important for precise completion of the procedure.

REFERENCES

1. Matsumoto T, Kar S. Latest advances in transseptal structural heart interventions-percutaneous mitral valve repair and left atrial appendage occlusion. Circ J. 2014;78:1782-90.
2. Faletra FF, Pedrazzini G, Pasotti E, et al. 3D TEE during catheter-based interventions, JACC Cardiovasc Imag. 2014;7:292-308.
3. Makkar RR, Fontana GP, Jilaihawi H, et al. Transcatheter aortic-valve replacement for inoperable severe aortic stenosis. N Engl J Med. 2012;366:1696-704.
4. Smith CR, Leon MB, Mack MJ, et al. Transcatheter versus surgical aortic-valve replacement in high-risk patients. N Engl J Med. 2011;364:2187-98.
5. Feldman T, Foster E, Glower DD, et al. Percutaneous repair or surgery for mitral regurgitation. N Engl J Med. 2011;364:1395-406.
6. Mookadam F, Raslan SF, Jiamsripong P, et al. Percutaneous closure of mitral paravalvular leaks: a systematic review and meta-analysis. J Heart Valve Dis. 2012;21:208-17.
7. Lee MS, Naqvi TZ. A practical guide to the use of echocardiography in assisting structural heart disease interventions. Cardiol Clin. 2013;31:441-54.
8. Tsang W, Lang RM, Kronzon I. Role of real-time three dimensional echocardiography in cardiovascular interventions. Heart. 2011;97:850-7.
9. Carminati M, Agnifili M, Arcidiacono C, et al. Role of imaging in interventions on structural heart disease. Expert Rev Cardiovasc Ther. 2013;11:1659-76.
10. Biaggi P, Fernandez-Golfin C, Hahn R, et al. Hybrid imaging during transcatheter structural heart interventions. Curr Cardiovasc Imaging Rep. 2015;8:33.
11. Jungen C, Zeus T, Balzer J, et al. Left atrial appendage closure guided by integrated echocardiography and fluoroscopy imaging reduces radiation exposure. PLoS One. 2015;10:e0140386.
12. Balzer J, Seus T, Hellhammer K, et al. Initial clinical experience using the EchoNavigator®-system during percutaneous interventions in structural heart disease. World J Cardiol. 2015;7:1-9.
13. Zamorano JL, Badano LP, Bruce, C, et al. EAE/ASE recommendations for the use of echocardiography in new transcatheter interventions for valvular heart disease. Eur Heart J. 2011;32:2189-214.
14. Jilaihawi H, Doctor N, Kashif M, et al. Aortic annular sizing for transcatheter aortic valve replacement using cross-sectional 3-dimensional transesophageal echocardiography. J Am Coll Cardiol. 2013;61:908-16.
15. Gonzalez Gomez A, Hernandez-Antolin R, Zamorano JL. Eco-X Ray Fusion for Transseptal Puncture. Rev Esp Cardiol (Engl Ed). 2015;68:714.
16. Gaemperli O, Schepis T, Kalff V, et al. Validation of a new cardiac image fusion software for three-dimensional integration of myocardial perfusion SPECT and stand-alone 64-slice CT angiography. Eur J Nucl Med Mol Imag. 2007;34:1097-106.
17. Casas RE, Fernandez-Golfin C, Zamorano J. Hybrid imaging with coronary tomography and 3D speckle-tracking stress echocardiography fusion. Eur Heart J Cardiovasc Imag. 2014;15:555.
18. White JA, Fine N, Gula LJ, et al. Fused whole-heart coronary and myocardial scar imaging using 3-T CMR. Implications for planning of cardiac resynchronization therapy and coronary revascularization. JACC Cardiovasc Imag. 2010;3:921-30.
19. Prior JO, Farhad H, Muller O. Multimodality imaging in ischemic cardiomyopathy. Curr Cardiovasc Imaging Rep. 2014;7:9285.
20. Tanis W, Scholtens A, Habets J, et al. CT angiography and (1)(8)F- FDG-PET fusion imaging for prosthetic heart valve endocarditis. JACC Cardiovasc Imag. 2013;6:1008-13.
21. Fagan TE, Truong UT, Jone PN, et al. Multimodality 3-dimensional image integration for congenital cardiac catheterization. Methodist Debakey Cardiovasc J. 2014;10:68-76.
22. Garcia JA, Bhakta S, Kay J, et al. On-line multi-slice computed tomography interactive overlay with conventional X-ray: a new and advanced imaging fusion concept. Int J Cardiol.
23. Kliger C, Eiros R, Isasti G, et al. Review of surgical prosthetic paravalvular leaks: diagnosis and catheter-based closure. Eur Heart J. 2013;34:638-49.
24. Kliger C, Al-Badri A, Wilson S, et al. Successful first-in-man percutaneous transapical-transseptal Melody mitral valve-in-ring implantation after complicated closure of a para-annular ring leak. Euro Intervention. 2014;10:968-74.

25. Kliger C, Jelnin V, Sharma S, et al. CT angiography-fluoroscopy fusion imaging for percutaneous transapical access. JACC Cardiovasc Imag. 2014;7:169-77.
26. Reddy VY, Mobius-Winkler S, Miller MA, et al. Left atrial appendage closure with the Watchman device in patients with a contraindication for oral anticoagulation: the ASAP study (ASA Plavix Feasibility Study With Watchman Left Atrial Appendage Closure Technology). J Am Coll Cardiol. 2013;61:2551-6.
27. Corti R, Biaggi P, Gaemperli O, et al. Integrated x-ray and echocardiography imaging for structural heart interventions. Euro Intervention. 2013;9:863-9.
28. Sommer M, Roehrich A, Boenner F, et al. Value of 3D TEE for LAA Morphology. JACC Cardiovasc Imag. 2015;8:1107-10.
29. Schubert S, Kainz S, Peters B, et al. Interventional closure of atrial septal defects without fluoroscopy in adult and pediatric patients. Clin Res Cardiol. 2012;101:691-700.
30. Cheung A, Stub D, Moss R, et al. Transcatheter mitral valve implantation with Tiara bioprosthesis. Euro Intervention. 2014;10(Suppl U):U115-9.
31. Bouleti C, Fassa AA, Himbert D, et al. Transfemoral implantation of transcatheter heart valves after deterioration of mitral bioprosthesis or previous ring annuloplasty. JACC Cardiovasc Interv. 2015;8:83-91.
32. Krishnaswamy A, Tuzcu EM, Kapadia SR. Three-dimensional computed tomography in the cardiac catheterization laboratory. Catheter Cardiovasc Interv. 2011;77:860-5.

CHAPTER 80

Interpreting a Nuclear Stress Test

GN Mahapatra

INTRODUCTION

Interpretation of a nuclear stress test most commonly known as myocardial perfusion single-photon emission computed tomography (SPECT) and stress positron emission tomography (PET) myocardial perfusion scintigraphy (MPS) are the most important and commonly performed noninvasive cardiac imaging test. The investigation plays an important role in the diagnosis of cardiovascular disease, establishing prognosis, assessing the effectiveness of therapy, and evaluating myocardial viability. Advancing technology and continuous improvements have been largely responsible for the success of the nuclear stress test. These include progressive hardware improvement of SPECT technologies, newer radiopharmaceuticals and new quantitative software. At present, a majority of stress MPS are performed with electrocardiogram (ECG)-gated SPECT which helps in evaluating both myocardial perfusion and cardiac function simultaneously. Although a variety of stress techniques are available, but exercise stress test is the preferred method because it provides several important prognostic data in addition to increasing coronary blood flow. Nuclear pharmacological stress must be considered if there is a contraindication to exercise stress testing. Thallium-201 (Chloride Tl-201), technetium-99m (Tc-99m)-sestamibi and Tc-99m tetrofosmin, N-13 ammonia, rubidium-82 (Rb-82) and very recently F-18-flurpiridaz stress PET myocardial perfusion studies are the currently used radiopharmaceuticals.[1,2] It should be noted that many artifacts and pitfalls in interpretation can potentially compromise nuclear stress test. It is therefore important that the technologist and the interpreting physician should be aware of potential sources of error to take appropriate steps to limit them beforehand, whenever possible. These can help preempt them or else correct them if they occur and if they cannot be eliminated, recognize their potential impact and factor it in the interpretation of the study.[3]

The major indications for nuclear stress test either of single photon emission computed tomography and computed tomography (SPECT-CT) or MPS, SPECT-CT are for the diagnosis of coronary artery disease (CAD) risk stratification in patients with known CAD, assessment of therapy and interpretation and assessment of myocardial viability before percutaneous intervention or bypass surgery. Therefore, it is essential the referring and interpreting physicians are in close collaboration to ensure appropriate indication for the study, optimal patient preparation and effective use of the test results in patient clinical management.

APPROACH TO INTERPRETATION

A systematic and consistent approach should be taken for the interpretation of MPS-SPECT images and should incorporate the following:

- Identify the presence of potential sources of image artifact and the distribution of extracardiac tracer activity during the evaluation of raw images in cine mode
- Ensure that the rest and poststress images are properly aligned
- Interpretation of images with respect to the location size, severity and reversibility of perfusion defects as well as cardiac chamber sizes and especially for Tl-201, presence or absence of increased pulmonary uptake
- Incorporation of the results of quantitative perfusion analysis
- Functional data obtained from gated images should also be considered
- Consideration of clinical factors that may influence the final interpretation of the study.

Normal Myocardial Perfusion Scan and Variants

Both rest and stress images must be evaluated carefully for any recognized artifacts before visual interpretation.[4]

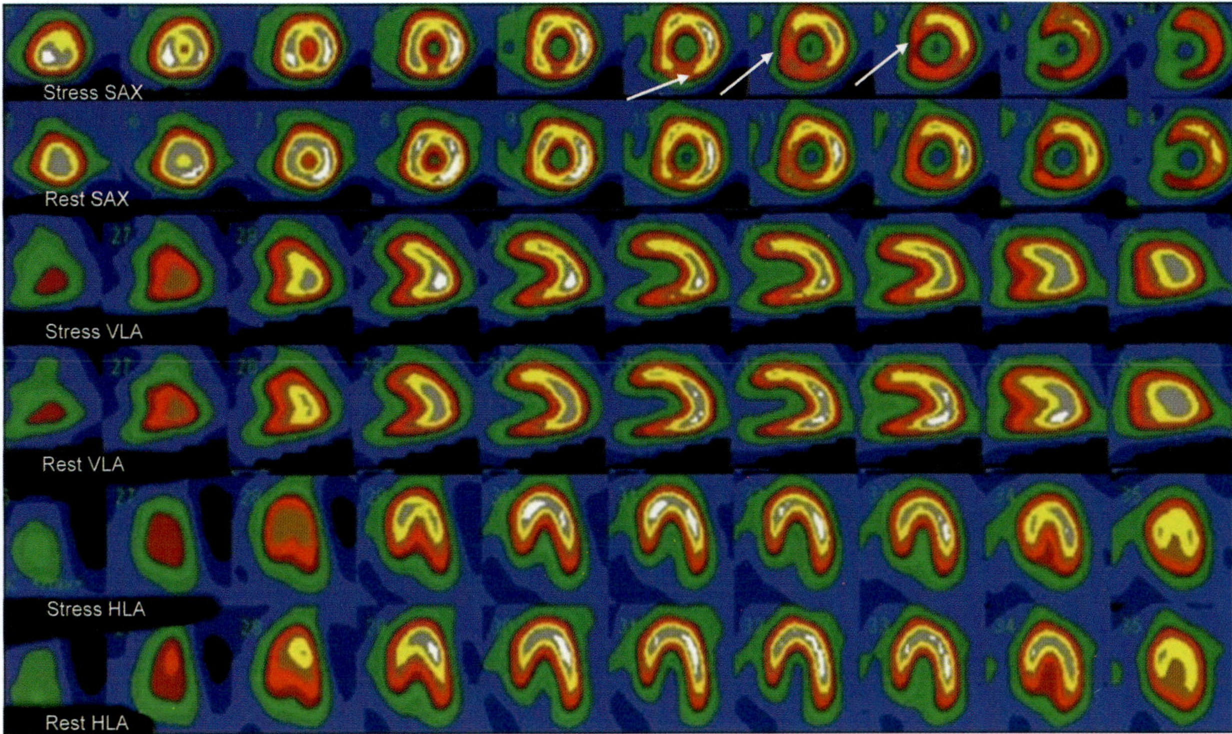

HLA, horizontal long axis; SAX, short axis; VLA, vertical long-axis.

FIG. 1: Normal myocardial perfusion single-photon emission computed tomography (myocardial perfusion scintigraphy) in a 55-year-old man referred because of positive exercise stress test. Both stress and rest images demonstrate normal radiotracer distribution. A mild decreased uptake in basal inferior wall and septum is normal due to membranous septum (white arrows). The top two rows are short-axis (SAX) images of the left ventricle at stress and the second row the corresponding SAX images at rest. The next two rows are vertical long-axis images at stress and rest. The bottom two rows are horizontal long axis at stress and rest.

A normal myocardial perfusion study is characterized by homogeneous radiotracer distribution in both stress and rest images. Slightly diminished activity in the apex may be observed and can be accounted for physiological apical thinning usually limited to the apex and not extending to the anterior wall. Normal thinning of the basal membranous septum and basal inferior wall causes perfusion defect in the corresponding segments. Focal increased activity in and at insertion of papillary muscle (2 o'clock and 6 o'clock position) may give a false impression of a defect adjacent to or between them showing these in long-axis images.

Attenuation Correction and Artifacts

A long recognized major factor limiting the specificity of SPECT for the detection of myocardial perfusion defects is attenuation of photons within the body. The impact of attenuation artifacts depends on the attenuation characteristics of the tissues imaged with the energy of the radio tracer. Various attenuation correction methods have been used.[5] When used in conjunction with quantitative analysis, they can significantly increase the specificity of SPECT myocardial perfusion imaging.[6]

Artifacts of Soft Tissue Attenuation

Soft tissue attenuation for example in the breast is a common reason for artifactual decrease in radio tracer activity in the anterior myocardial wall and may affect the depiction of activity in the septal and lateral walls as well depending on the patient's body habitus. If the breast is in the same position during stress and rest imaging, the apparent perfusion defects will be present on both sets of images. ECG-gated SPECT perfusion images in such case demonstrate normal wall motion and normal wall thickness, the apparent fixed defect is an artifact of soft tissue attenuation instead of an area of myocardial infarction. Other clues to the nature of such a defect may include a noncoronary distribution of the abnormality and the observation of large, dense breasts at cinematic review of the raw images.

Another attenuation artifact observed commonly in the inferior myocardial wall is a common-site of fixed or variable attenuation artifacts produced by the left hemidiaphragm. Again, the ECG-gated SPECT perfusion images will demonstrate normal wall motion and thickness if no perfusion defects are present, confirming the artifactual nature of the abnormalities.[7-10]

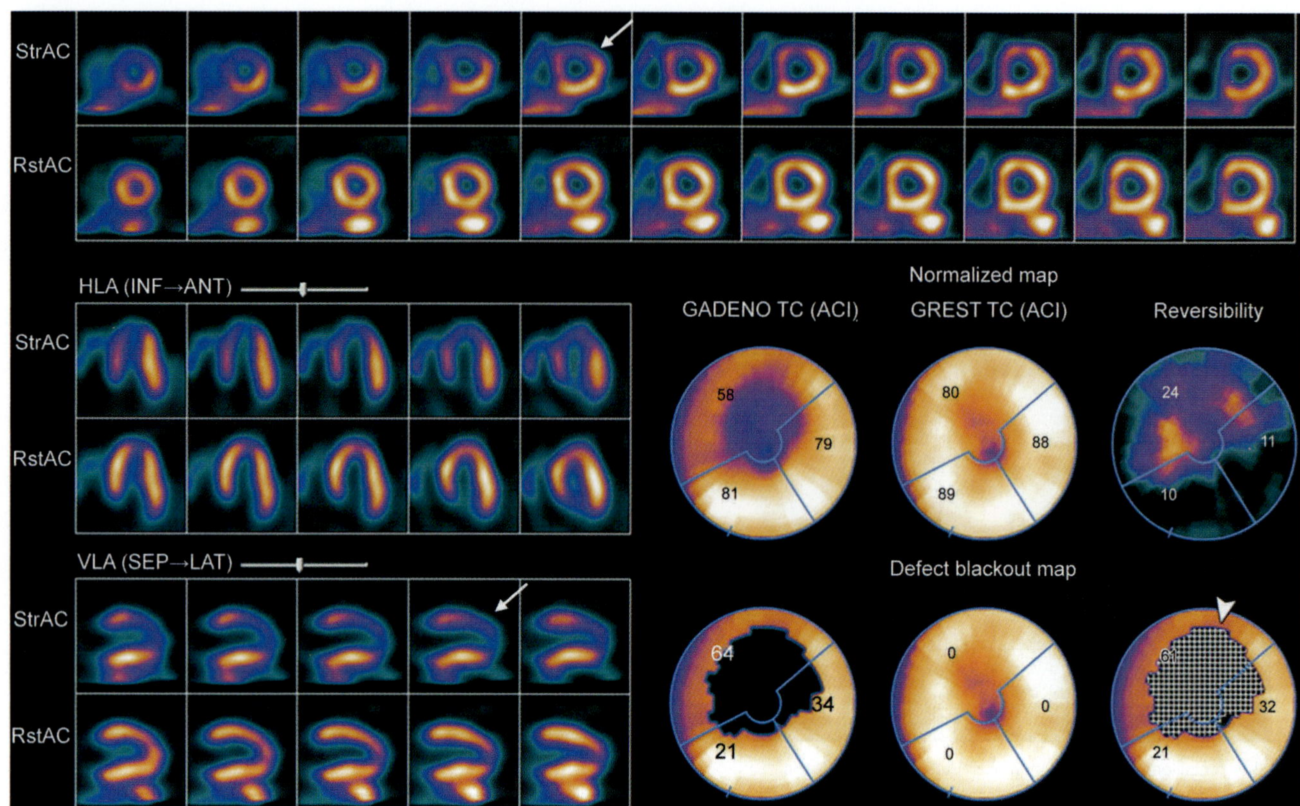

ACI, attenuation-corrected images; ANT, anterior; GADENO TC, electrocardiogram-gated stress imaging with regadenoson and a technetium-99m-labeled tracer; GREST TC, electrocardiogram-gated rest imaging with a technetium-99m-labeled tracer; HLA, horizontal long axis; INF, inferior; LAT, lateral wall; RstAC, attenuation-corrected rest; SEP, septum wall; StrAC, attenuation-corrected stress; VLA, vertical long axis.

FIG. 2: An attenuation-corrected stress and rest myocardial perfusion imaging examination performed with single-photon emission computed tomography or computed tomography showing a large reversible perfusion defect in the territory of the left anterior descending artery.

A substantial number of these artifacts can be corrected with the use of an attenuation correction technique like low-dose breath hold CT scan obtained on a hybrid SPECT-CT system. It would then be possible to compare attenuation corrected images from a particular patient both quantitatively and qualitatively with attenuation corrected images in data bases from patients with normal cardiac perfusion. In addition, if breast attenuation degrades the quality of cardiac perfusion images, the imaging examination can be repeated with patient in the prone position.[5,6]

Artifacts of Subdiaphragmatic Radiotracer Activity

Prominent subdiaphragmatic activity may be seen in organ adjacent to the heart due to hepatobiliary excretion of Tc-99m labeled radiotracers. This is seen predominantly in the liver and bowel but also occasionally in the stomach. Subdiaphragmatic radiotracer activity can affect myocardial perfusion images in several ways. First the scatter radiation from the radiotracer can lead to an appearance of increased perfusion in the inferior myocardial wall that might mask a true perfusion defect in this region especially when the effect of scatter is combined with partial volume effects. Secondly if the highest count is artificially elevated because of scatter, the remainder of the left ventricle may appear to have relatively low activity simulating an extensive perfusion defect.[11,12]

It may be difficult to eliminate the artifacts related to subdiaphragmatic radiotracer activity but several options are available. A repeat image acquisition may be attempted after a delay to allow clearance of the radiotracer from regions adjacent to heart. As with soft tissue attenuation artifacts, repeat imaging with the patient in the prone position can help minimize artifacts caused by—subdiaphragmatic radiotracer activity because the distance between the heart and the subdiaphragmatic organs may be decreased.

Last for patients who are unable to achieve symptom limited maximal exercise-induced stress, it may be helpful to combine the administration of a vasodilator with a low-level exercise protocol tailored to the abilities of the individual patient. The additional exercise induced stress even induced by low-level exercise may prevent subdiaphragmatic activity by reducing splanchnic blood flow to the viscera.

Motion Artifacts

One of the most common sources of artifacts of myocardial perfusion imaging is patient motion usually related to respiration. A careful review of raw images with a rotating cinematic display is best to detect these artifacts. Evaluation

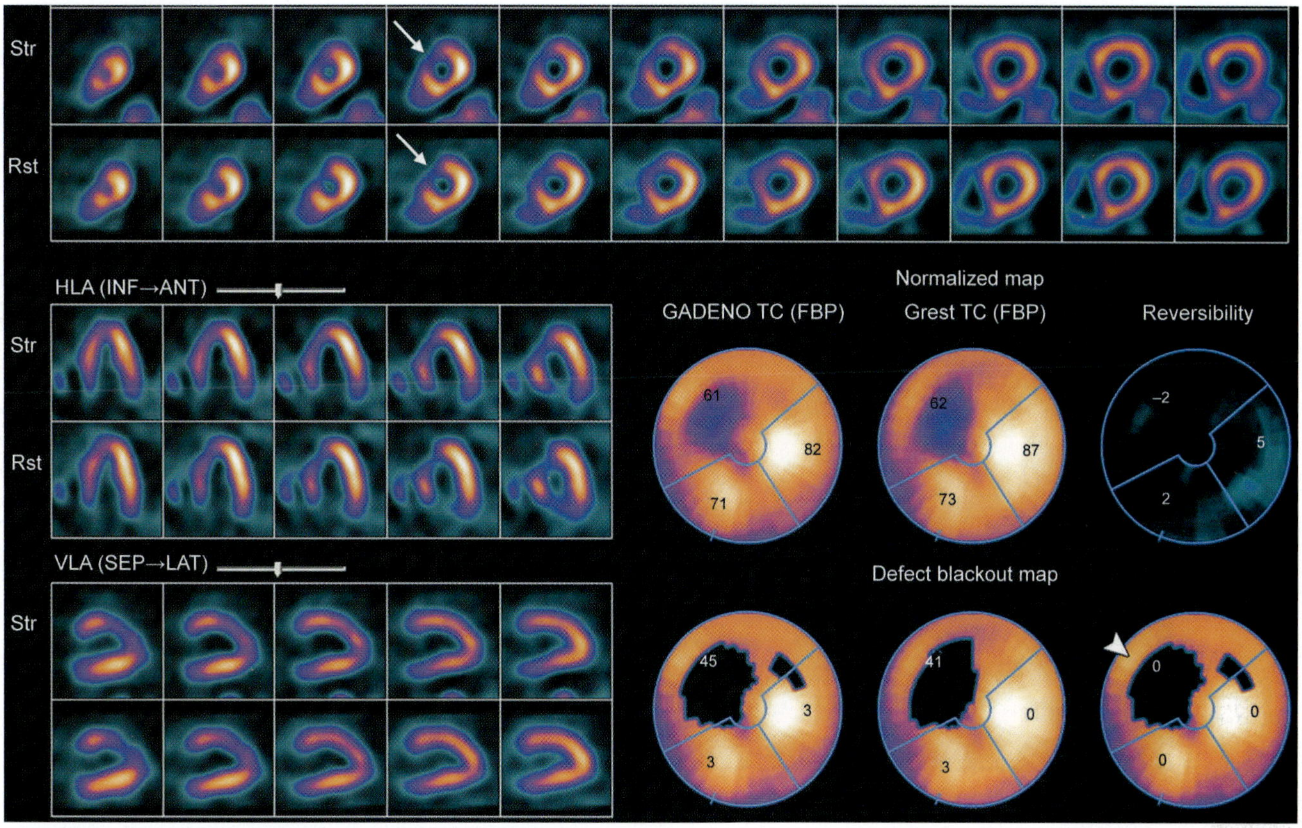

ANT, anterior; FBP, filtered back projection images; GADENO TC, electrocardiogram-gated stress imaging with regadenoson and a technetium-99m-labeled tracer; REST TC, rest imaging with a technetium-99m-labeled tracer; HLA, horizontal long axis; INF, inferior; LAT, lateral wall; Rst, rest; SEP, septum wall; Str, stress; VLA, vertical long axis.

FIG. 3: Shows stress and rest myocardial perfusion imaging performed with single-photon emission computed tomography or computed tomography. Perfusion images and polar maps demonstrate a large fixed anteroseptal perfusion defect, a finding indicative of an infarct in the territory of the left anterior descending artery (arrows). Defect blackout map shows a blackened region. A feature indicative of a fixed perfusion defect (infarction).

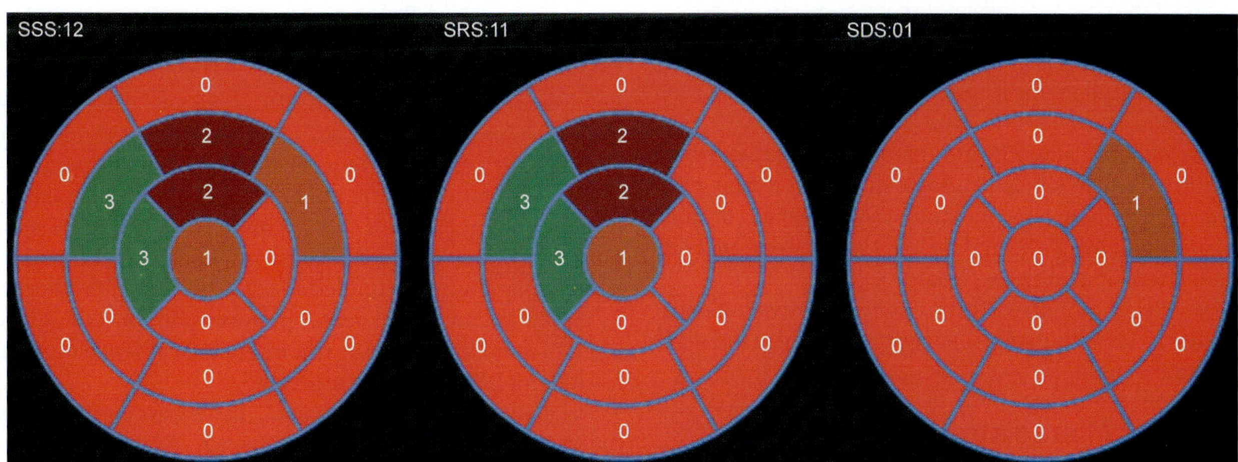

SDS, summed difference score; SRS, summed rest score; SSS, summed stress score.

FIG. 4: Shows the summed stress score, summed rest score, and summed difference score from the same single-photon emission computed tomography or computed tomography myocardial perfusion imaging examination as in figure 6. A summed stress score of 12 indicates an intermediate risk for a hard cardiac event over the subsequent 12 months. Summed stress scores of less than 3 are considered normal, whereas scores of 4–7, 8–12, and 13 or higher are indicative of low, intermediate, and high risk for a hard cardiac event.

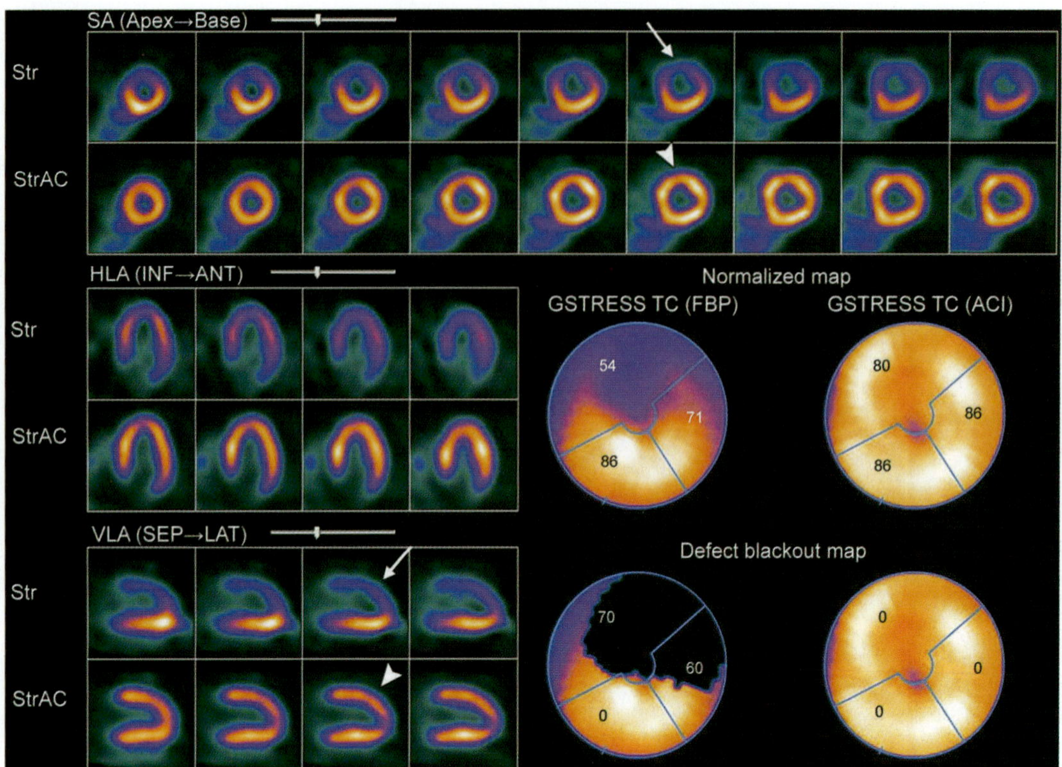

ACI, attenuation-corrected images; ANT, anterior; FBP, filtered back projection images; GSTRESS TC, electrocardiogram-gated stress imaging obtained with technetium-99m-labeled tracer; HLA, horizontal long axis; INF, inferior; LAT, lateral wall; SA, short axis; SEP, septum wall; Str,attenuation correction; StrAC, attenuation-corrected images; VLA, vertical long axis.

FIG. 5: Shows stress-only myocardial perfusion imaging performed with single-photon emission computed tomography or computed tomography in a heavy weight female patient shows a large apparent perfusion defect in the anterolateral myocardial wall (arrows) on images obtained without attenuation correction, whereas attenuation-corrected images show no evidence of a defect at this site (arrowheads).

of the sinogram for discontinuities may be especially useful for detecting movement. In the presence of a motion artifact, the heart will be seen in different location on adjacent SPECT projection images.[13] When the raw projection data are back projected on to the volume reconstruction matrix, there will be inconsistencies that the algorithm cannot correct for and the resultant artifactual defects mimic perfusion abnormalities.[14]

If a substantial amount of motion is detected during a study with a Tc-99m labeled radiotracer, repeat imaging can be performed without a second radiotracer injection became the distribution of Tc-99m labeled radiotracers remains relatively fixed for as early as 2 hours.

Alternatively, motion correction software is available that may be useful for eliminating misregistration due to the slight or moderate motion.

Artifacts of Misregistration

The low-dose CT data obtained for attenuation correction and the SPECT image data are acquired sequentially in the current SPECT-CT system, and patient movement may occur between the two types of acquisitions. Although, the new SPECT-CT system have software to align the SPECT and CT data sets, misregistration may occur if care is not taken in the acquisition and processing of the data sets and may lead to new and unexpected kinds of artifacts. In order to avoid this misregistration, the importance of a careful review of the CT attenuation map and verification of its accurate coregistration with the SPECT images.[13]

Artifacts of Left Bundle Branch Block

Left bundle branch block (LBBB) patients who undergo perfusion imaging during exercise or dobutamine-induced stress may appear to have a reversible or fixed septal perfusion defect. This results in the apparent septal defect appearing more pronounced when stress is induced, which pushes the heart rate higher than when stress is induced by vasodilators which generally have a limited effect on heart rate. In addition to the appearance of a septal perfusion defect, ECG-gated SPECT studies often demonstrate paradoxical septal motions as clues for LBBB-induced artifacts[12]

In patients with hypertrophic cardiomyopathy, asymmetrical septal thickness may create false widespread perfusion defect because of normalization to the hottest pixel in the septum. In balanced ischemia, MPS can only measure relative perfusion, not absolute quantification. The perfusion abnormalities may not be recognized if there is decreased perfusion to all cardiac walls. Decreased post-stress ejection fraction (EF) and new regional wall motion abnormality compared to rest scan, abnormal transient ischemic dilation

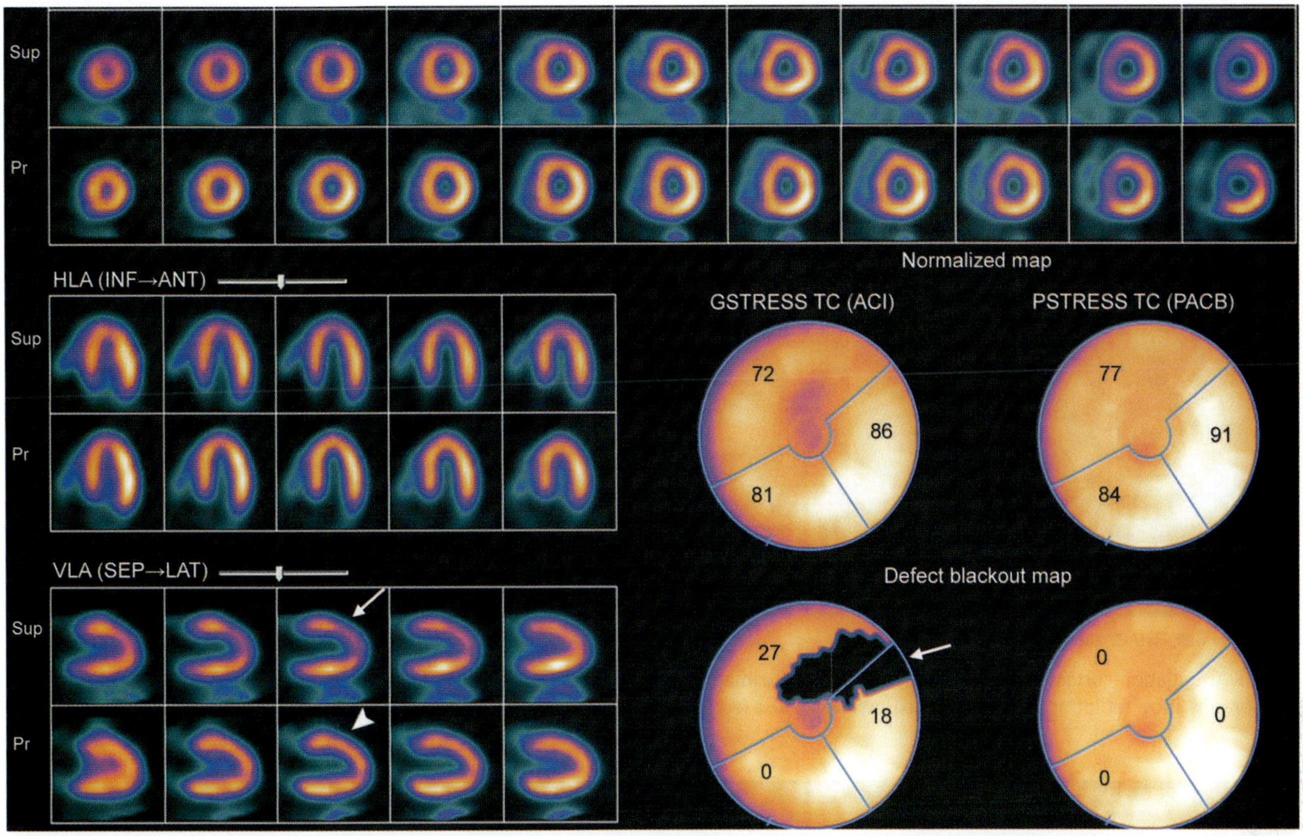

ACI, attenuation-corrected images; ANT, anterior; GSTRESS TC, supine electrocardiogram-gated stress imaging with a technetium-99m-labeled tracer; PSTRESS TC, prone free-breathing stress imaging with a technetium-99m-labeled tracer; HLA, horizontal long axis; INF, inferior, LAT, lateral wall; Pr, prone; Sup, supine; VLA, vertical long axis.

FIG. 6: Shows attenuation-corrected stress-only myocardial perfusion imaging performed with single-photon emission computed tomography or computed tomography) in a normal subject shows different results with the subject supine and prone: an area of reduced perfusion defect is seen in the anterior myocardial wall on supine images (arrows), whereas perfusion appears normal at this site on prone images (arrowhead). The apparent perfusion defect seen in this case is an artifact of soft tissue (breast) attenuation.

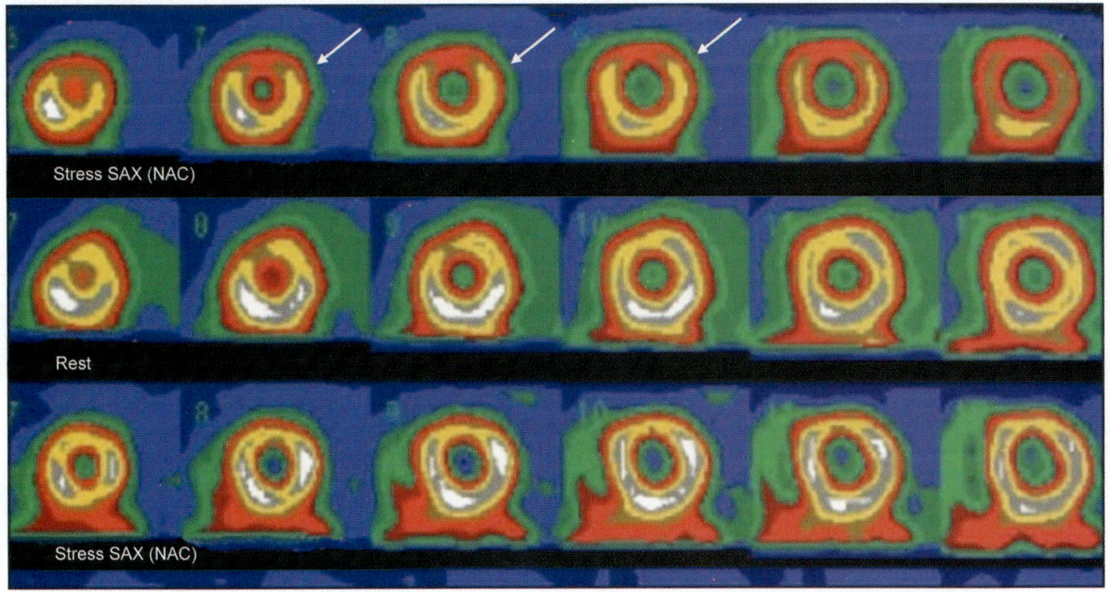

NAC, nonattenuation-corrected; SAX, short axis.

FIG. 7: Shifting breast attenuation in 60-year-old women came with chest pain, the myocardial perfusion scintigraphy was performed with dipyridamole because patient could not exercise owing to severe arthritis. Stress nonattenuation correction (NAC) images show anterior wall perfusion defect (white arrows) with normalization at rest. In the attenuation correction images (lower row) the perfusion defect disappears. Based on this finding the study was interpreted as normal with breast attenuation on NAC images.

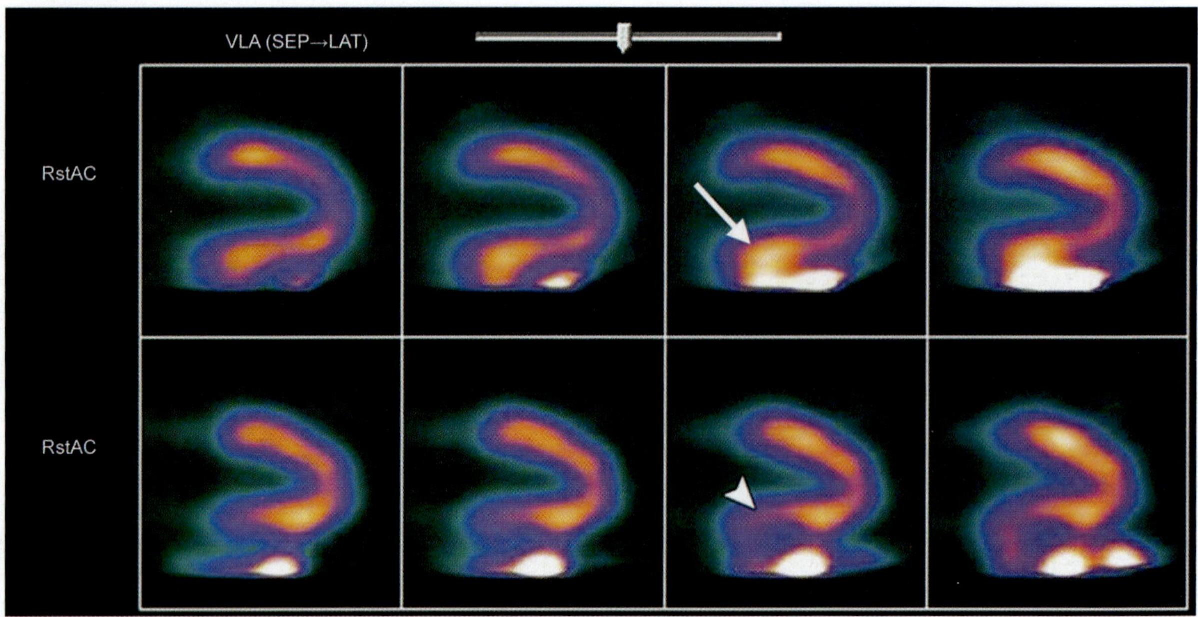

LAT, lateral wall; RstAC, attenuation-corrected resting; SEP, septum wall, VLA, vertical long axis.

FIG. 8: Attenuation-corrected resting myocardial perfusion images obtained with single-photon emission computed tomography or computed tomography show radiotracer activity in the bowel (arrow), a feature that masks the inferior wall defect evident on delayed images (arrowhead).

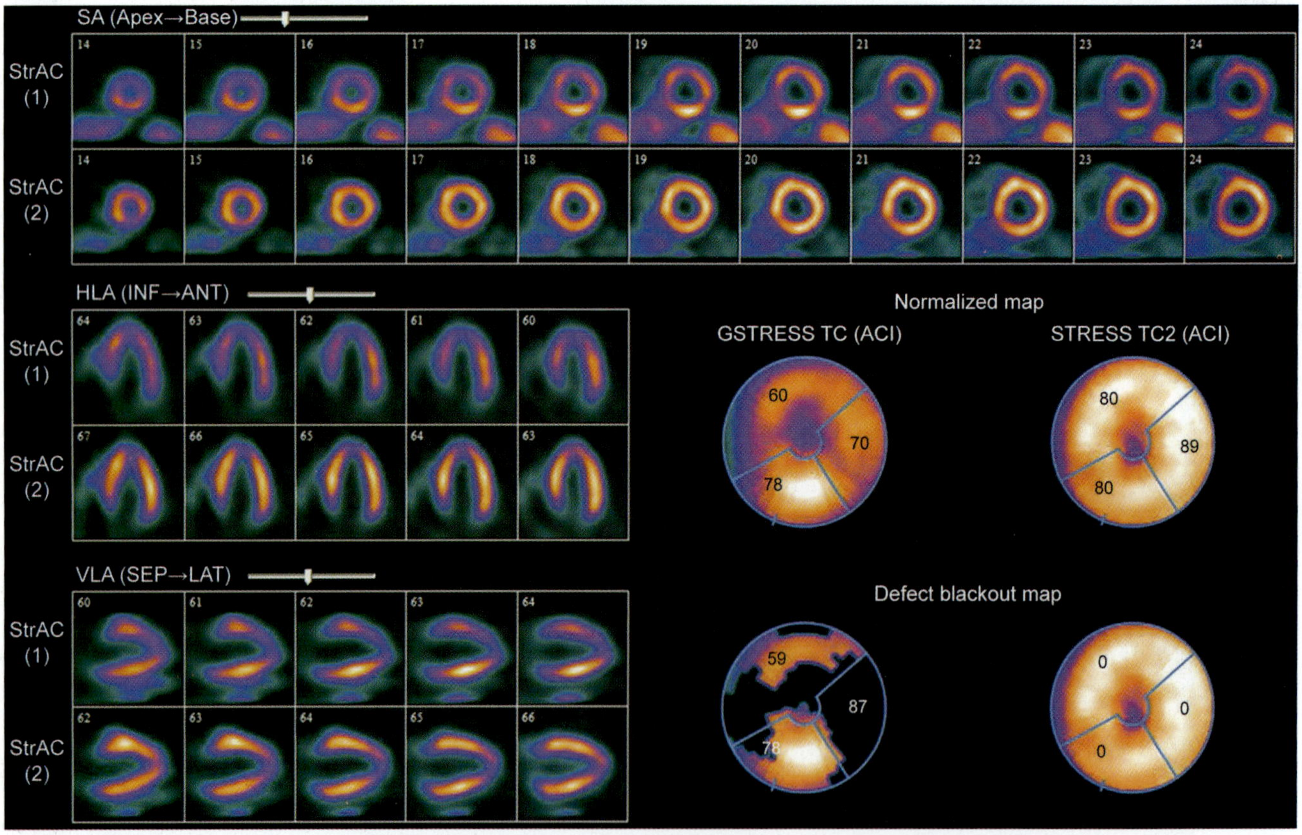

ACI, attenuation-corrected images; ANT, anterior; GSTRESS TC, electrocardiogram-gated stress imaging with a technetium-99m-labeled tracer; HLA,horizontal long axis; INF, inferior; LAT, lateral wall; SEP, septum wall; SA, short axis; StrAC, attenuation-corrected stress; STRESS TC2, delayed stress imaging after clearance of the radiotracer from abdominal organs; VLA, vertical long axis

FIG. 9: Shows an attenuation-corrected stress myocardial perfusion imaging examination (StrAC[1]) performed with single-photon emission computed tomography or computed tomography shows an extensive artifact in the inferior wall on images and polar maps. The artifact was caused by normalization errors produced by subdiaphragmatic scatter radiation. Repeat imaging (StrAC[2]) after clearance of the radiotracer from abdominal organs showed normal perfusion at the site of the apparent defect.

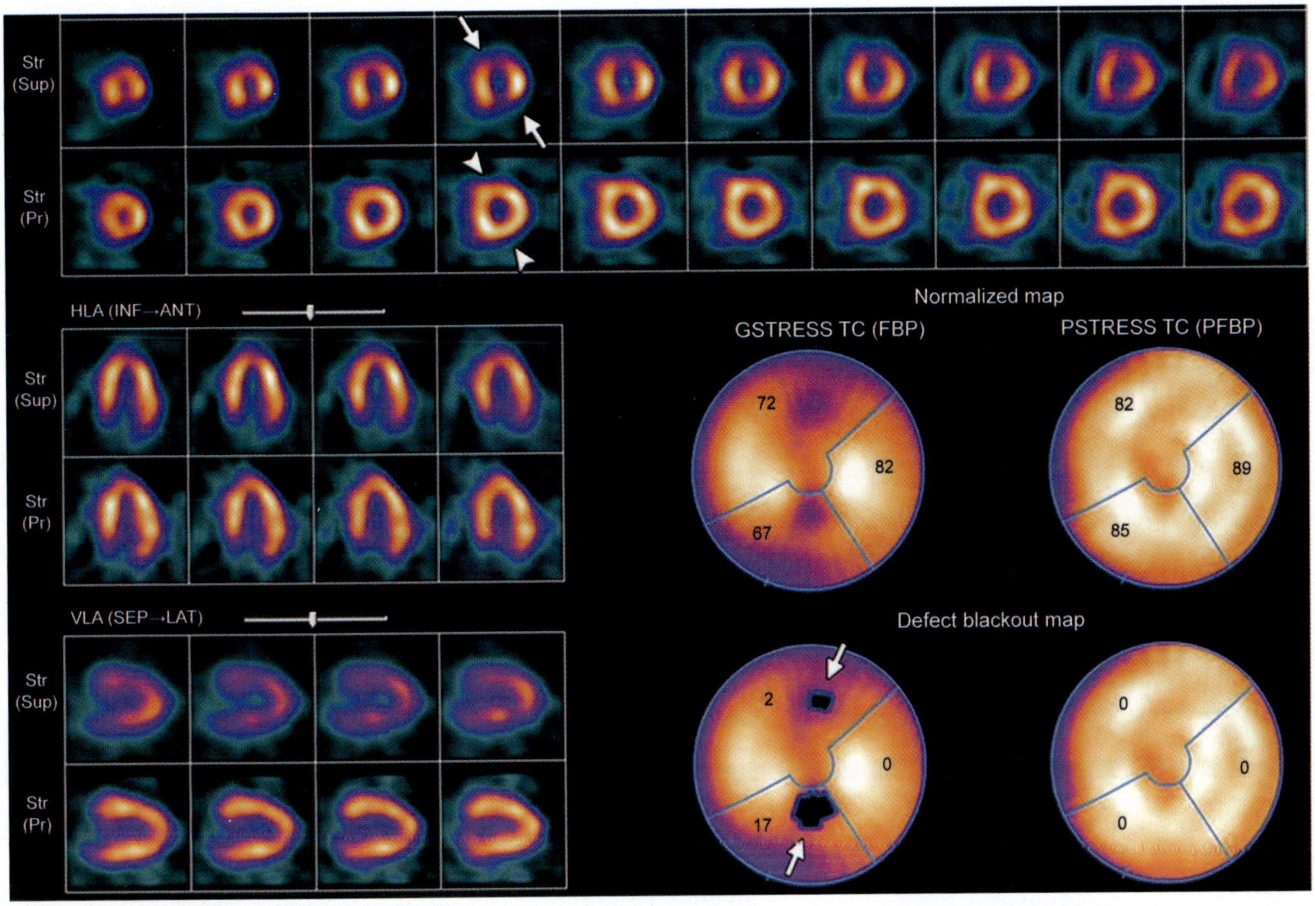

ANT, anterior; GSTRESS TC (FBP), supine electrocardiogram-gated stress imaging with a technetium-99m-labeled tracer and filtered back projection; HLA, horizontal long axis; INF, inferior; LAT, lateral wall; Pr, prone; PSTRESS TC (PFBP), prone free-breathing stress imaging with a technetium-99m-labeled tracer and prone filtered back projection; SEP, septum wall; Str, stress; Sup, supine; VLA, vertical long axis.

FIG. 10: Shows an attenuation-corrected stress and rest myocardial perfusion imaging examination performed with single-photon emission computed tomography or computed tomography (SPECT/CT) in a patient with chest pain. Initial screen shows a large reversible perfusion defect in the lateral and anterolateral wall (arrow in *a*), an artifact that is due to misregistration of the CT attenuation map and SPECT image dataset. Repeat analysis obtained after reregistration of the SPECT and CT datasets (*b*) shows normal perfusion at the site of the apparent perfusion defect.

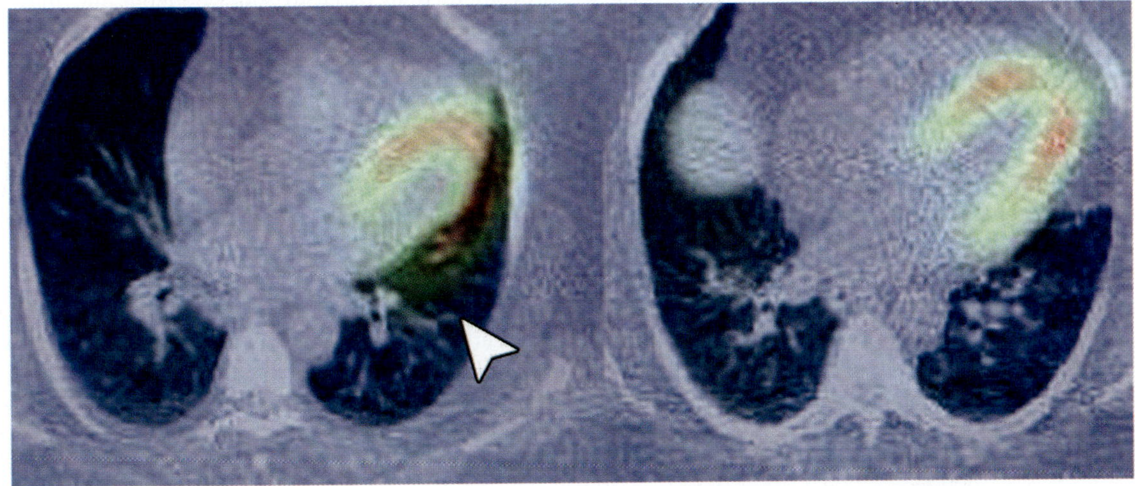

FIG. 11: Fused single-photon emission computed tomography or computed tomography (SPECT/CT) image obtained after the first post processing attempt (left) shows a defect in coregistration, with projection of the lateral wall of myocardium over the lung field (arrowhead). Fused image obtained after proper coregistration of the SPECT and CT datasets (right) shows normal perfusion.

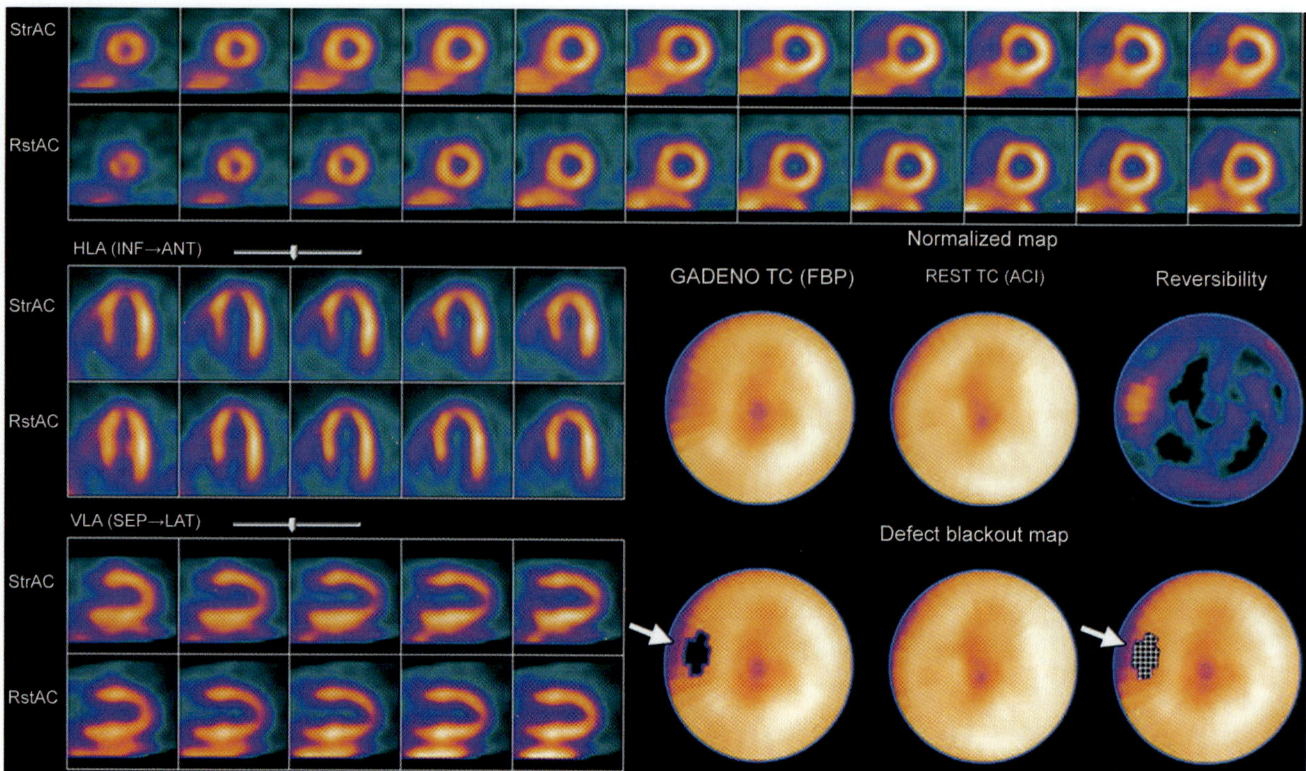

ACI, attenuation-corrected images; ANT, anterior; GADENO TC, electrocardiogram-gated stress imaging with regadenoson and a technetium-99m-labeled tracer; REST TC, rest imaging with a technetium-99m-labeled tracer; HLA, horizontal long axis; INF, inferior; LAT, lateral wall; RstAC, attenuation-corrected rest; SEP, septum wall; StrAC, attenuation-corrected stress; VLA, vertical long axis.

FIG. 12: Shows an attenuation-corrected stress and rest myocardial perfusion imaging examination performed with single-photon emission computed tomography or computed tomography in a patient with a left bundle branch block. Defect blackout maps from stress imaging show a small reversible perfusion defect in the midseptum (arrows), but this region appears normal on the rest images, and the septum is an unusual location for isolated coronary artery disease. Septal perfusion defects, whether reversible or fixed, are most likely to represent left bundle branch block-related artifacts.

(TID) and abnormal increased lung uptake Tl-201 are some clues pointing toward the possibility of balanced ischemia. Very recently calculation of coronary flow reserve (CFR) in three major arteries holds the key.

Artifact Related to Nuclear Medicine Equipment

Flood-field nonuniformity may be secondary to a defect in the photo multiplier tube, damage in collimator or faulty camera electronics. A daily intrinsic and weekly extrinsic flood field should be obtained in order to detect such abnormalities. SPECT acquisition using a camera with one or more source of nonuniformity typically produces ring artifacts which may create a false myocardial ischemia. Other sources of instrumentation artifacts include error in center rotation, camera head tilt and increased detector to patient distance. Both technologist and physician should be familiar with these potential artifacts and be able to detect and correct them.

Effect of Normal Apical Thinning

A normal anatomic finding, apical thinning is seen commonly and has a multifactorial etiology. Thinning may be more prominent than usual in some patients and may simulate a perfusion defect. Apical thinning is more apparent on attenuation corrected images and may be accentuated by the scatter correction and resolution recovery process that is commonly incorporated in the reconstruction of attenuation corrected images. Due to the proximity of the apex to the detector, the spatial resolution of the normally thin apical segments of the left ventricle is greater than that of other segments. Vertical and horizontal long-axis cardiac images and polar map displays are best to visualize apparent perfusion defect resulting from apical thinning. ECG-gated stress and rest SPECT images in such cases will show normal wall motion and normal wall thickening. With matching stress and rest perfusion patterns, recognition of preserved wall motion confirms that the apparent perfusion defect is prominent apical thinning and not an infarcted myocardium.[6]

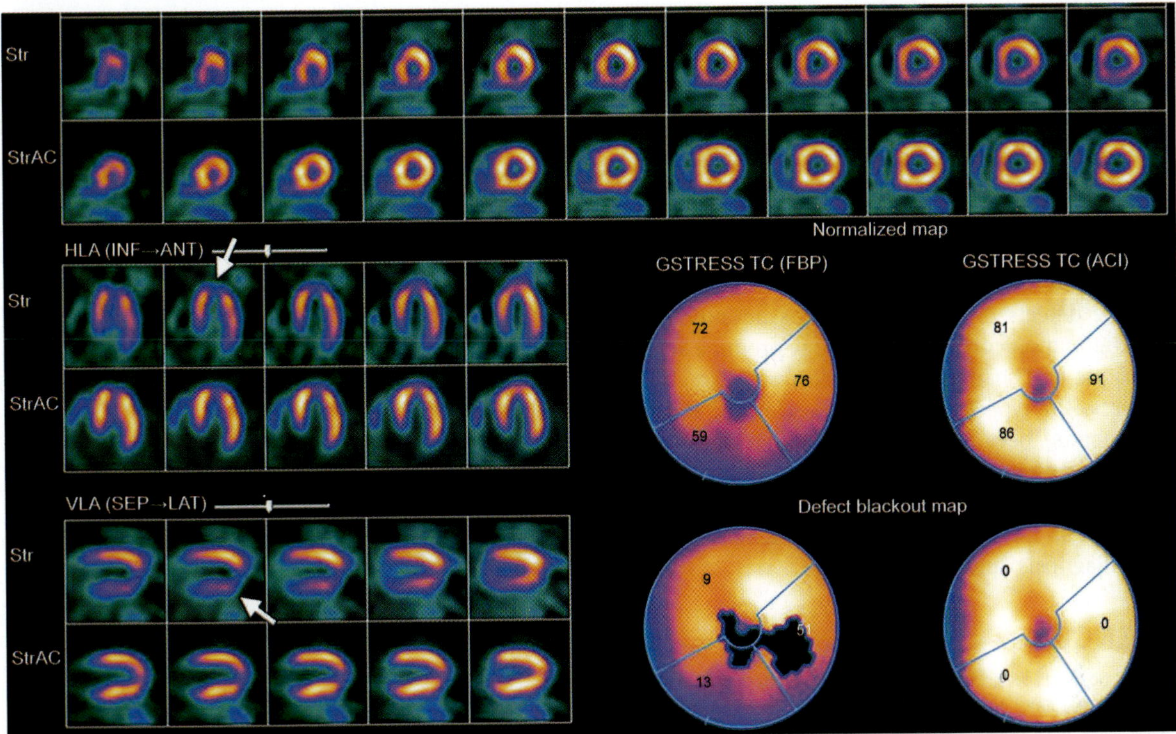

ACI, attenuation-corrected images; ANT, anterior; FBP, filtered back projection images; GSTRESS TC, electrocardiogram-gated stress imaging with a technetium-99m-labeled tracer; HLA, horizontal long axis; INF, inferior; LAT, lateral wall; SEP, septum wall; Str, stress; StrAC, attenuation-corrected stress; VLA, vertical long axis.

FIG. 13: Shows a stress-only myocardial perfusion imaging examination performed with single-photon emission computed tomography or computed tomography, with (StrAC) and without (Str) attenuation correction, shows an apparent small perfusion defect at the cardiac apex on both sets of images (arrows). This commonly observed feature is produced by apical thinning, and it should not be confused with a true perfusion defect; note that left ventricular wall motion and thickness appear normal.

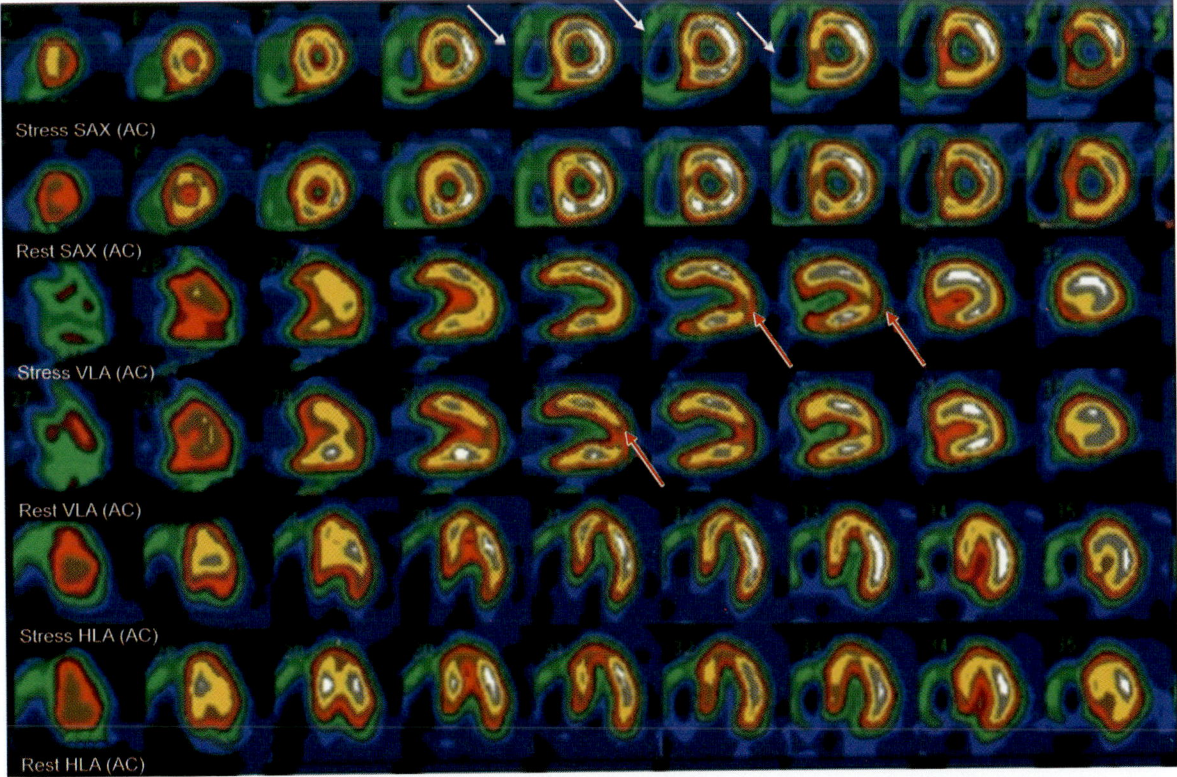

AC, attenuation correction; HLA, horizontal long axis; SAX, short axis; VLA, vertical long axis.

FIG. 14: Normal attenuation correction (AC) myocardial perfusion scintigraphy in 62-year-old women was performed for risk assessment before vascular surgery. In the AC images the right ventricle is clearly visualized, not to be confused with right ventricular hypertrophy (white arrows). The normal apical thing is more severe in AC images, and sometimes appears as a true perfusion defect (red arrows).

CONCLUSION

Accurate interpretation of nuclear stress test particularly of gated SPECT or SPECT-CT myocardial perfusion imaging studies requires both a working knowledge of potential abnormalities and a thorough understanding of the artifacts that can occur in image data acquisition and processing. Factors such as patient motion and improper alignment of the raw SPECT and CT image data sets can lead to propagation of artifacts on the final images. The attenuation corrected images can eliminate defects produced by soft tissue attenuation. However, attenuation correction itself may produce artifacts if the anatomic and scintigraphic images are misregistered in the process. The type of stress study performed also may affect the outcome, because left bundle branch block related artifacts are accentuated by physical stress and minimized by pharmacological stress. Review of the raw SPECT and CT images as well as the final reconstructed images can help prevent misdiagnosis due to artifacts.

REFERENCES

1. Albro PC, Gould KL, Westcott RJ, et al. Noninvasive assessment of coronary stenoses by myocardial imaging during pharmacologic coronary vasodilatation III. Clinical trial. Am J Cardiol. 1978;42(5):751-60.
2. Weich HF, Strauss HW, Pitt B. The extraction of thallium-201 by the myocardium. Circulation. 1977;56(2):188-91.
3. Beller GA, Watson DD. Physiological basis of myocardial perfusion imaging with technetium 99m agents. Semin Nucl Med. 1991;21(3):173-81.
4. Husain SS. Myocardial perfusion imaging protocols: is there an ideal protocol? J Nucl Med Technol. 2007;35(1):3-9.
5. Holly TA, Abbott BG, Al-Mallah M, et al. (2010). Imaging guidelines for nuclear cardiology procedure. Menu: Manage your practice: Guidelines and standards. [online] Available from http://www.asnc.org. [Accessed October, 2018].
6. Hendel RC, Corbett JR, Cullom SJ, et al. The value and practice of attenuation correction for myocardial perfusion SPECT imaging: a joint position statement from the American Society of Nuclear Cardiology and the Society of Nuclear Medicine. J Nucl Cardiol. 2002;9(1):135-43.
7. Cullom SJ, Case JA, Bateman TM. Electrocardiographically gated myocardial perfusion SPECT: technical principles and quality control considerations. J Nucl Cardiol. 1998;5(4):418-25.
8. Burrell S, MacDonald A. Artifacts and pitfalls in myocardial perfusion imaging. J Nucl Med Technol. 2006;34(4):193-211.
9. Cooper JA, Neumann PH, McCandless BK. Effect of patient motion on tomographic myocardial perfusion imaging. J Nucl Med. 1992;33(8):1566-71.
10. van Dongen AJ, van Rijk PP. Minimizing liver, bowel, and gastric activity in myocardial perfusion SPECT. J Nucl Med. 2000;41(8):1315-7.
11. Miles J, Cullom SJ, Case JA. An introduction to attenuation correction. J Nucl Cardiol. 1999;6(4):449-57.
12. Burns RJ, Galligan L, Wright LM, et al. Improved specificity of myocardial thallium-201 single-photon emission computed tomography in patients with left bundle branch block by dipyridamole. Am J Cardiol. 1991;68(5):504-8.
13. Galt JR, Germano G. Advances in instrumentation for cardiac SPECT. In: Depuey EG, Berman DS, Garcia EV, (Eds). Cardiac SPECT Imaging. New York: Raven Press; 1995. pp. 91-102.
14. Friedman J, Berman DS, Van Train K, et al. Patient motion in thallium-201 myocardial SPECT imaging. An easily identified frequent source of artifactual defect. Clin Nucl Med. 1988;13(5):321-4.

CHAPTER 81

Myocardial Viability Assessment: How Do We Apply in Clinical Practice?

Nagendra Boopathy Senguttuvan, Kewal C Goswami

INTRODUCTION

The term "viable" means things that are alive. At the cellular level, the term viable is defined by preserved metabolic, cellular, and contractile functions. According to Cambridge English Dictionary, the meaning of the word viable is "ability to work as intended or to succeed". The concepts discussed in this chapter are about the myocardial viability, different types of myocardial viability, pathophysiology, and assessment of myocardial viability in the current era.

ENERGY AND ISCHEMIA

When the total coronary artery occlusion duration lasts for less than 15–20 minutes, it does not cause necrosis. The amount of adenosine triphosphate (ATP) in the central region is reduced. In 3 minutes after occlusion, the ATP level is decreased to less than 50% of the preischemic level. The ATP levels are 22% of preischemic level after 3 days of reperfusion. Seven days are required for the ultrastructural changes to occur due to ischemia. There is shortage of the creatine phosphate stores from which ATP is formed. Plasma permeability is increased due to decrease in ATP leading to washout of the metabolites of ATP. This results in shortage of ATP after ischemia. ATP shortage causes decreased myocardial contractility. Myocardial dysfunction is also caused by the calcium influx postischemic reperfusion.[1]

After acute coronary occlusion, the ischemic cascade starts with reversible myocardial contractile dysfunction within seconds. In 20–30 minutes, intracellular edema occurs followed by irreversible myocyte injury in 30–60 minutes and, in 60–90 minutes, vascular endothelial cell injury occurs followed by cellular necrosis and apoptosis.[2] In myocardial necrosis, transmurality is time dependent as progression is from subendocardium toward subepicardium over 3–6 hours.[2]

Types of Viable Myocardium

Viable myocardium is referred to as "alive myocardium" and the reference in irrespective of the contractile status of the myocardium.[3] When blood flow is abruptly reduced, contractile dysfunction occurs, which persists even after the blood flow is restored, it is called "hit, run, and stun" phenomenon.[1] Viable dysfunctional myocardium is classified into hibernating myocardium and stunned myocardium. In patients with ischemic cardiomyopathy, the cellular changes are not uniform in the viable myocardium. The ultrastructural damage reflects concurrent process of myocardial hibernation and myocardial stunning.[4]

Hibernating Myocardium

Hibernating myocardium occurs due to persistently impaired coronary blood flow. The function of the myocardium may be completely or partially restored by improving the coronary blood flow. Myocardial function is also restored by reducing oxygen demand or by inotropic stimulation.[4] Hibernating myocardium is an adaptive mechanism to prevent myocyte death and preserve structural integrity of myocardium.[5] Metabolically, there is activation of the fetal gene program in the hibernating myocardium. Innate mechanism of myocardial protection causes similarities in hibernating myocardium and fetal myocardium.[6] At cellular level, there is dedifferentiation to embryonic phenotype with loss of myofibrils and sarcomeres, fibrotic changes in extracellular matrix, and increased glycogen storage.[7] There is switch in the metabolism from fat to glucose metabolism. Glycogen content of hibernating myocardium is increased dramatically. Time taken for recovery may be 6 months or more for severe ultrastructural derangement and 10 days for minor structural abnormalities.[8] Resting blood flow is reduced in hibernating myocardium. The spectrum of abnormalities assessed from a cellular, metabolic, and functional myocardial perfusion, and global left ventricular (LV) perspective is described in figure 1.[5]

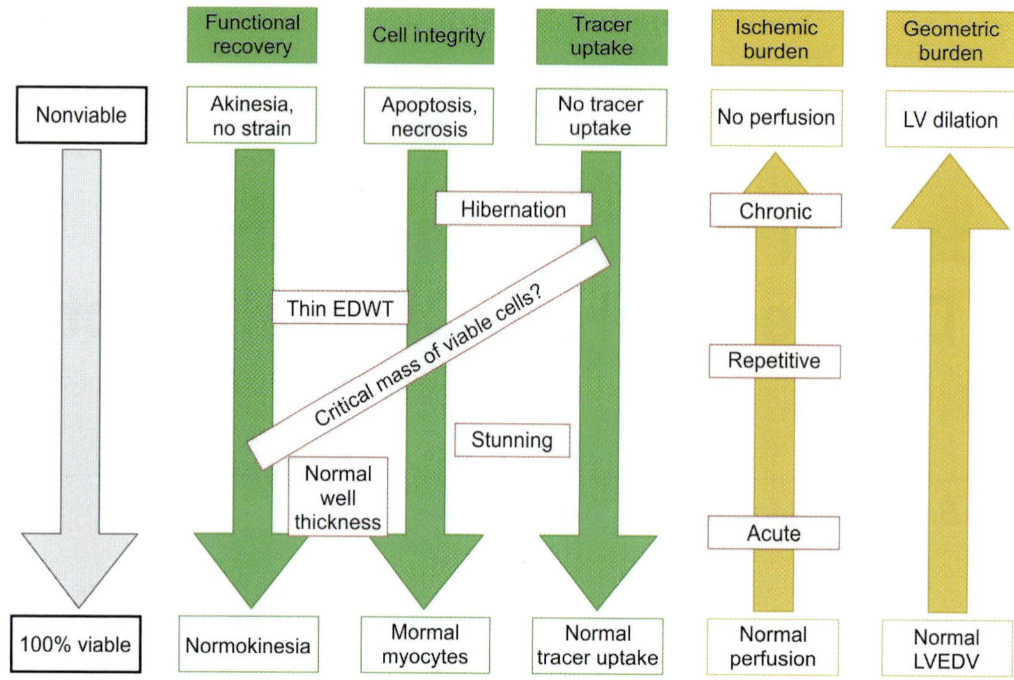

FIG. 1: Spectrum of abnormalities assessed from a cellular, metabolic and functional myocardial perfusion, and global left ventricular perspective.

Stunning Myocardium

The phenomenon of stunning myocardium in dogs was first observed by Heyndrickx.[9] Heyndrickx observed that ischemic myocardial cells that have been perfused, there is prolonged depression of the regional myocardial function. When myocardium undergoes repetitive ischemic episodes with stress, there is depressed cardiac function known as repetitive myocardial stunning. There is contractile dysfunction in stunned heart with normal perfusion. Myocardial function improves with revascularization.[10] The resting blood flow is preserved and the flow reserve is reduced.[11] Hence, myocardial stunning physiology is referred to as "perfusion contraction mismatch". Incomplete functional recovery of stunning segments between consecutive ischemia episodes results in permanently depressed myocardial function.

REVASCULARIZATION

Depressed LV function in patients with ischemic cardiomyopathy can be reversed using revascularization. Benefits of revascularization are increase in the resting left ventricular ejection fraction (LVEF) and reducing the inducible ischemia, thereby decreasing ventricular remodeling and diastolic dysfunction and thus reducing the symptoms of congestive heart failure (CHF).[12] STICHES (Surgical Treatment for IsCHemic heart failure Extension Study) is a 10-year follow-up study of patients with coronary artery disease (CAD), LV dysfunction (LVEF <335%) and ischemic cardiomyopathy amenable to coronary artery bypass grafting (CABG). Mortality of patients was reduced by 8% in patients who had CABG along with optimal medical therapy (OMT) when compared to those only on optimal contemporary medical treatment.

MODALITIES OF VIABILITY TESTING

Myocardial viability is tested using ultrasound, nuclear, and magnetic resonance based techniques (Table 1).

- Low-dose dobutamine stress echocardiography (DSE)—LV contractile reserve
- Late gadolinium enhancement with cardiac magnetic resonance (CMR)—identification of scarred myocardium
- Single-photon emission computed tomography (SPECT)—assess myocardial perfusion
- Positron emission tomography (PET)—assess myocardial perfusion, mitochondrial, sarcolemma, inner membrane integrity, intracellular glucose and fatty acid metabolism.

Echocardiography

Echocardiography is used to assess both LV and right ventricular (RV) systolic and diastolic function. Echocardiography can delineate contractile reserve with low dose of dobutamine. Patients with LV end-diastolic wall thickness more than 0.5–0.6 cm with hypokinetic rather than dyskinetic or akinetic myocardium indicates chances of improvement in LV function after revascularization.

TABLE 1: Comparison of diagnostic accuracy of noninvasive cardiac modalities in the diagnosis of myocardial viability

Imaging modality	Number of patients	Number of studies included	Specificity	Sensitivity	Negative predictive value	Positive predictive value
^{99}Tc labeled	721	25	65%	83%	76%	74%
^{201}Tl imaging	1119	40	54%	87%	79%	67%
DSE	1421	41	78%	80%	83%	75%
FDG PET	598	20	58%	93%	77%	85%
Cardiac magnetic resonance						
DSMR	272	9	82%	74%	78%	78%
EDWT	100	3	41%	95%	92%	56%
LGEMR	178	5	63%	84%	78%	72%

^{99}Tc, technetium-99m; ^{201}Tl, thallium-201, DSE, dobutamine stress echocardiography; DSMR, dobutamine stress magnetic resonance; FDG PET, fluorodeoxyglucose positron emission tomography; EDWT, end-diastolic wall thickness; LGEMR, late gadolinium enhancement magnetic resonance.

Tissue Doppler Imaging

Viable myocardium demonstrates positive velocities in tissue Doppler imaging. Deceleration time (DT) and strain rate are used to assess viability. A DT more than 150 ms predict an increase in LVEF by 5% after revascularization by CABG. Viable myocardium is indicated by increase in peak systolic strain rate from rest to dobutamine stimulation by more than 0.231/s.

Dobutamine Stress Imaging

Contractility reserve and myocardial viability can be assessed with low-dose dobutamine stress imaging. Regional and global LV functional recovery in acute postmyocardial infarction setting and chronic coronary revascularization can be assessed using dobutamine stress imaging. The maximum benefit after revascularization can be seen in the biphasic response. Low-dose dobutamine causes initial improvement in contraction due to the inotropic action and, later at higher doses, chronotropic action of dobutamine causes decrease in contractility. For predicting recovery of contractile function following coronary vascularization, the positive predictive value is 83% and negative predictive value is 81%.[10]

Speckle-tracking Echocardiography

It provides reproducible and objective quantification of regional and global myocardial function and detection of myocardial viability. Myocardial viability is assessed by determining the strain and strain rate from the short and long axis of LV myocardial deformation.[13]

Myocardial Contrast Echocardiography

Acoustically reflective high molecular weight inert gases are used in myocardial contrast echocardiography (MCE). The gases form microbubbles in intravascular space and acts as a contrast medium. Segments of myocardium showing homogeneity of contrast intensity indicate viable myocardium. Lack of contrast enhancement indicates nonviable segments due to obstruction or collapse of microvasculature caused by necrotic myocardial cells. The sensitivity and specificity to predict the recovery postrevascularization are 78–90% and 51–72%, respectively. Combination of DSE and MCE in assessment of myocardial viability has a sensitivity of 96% and specificity of 63%.[14] Likelihood of global LV function improvement following revascularization is indicated by presence of more than three viable segments in MCE.[3]

Positron Emission Tomography

Positron emission tomography viability assesses both myocardial perfusion and myocardial glucose metabolism.[13] N-NH_3 (ammonia) and ^{82}Rb (rubidium) are used to assess myocardial perfusion and fluorine-18-fluorodeoxyglucose (^{18}F-FDG) for myocardial glucose metabolism. In centers where PET perfusion tracers are not available, SPECT perfusion tracers can be used instead. ^{18}F-FDG tracer is glucose analog and its uptake in the myocardium reflects cardiac glucose utilization. Only the viable myocytes will show uptake of ^{18}F-FDG, but unlike glucose, FDG is not metabolized further and retention of the ^{18}F-FDG in the myocytes enables imaging (Table 2).

Oral glucose loading and nicotinic derivatives are used to achieve high glucose level and low free fatty acid level required for maximum cardiac glucose uptake.[12] More than 50% uptake of FDG in PET enables identification of 85% of myocardial LV segments which recovered function 1 year after revascularization.[15] Normal perfusion and FDG uptake indicates stunning. Reduced perfusion and preserved FDG uptake indicates hibernating myocardium (Fig. 2). Scar tissue is reflected by reduced (nontransmural scar) or absent (transmural scar) perfusion and FDG uptake (Fig. 3).

Single-photon Emission Computed Tomography

It is used to assess ischemia and viability. Thallium-201 and technetium-99m (Tc-99m) labeled tracers like Tc-99m sestamibi and Tc-99m tetrofosmin are the commonly used radiotracers for myocardial perfusion SPECT.

For the assessment of myocardial viability with thallium-201, rest-redistribution protocol is followed. After

TABLE 2: Flow metabolism patterns in ^{18}F-fluorodeoxyglucose positron emission tomography to assess myocardial viability[16]

Perfusion	Glucose metabolism	Category
Preserved	Preserved	• Viable – normal/stunned heart • Dilated ventricle in a remodeled heart
Preserved	Reduced	Reverse mismatch (altered glucose metabolism) • Revascularization early after myocardial infarction (MI) • Left bundle branch block • Right ventricular pacing • Nonischemic cardiomyopathy • Diabetes mellitus
Reduced	Reduced	• Match (nonviable scar)
Reduced	Preserved or increased fluorodeoxyglucose (FDG) uptake	• Mismatch (viable myocardium in hibernation)

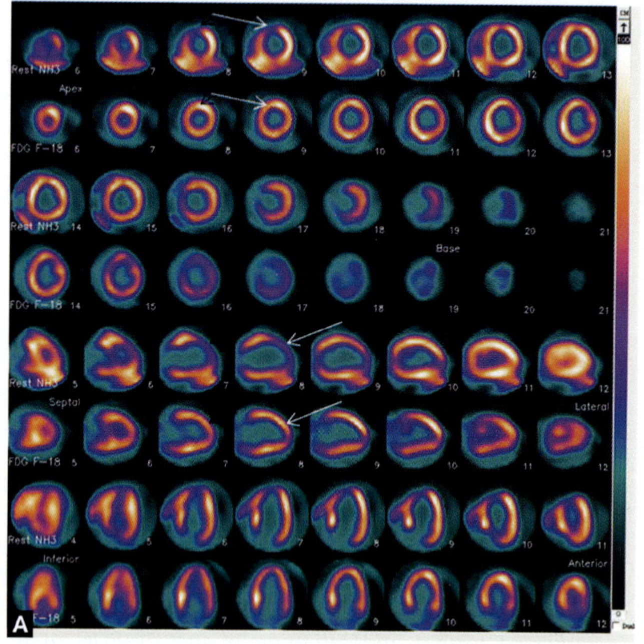

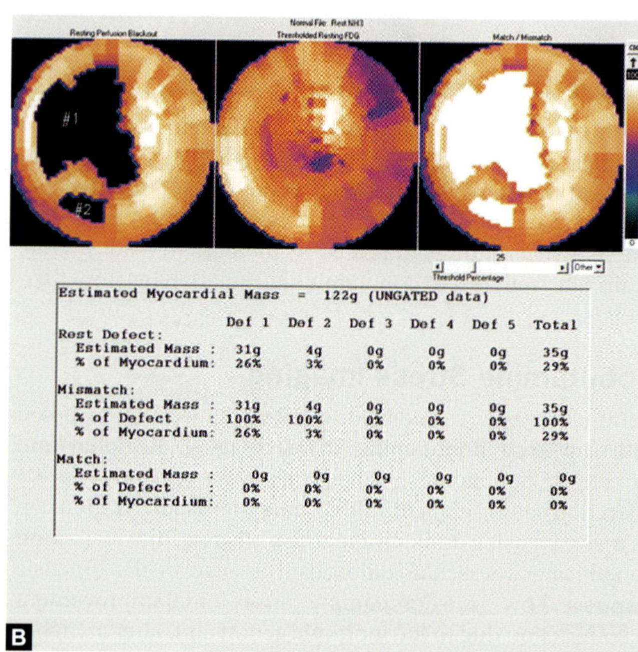

FIG. 2: N-13 NH3 (ammonia) perfusion and F-18-fluorodeoxyglucose study at rest shows "Mismatch" perfusion and metabolic defect in the anteroseptal wall and apex, consistent with hibernating myocardium.

administration of thallium-201, initial images are acquired after about 20 minutes followed by rest-redistribution images after about 3–4 hours.[12] The initial uptake of thallium is flow dependent and the uptake in the viable myocyte is via sodium potassium adenosine triphosphatase dependent active process. Thallium-201 has unique property of redistribution, a process which is flow independent and the redistribution takes place between the thallium-201 in the blood pool and the viable myocardium till equilibrium is reached. This is particularly important as this flow independent process allows thallium-201 to be taken up by chronically hypoperfused but viable myocardial segments.

Technetium-99m has shorter half-life and better tissue penetration. Tc-99m labeled tracers underestimate myocardial viability when compared to thallium-201 and ^{18}F-FDG PET. However, quantification of regional radiotracer uptake and nitrate administration before Tc-99m labeled radiotracer injection improves the assessment of myocardial viability.

Quantitative assessment of viability using either thallium-201 or technetium-labeled tracers can be performed using commercially available softwares that can quantify the size of scarred myocardium. A myocardial segment with uptake more than 50% of the uptake in the normal myocardial segments is considered viable myocardium and segments with less than 50% considered as nonviable. Size of the scar can be expressed as percentage of individual coronary territories or as percentage of total LV myocardium.

Cardiac Magnetic Resonance

Cardiac magnetic resonance gives information about myocardial contractility reserve, small myocardial scars and wall thickness. Different techniques used are measurement of wall thickness, late gadolinium enhancement magnetic resonance (LGEMR) and dobutamine stress magnetic resonance (DSMR). The gold standard technique for myo-

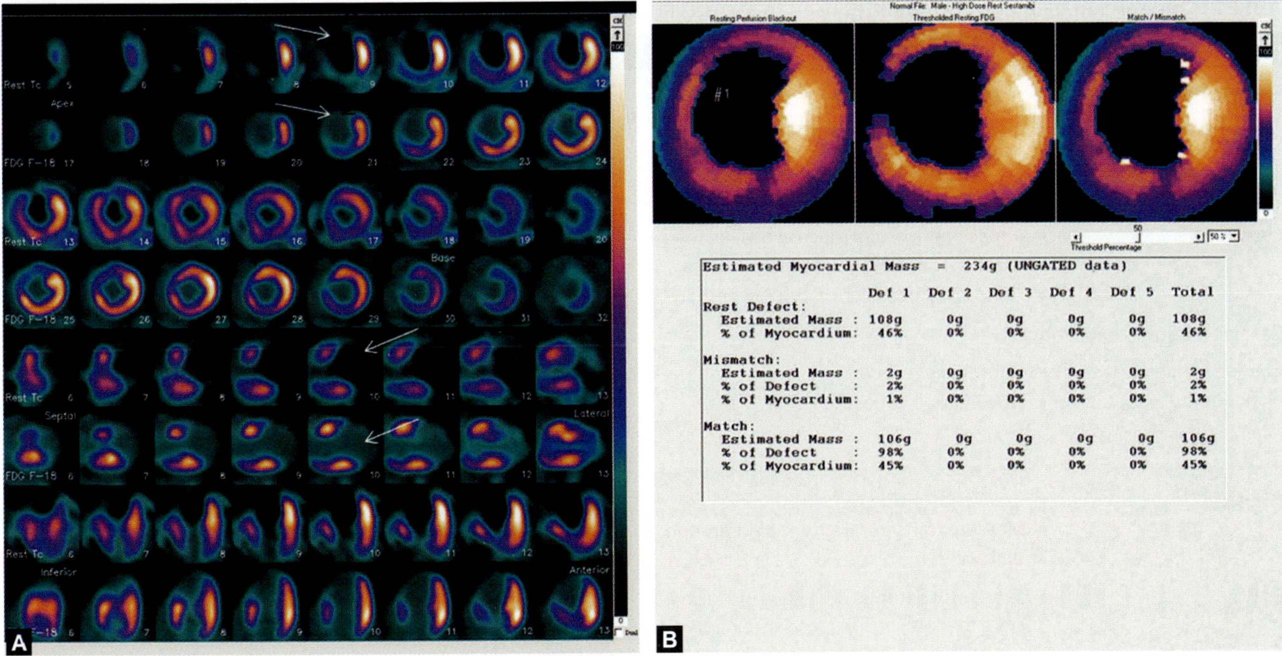

FIG. 3: Tc-99m MIBI perfusion and F-18-fluorodeoxyglucose study at rest shows "Match" perfusion and metabolic defect in the mid and distal anterior wall, distal septum and apex, consistent with scarred myocardium.

cardial scar imaging is LGEMR. Five to ten minutes after gadolinium contrast injection, basic sequence of inversion recovery imaging is done. Nonviable myocardium appears enhanced or bright and normal region appears black or null. Scar tissues have increased extracellular space resulting in increased gadolinium concentration and thereby signal enhancement. Large transmural infarcts due to microvascular obstruction appear as dark core within bright regions of late enhancement. Extent of LGEMR assessed at 12–48 hours post myocardial infarction is related with decreased functional recovery after 6 months. Sensitivity of LGEMR in detecting acute myocardial infarction is 99% and chronic myocardial infarction is 94%.[17] With each gram of scar measured by LGE, the increased risk of major adverse cardiovascular event (MACE) is 5% and death is 4%.[18] Low-dose dobutamine stress is combined with LGEMR to assess contractile reserve. Following administration of low-dose dobutamine, if there is increase in the systolic wall thickness by 2 mm or more, then the myocardium is considered viable. Biphasic response is seen in chronic LV dysfunction and hibernating myocardium. CMR helps in identifying the myocardial necrosis complications like hemorrhage, myocardial edema, LV thrombi, and microvascular obstruction. Limitations of CMR are lower temporal resolution, limited image quality with irregular rhythm, and the need for breath-holding sequence during acquisition (Table 3).

Coronary Computed Tomography

Coronary computed tomography is excellent tool to in ruling out CAD. Its use in assessing myocardial viability is still experimental.[19]

ROLE OF VIABILITY TESTING IN THE MANAGEMENT OF ISCHEMIC CARDIOMYOPATHY

Presence of 20–30% of the left ventricle needs to be hibernating or viable in order to have improvement in LVEF. Reverse remodeling after revascularization was found in patients with residual viability—20% resulting in increase in both end-diastolic and end-systolic volumes. Knowledge gaps are present regarding the application of noninvasive viability testing in patients with LV dysfunction and complex CAD. When ischemic cardiomyopathy patients are treated only with medical therapy, the outcomes are worse. Survival rate is improved with revascularization, when compared to medical treatment only. In a study where 144 patients underwent delayed enhanced CMR, patients with viable myocardium who underwent revascularization had better outcome when compared to medical therapy only.[20] Improvement in the regional LV function, exercise capacity, and heart failure symptoms may be predicted by the presence of viable myocardium in noninvasive testing. Positron emission tomography and recovery following revascularization (PARR)-1 study indicated that the scar extent was an independent predictor of recovery of ventricular function after revascularization. Smaller scar have better improvement in LVEF. Combined PET and clinical parameters predict degree of recovery.[21] PARR-2 study did not show statistically significant reduction in cardiac events in LV dysfunction and coronary disease patients with FDG PET directed therapy when compared to standard care. The limitation of PARR-2 study was that 25% of patients in FDG

TABLE 3: Comparison of imaging modalities used to assess viability of myocardium and their limitations[5]

Imaging modality	Viability assessment	Limitations
Nuclear medicine		
^{201}Thalium SPECT	• Integrity of sarcolemma • Widely used and good sensitivity	• Highest radiation exposure • Limited spatial resolution
^{99m}Technetium SPECT	• Integrity of mitochondrial membrane	• Limited spatial resolution
Cardiac PET	• Capacity of cellular glucose uptake • Excellent sensitivity, quantitative data • Good spatial resolution but lower than CMR	• Not widely available • Expensive • Radiation exposure
Cardiac magnetic resonance		
Cardiac magnetic resonance	• Contractile reserve • No radiation exposure	• Avoided in GFR <30 mL/min/1.72 m^2 • Body habitus • Avoided in patients with cardiac devices • Not available widely
LGE-CMR	• Excellent sensitivity • Measure transmural extent of infarction • Well validated	• No information regarding the contractile reserve of nonenhanced rim is got • Low specificity
EDWT	• Excellent anatomic detail got using steady state free precession cine sequence	• Reversed remodeling in 20% patients (tinned myocardium) • Low specificity
Dobutamine stress	• Better left ventricular coverage when compared to DSE • High-dose dobutamine— myocardial ischemia imaging • Good specificity and sensitivity	• Contraindicated in patients with implanted devices • Not a part of routine CMR examination • Trained personnel and resuscitation equipment required
Echocardiography		
DSE	• Good specificity and sensitivity • Well validated	• Adequate acoustic window required • Operator dependent
EDWT	• Easy to use	• Relation between viability and wall thickness is not straightforward • Low specificity
Myocardial strain imaging	• Good sensitivity	• Limited clinical use
CCT	• Potential merging of coronary imaging with viability imaging and myocardial perfusion study	• High radiation dose • Iodinated contrast material is necessary • High calcium scores impede evaluation of coronary patency
PET-CMR	• Contractile reserve • Cellular glucose uptake capacity • Advantages of combining function perfusion viability and metabolism imaging • Determines viability in the nonenhancing rim	• High cost, radiation exposure • Lack of integrated software • Inherent technical challenges • Need further studies

SPECT, single-photon emission computed tomography; PET, positron emission tomography; CMR, cardiac magnetic resonance; GFR, glomerular filtration rate; LGE, late gadolinium enhancement; EDWT, end-diastolic wall thickness; DSE, dobutamine stress echocardiography; CCT, cardiac computed tomography.

PET study group were not treated according to PET-guided recommendations. Adherence to PET recommendations for treatment showed significant benefit for FDG PET in group without recent coronary angiography.[22] The Ottawa-FIVE study of PARR trial compared the outcome of patients undergoing the FDG-directed therapy and standard therapy. Patients who underwent FDG PET-assisted management had statistically significant reduction in the cardiac events when compared with the standard treatment patients. Patients experiencing the composite endpoints (compared between the groups were myocardial infarction, cardiac death, and hospitalization in 1 year) was 19% in FDG PET-assisted group versus 41% in standard treatment group.[23] This underscores the importance of experienced, high volume centers where PET-based revascularization was better than standard treatment protocol. According to CHRISTMAS (carvedilol hibernation reversible ischemia trial), the improvement of LV function with carvedilol treatment in ischemic cardiomyopathy patients is dependent on the volume of myocardium affected by ischemia, hibernation or both. There was no or little improvement in LV function with carvedilol treatment in the absence of viable myocardium.[24] STICH (Surgical Treatment for IsCHemic heart failure) was done to compare the outcome of OMT alone or OMT plus CABG in patients with LV dysfunction and CAD.[25] Patients in OMT plus CABG group had lower rates of mortality.[26] Substudy of STICH assessed the role of viability based revascularization.[27] Almost 50% of patients had viability based revascularization in a nonrandomized fashion. Though, myocardial viability based revascularization strategy was found to have significant benefit as compared to other strategy in univariate analysis and multivariate analysis after adjustment of baseline variables like ejection fraction and LV end-diastolic volume did not show significant difference. There are lots of limitations of this particular trial. They include utility of SPECT and DSE used to assess myocardial viability which are not the gold standard to assess viability. The result of the substudy was done in a nonrandomized fashion. This emphasized that there exists a lacunae in the field of viability assessment, which needs to be addressed by future large volume randomized studies.

FUTURE DIRECTION

Myocardial viability assessment is important in a patient with multivessel disease and delayed presentation of myocardial infarction. Assessment of viable myocardium helps in decision making of need for revascularization. Its role is not clear in patient with severe LV dysfunction and CAD pending a large patient-based randomized study comparing the role of myocardial viability assessment in revascularization of such patients. Till then, we presume a heart team-based approach where patient remains the cornerstone in making informed decision about the need and kind of revascularization strategy.

ACKNOWLEDGMENTS

We acknowledge the role of Dr Balakrishna, Dr Chetan Patel, and Dr Nitish Naik in helping us in preparing this manuscript.

REFERENCES

1. Braunwald E, Kloner RA. The stunned myocardium: prolonged, postischemic ventricular dysfunction. Circulation. 1982;66(6):1146-9.
2. Jamiel A, Ebid M, Ahmed AM, et al. The role of myocardial viability in contemporary cardiac practice. Heart Fail Rev. 2017;22(4):401-13.
3. Bax JJ, Delgado V. Myocardial viability as integral part of the diagnostic and therapeutic approach to ischemic heart failure. J Nucl Cardiol. 2015;22(2):229-45.
4. Partington SL, Kwong RY, Dorbala S. Multimodality imaging in the assessment of myocardial viability. Heart Fail Rev. 2011;16(4):381-95.
5. Bogaert J, Gheysens O, Dymarkowski S, et al. Comprehensive Evaluation of Hibernating Myocardium: Use of Noninvasive Imaging. J Thorac Imaging. 2014;29(3):134-46.
6. Taegtmeyer H. Tracing Cardiac Metabolism in vivo: One Substrate at a Time. J Nucl Med Off Publ Soc Nucl Med. 2010;51(0 1):80S-7S.
7. Lim SP, Mc Ardle BA, Beanlands RS, et al. Myocardial viability: it is still alive. Semin Nucl Med. 2014;44(5):358-74.
8. Bax JJ, Visser FC, Poldermans D, et al. Time Course of Functional Recovery of Stunned and Hibernating Segments After Surgical Revascularization. Circulation. 2001;104(suppl 1):I314-8.
9. Heyndrickx GR, Millard RW, McRitchie RJ, et al. Regional myocardial functional and electrophysiological alterations after brief coronary artery occlusion in conscious dogs. J Clin Invest. 1975;56(4):978-85.
10. Bonow RO. Identification of Viable Myocardium. Circulation. 1996;94(11):2674-80.
11. Schinkel AFL, Bax JJ, Delgado V, et al. Clinical relevance of hibernating myocardium in ischemic left ventricular dysfunction. Am J Med. 2010;123(11): 978-86.
12. Anavekar NS, Chareonthaitawee P, Narula J, et al. Revascularization in Patients With Severe Left Ventricular Dysfunction: Is the Assessment of Viability Still Viable? J Am Coll Cardiol. 2016;67(24):2874-87.
13. Cong T, Sun Y, Shang Z, et al. Prognostic Value of Speckle Tracking Echocardiography in Patients with ST-Elevation Myocardial Infarction Treated with Late Percutaneous Intervention. Echocardiography. 2015;32(9):1384-91.
14. Bhat A, Gan GCH, Tan TC, et al. Myocardial Viability: From Proof of Concept to Clinical Practice. Cardiol Res Pract. 2016;2016:1020818.
15. Schindler TH, Dilsizian V. Cardiac positron emission tomography/computed tomography imaging of the Renin-Angiotensin system in humans holds promise for image-guided approach to heart failure therapy. J Am Coll Cardiol. 2012;60(24):2535-8.
16. Ghosh N, Rimoldi OE, Beanlands RSB, et al. Assessment of myocardial ischaemia and viability: role of positron emission tomography. Eur Heart J. 2010;31(24):2984-95.
17. Kim RJ, Fieno DS, Parrish TB, et al. Relationship of MRI Delayed Contrast Enhancement to Irreversible Injury, Infarct Age, and Contractile Function. Circulation. 1999;100(19):1992-2002.
18. Zemrak F, Petersen SE. Late gadolinium enhancement CMR predicts adverse cardiovascular outcomes and mortality in patients with coronary artery disease: systematic review and meta-analysis. Prog Cardiovasc Dis. 2011;54(3):215-29.
19. Mahnken AH, Koos R, Katoh M, et al. Assessment of myocardial viability in reperfused acute myocardial infarction using 16-slice computed tomography in comparison to magnetic resonance imaging. J Am Coll Cardiol. 2005; 45(12):2042-7.
20. Gerber BL, Rousseau MF, Ahn SA, et al. Prognostic value of myocardial viability by delayed-enhanced magnetic resonance in patients with coronary artery disease and low ejection fraction: impact of revascularization therapy. J Am Coll Cardiol. 2012;59(9):825-35.
21. Beanlands RSB, Ruddy TD, deKemp RA, et al. Positron emission tomography and recovery following revascularization (PARR-1): the importance of scar and the development of a prediction rule for the degree of recovery of left ventricular function. J Am Coll Cardiol. 2002;40(10):1735-43.
22. Beanlands RSB, Nichol G, Huszti E, et al. F-18-fluorodeoxyglucose positron emission tomography imaging-assisted management of patients with severe left ventricular dysfunction and suspected coronary disease: a randomized, controlled trial (PARR-2). J Am Coll Cardiol. 2007;50(20):2002-12.
23. Abraham A, Nichol G, Williams KA, et al. 18F-FDG PET imaging of myocardial viability in an experienced center with access to 18F-FDG and integration with clinical management teams: the Ottawa-FIVE substudy of the PARR 2 trial. J Nucl Med Off Publ Soc Nucl Med. 2010;51(4):567-74.
24. Cleland JGF, Pennell DJ, Ray SG, et al. Myocardial viability as a determinant of the ejection fraction response to carvedilol in patients with heart failure (CHRISTMAS trial): randomised controlled trial. Lancet. 2003;362(9377):14-21.
25. Velazquez EJ, Lee KL, Deja MA, et al. Coronary-Artery Bypass Surgery in Patients with Left Ventricular Dysfunction. N Engl J Med. 2011;364(17):1607-16.
26. Velazquez EJ, Lee KL, Jones RH, et al. Coronary-Artery Bypass Surgery in Patients with Ischemic Cardiomyopathy. N Engl J Med. 2016;374(16):1511-20.
27. Bonow RO, Maurer G, Lee KL, et al. Myocardial viability and survival in ischemic left ventricular dysfunction. STICH Trial Investigators. N Engl J Med. 2011;364(17):1617-25.

CHAPTER 82

Computed Tomography Coronary Angiography—Essentials for Cardiologists

Priya Jagia, Arun Sharma

INTRODUCTION

Computed tomography coronary angiography (CTCA) is increasingly being used in clinical context with the advent of technical refinements and introduction of third-generation CT scanners. It has established itself as the investigation of choice to rule out significant coronary artery disease (CAD) in low to intermediate risk symptomatic patients. Its use has now expanded beyond classic coronary stenosis detection to encompass plaque characterization, vulnerability detection, detection of coronary anomalies, patency of grafts and stents, treatment planning, and follow-up of patients, depending upon different clinical scenarios. This has reduced the negative catheter angiography in low to intermediate risk patients and resulted in substantial decrease in unnecessary radiation exposure to the cardiologists in catheterization laboratory.

CONVENTIONAL ANGIOGRAPHY OR COMPUTED TOMOGRAPHY CORONARY ANGIOGRAPHY

Coronary catheter angiography (CA) remains the gold standard for luminal assessment of coronary vasculature, but it carries some risks due to its invasive nature and exposure to ionizing radiation. Moreover, the cardiologist is also exposed to the aforementioned radiation repetitively, every time he performs a catheter study. Nearly up to 15–30% of patients undergoing CA turn out to be normal studies[1,2] adding unnecessary radiation to both the patient and the operator alike. Hence, using CT angiography (CTA) for even a select group of patients will result in substantial reduction in the radiation dose. Use of CTA for obtaining anatomical information noninvasively is very attractive for this reason besides being a much safer noninvasive alternative to CA.

Technical Advancements

At present, CTCA is considered the most robust imaging technique for noninvasive visualization of coronary atherosclerosis. The challenges in evaluation of coronary arteries by CT (cardiac and respiratory motion, temporal resolution, etc.) have now been largely overcome with various advancements of CT technology, most notably being the introduction of dual source CT.[3-6] The newer third-generation dual source CT scanners provide excellent image quality over a wide range of body sizes and heart rates at much lower radiation doses than the previous generation CT scanners. Extremely fast gantry rotation time combined with larger Z-axis volume coverage per rotation, have enabled single-heartbeat acquisitions in most patients with heart rates of up to 75–85 beats/min.

Low contrast protocols described in various studies have resulted in significant reduction in contrast medium requirements, without any difficulties in contrast medium timing or unsatisfactory vessel enhancement. Moreover, volumetric acquisition has enabled extensive image postprocessing, including multiplanar reformatted and maximum-intensity projection images to create virtual images similar to those obtained with CA.[5,6]

Diagnostic Performance of Computed Tomography Coronary Angiography

Various studies have demonstrated excellent diagnostic accuracy of CTCA for the detection of coronary stenosis, with a sensitivity of 86–99%, specificity of 92–98% and negative predictive value reaching almost up to 100%.[7] It can provide detailed information on coronary artery anatomy, and assess both coronary artery atherosclerosis as well as resultant luminal stenosis. Nonobese patients in sinus rhythm (heart rate <65 beats/min) with adequate breath hold and favorable coronary artery calcium (CAC) score provide best quality images which are comparable to coronary catheter angiogram. Most importantly, it detects early nonobstructive disease which allows for the early institution of medical therapy and lifestyle modifications. It is a rapid and low-cost modality which is usually available round the clock for noninvasive evaluation.

Limitations

Despite being noninvasive study with high accuracy, CTCA still has some limitations in the form of poor visualization of extensively calcified arteries and a poorer spatial resolution in distal most coronary artery segment. Moreover, evaluation may be suboptimal in obese patients and in patients with very high or irregular heart rates.

Patient Selection and Preparation

Optimal CTCA imaging requires proper patient selection and preparation. It depends on multiple factors like clinical indication, pretest probability of CAD and clinical and biochemical test results. A number of risk algorithms are available that can be used to calculate probability of CAD. Patients should be informed about the benefits and potential risks of the procedure. General instructions may include avoidance of caffeine 12 hours prior to the procedure to avoid cardiac stimulation, ruling out history of prior contrast allergy, and ruling out renal dysfunction. They should be instructed to avoid eating solid food 6 hours prior to the study and to maintain adequate hydration both pre- and postprocedure. Beta-blockers or nitroglycerine may be given as per the requirement and the necessary caution must be exercised during their administration. However, with use of third-generation CT scanners, administration of these pharmacologic drugs is relatively lesser.

Coronary Artery Calcium Scoring

High CAC score has been associated with increased mortality and adverse cardiovascular events, independent of other risk factors.[7,8] Moreover, absence of coronary calcium portends a remarkably favorable prognosis, with almost no patients experiencing adverse cardiac events in next 5 years. CAC scoring is now established as a risk stratification tool to identify high-risk patients who might benefit from further investigation. It can characterize the location as well as the burden of CAD (Fig. 1).

Applications of Computed Tomography Coronary Angiography

Computed tomography coronary angiography has wider applications in current cardiology practice. Knowledge of these applications is essential for judicious use of the technique over and above CA. These indications are briefly described here.

Evaluation of Coronary Artery Disease

Coronary Artery Disease Detection, Characterization, and Quantification

Computed tomography coronary angiography can be optimally used to rule out significant CAD (Fig. 2) in patients with low to intermediate pretest probability of CAD.[7-10] It has become possible due to its high negative predictive value. It is also helpful in cases of suspected left main ostial disease as the CA may not able to differentiate between spasm and true stenosis. Coronary evaluation may be needed prior to any major surgical procedure in patients at risk of CAD. It is also helpful in planning percutaneous coronary interventions in chronic total occlusion and evaluation of coronary arteries in post cardiac transplant patients.

Knowledge of normal coronary anatomy (origin, course, branches, and termination) and variants helps in accurate interpretation and reporting of CTCA. Normally, left anterior descending and posterior descending artery run in interventricular groove, while the circumflex and right coronary arteries run in the atrioventricular groove. Hypoplasia of one vessel is generally accompanied by

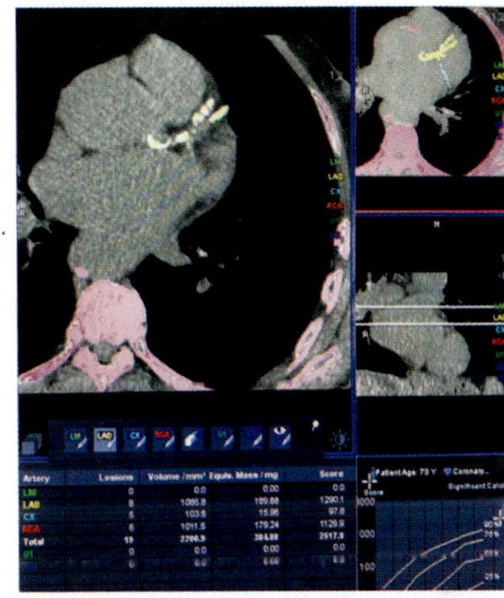

FIG. 1: Computed tomography angiography-derived coronary artery calcium score in a patient with significantly calcified coronary arteries. Color coding of plaque according to each coronary artery helps quantify calcium in each vessel.

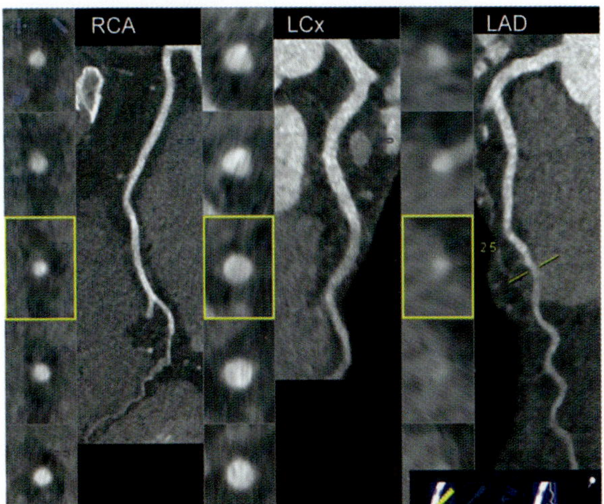

LAD, left anterior descending; LCx, left circumflex artery; RCA, right coronary artery.

FIG. 2: Curved multiplanar computed tomography angiography images showing normal coronary arteries. Side panels show the axial cross-sections with diameter and area.

prominence of another vessel. In cases where left anterior descending is small and does not extend to the apex, the posterior descending artery is typically prominent and extends to the apex. If the circumflex is small, there are typically prominent posterolateral branches from right coronary artery. If case of a large ramus intermedius, the diagonals may be small.

Degree of stenosis should be graded and mentioned in the report for baseline and follow-up. Various methods including visual assessment, "end-on" view assessment, diameter on maximum intensity projection images and software calculation of diameter or area. Highest correlation with quantitative CA is seen with cross-sectional area technique with smallest interobserver variability with maximum intensity projection technique.

It is to be borne in mind that stenosis is typically overestimated in areas where heavily calcified plaques are present, and significant decrease in specificity, positive predictive value, and accuracy of CTCA is seen when calcification is greater than 50% of the luminal diameter. Reconstruction of additional dataset using a sharper convolution kernel and use of bone window setting is advocated in such cases to reduce blooming artifacts from calcification.

Plaque Characterization

Characterization and quantification of atherosclerotic plaques may be useful to improve individualized risk stratification. Intravascular ultrasound remains the test of choice in this regard. CTCA using latest scanners is also helpful in characterizing coronary atherosclerotic plaques (Figs. 3 and 4) as it can identify lipid, fat, or calcium depending upon attenuation difference.[11-13] Further, it helps in ascertaining the vulnerability of the plaque as plaques with high lipid content have been shown to be more vulnerable and prone to rupture, whereas calcified plaques are thought to be more stable.

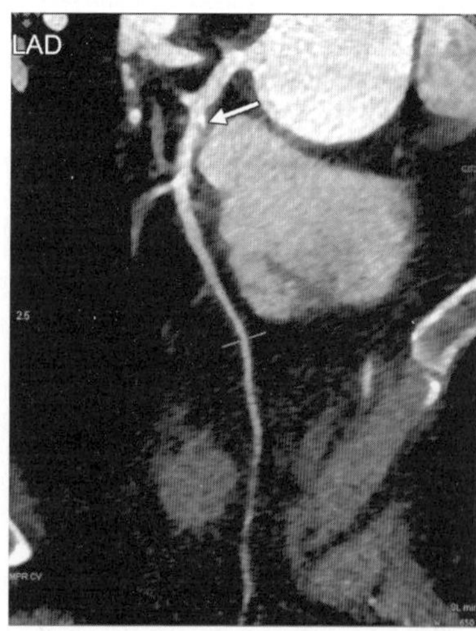

FIG. 3: Computed tomography angiography image showing mild disease with eccentric calcific plaque in proximal left anterior descending artery (arrow).

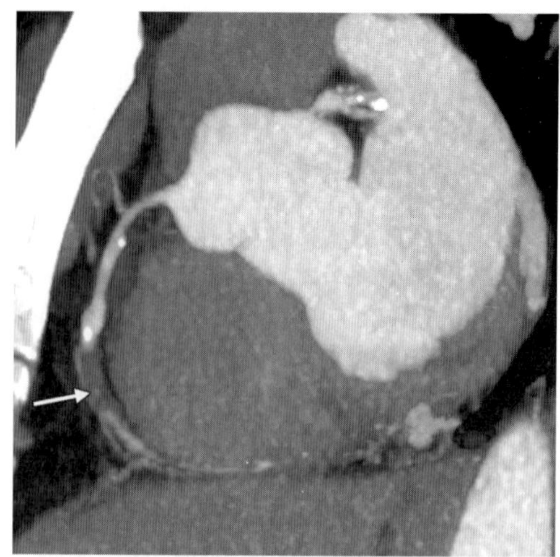

FIG. 4: Computed tomography angiography image showing complete occlusion of mid right coronary artery (arrow) with calcific plaques in proximal and mid-part.

Computed Tomography Fractional Flow Reserve

Conventional CA with measurement of FFR by means of a pressure wire technique is the established reference standard for the functional assessment of CAD.[14,15] Computed tomography fractional flow reserve (CT-FFR) has emerged as a noninvasive method for direct assessment of CAD and plaque characterization with high (75% vs. 44%) diagnostic accuracy.[16,17] Growing CT-evidence has validated the diagnostic accuracy of CT-FFR techniques compared with invasive FFR. The technique uses computational fluid dynamics to calculate "3-vessel" FFR from already acquired coronary CTA images. Its advantage over CA-derived FFR is that it is entirely noninvasive and no vasodilators are required as computational models allow CT-FFR to be calculated across a physiologically realistic range. CT-FFR has the potential to streamline and rationalize the care of patients suspected of having CAD and improve outcomes while reducing overall healthcare costs.

Myocardial Perfusion

Recently, the ability of dual-energy CT (DECT) to characterize tissue composition and organ perfusion has been demonstrated. Moreover, cardiac perfusion-imaging with DECT seems to correlate with fixed perfusion defects in technetium-99m (99mTc) sestamibi single photon emission computed tomography (SPECT).[18,19] Evaluation of myocardial perfusion using DECT may complement anatomic evaluation of the coronary arteries by gauging the hemodynamic significance of detected stenosis. However, further studies are needed to determine the diagnostic accuracy of these perfusion defects detected by DECT, their predictive value, and their impact on patient care.

Evaluation of Bypass Grafts

Computed tomography coronary angiography is the investigation of choice (sensitivity of 96.1%, specificity of 96.3%)

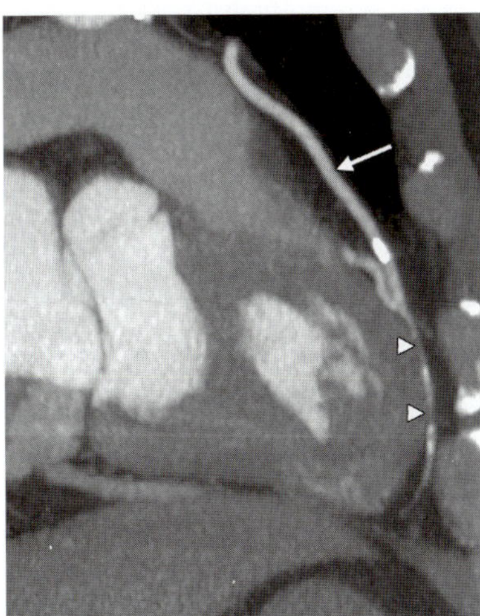

FIG. 5: Computed tomography angiography of a post coronary artery bypass graft patient showing patent left internal mammary artery—left anterior descending artery (LAD) graft (arrow) with diffuse distal LAD disease (arrowheads).

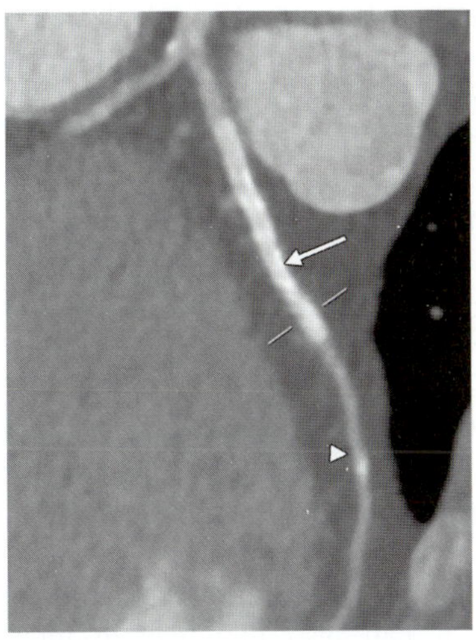

FIG. 6: Computed tomography angiography image showing patent stent in left anterior descending artery (arrow) with normal distal artery (arrowhead).

for evaluation of bypass graft patency (Fig. 5) in acutely symptomatic post coronary artery bypass graft (CABG) patients.[20-22] Another potential indication of CTCA in the setting of prior bypass grafting is surgical planning, providing a road-map on graft location, anatomic landmarks, and anastomotic sites before redo CABG surgery.[20-22] In patients with internal mammary grafts, the scan should extend superiorly to the level of the clavicle to rule out subclavian stenosis. Proximity of the grafts to the sternum should be mentioned in the report to avoid damage during a redo sternotomy. However, artifacts from surgical clips may limit graft evaluation by cardiac CTA (CCTA) and the distal anastomosis in particular is difficult to assess at times. Still, the evaluation of the native vessels, often calcified, remains the most challenging aspect of CCTA in post-CABG patients.

Evaluation of Coronary Stents

Computed tomography coronary angiography is also helpful in evaluation of patency of coronary stents (Fig. 6). Moreover, stent fracture can also be delineated well. Studies have reported high diagnostic accuracy (negative predictive value: 97–98%, accuracy: 84–93%) of CTCA for in-stent restenosis of stents greater than 3 mm diameter.[23,24] However, depiction of in-stent intimal hyperplasia, particularly in small vessels still remains a challenge for CTCA. Beam-hardening and streak artifacts caused by metallic stent struts significantly impair the visualization of the coronary artery lumen and make it difficult to diagnose in-stent intimal hyperplasia by means of CTCA.[25] Artifacts caused by metallic stent struts provoke attenuation defects that may mimic in-stent restenosis. Obesity, smaller stent diameter (<3 mm), increased strut thickness and thicker stent material have been shown to adversely affect the accuracy of CTCA. Iterative image reconstruction further improves in-plane stent visualization in cases of smaller stents and should preferably be used in combination with thinner collimation.[26]

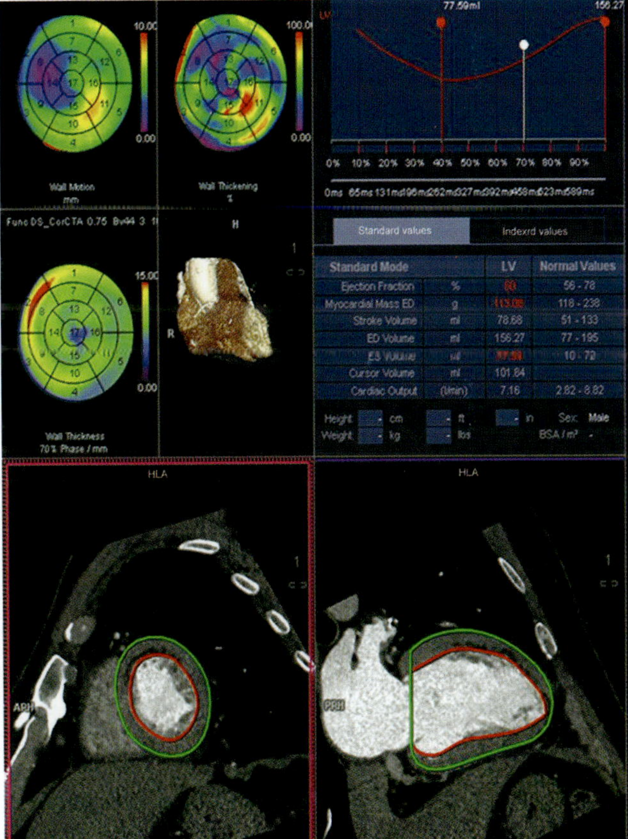

FIG. 7: Functional assessment using computed tomography which shows decreased ejection fraction (50%) in a patient earlier ischemic insult. Dark areas of hypoperfusion are seen in the anterior wall of left ventricle myocardium.

Ischemic Heart Disease and Cardiac Function

With the use of current postprocessing techniques, regional wall motion abnormalities and ejection fraction calculation (Fig. 7) can be ascertained from retrospective CTCA without doing any additional data acquisition.[18,19,27,28] Hence, early detection of subclinical functional abnormalities is possible in asymptomatic patients with myocardial dysfunction, especially those with diabetes. However, it is important to note that magnetic resonance imaging still remains the investigation of choice for functional and myocardial assessment.

Computed Tomography Coronary Angiography for Coronary Evaluation in Congenital Heart Disease

Computed tomography coronary angiography is extremely helpful in excluding anomalous coronary origins in pediatric population with simultaneous evaluation of cardiac and extracardiac morphology and airway or lung parenchymal changes.[29-31] It can also demonstrate interarterial anomalous coronary course which has therapeutic implications. Moreover, demonstration of the course of coronary artery can be helpful to avoid coronary injury during surgical reimplantation. It is also useful in diagnosis and follow-up of patients with Kawasaki disease, where it delineates exact morphology of coronary aneurysms and associated changes. All the possible recommended indications for doing coronary CTA are summarized in box 1.

BOX 1 Appropriate clinical indications for doing computed tomography coronary angiography

Nonacute chest pain patients suspected of ischemic chest pain:
- In low and intermediate pretest CAD probability when patients are unable to exercise/ECG results are uninterpretable

Acute chest pain patients suspected of acute coronary syndrome:
- Acute chest pain with normal ECG/enzymes
- For low or intermediate pretest probability patients with uninterpretable ECG/nondiagnostic ECG or with unclear myocardial enzymes

Patients suspected of ischemic chest pain after coronary revascularization:
- Graft patency evaluation after coronary artery bypass graft

Symptomatic patients with coronary artery stents:
- With coronary stent greater than 3 mm in diameter

CT coronary angiography in pediatric population:
- Coronary artery congenital anomalies
- Complex congenital heart disease
- Postoperative evaluation in congenital heart diseases
- Symptomatic Kawasaki heart disease patients with no prior testing
- For follow-up of patients with Kawasaki disease

Evaluation of the ventricular structure and systolic function:
- Assessment of left ventricular function in patients with acute MI / heart failure if other noninvasive imaging tests are inadequate
- Quantitative assessment of right ventricular function
- Assessment of right ventricular morphology in ARVC

Heart failure newly developed or newly diagnosed in patients with no history of CAD in low- to intermediate-risk
- Coronary artery assessment prior to noncoronary cardiac surgery

ARVC, arrhythmogenic right ventricular cardiomyopathy; CAD, coronary artery disease; CT, computed tomography; ECG, electrocardiogram; MI: myocardial infarction.

CONCLUSION

Computed tomography coronary angiography has gained wider application and acceptance in current cardiology practice. One must be acquainted with native radiological appearances and postoperative imaging findings of various cardiac pathologies for optimal interpretation of test results. Further advancements in evaluation of coronary plaque morphology, plaque vulnerability, myocardial perfusion, and CT-FFR may allow even more complete noninvasive cardiac assessment in future. Moreover, it may provide a highly effective method of cardiac risk stratification to facilitate early implementation of preventive cardiac care.

REFERENCES

1. Farrehi PM, Bernstein SJ, Rasak M, et al. Frequency of negative coronary arteriographic findings in patients with chest pain is related to community practice patterns. Am J Manag Care. 2002;8(7):643-8.
2. Jong P, Mohammed S, Sternberg L. Sex differences in the features of coronary artery disease of patients undergoing coronary angiography. Can J Cardiol. 1996;12(7):671-7.
3. Stein PD, Beemath A, Kayali F, et al. Multi-detector computed tomography for the diagnosis of coronary artery disease: a systematic review. Am J Med. 2006;119:203-16.
4. Danad I, Fayad ZA, Willemink MJ, et al. Recent advances in cardiac computed tomography: dual energy, spectral and molecular CT imaging. JACC Cardiovasc Imaging. 2015;8(6):710-23.
5. Yoon YE, Lim TH. Current roles and future applications of cardiac CT: Risk stratification of coronary artery disease. Korean J Radiol. 2014;15(1):4-11.
6. Machida H, Tanaka I, Fukui R, et al. Current and novel imaging techniques in coronary CT. Radiographics. 2015;35(4):991-1010.
7. Bax JJ, Schuijf JD. Which role for multislice computed tomography in clinical cardiology? Am Heart J. 2005;149(6):960-1.
8. Paech DC, Weston AR. A systematic review of the clinical effectiveness of 64-slice or higher computed tomography angiography as an alternative to invasive coronary angiography in the investigation of suspected coronary artery disease. BMC Cardiovasc Disord. 2011;11:32.
9. Hoffmann U, Truong QA, Schoenfeld DA, et al. Coronary CT angiography versus standard evaluation in acute chest pain. N Engl J Med. 2012;367(4):299-308.
10. Ghostine S, Caussin C, Daoud B, et al. Non-invasive detection of coronary artery disease in patients with left bundle branch block using 64-slice computed tomography. J Am Coll Cardiol. 2006;48(10):1929-34.
11. Schmermund A, Magedanz A, Voigtlander T. The role of CT angiography in risk stratification for atherosclerosis. Curr Atheroscler Rep. 2009;11(2):111-7.
12. Achenbach S. Can CT detect the vulnerable coronary plaque? Int J Cardiovasc Imaging. 2008;24(3):311-2.
13. Motoyama S, Sarai M, Harigaya H, et al. Computed tomographic angiography characteristics of atherosclerotic plaques subsequently resulting in acute coronary syndrome. J Am Coll Cardiol. 2009;54(1):49-57.
14. De Bruyne B, Fearon WF, Pijls NH, et al. Fractional flow reserve-guided PCI for stable coronary artery disease. N Engl J Med. 2014;371(13):1208-17.
15. Tonino PA, De Bruyne B, Pijls NH, et al. Fractional flow reserve versus angiography for guiding percutaneous coronary intervention. N Engl J Med. 2009;360(3):213-24.
16. Chow BJ, Small G, Yam Y, et al. Incremental prognostic value of cardiac computed tomography in coronary artery disease using CONFIRM: COroNary computed tomography angiography evaluation for clinical outcomes: an International Multicenter registry. Circ Cardiovasc Imaging. 2011;4(5):463-72.

17. Tesche C, De Cecco CN, Caruso D, et al. Coronary CT angiography derived morphological and functional quantitative plaque markers correlated with invasive fractional flow reserve for detecting hemodynamically significant stenosis. J Cardiovasc Comput Tomogr. 2016;10(3):1997-206.
18. Johnson TR, Krauss B, Sedlmair M, et al. Material differentiation by dual energy CT: initial experience. Eur Radiol. 2007;17(6):1510-7.
19. Ruzsics B, Lee H, Powers ER, et al. Images in cardiovascular medicine. Myocardial ischemia diagnosed by dual-energy computed tomography: correlation with single-photon emission computed tomography. Circ. 2008;117(9):1244-5.
20. Ohtsuka T, Takamoto S, Endoh M, et al. Ultrafast computed tomography for minimally invasive coronary artery bypass grafting. J Thorac Cardiovasc Surg. 1998;116(1):173-4.
21. Yamaguchi A, Adachi H, Ino T, et al. Three-dimensional computed tomographic angiography as preoperative evaluation of a patent internal thoracic artery graft. J Thorac Cardiovasc Surg. 2000;120(4):811-2.
22. Gulbins H, Reichenspurner H, Becker C, et al. Preoperative 3D-reconstructions of ultrafast-CT images for the planning of minimally invasive direct coronary artery bypass operation (MIDCAB). Heart Surg Forum. 1998;1(2):111-5.
23. Hamon M, Champ-RL, Morello R, et al. Diagnostic accuracy of in-stent coronary restenosis detection with multislice spiral computed tomography: a meta-analysis. Eur Radiol. 2008;18(2):217-25.
24. Amanuma M, Kondo T, Sano T, et al. Assessment of coronary in-stent restenosis: value of subtraction coronary computed tomography angiography. Int J Cardiovasc Imaging. 2016;32(4):661-70.
25. Maintz D, Seifarth H, Raupach R, et al. 64-slice multidetector coronary CT angiography: in vitro evaluation of 68 different stents. Eur Radiol. 2006;16(4): 818-26.
26. Geyer LL, Glenn GR, De Cecco CN, et al. CT evaluation of small-diameter coronary artery stents: Effect of an integrated circuit detector with iterative reconstruction. Radiology. 2015;276(3):706-14.
27. Schuijf JD, Bax JJ, Salm LP, et al. Noninvasive coronary imaging and assessment of left ventricular function using 16-slice computed tomography. Am J Cardiol. 2005;95:571-4.
28. van der Vleuten PA, de Jonge GJ, et al. Evaluation of global left ventricular function assessment by dual-source computed tomography compared with MRI. Eur Radiol. 2009; 19:271-7.
29. Dillman JR, Hernandez RJ. Role of CT in the evaluation of congenital cardiovascular disease in children. AJR Am J Roentgenol. 2009;192:1219-31.
30. Siegel MJ. Congenital heart disease. Pediatr Radiol. 2008;38 Suppl 2:S200-4.
31. Goo HW, Park IS, Ko JK, et al. Computed tomography for the diagnosis of congenital heart disease in pediatric and adult patients. Int J Cardiovasc Imaging. 2005;21:347-65.

CHAPTER 83

Current Indications for Cardiac Magnetic Resonance Imaging

Mona Bhatia, Shashank Jain

INTRODUCTION

Cardiac diseases are among the leading causes of death worldwide. While echocardiography has stood the test of time being noninvasive, nonionizing, easily available, portable and relatively cost-effective, its dependence on operators and acoustic window are among some of its limitations. Cardiac magnetic resonance imaging (MRI) is an excellent tool, nonionizing, currently capable of exceptional spatial, and temporal resolution. Cardiac MRI is capable of not only assessing cardiac structures, but ventricular volumes, function, myocardial perfusion, and tissue characterization with specific sequences to enable diagnosis of edema, ischemia, infarction, scars, myocardial iron content, and flow parameters through different pulse sequences. Hence, cardiac MRI is rapidly growing in the field of cardiac imaging, with a growing number of clinical applications for diagnosis, prognostication, to guide management and follow-up patients to improve clinical outcome. Recent years have seen cardiac MRI play a pivotal role in assessment of myocardial viability, distinguishing different cardiomyopathies, pericardial disease, cardiac masses, congenital and valvular heart diseases, and aortic and pulmonary vessel evaluation.[1,2] Emerging applications include coronary artery, plaque imaging, and vessel analysis besides guiding therapeutic electrophysiology and interventional procedures.[1]

TECHNICAL ASPECTS OF CARDIAC MRI

Image Acquisition

Cardiac MRI can be performed on both 1.5T and 3T scanners. During cardiac image acquisition, respiratory and cardiac motion are the prime culprits for image degradation. Hence, breath-holding and electrocardiogram (ECG)/vector cardiogram gating are essential to ensure optimal image acquisition and quality during a specific phase of the cardiac cycle.[3]

Imaging Planes

While majority of MRI is obtained in the axial, coronal, and sagittal planes, cardiac imaging is often acquired in specific planes as the vertical long axis (two-chamber view), horizontal long axis (four-chamber view), short axis, and three-chamber view.

Imaging Protocols and Sequences

Imaging protocols and sequences need to be tailored to the clinical question. Each pulse sequence is specific, broadly being divided into black-blood or bright-blood sequences. The black-blood spin-echo sequences have higher resolution and are preferred for morphological and anatomic evaluation. The stack of short-axis cine images, from base to apex are used for volumetric analysis and functional evaluation.[4] The high accuracy and reproducibility of MRI is responsible for making cardiac MRI the "gold standard" in the calculation of ventricular volumes, as end-diastolic, end-systolic and stroke volumes, besides determination of ejection fraction (EF) (Table 1), cardiac output, and myocardial mass assessment.[3,4] The excellent contrast between the blood and myocardium on steady-state free precession sequences enables high temporal resolution for accurate and reproducible evaluation of wall motion and ventricular wall thickness. Myocardial tagging with dark grid lines is capable of accurately analyzing cardiac rotation, strain, displacement and deformation of myocardial layers, subendocardial, mid-wall and subepicardial, through the entire cardiac cycle thus evaluating regional myocardial function.[1,5]

The T2-weighted and short inversion time inversion recovery (STIR) sequences are useful for evaluating myocardial edema. Postadministration of IV injection of 0.2 mmol/kg of a gadolinium-based contrast agent, the initial first-pass perfusion imaging is a reliable indicator of ischemia while T1-weighted fast-field echo inversion recovery sequences 10–15 minutes post-IV gadolinium, generate the late-enhancement images useful for myocardial tissue

TABLE 1: Left ventricle analysis results

End diastolic volume	42.4	mL
End systolic volume	10.9	mL
Ejection fraction	74.3	%
Stroke volume	31.5	mL
Stroke index	19.3	$mL/beat/m^2$
Cardiac output	2.3	L/min
Cardiac index	1.4	$L/min/m^2$
Right Ventricle Analysis Results		
End diastolic volume	43.6	mL
End systolic volume	16.2	mL
Ejection fraction	62.8	%
Stroke volume	27.4	mL
Stroke index	16.8	$mL/beat/m^2$
Cardiac output	2.0	L/min
Cardiac index	1.2	$L/min/m^2$

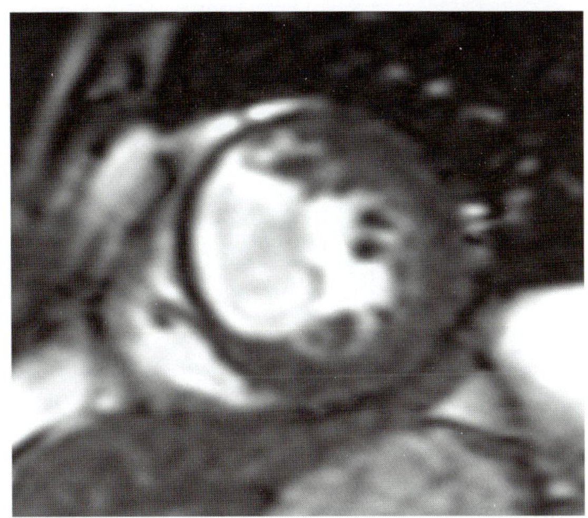

CMR, cardiac magnetic resonance; LAD, left anterior descending.

FIG. 1: Short-axis CMR image demonstrating septal wall thinning in the LAD territory in a case of ischemic cardiomyopathy.

characterization, scar assessment, and prognostication. It is also useful in the evaluation of myocardial infarctions, infiltrative processes and in differentiating masses from thrombi.[3] Phase-contrast sequences are used for quantifying flow and are valuable in stenosis, regurgitation, transvalvular flow, and evaluation of cardiac shunts. Even pressure gradient across lesions are calculated based on blood velocities.

INDICATIONS AND APPLICATIONS

The most frequent clinical applications for cardiac MRI include the following described here.

Ischemic Heart Disease

The three critical questions in evaluation of ischemic heart disease (IHD) are function, ischemia, and viability followed by evaluation of complications, all of which are essential for prognosticating the patient, guiding therapy and follow-up to improve overall patient outcome. Cardiac magnetic resonance (CMR), based on specific sequences can differentiate acute from chronic infarcts, and both qualitatively and quantitatively assess ischemia, distinguish hibernating and stunned myocardium from infarcted myocardium and determine viability.[3]

In the evaluation of cardiac function, cardiac MRI is today considered the gold standard for both regional and global myocardial function. Cardiac MRI can reliably assess both left and right ventricular volumes, and quantify end-diastolic, end-systolic, stroke volume, EF, and ventricular mass. Myocardial wall motion and wall thickness (Fig. 1) can be assessed both visually and quantitatively. Myocardial tagging can further be used for depicting strain. Regional wall motion abnormalities may be seen in both acute and chronic myocardial infarctions.

Acute infarctions demonstrate increased signal on T2-weighted imaging due to myocardial edema. Following IV

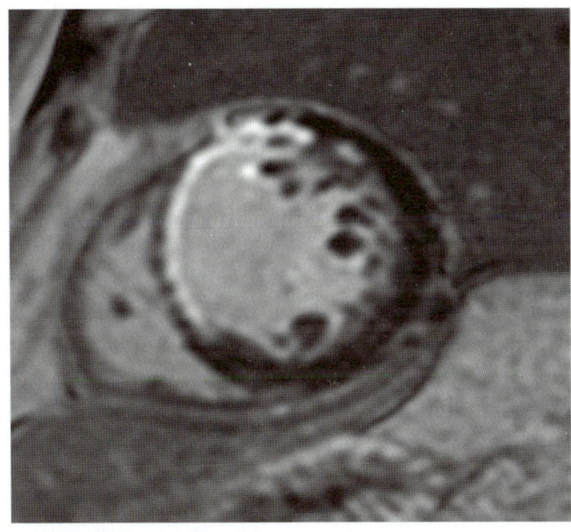

CMR, cardiac magnetic resonance; LAD, left anterior descending.

FIG. 2: Short-axis CMR image demonstrating subendocardial late gadolinium enhancement consistent with myocardial infarction in the LAD territory in a case of ischemic cardiomyopathy.

gadolinium administration, first-pass myocardial perfusion is used to delineate areas of ischemia. Delayed hyper-enhancement (DHE) is a reliable indicator of infarction as it is associated with myocyte necrosis (Fig. 2). A bull's eye mapping of all 17 segments of the left ventricle is possible for wall thickness, wall motion, ischemia, infarction, and viability (Fig. 3). Presence of perfusion defects with delayed-enhancement on the MRI study is highly predictive of scar formation.[2] Combining first-pass and delayed imaging is an indicator of ischemia and viability and predict functional recovery.[4]

Extent and transmurality of delayed enhancement has prognostic implications (Fig. 2) and is inversely proportional to the degree of functional recovery after acute myocardial infarction.[2] Extent of delayed enhancement in excess of 50%

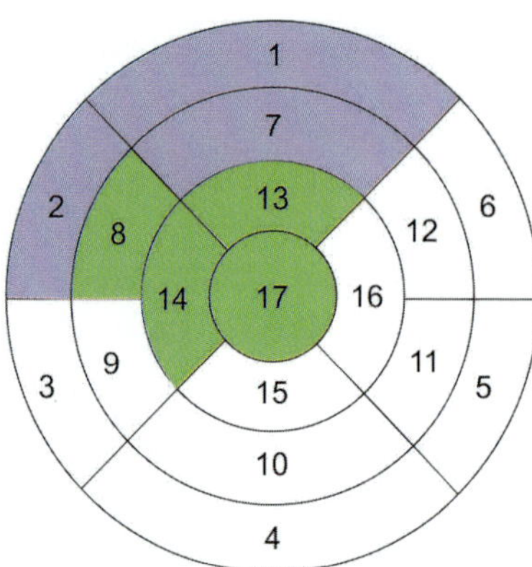

FIG. 3: Bulls eye view of the 17-segment cardiac model depiction percentage of involvement in different segments in a case of ischemic cardiomyopathy.

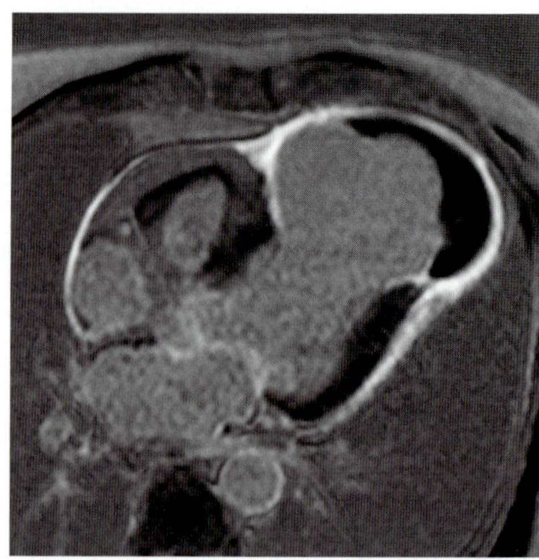

CMR, cardiac magnetic resonance; PSIR, phase sensitive inversion recovery.

FIG. 4: Four-chamber postgadolinium-enhanced PSIR CMR image demonstrating extensive transmural late gadolinium enhancement consistent with myocardial infarction in the LAD territory with aneurysmal change in the apex and intracavitary apical thrombus in a case of ischemic cardiomyopathy.

transmurality of the myocardium can predict segments that are less likely to improve function following revascularization or beta-blocker therapy (Fig. 2).

Magnetic resonance imaging today plays a lead role in identifying acute infarction with myocardial edema, ischemia, and differentiating viable myocardium from nonviable myocardium. Wall motion abnormality may be seen in the setting of ischemia, with transient hypoperfusion which can cause myocardial stunning. Adding myocardial delayed enhancement sequences to the cine MRI protocol, helps to differentiate wall motion abnormalities of myocardial stunning, which are reversible, from myocardial infarction and scarring, which are often irreversible.[2] While both stunning and infarction cause wall motion abnormality, delayed enhancement occurs only with infarcts. Lack of delayed enhancement is seen in stunning.

Similar to stress echocardiography, cine-stress MRI can be used to assess viability without contrast administration during a low-dose infusion of dobutamine (5–10 µg/kg/min).[1] Improvement in left ventricular wall thickening following stress in a poorly functioning segment at rest indicates viability.[2] Dobutamine and adenosine stress MRI can also be used to detect ischemic myocardium.[2] DHE can be seen in diseases as myocarditis, cardiomyopathy, sarcoidosis, amyloidosis, and arrhythmogenic right ventricular dysplasia besides acute and chronic infarcts.[6]

The pattern and distribution of enhancement in these disorders helps to differentiate ischemic from nonischemic cardiomyopathy. While ischemic cardiomyopathy starts in the subendocardial zone and extends like a wavefront, to become transmural, in a coronary artery territory, nonischemic cardiomyopathies demonstrate delayed enhancement, which may be linear, patchy or nodular with a preponderance for the mid-wall, epicardial or global endocardial regions, not following a coronary artery territory.[4]

In severe acute myocardial infarctions, the subendocardium may depict an area of nonenhancement surrounded by enhancement. This central region represents microvascular obstruction (MVO). While this may resolve by 2 weeks, leaving only a scar with DHE, the presence of MVO on delayed enhanced images is indicative of a poor clinical prognosis.[3] Intramyocardial hematomas may also occur as sequelae to severe infarction or reperfusion. Myocardial infarction may progress to myocardial thinning (<6 mm) (Fig. 1) with hypertrophy of the noninfarcted myocardium. Subsequent ventricular dilation, aneurysms, pseudoaneurysms, intraventricular thrombi adjacent to akinetic myocardium after infarction are complications that need further evaluation (Fig. 4).[3] Perfusion MRI following infusion of pharmacologic agents as adenosine and persantine, at rest and stress, when compared to standard methods as angiography or radionuclide scintigraphy, have a sensitivity of 67–83% and specificity of 75–100%.[1] Delayed-enhancement MRI has superior spatial resolution for assessment of scar and viability, in particular, for detecting subendocardial infarction, besides additional information on simultaneous anatomic and cine imaging for wall motion abnormalities.[2]

Myocardial delayed-enhancement cardiac MRI has a good correlation with dobutamine stress echocardiography.[7] On comparison with single-photon emission computed tomography (SPECT), CMR is superior. While there is good agreement between SPECT and CMR, SPECT depicted all of the nearly transmural infarctions but missed 47% of subendocardial infarctions in a study that were depicted on myocardial delayed-enhancement MRI.[2,8] On comparison with 18F-fluorodeoxyglucose positron emission tomography (PET) as the standard, myocardial delayed-enhancement MRI demonstrated 96% sensitivity and 84% specificity.[9]

Nonischemic Cardiomyopathy and Myocarditis

Magnetic resonance imaging can accurately assess ventricular morphology, wall motion abnormalities, function and myocardial wall enhancement pattern which help to characterize cardiomyopathy and myocarditis.[1] Cardiomyopathies may be classified as dilated, hypertrophic, restrictive, arrhythmogenic right ventricular, and other specific cardiomyopathies.

Dilated Cardiomyopathy

Dilated cardiomyopathy (DCM) is associated with dilatation and functional impairment of the left ventricle (LV) or of both ventricles in the absence of significant coronary artery disease (CAD).[10] The cause may be unclear hence a large number are considered idiopathic. Recognized cases include ischemic, genetic or familial, viral, immune, or toxic origin, or secondary to myocardial dysfunction not attributed to ischemic damage or volume overload.[11,12] Patients present with progressive cardiac failure, and the long-term prognosis is poor.[13] Affected ventricles may have normal or thinned walls with hypokinesia, increased cavitary volumes, impaired diastolic function,[14,15] and low EFs. Associated atrial dilatation and valvular dysfunction may occur. CMR is an ideal method to assess DCM[16] to analyze wall thickness, ventricular volumetrics, and delayed-enhancement characteristics to ascertain diagnosis, prognosis, management, and follow-up.[1]

The late gadolinium-enhanced sequences in cardiac MRI, in particular, are extremely useful as they help differentiate between dilated cardiomyopathy (CMP) secondary to CAD and other causes of dilated CMP, besides evaluating the degree of fibrosis which might predict outcome. The progressive replacement interstitial fibrosis in DCM is frequently mid-wall in the circumferential fiber layer rather than subendocardial as seen in IHD (Fig. 5).[10] This mid-wall myocardial fibrosis, a predictor of all-cause mortality, cardiovascular hospitalization, sudden cardiac death, and ventricular tachycardia. Thus, cardiac MRI is useful in risk stratification of patients with dilated CMP (Fig. 5).

Studies have demonstrated that mid-wall and basal anterolateral wall late gadolinium enhancement (LGE) is an independent predictor of major adverse cardiac events (MACE) in clinically diagnosed DCM patients, with normal coronary angiograms.[17,18]

Myocarditis

Myocarditis is inflammation of the myocardium due to various etiologies as viral, toxins, drugs, and autoimmune processes.[19] Myocarditis manifests as myocardial edema on T2-weighted images on CMR with associated wall-motion abnormalities, and patchy early and delayed myocardial enhancement postgadolinium contrast administration.[19] In myocarditis, LGE typically spares the endocardium and involves the mid-myocardial and subepicardial layers (Fig. 6).[20] The lateral free wall is more commonly involved in Parvovirus B.[21]

Hypertrophic Cardiomyopathy

Hypertrophic CMP is often genetic or familial, with a 50% autosomal-dominant hereditary pattern, and variable expression.[22] Patients are usually asymptomatic or mildly symptomatic, even sudden death may occur.[23-25] Hypertrophic CMP involves LV wall thickening, concentric, apical, asymmetric or papillary muscle involvement, although most often it is asymmetric with involvement of the interventricular septum (Fig. 7).[11] LV outflow tract obliteration may occur as a consequence, with systolic gradients (obstructive form). Left ventricle ejection fraction (LVEF) can be normal or increased, whereas cavitary volumes can be normal or reduced. Altered ventricular compliance may cause diastolic function impairment and valve insufficiency may coexist. Cardiac MRI is excellent in evaluating all these parameters.[14]

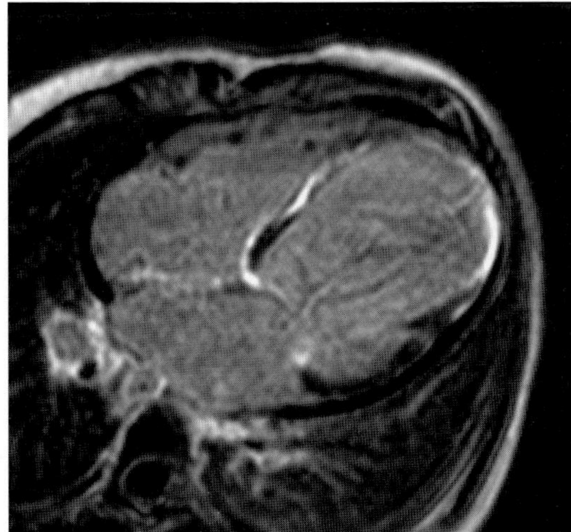

CMR, cardiac magnetic resonance; LV, left ventricle; PSIR, phase sensitive inversion recovery.

FIG. 5: Four-chamber postgadolinium-enhanced PSIR CMR image demonstrating dilated LV with global wall thinning, and mid-wall to transmural late gadolinium enhancement in a case of dilated cardiomyopathy.

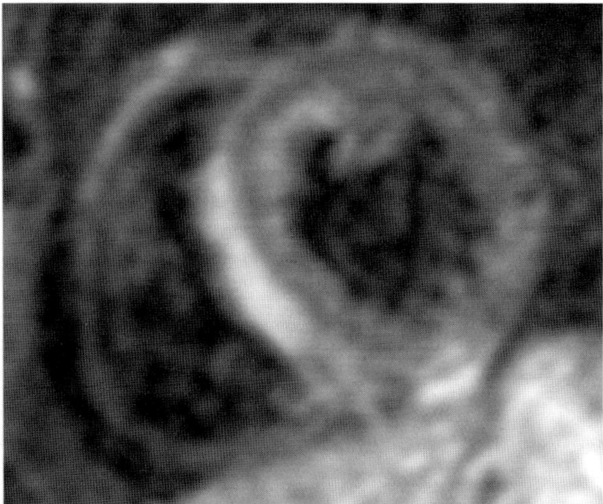

CMR, cardiac magnetic resonance.

FIG. 6: Short-axis T2-weighted CMR image demonstrating myocardial hyperintensity, suggestive of edema in a case of acute myocarditis.

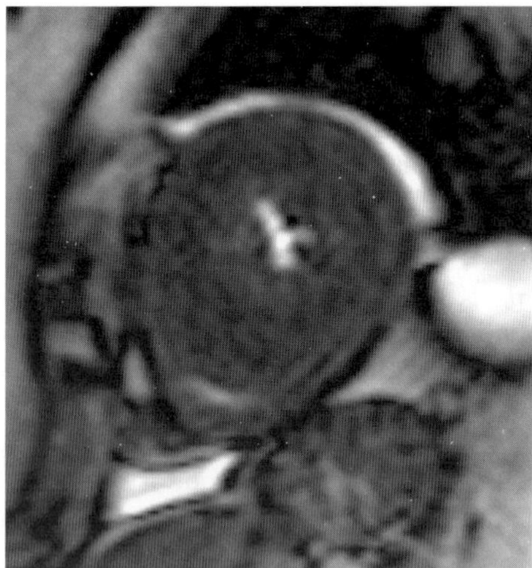

CMR, cardiac magnetic resonance; LV, left ventricle.

FIG. 7: Short-axis CMR image demonstrating concentric LV myocardial thickening in a case of hypertrophic cardiomyopathy.

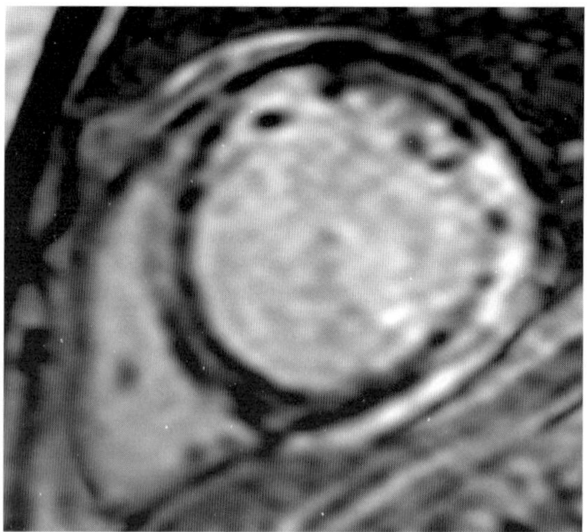

CMR, cardiac magnetic resonance.

FIG. 8: Postgadolinium-enhanced short axis CMR image depicting mid-wall and epicardial enhancement in a case of nonischemic cardiomyopathy.

Myocyte disarray and interstitial plus replacement fibrosis occur in hypertrophic CMP.[26] The myocardium in hypertrophic CMP demonstrates fibrotic scars and signs of myocardial microischemia[23] on late-enhancement images, the extent of which is associated with risk stratification for sudden cardiac death with important prognostic and therapeutic implications[26] as these scars act as a substrate for fatal arrhythmia.[23-25] As fibrosis detected by LGE is an independent predictor of adverse outcome[27,28] it has a role in diagnosing and identifying high-risk patients.[29] Cardiac MRI is also useful in the follow-up of patients after ventricular septal resection or percutaneous ablation.[1,3]

Restrictive Cardiomyopathy

Restrictive CMP manifests as reduced ventricular filling and diastolic volume, with resultant atrial dilatation and venous stasis, and usually preserved systolic function.[11] The condition may be idiopathic, or secondary to infiltrative or storage diseases (amyloidosis and sarcoidosis), or associated with myocardial disorders as hypereosinophilic syndrome (HES).[30] The RV may be enlarged if there is coexistent pulmonary hypertension. LV may demonstrate preserved or reduced systolic function.

One of the important differentials of restrictive CMP is constrictive pericarditis, where reduced ventricular filling and diastolic volumes may be seen in both diseases. Cardiac MRI is extremely useful as it can demonstrate pericardial thickening (>4 mm) typical of constrictive pericarditis, while real time cine images are useful in evaluating diastolic ventricular septal movements and septal motion during respiration.[31,32] While in restrictive CMP, septal convexity is maintained in all respiratory phases, in constrictive pericarditis, septal flattening may be seen in early inspiration.

Sarcoidosis

Sarcoidosis is a systemic granulomatous disease where cardiac involvement may occur with noncaseating granulomatous infiltration in 5–20% patients.[33,34] Myocardial thickening in sarcoid may resemble hypertrophic CMP. Typical granulomatous changes most often affect the LV lateral wall, papillary muscles, basal interventricular septum, RV subendocardial surface, and RV free wall. The distribution patterns may be patchy or striae-like sparing the subendocardium; while diffuse and transmural patterns occur in advanced disease.[35] Associated LV hypertrophy, LV or RV dilatation, septal thinning, systolic and diastolic left ventricular dysfunction, and pericardial effusion may be seen on CMR.[2]

Sarcoid lesions vary in different stages of the disease. Infiltrates may be diffuse or focal with hyperintensity due to myocardial edema in T2-weighted fat-saturated or STIR images. The lesions may vary from high intensity on T2-weighted sequences to central low intensity on T1- and T2-weighted imaging surrounded by a high-signal ring in different stages.[1] Postgadolinium administration, contrast enhancement may be seen as patchy mid-wall and epicardial in distribution with a predilection for the basal and lateral segments of the left ventricle (Fig. 8). These may represent fibrotic replacement of the myocardium. Cine images may demonstrate LV altered filling patterns consistent with secondary restrictive CMP. Segmental wall motion abnormalities corresponding to the distribution of late-enhancement areas may be seen.[35]

Hemochromatosis

Myocardial iron deposition may occur due to primary (genetic) hemochromatosis or secondary (transfusion dependent) iron overload.[19] Iron deposition is predominantly subepicardial. CMR can demonstrate extensive signal loss in native T1- and T2-weighted images in a dysfunctional myocardium. An associated abnormally "dark" liver confirms the diagnosis of iron deposition and systemic hemochromatosis.[1] CMR is superior to serum ferritin and liver iron in assessing patients at high risk of

HF and arrhythmia from myocardial siderosis, to guide management, monitor response to iron-chelating agents and prognosticate[36] as treatments differ depending on whether the prime target is extraction of iron from the heart or the liver.

Amyloidosis

Amyloidosis is characterized by deposition of amyloid—an extracellular insoluble fibrillar proteins deposition that results from protein misfolding—in tissue. Amyloidosis may be systemic or organ specific. Cardiac amyloid manifests classically as concentric myocardial thickening, similar to that in hypertrophic CMP, with normal or reduced contractility, thickened atrial walls, interatrial septum, biatrial dilation, altered transvalvular flow patterns, pericardial, and pleural effusions.

Thickness of the atrial septum or the right atrial posterior wall of 6 mm is fairly specific for amyloid infiltration.[1,37]

Postadministration of gadolinium, the wash-in wash-out is abnormal as amyloid fibrils accumulate gadolinium. CMR in amyloidosis has unique LGE appearances with circumferential enhancement, preferentially involving the subendocardium but sometimes extending transmurally, diffuse, and heterogeneous (Fig. 9).[38] Less often there is patchy focal LGE. The blood pool is atypically dark, reflecting high myocardial contrast uptake and fast blood pool wash-out. Depressed systolic ventricular function and reduced wall compliance manifest as overt restrictive CMP in advanced stages. Characteristic CMR LGE is a stronger predictor of mortality in cardiac amyloidosis compared to ECG and echocardiography.[39]

Endomyocardial Fibrosis

Hypereosinophilic syndrome with increased eosinophils can be a primary (myeloid or eosinophilic neoplasm), secondary (parasitic infections i.e. Loeffler's syndrome, or other non-stem cell tumors), or an idiopathic condition. Endomyocardial fibrosis (also termed Loeffler endocarditis) is characterized by fibrosis of the apical endomyocardium (Fig. 10). CMR demonstrates extensive subendocardial fibrosis, obliteration of the ventricular apices, apical thrombus formation, and progressive diastolic dysfunction manifesting as restrictive cardiomyopathy (Fig. 10).[19,40] The morphologic and functional features can be well quantified by MRI.

Arrhythmogenic Right Ventricular Dysplasia

Arrhythmogenic RV CMP is characterized by progressive fibrous or fibrofatty replacement of the myocytes of the ventricular wall, primarily RV, and clinically manifests as life-threatening ventricular arrhythmias, left bundle-branch block, heart failure, and sudden cardiac death.[26,41,42] Early diagnosis is key and CMR is the technique of choice. Fatty infiltration, fibrofatty replacement of the RV free walls, wall thinning with systolic and diastolic dysfunction, reduced EF and RV dilatation are seen. Associated regional wall motion abnormalities, with systolic and localized early diastolic bulging, gross dyskinesia, aneurysms of the RV free wall and outflow tract, dysplastic trabecular structures,[11] may be seen (Fig. 11).[1] Delayed enhancement of the right ventricular myocardium may have a diagnostic role.[2,3,43,44]

Left Ventricular Noncompaction

Left ventricular noncompaction (LVNC) is a congenital disorder of endomyocardial embryogenesis with arrest in normal process of myocardial compaction characterized by prominent LV trabeculations with deep intertrabecular recesses, resulting in a distinct noncompacted layer lining the LV cavity.[45] A ratio of noncompacted to compacted myocardium greater than 2.3 has a high specificity and sensitivity.[46] Findings are most prominent in the left ventri-

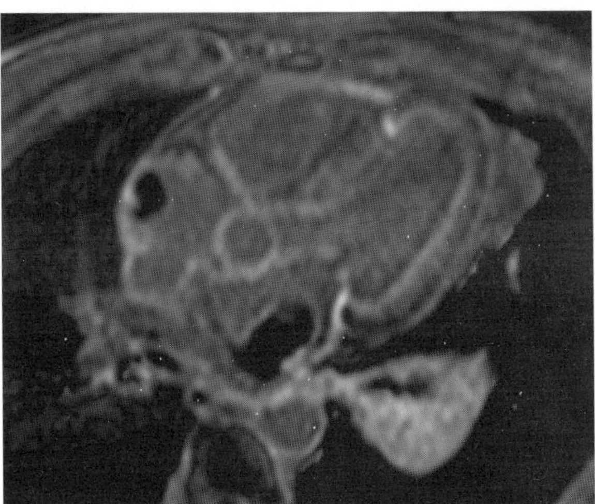

CMR, cardiac magnetic resonance.

FIG. 9: Four-chamber CMR image demonstrating global subendocardial enhancement and biatrial thrombi in a case of cardiac amyloidosis.

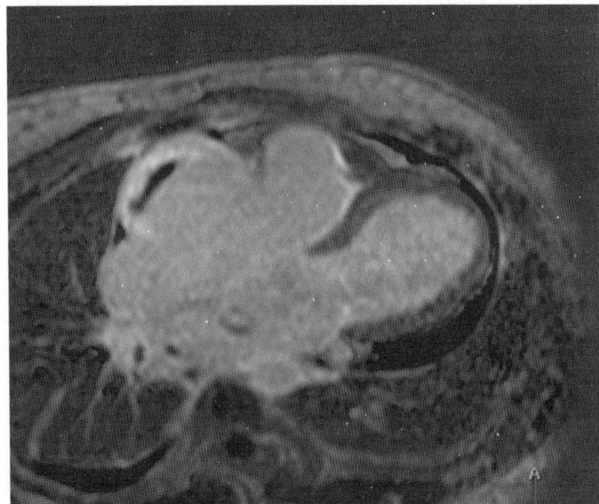

CMR, cardiac magnetic resonance.

FIG. 10: Four-chamber CMR view depicting right ventricular apical obliteration with endocardial fibrosis and dilated right atrium in a case of endomyocardial fibrosis.

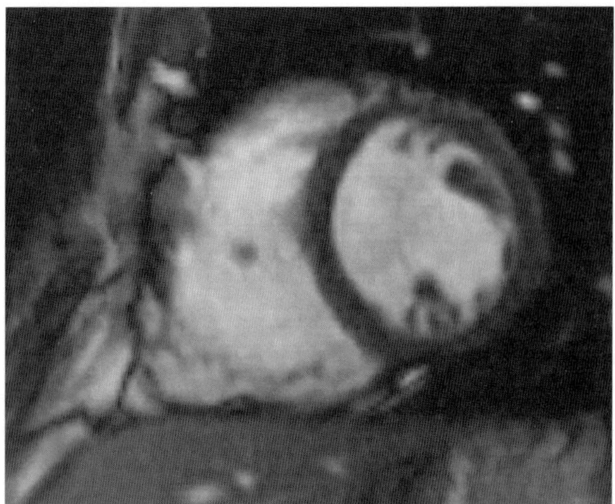

CMR, cardiac magnetic resonance; ARVC, arrhythmogenic right ventricular cardiomyopathy.

FIG. 11: Short-axis CMR image demonstrating dilated RV with wall thinning, irregularity, trabeculations, sacculations, and aneurysms in a case of ARVC.

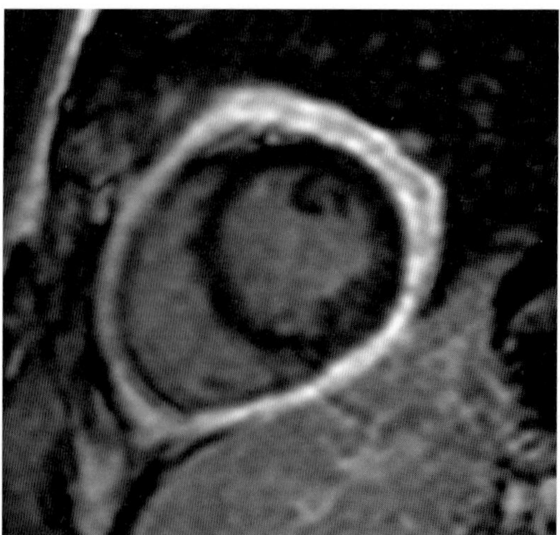

CMR, cardiac magnetic resonance.

FIG. 12: Postgadolinium contrast short-axis CMR image demonstrating a thickened enhancing pericardium in a case of constrictive pericarditis.

cular apex. LVNC may lead to heart failure, malignant arrhythmias, and thromboembolism.[10]

Takotsubo Cardiomyopathy

Takotsubo cardiomyopathy (stress cardiomyopathy) is a transient left ventricular ballooning with wall motion abnormalities, including apical akinesia in the absence of CAD.[47] CMR typically demonstrates myocardial edema but no LGE or fibrosis is seen and cardiac function fully recovers over time.[16]

Anderson-Fabry Disease

Fabry's disease is an X-linked inherited disorder of lysosomal metabolism with glycosphingolipid deposition in multiple organs.[19] Cardiac manifestations include LV hypertrophy, increased LVEF, reduced volume, and fibrosis. LGE occurs in specific locations (midbasal lateral LV wall) and the distribution pattern (subepicardial and mesocardial) in patients with Anderson-Fabry disease who have cardiac symmetric hypertrophy.[19]

Pericardial Disease

The most common indications for pericardial disease evaluation are constrictive pericarditis, effusion, and tamponade. CMR demonstrates normal pericardium as a thin band (2 mm) of low signal on T1-weighted images, bordered by epicardial and pericardial fat. MRI reliably assesses pericardial thickening, effusion, and fibrous pericarditis (Fig. 12).[1,4] CMR demonstrates effusions complicated with adhesions, loculations and aids differentiating transudative from exudative, hemorrhagic or chylous effusion based on signal characteristics and contrast enhancement.[1] Associated finding in the ventricles and cardiac valves[1] can be evaluated on cine MRI as small right ventricular chamber, restriction of diastolic filling, biatrial dilation, ventricular or septal alterations, septal bounce, adhesions between the pericardium and epicardium[3] with diastolic collapse of chambers in tamponade. MRI has high sensitivity in differentiating constrictive pericarditis from restrictive cardiomyopathy.[4]

Cardiac Masses, Thrombi, and Infections

Magnetic resonance imaging today is extremely useful in delineation of extent, origin, hemorrhage, vascularity, and calcification in cardiac masses[2] with clear delineation of relationship to other cardiac and neighboring structures.[1] On account of the superior soft tissue contrast and tissue characterization, MRI is useful in the evaluation of cardiac tumors as myxomas, lipomas, metastasis, fibroma, rhabdomyoma, hemangioma, pheochromocytoma, lymphoma, malignant fibrous histiocytoma, and angiosarcoma.[4]

A particular advantage of MRI is in its ability to distinguish thrombus from tumor. Unlike a tumor, a thrombus has low-signal intensity on gradient echo images because of the presence of deoxyhemoglobin.[4,48] In the event of a diagnostic dilemma where a myxoma appears hypointense secondary to calcification or hemorrhage, the differentiation is easily done postcontrast, as enhancement occurs in the tumor but not in the thrombus (Fig. 9).[4] Lipomas and lipomatous hypertrophy appear brighter on spin-echo T1-weighted sequences. The malignant tumors are more likely to be necrotic, inhomogeneous, heterogeneously enhancing with associated edema and invasion of surrounding structures.

Valvular Disease

Cardiac MRI can be used to evaluate stenotic or regurgitant lesions and quantify the same while also assessing aberrant valvular anatomy. Associated findings as ventricular dilation, dysfunction, and myocardial hypertrophy can also be assessed, which influence the decision and timing of valve replacement surgery.[3]

Postcardiac Transplantation

Post heart transplantation, acute cellular rejection with systolic dysfunction and myocardial edema and cardiac allograft vasculopathy are causes of early and late morbidity and mortality, respectively. CMR can be used for the identification of systolic dysfunction and myocardial edema in cardiac transplant recipients allowing early detection of cardiac rejection.[49] Moreover, LGE-CMR is useful indirectly in the detection of cardiac allograft vasculopathy based on the ability to detect silent myocardial infarctions. Overall, the role of CMR in the transplanted heart is still evolving.

FUTURE DEVELOPMENTS

In the future, contrast-enhanced MRI may be used to guide interventions. These include real-time monitoring of electromagnetic catheter-directed radiofrequency (RF) ablations (e.g., for treatment of atrial fibrillation) within the heart with the potential to provide more.

New treatments for heart failure involve the transplantation of primitive cell types (e.g., stem cells or myoblasts) into the damaged tissue, where they can transdifferentiate into functional tissue.[50] Stem cell therapy in the heart might further benefit from the combination of molecular imaging methods with interventional MRI techniques.

CONCLUSION

Magnetic resonance imaging is fast emerging as a dominant noninvasive imaging modality in the assessment of cardiovascular diseases.

Cardiac magnetic resonance has the unique capability of delineating detailed anatomical and myocardial functional assessment ensuring differentiation of ischemic from nonischemic cardiomyopathy, with additional features in the characterization of nonischemic cardiomyopathy. CMR is neither operator dependent nor limited by the acoustic window, problems commonly faced in echocardiography. CMR should hence be routinely integrated in the diagnostic workup of patients suspected of nonischemic cardiomyopathies for superior diagnosis, prognostication, management, and follow-up.

REFERENCES

1. Lima JA, Desai MY. Cardiovascular magnetic resonance imaging: Current and emerging applications. J Am Coll Cardiol. 2004;44:1164-71.
2. Edelman RR. Contrast-enhanced MR imaging of the heart: Overview of the literature. Radiology. 2004;232:653-68.
3. Norton PT, Nacey NC, Caovan DB, et al. Cardiac MRI: The basics. [online] Available from http:// www.med-ed.virginia.edu/courses/rad/cardiacmr/index.html [Accessed August 2018].
4. Lin EC. (2013). Cardiac MRI, technical aspects primer. [online] Medscape website. Available from http://emedicine.medscape.com/article/352250-overview [Accessed June 2018].
5. Kim HW, Crowley AL, Kim RJ. A clinical cardiovascular magnetic resonance service: Operational considerations and the basic examination. Cardiol Clin. 2007;25(1):1-13.
6. Weinsaft JW, Klem I, Judd RM. MRI for the assessment of myocardial viability. Cardiol Clin. 2007;25(1):35-56, v.
7. Zamorano J, Delgado J, Almeria C, et al. Reason for discrepancies in identifying myocardial viability by thallium-201 redistribution, magnetic resonance imaging, and dobutamine echocardiography. Am J Cardiol. 2002;90:455-9.
8. Wagner A, Mahrholdt H, Holly TA, et al. Contrast-enhanced MRI and routine single photon emission computed tomography (SPECT) perfusion imaging for detection of subendocardial myocardial infarcts: An imaging study. Lancet. 2003;361:374-9.
9. Kuhl HP, Beek AM, van der Weerdt AP, et al. Myocardial viability in chronic ischemic heart disease: A comparison of contrast-enhanced magnetic resonance imaging with (18F)-fluorodeoxyglucose positron emission tomography. J Am Coll Cardiol. 2003;41:1341-8.
10. Assomull R, Pennell D, Prasad S. Cardiovascular magnetic resonance in the evaluation of heart failure. Heart. 2007;93(8):985-92.
11. Richardson PJ, McKenna W, Bristow M, et al. Report of the 1995 World Health Organization/International Society and Federation of Cardiology Task Force on the Definition and Classification of Cardiomyopathies. Circulation. 1996;93:841-2.
12. Caforio ALP, Mahon NJ, Tona F, et al. Circulating cardiac autoantibodies in dilated cardiomyopathy and myocarditis: Pathogenetic and clinical significance. Eur J Heart Fail. 2002;4:411-7.
13. Juilliere Y, Danchin N, Briancon S, et al. Dilated cardiomyopathy: Long-term follow-up and predictors of survival. Int J Cardiol. 1988;21:269-77.
14. Mandinov L, Eberli FR, Seiler C, et al. Diastolic heart failure. Cardiovasc Res. 2000;45:813-25.
15. Fujimoto S, Nakagawa Y, Mizuno R, et al. Reduced early diastolic inflow velocities in the antero-posterior transverse direction in the left ventricle of patients with dilated cardiomyopathy. Int J Card Imaging. 2000,16:43-8.
16. Karamitsos T, Neubauer S. Cardiovascular magnetic resonance in heart failure. Curr Cardiol Rep. 2011;13(3):210-9.
17. Assomull RG, Prasad SK, Lyne J, et al. Cardiovascular magnetic resonance, fibrosis, and prognosis in dilated cardiomyopathy. J Am Coll Cardiol. 2006;48:1977-85.
18. McCrohon J. Differentiation of heart failure related to dilated cardiomyopathy and coronary artery disease using gadolinium-enhanced cardiovascular magnetic resonance. Circulation. 2003;108(1):54-9.
19. Wellnhofer E. Magnetic resonance low-dose dobutamine test is superior to scar quantification for the prediction of functional recovery. Circulation. 2004;109(18):2172-4.
20. Abdel-Aty H. Diagnostic performance of cardiovascular magnetic resonance in patients with suspected acute myocarditis: Comparison of different approaches. J Am Coll Cardiol. 2005;45:1815-22.
21. Mahrholdt H, Goedecke C, Wagner A. Cardiovascular magnetic resonance assessment of human myocarditis. A comparison to histology and molecular pathology. ACC Curr J Rev. 2004;13(6):25.
22. Schoen FJ. Heart. In: Cotran RS, Kumar V, Collins T, eds. Robbins Pathologic Basis of Disease [Italian version]. Philadelphia, PA: Saunders, 1999:681.
23. Basso C, Thiene G, Corrado D, et al. Hypertrophic cardiomyopathy and sudden death in the young: Pathologic evidence of myocardial ischemia. Hum Pathol. 2000;31:988-98.
24. Maron BJ, Olivotto I, Spirito P, et al. Epidemiology of hypertrophic cardiomyopathy-related death: Revisited in a large non-referral-based patient population. Circulation. 2000;102:858-64.
25. Choudhury L, Mahrholdt H, Wagner A, et al. Myocardial scarring in asymptomatic or mildly symptomatic patients with hypertrophic cardiomyopathy. J Am Coll Cardiol. 2002;40:2156-64.
26. Moon JCC, McKenna WJ, McCrohon JA, et al. Toward clinical risk assessment in hypertrophic cardiomyopathy with gadolinium cardiovascular magnetic resonance. J Am Coll Cardiol. 2003;41:1561-7.
27. Maron MS. The current and emerging role of cardiovascular magnetic resonance imaging in hypertrophic cardiomyopathy. J Cardiovasc Transl Res. 2009;2:415-25.

28. Bruder O, Wagner A, Jensen CJ, et al. Myocardial scar visualized by cardiovascular magnetic resonance imaging predicts major adverse events in patients with hypertrophic cardiomyopathy. J Am Coll Cardiol. 2010;56:875-87.
29. O'Hanlon R, Grasso A, Roughton M, et al. Prognostic significance of myocardial fibrosis in hypertrophic cardiomyopathy. J Am Coll Cardiol. 2010;56:867-74.
30. Kushwaha SS, Fallon JT, Fuster V. Restrictive cardiomyopathy. N Engl J Med. 1997;336:267-76.
31. Giorgi B, Mollet NRA, Dymarkowski S, et al. Clinically suspected constrictive pericarditis: MR imaging assessment of ventricular septal motion and configuration in patients and healthy subjects. Radiology. 2003;228:417-24.
32. Francone M, Dymarkowski S, Kalantzi M, et al. Real-time cine MRI of ventricular septal motion: A novel approach to assess ventricular coupling. J Magn Reson Imaging. 2005;234:542-7.
33. Kirk P, Roughton M, Porter JB, et al. Cardiac t2* magnetic resonance for prediction of cardiac complications in thalassemia major. Circulation. 2009;120:1961-8.
34. Matsui Y, Iway K, Tachibana T, et al. Clinicopathological study of fatal myocardial sarcoidosis. Ann N Y Acad Sci. 1976;278:455-69.
35. Vignaux O. Cardiac sarcoidosis: Spectrum of MRI features. AJR. 2005;184:249-54.
36. Austin BA, Tang WH, Rodriguez ER, et al. Delayed hyperenhancement magnetic resonance imaging provides incremental diagnostic and prognostic utility in suspected cardiac amyloidosis. JACC Cardiovasc Imaging. 2009;2:1369-77.
37. Fattori R, Rocchi G, Celletti F, et al. Contribution of magnetic resonance imaging in the differential diagnosis of cardiac amyloidosis and symmetric hypertrophic cardiomyopathy. Am Heart J. 1998;136:824-30.
38. Paulus WJ, Tschope C, Sanderson JE, et al. How to diagnose diastolic heart failure: A consensus statement on the diagnosis of heart failure with normal left ventricular ejection fraction by the Heart Failure and Echocardiography Associations of the European Society of Cardiology. Eur Heart J. 2007;28:2539-50.
39. Syed IS, Glockner JF, Feng D, et al. Role of cardiac magnetic resonance imaging in the detection of cardiac amyloidosis. JACC Cardiovasc Imaging. 2010;3:155-64.
40. Friedrich MG. Magnetic resonance imaging in cardiomyopathies J Cardiovasc Magn Reson. 2000;2:67-82.
41. Thiene G, Basso C, Danieli G, et al. Arrhythmogenic right ventricular cardiomyopathy. Trends Cardiovasc Med. 1997;7:84-90.
42. Kayser HWM, van der Wall EE, Sivananthan MU, et al. Diagnosis of arrhythmogenic right ventricular dysplasia: A review. RadioGraphics. 2002;22:639-50.
43. Sen-Chowdhry S. Arrhythmogenic right ventricular cardiomyopathy: Clinical presentation, diagnosis, and management. Am J Med. 2004;117:68595.
44. Sen-Chowdhry S, Syrris P, Prasad SK, et al. Left-dominant arrhythmogenic cardiomyopathy: An under-recognized clinical entity. J Am Coll Cardiol. 2008;52:2175-87.
45. Karamitsos T, Francis J, Myerson S, et al. The role of cardiovascular magnetic resonance imaging in heart failure. J Am Coll Cardiol. 2009;54(15):1407-24.
46. Petersen SE, Selvanayagam JB, Wiesmann F, et al. Left ventricular noncompaction: Insights from cardiovascular magnetic resonance imaging. J Am Coll Cardiol. 2005;46:101-5.
47. Friedrich MG, Sechtem U, Schulz-Menger J, et al. Cardiovascular magnetic resonance in myocarditis: A JACC white paper. J Am Coll Cardiol. 2009;53:1475-87.
48. Grizzard JD, Ang GB. Magnetic resonance imaging of pericardial disease and cardiac masses. Cardiol Clin. 2007;25(1):111-40, vi.
49. Storkecky S, Suter TM. Insights into cardiovascular side-effects of modern anticancer therapeutics. Curr Opin Oncol. 2010;22:312-7.
50. Orlic D, Hill JM, Arai AE. Stem cells for myocardial regeneration. Circ Res. 2002;91:1092-1102.

SECTION 12

Cardiovascular Pharmacology

CHAPTER 84

Newer Antianginals

Kewal C Goswami, Anunay Gupta

INTRODUCTION

Due to increased number of cases of coronary artery disease (CAD) over few decades, more and more patients are on antianginal medicines. Despite advances in percutaneous coronary intervention (PCI) and coronary artery bypass surgery (CABG) for ischemic heart disease (IHD), many patients with angina pectoris continue to have angina post-PCI or CABG. Many patients, who are not candidate of either PCI or CABG, continue to have refractory angina despite on maximal doses of conventional therapy such as long-acting nitrates, β-blockers or calcium channel blockers. This chapter reviews newer antianginal drugs (Table 1) available for such patients.

RANOLAZINE

Among all the newer antianginals that will be discussed here only ranolazine is approved by Food and Drug Administration (FDA).

Ranolazine was initially thought to be acting through partial inhibition of fatty acid oxidation, but its antianginal action is due to prevention of calcium overload and the subsequent increase in diastolic tension due to inhibition of late inward sodium channel (Flowchart 1). Initial dosing of ranolazine is 500 mg bd followed by 1,000 mg bd if patient remains symptomatic.

TABLE 1: Newer antianginals

Approved	Not approved/Investigational
• Ranolazine • Ivabradine • Nicorandil • Trimetazidine	• Fasudil • Testosterone • Allopurinol • Endothelin receptor blockers: Bosentan • High-dose statins • Molsidomine • L-arginine • GLP-1 analogs

GLP-1, glucagon-like peptide 1.

Ranolazine was found to be beneficial in stable angina in MARISA (Monotherapy Assessment of Ranolazine In Stable Angina), CARISA (Combination Assessment of Ranolazine In Stable Angina), and ERICA (Efficacy of Ranolazine in Chronic Angina) trials.[1-3] In MERLIN-TIMI 36 (Metabolic Efficiency With Ranolazine for Less Ischemia in Non-ST-Elevation Acute Coronary Syndromes) trial patients with an acute coronary syndrome (ACS), in the subset of 3,565 patients who had prior chronic angina, ranolazine significantly reduced the primary end point of cardiovascular (CV) death, myocardial infarction (MI), and recurrent ischemia due entirely to a significant reduction in recurrent ischemia [hazard ratio (HR) 0.78, 95% confidence interval (CI) 0.67–0.91].[4,5] Ranolazine was associated with lower rate of worsening angina (HR 0.77, 95% CI 0.55–1.00) and a significant improvement in exercise duration on a treadmill (514s vs. 482 s).[4,5] Ranolazine failed to improve outcomes in patients who had incomplete revascularization in RIVER-PCI (Ranolazine in patients with incomplete revascularization after percutaneous coronary intervention) trial.[6] In this trial 2,651 patients were randomized to ranolazine or placebo after incomplete revascularization with PCI. There was no difference in the rate of the primary efficacy end point (time to first occurrence of ischemia-driven revascularization or ischemia-driven hospitalization without revascularization) between the two groups (26% vs. 28%; HR 0.95, 95% CI 0.82–1.10) after a median follow-up of 643 days.

Ranolazine has antiarrhythmic effects also. Its antiarrhythmic properties are based on the frequency-dependent blockade of peak sodium channel current (peak INa) and rapidly activating delayed rectifier potassium current (IKr) in the atria and blockade of late phase of the inward sodium current (late INa) in the ventricles.[7] In MERLIN-TIMI 36 trial, it was associated with 3% lower frequency of ventricular tachycardia (VT), a 10.3% lower incidence of supraventricular tachycardia, and a 0.7% reduction in the onset of new atrial

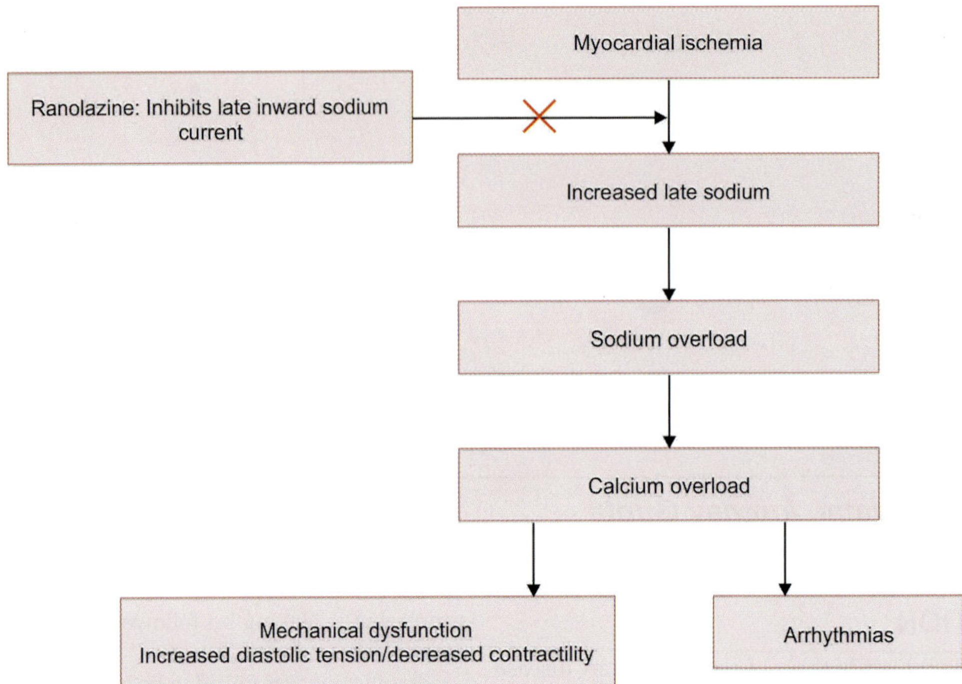

FLOWCHART 1: Mechanism of action of ranolazine.

fibrillation (AF).[8] Ranolazine is effective in prevention of AF in patients with ACSs, prevention as well as conversion of postoperative AF after cardiac surgery, conversion of recent-onset AF, and maintenance of sinus rhythm in recurrent AF.[7] Ranolazine significantly improved glycated hemoglobin (HbA1c) (fall of 0.3%) and recurrent ischemia in patients with diabetes mellitus and reduced the incidence of increased HbA1c in those without evidence of previous hyperglycemia.[9]

Most important adverse effect with use of ranolazine is increase in QTc interval. In a review of 746 patients, ranolazine was associated with mean QTc prolongation of 2.4 ms in patients who were treated for almost 3 years. Even though there is a dose-dependent increase in QTc interval, torsade de pointes has not been reported due to lack of reverse use dependence seen with ranolazine.[10]

NICORANDIL

Nicorandil is a nicotinamide derivative and an efficacious antianginal drug with a nitrate moiety in its chemical structure. Its efficacy is similar to that of nitrates, with several unique effects on the CV system. Nicorandil causes sustained dilation of both the arterial resistance and conductive vessels, hence causing significant dilation of the coronary artery and increasing coronary blood flow. The mechanism causing coronary vasodilation is dual first is nitrate donor and second appears to be due to activation of adenosine triphosphate (ATP)-dependent potassium channels (Flowchart 2). Dose is 5–20 mg bd.

The effect of nicorandil (20 mg twice per day) on coronary events was evaluated in the IONA (Impact Of Nicorandil in Angina) trial of 5,126 patients with chronic stable angina who were receiving other standard therapies.[11] After a mean follow-up of 1.6 years, nicorandil reduced the primary end point (coronary death, nonfatal MI, or unplanned hospitalization for angina) by 17% (13 vs. 15.5 for placebo, HR 0.83, 95% CI 0.72–0.97). There was significant reduction in the secondary end point of death and nonfatal MI (4.2% vs. 5.2%) and significant reductions in the incidence of an ACS (6% vs. 7.6%) and all CV events (14.7% vs. 17%). However, a point to highlight was that IONA was an outcome study and worsening of anginal status was not significantly different in patients taking nicorandil compared to those on placebo (22% vs. 24%, respectively).[11]

Common adverse effects include headache (>10% of cases; especially on initiation of treatment), flushing, and dizziness. Mucosal ulceration is rare (<0.01%), ranges from multiple intractable oral aphthous ulcers to anal fissure and rectovaginal fistula.[12]

IVABRADINE

Ivabradine, a selective sinus node If channel inhibitor, is a therapeutic innovation in the treatment of ischemia. Ivabradine can reduce heart rate (HR) without affecting cardiac systolic function, hence was recommended as a second-line antianginal agent. It has been shown to increase exercise capacity and reduce anginal frequency and severity. Its dose is 5–7.5 mg bd.

In a recently published landmark SIGNIFY (Study Assessing the Morbidity–Mortality Benefits of the *If* Inhibitor Ivabradine in Patients with Coronary Artery Disease) trial randomly assigned 19,102 patients with stable CAD without clinical heart failure (HF) and a HR of 70 beats/min or more to

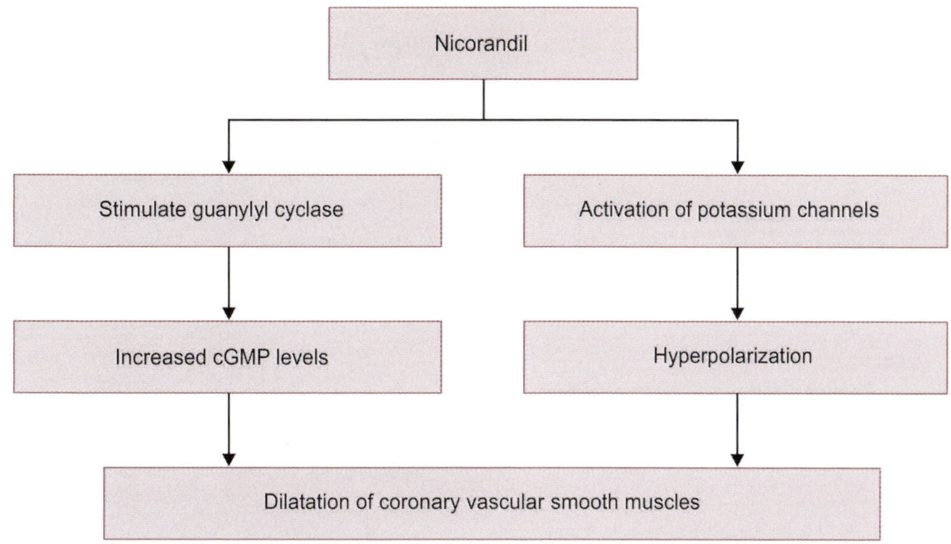

cGMP, cyclic guanosine monophosphate.

FLOWCHART 2: Mechanism of action of nicorandil.

ivabradine or placebo.[13] All patients were treated with optimal medical therapy including aspirin, statin, angiotensin-converting enzyme inhibitor, and a β-blocker. The majority of patients (63%) had Canadian Cardiovascular Society (CCS) class II or higher angina. It was seen that ivabradine group had a HR that was about 10 beats/min lower than those in the placebo group. CCS class II angina or higher, patients in the ivabradine group more frequently improved their CCS angina class (24.0% vs. 18.8%; p = 0.01). Among patients with angina CCS II angina or higher, there was an increase in the incidence of the primary end point which was a composite of death from CV causes or nonfatal MI (7.6% vs. 6.5%; HR 1.18, 95% CI 1.03–1.35). Ivabradine failed to improve outcomes cardiac outcomes in all patients with stable CAD and left-ventricular systolic dysfunction in BEAUTIFUL (morBidity-mortality EvAlUaTion of the If inhibitor ivabradine in patients with coronary disease and left-ventricULar dysfunction) trial.[14] In a subgroup analysis it was seen that in patients with HR more than or equal to 70 beats/min with limiting angina, there was a 73% reduction in hospitalization for MI (HR, 0.27, 95% CI, 0.11-0.66) and a 59% reduction in coronary revascularization (HR, 0.41, 95% CI, 0.17–0.99). Hence, ivabradine should not be used in stable angina patients who do not have clinical HF.[15]

Adverse effects seen with ivabradine include visual "flashing lights" known as phosphenes which are seen in up to 16% of patients, which are usually only mild-to-moderate in intensity and transient. They result from blockage of the Ih current in the retina, which is similar to the cardiac If current.[16] Other side effect is sinus bradycardia which may require discontinuation.

TRIMETAZIDINE

It acts by metabolic modulation. It is fatty acid oxidation inhibitor and acts via selective inhibition of 3-ketoacyl coenzyme A thiolase, therefore increases the efficiency of myocardial energy production (Flowchart 3). It inhibits reduction of intracellular ATP levels via conservation of cellular metabolism in ischemic regions and stimulates myocardial glucose consumption through inhibition of fatty acid metabolism. Its dose is 35 mg bd.

A Cochrane collaboration meta-analysis of trimetazidine use in stable angina found that trimetazidine significantly reduced attacks of angina, use of nitrates, and time to onset of ST-segment depression in patients.[17] It is also beneficial in patients with HF. In a meta-analysis on its role in HF, trimetazidine lead to left ventricular end-systolic volume reduction [weighted mean difference (WMD) 10.37 mL; 95% CI 15.46–5.29; p <0.01], improvement in the New York Heart Association (NYHA) class (WMD 0.41; 95% CI 0.51–0.31; p <0.01), and exercise duration (WMD, 30.26; 95% CI 8.77–51.75; p <0.01). Trimetazidine also had a significant protective effect for all-cause mortality (RR 0.29; 95% CI 0.17–0.49; p <0.00001) and CV events and hospitalization (RR 0.42; 95% CI 0.30–0.58; p <0.00001).[18]

Common side effects are gastrointestinal disturbances, dizziness, and headache. It can uncommonly cause reversible movement disorders.[12] Table 1 summarizes mechanism of action, dosing, and side effects newer antianginals.

FASUDIL

It is an inhibitor of Rho-kinase that is involved in the vascular smooth muscle contractile response and may be of benefit in patients with stable and microvascular angina (i.e., angina with normal coronary arteries). In a multicenter, placebo-controlled trial, 84 patients with stable angina were randomly assigned to fasudil (titrated to a dose of 80 mg twice daily) or placebo.[19] Fasudil leads to a significantly greater time to more than or equal to 1 mm ST-segment depression at both peak (172 s vs. 44 s with placebo) and trough (93 s vs. 24 s) but there was no difference in time to angina, frequency of angina or nitroglycerin use, or CCS functional class. Fasudil is not available in India.

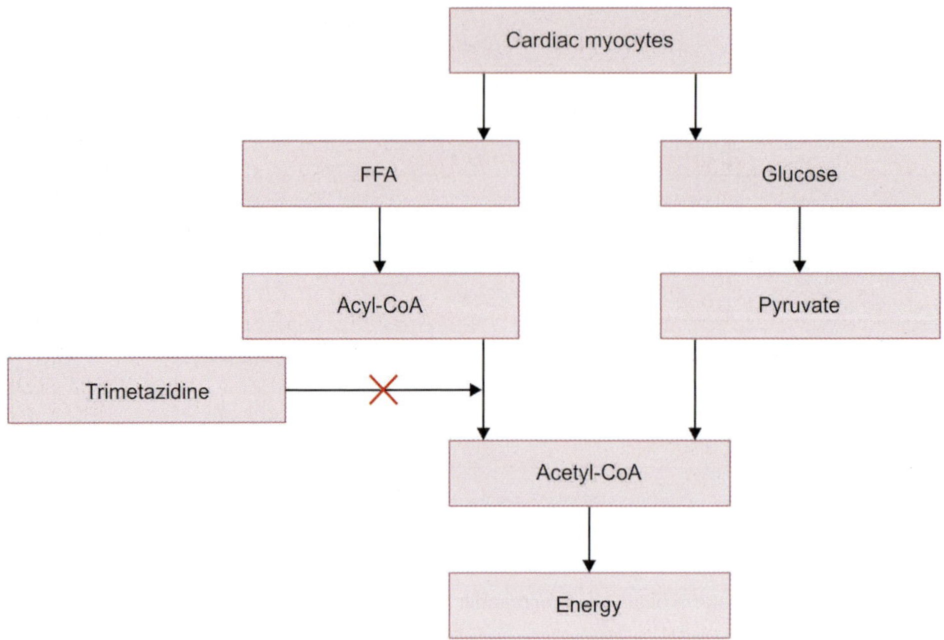

CoA, coenzyme A; FFA, free fatty acid.

FLOWCHART 3: Mechanism of action of trimetazidine.

TABLE 2: Mechanism of action, dose, and adverse effects of available newer antianginals

Drug	Dose	Mechanism of action	Adverse effects
Ranolazine	500–2000 mg bd	Inhibition of late inward sodium channel	Nausea, prolongation of QT interval
Nicorandil	20 mg bd	ATP sensitive potassium channel activator	Headache , mucosal ulcers
Ivabradine	5–7.5 mg bd	Inhibition of funny If channel in sinus node	Phosphenes, sinus bradycardia
Trimetazidine	35 mg bd	Metabolic modulator	Gastrointestinal side effects, movement disorders

ALLOPURINOL

It is a xanthine oxidase inhibitor. It is used in the prevention of recurrent gout. Its mechanism of action is inhibiting xanthine oxidase in vascular endothelium and hence preventing formation of superoxide free radicals formation. By reducing oxidative stress and improving endothelial-dependent vasodilation it decreases myocardial oxygen demand in patients with HF. However, it is rarely used to treat angina.

In a crossover study, allopurinol (600 mg/day) was compared to placebo, it significantly increased the median time to ST depression (298 s vs. 249 s, respectively, from a baseline of 232 s) and median total exercise time (393 s vs. 307 s, respectively, from a baseline of 301 s).[20] However, in view of lack of definitive evidence further evaluation of allopurinol is must before it can be used as an antianginal agent.

ENDOTHELIN RECEPTOR BLOCKERS

Endothelin (ET) receptor blockers act by producing vasodilation by inhibiting vasoconstriction produced by ET. They block ET-A and ET-B receptors. Because of vasodilator effect these agents help in relieving angina.

However, no clinical trials to date have examined the role of ET receptor blockers for reducing anginal symptoms. Furthermore, selective ET-A receptor blockade may have an adverse effect. In a small report of 30 patients undergoing PCI, it was seen that compared with intracoronary saline, an intracoronary injection of a selective ET-A receptor blocker prevented the normal reduction in myocardial ischemia on repeat balloon inflations.[21]

TESTOSTERONE

Testosterone act by improving endothelial dysfunction and may be used as an effective antianginal agent. In a trial of 46 men with stable angina a daily low dose (5 mg) transdermal testosterone patch for 12 weeks, significantly increased the time to 1 mm ST-segment depression on treadmill exercise testing compared to placebo (309 vs. 361 seconds at 12 weeks).[22] But there are multiple side effects of long-term use of aldosterone; further evidence is needed before testosterone can be considered as a therapy for angina.

HIGH-DOSE STATINS

Statins are used in all patients with stable IHD. There is increasing evidence that high-dose statin therapy reduces the incidence of anginal episodes in patients with stable IHD. AVERT (A Very Early Rehabilitation Trial after stroke) trial aggressive lipid lowering therapy with atorvastatin 80 mg led to a reduction in the rate of hospitalization for worsening angina compared to patients treated with angioplasty.[23] Similarly in the DUAAL (Double Blind Atorvastatin Amlodipine Study) trial, 311 patients with stable IHD, were randomly assigned to one of three treatment arms: amlodipine 10 mg/day, atorvastatin 80 mg/day, or amlodipine 10 mg/day plus atorvastatin 80 mg/day.[24] The primary efficacy end point, the number of ischemic episodes during 48-hour ambulatory electrocardiographic monitoring, decreased significantly from baseline (>66%) in all three groups. There was no significant difference in outcome among the three groups, with more than 50% of patients becoming free of episodes of transient myocardial ischemia at 26 weeks.

MOLSIDOMINE

Molsidomine dilates venous capacitance vessels (reducing preload), dilates coronary arterial segments, exerts a platelet stabilizing effect by inhibiting thromboxane, and has a nitric oxide-donating effect. It has been available in Europe since 1977 but has not been approved by the US FDA.

INVESTIGATIONAL DRUGS

The L-arginine, glucagon-like peptide 1 (GLP-1) mimetics and dipeptidyl peptidase-4 (DPP-4) analogs, mildronate, and estrogen/progesterone are other investigational drugs for angina and at present do not have a role in clinical practice.

CONCLUSION

Newer antianginals (Table 2) as discussed earlier are effective therapy in patients with CAD. They can be used as an add-on therapy in patients over conventional antianginals. Ivabradine should not be used as an antianginal in patients without HF in view of results of SIGNIFY trial. The choice of newer antianginals should be individualized and based on the severity of symptoms, drug tolerance, and comorbidities.

REFERENCES

1. Stone PH, Gratsiansky NA, Blokhin A, et al. ERICA Investigators. Antianginal efficacy of ranolazine when added to treatment with amlodipine: the ERICA (Efficacy of Ranolazine in Chronic Angina) trial. J Am Coll Cardiol. 2006;48(3):566-75.
2. Chaitman BR, Skettino SL, Parker JO, et al. Anti-ischemic effects and long-term survival during ranolazine monotherapy in patients with chronic severe angina. J Am Coll Cardiol. 2004;43(8):1375-82.
3. Chaitman BR, Pepine CJ, Parker JO, et al. Effects of ranolazine with atenolol, amlodipine, or diltiazem on exercise tolerance and angina frequency in patients with severe chronic angina: a randomized controlled trial. JAMA. 2004;291(3):309-16.
4. Morrow DA, Scirica BM, Karwatowska-Prokopczuk E, et al. Effects of ranolazine on recurrent cardiovascular events in patients with non-ST-elevation acute coronary syndromes: the MERLIN-TIMI 36 randomized trial. JAMA. 2007;297(16):1775-83.
5. Wilson SR, Scirica BM, Braunwald E, et al. Efficacy of ranolazine in patients with chronic angina observations from the randomized, double-blind, placebo-controlled MERLIN-TIMI (Metabolic Efficiency With Ranolazine for Less Ischemia in Non-ST-Segment Elevation Acute Coronary Syndromes) 36 Trial. J Am Coll Cardiol. 2009;53(17):1510-6.
6. Weisz G, Généreux P, Iñiguez A, et al. Ranolazine in patients with incomplete revascularisation after percutaneous coronary intervention (RIVER-PCI): a multicentre, randomised, double-blind, placebo-controlled trial. Lancet Lond Engl. 2016;387(10014):136-45.
7. Gupta T, Khera S, Kolte D, et al. Antiarrhythmic properties of ranolazine: A review of the current evidence. Int J Cardiol. 2015;187:66-74.
8. Scirica BM, Morrow DA, Hod H, et al. Effect of ranolazine, an antianginal agent with novel electrophysiological properties, on the incidence of arrhythmias in patients with non ST-segment elevation acute coronary syndrome: results from the Metabolic Efficiency With Ranolazine for Less Ischemia in Non ST-Elevation Acute Coronary Syndrome Thrombolysis in Myocardial Infarction 36 (MERLIN-TIMI 36) randomized controlled trial. Circulation. 2007;116(15):1647-52.
9. Morrow DA, Scirica BM, Chaitman BR, et al. Evaluation of the glycometabolic effects of ranolazine in patients with and without diabetes mellitus in the MERLIN-TIMI 36 randomized controlled trial. Circulation. 2009;119(15):2032-9.
10. Hondeghem LM, Snyders DJ. Class III antiarrhythmic agents have a lot of potential but a long way to go. Reduced effectiveness and dangers of reverse use dependence. Circulation. 1990;81(2):686-90.
11. IONA Study Group. Effect of nicorandil on coronary events in patients with stable angina: the Impact Of Nicorandil in Angina (IONA) randomised trial. Lancet Lond Engl. 2002;359(9314):1269-75.
12. Jones DA, Timmis A, Wragg A. Novel drugs for treating angina. BMJ. 2013;347: f4726.
13. Fox K, Ford I, Steg PG, et al. Ivabradine in stable coronary artery disease without clinical heart failure. N Engl J Med. 2014;371(12):1091-9.
14. Fox K, Ford I, Steg PG, et al; BEAUTIFUL Investigators. Ivabradine for patients with stable coronary artery disease and left-ventricular systolic dysfunction (BEAUTIFUL): a randomised, double-blind, placebo-controlled trial. Lancet Lond Engl. 2008;372(9641):807-16.
15. Fox K, Ford I, Steg PG, et al. Relationship between ivabradine treatment and cardiovascular outcomes in patients with stable coronary artery disease and left ventricular systolic dysfunction with limiting angina: a subgroup analysis of the randomized, controlled BEAUTIFUL trial. Eur Heart J. 2009;30(19):2337-45.
16. Savelieva I, Camm AJ. I f inhibition with ivabradine : electrophysiological effects and safety. Drug Saf. 2008;31(2):95-107.
17. Ciapponi A, Pizarro R, Harrison J. WITHDRAWN: Trimetazidine for stable angina. Cochrane Database Syst Rev. 2017;3:CD003614.
18. Gao D, Ning N, Niu X, et al. Trimetazidine: a meta-analysis of randomised controlled trials in heart failure. Heart Br Card Soc. 2011;97(4):278-86.
19. Mohri M, Shimokawa H, Hirakawa Y, et al. Rho-kinase inhibition with intracoronary fasudil prevents myocardial ischemia in patients with coronary microvascular spasm. J Am Coll Cardiol. 2003;41(1):15-9.
20. Noman A, Ang DSC, Ogston S, et al. Effect of high-dose allopurinol on exercise in patients with chronic stable angina: a randomised, placebo controlled crossover trial. Lancet Lond Engl. 2010;375(9732):2161-7.
21. Kyriakides ZS, Kremastinos DT, Kolettis TM, et al. Acute endothelin-A receptor antagonism prevents normal reduction of myocardial ischemia on repeated balloon inflations during angioplasty. Circulation. 2000;102(16):1937-43.
22. English KM, Steeds RP, Jones TH, et al. Low-dose transdermal testosterone therapy improves angina threshold in men with chronic stable angina: A randomized, double-blind, placebo-controlled study. Circulation. 2000;102(16):1906-11.
23. Pitt B, Waters D, Brown WV, et al. Aggressive lipid-lowering therapy compared with angioplasty in stable coronary artery disease. Atorvastatin versus Revascularization Treatment Investigators. N Engl J Med. 1999;341(2):70-6.
24. Deanfield JE, Sellier P, Thaulow E, et al. Potent anti-ischaemic effects of statins in chronic stable angina: incremental benefit beyond lipid lowering? Eur Heart J. 2010,31(21).2650-9.

CHAPTER 85

Newer Antihypertensives

TK Mishra

INTRODUCTION

Hypertension (HTN) is the single most common preventable risk factor for cardiovascular disease (CVD) and the number one cause of all cause mortality and morbidity globally. Affecting more than a billion people worldwide, HTN is responsible for 9.4 million deaths per year.[1] The morbidity due to the disease (measured by healthy life-years lost) has surged by 43% over the last 30 years owing to the aging of the population, and a 10% rise in the prevalence in HTN. The economic burden to society in the US alone is a staggering 46 billion dollars. Moreover, with the recent American College of Cardiology/American Heart Association (ACC/AHA) guideline redefining HTN as blood pressure (BP) more than 130/90 mm Hg, an additional 15% of the general adult population is labeled as hypertensive.

About 75% of the world's burden of HTN (639 million people) is found in the developing world. The crude prevalence of HTN in India has been found to be 25.3% including a disconcerting 12.1% in the 18–25 years age group. Gupta et al. found a steady increase in age-adjusted HTN prevalence in an urban population over the past 25 years.[2] The incidence in rural and urban India is 25% and 33%, respectively. From this pool, only about one-fourth of rural and half of the urban patients are aware of their condition. Again, only 25% of rural and 38% of urban Indians are being treated for HTN. Soberingly, an abysmal 10% rural and 20% urban patients have HTN under control.

The four major classes of antihypertensive drugs represented by the acronym "ABCD" [A = angiotensin-converting-enzyme inhibitors (ACEi) or angiotensin-receptor blockers (ARBs); B = β-blockers; C = calcium channel blockers (CCBs); D = diuretics] continue to be the bulwark of therapy. Yet, due to various reasons, HTN remains uncontrolled in 50% of patients worldwide and up to 70% in Asian countries. In select clinical or trial settings, 70–80% reach target BP levels, many of whom find it difficult to adhere to cumbersome multidrug regimens. Besides, an unmet need for therapy exists in certain groups such as treatment resistant hypertension (TRH), patients with comorbidities and those unable to tolerate the conventional drugs. Even after accounting for noncompliance, 10–15% of patients remain in the category of TRH defined as office BP more than 140/90 mm Hg, in spite of treatment with three or more antihypertensive drugs (inappropriate dose) including a nonpotassium sparing diuretic, and not due to secondary HTN. About 0.5% suffer from refractory HTN where BP is uncontrolled on five or more drugs. Suboptimal management of comorbidities like heart failure (HF) and renal failure contributes to uncontrolled HTN. Hence, the need for newer efficacious drugs with additional benefits of target organ protection to uniformly achieve the HTN control target of 50% set by the World Health Organization (WHO) global monitoring framework.

NEWER DRUGS FOR HYPERTENSION

The mineralocorticoid receptor antagonists (MRA) have emerged as an option in TRH where the putative mechanism is salt retention due to aldosterone breakthrough in patients on ACEi or ARB. The strongest evidence came from the PATHWAY-2 trial which compared spironolactone with bisoprolol (β-blocker), doxazosin (α-blocker), and placebo as a fourth add-on drug in patients of TRH.[3] Over a 3-month follow-up, the reduction in home BP recordings by spironolactone was twice that of the other drugs with the greatest benefit in patients with low renin levels. Other long-term observational studies confirm that this BP-lowering effect is sustained and durable. Bobrie et al. in a study of 167 patients of TRH displayed that sequential nephron blockade (spironolactone followed by loop diuretic) causes greater fall in BP than sequential ACEi-β-blocker therapy. Spironolactone acts best when serum potassium is less than 4.5 mEq/L and also reduces albuminuria in diabetics independent of its hemodynamic effect. Major side effects are type 4 renal tubular acidosis, gynecomastia, impotence, and hyperkalemia. However, the incidence of hyperkalemia in PATHWAY-2 was low-allaying apprehension about combining it with ACEi or ARB. For patients who experience gynecomastia with spironolactone, amiloride is a viable alternative. Amiloride is an indirect aldosterone inhibitor acting on the epithelial sodium channel (ENaC) in the collecting duct. Unlike the target sites of thiazide and high ceiling diuretics, this distal most channel has no further downstream channels to neutralize increased sodium resorption. Hence, small increments in ENaC activity can elevate BP considerably. In a study of 98 patients of TRH, introduction of either spironolactone or amiloride reduced BP significantly with a greater reduction by amiloride. The second generation MRA eplerenone is more selective for mineralocorticoid receptors but is less potent as an antihypertensive and needs twice daily dosing.

Sacubitril or valsartan (LCZ696), a first in class combination of ARB and neprilysin inhibitor (ARNi), is emerging as promising therapy for HTN. While valsartan reduces BP by inhibiting the RAS, the neprilysin inhibitor promotes salt excretion by the natriuretic peptides, hence acting as a diuretic without undesirable effects like hypokalemia or hyperuricemia. The landmark trials, Prospective Comparison of ARNi and ACEi to determine Impact on Global Mortality and Morbidity in Heart Failure (PARADIGM-HF) and PARAMOUNT that established the role of ARNi in HF also revealed that LCZ696 caused greater BP reduction than the comparator drug (enalapril or valsartan). The PARAMETER study compared the efficacy of LCZ696 (200 mg/day uptitrated to 400 mg/day) and olmesartan (20 mg/day uptitrated to 40 mg/day) in 454 elderly patients of HTN.[4] After 52 weeks of follow-up, both drugs were equally efficacious in reducing central aortic systolic pressure (CASP), central aortic pulse pressure (CAPP), and nocturnal BP. Moreover, while 47% of patients taking olmesartan required add-on drugs to achieve BP control, only 32% receiving LCZ696 did so. LCZ696 caused a greater fall in N-terminal pro b-type natriuretic peptide (NT-proBNP) implying greater distensibility of the arteries. It has also been shown to effect a greater reduction in left ventricular mass than olmesartan. In an Asian study comparing various doses of LCZ696 with placebo, Kario et al. demonstrated the greater BP lowering effect of the drug as compared to a Western population especially at lower doses along with an excellent tolerability and safety profile. High salt consumption in Asians possibly renders them more sensitive to the natriuretic effect of the drug. Subsequently, in a study of 261 Asian patients of systolic HTN, Wang et al. confirmed the superiority of LCZ696 over placebo as a second drug in patients uncontrolled on amlodipine (5 mg). In the light of the mounting evidence, LCZ696 could be a viable option in certain subgroups such as elderly with resistant HTN especially with systolic or nocturnal or salt sensitive HTN with the added benefit of prevention of HF. However, a possible concern with long-term use of the drug is decreased catabolism of amyloid beta (Aβ) peptide leading to Alzheimer's disease. While the short survival of HF patients precludes such events, the long duration of treatment coupled with a compromised blood brain barrier in hypertensive patients will necessitate prolonged neurological monitoring.

Clevidipine is a parenteral ultra-short-acting latest generation dihydropyridine CCB with high arteriolar selectivity, small volume of distribution and rapid clearance resulting in a half-life of about 1 minute. In the VELOCITY trial of 126 patients presenting with acute HTN [systolic blood pressure (SBP) >180 mm Hg], clevidipine effected a reduction of SBP by 6% at 3 minutes followed by 27% reduction at 18 hours without any major adverse effects. Subsequent subset analysis of renal failure and acute HF patients reproduced the favorable results of the overall trial. The study concluded that clevidipine is a safe and effective drug in management of acute severe HTN at a dose of 2 mg/hr followed by target BP based titration of infusion for 18 hours or more. The ECLIPSE trial compared clevidipine with nitroglycerine, nitroprusside, and nicardipine and concluded that it is not only a safe and effective drug but also provides more precise BP control than nitroglycerine and nitroprusside.[5] Clevidipine is administered as a nonweight based initial dose of 1–2 mg followed by doubling of dose every 90 seconds till target BP is reached. The required dose in most patients is 4–6 mg/h. An ongoing trial of parenteral clevidipine versus urapidil in hypertensive patients of intracerebral hemorrhage will further clarify the efficacy of clevidipine as compared to conventional antihypertensives.

The premium placed by regulatory authorities on CV safety data of novel antidiabetic drugs has spurred investigators to uncover CV benefits of such drugs. The sodium-glucose cotransporter-2 (SGLT2) inhibitors (empagliflozin, canagliflozin, and dapagliflozin) all reduce BP by 3–5/2–3 mm Hg without any increase in incidence of orthostatic hypotension. In the EMPA-REG OUTCOME trial, use of empagliflozin resulted in a 38% reduction in CV death and 39% reduction of incident or worsening nephropathy.[6] The SGLT2 inhibitors cause weight and BP reduction by promoting sodium and water loss. Hence, diuretics are to be used cautiously in combination. In a meta-analysis comparing glucagon-like peptide-1 receptor antagonists (GLP1-RA) with insulin and glimepiride, exenatide, and liraglutide lowered BP by 1–5 mm Hg. Dipeptidyl peptidase-4 (DPP-4) inhibitors, sitagliptin, and vildagliptin have been shown to have mild antihypertensive effect. The combination of GLP1-RA with SGLT2 inhibitors was tested in the DURATION-8 trial. Exenatide plus dapagliflozin reduced SBP by 4.2 mm Hg as compared to 1.3 mm Hg with exanetide and 1.8 mm Hg with dapagliflozin alone. A large meta-analysis of 61 observational studies in healthy adults concluded that even a 2 mm Hg reduction in SBP lessens stroke mortality by 10% and mortality from ischemic heart disease and other vascular causes by 7%.[7] Considering the heightened CV risk of diabetics, the BP lowering effects of the newer antidiabetics should strongly influence choice of antihyperglycemic therapy.

Azilsartan medoxomil is the eighth ARB approved by the FDA for the treatment of HTN. It is highly selective with a 10,000 times higher affinity for angiotensin 1 (AT1) receptor than for angiotensin II (AT2) receptor. Time course studies show that compared to other ARBs, the drug-AT receptor dissociation is more gradual. Experimental evidence indicates that azilsartan may exert some of its beneficial effect through peroxisome proliferator-activated receptors gamma (PPARγ) pathway activation. In a meta-analysis of 17 trials, azilsartan was shown to provide superior and sustained 24 hours antihypertensive effect as compared to ramipril, candesartan, valsartan, or olmesartan (at their highest approved doses) with similar safety profile. Confirming its efficacy in Asian patients, a Korean study found satisfactory BP reduction with a favorable benefit risk profile. It is the only drug approved as a fixed drug combination (FDC) with chlorthalidone on the basis of a titrate to target study that found this combination to be more effective than Olmesartan and hydrochlorothiazide.[8] The starting dose of azilsartan is 40 mg once daily (20 mg for patients >75 years of age) which may be increased to 80 mg once daily with full effect reached by 4 weeks.

A FDC of nebivolol and valsartan (5/80 mg tablet—Byvalson) was approved by the FDA in 2016 on the basis of a phase III double blind dose-escalating placebo controlled trial. Treatment with the combination lowered both SBP and diastolic blood pressure (DBP) more than each individual drug with similar adverse effect profile.

EMERGING MOLECULES

A number of research molecules with novel mechanisms of action are in various stages of preclinical or clinical development (Table 1). Activation of the renin–angiotensin system (RAS) in the brain is postulated to be contributory to HTN. Aminopeptidase A (APA) converts angiotensin II to angiotensin III which stimulates central sympathetic drive and vasopressin release. RB150, a selective APA inhibitor, is being investigated as a centrally acting antihypertensive and has been found to be safe in healthy volunteers without any change in heart rate or BP.[9] It is the subject of a phase IIa placebo controlled trial to assess its efficacy in stage 1 and 2 HTN. The angiotensin III/AT2 receptor arm of the RAS has vasodilator and natriuretic effects, actions antagonistic to the AT2/AT1 receptor arm. Compound 21 (C21) is a potent and highly selective AT2 receptor agonist which on account of its anti-inflammatory and antiapoptotic effect may also be useful in preventing target organ damage especially diabetic nephropathy (DN). Phase 1 testing in healthy volunteers is currently underway. The carboxypeptidase enzyme ACE2 converts AT2 to angiotensin (1–7), which antagonizes HTN induced target organ damage via Mas receptor. Agents that promote this conversion include ACE2 activators, Mas receptor, and AT2 receptor agonists. Diminazene aceturate (DIZI) is an ACE2 activator currently used in treatment of African trypanosomiasis but remains to be investigated in HTN. A Mas receptor modulator, CGEN-856 is still in the preclinical stage. An ACE2 modulator, recombinant human ACE2 (rhACE2) induced a sustained (>24 h) fall in AT2 with a good safety profile in a phase I clinical study on healthy subjects and is undergoing phase II studies.[10] A new renin inhibitor VTP-27999 is the subject of a phase II clinical trial.

Finerenone is a nonsteroidal mineralocorticoid antagonist with higher selectivity than spironolactone and higher affinity than eplerenone. Two class IIb trials in HF and DN [mineralocorticoid receptor antagonist tolerability study-HF (ARTS-HF) and ARTS-DN] found it to be equally effective

TABLE 1: Emerging molecules

Drug class	Drug	Stage of development
Aminopeptidase inhibitor	RB150	Phase IIa
AT2 receptor agonist	C21	Phase I
Mas receptor modulator	CGEN-856	Preclinical
ACE2 modulator	rhACE2	Phase II
Renin inhibitor	VTP-27999	Phase II
Mineralocorticoid receptor antagonist	Finerenone	Phase III
Aldosterone synthase inhibitor	LCI699	Phase II
Dual-acting endothelin-converting enzyme-neprilysin inhibitor	Daglutril	Phase II
Natriuretic peptide receptor agonist	PL-3994	Phase II
NO releasing COX inhibitor	Naproxcinod	Phase III
Soluble guanylate cyclase inhibitor	Riociguat	Phase III
Intestinal Na^+/H^+ exchanger 3 inhibitor	Tenapanor	Phase II
VIP receptor agonist	Vasomera	Phase I
PDE5 inhibitors	Tadalafil KD027	Marketed Phase II
Imidazoline receptor blocker	Moxonidine	Marketed

AT2, angiotensin II type 2; ACE2, angiotensin-converting enzyme 2; NO, nitric oxide; COX, cyclooxygenase; VIP, vasoactive intestinal peptide; PDE5, phosphodiesterase type 5.

as spironolactone in reducing BNP and albuminuria with lower incidence of hyperkalemia.[11] Two phase III studies on efficacy and safety of finerenone in DN are currently recruiting (FIDELIO-DKD and FIGARO-DKD). The aldosterone synthase inhibitor LCI699 is being examined for antihypertensive effect in a phase II trial. Daglutril is a dual endothelin converting enzyme and neprilysin inhibitor which was studied in a cohort of diabetic and hypertensive patients with nephropathy on losartan therapy. It was found to be safe and reduced BP but had no effect on albuminuria. PL-3994, a natriuretic peptide receptor agonist, was found useful in combination with ACEi in a phase II clinical study. Drugs acting on nitric oxide and soluble guanylate cyclase pathway have been tried in HTN. Naproxcinod is a cyclooxygenase inhibiting nitric oxide donating (CINOD) compound derived from naproxen that reduced BP in hypertensive patients and is currently being tested in phase III trials. Riociguat, approved for use in pulmonary HTN, has been shown to reduce systemic BP in experimental studies. Tenapanor, a small molecule inhibitor of the Na^+/H^+ exchanger isoform 3, lowers gastrointestinal absorption of sodium and thereby, may be useful in HTN. A phase II clinical trial found tenapanor useful in treatment of hyperphosphatemia in patients on hemodialysis.[12] Vasomera (a VIP receptor agonist) is a potent vasodilator that reduced BP in early phase I clinical studies. The phosphodiesterase type 5 (PDE5) inhibitors, tadalafil and KD027, have vasodilatory effect and are being investigated for HTN therapy. Stimulation of imidazoline receptor I1 in the medulla oblongata inhibits the sympathetic nervous system to reduce BP. Moxonidine is a second generation centrally acting antihypertensive with low toxicity on account of greater selectivity for I1 receptor as compared to α_2-receptor.

FUTURE PROSPECTS

Nanoparticles are a recent technological innovation to bypass various constraints in oral absorption and improve bioavailability of a drug. Most of the antihypertensives have low bioavailability due to low solubility and high permeability. In a nanoparticulate drug delivery system, the drug is combined with a nontoxic and biodegradable excipient enabling it to surpass impediments such as unfavorable pH, poor intestinal permeability, cytochrome P450 (CYP450)-mediated first pass metabolism and p-glycoprotein-mediated efflux. This complex is absorbed by various mechanisms such as paracellular transport (tight junctions), clathrin-mediated transport and caveolae-mediated endocytosis. In a murine model, combination of candesartan with soy lecithin sequestered the drug from acidic pH of stomach and increased bioavailability by 12 times.[13] Nanoparticles may also be used to deliver increased drug concentration in specific target organs. Chronotherapeutics aims to achieve maximal drug concentration at a specific time in keeping with the circadian rhythm of the disease determinant. Used in conjunction with nanotechnology, it can enhance drug efficacy and optimize outcomes.

Nanoparticle mediated gene therapy of HTN entails gene silencing through cleavage of target mRNA by small interfering RNA (siRNA) and disrupting protein synthesis. Vasquez et al. employed AT 1147 siRNA to silence AT1a receptor and preventing AT2 activity. When administered alone, the siRNA are rapidly catabolized by the nucleases in blood and cells. The combination of siRNA with nanoparticles protects it from degradation and allows it to reach the target site. Nolte et al. used an intravenous liposomal nanoparticle, lipoplex to target β1-adrenoceptor synthesis and achieved sustained BP reduction for 12 days.[14]

CONCLUSION

In spite of this plethora of molecules in the pipeline, no new molecule with a unique mechanism of action has entered the market in the last 20 years. The availability of a repertoire of time tested antihypertensive drugs (often generic) with high efficacy and placebo-like tolerability necessitates that any new drug will have to be more effective and equally safe to secure a place in the antihypertensive basket. The cost of introducing a new drug in the market (about 750 million to 1.5 billion dollars) has also dampened the enthusiasm of the industry and veered its interest toward nonpharmacological therapy of HTN. However, with sustained efforts toward study of newer candidate molecules and increasing emphasis on end organ, protection beyond BP control, it is hoped that the future will provide newer drugs for the hypertensive population in general and high-risk subgroups in particular.

REFERENCES

1. Forouzanfar MH, Afshin A, Alexander LT, et al. Global, regional, and national comparative risk assessment of 79 behavioural, environmental and occupational, and metabolic risks or clusters of risks, 1990-2015: a systematic analysis for the Global Burden of Disease Study 2015. Lancet. 2016;388(10053):1659-724.
2. Gupta R, Gupta VP, Prakash H, et al. 25-Year trends in hypertension prevalence, awareness, treatment, and control in an Indian urban population: Jaipur Heart Watch. Indian Heart Journal. 2017.
3. Williams B, MacDonald TM, Morant S, et al. Spironolactone versus placebo, bisoprolol, and doxazosin to determine the optimal treatment for drug-resistant hypertension (PATHWAY-2): a randomised, double-blind, crossover trial. Lancet. 2015;386:2059-68.
4. Williams B, Cockcroft JR, Kario K, et al. Effects of sacubitril/valsartan versus olmesartan on central hemodynamics in the elderly with systolic hypertension: the PARAMETER study. Hypertension. 2017;69:411-20.
5. Aronson S, Dyke CM, Stierer KA, et al. The ECLIPSE trials: comparative studies of clevidipine to nitroglycerin, sodium nitroprusside, and nicardipine for acute hypertension treatment in cardiac surgery patients. Anesth Analg. 2008;107:1110-21.
6. Zinman B, Wanner C, Lachin JM, et al. Empagliflozin, cardiovascular outcomes, and mortality in type 2 diabetes. N Engl J Med. 2015;373(22):2117-28.
7. Lewington S, Clarke R, Qizilbash N, et al. Age-specific relevance of usual blood pressure to vascular mortality: A meta-analysis of individual data for one million adults in 61 prospective studies. Lancet. 2002;360(9349):1903-13.
8. Cushman WC, Bakris GL, White WB, et al. A randomized titrate-to-target study comparing fixed-dose combinations of azilsartan medoxomil and chlorthalidone with olmesartan and hydrochlorothiazide in stage-2 systolic hypertension. J Hypertens. 2018;36(4):947-56.

9. Balavoine F, Azizi M, Bergerot D, et al. Randomised, double-blind, placebo controlled, dose-escalating phase I study of QGC001, a centrally acting aminopeptidase a inhibitor prodrug. Clin Pharmacokinet. 2014;53(4):385-95.
10. Haschke M, Schuster M, Poglitsch M, et al. Pharmacokinetics and pharmacodynamics of recombinant human angiotensin-converting enzyme 2 in healthy human subjects. ClinPharmacokinet. 2013;52(9):783-92.
11. Pitt B, Kober L, Ponikowski P, et al. Safety and tolerability of the novel nonsteroidal mineralocorticoid receptor antagonist BAY 94-8862 in patients with chronic heart failure and mild or moderate chronic kidney disease: a randomized, double-blind trial. Eur Heart J. 2013;34(31):2453-63.
12. Block GA, Rosenbaum DP, Yan A, et al. The effects of tenapanor on serum fibroblast growth factor 23 in patients receiving hemodialysis with hyperphosphatemia. Nephrol Dial Transplant. 2018.
13. Koziolek M, Grimm M, Becker D, et al. Investigation of pH and temperature profiles in the GI tract of fasted human subjects using the Intellicap(®) system. J Pharm Sci. 2015;104(9):2855-63.
14. Nolte A, Schneider M, Walker T, et al. Gene-silencing for treatment of cardiovascular diseases. In: Eberli D (Ed). Regenerative Medicine and Tissue Engineering—Cells and Biomaterials. Rijeka: Croatia; 2011.

CHAPTER 86

Newer Agents for Dyslipidemia

Iyengar SS, Saleha N

"Whenever science makes a discovery, the devil grabs it, while the angels are debating the best way to use it"

—French Quotes

INTRODUCTION

Atherosclerotic cardiovascular disease (ASCVD) is the leading cause of mortality and morbidity globally and locally. There is a significant increase in mortality rates from cardiovascular disease (CVD) and ischemic heart disease (IHD) in India. There is a 32.7% increase in years of life lost (YLL) from 1990 until 2016.[1] In contrast to this increase in mortality in India, USA, developed countries in Europe and most middle-income countries, including China have shown a 30–70% decline in CVD mortality in the past 50 years.[2,3]

Dyslipidemia, which is a disorder of lipid and lipoprotein metabolism, constitutes one of the major modifiable risk factors for ASCVD. It includes primarily three abnormalities, namely elevated low-density lipoprotein cholesterol (LDL-C), elevated triglycerides (TGs), and low high-density lipoprotein cholesterol (HDL-C).

Statins continue to reign supreme and remain a major cornerstone for treatment of atherogenic dyslipidemia (AD). However, they reduce the ASCVD risk by only 15–37%.[4] Continued research to meet the unmet needs of statin therapy has led to the development and emergence of various newer and nonstatin group of drugs to tackle the residual risk of ASCVD in patients who do not reach the target goals of treatment. Nonstatin drugs are also needed in those who do not tolerate statins, and usually have to be added in subjects or patients who have very high LDL-C, as is seen in familial hypercholesterolemia (FH).

In this chapter, we review the newer agents for treating dyslipidemia.

EZETIMIBE

It was one of the first new class of agents which was approved by the US Food and Drug Administration in October 2002. It reduces plasma cholesterol by inhibiting its absorption from the small intestine via Niemann-Pick C1-L 1 (NPC1L1) protein; this leads to decreased amount of cholesterol normally available to liver cells, leading them to absorb more from circulation and thus lowering levels of circulating cholesterol.

As an adjunct to diet, it may be used to reduce total cholesterol (TC), LDL-C, apolipoprotein B (apoB), and non-HDL-C in patients with hyperlipidemia on statin not reaching the target goal. In statin intolerant patients, it may be used singly. It is frequently used with statin in patients with FH. Ezetimibe is also used to reduce sitosterol and campesterol in patients with homozygous (Ho) sitosterolemia (phytosterolemia).

It is to be used in the dosage of 10 mg PO daily, to be taken either more than 2 hours before or more than 4 hours after bile acid sequestrants (BAS) if used in combination. Mean reduction of LDL-C is 18% with monotherapy and around 25% when combined with statins.[5] It is generally well tolerated, adverse effects include upper respiratory tract infection, diarrhea, arthralgia, sinusitis, and pain in extremity.

In the IMPROVE-IT trial, which was a large, double blind, randomized trial involving 18,144 patients with recent acute coronary syndrome (ACS), addition of ezetimibe to moderate intensity statin resulted in incremental lowering of LDL-C and reduced primary composite endpoint of cardiovascular (CV) death, nonfatal myocardial infarction (MI), unstable angina (UA) requiring rehospitalization, coronary revascularization more than 30 days after randomization, or nonfatal stroke. The median follow-up was 6 years.[6]

The SHARP trial, which was a randomized double blind trial of 9,270 patients with chronic kidney disease, with no known history of MI or coronary revascularization, simvastatin plus ezetimibe reduced LDL-C and reduced primary endpoint of first major ASCVD event compared to placebo over a median follow-up of 4.9 years.[7]

A prespecified analysis of IMPROVE-IT trial focused on the 4,933 (27%) patients with diabetes. They were compared to 13,202 nondiabetic patients. The beneficial effects of adding ezetimibe to statin therapy was "enhanced" in patients with diabetes and also in those who were not diabetics but were at high risk for ASCVD.[8]

PROPROTEIN CONVERTASE SUBTILISIN/KEXIN TYPE 9 INHIBITORS

Proprotein convertase subtilisin/kexin type 9 (PCSK9) inhibitors are a critical addition to the LDL-lowering armamentarium. In 2015, two of these agents, namely alirocumab and evolocumab, were approved in the USA and Europe for clinical use. Evolocumab received approval for HoFH, whereas both drugs were approved for heterozygous FH (HeFH) and clinical ASCVD. Bococizumab was studied in two randomized trials comparing it with placebo.[9] Bococizumab had no benefit with respect to major adverse CV events involving lower-risk patients but did have a significant benefit in the trial involving higher-risk patients. Bococizumab is not a fully humanized monoclonal antibody (mAb) and its further development has currently been given up.

They are mAbs against PCSK9 and act by binding to it, thereby increasing the number of LDL receptors available to clear circulating LDL as shown in figure 1.

FOURIER trial[10] a randomized, controlled study involved 27,564 patients with ASCVD and LDL cholesterol levels of 70 mg% or more on statin therapy. They were randomized to receive evolocumab or placebo. The primary efficacy endpoint was the composite of CV death, MI, stroke, hospitalization for UA, or coronary revascularization. The secondary efficacy endpoint was the composite of CV death, MI, or stroke. The patients were followed up for a median duration of 2.2 years. Evolocumab added to statin therapy lowered LDL cholesterol levels to a median of 30 mg% and reduced the risk of CV events. The study concluded that patients with ASCVD benefit from lowering of LDL cholesterol levels below currently recommended targets. ODYSSEY trial[11] enrolled 18,924 patients with recent ACS (1–12 months prior to randomization), on high-intensity statin therapy, but with LDL-C more than or equal to 70 mg%, non-HDL-C more than or equal to 100 mg%, or apoB more than or equal to 80 mg%. Patients were randomly assigned to alirocumab 75 mg subcutaneous (SQ) every 2 weeks or placebo, targeting LDL-C levels between 25 mg% and 50 mg%. After a median follow-up of 2.8 years, alirocumab reduced major adverse cardiovascular events, MI, and ischemic stroke. Alirocumab was also associated with a lower rate of all-cause death.

GLAGOV study,[12] a randomized control trial looked at the effects of PCSK9 inhibition with evolocumab on coronary atherosclerosis in statin-treated patients 968 patients who

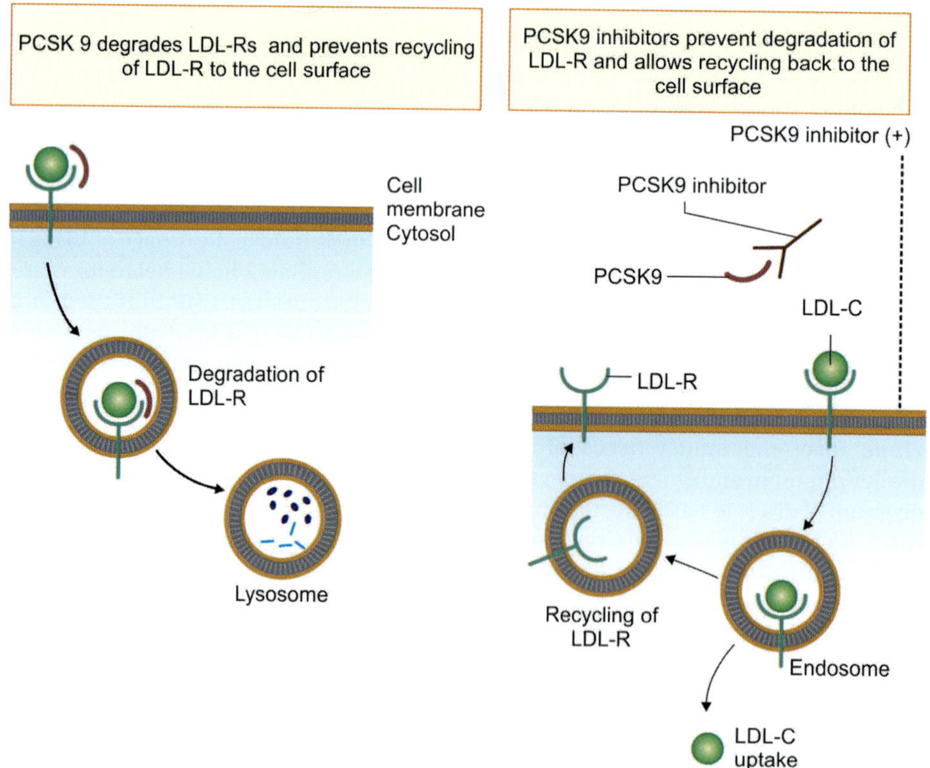

PCSK9, proprotein convertase subtilisin/kexin type 9; LDL-R, low-density lipoprotein receptor; LDL-C, low-density lipoprotein cholesterol.

FIG. 1: Mechanism of action of PCSK 9 inhibitors.

Source: Ahn CH, Choi SH. New drugs for treating dyslipidemia: beyond statins. Diabetes Metab J. 2015;39(2):87-94.

underwent coronary angiography. Among patients with angiographic coronary disease treated with statins, addition of evolocumab, compared with placebo, resulted in a greater decrease in percent atheroma volume (PAV) after 76 weeks of treatment, based on the findings of serial intravascular ultrasound (IVUS).

In the following group of patients, use of PCSK9 inhibitors is recommended by the European Society of Cardiology/ European Atherosclerosis Society (ESC/EAS) task force:[13]

- Patients with ASCVD, who are at very high-risk, who have substantially elevated LDL-C levels despite maximally tolerated statin with or without ezetimibe therapy, and thus are considered at particularly high risk of an adverse prognosis
- Patients with ASCVD and at very high-risk who do not tolerate appropriate doses of at least three statins and thus have elevated LDL-C levels
- Familial hypercholesterolemia patients without clinically diagnosed ASCVD, at high or very high CV risk, and with substantially elevated LDL-C levels despite maximally tolerated statin plus ezetimibe therapy.

Dosage and Administration

Alirocumab

Initiate 75 mg SQ every 2 weeks. If more LDL reduction needed, may increase dose to 150 mg every 2 weeks. Alternative starting dose is 300 mg SQ every 4 weeks.

Evolocumab

In primary hypercholesterolemia with established clinical ASCVD or HeFH, give 140 mg SQ every 2 weeks or 420 mg SQ once monthly in abdomen, thigh, or upper arm. In HoFH, give 420 mg SQ once monthly. To administer 420 mg, give three (140 mg) injections consecutively within 30 minutes.

Drug Interaction with Statins

Proprotein convertase subtilisin/kexin type 9 inhibitors have an interesting and beneficial drug interaction with statins. Statins reduce synthesis of cholesterol. This leads to setting up of a counterregulatory process wherein sterol regulatory element-binding protein-2 (SREBP-2), a membrane-bound transcription factor that regulates cholesterol homeostasis in cells. SREBP-2 increases LDL-receptor density, and at the same time it stimulates the secretion PCSK9. If PCSK9 inhibitors are administered along with statins, it will counteract the action of PCSK9 and increases LDL receptors recycling (Fig. 2).

INCLISIRAN

Inclisiran is a chemically synthesized short interfering RNA molecule that produces sustained hepatocyte-specific, PCSK9-specific RNA silencing, thereby decreasing translation of the PCSK9 protein. In a phase II trial, ORION-1, inclisiran was found to lower PCSK9 and LDL cholesterol levels among patients at high CV risk who had elevated LDL cholesterol levels.[14]

In a prespecified analysis of secondary endpoints from the ORION-1 phase II study which was presented at the 86th European Atherosclerosis Society Congress (EAS, 2018), inclisiran showed effects beyond LDL-C and showed that it also reduces other atherogenic lipoproteins—non-HDL-C, apoB, very-low-density lipoprotein cholesterol (VLDL-C) and lipoprotein(a) [Lp(a)]—significantly and in a sustained manner.[15]

ORION program is running about 15 studies in various clinical scenarios (e.g., ORION-9 in HeFH and ORION-10 in ASCVD) and the studies are actively enrolling the subjects.

Inclisiran appears quite a promising therapy for AD. It eliminates LDL-C variability, reduces injection burden with

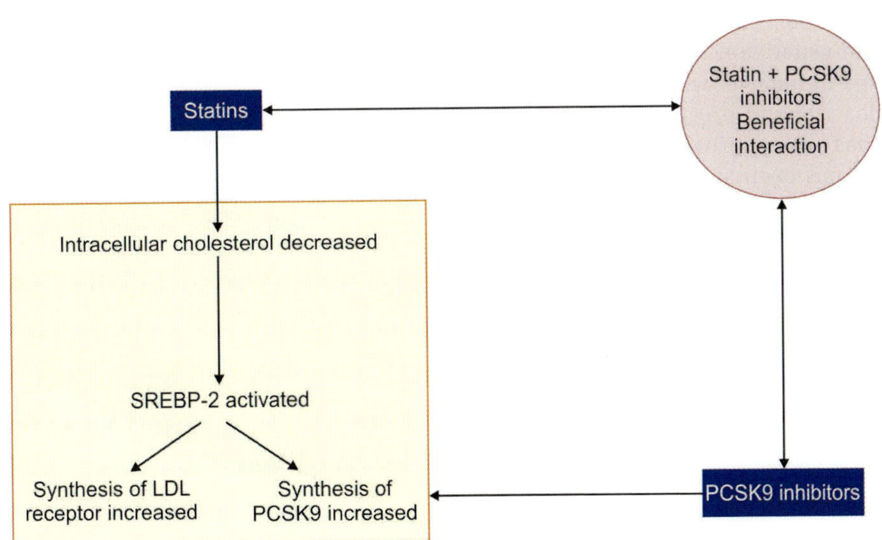

SREBP-2, sterol regulatory element-binding protein 2; PCSK9, proprotein convertase subtilisin/kexin type 9; LDL, low-density lipoprotein.

FIG. 2: Synergistic action between statins and PCSK9 inhibitors.

consequent better adherence to treatment and so far has shown robust efficacy and no safety issues.

In the meanwhile, FDA has granted "Orphan Drug Designation" to inclisiran for the treatment of HoFH.

MICROSOMAL TRIGLYCERIDE TRANSFER PROTEIN INHIBITOR: LOMITAPIDE

Lomitapide has been approved to reduce LDL-C, TC, apoB, and non-HDL-C in patients HoFH. It is an oral inhibitor of the microsomal triglyceride transport protein (MTP).

Microsomal triglyceride transport protein is an intracellular lipid-transfer protein that plays an important role in transport of TGs, cholesterol esters and phospholipids to apoB molecules and synthesis of VLDL and chylomicrons in the hepatocytes and enterocytes, respectively. Hence its inhibition provides a therapeutic target. Clinical trials have shown efficacy of lomitapide in reducing LDL-C. In a multinational single-arm, open-label, 78-week, phase III trial, lomitapide reduced mean plasma LDL-C levels by 50% from baseline in 23 evaluable adults with HoFH over a 26 weeks treatment period. Reductions from baseline in LDL-C levels were sustained for up to 78 weeks with continued lomitapide treatment.[16]

The recommended starting dose is 5 mg once daily and the dose should be escalated gradually up to a maximum recommended dose of 60 mg. Adverse effects include nausea, flatulence, diarrhea and fecal urgency, increase of transaminases, and hepatic fat content. It is contraindicated in patients with moderate or severe hepatic impairment, and in patients with mild hepatic impairment, dose should not exceed 40 mg daily. Regular liver monitoring should be performed at baseline and on an annual basis using both imaging and biomarker evaluations.

ANTISENSE OLIGONUCLEOTIDE AGAINST APOLIPOPROTEIN B—MIPOMERSEN

Mipomersen, a second-generation antisense oligonucleotide (ASO), acts mainly in the liver where it binds to apoB mRNA causing its cleavage and prevents the synthesis of apoB-100 protein. It has been approved by the FDA for the treatment of HoFH. It has been shown to reduce LDL-C, Lp(a), and apoB (Fig. 3). It is administered SQ in a dose of 200 mg weekly. The most common adverse effect is injection site reactions, flu like symptoms, and increase in hepatic fat content.[17,18]

BEMPEDOIC ACID

It is a once-daily, oral LDL-C lowering drug that significantly reduces elevated LDL-C levels.

In the liver, bempedoic acid is converted to a coenzyme A (CoA) derivative, or ETC-1002-CoA, which directly inhibits ATP citrate lyase (ACL), a key enzyme that supplies substrate for cholesterol and fatty acid synthesis in the liver. Inhibition of ACL by ETC-1002-CoA results in reduced cholesterol synthesis and upregulation of LDL receptor activity in the liver. However, unlike statins, bempedoic acid does not inhibit the cholesterol biosynthesis pathway in skeletal muscle, so it is unlikely to lead to muscle-related side effects. Bempedoic acid is inactive until it enters the liver where it is converted to its active form by the enzyme, ACSVL1, an enzyme not found in skeletal muscle cells.

It has completed phase I and phase II clinical studies, which have demonstrated efficacy and safety of the drug. CLEAR Serenity is an ongoing phase III trial using this drug in patients with hypercholesterolemia, expected to be completed by July 2018.[19]

GEMCABENE

This is a novel drug which has multiple level targets that lower LDL-C, TG, and high sensitivity C-reactive protein (hsCRP) in plasma. It inhibits acetyl CoA carboxylase (ACC) and 3-hydroxy-3-methylglutaryl-coenzyme A (HMG-CoA) synthase in the liver, thereby resulting in reduced production of cholesterol and TGs. Gemcabene has also been shown to enhance clearance of VLDL in the plasma by reduction of apoC-3 gene expression and thus plasma apoC-3 levels, which may facilitate the uptake of VLDL remnants via hepatic remnant receptors. Gemcabene's effects on hsCRP may be due to its effect on reduction of interleukin-6 expression.

Gemcabene was observed to be well tolerated in 895 subjects across 18 phase I and phase II trials both as monotherapy and in combination with statins.

In a phase II study in men and postmenopausal women more than 18 years old and less than 65 years of age with LDL-C 130 mg% or more while on low-intensity to high-intensity stable statin (the majority on moderate intensity) therapy. Sixty six patients were randomized 1:1:1 to gemcabene 300 mg, 900 mg, or placebo QD. It was concluded that gemcabene as add-on to stable statin therapy produces significant reductions in LDL-C of more than 20% and CRP more than 40% compared to placebo.[20]

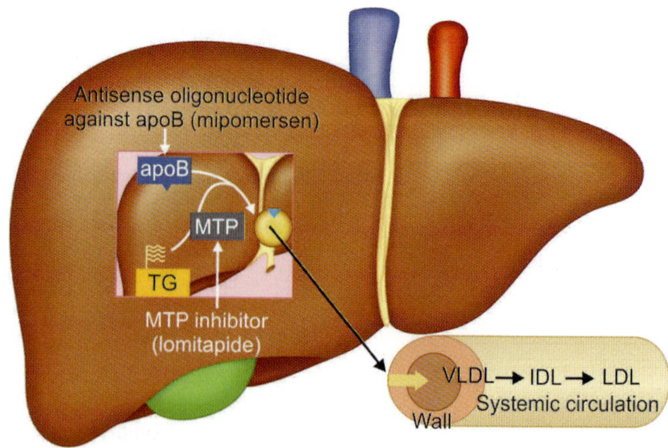

apoB, apolipoprotein B; MTP, microsomal triglyceride transfer protein; TG, triglycerides; LDL, low-density lipoprotein; VLDL, very low-density lipoprotein; IDL, intermediate-density lipoprotein.

FIG. 3: Mechanism of action of mipomersen and lomitapide.

CAT-2054

It is a novel oral product candidate designed to modulate SREBP in the liver. SREBP is a master regulator of lipid metabolism and controls the metabolism of both LDL-C and TGs, through effects on multiple downstream proteins including PCSK9 and HMG-CoA reductase. It is a conjugate of eicosapentaenoic acid and niacin by proprietary linkers that can be cleaved by the intracellular enzyme fatty acid amide hydrolase (FAAH). It has completed phase I trials and entering phase II studies.[21]

NOVEL DRUGS TARGETING HIGH-DENSITY LIPOPROTEIN CHOLESTEROL

Cholesteryl Ester Transfer Protein Inhibitors

Although it is well known that HDL-C plays a protective role against ASCVD, until recently there is no established data that raising HDL level is beneficial in terms of CV outcomes. Studies with niacin Atherothrombosis Intervention in Metabolic Syndrome With Low HDL/High Triglycerides (AIM-HIGH),[22] The Heart Protection Study 2-Treatment of HDL to Reduce the Incidence of Vascular Invents (HPS-2-THRIVE)[23] and CETP inhibitors dalcetrapib in Dal-OUTCOMES,[24] torcetrapib in Investigation of Lipid Level Management to Understand its Impact in Atherosclerotic Events (ILLUMINATE)[25] failed to show any CV benefit despite increasing HDL levels.

Cholesteryl ester transfer protein (CETP) transfers cholesterol from HDL-C to VLDL or LDL-C. Inhibition of this process results in higher HDL levels and reduces LDL levels.

However, the recently published Randomized Evaluation of the Effects of Anacetrapib Through Lipid-modification (REVEAL) trial, which was a randomized, double blind, placebo-controlled trial involving 30,449 adults with ASCVD on intensive atorvastatin therapy and who had a mean LDL cholesterol level of 61 mg/dL, a mean non-HDL-C level of 92 mg/dL and a mean HDL-C level of 40 mg/dL were randomized to receive 100 mg anacetrapib daily versus placebo. Follow-up period was 4.1 years. Primary outcome, which was first major coronary event, a composite of coronary death, MI, or coronary revascularization occurred in significantly fewer patients in the anacetrapib group than in the placebo group (10.8% vs. 11.8%, $p = 0.004$). It also demonstrated increase in mean HDL-C level and decrease in non HDL-C compared to placebo.[26] Despite this, the manufacturer felt that the clinical profile for anacetrapib does not support regulatory filings.

Upregulators of Apolipoprotein A-1 Transcription

Apolipoprotein A-1 (apo A-1) is the major and critical component of HDL particles and responsible for reverse cholesterol transport. Therefore enhancing the endogenous expression of apo A-1 forms a potential therapeutic target against atherosclerosis.

Overexpression of human apo A-1 in transgenic mice has elucidated that increased apo A-1 and HDL-C reduced atherosclerosis progression. On the basis of these observations, the development of new therapies targeting apo A-1 is ongoing. Several known drugs, like fenofibrate, pioglitazone, and 9-cis-retinoic acid, have been reported to regulate apo A-I gene transcription by activating peroxisome proliferator-activated receptor α (PPARα) or retinoid X receptor (RXR), and retinoic acid receptor (RAR) heterodimer; however, they have not been as potent as expected, so identification of effective small molecules that raise the apo A-1 production by increasing its transcription is highly desired.[27]

High-density Lipoprotein Cholesterol Infusion Therapy

Newly developed HDL infusions including reconstituted HDL (rHDL) are currently being tested in clinical trials to determine their effect on the amount and the composition of the plaque and the general state of inflammation. HDL infusions achieve stable levels rapidly in the plasma, making them most suitable in the post ACS stage when most ischemic events are likely to recur. rHDL has been shown to effectively induce cholesterol reflux and inhibit proinflammatory changes and platelet aggregation.[28] In the Effect of rHDL on Atherosclerosis-Safety and Efficacy (ERASE) trial, it was shown that short-term rHDL infusions can induce plaque regression within 4 weeks of treatment in ACS patients.[29]

Triglyceride Reduction

Apolipoprotein C-3 Antisense Oligonucleotide-Volanesorsen

Apolipoprotein C-3 (apo C-3) is a multifaceted protein which plays a key role in TGs metabolism, but recent evidence also suggests that it also participates in the atherosclerotic lesion formation and several other pathological processes involved in atherosclerosis. Genetic observations have shown that loss-of-function mutations in the gene encoding apo C-3 leading to reduced TG levels are associated with decreased CVD risk.

Species-specific antisense suppression of apo C-3 has produced robust reduction in serum apo C-3 and TG and demonstrated good tolerance in various phase I and II trials.

Ongoing phase III trials about volanesorsen include the APPROACH (the APPROACH study: A Study of ISIS-APOCIIIRx in Patients with Familial Chylomicronemia Syndrome, NCT02211209), the COMPASS (the COMPASS study: A Study of Volanesorsen in Patients with Hypertriglyceridemia, NCT02300233), and the BROADEN (the BROADEN study: A Study of Volanesorsen in Patients with Partial Lipodystrophy, NCT02527343).[30] These studies aim to evaluate the efficacy and safety of 300 mg volanesorsen versus placebo. Thus to lower the apo C-3 levels in circulation via specific intervention seems to be an intriguing therapy for CV protection.

Angiopoietin-like Proteins Inhibitors

Angiopoietin-like proteins (ANGPTLs) are proteins that are related structurally to angiopoietins. Of these, ANGPTL 3 and 4 have recently been identified to play a role in regulating plasma lipid levels acting via lipoprotein lipase- and endothelial lipase-mediated hydrolysis of TGs and phospholipids, with more data available for ANGPTL 3 than 4. Loss-of-function variants in ANGPTL3 were associated with a reduced risk of coronary artery disease making it a potential therapeutic target to treat combined hyperlipidemia.

Inhibition of this protein has been shown to reduce plasma lipid levels in both animals and human studies. Strategies to inactivate ANGPTL3 include mAbs against it, namely evinacumab and selective antisense inhibition of *ANGPTL3* expression in the liver.

In human volunteers, inhibition of ANGPTL3 with evinacumab was associated with dose-dependent reductions in LDL cholesterol (29%) and TG levels (76%).[31]

New PPARα Agonists

Peroxisome proliferator-activated receptors are members of the nuclear receptor superfamily of ligand-activated transcription factors. PPARs contain three isotypes encoded by PPARα (NR1C1), PPARβ/δ (NR1C2), and PPARγ (NR1C3) genes. PPARα plays a role in regulation of fatty acid transport as well as peroxisomal and mitochondrial β-oxidation in the liver. Fibrates are PPARα-agonists. The next generation of PPARα agonists is called "selective PPARα modulators" (SPPARMα). They maximize the beneficial effects and minimize the adverse effects of fibrates.

Pemafibrate

It is the first of the SPPARMα to be developed, and has been shown to be safe and efficacious against dyslipidemia in a phase II study.[32]

Pemafibrate to Reduce Cardiovascular OutcoMes by Reducing Triglycerides IN patiENts With diabeTes (PROMINENT) is ongoing study with the primary objective of the study being to determine whether pemafibrate administered twice daily will delay the time to first occurrence of any component of the clinical composite endpoint of nonfatal MI, nonfatal ischemic stroke hospitalization for UA requiring unplanned coronary revascularization, or CV death in diabetics with well-controlled sugars and LDL-C, but having raised TGs and low HDL-C.[33]

Saroglitazar

Saroglitazar is novel first in class drug which acts as a dual PPARα and γ agonist. Agonist action at PPARα lowers high blood TGs, and agonist action on PPARγ improves insulin resistance and consequently lowers blood sugar.[34]

Saroglitazar is indicated for the treatment of diabetic dyslipidemia and hypertriglyceridemia with type 2 diabetes mellitus not controlled by statin therapy. It is approved for clinical use in India, though outcome data are awaited.

TABLE 1: Safety of PCSK 9 inhibitors, evolocumab[10]

Adverse event (AE)	Evolocumab (13,769 patients)	Placebo (3,756 patients)
Any AE	77	77
Serious AE	25	25
Reaction at injection site	2.1	3.6
Discontinuation of drug due to AE	1.6	1.5
Allergic reactions	3.1	2.9
Myalgia/myositis	5.0	4.8
New onset diabetes	8.1	7.7
Defective cognition	1.6	1.5

WHAT ARE THE RECOMMENDATIONS OF THE MEDICAL SOCIETIES ON NEW NONSTATIN MEDICATIONS?

2016 ACC Expert Consensus Statement[35]

1. Ezetimibe is the first nonstatin medication that should be considered in most of the case scenarios, since it has established its safety and efficacy
2. Bile acid sequestrants may be considered as second-line therapy for patients in whom ezetimibe is not tolerated, but they should be avoided in patients with TGs greater than 300 mg/dL
3. Alirocumab and evolocumab may be considered if the goals of therapy have not been achieved on maximally tolerated statin and ezetimibe in higher-risk patients with clinical ASCVD or FH. They are not recommended for use in primary prevention patients in the absence of FH
4. For patients with HoFH, other options are use of lomitapide, mipomersen, and LDL apheresis as necessary.

2016 ESC/EAS Guidelines for the Management of Dyslipidemias[36]

1. In the case of statin intolerance, ezetimibe, or BAS, or these combined, should be considered (IIa)
2. If the goal is not reached, statin combination with a cholesterol absorption inhibitor should be considered (IIa)
3. If the goal is not reached, statin combination with a BAS may be considered (IIb)
4. In patients at very high-risk, with persistent high LDL-C despite treatment with maximal tolerated statin dose, in combination with ezetimibe or in patients with statin intolerance, a PCSK9 inhibitor may be considered (IIb).

Lipid Association of India Expert Consensus Statement on Management of Dyslipidemia in Indians 2016: Part 1[37]

Nonstatin drugs may be used in the following settings:

1. As an alternative to statins when the patient is completely statin intolerant
2. In combination with statins when the desired dose of statin cannot be used due to intolerance.

SAFETY OF VERY LOW LOW-DENSITY LIPOPROTEIN CHOLESTROL

There is a concern in the minds of many a clinicians and amongst general population about the safety of very low LDL-C. However, the evidence from the clinical trials to the contrary, is reassuring.

Further Cardiovascular Outcomes Research with PCSK9 Inhibition in Subjects with Elevated Risk (FOURIER)[10] trial where median LDL-C achieved was 30 mg%, no difference was noted between the evolocumab group and the placebo group, except that injection site reactions were more common in the evolocumab group (Table 1). Even those patients who achieved LDL-C below 20 mg% showed no increased adverse effects, including neurocognitive functions as compared to the placebo.

In the Evaluating PCSK9 Binding Antibody Influence on Cognitive Health in High Cardiovascular Risk Subjects (EBBINGHAUS) study, a subgroup of patients from FOURIER trial, numbering 1,204 patients were followed for a median of 19 months. They were prospectively assessed for cognitive function more objectively, using the Cambridge Neuropsychological Test Automated Battery (CANTAB). The conclusion was that patients who received either evolocumab or placebo in addition to statin therapy, no significant difference in cognitive function between the groups was observed over a follow-up of a median of 19 months.[38]

"HIGHEST RISK-HIGHEST BENEFIT STRATEGY"

Since PCSK 9 inhibitors are pricey, "Highest Risk-Highest Benefit' Strategy" is a pragmatic, cost-effective approach to targeting use of PCSK9 inhibitor therapies. The addition of ezetimibe or PCSK9 mAbs to maximally tolerated statin therapy is expected to be cost-effective in very high-risk and high-risk patients. Clinical ASCVD in a diabetic with or without CKD, ASCVD with CKD, recent ACS (<3 months), coronary heart disease (CHD) with poorly controlled risk factors, CHD with peripheral vascular disease, CAD in patients more than 65 years old, stroke in a male subject, and FH fall into high or very high-risk for ASCVD.[39]

CONCLUSION

Statins continue to stay as the first-line pharmacologic therapy for treating AD to reduce risk of ASCVD. However, there are situations when it becomes necessary to introduce nonstatins in addition or as a substitute to statins. At present, approved newer agents are ezetimibe which is already available in our country and PCSK 9 inhibitors which would be available shortly. Judicious use of these agents would effectively address the issue of residual cholesterol risk.

REFERENCES

1. Global Health Data Exchange. (2015). Global Burden of Disease Study Health Data. [online] Available from http://ghdx.healthdata.org/gbd-data-tool. [Accessed August 2018].
2. Gupta R, Guptha S, Joshi R, et al. Translating evidence into policy for cardiovascular disease control in India. Health Res Policy Syst. 2011;9:8.
3. Roth GA, Johnson C, Abajobir A, et al. Global, regional, and national burden of cardiovascular diseases for 10 causes, 1990 to 2015. J Am Coll Cardiol. 2017;70(1):1-25.
4. Ahn CH, Choi SH. New drugs for treating dyslipidemia: beyond statins. Diabetes Metab J. 2015;39(2):87-94.
5. Lloyd-Jones DM, Morris PB, Ballantyne CM, et al. 2017 Focused Update of the 2016 ACC Expert Consensus Decision Pathway on the Role of Non-Statin Therapies for LDL-Cholesterol Lowering in the Management of Atherosclerotic Cardiovascular Disease Risk. J Am Coll Cardiol. 2017;70(14):1785-822.
6. Cannon CP, Blazing MA, Giugliano RP, et al. Ezetimibe added to statin therapy after acute coronary syndromes. N Engl J Med. 2015;372(25):2387-97.
7. Baigent C, Landray MJ, Reith C, et al. The effects of lowering LDL cholesterol with simvastatin plus ezetimibe in patients with chronic kidney disease (Study of Heart and Renal Protection): a randomized placebo-controlled trial. Lancet. 2011;377(9784):2181-92.
8. Giugliano RP, Cannon CP, Blazing MA, et al. Benefit of adding ezetimibe to statin therapy on cardiovascular outcomes and safety in patients with versus without diabetes mellitus: results from IMPROVE-IT (Improved Reduction of Outcomes: Vytorin Efficacy International Trial). Circulation. 2018;137(15):1571-82.
9. Ridker PM, Revkin J, Amarenco P, et al. Cardiovascular efficacy and safety of bococizumab in high-risk patients. N Engl J Med. 2017;376:1527-39.
10. Sabatine MS, Giugliano RP, Keech AC, et al. Evolocumab and clinical outcomes in patients with cardiovascular disease. N Engl J Med. 2017;376(18):1713-22.
11. Steg P, Szarek M, Bhatt D. Late-breaking clinical trial: cardiovascular outcomes with alirocumab after acute coronary syndrome: results of the ODYSSEY Outcomes trial. ACC. 2018. 2018;401-8.
12. Nicholls SJ, Puri R, Anderson TA, et al. Effect of evolocumab on progression of coronary disease in statin-treated patients: The GLAGOV randomized clinical trial. JAMA. 2016;316(22):2373-84.
13. Landmesser U, Chapman MJ, Stock JK, et al. 2017 Update of ESC/EAS Task Force on practical clinical guidance for proprotein convertase subtilisin/kexin type 9 inhibition in patients with atherosclerotic cardiovascular disease or in familial hypercholesterolaemia. Eur Heart J. 2018;39(14):1131-43.
14. Ray KK, Landmesser U, Leiter LA, et al. Inclisiran in patients at high cardiovascular risk with elevated LDL cholesterol. N Engl J Med. 2017;376(15):1430-40.
15. Ray KK, Stoekenbroek RM, Kallend D, et al. Effect of a siRNA therapeutic targeting PCSK9 on atherogenic lipoproteins: pre specified secondary end points in ORION 1. Circulation. 2018.
16. Cuchel M, Meagher EA, du Toit Theron H, et al. Efficacy and safety of a microsomal triglyceride transfer protein inhibitor in patients with homozygous familial hypercholesterolaemia: a single-arm, open-label, phase 3 study. Lancet. 2013;381(9860):40-6.
17. Raal FJ, Santos RD, Blom DJ, et al. Mipomersen, an apolipoprotein B synthesis inhibitor, for lowering of LDL cholesterol concentrations in patients with homozygous familial hypercholesterolemia: a randomised, double-blind, placebo-controlled trial. Lancet. 2010;375(9719):998-1006.
18. McGowan MP, Tardif JC, Ceska R, et al. Randomized, placebo-controlled trial of mipomersen in patients with severe hypercholesterolemia receiving maximally tolerated lipid-lowering therapy. PLoS One. 2012;7(11):e49006.
19. US National Library of Medicine. Evaluation of the efficacy and safety of bempedoic acid (ETC-1002) in patients with hyperlipidemia and statin intolerant (CLEAR serenity). [online] Available from https://clinicaltrials.gov/ct2/show/NCT02988115. [Accessed August, 2018].

20. Stein E, Bays H, Koren M, et al. Efficacy and safety of gemcabene as add-on to stable statin therapy in hypercholesterolemic patients. J Clin Lipidol. 2016;10(5):1212-22.
21. Donovan JM, Mancini M, Sanabria S, et al. Phase 1 study of CAT-2054, an oral novel modulator of SREBP. J Clin Lipidol. 2015;9:474-5.
22. AIM-HIGH Investigators; Boden WE, Probstfield JL, Anderson T, et al. Niacin in patients with low HDL cholesterol levels receiving intensive statin therapy. N Engl J Med. 2011;365(24):2255-67.
23. HPS2-THRIVE Collaborative Group; Landray MJ, Haynes R, Hopewell JC, et al. Effects of extended-release niacin with laropiprant in high-risk patients. N Engl J Med. 2014;371(3):203-12.
24. Schwartz GG, Olsson AG, Abt M, et al. Effects of dalcetrapib in patients with a recent acute coronary syndrome. N Engl J Med. 2012;367(22):2089-99.
25. Barter PJ, Caulfield M, Eriksson M, et al. Effects of torcetrapib in patients at high risk for coronary events. N Engl J Med. 2007;357(21):2109-22.
26. HPS3/TIMI55-REVEAL Collaborative Group; Bowman L, Hopewell JC, Chen F, et al. Effects of anacetrapib in patients with atherosclerotic vascular disease. N Engl J Med. 2017;377(13):1217-27.
27. Zannis VI, Duka A, Drosatos K, et al. Regulation of apo A-I gene expression and prospects to increase plasma apo A-I and HDL levels. Schaefer EJ (Ed). High Density Lipoproteins, Dyslipidemia, and Coronary Heart Disease; 2010. pp. 15-24.
28. Newton RS, Krause BR. HDL therapy for the acute treatment of atherosclerosis. Atheroscler. 2002;3:31-8.
29. Tardif JC, Grégoire J, L'Allier PL, et al. Effects of reconstituted high-density lipoprotein infusions on coronary atherosclerosis: a randomized controlled trial. JAMA. 2007;297:1675-82.
30. Schmitz J, Gouni-Berthold I. APOC-III antisense oligonucleotides: a new option for the treatment of hypertriglyceridemia. Curr Med Chem. 2018;25(13):1567-76.
31. Dewey FE, Gusarova V, Dunbar RL, et al. Genetic and pharmacologic inactivation of ANGPTL3 and cardiovascular disease. N Engl J Med. 2017;377:211-22.
32. Ishibashi S, Yamashita S, Ara H, et al. Effects of K-877, a novel selective PPARα modulator (SPPARMα), in dyslipidaemic patients: A randomized, double blind, active- and placebo-controlled, phase 2 trial. Atherosclerosis. 2016;249:36-43.
33. ClinicalTrials.gov. (2017). Pemafibrate to reduce cardiovascular outcomes by reducing triglycerides in patients with diabetes (PROMINENT). [online] Available from https://clinicaltrials.gov/ct2/show/NCT03071692?cond=Pemafibrate+to+reduce+cardiovascular+outcomes+by+reducing+triglycerides+in+patients+with+diabetes&rank=1 [Accessed August 2018].
34. Joshi SR. Saroglitazar for the treatment of dyslipidemia in diabetic patients. Expert Opin Pharmacother. 2015;16(4):597-606.
35. Lloyd-Jones DM, Morris PB, Ballantyne CM, et al. 2016 ACC Expert Consensus Decision Pathway on the role of non-statin therapies for LDL-cholesterol lowering in the management of atherosclerotic cardiovascular disease risk. J Am Coll Cardiol. 2016;68(1):92-125.
36. Catapano AL, Graham I, De Backer G, et al. 2016 ESC/EAS guidelines for the management of dyslipidaemias. Eur Heart J. 2016;37(39):2999-3058.
37. Iyengar SS, Puri R, Narasingan SN, et al. Lipid Association of India Expert Consensus Statement on management of dyslipidemia in Indians 2016: Part 1. J Assoc Physicians India. 2016;64(3):7-52.
38. Giugliano RP, Mach F, Zavitz, K, et al. Cognitive function in a randomized trial of evolocumab. N Engl J Med. 2017;377(7):633-43.
39. Robinson JG, Huijgen R, Ray K, et al. Determining when to add nonstatin therapy: a quantitative approach. J Am Coll Cardiol. 2016;68(22):2412-21.

CHAPTER 87

Choosing Between NOACS Wisely: Are They all the Same?

Sandeep Bansal, Anunay Gupta

INTRODUCTION

For over half a century, we have been using vitamin K-based drugs as oral anticoagulants. The vitamin K anticoagulants (VKAs) as oral anticoagulant (OAC) drugs act indirectly on the process of glutamic acid (Glu) carboxylation of the vitamin K-dependent coagulation factor proteins. They have been used for several indications like:

- Stroke prevention in atrial fibrillation (SPAF)
- Coronary artery disease (CAD)
- Prevention and treatment of deep vein thrombosis and pulmonary embolism in surgical or medical conditions
- Ischemic stroke
- Rare hypercoagulable states (e.g., factor-V Leiden or protein C and S deficiency).

They have been very successful in what they are meant for, i.e., anticoagulation and prevention of thrombosis. They reduce incidence of non-valvular atrial fibrillation (NVAF) by nearly two-thirds. However, they do have several shortcomings, viz. slow onset or offset, need for monitoring international normalized ratio (INR), significant drug and food interactions and high incidence of bleeding. This necessitated the development of non-vitamin K antagonist oral anticoagulants (NOACs) or directly-acting oral anticoagulants (DOACs).

Non-vitamin K antagonist oral anticoagulants have undergone phase three trials in prevention or treatment of venous thromboembolism following orthopedic surgeries, prevention or treatment of venous thromboembolism following general surgeries or medical conditions, prevention, and treatment of pulmonary embolism, SPAF and lately in treatment of CAD both with and without atrial fibrillation (AF). They are now widely being used for all these indications. However, the current discussion would largely be dedicated to choosing a NOAC in SPAF.

Currently, four NOACs are approved by the US Food and Drug Administration (FDA), i.e., Dabigatran [direct thrombin inhibitor (DTI)], apixaban, edoxaban, and rivaroxaban (factor-Xa inhibitors).

Although there is a lot of data available on these agents. But still clinicians find it difficult to choose most appropriate NOACs for their individual patient. Dienner HC et al. had recently reviewed this issue in two papers which are worth reading for every clinician prescribing NOACs for various indications.[1,2] This review is intended to highlights practical points related to everyday use of NOACs in clinical practice. Several factors determine a physician's choice, viz:

- Medical conditions like kidney and liver functions
- Age of the patient
- Patient's profile, e.g., which is a greater consideration high risk of ischemic stroke or high-risk of bleeding
- Concomitant medications
- Adherence – likelihood of using once or twice daily regimen
- Cost
- Trial designs of phase three SPAF trials.

PHARMACOKINETICS AND PHARMACODYNAMICS DIFFERENCES

All NOACs differ from VKAs as a group and have many similarities. They have rapid onset of action, hence do not require bridging parental anticoagulation. They do not require monitoring.[3] Their half-life is also similar (5–7 h). Table 1 highlights major difference among NOACs. As mentioned in the table dabigatran has a very low bioavailability 6–7% and its absorption depends on gastrointestinal (GI) pH and comes formulated with tartaric acid, which is considered responsible for GI side effects seen. Dabigatran capsules are hygroscopic, hence medication should be stored in bottles. Rivaroxaban bioavailability is high when taken with food (66–80%), hence it should be preferably taken with food. Although, drug interactions seen with NOACs are much less as compared to warfarin, there are few important interactions of which clinician should be aware of. All NOACs are impacted by permeability glycoprotein (P-glycoprotein) system. Similarly, cytochrome P450 metabolizes all NOACs except dabigatran. Hence, drugs which are inducers of

TABLE 1: General pharmacological characteristics of NOACs

Characteristics	Dabigatran	Rivaroxaban	Apixaban	Edoxaban
Bioavailability	pH dependent	Food dependent 60–80%	50%; food independent	62%; food independent
Renal clearance	80%	35%	25%	50%
CYP3A4 metabolism	No	Yes	Minor	Minor
P-glycoprotein	Yes	Yes	Yes	Yes

CYP3A4, cytochrome P450 3A4; NOACs, non-vitamin K antagonist oral anticoagulants; P-glycoprotein, permeability glycoprotein.

TABLE 2: Main characteristic features of four pivotal trials of NOACs*

	RE-LY		Rocket AF	Aristotle	Engage AF	
Drug	Dabigatran		Rivaroxaban	Apixaban	Edoxaban	
Patients	18,113		14,264	18,201	21,105	
Age (y)	71		73	70	72	
Mean $CHADS_2$ Score	2.1		3.5	2.1	2.8	
Dose	110 mg BD	150 mg BD	20 mg OD	5 mg BD	60 mg OD	30 mg OD
Prior VKA(%)	50		62	57	58.8	59.2
Mean TTR(%)	64		55	62	68.4	
RR of ischemic stroke	1.1	0.76	0.94	0.92	1.141	1.0
RR of stroke or systemic embolism	0.91	0.66	0.88	0.79	1.13	0.87
RR of major bleed	0.80	0.93	1.04	0.69	0.80	0.47
RR of hemorrhagic stroke	0.31	0.40	0.67	0.42	0.47	0.30
RR of GI bleed	1.09	1.49	1.47	0.88	1.23	0.67
RR of myocardial infarction	1.29	1.27	0.81	0.88	0.94	1.19
RR of death	0.91	0.88	0.85	0.89	0.92	0.87

*Modified and adapted from multiple sources.

AF, atrial fibrillation; GI, gastrointestinal; NOACs, non-vitamin K antagonist oral anticoagulants; RR, relative risk; TTR, time in therapeutic range; VKA, vitamin K anticoagulants.

P-glycoprotein should be used cautiously or not used with NOACs. Such drugs commonly used in clinical practice are antifungals, antituberculars, and antiepileptic drugs.

MAJOR DIFFERENCES IN TRIALS

To know the differences between the available NOACs, it is important to review the differences between those four major studies (Table 2). The Randomized Evaluation of Long-Term Anticoagulation Therapy (RE-LY study)[4] was an open, blinded study that compared blinded doses of dabigatran 110 or 150 mg twice daily to open-label dose-adjusted warfarin. The other three trials were double-blinded, double-dummy trials comparing a once daily 20 mg dose of rivaroxaban (ROCKET AF),[5] twice daily, 5 mg dose of apixaban (ARISTOTLE),[6] and two doses (30 and 60 mg) of edoxaban, once daily (ENGAGE AF-TIMI),[7] respectively, to warfarin.

One thing to always remember is that even though dabigatran 150 BD was superior to warfarin but confidence interval (CI) margin was just 0.98 means 24% relative reduction (RR) was with odds ratio (OR) 0.76 (0.60 - 0.98) and probability (p) value of 0.03. Hence, it can be said theoretically all NOACs were non inferior to warfarin, if it comes to efficacy except high-dose dabigatran wherein a statistical significant superiority was noted. They were importantly superior over warfarin predominantly on the basis of improved safety margin.

Which NOACS to use?

It is difficult to directly compare NOACs from each other due to differences in the trial characteristics as summarized in Table 2. Table 3 summarizes individual patient group in which one NOACs can be used preferably over on the basis of multiple subgroup and post hoc analysis, and meta-analysis.[8]

Asian Patients

Asian patients are at high-risk of stroke due to increased prevalence of stroke risk factors. But they are also at increased risk of intracranial bleed, this fear leads to under treatment of AF patients with anticoagulation. In Asian patients, there was no excess bleeding when NOACs were used and superiority of NOACs to warfarin in reducing thromboembolism was maintained. Hence, NOACs are preferentially indicated in Asians in terms of both efficacy and safety.[9]

TABLE 3: Choosing the right NOACs for right patient

Factor	Features	NOACs
Patient compliance and preference	OD dosing	Rivaroxaban, edoxaban 60 mg
Renal dysfunction	Least renal clearance	Apixaban (preferred), rivaroxaban
Increased GI bleeding risk	Least incidence of GI bleeding	Apixaban, low-dose edoxaban
High-risk of bleeding (HAS-BLED >3)	Least bleeding risk	Dabigatran 110 BD and apixaban
Stable CAD	Evaluated in trial	Rivaroxaban low dose (not FDA approved)
Post PCI	Evaluated in trial	Rivaroxaban and dabigatran
Elderly (age >75 years)	Lesser risk of extracranial bleeding	Rivaroxaban or apixaban
High-risk of ischemic stroke, less risk of bleeding	Best reduction in ischemic stroke	Apixaban

CAD, coronary artery disease; FDA, Food and Drug Administration; NOACs, non-vitamin K antagonist oral anticoagulants; PCI, percutaneous coronary intervention.

Elderly Patients

Elderly patients (age >75 years) well participated in all the major NOAC trials. Meta-analysis of the trials in elderly population had shown that NOACs were more effective than conventional warfarin therapy in the prevention of stroke and systemic embolism, and they were not associated with any increase in major or clinically relevant bleeding events in patients over 75 years of age.[10] However, in elderly patients intracranial bleeding risk was lower but extracranial bleeding risk was similar or higher with both doses of dabigatran compared with warfarin.[11] Hence, direct factor-Xa inhibitors should be preferably used in elderly.

Patient at High-risk of Bleed

The HAS-BLED (Hypertension, abnormal renal and liver function, stroke, bleeding, labile INR, elderly, drugs or alcohol) score can be used to predict patients at high risk of hemorrhage, with a score of 3 or greater signifying significant risk.[12] Low-dose Dabigatran (RR 0.80, 95%; CI 0.69–0.93; p = 0.003), apixaban (RR 0.69, 95%; CI 0.60–0.80; p <0.001) and edoxaban at high (RR 0.80, 95%; CI 0.70–0.91; p <0.001) and low-dose (RR 0.47, 95%; CI 0.41–0.55; p <0.001) have shown significantly reduced rates of major hemorrhage compared to warfarin as shown in table 2. However, there was no significant difference in the incidence of major bleeding in high-dose dabigatran (150 mg BD) and rivaroxaban versus warfarin (Table 2). Patients in ROCKET-AF trial who were in time in therapeutic range (TTR) were lower (only 55%), hence might have affected the rate of hemorrhage in warfarin arm. It should be remembered that rate of intracranial bleeding was significantly lower among all the doses tested of all NOACs. Hence, low-dose dabigatran, apixaban, and edoxaban may be used preferably in patients who are at high-risk of bleeding.

Increased Risk of Gastrointestinal Hemorrhage

Dabigatran 150 BD (RR 1.50) and rivaroxaban (3.2 vs. 2.2% p value <0.001) have higher risk of GI bleed, hence should be avoided in patient at risk of GI bleed. All NOACs except low-dose edoxaban are associated with similar or increased risk of GI hemorrhage compared to warfarin. Apixaban and low-dose dabigatran have similar risk of GI bleed as compared to warfarin. Important point to remember is that GI bleeding, even in the setting of anticoagulation, does usually not cause death or permanent major disability and identifying and treating the cause is mandatory. Thus, the choice of OAC should be driven mainly by stroke prevention considerations. Hence, it would be suggested to use dabigatran 110 BD and apixaban 5 BD in such patients. Even though low-dose edoxaban was associated with low-risk of GI bleed but with reduced efficacy of stroke prevention.

Chronic Kidney Disease

Patients with renal impairment requires dose modification of all NOACs as they all are excreted by kidney (Table 4).

There are no clinical outcome data regarding the use of NOACs for patients with creatinine clearance (calculated by the Cockcroft–Gault equation) of less than 30 mL/min and also patients on hemodialysis. Hence, warfarin is the preferred anticoagulant for these patient subgroups.

TABLE 4: Summarizes dose modification criteria in patients with renal disease

Drugs	Criteria	Dose modification
Dabigatran	Creatinine clearance <50 mL/min <30 mL/min	110 mg BD as per ESC guidelines should not be used
Rivaroxaban	Creatinine clearance <50 mL/min	15 mg OD
Apixaban	Two of these factors: Age >80, creatinine >1.5, weight <60	2.5 BD
Edoxaban	Creatinine clearance <50 mL/min	30 OD

ESC, European Society of Cardiology.

Coronary Artery Disease Patients

Patients with stable CAD with AF is common and constituted up to 30% of patients in major NOACs trials. Incidence of CAD in more than 70 years of AF was 41%.[13] Use of antiplatelet along with NOACs therapy is associated with increased risk of bleeding. Increased risk of myocardial infarction (MI) with dabigatran as was initially thought, was not supported by large FDA Medicare analysis.[14] The COMPASS (Cardiovascular outcomes for people using anticoagulation strategies) trial evaluated role of rivaroxaban (low-dose) in stable CAD.[15] Among patients with stable atherosclerotic vascular disease, patients who were randomized to rivaroxaban (2.5 mg twice daily) plus aspirin had better cardiovascular outcomes, but more major bleeding events versus those who were randomized to aspirin alone. Rivaroxaban (5 mg twice daily) dose alone did not result in better cardiovascular outcomes versus aspirin alone and resulted in more major bleeding events. Monotherapy with an NOAC is preferable for patients with AF and stable CAD. This suggestion is applicable to all NOACs.[1]

Patient with AF undergoing percutaneous coronary intervention (PCI) and stenting need dual anti-platelet therapy (DAPT) for preventing stent thrombosis and Oral anticoagulation for preventing stroke. But it comes at the cost of increased risk of bleeding. In the PIONEER AF-PCI trial[16] two rivaroxaban-based dual therapy (rivaroxaban 15/20 OD with P2Y12 inhibitor) treatment regimens significantly reduced bleeding complications compared to conventional triple therapy (DAPT plus oral anticoagulation) without increasing embolic or ischemic complications following PCI. Dual therapy with rivaroxaban and clopidogrel appeared to provide an optimal risk-benefit ratio.[17] Similarly in the RE-DUAL PCI trial[18] dual therapy with dabigatran (110 BD/150 BD) also reduced bleeding complications compared to conventional triple therapy in patients with AF undergoing PCI.

Single Risk Factor (CHA_2DS_2-VASc Score of 1 in Males or 2 in Females)

Patient with single-stroke risk factor increased risk of stroke varies from 0.5 to 3 %, but risk is lower compared to those with multiple risk factors. The CHA_2DS_2-VASc 2 score is used to assess risk of stroke in AF patients. The risk of embolization attributable to the individual risk factors (that might lead to a score of 1) is not equal. Female sex and vascular disease carry a lower risk than diabetes, hypertension, or age of 65–74 years.[19]

Women with a CHA_2DS_2-VASc score of 1 (or 0 for males) are at low-risk, and no antithrombotic therapy is recommended.[20] Anticoagulation should be considered for patients with AF and one or more additional stroke risk factors (i.e., men with a CHA_2DS_2-VASc score of ≥1 or women with a score of ≥2).[21] There has been no randomized controlled trial (RCT) with NOACs with only one risk factor as event rates will be very low. In the ROCKET AF trial, the proportion of enrolled patients with $CHADS_2$ scores of 2 was capped at 10%. Mean $CHADS_2$ score was 3.5 in ROCKET-AF and 2.8 in ENGAGE-AF. Only dabigatran and apixaban have been studied in such patients and hence should be preferably used.

COMPLIANCE

Once daily dosing has been shown to improve compliance and adherence over medications requiring multiple daily dosing. To promote adherence rivaroxaban or edoxaban should be considered due to their convenient OD dosing.[3]

CONCLUSION

We would like to suggest a patient-centered, individualized approach to manage thromboembolic risk in patients with AF. With the availability of several NOAC drugs now available, we can fit the drug to the patient profile. As discussed above, there are no head-to-head trials available for comparing NOACs. However, as summarized above we can carefully choose one NOACs over the other depending on the patient specific factors and shared decision making.

REFERENCES

1. Diener HC, Aisenberg J, Ansell J, et al. Choosing a particular oral anticoagulant and dose for stroke prevention in individual patients with non-valvular atrial fibrillation: part 1. Eur Heart J. 2017;38(12):852-9.
2. Diener HC, Aisenberg J, Ansell J, et al. Choosing a particular oral anticoagulant and dose for stroke prevention in individual patients with non-valvular atrial fibrillation: part 2. Eur Heart J. 2017;38(12):860-8.
3. Schaefer JK, McBane RD, Wysokinski WE. How to choose appropriate direct oral anticoagulant for patient with nonvalvular atrial fibrillation. Ann Hematol. 2016;95(3):437-49.
4. Nagarakanti R, Ezekowitz MD, Oldgren J, et al. Dabigatran versus warfarin in patients with atrial fibrillation: an analysis of patients undergoing cardioversion. Circulation. 2011;123(2):131-6.
5. Cappato R, Ezekowitz MD, Klein AL, et al. Rivaroxaban vs. vitamin K antagonists for cardioversion in atrial fibrillation. Eur Heart J. 2014;35(47):3346-55.
6. Connolly SJ, Eikelboom J, Joyner C, et al. Apixaban in patients with atrial fibrillation. N Engl J Med;364: 806-17.
7. Giugliano RP, Ruff CT, Braunwald E, et al. Edoxaban versus warfarin in patients with atrial fibrillation. N Engl J Med. 2013;369:2093-104.
8. Shields AM, Lip GYH. Choosing the right drug to fit the patient when selecting oral anticoagulation for stroke prevention in atrial fibrillation. J Intern Med. 2015;278(1):1-18.
9. Chiang CE, Wang KL, Lip GYH. Stroke prevention in atrial fibrillation: an Asian perspective. Thromb Haemost. 2014;111(5):789-97.
10. Sardar P, Chatterjee S, Chaudhari S, et al. New oral anticoagulants in elderly adults: evidence from a meta-analysis of randomized trials. J Am Geriatr Soc. 2014;62(5):857-64.
11. Eikelboom JW, Wallentin L, Connolly SJ, et al. Risk of bleeding with 2 doses of dabigatran compared with warfarin in older and younger patients with atrial fibrillation: an analysis of the randomized evaluation of long-term anticoagulant therapy (RE-LY) trial. Circulation. 2011 ;123(21):2363-72.
12. Pisters R, Lane DA, Nieuwlaat R, et al. A novel user-friendly score (HAS-BLED) to assess 1-year risk of major bleeding in patients with atrial fibrillation: the Euro Heart Survey. Chest. 2010;138(5):1093-100.
13. Kralev S, Schneider K, Lang S, et al. Incidence and severity of coronary artery disease in patients with atrial fibrillation undergoing first-time coronary angiography. PloS One. 2011;6(9):e24964.
14. Graham DJ, Reichman ME, Wernecke M, et al. Cardiovascular, bleeding, and mortality risks in elderly Medicare patients treated with dabigatran or warfarin for nonvalvular atrial fibrillation. Circulation. 2015;131(2):157-64.
15. Eikelboom JW, Connolly SJ, Bosch J, et al. Rivaroxaban with or without Aspirin in Stable Cardiovascular Disease. N Engl J Med. 2017;377(14):1319-30.

16. Gibson CM, Mehran R, Bode C, et al. Prevention of Bleeding in Patients with Atrial Fibrillation Undergoing PCI. N Engl J Med. 2016;375(25):2423-34.
17. Duerschmied D, Brachmann J, Darius H, et al. Antithrombotic therapy in patients with non-valvular atrial fibrillation undergoing percutaneous coronary intervention: should we change our practice after the PIONEER AF-PCI and RE-DUAL PCI trials? Clin Res Cardiol. 2018;107(7):533-8.
18. Cannon CP, Bhatt DL, Oldgren J, et al. Dual Antithrombotic Therapy with Dabigatran after PCI in Atrial Fibrillation. N Engl J Med. 2017;377(16):1513-24.
19. Huang D, Anguo L, Yue WS, et al. Refinement of ischemic stroke risk in patients with atrial fibrillation and CHA2 DS2 -VASc score of 1. Pacing Clin Electrophysiol PACE. 2014;37(11):1442-7.
20. Lip GYH, Skjøth F, Rasmussen LH, et al. Net Clinical Benefit for Oral Anticoagulation, Aspirin, or No Therapy in Nonvalvular Atrial Fibrillation Patients With 1 Additional Risk Factor of the CHA2DS2-VASc Score (Beyond Sex). J Am Coll Cardiol. 2015;66(4):488-90.
21. Lip GYH, Lane DA. Stroke prevention in atrial fibrillation: a systematic review. JAMA. 2015;313(19):1950-62.

CHAPTER 88

Newer Antihyperkalemic Drugs

AK Pancholia

INTRODUCTION

Hyperkalemia is the common electrolyte imbalance in clinical practice. Moderate-to-severe hyperkalemia leads to potentially fatal cardiac conduction abnormalities or arrhythmias. Risk factors for hyperkalemia include excess intake or supplementation of potassium, type 2 diabetes, liver cirrhosis, congestive heart failure (CHF), and chronic kidney disease (CKD). Ninety to ninety-five percent of ingested potassium is excreted through kidneys while rest excreted through gut. Normal kidneys take 6–12 hours to excrete an acute potassium load. Thus when kidney function decreases, risk for hyperkalemia increases.[1] Hyperkalemia has been observed in 26% of patients with CKD stages 3–5 [glomerular filtration rate (GFR) <60 mL/min].[2] Renin-angiotensin-aldosterone system (RAAS) inhibitors, including angiotensin-converting enzyme inhibitors (ACEIs), angiotensin receptor blockers (ARBs), and aldosterone antagonists are associated with hyperkalemia. Though RAAS blockers can play an important role in the management of CKD and cardiovascular disease (CVD), the development of hyperkalemia leads to a dose reduction or discontinuation of these medications, limiting their therapeutic benefit. Nonpharmacological therapeutic options for treatment of hyperkalemia are limited. In addition to reducing or discontinuing related medications, strategies include use of diuretics (as appropriate), treatment of metabolic acidosis, and dietary restrictions (i.e., limiting high-potassium foods).[1] Even pharmacologically, there has been no better option for correcting hyperkalemia.

Recent approval of the new heart failure (HF) medication entresto (LCZ696; sacubitril or valsartan) has further enhanced an interest by the healthcare community to optimize treatment regimens that include life-saving therapies such as ACEIs and ARBs. These agents are known in some patients to increase serum potassium to dangerously high levels that can lead to life-threatening arrhythmias. Patients who have CKD, advanced age, HF, and/or diabetes mellitus are particularly prone to developing hyperkalemia. In the nephrology community, hyperkalemia has been reported in over half of all CKD patients. Thus monitoring and control of hyperkalemia is of paramount importance.

For last several years sodium polystyrene sulfonate (SPS), the US FDA-approved drug, is being used in treatment for hyperkalemia. Because of the variability in its time to onset of effect and high-sodium content make it a poor choice in acute hyperkalemia and sodium-restricted patient populations.[3] To overcome these limitations the newer drugs patiromer sorbitex calcium (patiromer) and sodium zirconium cyclosilicate (ZS-9) have been developed.[4,5]

CLINICAL MANIFESTATIONS OF HYPERKALEMIA

Increase in plasma potassium concentration has a several adverse clinical effects which may be magnified in the critically ill patient.

Cardiac Effects

Depolarization of cell membrane and decrease in duration of action potential due to hyperkalemia lead to some classical ECG changes (Fig. 1).[6]

Hospitalized patients with hyperkalemia have a higher mortality rate than those without hyperkalemia.[7,8] The first cardiac manifestation of hyperkalemia may be ventricular fibrillation.[9]

Neuromuscular Effects

Hyperkalemia causes muscle weakness progressing to a flaccid paralysis and paresthesia. Deep tendon reflexes are depressed or absent, sensory changes are minimal.[10,11]

Metabolic Effects

Hyperkalemia may produce a mild hyperchloremic metabolic acidosis,[12] and will limit the kidney's ability to excrete an acid load and thus prevent correction of a metabolic acidosis.[13]

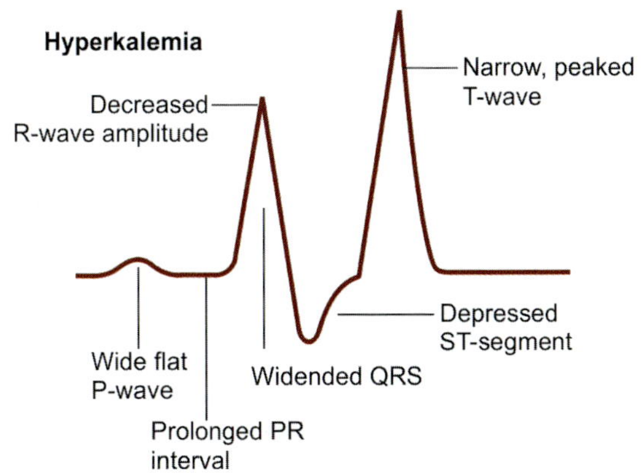

FIG. 1: Electrocardiography changes of hyperkalemia.

TABLE 1: Old drugs for hyperkalemia and their mechanism of action

Therapy	Start	Mechanism
Calcium gluconate	Fast	Antagonize excitation of membrane
Insulin and dextrose	Intermediate	Moves potassium inside the cell
Beta-adrenergic antagonists	Intermediate	Moves potassium inside the cell
Sodium bicarbonate	Intermediate	Moves potassium inside the cell
Diuretics	Late	Increases potassium urine excretion
Resins	Late	Increases potassium gastrointestinal excretion
Dialysis	Late	Potassium extracorporeal elimination

THERAPY FOR HYPERKALEMIA

Older Drugs for Hyperkalemia

Old drugs for hyperkalemia and their mechanism of action are shown in table 1.

Newer Drugs for Hyperkalemia

Limitations of the old therapy for hyperkalemia have paved the way for newer, effective, and safe drugs.

Sodium Polystyrene Sulfonate

Sodium polystyrene sulfonate, an organic enteral potassium-sodium exchange resin, nonselectively binds potassium and other cations, is commonly given with sorbitol, which results in diarrhea.[14] Diarrhea lowers potassium via colonic epithelial cells that upregulate their ability to facilitate luminal losses of potassium in CKD, but it is a potentially dangerous side effect for hospitalized patients who are at risk for volume loss. It is also associated with frequent adverse effects and carries the risk of acute bowel necrosis as both an oral solution and as a retention enema, particularly in critically ill and postsurgical patients. It also causes hypernatremia.[15] Thus, SPS is not routinely prescribed as an outpatient, chronic oral therapy because of diarrhea and concerns about its unknown efficacy and poor tolerability.

Sodium Zirconium Cyclosilicate

It is a new oral agent used in the management of hyperkalemia. ZS-9 binds the potassium selectively. It is taken as an oral powder in liquid which is insoluble and not absorbed by the gut. Zirconium is a trace element, biologically inert, used in dental and medical processes, including as part of renal dialysis to remove ammonium. As a crystalline lattice, ZS-9 has many micropores with a specific size and negatively charged selectivity filter (Fig. 2).

The dietary potassium incorporates through micropores, with counter ions of sodium and hydrogen exchanged from within the latticework, with excretion of potassium-rich compound rather than absorbed. The pores are selective for potassium over both sodium ions and divalent ions like calcium and magnesium.[16] ZS-9 has a low-risk of toxic effects because of lack of absorption. Its insolubility also prevents water absorption, which has led to constipation in polystyrene-based resins. ZS-9 is approved for clinical use in Europe but has not yet been approved by the FDA in the US.

Mechanism of Action

Figure 3 shows the mechanism of action of sodium zirconium cyclosilicate.

Clinical Trial with Sodium Zirconium Cyclosilicate

The HARMONIZE study (Fig. 4) was a phase 3, multicenter, double-blind, randomized controlled trial in hyperkalemic patients in outpatients for 28 days.[17] Total 258 patients were given 10 g of ZS 9 with meals three times a day for 48 hours, then the 237 subjects who achieved normokalemia were randomized into receiving 28 days of a once-daily preparation of different doses (5 g, 10 g, 15 g) or placebo in each of the treatment groups patients maintain normokalemia (K^+ <5.1 mmol/L) at 28 days with comparable adverse effects with placebo.

Patiromer Sorbitex Calcium

Patiromer is a nonabsorbed potassium-binding polymer, available in powder form to be taken orally as suspension in water, and a calcium-sorbitol counter ion that binds potassium in the gastrointestinal lumen and increases fecal potassium excretion, leading to removal of potassium from the body and lowering of serum potassium levels.

Preclinical Studies

In balance studies[18] in dogs given C13-patiromer, 99.9% of the administered dose was found in the feces with less than 0.1% in the urine and 0.002% in the plasma.

Phase I Studies

In these studies patiromer was found to increase the fecal contents of sodium and magnesium, reduced the fecal content of calcium in a dose-dependent manner.[19] In the

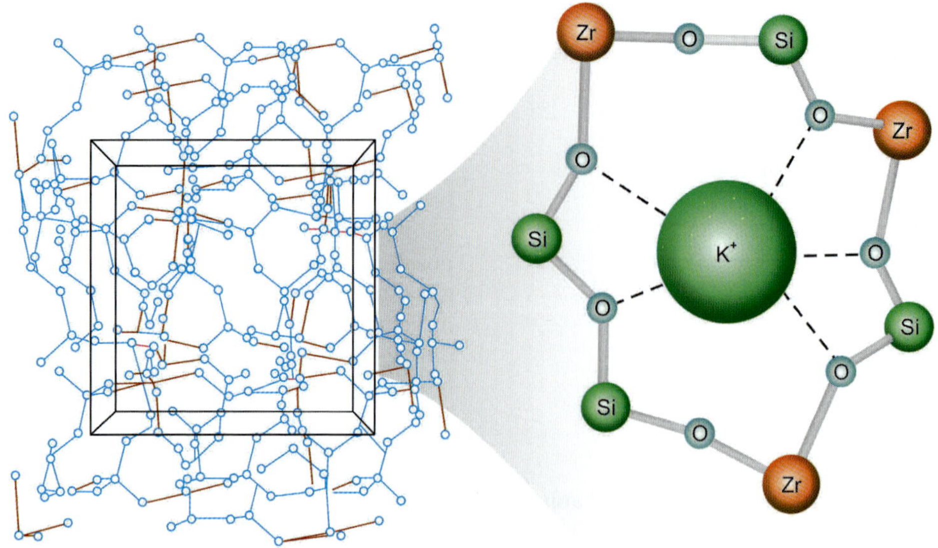

FIG. 2: Sodium zirconium cyclosilicate.

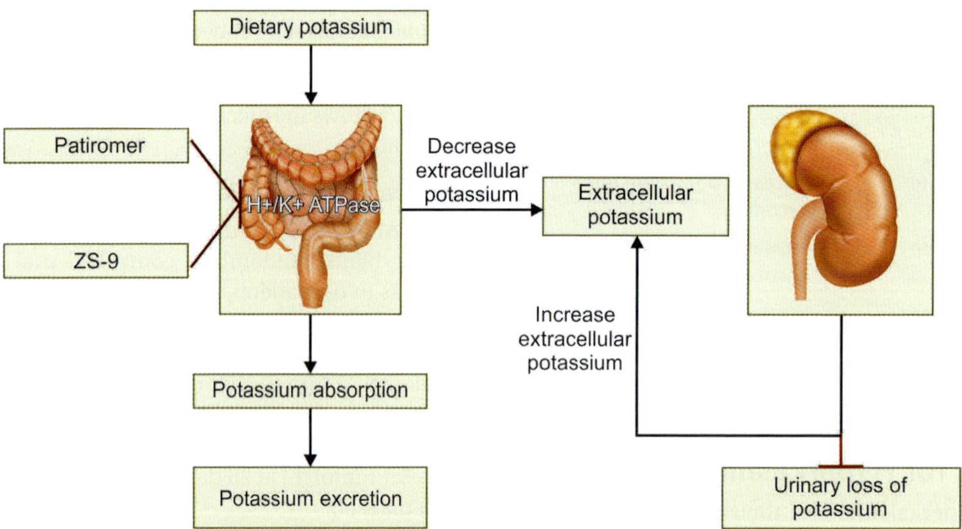

ZS-9, sodium zirconium cyclosilicate; ATPase, adenosine triphosphatase.

FIG. 3: Mechanism of action of sodium zirconium cyclosilicate.

Source: van der Meer P, van Veldhuisen DJ. To bind or not to bind: potassium-lowering drugs in heart failure. Eur Heart J. 2011;32(7):791-2.

phase I clinical study,[20] subjects with established CKD and HF, and with serum potassium levels in the range of 4.3-5.1 mmol/L were given either patiromer (30 g/day) or a placebo. Patiromer significantly reduced serum potassium; this was also demonstrated in patients with CKD.[21] Patiromer was administered in a dose of 8.4 g twice daily for 2 days (at 0, 10, 24, and 34 hours). After 7 hours there was a significant reduction in the mean serum potassium level. Twenty-four hours after the first dose, 80% of subjects had a serum potassium level of less than 5.6 mmol/L in the mild hyperkalemia range. When the fourth and last dose was given after 34 hours, the mean serum potassium was 5.27 mmol/L. The mean serum potassium level continued to decline for 7–10 hours after this last dose.

Phase II and III Studies—The AMETHYST-DN Trial

In this phase II trial,[22] a study was made of the effect of different doses of patiromer on serum potassium levels. All subjects had type 2 diabetes, CKD [estimated GFR (eGFR) 15–<60 mL/min/1.73 m^2] and were taking a RAAS inhibitor (RAASI) before and during the trial. Subjects were stratified into two groups; those with mild hyperkalemia with serum potassium levels 5-5.5 mmol/L and those with moderate hyperkalemia with serum potassium levels 5.6-5.9 mmol/L.

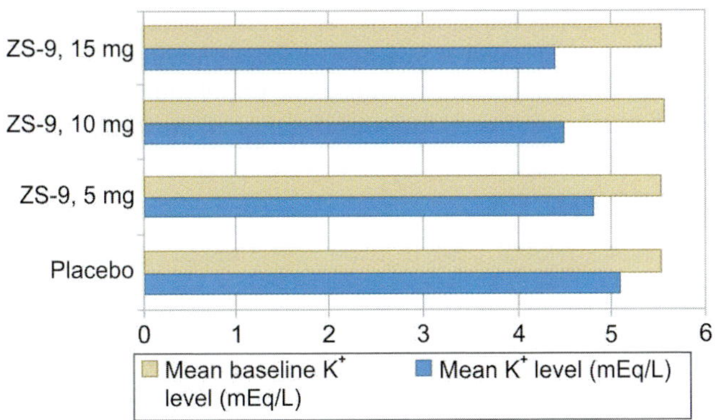

FIG. 4: HARMONIZE trial.

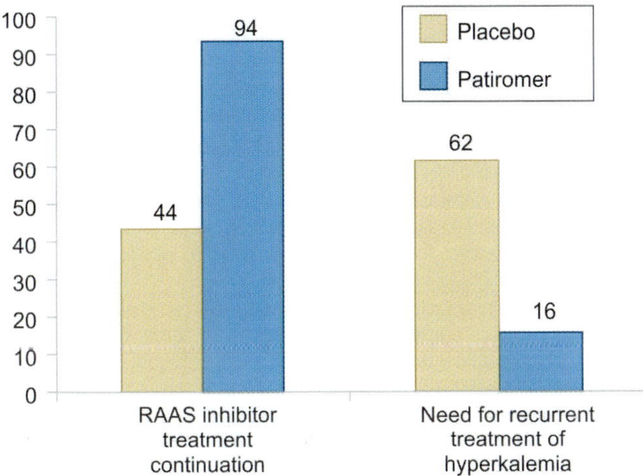

CKD, chronic kidney disease; RAAS, renin–angiotensin–aldosterone system.

FIG. 5: The OPAL-K trial.

Subjects received one of three dosage schedules for 8 weeks. All doses used caused significant reductions in serum potassium levels after 28 days on patiromer. On the basis of these findings the lowest starting doses were chosen. Those with mild hyperkalemia were to receive 8.4 g/day (which caused a fall in serum potassium of 0.35 mmol/L in the first phase) and those with moderate hyperkalemia were to receive 16.8 g/day (which caused a fall in serum potassium of 0.87 mmol/L in the first phase) as starting doses. Subjects then continued on patiromer for a further 44 weeks for a total of 52 weeks on patiromer. From week 4 to week 52, significant ($p < 0.001$) mean decreases from baseline in serum potassium were found at each monthly time point in subjects with mild or moderate hyperkalemia.

The OPAL-K Trials (Fig. 5)

In the OPAL-K study[23,24] the effects of patiromer were studied in patients with CKD. Eligible subjects for the study had to have stage 3 or 4 CKD (eGFR 15–<60 mL/min/1.73 m^2), have a serum potassium level of 5.1–6.4 mmol/L and have been on at least one RAASI for at least 28 days. There were two parts to the OPAL-K study. In the first, a study was made of the effects of patiromer in subjects with CKD.[23] In the second part of the study, the effects of patiromer were examined in subjects with both CKD and HF.[24] In the initial 4-week phase of the OPAL-K study of subjects with CKD,[23] those with mild hyperkalemia (serum potassium, 5.1–6.4 mmol/L) received patiromer 8.4 g/day, while those with moderate-to-severe hyperkalemia (serum potassium, 5.5–6.4 mmol/L) received patiromer 16.8 g/day; these doses were increased if the target potassium level had not been reached or maintained. The mean daily doses actually taken were 12.8 g/day and 21.4 g/day in the mild and moderate hyperkalemia groups. At the end of the initial treatment phase after 4 weeks, the mean potassium level had fallen by 0.65 ± 0.05 mmol/L in the mild hyperkalemia group, and by 1.23 ± 0.04 mmol/L in the moderate hyperkalemia group. After only 2 days, patiromer had caused a fall in serum potassium. After 4 weeks 74% of those in the mild and 77% of those in the moderate-to-severe hyperkalemia groups were in the target serum potassium range (3.8–5 mmol/L).[23] Furthermore, 94% of subjects who continued on patiromer were able to continue taking a RAASI compared to 74% of subjects on a placebo.

In the second OPAL-HK trial (Fig. 6),[24] subjects were studied in two groups in the withdrawal phase; those with HF and those without HF. After the initial phase, subjects were eligible to continue to the randomized withdrawal phase if they had had moderate-to-severe hyperkalemia at baseline (>5.5 mmol/L at baseline), and if they now had a normal serum potassium level (3.8–5.0 mmol/L) after the initial 4 weeks on patiromer, and were still taking an RAASI and had HF. Subjects meeting these criteria were randomly assigned to receive either placebo or to carry on taking patiromer at the same dose as in the previous 4 weeks. At the start of this new phase, the mean serum potassium levels did not differ in these two groups. Subjects continuing on placebo had a mean increase of 0.74 mmol/L in their serum potassium levels, whereas those on patiromer had a mean increase of 0.10 mmol/L in their potassium levels. Those on patiromer were markedly less likely to redevelop hyperkalemia (serum

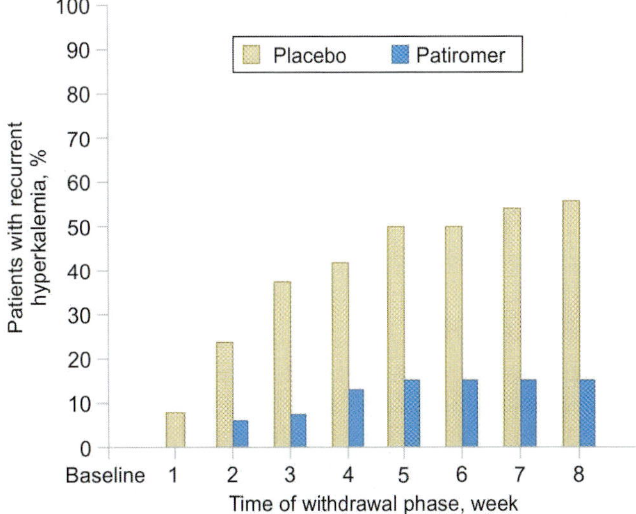

FIG. 6: The OPAL-HK trial.

BOX 1 Adverse effects of patiromer

- Common adverse effects:
  - Constipation (7.2%)
  - Hypomagnesemia (5.3%)
  - Diarrhea (4.8%)
  - Nausea (2.3%)
- Common laboratory abnormalities:
  - Hypomagnesemia <1.4 mg/dL (9%)
  - Hypokalemia <3.5 mEq/L (4.7%)

potassium >5.5 mmol/L) as only 8% had at least one episode of mild or moderate hyperkalemia compared to 52% of those on placebo.

The PEARL-HF Trial

In the PEARL-HF trial,[25,26] the effects of patiromer were studied in subjects with a history of chronic HF. To enter the trial, subjects had to have CKD (eGFR <60 mL/min/1.73 m^2) and be on one or more therapies for HF, or had to have a history of hyperkalemia that had led to the stopping of therapy for HF within the last 6 months. Subjects were randomly assigned to receive either placebo or patiromer (30 g/day). All subjects were also started on spironolactone (25 mg/day). After 14 days the dose of spironolactone was raised to 50 mg/day if their serum potassium level was 3.5–5.0 mmol/L. After 14 days the dose of spironolactone was left unchanged if the potassium level was 5.1–5.5 mmol/L, but spironolactone was stopped if the level was less than 3.5 or more than 5.5 mmol/L. At the start of the trial the mean serum potassium levels of the two groups did not differ significantly. The two groups differed significantly after 48 hours with the serum potassium level being lower in the group receiving patiromer; the difference remained significant thereafter until the end of the trial. After 2 weeks of treatment the group receiving patiromer had a mean serum potassium level that was 0.45 mmol/L lower than those on placebo and this was also the difference after 4 weeks.

Adverse Effects of Patiromer

Box 1 shows adverse effects of patiromer.

Dosage and Administration

The recommended starting dose of patiromer is 8.4 g once daily, monitor the serum potassium level and dose can be increased to maximum up to 25.2 g once daily. It should not be used in emergency life-threatening situation because of slow onset of action. It can be taken with food but food should not be heated. It should not be taken in dry form.

CONCLUSION

Management of CKD, HF, and acute kidney disease is complicated by both acute and chronic hyperkalemia. Use of RAASI in these conditions further aggravate the problem and is challenging. Newer drugs like polymer patiromer sorbitex calcium and ZS-9 showed promise in both as acute remedies and as adjunctive therapies for hyperkalemia, and may allow greater use of ACEIs, ARBs, and mineralocorticoid receptor antagonists in the vulnerable populations who have an especially great need for neurohormonal blockade.

REFERENCES

1. Gilbert S, Weiner D, Gipson D. National Kidney Foundation. Primer on kidney diseases. Philadelphia: Saunders Elsevier; 2014.
2. Einhorn LM, Zhan M, Hsu VD, et al. The frequency of hyperkalemia and its significance in chronic kidney disease. Arch Intern Med. 2009;169(12):1156-62.
3. Emmett M, Hootkins RE, Fine KD, et al. Effect of three laxatives and a cation exchange resin on fecal sodium and potassium excretion. Gastroenterology. 1995;108(3):752-60.
4. Packham DK, Rasmussen HS, Lavin PT, et al. Sodium zirconium cyclosilicate in hyperkalemia. N Engl J Med. 2015;372(3):222-31.
5. Weir MR, Bakris GL, Bushinsky DA, et al. Patiromer in patients with kidney disease and hyperkalemia receiving RAAS inhibitors. N Engl J Med. 2015;372(3):211-21.
6. Veltassa (Patiromer) [package insert]. Redwood City, CA: Relypsa, Inc. 2015.
7. Montaperto AG, Gandhi MA, Gashlin LZ, et al. Patiromer: a clinical review. Curr Med Res Opin. 2016;32(1):155-64.
8. Epstein M, Palmer B, Mayo M, et al. (2015). Mechanism of action of patiromer for oral suspension: increases fecal K+ excretion in healthy volunteers independent of race. [online] Available from http://www.posters2view.eu/wcn2015/view.php?nu=3287 [Accessed August 2018].
9. Kosiborod M, Rasmussen HS, Lavin P, et al. Effect of sodium zirconium cyclosilicate on potassium lowering for 28 days among outpatients with hyperkalemia: the HARMONIZE randomized clinical trial. JAMA. 2014;312(21):2223-33.
10. Center for Drug Evaluation and Research. Clinical pharmacology and biopharmaceutics review(s). [online] Available from https://www.accessdata.fda.gov/drugsatfda_docs/nda/2017/761049Orig1s000ClinPharmR.pdf [Accessed August 2018].
11. US Food and Drug Administration. (2015). FDA drug safety communication: FDA requires drug interaction studies with potassium-lowering drug Kayexalate (sodium polystyrene sulfonate). [online] Available from http://www.fda.gov/Drugs/DrugSafety/ucm468035.htm [Accessed August 2018].
12. Bakris GL, Pitt B, Weir MR, et al. Effect of patiromer on serum potassium level in patients with hyperkalemia and diabetic kidney disease: the AMETHYST-DN randomized clinical trial. JAMA. 2015;314(2):151-61.
13. Pitt B, Anker SD, Bushinsky DA, et al. Evaluation of the efficacy and safety of RLY5016, a polymeric potassium binder, in a double-blind, placebo-controlled study in patients with chronic heart failure (the PEARL-HF) trial. Eur Heart J. 2011;32(7):820-8.
14. Flinn RB, Merrill JP, Welzant WR. Treatment of the oliguric patient with a new sodium-exchange resin and sorbitol; a preliminary report. N Engl J Med. 1961;264:111-5.
15. Nepal M, Bucaloiu ID, Norfolk ER. Hypernatremia in a patient treated with sodium polystyrene sulfonate. Int J Nephrol Renovasc Dis. 2010;3:141-3.
16. Stavros F, Yang A, Leon A, et al. Characterization of structure and function of ZS-9, a K+ selective ion trap. PLoS One. 2014;9(12):e114686.
17. Kosiborod M, Rasmussen HS, Lavin P, et al. Effect of sodium zirconium cyclosilicate on potassium lowering for 28 days among outpatients with hyperkalemia: the HARMONIZE randomized clinical trial. JAMA. 2014; 312(21):2223-33.
18. Huang IZ, Blok T, Burdick M, et al. RLY5016: a novel, non-absorbed, therapeutic polymer for the control of serum potassium. J Am Soc Nephrol. 2010;21:p482A.
19. Cope J, Ciaravino V, Du X, et al. RLY5016: a new, effective, non-absorbed, therapeutic polymer to control serum potassium. J Am Soc Nephrol. 2010;21:Abst F-PO1616.
20. Bushinsky A, Huang IZ, Stefan D, et al. RLY5016: a novel, effective, non-absorbed polymer for the control of serum potassium in heart failure and chronic kidney disease. J Am Soc Nephrol. 2010;21:Abst F-PO1617PO1615.

21. Bushinsky DA, Williams GH, Pitt B, et al. Patiromer induces rapid and sustained potassium lowering in patients with chronic kidney disease and hyperkalemia. Kidney Int. 2015;88(6):1427-33.
22. Bakris GL, Pitt B, Weir MR, et al. Effect of patiromer on serum potassium level in patients with hyperkalemia and diabetic kidney disease: The AMETHYST-DN randomized clinical trial. JAMA. 2015;314(2):151-61.
23. Weir MR, Bakris GL, Bushinsky DA, et al. Patiromer in patients with kidney disease and hyperkalemia receiving RAAS inhibitors. N Engl J Med. 2015;372(3):211-21.
24. Pitt B, Bakris GL, Bushinsky DA, et al. Effect of patiromer on reducing serum potassium and preventing recurrent hyperkalaemia in patients with heart failure and chronic kidney disease on RAAS inhibitors. Eur J Heart Fail. 2015;17(10):1057-65.
25. Pitt B, Anker SD, Bushinsky DA, et al. Evaluation of the efficacy and safety of RLY5016, a polymeric potassium binder, in a double-blind, placebo-controlled study in patients with chronic heart failure (the PEARL-HF) trial. Eur Heart J. 2011;32(7):820-8.
26. Buysse JM, Huang IZ, Pitt B. PEARL-HF: prevention of hyperkalemia in patients with heart failure using a novel polymeric potassium binder, RLY5016. Future Cardiol. 2012;8(1):17-28.

CHAPTER 89

Drug Interactions in Cardiology

Arunangshu Ganguly

INTRODUCTION

With increasingly more drugs, supplements, alternative therapies thronging the armamentarium of medical treatment the interactions between various forms of therapy are gaining increasing importance in field of medicine of which cardiovascular pharmacotherapeutics form an inseparable part. The interactions may potentiate or suppress the various drug effects, can cause harmful consequences or lead to a therapy being ineffective. So, a ready knowledge would be very comforting in choosing the drugs for use in different setting.

When two or more drugs interact to alter the effectiveness or toxicity of one or more drugs, drug-drug interactions (DDI) may be observed.[1-4] In patients receiving multidrug therapy, DDI is a major concern as it leads to an increased risk of hospitalization. Healthcare costs also rise considerably.[5] Besides DDI, food-drug interaction is also an important component of drug interactions. They are caused by food nutrient supplements interacting with drug, such that body is unable to utilize the food or drug. The lack of knowledge about the active ingredients is the most common cause besides inadvertent usage. Alcohol, commonly used herbs and fruits may change the effects of drug causing serious health effects.

INCIDENCE

Actual incidence of DDI is around 1.3%.[6,7] According to few other studies, the incidence is up to 11%. They constitute 2.8% patients admitted to hospital.[8,9] Increased healthcare availability has increased DDI.[10] In a recent study, it was reported that 1% of all the admission to the hospital is caused by DDIs. Adverse drug reactions (ADR), account for 0.6% admissions in hospital, 0.05% of visits to emergency department, and 0.1 % of rehospitalizations.[11,12]

The incidence of cardiovascular disease (CVD) has already reached the top of the charts among all diseases. So, CV drugs are one of the most popularly prescribed drugs in medicine. The drug interactions with CV drugs is more common as the patients are aged, have multiple ailments requiring treatment, hence, polypharmacy is the rule than exception. There is paucity of Indian data as to the incidence of this innocuous yet important happening. However, Mateti et al. reported that clinically important DDI in cardiology patients who have been admitted is 14.66%. Another study in the same setting reported DDI incidence to be 30%.[13] Higher incidence of DDIs was reported in women and elderly men above 60 years. This was supported by others also.[5,14,15]

The maximum DDIs were noted with antiplatelet and anticoagulant drugs around 76.13% and 72.72%, respectively. Drug pairs which are responsible for most DDIs were between heparin and aspirin (37.54%), clopidogrel and heparin (12.5%), clopidogrel and torsemide (12.5%), and heparin and warfarin (9.09%). Bleeding was the most common complication.[16] In a separate study by Sharma et al. from Western Nepal a DDI of 21.3% was noted. Of the drugs that caused most of the interactions were clopidogrel, warfarin, atorvastatin, digoxin, furosemide and enalapril. Most interactions were of moderately severe category.

MECHANISM OF DRUG–DRUG INTERACTION

- Pharmacokinetic interaction—How body treats the drugs
- Pharmacodynamic interaction—What the drug does to your body
- Effect of genetic polymorphism—How the pharmacokinetics vary with it.

Pharmacokinetic Interactions

It depends on drug absorption, drug distribution, and drug metabolism.

- *Drug absorption*: Occurs in mucous membrane of gastrointestinal (GI) tract. Most mechanism leads to decreased absorption. However, one must remain more concerned with rate of absorption. In drugs like oral anticoagulants if the total absorbed dose remains less affected it matters little if the rate of absorption slows down. But in drugs that requires instant action the rate of absorption is important. Changes in gastric pH, adsorption and chelation, gastric motility, inhibition of drug transporter proteins, and malabsorption are the important mechanisms associated with drug absorption. Digoxin is metabolized by P glycoprotein (the most characterized transporter protein). Hence the drugs that induce P-glycoprotein like rifampicin, may decrease the bioavailability of digoxin. Digoxin absorption is also affected by binding agents like cholestyramine. The tricyclic antidepressants increase the absorption of dicoumarol by decreasing gastric motility

- *Drug distribution*: Drug distribution interactions occur mainly through two principles—
  - Protein-binding interactions and
  - Induction or inhibition of drug transport proteins.

Following absorption there is rapid distribution through circulation which may be in plasma dissolved state or bound to plasma proteins. In protein bound state, the degree of displacement, clearance, and excretion ratio determine the augmentation or decrease in drug effects. The importance of this interaction mechanism has been grossly overemphasized.[10] As many drugs which are displaced in *in vitro* interactions are effectively buffered when the same happens *in vivo*. The distribution of drugs into the organs like brain, testis, etc. is limited by actions of P-glycoprotein like drug transporter proteins. Evidence is accumulating that DDI occurs due to interference with the activity of P-glycoprotein. P-glycoproteins are found in some cell membranes. They are responsible in expelling drugs and metabolites from cells. This has an impact on absorption, distribution, and elimination of drugs. The drugs inhibiting the transporters can therefore modify the actions of drugs according to which process the transporter is involved with the drug. For example, if the transporter acts by expunging some already absorbed drugs then its inhibition will increase the quantum of absorption of drugs leading to increased effects. Similarly, drugs like rifampicin which induces the activity of glycoprotein transporter causes vigorous expulsion of drugs like digoxin reducing the serum levels of digoxin in DDI with rifampicin[17-19]

- *Drug metabolism*: Though some drugs are cleared from the body by direct elimination by kidneys, most are metabolized to less lipid soluble entities which are easily eliminated by the kidneys. This chemical change is called "metabolism", "biotransformation", "biochemical degradation", or sometimes "detoxification". Some drug metabolism occurs in serum, kidneys, and skin; however, the major degradation occurs in liver microsomal enzymes. Drug metabolism entails two major reactions:
  - Phase I reactions (which involves oxidation, reduction, hydrolysis), turn drugs into more polar compounds, while
  - Phase II reactions which involve coupling of drugs with some other substances (e.g., glucuronic acid, known as glucuronidation) to make usually inactive compounds.

Most phase 1 oxidation reactions are done by cytochrome P450, a heme-containing enzyme, which comprise of around 30 isoenzymes of which a few specific ISO enzymes of the family is of practical importance being involved in around 90% of the reactions. The most important isoenzymes are: cytochrome P (CYP)1A2, CYP2C9, CYP2C19, CYP2D6, CYP2E1, and CYP3A4. Other enzymes involved in phase I metabolism include monoamine oxidases and epoxide hydrolases. Less is known about the enzymes responsible for phase II conjugation reactions. However, UDP-glucuronyltransferases (UGT), methyltransferases, and N-acetyltransferases (NAT) are examples. Although metabolism is very important in the body removing drugs, it is increasingly recognized that drugs can be adsorbed, distributed, or eliminated by transporters, the most well understood at present being "P-glycoprotein." So, the drug metabolism acts through changes in first-pass metabolism, enzyme induction, enzyme inhibition, and genetic factors like polymorphism. Changes in first-pass metabolism occur by regulating porto hepatic blood flow and/or induction of first-pass metabolism. Polymorphism explains the difference in metabolism of the same drug in different individuals[20-25]

- *Drug excretion interaction*: Drugs are mostly excreted in bile or urine. In renal circulation, the smaller molecules like salts water and some drugs get filtered through the pore of the glomerular membrane into the lumen of the tubules. The larger molecules like plasma proteins, blood cells are retained. The blood then passes through the remaining parts of the kidney where active energy transport mechanism removes drugs and their metabolites from the blood and secretes them into tubular filtrate (Fig. 1).

The drug interactions occur by means of changes in renal blood flow, changes in urinary pH, changes in tubular secretion, and changes in enterohepatic circulation.[26,27]

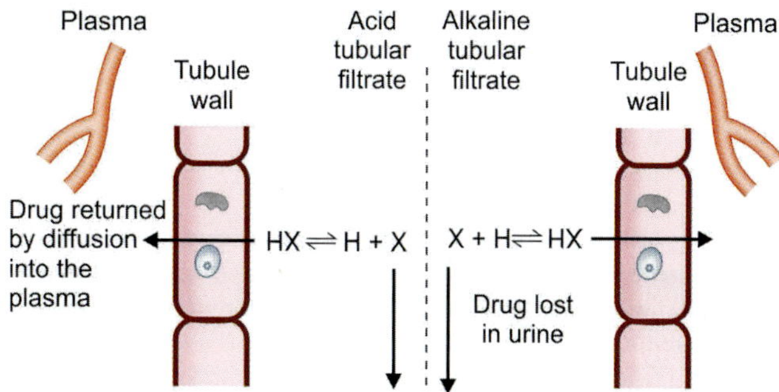

FIG. 1: An excretion interaction. If the tubular filtrate is acidified, most of the molecules of weakly acid drugs (HX) exist in a unionized lipid-soluble form and are able to return through the lipid membranes of the tubule cells by simple diffusion. Thus, they are retained. In alkaline urine most of the drug molecules exist in an ionized nonlipid soluble form (X). In this form the molecules are unable to diffuse freely through these membranes and are therefore lost in the urine.

Pharmacodynamic Interactions

When the effects of one drug are changed by the presence of another drug at its site of action, the interaction is called dynamic interaction. Sometimes the drug directly competes for particular receptors (e.g., β_2 agonists). At other times it is indirect involving physiological processes. These interactions are much less easy to classify neatly than those of a pharmacokinetic type. They are basically of these types: synergistic (additive); antagonistic (opposing); drug or neurotransmitter uptake interactions (Tables 1 and 2).

- *Synergistic*: When drugs with same effect are given together the result is additive. This can occur with main as well as adverse effects. Sometimes effects are solely toxic like—ototoxicity, nephrotoxicity, QT interval prolongation
- *Antagonistic or opposing reactions*: Certain pairs of drugs have activities that are opposed to one another. For example, the coumarins prolong the prothrombin time by competitively inhibiting the effects of dietary vitamin K. If the intake of vitamin K is increased, the effects of the oral anticoagulant are opposed, and the prothrombin time does not increase to produce therapeutic benefits
- *Drug or neurotransmitter uptake reactions*: Presence of other drugs to prevent drugs acting on adrenergic neurons to reach the required sites of action. The tricyclic antidepressants prevent the reuptake of noradrenaline into peripheral adrenergic neurons. Thus, patients taking tricyclics and given parenteral noradrenaline have a markedly increased response (hypertension, tachycardia); similarly, the uptake of guanethidine (and related drugs guanoclor, betanidine, debrisoquine, etc.) is blocked by "chlorpromazine, haloperidol, and thiothixene", a number of "amphetamine-like drugs", so that the antihypertensive effect is prevented. The antihypertensive effects of clonidine are also prevented

TABLE 1: Additive, synergistic, or summation reactions

Drugs	Result of interaction
Antipsychotics + antimuscarinics	Increased antimuscarinic effects; heat stroke in hot and humid Conditions, adynamic ileus, toxic psychoses
Antihypertensives + drugs that cause hypotension (e.g., phenothiazines, and sildenafil)	Increased antihypertensive effects; orthostasis
Beta-agonist bronchodilators + potassium-depleting drugs	Hypokalemia
CNS depressants + CNS depressants Alcohol + antihistamines benzodiazepines + anaesthetics, general opioids + benzodiazepines	Impaired psychomotor skills, reduced alertness, drowsiness, stupor, respiratory depression, coma, and death
Drugs that prolong the QT interval + other drugs that prolong the QT interval Amiodarone + disopyramide	Additive prolongation of QT interval, increased risk of torsade de pointes
Methotrexate + co-trimoxazole	Bone marrow megaloblastosis due to folic acid antagonism
Nephrotoxic drugs + nephrotoxic drugs (e.g., aminoglycosides, ciclosporin, cisplatin, and vancomycin)	Increased nephrotoxicity
Neuromuscular blockers + drugs with neuromuscular blocking effects (e.g., aminoglycosides)	Increased neuromuscular blockade; delayed recovery, prolonged apnea
Potassium supplements + potassium-sparing drugs (e.g., ACE inhibitors, angiotensin II receptor antagonists, potassium-sparing diuretics)	Hyperkalemia

ACE, angiotensin-converting enzyme; CNS, central nervous system.

TABLE 2: Antagonistic or opposing interactions

Drug affected	Interacting drugs	Results of interaction
ACE inhibitors or loop diuretics	NSAIDs	Antihypertensive effects opposed
Anticoagulants	Vitamin K	Anticoagulant effects opposed
Antidiabetics	Glucocorticoids	Blood glucose-lowering effects opposed
Antineoplastics	Megestrol	Antineoplastic effects possibly opposed
Levodopa	Antipsychotics (those with dopamine antagonist effects)	Antiparkinsonian effects opposed
Levodopa	Tacrine	Antiparkinsonian effects opposed

ACE, angiotensin-converting enzyme; NSAIDs, nonsteroidal anti-inflammatory drugs.

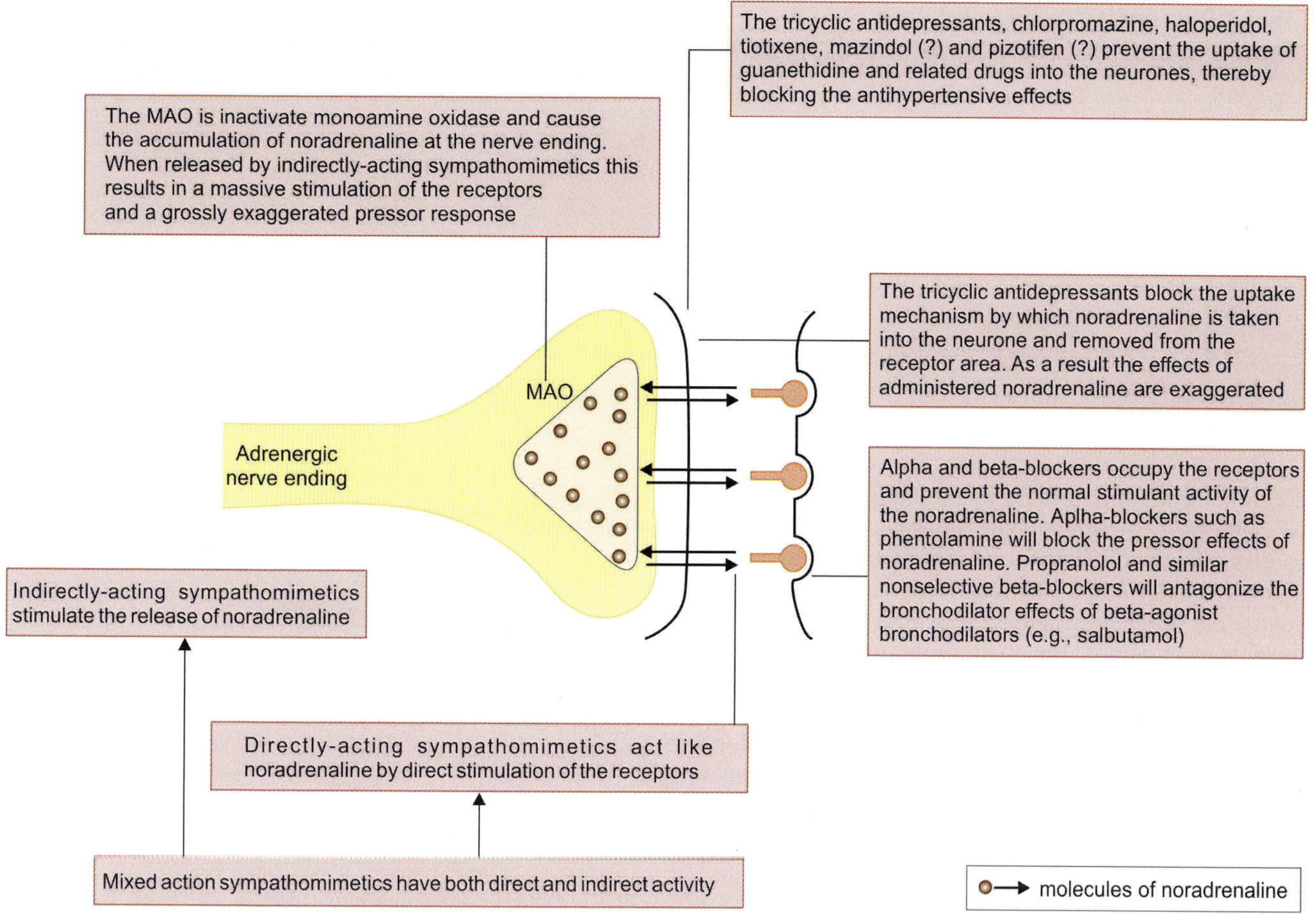

FIG. 2: Interactions at adrenergic neurons.

by the tricyclic antidepressants, one possible reason being that the uptake of clonidine within the central nervous system is blocked. Some of these interactions at adrenergic neurons are illustrated in figure 2.

Some Common Drug–Drug Interactions

Drugs commonly used in cardiology:

- *Antihypertensive*: Angiotensin receptor blockers (ARBs), calcium channel blockers (CCBs), angiotensin-converting enzyme inhibitors (ACEIs), and diuretics
- *Antidyslipidemic*: Statin, nicotinic acid
- *Antiplatelet drug*: Aspirin, glycoprotein IIb/IIIa antagonist
- *Anticoagulants*: Coumadin, heparin
- *Antiarrhythmic*: Amiodarone
- *Antiheart failure*: Beta-blocker, ACEI.

Angiotensin-converting enzyme inhibitor and ARB: Usually do not have very significant interactions with other drugs. Aluminum hydroxide in antacids causes decreased absorption; however, H2 blockers do not have synergistic effects of blood pressure reduction with CCBs and β-blockers. With aspirin; however, there is some controversy. Prostaglandin (PG) inhibition effects are not so prominent in patients who are euvolemic and normotensive. However, it affects the action of all antihypertensive drugs including ACEI in patients having hypertension. ACEI plays a vital role in remodeling of heart and thereby decreases heart failure (HF). The use of aspirin and ACEI together in moderate-to-severe HF patients is detrimental as ACEI actions are suppressed (Hall et al., 2000). But this was countered by Latini et al. (2000). Low-dose aspirin (≤100 mg daily) appears to have little effect. It is not clear if aspirin really attenuates the benefits of ACE in HF. The likelihood of an interaction may depend on disease state and its severity. With diuretics some enhancements of first dose hypotension occur. However, chance of hypokalemia is not totally allied with concomitant use of ACEI and diuretics.

Alpha blockers: Selective α1 blockers in cardiac use are mainly prazosin and doxazosin. With ACEI, β-blockers, and CCBs they have a propensity of accentuated postural hypotension symptoms which need to be explained properly to patients.

Antiarrhythmic: Two arrhythmic of same class are to be cautiously coadministered if obligatory otherwise to be avoided for risk of precipitation of adverse effects. Two class 1 antiarrhythmic drugs prolong QT to precipitate torsade. Similarly, two antiarrhythmic with effects on either sinoatrial node or atrioventricular (AV) node leads to symptomatic bradycardia or increased AV nodal delay leading to syncope.

The effects of adenosine is unduly accentuated if patient is on dipyridamole leading to cardiac arrest, whereas its

TABLE 3: Drug interactions of amiodarone

Drug	Result of interaction
Digoxin	Elevated digoxin plasma concentration
Warfarin	Elevated prothrombin time
Simvastatin	Increased incidence of myopathy when simvastatin dosage is higher than 20 mg per day
Sildenafil	Increased sildenafil plasma concentration
Cyclosporine	Increased cyclosporine plasma concentration
Antiarrhythmic drugs	Additive effects: possible elevated plasma concentrations of quinidine, disopyramide, flecainide, propafenone, and dofetilide
Quinolones	Additive QT effect: possible increased risk of proarrhythmia
Antidepressants	Increased plasma concentration of drugs metabolized in liver: possible increased iisk of proarrhythmia

accentuons are diminished by simultaneous administration of xanthines. So while doing nuclear magnetic imaging studies one must be careful to discontinue xanthines for at least 24 hours prior to the test. Hypotension, bradycardia, ventricular fibrillation, and asystole have been seen in a few patients given amiodarone with propranolol, metoprolol or sotalol due to extreme QT prolongation. However, analysis of clinical trials suggests that the combination can be beneficial. Amiodarone may inhibit the metabolism of β-blockers metabolized by CYP2D6, such as metoprolol, which might be a factor in the interaction (Table 3). Verapamil and β-blockers often cause additive inhibitory action which however is helpful in controlling symptomatic atrial fibrillation with fast ventricular rate and left ventricular dysfunction.

Beta-blockers (especially propranolol and metoprolol) are generally metabolized by first-pass metabolism in liver. So drugs increasing this, like cimetidine and hydralazine, decrease effects of β-blockers.

Anticoagulants: The effects of acenocoumarol and warfarin are enhanced by amiodarone resulting in bleeding. It has been noted that although the maximal effects of interaction occur between 2 and 7 weeks, the effect may last long after withdrawal. Altered (usually enhanced) coumarin response has been reported with virtually every class of antibacterial. While some such as sulfamethoxazole, clearly have a pharmacokinetic interaction, for others there is no clear explanation for which an interaction might be expected. Theoretical mechanisms include reduction in production of vitamin K2 substances by intestinal bacteria or reduced enterohepatic recycling. Possible confounding mechanisms include a reduction in dietary vitamin K1 intake because of illness, or the effect of fever or infection on coagulation or drug metabolism. Cephalosporins and related β-lactams that have caused increases in prothrombin times when used alone, and might therefore be predicted to interact, include aztreonam, cefalotin, cefoperazone, ceftriaxone, and latamoxef. Other cephalosporins with a related side-chain include cefmenoxime, cefmetazole, cefminox, ceforanide, cefotetan, and cefpiramide. The macrolides, linezolid, chloramphenicol on the other hand have little interactions with coumarins. Penicillins and metronidazole report anecdotal cases whereas unpredictable response of increase

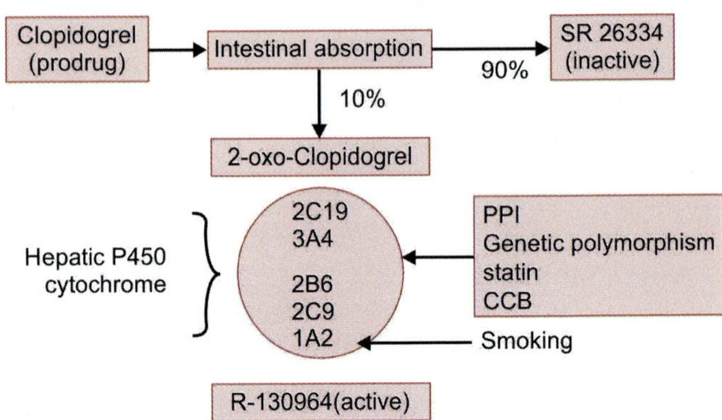

CCB, calcium channel blockers; PPI, proton pump inhibitors.

FIG. 3: Different clopidogrel interactions.

international normalized ratio (INR) may be observed with Quinolones. Rifamycins on the other hand reduce the effects of coumarins and the dose of coumarins may be required to increase 2–5-fold to maintain the INR. Most antidiabetic drugs do not have significant interactions except that older generation sulfonylurea actions are potentiated by coumarins causing hypoglycemia although the same has been rarely reported with newer generation sulfonylureas. Low-dose aspirin (75–325 mg daily) increases the risk of bleeding when given with warfarin by about 1.5–2.5-fold, although, in most studies the absolute risks have been small. The overall benefits of concurrent use outweigh the risks in certain patient groups; however, for some warfarin indications, there is not enough data to assess this. In addition to increased bleeding, high doses of aspirin (4 g daily or more) can increase prothrombin times. Therefore, aspirin is not considered a suitable analgesic or anti-inflammatory drug for those taking oral anticoagulants. However, clopidogrel, ticlopidine, and cilostazol do not have significant interactions with coumarins (Fig. 3). With antifungals, fluconazole and miconazole significantly potentiates actions of coumarins however with itraconazole and voriconazole the incidents are few. Griseofulvin decreases the effects of coumarins. Fibrates enhance the action of coumarins leading to blending complications whereas ezetimibe is neutral in interaction. Heparin may prolong the prothrombin time; therefore a sufficient time interval should be allowed after the last heparin dose in a patient taking a coumarin to obtain a valid prothrombin time. Combined use of nonsteroidal anti-inflammatory drugs (NSAIDs) and coumarin anticoagulants increases the risk of GI hemorrhage. Care is needed with the combination. Some individual NSAIDs also alter the pharmacokinetics of warfarin like benzydamine and coxibs. Studies have suggested that fluvastatin and rosuvastatin can increase warfarin levels and/or effects. Other studies with atorvastatin, lovastatin, pravastatin, and simvastatin suggest that they do not usually significantly alter the effects of warfarin, although cases of bleeding have been seen when these statins were given with coumarins and fluindione. Neither aspirin nor piroxicam altered the pharmacokinetics of fondaparinux, and there was no significant change in bleeding time during concurrent use. In a pharmacodynamic study, the dose of heparin did not need changing when clopidogrel was also given, and the antiplatelet effects of clopidogrel were unaltered. Nevertheless, concurrent use of heparin or low-molecular weight heparins (LMWH) and antiplatelet drugs like clopidogrel and ticlopidine has the potential to increase bleeding risk and increased monitoring would be prudent. The combined use of aspirin with heparin or LMWH slightly increases the risk of hemorrhage. Combined use may be a contributing factor to the very rare complication of epidural or spinal hematoma. The bleeding time was prolonged by the concurrent use of dalteparin and ketorolac in healthy subjects, but not using heparin and ketorolac. Parecoxib did not alter the effect of heparin on activated partial thromboplastin time (aPTT). In a small clinical study, intramuscular ketorolac and subcutaneous enoxaparin appeared not to increase measures of postoperative bleeding when compared with opioids. Cases of spinal hematomas have been reported with concurrent use of heparin or LMWH and NSAIDs. Note that ketorolac may possibly cause serious GI bleeding and in the UK it is considered to be contraindicated in patients taking anticoagulants.

Aspirin: When aspirin and NSAIDs are given together, the effect of aspirin decreases, so, one should use analgesic with caution in HF patients.

Aspirin and ACEI are often coprescribed. Aspirin acts by inhibiting the production of thromboxane A2 (TXA2) and thus prevent the PG activity. The problem is aspirin acts by inhibiting PG production while ACEI needs PGs for its optimal action.

Effect of inhibition of PG is not so pronounced in normotensive and euvolemic subjects. In hypertensive subjects, inhibition of PG hampers the effect of nearly every antihypertensive drug including ACEI. As ACEI is immensely effective in controlling remodeling of heart and thus reduce the HF, concurrent use of aspirin and ACEI in moderate-to-high degree of HF patient will reduce the effect of ACEI (Hall et al., 2000), though it was countered by Latini et al. (2000).

Studies like SOLVD (Studies of Left Ventricular Dysfunction) and CONSENSUS II (the Cooperative New Scandinavian Enalapril Survival Study II) suggested that ACEI response was

TABLE 4: Different CYP3A4 inhibitor drug stratified according to their potency

High	• Antibiotics • Antifungal • Antidepressant	• Clarithromycin, telithromycin, chloramphenicol • Azole • Nefazodone
Moderate	• CCB • Antibiotics • Herbal therapy	• Verapamil, diltiazem • Erythromycin • Grapefruit juice
Unspecified potency	• Amiodarone • Ciprofloxacin • Norfloxacin • Dithiocarbamate	–

CCB, calcium channel blockers.

TABLE 5: Profile of reports of rhabdomyolysis associated with selected statins

Statin	Frequency of reports	Unique cases	No. of cases associated with potentially interacting drugs (n)	
Simvastatin	321	215	• Fusidic acid (1) • Fibrates (33) • Cyclosporine (31) • Warfarin (12) • Macrolide antibi otics (10) • Digoxin (9)	• Azole antifungals (4) • Chlorzoxazone (2) • Nefazodone (2) • Niacin (2) • Tacrolimus (1)
Cerivastatin	231	192	• Fibrates (22) • Digoxin (7) • Warfarin (6) • Macrolide antibiotics (2) • Cyclosporine (1)	–
Lovastatin	51	40	• Cyclosporine (12) • Macrolide antibiotics (2) • Azole antifungals (6) • Fibrates (5)	• Digoxin (2) • Nefazodone (2) • Niacin (1) • Warfarin (I)

attenuated when used simultaneously with aspirin. So low-dose aspirin or short-term aspirin, other antiplatelet agents like clopidogrel, etc. were suggested by Peterson and Laurer (2011) as methods to prevent this conflict.

Statins: Commonly exert their lipid lowering action by decreasing the functions of HMG-CoA (3-hydroxy-3-methyl-glutaryl-coenzyme A) reductase enzyme which modulates a principal rate-limiting step in cholesterol biosynthesis.

How statin problems supposedly occur:

- Statins are transported to liver via the enzyme organic anion-transporter polypeptide 1 B1 (OATP1B1) which is encoded by the gene *SLCO1B1* (solute carrier organic anion transporter family, member 1B1). Now even if there is a single nucleotide polymorphism in the encoding gene stain transport to liver is hampered leading to increased statins in blood causing rhabdomyolysis
- The CYP isoenzymes in liver metabolize most of the statins like simvastatin, atorvastatin, mevastatin and lovastatin. The statins like fluvastatin and rosuvastatin are metabolized by CYP2C19 and CYP2C9. Pravastatin is the only statin metabolized through non-CYP pathway. When CYP3A4 inhibitor is used simultaneously with simvastatin rhabdomyolysis occurs (Rowan et al., 2010) (Tables 4 and 5). Although, in case of other statins using the same pathway there is no data however the same caution should be maintained for atorvastatin, lovastatin, and mevastatin.

  Measures to be taken:
- To rule out statin toxicity, genetic testing is usually not required
- If one has to us CYP3A4 inhibitor statin therapy should stop. If statins are required to be used then rosuvastatin or pravastatin should be used.

Clopidogrel: Only 10% of total infused clopidogrel is absorbed in system and then they are metabolized into active form by several P450 group of enzymes, e.g., CYP2C19, CYP1A2, CYP2B6, and CYP3A4. Worsening of pharmacokinetic response of clopidogrel is a common problem. The various postulations to predict:

- Poor metabolism of clopidogrel may be due to polymorphism in CYP219 enzyme. This is accepted in epidemiological studies. A single nucleotide polymorphisms (SNP) CYP2C19*2 (or 681 G>A) can cause an increased risk of major adverse cardiovascular events (MACE) in the follow up [relative risk (RR): 1.96 (1.14–3.37); p = 0.02). In the studies where stent thrombosis was evaluated (n = 4, total patients = 4,975), there was increased risk where the variant allele was present. [RR: 3.82 (2.23–6.54); p = 0.0001] (Sofi et al., 2011)
- Clopidogrel uses CYP3A4 enzyme for its metabolism. Stains and CCBs compete with clopidogrel for metabolism by the same enzyme. Hence, they reduce the activity of both statins and CCBs (Clarke et al., 2003; Jolanta et al., 2008). However, epidemiological studies by Mukherjee et al. in 2205; Saw et al. in 2007; and Schmidt et al. in 2011 show that there is no competitive interaction between clopidogrel and statin
- There was a remarkable interaction with smoking. Smoking increases the activity of CYP1A2 and hence increases the metabolism of clopidogrel. Since clopidogrel is a prodrug, the increased metabolism increases the utility of clopidogrel. Although some epidemiological studies by Jae Kean Ryu, 2010 and Berger et al., 2009, agree to this hypothesis but there are other studies like Sibbald et al. in 2010 which contradict it
- The interaction of proton pump inhibitors (PPI) and clopidogrel is a bit elaborate. PPI gets metabolized through CYP3A4 whereas clopidogrel uses CYP2C19. So as such they do not interact with each other. However, when they are taken with grapefruit juice, the juice uses CYP3A4 for its metabolism and displaces PPI to be metabolized by CYP2C19. This diminishes the clopidogrel response. Similarly, when St John's Wort is taken it induces both the enzymes—CYP3A4 and CYP2C19 and so when PPI's, clopidogrel and St John's Wort are taken together significant drug interactions occur.

  Measures to be taken:
- Due to significant interactions on concomitant usage, grapefruit juice and St John's wort should not be taken along with clopidogrel and PPI
- Similarly as there is no definite data to support statin and clopidogrel interaction; they can be coadministered. However, in high-risk patients one may avoid this. In that case a non-CYP statin like pravastatin or a different antiplatelet like prasugrel may be used instead
- When CCBs and clopidogrel are simultaneously administered their response should be closely monitored and in case there is a possible interaction ongoing, any alternative molecule may be used.

Drug Food Interactions

Interaction between cardiac drugs and food occur mainly with grapefruit juice, monoamine oxidase inhibitors, antihypertensive and warfarin/acitrom, i.e., coumarin derivatives (Table 6).

TABLE 6: Food-drug interaction

Drug	Food	Interactions
Warfarin	High protein diet	Decrease INR raising serum albumin
	Green leafy vegetables	Decrease INR
	Vegetables containing vitamin K	Decrease INR
	Charbroiled	Decrease INR
	Cooked onions	Increase INR
	Cranberry juice	Increase INR without bleeding in elderly
Propranolol	Rich protein food	Increase serum levels
Celiprolol	Orange juice	Intestinal absorption inhibited
ACEIs	Empty stomach	Increase absorption
CCBs	Grapefruit juice	Increase bioavailability

ACEIs, angiotensin-converting enzyme inhibitors; CCB, calcium channel blockers; INR, international normalized ratio.

REFERENCES

1. Hartshorn EA. Handbook of Drug Interactions. Hamilton, Illinois: Drug Intelligence Publications; 1973.
2. Peterson JF, Bates DW. Preventable medication errors: Identifying and eliminating serious drug interactions. J Am Pharma Assoc. 2001;41:159-60.
3. Ray WA, Murray KT, Meredith S, et al. Oral erythromycin and the risk of sudden death from cardiac causes. N Engl J Med. 2004;351:1089-96.
4. Jonsson AK, Spigset O, Jacobson I, et al. Cerebral haemorrhage induced by warfarin - the influence of drug-drug interactions. Pharmaco Drug Safety. 2007;16:309-15.
5. Hamilton RA, Briceland LL, Andritz, MH. Frequency of hospitalization after exposure to known drug-drug interaction in a medical population. Pharmacotherapy. 1998;18:112-20.
6. Kurfees JF, Dotson RL. Drug interactions in elderly. J Fam Pract. 1987;25:477-88.
7. Ho YF, Huang SH, Lin HN. Detecting drug-drug interactions in medication profiles of psychiatric inpatients: A two stage approach. J Formosan Med Assoc. 2002;101:294-7.
8. Grymonpre RE, Mitenko PA, Sitar DS, et al. Drugs-associated hospital admissions in older medical patients. J Am Geriatr Soc. 1988;36:1092-8.
9. Jankel CA, Speedie SM. Detecting drug interactions: A review of the literature. DICP. 1990;24:982-9.
10. Jankel CA, McMillan JA, Martin BC. Effect of drug interactions on outcomes of patients receiving warfarin or theophylline. Am J Hosp Pharm. 1994;51:661-6.
11. Pirmohamed M, James S, Meakin S, et al. Adverse drug reactions as cause of admission to hospital: Prospective analysis of 18820 patients. BMJ. 2004;329:15-29.
12. Becker ML, Kallewaard M, Caspers PW, et al. Hospitalization and emergency department visits due to drug-drug interactions: A literature review. Pharmaco Drug Saf. 2007;16:641-51.
13. Mateti UV, Rajakannan T, Nekkanti H, et al. Drug-drug interactions in hospitalized cardiac patients. J Young Pharmacists. 2011;3:329-33.
14. Bjorkman IK, Fastbom J, Schmidt IK, et al. Drug-drug interactions in the elderly. Ann Pharmacother. 2002;36:1675-81.
15. Kohler G, Bode-Boger S, Busse R, et al. Drug-drug interactions in medical patients: Effect of in-hospital treatment and relation to multiple drug use. Int J Clin Pharmacol Ther. 2000;38:504-13.
16. UK National Patient Safety Agency. Risk assessment of anticoagulants the-rapy.Available from: http://www.npsa.nhs.uk/site/media/docouments/1773_anticoagulantreport.pdf.
17. MacKichan JJ. Protein binding drug displacement interactions: Fact or fiction? Clin Pharmacokinet. 1989;16:65-73.
18. Sansom LN, Evans AM. What is the true clinical significance of plasma protein binding displacement interactions? Drug Safety. 1995;12:227-33.
19. Benet LZ, Hoener B-A. Changes in plasma protein binding have little clinical relevance. Clin Pharmacol Ther. 2002;71:115-21.
20. Phillips KA, Veenstra DL, Oren E, et al. Potential role of pharmacogenomics in reducing adverse drug reactions: A systematic review. JAMA. 2001;286:2270-9.
21. Bjornsson TD, Callaghan JT, Einolf HJ, et al. The conduct of in vitro and in vivo drug-drug interaction studies: A PhRMA perspective. J Clin Pharmacol. 2003;43:443-69.
22. Bachmann KA, Ghosh R. The use of in vitro methods to predict in vivo pharmacokinetics and drug interactions. Curr Drug Metab. 2001;2:299-314.
23. Yao C, Levy RH. Inhibition-based metabolic drug–drug interactions: Predictions from in vitro data. J Pharm Sci. 2002;91:1923-35.
24. Worboys PD, Carlile DJ. Implications and consequences of enzyme induction on preclinical and clinical drug development. Xenobiotica. 2001;31:539-56.
25. Venkatakrishnan K, von Moltke LL, Obach RS, et al. Drug metabolism and drug interactions: Application and clinical value of in vitro models. Curr Drug Metab. 2003;4:423-59.
26. Lee W, Kim RB. Transporters and renal drug elimination. Annu Rev Pharmacol Toxicol. 2004;44:137-66.
27. Faber KN, Müller M, Jansen PLM. Drug transport proteins in the liver. Adv Drug Deliv Rev. 2003;55:107-24.

CHAPTER 90

Unsuspected Drug Toxicity in Cardiology Practice

Ashish Tiwari, Sharad Chandra

INTRODUCTION

Cardiotoxicity is the occurrence of damage of myocardium cell leading to cardiac dysfunction. The heart becomes weaker and less efficient in pumping and therefore circulating blood to different part of body. Cardiotoxicity may be caused by chemotherapy and other drug treatment, complications from anorexia nervosa, adverse effects of heavy metals intake, or an incorrectly administered drug such as bupivacaine. Cardiotoxicity, if severe, leads to cardiomyopathy which is a serious disease in which the heart muscle becomes inflamed and lead to dysfunction of same.

CARDIOTOXICITY OF CYTOTOXIC DRUGS

Cardiotoxicity is a side effect of several cytotoxic drugs, mainly of the anthracyclines, can lead to long-term morbidity. The mechanism of toxicity in case of anthracyclines seems to involve the formation of free radicals leading to oxidative stress. This may cause apoptosis of cardiac cells or immunologic reactions. Cardiac protection can be achieved by limitation of the cumulative dose. Cytotoxic drugs causing cardiotoxicity includes anthracyclines, trastuzumab and HER2 agents, cyclophosphamide, bleomycin, vinca alkaloids, 5-fluorouracil, interferons, interleukins, paclitaxel, bortezomib and other cytotoxic drugs are associated with cardiotoxicity as well although little is known about the possible mechanisms.

Among all cytotoxic drugs, anthracyclines has a prominent role in treating many malignancies. All anthracyclines are cardiotoxic though their relative cardiotoxicity varies with different drugs (Doxorubicin > epirubicin > idarubicin > liposomal doxorubicin in that order).

There are three mechanisms which are involved in the cytotoxic action of anthracyclines—(1) high affinity binding to DNA (via nucleic intercalation causing inhibition of DNA and RNA synthesis and cleavage of DNA strands by alterations of topoisomerase II); (2) binding to the cell membrane which alters its normal fluidity and transport of ions semiquinonic; and (3) oxygen free radical production (via reduction of enzymatic reaction).

Incidence of anthracycline cardiotoxicity ranges from 5 to 65% of treated cases, in relation to the total dose of drugs administered and over the duration of follow-up. Pathophysiological mechanism of drug toxicity includes formation of oxygen free radicals, calcium overload in myocytes, deficiency of antioxidant systems as catalase and superoxide dismutase and possible immunological reaction induced by the drug.[1]

Clinical feature of anthracycline cardiotoxicity manifests as congestive heart failure (CHF) which includes pulmonary edema, fluid overload and dyspnea on exertion. Patient can be minimally symptomatic in form of tachypnea to severely symptomatic like in pulmonary edema.

Apart from cardiomyopathy, other cardiovascular (CV) complications of cancer therapy include systemic hypertension, pulmonary hypertension, pericardial disease, thromboembolism, QT prolongation and dysrhythmias. In fact, hypertension is commonest CV comorbidity seen in cancer registry. Anticancer drugs causing hypertension are mainly vascular endothelial growth factor (VEGF) inhibitors (bevacizumab, sorafenib and sunitinib) and proteasome inhibitors (carfilzomib). Dasatinib, which is used for chronic myeloid leukemia, causes pulmonary hypertension in estimated 0.45% of cases. Drugs associated with pericardial disease include cyclophosphamide, anthracyclines, cytarabine, imatinib, dasatinib, interferon-α, docetaxel and 5-fluorouracil. Chemotherapy causing thromboembolism includes thalidomide and lenalidomide, cisplatin, bevacizumab and everolimus (Tables 1 and 2).

Types of Cardiotoxicity

Acute or Subacute Cardiotoxicity

Alteration of ventricular repolarization phase, duration of QT, arrhythmias, acute heart failure (HF), myocarditis-pericarditis like syndrome.

TABLE 1: Anticancer agents associated with hypertension

Chemotherapy agents	Frequency	Incidence (%)	Comments of Use
Monoclonal antibody-based tyrosine kinase inhibitors			**Pretreatment risk assessment**
Bevacizumab	+++	4–35	BP goal <140/90 mm Hg
Ado-trastuzumab emtansine	+	5.1	
Monoclonal antibodies			
Alemtuzumab	+	14	Weekly BP monitoring in 1st cycle
Ibritumomab	NA	7	Every 2–3 weeks BP monitoring for duration of therapy
Ofatumumab	+	5–8	
Rituximab	+++	6–12	
mTOR inhibitors			
Everolimus	++++	4–13	Initiate BP treatment when diastolic BP increases by 20 mm Hg
Temsirolimus	++	7	
Small molecule tyrosine kinase inhibitors			
Pazopanib	++++	42	More than 1 anti-HTN medication may be needed
Ponatinib	+	68	
Sorafenib	++++	7–43	Avoid diltiazem and verapamil with sorafenib
Sunitinib	++++	5–24	
Axitinib	++++	4	Hold chemotherapy as the last resort
Cabozantinib	NA	33–61	
Ibrutinib	++++	17	
Nilotinib	++++	10–11	Hold bevacizumab if systolic BP >160 mm Hg or diastolic
Ramucirumab	+	16	
Regorafenib	++++	30 59	BP >100 mm Hg
Trametinib	++++	15	
Vandetanib	NA	33	Early consultation with cardiologist
Ziv-aflibercept	+	41	
Proteasome inhibitors			
Bortezomib	++	6	
Carfilzomib	++	11-17	
Antimetabolites			
Decitabine	++	6	

Frequency of use was determined using inpatient and outpatient doses dispensed at MD Anderson Cancer Center during the time period of January 1, 2014 through December 21, 2014.

Key: + = <1,000 doses dispensed; ++ = 1,000–5,000 doses dispensed; +++ = 5,000–10,000 doses dispensed

BP, blood pressure; HTN, hypertension; mTOR, mammalian target of rapamycin.

Chronic Cardiotoxicity

Asymptomatic left ventricular dysfunction (LVD), systolic and/or diastolic dysfunction, severe form of dilated cardiomyopathy, cardiac death.

Symptoms of Cardiac Toxicity

Symptoms of cardiotoxicity includes feature of HF like shortness of breath on exertion, worsening to shortness of breath at rest, discomfort lying on your back, swelling of the ankles and fatigue. As the disease progresses, condition deteriorates and can lead to pulmonary edema and shock. Cardiomyopathy has a high mortality and morbidity.

Prevention of Cardiac Toxicity

Heart problems may be prevented by altering the amount of drug administered (dose), method of administration and type of anthracycline. Also, some medications that can prevent damage from doxorubicin have been developed. Cardiac toxicity can often be prevented by giving less of the cancer drug or the schedule of the drug can be changed

TABLE 2: Anticancer agents associated with QT prolongation

Chemotherapy agents	Frequency	Incidence (%)	Comments of use
Histone deacetylase inhibitors	+	4–11	Tangent method of QT measurement
Belinostat	++++	3.5–6.0	–
Vorinostat	–	–	Fridericia correction formula
Chemicals Arsenic trioxide	++	26–93	–
Small molecule tyrosine kinase	Inhibitors	–	–
Dabrafenib	++++	2–13	Correct low K or Mg
Dasatinib	++++	<1–3	–
Lapatinib	++++	10–16	Remove QTc prolonging medications
Nilotinib	++++	<1–10	QTc >500 ms or >60 ms above baseline associated with TdP
Vandetanib	++++	8–14	–
BRAF inhibitor	–	–	–
Vemurafenib	++++	3	TdP reported fore arsenic trioxide, sunitinib, pazopanib, vandetanib, and vemurafenib

See table 1 for frequency of use description.
K, potassium; Mg, magnesium; Qtc, corrected QT interval; TdP, torsades de pointes.

so that you get lower doses more often (rather than larger doses less often). There are also forms of drugs that may be less toxic, for example, liposomal anthracyclines might have less cardiac toxicity than regular anthracyclines. Various agents and strategies have been tried over the years for cardioprotection which includes antioxidants, free radical scavenger, cardioselective β-blocker, statins, and modified anthracycline preparation (liposomal doxorubicin). Some of these are effective like modified anthracycline preparation, dexrazoxane, enalapril, candesartan, and β-blocker, while others like N-acetylcysteine and calcium antagonist did not show any improvement in trials.

Unsuspected Drugs Causing Cardiotoxicity (Other than Cytotoxic Drugs)

Analgesics

Nonsteroidal anti-inflammatory drugs (NSAIDs) are among the most commonly prescribed over-the-counter (OTC) medicine prescribed all over world. Traditional NSAIDs have the potential to trigger HF through sodium and water retention, increased systemic vascular resistance and blunted response to diuretics. Observational studies suggest an association between traditional NSAIDs use and HF precipitation and exacerbation. In an evaluation of 7,277 long-term NSAID users over 72 months, the Rotterdam study results found a trend to an increased risk of HF.[2-5]

Anesthetic Medications

Inhalational or volatile anesthetics (desflurane, enflurane, halothane, isoflurane, and sevoflurane) can cause myocardial depression, peripheral vasodilation, and attenuated sympathetic activity with immediate effect. Intravenous anesthetics like ketamine and propofol are associated with negative inotrope effect, while Dexmedetomidine is associated with alpha-2 adrenergic agonist action.[6]

Diabetes Mellitus Medication

As diabetes mellitus remains a major problem in most of the world and commonly associated with coronary artery disease (CAD) patients, side effects of these medications sometimes lead to adverse cardiac effects. Thiazolidinediones are associated with possible calcium channel blocker (CCB), metformin is associated with elevated lactic acid level and increased anaerobic metabolism. Recently dipeptidyl peptidase-4 inhibitors are also associated with HF.[6]

Cardiac Effects of Glitazones

Nissen et al. published meta-analysis in 2007 suggested 64% increase in death from CV cause and 43% increase in myocardial infarction (MI) after use of rosiglitazone. This meta-analysis has led to box warning and restricted access to rosiglitazone in the United States.[7] However, later on further meta RECORD (Rosiglitazone Evaluated for Cardiovascular Outcomes and Regulation of Glycemia in Diabetes) trial and later on Food and Drug Administration stated that was not associated with excess CV risk. Recent data suggests that glitazones are relatively safe.[8]

Antiarrhythmic Medication

Antiarrhythmic medication can itself have cardiotoxic effects. Class I antiarrhythmics have negative inotrope and proarrhythmic effects. Sotalol, which is a class III agent, has proarrhythmic property and β-blocker property.[6]

Antihypertensive Medications

Among antihypertensive drugs, calcium channel blockers have negative inotropic effect while α_1 blockers can stimulate β_1 receptors with increase in renin and aldosterone.[6]

TABLE 3: Drugs causing prolong QT

Antipsychotics	Antiarrhythmics	Tricyclic antidepressents	Other antidepressents	Antihistamines	Others
Chlorpromazine	Quinidine	Amitriptyline	Mianserin	Diphenhydramine	Quinine
Haloperidol	Procainamide	Doxepin	Citalopram	Astemizole	Chloroquine
Droperidol	Disopyramide	Imipramine	Escitalopram	Loratadine	Hydroxychloroquine
Quetiapine	Flecainide	Nortriptyline	Venlafaxine	Terfenadine	Erythromycin
Olanzapine	Encainide	Desipramine	Bupropion	–	Ranolazine
Amisulpride	Sotalol	–	Moclobemide	–	–
Thioridazine	Amiodarone	–	–	–	–

Antifungal Medicines

Itraconazole, a commonly used antifungal medicine has negative inotropic action and should be cautiously used in patient with LVD. Amphotericin B can cause LVD on prolong use but function generally improves after discontinuation of drugs.[6]

Hematological Medication

Anagrelide can cause inhibition of phosphodiesterase-4 while cilostazol causes inhibition of phophodiesterase-3 resulting in arrhythmias. Cilostazol is contraindicated in HF patient.

Neurological and Antipsychiatry Medication

Among the antiepileptics, carbamazepine has negative inotropic and chronotropic action. It also depresses phase 2 repolarization and suppresses sinus node automaticity and atrioventricular conduction. Pregabalin causes L-type CCB which leads to negative inotropic action.

In antidepressent group of medication, citalopram causes dose-dependent QT prolongation, while tricyclic antidepressants have negative inotropic and proarrhythmic properties. Antimigrainal medicines like ergotamine and methysergide causes valvular damge due to excessive serotonin activity. Lithium which is commonly used in bipolar disorders can cause direct myofibril degeneration and adrenergic stimulation.[6]

Urological Agents

Urological agents like tamsulosin, doxazosin, and prazosin causes beta-1 receptor stimulation with increase in renin and aldosterone.

Cardiac Effects of Antiretroviral Drugs

Premature atherosclerosis is a known complication of highly active antiretroviral therapy (HAART) mainly related to use of protease inhibitor component. HAART therapy can lead to dyslipidemia, insulin resistance and risk of diabetes, Lipodystrophy and increased risk of MI. Among all deaths in HIV patients, CV death attributes to more than 10% and this further increases if exposure to HAART prolongs. Large studies showed that protease inhibitors are associated with increased risk of MI while nucleoside reverse transcriptase inhibitors (NRTI) and non-nucleoside reverse transcriptase inhibitor (NNRTI) are not. Despite all these effects of HAART, CV events can be controlled up to certain extent by tight control of metabolic derangement. So comprehensive evaluation of the absolute coronary risk of HIV patients before starting antiretroviral therapy is strongly advisable.[9]

Drugs Causing Prolong QT

These are listed in table 3.

CONCLUSION

Cardiotoxicity is a well-known side effect of many drugs including cytotoxic drugs. Apart from cytotoxic drugs where cardiotoxicity is common, drugs like analgesic, anesthetics, antiarrhythmics, antifungal medicines, hematological and neurological medicines can also cause cardiotoxicity. Cardiotoxicity presentation may vary from entirely asymptomatic patient to severely symptomatic HF. Hence, all cardiotoxic drugs should be judiciously used for the indicated purpose.

REFERENCES

1. McGowan JV, Chung R, Maulik A, et al. Anthracycline Chemotherapy and Cardiotoxicity. Cardiovasc Drugs Ther. 2017;31(1):63-75.
2. Feenstra J, Heerdink ER, Grobbee DE, et al. Association of nonsteroidal anti-inflammatory drugs with first occurrence of heart and with relapsing heart failure: The Rotterdam Study. Arch Intern Med. 2002;162:265-70.
3. Heerdink ER, Leufkens HG, Herings RM, et al. NSAIDs associated with increased risk of congestive heart failure in elderly patients taking diuretics. Arch Intern Med. 1998;158:1108-12.
4. Page J, Henry D. Consumption of NSAIDs and the development of congestive heart failure in elderly patients: an underrecognized public health problem. Arch Intern Med. 2000;160:777-84.
5. Huerta C, Varas-Lorenzo C, Castellsague J, et al. Non-steroidal anti-inflammatory drugs and risk of first hospital admission for heart failure in the general population. Heart. 2006;92:1610-5.
6. Page RL 2nd, O'Bryant CL, Cheng D, et al. Drugs That May Cause or Exacerbate Heart Failure: A Scientific Statement from the American Heart Association. Circulation. 2016;134(6):e32-69.
7. Nissen SE, Wolski K. Effect of rosiglitazone on the risk of myocardial infarction and death from cardiovascular causes. N Engl J Med. 2007;356(24): 2457-71.
8. Hiatt WR, Kaul S, Smith RJ. The cardiovascula safety of diabetes drugs--insights from the rosiglitazone experience. N Engl J Med. 2013;369(14):1285-7.
9. Filardi PP, Paolillo S, Marciano C, et al. Cardiovascular effects of antiretroviral drugs: clinical review. Cardiovasc Hematol Disord Drug Targets. 2008;8(4): 238-44.

SECTION 13

Heart Failure

CHAPTER 91

Heart Failure in India

Sandeep Seth, Karishma Landge

HEART FAILURE IN INDIA IS REACHING EPIDEMIC PROPORTIONS

Heart failure (HF) affects 26 million people worldwide and the burden of HF in India is about 1% of the population which comes to about 5–10 million patients. The rural community could have a lower burden and an actual survey found the HF prevalence about 1.2 per 1,000 adult population. The mortality is also high with almost one-third patients getting readmitted or dying soon after an acute HF event. Indian patients are younger, sicker and get less medication as compared to what is recommended by the guidelines.[1-12]

CAUSES

Estimates suggest that the causes of HF contributing to this large number include rheumatic heart disease (13–52%), ischemic heart disease (27–55%), hypertension (6–23%), dilated cardiomyopathy (10%) and congenital heart disease (6%).[13-15] A study from a rural community which screened for symptomatic HF,[14] shortness of breath with or without pedal edema, found a prevalence of 1.2 per 1,000 population after screening an adult population of about 10,000 villagers and the causes were uncontrolled hypertension or ischemic heart disease.[14] Hospital registries show a higher number of rheumatic heart disease. About 20% of the patients coming to cardiology outpatient departments (OPDs) have HF and the causes are more equally distributed between rheumatic heart disease and ischemic heart disease.[13-23]

SEVERITY OF DISEASE

The mortality is 20–30% over 6 months[24-26] (after an episode of acute decompensation) and use of guideline-based medical therapy is only 25–50%.[16,25]

In the Trivandrum Heart Failure Registry,[15,16] one of three HF patients died within 1 year of follow-up. They had taken patients of two groups, one with ejection fraction (EF) less than 45% and the other with EF more than 45% with most common etiology being ischemic heart disease, hypertension, chronic kidney disease (CKD), diabetes mellitus (DM), and stroke. Among 1,103 participants, 269 patients were readmitted once, 64 of them were readmitted more than once, and 75 of them underwent invasive procedure. One out of every three HF patients died and the cause of death was determined by verbal autopsy, i.e., patient who died prior to reach hospital and the patients who died within 24 hours of hospital admission were considered to be sudden cardiac death. And the participants who died in hospital after 24 hours of admission with required inotropic support were considered to have died with cardiogenic shock. The increased mortality in India is due to lack of optimal guideline-based medical treatment and increased hospital readmissions. According to the data 30% HF with reduced EF (HFrEF) patients received appropriate medication i.e., angiotensin-converting enzyme inhibitor or angiotensin receptor blocker (ACEI/ARB) and beta-blockers. (These medications are underused in India despite having scientific evidence which shows reduction in hospitalization and mortality in HF patients, due to lack of postdischarge transitional care and also due to lack of electronic medical records, nonexistent outpatient record keeping, and also difficulty in engaging physicians due to a hectic schedule.

The International Congestive Heart Failure (INTER-CHF)[26] study enrolled patients from rural parts of India, with history of hypertension 29%, DM 8%, CKD and 50% participants of left ventricular ejection fraction (LVEF) less than 40% and the cause of HF was ischemia 39%, hypertension 17%, idiopathic dilated cardiomyopathy 12% and primary valve disease 11% out of which 66% patients were from outpatient and 34% were inpatient. Of the 858 deaths within 1 year, the cardiac deaths were 46%, noncardiac deaths were 16% and unknown causes 38%. The all-cause mortality within 1 year was 16.5% with a mean age of 59 years. The study done in 16 different countries with total number of patients being 5,823 and overall mortality was Africa 34%, India 23%, Southeast Asia 15%, Middle East 9%, and China 7%. The highest mortality was seen in Africa and India.

In the Acute Failure Registry (AFAR) study from All India Institute of Medical Sciences (AIIMS),[25] almost one-third of the patients died during the hospital admission and after discharge, over the next 3–6 months, another one-third either died or got readmitted. From this, we developed the Rule of Three, i.e., in acute HF, one-third die in hospital, at discharge one-third will have an event within 3 months. This study reports a higher in-hospital and follow-up mortality rates in acute decompensated heart failure (ADHF) patients of a younger age when compared to the western world. Total number of patients enrolled were 90 with left ventricular (LV) systolic dysfunction and leading cause being ischemic cardiomyopathy (53.9%), idiopathic cardiomyopathy (18.5%), and rheumatic heart disease (10.8%). Hospital care was given according the HF guideline-based treatment. During the 6 months period of study 1-month mortality rate was 15.8%, 3-month mortality was 26.3%, and 6-month mortality was 26.3%. At the end of 6-month 42 patients survived and 6-month rehospitalization ratio in patients were 39.5%. The overall in-hospital mortality was 30.8%.

Therefore, the target for interventions in acute HF has to be from the time of intervention to the first 3 months of discharge.

Some of the interventions that we suggest for reducing the high mortality of acute HF in India are as follows:

- At admission appropriate use of high-dose diuretics and avoidance of excess inotropes to manage acute HF. Taking care of precipitating factors like anemia and infections, correcting causes like ischemia
- Appropriate addition of vasodilators like ACEI or ARB or hydralazine-nitrate combinations and titration
- Addition of beta-blockers or ivabradine for rate control
- Adequate decongestant before discharge and addition of spironolactone or eplerenone
- Adequate discharge planning and OPD visit planning on day 3 or 7 depending on patient condition at discharge
- Creating HF clinics or disease management programs to manage such patients.

TACKLING THE PROBLEM IN INDIA

Heart failure is a problem which needs to be tackled at multiple levels starting from primary prevention, to controlling the risk factors like diabetes, hypertension, and all the risk factors for coronary artery disease. We need to focus strongly on ensuring prescription of guideline-based medication comprising of ACEI, beta-blockers and mineralocorticoid receptor inhibitors to all patients. Patients with indications for anticoagulation (atrial fibrillation) and resynchronization therapy [left bundle branch block (LBBB)] should be appropriately advised. End-stage HF patients should be advised and guided to centers doing LV assist device implants and heart transplants. Creating a cadre of HF nurses, HF management programs and HF clinics will help organize some of these efforts.[27-33]

Some of the efforts made in this direction by various centers in India include the use of checklists, smartphone apps developed in India and doing small workshops focusing on training doctors on the better use of guideline-based therapy for HF. More efforts are needed for this.

At AIIMS, we are regularly using all these to help the HF patients. There is a HF clinic. The heart transplant program started on 3rd August 1994 and Prof P Venugopal and his team did the first successful heart transplant in India on that day. Till date we have done 66 heart transplants. In India about 500 heart transplants have been done in the past 25 years. We also started the LV assist device program in India starting initially with the HeartMate first-generation devices which were implanted and then patients switched to a transplant and now the third-generation devices which can be used to bridge to a transplant or as destination therapy. We are currently using the HeartWare device.

India-specific guidelines are available and were published in 2015 and recently updated and are summarized here:[27-33]

- All patients of HF should be advised diet modification with salt and water restriction
- All patients should be taught how to monitor their weight and how to respond to water accumulation by increasing their diuretics and restricting water
- All patients should receive influenza and pneumococcal vaccine
- Simple innovative techniques like checklists have been developed like the Dhadkan app available on Google Play Store and Hriday card checklist which are being used at AIIMS and are available on request (Fig. 1)
- Heart failure clinics and management programs are being set-up all over India and the initial data coming in is already showing promise
- Vasodilators should be given to all. ACEI are preferred. ARBs are the alternative. If neither can be given then a combination of hydralazine-nitrate should be used. If the patients are still symptomatic on ACEI then the patients should be started on angiotensin receptor neprilysin inhibitor (ARNI). These are started after stopped ACE or ARB and at low doses which is especially important for Indian patients. The usual starting dose has been 50 mg twice daily, though in patients with borderline blood pressure it has been found that start with lower doses like half a tablet (half of 50 mg), i.e., 25 once a day and then gradually building up the dose is more tolerated (JPCS HF guidelines 2017)
- Beta-blockers should be given to all and uptitrated. These are not uptitrated in Indian patients. Ivabradine should be used if adequate heart rate control is not achieved
- Diuretics should be used in adequate doses to reduce shortness of breath and eliminate pedal edema. Torsemide and metolazone is sometimes more useful here since better diuresis and higher doses are achievable. Torsemide has better absorption and higher doses up to 100 mg are available. Spironolactone or eplerenone should be added to all patients

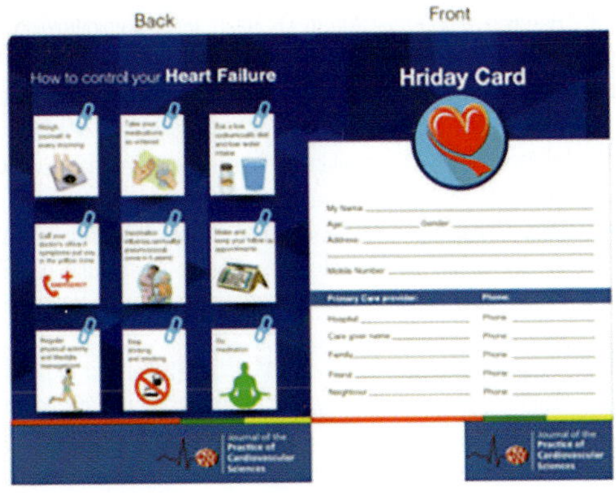

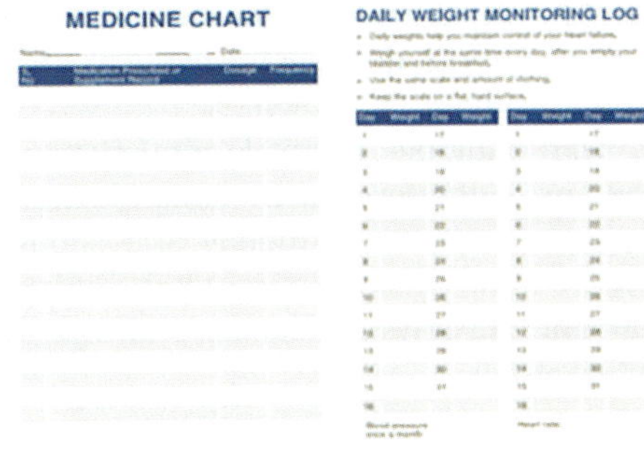

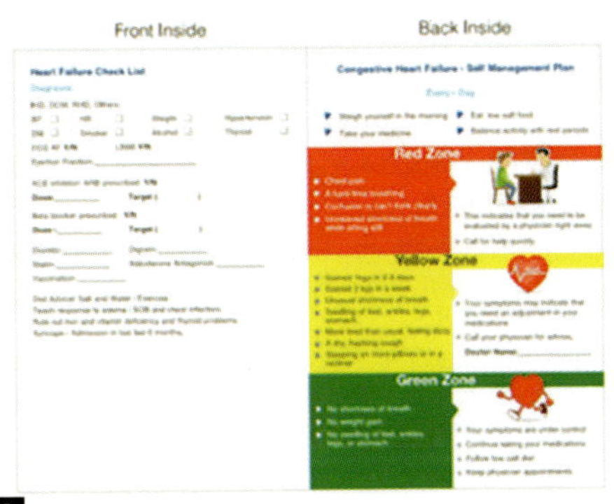

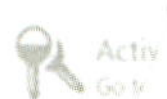

A

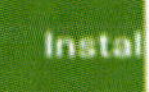

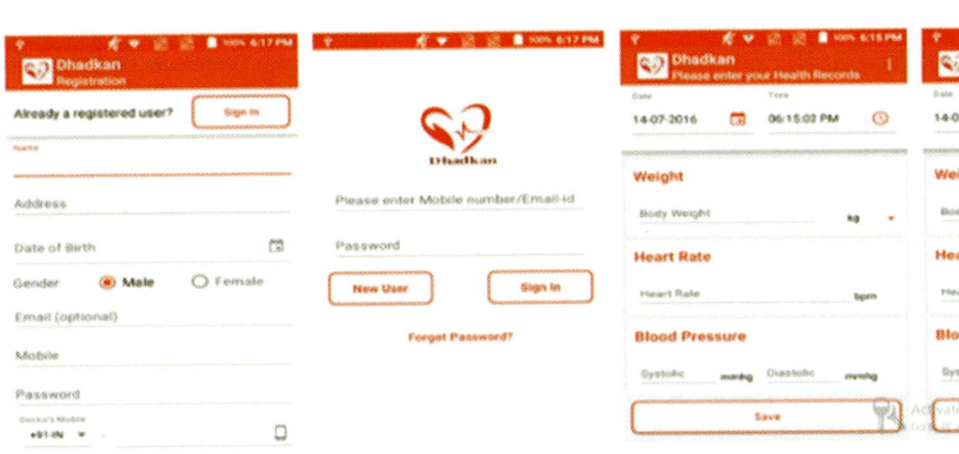

B

FIG. 1: **A,** The Hriday card; **B,** The Dhadkan app.

- Beyond drugs, patients should be assessed for need for devices in terms of implantable cardioverter defibrillators and cardiac resynchronization therapy in the presence of LBBB and an EF less than 35%
- In patients with multiple hospital admissions, end-stage HF therapy in the form of LV assist devices and heart transplant are practical options and should be offered. They are now available in most parts of India in both government and private hospitals with options of government aid also.

CONCLUSION

In conclusion, HF today can be treated and we are in a position to take failure out of HF.

REFERENCES

1. Ponikowski P, Voors AA, Anker SD, et al. 2016 ESC Guidelines for the diagnosis and treatment of acute and chronic heart failure: The Task Force for the diagnosis and treatment of acute and chronic heart failure of the European Society Of Cardiology (ESC) Developed with the special contribution of the Heart Failure Association (HFA) of the ESC. Eur Heart J. 2016;37(27):2129-200.
2. Reddy KS. Rising burden of cardiovascular disease in Indians. In: Sethi KK (Ed). Coronary Artery Disease in Indians: A Global Perspective. Mumbai: Cardiological Society of India; 1998.
3. Swedberg K, Cleland J, Dargie H, et al. Guidelines for the diagnosis and treatment of chronic heart failure: executive summary (update 2005): the task force for the diagnosis and treatment of chronic heart failure of the European Society Of Cardiology. Eur Heart J. 2005;26(11):1115-40.
4. McMurray JJ, Stewart S. Epidemiology, aetiology, and prognosis of heart failure. Heart. 2000;83(5):596-602.
5. Cowie MR, Mosterd A, Wood DA, et al. The epidemiology of heart failure. Eur Heart J. 1997;18(2):208-25.
6. Lloyd-Jones DM, Larson MG, Leip EP, et al. Lifetime risk for developing congestive heart failure: the Framingham heart study. Circulation. 2002;106(24):3068-72.
7. Joshi R, Chow CK, Raju PK, et al. Fatal and nonfatal cardiovascular disease and the use of therapies for secondary prevention in a rural region of India. Circulation. 2009;119(14):1950-5.
8. Jafary FH, Kumar M, Chandna IE. Prognosis of hospitalized new-onset systolic heart failure in indo-Asians—A lethal problem. J Card Fail. 2007;13(10):855-60.
9. Seow SC, Chai P, Lee YP, et al. Heart failure mortality in Southeast Asian patients with left ventricular systolic dysfunction. J Card Fail. 2007;13(6):476-81.
10. Ng TP, Niti M. Trends and ethnic differences in hospital admissions and mortality for congestive heart failure in the elderly in Singapore, 1991 to 1998. Heart. 2003;89(8):865-70.
11. Joshi PP, Mohanan CJ, Sengupta SP, et al. Factors precipitating congestive heart failure—role of patient non-compliance. J Assoc Physicians India. 1999;47(3):294-5.
12. Docherla M, Manjunath H, Kavitha S, et al. Comparative study of systolic and diastolic cardiac failure in elderly hospitalized patients in a tertiary care hospital in Southwest India. J Clin Diagn Res. 2009;3:1529-36.
13. Huffman MD, Prabhakaran D. Heart failure: epidemiology and prevention in India. The Natl Med J India. 2010;23(5):283-8.
14. Chaturvedi V, Parakh N, Seth S, et al. Heart failure in India: The INDUS (India Ukieri Study) study. J Pract Cardiovasc Sci. 2016;2(1):28-35.
15. Harikrishnan S. Heart failure in India—iceberg tsunami? J Pract Cardiovasc Sci. 2016;2(1):2-3.
16. Harikrishnan S, Sanjay G, Anees T, et al. Clinical presentation, management, in hospital and 90 day outcomes of heart failure patients in Trivandrum, Kerala, India: the Trivandrum Heart Failure Registry. Eur J Heart Fail. 2015;17(8):794-800.
17. Lopez AD, Mathers CD, Ezzati M, et al. Global and regional burden of disease and risk factors, 2001: Systematic analysis of population health data. Lancet. 2006;367(9524):1747-57.
18. Strasser T, Dondog N, El Kholy A, et al. The community control of rheumatic fever and rheumatic heart disease: Report of a WHO international cooperative project. Bull World Health Organ. 1981;59(2):285-94.
19. Rizvi SF, Khan MA, Kundi A, et al. Status of rheumatic heart disease in rural Pakistan. Heart. 2004;90(4):394-9.
20. Arora R, Subramanyam G, Khalilullah M, et al. Clinical profile of rheumatic fever and rheumatic heart disease: A study of 2,500 cases. Indian Heart J. 1981;33(6):264-9.
21. Meenakshisundaram R, Thirumalaikolundusubramanian P. Valvular heart disease in Indian subcontinent: Social issues. Indian J Community Med. 2009;34(1):57-8.
22. Kumar R, Raizada A, Aggarwal AK, et al. A community-based rheumatic fever/rheumatic heart disease cohort: twelve-year experience. Indian Heart J. 2002;54(1):54-8.
23. Grover A, Dhawan A, Iyengar SD, et al. Epidemiology of rheumatic fever and rheumatic heart disease in a rural community in Northern India. Bull World Health Organ. 1993;71(1):59-66.
24. Jose VJ, Gupta SN. Mortality and morbidity of acute ST segment elevation myocardial infarction in the current era. Indian Heart J. 2004;56(3):210-4.
25. Seth S, Khanal S, Ramakrishnan S, et al. Epidemiology of acute decompensated heart failure in India: The AFAR study (Acute failure registry study). J Pract Cardiovasc Sci. 2015;1(1):35-8.
26. Dokainish H, Teo K, Zhu J, et al. Heart failure in Africa, Asia, the Middle East and South America: the INTER-CHF study. Int J Cardiol. 2016;204:133-41.
27. Ramachandran K, Husain N, Maikhuri R, et al. Impact of a comprehensive telephone-based disease management programme on quality-of-life in patients with heart failure. Natl Med J India. 2007;20(2):67-73.
28. Rai M, Sharma KK, Seth S, et al. A randomized controlled trial to assess effectiveness of a nurse-led home-based heart failure management program. J Prac Cardiol Sci. 2017;3(1):28-33.
29. Seth S. "Dhadkan," an indigenous smartphone app for heart failure patients. J Prac Cardiol Sci. 2016;2(3):141.
30. Seth S, Vashista S. The Hriday Card: A checklist for heart failure. J Prac Cardiovas Sci. 2017;3(1):5.
31. Seth S, Bhargava B, Maulik S K, et al. Consensus statement on management of chronic heart failure in India. J Pract Cardiovasc Sci. 2015;1(2):105-12.
32. Seth S, Ramakrishnan S, Parekh N, et al. Heart failure guidelines for India: Update 2017. J Pract Cardiovasc Sci. 2017;3(3):133-8.
33. Ramakumar V, Naik N. Current status of the ICD in nonischemic cardiomyopathy. J Pract Cardiovasc Sci. 2018;4(1):6-9.

CHAPTER 92

Biomarkers for Heart Failure: Current Role and Relevance

Anunay Gupta, Ambuj Roy

CASE VIGNETTE

Mr AS, a 72-year-old man presents to the emergency with increasing cough and breathlessness. His pulse rate is 98 beats/min and blood pressure is 162/68 mm Hg. He is a known case of chronic obstructive airway disease (COAD), chronic kidney disease stage 3A and heart failure with preserved ejection fraction (HFpEF) on treatment. Important clinical decisions to be taken are whether it is heart failure (HF) or acute exacerbation of COAD. If its HF then how severe and what is the prognosis? Are there biomarkers to guide the management and discharge of the patient beyond usual clinical care?

INTRODUCTION

Heart failure burden has increased by many folds due to changing demographics, increasing burden of its risk factors like hypertension and diabetes and also better management coronary artery disease leading to higher number of its survivors but with impaired heart function. Despite improvements in therapy, the mortality rate in patients with HF has remained unacceptably high. However, the survival varies by countries and in the recent INTERCHF registry Indian patients had a very high mortality rate of 23% at one year which was lower than African countries but much higher than China and countries in Latin American and Middle East.[1]

The diagnosis of HF has largely been a clinical diagnosis aided by investigations such as ECG, chest X-ray, and echocardiography. However, with increasing prevalence of multiple comorbidities as in the above case there has been a need for additional diagnostic aids for diagnosis of HF. In this respect many biomarkers of HF have been developed over the years, some of which have helped in improved diagnostic accuracy and also management of HF and have been mainstreamed in clinical care. There are others that have some varying promise and others which are in the pipeline. This review provides a focused update on current role and recent advances of biomarkers in HF.

What is an ideal biomarker?

An ideal biomarker of HF is that which will help in the diagnosis of HF, its prognosis, risk stratification, and guiding therapy. Therapy should alter its levels so as be a marker of the state of HF in the individual patient.

NATRIURETIC PEPTIDES: B-TYPE NATRIURETIC PEPTIDE AND N-TERMINAL PROHORMONE B-TYPE NATRIURETIC PEPTIDE

Natriuretic peptide is the most widely tested and established biomarker in the management of HF. The natriuretic peptide system impacts salt and water handling and pressure regulation and may influence myocardial structure and function. B-type natriuretic peptide (BNP) is a natriuretic hormone initially identified in the brain but released primarily from the heart, particularly the ventricles. Cleavage of the prohormone proBNP produces biologically active 32 amino acid BNP as well as biologically inert 76 amino acid N-terminal proBNP (NT-proBNP). BNP have diuretic, natriuretic, and hypotensive effects. They inhibit the renin–angiotensin system, endothelin secretion, and systemic and renal sympathetic activity. Among patients with HF, increased secretion of BNP partially counteract the effects of norepinephrine, endothelin, and angiotensin II, limiting the degree of vasoconstriction and sodium retention.

In breathing not properly study, a plasma BNP more than 100 pg/mL diagnosed HF with a sensitivity, specificity, and predictive accuracy of 90%, 76%, and 83%, respectively.[2] NT-proBNP in the PRIDE study had similar sensitivity for excluding HF at cutoff of 300 pg/mL.[3] NT-proBNPs have a varying sensitivity and specificity based on age, with age-related cutoffs of 450 pg/mL for less than 50 years, 900 pg/mL for 50–75 years, and 1,800 pg/mL for more than 75 years.[4] Table 1 highlights the impact of other associated conditions on NT-proBNP levels. In a systematic review of 42 studies at a

TABLE 1: Impact of other conditions which can lead to variability in B-type natriuretic peptide (BNP) levels

Increased levels	Decreased levels
Increasing age	Obesity
Acute coronary syndrome	Flash pulmonary edema
Renal failure	Burnt out cardiomyopathy
Pulmonary hypertension	–
Pulmonary embolism	–
Atrial fibrillation	–
Anemia	–

threshold of 100 ng/L for BNP and 300 ng/L for NT-proBNP, the natriuretic peptides had sensitivities of 95% and 99%, and negative predictive values of 94% and 98%, respectively for a diagnosis of acute HF.[5]

Elevations in plasma BNP can establish the presence of HFpEF with similar accuracy to HF with reduced ejection fraction (HFrEF), though values are generally higher with HFrEF.[6] However, the values do not adequately differentiate between HFrEF and HFpEF.[7]

It is important to note that not all patients with symptomatic HF have high plasma BNP concentrations and not all asymptomatic patients have low values. This was demonstrated in a review of 558 consecutive ambulatory patients with treated stable HF in a specialized outpatient HF clinic.[8] In this study, 60 patients were considered asymptomatic, and their plasma BNP levels ranged from 5 pg/mL to 572 pg/mL (median, 147 pg/mL). Of the remaining 498 symptomatic (NYHA functional class II-III) patients, 106 (21.3%) had plasma BNP levels were normal (<100 pg/mL). These patients were more likely to be young and female and to have a nonischemic cardiomyopathy. While patients with raised levels without clinical HF may seem false positive cases, there is usually some pathophysiological cause for ventricular stress. Similarly, the other way round natriuretic levels may be normal in flash pulmonary edema at presentation but may rise subsequently over hours despite therapy. Another classical case of raised venous pressure without rise in natriuretic levels may be cardiac tamponade since it is not a ventricular failure.

There has been enthusiasm to use these biomarkers to guide therapy in HF patients so as to reduce clinical events and hospitalization. A patient-level meta-analysis of data from 2,431 patients from 11 trials showed a significant 38% reduction in all-cause mortality with natriuretic peptide-guided therapy compared with usual care.[9] However, more recent Guide-IT trial using NT-proBNP-guided strategy failed to improve outcomes in HF with reduced ejection fraction. Patients with EF of 40% or less with elevated natriuretic peptide within 30 days of enrollment and history of a prior hospitalization for HF were recruited. The patients were assigned to a guided strategy in which HF therapy was titrated with the goal of NT-proBNP less than 1,000 pg/mL or to the usual guideline-directed care. There was no difference in the outcomes such as cardiovascular mortality, all-cause mortality and time to first HF hospitalization at 15 months of follow up. There was no significant difference at 12 months in achieved NT-proBNP levels; the intervention group declined 53% to a median of 1,209 pg/mL and the control group declined 48% to a median of 1,397 pg/mL. The target of less than 1,000 pg/mL was achieved in 46% of the intervention group versus 40% of the control group ($p = 0.21$). This result highlights that when guideline-directed therapy is practiced, biomarkers-guided therapy do not make a difference and that guideline-directed care can lead to outcomes similar or to biomarker-guided care if achieved.[10] The difference between this study and other trials was the excellent management of the control group which probably negated the benefits of biomarker driven therapy.

In PARADIGM-HF trial, angiotensin receptor-neprilysin inhibitor (ARNI) showed improved outcomes compared to enalapril. ARNI inhibits the degradation of BNP resulting in elevated BNP levels. Thus, monitoring of chronic HF patients on sacubitril-valsartan treatment with BNP testing may be impaired. This is especially true in the first few weeks of ARNI therapy after which levels of BNP are stabilized and could be used in future management. The interpretation of NT-proBNP testing in HF appears to be unaffected by ARNI.[11] In a subset analysis it was seen that treatment with ARNI was nearly twice as likely as enalapril to reduce NT-proBNP to values less than or equal to 1,000 pg/mL and reduction in NT-proBNP levels was associated with reduced clinical events.[12]

Soluble ST2

Soluble ST2 (sST2) is a member of the interleukin (IL)-1 receptor-like family of proteins. It is expressed in response to mechanical stress on fibroblasts and cardiomyocytes. It is expressed in a transmembrane form (ST2L) and a soluble circulating form (sST2). Current assays measure sST2 and is the one in use in clinical studies.[13] Soluble ST2 lacks disease specificity and, therefore, is not a valuable marker for the diagnosis of HF. Soluble ST2 is associated with adverse outcomes in HF, myocardial infarction, pulmonary disease, infection, and rheumatologic disorders. Higher levels of sST2 reflect increased inflammation, fibrosis, and wall stress and hence have the ability to be used as a composite marker like the "hemoglobin A1c (HbA1c)" for HF.[13] The recommended cutoff for sST2 in chronic HF is 35 ng/mL. It is a prognostic marker for both HFpEF and HFrEF. In the PRIDE study, sST2 values were significantly higher in patients with HF and it was a powerful predictor of outcome. It has been shown that β-blockers can mitigate the risk associated with elevated sST2 in HF.[8] Similarly, mineralocorticoid antagonist have been found to be beneficial in patients with elevated sST2.[14] It is not known that whether sST2 can be used as a biomarker-guided strategy as seen with NT-proBNP.

High-sensitivity Troponin

The latest generation of high-sensitivity troponin (hsTn) assays are able to detect troponin in more than 50% of healthy subjects and ideally more than 95%.[15] Recent American Heart Association/American College of Cardiology Foundation guidelines endorse measuring troponin in acute HF to rule out acute coronary syndrome and risk stratification.[16] Elevated hsTn is associated with increased in hospital mortality and can be used for risk stratification in HF.[17] Serial measurements of hsTn during hospitalization for acute HF has shown to risk-stratify patients for 90-day mortality and readmission. It can also identify patients who are at high risk of developing clinical HF in the future in patients with stage A and B HF.[18]

NEWER BIOMARKERS

Even though natriuretic peptides have proven their usefulness in management of HF, limitations of natriuretic peptides measurement such as multiple comorbidities of HF patients that effect concentrations of BNP or NT-proBNP (e.g., sepsis, renal disease, and obesity), demand for other biomarkers.

Galectin 3

Galectin-3 (LGALS3) is a lectin expressed at low levels in body; however, upon injury or stress, its production is substantially increased. It is considered as a marker of myocardial fibrosis.[19] In PRIDE study galectin-3 was a stronger prognostic marker for 60-day mortality compared to NT-proBNP. Moreover, the combination of galectin-3 with NT-proBNP was the best predictor for prognosis in subjects with acute HF.[20] Similarly in COACH study galectin-3 was associated with 18-month mortality and hospitalization rates.[21] In a recent meta-analysis, pooled data from 8,419 patients with acute and chronic HF with a follow-up of 1–8.7 years, it was shown that an increase of 1% in circulating galectin-3 was associated with a 28% increased risk for all-cause mortality and a 59% increase in CV mortality, in fully adjusted models including estimated glomerular filtration rate and NT-proBNP.[22] As with ST2, it is not known whether galectin-3 could have a role in guiding therapy. Similarly it is not known whether therapy targeting galectin-3 as an antifibrotic agent can be beneficial or not.

Procalcitonin

Procalcitonin (PCT) is a protein whose expression in parenchymal tissue is induced by bacterial infection, either by endotoxin or via cytokines (e.g., IL-6). It acts as a function of infection in patients presenting with acute dyspnea. Maisel et al. showed that patients with a diagnosis of acute HF and an elevated PCT concentration (>0.21 ng/mL) had a worse outcome if not treated with antibiotics ($p = 0.046$), while patients with low PCT values (<0.05 ng/mL) had a better outcome if they did not receive antibiotic therapy ($p = 0.049$). Therefore, PCT may aid in the decision to administer antibiotic therapy to patients presenting with acute HF in which clinical uncertainty exists regarding a superimposed bacterial infection.[23]

Growth Differentiation Factor-15

Growth differentiation factor-15 (GDF-15) is a stress-response cytokine. In cardiomyocytes, it is produced and released in the setting of oxidative stress or in response to stimulation with cytokines or angiotensin II.[19] Increased levels are associated with worse outcomes in both acute HF and chronic HF.[24] GDF-15 offers additional prognostic value over and above natriuretic peptides.[19]

Mid-regional Proatrial Natriuretic Peptide

Mid-regional-proatrial natriuretic peptide (MR-proANP) provides both diagnostic and prognostic information that is additive to BNP or NT-proBNP, and has been shown in multiple HF studies.[25,26]

CONCLUSION

Heart failure burden has rapidly increased and likely to worsen due to current demographic and disease patterns. Heart failure diagnosis and prognostication can be a challenge to clinicians. The biomarkers are envisioned to fill this void. Natriuretic peptides have become an integral part in the diagnosis and management of HF patients. Other biomarkers like sST2, hsTn, and PCT have also shown promise and are increasingly being used in HF patients in various settings. Role of newer biomarkers in the management of HF is still not well known and is evolving.

REFERENCES

1. Dokainish H, Teo K, Zhu J, et al. Global mortality variations in patients with heart failure: results from the International Congestive Heart Failure (INTER-CHF) prospective cohort study. Lancet Glob Health. 2017;5:e665-72.
2. Maisel AS, Krishnaswamy P, Nowak RM, et al. Rapid measurement of B-type natriuretic peptide in the emergency diagnosis of heart failure. N Engl J Med. 2002;347:161-7.
3. Januzzi JL, Camargo CA, Anwaruddin S, et al. The N-terminal Pro-BNP investigation of dyspnea in the emergency department (PRIDE) study. Am J Cardiol. 2005;95:948-54.
4. Januzzi JL, van Kimmenade R, Lainchbury J, et al. NT-proBNP testing for diagnosis and short-term prognosis in acute destabilized heart failure: an international pooled analysis of 1256 patients: the International Collaborative of NT-proBNP Study. Eur Heart J. 2006;27:330-7.
5. Roberts E, Ludman AJ, Dworzynski K, et al. The diagnostic accuracy of the natriuretic peptides in heart failure: systematic review and diagnostic meta-analysis in the acute care setting. BMJ. 2015;350:h910.
6. Krishnaswamy P, Lubien E, Clopton P, et al. Utility of B-natriuretic peptide levels in identifying patients with left ventricular systolic or diastolic dysfunction. Am J Med. 2001;111:274-9.
7. Lubien E, DeMaria A, Krishnaswamy P, et al. Utility of B-natriuretic peptide in detecting diastolic dysfunction: comparison with Doppler velocity recordings. Circulation. 2002;105:595-601.
8. Gaggin HK, Motiwala S, Bhardwaj A, et al. Soluble concentrations of the interleukin receptor family member ST2 and β-blocker therapy in chronic heart failure. Circ Heart Fail. 2013;6:1206-13.
9. Troughton RW, Frampton CM, Brunner-La Rocca HP, et al. Effect of B-type natriuretic peptide-guided treatment of chronic heart failure on total mortality and hospitalization: an individual patient meta-analysis. Eur Heart J. 2014;35:1559-67.
10. Felker GM, Anstrom KJ, Adams KF, et al. Effect of Natriuretic Peptide-Guided Therapy on Hospitalization or Cardiovascular Mortality in High-Risk Patients With Heart Failure and Reduced Ejection Fraction: A Randomized Clinical Trial. JAMA. 2017;318:713-20.
11. Mair J, Lindahl B, Giannitsis E, et al. Will sacubitril-valsartan diminish the clinical utility of B-type natriuretic peptide testing in acute cardiac care? Eur Heart J Acute Cardiovasc Care. 2017;6:321-8.

12. Zile MR, Claggett BL, Prescott MF, et al. Prognostic Implications of Changes in N-Terminal Pro-B-Type Natriuretic Peptide in Patients With Heart Failure. J Am Coll Cardiol. 2016;68:2425-36.
13. Wettersten N, Maisel AS. Biomarkers for Heart Failure: An Update for Practitioners of Internal Medicine. Am J Med. 2016;129:560-7.
14. Maisel A, Xue Y, van Veldhuisen DJ, et al. Effect of spironolactone on 30-day death and heart failure rehospitalization (from the COACH Study). Am J Cardiol. 2014;114:737-42.
15. Apple FS, Collinson PO, IFCC Task Force on Clinical Applications of Cardiac Biomarkers. Analytical characteristics of high-sensitivity cardiac troponin assays. Clin Chem. 2012;58:54-61.
16. Eckel RH, Jakicic JM, Ard JD, et al. 2013 AHA/ACC guideline on lifestyle management to reduce cardiovascular risk: a report of the American College of Cardiology/American Heart Association Task Force on Practice Guidelines. J Am Coll Cardiol. 2014;63:2960-84.
17. Pascual-Figal DA, Casas T, Ordonez-Llanos J, et al. Highly sensitive troponin T for risk stratification of acutely destabilized heart failure. Am Heart J. 2012;163:1002-10.
18. Saunders JT, Nambi V, de Lemos JA, et al. Cardiac troponin T measured by a highly sensitive assay predicts coronary heart disease, heart failure, and mortality in the Atherosclerosis Risk in Communities Study. Circulation. 2011;123:1367-76.
19. de Boer RA, Daniels LB, Maisel AS, et al. State of the Art: Newer biomarkers in heart failure. Eur J Heart Fail. 2015;17:559-69.
20. van Kimmenade RR, Januzzi JL, Ellinor PT, et al. Utility of amino-terminal pro-brain natriuretic peptide, galectin-3, and apelin for the evaluation of patients with acute heart failure. J Am Coll Cardiol. 2006;48:1217-24.
21. de Boer RA, Lok DJA, Jaarsma T, et al. Predictive value of plasma galectin-3 levels in heart failure with reduced and preserved ejection fraction. Ann Med. 2011;43:60-8.
22. Chen A, Hou W, Zhang Y, et al. Prognostic value of serum galectin-3 in patients with heart failure: a meta-analysis. Int J Cardiol. 2015;182:168-70.
23. Maisel A, Neath SX, Landsberg J, et al. Use of procalcitonin for the diagnosis of pneumonia in patients presenting with a chief complaint of dyspnoea: results from the BACH (Biomarkers in Acute Heart Failure) trial. Eur J Heart Fail. 2012;14:278-86.
24. Wollert KC, Kempf T. Growth differentiation factor 15 in heart failure: an update. Curr Heart Fail Rep. 2012;9:337-45.
25. Maisel A, Mueller C, Nowak R, et al. Mid-region pro-hormone markers for diagnosis and prognosis in acute dyspnea: results from the BACH (Biomarkers in Acute Heart Failure) trial. J Am Coll Cardiol. 2010;55:2062-76.
26. Shah RV, Truong QA, Gaggin HK, et al. Mid-regional pro-atrial natriuretic peptide and pro-adrenomedullin testing for the diagnostic and prognostic evaluation of patients with acute dyspnoea. Eur Heart J. 2012;33:2197-205.

CHAPTER **93**

Practical Tips for using Beta-blockers, ACEI, ARBs, ARNI, Diuretics, Aldosterone Antagonists in Heart Failure

Vijay Kumar Chopra, Sanjay Mittal

INTRODUCTION

With the onset of heart failure (HF), there is activation of various neurohormonal systems as an adaptive response. However, over the course of time, this response becomes maladaptive and is responsible for perpetuation of HF. It follows, therefore, that the beneficial effects in terms of mortality and morbidity will occur with modification of neurohormonal systems and indeed, i.e., what has been shown in several HF trials. Beneficial as these agents are, for an optimal response it is important to use them in doses which have been shown to be beneficial in clinical trials or at least to use the maximally tolerated doses. It is also important to use them judiciously while watching for their side effects and drug interactions. This brief review focuses on some practical tips for the appropriate use of these drugs in HF (Table 1).

BETA-BLOCKERS

Heart failure is characterized by sympathetic activation. Most of the deleterious effects are mediated by beta-blockers (BBs) and adrenergic receptors.[1] This results in tachycardia,

TABLE 1: Drugs for the prevention and treatment for chronic heart failure

Agent	Initiating daily dose	Maximal daily dose
Angiotensin-converting enzyme inhibitors		
Captopril	6.25 mg thrice	50 mg thrice
Enalapril	2.5 mg twice	10 mg twice
Lisinopril	2.5–5.0 mg once	20 mg once
Ramipril	1.25–2.5 mg once	10 mg once
Angiotensin receptor blockers		
Valsartan	40 mg twice	160 mg twice
Candesartan	4–8 mg once	32 mg once
Losartan	12.5–25 mg once	50 mg once
Beta-blockers		
Carvedilol	3.125 mg twice	25 mg twice (50 mg twice in patients weighing > 85 kg)
Carvedilol-CR	10 mg once	80 mg once
Bisoprolol	1.25 mg once	10 mg once
Metoprolol succinate CR	12.5–25 mg qd	200 mg once
Aldosterone antagonists		
Spironolactone	12.5–25 mg once	25–50 mg once
Eplerenone	25 mg once	50 mg once

fluid retention, and increased metabolic demands by the myocardium. Sympathetic activation also perpetuates remodeling of the ventricles resulting in hypertrophy and dilatation of ventricular cavities, which in turn places greater strain on the myocardium. By reducing heart rate (HR), BB when given in concert with angiotensin-converting enzyme inhibitor (ACEI), reverse this process, resulting in reverse remodeling, amelioration of symptoms, and prolongation of life. All patients of HF with ejection fraction (EF) less than 40%, whether symptomatic or not, should be on BB.

- Ensure that the patient does not have bronchial asthma, as it can get worse with BB. However, several patients of chronic bronchitis can tolerate BB and derive equal benefit. One has to watch for bronchospasm, however, which will necessitate withdrawal of BB
- Beta-blockers should not be started in grossly volume overloaded patients. Ideally a euvolemic status should be achieved before starting BB
- Initial dose should be relatively small depending upon the HR and blood pressure (BP). Uptitration should be done not earlier than 2 weeks depending upon the clinical status of the patient as each increment of dose may result in fluid retention. This can be managed by diuretics HR and BP in sitting and standing position should be checked at every visit and chest should be auscultated
- Recommended BB are carvedilol, metoprolol succinate, and bisoprolol with some evidence emerging for nebivolol. If the BP is on the lower side, one may like to avoid carvedilol as it is both alpha- and beta-blocker and may result in a greater drop in BP. As far as possible, BB should be started before discharge from the hospital. Nearly 85% of HF patients tolerate BB, including those with diabetes mellitus, peripheral vascular disease (PVD), and chronic obstructive pulmonary disease (COPD). Over a period of weeks and months, one after find a gradual increase in BP as a result of reverse remodeling allowing for further increase in the doses
- During acute decompensation, the dose of BB may have to be reduced at times[2] but not always, especially with gross fluid overload, bradycardia, and hypotension (Box 1). In case of fluid overload, the first attempt should be to identify and reverse any factors responsible for the same, i.e., hypertension, high salt intake, nonsteroidal anti-inflammatory drugs (NSAIDs), other fluid retaining drug or missing the dose of diuretics. Increase of diuretics dose may help in reversing fluid overload in most patients and reducing BB may not be necessary. In case of bradycardia, the first attempt should be to reduce or stop concomitant rate reducing agents like digoxin, amiodarone, or diltiazem. HR of 50 should be acceptable if hemodynamically stable. Dose of BB should be reduced if the HR falls below this level. Similar approach should be reduced in case of hypotension. Reducing diuretics or other concomitant antihypertensives like dihydropyridines should be the first step
- Symptoms of fatigue are common with BB, but generally resolve over time

BOX 1 Factors that may precipitate acute decompensation in patients with chronic heart failure

- Dietary indiscretion
- Inappropriate dose reduction/discontinuation of HF medications
- Myocardial ischemia/infarction
- Arrhythmias (tachycardia or bradycardia)
- Infection
- Anemia
- Initiation of medications that worsen the symptoms of HF
  - Calcium antagonists (verapamil and diltiazem)
  - Beta-blockers
  - NSAIDs
  - Thiazolidinediones
  - Antiarrhythmic agents [all class I agents, sotalol (class III)]
  - Anti-TNF antibodies
- Alcohol consumption
- Pregnancy
- Worsening hypertension
- Acute valvular insufficiency

HF, heart failure; NSAIDs, nonsteroidal anti-inflammatory drugs; TNF, tumor necrosis factor.

- Dose of BB should be decreased if HR is less than 50/min or if second or third degree heart block or hypotension develops.

ANGIOTENSIN-CONVERTING ENZYME INHIBITOR

In HF, activation of renin-angiotensin-aldosterone (RAS) axis has been well documented. This results in increase in peripheral resistance, salt and water retention, remodeling, endothelial dysfunction, and a host of other adverse hemodynamic and metabolic effects. Several ACEIs have been tried in landmark clinical trials[3-5] with gratifying results and as a result they have established their place firmly as class I drugs in patients of symptomatic and asymptomatic HF. Enalapril, captopril, ramipril, and perindopril have all shown benefit in several studies. They relieve symptoms, prevent hospitalization, and prolong life.

Fluid retention can attenuate their effects. So it is preferable to optimize the dose of diuretics first (Table 2). There are certain precautions to be observed in their appropriate use:

- As with other vasoactive drugs, the initial dose should be relatively small depending upon the BP. The dose can be stepped up every 3–5 days depending upon the BP which should also be checked in standing position. Diuretics should be simultaneously reduced to prevent hypotension. BB can be started before the full dose of ACEI has been achieved
- Abrupt withdrawal of ACEI should be avoided in the absence of angioneurotic edema and hyperkalemia
- Majority of the adverse effects of ACEI are related to suppression of renin angiotensin system. Initial decrease

TABLE 2: Diuretics for treating fluid retention in chronic heart failure

Drug	Initial daily dose (s)	Maximum total daily dose	Duration of action
Loop diuretics			
Furosemide	20–40 mg once or twice	600 mg	6–8 h
Torsemide	10–20 mg once	200 mg	12–16 h
Thiazide diuretics			
Chlorthalidone	12.5–25 mg once	100 mg	24–72 h
Hydrochlorothia-zide	25 mg once or twice	200 mg	6–12 h
Indapamide	2.5 mg once	5 mg	36 h
Metolazone	2.5–5.0 mg once	20 mg	12–24 h

in BP and mild azotemia seen during initiation of therapy is generally well tolerated, unless it becomes severe or symptomatic. While using ACEI, it is important to periodically monitor renal function test (RFT), as rise in creatinine and hyperkalemia may occur. A set of values should be obtained before starting these drugs and subsequently should be checked after 1-2 weeks at the time of stepping up the dose and every 2-3 months subsequently especially in patients of renal dysfunction, in those receiving aldosterone antagonists (AAs) and potassium sparing diuretics and in those with pre-existing hyponatremia, azotemia, and hypotension

- Precautionary measures should be taken to reduce the risk of worsening renal function which include avoiding concomitant nephrotoxic drugs (e.g., NSAIDs), evaluating and treating other causes of worsening renal function (e.g., intrinsic kidney disease), and avoiding volume depletion (i.e., if no congestion is present, reducing or suspending diuretic) at the time of ACEI initiation
- If serum creatinine increases by more than 50% above baseline or if serum creatinine is more than 3 mg/dL dose of ACEI should be decreased by one-half. Volume status should be evaluated the appropriateness of decreasing the diuretic dose should be considered tests. Serum creatinine, blood urea nitrogen (BUN), and serum potassium should be rechecked frequently (at least weekly) until levels have stabilized. After renal functions have stabilized, the appropriateness of uptitrating ACEI dose should be assessed
- If serum creatinine is more than 3.5 mg/dL, ACEI should be stopped and volume statues evaluated to determine the appropriateness of decreasing the diuretic dose. Serum creatinine, BUN, and serum potassium should be rechecked frequently (at least weekly) until levels have stabilized
- Caution should be taken in starting ACEI in patients with resting potassium levels above 5 mEq/L. The risk of hyperkalemia is increased if an AA is administered concomitantly. On the other hand, concomitant potassium-wasting diuretic therapy can cause hypokalemia. It is advisable to check serum electrolytes and renal function at 1 week and at 1 month following increases in ACEI dose and then periodically (e.g. event 3-6 months), depending on the patient's stability and baseline renal function
- Cough and throat irritation occurs in about 10% of patients receiving ACEI. It is important to note that in patients receiving ACEI there may be other causes of cough such as bronchitis or HF. A careful history will establish the causality. If so suspected, ACEI should be discontinued and substituted with an angiotensin receptor blocker (ARB). Skin rash and itching also occurs in some patients due to elevated histamine levels
- Angioneurotic edema has been reported with ACEI, though it is uncommon (less than 1%).

ANGIOTENSIN RECEPTOR BLOCKERS

They should be used in symptomatic and asymptomatic patients with EF less than 40% in patients intolerant to ACEI due to cough, rash or angioneurotic edema but not in those with hyperkalemia. In ACEI intolerant patients, ARBs have shown improvement in outcomes.[6-9] Like other drugs for HF, they too should be started in lower doses which should be gradually stepped up. The precautions in their use are identical to ACEI. An occasional patient can have cough or angioedema even with ARBs though the incidence is much less than with ACEI. ARBs approved for HF are losartan, valsartan and candesartan. Generally, ACEI and ARBs should not be combined except in certain specific situations. These will include difficult to control HF[10] and heavy albuminuria. This decision is best left to the HF specialists and nephrologists.

ANGIOTENSIN RECEPTOR NEPRILYSIN INHIBITOR

This is a new class of drug which came into clinical use about 2 years ago after the remarkable success of the landmark PARADIGM (Prospective comparison of ARNI with ACEI to Determine Impact on Global Mortality and Morbidity) trial, which was prematurely stopped due to overwhelming superiority of the drug as compared to enalapril in treatment of chronic congestive HF. So strong was the evidence that on the basis of a single trial, both Food and Drug Administration (FDA) and the European Society of Cardiology (ESC) gave it a class I recommendation. The first in class drug is sacubitril/valsartan. This is a combination of an ARB valsartan and sacubitril, which is an inhibitor of neprilysin. Neprilysin is responsible for the breakdown of brain-type natriuretic peptide (BNP), other natriuretic peptides (NPs), and angiotensin II. Its inhibitor results in the elevation of NP levels, while valsartan blocks the effects angiotensin II despite at elevated levels. Following are some of the important tips for its use:

- American College of Cardiology/American Heart Association (ACC/AHA) recommend the use of angiotensin

receptor neprilysin inhibitor (ARNI) in patients with chronic congestive heart failure (CHF) even among those who are stable on ACEI or ARBs to improve cardiovascular outcomes, while ESC recommends the use of ARNI in patients who continue to be symptomatic or in HF despite adequate doses of ACEI/ARBs
- Patients on ARBs can be switched to ARNI straight away, if so required. Patients on ACEIs should have a gap of at least 36 hours between the last dose of ACEI and the first dose of ARNI to avoid angioneurotic edema. ARNI should never be combined with ACEI or other ARBs
- In ACEI/ARB naïve patients the starting dose of ARNI is 50 mg twice daily while patients already on a good dose of ARBs or ACEIs can be started on 100 mg twice daily if the BP is over 100 mm Hg. Clinical judgment should be exercised to avoid hypotension. The dose can be gradually stepped up every 2–4 weeks till 200 mg twice daily or a maximally tolerated dose has been achieved
- The ARNI should be started only if the BP is over 100 mm Hg systolic. If during the course of treatment the systolic BP falls to below 95 mm Hg then one should try to reduce other drugs which may be contributing to hypotension including reducing the dose of diuretics. If nothing else works, then the dose of ARNI can also be reduced. After correction of other factors, one should again try to increase the dose of ARNI if clinically possible.
- Reverse remodeling has been documented with ARNI. This means that after a few weeks or months of treatment the BP may actually come up with or without improvement in EF. This allows further uptitration of ARNI and BBs
- As with ACEI and ARBs, RFT should be monitored and the dose of diuretics should be gradually reduced to the minimum required to keep a patient euvolemic
- As with ACEI and ARBs, angioneurotic edema could occur and patients should be prewarned about it.

DIURETICS

In volume overloaded patients, diuretics play a critical role in improving symptoms of dyspnea and congestion. Depending upon the degree of congestion the starting dose could be oral or intravenous (IV). Loop diuretics, of which are extremely effective and fast acting. As HF improves, the dose of diuretics should be gradually reduced to the minimum required to maintain euvolemia.

- In patients with acute dyspnea and fluid overload, IV loop diuretics are the drugs of choice. They can be given in doses of 20–40 mg 1–3 times a day, depending upon the clinical condition. The dose should be increased or decreased, depending upon the response of the patient. A commonly used method for dose titration in case of inadequate response is to double the dose till desired effect is achieved or the maximal dose is reached
- If diuresis is inadequate, one can use loop diuretics as an infusion, starting with 5 mg/hour and double the dose every 3–4 hours, depending upon the response. There is some evidence that this may be more effective than IV bolus doses, though some studies did not find any difference[11]
- Loop diuretics can be combined with AAs or thiazide diuretics for enhancing the response.
- With IV diuretics, a close monitoring of BP, electrolytes and renal functions is needed. Hypokalemia, hyponatremia, azotemia, and hypomagnesemia are important. In patients receiving potassium sparing diuretics, hyperkalemia should be looked for especially in those receiving ACEI/ARBs and ARNI.[12] This is especially important in diabetics who may have occult renal dysfunction. Serum K levels between 4 mg/dL and 5 mg/dL are considered ideal administration of AA prevents low potassium. Hyperuricemia and metabolic alkalosis are the other complication of diuretics
- As euvolemia is achieved, the doses should be reduced and changed to oral route. At each subsequent visit the need and the dose of diuretics should be evaluated. When euvolemia is achieved, the patient in dry weight should be recorded. Subsequently patients should weigh themselves daily to maintain their ideal weight and to avoid fluid overload
- Bioavailability of frusemide is about 40–79% resulting in variable response. Bumetanide and torsemide have a better bioavailability
- Aggressive diuretic use can result in severe hyponatremia, especially in people with high RAS activation and high arginine vasopressin (AVP) levels and requires stringent water restriction
- Ototoxicity resulting in temporary or permanent hearing loss can be seen with rapid IV frusemide injections, it is much less with oral use
- Diuretics resistance refers to progressively diminishing response to diuretics and is associated with excessive salt intake, hypotension,[13] advanced HF, and abrupt decline in cardiac or renal functions. One should enquire if any drugs are responsible, e.g., COX-2 inhibitors, NSAIDs, thiazolidinediones, trimethoprim, and other nephrotoxic drugs
- To treat diuretics resistance, on can add a proximal tubule diuretic or a distal collecting tubule diuretic, e.g., metolazone without reducing the loop diuretic
- Ultrafiltration should be considered if diuresis is inadequate despite all the measures.

ALDOSTERONE ANTAGONISTS

They are not only K-sparing diuretics, but have beneficial effects that are independent of their diuretic actions. They are recommended for New York Heart Association (NYHA) class II–IV patients with EF less than 35% who are receiving standard therapy with diuretics, ACEI, and BB.[6] Spironolactone and eplerenone are the two AA available and have shown efficacy in clinical trials.[14]

- Start with a small dose and gradually increase
- Generally K supplementation should be stopped when starting AA
- Watch for hyperkalemia, especially in diabetics, and those receiving ACEI/ARBs/ARNI
- Check K and RFT after 3 days and 1 week after starting AA and subsequently once a month

- Aldosterone antagonists are not recommended in patients with serum creatinine more than 2.5 mg/dL or K more than 5.5 mEq/L
- Painful gynecomastia occurs in 10–15% of patients receiving spironolactone. These patients should be switched to eplerenone and gynecomastia usually resolves in 2–4 weeks.

REFERENCES

1. Mann DI, Bristow MR. Mechanisms and models in heart failure: the biomechanical model and beyond. Circulation. 2005;111:2837.
2. Jondeau G, Neuder Y, Eicher JC, et al. B-CONVINCED: Beta-blocker CONtinuation Vs. INterruption in patients with Congestive heart failure hospitalizED for a decompensation episode. Eur Heart J. 2009;30:2186-92.
3. McMurray JJ, Adamopoulos S, Anker SD, et al. ESC guidelines for the diagnosis and treatment of acute and chronic heart failure 2012: The Task Force for the Diagnosis and Treatment of Acute and Chronic Heart Failure 2012 of the European Society of Cardiology. Developed in collaboration with the Heart Failure Association (HFA) of the ESC. Eur Heart J. 2012;33:1787-847.
4. Yusuf S, Pitt B, Davis CE, et al. Effect of enalapril on survival in patients with reduced left ventricular ejection fractions and congestive heart failure. N Engl J Med. 1991;325:293-302.
5. A randomised clinical trial investigating the effect of enalapril versus placebo in severe congestive heart failure (New York Heart Association [NYHA] functional class IV). N Engl J Med. 1987;316:1429-35.
6. Jessup M, Abraham WT, Casey DE, et al. 2009 focused update: ACCF/AHA Guidelines for the Diagnosis and Management of Heart Failure in Adults: a report of the American College of Cardiology Foundation/American Heart Association Task Force on Practice Guidelines: developed in collaboration with the International Society for Heart and Lung Transplantation. Circulation. 2009;119:1977-2016.
7. Granger CB, McMurray JJ, Yusuf S, et al. Effects of candesartan in patients with chronic heart failure and reduced left-ventricular systolic function intolerant to angiotensin-converting enzyme inhibitors: The CHARM-Alternative trial. Lancet. 2003;362:772-6.
8. Cohn JN, Tognoni G. A randomized trial of the angiotensin-receptor blocker valsartan in chronic heart failure. N Engl J Med. 2001;345:1667-75.
9. Pfeffer MA, McMurray JJ, Velazquez EJ, et al. Valsartan, captopril, or both in myocardial infarction complicated by heart failure, left ventricular dysfunction, or both. N Engl J Med. 2003;349:1893-906.
10. McMurray JJ, Ostergren J, Swedberg K, et al. Effects of candesartan in patients with chronic heart failure and reduced left-ventricular systolic function taking angiotensin-converting enzyme inhibitors. The CHARM-added trial. Lancet. 2003;362:767-71.
11. Felker GM, Lee KL, Bull DA, et al. Diuretic strategies in patients with acute decompensated heart failure. N Engl J Med. 2011;364:797-805.
12. Juurlink DN, Mamdani MM, Lee DS, et al. Rates of hyperkalemia after publication of the Randomized Aldactone Evaluation Study. N Engl J Med. 2004;351:543-51.
13. Dupont M. Mukkens W, Finucan M, et al. Determinants of dynamic changes in serum creatinine in acute decompensated heart failure: The importance of the blood pressure reduction during treatment. Eur J Heart Fail. 2013;15:433-40.
14. Zannad F. Gattis SW, Rossignol P, et al. Mineralocorticoid receptor antagonists for heart failure with reduced ejection fraction: Integrating evidence into clinical practice. Eur heart J. 2012;33.2782-95.

CHAPTER 94

HFpEF—How to Diagnose and Manage?

Sanjeev Sanghvi, Swati Mahajan

INTRODUCTION

Heart failure (HF) with preserved ejection fraction (HFpEF) accounts for up to 50% of all HF cases in the developed countries.[1] The prevalence of HFpEF ranges from 1% to 3%, and is expected to rise further with increasing life expectancy, better diagnostic awareness, and increasing prevalence of comorbidities like obesity, diabetes, hypertension, and atrial fibrillation (AF).[1] HFpEF was previously referred to as "diastolic" HF. This was in comparison to "systolic" HF, which corresponded to HF with reduced ejection fraction (HFrEF). However, diastolic dysfunction is not unique to HFpEF, as evidenced by presence of diastolic dysfunction in systolic HF also. The term "HF with normal ejection fraction" (HFnEF) was used briefly; however newer imaging techniques have confirmed that systolic function in HFpEF patients is not completely normal, with mildly reduced left ventricular (LV) systolic function by global longitudinal strain.[2] As the exact normal range of function is difficult to define and the LV function may not be entirely normal, the term "HFpEF" is now used.

In observational studies, rates of hospitalization and death among patients with HFpEF are similar to those among patients with HFrEF, but in clinical-trial populations, outcomes are better in patients who have HFpEF.[3] Death from noncardiovascular causes is more common in patients who have HFpEF than in those with HFrEF.[4,5] Long-term mortality trends in HFpEF is similar to HFrEF, with less than 50% 5-year survival in HFpEF cohorts.[6,7] Outcomes following hospitalization for decompensated HFpEF are quite poor, with more than one-third of patients dead or rehospitalized within 60–90 days of discharge.[8]

PATHOPHYSIOLOGY OF HFpEF

Despite its burden, the pathophysiological mechanisms of HFpEF remain controversial and are likely to be multifactorial.[9] The lack of a comprehensive paradigm applicable to all patients suggests that hemodynamic derangements responsible for this disorder may be quite heterogeneous. Hemodynamic features of HFpEF involve both cardiac and extracardiac mechanisms (Fig. 1).

DIAGNOSIS OF HFpEF

The diagnosis of HFpEF remains challenging due to the advanced age of the patient and concomitant multiple illnesses. In fact, multiple comorbidities are the rule in HFpEF rather than the exception,[10] and significantly influence cardiovascular structure and function as well as long-term prognosis.[11] Depending upon the LV ejection fraction (LVEF), HF can be defined as those with normal LVEF (typically considered as ≥50%: HFpEF) and those with reduced LVEF (typically considered as <40%: HFrEF). Patients with an LVEF in the range of 40–49% represent a "grey area", which is now defined as HF with midrange ejection fraction (HFmrEF).[12] Current guidelines advocate using LVEF as one component of a diagnostic algorithm for HFpEF, alongside detection of additional myocardial abnormalities to implicate a cardiac cause for symptoms (Table 1).[12,13]

HISTORY AND CLINICAL EXAMINATION

A detailed history should always be obtained. At each visit, symptoms and signs of HF should be assessed, with particular attention to the evidence of congestion. Symptoms and signs for HF are usually nonspecific and hence may not discriminate well between HF and other clinical conditions. The diagnosis of chronic HFpEF, especially in elderly patients with comorbidities and no signs of central fluid overload, becomes difficult. In order to improve the specificity, the clinical diagnosis of HFpEF should be supported by objective measures of cardiac dysfunction at rest or during exercise. Symptoms and signs are important to monitor the response to the treatment.

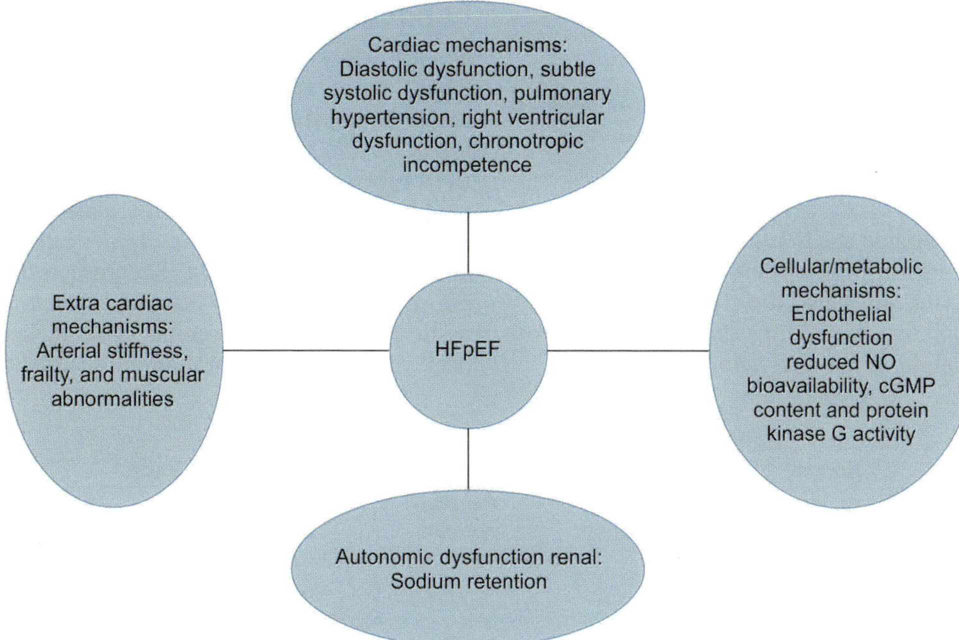

cGMP: cyclic guanosine monophosphate; HFpEF: heart failure with preserved ejection fraction; NO: nitric.

FIG. 1: Pathophysiology of heart failure with preserved ejection fraction.

TABLE 1: Diagnosis of heart failure with preserved ejection fraction

	ESC guidelines 2016[12]	AHA guidelines 2013[13]
History and examination	Symptoms and signs of HF	Symptoms and signs of HF
Ejection fraction	≥50%	≥50%
Natriuretic peptides	BNP >35 pg/mL and/or NT-proBNP >125 pg/mL	Elevated levels are supportive
Imaging	Cardiac structural alterations: • LAVI >34 mL/m2 • LVMI ≥115 g/m^2 (males) ≥95 g/m^2 (females) And/or cardiac functional alterations: • E/e' mean septal/lateral ≥13 e'septal/lateral wall <9 Other indirect measures: • Decreased global longitudinal strain, increased PASP	Abnormalities in LV diastolic function
ECG (electrocardiogram)	Findings like AF, repolarization abnormalities and LVH	Not specified
Exclusions	Exclusion of other causes of HF	Exclusion of other causes of HF
Further testing in case of uncertainty	• Diastolic stress test, invasive LV pressure assessment • Resting PCWP ≥15 mm Hg with change to ≥25 mm Hg with exercise or LVEDP ≥16 mm Hg	

AF, atrial fibrillation; AHA, American Heart Association; BNP, B-type natriuretic peptide; ESC, European Society of Cardiology; HF, heart failure; NT-proBNP, N-terminal proBNP; LAVI, left atrial volume index; LV, left ventricular; LVEDP, left ventricular end-diastolic pressure; LVH, left ventricular hypertrophy; LVMI, left ventricular mass index; PASP, pulmonary artery systolic pressure; PCWP, pulmonary capillary wedge pressure.

INVESTIGATIONS

Electrocardiogram

The electrocardiogram (ECG) may reveal abnormalities like repolarization abnormalities, AF, and LV hypertrophy.

Chest X-Ray

A chest X-ray is of limited use in the diagnosis of HFpEF. It is most useful in identifying an alternative explanation for a patient's symptoms and signs. The chest X-ray may show evidence of pulmonary venous congestion in a patient with HF, and is more helpful in the acute setting.

Echocardiography

Echocardiography has an important role in the diagnosis of HFpEF and is considered one of the most useful investigations in this setting. As diastolic dysfunction, which is graded from I to IV (Fig. 2), is the hallmark pathophysiological process in HFpEF, it is not surprising that echocardiography in HFpEF mainly focuses on markers of diastolic dysfunction. The key echocardiographic measurement in the assessment of diastolic dysfunction is E/e'. E represents the peak velocity of transmitral flow in early diastole, whereas e' represents the tissue Doppler early diastolic septal or lateral lengthening peak velocity of the mitral annulus. E/e' is thought to be a

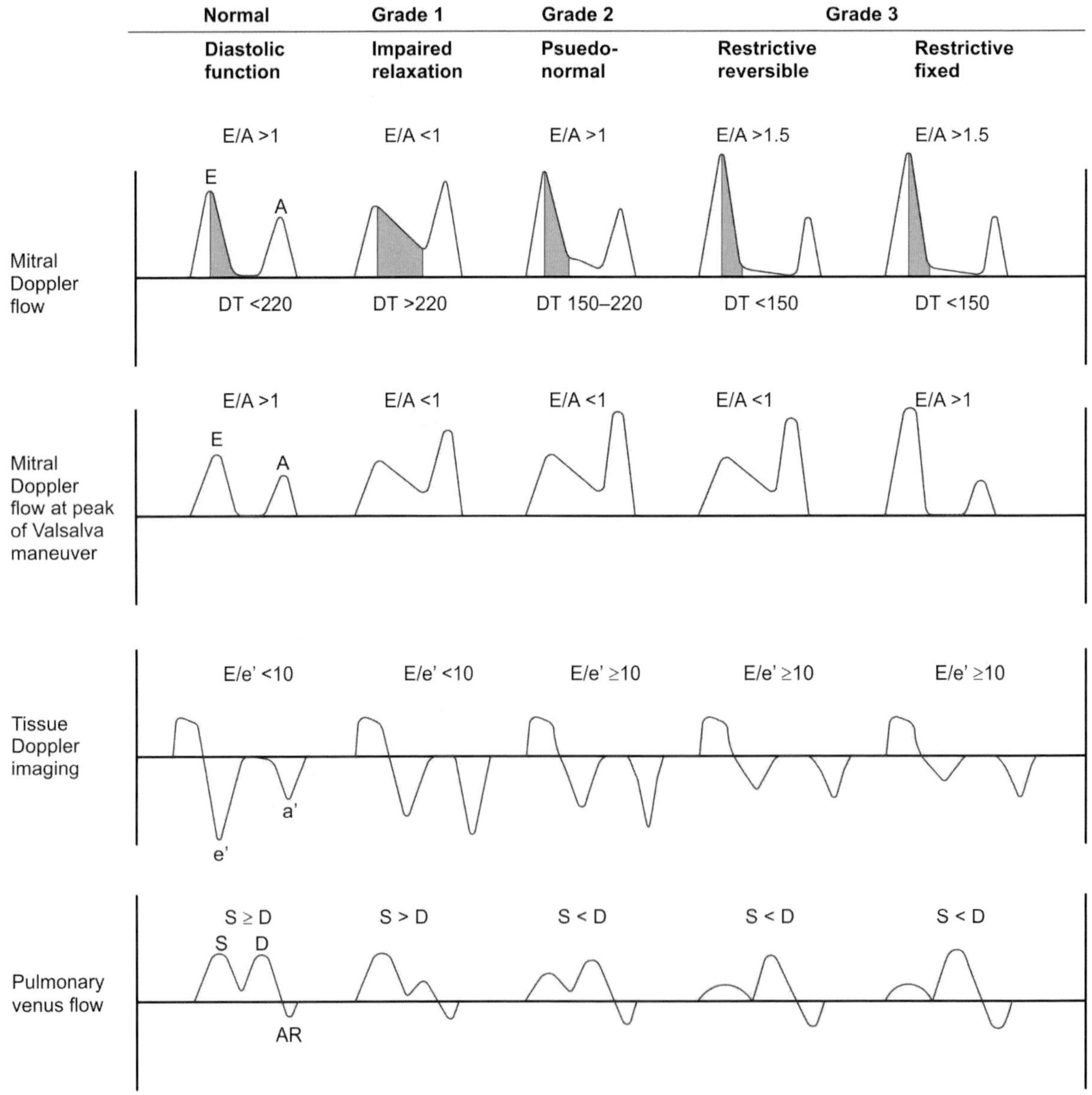

A, transmitral flow velocity with atrial contraction, a': velocity of mitral annular motion with atrial contraction; AR: flow into pulmonary vein during atrial contraction; D: diastolic; E: early diastolic flow velocity; e': velocity of early diastolic mitral annular motion; S: systolic.

FIG. 2: Classification of diastolic dysfunction.

reflection of left atrial pressures and thus of LV end-diastolic pressure (LVEDP). To date, an elevated E/e' (reflecting filling pressures ≥13 mm Hg) has been incorporated in guidelines as sufficient evidence of diastolic dysfunction.[12] However, only 25% of HFpEF patients have an elevated E/e', thereby suggesting low specificity and sensitivity of this parameter, even in combination with additional echo markers of diastolic dysfunction. Therefore, absence of an elevated E/e' does not rule out the presence of diastolic dysfunction.

Biomarkers

Normal levels of brain natriuretic peptide (BNP) are reported in up to 30% of patients, despite clinical, echocardiographic, and invasive hemodynamic evidence of HFpEF.[14] The absence of LV dilatation in HFpEF yields lower BNP concentrations and therefore less sensitive discrimination between the normal and HF state. Further ambiguity may be introduced by obesity, which is associated with lower plasma BNP concentrations, and by AF, which is associated with raised plasma BNP concentrations.[15] Other biomarkers like galectin-3, ST2, tissue inhibitor of metalloproteinases (TIMPs), amino-terminal propeptide of type III procollagen (PIIINP), homocysteine and resistin are particularly upregulated in HFpEF.[16]

Invasive Testing

Invasive hemodynamics at rest with assessment of filling pressures pulmonary capillary wedge pressure (PCWP) more than or equal to 15 mm Hg or LVEDP more than or equal to 16 mm Hg, followed by exercise hemodynamics if below these thresholds, with assessment of changes in filling pressures, pulmonary artery systolic pressure (PASP), stroke volume and cardiac output, can be performed.[17]

Diastolic Stress Testing

Exercise testing has been shown to enhance the diagnosis of HFpEF in patients with no overt signs of volume overload and normal filling pressures at rest and it holds promise for novel diagnostic strategies.[17]

One of the first studies addressing markedly elevated filling pressures during moderate exercise in patients with normal resting hemodynamics was by Borlaug et al.[17] They showed that more than 50% of patients with dyspnea on exertion had increased LV filling pressures only during exercise. Different dynamic exercise protocols are available, with semisupine bicycle ergometry and echocardiography at rest and submaximal exercise being used most often.[18] Exercise-induced increase in E/e' beyond diagnostic cut-offs (i.e. 13) and other indirect measures of systolic and diastolic function, such as longitudinal strain, are used.

Additional Role of Cardiac Magnetic Resonance Imaging

Over the last decade, attention has been given to the potential utility of cardiac magnetic resonance (CMR) and it is among the most promising noninvasive modalities. It provides good spatial resolution, and helps in the assessment of global as well as regional cardiac anatomy. Furthermore, information on left atrial volume and function, blood flow velocities, as well as myocardial tissue characteristics can be obtained. T1-mapping is used to quantify the degree of diffuse myocardial fibrosis.[19] In addition, CMR is considered the gold standard for the assessment of the right ventricle.[20] CMR may also be useful in the diagnosis of infiltrative cardiomyopathy (amyloidosis) or inflammatory cardiomyopathy (sarcoidosis).

TREATMENT (FIG. 3)

Pharmacological Treatment

Neurohormonal Antagonists

Angiotensin-converting Enzyme Inhibitors/ Angiotensin Receptor Blockers

Various studies have evaluated the role of angiotensin-converting enzyme (ACE) inhibitors and angiotensin receptor blockers (ARBs) for the treatment of HFpEF, including perindopril in elderly people with chronic HF (PEP-CHF),[21] CHARM-Preserved,[22] and irbesartan in patients with HF and preserved systolic function (I-Preserve).[23] No improvement was detected among patients randomized to the ACE-inhibitor or ARB in these trials, but the studies were limited by high crossover rates and, in part, insufficient power. Trials employing a low ejection fraction (EF) cut-off for HFpEF (e.g., >40% CHARM-Preserved, >45% I-Preserve) insufficiently represented symptomatic HFpEF, as defined by current guidelines.[13] The recent American College of Cardiology/ American Heart Association (ACC/AHA) 2013 HF guidelines recommend the use of ACE-inhibitors, ARBs, or beta-blockers in hypertensive patients with HFpEF with the goal of

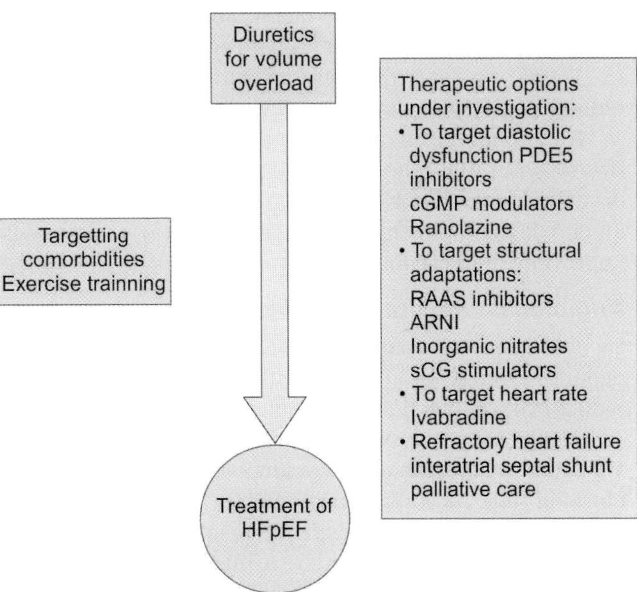

ARNI, angiotensin receptor-neprilysin inhibitor; cGMP, cyclic guanosine monophosphate; HFpEF, heart failure with preserved ejection fraction; PDE5, phosphodiesterase-5; RAAS, renin-angiotensin-aldosterone system.

FIG. 3: Treatment of heart failure with preserved ejection fraction.

controlling blood pressure (class IIa recommendation, level of evidence C), but data on beneficial outcomes, beyond risk factor control are inadequate to recommend the use of these agents specifically for the treatment of HFpEF.[13]

Beta-blockers

The effect of beta-blockers in patients with HFpEF has not been evaluated in an adequately powered study. Randomized trial to determine the effect of nebivolol on mortality and cardiovascular hospital admission in elderly patients with HF (SENIORS)[24] concluded that nebivolol, a beta-blocker with vasodilating properties, is an effective and well-tolerated treatment for HF in the elderly, however recruiting few patients with EF more than or equal to 50%, SENIORS insufficiently represented symptomatic HFpEF, as defined by current guidelines.

Mineralocorticoid Receptor Antagonist

Animal studies showed that mineralocorticoid receptor antagonist (MRA) prevent collagen synthesis and remodeling.[25] Small studies in HFpEF patients showed improvement in diastolic dysfunction parameters after treatment with MRA.[26] The Aldosterone Receptor Blockade in Diastolic Heart Failure (Aldo-DHF) trial was conducted in patients with chronic HF, New York Heart Association (NYHA) class II or III. It was a randomized, double-blinded, placebo-controlled trial.[27] It was observed that the co-primary endpoint E/e′ was significantly reduced in the spironolactone group. However, peak volume of oxygen (VO_2) was not affected by spironolactone. There was improvement in LVEF, with significant decrease in LV mass index (LVMI), and N-terminal pro B-type natriuretic peptide (NT-proBNP) from baseline in the spironolactone group. Treatment of preserved cardiac function HF with an aldosterone antagonist (TOPCAT), a phase-III trial found no reduction in the composite of cardiovascular death, aborted cardiac arrest, or HF hospitalization in patients with symptomatic HF and a LVEF 45% or more with the use of spironolactone, however, reduction in HF hospitalization was observed.[28]

The Randomized aldosterone antagonism in HFpEF (RAAM-PEF) trial randomized HFpEF patients to 6 months of eplerenone versus placebo, and showed reductions in circulating markers of collagen turnover and modest improvement in diastolic function.[29]

Angiotensin Receptor-Neprilysin Inhibitor

Sacubitril, a neprilysin inhibitor, increases the levels of peptides which promote natriuresis, vasodilation, and reduce extracellular fluid (ECF) volume via sodium excretion; eventually reducing preload and ventricular remodeling. Valsartan inhibits the effects of angiotensin-II by selectively blocking the receptor type-1 (AT_1), and concomitantly inhibits angiotensin-II-dependent aldosterone release. LCZ696 (sacubitril/valsartan) is a member of a new class of agents called angiotensin receptor-neprilysin inhibitor (ARNI), which combines a neprilysin inhibitor and an ARB. Prospective comparison of ARNI with ARB on examination of HFpEF (PARAMOUNT) trial randomized patients with LVEF more than or equal to 45%, signs and symptoms of HF, and elevated NT-proBNP plasma levels to LCZ696 or valsartan for 12 weeks.[30] The primary endpoint was change in NT-proBNP levels from baseline to 12 weeks. There was significant decrease in NT-proBNP levels from the baseline in LCZ696 group compared to valsartan group. There was significant reduction in left atrial volumes and dimensions after 36 weeks in the LCZ696 group. PARAGON-HF (NCT01920711) is an ongoing trial to determine the efficacy of sacubitril/valsartan compared with valsartan in patients with chronic HFpEF.

Other Pharmacological Agents

Diuretics

Diuretics are used to relieve the symptoms of congestion in patients with HFpEF.

Phosphodiesterase-5 Inhibitors

Phosphodiesterase-5 (PDE5) inhibition leads to accumulation of intracellular cyclic guanosine monophosphate (cGMP)- and nitric oxide (NO) induced pulmonary vasodilation in patients with pulmonary arterial hypertension.[31] PDE5 inhibition to improve clinical status and exercise capacity in HFpEF (RELAX) trial determined the effect of the PDE5 inhibitor sildenafil on exercise capacity and clinical status in HFpEF.[32] Sildenafil (n = 113) or placebo (n = 103) was administered orally at 20 mg, 3 times daily for 12 weeks, followed by 60 mg, 3 times daily for 12 weeks. PDE5 inhibition with sildenafil, compared with placebo, did not result in significant improvement in exercise capacity or clinical status in patients with HFpEF.

Cyclic Guanylate Monophosphate Stimulators

Modulation of NO-cGMP-protein kinase G signaling pathway, by various pharmacological agents, may increase cGMP content and reduce myocardial stiffness in HFpEF.

Oral Soluble Guanylate Cyclase Stimulators

Acute hemodynamic effects of riociguat in patients with pulmonary hypertension associated with diastolic HF (DILATE-1) evaluated riociguat in patients with pulmonary hypertension with LV diastolic dysfunction. Improvement in hemodynamics was observed with the use of riociguat.[33]

The SOCRATES-PRESERVED was a prospective, randomized, placebo-controlled double blind, phase 2b dose-finding study in patients with HFpEF (EF ≥45%), to determine tolerability and the optimal dose regimen of the soluble guanylate cyclase stimulator vericiguat in patients with chronic HF and preserved EF. Patients received vericiguat once daily at 1.25 or 2.5 mg fixed doses, or 5 or 10 mg titrated from a 2.5 mg starting dose or placebo for 12 weeks. Vericiguat was well tolerated, was associated with improvements in quality of life in patients with HFpEF but with no change in NT-proBNP at 12 weeks compared with placebo.[34]

Others

Use of isosorbide mononitrate (ISMN) has not shown any improvement in HFpEF trials.[35] Nitrate's effect on activity tolerance in HFpEF (NEAT-HFpEF) trial demonstrated decrease in patient's activity with the use of ISMN, possibly because of excess hypotension.[35]

Inorganic nitrate delivers NO during hypoxia and acidosis and avoids hypotension as seen with ISMN. Beetroot juice (dietary inorganic nitrate) has been evaluated in a phase II study where it led to improvement in exercise endurance in patients with HFpEF.[36] Presently, there are ongoing studies with inhaled nitrite preparation, to evaluate its benefits in HFpEF patients.

Ivabradine

Heart rate (HR) is one of the major determinant of diastolic function. Slow incomplete relaxation can be induced by increased afterload to such an extent that it leads to marked increase in filling pressures. Also the myocardium of HF patients may exhibit a flat or negative myocardial relaxation velocity to HR relationship, even at a lower range of HR, when compared to a normal heart. Hence, lowering the HR would prevent the clinical expression of this HR-dependent relaxation impairment. Reil et al. showed that ivabradine decreases arterial elastance by enhancing arterial compliance and reducing HR.[37] Effect of ivabradine in patients with HFpEF (EDIFY) trial showed that HR reduction with ivabradine did not improve outcomes.[38]

Late Sodium (Na^+) Current Inhibition

Ranolazine inhibits the late Na^+ current, thereby minimizing intramyocyte Na^+ accumulation and the resultant Ca^{2+} overload. The ranolazine for the treatment of diastolic HF (RALI-DHF) study evaluated the effect of ranolazine versus placebo on hemodynamics, measures of diastolic dysfunction, and biomarkers in 20 patients with HFpEF and diastolic dysfunction.[39] After 30 minutes of infusion, significant decrease from baseline were observed in LVEDP and PCWP in the ranolazine group, but not in the placebo group. RAZE trial, is an ongoing trial to evaluate the effects of ranolazine compared with placebo on exercise capacity in patients with HFpEF [NCT01505179].

Other Novel Therapies

Functional Iron Deficiency and Anemia

In a small study, functional iron deficiency was present in almost 50% of HFpEF patients; however, it did not correlate with diastolic dysfunction or exercise capacity.[40] FAIR-HFpEF [NCT03074591] is an ongoing trial to see the effect of intravenous (IV) iron (ferric carboxymaltose) on exercise tolerance, symptoms, and quality of life in patients with HFpEF and iron deficiency with and without anemia.

Bendavia

Bendavia (mitochondrial enhancer) is being evaluated in Mito-HFpEF trial, an ongoing study.

Treatment of co-morbidities

Comorbidities, such as hypertension, AF, diabetes, renal or pulmonary disease, anemia, obesity, and deconditioning, may contribute to the HFpEF. Management of comorbidities in the patients with HFpEF is class IB or C according to AHA 2013 guidelines.[13]

Nonpharmacological Treatment

Exercise Training

To date, exercise training is the only intervention that has shown symptomatic benefit in relatively young patients with HFpEF. Exercise training in Diastolic HF Pilot study (Ex-DHF-P) evaluated the benefit of combined endurance or resistance exercise training compared with usual care in symptomatic (NYHA class II-III) HFpEF patients.[41] There was significant improvement in peak VO_2 after 3 months in the training group. The ongoing phase II Ex-DHF study (ISRCTN 86879094) will evaluate the role of exercise training in patients with HFpEF.

Autonomic Modulation and Chronotropic Incompetence

Autonomic dysfunction is one of the factors implicated in the pathophysiology of HFpEF. Modulation of autonomic function, e.g., by baroreceptor activation, vagal nerve stimulation, and renal artery denervation, is under investigation for treating the patients with HFpEF.[42]

Controlled Left to Right Interatrial Shunt

In patients with HF and EF more than or equal to 40% creation of an interatrial shunt with the interatrial shunt device (IASD) leads to unloading of left atrium and reduction in PCWP during exercise.

The REDUCE LAP-HF I was a phase II randomized, parallel-group, blinded multicenter trial. Patients were randomized (1:1) to the IASD versus a sham procedure. IASD treatment led to reduction in PCWP during exercise.[43]

CONCLUSION

Patients who have signs and symptoms of HF but a preserved EF, objective evidence of abnormal cardiac structure and function should be confirmed. Natriuretic peptide levels may be normal in patients with HFpEF, particularly in obese patients. Medications that improve outcomes in patients with HFrEF have not shown to be of benefit in those who have HFpEF. Since, no therapy has been shown to improve outcomes in patients with HFpEF, current therapy mainly relies on the relief of volume overload (when present) and treatment of coexisting conditions. Certainly, our current knowledge base is still inadequate to the task of managing this increasing clinical problem.

REFERENCES

1. Dunlay SM, Roger VL, Redfield MM. Epidemiology of heart failure with preserved ejection fraction. Nat Rev Cardiol. 2017;14:591-602.
2. Sanderson JE. HFNEF, HFpEF, HF-PEF, or DHF: What is in an Acronym? JACC Heart Fail. 2014;2:93-4.
3. Campbell RT, Jhund PS, Castagno D, et al. What have we learned about patients with heart failure and preserved ejection fraction from DIG-PEF, CHARM-preserved, and I-PRESERVE? J Am Coll Cardiol. 2012;60:2349-56.
4. Chan MM, Lam CS. How do patients with heart failure with preserved ejection fraction die? Eur J Heart Fail. 2013;15:604-13.

5. Lee DS, Gona P, Albano I, et al. A systematic assessment of causes of death after heart failure onset in the community: impact of age at death, time period, and left ventricular systolic dysfunction. Circ Heart Fail. 2011;4:36-43.
6. Owan TE, Hodge DO, Herges RM, et al. Trends in prevalence and outcome of heart failure with preserved ejection fraction. N Engl J Med. 2006;355(3):251-9.
7. Tribouilloy C, Rusinaru D, Mahjoub H, et al. Prognosis of heart failure with preserved ejection fraction: a 5 year prospective population-based study. Eur Heart J. 2008;29(3):339-47.
8. Fonarow GC, Stough WG, Abraham WT, et al. Characteristics, treatments, and outcomes of patients with preserved systolic function hospitalized for heart failure: a report from the OPTIMIZE-HF Registry. J Am Coll Cardiol. 2007;50(8):768-77.
9. Senni M, Paulus WJ, Gavazzi A, et al. New strategies for heart failure with preserved ejection fraction: the importance of targeted therapies for heart failure phenotypes. Eur Heart J. 2014;35:2797-815.
10. Lam CSP, Lyass A, Kraigher-Krainer E, et al. Cardiac Dysfunction and Noncardiac Dysfunction as Precursors of Heart Failure with Reduced and Preserved Ejection Fraction in the Community/Clinical Perspective. Circulation. 2011;124(1):24-30.
11. Mohammed SF, Borlaug BA, Roger VL, et al. Comorbidity and ventricular and vascular structure and function in heart failure with preserved ejection fraction: a community based study. Circ Heart Fail. 2012;5:710-9.
12. Ponikowski P, Voors AA, Anker SD, et al. 2016 ESC Guidelines for the diagnosis and treatment of acute and chronic heart failure: The Task Force for the diagnosis and treatment of acute and chronic heart failure of the European Society of Cardiology (ESC) Developed with the special contribution of the Heart Failure Association (HFA) of the ESC. Eur Heart J. 2016;37:2129-200.
13. Yancy CW, Jessup M, Bozkurt B, et al. 2013 ACCF/AHA Guideline for the management of heart failure: a report of the American college of cardiology foundation/American heart association task force on practice guidelines. Circulation. 2013;128:1810-52.
14. Anjan VY, Loftus TM, Burke MA, et al. Prevalence, clinical phenotype, and outcomes associated with normal B-type natriuretic peptide levels in heart failure with preserved ejection fraction. Am J Cardiol. 2012;110:870-6.
15. Zakeri R, Borlaug BA, McNulty SE, et al. Impact of atrial fibrillation on exercise capacity in heart failure with preserved ejection fraction: a RELAX trial ancillary study. Circ Heart Fail. 2014;7:123-30.
16. Meijers WC, van der Velde AR, de Boer RA. Biomarkers in heart failure with preserved ejection fraction. Neth Heart J. 2016;24(4):252-8.
17. Borlaug BA, Nishimura RA, Sorajja P, et al. Exercise hemodynamics enhance diagnosis of early heart failure with preserved ejection fraction. Circ Heart Fail. 2010;3:588-95.
18. Erdei T, Smiseth OA, Marino P, et al. A systematic review of diastolic stress tests in heart failure with preserved ejection fraction, with proposals from the EU-FP7 MEDIA study group. Eur J Heart Fail. 2014;16:1345-61.
19. Su M-YM, Lin L-Y, Tseng Y-HE, et al. CMR-verified diffuse myocardial fibrosis is associated with diastolic dysfunction in HFpEF. JACC Cardiovasc Imaging. 2014;7:991-7.
20. Champion HC, Michelakis ED, Hassoun PM. Comprehensive invasive and noninvasive approach to the right ventricle–pulmonary circulation unit state of the art and clinical and research implications. Circulation. 2009;120:992-1007.
21. Cleland JG, Tendera M, Adamus J, et al. The perindopril in elderly people with chronic heart failure (PEP-CHF) study. Eur Heart J. 2006;27:2338-45.
22. Yusuf S, Pfeffer MA, Swedberg K, et al. CHARM Investigators and Committees. Effects of candesartan in patients with chronic heart failure and preserved left-ventricular ejection fraction: the CHARM-Preserved Trial. Lancet. 2003; 362:777-81.
23. Massie BM, Carson PE, McMurray JJ, et al. Irbesartan in patients with heart failure and preserved ejection fraction. N Engl J Med. 2008;359:2456-67.
24. van Veldhuisen DJ, Cohen-Solal A, Böhm M, et al. Beta-blockade with nebivolol in elderly heart failure patients with impaired and preserved left ventricular ejection fraction: data from SENIORS (Study of effects of nebivolol intervention on outcomes and rehospitalization in Seniors with heart failure). J Am Coll Cardiol. 2009;53:2150-8.
25. Brilla CG, Zhou G, Matsubara L, et al. Collagen metabolism in cultured adult rat cardiac fibroblasts: response to angiotensin II and aldosterone. J Mol Cell Cardiol. 1994;26:809-20.
26. Mottram PM, Haluska B, Leano R, et al. Effect of aldosterone antagonism on myocardial dysfunction in hypertensive patients with diastolic heart failure. Circulation. 2004;110:558-65.
27. Edelmann F, Schmidt AG, Gelbrich G, et al. Rationale and design of the 'aldosterone receptor blockade in diastolic heart failure' trial: a double-blind, randomized, placebo controlled, parallel group study to determine the effects of spironolactone on exercise capacity and diastolic function in patients with symptomatic diastolic heart failure (Aldo-DHF). Eur J Heart Fail. 2010;12:874-82.
28. Desai AS, Lewis EF, Li R, et al. Rationale and design of the treatment of preserved cardiac function heart failure with an aldosterone antagonist trial: a randomized, controlled study of spironolactone in patients with symptomatic heart failure and preserved ejection fraction. Am Heart J. 2011;162:966-72.
29. Deswal A, Richardson P, Bozkurt B, et al. Results of the randomized aldosterone antagonism in heart failure with preserved ejection fraction trial (RAAM-PEF). J Card Fail. 2011;17(8):634-42.
30. Solomon SD, Zile M, Pieske B, et al. The angiotensin receptor neprilysin inhibitor LCZ696 in heart failure with preserved ejection fraction: a phase 2 double-blind randomised controlled trial. Lancet. 2012;380:1387-95.
31. Galie N, Hoeper MM, Humbert M, et al. Guidelines for the diagnosis and treatment of pulmonary hypertension: the task force for the diagnosis and treatment of pulmonary hypertension of the European Society of Cardiology (ESC) and the European Respiratory Society (ERS), endorsed by the International Society of Heart and Lung Transplantation (ISHLT). Eur Heart J. 2009;30:2493-537.
32. Redfield MM, Borlaug BA, Lewis GD, et al. Phosphdiesterase-5 Inhibition to Improve CLinical Status and EXercise Capacity in Diastolic Heart Failure (RELAX) Trial: Rationale and Design. Circ Heart Fail. 2012;5:653-9.
33. Bondermann D, Pretsch I, Steringer-Mascherbauer R, et al. Acute hemodynamic effects of riociguat in patients with pulmonary hypertension associated with diastolic heart failure (DILATE-1): a randomized, double-blind, placebo-controlled, single-dose study[abstract P3321]. Eur Heart J (Suppl). 2013;34:620.
34. Burkert P, Aldo PM, Carolyn SP, et al. Vericiguat in patients with worsening chronic heart failure and preserved ejection fraction: results of the Soluble guanylate Cyclase stimulator in heart failure patients with PRESEVED EF (SOCRATES-PRESERVED) study. Eur Heart J. 2017;38(15):1119-27.
35. Redfield MM, Anstrom KJ, Levine JA, et al. Isosorbide mononitrate in heart failure with preserved ejection fraction. N Engl J Med. 2015;373:2314-24.
36. Zamani P, Rawat D, Shiva-Kumar P, et al. Effect of inorganic nitrate on exercise capacity in heart failure with preserved ejection fraction. Circ. 2015;131: 371-80.
37. Reil JC, Tardif JC, Ford I, et al. Selective heart rate reduction with ivabradine unloads the left ventricle in heart failure patients. J Am Coll Cardiol. 2013;62:1977-85.
38. Komajda M, Isnard R, Cohen-Solal A, et al. Effect of ivabradine in patients with heart failure with preserved ejection fraction: the EDIFY randomized placebo-controlled trial. Eur J Heart Fail. 2017;19(11):1495-503.
39. Jacobshagen C, Belardinelli L, Hasenfuss G, et al. Ranolazine for the treatment of heart failure with preserved ejection fraction: background, aims, and design of the RALI-DHF study. Clin Cardiol. 2011;34:426-32.
40. Kasner M, Aleksandrov AS, Westermann D, et al. Functional iron deficiency and diastolic function in heart failure with preserved ejection fraction. Int J Cardiol. 2013;168:4652–7.
41. Edelmann F, Gelbrich G, Düngen HD, et al. Exercise training improves exercise capacity and diastolic function in patients with heart failure with preserved ejection fraction: Results of the Ex-DHF (Exercise training in Diastolic Heart Failure) Pilot Study. J Am Coll Cardiol. 2011;58(17):1780-91.
42. Zile MR, Little WC. Effects of autonomic modulation: more than just blood pressure. J Am Coll Cardiol. 2012;59:910-2.
43. Feldman T, Mauri L, Kahwash R, et al. Transcatheter Interatrial Shunt Device for the Treatment of Heart Failure with Preserved Ejection Fraction (REDUCE LAP-HF I):A Phase 2, Randomized, Sham-Controlled Trial. Circ. 2018;137:364-75.

CHAPTER 95

Heart Failure with Midrange Ejection Fraction—What is This?

Arup Dasbiswas

INTRODUCTION

In heart failure (HF) cases, we find the ejection fraction (EF) as a continuum between reduced and preserved EF. Initially, studies were conducted mainly in HF with reduced EF (HFrEF) patients having a left ventricle ejection fraction (LVEF) less than 35–40%. Subsequently, focus was shifted to the cohort of patients having HF with preserved EF (HFpEF), i.e., on patients with HF symptoms, but with a LVEF exceeding 50%. The recent guidelines from the American Heart Association/American College of Cardiology Foundation (AHA/ACCF) and the European Society of Cardiology (ESC) have defined HFrEF as having symptoms and signs of HF with an LVEF less than 40%, whereas HFpEF is defined as HF with an LVEF more than or equal to 50%.[1,2]

The OPTIMIZE-HF (Organized Program to Initiate Lifesaving Treatment in Hospitalized Patients with Heart Failure)[3] and the ADHERE (Acute Decompensated Heart Failure Registry)[4] studies started to explore the characteristics, treatment patterns, and outcomes of patients with mildly reduced LVEF, suggesting these patients might have notable differences from those patients with HFrEF and HFpEF. Therefore, in-between HFrEF and HFpEF a less studied and a less characterized cohort remains, which fills in the gap of EF continuum with HF. The 2013 ACCF/AHA guidelines classified this range of LVEF 41–49% as borderline HFpEF[1], whereas the 2016 ESC guidelines have identified patients with HF and an LVEF 40–49% as having heart failure with midrange ejection fraction (HFmrEF).[2]

Considered as a grey area, the HFmrEF is gaining increasing attention in recent studies. Though, it is known that the patients with HFmrEF have higher readmission rates than patients with HFpEF and mortality rates comparable to HFrEF and HFpEF,[5] HFmrEF remains insufficiently characterized compared with the other groups. Therapy for patients with HFmrEF is also unclear, as clinical trials have not directly targeted this sizeable HF population. However, targeting this group to improve the outcome may lead to achieving success in a sizeable proportion of HF patients, because this group forms a good chunk of the population having HF, as the prevalence of HFmrEF is estimated to be in the range of 10–20% of all HF patients.[6,7]

CLINICAL CHARACTERISTICS

Four elements are simultaneously required for a positive diagnosis of HFmrEF: (1) symptoms with or without signs of HF, (2) LVEF of 40–49%, (3) elevated natriuretic peptides [B-type natriuretic peptide ≥35 pg/mL or N-terminal pro b-type natriuretic peptide (NT-proBNP) ≥125 pg/mL], and (4) relevant structural heart disease—left ventricle hypertrophy (left ventricular mass index ≥115 g/m^2 for males and ≥95 g/m^2 for females) or left atrial enlargement (>34 mL/m^2) or diastolic dysfunction (E/e' ≥13 and a mean e' septal and lateral wall <9 cm/s).[2]

Characteristics of patients with HFmrEF are largely intermediate between those of HFpEF and HFrEF.[8] The exception to this statement is cases in which ischemia is an etiology or a precipitating factor for HF decompensation, which is at least as common in HFmrEF as HFrEF.[9,10]

Outcome Data

Reported outcomes are variable, with some studies reporting similar long-term event rates, others reporting intermediate medium-term outcomes, and yet others reporting lower in-hospital mortality rates in HFmrEF.

Rickenbacher et al.[11] studied 622 patients with HF. The analysis was based on the Trial of Intensified versus standard Medical therapy in Elderly patients with Congestive Heart Failure (TIME-CHF) comprising a population with established HF including the whole spectrum of LVEF. Of the 622 patients, 108 (17%) were classified as having HFmrEF. During a median follow-up of 794 days, mortality was 39.7% without significant differences between groups. NT-proBNP—guided as compared with standard therapy resulted in improved survival free of HF hospitalizations in HFrEF and HFmrEF, but not in HFpEF.

Chioncel et al.[12] followed up 9,134 patients' data for 1 year. They found that The HFmrEF group resembled the HFrEF group in some features, including age, gender, and ischemic etiology, but had less left ventricular and atrial dilation. Mortality at 1 year differed significantly between HFrEF and HFpEF (8.8% vs. 6.3%); HFmrEF patients experienced intermediate rates (7.6%). Age, New York Heart Association (NYHA) class III/IV status, and chronic kidney disease (CKD) predicted mortality in all LVEF groups. Low systolic blood pressure and high heart rate were predictors for mortality in HFrEF and HFmrEF.

Kapoor et al.[9] analyzed the factors potentially contributing to HF hospitalization among 99,825 HF admissions from 305 hospitals in the Get With The Guidelines-HF (GWTG-HF) database between January 2005 and September 2013 and assessed their association with length of stay and in-hospital mortality. In patients with borderline EF (EF, 40–49%), pneumonia was associated with longer hospital stay, whereas dietary and medication noncompliance were associated with reduced length of stay.

PREDICTORS AND OUTCOMES OF HEART FAILURE WITH MIDRANGE EJECTION FRACTION

The majority of aforementioned data have been taken from prevalent cases of HF. Whereas, Bhambhani et al.[13] sought to examine clinical and biochemical predictors of incident HFmrEF in the community. They pooled data from four community-based longitudinal cohorts, with ascertainment of new HF classified into HFmrEF (EF 41–49%), HFpEF (EF ≥50%), and HFrEF (EF ≤40%). Predictors of incident HF subtypes were assessed using multivariable Cox models. Among 28,820 participants free of HF followed for a median of 12 years, there were 200 new HFmrEF cases, compared with 811 HFpEF and 1,048 HFrEF. Clinical predictors of HFmrEF included age, male sex, systolic blood pressure, diabetes mellitus, and prior myocardial infarction (multivariable adjusted p ≤0.003 for all). Biomarkers that predicted HFmrEF included natriuretic peptides, cystatin-C, and high-sensitivity troponin (p ≤0.0004 for all). Natriuretic peptides were stronger predictors of HFrEF [hazard ratio (HR) 2.00 per 1 standard deviation increase, 95% confidence interval (CI) 1.81–2.20] than of HFmrEF (HR 1.51, 95% CI 1.20–1.90, p = 0.01 for difference), and did not differ in their association with incident HFmrEF and HFpEF (HR 1.56, 95% CI 1.41–1.73, p = 0.68 for difference). All-cause mortality following the onset of HFmrEF was worse than that of HFpEF (50 vs. 39 events per 1,000 person-years, p = 0.02), but comparable to that of HFrEF (46 events per 1,000 person-years, p = 0.78). They found overlap in predictors of incident HFmrEF with other HF subtypes. In contrast, mortality risk after HFmrEF was worse than HFpEF, and similar to HFrEF.

Therapeutic Implications

Patients with LVEF between 40 and 50% were sometimes included in HFpEF trials, when the cut-off point for inclusion was LVEF more than 45%, but the patients with HFmrEF were not studied as a separate entity. Therefore, specific therapeutic evidence for this group of patients with HFmrEF is lacking. As the patients with HFmrEF, have to some extent, been included in trials of HFpEF, rather than in HFrEF, the 2016 ESC guidelines for the diagnosis and treatment of acute and chronic heart failure[2] recommended that they should be treated as patients with HFpEF, until further evidence demonstrating a prognostic difference between these two categories emerge.

Comorbidity control should be the prime target for the management of HFmrEF. Both cardiovascular diseases (CVD) (atrial fibrillation, hypertension, coronary artery disease, and pulmonary hypertension) and noncardiovascular diseases [diabetes, CKD, anemia, iron deficiency, chronic obstructive pulmonary disease (COPD), and obesity] should be looked into and managed optimally.

Similarly, precipitating factors should be prevented and/or rapidly managed. In the GWTG-HF registry of patients hospitalized for HF the most common precipitants for hospitalization were pneumonia/respiratory process (28%), arrhythmia (22%), medication noncompliance (16%), worsening renal failure (15%), and uncontrolled hypertension (15%), regardless of the baseline EF group.[5]

Diuretics should be used only if signs or symptoms of congestion are present; they represent the hallmark of symptom relief therapy, but have no influence on mortality. There is no specific recommendation for diuretic usage depending on LVEF, but rather a clinical judgment, depending on symptoms.

As the HFmrEF patients often have comorbidities such as hypertension, atrial fibrillation or ischemic heart disease (IHD), they often receive β-blockers and angiotensin-converting enzyme (ACE) inhibitors or angiotensin-receptor blockers (ARBs), and rarely mineralocorticoid receptor antagonist (MRA), in different combinations.[14] These are the drugs known to have prognostic impact on HFrEF, and same expectation is there while treating patients with HFmrEF. However, future studies on this subset of patients are needed.

In diabetes mellitus, sodium-glucose co-transporter type 2 (SGLT2) inhibitors modestly lower glycated hemoglobin A1c (HbA1c). But in EMPA-REG (10% HF at baseline), empagliflozin reduced HF hospitalization by 35%,[15] and in CANVAS (14% HF at baseline), canagliflozin reduced HF hospitalization by 33%.[16] This has generated considerable interest in SGLT2 and also SGLT2/1 inhibition in HF[17,18] and several trial programs are underway[19] to address whether SGLT2/1 inhibitors in combination with diuretics can improve outcomes in prevalent HF with HFrEF, HFmrEF, and/or HFpEF, in patients with and without diabetes.

Heart Failure with Recovered Ejection Fraction[20]

For patients with HFrEF, improving left ventricular (LV) reverse remodeling is an important goal. This may be achieved via multiple measures, including neurohormonal blockade, revascularization, resynchronization therapy, and mechanical unloading, etc. Not every patient responds to these measures in the same manner. Factors that are associated with better reverse remodeling include female sex, younger age, shorter HF duration, lack of a left bundle branch block, higher baseline BP, a nonischemic etiology, etc. These treatment responders may achieve improvement in the EF and reduced LV size. They may improve from HFrEF to HFmrEF and even normalized EF to more than or equal to 50%.

CONCLUSION[21]

The 2016 ESC guidelines introduced the term HFmrEF, corresponding to the previously denoted "grey area" EF 40–49%. But, one should remember EF is not the ideal marker to classify HF. EF also may change with time and treatment. Around 17–34% of patients with HF may improve to a higher category with appropriate management, more common in absence of IHD.[22] Other modalities may better characterize HF, e.g., global longitudinal strain, but their impact and feasibility in routine clinical practice are yet to be seen. Utilizing multiple markers and personalized approaches to HF may improve characterization and classification in HF.

Heart failure with midrange EF is intermediate regarding certain characteristics, and it resembles HFrEF regarding age, preponderance of male sex, greater prevalence of IHD, and greater prognostic impact of CKD.

In an individual patient-level meta-analysis from RCTs, β-blockers were not effective in atrial fibrillation (AF), but in sinus rhythm, they reduced all-cause and CV mortality in HFrEF and HFmrEF but not HFpEF.[23] In a post-hoc analysis from CHARM (Candesartan in Heart failure: Assessment of Reduction in Mortality and Morbidity), candesartan reduced the composite of CV death and HF hospitalization in HFrEF (where 57% received concomitant ACE inhibitor), and HFmrEF (27% ACE inhibitor) but not HFpEF (16% ACE inhibitor).[24]

Despite significant research done in the field of HFmrEF, further data collection and pragmatic and well-designed trials are needed to form appropriate guidelines.

REFERENCES

1. Yancy CW, Jessup M, Bozkurt B, et al. 2013 ACCF/AHA guideline for the management of heart failure: A report of the American College of Cardiology Foundation/American Heart Association Task Force on Practice Guidelines. J Am Coll Cardiol. 2013;62:e147-239.
2. Ponikowski P, Voors AA, Anker SD, et al. 2016 ESC guidelines for the diagnosis and treatment of acute and chronic heart failure: The Task Force for the diagnosis and treatment of acute and chronic heart failure of the European Society of Cardiology (ESC) developed with the special contribution of the Heart Failure Association (HFA) of the ESC. Eur Heart J. 2016;37:2129-200.
3. Fonarow GC, Stough WG, Abraham WT, et al. Characteristics, treatments, and outcomes of patients with preserved systolic function hospitalized for heart failure: A report from the OPTIMIZE-HF Registry. J Am Coll Cardiol. 2007;50:768-77.
4. Sweitzer NK, Lopatin M, Yancy CW, et al. Comparison of clinical features and outcomes of patients hospitalized with heart failure and normal ejection fraction (> or = 55%) versus those with mildly reduced (40% to 55%) and moderately to severely reduced (<40%) fractions. Am J Cardiol. 2008;101:1151-6.
5. Cheng RK, Cox M, Neely ML, et al. Outcomes in patients with heart failure with preserved, borderline, and reduced ejection fraction in the Medicare population. Am Heart J. 2014;168:721-30.
6. Lam CS, Solomon SD. The middle child in heart failure: Heart failure with mid-range ejection fraction (40–50%). Eur J Heart Fail. 2014;16(10):1049-55.
7. Solomon SD, Anavekar N, Skali H, et al. Influence of ejection fraction on cardiovascular outcomes in a broad spectrum of heart failure patients. Circulation. 2005;112:3738-44.
8. Tromp J, Voors AA, Lam CSP. Heart failure with mid-range ejection fraction: Causes and consequences. Eur J Heart Fail. 2018;20:660-2.
9. Kapoor JR, Kapoor R, Ju C, et al. Precipitating clinical factors, heart failure characterization, and outcomes in patients hospitalized with heart failure with reduced, borderline, and preserved ejection fraction. JACC Heart Fail. 2016;4:464-72.
10. Koh AS, Tay WT, Teng TH, et al. A comprehensive population-based characterization of heart failure with mid-range ejection fraction. Eur J Heart Fail. 2017;19:1624-34.
11. Rickenbacher P, Kaufmann BA, Maeder MT, et al. Heart failure with mid-range ejection fraction: A distinct clinical entity? Insights from the Trial of Intensified versus standard Medical therapy in Elderly patients with Congestive Heart Failure (TIME-CHF). Eur J Heart Fail. 2017;19(12):1586-96.
12. Chioncel O, Lainscak M, Seferovic PM, et al. Epidemiology and one-year outcomes in patients with chronic heart failure and preserved, mid-range and reduced ejection fraction: An analysis of the ESC Heart Failure Long-Term Registry. Eur J Heart Fail. 2017;19(12):1574-85.
13. Bhambhani V, Kizer JR, Lima JAC, et al Predictors and outcomes of heart failure with mid-range ejection fraction. Eur J Heart Fail. 2018;20(4):651-9.
14. Lauritsen J, Gustaffsson,F, Abdulla J. Characteristics and long-term prognosis of patients with heart failure and mid-range ejection fraction compared with reduced and preserved ejection fraction: A systematic review and meta-analysis. ESC Heart Fail. 2018;5(4):685-94.
15. Zinman B, Wanner C, Lachin JM, et al. Empagliflozin, cardiovascular outcomes, and mortality in type 2 diabetes. N Engl J Med. 2015;373:2117-28.
16. Neal B, Perkovic V, Mahaffey KW, et al. Canagliflozin and cardiovascular and renal events in type 2 diabetes. N Engl J Med. 2017;377:644-57.
17. Savarese G, D'Amore C, Federici M, et al. Effects of dipeptidyl peptidase 4 Inhibitors and Sodium-Glucose Linkedco Transporter-2 Inhibitors on cardiovascular events in patients with type 2 diabetes mellitus: A meta-analysis. Int J Cardiol. 2016;220:595-601.
18. Fitchett DH, Udell JA, Inzucchi SE. Heart failure outcomes in clinical trials of glucose-lowering agents in patients with diabetes. Eur J Heart Fail. 2017;19:43-53.
19. Butler J, Hamo CE, Filippatos G, et al. The potential role and rationale for treatment of heart failure with sodium-glucose co-transporter 2 inhibitors. Eur J Heart Fail. 2017;19:1390-400.
20. Unkovic P, Basuray A. Heart failure with recovered EF and heart failure with mid-range EF: Current recommendations and controversies. Curr Treat Options Cardio Med. 2018;20:35.
21. Lund LH, Køber L, Swedberg K, et al. The year in cardiology 2017: Heart failure. Eur Heart J. 2018;39:832-9.
22. Vedin O, Lam CSP, Koh AS, et al. Significance of ischemic heart disease in patients with heart failure and preserved, midrange, and reduced ejection fraction: A nationwide cohort study. Circ Heart Fail. 2017;10:e003875.
23. Tsuji K, Sakata Y, Nochioka K, et al. Characterization of heart failure patients with mid-range left ventricular ejection fraction—a report from the CHART-2 Study. Eur J Heart Fail. 2017;19:1258-69.
24. Lund LH, Claggett B, Liu J, et al. Heart failure with mid ejection fraction in CHARM: Characteristics, outcomes and effect of candesartan across the entire EF spectrum. Eur J Heart Fail. 2018;20(8):1230-9.

CHAPTER 96

Monitoring Therapy in Heart Failure with Reduced Ejection Fraction

Soura Mookerjee

INTRODUCTION

Once any difficulties regarding the diagnosis of heart failure (HF) have been overcome, the question of how best to manage patients in the long-term arises. Successful management includes monitoring in addition to treatment of HF.

Nothing can substitute for a careful history and physical examination. However, it necessitates adequate time available for well-trained health professionals and full examination of each patient's chest, jugular venous pressure (JVP), abdomen, and periphery as well as measurement of arterial pressure in the supine and standing positions. Especially useful are accurate examination of the JVP and auscultation for a third heart sound, both necessitating observer experience. A low blood pressure that falls further with upright posture indicates deterioration in left ventricular (LV) function and/or volume depletion, the latter necessitating reduction in diuretic dose or relaxation of restriction on dietary sodium intake. Uncontrolled hypertension, on the other hand, is one precipitant of hospital readmission for HF.

Body weight standardized to time of day and clothing, should preferably be recorded regularly by the patient at home as well as in the clinic. This can detect sodium and water retention (increased weight) and overdiuresis or cardiac cachexia (weight loss). Plasma electrolytes and renal function should be measured every few months and more frequently when there is clinical deterioration.

TRIALS OF BIOMARKER-GUIDED THERAPY FOR HEART FAILURE (TABLE 1)

Since 2000, several randomized controlled trials have reported the efficacy of serial measurements of plasma B-type peptides in titration of therapy for chronic HF.[1] Trials were heterogeneous with respect to design, patient characteristics duration of follow-up, end points, and target peptide concentrations. However, there was an overall consistency as supported by two meta-analyses.[2,3]

The first of these was a pilot study from Christchurch, New Zealand reported in 2000 with 69 patients. Significantly, fewer deaths or admissions with newly decompensated HF were observed in the hormone-guided group. This small, but positive, study was the sole contribution to the field until 2007, when the French multicenter STARS-BNP was reported.[4]

The GUIDE-IT (Guiding Evidence Based Therapy Using Biomarker Intensified Treatment in Heart Failure) study[5] was planned for 1,100 patients with ejection fraction (EF) of 40% or less, elevated natriuretic peptide and history of a prior HF event. Patients were assigned patients to a guided strategy in which HF therapy was titrated with the goal of N-terminal prohormone of brain natriuretic peptide (NT-proBNP) less than 1,000 pg/mL or to the usual guideline-directed care. The primary endpoint was a composite of time to first HF hospitalization or cardiovascular (CV) mortality.

The trial was stopped for futility by the data safety and monitoring board after 864 patients were enrolled due to a lack of benefit in the biomarker guided arm. As quoted from an editorial "Perhaps the most likely explanation for the outcomes observed in the GUIDE-IT trial is that when clinical care follows guidelines and addresses the key issues, biomarkers do not make a difference and that guideline-directed care, if achieved, is more efficient and can lead to outcomes similar to biomarker-guided care".

Thus the failure of the GUIDE-IT was a big blow to the biomarker-guided approach to tailor HF medications.

MULTIDISCIPLINARY CARE APPROACH TO THE MANAGEMENT OF HEART FAILURE PATIENTS

The multidisciplinary HF care approach includes:

- Standard care (i.e., in person follow-up visits) and
- Alternative approaches (regularly scheduled telephone contact between patient and health care specialist by electronic transfer of physiological data using remote

TABLE 1: Trials of biomarker-guided therapy for heart failure

Trials	Year	No. of patients	Follow up	Target proBNP	Primary endpoint	Result
New Zealand	2000	69	9 months	<1,700 pmol/L	Death + admissions	+
STARS-BNP	2006	220	15 months	<1,000 pg/mL	Death due to HF Death + hospitalizations All-cause mortality	+ + –
TIME-CHF	2009	499	18 months	BNP level 2 times less ULN and NYHA to II	Event free survival and QoL	–
BATTLESCARRED	2009	364	3 years	NT-proBNP <1,300 pg/mL	Mortality	+ (for age <75 years)
PRIMA	2010	345	702 days	NT-proBNP <2,491 pg/mL	Days alive out of hospital	–
PROTECT	2010	151	10 months	NT-proBNP <1,000 pg/mL	Total cardiovascular events	+
SIGMA-HF	2010	252	9 months	NT-proBNP <800 male <1,000 female	Days alive, days out of hospital and symptom score	–
STARBRITE	2011	130	90 days	BNP level. Congestion score	Death/hospitalizations	–
GUIDE-IT	2017	864	15 months	NT-proBNP <1,000 pg/mL	Time to first HF hospitalization and CV mortality	(Halted)

BNP, brain natriuretic peptide; HF, heart failure; NYHA, New York Heart Association; QoL, quality of life; ULN, upper level of normal; NT-proBNP, N-terminal prohormone of brain natriuretic peptide; CV, cardiovascular.

access technology. These alternative approaches may decrease the number of office visits and increase the efficiency of treatment of HF).

REMOTE MONITORING OF HEART FAILURE: TOOLS AND RESULTS

Structured Transtelephonic Support and Telemonitoring of Heart Failure Patients

Inglis et al. analyzed 41 randomized clinical trials comparing structured telephone support (25 studies, 9,332 patients) and telemonitoring (18 studies, 3,860 patients) with standard care for HF.[6] A significant reduction in all-cause mortality and HF hospitalizations was achieved with telemonitoring.

Telemonitoring involved an interactive voice-response system that transmitted daily information about symptoms and weight to the clinicians. Just over half of patients in the telemonitoring group actually used the system. Fourteen percent of patients never used the system.

However, the TIM-HF (Telemedical Interventional Monitoring in Heart Failure) study[7] failed to show a benefit.

Thus telemonitoring for HF though promising has not yet conclusively proven to be of benefit.

Remote Monitoring with Implanted Therapeutic Devices

The number of HF patients with cardiac implantable electronic devices (CIEDs) has increased in recent decades. A substantial number of modern CIEDs are equipped with remote monitoring capabilities. Remote monitoring of implantable cardioverter defibrillators (ICDs) and cardiac resynchronization therapy (CRT) devices allow wireless download and stored diagnostic information from device to an external transmitter and transfer to the manufacturer's database and available to the clinician through a specific interface.

Furthermore, technical features of the devices [anti-tachycardia pacing, direct current (DC) shock, ventricular pacing percentage] and so-called "HF diagnostic" parameters, such as thoracic impedance, heart rate variability, presence of arrhythmias, patients' activity level, mean heart rate at rest and exertion, can also be remotely monitored.

Remote monitoring may play an important role in the early diagnosis and management of system-related complications in patients with implanted CIEDs.[8] The majority of which are lead-related complications (insulation defect or conductor disruption). The TRUST (The Lumos-T Safely RedUceS RouTine Office Device Follow-Up) trial[9] and ECOST trial[10] have shown the beneficial effect of remote monitoring. Spencker et al. in a retrospective cohort analysis of 54 patients with an ICD lead failure[11] have shown that in 91% of all lead-related ICD complications, the diagnosis could be established correctly by an alert from the remote monitoring system.

Detection of Hemodynamic Deterioration in Heart Failure Patients

Many commercially available CIEDs can measure intrathoracic impedance which changes with volume overload in the pulmonary circulation caused by an elevated LV filling pressure.

While Yu et al.[12] and Abraham et al.[13] demonstrated the superiority of impedance monitoring, the SENSE-HF (Sensitivity of the InSync Sentry OptiVol feature for the prediction of Heart Failure) trial (501 patients) showed that an intracardiac impedance-derived fluid index had low sensitivity and positive predictive value.[14] Similar disappointing results have been demonstrated in the DOT-HF (Diagnostic Outcome Trial in Heart Failure) study.[15]

The PARTNERS-HF (Program to Access and Review Trending Information and Evaluate Correlation to Symptoms in Patients With Heart Failure) trial[16] showed that in patients with implanted CRT-Ds reduced impedance was the most sensitive parameter to predict HF hospitalizations. Cowie et al. developed and validated a dynamic HF score based on the following parameters monitored by implanted ICDs or CRTs: intrathoracic impedance, heart rate variability, arrhythmia burden, and patient activity.[17] The IN-TIME (Implant-Based Multiparameter Telemonitoring of Patients with Heart Failure) trial[18] also showed that composite clinical score and mortality were significantly lower in the telemonitoring group versus standard monitoring group. However, the world's largest remote monitoring study REM-HF (Remote Management of Heart Failure Using Implantable Electronic Devices) trial[19] presented at the ESC Congress 2016 and the MORE-CARE (The MOnitoring Resynchronization dEvices and CARdiac patiEnts) trial with biventricular ICD[20] turned out to be negative trials.

A meta-analysis of the TRUST, ECOST, and IN-TIME trials[21] demonstrated that remote monitoring with BIOTRONIK Home Monitoring was associated with a 38% reduction in all-cause mortality compared to conventional office follow-ups. The combined risk of all-cause mortality or hospitalization for HF decompensation was 36% lower in the remote monitoring group.

The presented results demonstrate that significant differences exist between devices from different manufacturers which can have an impact on their effectiveness.

Detection of Sleep Disorders in Heart Failure by Remote Monitoring (Table 2)

Patients with HF often complain of sleep disorders such as sleep fragmentation or nonrestorative sleep, difficulties in initiating sleep, or waking up too early in the morning.[22] Additionally, HF patients can have secondary insomnia due to HF itself or from the adverse effects of prescribed medications.[23] CIEDs with incorporated sleep apnea monitoring (SAM) system can detect, count, and report breathing disorders during the night.

Remote Monitoring by Implanted Monitoring-only Devices (Table 2)

Implanted monitoring-only devices are hemodynamic monitors measuring intracardiac or intravascular pressures. Examples are:

- Chronicle (Medtronic) studied in COMPASS-HF (Chronicle Offers Management to Patients with Advanced Signs and Symptoms of Heart Failure)[24]
- Cardio-MEMS (St Jude Medical, acquired by Abbott) studied in CHAMPION (The CardioMEMS Heart Sensor Allows Monitoring of Pressure to Improve Outcomes in NYHA Class III Heart Failure Patients)[25]
- HeartPOD device (St Jude Medical) studied in HOMEOSTASIS.[26]

TABLE 2: Major studies demonstrating role of remote monitoring in heart failure

Study	No. of patients	Study protocol	Results
Structured transtelephonic support and telemonitoring of HF patients			
Tele-HF	1,653	Telemonitoring care vs. usual care	• Readmission rates – NS • Deaths – NS
TIM-HF	710	Telemedical care vs. usual care	Hospitalization rates – NS
Remote monitoring with implanted therapeutic devices—detection of heart rhythm disorders			
ASSERT	2,580	Patients with implanted CIEDs, 2.5 years of follow-up. Newly detected AF episodes (with >6 min of duration) were counted	Newly detected AF episode detected in 34.7%
TRENDS	1,368	Patients without history of AF enrolled. Newly detected AF episodes (with >5 min of duration) were counted	Newly detected AF episode detected in 30%
TRUST	1,339	Remote monitoring vs. standard care	AF detection earlier (5.5 days) in remote monitoring group vs. 40 days with standard care
CONNECT	1,997	ICD implanted patients	Patients with implanted ICDs were involved 3 vs. 24 days interval between AF episodes detection and clinical response in the remote monitoring vs. standard follow-up groups

Continued

Continued

Study	No. of patients	Study protocol	Results
COMPAS	538	Remote monitoring vs. standard care (18.3 months)	• 17.3% vs. 19.1% (p <0.01 for noninferiority) patients experienced at least one major adverse event (all-cause death, hospitalizations for device-related or CV events) in remote monitoring standard care • Fewer hospitalizations for atrial arrhythmias (6 vs. 18) and strokes (2 vs. 8) (p <0.05) • 56% less interim ambulatory visits in the remote monitoring vs. standard care group (p <0.001)
Detection and management of system-related complications in patients with implanted CIEDs			
ECOST	40	Patients with high-voltage leads with 22 ± 4 months of follow-up	Lead failure registered in 7.5%
Detection of heart failure worsening in hemodynamics			
SENSE-HF	501	Intracardiac impedance-derived fluid index measurement	Low-sensitivity and positive predictive value in the early period after implantation (6 months), though sensitivity improved within the first 6 months after implantation
DOT-HF	335	Patients with implanted CIEDs. Randomized to have information available to physicians and patients as an audible alert in case of preset threshold crossings (access arm) or not (control arm)	Routine monitoring of intrathoracic impedance did not show better outcome and associated with more HF hospitalization
PARTNERS-HF	694	Patients with implanted CRT-Ds followed-up for 11.7 ± 2 months	Reduced impedance/increased fluid index was the most sensitive parameter to predict HF hospitalizations
IN-TIME	664	NYHA II and III patients with implanted ICDs and CRTDs randomized to standard vs. remote monitoring (in response to telemonitoring observations the investigators did a standardized telephone interview to confirm worsening of patient's overall condition or symptoms, or sudden increase in body weight (>2 kg in preceding 3 days) or scheduled visit to family doctor arms	• 63 patients (18.9%) with worsened composite clinical score in the telemonitoring group vs. 90 patients (27.2%) in the control group (p = 0.013) • Mortality lower in telemonitoring vs control group(n = 10 vs. 27) • No significant differences in hospitalization
REM-HF	1,650	Patients with implanted CIEDs (ICD, CRTP, and CRT-D) with remote monitoring facility randomized to usual care or remote monitoring, with follow-up of 2.8 years. Management of patients with remote monitoring was based on the data healthcare professional received on a weekly basis. Patients in usual care group had a usual care from heart failure service and remote monitoring of the device (once per 3–6 months)	No significant difference in the primary (death from any cause or unplanned CV hospitalization) and secondary (death from any cause, CV death) unplanned hospitalization) end points
MORE-CARE	865	Patients with implanted CRT-Ds randomized into remote and standard follow-up arms	• No significant different in the composite of death and hospitalization due to CV and device-related reasons between these two groups • Sign 38% reduction in healthcare resources use in the remote arm (2-year rates of CV hospital, CV emergency admissions, and CV in-office follow up) compared with the standard arm
Detection of sleep disorders: the potential implementation of remote monitoring			
DREAM	40	Patients with implanted CIEDs and incorporated sleep apnea monitoring (SAM) algorithm were enrolled. Sleep apnea diagnosis was confirmed by polysomnography as a gold standard diagnostic technique and compared with the respiratory disturbances index evaluated by the SAM algorithm	• 88.9% sensitivity (95% CI 65.3–98.6%) • 88.9% positive predictive value (95% CI 65.3–98.6%) • 84.6% specificity (95% CI 54.6–98.1%)

Continued

Continued

Study	No. of patients	Study protocol	Results
Remote monitoring with implanted monitoring-only devices			
COMPASS-HF	274	Patients were randomized into chronicle device and standard groups	• Reduction in HF admissions or urgent follow-up visits in chronicle group by 21% (p = 0.33) ns • Statistically significant 36% reduction in relative risk of time to first hospitalization
REDUCE-HF	1,300	Patients with an indication of ICD implantation evaluated (ICD implantation with an RV pressure monitoring)	• The trial was prematurely terminated due to technical complications • No benefit from hemomonitor
CHAMPION	550	NYHA Class III patients randomized into the CardioMEMs and usual monitoring groups	• Statistically significant reduction in HF hospitalization (regardless of LV ejection fraction) by 28% and 37% in the CardioMEMS group over 6- and 15-month follow up respectively • Non-HF-related hospitalizations were similar. • CardioMEMS group had a significant reduction in the mean PAP and better QoL during the 6-month follow up (Minnesota Living with Heart Failure Questionnaire)
HOMEO-STASIS	40	NYHA class III-IV HF patients received a HeartPOD device to directly measure LA pressure The follow-up period was divided into the first blinded (3 months), the second titration (3 months) and the third stability periods (19 months)	HeartPOD group had statistically significant: • Improved control of LA pressure • Improved NYHA class • More optimal neurohormonal antagonist dosing • 59% reduction of clinical events in the titration and stability period vs. observation period

AF, atrial fibrillation; CIED, cardiac implantable electronic device; CI, confidence interval; CV, cardiac vascular; CRTD, cardiac resynchronization therapy defibrillator; CRTP, cardiac resynchronization therapy pacemaker; HF, heart failure; ICD, implantable cardioverter defibrillator; LA, left atrial; NYHA, New York Heart Association; QoL, quality of life; RV, right ventricle.

Despite the theoretical advantage of implantable hemodynamic monitoring devices, the sensitivity for such approach needs to be validated in large randomized trials.

CONCLUSION

- Biomarker-guided therapy for HF is a new avenue to tailor HF medications
- Telemonitoring of HF patients can obviate the need for frequent physical examination of heart failure patients
- Remote monitoring through implanted devices can provide valuable information regarding hemodynamic parameters, sleep disorders, and implanted device-related complications
- None of the above approaches have till date unequivocally demonstrated their efficacy in randomized trials and presently do not supercede a meticulous clinical evaluation of heart failure patients.

REFERENCES

1. Troughton RW, Frampton CM, Yandle TG, et al. Treatment of heart failure guided by plasma amino-terminal brain natriuretic peptide (N-BNP) concentrations. Lancet. 2000;355(9210):1126-30.
2. Felker GM, Hasselblad V, Hernandez AF, et al. Biomarker-guided therapy in chronic heart failure: A meta-analysis of randomized controlled trials associated with a significant reduction in all-cause mortality compared to usual care in patients with chronic heart failure. Am Heart J. 2009;158:422-30.
3. Porapakkham P, Porapakkham P, Zimmet H, et al. B-type natriuretic peptide guided heart failure therapy: A meta-analysis. Arch Intern Med. 2010;170:507-14.
4. Jourdain P, Jondeau G, Funck F, et al. Plasma brain natriuretic peptide-guided therapy to improve outcome in heart failure. The STARS-BNP Multicenter Study. J Am Coll Cardiol. 2007;49:1733-9.
5. Felker GM, Anstrom KJ, Adams KF, et al. Effect of natriuretic peptide–guided therapy on hospitalization or cardiovascular mortality in high-risk patients with heart failure and reduced ejection fraction: A randomized clinical trial. JAMA. 2017;318:713-20.
6. Inglis SC, Clark RA, Dierckx R, et al. Structured telephone support or non-invasive telemonitoring for patients with heart failure. Cochrane Database Syst Rev. 2015;10:CD007228.
7. Koehler F, Winkler S, Schieber M, et al. Telemedical Interventional Monitoring in Heart Failure (TIM-HF), a randomized, controlled intervention trial investigating the impact of telemedicine on mortality in ambulatory patients with heart failure: study design. Eur J Heart Fail. 2010;12:1354-62.
8. Theuns DAMJ, Jordaens L. Use of remote monitoring in the management of system-related complications in implantable defibrillator patients. Neth Heart J. 2012;20:82-5.
9. Varma N, Epstein AE, Iripmen A, et al. Efficacy and safety of automatic remote monitoring for implantable cardioverter-defibrillator follow-up: The Lumos-T Safely Reduces Routine Office Device Follow-up (TRUST) trial. Circulation. 2010;122:325-32.
10. Guedon-Moreau L, Chevalier P, Marquie C, et al. Contributions of remote monitoring to the follow-up of implantable cardioverter defibrillator leads under advisory. Eur Heart J. 2010;31:2246-52.
11. Spencker S, Coban N, Koch L, et al. Potential role of home monitoring to reduce inappropriate shocks in implantable cardioverter defibrillator patients due to lead failure. Europace. 2009;11(4):483-8.
12. Yu CM, Wang L, Chau E, et al. Intrathoracic impedance monitoring in patients with heart failure: correlation with fluid status and feasibility of early warning preceding hospitalization. Circulation. 2005;112:841-8.

13. Abraham WT, Compton S, Haas G, et al. Intrathoracic impedance vs. daily weight monitoring for predicting worsening heart failure events: results of the Fluid Accumulation Status Trial (FAST). Congest Heart Fail. 2011;17:51-5.
14. Conraads VM, Tavazzi L, Santini M, et al. Sensitivity and positive predictive value of implantable intrathoracic impedance monitoring as a predictor of heart failure hospitalizations: the SENSE-HF trial. Eur Heart J. 2011;32:2266-73.
15. Van Veldhuisen DJ, Braunschweig F, Conraads V, et al. Intrathoracic impedance monitoring, audible patient alerts, and outcome in patients with heart failure. Circulation. 2011;124:1719-26.
16. Whellan DJ, Ousdigin KT, Al-Khatib SM, et al. Combined heart failure device diagnostics identify patients at higher risk of subsequent heart failure hospitalizations: results from PARTNERS HF (Program to Access and Review Trending Information and Evaluate Correlation to Symptoms in Patients With Heart Failure) study. J Am Coll Cardiol. 2010;55(17):1803-10.
17. Cowie MR, Sarkar S, Koehler J, et al. Development and validation of an integrated diagnostic algorithm derived from parameters monitored in implantable devices for identifying patients at risk for heart failure hospitalization in an ambulatory setting. Eur Heart J. 2013;34(31):2472-80.
18. Hindriks G, Taborsky M, Glikson M, et al. Implant-based multiparameter telemonitoring of patients with heart failure (IN-TIME): a randomised controlled trial. The Lancet. 2014;384(9943):583-90.
19. Morgan JM, Kitt S, Gill J, et al. Remote management of heart failure using implantable electronic devices. Eur Heart J. 2017;38(30);2352-60.
20. Boriani G, Da Costa A, Quesada A, et al. Effects of remote monitoring on clinical outcomes and use of healthcare resources in heart failure patients with biventricular defibrillators: Results of the MORE-CARE multicentre randomized controlled trial. Eur J Heart Fail. 2017;19(3):416-25.
21. Hindricks G, Varma N, Kacet S, et al. Daily remote monitoring of implantable cardioverter-defibrillators: insights from the pooled patient-level data from three randomized controlled trials (IN-TIME, ECOST, TRUST). Eur Heart J. 2017; 38(22):1749-55.
22. Parati G, Lombardi C, Castagna F, et al. Heart failure and sleep disorders. Nat Rev Cardiol. 2016;13(7):389-403.
23. Jimenez JA, Greenberg BH, Mills PJ. Effects of heart failure and its pharmacological management on sleep. Drug Discov Today DisModels. 2011;8: 161-6.
24. Bourge RC, Abraham WT, Adamson PB, et al. Randomized controlled trial of an implantable continuous hemodynamic monitor in patients with advanced heart failure: The COMPASS-HF study. J Am Coll Cardiol. 2008;51(11): 1073-9.
25. Abraham WT, Adamson PB, Hasan A, et al. Safety and accuracy of a wireless pulmonary artery pressure monitoring system in patients with heart failure. Am Heart J. 2011;161:558-66.
26. Ritzema J, Troughton R, Melton I, et al. Physician-directed patient self-management of the left atrial pressure on advanced chronic heart failure. Circulation. 2010;121(9):1086-95.

CHAPTER 97

Stepwise Approach to Acute Decompensated Heart Failure

BP Singh, Ravi V Prasad, Nirav Kumar

INTRODUCTION

Acute heart failure (AHF) is defined as new-onset or recurrence of sign and symptoms of heart failure (HF) requiring emergent therapy and hospitalization.[1] In most cases, it is due to deterioration of symptoms in previous HF. Acute coronary syndrome (ACS), myocarditis, acute valve regurgitation, and cardiac tamponade are some important causes of AHF diagnosed for the first time.[2] Many terms have been used to characterize AHF which include AHF syndromes, acute decompensated heart failure (ADHF), and acute decompensation of chronic HF requiring hospitalization. The term ADHF will be used in this review. Despite marked improvement in treatment and survival of chronic HF, outcomes of ADHF remain still poor with recurrent rehospitalization and 1-year mortality rates reaching 10–30%.[3]

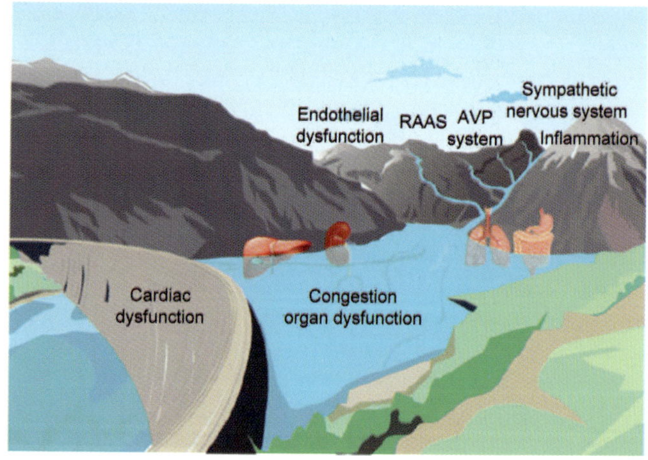

AVP, arginine-vasopressin; RAAS, renin–angiotensin–aldosterone system.

FIG. 1: Congestion in heart failure.

PATHOPHYSIOLOGY

In ADHF patients, three neurohormonal pathways viz., sympathetic nervous system, renin–angiotensin–aldosterone system and arginine-vasopressin system, are activated to counteract the negative effects of HF. There is impaired excretion of sodium through the kidneys resulting in sodium and water retention (Fig. 1).[4] Raised cardiac filling pressures and venous congestion are observed prior to the frank features of clinical decompensation.[5]

EVALUATION OF THE PATIENT WITH ACUTE DECOMPENSATED HEART FAILURE

Acute decompensated heart failure is a life-threatening condition and treatment should be initiated at the earliest after the hospitalization of these patients.[6] The initial evaluation of ADHF includes:

- Establishing diagnosis as rapidly and effectively
- Emergent treatment for potentially life-threatening conditions (e.g., circulatory failure, respiratory failure)
- Identifying any precipitating causes and their treatment (Box 1)
- Risk stratification for triage of patients (Fig. 2).

History and physical examination should primarily focus on the presence of congestion which is the typical feature of ADHF. Left-sided congestion may cause dyspnea, cough, orthopnea, paroxysmal nocturnal dyspnea, tachypnea, abnormal lung auscultation (rales, crackles, and wheezing) and finally, hypoxia.[7,8] Right-sided congestion may cause bilateral peripheral edema, decreased urine output, abdominal pain, nausea, and vomiting, jugular vein distention or positive hepatojugular reflux, ascites, hepatomegaly and/or icterus.[7] Hypotension, tachycardia, weak pulse, mental confusion, anxiety, fatigue, cold sweated extremities, and decreased urine output indicate signs and symptoms of hypoperfusion and thus, severity of the condition. Cardiogenic shock is the most severe form of ADHF characterized by reduced stroke volume, decreased systolic blood pressure (SBP), and clinical

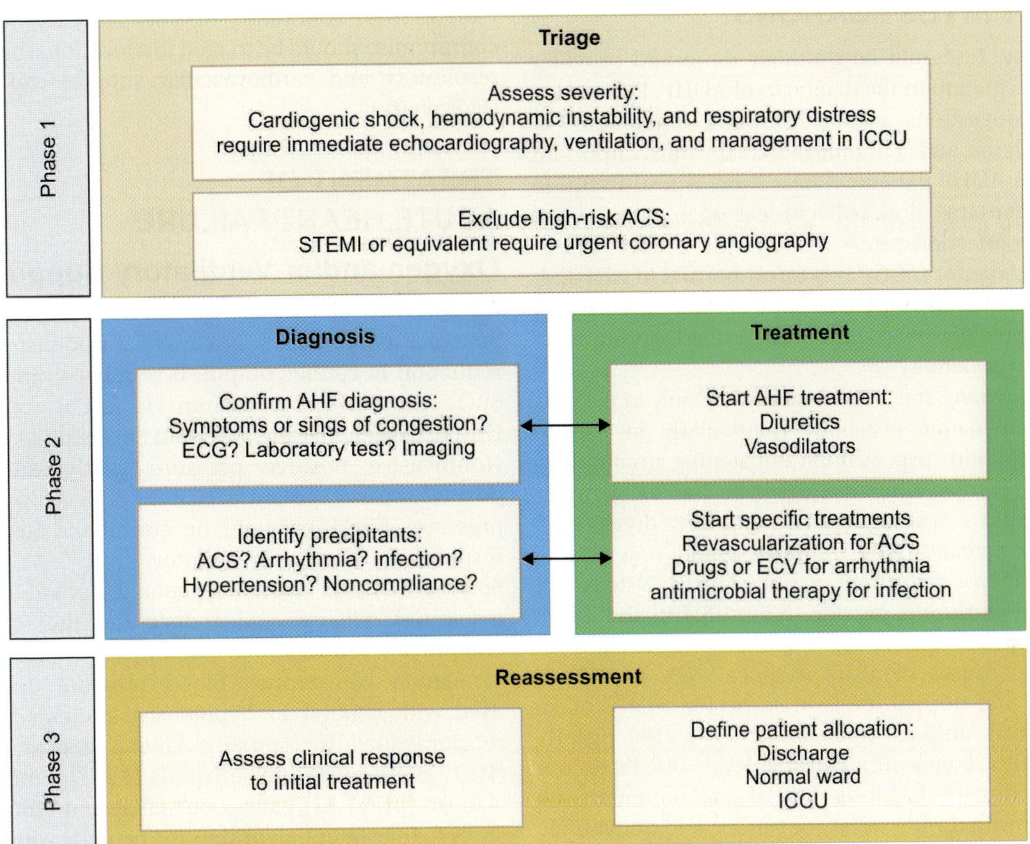

ACS, acute coronary syndrome; ECV, electrical cardioversion; ECG, electrocardiograph; ICCU, intensive cardiac care unit; STEMI, ST-elevation myocardial infarction.

FIG. 2: Early management and triage of acute decompensated heart failure.

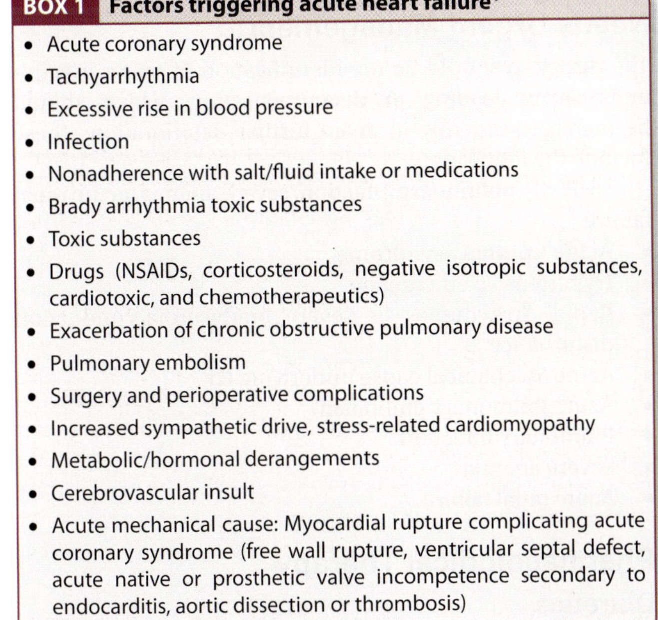

BOX 1 Factors triggering acute heart failure[1]

- Acute coronary syndrome
- Tachyarrhythmia
- Excessive rise in blood pressure
- Infection
- Nonadherence with salt/fluid intake or medications
- Brady arrhythmia toxic substances
- Toxic substances
- Drugs (NSAIDs, corticosteroids, negative isotropic substances, cardiotoxic, and chemotherapeutics)
- Exacerbation of chronic obstructive pulmonary disease
- Pulmonary embolism
- Surgery and perioperative complications
- Increased sympathetic drive, stress-related cardiomyopathy
- Metabolic/hormonal derangements
- Cerebrovascular insult
- Acute mechanical cause: Myocardial rupture complicating acute coronary syndrome (free wall rupture, ventricular septal defect, acute native or prosthetic valve incompetence secondary to endocarditis, aortic dissection or thrombosis)

NSAIDs, nonsteroidal anti-inflammatory drugs.

signs of hypoperfusion.[9] This form of ADHF carries very high in-hospital motility rate of about 40–50%.[10]

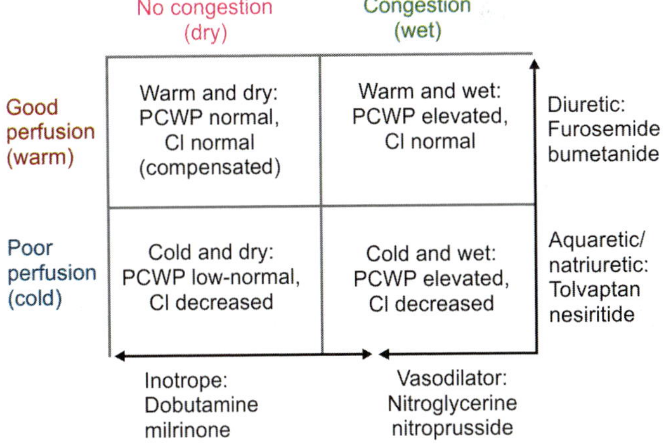

PCWP, pulmonary capillary wedge pressure; CI, cardiac index.

FIG. 3: Classification of patients presenting with acutely decompensated heart failure.

Based on presence/absence of congestion and hypoperfusion, patients are classified into four groups (Fig. 3).[11] They are "wet-warm" (congested but well perfused), "wet-cold" (congested and hypoperfused), "dry-cold" (not congested and hypoperfused) and lastly, "dry-warm" (decongested, well-perfused). This classification may help to guide initial therapy (mostly vasodilators and/or diuretics) and carries prognostic information.[12]

RELEVANT INVESTIGATIONS

- *Chest X-ray*: It should be routinely done and provides useful information in the diagnosis of ADHF. Pulmonary venous congestion, pleural effusion, interstitial or alveolar edema, and cardiomegaly are the most important findings in ADHF patients. Chest X-ray is also useful to identify alternative noncardiac diseases i.e., pneumonia, pulmonary infections, etc.[8]
- *Electrocardiogram (ECG)*: It is rarely normal in ADHF. It is helpful in identifying underlying cardiac disease and potential precipitants (rapid atrial fibrillation and acute myocardial ischemia)[13]
- *Echocardiography*: It is done immediately only in patients with hemodynamic instability (particularly in cardiogenic shock) and suspected life-threatening structural or functional cardiac abnormalities (mechanical complications, acute valvular regurgitation, and aortic dissection)[1]
- *Natriuretic peptides (NP):* Upon presentation, a plasma NP level [B-type natriuretic peptide (BNP), N-terminal pro-B-type natriuretic peptide (NT-proBNP)] should be measured in all patients for differentiating ADHF from noncardiac causes of acute dyspnea. NPs have high sensitivity and normal levels in suspected ADHF make the diagnosis unlikely (thresholds: BNP <100 pg/mL, NT-proBNP <300 pg/mL). Elevated levels of NPs do not always confirm the diagnosis of ADHF, as they may also be associated with a wide variety of cardiac and noncardiac causes[14]
- *Other laboratory tests should be performed at admission on all patients with ADHF*: Cardiac troponin, blood urea nitrogen, creatinine, electrolytes, liver function tests, thyroid stimulating hormone, glucose, and complete blood count. D-dimer is indicated in patients with a suspicion of acute pulmonary embolism.[1]

Routine arterial blood gas (ABG) is not needed and should be restricted to patients in whom oxygenation cannot be readily assessed by pulse oximetry.[1]

Cardiac troponins measurement is useful for detection of ACS as the underlying cause of ADHF. However, elevated concentrations of cardiac troponins are detected in ADHF, even without obvious myocardial ischemia or an acute coronary event, suggesting ongoing myocyte injury or necrosis in these patients. Also in acute pulmonary embolism, elevated troponins are seen.[15]

Routine invasive hemodynamic evaluation with a pulmonary artery catheter is not indicated for the diagnosis of ADHF. It may be helpful in selected cases of hemodynamically unstable patients with an unknown mechanism of deterioration.[1]

MANAGEMENT GOALS

All ADHF patients require rapid transfer to the nearest hospital preferably to a site with a cardiology department with intensive care unit. Early diagnosis is important in ADHF. All patients with suspected ADHF should have a diagnostic workup, appropriate pharmacological, and nonpharmacological treatment started promptly and in parallel.

Patients with respiratory distress/failure or hemodynamic compromise should be triaged to a location where immediate respiratory and cardiovascular support can be provided (Flowchart 1).

TREATMENT OF ACUTE HEART FAILURE

Oxygen and/or Ventilatory Support

In ADHF, oxygen should not be used routinely in nonhypoxemic patients, as it causes vasoconstriction and a reduction in cardiac output. It is only recommended when SpO_2 <90% or PaO_2 <60 mm Hg to correct hypoxemia.[16] During oxygen therapy, ABG and SpO_2 should be monitored. Noninvasive positive pressure ventilation [continuous positive airway pressure (CPAP), bilevel positive airway pressure (BiPAP)] should be considered in patients with respiratory distress (respiratory rate >25 breaths/min, SpO_2 <90%) and started as soon as possible to decrease respiratory distress and reduce the rate of mechanical endotracheal intubation. Noninvasive positive pressure ventilation can reduce blood pressure and should be used with caution in hypotensive patients. Intubation is recommended, if respiratory failure, leading to hypoxemia (PaO_2 <60 mm Hg), hypercapnia ($PaCO_2$ >50 mm Hg) and acidosis (pH <7.35), cannot be managed noninvasively.[17]

A management algorithm for patients with ADHF based on the clinical profile during an early phase is presented in flowchart 2.

Identification of Precipitants/Causes Leading to Decompensation that Needs Urgent Management[1]

The next step should be the identification of major precipitants/causes leading to decompensation, which should be managed urgently to avoid further deterioration. These include the following:

CHAMP, pulmonary infection, severe anemia, acute renal failure.[1]

- Acute **C**oronary syndrome
- **H**ypertensive emergency
- Rapid **A**rrhythmias or severe bradycardia/conduction disturbance
- Acute **M**echanical cause underlying HF
- Acute **P**ulmonary embolism
- Pulmonary infection
- Severe anemia
- Acute renal failure.

Pharmacological Therapy

Diuretics

Diuretics play important role in the treatment of ADHF especially with signs of fluid overload and congestion. Diuretics increase salt and water excretion. In patients with signs of hypoperfusion, diuretics should be avoided. Intravenous loop diuretics are recommended to improve symptoms rapidly.[18] It

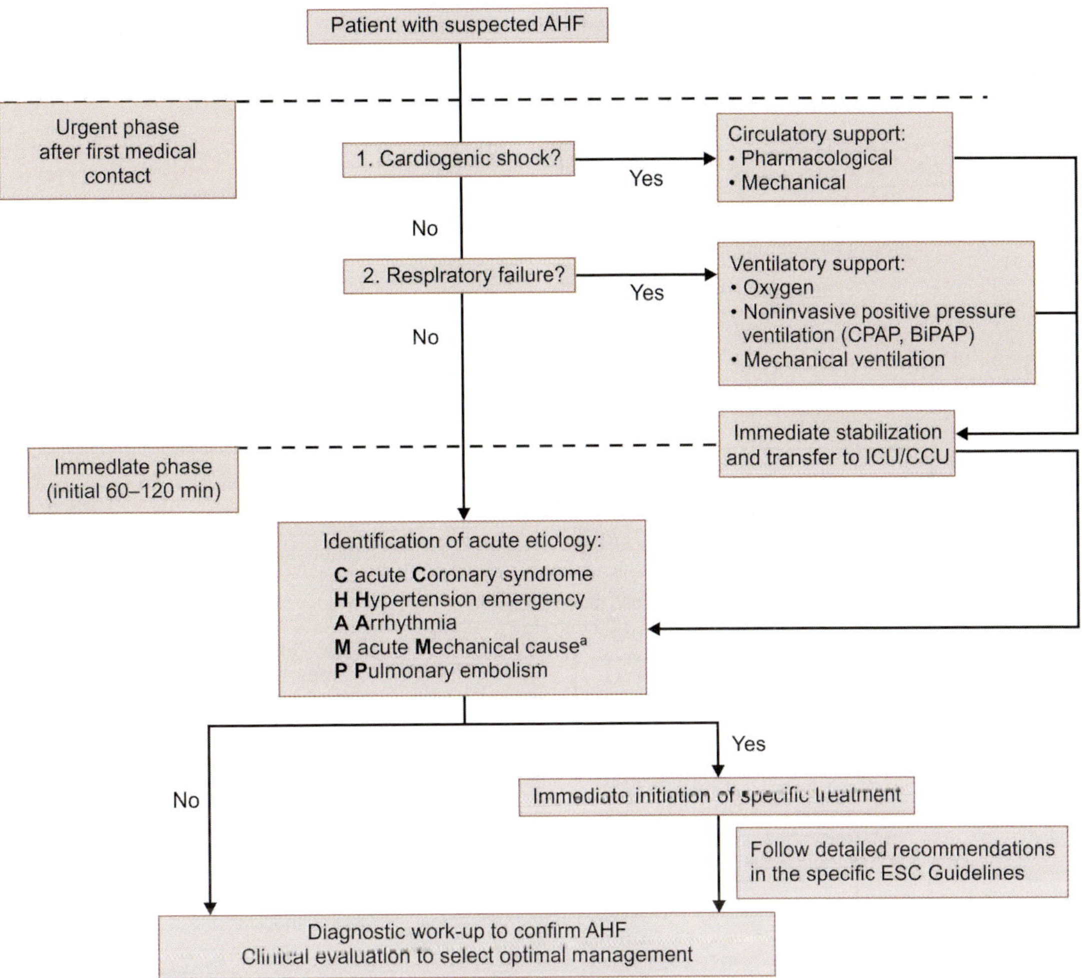

AHF, acute heart failure; BiPAP, bilevel positive airway pressure; CPAP, continuous positive airway pressure; CCU, coronary care unit; ESC, European Society of Cardiology; ICU, intensive care unit.

FLOWCHART 1: Overall management of a patient with acute heart failure.[1]

is recommended to regularly monitor symptoms, urine output, renal function, and electrolytes during use of intravenous diuretics. Current evidence demonstrates that there is no significant difference in symptoms or changes in renal function when loop diuretics are administered as a bolus compared to continuous infusion or at a high dose compared to a low dose. Furthermore, no difference appears to exist in the safety and efficacy of bolus injection compared to continuous infusion of loop diuretics.[19] Combination of loop diuretic with either thiazide-type diuretic or spironolactone may be considered in patients with resistant edema or insufficient symptomatic response.

Vasodilators

Intravenous vasodilators are the second most often used agents in ADHF for symptomatic relief. They have dual benefit by decreasing venous tone (to optimize preload) and arterial tone (decrease afterload). Consequently, they also increase stroke volume. Vasodilators are especially useful in patients with hypertensive ADHF, whereas in those with SBP <90 mm Hg (or with symptomatic hypotension), they should be avoided. Dosing should be carefully controlled to avoid excessive decreases in blood pressure.[20-22] They should be used with caution in patients with significant mitral or aortic stenosis (Table 1).

Inotropic Agents

Use of inotropes like dobutamine, dopamine, levosimendan, phosphodiesterase III (PDE III) inhibitors should be reserved for patients with a severe reduction in cardiac output resulting in compromised vital organ perfusion, which occurs most often in hypotensive ADHF.[23] Levosimendan is preferable over dobutamine to reverse the effect of beta-blockade if beta-blockade is thought to be contributing to hypoperfusion.[24] Inotropes, especially those with adrenergic mechanisms may cause myocardial ischemia and arrhythmias, thus, ECG monitoring is required. There is long-standing concern that they may increase mortality. In any case, inotropes must be used with caution starting from rather low doses and up-titrating with close monitoring (Table 2).[25]

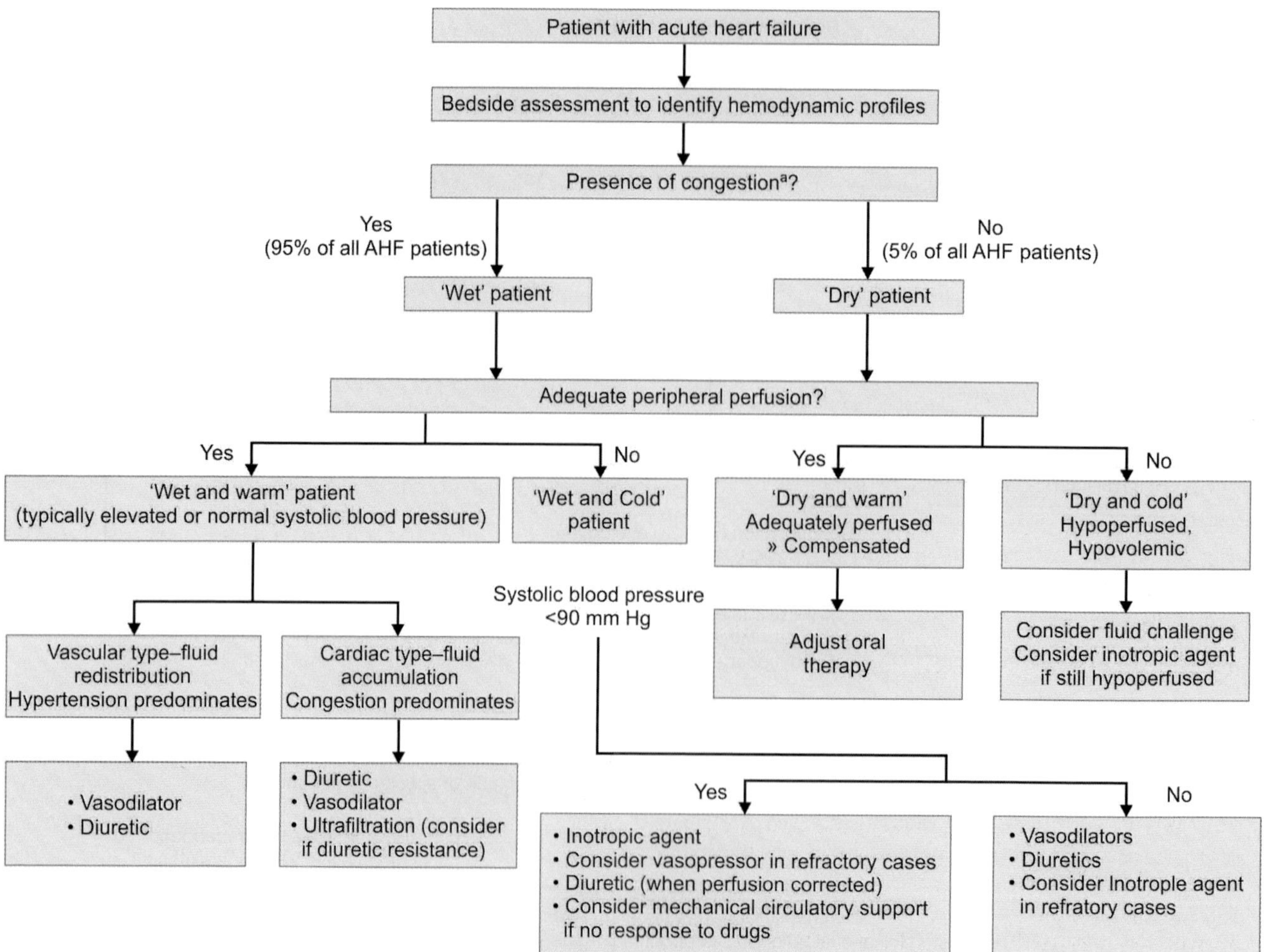

AHF, acute heart failure.

FLOWCHART 2: Management of patients with acute heart failure based on clinical profile during an early phase 1.

TABLE 1: Intravenous vasodilators used to treat acute decompensated heart failure (ADHF)[1]

Vasodilator	Dosing	Main side effects	Other
Nitroglycerine	Start with 10–20 µg/min increase up to 200 µg/min	Hypotension, headache	Tolerance on continuous use
Isosorbide dinitrate	Start with 1 mg/h, increase up to 10 mg/h	Hypotension, headache	Tolerance on continuous use
Nitroprusside	Start with 0.3 µg/kg/min, increase up to 5 µg/kg/min	Hypotension, isocyanate toxicity	Light sensitive
Nesiritide	Bolus 2 µg/kg + infusion 0.01 µg/kg/min	Hypotension	–

TABLE 2: Positive inotropes and/or vasopressors used to treat acute decompensated heart failure[1]

Vasodilator	Bolus	Infusion rate
Dobutamine	No	2–20 µg/kg/min (β+)
Dopamine	No	3–5 µg/kg/min: inotropic (β+)
Milrinone	25–75 µg/kg over 10–20 min	0.375–0.75 µg/kg/min
Enoximone	0.5–1.0 mg/kg over 5–10 min	5–20 µg/kg/min
Levosimendan	12 µg/kg over 10 min(optical)	0.1 µg/kg/min which can be decreased to 0.05 or increased to 0.2 µg/kg/min
Norepinephrine	No	0.2–1.0 µg/kg/min
Epinephrine	Bolus: 1 mg can be given IV during resuscitation, repeated every 3–5 min	–

Vasopressors

Drugs with prominent peripheral arterial vasoconstrictor action such as norepinephrine or dopamine in higher doses (>5 mg/kg/min) are given to patients with marked hypotension. These agents raise blood pressure and redistribute blood to the vital organs at the expense of an increase in left ventricle (LV) afterload. Dopamine was compared with norepinephrine in the treatment of various shock patients.[26] A subgroup analysis suggested that norepinephrine would have fewer side effects and lower mortality. Epinephrine (adrenaline) should be restricted to patients with persistent hypotension despite adequate cardiac filling pressures and the use of other vasoactive agents, as well as for resuscitation protocols (Table 2).[27]

Conventional Guideline-directed Medical Therapy

During admission, all previous guideline-directed medical therapy should be evaluated and adjusted based on patient presentation. If hypotension is present, holding beta-blockers and angiotensin-converting enzyme inhibitors (ACEIs) or angiotensin receptor blockers may be beneficial to allow for adequate diuresis and ensure target organ perfusion. ACEI therapy should be started at low doses as early as possible during the index hospitalization in the absence of significant renal dysfunction or hypotension. Beta-blockers doses should also be started in low dose and titrated to achieve target doses. They are avoided in presence of hypotension, bronchospasm, or symptomatic bradycardia. Caution should be used when administering beta-blockers to patients who have required inotropic therapy during their index hospitalization and to patients with newly diagnosed HF.[28]

Thromboembolism Prophylaxis

Thromboembolism prophylaxis is recommended to reduce the risk of deep venous thrombosis and pulmonary embolism.[29]

Digoxin

It should be used in patients with AF and fast ventricular rate (>110 bpm) and can be given in boluses of 0.25–0.5 mg intravenous; if there is urgency, 0.0625–0.125 mg may be an adequate dose in patients with moderate-to-severe renal dysfunction.[30]

Opiates/Anxiolytics and Sedatives

Opiates relieve dyspnea and anxiety. In ADHF, routine use of opiates is not recommended and only be cautiously considered in patients with severe dyspnea, mostly with pulmonary edema. Side effects include nausea, vomiting, hypotension, bradycardia, and respiratory depression may be observed with use of opiates. Anxiolytics or sedatives may be needed in a patient with agitation or delirium.[31]

Renal Replacement Therapy

Ultrafiltration involves the removal of plasma water across a semipermeable membrane in response to a transmembrane pressure gradient.[1] Routine use of ultrafiltration is not recommended and should be confined to patients who fail to respond to diuretic based strategies.[32] The following criteria may indicate the need for initiation of renal replacement therapy in patients with refractory volume overload: oliguria unresponsive to fluid resuscitation measures, severe hyperkalemia (K^+ > .6.5 mmol/L), severe acidemia (pH <7.2), serum urea level (>150 mg/dL), and serum creatinine (>3.4 mg/dL).[33]

Mechanical Circulatory Support in Acute Heart Failure

To manage patients with ADHF with cardiogenic shock, short-term mechanical support systems like percutaneous cardiac support devices, extracorporeal life support (ECLS), and extracorporeal membrane oxygenation (ECMO) may be used to support patients with left or biventricular failure until cardiac and other organ function have recovered. Typically, the use of these devices is restricted to a few days to weeks. Evidence regarding the benefits of temporary percutaneous support system in patients not responding to standard therapy, including inotropes is limited.[34]

Intra-aortic Balloon Pump

The indications for an intra-aortic balloon pump (IABP) are to support the circulation before surgical correction of specific acute mechanical problems like rupture of ventricular septum, acute regurgitation of mitral valve, severe acute myocarditis and in selected cases of acute myocardial ischemia or infarction before, during and after percutaneous or surgical revascularization.[35]

Other Interventions

In patients with ADHF and pleural effusion, pleurocentesis may be considered to alleviate dyspnea. In patients with ascites, ascitic tapping may be considered to relieve symptoms. This procedure leads to reduction in intra-abdominal pressure, may partially normalize the transrenal pressure gradient, thus improving renal filtration.[36]

MANAGEMENT OF PATIENTS WITH CARDIOGENIC SHOCK

In patients with suspected cardiogenic shock, immediate ECG, and echocardiography are recommended. These patients should be referred to a higher center with facility of cardiac catheterization Lab and a dedicated coronary care unit (CCU) with availability of mechanical circulatory support. In patients with cardiogenic shock complicating ACS, an immediate coronary angiography is recommended (within 2 h from hospital admission) with intent to perform coronary revascularization.[37] Continuous ECG, blood pressure, and invasive arterial monitoring are recommended. Intravenous inotropic agents (dobutamine) may be considered to increase cardiac output. Vasopressors (norepinephrine preferable over dopamine) may be considered if there is a need to maintain systolic pressure in the presence of persistent hypoperfusion. IABP is not routinely recommended in cardiogenic shock. Short-term mechanical circulatory support may be considered in refractory cardiogenic shock.[34]

When to Discharge Acute Decompensated Heart Failure Patients

Patients admitted with ADHF are medically fit for discharge when they are hemodynamically stable, euvolemic, put on evidence-based oral medication and with stable renal function for at least 24 hours before discharge (Box 2).[38]

Goals of Treatment During the Different Stages of Management of Acute Heart Failure

The goals of treatment during the different stages of management of acute heart failure as shown in box 3.[39]

BOX 2 Discharge checklist-discharge planning goals[1]

- Guideline-directed medical therapy has been reviewed and patient has been stable for 24 h
- Potential exacerbating/confounding comorbidities have been addressed
- Exercise tolerance has returned to New York Heart Association Class II
- Volume status has been optimized
- Education has been provided
- Clinic follow-up has been scheduled

BOX 3 Goals of treatment in acute decompensated heart failure[1]

Immediate (ED/ICU/CCU):

- Improve hemodynamic and organ perfusion
- Restore oxygenation
- Alleviate symptoms
- Limit cardiac and renal damage
- Prevent thromboembolism
- Minimize ICU length of stay

Intermediate (in hospital):

- Identify etiology and relevant comorbidities
- Titrate therapy to control symptoms and congestion and optimize blood pressure
- Initiate and up-titrate disease – modifying pharmacological therapy
- Consider device therapy in appropriate patients

Predischarge and long-term management:

- Develop a care plan that provides:
    - A schedule for up-titration and monitoring of pharmacological therapy
    - Need and timing for review for device therapy
    - Who will see the patient for follow-up and when
- Enroll in disease management program, educate, and initiate appropriate lifestyle adjustments
- Prevent early readmission
- Improve symptoms, quality of life, and survival

CCU, coronary care unit; ED, emergency department; ICU, intensive care unit.

CONCLUSION

Inpatient therapy for patients with ADHF should be directed at decongestion and symptom improvement. Always treat possible precipitating events, identify comorbid conditions that exacerbate HF, evaluate and update current guideline-directed medical therapy, and perform risk stratification for all patients. Effort should be made to educate patients about the importance of restricting sodium and fluid, monitoring daily weights, and adhering to a graded exercise program. Early discharge follow-up and continued optimization of guideline-directed medical therapy are key to preventing future ADHF readmissions.

REFERENCES

1. Ponikowski P, Voors AA, Anker SD, et al. 2016 ESC Guidelines for the diagnosis and treatment of acute and chronic heart failure: The Task Force for the diagnosis and treatment of acute and chronic heart failure of the European Society of Cardiology (ESC). Eur Heart J. 2016;37(27):2129-200.
2. Nieminen MS, Brutsaert D, Dickstein K, et al. EuroHeart Failure Survey II (EHFS II): a survey on hospitalized acute heart failure patients: Description of population. Eur Heart J. 2006;27:2725-36.
3. Ambrosy AP, Fonarow GC, Butler J, et al. The global health and economic burden of hospitalizations for heart failure: Lessons learned from hospitalized heart failure registries. J Am Coll Cardiol. 2014;63:1123-33.
4. Arrigo M, Parissis JT, Akiyama E, et al. Understanding acute heart failure: pathophysiology and diagnosis. Eur Heart J. 2016;18(Suppl G):G11-8.
5. Chaudhry SI, Wang Y, Concato J, et al. Patterns of weight change preceding hospitalization for heart failure. Circulation. 2007;116:1549-54.
6. Mebazaa A, Yilmaz MB, Levy P, et al. Recommendations on pre-hospital and early hospital management of acute heart failure: A consensus paper from the Heart Failure Association of the European Society of Cardiology, the European Society of Emergency Medicine and the Society of Academic Emergency Medicine - short version. Eur Heart J. 2015;36:1958-66.
7. Gheorghiade M, Follath F, Ponikowski P, et al. Assessing and grading congestion in acute heart failure: A scientific statement from the acute heart failure committee of the heart failure association of the European Society of Cardiology and endorsed by the European Society of Intensive Care Medicine. Eur J Heart Fail. 2010;12:423-33.
8. Chakko S, Woska D, Martinez H, et al. Clinical, radiographic, and hemodynamic correlations in chronic congestive heart failure: conflicting results may lead to inappropriate care. Am J Med. 1991;90:353-9.
9. Nohria A, Tsang SW, Fang JC, et al. Clinical assessment identifies hemodynamic profiles that predict outcomes in patients admitted with heart failure. J Am Coll Cardiol. 2003;41:1797-804.
10. Rudiger A, Harjola VP, Müller A, et al. Acute heart failure: Clinical presentation, one-year mortality and prognostic factors. Eur J Heart Fail. 2005;7:662-70.
11. Nohria A, Lewis E, Stevenson LW. Medical management of advanced heart failure. JAMA. 2002;287:628-40.
12. Drazner MH, Hellkamp AS, Leier CV, et al. Value of clinician assessment of hemodynamics in advanced heart failure: The ESCAPE trial. Circ Heart Fail. 2008;1:170-7.
13. Wang CS, FitzGerald JM, Schulzer M, et al. Does this dyspneic patient in the emergency department have congestive heart failure? JAMA. 2005;294: 1944-56.
14. Kelder JC, Cowie MR, McDonagh TA, et al. Quantifying the added value of BNP in suspected heart failure in general practice: an individual patient data meta-analysis. Heart. 2011;97:959-63.
15. Felker GM, Mentz RJ, Teerlink JR, et al. Serial high sensitivity cardiac troponin T measurement in acute heart failure: Insights from the RELAX-AHF study. Eur J Heart Fail. 2015;17:1262-70.
16. Rawles JM, Kenmure AC. Controlled trial of oxygen in uncomplicated myocardial infarction. Br Med J. 1976;1:1121-3.
17. Weng CL. Zhao YT, Liu QH, et al. Meta-analysis: Noninvasive ventilation in acute cardiogenic pulmonary edema. Ann Intern Med. 2010;152:590-600.

18. Mentz RJ, Kjeldsen K, Rossi GP, et al. Decongestion in acute heart failure. Eur J Heart Fail. 2014;16:471-82.
19. Felker GM, Lee KL, Bull DA, et al. Diuretic strategies in patients with acute decompensated heart failure. N Engl J Med. 2011;364:797-805.
20. Wakai A, McCabe A, Kidney R, et al. Nitrates for acute heart failure syndromes. Cochrane Database Syst Rev. 2013;8:CD005151.
21. Publication Committee for the VMAC Investigators (Vasodilatation in the Management of Acute CHF). Intravenous nesiritide vs nitroglycerin for treatment of decompensated congestive heart failure: A randomized controlled trial. JAMA. 2002;287:1531-40.
22. Cohn JN, Franciosa JA, Francis GS, et al. Effect of short-term infusion of sodium nitroprusside on mortality rate in acute myocardial infarction complicated by left ventricular failure: Results of a Veterans Administration cooperative study. N Engl J Med. 1982;306:1129-35.
23. Elkayam U, Tasissa G, Binanay C, et al. Use and impact of inotropes and vasodilator therapy in hospitalized patients with severe heart failure. Am Heart J. 2007;153:98-104.
24. Mebazaa A, Nieminen MS, Filippatos GS, et al. Levosimendan vs. dobutamine: Outcomes for acute heart failure patients on b-blockers in SURVIVE. Eur J Heart Fail. 2009;11:304-11.
25. Belletti A, Castro ML, Silvetti S, et al. The effect of inotropes and vasopressors on mortality: A meta-analysis of randomized clinical trials. Br J Anaesth. 2015;115:656-75.
26. De Backer D, Biston P, Devriendt J, et al. Comparison of dopamine and norepinephrine in the treatment of shock. N Engl J Med. 2010;362:779-89.
27. Monsieurs KG, Nolan JP, Bossaert LL, et al. European Resuscitation Council Guidelines for Resuscitation 2015: Section 1. Executive summary. Resuscitation. 2015;95:1-80.
28. Krim SR, Campbell PT, Desai S, et al. Management of patients admitted with acute decompensated heart failure. Ochsner J. 2015;15:284-9.
29. Dentali F, Douketis JD, Gianni M, et al. Meta-analysis: Anticoagulant prophylaxis to prevent symptomatic venous thromboembolism in hospitalized medical patients. Ann Intern Med. 2007;146:278-88.
30. Delle Karth G, Geppert A, Neunteufl T, et al. Amiodarone versus diltiazem for rate control in critically ill patients with atrial tachyarrhythmias. Crit Care Med. 2001;29:1149-53.
31. Peacock WF, Hollander JE, Diercks DB, et al. Morphine and outcomes in acute decompensated heart failure: An ADHERE analysis. Emerg Med J. 2008;25:205-9.
32. Costanzo MR, Guglin ME, Saltzberg MT, et al. Ultrafiltration versus intravenous diuretics for patients hospitalized for acute decompensated heart failure. J Am Coll Cardiol 2007; 49:675-83.
33. Costanzo MR, Guglin ME, Saltzberg MT, et al. Ultrafiltration is associated with fewer rehospitalization than continuous diuretic infusion in patients with decompensated heart failure: Results from UNLOAD. J Card Fail. 2010;16:277-84.
34. Stewart GC, Givertz MM. Mechanical circulatory support for advanced heart failure: Patients and technology in evolution. Circulation. 2012;125:1304-15.
35. Thiele H, Zeymer U, Neumann FJ, et al. Intra-aortic balloon counterpulsation in acute myocardial infarction complicated by cardiogenic shock (IABP-SHOCK II): Final 12-month results of a randomised, open-label trial. Lancet. 2013;382:1638-45.
36. Mullens W, Abrahams Z, Francis GS, et al. Prompt reduction in intra-abdominal pressure following large-volume mechanical fluid removal improves renal insufficiency in refractory decompensated heart failure. J Card Fail. 2008;14:508-14.
37. Steg PG. James SK, Atar D, et al. ESC Guidelines for the management of acute myocardial infarction in patients presenting with ST-segment elevation. Eur Heart J. 2012;33:2569-619.
38. Mebazaa A, Parissis J, Porcher R, et al. Short-term survival by treatment among patients hospitalized with acute heart failure: The global ALARM-HF registry using propensity scoring methods. Intensive Care Med. 2011;37:290-301.
39. Lainscak M, Blue L, Clark AL, et al. Self-care management of heart failure: Practical recommendations from the Patient Care Committee of the Heart Failure Association of the European Society of Cardiology. Eur J Heart Fail. 2011;13:115-26.

CHAPTER 98

Advanced Heart Failure Therapies—An Overview

Rishi A Bhargava, Prafulla G Kerkar

INTRODUCTION

Therapy for cardiac disease could be considered as the best example of triumph of mankind over the disease. Heart failure (HF), however, still exists in the scale of an epidemic across the world with significant impact on lives and economy of the people. Most HF-related hospitalizations and deaths are incurred by a subgroup of patients that is refractory to guideline-based medical management, a group categorized as having "advanced HF" [stage D, as per the American College of Cardiology (ACC)/American Heart Association (AHA) classification of HF] (Flowchart 1).[1] For these individuals, average survival is less than 6 months[2] and until recently, there was little available to support these patients, to extend life, and to improve functional status. However, advances in therapies like transplantation, emerging mechanical technologies, and novel, multidisciplinary approaches have all contributed substantially to the care of this growing patient population.

This chapter intends to present a comprehensive review of various treatment modalities available for the management of end-stage HF.

ESTIMATING PROGNOSIS IN ADVANCED HEART FAILURE

Assessment of prognosis is the basis for selecting therapies for most life-threatening diseases, but this is particularly challenging for HF. The clinical course varies dramatically across the spectrum of disease severity and is relatively unpredictable for individual patients.[3,4] This contrasts with the more linear decline of patients with advanced cancer, which has traditionally been the model for approaches to end-stage disease. Even late in HF, patients often enjoy "good days" and brief interludes of apparent stability, which can lull them and their care providers into postponing vital decisions. Prognosis is further clouded by the unique contrast between unexpected sudden death (i.e., lethal arrhythmia) and lingering death with congestive symptoms (i.e., progressive pump failure). Many models, comprising of multiple variables, have been published in an effort to provide more accurate predictions of prognosis in patients with HF. These models have shown the importance of natriuretic peptides, renal function, and low blood pressure as predictors of survival in patients with advanced HF.[5-8]

ADVANCED HEART FAILURE—TREATMENT STRATEGIES

As duration of disease and treatment options have increased, decision making for advanced HF has become both more critical and more challenging. Medically reasonable options are analyzed to make suitable decision, in alignment with preferences, values, and goals of informed patients and relatives.

Following are the key areas:

- Communication about treatment options
- Pharmacotherapy
- Interventions and surgeries
- Pacing device therapy
- Mechanical circulatory support (MCS)
- Heart transplant
- Palliative care.

Communication about Treatment Options

It is the onus of the treating physician to define the range of options that are medically appropriate. Following aspects need to be considered:[9]

- Counseling about major interventions should always include specific description of alternative approaches, including withdrawal or continuation of ongoing treatments and focus on symptomatic care
- Discussions should include various anticipated outcomes, including, not only, survival but also adverse events, independence, functional capacity, and quality of life for both patient and caregiver. There should be no

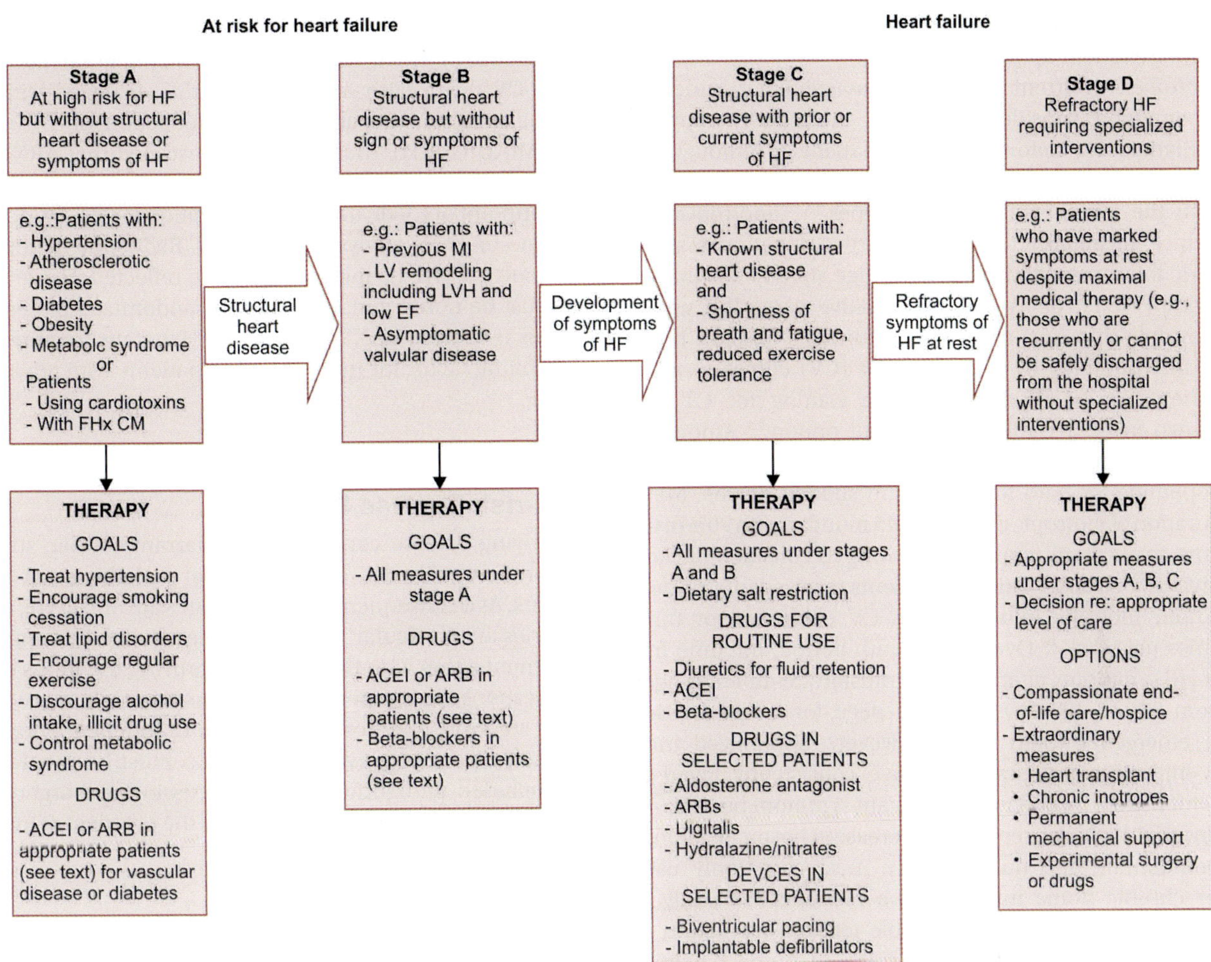

ACEI, angiotensin-converting enzyme inhibitor; ARBs, angiotensin receptor blockers; EF, ejection fraction; HF, heart failure; LVH, left ventricular hypertrophy; MI, myocardial infarction.

FLOWCHART 1: American College of Cardiology/American Heart Association classification of heart failure.

Source: Hunt SA, Abraham WT, Chin MH, et al. ACC/AHA 2005 guideline update for the diagnosis and management of chronic heart failure in the adult: a report of the American College of Cardiology/American Heart Association Task Force on Practice Guidelines (Writing Committee to Update the 2001 Guidelines for the Evaluation and Management of Heart Failure). Circulation. 2005;112:e154-235.

hesitation to even acknowledge lack of this information for some interventions

- Some therapies may lead to dependence [e.g., intravenous (IV) inotropes, renal replacement therapy, and intubation] and need to be weighed and discussed carefully before initiation even when anticipated to be temporary
- Risk-benefit of noncardiac procedures (e.g., hip replacement, repair of asymptomatic aortic aneurysm, or screening tests) should be analyzed in the context of competing risks of functional limitation and death caused by HF
- Major cardiac and noncardiac interventions discussion should include consideration of unanticipated adversities and options to deal with them ("what if" situation discussion)
- Palliative care team should be considered for assistance with symptom management in advanced disease, difficult decision-making, and caregiver support even as patients continue to receive supportive or disease-modifying therapies.

Management discussion should not be a one-time process and needs to be carried out at different steps of the disease stages.

Pharmacotherapy

- Medical therapy generally comprise of all stage C therapies like angiotensin-converting enzyme inhibitor (ACEI)/angiotensin receptor blocker (ARB), mineralocorticoid receptor antagonist (MRA), beta-blocker and diuretics.[10,11] The initial approach to advanced HF is optimization of these treatments to attain maximum tolerated dose. Some patients with end-stage HF with reduced ejection fraction (HFrEF) may tolerate little, if any, of the oral medications proven to reduce morbidity or prolong life. In other instances, patients may develop symptoms that are refractory to these oral therapies. Advanced therapies like left ventricular assist device

(LVAD) and cardiac transplantation (CT) remain the only valid treatment options for them

- *Inotropes*: Current HFrEF management guidelines recommend consideration of IV inotrope therapy for palliation of symptoms in stage D patients.[12] Although two meta-analyses have reported that mortality is not reduced with the administration of inotropes,[13,14] inotropes can reduce hospitalizations and improve functional status and, thus, are often used as bridge to CT, destination therapy (DT), or as part of palliative care. The use of inotropic infusions either on continuous basis at home or intermittently in cardiovascular (CV) clinics to allow patients to be discharged home waiting for CT was shown to be a viable management option.[15] Among 20 patients with continuous home infusions of dobutamine, dopamine, or both there were no sudden deaths. Mean duration of inotropic therapy was 5 months, with 70% of the time spent as an outpatient, leading to considerable cost savings. In a larger study, 73 patients received intermittent 4-hour inotrope infusions in a CV clinic two or three times per week.[16] Over a 49-month period, the time free of HF symptoms after the final infusion treatment ranged from 201 to 489 days, with no need for hospitalization or emergency room visits. However, randomized trials of intermittent dobutamine have consistently failed to demonstrate mortality or significant symptom benefit.[17,18] One trial, however, reported a decrease in hospitalization.[18] Dobutamine and milrinone are most commonly used for chronic home infusion. In a retrospective study of 112 patients considered ineligible for transplantation or LVAD implantation and discharged to home palliative care receiving continuous dobutamine or milrinone, the mean dose for dobutamine was 5.4 ± 2.5 μg/kg/min and milrinone was 0.4 ± 0.2 μg/kg/min. There was no difference in the likelihood of death or hospitalization with the use of either inotrope. Dobutamine overall demonstrated a cost-saving effect at 1 year, while milrinone was costlier than the standard therapy.[19] The ACC/AHA guidelines, given the lack of survival benefit, classify IV inotropes as a class IIB indication for end-stage HF
- *Newer agents*: Angiotensin receptor-neprilysin inhibitor (ARNI) (sacubitril-valsartan; or LCZ696) is a combination of ARB (valsartan) and neprilysin inhibitor (sacubitril), and is indicated for use in symptomatic HFrEF [with left ventricular ejection fraction (LVEF) ≤35%]. The Prospective Comparison of ARNI with Angiotensin Converting Enzyme Inhibitors to Determine Impact on Global Mortality and Morbidity in Heart Failure (PARADIGM-HF) trial was a landmark study comparing the novel agent ARNI with the standard of care ACEI, enalapril in symptomatic New York Heart Association (NYHA) Class II–IV patients.[20] The primary objective of the trial was to determine whether sacubitril-valsartan (ARNI) was superior to a renin-angiotensin inhibitor (enalapril—an ACEI) alone in reducing the risk of the combined endpoint of CV death or hospitalization for HF. The trial was stopped prematurely at 27 months of a planned 4-year duration in light of the significant benefit with use of ARNI. There was a 20% incremental reduction in CV death with ARNI beyond that achieved with the enalapril and an absolute risk reduction of 4.7%. The PARADIGM-HF trial, thus, demonstrated that ARNI was superior to enalapril in reducing the risk of the combined endpoint of CV death or hospitalization for HF, based on a time-to-event analysis ($p < 0.0001$). Reduction in both CV death and HF hospitalization were reflected. However, it must be noted that only 1.5% of randomized patients in this trial were in NYHA class IV. Hypotension may be a limiting factor for use of ARNI in patients with advanced HF.

Intervention and Surgeries

High-risk Cardiac Surgery

Underlying disease condition may warrant cardiac surgery for coronary, valvular, and pericardial pathologies in these patients. As a consequence of the patient's advanced HF, these surgeries are particularly high-risk. These procedures may be performed either with the hope of improving the status of HF or in response to a superimposed diagnosis such as acquired aortic stenosis. The potential for loss of independence and protracted postoperative rehabilitation must be considered and included thoughtfully in the discussion, as surgery can inherently increase short-term risk for the prospect of longer-term benefit.

Percutaneous Interventions

Percutaneous approaches for the treatment of coronary and valvular diseases seems appealing in advanced HF because of the increased surgical risk among these patients. Catheter approaches to both aortic[21] and mitral valve[22] disease [transcatheter aortic valve replacement (TAVR) and MitraClip, respectively] have now gained reputation as reasonable alternatives to surgery in certain populations. Discussion regarding percutaneous interventions should also give due consideration to whether "bail out" surgery (in case of adverse event) would be appropriate and feasible.

Electrophysiological Device Therapy

Cardiac Resynchronization Therapy and Implantable Cardioverter Defibrillators

Cardiomyopathy patients are prone to cardiac dyssynchrony. It is complex and multifaceted phenomenon. Due to prolongation of the atrioventricular (AV) interval, systolic contraction of the ventricle is delayed, which then might encroach on early diastolic filling. Also, if ventricular contraction is delayed and occupies the diastolic filling, the LV diastolic pressures will exceed atrial pressure, causing diastolic mitral regurgitation (MR). This leads to underfilling of the ventricle, causing loss of ventricular preload and ultimately leading to reduction in LV contractility, due to loss of the Starling mechanism. Inter- and intraventricular conduction delays lead to asynchronous contraction of LV wall regions (ventricular dyssynchrony), thereby impairing cardiac efficiency and reducing stroke volume and systolic blood pressure. Also, poorly coordinated papillary muscle function may cause or aggravate functional systolic MR. Impaired performance enhances adverse LV remodeling.

Cardiac resynchronization therapy (CRT) intends to pace both the left and right ventricles simultaneously with the aim of restoring synchrony, thus improving cardiac function with the aim of achieving symptomatic improvement.

Implantable cardioverter defibrillators (ICDs) are effective in correcting potentially lethal ventricular arrhythmias and preventing bradycardia, thus reducing the risk of sudden death.

These treatment options are recommended for patients with HF who have LV dysfunction with an ejection fraction (EF) of less than 35% according to NYHA class, QRS duration, and presence of bundle branch block. Type of device to be implanted is decided as per clinical presentation (HF with/without ventricular arrhythmia). In cases with left bundle branch block (LBBB), QRS duration more than 150 ms, LVEF less than 35%, and who remains in NYHA functional class II, III, or ambulatory IV, CRT is class I indication.[23]

Mechanical Circulatory Support (MCS)

Mechanical circulatory support devices (Fig. 1) are mechanical pumps designed to assist or replace the function of either the left or right ventricle, or both ventricles, of the heart. Important characteristics of MCS devices include: (1) location of the pumping chamber; (2) specific ventricle(s) supported; (3) pumping mechanism; and (4) indicated duration of support, for either temporary (days to weeks) or long-term (months to years) use.

Typically, short-term devices are extracorporeal or paracorporeal pumps (located outside the body), whereas durable devices are implantable (intracorporeal) systems.

There are several different CV circuits available for MCS (Box 1):

- Short-term right atrium (RA) to artery support can be provided by central or peripheral venoarterial extracorporeal membrane oxygenation (VA-ECMO) or extracorporeal life supports (ECLSs)
- The primary left atrium (LA) to aorta support system is the TandemHeart percutaneous LVAD (CardiacAssist, Inc., Pittsburgh, Pennsylvania)

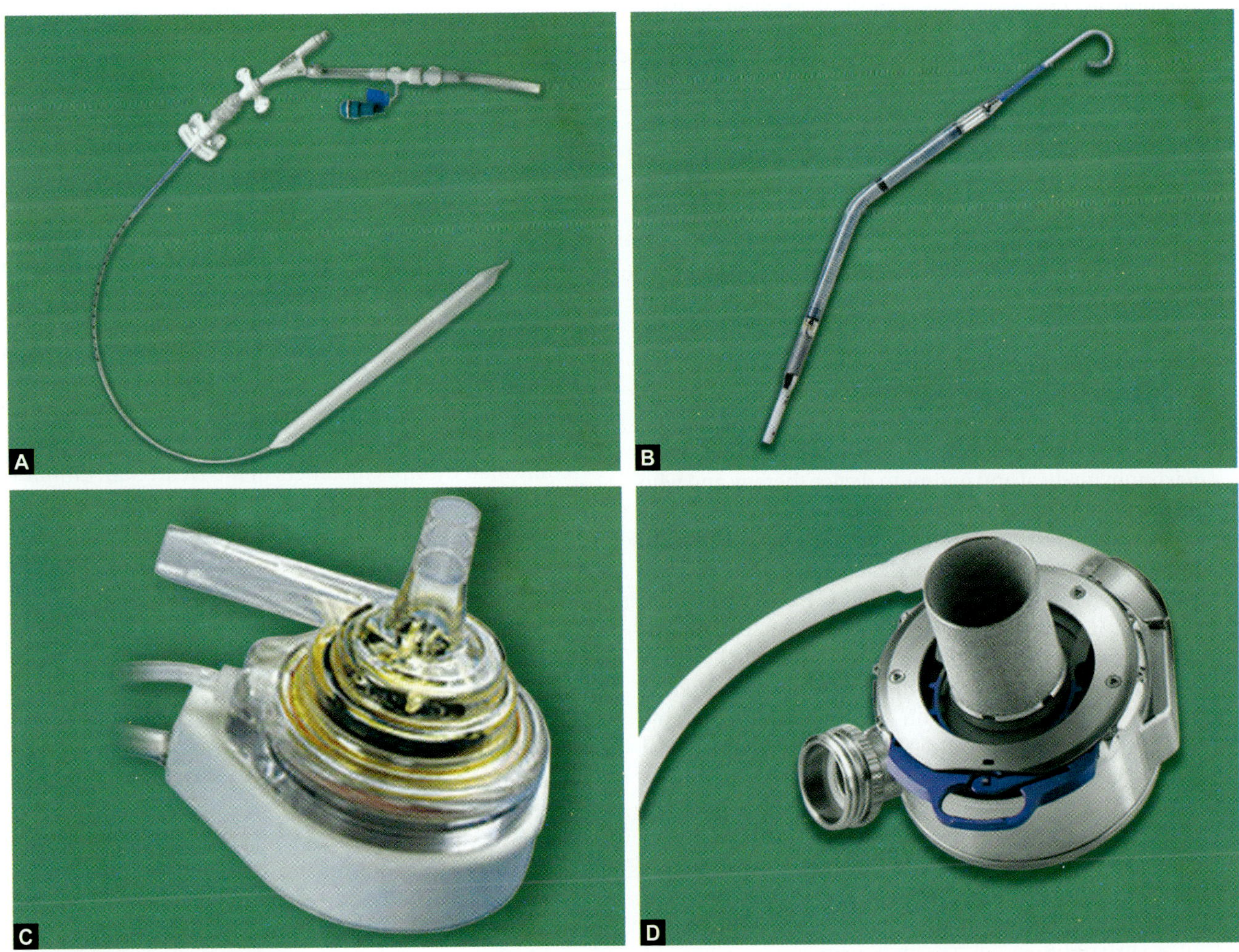

FIG. 1: Examples of commonly used mechanical circulatory support systems. **A,** Intra-aortic balloon pump; **B,** Impella; **C,** TandemHeart; **D,** HeartMate 3.

BOX 1 Types of mechanical circulatory support devices

- Short-term right atrium to artery support
- Short-term left atrium to aorta support
- Short-term left ventricle (LV) to aorta support: Percutaneous and central/surgical
- Long-term LV to aorta support.

- Short-term percutaneous LV to aorta support devices includes the Impella devices (Abiomed, Danvers, Massachusetts) and the percutaneous heart pump (PHP, Thoratec, Pleasanton, California)
- Short-term central LV to aorta support can be provided in the form of CentriMag ventricular assist device (Thoratec, Pleasanton, California)
- Multiple LV to aorta devices are available for durable, long-term support, commonly known as LVADs. LVADs currently available in the United States include the HeartMate II (St Jude Medical, St Paul, Minnesota) and HeartWare ventricular assist device (HVAD) (HeartWare International, Framingham, Massachusetts)
- Additionally, the HeartMate 3 (St Jude Medical, St Paul, Minnesota), Jarvik 2000 (Jarvik Heart Inc., New York, New York), and HeartAssist5 (ReliantHeart Inc., Houston, Texas) are investigational through clinical trials.

Nondurable mechanical circulatory support (MCS), including the use of percutaneous and extracorporeal ventricular assist devices (VADs), is reasonable as a "bridge to recovery" or "bridge to decision" for carefully selected patients with HFrEF with acute, profound hemodynamic compromise. As per Indian guidelines for management of HF, LVAD should be considered in the following scenarios:[24]

- Patients who have symptomatic advanced HF with reduced EF, despite optimal medical and device therapy, and who are eligible for heart transplantation, as bridge to transplant
- As DT in patients who have end-stage HFrEF despite maximum medical and optimum device therapy and who are not eligible for heart transplantation
- Patients with severe symptoms of more than 2 months duration despite optimal medical and device therapy and one or more of the following: (1) LVEF less than 25%, and if measured, peak VO_2 less than 12 mL/kg/min; (2) more than or equal to three HF hospitalizations in previous 12 months without an obvious precipitating cause; (3) dependence on IV inotropic therapy; (4) progressive end-organ dysfunction (worsening renal and/or hepatic function) due to reduced perfusion and not due to inadequate ventricular filling pressure [pulmonary capillary wedge pressure (PCWP) more than or equal to 20 mm Hg and systolic BP less than or equal to 80–90 mm Hg or cardiac index (CI) less than or equal to 2 L/min/m^2]; and (5) absence of severe right ventricular (RV) dysfunction together with severe tricuspid regurgitation.

For implanted MCS, patients are dependent on a device with possible complications of infection and stroke. Also, there are chances of continued symptoms and need of therapies for right-sided HF symptoms. Thus, whether to initiate these therapies represents one of the most crucial decisions that patients and clinicians can make. There may be an increase in the use of MCS as the technology improves but is likely to remain less commonly employed for the majority of patients with HF because of the large number of patients of HF with normal EF, multiple comorbidities, very advanced age, and lack of availability.[25,26]

Heart Transplant

The true "cure" for refractory or end-stage HFrEF is CT. The first CT using a cadaveric donor was performed on December 3, 1967 by Dr Christian Barnard in Cape Town, South Africa. Within 1 year of this event, Dr P K Sen performed first CT (heterologous) in India at Municipal-run King Edward Memorial (KEM) Hospital, Mumbai.[27] Considering the increasing incidence of advanced HF and need of CT, the Government of India has drafted a policy to determine suitable donor and recipient.[28]

Categorization of Potential Cardiac Recipients

Three categories are proposed:

1. *Priority 1 (emergency)*: These are patients on VADs, but still critical, like those on intra-aortic balloon pump (IABP) waiting for heart/heart lung transplantation. These recipients will get priority based on blood group and size matching. Their status needs to be confirmed on weekly basis
2. *Priority 2 (semi-emergency)*: These are patients in intensive care unit dependent on inotropic support for at least a week and not maintaining hemodynamics if inotropes are being weaned off. Their category needs to be updated every 48 hours. Based on their progress, they may stay in priority 2 or change to other priorities. If a deceased donor organ is available, their status needs to be confirmed by three members of the Heart Subcommittee as appointed by the Chairman of the Subcommittee
3. *Priority 3 (elective)*: These are patients electively waiting for transplantation. Their status needs to be confirmed or changed as per their progress on monthly basis.

Criteria for Suitable Donors for Heart

Apart from the general criteria for donors, the following criteria are needed:

- Age less than 60 years. If donor is more than 40 years, coronary angiogram is desirable to exclude asymptomatic coronary artery disease
- No history of heart disease and echocardiogram showing good cardiac function and no anatomical abnormalities
- Maintaining good hemodynamics and not on high doses of inotropes (dopamine less than 10 µg/kg/min; epinephrine, norepinephrine less than 0.1 µg/kg/min; and dobutamine less than 10 µg/kg/min)

- *Cardiac arrest*: Donors revived after a brief cardiac arrest must be assessed more carefully; but can be considered if the cardiac function is absolutely normal.

Cardiac transplantation and MCS can fundamentally alter the clinical course of HF by exchanging it for an invasive therapy and the need to adjust to living with a different set of risks, benefits, burdens, and complications. In the case of CT, patients must adapt to the risks of surgical procedure, immunosuppression, its side effects, and threat of organ rejection. The use of CT is constrained by a limited supply of donor hearts, a situation that likely will not change in the near future. An appropriate policy for equitable and judicious allocation of any available donated organ (heart and lungs) is mandatory and needs systematic efforts to promote awareness about organ donation among citizens.

Palliative Care

The word "palliative" is derived from the Latin word palliare, which means to cloak. Palliative care aspires to relieve suffering by a holistic and multidisciplinary approach that addresses patient's and caregiver's physical, emotional, logistical, and spiritual needs.

The natural course of HF is marked by acute exacerbations, usually requiring inpatient treatment, followed by periods of moderate symptoms, with gradual overall deterioration in health status. This pattern of stuttering decline often results in significant confusion among providers when considering the timing of palliative care and advanced directive discussions. Nevertheless, physicians treating patients with NYHA class IV, stage D HF should establish goals-of-care with their patients.

Following are the points related with palliation in the advanced HF:

- Liaison between the specialist palliative care and HF teams, or the primary care physician in a shared care approach, is encouraged to optimally address and coordinate the patient's needs
- Dyspnea, pain, depression, fatigue, and edema constitutes the most common symptoms and comorbidities among patients with end-stage HF.[3,29,30] Effective palliative approaches based on evidences should be advised[31]
- In patients with ICD implanted, as HF worsens, they are likely to receive more frequent shocks, which cause significant pain and anxiety. If the stage diagnosed as near end of life, turning off the ICD is a viable option after discussion among the caregivers and the treating physician
- Near the end of life, the management of VAD presents serious challenges to the patient, treating physician, and the family. Patients may have sudden VAD mechanical dysfunction causing fall in cardiac output and rapid decompensation. Alternatively, patient develops other serious and potential life-threatening complications or pathologies (e.g., infections, embolic, or renal) while the device is still functional. The decision making is challenging in both the scenarios and should take into account patient's and relative's choices along with the guidelines
- If a patient is deemed to be ineligible for LVAD/CT, a more focused discussion regarding palliative care options should be pursued.

ADVANCED HEART FAILURE THERAPIES—INDIAN SCENARIO

Advanced HF is increasing rapidly in India and need dedicated efforts at every level to timely provide suitable treatment to these patients. Pertaining to Indian scenario, following points are noteworthy:

- *Delay in seeking treatment*: Many patients do not report symptoms at initial stages and seek treatment during refractory HF. Delayed referral to higher-level health facility further adds to the problems
- *Lack of resources at peripheral health centers*: Primary health centers (PHCs) and urban health centers continues to be the first medical contact for significant numbers of Indians. These centers are not fully equipped with diagnostic armamentarium and therapeutic capabilities to treat HF patients and its risk factors
- *Empirical use of inotropes*: Though not supported by the evidences and guidelines, inotropes still considered to be a necessary treatment for all patients of HF with hypotension irrespective of the etiology. Nonavailability of MCS is one of the reasons behind the frequent use of the inotropic drugs. Individualized approach needs to be followed
- *Financial constraints*: A large number of people in India are not under cover of government health schemes and private health insurance plans and end up spending money for health care from their own pockets. Advanced HF therapies are expensive and financial issues poses significant constraint in their uses
- *Lack of availability of MCS*: Many tertiary care facilities in India lacks necessary expertise and infrastructure for the use of MCS and hence not commonly used
- *Cardiac transplantation*: Lack of awareness about the organ donation leads to unmet need of CT. Also, the expenses of the preprocedural assessment, procedure, medications, and follow-up costs in lakhs and puts significant financial burden on nonaffording patients.

CONCLUSION

Management of the advanced HF patient can be complex. Along with approved HF medications, therapies include CT, MCS, and inotropic agents for the short duration. Despite an ever-increasing armamentarium of resources, the physician must critically weigh the risks and benefits of each therapy to develop an optimal treatment approach, which necessarily be individualized. While CT remains the only true "cure" for advanced stage disease, its application is limited and the demand continues to outpace the supply. VAD therapy has emerged as a feasible option for improving morbidity and mortality for patients who are transplant ineligible or likely to succumb to their illness prior to transplant. IV inotropes can be used for symptom control in patients who are nonoperable or for treatment prior to surgery. Management of the HF patient requires, irrespective of the treatment strategy chosen, thoughtful discussion, multidisciplinary approach, and individualized care. Though the survival is crucial, most patients desire improved quality of life above all outcomes. Adding life to years rather than years to life may be more relevant.[32] It is important that clinicians make goals-of-care discussions a priority when seeing patients with advanced HF. Palliative care consultation facilitates these difficult conversations to ensure that all patient needs, curative or supportive, are ultimately met.

Although there are exciting developments in the field of advanced HF therapies, invasive as well as noninvasive, changing the paradigm will take time. It is, thus, the duty of every caregiver to strive hard and provide the best available treatment at the moment that sometimes may be palliative at best.

REFERENCES

1. Hunt SA, Abraham WT, Chin MH, et al. ACC/AHA 2005 guideline update for the diagnosis and management of chronic heart failure in the adult: a report of the American College of Cardiology/American Heart Association Task Force on Practice Guidelines (Writing Committee to Update the 2001 Guidelines for the Evaluation and Management of Heart Failure). Circulation. 2005;112:e154-235.
2. Stevenson LW, Rose EA. Left ventricular assist devices: bridges to transplantation, recovery, and destination for whom? Circulation. 2003;108:3059-63.
3. Goodlin SJ, Hauptman PJ, Arnold R, et al. Consensus statement: palliative and supportive care in advanced heart failure. J Card Fail. 2004;10:200-9.
4. Lanken PN, Terry PB, Delisser HM, et al. An official American Thoracic Society clinical policy statement: palliative care for patients with respiratory diseases and critical illnesses. Am J Respir Crit Care Med. 2008;177:912-27.
5. Aaronson KD, Schwartz JS, Chen TM, et al. Development and prospective validation of a clinical index to predict survival in ambulatory patients referred for cardiac transplant evaluation. Circulation. 1997;95:2660-7.
6. Levy WC, Mozaffarian D, Linker DT, et al. The Seattle Heart Failure Model: prediction of survival in heart failure. Circulation. 2006;113:1424-33.
7. Fonarow GC, Adams KF, Abraham WT, et al. Risk stratification for in-hospital mortality in acutely decompensated heart failure: classification and regression tree analysis. JAMA. 2005;293:572-80.
8. Krumholz HM, Wang Y, Mattera JA, et al. An administrative claims model suitable for profiling hospital performance based on 30-day mortality rates among patients with heart failure. Circulation. 2006;113:1693-701.
9. Allen LA, Stevenson LW, Grady KL, et al. Decision Making in Advanced Heart Failure—A Scientific Statement From the American Heart Association Endorsed by Heart Failure Society of America, American Association of Heart Failure Nurses, and Society for Medical Decision Making. Circulation. 2012;125:1928-52.
10. Lindenfeld J, Albert NM, Boehmer JP, et al. HFSA 2010 comprehensive heart failure practice guideline. J Card Fail. 2010;16:e1-94.
11. Dickstein K, Cohen-Solal A, Filippatos G, et al. ESC guidelines for the diagnosis and treatment of acute and chronic heart failure 2008: the Task Force for the Diagnosis and Treatment of Acute and Chronic Heart Failure 2008 of the European Society of Cardiology: developed in collaboration with the Heart Failure Association of the ESC (HFA) and endorsed by the European Society of Intensive Care Medicine (ESICM). Eur Heart J. 2008;29:2388-442.
12. Hunt SA, Abraham WT, Chin MH, et al. 2009 Focused update incorporated into the ACC/AHA 2005 Guidelines for the Diagnosis and Management of Heart Failure in Adults. A Report of the American College of Cardiology Foundation/American Heart Association Task Force on Practice Guidelines Developed in Collaboration With the International Society for Heart and Lung Transplantation. J Am Coll Cardiol. 2009;53:e1-90.
13. Thackray S, Easthaughb J, Freemantleb N, et al. The effectiveness and relative effectiveness of intravenous inotropic drugs acting through the adrenergic pathway in patients with heart failure—a meta-regression analysis. Eur J Heart Fail. 2002;4:515-29.
14. Tacon CL, McCaffrey J, Delaney A. Dobutamine for patients with severe heart failure: a systematic review and meta-analysis of randomized controlled trials. Intensive Care Med. 2012;38:359-67.
15. Sindone AP, Keogh AM, Macdonald PS, et al. Continuous home ambulatory intravenous inotropic drug therapy in severe heart failure: safety and cost efficacy. Am Heart J. 1997;134:889-900.
16. López-Candales AL, Carron C, Schwartz J. Need for hospice and palliative care services in patients with end-stage heart failure treated with intermittent infusion of inotropes. Clin Cardiol. 2004;27:23-8.
17. Elis A, Bental T, Kimchi O, et al. Intermittent dobutamine treatment in patients with chronic refractory congestive heart failure: a randomized, double-blind, placebo-controlled study. Clin Pharmacol Ther. 1998;63:682-5.
18. Oliva F, Latini R, Politi A, et al. Intermittent 6-month low-dose dobutamine infusion in severe heart failure: DICE multicenter trial. Am Heart J. 1999;138:247-53.
19. Gorodeski ED, Chu EC, Reese JR, et al. Prognosis on Chronic Dobutamine or Milrinone Infusions for Stage D Heart Failure. Circ Heart Fail. 2009;2:320-4.
20. McMurray JJ, Packer M, Desai AS, et al. Angiotensin-neprilysin inhibition versus enalapril in heart failure. N Engl J Med. 2014;371:993-1004.
21. Smith C. Transcatheter Valve Implantation Compared to Surgical Valve Replacement for Severe Aortic Stenosis: the PARTNER Cohort A Study. New Orleans: American College of Cardiology; 2011.
22. Feldman T, Foster E, Glower DG, et al. Percutaneous repair or surgery for mitral regurgitation. N Engl J Med. 2011;364:1395-406.
23. Tracy CM, Epstein AE, Darbar D, et al. 2012 ACCF/AHA/HRS focused update of the 2008 guidelines for device-based therapy of cardiac rhythm abnormalities: a report of the American College of Cardiology Foundation/American Heart Association Task Force on Practice Guidelines. Circulation. 2012;126:1-17.
24. Mishra S, Mohan JC, Nair T, et al. Management protocols for chronic heart failure in India. Indian Heart J. 2018;70:105-27.
25. Roger VL, Go AS, Lloyd-Jones DM, et al. Heart disease and stroke statistics—2012 update: a report from the American Heart Association. Circulation. 2012;125:e2-220.
26. Cubbon RM, Gale CP, Kearney LC, et al. Changing characteristics and mode of death associated with chronic heart failure caused by left ventricular systolic dysfunction: a study across therapeutic eras. Circ Heart Fail. 2011;4:396-403.
27. Das MK, Kumar S, Deb PK, et al. History of Cardiology in India. Indian Heart J. 2015;67:163-9.
28. National Organ and Tissue Transplant Organisation (NOTTO). (2017). Allocation Criteria for Heart, Lung and Heart-Lung Contents. [online] Available from http://www.notto.gov.in/WriteReadData/Portal/News/418_1_29082016FinalHeartAllocationPolicy.pdf. [Accessed September, 2018].
29. Lorenz KA, Lynn J, Dy SM, et al. Evidence for improving palliative care at the end of life: a systematic review. Ann Intern Med. 2008;148:147-59.
30. Nordgren L, Sorensen S. Symptoms experienced in the last six months of life in patients with end-stage heart failure. Eur J Cardiovasc Nurs. 2003;2:213-7.
31. Faris R, Flather MD, Purcell H, et al. Diuretics for heart failure. Cochrane Database Syst Rev. 2006;1:CD003838.
32. Kar S. Percutaneous transcatheter mitral valve repair. JACC. 2013;62:1062-4.

CHAPTER 99

Takotsubo Cardiomyopathy—An Update

Pintu Nahata

INTRODUCTION

Takotsubo cardiomyopathy (TCM) is a syndrome characterized by transient left ventricular (LV) dysfunction in the absence of angiographic evidence of significant obstructive disease in the coronary arteries, most commonly occurring after sudden emotional breakdown.[1] Usually, the regional wall motion abnormality (RWMA) extends beyond the supply area of a single coronary artery.

The term "Takotsubo" is taken from the Japanese name for an octopus trap. The shape of the Octopus trap is similar to the LV angiographic appearance seen in this disease characterized by systolic apical ballooning of the LV along with depressed mid and apical segments of the LV, and hyperkinesis of the basal walls.[2]

This disorder is also known as stress cardiomyopathy, broken heart syndrome, and transient apical ballooning syndrome.

HISTORY

The first case of its type was reported by Iga et al. in which they noted transient LV dysfunction which was reversible with characteristic takotsubo appearance in the patient of pheochromocytoma, but the term takotsubo was not used by them. They also noted high level of circulating catecholamines in the patient.[3] However, only in 1990 Sato et al. first described this reversible cardiomyopathy as *takotsubo* like LV dysfunction. This phenomenon was labelled as apical ballooning or stress cardiomyopathy outside Japan.[4-6]

DIAGNOSTIC CRITERIA

The diagnostic criteria are proposed by Mayo clinic (Table 1).[7]

All the criteria must be satisfied to establish the diagnosis of TCM.

EPIDEMIOLOGY

Takotsubo cardiomyopathy is more common in women than in men; postmenopausal women are more commonly affected. Frequently preceded by an emotional and physical trigger. In the International Takotsubo registry (a consortium of 26 centers in Europe and the United States), out of 1,750 patients with TCM, a vast majority were women (89.9%) and mean age was 66.4 years.[8] Most of the patients are Asian or Caucasian. Condition probably accounts for 1–2% of all cases of suspected acute myocardial infarction.[9]

ETIOPATHOGENESIS

The pathogenesis of this disorder is not well-understood. Why the condition has strong predilection for postmenopausal women is not clear? Further, why predominantly the LV mid-cavity and apex are affected is also not fully understood. Several mechanisms have been proposed:[10]

TABLE 1: Diagnostic criteria proposed by Mayo clinic

1.	Transient hypokinesis, akinesis, or dyskinesis in the left ventricular midsegments with or without apical involvement; regional wall motion abnormalities that extend beyond a single epicardial vascular distribution; and frequently, but not always, after a stressful trigger
2.	The absence of obstructive coronary disease or angiographic evidence of acute plaque rupture
3.	New ECG abnormalities (ST-segment elevation and/or T-wave inversion) or modest elevation in cardiac troponin
4.	The absence of pheochromocytoma and myocarditis

ECG, electrocardiogram.

- Multi vessel epicardial coronary artery spasm
- Coronary microvascular impairment
- Catecholamine cardiotoxicity
- Neurogenic stunned myocardium.

At rest and during aerobic activity, our heart utilizes major portion (approximately 90%) of energy by fatty acid metabolism. However, when the heart is subjected to ischemia glucose is utilized largely, and fatty acid metabolism is suppressed. This may result in cardiac dysfunction. In patients with TCM despite the lack of ischemia the glucose pathway as a source of energy is activated and this is detrimental to cardiac function.

The most commonly discussed mechanism for TCM is stress-induced catecholamine release, which may result in myocardial toxicity and subsequent stunning of the myocardium. The apical parts of the heart have very high concentration of sympathetic receptors, which may explain why these excess catecholamines affect the apices more.[11]

Myocardial biopsy often shows interstitial infiltrates consisting predominantly of mononuclear lymphocytes, leukocytes, and macrophages; along with myocardial fibrosis; and contraction bands with or without myocardial necrosis. The inflammation and contraction bands characterize TCM, as compared to coagulation necrosis seen in acute myocardial infarction.

CLINICAL FEATURES

The most common presenting symptom is acute substernal chest pain, but some patients present with dyspnea or syncope. In the International Takotsubo Registry study, the most common symptoms were chest pain, dyspnea, and syncope (75.9%, 46.9%, and 7.7%, respectively).[8]

Minority of patients may develop signs of heart failure, tachyarrhythmia as ventricular tachycardia (VT) or ventricular fibrillation (VF), bradyarrhythmias, significant mitral regurgitation (MR) or sudden cardiac arrest. 10% patients may develop shock also.

Takotsubo cardiomyopathy is often preceded by emotional or physical stress such as an unexpected death in the family, physical, or emotional outbursts exhausting work, however, in some patients no such precipitant stressor could be found.

Electrocardiography

Electrocardiography (ECG) findings in TCM resemble that of ST-elevation myocardial infarction (STEMI) and most of the times it is impossible to distinguish between two conditions on the basis of ECG.[12]

Following are the varied ECG findings:[8]

- ST-segment elevation is frequent (43.7% in the International Takotsubo Registry study). ST-segment elevation involves the anterior precordial leads and is often similar to that seen with an acute anterior wall STEMI
- ST-depression is a less common finding (7.7%) among patients with TCM
- Other findings include QT interval prolongation, T-wave inversion, abnormal Q waves, and nonspecific abnormalities.

In a retrospective study of 33 patients with TCM, the authors proposed ECG criteria to distinguish TCM from anterior acute myocardial infarction in those who presented within 6 hours of symptom onset. The combination of absent abnormal Q waves, absent reciprocal changes, lack of ST-segment elevation in lead V_1, and presence of ST-segment elevation in lead augmented vector right (aVR) had more than 91% sensitivity and 96% specificity for TCM.[13]

Various ECG criteria have been evaluated for differentiating TCM from acute STEMI. In one of the retrospective study involving 33 patients of TCM within 6 hours of symptom onset, a combination of absent Q waves, absent reciprocal ST changes, ST elevation in aVR and absence of ST elevation in V1 had a 91% sensitivity and specificity for TCM (Fig. 1).

Biomarkers

Patients with TCM have high levels of circulating catecholamines and B-type natriuretic peptide (BNP), also these patients have slight elevation of creatinine kinase and troponin. BNP elevation pattern in TCM is often similar to that of STEMI patients.[14]

In one of the studies, a higher values of following ratios were capable of distinguishing TCM from STEMI at an early stage:

- Ratio of N-terminal pro-BNP (NT-proBNP) to troponin I (TnI)
- Ratio of NT-proBNP to creatine kinase-MB (CK-MB) mass
- Ratio of NTproBNP to ejection fraction (EF)
- Of all these, NT-proBNP-to-TnI ratio showed greater accuracy.[15]

Echocardiography

Transthoracic echocardiography is an easy and quick method of diagnosing RWMA, especially hypokinesia and akinesia of mid and apical segment of LV along with hypercontractile basal segments. Characteristically, the RWMA extends beyond a supply territory of any single coronary artery. Basal hyperkinesia might be related with LV end-diastolic pressure and BNP release (Figs. 2 and 3).[16]

Coronary Angiography

Coronary angiography is the best tool to diagnose TCM as most of the patients lack significant obstruction in spite of having severe LV dysfunction. In the International Takotsubo Registry study, concurrent obstructive coronary artery disease was found in coronary angiography among 15.3% of patients with TCM.[8]

Left ventriculogram is considered as the best imaging modality for showing the pathognomonic RWMA as seen in TCM (Fig. 4).

Cardiac Magnetic Resonance Imaging

Cardiac magnetic resonance imaging (MRI) can be a useful tool in differentiating TCM from myocardial infarction and

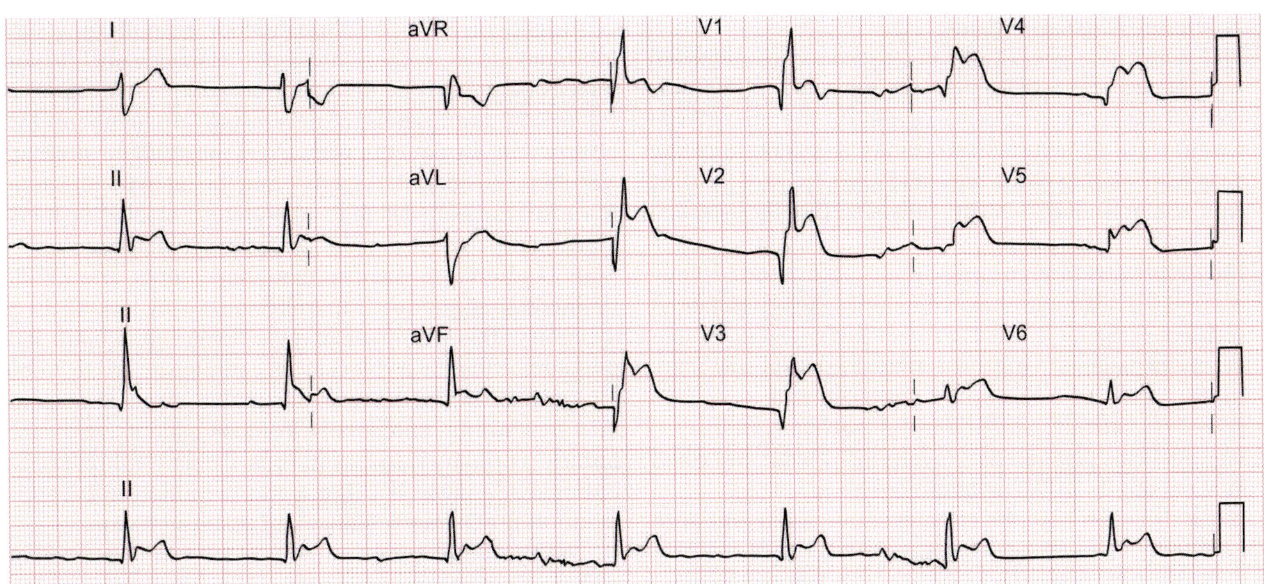

aVF, augmented vector foot; aVL, augmented vector left; aVR, augmented vector right. aVF, augmented vector foot; aVL, augmented vector left; aVR, augmented vector right.

FIG. 1: Electrocardiogram showing ST elevation in Takotsubo cardiomyopathy.

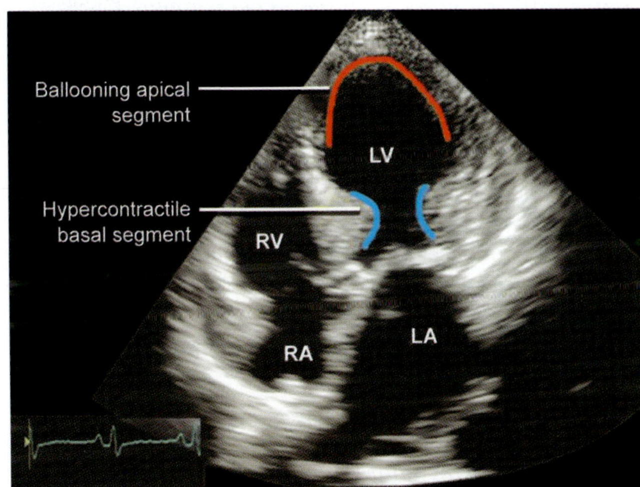

LA, left atrium; RA, right atrium; RV, right ventricle; LV, left ventricle.

FIG. 2: Left ventricle Takotsubo cardiomyopathy showing characteristic apical ballooning.

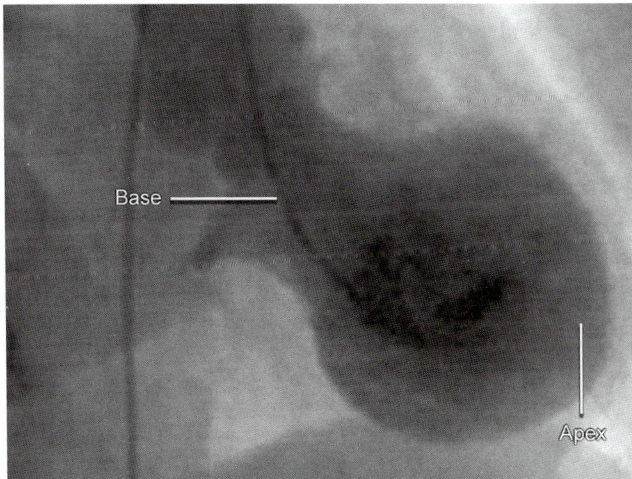

FIG. 4: Left ventriculogram—morphology of left ventricle with typical appearance of apical ballooning.

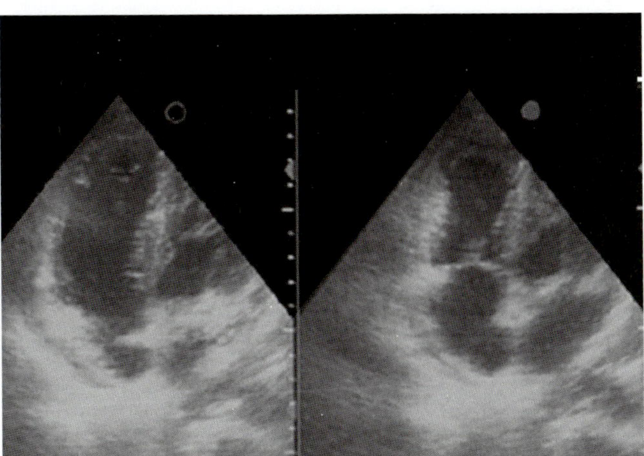

FIG. 3: Right ventricle Takotsubo cardiomyopathy showing RV Apical ballooning and hypercontractile basal segment.

also from myocarditis. Late gadolinium enhancement (LGE) subendocardial or transmural which is typically present in myocardial infarction is not seen in TCM. Also in myocarditis there is patchy LGE which is not there in TCM.[17]

Positron Emission Tomography

Inverse flow metabolism mismatch is seen, i.e., normal perfusion and decreased glucose utilization.[18]

VARIANT[8]

Apical type: This type was present in 81.7% of patients in the International Takotsubo Registry study. In the typical form, there is systolic apical ballooning of the LV, due to severely depressed mid and apical segments, along with hyperkinesia of the basal walls.

Less common (atypical) variants:

- *Mid-ventricular type (14.6%)*: In the second most common type, ventricular hypokinesia was restricted to the mid-part of the LV with relative sparing of the apex. Basal type reverse or inverted takotsubo—hypokinesia of the base with sparing of the mid- and apical part of LV. This type was present in 2.2% of patients in the International Takotsubo Registry study
- *Focal type*: Very rarely a focal variant is also reported. Only an isolated segment, most commonly the anterolateral segment of the LV via only affected. This type was present in 1.5% of patients in the International Takotsubo Registry study
- *Global type*: Rarely, patients have global hypokinesia
- Variants with biventricular involvement were described in about one-fourth of patients
- It has also been described as one of the case report after transcatheter aortic valve replacement (TAVR)[19]
- Isolated right ventricle TCM has also been illustrated without simultaneous involvement of left ventricle.[20]

MANAGEMENT

Patients with TCM are managed on supportive therapy. Measures to relieve stress and anxiety may help in arresting the disease process. But some patients may develop complications in the form of heart failure or shock. Heart failure is managed as per standard protocols. Mainstay of treatment includes supplemental oxygen, assisted ventilation, diuretics, β-blockers, and ace inhibitors or angiotensin II receptor blockers (ARBs).

Approximately, 10% of patients are complicated by shock. Urgent echo is warranted to rule out LV outflow tract (LVOT) obstruction which can be seen in 10–25% of patients with shock. In the patients without LVOT obstruction management includes fluid resuscitation, inotropes with close watch to whether out flow obstruction is setting in. In extremes of LV dysfunction vasopressors and intra-aortic balloon pump (IABP) remains the bailout methods.

In patients with LVOT obstruction complicating shock, inotropes are contraindicated. Management includes increasing preload by fluid support and passive leg raising, β-blockers are useful in decreasing gradients of LVOT obstruction. In patients with LVOT obstruction presenting with hypotension an α-agonist may be added with caution, if the patient is not able to tolerate a β-blocker or there is inadequate response to a β-blocker. Phenylephrine is a pure β-adrenergic agonist that may reduce the gradient by increasing afterload, thereby improving overall hemodynamics. This treatment may be helpful to support blood pressure while a β-blocker is administered to reduce inotropy. However, the vasoconstrictive effects of α-agonists may be harmful, particularly in those patients who can be prone to coronary vasospasm. Thus, if phenylephrine is used, it should be done with a high degree of caution and very close monitoring of hemodynamics and tissue perfusion.

Patients developing thrombus in left ventricle are treated with warfarin as standard anticoagulant therapy.

Because of the occasional association with acute QT prolongation, care should be taken to avoid using QT-prolonging medications, such as macrolide antibiotics or certain antiarrhythmic agents (Table 2).

PROGNOSIS

The prognosis in TCM is usually considered as excellent, with nearly 95% of patients recover completely within 4–8 weeks. Mortality ranges from 1 to 3.2%. Annual recurrence rate is approximately 1.5%.[21,22]

Complications can occur in approximately 20% of cases. They are more common in early stage. Following can be the complications:[23,24]

- Left heart failure with and without pulmonary edema
- Cardiogenic shock
- LV outflow obstruction
- Mitral regurgitation
- Ventricular arrhythmias
- LV mural thrombus formation

TABLE 2: American Heart Association Guidelines for management of Takotsubo cardiomyopathy

COR		LOE
I	Stress (Takotsubo) cardiomyopathy should be considered in patients who present with apparent ACS and nonobstructive CAD at angiography	C
I	Imaging with ventriculography, echocardiography, or magnetic resonance imaging should be performed to confirm or exclude the diagnosis of stress (Takotsubo) cardiomyopathy	B
I	Patients should be treated with conventional agents (ACE inhibitors, β-blockers, aspirin, and diuretics) as otherwise indicated if hemodynamically stable	C
I	Anticoagulation should be administered in patients who develop LV thrombi	C
IIa	It is reasonable to use catecholamines for patients with symptomatic hypotension if outflow tract obstruction is not present	C
IIa	The use of IABP is reasonable for patients with refractory shock	C
IIa	It is reasonable to use β-blockers and α-adrenergic agents in patients with outflow tract obstruction	C
IIb	Prophylactic anticoagulation may be considered to inhibit the development of LV thrombi	C

ACE, angiotensin-converting enzyme; ACS, acute coronary syndrome; CAD, coronary artery disease; COR, class of recommendation; IABP, intra-aortic balloon pump; LOE, level of evidence; LV, left ventricular.

- LV free-wall rupture
- Death.

CONCLUSION

To conclude, stress cardiomyopathy or TCM is a fascinating disease characterized by transient regional LV dysfunction in the absence of significant coronary artery disease. The pathogenesis and diagnostic criteria are evolving. Conservative treatment and resolution of physical or emotional stress usually results in rapid resolution of symptoms. To understand the pathogenesis and to devise rational treatment and prevention strategies, more attention should be paid not only to the myocardium and coronary arteries but also to the integration of central neural, autonomic, endocrine, and circulatory systems in emotional distress.[25]

REFERENCES

1. Zamir M. The Physics of Coronary Blood Flow. USA: Springer Science and Business Media. 2005; p. 387.
2. Akashi YJ, Nef HM, Möllmann H, et al. Stress cardiomyopathy. Annu Rev Med. 2010;61:271-86.
3. Iga K, Gen H, Tomonaga G, et al. Reversible left ventricular wall motion impairment caused by pheochromocytoma: a case report. Jpn Circ J. 1989;53:813-8.
4. Sato H, Tateishi H, Uchida T. Takotsubo-type Cardiomyopathy due to Multivessel Spasm. In: Kodama K, Haze K, Hon M (eds). Clinical Aspect of Myocardial Injury: From Ischemia to Heart Failure. Tokyo, Japan: Kagakuhyouronsha; 1990. pp. 56-64.
5. Bybee KA, Prasad A, Barsness GW, et al. Clinical characteristics and thrombolysis in myocardial infarction frame counts in women with transient left ventricular apical ballooning syndrome. Am J Cardiol. 2004;94:343-6.
6. Sharkey SW, Lesser JR, Zenovich AG, et al. Acute and reversible cardiomyopathy provoked by stress in women from the United States. Circulation. 2005;111:47-9.
7. Prasad A, Lerman A, Rihal CS. Apical ballooning syndrome (Tako-Tsubo or stress cardiomyopathy): a mimic of acute myocardial infarction. Am Heart J. 2008;155:408-17.
8. Templin C, Ghadri JR, Diekmann J, et al. Clinical features and outcomes of takotsubo (stress) cardiomyopathy. N Engl J Med. 2015;373:929.
9. Kurowski V, Kaiser A, von Hof K, et al. Apical and midventricular transient left ventricular dysfunction syndrome (tako-tsubo cardiomyopathy): frequency, mechanisms, and prognosis. Chest. 2007;132:809-16.
10. Yoshihiro JA, David SG, Giuseppe B, et al. Takotsubo cardiomyopathy: A New Form of Acute, Reversible Heart Failure. Circulation. 2008;118(25):2754-62.
11. Dorfman TA, Iskandrian AE. Takotsubo cardiomyopathy: State-of-the-art review. J Nucl Cardiol. 2009;16(1):122-34.
12. Bybee KA, Motiei A, Syed IS, et al. Electrocardiography cannot reliably differentiate transient left ventricular apical ballooning syndrome from anterior ST-segment elevation myocardial infarction. J Electrocardiol. 2007;40:38.e1-6.
13. Kosuge M, Ebina T, Hibi K, et al. Simple and accurate electrocardiographic criteria to differentiate takotsubo cardiomyopathy from anterior acute myocardial infarction. J Am Coll Cardiol. 2010;55(22):2514-6.
14. Nef HM, Mollmann H, Weber M, et al. Release pattern of cardiac biomarkers in left ventricular apical ballooning. Int J Cardiol. 2007;115:128-9.
15. Budnik M, Kochanowski J, Piatkowski R, et al. Simple markers can distinguish Takotsubo cardiomyopathy from ST segment elevation myocardial infarction. Int J Cardiol. 2016;219:417-20.
16. Akashi YJ, Musha H, Nakazawa K, et al. Plasma brain natriuretic peptide in takotsubo cardiomyopathy. Q J Med. 2004;97:599-607.
17. Eitel I, von Knobelsdorff-Brenkenhoff F, Bernhardt P, et al. Clinical characteristics and cardiovascular magnetic resonance findings in stress (takotsubo) cardiomyopathy. JAMA. 2011;306:277.
18. Testa M, Feola M. Usefulness of myocardial positron emission tomography/ nuclear imaging in Takotsubo cardiomyopathy. World J Radiol. 2014;6:502.
19. Ahmed H, Konstantinos PK, Leo M, et al. Takatsubo cardiomyopathy after transcatheter aortic valve replacement. JACC. 2016;9(12).
20. Igor M, Jasna K, Jovan P, et al. Right ventricular takotsubo cardiomyopathy. JACC 2010;55(16).
21. Donohue D, Movahed MR. Clinical characteristics, demographics and prognosis of transient left ventricular apical ballooning syndrome. Heart Fail Rev. 2005;10(4):311-6.
22. Gianni M, Dentali F, Grandi AM, et al. Apical ballooning syndrome or takotsubo cardiomyopathy: a systematic review. Eur Heart J. 2006;27(13): 1523-9.
23. Bybee KA, Kara T, Prasad A, et al. Systematic review: transient left ventricular apical ballooning: a syndrome that mimics ST-segment elevation myocardial infarction. Ann Intern Med. 2004;141(11):858-65.
24. Merchant EE, Johnson SW, Nguyen P, et al. Takotsubo cardiomyopathy: a case series and review of the literature. West JEM. 2008;9:104-11.
25. Goldstein DS. Adrenaline and the Inner World: An Introduction to Scientific Integrative Medicine. Baltimore, Md: Johns Hopkins Univers Press; 2006.

SECTION 14

Syncope

CHAPTER 100

Syncope: What is New?

Satish K Kaushik, Surendra K Chutani

INTRODUCTION

The European Society of Cardiology (ESC) 2018 guidelines[1] for diagnosis and management of syncope have been published. In this chapter we are going to discuss what is new or revised as compared to 2009 edition.[2]

Syncope is a common potentially high-risk complaint in emergency department (ED). Lifetime risk for syncope is 50% in the general population.

DEFINITION

Syncope is a transient loss of consciousness due to cerebral hypoperfusion with rapid onset, short duration, and complete spontaneous recovery.

Compared to previous version, 2018 ESC guidelines include separate supplementary data for further explanation on specific points and web practical instructions where advice is given on how to evaluate patients with loss of consciousness (LOC), and how to perform and interpret tests properly; whenever possible, they have provided relevant tracings, videos, flow charts, and checklists. The document aims to be patient-orientated and focused on therapy.

THE NEW OR REVISED CONCEPTS

New Revised Clinical Settings and Tests

- *Tilt testing*: Concept of hypotensive susceptibility has been highlighted
- *Increased role of prolonged electrocardiographic (ECG) monitoring*: External loop recorder (ELR) or internal loop recorder (ILR); especially ILR in early phase of evaluation of unexplained syncope, patients with bundle branch block (BBB) in whom atrioventricular (AV) block is likely despite electrophysiological studies (EPS) is negative, patients with suspected unproven epilepsy where treatment is ineffective, in patients with primary cardiomyopathy or inherited arrhythmogenic disorders who are at low risk of sudden cardiac death (SCD) as an alternate to implantable cardioverter defibrillator (ICD).In this way it has eclipsed EPS to some extent
- *Video recording* at home or hospital in suspected syncope, especially useful to diagnose psychogenic nonepileptic seizures (PNES) and psychogenic pseudosyncope (PPS). This can also be added to tilt test
- Assess *adenosine sensitive syncope*: Syncope without prodrom, normal ECG and normal heart
- *Neurological causes*: "Ictal asystole"
- *Electrophysiological studies-guided pacemaker implantation*: In patients with prolonged sinus node recovery time (SNRT), HV interval more than 70 ms.

New Revised Indications of Treatment

- Reflex syncope:
  1. Algorithms for selection of appropriate therapy based on age, severity of syncope, and clinical forms have been given
  2. Algorithms for selection of best candidates for pacemaker therapy, primarily patients with cardioinhibitory syncope will respond better to pacemaker rather than patients with vasodepressor or hypotensive susceptibility this has been clearly made out
- *Patients at risk of SCD*: Definition of unexplained syncope and indication of ICD has been given
- Implantable loop recorder as alternative to ICD in selected cases has been recommended.

Guidelines for Management in Emergency Department are Clearly Defined

- List of low-risk and high-risk features has been defined
- Risk stratification flowchart has been given
- Indications for management in ED or fast track to syncope unit (SU) have been mentioned
- Restricted admission criteria "Who should be admitted?" is defined. Thus as per these guidelines low-risk patients

should be discharged from ED, while high-risk patient should have intensive evaluation in ED or SU or hospitalized as per guidelines. Those patients who are neither high nor low risk are observed in ED or SU instead of being hospitalized
- Limited usefulness of risk stratification scores has been highlighted and they are not recommended to be used alone for risk stratification in ED.

Details on creating an outpatient SU with details of staff, equipment, tests, referrals, role of clinical nurse specialist, etc. is defined.

Multiple elements have been downgraded, e.g., discussion on contraindications of carotid sinus massage (CSM), tilt testing indications, and Holter monitoring.

These guidelines propose a care pathway for the management of patients with transient loss of consciousness (TLOC) from their arrival in the ED, and give practical instructions on how to set up outpatient syncope clinics (SU) aimed at reducing hospitalization, under- and misdiagnoses.

Syncope shares many clinical features with other disorders; it therefore presents in many differential diagnoses. This group of disorders is labeled as TLOC.

Transient Loss of Consciousness

Transient loss of consciousness is defined as a state of real or apparent LOC with loss of awareness, characterized by amnesia for the period of unconsciousness, abnormal motor control, loss of responsiveness, and a short duration.

The two main groups of TLOC are "TLOC due to head trauma" and "nontraumatic TLOC".

Classification of Transient Loss of Consciousness

A. Traumatic

B. Nontraumatic:

1. Syncope, e.g., reflex syncope, orthostatic hypotension (OH), and cardiac
2. *Epileptic seizures:* Generalized—tonic, clonic, and atonic
3. *Psychogenic:* PPS and PNES.

These guidelines have discussed only nontraumatic TLOC. Transient loss of consciousness groups have following characteristics:

- Syncope is characterized by cerebral hypoperfusion
- Epileptic seizures are characterized by abnormal excessive brain activity.
- Psychogenic TLoC has psychological cause.

Syncope can be classified as:

- *Reflex syncope:* which includes vasovagal, carotid sinus syndrome, or situational (cough/micturition)
- *Orthostatic hypotension leading to syncope*: Volume depletion, drug induced, autonomic failure, etc.
- *Cardiac causes leading to syncope*: Arrhythmias, structural diseases of heart, pulmonary embolism, etc.

The guidelines have framed clear questions, which should be answered by attending clinician for evaluation and management of TLOC.

At the time of initial evaluation clinician should answer the following key questions:

- Was the event TLOC?
- In case of TLOC, is it of syncopal or nonsyncopal origin?
- In case of suspected syncope, is there a clear etiology?
- Is there evidence to suggest a high risk of cardiovascular events or death?

Transient loss of consciousness has four specific characteristics: short duration, abnormal motor control, loss of responsiveness, and amnesia for the period of LOC.

Transient loss of consciousness is probably syncope when: (1) there are signs and symptoms specific for reflex syncope, syncope due to OH, or cardiac syncope, and (2) signs and symptoms specific for other forms of TLOC (head trauma, epileptic seizures, psychogenic TLOC, and/or rare causes) are absent.

Diagnosis of Syncope

Initial syncope evaluation of suspected syncope includes:

- Careful history-taking concerning present and previous attacks, as well as eyewitness accounts, in person or through a telephone interview
- Physical examination, including supine and standing blood pressure (BP) measurements
- Electrocardiogram.

Based on history, physical examination, and ECG they have been classified into low-risk and high-risk category. Following investigations as indicated should be done:

- Electrocardiographic monitoring, if arrhythmia is suspected
- Echocardiogram, if structural heart disease is suspected
- Carotid sinus massage in persons above 40 years age where cause of syncope is not known
- Tilt test if orthostatic hypotension or reflex syncope is suspected.

Patients coming to emergency should have risk stratification:

- Patient with low-risk condition can be identified and can be discharged from emergency with adequate counseling.
- High-risk patients will require urgent investigation and hospitalization.

Syncope Severity

Cardiac syncope is associated with high morbidity and considerable mortality, meaning that any syncope due to a proven cardiac cause is classified as severe syncope, even if the actual episode was short-lived and had no adverse effects. High-risk patients are more likely to have cardiac syncope.

High-risk or low-risk features are decided by features of syncopal event, past medical history, physical examination, and ECG pattern.

Syncopal Event

- *High-risk features*: Syncopal event, with new onset chest pain, breathlessness, syncope during exertion or when supine, sudden onset of palpitation immediately followed by syncope. Minor or high risk if associated with structural heart disease or abnormal ECG, no warning symptoms or short prodrome, family history of SCD at young age, syncope in sitting position
- *Low-risk features*: Associated with prodrome typical of reflex syncope, after sudden unexpected unpleasant

sight, sound smell, pain; after prolonged standing, during or after meal.

Triggered by cough, defecation, micturition, with head rotation or pressure on carotid sinus, and standing from sitting or supine position.

Past Medical History

- *High-risk features*: Severe structural or coronary artery disease, heart failure, and low left ventricular ejection fraction (LVEF)
- *Low-risk features*: Long history of recurrent syncope with low-risk features with same characteristics of the current syncope

Physical Examination

- *High-risk features*: Unexplained systolic BP in ED less than 90 mm Hg, gastrointestinal (GI) bleed, bradycardia, and undiagnosed systolic murmur
- *Low-risk features*: Normal examination.

Electrocardiogram

- *High-risk features*: ECG changes consistent with acute ischemia, Mobitz II or III degree AV block, atrial fibrillation (AF) with slow ventricular response (VR) <40 beats/min, sinus pauses more than 3 seconds, persistent bradycardia, BBB, intraventricular conduction disturbance, ventricular hypertrophy, Q waves, ventricular tachycardia, pacemaker or ICD malfunction, Brugada syndrome type I, long QT
- *Low-risk features*: Normal ECG.

Patients with Low risk Features

These patients do not need further diagnostic tests in the ED as they are likely to have reflex, situational, or orthostatic syncope. They will benefit from reassurance and counseling.

Patients with High-risk Features

- These patients require an intensive diagnostic approach and may need urgent treatment and admission. High-risk patients should be monitored 6–24 hours in ED
- *External loop recorder or internal loop recorder*: For recurrent and unexplained syncope if features suggest arrhythmic syncope
- Electrophysiological studies are indicated in patients with bifascicular BBB or if tachycardia is suspected
- Treadmill/other stress test should be done in patients who have syncope during or shortly after exertion
- Ambulatory blood pressure monitoring (ABPM) and autonomic function evaluation in patients where neurogenic orthostatic hypotension is suspected
- If TLOC is suspected of nonsyncopal in nature then video recording is recommended

Patients with intermediate risk can probably be managed in OPD setting.

Treatment

Treatment is based on identification of specific mechanism and risk stratification. Effectiveness of treatment to prevent recurrences is determined by mechanisms of syncope rather than its etiology, e.g., treatment of symptomatic bradycardia is pacemaker but it will be less effective if hypotension coexists. Often therapy to prevent recurrence differs from that for underlying disease.

Reflex Syncope

Algorithm based on age, severity of syncope, and clinical forms has been given. Overlap between subgroup is expected.

- Education and lifestyle measures
- Severe or recurrent form:
  - Low BP (chronic systolic BP <110 mm Hg) phenotype younger patient (40 years) can be prescribed drugs, e.g., fludrocortisone, midodrine
  - Patients with prodrome are advised counter pressure measures/tilt training
  - Patients with no or very short prodromes should have ILR-guided management
  - In patients on hypotensive drugs, we can stop or reduce dose of drugs
  - Patients with dominant cardioinhibition, especially older patients more than 60 years are advised pacemaker.

To all patients with reflex syncope and OH, explain the diagnosis, reassure, explain the risk of recurrence, and give advice on how to avoid triggers and situations. These measures are the cornerstone of treatment and have a high impact in reducing the recurrence of syncope.

Orthostatic Hypotension

- Educate patients regarding lifestyle maneuvers including adequate salt intake and hydration
- Stop or reduce antihypertensive therapy
- Counter pressure maneuvers
- Supportive stocking or abdominal binders
- Sleeping in head uptilt position.
- Drugs-Fludrocortisone midodrine can be prescribed.

Cardiac Syncope

All patients with cardiac syncope should receive the specific treatment for arrhythmia/or of the underlying disease causing syncope. ICD may be considered in high-risk patients with unexplained syncope.

CONCLUSION

In conclusion, syncope is a common presentation in ED, majority of cases are low risk and can be identified and discharged form ED with reassurance, education and advice, while high-risk patients should be identified and have intensive diagnostic workup and monitored for 6-24 hrs in ED, SU or hospitalized and treated promptly as per guidelines. The new points of 2018 guidelines have been discussed.

REFERENCES

1. Brignole M, Moya A, de Lange FJ, et al. 2018 ESC guidelines for diagnosis and management of syncope. Eur Heart J. 2018;39(21):1843-948.
2. Moya A, Sutton R, Ammirati F, et al. Guidelines for diagnosis and management of syncope (Version 2009). Eur Heart J. 2009;30:2631-71.

CHAPTER 101

Tilt Table Testing in Syncope

Surender Deora, Kewal C Goswami

INTRODUCTION

Syncope is one of the differential diagnoses of group of disorders known as transient loss of consciousness (TLOC). TLOC is defined as per the European Society of Cardiology (ESC) guidelines as a state of real or apparent loss of consciousness with loss of awareness, characterized by amnesia for the period of unconsciousness, abnormal motor control, loss of responsiveness, and a short duration.[1] Essential within this diagnosis are two key facts: that the loss of consciousness is brief in duration and that recovery is complete. There are various differential diagnoses of TLOC including syncope, seizure disorder, blunt trauma head, psychogenic pseudosyncope (PPS), cataplexy, transient ischemic attack (TIA), and metabolic disturbances like hypoglycemia. Syncope is defined as TLOC due to cerebral hypoperfusion characterized by rapid onset, short duration, and spontaneous complete recovery. The *sine qua non* of syncope pathophysiology is transient cerebral hypoperfusion due to fall in systemic arterial blood pressure (BP) below cerebral perfusion pressure. Sudden fall of systolic BP in upright position below 50–60 mm Hg (cardiac level; 30–45 mm Hg at brain level) for 6–8 seconds can cause complete loss of consciousness.[1] Syncope is mainly classified based on the mechanism leading to cerebral hypoperfusion as neurally mediated (reflex mediated), cardiac syncope or due to orthostatic hypotension. The approach to the patient with syncope includes meticulous history given by patient as well as eye witness if available. If the diagnosis of syncope is suspected then further investigations are warranted. Measurement of BP in both supine and standing, Electrocardiogram (ECG) and echocardiogram are initially done in the evaluation of syncope. Head-up tilt test (HUTT) has been performed for evaluation of patients of reflex syncope [most common vasovagal syncope (VVS)]. The clinical utility of this test in diagnosis and management of the patients with reflex syncope is limited. The purpose of this test has been changed recently from diagnosing the reflex syncope to know the susceptibility for reflex or postural hypotension.[1]

PATHOPHYSIOLOGY OF VASOVAGAL SYNCOPE

During tilted position there is redistribution of 750–1000 mL of venous blood from central blood compartment to lower limb and splanchnic organs.[2] This results in decrease in ventricular preload, stroke volume, and systolic BP. In response to this and to provide adequate perfusion pressure to vital organs, the nervous system gets activated and releases catecholamines and activates the renin–angiotensin–aldosterone system releasing various neuropeptides like endothelin, etc. which increases the peripheral vascular resistance and increase in rate and force of left ventricular contraction. Patients with autonomic dysfunction and neurohormonal deficiency, the compensatory mechanism to increase the heart rate (HR) and peripheral resistance are insufficient which leads to cerebral hypoperfusion and TLOC. Neurocardiogenic reflex also contributes to the symptoms but the mechanism is not very well understood.

HEAD-UP TILT TEST

The tilt table was used earlier for the evaluation of HR and BP in upright position. While evaluating these parameters, some patients developed faintness or TLOC with hypotension which was associated with bradycardia in some patients mimicking the vasovagal reaction.[3,4] These initial observation in case studies formed the basis for further evaluation of syncope patient with HUTT. The first report of HUTT as a tool to diagnose syncope was reported by Kenny et al. in a landmark study published in Lancet.[5] They studied 15 patients with undiagnosed recurrent syncope despite complete clinical and electrophysiological assessment. During HUTT with 40° elevation for 60 minutes, ten patients developed significant bradycardia with hypotension and reproduced similar clinical symptoms as previously experienced. Since then the test is used in assessment of VVS if the diagnosis is doubtful after thorough clinical examination. Thereafter, various parameters have been adapted regarding the angle of tilt, duration of tilt and if any provocative stimulus is needed. Fitzpatrick et al. studied 71 patients with recurrent unexplained syncope for the angle of tilt, duration of tilt, and method of tilt support. The authors first time defined standard protocol for HUTT. They concluded tilt angle of 60° with tilt timing of 45 minutes is sufficient and use of foot board for support increases the specificity as compared to bicycle saddle or seat.[6] The use of isoproterenol as a provocative agent is based on studies showing excess catecholamine before the syncopal episode may paradoxically increase the susceptibility to bradycardia and hypotension.[7,8] The studies by Alquist et al. and Waxman et al. showed the clinical use of isoproterenol in provoking neurally mediated syncope during tilt testing.[9,10] Because of provocation agents, the duration of the tilt was reduced to 20 minutes in some studies. Although isoproterenol in dosage up to 5 µg/min increases the sensitivity of the test but it decreases the specificity (45–65%) and its use as a provocative agent became questionable.[11] But with reduced dosage of isoproterenol up to 3 µg/min, the specificity of the test was found up to 93%.[12] Because of significant risk of arrhythmia and ischemia in patients with coronary artery disease the use of isoproterenol is gradually decreased. Moreover, it is time consuming to infuse it through syringe pump. Therefore, nitroglycerine (NTG) given as sublingual dosage became more preferred choice. Raviele et al. first introduced the NTG in HUTT protocol as an infusion.[13] Later the same group evaluated sublingual NTG in 235 patients with syncope of unknown origin and no evidence of organic heart disease. All patients underwent HUTT with 60° tilt for 45 minutes followed by 300 µg sublingual NTG in next 20 minutes. They concluded the addition of NTG maintained the high specificity (94%) and doubled the rate of positive test.[14]

The following are the standard protocols for HUTT:

- Patients should be NPO (nil per orally) for 3–4 hours before the test. The longer fasting period may leads to dehydration which may affect the test result. If the patients are fasting for more than 4 hours intravenous (IV) saline may be infused prior to the test according to the volume status of patients
- The room should be equipped with emergency crash cart, defibrillator nearby and trained nurse, technician, and physician assistant should be available. Physician may not be needed all time but should be in the premises if emergency occurs[15]
- Patient should be gently wrapped and supported by footboard to avoid fall in case syncope occurs
- Electrocardiogram leads (minimum three) should be recorded continuously with continuous noninvasive beat-to-beat BP monitoring. If continuous noninvasive beat to beat monitoring of BP is not possible, then BP may be monitored by arm cuff though this is less desirable
- The tilt table should be capable of achieving tilt angle between 60° and 70° (Fig. 1)
- Pretilt a resting supine period of 5–10 minutes should be ensured in which the patient is monitored. If any venous or arterial cannulation beyond a routine peripheral IV line is required then a longer period of rest of at least 20 minutes is required (so that endogenous catecholamine levels settle back to baseline). We advise venous cannulation for all patients for HUTT
- Passive phase of tilt of 20–45 minutes depending on patient's clinical parameters and symptoms.
- If the passive phase is negative, a drug provocation with either sublingual NTG (300–400 µg) or IV isoproterenol (1–3 µg/min to increase HR ~20–25% above baseline) may be done
- The test should be continued until either the test is positive or the protocol is completed.

RESPONSE TO HEAD-UP TILT TEST

- Normal response is defined as no change in BP or HR or increase of less than or equal to 10% till patient is brought to supine position
- In patients with reflex syncope, BP falls after a latent period of tilt with rate of fall increasing (convex curve) associated with decrease in HR (Fig. 2)
- In patients with orthostatic hypotension, BP starts falling just after tilt with rate of fall decreases progressively (concave curve) associated with increase in HR
- In patients with psychogenic pseudosyncope, both BP and HR do not change or rather may increase. The event (pseudosyncope) occurs at variable interval after head-up tilt

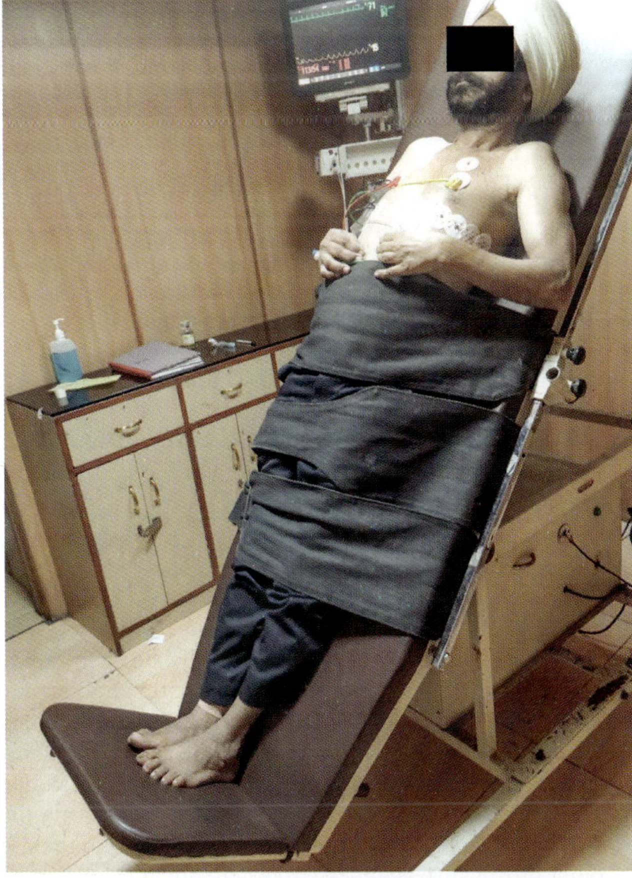

FIG. 1: Head-up tilt test: Patient is first monitored in a supine position for 5–10 minutes and is then tilted to 70°. If there is no drop in heart rate or blood pressure then drug provocation is performed.

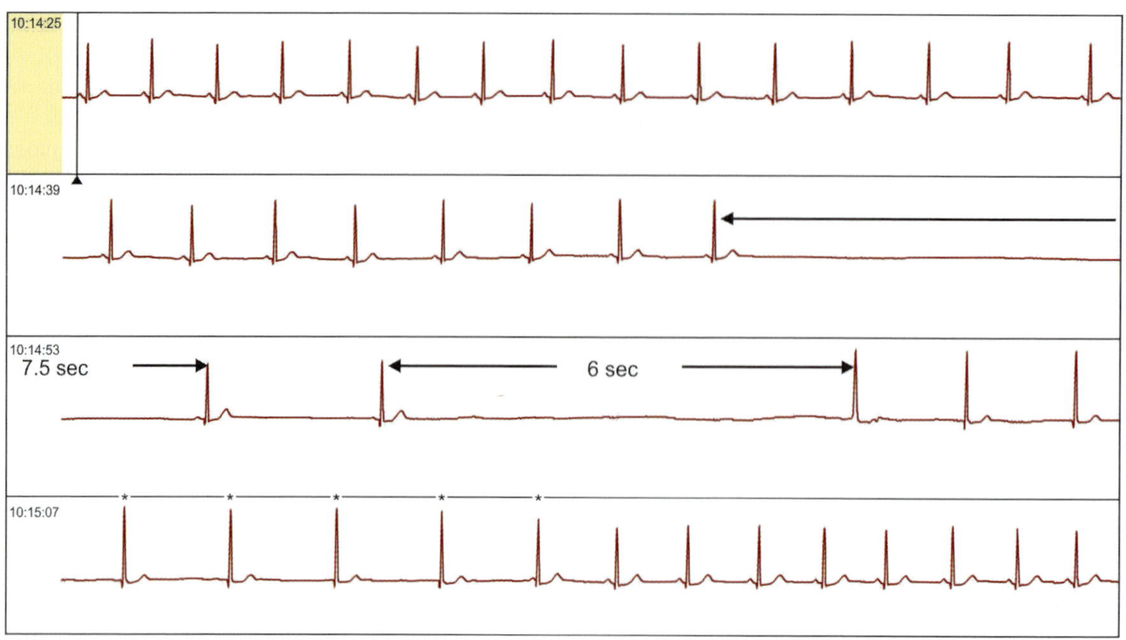

*Junctional beat.

FIG. 2: Positive head-up tilt test: With a 70° and on drug provocation (nitroglycerine) there is a drop in blood pressure (not shown) and progressive bradycardia culminating in asystole and syncope. The patient was quickly brought back to supine position. The blood pressure and heart rate gradually returned to baseline.

- Patients with postural orthostatic tachycardia syndrome (POTS) manifest increase in HR more than or equal to 30 beats/min or a HR of more than or equal to 120 beats/min during the tilt without a fall in BP.

INDICATIONS

Before HUTT all patients should be thoroughly evaluated by history taking, clinical examination, orthostatic BP measurement, ECG, and echocardiography. The following are the indications for HUTT:
- Recurrent reflex syncope of unknown origin
- Recurrent orthostatic hypotension
- Postural orthostatic tachycardia syndrome
- Psychogenic pseudosyncope
- To diagnose convulsive syncope and to differentiate it from seizure disorder
- Unexplained falls.

COMPLICATIONS AND CONTRAINDICATIONS

Head-up tilt test is a safe procedure and till date no mortality has been reported. Patients should be informed about the test and explained about the headache and fatigue which may appear after the syncopal episode. Most of the problems experienced by the patients are relieved once the supine position is achieved. NTG may cause headache during the test. There are reports of ventricular arrhythmia with the use of other provocative agent like isoproterenol in patients with ischemic heart disease (IHD) and sick sinus syndrome.[16,17] Patients may develop transient atrial fibrillation during or post-HUTT.[18] Prolonged asystole may occur during the tilt and mostly is resolved on returning the patient to supine position. It hardly ever needs any resuscitation measures like atropine, pacing or cardiopulmonary resuscitation. Very rarely, the syncopal episode may be associated with myoclonic jerks which may be confused with seizure disorder.

There are no absolute contraindications for HUTT except if provocative test with isoproterenol is required. Patients with aortic stenosis, subvalvular obstruction [e.g., hypertrophic obstructive cardiomyopathy (HOCM)], IHD or uncontrolled hypertension, past history of ventricular arrhythmias with exertion should not be given isoproterenol as provocative agents.

FUTURE PROSPECTS

The role cardiac pacing in prevention of recurrent event in patients with reflex syncope is always controversial.[19,20] There are two components in the pathophysiology of reflex syncope: (1) cardioinhibition, and (2) vasodepressor. In most of the cases, it is mixed type of mechanisms and therefore cardiac pacing has controversial benefit. The ISSUE-2 (International Study on Syncope of Uncertain Etiology 2) was prospective observational study in patients with reflex syncope and implantable loop recorder (ILR) for studying the mechanism of syncope. It revealed that half of the patients with reflex syncope had asystolic event and cardiac pacing resulted in 80% relative risk reduction in syncope recurrence.[21] The ISSUE-3 was double blinded, randomized, multicentric trial in patients with recurrent syncope to assess the apparent pacing benefit in ISSUE-2 trial. It concluded that dual chamber cardiac pacing in patients of reflex syncope with significant asystolic component showed 32% absolute risk reduction and 57% relative risk reduction in symptom recurrence.[22] Therefore, the combination of ILR and HUTT is proposed for evaluating the patients with reflex syncope for risk stratification and selecting those who will be benefitted with cardiac pacing.

CONCLUSION

Vasovagal syncope is a clinical diagnosis and careful history taking with thorough clinical examination is of utmost importance. There is no gold standard investigation for the diagnosis of reflex syncope. HUTT with or without provocation is a low cost, noninvasive, readily available modality for assessment of hypotensive susceptibility in patients with syncope. The HUTT has clinical value only when it reproduces the similar symptoms as during the event. The interpretation of HR and BP response during tilt helps in differentiating VVS from other similar presenting diagnosis. Its role in assessment of therapeutic options is limited at present but is an evolving opportunity.

REFERENCES

1. Brignole M, Moya A, de Lange FJ, et al. 2018 ESC Guidelines for the diagnosis and management of syncope. Eur Heart J. 2018;39:1883-948.
2. McMichael J, Sharpey-Schafer EP. Cardiac output in man by a direct Fick method: Effects of posture, venous pressure change, atropine, and adrenaline. Br Heart J. 1944;6:33-40.
3. Allen SC, Taylor CL, Hall VE. A study of orthostatic insufficiency by the tilt-board method. Am J Physiol. 1945;143:11-20.
4. Hammill SC, Holmes DR, Wood DL, et al. Electrographic testing in the upright position: Improved evaluation of patients with rhythm disturbances using a tilt table. J Am Coll Cardiol. 1984;4:65-71.
5. Kenny RA, Ingram A, Bayliss J, et al. Head-up tilt: A useful test for investigating unexplained syncope. Lancet. 1986;1:1352-5.
6. Fitzpatrick AP, Theodorakis G, Vardas P, et al. Methodology of head-up tilt testing in patients with unexplained syncope. J Am Coll Cardiol. 1991;17:125-30.
7. Chosy JJ, Graham DT. Catecholamines in vasovagal fainting. J Psychosom Res. 1965;9:189-94.
8. Vingerhoets AJ. Biochemical changes in two subjects succumbing to syncope. Psychosom Med. 1984;46:95-103.
9. Almquist A, Goldenberg IF, Milstein S, et al. Provocation of bradycardia and hypotension by isoproterenol and upright posture in patients with unexplained syncope. N Engl J Med. 1989;320:346-51.
10. Waxman MB, Yao L, Cameron DA, et al. Isoproterenol induction of vasodepressor-type reaction in vasodepressor prone persons. Am J Cardiol. 1989;63:58-65.
11. Kapoor WN, Brant N. Evaluation of syncope by upright tilt testing with isoproterenol. A nonspecific test. Ann Intern Med. 1992;116:358-63.
12. Morillo CA, Klein GJ, Zandri S, et al. Diagnostic accuracy of a low-dose isoproterenol head-up tilt protocol. Am Heart J. 1995;129:901-6.
13. Raviele A, Gasparini G, Di Pede F, et al. Nitroglycerin infusion during upright tilt: A new test for the diagnosis of vasovagal syncope. Am Heart J. 1994;127:103-11.
14. Raviele A, Menozzi C, Brignole M, et al. Value of head-up tilt testing potentiated with sublingual nitroglycerin to assess the origin of unexplained syncope. Am J Cardiol. 1995;76:267-72.
15. Haines DE, Beheiry S, Akar JG, et al. Heart rhythm society expert consensus statement on electrophysiology laboratory standards: Process, protocols, equipment, personnel, and safety. Heart Rhythm. 2014;11:e9-51.
16. Leman RB, Clarke E, Gillette P. Significant complications can occur with ischemic heart disease and tilt table testing. Pacing Clin Electrophysiol. 1999;22:675-7.
17. Kenny RA, O'Shea D, Parry SW. The Newcastle protocols for head-up tilt table testing in the diagnosis of vasovagal syncope, carotid sinus hypersensitivity, and related disorders. Heart. 2000;83:564-9.
18. de Castro RR, Mesquita ET, da Nobrega AC. Parasympathetic-mediated atrial fibrillation during tilt test associated with increased baroreflex sensitivity. Europace. 2006;8:349-51.
19. Connolly SJ, Sheldon R, Thorpe KE, et al. Pacemaker therapy for prevention of syncope in patients with recurrent severe vasovagal syncope: Second Vasovagal Pacemaker Study (VPS II): A randomized trial. JAMA. 2003;289:2224-9.
20. Raviele A, Giada F, Menozzi C, et al. A randomized, double-blind, placebo-controlled study of permanent cardiac pacing for the treatment of recurrent tilt-induced vasovagal syncope. The vasovagal syncope and pacing trial (SYNPACE). Eur Heart J. 2004;25:1741-8.
21. Brignole M, Sutton R, Menozzi C, et al. Early application of an implantable loop recorder allows a mechanism-based effective therapy in patients with recurrent suspected neurally-mediated syncope. Eur Heart J. 2006;27:1085-92.
22. Brignole M, Menozzi C, Moya A, et al. Pacemaker therapy in patients with neurally-mediated syncope and documented asystole. Third international study on syncope of unknown etiology (ISSUE-3): A randomized trial. Circulation. 2012;125:2566-71.

CHAPTER 102

Implantable and External Loop Recorders: Indications in My Practice

Praloy Chakraborty

INTRODUCTION

Arrhythmia can present as sudden cardiac arrest, syncope [with total loss of consciousness (TLoC)], presyncope, and palpitation. The gold standard procedure to diagnose arrhythmia is symptom-electrocardiogram (ECG) correlation. The ECG recordings during symptoms allow physicians to either confirm or exclude an arrhythmia as the mechanism of symptom. Recording of ECG during symptom is the most challenging task in clinical practice. Most of cardiac arrhythmias are intermittent and are of unpredictable frequency. The frequency may vary from few episodes in an hour to minimal episodes in years. Recent guidelines for the management of patients with cardiac arrhythmias recommend the use of prolonged electrocardiogram monitoring techniques for better correlation between the symptoms and the arrhythmias and to detect asymptomatic significant rhythm disturbances. There are several prolong ECG monitoring systems depending on the duration of monitoring, the duration varies from 24 hours to 3 years. Choice of each system depends on frequency of symptoms.

Features of different prolong ECG monitors are described in table 1.[1] Conventional Holter monitoring can record ECG for 24 hours to few days. If the symptoms are less frequent, Holter monitoring is unlikely to be effective in detecting events. ECG loop recorders can continuously record and deletes the patient's ECG. They are either activated by patient-activation function as a result of symptoms or an autoactivation feature allowing the capture of arrhythmic events without relying on patient compliance or perception of symptoms. Loop recorders can be implantable (ILR) and external (ELR). Presence of retrospective memory differentiates loop recorders from prospective-only event recorders. While event recorders have some usefulness in patients with intermittent palpitations, they have no indication to detect syncope. In the current chapter use of ECG loop recorder in clinical practice will be discussed.

PATIENTS WITH SYNCOPE

Prolong ECG monitoring, in the form of loop recorder (ILR or ELR), is required in investigating arrhythmic syncope. Although syncope is a very common presenting symptom[1] (more than 50% of general population complains of an episode of suspected syncope in life time), reflex syncope being the most common, arrhythmic syncope is less common.[2] Initial clinical history including the clinical settings, examinations, and base line ECG can diagnose the etiology of a syncope in about half of the patient population.[3] A smaller proportion of patients require specialized evaluation. The clinical clues to arrhythmic etiology of syncope include:[4]

- Syncope at rest or exertion
- Brief or absent prodrome
- Rapid recovery (<5 min)
- May be preceded by palpitations
- Abnormality in baseline ECG.

In patients with suspected arrhythmic syncope, an initial attempt should be made to identify those patients who are at high risk of sudden cardiac death with subsequent attack. The "high-risk" features consist of presence of external bleeding, persistent hypotension [systolic blood pressure (SBP) <90 mm Hg] or bradycardia [heart rate (HR) <40 beats/min], evidence of structural [heart failure, old or new myocardial infarction (MI), low ejection fraction] or electrical [short or long QT, Brugada pattern, epsilon wave, fascicular or atrioventricular (AV) nodal block, intraventricular conduction delay (IVCD), etc.] cardiac disorders.[5]

For all other patient with high-risk feature initial evaluation can be done in emergency department or syncope unit. These patients should be managed with standard guideline instead of extensive investigations. If ECG monitoring is required, they should be subjected to in hospital ECG monitoring. In patients with suspected arrhythmic syncope and who are at low risk, besides baseline ECG, echocardiography and Holter monitoring are to be done. Besides that, few specific tests should also be done like.

TABLE 1: Salient features of prolong electrocardiogram monitoring[1]

Name	Holter monitoring	External event recorder	External loop recorder	Implantable loop recorder
Duration of monitoring	Usually 24–48 h, may be up to 7 days	Specific time for single even (for example up to 30 s) of even. Total number of events depends on capacity of memory card	Up to 4 weeks	Up to 3 years
Noninvasive/invasive	Noninvasive	Noninvasive	Noninvasive	Invasive
Autodeletion of records	No	No	Yes	Yes
Storage memory of retrospective ECG	Not required	No	Yes	Yes
Total memory	Usually whole monitoring time	Depends on capacity of memory card	Few hours to 4 weeks	40–45 min
Patient activation	Yes	Yes	Yes	Yes
Auto activation	No	No	Yes	Yes
Clinical indication	Palpitations and syncope	Palpitations	Palpitations and syncope	Palpitations and syncope
Cost	Inexpensive	Inexpensive	Inexpensive	expensive

- Exercise testing (for exertional syncope)
- Carotid sinus massage
- Head-up tilt test (HUTT for suspected neurocardiogenic syncope).

Early use of electrophysiological studies should be considered in clinical situations listed here.

- Presence of asymptomatic sinus bradycardia (<50 beats/min) or sinoatrial block, documented by 12-lead ECG or 24 hours ECG monitoring[6]
- In patients with syncope preceded by sudden-onset brief palpitations suggesting supraventricular tachycardia (SVT), if only curative catheter ablation is planned
- Presence of pre-excited QRS complex
- In patients with previous MI and preserved left ventricular ejection fraction (LVEF), induction of sustained monomorphic ventricular tachycardia (VT) is strongly predictive of the cause of syncope.[7] The absence of inducible ventricular arrhythmias identifies a group of patients at lower risk of arrhythmic syncope[8,9]
- *Syncope in patients with bundle branch block*:[10,11] Prolonged HV interval or induction of AV block by pacing or by pharmacological stress identifies a group of patients at higher risk of developing AV block in follow-up, but the absence of abnormal findings does not exclude the development of AV block.

If the mechanism of syncope is unexplained after initial evaluation, prolong ECG monitoring is required for symptom and arrhythmia correlation. The usage of particular loop recorder depends on the expected frequency of recurrence of syncope.

In the initial clinical experience, where ILR was used for diagnosis in patients with unexplained syncope at the end of unsuccessful full conventional work-up, ILR was found to diagnose the etiology of syncope in 35% cases.[1] Consequently, early implantation with ILR was found to be more effective compared to the conventional strategy.[11,12] Early implantation of ILR is cost effective,[11] associated with improved quality of life[13] and does not increase the mortality.[11,13] Apart from diagnosis of unexplained, low risk, infrequent syncope ILR can also be used in some specific situations:

- *Unexplained syncope in presence of detectable cardiac disease*:
  - Syncope, bundle branch block, and normal electrophysiological studies.[14] About one-third of patients with negative electrophysiological study in whom an ILR was implanted, developed intermittent or permanent AV block on follow-up[15]
  - Patients with definite structural heart disease in whom an arrhythmia is likely despite a negative work-up.[16] For example, patient with old MI and nonsustained VT when electrophysiological study failed to induce sustained monomorphic VT
  - Patients with cardioinhibitory carotid sinus hypersensitivity when the understanding of the exact mechanism of spontaneous syncope is needed to guide a specific therapy[17]
  - Pediatric patients in whom a cardiac cause of syncope is suspected due to structural heart disease or electrocardiographical abnormalities.[18]
- *Where justification of therapy is required*: In patients with suspected neurocardiogenic syncope, even if tilt test is positive, in order to capture an asystolic event when cardiac pacing would be justified by the severity and unpredictability of symptoms and lack of alternative therapies[19]
- *Suspected but not established syncope*:
  - Patients in whom epilepsy was suspected but the treatment has proved ineffective[20]
  - Patients with established epilepsy in order to detect peri-ictal cardiac arrhythmias that require treatment[21]
  - Patients with major depressive diseases and frequent recurrent unexplained episodes of LoC in order to exclude an arrhythmic cause of syncope[22]
  - In older patients with nonaccidental falls to establish the syncopal nature of the event.[23]

Although studies suggest that ELR has similar diagnostic yield like ILR in the same timeframe,[24-26] usage of ELR is limited by patient compliance, failure to operate the device correctly and difficulties in handling cutaneous patch electrodes.[25] A cost-effective analysis has indicated that ELRs are an economically attractive alternative when compared to Holter.[27] The ELR appears to have its greatest role in motivated patients with frequent syncope where spontaneous symptoms are likely to recur within 4–6 weeks.

Although documentation of arrhythmia during spontaneous syncope is considered as diagnostic gold standard, however presence of some asymptomatic significant arrhythmias like prolonged asystole (3 seconds or more), rapid SVTs (160 beats/min for 32 beats), or VT, are also considered by several authors as a diagnostic finding.[1] Absence of documented arrhythmia during a syncopal episode allows exclusion of an arrhythmia as the mechanism of the syncope.

There are specific criteria to diagnose arrhythmias in loop recorders.[28] The diagnostic yield of ILR was hampered by the failure to document a syncopal relapse in further 5–9% of the patients (16% of the events) despite the manual and automated features of the device[29] and by false-positive arrhythmia detection even in the most recent devices.

As per guidelines, loop recorders can be used in following conditions:[5]

- *Implantable loop recorder*: It is useful in any of the following conditions:
  - In patients with recurrent syncope if high-risk features are absent and recurrence rate is low
  - In patients with high-risk features, if immediate comprehensive evaluation failed to demonstrate any cause and there is no indication of immediate implantation of implantable cardioverter defibrillator (ICD) or pacemaker
  - In patients with suspected or definitive reflex syncope to understand the mechanism in presence of frequent or severe episodes
  - In patients with unexplained falls
  - If epilepsy is suspected but the patient does not respond to treatment.
- *External loop recorder*: It may be used instead of ILR in patients with nonhigh-risk unexplained syncope of suspected arrhythmic origin if intersymptom interval of 4 weeks.

PATIENTS WITH PALPITATIONS

Palpitations resulting from either primary cardiac arrhythmias or due to sinus tachycardia secondary to noncardiac disorders are one of the most common clinical symptoms. If symptoms a less frequent, it is difficult to establish symptom-ECG correlation despite careful evaluation that includes standard ECG and Holter monitoring. Event recorders are unable to detect the mechanism of onset of episodes and some short-lasting episodes due to lack of automatic detection.[1] Like syncope, high-risk patients may need aggressive interventions, including hospitalization and invasive tests to rule out life-threatening arrhythmias. The patients at low risk with frequent and/or severe symptoms are the best candidates for loop recorders. ILR, due to their invasive nature and costs, play a minor role in patients with recurrent unexplained palpitations when compared with those with syncope. In patients with infrequent (1 episode/month) and sustained (>1 min) palpitations, ILR implantation with 1-year monitoring was found to be more effective.[30]

External loop recorders can be more useful for palpitation than for syncope evaluation. In a consecutive series of 125 patients all with an intersymptom interval of 4 weeks, ELR was found to be effective.[31]

As per guideline,[1] ELRs can be used in patients with recurrent palpitations, normal baseline ECG, frequent symptoms (intersymptom interval <4 weeks), and absence of high-risk criteria. ILRs may be indicated if symptoms are infrequent and normal result in ELRs and other ECG monitoring systems. The specificity of the technique is high when an arrhythmia is documented during symptoms. Normal ECG recording during palpitations excludes an arrhythmic cause. The outcome of asymptomatic arrhythmias remains uncertain.

NONESTABLISHED INDICATIONS

Although the current guideline approves usage of loop recorders only for unexplained syncope and palpitations, there are fewer emerging indications in clinical practice:

- In rhythm control trial, when intermittent or continuous capturing of symptomatic or asymptomatic atrial fibrillation is required[1]
- In cryptogenic ischemic stroke in presence of minimal or no structural heart disease, to look for atrial fibrillation
- To detect asymptomatic arrhythmias in patients after MI, most commonly in clinical research[32]
- Documentation of arrhythmic origin of syncope or presyncope in patients with phenotypic or genotypic evidence of inherited arrhythmias. In this setting syncope is usually considered as high risk of sudden cardiac death and ICD implantation is indicated. The mechanism of syncope may be heterogeneous and most of the patients have inherited arrhythmias, who received ICD for syncope, are not at risk of recurrent ICD discharge in follow-up studies.[33] In many patients, ILR can be used to identify the mechanism of syncope before embarking in ICD therapy. This hypothesis requires to be validated by clinical trials.[34]

Loop recorders are increasingly used to detect symptomatic and asymptomatic arrhythmias. Ultimate goal of using loop recorders should be prevention of syncopal recurrences, severe injuries, and death. Further research is required to minimize artifact as well as to reduce the device size. Device miniaturization could increase the use of cardiac monitors, which could become the new standard of care for serious adverse event prevention and long-term monitoring of patients with chronic cardiac diseases.

REFERENCES

1. Brignole M, Vardas P, Hoffman E, et al. Indications for the use of diagnostic implantable and external ECG loop recorders. Europace. 2009;11(5):671-87.
2. Colman N, Nahm K, Ganzeboom KS, et al. Epidemiology of reflex syncope. Clin Auton Res. 2004;14(Suppl 1):i9-17.
3. Croci F, Brignole M, Alboni P, et al. The application of a standardized of evaluation in patients with syncope referred to three Syncope Units. Europace. 2002;4:351-6.
4. Saklani P, Krahn A, Klein G. Syncope. Circulation. 2013;127(12):1330-9.
5. Brignole M, Moya A, de Lange FJ, et al.; ESC Scientific Document Group. 2018 ESC Guidelines for the diagnosis and management of syncope. Eur Heart J. 2018;39(21):1883-948.
6. Gann D, Tolentino A, Samet P. Electrophysiologic evaluation of elderly patients with sinus bradycardia. A long-term follow-up study. Ann Intern Med 1979;90: 24–29.
7. Gann D, Tolentino A, Samet P. Electrophysiologic evaluation of elderly patients with sinus bradycardia. A long-term follow-up study. Ann Intern Med. 1979;90:24-9.
8. Olshansky B, Hahn EA, Hartz VL, et al. Clinical significance of syncope in the electrophysiologic study versus electrocardiographic monitoring (ESVEM) trial. The ESVEM Investigators. Am Heart J. 1999;137:878-86.
9. McAnulty JH, Rahimtoola SH, Murphy E, et al. Natural history of "high-risk" bundle-branch block: final report of a prospective study. N Engl J Med. 1982;307(3):137-43.
10. McAnulty JH, Rahimtoola SH, Murphy E, et al. Natural history of 'high risk' bundle branch block. Final report of a prospective study. N Engl J Med. 1982;307:137-43.
11. Scheinman MM, Peters RW, Suave MJ, et al. Value of the H–Q interval in patients with bundle branch block and the role of prophylactic permanent pacing. Am J Cardiol. 1982;50:1316-22.
12. Krahn AD, Klein GJ, Yee R, et al. Randomized assessment of syncope trial: conventional diagnostic testing versus a prolonged monitoring strategy. Circulation. 2001;104:46-51.
13. Edvardsson N, Frykman V, van Mechelen R, et al. Use of an implantable loop recorder to increase the diagnostic yield in unexplained syncope: Results from the PICTURE registry. Europace. 2011;13:262-9.
14. Farwell DJ, Freemantle N, Sulke N. The clinical impact of implantable loop recorders in patients with syncope. Eur Heart J. 2006;27:351-6.
15. Brignole M, Menozzi C, Moya A, et al. The mechanism of syncope in patients with bundle branch block and negative electrophysiologic test. Circulation. 2001;104:2045-50.
16. Brignole M, Menozzi C, Moya A, et al. Mechanism of syncope in patients with bundle branch block and negative electrophysiological test. Circulation. 2001;104:2045-50.
17. Solano A, Menozzi C, Maggi R, et al. Incidence, diagnostic yield and safety of the implantable loop-recorder to detect the mechanism of syncope in patients with and without structural heart disease. Eur Heart J. 2004;25:1116-9.
18. Maggi R, Menozzi C, Brignole M, et al. Cardioinhibitory carotid sinus hypersensitivity predicts an asystolic mechanism of spontaneous neurally mediated syncope. Europace. 2007;9:563-7.
19. Frangini P, Cecchin F, Jordao L, et al. How revealing are insertable loop recorders in pediatrics? Pacing Clin Electrophysiol. 2008;31:338-43.
20. Brignole M, Sutton R, Menozzi C, et al. Early application of an implantable loop recorder allows effective specific therapy in patients with recurrent suspected neurally mediated syncope. Eur Heart J. 2006;27:1085-92.
21. Zaidi A, Clough P, Cooper P, et al. Misdiagnosis of epilepsy: Many seizure-like attacks have a cardiovascular cause. J Am Coll Cardiol. 2000;36:181-4.
22. Rugg-Gunn F, Simister R, Squirrel M, et al. Cardiac arrhythmias in focal epilepsy: A prospective long-term study. Lancet. 2004;364:2212-9.
23. Pezawas T, Stix G, Kastner J, et al. Implantable loop recorder in unexplained syncope: Classification, mechanism, transient loss of consciousness and role of major depressive disorder in patients with and without structural heart disease. Heart. 2008;94:17-24.
24. Armstrong L, Lawson J, Kamper A, et al. The use of implantable loop recorder in the investigation of unexplained syncope in older people. Age Ageing. 2003;32:185-8.
25. Brignole M, Menozzi C, Bartoletti A, et al. A new management of syncope: Prospective systematic guideline-based evaluation of patients referred urgently to general hospitals. Eur Heart J. 2006;27:76-82.
26. Sivakumaran S, Krahn AD, Klein GJ, et al. A prospective randomized comparison of loop recorders versus Holter monitors in patients with syncope or presyncope. Am J Med. 2003;115:1-5.
27. Gula LJ, Krahn AD, Massel D, et al. External loop recorders: Determinants of diagnostic yield in patients with syncope. Am Heart J. 2004;147:644-8.
28. Schuchert A, Maas R, Kretzschmar C, et al. Diagnostic yield of external electrocardiographic loop recorders in patients with recurrent syncope and negative tilt table test. Pacing Clin Electrophysiol. 2003;26:1837-40.
29. Brignole M, Moya A, Menozzi C, et al. Proposed electrocardiographic classification of spontaneous syncope documented by an Implantable Loop Recorder. Europace. 2005;7:14-8.
30. Krahn AD, Klein GJ, Yee R, et al. Use of an extended monitoring strategy in patients with problematic syncope. Reveal Investigators. Circulation. 1999;99: 406-10.
31. Giada F, Gulizia M, Francese M, et al. Recurrent unexplained palpitations (RUP) study. Comparison of implantable loop recorder versus conventional diagnostic strategy. J Am Coll Cardiol. 2007;49:1951-6.
32. Brignole M. Indications and utility of external loop recorders. e-Journal Cardiol Pract. 2008;75.
33. Huikuri HV, Raatikainen MJP, Moerch-Joergensen R, et al. Prediction of fatal or near fatal cardiac arrhythmia events in patients with depressed left ventricular function after an acute myocardial infarction. Results of the Cardiac Arrhythmias and Risk Stratification after Acute Myocardial Infarction (CARISMA) Study. Eur Heart J. 2009;30(6):689-98.
34. Sacher F, Probst V, Iesaka Y, et al. Outcome after implantation of a cardioverter-defibrillator in patients with Brugada syndrome: A multicenter study. Circulation. 2006;114:2317-24.

CHAPTER 103

Sudden Death in Dilated Cardiomyopathy—What is New in 2018?

Kamal K Sethi, Ashish K Govil

INTRODUCTION

Sudden cardiac death (SCD) is one of the leading causes of morality in dilated cardiomyopathy (DCM) apart from terminal pump failure. Defined as natural death heralded by abrupt loss of consciousness within 1 hour of the onset of an acute change in cardiovascular status, its key elements are natural, rapid, and an unexpected event.[1] The risk of SCD is most pronounced in patients with heart failure (HF); 1-year absolute risk between 4 and 13%.[2]

The term DCM refers to a spectrum of heterogeneous myocardial disorders that are characterized by ventricular dilation and depressed myocardial performance in the absence of hypertension, valvular, congenital, or ischemic heart disease.[3] The term nonischemic cardiomyopathy (NICM) has been interchangeably used with DCM. Although this approach might be practical, it fails to recognize that NICM can include cardiomyopathies caused by volume or pressure overload (such as hypertension or valvular heart disease) that are not conventionally accepted under the definition of DCM.[4]

In general, ventricular tachyarrhythmias (VTs), including ventricular fibrillation and pulseless ventricular tachycardia, are the most common electrophysiological mechanisms leading to SCD.[5,6] Other physiological events that can result in SCD include pulseless electric activity, bradyarrhythmias, and asystole.[7] The risk of SCD has almost halved over the past two decades among patients with symptomatic heart failure and reduced ejection fraction (HFrEF).[8] The primary contribution in this paradigm shift is of the sequential introduction of medications including angiotensin-converting enzyme inhibitors (ACEIs), angiotensin receptor blockers (ARBs), β-blockers, mineralocorticoid receptor antagonists (MRAs) and the latest, angiotensin receptor-neprilysin inhibitor (ARNI).[9]

Implantable cardioverter defibrillators (ICDs) play an important role in reducing arrhythmogenic events and have a clear indication in secondary prevention of SCD. However, their benefit in primary prevention in DCM has become a matter of debate in the era of improved medical treatment and application of cardiac resynchronization therapy (CRT).[10]

PATHOPHYSIOLOGY OF DILATED CARDIOMYOPATHY

The dilatation of left ventricle (LV) is a result of the maladaptive changes in surviving myocytes and extracellular matrix which leads to pathological remodeling and impaired contractility. This activates the sympathetic and renin-angiotensin-aldosterone system which in turn produces syndrome of HF and myocardial electrical instability, the substrate for ventricular arrhythmias.[11,12]

ROLE OF DRUG THERAPY IN SUDDEN CARDIAC DEATH

Pharmacological treatment is the backbone for prevention of disease progression in DCM. Drugs which modify the underlying substrate for LV remodeling not only prevent progression to terminal HF but also reduce the arrhythmic burden (Figs. 1 to 4).

Beta-blockers

Beta-blockers reduce myocardial oxygen demand and electrical excitability. Their antiarrhythmic efficacy is related to adrenergic blockade on sympathetically mediated triggering mechanisms, slowing of the sinus rate and inhibition of excess calcium release by the ryanodine receptors. Beta-blockers reduce the risk of SCD by 31%, cardiovascular disease (CVD) by 29%, and all-cause mortality by 33%.[13]

Three β-blockers (i.e., bisoprolol, carvedilol, sustained-release metoprolol succinate) have been proven to reduce mortality in patients with current or prior symptoms of HFrEF, with almost similar reductions in SCD. There is some evidence for greater benefit of vasodilating β-blockers compared with the nonvasodilating agents in patients with NICM.[14]

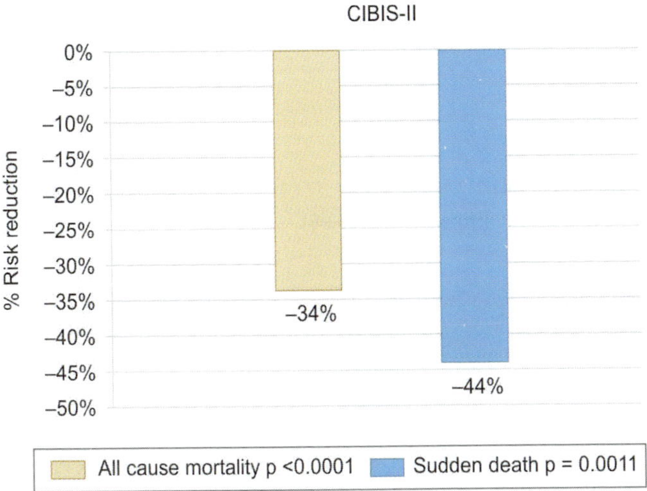

CIBIS-II, Cardiac Insufficiency Bisoprolol Study II.

FIG. 1: CIBIS-II.

Source: The Cardiac Insufficiency Bisoprolol Study II (CIBIS-II): a randomised trial. Lancet. 1999 Jan 2;353(9146):9-13.

MERIT-HF

Mortality	Number of deaths	Metoprolol CR/XL better	Risk reduction (%)
Total mortality	362		34
Cardiovascular mortality	331		38
Sudden death	211		41
Death from worsening heart failure	88		49

0 0.5 1.0 1.5
Relative risk (95% CI)

CR, controlled release; HF, heart failure; XL, extended release ; CI, confidence interval; MERIT-HF, Metoprolol CR/XL Randomised Intervention Trial in Congestive Heart Failure.

FIG. 2: MERIT heart failure.

Source: Effect of metoprolol controlled release/extended release (CR/XL) in chronic heart failure: Metoprolol CR/XL Randomised Intervention Trial in Congestive Heart Failure (MERIT-HF)Lancet. 1999 Jun 12;353(9169):2001-7.

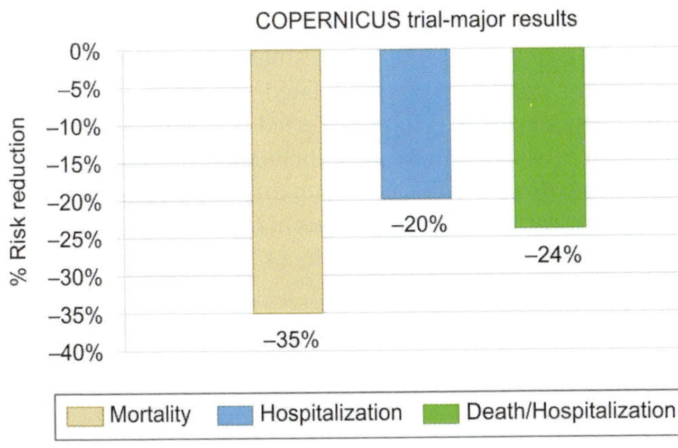

FIG. 3: Major results of copernicus trial.

Source: Eichhorn EJ, Bristow MR. The Carvedilol Prospective Randomized Cumulative Survival (COPERNICUS) trial. Current Controlled Trials in Cardiovascular Medicine. 2001;2(1):20-3.

Mineralocorticoid Receptor Antagonists

The therapeutic effect of SCD prevention with MRAs are derived from a variety of mechanisms. MRAs limit potassium and magnesium loss and decrease myocardial fibrosis and hypertrophy. They also decrease stimulation of central adrenergic system, reduce the release of norepinephrine from sympathetic nerve terminals through enhanced parasympathetic activity and increase myocardial uptake of norepinephrine.[15] Therapies with the MRAs, spironolactone, and eplerenone, have demonstrated reductions in both all-cause mortality and SCD.[16]

Angiotensin-converting Enzyme Inhibitors and Angiotensin Receptor Blockers

Local renin–angiotensin system (RAS) expression contributes substantially to myocardial structural changes that favor cardiac arrhythmias.[17] ACEI have been postulated to reduce SCD by their sympatholytic activity and reduction in angiotensin II which is a facilitator of adrenergic transmission.[18] Similarly, ARBs are indicated in patients who require RAS inhibition but are intolerant to ACEI. Both the drugs conserve potassium which is also involved in suppression of VAs.

Angiotensin Receptor-Neprilysin Inhibitor

The newest drug in the armamentarium for the management of HF has proved superior to enalapril in reducing the risks of death and of hospitalization for HF.[19] The benefit was observed in both SCDs and deaths from worsening HF, which accounted for the majority of cardiovascular deaths.[20]

ROLE OF IMPLANTABLE CARDIOVERTER DEFIBRILLATOR

The evidence supporting prophylactic ICD implantation in patients with nonischemic DCM has been inconclusive from the very beginning. The initial trials which compared ICD to either medical therapy or amiodarone showed no significant benefit in primary end point of all-cause mortality.

In the Cardiomyopathy Trial (CAT), 104 patients having recent onset DCM with an ejection fraction of less than or equal to 30% were randomly assigned to an ICD or control. With a mean follow up of 5.5 + 2.2 years there was no significant difference in cumulative survival between control and ICD groups at 2 and 4 years, respectively. However, in this trial there were no sudden deaths in either group during the initial 2 years and only 4% of the population received β-blockers. This trial was limited by small number of patients and overall low observed mortality rates.[21]

The amiodarone versus implantable cardioverter-defibrillator randomized trial in patients with nonischemic DCM and asymptomatic nonsustained ventricular tachycardia (AMIOVIRT) randomized 103 patients with DCM, left ventricular ejection fraction (LVEF) of less than or equal to 35% and NSVT to either amiodarone or ICD. There was no significant difference in the primary end point of

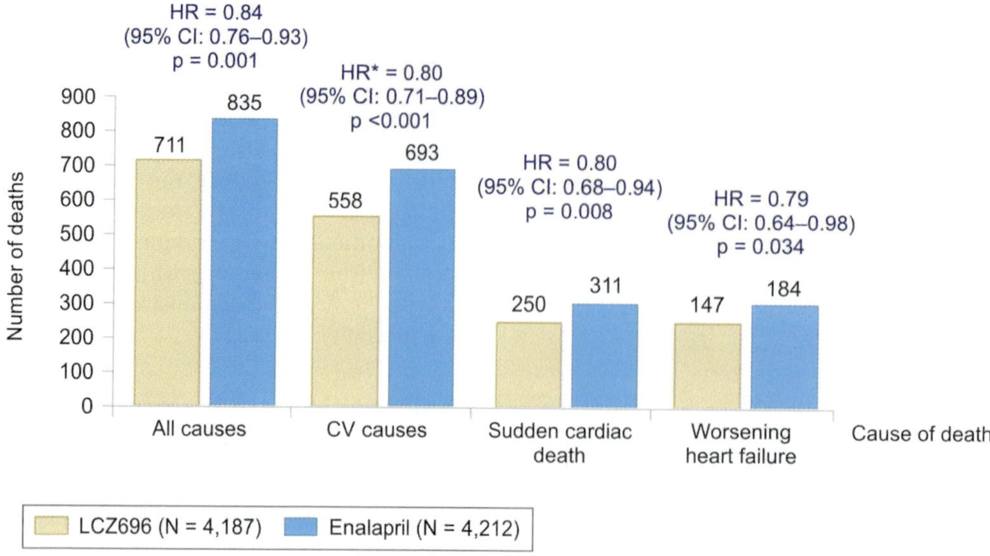

CI, confidence interval; CV, cardiovascular; HR, hazard ratio.

FIG. 4: Modes of death in Paradigm-heart failure: The Mortality benefit of LCZ696 is related to the observed reduction in sudden cardiac death and death due to worsening heart failure.

Source: Desai AS, McMurray JJ, Packer M, et al. Effect of the angiotensin-receptor-neprilysin inhibitor LCZ696 compared with enalapril on mode of death in heart failure patients. Eur Heart J. 2015;36:1990-7.

3-year survival rate which was approximately 89% in both the groups. However, there was a trend towards improved arrhythmia-free survival and up-to 60% cost savings with amiodarone therapy. Again, the trial was limited by a small sample size and absence of control group.[22]

The third trial in succession was DEFINITE which randomized 458 patients with nonischemic DCM, a LVEF of less than or equal to 36%, and PVCs or nonsustained ventricular tachycardia (NSVT) to receive either standard medical therapy or standard medical therapy plus a single chamber ICD. In this trial therapy with an ICD significantly reduced the risk of sudden death from arrhythmia (hazard ratio, 0.20; p = 0.006) and a nonsignificant trend towards reduction in all-cause mortality. Patients in New York Heart Association (NYHA) class III derived the largest survival benefit from ICD therapy. This was the first trial which laid the foundation of role of ICD in primary prevention of SCD.[23]

The sudden cardiac death in heart failure trial (SCD-HeFT) which randomized 2,521 patients with congestive heart failure (CHF) (both ischemic and nonischemic etiologies) and LVEF of 35% or less to therapy with shock only ICD, amiodarone, or placebo. ICD therapy had a significant benefit in patients in NYHA class II with an overall reduction in mortality by 23% but not in those in NYHA class III CHF. In the subgroup of patients with NICM the hazard ratio for all-cause death was 0.73 with a 95% confidence interval (CI) between 0.50 and 1.04.[24]

Pooling these and three other secondary prevention trials, a meta-analysis by Desai et al. found an overall 31% mortality reduction with ICD in patients having nonischemic DCM.[25] The present American College of Cardiology/American Heart Association (ACC/AHA) guidelines for primary prevention of SCD in nonischemic DCM is largely based on the data from these trials and meta-analysis,[1] and recommend ICDs as a class I A indication for prevention of SCD in DCM.

However, with the trials in present era of CRTs and improved medical therapy, more controversy has erupted than a sound consensus. The Danish study to Assess the Efficacy of ICDs in Patients with Nonischemic Systolic Heart Failure on Mortality (DANISH) randomized 1,116 patients without ischemic heart disease having NYHA class II or III HF symptoms or NYHA class IV symptoms if CRT planned, LVEF of less than or equal to 35%, and an increased N-terminal pro B-type natriuretic peptide (NT-proBNP) despite guideline-directed medical therapy to an ICD or medical therapy alone. There was a significant reduction in secondary outcome of SCD but a neutral effect on primary outcome of all-cause mortality over a median follow up of 5.6 years with the use of an ICD. Younger patients fared much better with an ICD than those over 70 years.[26] The reasons behind nonachievement of primary endpoints as speculated are primarily due to overall low risk of SCD in the selected population attributed to robust medical management including full throttle use of β-blockers, ACEI or ARBs and in up to two-thirds, addition of MRA. However, 58% of the patients in both the arms received CRT, thus confounding the results as it was not a pure ICD trial.

As the results were directly in confrontation with the recommended American and European guidelines, more meta-analyses including or excluding DANISH trial have been done in an attempt to resolve the dilemma.

A meta-analysis done by Barakat A et al.[27] which included five multicenter randomized controlled trials (RCTs) with 2,573 patients found that ICD therapy for primary prevention

Study	Years	HR (95% CI)	Weight %
CAT	2002	0.83 (0.45, 1.82)	4.72
AMIOVIRT	2003	0.87 (0.31, 2.42)	1.99
DEFINITE	2004	0.65 (0.40, 1.06)	20.32
SCD-HeFT	2005	0.73 (0.50, 1.07)	27.25
DANISH	2016	0.87 (0.68, 1.12)	45.73
Overall (I-squared = 0.0%, p = 0.844)		0.79 (0.64, 0.93)	100.00

Note: Weights are from random effects analysis

0.1 1 5

ICD is associated with lower all-cause mortality ICD is associated with higher all-cause mortality

AMIOVIRT, Amiodarone Versus Implantable Defibrillator Trial; CAT, Cardiomyopathy Trial; DANISH, Danish Study to Assess the Efficacy of ICDs in Patients with Non-ischaemic Systolic Heart Failure on Mortality; DEFINITE, Defibrillators in non-ischemic cardiomyopathy treatment evaluation; ICD, implantable cardioverter defibrillator; SCD-HeFT: Sudden Cardiac Death in Heart Failure Trial.

FIG. 5: Summary forest plot of all-cause mortality. The relative size of the data markers indicates the weight of the sample size from each study.

Source: Adapted from Barakat AF, Saad M, Elgendy AY, et al. Primary prevention implantable cardioverter defibrillator in patients with non-ischaemic cardiomyopathy: a meta-analysis of randomised controlled trials. BMJ Open. 2017;7:e016352.[27]

in patients with nonischemic DCM was associated with 21% relative risk reduction and 3% absolute risk reduction in all-cause mortality (number needed to treat = 33) compared with medical therapy alone, at a mean follow-up of approximately 4 years. The benefit was seen across a wide spectrum of nonischemic DCM patients, with diverse demographics and clinical presentations. There was a suggestion of possible effect modification by age, with more benefit in patients less than 60 years (Fig. 5).[28]

The COMPANION trial was excluded from this meta-analysis due to unbalanced use of CRT between the intervention and control arms. Pooled data from another meta-analysis done by Al-Khatib et al. which included four RCTs of nonischemic DCM with 1,874 unique patients equally divided into ICD and control group, showed a significant reduction in all-cause mortality with an ICD (hazard ratio, 0.75; 95% CI, 0.61–0.93; p = 0.008; p = 0.87 for heterogeneity).

The strength of this meta-analysis was a more robust approach to reduce heterogeneity by excluding trials of CRT and anti-arrhythmic medications. However, actual mortality rates were available for only DEFINITE and SCD-HeFT trials due to nonavailability of patient level data from the CAT and DANISH trials which was a major limitation here.

An updated meta-analysis by Golwalla H et al. enrolled 2,970 patients from six RCTs (including those with CRT defibrillator) to study the efficacy of ICD in primary prevention. Pooled analysis demonstrated a statistically significant 23% reduction in all-cause mortality in favor of ICD therapy (hazard ratio, 0.77; 95% CI, 0.64–0.91).[29]

Even on doing a separate analysis by excluding trials of CRTs there was still a 24% reduction in all-cause mortality. Also, despite the individual subgroup analysis of COMPANION and DANISH trials demonstrating no incremental benefit of ICD in patients with CRT, when combined, it was found that ICDs may still reduce all-cause mortality in patients who are also candidates for CRT therapy, although the results did not meet statistical significance.

RISK STRATIFICATION

In the absence of better markers, LVEF continues to be used as a key criterion to select patients for primary prevention ICDs. However, LVEF has a low sensitivity and specificity for SCD prediction[30] as reflected by delivery of appropriate therapies from device follow up which are seen in only about 20% of patients with DCM who have ICDs for primary prevention.[23]

Registry data suggest that some of patients with DCM and an out-of-hospital cardiac arrest do not have a markedly reduced LVEF. In addition, many patients with reduced LVEF die of nonsudden causes of death.[31]

There are various risk stratification models which try to predict chances of SCD but none have been proven useful. There is a clear need to improve this prediction (Table 1).

Cardiac Magnetic Resonance Imaging

Late Gadolinium Enhancement as a Marker of Increased Risk

Ventricular fibrosis identified by cardiac magnetic resonance (CMR) with late gadolinium enhancement (LGE) has emerged as a promising tool for targeted stratification of SCD in nonischemic DCM. Patients with DCM have characteristic mid-wall fibrosis which can be detected by LGE-CMR[32] and have been associated with adverse cardiac events such as HF hospitalizations, appropriate ICD therapy, and SCD as well as all-cause mortality.[33-35]

In a recent systemic review and meta-analysis of the association between LGE-based myocardial scar and the

TABLE 1: Traditional and novel risk markers

Traditional risk markers	Novel risk markers
Left ventricular ejection fraction	Cardiac magnetic resonance imaging
NYHA class	PET
QRS duration, QT interval, and dispersion	SPECT
Cardiac autonomic modulation (BRS, HRT, HRV)	Left ventricular sphericity index
Microscopic T-wave alternans	Gene susceptibility
Signal averaged ECG	Serum protein biomarkers
EPS and Holter studies	–

BRS, baroreflex sensitivity; ECG, electrocardiogram; HRT, heart rate turbulence; HRV, heart rate variability; PET, positron-emission tomography; EPS, Electrophysiology Study; SPECT, single-photon emission computed tomography.

risk for VT in patients with DCM, it was found that LGE is a strong independent predictor of arrhythmic events and could improve risk stratification for SCD and appropriateness of ICD therapy. A total of 2,948 patients from 29 studies were included in this meta-analysis who were followed for an average of 3 years. LGE was found to be present in 44% of patients. The arrhythmic endpoint was defined as sustained ventricular arrhythmias, appropriate ICD intervention, or SCD. In this meta-analysis, LGE had the strongest association with the arrhythmic outcome (odds ratio: 7.8) in patients who were implanted ICDs for primary prevention. Patients with LGE had a relatively high annual event rate (17.2% per year) as compared to those without LGE (2.1% per year).[36]

However, in one study, myocardial scar assessed by LGE-CMR predicted only monomorphic VT, but not polymorphic VT/ventricular fibrillation (VF) in patients with nonischemic DCM, who remain at risk for potentially fatal polymorphic VT/VF.[37] Also, due to marked variability in methodology and interpretation of LGE, there is a need for standardization of qualitative and quantitative criteria to reinforce its role in decision making in patients with DCM.

CONCLUSION

While data on secondary prevention of SCD in DCM are robust, those in primary prevention are relatively handicapped by small number of patients in almost all studies making them unable to reach statistical significance in individual trials. The majority of meta-analysis, however, including those with or without CRT, show a reduction of mortality by ICDs in primary prevention. The current ACC/AHA/HRS (the Heart Rhythm Society) guidelines for prevention of SCD have retained ICDs as a class I indication in nonischemic DCM in primary prevention. Till we see a large RCT on primary prevention in nonischemic DCM proving otherwise, ICDs shall continue to be prescribed in patients with nonischemic DCM. In the absence of definite risk predictors, LVEF shall remain as the only deciding criterion for selection of patients for ICD. CMR imaging appears promising but only observational data is available in a relatively small number of patients. Clearly, there is a need for further research in this area.

REFERENCES

1. Al-Khatib SM, Stevenson WG, Ackerman MJ, et al. 2017 AHA/ACC/HRS Guideline for Management of Patients with Ventricular Arrhythmias and the Prevention of Sudden Cardiac Death, Heart Rhythm. 2017.
2. Piccini JP, Berger JS, O'Connor CM. Amiodarone for the prevention of sudden cardiac death: a meta-analysis of randomized controlled trials. Eur Heart J. 2009;30:1245-53.
3. Bozkurt B, Colvin M, Cook J, et al. Current diagnostic and treatment strategies for specific dilated cardiomyopathies: a scientific statement from the American Heart Association. Circulation. 2016;134:e579-646.
4. Richardson P, McKenna W, Bristow M, et al. Circulation. 1996; 93(5):841-842. Report of the 1995 World Health Organization/International Society and Federation of Cardiology Task Force on the Definition and Classification of cardiomyopathies. Circulation. 1996;93:841-2.
5. Bayes de Luna A, Coumel P, Leclercq JF. Ambulatory sudden cardiac death: mechanisms of production of fatal arrhythmia on the basis of data from 157 cases. Am Heart J. 1989;117(1):151-9.
6. Wood MA, Stambler BS, Damiano RJ, et al. Lessons learned from data logging in a multicenter clinical trial using a late-generation implantable cardioverter-defibrillator. The Guardian ATP 4210 Multicenter Investigators Group. J Am Coll Cardiol. 1994;24(7):1692-9.
7. Nichol G, Thomas E, Callaway CW, et al. Resuscitation Outcomes Consortium Investigators, Regional variation in out-of-hospital cardiac arrest incidence and outcome. JAMA. 2008;300:1423-31.
8. Shen L, Jhund PS, Petrie MC, et al. Declining Risk of Sudden Death in Heart Failure. N Engl J Med. 2017; 377(1): 41-51.
9. Desai AS, McMurray JJ, Packer M, et al. Effect of the angiotensin-receptor-neprilysin inhibitor LCZ696 compared with enalapril on mode of death in heart failure patients. Eur Heart J. 2015;36:1990-7.
10. Køber L, Thune JJ, Nielsen JC, et al. Defibrillator implantation in patients with nonischemic systolic heart failure. N Engl J Med. 2016;375:1221-30.
11. Francis GS, Goldsmith SR, Levine TB, et al. The neurohumoral axis in congestive heart failure. Ann Intern Med. 1984;101:370-7.
12. McMurray JJ. Clinical practice. Systolic heart failure. N Engl J Med. 2010;362(3): 228-38.
13. Al-Gobari M, Khatib CE, Pillon F, et al. Beta-blockers for the prevention of sudden cardiac death in heart failure patients: a meta-analysis of randomized controlled trials. BMC Cardiovascular Disorders. 2013;13:52.
14. Bonet S, Agustí A, Arnau JM, et al. Beta-adrenergic blocking agents in heart failure: Benefits of vasodilating and non-vasodilating agents according to patients' characteristics: a meta-analysis of clinical trials. Arch Intern Med. 2000;160:621-7.
15. Al Chekakie MO. Traditional heart failure medications and sudden cardiac death prevention: a review. J Cardiovasc Pharmacol Ther. 2013;18:412-26.
16. Bapoje SR, Bahia A, Hokanson JE, et al. Effects of mineralocorticoid receptor antagonists on the risk of sudden cardiac death in patients with left ventricular systolic dysfunction: A meta-analysis of randomized controlled trials. Circulation Heart Failure. 2013;6(2):166-73.
17. Iravanian S, Dudley SC Jr. The renin-angiotensin-aldosterone system (RAAS) and cardiac arrhythmias. Heart Rhythm. 2008; 5(6 Suppl):S12-7.
18. Grassi G, Cattaneo BM, Seravalle G, et al. Effects of chronic ACE inhibition on sympathetic nerve traffic and baroreflex control of circulation in heart failure. Circulation. 1997; 96:1173-9.
19. McMurray JJ, Packer M, Desai AS, et al. Angiotensin-neprilysin inhibition versus enalapril in heart failure. N Engl J Med. 2014;371(11): 993-1004.
20. Desai AS, McMurray JJ, Packer M, et al. Effect of the angiotensin-receptor-neprilysin inhibitor LCZ696 compared with enalapril on mode of death in heart failure patients. Eur Heart J. 2015;36(30):1990-7.
21. Bänsch D, Antz M, Boczor S, et al. Primary prevention of sudden cardiac death in idiopathic dilated cardiomyopathy: The cardiomyopathy trial (CAT). Circulation. 2002;105(12):1453-58.

22. Strickberger SA, Hummel JD, Bartlett TG, et al. Amiodarone Versus Implantable Cardioverter-Defibrillator: Randomized Trial in Patients With Nonischemic Dilated Cardiomyopathy and Asymptomatic Nonsustained Ventricular Tachycardia (AMIOVIRT). J Am Coll Cardiol. 2003;41:1707-12.
23. Kadish A, Dyer A, Daubert JP, et al. Prophylactic Defibrillator Implantation in Patients with Non-ischemic Dilated Cardiomyopathy: Defibrillators in Non-Ischemic Cardiomyopathy Treatment Evaluation (DEFINITE). N Engl J Med. 2004;350:2151-8.
24. Bardy GH, Lee KL, Mark DB, et al. Amiodarone or an implantable cardioverter–defibrillator for congestive heart failure. Sudden cardiac death in heart failure trial (SCD-HeFT). N Engl J Med. 2005;352:225-37.
25. Desai AS, Fang JC, Maisel WH, et al. Implantable defibrillators for the prevention of mortality in patients with nonischemic cardiomyopathy: a meta-analysis of randomized controlled trials. JAMA. 2004; 292(23): 2874-9.
26. Køber L, Thune JJ, Nielsen JC, et al. Defibrillator Implantation in Patients with Non-ischemic Systolic Heart Failure (DANISH). N Engl J Med. 2016;375(13):1221-30.
27. Barakat AF, Saad M, Elgendy AY, et al. Primary prevention implantable cardioverter defibrillator in patients with non-ischaemic cardiomyopathy: a meta-analysis of randomised controlled trials. BMJ Open. 2017;7:e016352.
28. Al-Khatib SM, Fonarow GC, Joglar JA, et al. Primary prevention implantable cardioverter defibrillators in patients with nonischemic cardiomyopathy: A Meta-analysis. JAMA Cardiol. 2017;2(6):685-8.
29. Golwala H, Bajaj NS, Arora G, et al. Implantable Cardioverter-Defibrillator for Non-ischemic Cardiomyopathy: An Updated Meta-Analysis. Circulation. 2017;135:201-3.
30. Buxton AE, Ellison KE, Lorvidhaya P, et al. Left ventricular ejection fraction for sudden death risk stratification and guiding implantable cardioverter-defibrillators implantation. J Cardiovasc Pharmacol2010;55:450-5.
31. Halliday BP, Cleland JGF, Goldberger JJ, et al. Personalizing Sudden Death Risk Stratification in Dilated Cardiomyopathy: Past, Present and Future. Circulation. 2017;136(2):215-31.
32. Iles LM, Ellims AH, Llewellyn H, et al. Histological validation of cardiac magnetic resonance analysis of regional and diffuse interstitial myocardial fibrosis. Eur Heart J Cardiovasc Imaging. 2015;16:14-22.
33. Wu KC, Weiss RG, Thiemann DR, et al. Late gadolinium enhancement by cardiovascular magnetic resonance heralds an adverse prognosis in nonischemic cardiomyopathy. J Am Coll Cardiol. 2008;51:2414-21.
34. Gulati A, Jabbour A, Ismail TF, et al. Association of fibrosis with mortality and sudden cardiac death in patients with non-ischemic dilated cardiomyopathy. JAMA. 2013;309:896-908.
35. Iles L, Pfluger H, Lefkovits L, et al. Myocardial fibrosis predicts appropriate device therapy in patients with implantable cardioverter-defibrillators for primary prevention of sudden cardiac death. J Am Coll Cardiol. 2011;57:821-8.
36. Di Marco A, Anguera I, Schmitt M, et al. Late gadolinium enhancement and the risk for ventricular arrhythmias or sudden death in dilated cardiomyopathy: systematic review and meta-analysis. J Am Coll Cardiol HF. 2017;5:28-38.
37. Piers SR, Everaerts K, van der Geest RJ, et al. Myocardial scar predicts monomorphic ventricular tachycardia but not polymorphic ventricular tachycardia or ventricular fibrillation in non-ischemic dilated cardiomyopathy. Heart Rhythm. 2015;12:2106-14.

CHAPTER 104

Orthostatic Hypotension

Siddharthan Deepti, Kewal C Goswami

INTRODUCTION

Orthostatic hypotension results from a sustained reduction in blood pressure (BP) upon standing and may present as a disabling condition. Most commonly seen in the elderly, orthostatic hypotension may cause postural instability, syncope, and falls and is associated with an increased risk of stroke, myocardial ischemia, and mortality.

DEFINITION

Orthostatic hypotension is a clinical sign defined as a sustained decrease in systolic BP of at least 20 mm Hg or diastolic BP of at least 10 mm Hg or both within 3 minutes of standing or head-up tilt to at least 60° on a tilt table.[1] A reduction in systolic BP of 30 mm Hg may be a considered a better criterion in patients with supine hypertension, because the extent of the postural fall in BP is dependent on the baseline BP. Orthostatic hypotension is a clinical sign by definition and therefore, may be symptomatic or not.

EPIDEMIOLOGY

The prevalence of orthostatic hypotension is variable in different epidemiological studies, depending on the definitions used, the population studied (age range, institutions) and the composition of the population (unselected healthy population versus select groups). Overall, in a population of unselected middle-aged subjects (>40 years), the cross-sectional prevalence is estimated to be approximately 5–6%.[2,3] There is a gradual increase in the prevalence with age ranging from 10 to 30% in older subjects,[4] with orthostatic hypotension affecting more than two-fifths of the population aged older than or equal to 80 years, more commonly in the institutionalized elderly.[5] Its prevalence is increased in certain neurological disorders and with use of certain drugs.

Orthostatic hypotension may cause postural instability, syncope, and falls. It is a negative prognostic factor, which has been shown in longitudinal studies to be associated with an increased risk of stroke, myocardial ischemia, and mortality.[6,7]

PHYSIOLOGY OF THE NORMAL ORTHOSTATIC RESPONSE

Assumption of the upright posture from supine or sitting positions leads to a series of changes. Due to the effect of gravity, there is pooling of 500–700 mL of blood from the upper body to the venous capacitance vessels of the lower limbs and splanchnic circulation within a few seconds of standing. Additionally, there is a shift of approximately 10% of the intravascular plasma toward the interstitial compartment due to increased hydrostatic pressure within 10–30 minutes of upright posture. The resultant decrease in venous return leads to a fall in right ventricular filling pressure, and ultimately cardiac output by approximately 20%. The ensuing reduction in BP would compromise perfusion of organs above heart level if not for the compensatory mechanisms that have evolved to counteract the gravitational stress, and thus allow humans to maintain an erect posture for prolonged periods of time. The compensatory mechanisms include the following.

Baroreflex

The autonomic nervous system is the main physiological system involved in maintenance of homeostasis upon assuming the upright posture. The reflex is primarily mediated via baroreceptors which are stretch-dependent mechanoreceptors located within the wall of vessels, that detect small variations in arterial pressure or central blood volume, through deformations of the vessel wall. There are two types of baroreceptor each having separate roles. Arterial or high-pressure baroreceptors are located in the carotid sinuses, the aortic arch and the origin of the right subclavian artery. They are the most significant players in the acute adaptation to the upright posture.

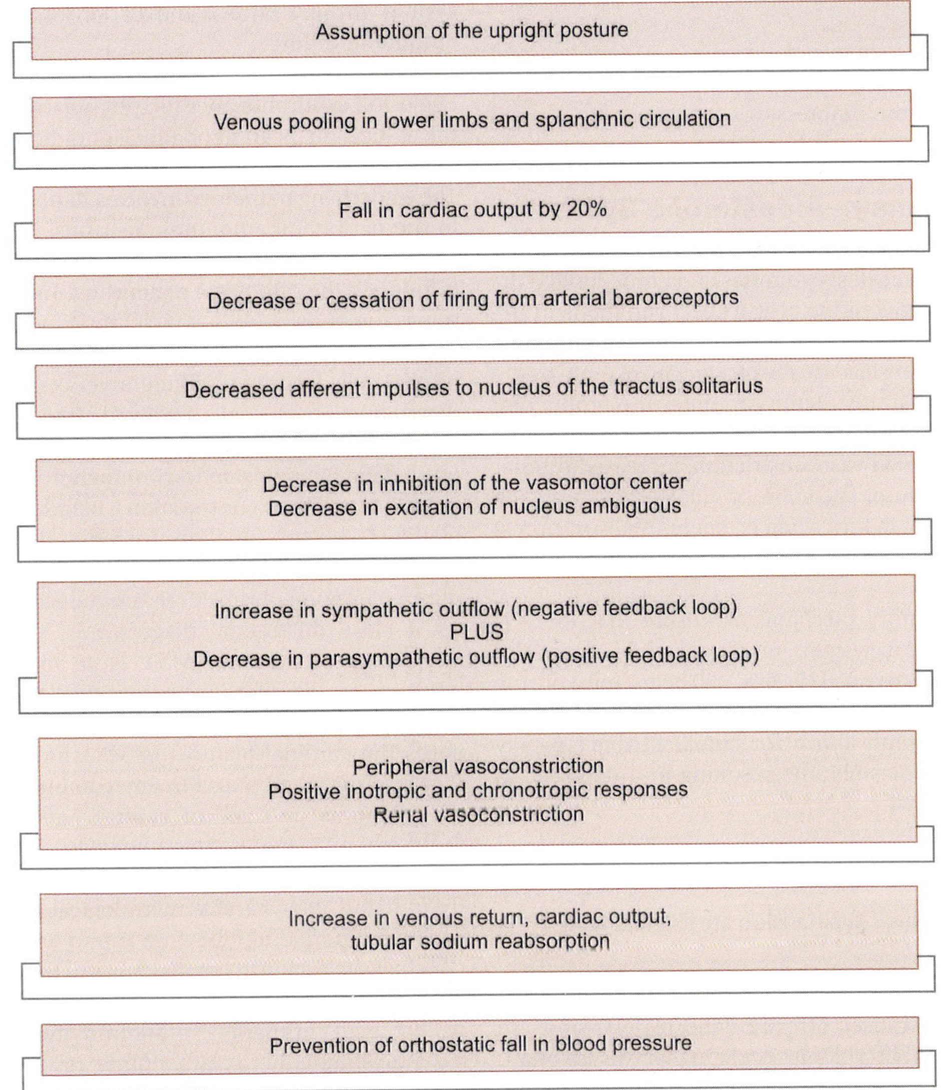

FLOWCHART 1: Baroreceptor reflex.

Cardiopulmonary or low-pressure baroreceptors are located in major cardiopulmonary vessels. They respond to changes in central blood volume and are involved in the control of renal sympathetic nerves.

Afferent impulses travel via the glossopharyngeal (IX) and vagus (X) nerves from carotid and aortic baroreceptors, respectively, and via nonmyelinated vagal nerve fibers from low-pressure baroreceptors to the nucleus of the tractus solitarius (NTS). The NTS sends inhibitory fibers to the vasomotor center in the caudal ventrolateral medulla and the rostral ventrolateral medulla, which controls sympathetic output to the arteries, veins, and heart through the intermediolateral column of the thoracic spinal cord. Additionally, the NTS sends excitatory fibers to the nucleus ambiguous, which controls parasympathetic output to the sinoatrial node of the heart.

Distension of a vessel with rise in BP leads to the activation of baroreceptors that generate action potentials increasing in frequency in correlation to the amount of stretch. The frequency of these potentials is taken as a surrogate measure of BP at the level of the NTS, with higher frequency correlating with higher BP. The high-pressure baroreceptors remain tonically active at a mean arterial pressure above 70 mm Hg, which is termed the baroreceptor set point. At a mean arterial pressure below this set point, the receptors become essentially silent.

A fall in BP upon standing leads to decrease or cessation of firing from the arterial baroreceptors, causing an increase in sympathetic outflow (negative feedback loop) and a decrease in parasympathetic outflow (positive feedback loop). These changes lead to peripheral vasoconstriction, positive inotropic and chronotropic responses, and renal vasoconstriction. All these homeostatic mechanisms in turn increase venous return, cardiac output, and tubular sodium reabsorption, thereby preventing orthostatic fall in BP. The baroreceptor reflex has been summarized in flowchart 1.

Muscle Pump

Muscle contractions involved in the assumption and maintenance of upright posture contribute to prevention of orthostatic fall in BP by compressing capacitance vessels and by increasing peripheral vascular resistance.

Renin–Angiotensin–Aldosterone System

The renin-angiotensin-aldosterone system enables long-term orthostatic homeostasis (minutes and hours) unlike the baroreflexes which govern the beat-to-beat variations in BP. The transient fall in glomerular afferent arteriole perfusion pressure upon standing leads to the production of renin by the juxtaglomerular apparatus. Renin promotes the production of angiotensin II via angiotensin converting enzyme. Angiotensin II results in vasoconstriction, increased tubular reabsorption of sodium, secretion of aldosterone from the adrenal cortex, which in turn again promotes reabsorption of water and sodium and finally, increase in central sympathetic outflow.

These compensatory mechanisms ensure that there is only a small decrease in systolic and diastolic BP (~5 mm Hg) and an increase in heart rate (15–30%, <30 beats/min) during the first 10 seconds after standing, followed by a return to baseline value (or slightly above) for systolic BP and typically a small increase in diastolic BP, resulting in a decrease in pulse pressure (5–10%).

ETIOLOGY

The causes of orthostatic hypotension are listed in table 1.

Drugs

The most common causes of orthostatic hypotension are drugs that cause either volume depletion or vasodilation. The most intuitive culprits are the antihypertensive drugs. But not all antihypertensive drugs cause orthostatic fall in BP to the same extent. The most notorious are the α-adrenergic blocking drugs, β-adrenergic blocking drugs, diuretics including spironolactone, centrally acting hypotensive drugs and peripheral vasodilators. The angiotensin-converting enzyme inhibitors, angiotensin receptor blockers, and calcium channel blockers are found to be less associated with orthostatic hypotension.

Apart from antihypertensive drugs, other classes including antidepressants, antipsychotic drugs, sedatives, pulmonary vasodilators, and dopamine agonists are associated with orthostatic hypotension.

Neurogenic Causes

Orthostatic hypotension may also be caused by autonomic nervous system dysfunction which may be primary or secondary.

Primary Autonomic Failure

Primary causes of autonomic dysfunction are usually idiopathic and include pure autonomic failure (PAF), multiple system atrophy (MSA), and Parkinson's disease (PD) with autonomic failure.

Pure autonomic failure, also known as Bradbury-Eggleston syndrome after the physicians who first described this condition, is an idiopathic sporadic disorder with onset in the fifth or sixth decades and a slowly progressive course. The underlying pathology involves deposition of α-synuclein in the peripheral autonomic neurons. Alpha-synuclein is a small, highly conserved and natively unfolded protein which is found in the cytoplasm of neurons. The exact physiological role is not known. In α-synucleinopathies, there is abnormal deposition of fibrillar α-synuclein in cytoplasm of neurons or glial cells leading to different yet overlapping syndromes depending on the cells involved. PAF is characterized by manifestations of widespread dysautonomia including orthostatic hypotension in conjunction with disturbances in bowel (diarrhea or constipation), bladder (urgency or atonic bladder), sexual function (erectile dysfunction), and/or thermoregulatory function (hypo or hyperhidrosis). Supine plasma norepinephrine levels are reduced.

A close differential diagnosis is MSA also known as Shy-Drager syndrome. MSA is a sporadic, progressive, adult-onset disorder occurring due to accumulation of α-synuclein in glial cells of basal ganglia, cortex, and spinal cord. The cardinal features of MSA include dysautonomia, Parkinsonism, and ataxia in any combination. The presence of symptoms or signs of central neurodegeneration and rapid eye movements, sleep behavior disorders favor MSA over PAF. Often, demonstration of an isolated autonomic dysfunction after careful neurological examination over a prolonged period of follow-up (up to 5 years) is required to conclusively establish the diagnosis of PAF.

A third cause of primary autonomic failure is a subset of PD with primarily autonomic dysfunction. Also, an α-synucleinopathy, dysautonomia results from deposition of α-synuclein in not only in brainstem nuclei, but also in peripheral autonomic neurons, unlike MSA. The parkinsonian form of MSA may be distinguished from PD with autonomic failure by good response of Parkinsonism to levodopa in PD, though this feature is not completely sensitive. An additional aspect of orthostatic hypotension in PD is the fact that most drugs used for treatment of Parkinsonism (levodopa, anticholinergic drugs, and monoamine oxidase inhibitors) can themselves cause orthostatic hypotension.

Secondary Neurogenic Causes

The secondary neurogenic causes of orthostatic hypotension are listed in table 1. The most important of these are discussed below:

- *Diabetes*: Orthostatic hypotension is more prevalent in diabetic patients than in age- and sex-matched control subjects and is associated with increasing age and chronic poor glycemic control. The prevalence of orthostatic hypotension in diabetes varies from 7–18% depending on the definitions used and populations sampled. This figure compares with the prevalence in unselected subjects above the age of 65 years. In diabetic patients, orthostatic

TABLE 1: Causes of orthostatic hypotension

	Drugs		
1.	Antihypertensive drugs	α-adrenergic blocking drugs	• Terazosin • Prazosin • Doxazosin
		β-adrenergic blocking drugs	• Acebutolol • Atenolol • Bisoprolol
		Diuretics	
		Adrenergic neuron blocking drugs	• Guanethidine
		Ganglion-blocking drugs	• Hexamethonium • Mecamylamine
		Centrally acting hypotensive drugs	• Methyldopa • Clonidine
		Peripheral vasodilators	• Hydralazine • Minoxidil
		Angiotensin-converting enzyme inhibitors	
		Angiotensin receptor blockers	
		Aldosterone antagonists	
		Calcium channel blockers	
	Antidepressants	Monoamine oxidase inhibitors	
	Antipsychotic drugs	Phenothiazines	
		Barbiturates	
	Miscellaneous	Phosphodiesterase 1 inhibitor	• Sildenafil
		Dopamine agonists	• Levodopa • Ropinirole • Bromocriptine
		Anticholinergics	• Oxybutynin • Ipratropium
2	Primary autonomic failure	Pure autonomic failure (Bradbury- Eggleston syndrome)	
		Multiple system atrophy (Shy–Drager syndrome)	
		Parkinson's disease with autonomic failure	
3	Secondary neurogenic causes	Aging	
		Alcoholism	
		General medical disorders	• Diabetes • Renal failure • Amyloid
		Metabolic disease	• Vitamin B12 deficiency • Porphyria • Fabry disease • Tangier disease
		Carcinomatosis autonomic neuropathy	
		Hereditary sensory neuropathies	
		Autoimmune disease	• Guillain–Barré syndrome • Lambert–Eaton syndrome • Systemic lupus erythematosus • Rheumatoid arthritis • Mixed connective-tissue disease

Continued.

Continued

	Drugs		
		Infections of the nervous system	• HIV infection • Chagas disease • Botulism • Syphilis
		Dopamine β-hydroxylase deficiency	
		Spinal cord lesions	
		Central brain lesions	• Multiple sclerosis • Wernicke encephalopathy • Vascular lesions or tumors involving the hypothalamus and midbrain
		Familial hyperbradykinism	

HIV, human immunodeficiency virus.

hypotension is usually associated with generalized polyneuropathy, with diabetes being the most common cause of autonomic dysfunction in developed countries.

- *Amyloidosis*: Mixed sensory and motor peripheral neuropathy and/or autonomic neuropathy account for 20% and 15% of cases of amyloid light-chain (AL) amyloidosis.[8] Nerve injury is attributed to direct compression by accumulation of fibrils in vasa nervorum walls. Autonomic dysfunction, including orthostatic hypotension, is frequently associated with polyneuropathy at an advanced stage and is associated with a poor prognosis.
- *Paraneoplastic autonomic neuropathies*: Dysautonomia leading to orthostatic hypotension may be the presenting feature of an underlying neoplasm. It is most often observed with neoplasms of the lung [more common with small-cell lung cancer (anti-Hu antibodies)] followed by cancers of gastrointestinal tract, prostate, breast, bladder, kidney, pancreas, testicle, and ovary.
- *Hereditary autonomic neuropathies*: Hereditary sensory and autonomic neuropathy (HSAN) type III (also called familial dysautonomia) is an autosomal recessive disorder seen primarily in Ashkenazi Jewish children. Orthostatic hypotension is associated with lack of sensitivity to pain and temperature stimuli, hyporeflexia, absence of tears (alacrima), and absence of lingual fungiform papillae.
- *Miscellaneous*: Other causes of peripheral autonomic dysfunction include infectious diseases like HIV/AIDS (human immunodeficiency virus/acquired immune deficiency syndrome) and Chagas disease, neurotoxic drugs like vincristine and azole antifungals, vitamin B12 deficiency and primary Sjögren's syndrome.

Non-neurogenic Causes

In the vast majority of cases, an obvious neurogenic cause is lacking. The main inciting factors in such cases include hypovolemia, either absolute (dehydration, diarrhea, bleeding, hemodialysis, adrenal insufficiency, and hypoaldosteronism) or relative, due to vasodilatation (alcohol, heat, carcinoid syndrome, and mastocytosis) or venous pooling (cirrhosis). Orthostatic hypotension is frequently seen in heart failure without involvement of the autonomic nervous system. Another important mechanism for non-neurogenic orthostatic hypotension is deconditioning, commonly seen in elderly hospitalized patients after prolonged bed rest.

CLINICAL PRESENTATION

Orthostatic hypotension, by definition, is a clinical sign and therefore, may be entirely asymptomatic. Symptoms will result if the postural reduction in BP is severe enough to cause cerebral hypoperfusion. Characteristic symptoms include dizziness, light-headedness, or even syncope in response to sudden postural changes. However, the symptoms may be nonspecific such as fatigue, altered mentation, generalized weakness, nausea, headache, pain in the neck and shoulders (the so-called "coat hanger pain", due to hypoperfusion of neck muscles), leg buckling, and low back pain. Retinal or occipital lobe ischemia may cause blurring of vision upon standing. Other less common forms of clinical presentation include orthostatic dyspnea (attributed to ventilation–perfusion mismatch due to inadequate perfusion of ventilated lung apices) or orthostatic angina (attributed to impaired myocardial perfusion even in patients with normal coronary arteries). These symptoms are aggravated by exercise, meals, in the mornings or in hot weather and are characteristically relieved with sitting or lying down.

ORTHOSTATIC TESTING AND VARIANTS OF ORTHOSTATIC HYPOTENSION

Testing for orthostatic hypotension should be done in a quiet room, at a temperature between 20 and 24°C after the patient has been resting for 5 minutes with an empty bladder. Orthostatic testing may be done either at the bedside or on a tilt table.

This mode of testing may miss two important variants of orthostatic hypotension listed below:

1. The first variant is initial orthostatic hypotension which is seen more commonly in young subjects. The orthostatic fall in BP occurs within 15 seconds of standing (more

than 40 mm Hg systolic or more than 20 mm Hg diastolic BP) and recovers quickly, though this might be enough to cause syncope. This is likely to be thought to be due to a transient mismatch between cardiac output and peripheral vascular resistance rather than autonomic failure. Beat-to-beat measurement of BP is required to diagnose this condition.

2. The second variant is delayed orthostatic hypotension, wherein orthostatic hypotension occurs after 3 minutes of standing. This variant may represent an early form of sympathetic dysfunction. Prolonged measurements may be necessary for diagnosis.

Simultaneous monitoring of heart rate enables differentiation between the neurogenic and non-neurogenic causes of orthostatic hypotension. Non-neurogenic hypotension is often accompanied by a compensatory increase in heart rate (approximately 15 beats/min) reflecting preserved autonomic function.

DIFFERENTIAL DIAGNOSIS

Orthostatic hypotension should be differentiated from the following closely related disorders:

- Orthostatic intolerance is a distinct entity seen most commonly in young women who present with symptoms similar to that of orthostatic hypotension. However, no drop in BP is observed on orthostatic testing. This condition is associated with problems of localized excess noradrenergic stimulation to abnormalities of the baroreflex response.
- Postural orthostatic tachycardia syndrome (POTS) is defined by symptoms of orthostatic intolerance accompanied by a sustained increase in heart rate of more than 30 beats/min upon assuming the upright posture. However, there is characteristic absence of significant hypotension, or sometimes even a mild increase in BP on standing. This condition is usually seen in the second or third decades of life and is far more common in women than men. POTS is believed to result from impaired sympathetic tone, resulting in a reduced venoconstriction and pooling of blood volume in the lower limb and splanchnic vascular beds or secondary to deconditioning after prolonged bed rest. Standing serum norepinephrine levels are increased. A hyperadrenergic form of POTS is also described which is associated with increase in BP upon standing.
- Neurally mediated or reflex syncope may present with symptoms similar to orthostatic hypotension but the autonomic function testing between the episodes is normal. The mechanism of reflex syncope differs from that of orthostatic hypotension and involves cardiac hypercontractility secondary to decreased venous return to the heart resulting from increased peripheral venous pooling of blood. In this condition, the reflex bradycardia and hypotension are similar to those evoked by the Bezold–Jarisch reflex and are not due to baroreceptor inactivation.

MANAGEMENT

The etiologic work-up should begin with the establishment of the diagnosis with orthostatic testing. A detailed treatment history should be taken to exclude the use of drugs causing orthostatic hypotension. If the postural fall in BP is associated with a compensatory increase in heart rate, non-neurogenic causes should be looked for (e.g., absolute or relative hypovolemia). If a heart rate response is absent, a neurogenic cause should be suspected. A structured history, physical and neurological examination, should be done in search of central and peripheral neurological symptoms and signs. Important investigations include blood glucose (diabetes), serum electrophoresis and urine protein (AL amyloid), and serum cortisol levels (Addison's disease) if no clue is found on clinical evaluation.

TREATMENT

The mainstay of treatment is education of the patient regarding the nature of the condition and nonpharmacological measures.[11]

Nonpharmacological Treatment

The obvious first measure should be stop any offending drugs after weighing the risk-benefit ratio. The nonpharmacologic measures include:

- Avoidance of triggering factors or situations like hot weather, prolonged standing, and abrupt standing
- Gradual staged movements with change from supine to standing positions, especially in the morning, when orthostatic tolerance is lowest
- Physical counter-maneuvers like leg-crossing, toe raising, stooping, squatting and tensing the muscles of the leg, abdomen, or buttocks or of the whole body
- Use of elastic compression stockings covering both lower limbs and lower abdomen or a separate binder for abdomen; however, these are poorly accepted by patients due to discomfort
- Sleeping after raising the head of the bed by 10–20°
- Avoiding prolonged recumbency
- Avoidance of large meals, foods rich in carbohydrates, and alcohol intake to minimize postprandial orthostatic hypotension. (Sudden standing or physical activity immediately after eating should be avoided)
- Performing isotonic exercises (recumbent or seated exercise may be preferable with avoidance of straining during exercise)
- Increasing intake of water (2–2.5 L/day) and salt (up to 6–10 g/day), if feasible
- Rapid ingestion of tap water or preferably intake of cold water.

Pharmacological Treatment

If there is inadequate response to nonpharmacologic measures, the following drugs are recommended.

- *Fludrocortisone acetate:* A potent synthetic mineralocorticoid analog, fludrocortisone increases renal sodium reabsorption and leads to expansion of intravascular volume. Additionally, it enhances the release of norepinephrine from sympathetic neurons thereby potentiating the vasoconstrictive effect of norepinephrine. However, though these effects are useful in decreasing orthostatic hypotension, they are also responsible for supine hypertension and decompensation in patients with heart failure. Accordingly, fludrocortisone was recommended by the European Federation of Neurological Societies in 2006 as the first-line drug for orthostatic hypotension refractory to nonpharmacologic measures provided supine hypertension and heart failure are absent.[9] Robust evidence for the use of this drug is however lacking. A Cochrane systematic review is currently underway to ascertain the efficacy of this drug in orthostatic hypotension.

  Dose is 50 µg/day at initiation with up-titration up to 300 µg/day depending on the clinical response. Adverse effects include exacerbation of heart failure, hypokalemia, hypomagnesemia, and supine hypertension. Additionally, mineralocorticoids have been shown to promote cardiac fibrosis through the induction of oxidative stress and endothelial dysfunction in animal models.
- *Midodrine:* Midodrine, a selective and direct α1-adrenoreceptor agonist, increases peripheral resistance. This drug is approved by the US Food and Drug Administration (FDA) in orthostatic hypotension. Evidence to recommend the use of midodrine in orthostatic hypotension is insufficient and low-quality.[10] The half-life is only 4 hours with increase in BP lasting for 2–3 hours. Therefore, dosing needs to be individualized according to patient's activities. The first dose is usually administered 30 minutes before morning rise. The drug should be avoided after 4 PM as it promotes nighttime supine hypertension. The daily dose varies greatly, from 2.5 to 37.5 mg depending on the degree of desensitization. Adverse events include piloerection, scalp pruritus, paresthesias, urinary hesitancy or retention, and supine hypertension
- *Droxidopa:* L-threo-3,4-dihydroxyphenylserine (L-DOPS) or droxidopa is an oral sympathomimetic amino acid which is metabolized into norepinephrine both peripherally and centrally by DOPA decarboxylase. This drug was approved by the US FDA in February 2014 for use in symptomatic orthostatic hypotension secondary to primary autonomic failure, dopamine β-hydroxylase deficiency (DBHD) or nondiabetic autonomic neuropathy. A recent meta-analysis concluded that there is moderate level of evidence for improvement with droxidopa in both dizziness and general orthostatic hypotension-related symptoms in patients with neurogenic orthostatic hypotension, in the short term. The starting dose is 100 mg three times a day with the final dose before 5 PM to avoid supine hypertension. The dose may be up-titrated to a maximum of 600 mg thrice daily depending on the clinical response. There are no significant adverse effects apart from supine hypertension
- *Atomoxetine:* It is a selective norepinephrine reuptake inhibitor that selectively inhibits the reuptake of norepinephrine with little to no activity at the other neuronal reuptake pumps or receptor sites. The role of this drug in the treatment of orthostatic hypotension has been explored recently. In a randomized study in patients with severe autonomic dysfunction, atomoxetine was shown to be a viable and possibly superior treatment option compared with midodrine. Before initiation, the possible adverse effects should be discussed, including suicidal ideation (though reported mainly in children and adolescents), depression, aggressive behavior, priapism, urination retention, and hepatotoxicity (requiring monitoring with liver function tests). This drug should be avoided in patients with serious structural heart disease because of risk of sudden death, stroke, and myocardial infarction
- *Miscellaneous:* Other agents that have been tried in orthostatic hypotension include pyridostigmine, erythropoietin, octreotide, phenylpropanolamine, pseudoephedrine, and arginine vasopressin. However, the evidence in support of their use is poor and low quality.

CONCLUSION

Orthostatic hypotension is a common yet underreported clinical sign, which is associated with an increased morbidity and mortality. A clear understanding of the pathophysiology is required for diagnosis. Treatment should always first rely on elimination of the causative mechanism and nonpharmacological measures, which are sufficient in a large number of patients. Pharmacologic treatment is based on a weak level of evidence.

REFERENCES

1. Freeman R, Wieling W, Axelrod FB, et al. Consensus statement on the definition of orthostatic hypotension, neurally mediated syncope and the postural tachycardia syndrome. Clin Auton Res. 2011;21(2):69-72.
2. Fedorowski A, Stavenow L, Hedblad B, et al. Consequences of orthostatic blood pressure variability in middle-aged men (The Malmo Preventive Project). J Hypertens. 2010;28(3):551-9.
3. Rose KM, Eigenbrodt ML, Biga RL, et al. Orthostatic hypotension predicts mortality in middle-aged adults: The Atherosclerosis Risk In Communities (ARIC) Study. Circulation. 2006;114(7):630-6.
4. Low PA. Prevalence of orthostatic hypotension. Clin Auton Res. 2008;15(Suppl 1):8-13.
5. Finucane C, O'Connell MDL, Fan CW, et al. Age-related normative changes in phasic orthostatic blood pressure in a large population study: findings from The Irish Longitudinal Study on Ageing (TILDA). Circulation. 2014;130(20):1780-9.
6. Rose KM, Tyroler HA, Nardo CJ, et al. Orthostatic hypotension and the incidence of coronary heart disease: the Atherosclerosis Risk in Communities study. Am J Hypertens. 2000;13(6 pt 1):571-8.
7. Ricci F, Fedorowski A, Radico F, et al. Cardiovascular morbidity and mortality related to orthostatic hypotension: a meta-analysis of prospective observational studies. Eur Heart J. 2015;36:1609-17.
8. Merlini G, Seldin DC, Gertz MA. Amyloidosis: Pathogenesis and new therapeutic options. J Clin Oncol. 2011;29:1924-33.
9. Lahrmann H, Cortelli P, Hilz M, et al. EFNS guidelines on the diagnosis and management of orthostatic hypotension. Eur J Neurol. 2006;13:930-6.
10. Parsaik AK, Singh B, Altayar O, et al. Midodrine for orthostatic hypotension: a systematic review and meta-analysis of clinical trials. J Gen Intern Med. 2013;28(11):1496-503.
11. Joseph A, Wanono R, Flamant M, et al. Orthostatic hypotension: A review. Nephrol Ther. 2017;13 Suppl 1:S55-67.

SECTION 15

Atrial Fibrillation

CHAPTER 105

Stroke Prevention in Atrial Fibrillation: New Oral Anticoagulants

Sharad Agrawal

INTRODUCTION

Stroke has long been recognized as a devastating complication of atrial fibrillation (AF). Long-term anticoagulation with warfarin (with all its inherent problems) has been the standard treatment for majority of such patients for many decades. Understandably, the patient with AF may well feel stuck between a devil and the deep sea, because of high risk of stroke associated with AF on one hand and the problems associated with standard warfarin therapy on the other.[1]

However, several new oral anticoagulants (NOACs), have now been approved for clinical use and offer much better efficacy and safety than the standard warfarin therapy even without the need for regular therapeutic monitoring.[1] The field of stroke prevention in AF is being revolutionized not just by NOACs but also by the development of new risk scoring systems for better identification of patients at higher risk of stroke and the bleeding complications.[1,2]

Most of the morbidity and mortality associated with AF is primarily due to thromboembolic complications resulting into ischemic strokes.[3] Mortality due to stroke can largely be mitigated by effective anticoagulation,[4] while other cardiovascular deaths, i.e., due to heart failure and sudden death, remain unaffected despite the contemporary evidence-based treatment.[5]

EPIDEMIOLOGY OF STROKE IN ATRIAL FIBRILLATION

Atrial fibrillation is quite common sustained cardiac arrhythmia. It is currently estimated to affect approximately 1–2% of general population, but its prevalence is expected to at least double in the next 50 years.[2] AF may often remain undiagnosed (silent AF) for a long time due to relative paucity of symptoms. The increase in prevalence of AF can be attributed to better detection of silent AF,[6] increasing average age of population as well as conditions predisposing to AF.[7]

Even if silent, AF is not a benign condition. It may confer a fivefold increase in the overall risk of stroke, and it is responsible for up to 15% of all strokes.[8] Strokes in AF have particularly higher significance as they are often large, likely recurrent and therefore result in long-term disability or death.[2,9] Mortality from AF-related stroke is doubled and the cost of care is also significantly increased.[9]

RISK STRATIFICATION TOOLS IN ATRIAL FIBRILLATION

Previously available schemes categorized the stroke risks with AF into a "low", "medium", or the "high" risk groups with overlapping features; and therefore, leading to inconsistent recommendations regarding the use of anticoagulants. Several risk stratification tools have now been developed to objectively assess the risk of stroke as well as the bleeding complications depending upon their associated clinical features.[10]

Estimation of Stroke Risk in Atrial Fibrillation

The risk of stroke is not homogeneous among all patients with AF and can vary up to 20-fold depending on presence of other associated clinical features.[11] The most consistent predictors of stroke in AF are previous history of stroke or transient ischemic attack (TIA) or systemic embolism, advanced age, hypertension, diabetes mellitus, and congestive heart failure.[11] Although a number of risk stratification tools are currently available, the CHA_2DS_2-VASc score is most widely used and recommended by the European Society of Cardiology (ESC) guidelines.[2,4]

The CHA_2DS_2-VASc score[12] is based on a point system in which 2 or 1 points are assigned for various associated clinical features as shown in table 1.

Several validation studies have shown incremental risk of stroke with increasing CHA_2DS_2-VASc scores as shown in table 2.[13]

TABLE 1: The CHA_2DS_2-VASc scoring system[12]

Letter	Clinical features	Score (points)
C	Congestive heart failure/LV dysfunction	1
H	Hypertension	1
A_2	Age >75 years	2
D	Diabetes mellitus	1
S_2	Previous stroke/TIA	2
V	Vascular disease (includes old MI, peripheral arterial disease)	1
A	Age 65–74 years	1
Sc	Sex category (i.e., female sex)	1

LV, left ventricular; MI, myocardial infarction; TIA, transient ischemic attack.

TABLE 2: The CHA_2DS_2-VASc score and the stroke rate[13]

CHA_2DS_2-VASc score	Number of patients (n = 7,329)	Adjusted stroke rate (% per year)
0	1	0%
1	422	1.3%
2	1,230	2.2%
3	1,730	3.2%
4	1,718	4.0%
5	1,159	6.7%
6	679	9.8%
7	294	9.6%
8	82	6.7%
9	14	15.2%

Estimation of Bleeding Risk for Anticoagulant Therapy in Atrial Fibrillation

Although several bleeding risk scores have been developed and validated, but most widely used risk score is *HAS-BLED* (Hypertension; Abnormal renal and liver function; Stroke; Bleeding; Labile INR; Elderly; Drugs or alcohol), which was developed using data from 3,978 European subjects with AF from the Euro Heart Survey (Table 3).[14]

A score of more than or equal to 3 indicates “high risk”, and some caution and regular review of the patient is needed following the initiation of antithrombotic therapy.[2]

Recent validation study has shown that HAS-BLED scores work better as compared to several other schemes tested (Table 4).[15]

ANTITHROMBOTIC MANAGEMENT OF ATRIAL FIBRILLATION

The currently available therapeutic options are:

- Antiplatelet agents (aspirin and clopidogrel)—mostly abandoned now
- Vitamin K antagonist (warfarin)—has been standard therapy but less popular

TABLE 3: The HAS-BLED bleeding risk score[14]

Letter	Clinical features	Score (points)
H	Hypertension	1
A	Abnormal renal and/or liver functions (1 point each)	1 or 2
S	Stroke	1
B	Bleeding	1
L	Labile INRs	1
E	Elderly (age >65 years)	1
D	Drugs and/or alcohol (1 point each)	1 or 2

INR, international normalized ratio.

TABLE 4: The HAS-BLED scores and the bleed rates[15]

HAS-BLED score	Number of patients (n = 3,071)	Bleeds/100 patients
0	798	1.13
1	1,286	1.02
2	744	1.88
3	187	3.74
4	46	8.70
5	8	12.50
Any score	3,071	1.56

- New oral anticoagulants—fast becoming treatment of choice:
  - Direct thrombin inhibitors—dabigatran
  - Factor Xa inhibitors—rivaroxaban, apixaban, and edoxaban.

Antiplatelet Therapy (As an Alternative to Oral Anticoagulants?)

Up until recently, aspirin has traditionally been used very widely in thromboprophylaxis for stroke prevention in patients with AF. This was partly because of the reluctance of patients to accept warfarin therapy.[1] In a recent meta-analysis of eight independent trials by Hart, aspirin compared with placebo showed only a nonsignificant effect or even no effect in reducing the risk of stroke in AF.[16] In another study aspirin appears to confer no benefit, but more bleeding events.[17]

Dual Antiplatelet Therapy in Stroke Prevention in Atrial Fibrillation

The possibility that dual antiplatelet therapy might represent a safe and simpler alternative to oral anticoagulation was evaluated in the prospective ACTIVE-W trial[18] in which 6,706 patients with AF at high risk of stroke were randomized to treatment with either aspirin + clopidogrel or warfarin [target international normalized ratio (INR) 2.0–3.0]. The trial was stopped early because of the superiority of warfarin therapy in stroke prevention with no significant difference in bleeding events between treatment arms.[18]

Latest ESC guidelines 2016 therefore conclude that the antiplatelet therapy cannot be recommended for stroke prevention in AF patients.[4]

Vitamin K Antagonist

Vitamin K antagonist (VKA), such as warfarin, has been in the clinical use for over 50 years and has been the most common oral anticoagulant agent, used in the prevention of stroke in patients with AF. Warfarin has shown unequivocal superiority over aspirin and reduces the risk of AF-related stroke by about 70%.[2] VKAs produce their anticoagulant effect by preventing the g-carboxylation of the vitamin K-dependent coagulation factors prothrombin and factors VII, IX, and X.[2]

Unfortunately, VKAs have a narrow therapeutic window. Therefore, regular blood tests and dose adjustments are necessary to maintain target intensity corresponding to INR 2.0–3.0.[19] Warfarin also has unpredictable pharmacokinetics and pharmacodynamics, which are affected by genetic factors, drug-drug interactions, and consumption of foods containing vitamin K.

New Oral Anticoagulants

The limitations and the problems associated with the use of warfarin exposed the unmet need for new anticoagulants in stroke prevention in patients with AF.[20] Serious efforts have been made over many years to develop specific inhibitors against factors in the coagulation cascade like thrombin and factor Xa (Fig. 1).[21] Four NOAC agents are now commercially available and have been approved for clinical use:

- Direct thrombin inhibitors—dabigatran
- Factor Xa inhibitors—rivaroxaban, apixaban, and edoxaban.

Direct Thrombin Inhibitors (Dabigatran)

Ximelagatran was the first direct thrombin inhibitor which underwent an extensive clinical trial program for prevention and treatment of venous thromboembolism (VTE) after orthopedic surgery,[21] but it had to be withdrawn from the market in February 2006, due to severe hepatotoxicity and major adverse cardiovascular events.

Dabigatran etexilate was then introduced which is a prodrug and is rapidly converted to active compound dabigatran, which is a direct thrombin (factor IIa) inhibitor. It has an absolute bioavailability of 6.5% and 80% of the given dose is excreted by the kidneys. Its serum half-life is 12–17 hours, and it does not require regular monitoring.[22] It needs to be given in twice daily dosage.

In the randomized evaluation of long-term anticoagulant therapy (RE-LY) study, dabigatran was compared head to head with warfarin in 18,113 patients with AF who were at increased risk of stroke.[22]

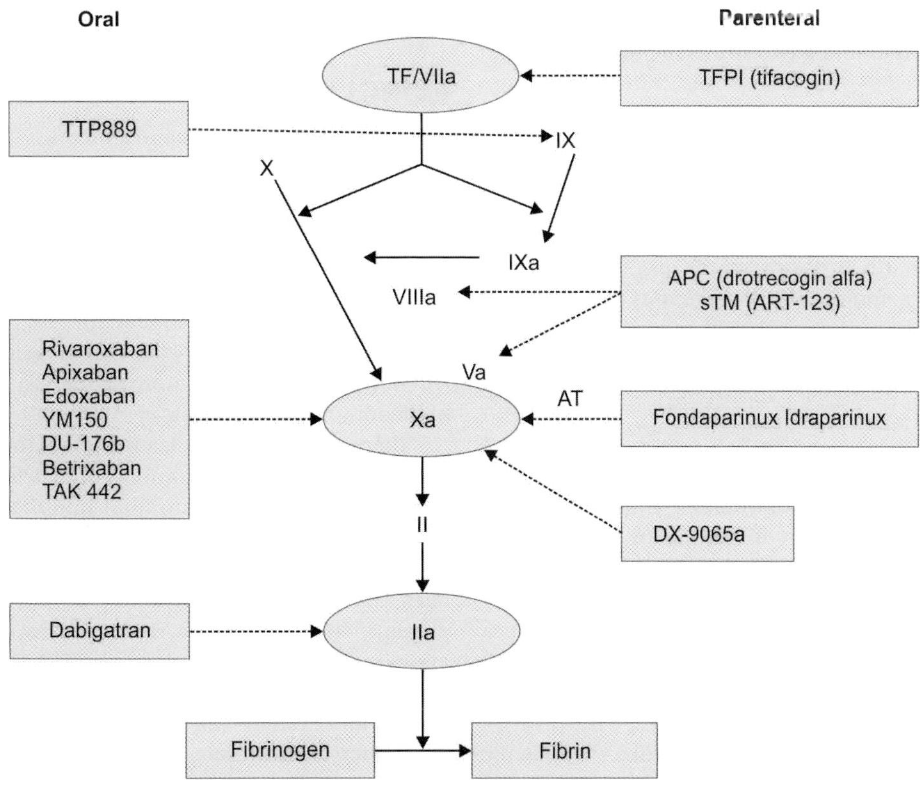

APC, activated protein C; TFPI, tissue factor pathway inhibitor.

FIG. 1: Various new anticoagulants and their target sites.

Dabigatran etexilate was administered in two different dose regimen either 110 mg or 150 mg twice daily, in a blinded fashion and compared with open-labeled warfarin with a target INR ratio of 2.0–3.0. Dabigatran 110 mg bid was noninferior to warfarin for the prevention of stroke and systemic embolism with lower rates of major bleeding (relative risk reduction 20%), while dabigatran 150 mg bid was associated with lower rates of stroke and systemic embolism (relative risk reduction by 35%) with similar rates of major hemorrhage, compared with warfarin.[22] Both the doses significantly reduced the relative risk of intracranial hemorrhage by 70% and 59%, respectively as compared to warfarin.[22]

Factor Xa Inhibitors—Rivaroxaban, Apixaban, Edoxaban

An attractive alternative to direct thrombin inhibition is selective inhibition of factor Xa. In fact, factor Xa may be a better target than thrombin (factor IIa) because it has fewer functions outside coagulation; thus, inhibition of factor Xa may cause fewer side-effects.[23] Numerous direct oral factor Xa inhibitors are currently at various stages of clinical development.[23] Crucial phase III studies of stroke prevention in patients with AF have been completed for rivaroxaban (ROCKET-AF), apixaban (AVERROES and ARISTOTLE) as well as edoxaban (ENGAGE AF-TIMI 48) and they have also been licensed for clinical use.

Rivaroxaban

It is an oral, direct factor Xa inhibitor with a rapid onset of action and a dual mode of elimination, (one-third eliminated by kidneys and the remaining two-thirds metabolized by the liver).[20] It can be used as once daily dose.

The ROCKET-AF is a randomized double blind multi-center trial, that compared rivaroxaban with warfarin for the prevention of stroke or systemic embolism among 14,264 patients with nonvalvular AF who were at moderate-to-high risk for stroke.[24] Results showed that rivaroxaban was noninferior to warfarin in terms of the primary endpoint [composite of stroke and non-central nervous system (CNS) embolism]. The rates of major and nonmajor clinically relevant bleeding were comparable in both groups, with less fatal bleeding and intracranial hemorrhage with rivaroxaban as compared to warfarin.[25]

Apixaban

It is also an oral direct factor Xa inhibitor which is a highly selective and potent inhibitor of free factor Xa and pro-thrombinase activity and needs to be given in twice daily dosage.[2]

The ARISTOTLE is a large randomized double-blind multi-center trial that compared apixaban (5 mg twice daily) with warfarin (target INR of 2.0–3.0) in 18,201 patients with AF and at least one additional risk factor for stroke.[26] The primary outcome was ischemic or hemorrhagic stroke or systemic embolism. Apixaban was not only noninferior, but actually superior to warfarin, reducing the risk of stroke or systemic embolism by 21% and the risk of major bleeding by 31%. Moreover, apixaban is the first of the newer anticoagulants to show a significant reduction in the risk of death from any cause by 11%, as compared with warfarin.[26]

Edoxaban

It is the latest factor Xa inhibitor which is used in once daily dosage. Phase III clinical trial on edoxaban (ENGAGE AF-TIMI 48) compared it with warfarin in a double-blind, double-dummy, randomized controlled noninferiority design for the prevention of thromboembolism in patients with AF.[24]

Two dose regimen of edoxaban 60 mg or 30 mg od were compared with warfarin. Edoxaban 60 mg once daily was noninferior to warfarin and significantly reduced stroke or systemic embolism by 21% and significantly reduced major bleeding events by 20% compared with warfarin. Edoxaban 30 mg once daily was also noninferior to warfarin for prevention of stroke and systemic embolism but significantly reduced major bleeding events by 53%.[24] Only the higher dose regimen has been approved for stroke prevention in AF.[4]

CURRENT RECOMMENDATIONS FOR ANTITHROMBOTIC THERAPY IN ATRIAL FIBRILLATION

Current ESC guidelines on the management of AF recommends oral anticoagulant should be considered for men with a CHA_2DS_2-VASc score of 1 and women with a score of 2, balancing the expected stroke reduction, bleeding risk, and patient preference.[4] Precautions in patients with high HAS-BLED score, include lower anticoagulation intensity, more careful dose regulation, or better control of hypertension.[2,4]

CONCLUSION

Atrial fibrillation significantly increases the risk of stroke by promoting thrombus formation particularly in the left atrium. New ESC guidelines for the management of AF recommend the use of formal risk scoring systems like CHA_2DS_2-VASc and HAS-BLED for the formal risk stratification of patients.[4] The routine use of these scores has proved extremely helpful for the patients and their clinicians alike to identify the correct group of patients who will benefit by long term anticoagulation without undue risk of bleeding complications.

There is a growing realization about the limited efficacy of aspirin and its use for thromboprophylaxis in AF is no longer recommended. Direct thrombin inhibitor (dabigatran) and factor Xa inhibitors (rivaroxaban, apixaban, and edoxaban) are among the several new anticoagulant agents which are currently licensed for clinical use for prevention of stroke in patients with nonvalvular AF. These new anticoagulants now appear to be all set to replace warfarin, which has been the standard medication for over 50 years to reduce the risk of strokes and systemic embolism in patients with AF. NOACs have shown favorable bleeding profiles as compared to warfarin and have also overcome the need for routine INR monitoring and frequent dose adjustments. A new era of anticoagulation seems to be emerging for patients with AF.[28]

These NOACs are not licensed for thromboprophylaxis in patients with prosthetic heart valves and or significant mitral stenosis, where warfarin remains the drug of choice.

REFERENCES

1. Agrawal S. Anti-coagulants in Atrial Fibrillation – Devil and the Deep Sea. In: Seth A (Ed). Cardiology Update 2011: IJCP Group of Publications for Cardiological Society of India, 1st edition. 2011; pp. 206-19.
2. Camm AJ, Kirchhof P, Lip GY, et al. ESC Guidelines for the management of atrial fibrillation. European Heart J. 2010;31:2369-429.
3. Hohnloser PSH, Duray GZ, Baber U, et al. Prevention of stroke in patients with atrial fibrillation: current strategies and future directions. European Heart J Supp. 2008;10:(H):H4-10.
4. Kirchhof P, Benussi S, Kotecha D, et al. 2016 ESC Guidelines for the management of atrial fibrillation developed in collaboration with EACTS. European Heart J. 2016;37:2893-962.
5. Kotecha D, Holmes J, Krum H, et al. Beta-Blockers in Heart Failure Collaborative Group. Efficacy of beta-blockers in patients with heart failure plus atrial fibrillation: an individual-patient data meta-analysis. Lancet. 2014;384:2235-43.
6. Kishore A, Vail A, Majid A, et al. Detection of atrial fibrillation after ischemic stroke or transient ischemic attack: a systematic review and meta-analysis. Stroke. 2014;45:520-6
7. Schnabel RB, Yin X, Gona P, et al. 50 year trends in atrial fibrillation prevalence, incidence, risk factors, and mortality in the Framingham Heart Study: a cohort study. Lancet. 2015;386:154-62.
8. Hart RG, Halperin JL. Atrial fibrillation and stroke: concepts and controversies. Stroke. 2001;32:803-8.
9. Lip GYH, Lim HS. Atrial fibrillation and stroke prevention. Lancet Neurol. 2007;6:981-93.
10. Fang MC, Go AS, Chang Y, et al. Comparison of risk stratification schemes to predict thromboembolism in people with nonvalvular atrial fibrillation. J Am Coll Cardiol. 2008;51:810-5.
11. The Stroke Risk in Atrial Fibrillation Working Group. Independent predictors of stroke in patients with atrial fibrillation. A systematic review. Neurol. 2007;69:546-54.
12. Lip GY, Nieuwlaat R, Pisters R, et al. Refining clinical risk stratification for predicting stroke and thromboembolism in atrial fibrillation using a novel risk factor-based approach: The Euro Heart Survey on atrial fibrillation. Chest. 2010;137:263-72.
13. Lip GY, Frison L, Halperin J, et al. Identifying patients at risk of stroke despite anticoagulation. Stroke. 2010;41:2731-8.
14. Pisters R, Lane DA, Nieuwlaat R, et al. A novel user friendly score (HAS-BLED) to assess one-year risk of major bleeding in atrial fibrillation patients: The Euro Heart Survey. Chest. 2010;138:1093-100.
15. Lip GYH, Frison L, Halperin JL, et al. Comparative validation of a novel risk score for predicting bleeding risk in anticoagulated patients with atrial fibrillation. J Am Coll Cardiol. 2011;57:173-80.
16. Hart RG, Pearce LA, Aguilar MI. Meta-analysis: antithrombotic therapy to prevent stroke in patients who have nonvalvular atrial fibrillation. Ann Intern Med. 2007;146(12):857-67.
17. Sato H, Ishikawa K, Kitabatake A, et al. Low-dose aspirin for prevention of stroke in low-risk patients with atrial fibrillation: Japan Atrial Fibrillation Stroke Trial. Stroke. 2006;37:447-51.
18. Connolly S, Pogue J, Hart R, et al. Clopidogrel plus aspirin versus oral anticoagulation for atrial fibrillation in the Atrial fibrillation Clopidogrel Trial with Irbesartan for prevention of Vascular Events (ACTIVE W): a randomised controlled trial. Lancet. 2006;367:1903-12.
19. Nieuwlaat R, Olsson SB, Lip GY, et al. Guideline-adherent anti-thrombotic treatment is associated with improved outcomes compared with under treatment in high-risk patients with atrial fibrillation. The Euro Heart Survey on Atrial Fibrillation. Am Heart J. 2007;153:1006-12.
20. Turpie AGG. New oral anticoagulants in atrial fibrillation. (Review) European Heart J. 2007;29:155-65.
21. Weitz JI, Bates SM. New anticoagulants. J Thromb Haemost. 2005;3:1843-53.
22. Connolly SJ, Ezekowitz MD, Yusuf S, et al. Dabigatran versus warfarin in patients with atrial fibrillation. N Engl J Med. 2009;361:1139-51.
23. Kubitza D, Haas S. Novel factor Xa inhibitors for prevention and treatment of thromboembolic diseases. Expert Opin Investig Drugs. 2006;15:843-55.
24. Giugliano RP, Ruff CT, Braunwald E, et al. Edoxaban versus warfarin in patients with atrial fibrillation (ENGAGE AF-TIMI 48). N Engl J Med. 2013;369:2093-104.
25. Patel MR, Mahaffey KW, Garg J, et al. Rivaroxaban versus warfarin in non-valvular atrial fibrillation. N Engl J Med. 2011;365:883-91.
26. Granger CB, Alexander JH, McMurray JJV, et al. Apixaban versus warfarin in patients with atrial fibrillation. N Engl J Med. 2011;365(11):981-92.
27. Mega JL. A New Era for Anticoagulation in Atrial Fibrillation (Editorial). N Engl J Med. 2011;365:1052-4.

CHAPTER 106

Catheter Ablation of Atrial Fibrillation

Dinkar Bhasin, Gautam Sharma

INTRODUCTION

Atrial fibrillation (AF) is the most common arrhythmia in clinical practice. The prevalence increases with age and up to 10% octogenarians having AF.[1] AF is associated with debilitating symptoms, poor quality of life (QoL), increased incidence of systemic embolism, vascular dementia, and heart failure (HF).[2,3] The risk of stroke with AF increases by 5-fold for patients with nonvalvular AF and 17-fold in patients with rheumatic heart disease (RHD).[4] Risk factors for developing AF include hypertension, diabetes mellitus, thyroid disorders, chronic lung disease, cardiac disease, and sleep apnea. Data derived from Indian cohorts of international registries has shown RHD to be the most common cause of AF in the Indian population. Traditionally the management of AF has focused on rate control with results of rhythm control being less satisfactory. However, the development of catheter ablation for AF has increased the management options available in the current era.

ADVANTAGES OF MAINTAINING SINUS RHYTHM

Maintenance of sinus rhythm in patients with AF has been long debated. Overall, data from studies that used antiarrhythmic drugs (AAD) for rhythm control suggested no difference in mortality and stroke risk when comparing rhythm control versus rate control. These studies were handicapped by the adverse effects and tolerability issues associated with AADs. However, several studies have shown that maintenance of sinus rhythm per se in patients with AF is associated with better symptom control and improvement of QoL.[5] Catheter ablation has offered a non-AAD option for the quest of sinus rhythm in patients with AF. A recent randomized control trial (RCT) evaluated the role of catheter ablation of AF in patients with HF with reduced ejection fraction (EF <35%) and showed that catheter ablation was associated with a 16.1% absolute risk reduction in the composite endpoint of death from any cause or hospitalization for worsening HF [28.5% vs. 44.6%; hazard ratio (HR) = 0.62; 95%; p = 0.007]. There was a significant reduction in death from any cause with catheter ablation (13.4% vs. 25.0%; HR, 0.53; p = 0.01) though the trial was not powered to study this outcome alone.[6] Another small RCT (n = 68) studied the effects of AF ablation in patients with unexplained left ventricular (LV) dysfunction and showed significant improvement in left ventricular ejection fraction (LVEF) in patients undergoing catheter ablation (18 ± 13% vs. 4.4 ± 13%; p <0.0001) with normalization of EF (LVEF >50%) in 58% patients undergoing ablation compared to 9% managed with medical therapy (p = 0.0002). Further, lack of ventricular late gadolinium enhancement on cardiac magnetic resonance imaging was associated with greater improvement in LVEF and normalization at 6 months suggesting that preprocedural screening with MRI may be useful to select patients for catheter ablation.[7]

The largest trial comparing catheter ablation with drug therapy in patients with AF is the CABANA (Catheter Ablation Versus Anti-arrhythmic Drug Therapy for Atrial Fibrillation Trial) trial (n = 2,204). The results from this trial were recently presented and showed that there was no difference in the primary outcome (death, disabling stroke, serious bleeding, or cardiac arrest) between ablation or drug therapy at 5 years (8% vs. 9.2% HR = 0.86, p = 0.3). However, the rates of death or cardiovascular hospitalization was lower in patients undergoing ablation (51.7% vs. 58.1%, HR = 0.83, p = 0.002) and the on treatment analysis showed significant reduction in primary endpoint with ablation (7.0% vs. 10.9%, p = 0.006).[8]

PATHOPHYSIOLOGY OF ATRIAL FIBRILLATION

Atrial fibrillation is a complex arrhythmia, and several mechanisms have been proposed to explain the pathogenesis of AF with both ectopic activity and reentrant mechanisms playing an important role. The three primary hypothesis are multiple reentrant wavelet theory, rapidly discharging automatic foci, and a single reentrant circuit with fibrillatory conduction.[9] However, crucial to the understanding was the observation that ectopic automatic firing from pulmonary vein (PV) foci can trigger and/or maintain AF. Such activity arises from muscle sleeves of left atrial musculature into the pulmonary veins. About 90% of paroxysmal AF originates from such PV foci.[10] Further, there is electrical remodeling of the left atrium producing a substrate for the maintenance of the arrhythmia. This remodeling starts within hours of AF onset and involves altered expression and function of ion channels leading to abbreviation of atrial refractoriness and changes in calcium handling. In the long run, this electrical and contractile remodeling leads to structural remodeling via atrial stretch and atrial fibrosis.[11]

A recent study has validated this hypothesis by electron microscopic demonstration of cardiomyocytes with depletion of the contractile elements (Z-bands), glycogen particle accumulation, and an increase in mitochondria. Majority of persistent AF cases showed interstitial collagen bundles and extensive fibrosis.[12] Hence, AF represents a continuum of pathophysiologic changes and initial paroxysmal episodes can progress into persistent and permanent AF. Nearly 25% of the patients with paroxysmal AF progress to persistent AF in 5 years and over 50% in 10 years.[13,14]

INDICATIONS FOR ATRIAL FIBRILLATION ABLATION (TABLE 1)

The latest guidelines for catheter ablation of AF are provided in the HRS/EHRA/ECAS/APHRS/SOLAECE expert consensus statement.[15] The strongest indication for AF ablation is the presence of symptoms despite adequate medical therapy as there is consistent evidence that ablation in this setting improves QoL. The level of evidence is highest for patients with paroxysmal AF who are symptomatic despite treatment with one class I or III antiarrhythmic drug as the likelihood of success is highest in these patients. It is reasonable to attempt catheter ablation in patients with persistent AF and can be considered in patients with long-standing AF even though the expected success rates are lower in these settings. However, increasingly catheter ablation is being considered for first-line therapy in patients with paroxysmal and persistent AF without use of antiarrhythmic therapy. Evidence from recent studies suggests that such an approach may be associated with a lower rate of AF recurrence and no difference in rates of symptomatic AF. Certain patient populations where this strategy may be particularly useful include patients with tachy-brady syndrome who have symptomatic pauses and competitive athletes with AF.

Catheter ablation may also be considered as a first-line therapy for patients with HF with reduced ejection fraction who have AF. Maintenance of normal sinus rhythm is associated with better LV performance in such patients and evidence from recent studies suggests that this may translate into a survival benefit.[6,16,17]

Patients with asymptomatic AF often have occult symptoms which are obvious once sinus rhythm is restored. Preprocedural cardioversion to sinus rhythm and reassessment of symptom status may help in decision making. Nonetheless, catheter ablation can be offered to select patients with asymptomatic with paroxysmal or persistent AF when procedural success rates are deemed to be high.

TECHNIQUE FOR PULMONARY VEIN ISOLATION

Catheter ablation can be done under conscious sedation or general anesthesia as per the preference of the operator. When general anesthesia is used, esophageal temperature monitoring is recommended to decrease the risk of esophageal injury. The procedure is done under fluoroscopic guidance and using a 3D electroanatomical map into which preacquired CT images can also be integrated. Standard septal puncture needles are used for left atrial access. Most centers prefer using both mapping catheters and radiofrequency ablation (RFA) catheters. Anticoagulation during the procedure is maintained with unfractionated heparin to maintain an activated clotting time of 300 seconds.

TABLE 1: Indications for catheter ablation of atrial fibrillation[15]

Symptomatic AF refractory or intolerant to at least one class I or III antiarrhythmic drug	
• Paroxysmal: Class Ia • Persistent: Class IIa • Permanent: Class IIb	
Symptomatic AF before trial of any anti-arrhythmic drug therapy	
• Paroxysmal: Class IIa • Persistent: Class IIb	
Specific patient groups	
Heart failure	Similar indications as for patients without heart failure
HCM	Similar indications as for patients without HCM
Tachy-brady syndrome	Catheter ablation may be offered as an alternative to pacemaker implantation (IIa)
Athletes with AF	Catheter ablation may be offered as first-line treatment (IIa)
Asymptomatic AF	Catheter ablation may be considered in selected asymptomatic patients with paroxysmal or persistent AF (IIb)

AF, atrial fibrillation; HCM, hypertrophic cardiomyopathy.

Cryoballoon ablation (CBA) is an alternative to RFA (Fig. 1). It isolates the PV by freezing the tissue to temperatures less than -80°C.[18] While the use of RFA requires point-by-point ablation, cryoablation with a balloon allows a single shot ablation at the PV level. Both RFA and CBA have similar success rates and overall rates of complications. However, CBA is associated with higher rates of phrenic nerve (PN) injury most of which are self-resolving with low rates of permanent injury (0.3%).[19]

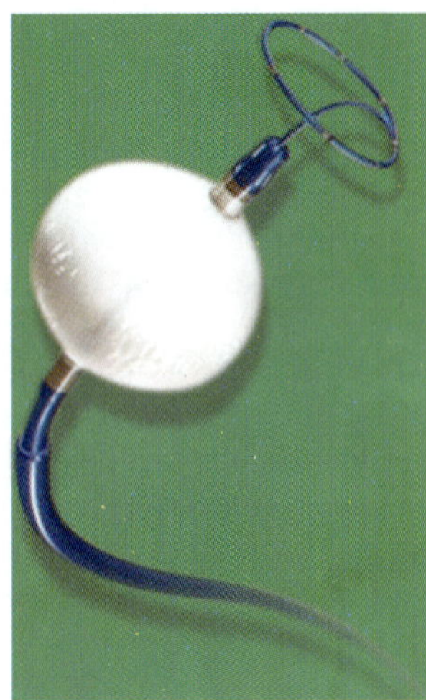

FIG. 1: Cryoablation balloon.
Source: Reproduced with permission from Medtronic, Inc.

The main objective of catheter ablation of AF is the permanent electrical isolation of the pulmonary veins by using either radiofrequency or cryoablation. In certain scenarios additional lesions may be used to target non-PV triggers and for substrate modification. By using mapping catheters circumferential mapping of PV potentials is done to define the activation sequence (Fig. 2). When such sites of earliest activity are ablated the technique is known as segmental PV isolation (Fig. 3). However, our current practice is to employ circumferential anatomic ablation around PV ostia either individually or by encircling both the ipsilateral veins (Fig. 4). The ablation site should ideally be in the antrum and not directly at the ostia or in the body of pulmonary veins which may increase the risk of PV stenosis. Ablation is often started at the posterior wall and then continued around the PV ostia. The endpoint of ablation is the elimination of PV vein potentials and demonstration of entrance block into the PVs. It is reasonable to monitor for 20–30 minutes after ablation for confirmation of PV isolation. Intravenous adenosine or pace-capture may be used to demonstrate isolation after this waiting period. When RFA is used, a force sensing catheter providing a minimum of 5–10 g of contact force is preferable. Use of such catheters is associated with lesser rates of dormant PV conduction and lower complications rates.

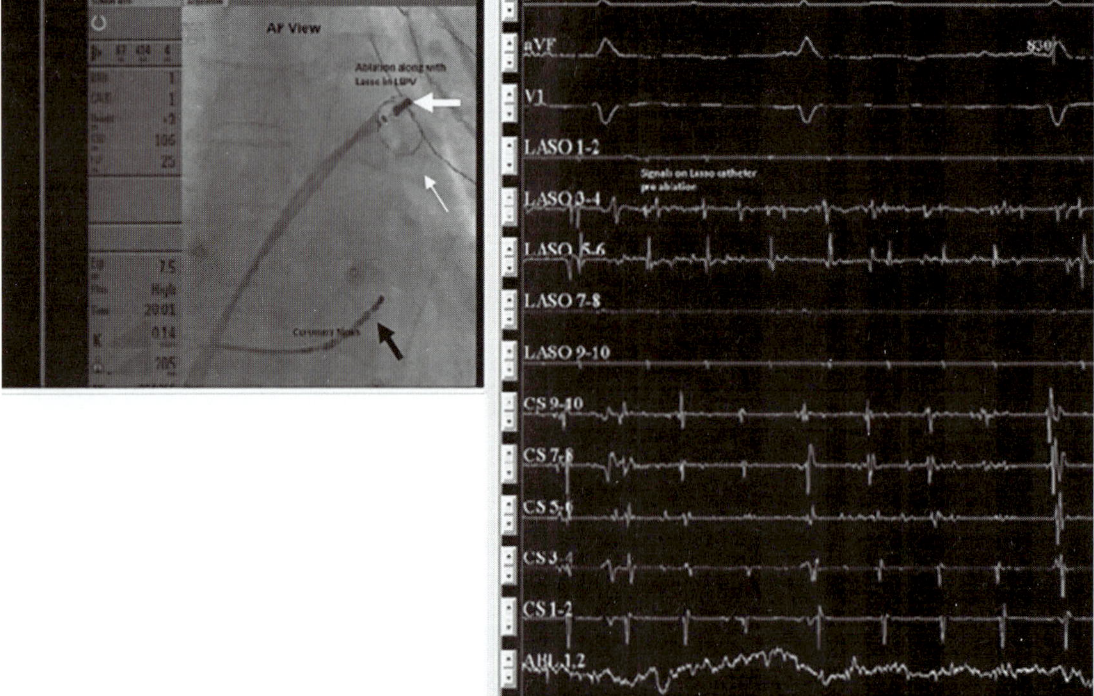

FIG. 2: Procedure for atrial fibrillation ablation. The mapping Lasso catheter has been positioned in the left superior pulmonary vein (PV) (thin white arrow) and the ablation catheter is at the PV antrum (thick white arrow). A decapolar catheter has been positioned in the coronary sinus (black arrow). Potentials picked by the 10 poles of the circular lasso catheter and the ablation catheter are used for mapping.

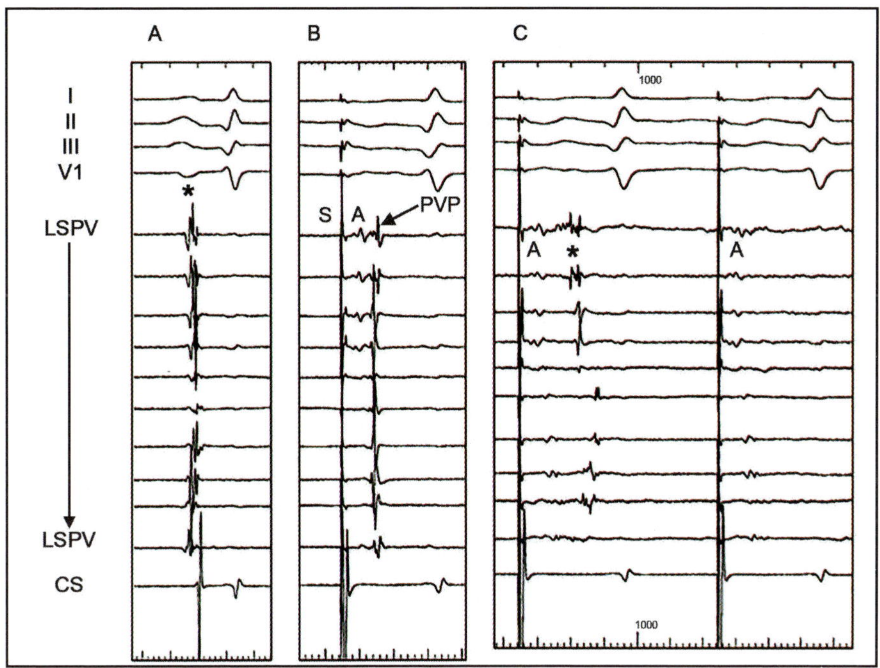

FIG. 3: Isolation of the left superior pulmonary vein (LSPV). **A,** Left atrial and pulmonary vein potentials (PVP) are superimposed; **B,** Pacing from the coronary sinus (CS) shows PVPs following the far-field atrial potential; **C,** PVPs disappear after radiofrequency ablation (RFA) demonstrating complete isolation.

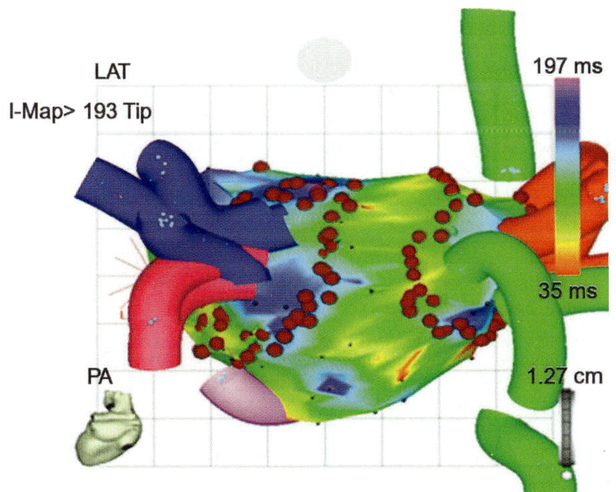

FIG. 4: Three-dimensional electroanatomical map of left atrium showing circumferential ablation points around pulmonary vein ostia.

ADJUNCTIVE ABLATION STRATEGIES

While pulmonary vein isolation (PVI) remains the cornerstone for ablation therapy for paroxysmal AF, additional strategies are often utilized in persistent or long-standing AF and those undergoing redo-ablation with the intent to increase success rates. Such additional lesions result in compartmentalization of the atria and prevent reentry. However, evidence in support of such additional techniques is limited. Hence, they are not universally recommended and the decision is made on a case to case basis depending upon operator preference and experience.

Focal triggers can be identified outside the PV in up to 10–30% cases. Common sites include the posterior wall of left atrium (LA), crista terminalis, and superior vena cava (SVC). These lesions are inducible with isoproterenol infusion and if provoked should be ablated. If typical atrial flutter is induced during AF ablation, additional linear lesions should be given at the cavotricuspid isthmus. Electrical isolation of the posterior wall involves linear lesions joining the superior PVs and the inferior PVs and can be considered in certain groups especially in patients with persistent AF and those undergoing repeat ablation. Linear lesions in LA roof and along the mitral valve have also been used in patients with persistent or long-standing AF. If such additional linear lesions are employed, pacing and mapping should be done to achieve complete isolation as incomplete ablation can be responsible for recurrence of AT. Complex fractionated atrial electrogram represent fractionated potentials which have a short cycle length. Ablation of such potentials has been hypothesized to decrease the recurrence rates. Mapping and ablating rotational activity and ablation of left atrial autonomic ganglia has also been proposed.

COMPLICATIONS OF ATRIAL FIBRILLATION ABLATION

Major complications associated with catheter ablation include cardiac tamponade, pulmonary vein stenosis, esophageal injury, PN injury, and periprocedural stroke. As per a multicenter survey of over 90,000 patients, the incidence of complications is estimated at 6.29% with an in-hospital mortality rate of 0.46%.[20] The rate of complications is associated with operator experience and hospital procedure volumes. The reported mortality risk with the procedure is less than 0.1% and 30-day all-cause mortality rates are less than 1%.[20,21]

The most common life-threatening complication is cardiac tamponade. Overall incidence is reported between 0.2 and 5% with an average of around 1.5%.[15,20] Pulmonary veins stenosis has been described with both RFA and cryoablation. The incidence has been variable reported between 0 and 40% depending upon the modality used for diagnosis but has markedly decreased with increasing operator awareness.[15] Esophageal injuries are infrequent but difficult to manage complications of AF ablation and include esophageal hematoma, esophageal ulcer, esophageal perforation and atrial-esophageal fistula. Prevention includes use of esophageal temperature monitoring while ablation, periprocedural use of proton pump inhibitors, and careful ablation along the posterior LA wall. PN palsy can be a significant complication of AF ablation. Rates of transient PN palsy vary from 3.5 to 11.2% but permanent injury beyond 1 year is rare (<0.5%). Management is conservative and most cases resolve spontaneously. Pacing to detect PN stimulation at the ablation site prior to delivery of the RF energy can reduce the risk of damage.

OUTCOMES

Atrial fibrillation ablation results in significantly higher success rates for maintaining sinus rhythm compared to antiarrhythmic drug therapy alone. Trials studying PV isolation for paroxysmal AF have reported success rates ranging from 59 to 89% at 12 months compared with drug therapy alone which had success rates of 5–23%. Trials studying AF ablation in patients with persistent and long-standing AF have utilized other strategies in addition to PV isolation and have reported success rates of 59–80% at 6–12 months.[15]

REFERENCES

1. Furberg CD, Psaty BM, Manolio TA, et al. Prevalence of atrial fibrillation in elderly subjects (the Cardiovascular Health Study). Am J Cardiol. 1994;74:236-41.
2. Krahn AD, Manfreda J, Tate RB, et al. The natural history of atrial fibrillation: Incidence, risk factors, and prognosis in the Manitoba Follow-Up Study. Am J Med. 1995;98:476-84.
3. Feinberg WM, Blackshear JL, Laupacis A, et al. Prevalence, age distribution, and gender of patients with atrial fibrillation. Analysis and implications. Arch Intern Med. 1995;155:469-73.
4. Wolf PA, Dawber TR, Thomas HE, et al. Epidemiologic assessment of chronic atrial fibrillation and risk of stroke: The Framingham study. Neurology. 1978;28:973-7.
5. Pappone C, Rosanio S, Augello G, et al. Mortality, morbidity, and quality of life after circumferential pulmonary vein ablation for atrial fibrillation: Outcomes from a controlled nonrandomized long-term study. J Am Coll Cardiol. 2003;42:185-97.
6. NEJM. [2018]. Catheter Ablation for Atrial Fibrillation with Heart Failure. [online] Available from https://www.nejm.org/doi/full/10.1056/NEJMoa1707855 [Accessed September 2018].
7. Prabhu S, Taylor AJ, Costello BT, et al. Catheter ablation versus medical rate control in atrial fibrillation and systolic dysfunction: The CAMERA-MRI study. J Am Coll Cardiol. 2017;70:1949-61.
8. Catheter ablation vs antiarrhythmic drug therapy in atrial fibrillation. American College of Cardiology. 2018. [online] Available from http%3a%2f%2fwww.acc.org%2flatest-in-cardiology%2fclinical-trials%2f2018%2f05%2f10%2f15%2f57%2fcabana
9. Yamazaki M, Jalife J. Pathophysiology of atrial fibrillation: From initiation to maintenance. J Arrhythmia. 2012;28:129-39.
10. Haïssaguerre M, Jaïs P, Shah DC, et al. Spontaneous initiation of atrial fibrillation by ectopic beats originating in the pulmonary veins. N Engl J Med. 1998;339:659-66.
11. Kourliouros A, Savelieva I, Kiotsekoglou A, et al. Current concepts in the pathogenesis of atrial fibrillation. Am Heart J. 2009;157:243-52.
12. Sharma S, Sharma G, Hote M, et al. Light and electron microscopic features of surgically excised left atrial appendage in rheumatic heart disease patients with atrial fibrillation and sinus rhythm. Cardiovasc Pathol Off J Soc Cardiovasc Pathol. 2014;23:319-26.
13. Padfield GJ, Steinberg C, Swampillai J, et al. Progression of paroxysmal to persistent atrial fibrillation: 10-year follow-up in the Canadian Registry of Atrial Fibrillation. Heart Rhythm. 2017;14:801-7.
14. Proietti R, Hadjis A, AlTurki A, et al. A systematic review on the progression of paroxysmal to persistent atrial fibrillation: Shedding new light on the effects of catheter ablation. JACC Clin Electrophysiol. 2015;1:105-15.
15. Calkins H, Hindricks G, Cappato R, et al. 2017 HRS/EHRA/ECAS/APHRS/SOLAECE expert consensus statement on catheter and surgical ablation of atrial fibrillation: Executive summary. Europace. 2018;20(1):157-208.
16. Hunter RJ, Berriman TJ, Diab I, et al. [2018]. A randomized controlled trial of Catheter Ablation Versus Medical Treatment of Atrial Fibrillation in Heart Failure (The CAMTAF Trial). [online] Available from https://www.ahajournals.org/doi/full/10.1161/CIRCEP.113.000806 [Accessed September 2018].
17. Al Halabi S, Qintar M, Hussein A, et al. Catheter ablation for atrial fibrillation in heart failure patients: A meta-analysis of randomized controlled trials. JACC Clin Electrophysiol. 2015;1:200-9.
18. Chierchia GB, Sorgente A, Sarkozy A, et al. The use of cryoballoon ablation in atrial fibrillation: simplifying pulmonary vein isolation? J Atr Fibrillation. 2010;3(4):294.
19. Kuck KH, Fürnkranz A, Julian Chun KR. [2018]. Cryoballoon or radiofrequency ablation for symptomatic paroxysmal atrial fibrillation: reintervention, rehospitalization, and quality-of-life outcomes in the FIRE AND ICE trial. [online] Available from https://academic.oup.com/eurheartj/article/37/38/2858/2336161 [Accessed September 2018].
20. Deshmukh A, Patel NJ, Pant S, et al. In-hospital complications associated with catheter ablation of atrial fibrillation in the United States Between 2000 and 2010: Analysis of 93,801 Procedures. Circulation. 20135;128:2104-12.
21. Piccini JP, Sinner MF, Greiner MA, et al. Outcomes of medicare beneficiaries undergoing catheter ablation for atrial fibrillation. Circulation. 2012;126:2200-7.

CHAPTER 107

Postoperative Atrial Fibrillation: Clinical Correlates and Management

Krishnarpan Chatterjee, Naveen Garg

INTRODUCTION

Atrial fibrillation (AF) and atrial flutter occur frequently after cardiac surgery. Most episodes occur by the third postoperative day. Potential adverse outcomes of these atrial arrhythmias include a longer length of stay, stroke, or death and worse long-term prognosis.

INCIDENCE AND TIME COURSE

Atrial fibrillation occurs in 15–40% of patients in the early postoperative period following coronary artery bypass graft surgery (CABG).[1-3] In a 2018 *post hoc* analysis of 1,812 patients without prior AF in the EXCEL trial, which compared CABG with percutaneous coronary intervention (PCI) for left main coronary artery disease, perioperative AF developed in 18.0% of those undergoing CABG (and 0.1% of those who received PCI). The incidence increases with increasing age.[4] AF occurs in 37–50% after valve surgery, and in as many as 60% undergoing valve replacement plus CABG.[1]

Atrial arrhythmias occur most often within the first few days after surgery.[1] In a prospective, multi-center study of 4,657 patients undergoing surgery, the majority of first episodes of AF occurred by day 2, while the majority of recurrent episodes occurred by day 3.[5] Among patients with postoperative AF with no prior history of atrial arrhythmias, the AF is usually self-limited, as 15–30% convert within 2 hours and up to 80% in 24 hours.[1,6,7] The mean duration of AF in one report was 12 hours and more than 90% are in sinus rhythm 6–8 weeks following surgery.[1,7]

Atrial fibrillation may also occur late after cardiac surgery and the incidence is likely higher than appreciated because many patients may have continued asymptomatic episodes of AF.[8] Late postoperative AF was associated with adverse outcomes, including heart failure and rehospitalization.

PATHOGENESIS

After cardiac surgery, AF and atrial flutter can occur early in the postoperative period or as a late complication. Postoperative AF is related to a combination of factors. These include preexisting degenerative changes in the atrial myocardium and perioperative conditions that result in abnormalities of several electrophysiologic parameters that promote the development of AF.[1]

Risk Factors

Most patients who develop AF after cardiac surgery have at least one clinical predictor.

- *Preoperative risk factors*:
  - Increasing age
  - Previous history of AF
  - Increased left atrial size or cardiomegaly
  - Mitral valvular disease, particularly mitral stenosis
  - Previous cardiac surgery
  - Chronic obstructive pulmonary disease (COPD)
  - Elevated preoperative HbA1c
  - Low-intensity physical activity in the year prior to surgery
  - Obesity
  - Caucasian race
  - Absence of β-blocker or angiotensin-converting enzyme inhibitor (ACEI) treatment or withdrawal of previous treatment
  - Preoperative digoxin use
  - Higher preoperative plasma concentration of brain natriuretic peptide (BNP)
  - Low-dose dopamine
  - Severe right coronary artery stenosis
  - Preoperative increase in P-wave duration on ECG
  - Hypokalemia and hypomagnesemia.
- *Perioperative risk factors*:
  - Pericarditis
  - Atrial injury from surgical handling, or cannulation, atrial suture lines
  - Acute atrial enlargement from pressure or volume overload
  - Atrial ischemia

- Long bypass and aortic cross-clamp times
- Inadequate myocardial protection during cardiopulmonary bypass
- Hyperadrenergic state (e.g., postoperative inotropes)
- Pulmonary complications causing hypoxemia
- Hypokalemia and hypomagnesemia
- Oxidative stress.

- *Protective factors*:
  - *Off-pump CABG*: It is associated with a lower rate of postoperative AF than conventional CABG in some but not all studies
  - Preservation of the anterior fat pad; some but not all studies have found lower rate of postoperative AF with preservation of the anterior fat pad.

However, these risk factors do not have adequate predictive accuracy to identify the individual patient at risk for postoperative AF. As a result, risk models that use several factors have been created that predict any postoperative AF as well as recurrent AF.[3] While these risk models are not routinely used, they highlight the individual risks.

CLINICAL MANIFESTATIONS AND DIAGNOSIS

No studies have systematically characterized the clinical manifestations of postoperative AF in cardiac surgery patients. About 90% of these individuals are symptomatic and about 15% are hemodynamically unstable. The diagnosis of AF is not difficult as most patients are on continuous monitoring. All patients should have documentation of the rhythm with a 12-lead electrocardiogram.

Adverse Outcomes Following Atrial Fibrillation

Potential adverse outcomes after the development of postoperative AF include stroke, death, and prolongation of hospital stay.

PREVENTION OF ATRIAL FIBRILLATION AND COMPLICATIONS

Therapies to prevent the development of postoperative AF in patients undergoing cardiac surgery are recommended to decrease the duration of hospitalization, to possibly decrease the risk of in-hospital stroke and death and to decrease the need for anticoagulation in some patients.

Prevention of Atrial Fibrillation

The use of β-blockers, sotalol, amiodarone, atrial pacing, or antioxidant vitamins lowers the risk of postoperative AF.[9] Beta-blockers are the best studied of these therapies and are preferred to sotalol or amiodarone based on their ease of use and better safety profile. Atrial pacing is not recommended in most cases. There has been no study comparing the traditional antiarrhythmic drugs to antioxidant vitamins.

Beta-blockers

Beta blocker administration is the most widely used prophylactic strategy based on numerous studies showing benefit, ease of use, and cost considerations.[1,6] Meta-analyses of randomized trials found that they reduced the risk of AF compared to placebo or no therapy [odds ratio (OR) 0.35, 95% confidence interval (CI) 0.26–0.49 and 0.39, 95% CI 0.28–0.52].[10] The issue of whether some β-blockers lower the risk of postoperative AF more successfully than others has not been well studied. In a meta-analysis of randomized trials with 601 patients that compared carvedilol to metoprolol (succinate and tartrate), carvedilol reduced the incidence of AF (OR 0.50, 95% CI 0.32–0.80).[11]

The benefit is seen when β-blockers are begun prior to or immediately after surgery. Evidence is not strong enough to recommend one β-blocker over another. When possible, β-blockers should be started at least 48 hours before surgery, due to concerns about the induction of excessive bradycardia. There are also concerns about the increased risk of stroke seen in patients undergoing noncardiac surgery who receive β-blockers soon before surgery.

The optimal duration of β-blocker therapy for prevention of postoperative atrial arrhythmias is uncertain, but often continued until the first postoperative visit. Many patients undergoing CABG though have a clear indication for the long-term use of β-blocker therapy (e.g., previous myocardial infarction, left ventricular systolic dysfunction with heart failure, or hypertension).

Sotalol

Sotalol is a class III antiarrhythmic agent that has β blocking activity. Meta-analysis of 15 randomized studies of patients undergoing cardiac surgery found that sotalol lowers the risk of AF compared to placebo (RR 0.55, 95% CI 0.45–0.66).[12] Compared to β-blocker, sotalol was more effective. There was no significant difference in the rates between sotalol and amiodarone. Risks of sotalol include torsade de pointes and bradycardia. Sotalol is effective when begun 24–48 hours before surgery or 4 hours after surgery.

Amiodarone

Amiodarone lowers the incidence of postoperative AF by about 40–50%.[10] Meta-analysis of 18 trials that included nearly 3,000 patients found that amiodarone lowers the risk of AF or atrial flutter compared to placebo (OR 0.48, 95% CI 0.40–0.57).[13] However, amiodarone is associated with more adverse cardiac events compared to placebo, including bradycardia requiring temporary pacing (5.7% vs. 2%), and QT prolongation (1.3% vs. 0%).[14] The rates of the development of AF were similar (23.9% and 24.8%, respectively) when metoprolol was directly compared to amiodarone in a trial of patients who underwent CABG or valve surgery.[15]

A number of different preoperative regimens of amiodarone have been tried. It has been given orally 1–7 days before surgery, intravenously immediately after surgery, or intravenously for 24 hours followed by oral therapy for 4 days.

Intravenous amiodarone begun on call to the operating room and continued for 48 hours, followed by oral amiodarone for 3 days has also significantly reduced postoperative AF.

Although, some have suggested that amiodarone might be more effective than a β-blocker for the prevention of AF after cardiac surgery, this was not confirmed in two meta-analyses.[10]

Antioxidant Vitamins

Oxidative stress contributes to ischemia-reperfusion injury, which occurs in open heart surgery and is involved in the pathogenesis of AF. Despite of limited supportive evidence, due to absence of side effects and low cost, antioxidant vitamins to lower the rate of postoperative AF may be considered.[16] Supplementation with vitamin C (1 g/day), and vitamin E (400 IU/day) 2 days before cardiac surgery have been studied. Treatment was continued until hospital discharge.

Atrial Pacing

Atrial pacing to prevent postoperative AF has been examined in a number of studies. Most studies, but not all showed benefit.

Ineffective or Possibly Effective Therapies

The following preventive strategies to prevent the development of atrial arrhythmias are not recommended:

- *Digoxin*: Digoxin, given preoperatively or postoperatively, does not appear to prevent AF[17]
- *Antiarrhythmic drugs*: Data about the prophylactic use of class I antiarrhythmic drugs to prevent postoperative AF are limited. Procainamide appears to reduce the number of episodes and duration of AF compared to placebo, but not the incidence of AF[18]
- *Calcium channel blockers*: These have uncertain utility in preventing AF after cardiac surgery[19]
- *Intravenous magnesium*: Based on the fact that hypomagnesemia is a risk factor for AF, magnesium supplementation has been evaluated as a possible therapy to reduce postoperative atrial arrhythmias. In a meta-analysis, supraventricular arrhythmia occurred significantly less often in patients treated with magnesium compared to controls.[13] However, there was no effect on hospital stay, perioperative myocardial infarction, or mortality.
- *Angiotensin inhibition*: Although ACEIs and angiotensin II receptor blockers (ARBs) have suggested benefit as a therapy of AF in nonsurgical settings. A significant reduction in the incidence of postoperative AF (20% vs. 34%) with ACEIs was seen in an observational study of 4,657 patients undergoing CABG.[5] A retrospective analysis of 8,889 patients undergoing CABG described an increase in major adverse events, including postoperative renal dysfunction as well as AF, in patients receiving preoperative ACEIs.[20] Given the inconsistency in the results among these studies, preoperative ACEIs specifically for prevention of AF in patients undergoing CABG are not recommended.
- *Statins*: Some, but not all studies have shown that statins lower the rate of postoperative AF. One meta-analysis of randomized trials that compared statin therapy with either placebo or no therapy prior to cardiac surgery (predominantly CABG surgery) found that such treatment reduced the incidence of postoperative AF but failed to influence short-term mortality or postoperative stroke.[21] The largest randomized trial of preoperative statin therapy was the STICS trial, showed a similar rate of the primary outcome of postoperative AF within 5 days of surgery was in both groups.[22] In addition, rosuvastatin was associated with a significant absolute excess in the rate of postoperative acute kidney injury. Based upon established benefits of statin therapy in patients with coronary heart disease, all patients should be on long-term statin. However, for patients not on statin therapy before CABG, it should be started after surgery, as there is no clear evidence of benefit from preoperative initiation and possible harm
- *N-acetylcysteine (NAC)*: It has the potential to protect against the development of perioperative AF due to its antioxidant and anti-inflammatory properties. But more data is required before advocating its routine clinical use
- *Colchicine*: It reduces the incidence of the postpericardiotomy syndrome. In the COPPS-2 trial, 360 patients scheduled for cardiac surgery were randomly assigned to oral colchicine or placebo before surgery.[23] The drug was continued for 1 month after surgery. At 3 months, there was no significant difference between the two groups in the secondary endpoint of postoperative AF. There is insufficient evidence to recommend the routine use of colchicine, due to concern that it may negatively impact wound healing and that it leads to gastrointestinal side effects
- *Naproxen*: The potential benefit from naproxen was evaluated in the NAFARM trial.[24] There was no significant difference in the rate of postoperative AF. The study was stopped early because of an increase in renal failure in the naproxen group
- *Glucocorticoid*: Based upon the hypothesis that perioperative inflammation may contribute to the development of AF, glucocorticoids have been suggested as prophylactic therapy. The large, randomized SIRS trial, found no difference in the rate of new AF.[25] Due to their potential adverse effects on glucose metabolism, wound healing, infection, and the absence of a lowering of the risk of death, the routine use of glucocorticoid therapy to prevent AF is not recommended.

Prevention of Complications of Atrial Fibrillation

While β-blockers, sotalol, amiodarone, and pacing decrease the risk of postoperative AF, the evidence is less robust that the risk of complications such as stroke, death, or length of stay can be prevented. It may be difficult to demonstrate a lowering of the risk of in-hospital stroke with these therapies, as AF is only one risk factor for stroke and as the incidence of stroke is low. The best available evidence of the impact of these interventions on the complications of AF comes from a meta-analysis of heterogeneous trials, which noted the following:[13]

- In 29 trials that evaluated length of stay, only amiodarone and pacing shortened the average length of stay
- In 25 trials that reported on the incidence of postoperative stroke, the risk of stroke was decreased with treatment. Amiodarone was the only single intervention that significantly lowered the risk of stroke compared to placebo.

Approach to Prevention

Preventive therapy to reduce the incidence of postoperative AF is recommended, especially in patients at high risk of its development. While the evidence is not robust, prevention of AF may lead to a lowering of the risk of in-hospital stroke and a shortened length of stay. In addition, successful prevention of AF will prevent the need for anticoagulation in some patients. Beta-blockers, sotalol, amiodarone, and atrial pacing are significantly more effective than placebo in lowering the rate of postoperative AF.[10,13] There is some evidence to support the use of antioxidant vitamins for this purpose. Beta-blockers are preferred to amiodarone or sotalol due to lower cost and lower risk of potential side effects and to pacing because of its relative complexity and cost. Amiodarone or sotalol is a reasonable alternative in patients who cannot tolerate β-blockade. If possible, β-blockers should be started before CABG.

MANAGEMENT

While prevention with β-blockers, amiodarone, sotalol, or pacing lowers the risk of postoperative AF, many patients still develop AF. There is uncertainty as to the optimal management of these patients, because it is not known whether postoperative AF has similar natural history in terms of future adverse events as AF occurring without cardiac surgery. The initial management should include correction of predisposing factors such as hypoxemia, electrolyte abnormalities, and hemodynamic instability as well as pain management and withdrawal of stimulating factors such as inotropic agents. Subsequent management relates to the issues of rate control versus rhythm control, cardioversion, and anticoagulation.

Rate Control

Given the transient nature of the arrhythmia, initial control of the ventricular response rate is an effective and relatively safe strategy in many patients who develop postoperative AF.[6] Rate control is most commonly achieved with β-blockers. Intravenous esmolol, a β-blocker with a short half-life, can be given for acute rate control if there is a concern for bradyarrhythmias, hypotension, or bronchospasm. Slowing of the ventricular rate in many AF patients receiving inotropic agents postoperatively can be achieved by lowering the dose or discontinuation of these agents.

The optimal rate goal for patients with AF after cardiac surgery has not been determined. As these patients vary widely in many clinical features (comorbidities, need for rapid ventricular rate, etc.), the optimal ventricular rate should be determined on a case by case basis. In many patients, a ventricular rate of less than 110 beats/minute will prevent symptoms such as palpitations and allow for optimal cardiac performance. Calcium channel blockers and digoxin are the other atrioventricular (AV) nodal blockers that can control the ventricular rate in AF, but they are not more effective than β-blockers. In patients in whom alternate agents have not been successful in rate control, intravenous amiodarone can be used to slow the ventricular response. Ivabradine is not effective, as it does not have any effect on AV node conduction.

Rhythm Control

Restoration of sinus rhythm from well-tolerated postoperative AF is usually not necessary but occasionally can be beneficial. Restoration of sinus rhythm is indicated in symptomatic patients or in those when rate control is difficult to achieve. An attempt at the restoration of sinus rhythm can be beneficial in patients with a low ejection fraction. In addition, cardioversion in asymptomatic patients may be reasonable when well-tolerated AF occurs near the time of anticipated hospital discharge or when it does not spontaneously terminate within 24 hours, so that oral anticoagulation can be avoided; especially in patients at high risk of bleeding.

An attempt at cardioversion with either electrical or pharmacologic therapy is reasonable. The choice between the two should be made on local practice and patient conditions. Electrical therapy of AF involves direct current external transthoracic cardioversion and it is effective in approximately 95% cases.[26] For patients where transthoracic cardioversion fails or is not feasible, pharmacologic therapy with intravenous sotalol or amiodarone is reasonable. The efficacy of antiarrhythmic drugs for reversion of postoperative AF is similar to that in AF not related to surgery.[27]

Rate Versus Rhythm Control

For patients who do not spontaneously revert to sinus rhythm within a few hours, rate control, and rhythm control (with or without electrical cardioversion) appear to be comparable strategies.[7] Advantages of a rate control strategy include the absence of side effects from drug therapy; disadvantages include a slower resolution of AF, thereby leading to a potentially greater need for anticoagulation at discharge.

ANTICOAGULATION

Patients on Long-term Anticoagulant

For AF patients on warfarin or direct oral anticoagulants, anticoagulation is stopped at least 3 days before surgery and restarted 3–5 days after surgery. Bridging with heparin therapy for patients at high risk of an embolic complication while off oral anticoagulant, must be balanced against increased bleeding risk.

Patients not Taking Anticoagulant Prior to Cardiac Surgery

Patients with AF or atrial flutter, regardless of the setting, are at risk for thromboembolic events. Thromboembolic risk is primarily limited to AF or atrial flutter of more than 48 hours duration and is greater in patients with certain high-risk features (rheumatic mitral valve disease, previous thromboembolism, hypertension, or heart failure, etc.).[27]

Patients who develop AF after cardiac surgery are at risk of thromboembolic events, including in-hospital stroke. However, in the individual postsurgical patient with an embolic event, the cause may be unclear, as underlying comorbidities are often responsible for such strokes, rather than the arrhythmia itself.[10] It is reasonable to believe that such therapy will lead to fewer embolic events in patients with postoperative AF but a reduction of events with anticoagulant therapy in this population has never been well studied.

The complications of anticoagulation were seen in observational studies of patients who were treated with intravenous heparin or oral anticoagulants.[28] When closely monitored, complication rates appear to be low. However, one report found a significant increase in large pericardial effusions and tamponade in patients treated with warfarin, particularly when the international normalized ratio (INR) was above the therapeutic target.[28] Thus, when anticoagulation is initiated, the patient must be monitored carefully. Similarly, the optimal duration of anticoagulation after hospital discharge is unknown. Among patients with new-onset AF after cardiac surgery, many will revert to and maintain sinus rhythm.[1,7]

As their therapeutic effect is not easily reversed, newer oral anticoagulants are not in routine clinical use in the early postoperative period. There are limited data at present, but this is an evolving strategy that may gain support as our understanding evolves.[29]

Evidence is emerging that the left atrial appendage may play a major role in the development of stroke and interventional/surgical elimination may obviate the need for anticoagulation. However, there are insufficient data at this time to support routine surgical elimination.

Approach to Postoperative Anticoagulation

Among patients who develop AF following cardiac surgery, the following approach to anticoagulation may be considered. For patients with multiple episodes of AF or one episode that lasts more than 24–48 hours, oral anticoagulant therapy should be started, but only if bleeding risks are considered acceptable. As the role of direct thrombin and factor Xa inhibitors has not been established for patients with postoperative AF, warfarin should be chosen for most patients (INR 2.0–3.0).

Anticoagulation should be continued for at least 4 weeks after return to sinus rhythm, particularly if the patient has risk factors for thromboembolism. Longer duration of anticoagulation is recommended by some in patients with high CHADS-VASc scores, at low-risk for bleeding based on the HAS-BLED score, or at high-risk of AF recurrence. Long-term anticoagulation should be considered for patients who remain in AF or who have paroxysmal AF at 4 weeks. Oral anticoagulation should be continued in patients in which a concomitant Cox–Maze procedure has been performed for at least 3 months, regardless of no postoperative atrial arrhythmias. After 3 months with no AF recurrence, anticoagulation may be interrupted, considering the patient risk profile for stroke by the CHADS-VASc score.[30]

In most cases, intravenous heparin is not used as a bridge to full oral anticoagulation, as the risk of postoperative bleeding outweighs the small benefit from stroke prevention. For patients with prior systemic or pulmonary embolization or those with a mechanical valve, bridging anticoagulation with heparin may be reasonable. Both intravenous and oral anticoagulation should be monitored closely, as bleeding complications, including pericardial effusion and tamponade increase with excessive anticoagulation.

REFERENCES

1. Maisel WH, Rawn JD, Stevenson WG. Atrial fibrillation after cardiac surgery. Ann Intern Med. 2001;135:1061-73.
2. Cox JL. A perspective of postoperative atrial fibrillation in cardiac operations. Ann Thorac Surg. 1993;56:405-9.
3. Amar D, Shi W, Hogue CW Jr, et al. Clinical prediction rule for atrial fibrillation after coronary artery bypass grafting. J Am Coll Cardiol. 2004;44:1248-53.
4. Kosmidou I, Chen S, Kappetein AP, et al. New-Onset Atrial Fibrillation After PCI or CABG for Left Main Disease: The EXCEL Trial. J Am Coll Cardiol. 2018;71:739-48.
5. Mathew JP, Fontes ML, Tudor IC, et al. A multicenter risk index for atrial fibrillation after cardiac surgery. JAMA. 2004;291:1720-9.
6. Soucier RJ, Mirza S, Abordo MG, et al. Predictors of conversion of atrial fibrillation after cardiac operation in the absence of class I or III antiarrhythmic medications. Ann Thorac Surg. 2001;72:694-7.
7. Lee JK, Klein GJ, Krahn AD, et al. Rate-control versus conversion strategy in postoperative atrial fibrillation: a prospective, randomized pilot study. Am Heart J. 2000;140:871-7.
8. Ambrosetti M, Tramarin R, Griffo R, et al. Late postoperative atrial fibrillation after cardiac surgery: a national survey within the cardiac rehabilitation setting. J Cardiovasc Med (Hagerstown). 2011;12:390-5.
9. Arsenault KA, Yusuf AM, Crystal E, et al. Interventions for preventing post-operative atrial fibrillation in patients undergoing heart surgery. Cochrane Database Syst Rev. 2013;(1):CD003611.
10. Crystal E, Garfinkle MS, Connolly SS, et al. Interventions for preventing post-operative atrial fibrillation in patients undergoing heart surgery. Cochrane Database Syst Rev. 2004;(4):CD003611.
11. DiNicolantonio JJ, Beavers CJ, Menezes AR, et al. Meta-analysis comparing carvedilol versus metoprolol for the prevention of postoperative atrial fibrillation following coronary artery bypass grafting. Am J Cardiol. 2014;113:565-9.
12. Kerin NZ, Jacob S. The efficacy of sotalol in preventing postoperative atrial fibrillation: a meta-analysis. Am J Med. 2011;124:875. e1-9.
13. Burgess DC, Kilborn MJ, Keech AC. Interventions for prevention of postoperative atrial fibrillation and its complications after cardiac surgery: a meta-analysis. Eur Heart J. 2006;27:2846-57.
14. Mitchell LB, Exner DV, Wyse DG, et al. Prophylactic Oral Amiodarone for the Prevention of Arrhythmias that Begin Early After Revascularization, Valve Replacement, or Repair: PAPABEAR: a randomized controlled trial. JAMA. 2005;294:3093-100.
15. Halonen J, Loponen P, Järvinen O, et al. Metoprolol versus amiodarone in the prevention of atrial fibrillation after cardiac surgery: a randomized trial. Ann Intern Med. 2010;153:703-9.

16. Harling L, Rasoli S, Vecht JA, et al. Do antioxidant vitamins have an anti-arrhythmic effect following cardiac surgery? A meta-analysis of randomised controlled trials. Heart. 2011;97(20):1636-42.
17. Weiner B, Rheinlander HF, Decker EL, et al. Digoxin prophylaxis following coronary artery bypass surgery. Clin Pharm. 1986;5:55-8.
18. Gold MR, O'Gara PT, Buckley MJ, et al. Efficacy and safety of procainamide in preventing arrhythmias after coronary artery bypass surgery. Am J Cardiol. 1996;78:975-9.
19. Davison R, Hartz R, Kaplan K, et al. Prophylaxis of supraventricular tachyarrhythmia after coronary bypass surgery with oral verapamil: a randomized, double-blind trial. Ann Thorac Surg. 1985;39:336-9.
20. Bandeali SJ, Kayani WT, Lee W, et al. Outcomes of preoperative angiotensin-converting enzyme inhibitor therapy in patients undergoing isolated coronary artery bypass grafting. Am J Cardiol. 2012;110:919-23.
21. Liakopoulos OJ, Kuhn EW, Slottosch I, et al. Preoperative statin therapy for patients undergoing cardiac surgery. Cochrane Database Syst Rev. 2012;(4):CD008493.
22. Zheng Z, Jayaram R, Jiang L, et al. Perioperative Rosuvastatin in Cardiac Surgery. N Engl J Med 2016; 374:1744-53.
23. Imazio M, Brucato A, Ferrazzi P, et al. Colchicine for prevention of postpericardiotomy syndrome and postoperative atrial fibrillation: the COPPS-2 randomized clinical trial. JAMA. 2014;312:1016-23.
24. Horbach SJ, Lopes RD, da C Guaragna JC, et al. Naproxen as prophylaxis against atrial fibrillation after cardiac surgery: the NAFARM randomized trial. Am J Med. 2011;124:1036-42.
25. Whitlock RP, Devereaux PJ, Teoh KH, et al. Methylprednisolone in patients undergoing cardiopulmonary bypass (SIRS): a randomised, double-blind, placebo-controlled trial. Lancet. 2015; 386:1243-53.
26. European Heart Rhythm Association, European Association for Cardio-Thoracic Surgery, Camm AJ, et al. Guidelines for the management of atrial fibrillation: the Task Force for the Management of Atrial Fibrillation of the European Society of Cardiology (ESC). Eur Heart J. 2010;31:2369-429.
27. European Heart Rhythm Association; Heart Rhythm Society, Fuster V, et al. ACC/AHA/ESC 2006 Guidelines for the Management of Patients With Atrial Fibrillation A Report of the American College of Cardiology/American Heart Association Task Force on Practice Guidelines and the European Society of Cardiology Committee for Practice Guidelines (Writing Committee to Revise the 2001 Guidelines for the Management of Patients With Atrial Fibrillation). J Am Coll Cardiol. 2006;48:854-906.
28. Malouf JF, Alam S, Gharzeddine W, et al. The role of anticoagulation in the development of pericardial effusion and late tamponade after cardiac surgery. Eur Heart J. 1993;14:1451-7.
29. Anderson E, Johnke K, Leedahl D, et al. Novel oral anticoagulants vs warfarin for the management of postoperative atrial fibrillation: clinical outcomes and cost analysis. Am J Surg. 2015;210:1095-102.
30. Dunning J, Nagendran M, Alfieri OR, et al. Guideline for the surgical treatment of atrial fibrillation. Eur J Cardiothorac Surg. 2013;44:777-91.

CHAPTER 108

Managing Antithrombotics after Percutaneous Coronary Intervention in Atrial Fibrillation: Current Recommendations

Sundeep Mishra

INTRODUCTION

The management of patients who have undergone percutaneous coronary intervention (PCI) and already have atrial fibrillation (AF) is a challenging problem but is quite common. Broadly, there are three issues in the management paradigm; risk of stent thrombosis (ST) poststent implantation, risk of ischemic stroke due to embolization of clot (formed commonly in left atrial appendage) as a result of irregular rate alterations in AF and risk of bleeding consequent to use of antiplatelets or anticoagulants. Optimal therapy in this group comprises of striking a balance between these three concerns (Fig. 1). These risks can vary depending on patient's condition, lesion condition, and time after procedure and thus therapy may require to be individualized according to individual patients and temporal profile. AF is the most common arrhythmia and nearly one-third of patients of AF have coronary artery disease (CAD) and nearly one-tenth of all AF patients undergo PCI.[1] On the other hand, it has been estimated that approximately 5–7% of patients undergoing PCI also have AF or other indications for chronic oral anticoagulant (OAC) therapy.[2-5] Thus the matter is not trivial but requires a careful consideration. The crux of the matter is that post PCI with stenting patients require dual antiplatelet therapy (DAPT) to prevent ST but those having AF require anticoagulation to prevent stroke and other thromboembolic events. Thus triple antithrombotic (TAT) is a logical outcome. However, TAT is associated with a significant bleeding risk. Thus the issue at hand is whether TAT is necessary? If necessary which anticoagulant to use; vitamin K antagonist (VKA) or nonvitamin K oral anticoagulant (NOAC)? Which antiplatelet to use aspirin (ASA), clopidogrel, prasugrel, or ticagrelor or a combination of them? If combination, which combination? Finally, how long should TAT be continued, and what next?

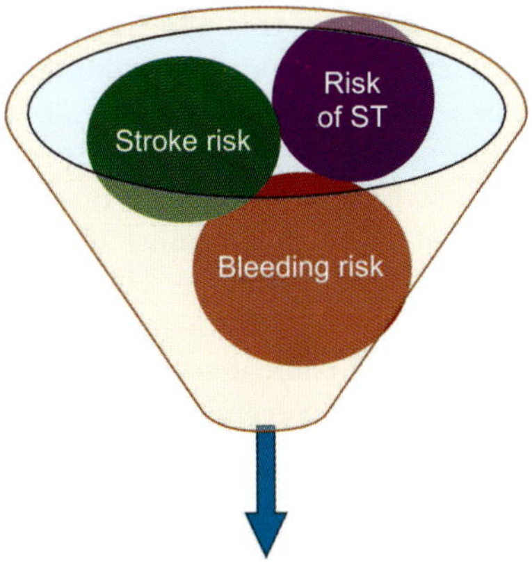

AF, atrial fibrillation; PCI, percutaneous coronary intervention; ST, stent thrombosis.

FIG. 1: Issues at stake in patients with atrial fibrillation undergoing percutaneous coronary intervention.

WHY RISK OF THROMBOSIS AFTER PERCUTANEOUS CORONARY INTERVENTION?

Currently PCI is invariably associated with stent or scaffold deployment. During the course of stent deployment, significant trauma and damage to the endothelium can occur during the procedure. Subsequently, struts of the stent or scaffold are exposed to flowing blood in the coronary artery promoting platelet activation and aggregation and thus contributing to a milieu of arterial thrombosis, the risk persisting till the time endothelialization of exposed struts happen. Finally, PCI is often carried out in the context of acute coronary syndrome or acute myocardial infarction (AMI), conditions per se which can increase risk of arterial thrombosis (Box 1).

BOX 1 Risk of vascular thrombosis after percutaneous coronary intervention

Risk of thrombosis associated with percutaneous coronary intervention
- Acute arterial vessel injury during percutaneous coronary intervention procedure
- Risk of stent thrombosis after procedure
- Risk of arterial thrombosis associated with accompanying acute coronary syndrome

WHY RISK OF STROKE AFTER ONSET OF ATRIAL FIBRILLATION?

Blood flow is usually sluggish in the venous chambers and top chambers of the heart (atrial part) which can lead to formation of blood clots, particularly in left atrial appendage. During onset of AF or with change in heart rate associated with AF, a piece of a clot can break off. This clot commonly travels to the brain to cause a stroke, but it can travel to other organs in body as well.

HOW TO PREVENT THROMBOSIS IN PATIENT UNDERGOING PERCUTANEOUS CORONARY INTERVENTION?

Potent antiplatelets are required to prevent ST. ASA (ASA) can inhibit both platelet activation and aggregation, the mechanism primarily involves irreversible inhibition of the platelet-dependent enzyme cyclooxygenase (COX). One of the isoenzymes COX-1 (inhibited by ASA) is a powerful inhibitor of thromboxane A2 (TxA2). TxA2 promotes platelet aggregation and vasoconstriction. During platelet activation, the hydrolysis of membrane phospholipids yields arachidonic acid, which is converted to prostaglandin H2 by the catalytic activity of the COX enzyme prostaglandin G/H synthase. By the selective and irreversible acetylation of a single serine residue within prostaglandin G/H synthase, ASA causes the inactivation of COX activity (Flowchart 1). In coronary tree platelet activation and aggregation lead to activation of clotting cascade contributing to acute vascular closure and myocardial infarction (MI). Besides inhibition of TxA2, ASA may act by many other favorable mechanisms as well; inhibition of COX-dependent vasoconstrictors, inhibition of endothelial dysfunction, inhibition of the production of endothelial-produced prostacyclin (a vasodilator and inhibitor of platelet aggregation), inhibition of inflammation and even inhibition of TxA2 biosynthesis (Box 2).[6] Unlike platelets, endothelial cells recover their ability to synthesize prostacyclin within a couple of hours. As a result of its potent action ASA has been widely accepted as a cornerstone therapy in reducing ischemic complications after balloon angioplasty or stent implantation. The therapy should be initiated before the advent of procedure and continued lifelong (preferably) after the procedure.[7-12] Regarding the optimal dose of ASA for prevention of MI, stroke, or vascular death following PCI, a narrow range of 75-160 mg/day seems enough as nearly complete inhibition of COX-1 can occur at this dose.[13,14] During PCI, platelet activation leads to platelet aggregation which can lead to activation of coagulation cascade. ASA inhibits platelet aggregation by inhibiting the production of TxA2. However, there could be other mechanisms of platelet aggregation besides COX dependant pathway; particularly adenosine diphosphate (ADP)-mediated pathways (Fig. 2). ASA alone has no effect on this pathway and thus platelet aggregation may still happen despite optimal ASA therapy. Furthermore, in certain instances inability of ASA to reduce TXA2 production culminating in inability to prolong bleeding time, or producing typical in vitro effects on platelet function resulting in lack of protection against thrombotic events, an effect known as ASA resistance.[15,16] The prevalence of ASA resistance is highly variable (5–60%) depending on the population studied, the clinical situation and the method employed for testing.[15-17] Several mechanisms have been implicated in development of ASA resistance; genetic polymorphisms of COX 1, enhanced platelet turnover, genetic polymorphism of other genes involved in Tx biosynthesis, upregulation of nonplatelet sources of Tx, and drug interactions (Box 3).[15,18,19] Thus it is clear that there is a requirement of other inhibitors of platelet function to achieve optimal antithrombotic effect. Dipyridamole interferes with platelet-stimulating factors like collagen through various mechanisms including the inhibition of phosphodiesterase and inhibition of cellular uptake of adenosine. However, its benefit in context

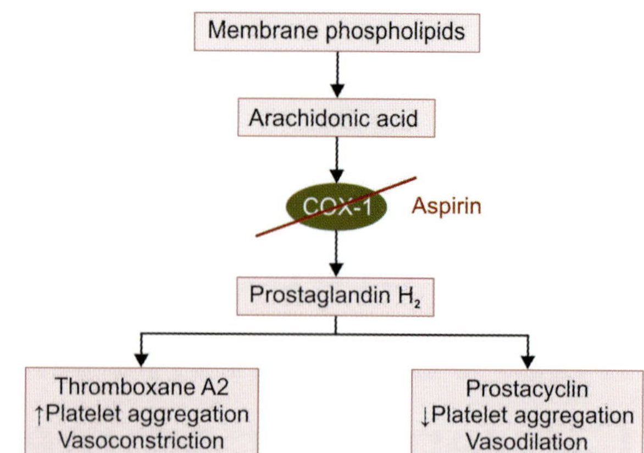

FLOWCHART 1: Mechanism of action of aspirin.

BOX 2 Mechanism of action of aspirin in preventing coronary ischemia

Mechanism of action of aspirin
- Inhibiting COX-1 mediated activation of TxA2 and thus inhibiting platelet aggregation
- Inhibiting COX mediated vasoconstrictors, reducing endothelial dysfunction
- Inhibition of the production of endothelial-produced prostacyclin (a vasodilator and inhibitor of platelet aggregation)
- Inhibition of inflammation
- Inhibiting TxA2 biosynthesis

COX, cyclooxygenase; TxA2, thromboxane A2.

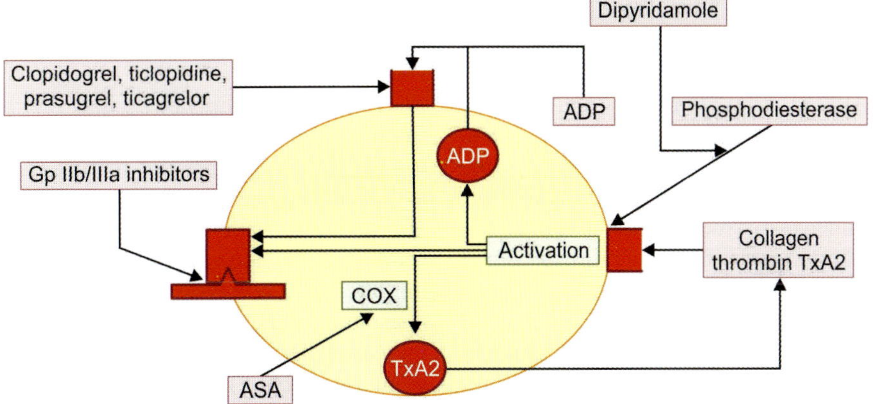

ASA, aspirin; ADP, adenosine diphosphate; COX, cyclooxygenase; TxA2, thromboxane A2.

FIG. 2: Mechanism of platelet activation and aggregation.

BOX 3 Mechanism of aspirin resistance

Mechanism of aspirin resistance
- Genetic polymorphisms of COX-1 upregulation of non-platelet sources of Tx and drug interactions
- Enhanced platelet turnover
- Genetic polymorphism of other genes involved in Tx biosynthesis
- Upregulation of nonplatelet sources of Tx
- Drug interactions

COX, cyclooxygenase; Tx, thromboxane.

of PCI is not established. Cochrane review of 29 randomized trials involving 23,019 patients could demonstrate no benefit for the combination of ASA with dipyridamole in context of CAD.[20] Cilostazol is another agent (2-oxoquinoline derivative) which possesses vasodilatory and antithrombotic effects as well as antiproliferative properties, useful in reducing smooth muscle cell proliferation and neointimal hyperplasia after endothelial injury. However, no large scale study is available demonstrating its usefulness in the current context. On the other hand, the P2Y12 receptor antagonists (clopidogrel, prasugrel, and ticagrelor) which bind and inhibit ADP receptors on platelets, thereby, inhibiting glycoprotein IIb/IIIa-receptor activation and subsequent platelet aggregation (Fig. 3). Ticlopidine was the first generation thienopyridine but its use was seriously limited as a result of bone marrow toxicity and was largely replaced by clopidogrel which till recently had become standard of care in patients undergoing PCI.[21] The level of platelet aggregation inhibition (via ADP-induced pathway), by usual doses of clopidogrel (50 100 mg), when steady state is reached is around 50–60% but this state is achieved only after 4–7 days. The clinical benefit of a combination of ASA and clopidogrel over ASA alone has been confirmed in various clinical situations after PCI; clopidogrel for the reduction of events during observation

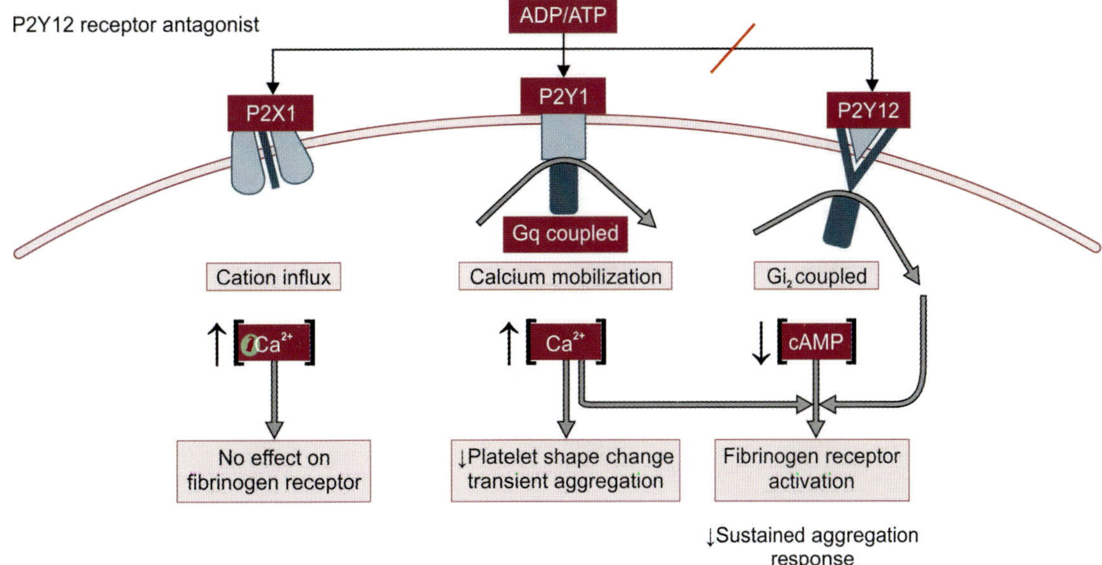

cAMP, cyclic adenosine monophosphate; ADP, adenosine diphosphate; ATP, adenosine triphosphate.

FIG. 3: Mechanism of action of P2Y12 receptor antagonists.

(CREDO), clopidogrel and metoprolol myocardial infarction trial (COMMIT) [within 12 hours of ST-elevation myocardial infarction (STEMI)], and clopidogrel as adjunctive reperfusion therapy (CLARITY) trial (within 24 hours of STEMI).[22-24] However, clopidogrel itself has its own set of limitations. One of them is slow onset of action. There is some evidence that use of a 600-mg rather than a 300-mg loading dose of clopidogrel would lead to a more rapid onset of action and greater platelet inhibition and reduce the rate of ST albeit at the cost of some increase in major bleeding.[25,26] Another limitation of clopidogrel therapy is high on-treatment platelet reactivity or platelet resistance. It is known to occur in nearly one-third of patients and has been associated with 1.5–5 times increased risk of ST. The prevalence varies according to presence of comorbidities (dyslipidemias, diabetes mellitus, etc.), use of proton pump inhibitors (omeprazole), and concomitant therapies (atorvastatin, calcium channel blockers, etc.). The mechanism of this resistance could be insufficient active metabolite generation (clopidogrel being a prodrug) particularly from effect on CYP450 isoenzymes (2C19, 1A2, 2B6, 2C9, 3A4), either extraneous influences or genetic polymorphisms.[27-29] Indeed in a meta-analysis of nine studies [9,685 patients with acute coronary syndrome (ACS) or undergoing PCI], Mega and co-worker demonstrated a 55% increase in risk of MI, stroke, or cardiovascular death in carriers with one loss of function CYP2C19 allele and an increase of 76% with two loss of function alleles, both statistically significant compared to noncarriers. Overall, more than 7/10 subjects were noncarriers, more than 1/4 had one reduced-function CYP2C19 allele, and more than 2% had two reduced-function CYP2C19 alleles.[30]

These limitations of clopidogrel therapy have led to an ongoing search for a better thienopyridine; more efficacious, faster onset of action and more predictable response. Prasugrel, another prodrug of the same group, has a more rapid onset of action, a complete inhibition of ADP-induced platelet aggregation and has a more consistent response compared with clopidogrel.[31,32] Prasugrel has been found efficacious and safe in clinical studies as well. The trial to assess improvement in therapeutic outcomes by optimizing platelet inhibition with prasugrel-thrombolysis in myocardial infarction 38 (TRITON-TIMI 38) demonstrated that there was a 19% reduction in the composite primary outcome of MI, stroke, or cardiovascular death [9.9% vs. 12.1%; 95% confidence interval (CI): 0.73–0.90] as well as a significant reduction of ST (1.1% vs. 2.4%, p = 0.001) without an increase in major, life-threatening, or fatal bleeding with prasugrel therapy compared with standard clopidogrel therapy (300 mg loading dose followed by 75 mg/day).[33] Interestingly this study revealed a greater benefit of this therapy in patients undergoing primary PCI, a contest where rapid and complete inhibition of platelets is of vital importance, also highlighting the limitation of clopidogrel in this setting. Another situation where prasugrel is remarkably effective vis-à-vis clopidogrel is diabetes mellitus, a context of high clopidogrel resistance as well as one where complete platelet inhibition is required. This drug is associated with increase of minor bleeding but is contraindicated in patients with active bleeding or history of stroke or transient ischemic attack (TIA) and used with caution in older (>75 years age) or thinner individuals (<60 kg weight).

Ticagrelor is the newest kid on the block among the thienopyridines. It scores in many ways above clopidogrel: it is an active drug (does not require biotransformation to be active); it has a significantly shorter delay of action (requiring only an hour to achieve maximal platelet reactivity inhibition vis-à-vis 6–12 hours with clopidogrel; it is a more potent inhibitor, has a very-low interpatient variability (ticagrelor resistance is ~3% only), has vasodilatory effects (mediated via increased ADP) and has a shorter duration of action (inhibition being reversible). The shorter duration of action (3 days vs. 5 days with clopidogrel) can be useful when the patient is due for emergency surgery or those experiencing bleeding.[34-37] In the Platelet Inhibition and Patient Outcomes (PLATO) trial testing efficacy of ticagrelor with clopidogrel standard therapy in patients of ACS and STEMI ticagrelor was associated with a significant reduction in ischemic events (MI, ST, and total mortality). Interestingly mortality reduction was to the tune of 22% (p <0.01), a first by any thienopyridine. However, the only limitation with ticagrelor Rx was increased rate of non-CABG-related major bleeding (2.8 vs. 2.2%; p = 0.03) although the overall rate of major bleeding remained same.[38] In another landmark trial, prevention of cardiovascular events in patients with prior heart attack using ticagrelor compared to placebo on a background of ASA (PEGASUS) trial the effect of different doses of ticagrelor (60 mg, 90 mg) was compared with placebo (the other drug in all arms being ASA) in a subset of patients with a higher risk. Over nearly 3 years of follow-up, both doses of ticagrelor (combined with ASA) were superior to ASA alone in preventing ischemic complications (MI, stroke, or death) over a prolonged duration of DAPT Rx. Expectedly, risk of nonCABG TIMI bleed was higher in ticagrelor groups but interestingly, the lower dose of ticagrelor had similar ischemic benefit but a reduced risk of bleeding.[39,40] This raises the possibility of prolonged use of DAPT with low-dose ticagrelor in patients with higher ischemic risk.

HOW TO PREVENT STROKE IN A PATIENT WITH ATRIAL FIBRILLATION?

Atrial fibrillation is the most common arrhythmia afflicting mankind (up to 2% of world suffers from it and after age of 40 years nearly one-fourth of the population will develop it).[41,42] It also one of the most important risk factor for stroke, which happens to be one of the leading causes of cerebrovascular mortality worldwide.[43] It is a common knowledge that the stroke rate among patients with nonvalvular AF is 5% per annum (with valvular AF particularly in context of severe mitral stenosis it is much higher) but what is not that well known is the fact that nearly 50% of patients with AF-related stroke die within 1-year.[44] Even if they survive, stroke has a devastating effect on patients, their families and careers and a significant financial impact on the national economy. Costs of this disease escalate far beyond mere cost of medication; cost of long-term care for the living and the financial impact of lost productivity. However, the

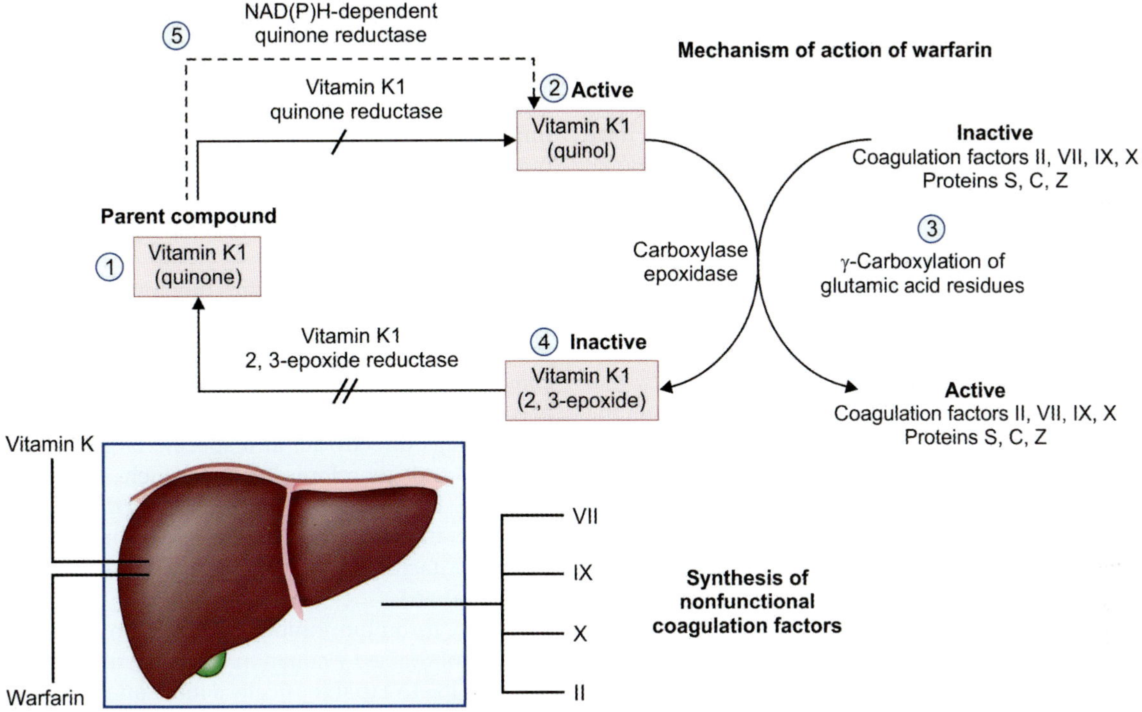

FIG. 4: Mechanism of action of vitamin K antagonists.

risk of stroke varies between different patient subgroups and associated comorbidities. Likewise the bleeding risk also varies among the patient groups and disease situations. The crux of optimal therapy is striking the right balance between ischemic risk of stroke and the underlying bleeding risk.

Vitamin K antagonists have remained the cornerstone of therapy for stroke prevention in AF till recently. They act by depleting the active form of the vitamin by inhibiting reversibly the enzyme vitamin K epoxide reductase and thus the recycling of the inactive vitamin K epoxide back to the active reduced form of vitamin K. Vitamin K is required for the carboxylation of clotting proteins II (carboxylate-specific glutamic acid residues on prothrombin), VII, IX, and X. Without adequate levels of vitamin K, the liver produces partially carboxylated and decarboxylated clotting proteins, which have reduced procoagulant activity. Vitamin K is required for the synthesis of certain proteins. Without these carboxylated residues, the protein will not form the appropriate conformation of thrombin (and other components of the pathway), an essential component of blood clotting process. Thus, no fibrin monomers will form that are polymerized to form blood clots (Fig. 4).[45] Being reversible (competitive inhibition) in nature, the action of this class of anticoagulants may be reversed by administering vitamin K for the duration of the anticoagulant's residence in the body, and the daily dose needed for reversal is the same for all drugs in the class. Coumarins or coumadins (more accurately 4-hydroxycoumarins) are the most commonly used VKAs, and warfarin is the most commonly used coumarin. Numerous trials have shown benefit of warfarin in stroke prevention in AF (SPAF) and a recent meta-analysis involving six randomized controlled trials (RCTs) of both primary and secondary patients, enrolling more than 2,500 individuals; atrial fibrillation ASA and anticoagulation (AFASAK), Boston area anticoagulation trial for atrial fibrillation (BAATAF), Canadian atrial fibrillation anticoagulation (CAFA), stroke prevention in atrial fibrillation (SPAF) I, stroke prevention in nonrheumatic atrial fibrillation (SPINAF), and European atrial fibrillation trial (EAFT) confirm the same. Overall, with use VKA the risk of nonfatal stroke was reduced by two-thirds and mortality by one-fourth (vs. no treatment).[46-52] However, since VKAs also increase the risk of bleeding, particularly major, nonfatal, noncranial bleeding its use in patients with low risk [$CHADS_2$ score (congestive heart failure, hypertension, age ≥75 years, diabetes mellitus, stroke) 0], may not be mandated. Acenocoumarol is another coumarin group of drugs available in some countries like India. It may have some pharmacokinetic and pharmacodynamic benefits over warfarin (Box 4).

Antiplatelets acts by inhibiting platelet aggregation, a step in coagulation cascade, active after formation of fibrin clots. Thus it is not surprising that several RCTs

BOX 4 **Difference of acenocoumarol compared with warfarin**

Acenocoumarol (acitrom)

Same as warfarin with following differences:

- Shorter half life 10–16 h
- More rapid onset of action on PT
- Shorter duration of action (2 days)
- Causes gastrointestinal disturbances, oral ulcerations, and dermatitis
- Total 4 mg on day one, 4–8 mg on the day 2nd then maintenance dose 1–8 mg according to response by PT test

have demonstrated that antiplatelet monotherapy could contribute to one-fifth reduction in risk of nonfatal stroke (vs. No Rx).[46,49,51,53-57] However, data from analysis of six primary prevention trials and a meta-analysis of 60 secondary prevention trials, enrolling nearly 200,000 patients have revealed that ASA increases the risk of nonfatal, noncranial bleeding by 50%.[58,59] On the other hand, adjusted-dose warfarin may be far superior to ASA for the prevention of stroke in patients with AF but at the same time is likely to be associated with a greater bleeding risk. A meta-analysis involving 11 RCTs and 6,526 patients (comparing adjusted-dose VKA therapy to antiplatelet monotherapy) has revealed that VKA therapy led to reduction in risk of stroke by half although it simultaneously increased risk of major bleeding 2–2.5-fold.[60-70] Thus, if ischemic risk is higher; $CHADS_2$ above 0, VKA may be preferred. On the other hand, if risk is low ($CHADS_2 = 0$), ASA may be preferred.

Use of DAPT in AF can be considered in patients who are unsuitable for oral anticoagulant therapy. A combination of ASA and clopidogrel (DAPT) versus ASA alone, in the atrial fibrillation clopidogrel trial with irbesartan for prevention of vascular events (ACTIVE) A trial enrolling 7,554 patients has revealed that DAPT is more effective in reducing the risk of nonfatal stroke, albeit with increased risk of nonfatal, noncranial major bleeding.[71]

Vitamin K antagonists are fairly effective in stroke prevention; however, there are many serious downsides to this therapy. The standard risk of major bleeding with this therapy is 1–4% per year (in ambulatory pts. 4–9% per year), with an intracranial bleeding (IC bleed) rate of 0.2–0.5% per year. Further, the bleeding risk increases dramatically when the international normalized ratio (INR) exceeds 4.0 and as a matter of fact warfarin-induced out-of-range INR is the most important risk factor for IC bleeds, thus entailing the need for frequent monitoring of INR. Thus VKAs are beset with so many serious issues that it is under use worldwide is not surprising and its use is considered "a disease in itself" by some physicians.

As a result anticoagulant therapy for AF is evolving rapidly with the development of newer oral anticoagulants that mechanistically directly target different levels of the coagulation pathway but at the same time have a more predictable efficacy, thus not requiring INR monitoring. These drugs directly act at a specific target on coagulation cascade and therefore have a much more predictable outcome (Fig. 5). Currently the following drugs are available:

- Direct thrombin inhibitors (dabigatran)
- Direct factor Xa inhibitors (apixaban, rivaroxaban, and edoxaban).

Direct thrombin inhibitor, dabigatran was found useful in the randomized evaluation of long-term a nticoagulation therapy (RE-LY) trial (basically a meta-analysis of three RCTs enrolling >18,000 patients and testing two doses of dabigatran; 110 mg and 150 mg) compared with dose adjusted warfarin (target INR 2.0–3.0). Data revealed that it was high-dose dabigatran (150 mg) which was associated with one-third reduction in nonfatal stroke with no increase in nonfatal, noncranial bleeding. Interestingly, there was even a trend

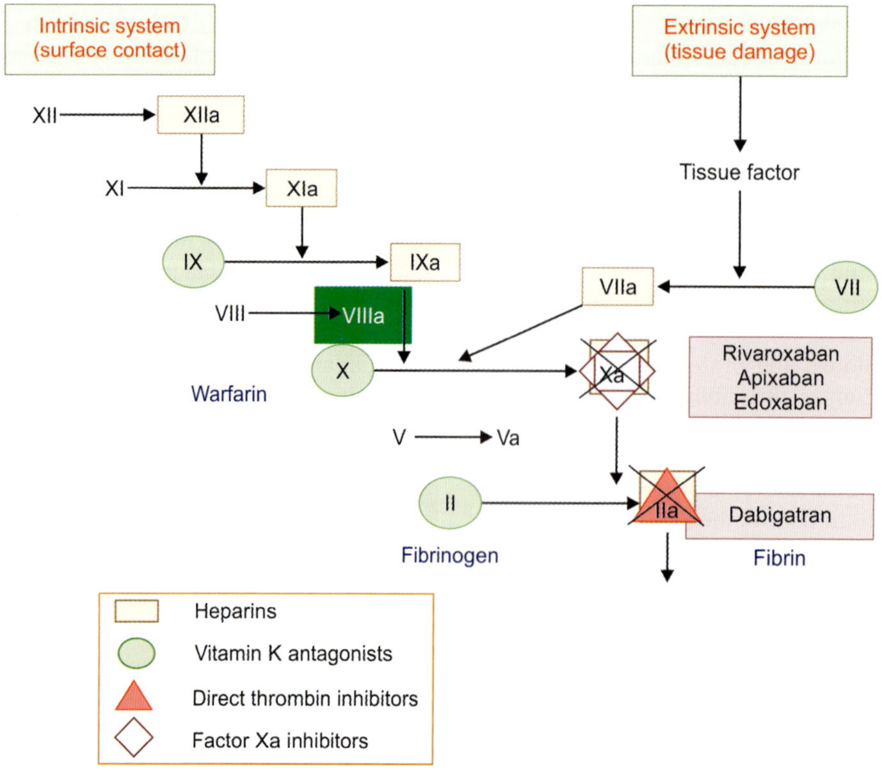

FIG. 5: Mechanism of action of anticoagulant drugs.

toward mortality reduction (11%) in these patients.[72] Likewise, apixaban for the prevention of stroke in subjects with atrial fibrillation (ARISTOTLE) trial, a double-blind, double-dummy RCT, enrolling >18,000 patients with AF, and comparing 10 mg daily apixaban to warfarin (target INR 2.0–3.0) revealed that a use of apixaban led to 21% reduction in risk of ischemic or hemorrhagic stroke but also 31% reduction in risk of major bleeding (vs. warfarin). Furthermore all-cause mortality was 11% lower with apixaban.[73] On the other hand, the rivaroxaban once daily oral direct factor Xa inhibition compared with vitamin K antagonism for prevention of stroke and embolism trial in atrial fibrillation (ROCKET-AF), a double-blind RCT, enrolling >14,000 was not superior to warfarin (INR 2–3) with an increased risk of major GI bleeding (3.2% and 2.2%, respectively, $p < 0.001$), although overall major bleeding was no different. There was no effect on mortality.[74] However, in all the three trials use of newer nonvitamin K oral coagulants versus warfarin, the rate of IC-hemorrhage was lower.[72-76]

HOW TO BALANCE RISKS AND BENEFITS IN PATIENT OF ATRIAL FIBRILLATION UNDERGOING PERCUTANEOUS CORONARY INTERVENTION

Since antiplatelet drugs have some anticoagulant effect and anticoagulant drugs have some antiplatelet effects, theoretically it might be reasonable to assume that using one class of drug may be sufficient for both activities (Fig. 6). However, it has to be understood that antithrombotic drugs act predominantly in reducing arterial thrombosis (consequent upon PCI) whereas anticoagulants are predominantly effective in reducing venous thrombosis [precursor of stroke and thromboembolic events (TE) complications of AF]. The effect of one therapeutic modality on the other one is very weak at best. It is thus clear that a combination of both agents would be required to appropriately address risk of this complex situation.[77,78] Indeed, early guidelines suggested TAT strategy for patient of AF undergoing PCI with stent implantation.[79,80] However, TAT, while vary efficacious for ischemic and thromboembolic complications, carries a nearly 3-fold increase in risk of bleeding. Indeed, several trails and later network meta-analysis revealed that risk of bleeding from TAT was the highest.[81-97] Analysis of RCTs in this area also revealed same general findings.[98-101]

It is clear that a combination will be required which will balance all the risks associated with arterial thrombosis, venous thrombosis and bleeding risks. Thus, it is important to understand the risk benefits associated with individual drugs; antiplatelet or anticoagulants. The comparison of these drugs for various risks (from highest to least) is as follows.

Anti-ischemic Risk

The anti-ischemic risk is as follows ASA > NOACs > VKA > clopidogrel > ticagrelor > prasugrel (Table 1 and Fig. 7).

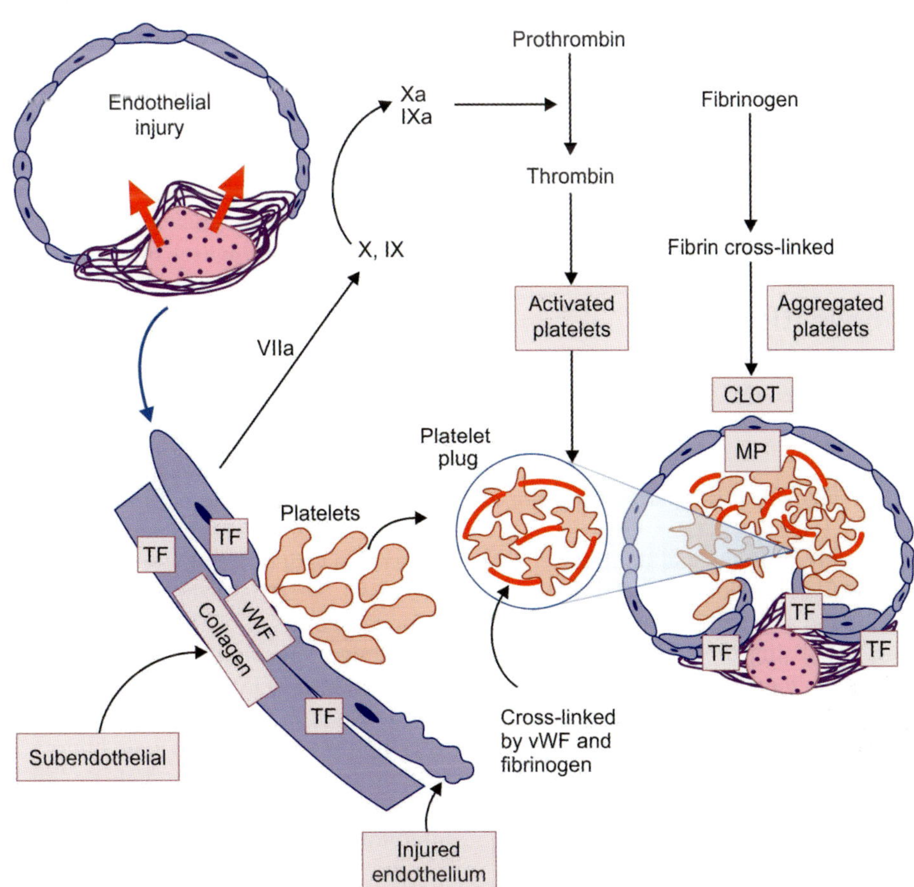

FIG. 6: Mechanism of formation of blood clot.

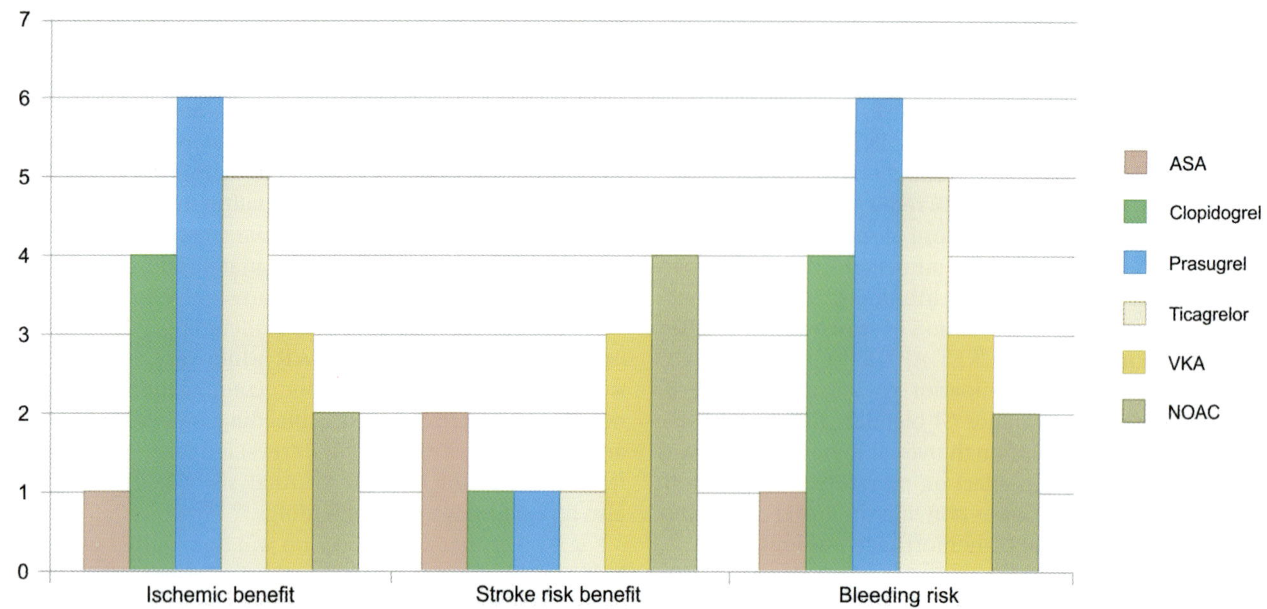

ASA, aspirin; NOAC, nonvitamin K oral anticoagulant; VKA, vitamin K antagonist.

FIG. 7: Risk and benefits of individual antiplatelet and anticoagulant agents.

TABLE 1: Risk and benefits of individual antiplatelet and anticoagulant agents

Drugs	Ischemic benefit	Thromboembolic benefit	Bleeding risk
Aspirin	+	++	+
Clopidogrel	++++	+	++++
Prasugrel	++++++	+	+ +++++
Ticagrelor	+++++	+	+++++
VKA	+++	+++	+++
NOAC	++	++++	++

VKA, vitamin K antagonist; NOAC, nonvitamin K antagonist oral anticoagulants.

Antithromboembolic Risk

The stroke risk and other thromboembolic risk as follows clopidogrel, ticagrelor, prasugrel > VKA > NOAC (Fig. 7).

Bleeding Risk

The bleeding risk is as follows: prasugrel > ticagrelor > clopidogrel > VKA > NOAC (Fig. 7).

While risk benefit profile of individual antiplatelet and anticoagulant may be useful in predicting the profile of their combinations, there could be some variations. For example, while TATs should be possessing most efficacy, in reality their efficacy can be lower than a combination of DAPT and low-dose NOAC. The reason could be that because of increased bleeding risk, during the time of bleeding, effective antithrombotic therapy may be discontinued contributing to increased ischemic risk. The anti-ischemic benefit and bleeding risk (from least to highest) are as follows.

Thrombotic Risk

The antithrombotic benefit (ST + stroke) is as follows:

DAPT < TAT < VKA + P2Y12 inhibitor < DAPT + low dose NOAC < NOAC (full dose) + P2Y12 inhibitor.

Bleeding Risk

The bleeding risk is as follows: DAPT< VKA + P2Y12 inhibitor < DAPT + low dose NOAC < NOAC (full dose) + P2Y12 inhibitor < TAT (Table 2 and Fig. 8).

It is clear from the above discussion that DAPT has the least antithrombotic efficacy (particularly low against stroke) and TAT has the highest bleeding risk (at least 505 more than any dual combination). As such both are not suitable for this complex subset. Full dose NOAC + P2Y12 inhibitor has a high bleeding risk as well (although this combination has the highest thrombotic efficacy). Low dose NOAC with DAPT has higher antithrombotic efficacy compared to VKA + P2Y12 inhibitor but it has higher bleeding risk as well. Thus a clinician has generally two options: If the risk of ST is high; left main disease, bifurcation disease, ACS, diabetes mellitus etc., low dose NOAC with DAPT may be chosen. On the other hand in a garden variety of PCI, VKA + P2Y12 inhibitor therapy may be chosen. [98,99] It has to be understood that as far as bleeding is concerned, VKA + P2Y12 inhibitor therapy only decreases risk of minor bleeding, so unless background bleeding risk is high low-dose NOAC with DAPT still remains a reasonable alternative in this group as well. On the other hand if risk of ST is inordinately high; left main bifurcation or bioresorbable scaffold or primary PCI in diabetic but bleeding risk is not inadvertently high a therapy of full dose NOAC + P2Y12 inhibitor may be chosen. The only difference in approach

TABLE 2: The risk and benefits of various antithrombotic combinations

Combination	Ischemic benefit	Bleeding risk
DAPT	+	+
NOAC (full dose) + P2Y12 Inhibitor	+++++	++++
DAPT+ low dose NOAC	++++	+++
TAT	++	+++++
VKA + P2Y12 Inhibitor	+++	++

DAPT, dual antiplatelet therapy; NOAC, nonvitamin K antagonist oral anticoagulants; TAT, triple antithrombotic; VKA, vitamin K antagonist.

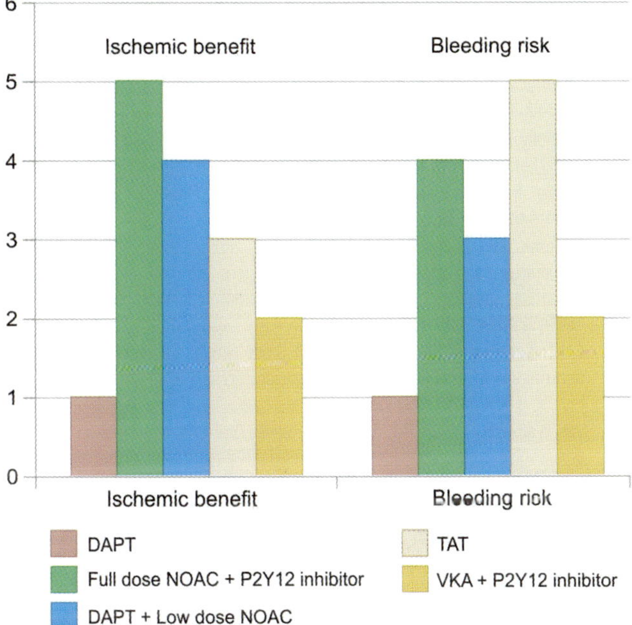

DAPT, dual antiplatelet therapy; NOAC, nonvitamin K oral anticoagulants; TAT, triple antithrombotic.

FIG. 8: The risk and benefits of various antithrombotic combinations.

would be that this combination therapy could be limited to 6 weeks or 6 months as the risk may be. The main limitation of low-dose NOAC with DAPT is a higher bleeding risk (vis-à-vis VKA + P2Y12 inhibitor). If instead of DAPT, only clopidogrel is used it may strike the right balance; sufficient efficacy with less bleeding risk (vis-à-vis DAPT or even prasugrel or ticagrelor). Thus a combination of clopidogrel with low-dose NOAC may be the ideal combination for the regular PCI.

A number of points can be made regarding the combination therapy:[100]

- Where NOAC is used along with clopidogrel or other P2Y12 inhibitors, a lower dose should be used
- In setting of ACS, dabigatran increases the risk of GI bleeding
- Rivaroxaban in very-low-doses (2.5 mg BD) possesses anti-ischemic properties although it may not be useful in stroke prevention at this dose.
- NOACs are associated with significantly lower intracranial bleeding versus VKA
- Newer P2Y12 inhibitors like prasugrel or ticagrelor should not be used with NOACs because of increased bleeding risk. There is especially a drug interaction between dabigatran and ticagrelor. Here is especially a drug interaction between dabigatran and ticagrelor

REFERENCES

1. Mirra M, Di Maio M, Vitulano G, et al. Management of Atrial Fibrillation in Patients Undergoing Percutaneous Coronary Intervention. Transl Med UniSa. 2014;9:33-7.
2. Rossini R, Musumeci G, Lettieri C, et al. Long-term outcomes in patients undergoing coronary stenting on dual oral antiplatelet treatment requiring oral anticoagulant therapy. Am J Cardiol. 2008;102:1618-23.
3. Wang TY, Robinson LA, Ou FS, et al. Discharge antithrombotic strategies among patients with acute coronary syndrome previously on warfarin anticoagulation: physician practice in the CRUSADE registry. Am Heart J. 2008;155:361-8.
4. Rubboli A, Colletta M, Valencia J, et al. WARfarin and Coronary STENTing (WAR-STENT) Study Group. Periprocedural management and in-hospital outcome of patients with indication for oral anticoagulation undergoing coronary artery stenting. J Interv Cardiol. 2009;22:390-7.
5. Capodanno D, Angiolillo DJ. Management of antiplatelet and anticoagulant therapy in patients with atrial fibrillation in the setting of acute coronary syndromes or percutaneous coronary interventions. Circ Cardiovasc Interv. 2014;7:113-24.
6. Dai Y, Ge J. Clinical use of aspirin in treatment and prevention of cardiovascular disease. Thrombosis. 2012;2012:245037
7. Kubota N, Kasai T, Miyauchi K, et al. Therapy with statins and aspirin enhances long-term outcome of percutaneous coronary intervention. Heart Vessels. 2008;23(1):35-9.
8. Njaman W, Miyauchi K, Kasai K, et al. Impact of aspirin treatment on long-term outcome (over 10 years) after percutaneous coronary intervention. Int Heart J. 2006;47(1):37-45.
9. Schwartz L, Bourassa MG, Lesperance J, et al. Aspirin and dipyridamole in the prevention of restenosis after percutaneous transluminal coronary angioplasty. N Engl J Med. 1988;318(26):1714-9.
10. Taylor RR, Gibbons FA, Cope GD, et al. Effects of low-dose aspirin on restenosis after coronary angioplasty. Am J Cardiol. 1991;68(9):874-8.
11. Lembo NJ, Black AJR, Roubin GS, et al. "Effect of pretreatment with aspirin versus aspirin plus dipyridamole on frequency and type of acute complications of percutaneous transluminal coronary angioplasty. Am J Cardiol. 1990;65(7):422-6.
12. Barnathan ES, Schwartz JS, Taylor L. Aspirin and dipyridamole in the prevention of acute coronary thrombosis thrombosis 7 complicating coronary angioplasty. Circulation. 1987;76(1):125-34.
13. Eikelboom JW, Hirsh J, Spencer FA, et al. Antithrombotic Therapy and Prevention of Thrombosis, 9th edition: American College of Chest Physicians Evidence-Based Clinical Practice Guidelines. CHEST. 2012;141(2)(Suppl):e89S-e119S.
14. Antithrombotic Trialists' Collaboration. Collaborative meta-analysis of randomised trials of antiplatelet therapy for prevention of death, myocardial infarction, and stroke in high-risk patients. BMJ. 2002;324(7329):71-86.
15. Airee A, Draper HM, Finks SW. Aspirin resistance: disparities and clinical implications. Pharmacotherapy.2008;28(8):999-1018.
16. Papathanasiou A, Guodevenos J, Tselepis AD. Aspirin resistance in cardiovascular disease: pathogenesis, diagnosis and clinical impact. Curr Pharmaceut Des. 2009;15(10):1085-94.
17. Lancaster Gl, Srinivasan J, Jain H, Aspirin resistance: an update. Curr Atheroscl Rep. 2009;11(2):105-110.
18. Blair P, Freedman JE. Aspirin resistance in atherosclerosis. Curr Atheroscl Rep. 2008;10(2):149-57
19. Tseeng S, Arora R. Reviews: aspirin resistance: biological and clinical implications. J Cardiovasc Pharmacol Therapeut. 2008;13(1)5-12.

20. De Schryver EL, Algra A, van Gijn J. Dipyridamole for preventing stroke and other vascular events in patients with vascular disease. An Update Stroke. 2008;39:1297-398.
21. Bhatt DL, Bertrand ME, Berger PB, et al. Meta-analysis of randomized and registry comparisons of ticlopidine with clopidogrel after stenting. J Am Coll Cardiol. 2002;39(1): 9-14.
22. Steinhubl SR, Berger PB, Mann JT III, et al. CREDO Investigators. Clopidogrel for the reduction of events during observation. Early and sustained dual oral antiplatelet therapy following percutaneous coronary intervention: a randomized controlled trial. JAMA. 2002;288 (19):2411-20.
23. Chen ZM, Jiang LX, Chen YP, et al.; COMMIT (ClOpidogrel and Metoprolol in Myocardial Infarction Trial) collaborative group. Addition of clopidogrel to aspirin in 45,852 patients with acute myocardial infarction: randomised placebocontrolled trial. Lancet. 2005;366 (9497):1607-21.
24. Sabatine MS, Cannon CP , Gibson CM, et al. CLARITY-TIMI 28 Investigators. Addition of clopidogrel to aspirin and fibrinolytic therapy for myocardial infarction with ST-segment elevation. N Engl J Med. 2005;352 (12):1179-89.
25. Angiolillo DJ, Gibson CM, Cheng S, et al. Differential effects of omeprazole and pantoprazole on the pharmacodynamics and pharmacokinetics of clopidogrel in healthy subjects: randomized, placebo-controlled, crossover comparison studies. Clin Pharmacol Ther. 2011;89(1):65-74.
26. Mehta SR, Tanguay JF, Eikelboom JW, et al. CURRENTOASIS 7 trial investigators. Double-dose versus standard dose clopidogrel and high-dose versus low-dose aspirin in individuals undergoing percutaneous coronary intervention for acute coronary syndromes (CURRENT-OASIS 7): a randomised factorial trial. Lancet. 2010;376 (9748):1233-43.
27. Bonello L, Tantry US, Marcucci R, et al.; Working Group on High On-Treatment Platelet Reactivity. Consensus and future directions on the definition of high on-treatment platelet reactivity to adenosine diphosphate. J Am Coll Cardiol. 2010;56(12): 919-33.
28. Zahno A, Brecht K, Bodmer M, et al. Effects of drug interactions on biotransformation and antiplatelet effect of clopidogrel in vitro. Br J Pharmacol. 2010;161(2):393-404.
29. Angiolillo DJ, Gibson CM, Cheng S, et al. Differential effects of omeprazole and pantoprazole on the pharmacodynamics and pharmacokinetics of clopidogrel in healthy subjects: randomized, placebo-controlled, crossover comparison studies. Clin Pharmacol Ther. 2011;89(1):65-74.
30. Mega JL, Simon T, Collet JP, et al. Reduced-function CYP2C19 genotype and risk of adverse clinical outcomes among patients treated with clopidogrel predominantly for PCI: a meta-analysis. JAMA. 2010;304 (16):1821-30.
31. Brandt JT, Payne CD, Wiviott SD, et al. A comparison of prasugrel and clopidogrel loading doses on platelet function: magnitude of platelet inhibition is related to active metabolite formation. Am Heart J. 2007;153(1):66.e9-16.
32. Jernberg T, Payne CD, Winters KJ, et al. Prasugrel achieves greater inhibition of platelet aggregation and a lower rate of non-responders compared with clopidogrel in aspirin-treated patients with stable coronary artery disease. Eur Heart J. 2006;27(10):1166-73.
33. Wiviott SD, Braunwald E, McCabe CH, et al. TRITONTIMI 38 Investigators. Prasugrel versus clopidogrel in patients with acute coronary syndromes. N Engl J Med. 2007;357(20): 2001-15.
34. Gurbel PA, Bliden KP, Butler K, et al. Randomized double-blind assessment of the ONSET and OFFSET of the antiplatelet effects of ticagrelor versus clopidogrel in patients with stable coronary artery disease: the ONSET/OFFSET study. Circulation. 2009;120:2577-85.
35. Hochholzer W, Trenk D, Frundi D, et al. Time dependence of platelet inhibition after a 600-mg loading dose of clopidogrel in a large, unselected cohort of candidates for percutaneous coronary intervention. Circulation. 2005;111:2560-4.
36. Storey RF, Angiolillo DJ, Patil SB, et al. Inhibitory effects of ticagrelor compared with clopidogrel on platelet function in patients with acute coronary syndromes: the PLATO (PLATelet inhibition and patient Outcomes) PLATELET substudy. J Am Coll Cardiol. 2010;56:1456-62.
37. Bonello L, Laine M, Kipson N, et al. Ticagrelor increases adenosine plasma concentration in patients with an acute coronary syndrome. J Am Coll Cardiol. 2014;63:872-7.
38. Wallentin L, Becker RC, Budaj A, et al. Ticagrelor versus clopidogrel in patients with acute coronary syndromes. N Engl J Med. 2009;361:1045-57.
39. Bonaca MP, Bhatt DL, Cohen M, et al. Long-term use of ticagrelor in patients with prior myocardial infarction. N Engl J Med. 2015;372:1791-800.
40. Levine GN, Bates ER, Bittl JA, et al. 2016 ACC/AHA guideline focused update on duration of dual antiplatelet therapy in patients with coronary artery disease: a report of the American College of Cardiology/American Heart Association task force on clinical practice guidelines. J Am Coll Cardiol. 2016;68(10):1082-115.
41. Lloyd-Jones DM, Wang TJ, Leip EP, et al. Lifetime risk for development of atrial fibrillation: the Framingham Heart Study. Circulation. 2004;110(9):1042-6.
42. Miyasaka Y, Barnes ME, Gersh BJ, et al. Secular trends in incidence of atrial fibrillation in Olmsted County, Minnesota, 1980 to 2000, and implications on the projections for future prevalence. Circulation. 2006;114(2):119-25.
43. Wolf PA, Abbott RD, Kannel WB. Atrial fibrillation as an independent risk factor for stroke: the Framingham Study. Stroke. 1991;22(8):983-8.
44. Risk factors for stroke and efficacy of antithrombotic therapy in atrial fibrillation. Analysis of pooled data from five randomized controlled trials. Arch Intern Med. 1994;154(13):1449-57.
45. Suttie JW. Mechanism of Action Of Vitamin K: Synthesis Of Y-Carboxyglutamic Acid. CRC Crit Rev Biochem. 1980;8(2):191-223.
46. Petersen P, Boysen G, Godtfredsen J, et al. Placebo-controlled, randomised trial of warfarin and aspirin for prevention of thromboembolic complications in chronic atrial fibrillation. The Copenhagen AFASAK study. Lancet. 1989;1(8631):175-9.
47. The Boston Area Anticoagulation Trial for Atrial Fibrillation Investigators. The effect of low-dose warfarin on the risk of stroke in patients with nonrheumatic atrial fibrillation. N Engl J Med. 1990;323(22):1505-11.
48. Connolly SJ, Laupacis A, Gent M, et al. Canadian Atrial Fibrillation Anticoagulation (CAFA) study. J Am Coll Cardiol. 1991;18(2):349-55.
49. Stroke Prevention in Atrial Fibrillation Study. Final results. Circulation. 1991;84(2):527-39.
50. Ezekowitz MD, Bridgers SL, James KE, et al. Veterans affairs stroke prevention in nonrheumatic atrial fibrillation investigators warfarin in the prevention of stroke associated with nonrheumatic atrial fibrillation. N Engl J Med. 1992;327(20):1406-12.
51. EAFT (European Atrial Fibrillation Trial) Study Group. Secondary prevention in non-rheumatic atrial fibrillation after transient ischaemic attack or minor stroke. Lancet. 1993;342(8882):1255-62.
52. van Walraven C, Hart RG, Singer DE, et al. Oral anticoagulants vs aspirin in nonvalvular atrial fibrillation: an individual patient meta-analysis. JAMA. 2002;288(19):2441-8.
53. Benavente O, Hart R, Koudstaal P, et al. Antiplatelet therapy for preventing stroke in patients with atrial fibrillation and no previous history of stroke or transient ischemic attacks. Cochrane Database Syst Rev. 2000;(2):CD001925.
54. Posada IS, Barriales V. LASAF Pilot Study Group. Alternate-day dosing of aspirin in atrial fibrillation. Am Heart J. 1999;138(1 pt 1):137-3.
55. Sato H, Ishikawa K, Kitabatake A, et al. Japan Atrial Fibrillation Stroke Trial Group. Low-dose aspirin for prevention of stroke in low-risk patients with atrial fibrillation: Japan Atrial Fibrillation Stroke Trial. Stroke. 2006;37(2):447-451.
56. Diener HC, Lowenthal A. Antiplatelet therapy to prevent stroke: risk of brain hemorrhage and efficacy in atrial fibrillation. J Neurol Sci. 1997;153(1):112.
57. Edvardsson N, Juul-Möller S, Omblus R, et al. Effects of low-dose warfarin and aspirin versus no treatment on stroke in a medium-risk patient population with atrial fibrillation. J Intern Med. 2003;254(1):95-101.
58. Baigent C, Blackwell L, Collins R, et al. Antithrombotic Trialists' (ATT) Collaboration. Aspirin in the primary and secondary prevention of vascular disease: collaborative meta-analysis of individual participant data from randomised trials. Lancet. 2009;373(9678):1849-60.
59. Antithrombotic Trialists' Collaboration, Baigent C, Blackwell L, et al. Collaborative meta-analysis of randomised trials of antiplatelet therapy for prevention of death, myocardial infarction, and stroke in high risk patients. BMJ. 2002;324(7329):71-86.
60. Vemmos KN, Tsivgoulis G, Spengos K, et al. Primary prevention of arterial thromboembolism in the oldest old with atrial fibrillation—a randomized pilot trial comparing adjusted-dose and fixed low-dose coumadin with aspirin. Eur J Intern Med. 2006;17(1):48-52.
61. Gulløv AL, Koefoed BG, Petersen P, et al. Fixed mini-dose warfarin and aspirin alone and in combination vs adjusted-dose warfarin for stroke prevention in atrial fibrillation: Second Copenhagen Atrial Fibrillation, Aspirin, and Anticoagulation Study. Arch Intern Med. 1998;158(14):1513-21.
62. Mant J, Hobbs FD, Fletcher K, et al. BAFTA Investigators Midland Research Practices Network (MidReC). Warfarin versus aspirin for stroke prevention in

an elderly community population with atrial fibrillation (the Birmingham Atrial Fibrillation Treatment of the Aged Study, BAFTA): a randomised controlled trial. Lancet. 2007;370(9586):493-503.

63. Pérez-Gómez F, Alegría E, Berjón J, et al. NASPEAF Investigators. Comparative effects of antiplatelet, anticoagulant, or combined therapy in patients with valvular and nonvalvular atrial fibrillation: a randomized multicenter study. J Am Coll Cardiol. 2004;44(8):1557-66.
64. Hellemons BS, Langenberg M, Lodder J, et al. Primary prevention of arterial thromboembolism in non-rheumatic atrial fibrillation in primary care: randomised controlled trial comparing two intensities of coumarin with aspirin. BMJ. 1999;319(7215):958-64.
65. Morocutti C, Amabile G, Fattapposta F, et al. SIFA (Studio Italiano Fibrillazione Atriale) Investigators. Indobufen versus warfarin in the secondary prevention of major vascular events in nonrheumatic atrial fibrillation. Stroke. 1997;28(5):1015-21.
66. Warfarin versus aspirin for prevention of thromboembolism in atrial fibrillation: Stroke Prevention in Atrial Fibrillation II Study. Lancet. 1994;343(8899):687-91.
67. Adjusted-dose warfarin versus low-intensity, fixed-dose warfarin plus aspirin for high-risk patients with atrial fibrillation: Stroke Prevention in Atrial Fibrillation III randomised clinical trial. Lancet. 1996;348(9028):633-8.
68. Rash A, Downes T, Portner R, et al. A randomised controlled trial of warfarin versus aspirin for stroke prevention in octogenarians with atrial fibrillation (WASPO). Age Ageing. 2007;36(2):151-6.
69. Anand SS, Yusuf S. Oral anticoagulants in patients with coronary artery disease. J Am Coll Cardiol. 2003;41(4) 62S-9S.
70. Chimowitz MI, Lynn MJ, Howlett-Smith H, et al. Warfarin-Aspirin Symptomatic Intracranial Disease Trial Investigators. Comparison of warfarin and aspirin for symptomatic intracranial arterial stenosis. N Engl J Med. 2005;352(13): 1305-16.
71. Connolly SJ, Pogue J, Hart RG, et al. ACTIVE Investigators Effect of clopidogrel added to aspirin in patients with atrial fibrillation. N Engl J Med. 2009;360(20):2066-78.
72. Connolly SJ, Ezekowitz MD, Yusuf S, et al. RE-LY Steering Committee and Investigators. Dabigatran versus warfarin in patients with atrial fibrillation. N Engl J Med. 2009;361(12):1139-51.
73. Granger CB, Alexander JH, McMurray JJ, et al. ARISTOTLE Committees and Investigators. Apixaban versus warfarin in patients with atrial fibrillation. N Engl J Med. 2011;365(11):981-92.
74. Patel MR, Mahaffey KW, Garg J, et al. ROCKET AF Investigators. Rivaroxaban versus warfarin in nonvalvular atrial fibrillation. N Engl J Med. 2011;365(10): 883-91.
75. Connolly SJ, Eikelboom J, Joyner C, et al. AVERROES Steering Committee and Investigators. Apixaban in patients with atrial fibrillation. N Engl J Med. 2011; 364(9):806-17.
76. Roskell NS, Lip GY, Noack H, et al. Treatments for stroke prevention in atrial fibrillation: a network meta-analysis and indirect comparisons versus dabigatran etexilate. Thromb Haemost. 2010;104(6):1106-15.
77. Holmes DR Jr, Kereiakes DJ, Garg S, et al. Stent thrombosis. J Am Coll Cardiol. 2010;56 (17):1357-65.
78. Lip GY, Huber K, Andreotti F, et al. Management of antithrombotic therapy in atrial fibrillation patients presenting with acute coronary syndrome and/or undergoing percutaneous coronary intervention/stenting. Thromb Haemost. 2010;103:13-28.
79. Faxon DP, Eikelboom JW, Berger PB, et al. Consensus document: antithrombotic therapy in patients with atrial fibrillation undergoing coronary stenting. A North-American perspective. Thromb Haemost. 2011;106:572-84.
80. Huber K, Airaksinen KJ, Cuisset T, et al. Antithrombotic therapy in patients with atrial fibrillation undergoing coronary stenting: similarities and dissimilarities between North America and Europe. Thromb Haemost. 2011;106:569-71.
81. Maegdefessel L, Schlitt A, Faerber J, et al. Anticoagulant and/or antiplatelet treatment in patients with atrial fibrillation after percutaneous coronary intervention. A single center experience. Med Klin (Munich). 2008;103(9): 628-32.
82. Dewilde WJ, Oirbans T, Verheugt FW, et al. Use of clopidogrel with or without aspirin in patients taking oral anticoagulant therapy and undergoing percutaneous coronary intervention: an open-label, randomised, controlled trial. Lancet. 2013;381(9872):1107-15.
83. Dąbrowska M, Ochała A, Cybulski W, et al. Balancing between bleeding and thromboembolism after percutaneous coronary intervention in patients with atrial fibrillation. Could triple anticoagulant therapy be a solution? Postepy Kardiol Interwencyjnej. 2013;9(3):234-40.
84. Fosbol EL, Wang TY, Li S, et al. Warfarin use among older atrial fibrillation patients with non-ST-segment elevation myocardial infarction managed with coronary stenting and dual antiplatelet therapy. Am Heart J. 2013;166(5):864-70.
85. Kawai H, Watanabe E, Yamamoto M, et al. Major bleeding complications related to combined antithrombotic therapy in atrial fibrillation patients 12 months after coronary artery stenting. J Cardiol. 2015;65(3):197-202.
86. Rubboli A, Schlitt A, Kiviniemi T, et al. One-year outcome of patients with atrial fibrillation undergoing coronary artery stenting: an analysis of the AFCAS registry. Clin Cardiol. 2014;37(6):357-64.
87. Suh SY, Kang WC, Oh PC, et al. Efficacy and safety of aspirin, clopidogrel, and warfarin after coronary artery stenting in Korean patients with atrial fibrillation. Heart Vessels. 2014;29(5):578-83.
88. Kang DO, Yu CW, Kim HD, et al. Triple antithrombotic therapy versus dual antiplatelet therapy in patients with atrial fibrillation undergoing drug-eluting stent implantation. Coron Artery Dis. 2015;26(5):372-80.
89. Lahtela HM, Kiviniemi TO, Puurunen MK, et al. Antithrombotic therapy for AF patients undergoing PCI. PLoS One. 2015;10(6):e0128492.
90. Hess CN, Peterson ED, Peng SA, et al. Use and outcomes of triple therapy among older patients with acute myocardial infarction and atrial fibrillation. J Am Coll Cardiol. 2015;66(6):616-27.
91. Mennuni MG, Halperin JL, Bansilal S, et al. Balancing the risk of bleeding and stroke in patients with atrial fibrillation after percutaneous coronary intervention (from the AVIATOR Registry). Am J Cardiol. 2015;116(1):37-42.
92. Sambola A, Mutuberría M, García Del Blanco B, et al. Effects of triple therapy in patients with non-valvular atrial fibrillation undergoing percutaneous coronary intervention regarding thromboembolic risk stratification. Circ J. 2016;80(2):354-62.
93. Sambola A, Mutuberría M, García Del Blanco B, et al. Impact of triple therapy in elderly patients with atrial fibrillation undergoing percutaneous coronary intervention. PLoS One. 2016;11(1):e0147245.
94. Sherwood MW, Cyr DD, Jones WS, et al. Use of dual antiplatelet therapy and patient outcomes in those undergoing percutaneous coronary intervention: The ROCKET AF Trial. JACC Cardiovasc Interv. 2016;9(16):1694-702.
95. Gibson CM, Pinto DS, Chi G, et al. Recurrent hospitalization among patients with atrial fibrillation undergoing intracoronary stenting treated with 2 treatment strategies of rivaroxaban or a dose-adjusted oral vitamin K antagonist treatment strategy. Circulation. 2017;135(4):323-33.
96. De Vecchis R, Cantatrione C, Mazzei D. Clinical relevance of anticoagulation and dual antiplatelet therapy to the outcomes of patients with atrial fibrillation and recent percutaneous coronary intervention with stent. J Clin Med Res. 2016;8(2):153-61.
97. Gong X, Tang S, Li J, et al. Antithrombotic therapy strategies for atrial fibrillation patients undergoing percutaneous coronary intervention: a systematic review and network meta-analysis. PLoS One. 2017;12(10):e0186449.
98. .Lamberts M, Gislason GH, Olesen JB, et al. Oral anticoagulation and antiplatelets in atrial fibrillation patients after myocardial infarction and coronary intervention. J Am Coll Cardiol. 2013;62:981-9.
99. Dewilde WJ, Oirbans T, Verheugt FW, et al. Use of clopidogrel with or without aspirin in patients taking oral anticoagulant therapy and undergoing percutaneous coronary intervention: an open-label, randomised, controlled trial. Lancet. 2013;381:1107-15.
100. Lip GY, Windecker S, Huber K, et al. Management of antithrombotic therapy in atrial fibrillation patients presenting with acute coronary syndrome and/or undergoing percutaneous coronary or valve interventions: a joint consensus document of the European Society of Cardiology Working Group on Thrombosis, European Heart Rhythm Association (EHRA), European Association of Percutaneous Cardiovascular Interventions (EAPCI) and European Association of Acute Cardiac Care (ACCA) endorsed by the Heart Rhythm Society (HRS) and Asia-Pacific Heart Rhythm Society (APHRS). Eur Heart J. 2014;35(45):3155-79.
101. Golwala HB, Cannon CP, Steg PG, et al. Safety and efficacy of dual vs. triple antithrombotic therapy in patients with atrial fibrillation following percutaneous coronary intervention: a systematic review and meta-analysis of randomized clinical trials. Eur Heart J. 2018;39:1726-35.

CHAPTER 109

Treatment of Atrial Fibrillation in Heart Failure: Is It Any Different?

Rajesh A Dhopeshwarkar

INTRODUCTION

Atrial fibrillation (AF) is a very common arrhythmia and is seen in a myriad of conditions.

Heart failure (HF) and AF have a hand in glove relationship with one frequently perpetuating the other. Besides numerous conditions are common for both of them.

Atrial fibrillation increases both morbidity and mortality by increasing thromboembolic risk and worsening HF. In a large database analysis of all patients admitted with AF and HF between 2001 and 2011, patients with HF and AF had greater in-hospital mortality compared with those without AF (4.6% vs. 3.3%, respectively, p <0.0001). Additionally, black, Hispanic, Asian, and white patients with HF and AF had a 24%, 17%, 13%, and 6% higher mortality, respectively, than if they did not have AF.[1]

GOALS OF TREATMENT IN ATRIAL FIBRILLATION

Symptom Control

Most of the symptoms due to AF are a result of fast ventricular rate. However, in patients with HF, loss of atrial kick also significantly contributes to symptoms and progression of HF (Flowchart 1).

Managing Heart Failure and Progression of Heart Failure

Atrial fibrillation significantly contributes to worsening of HF onset of a potent poor prognosis in HF patients where, management of HF fundamentally remains the same. AF causes significant challenges and needs meticulous understanding of disease processes and more aggressive approach in treating both (Flowchart 2).

Stroke Prevention

Presence of HF increases stroke risk in AF. Anticoagulation remains the mainstay in treatment. Associated organ dysfunction may imply modification of drug dosing. Besides, presence of intracavitary clot may preclude use of newer oral anticoagulants and may necessitate use of vitamin K antagonist (VKA).

Rate Control

Aggressive rhythm control strategy remains the mainstay for managing AF with congestive HF. Patients with permanent AF and congestive HF rate control may be attempted. Digoxin is a frontline drug in rate control strategy in HF with reduced ejection fraction (HFrEF) patients given its

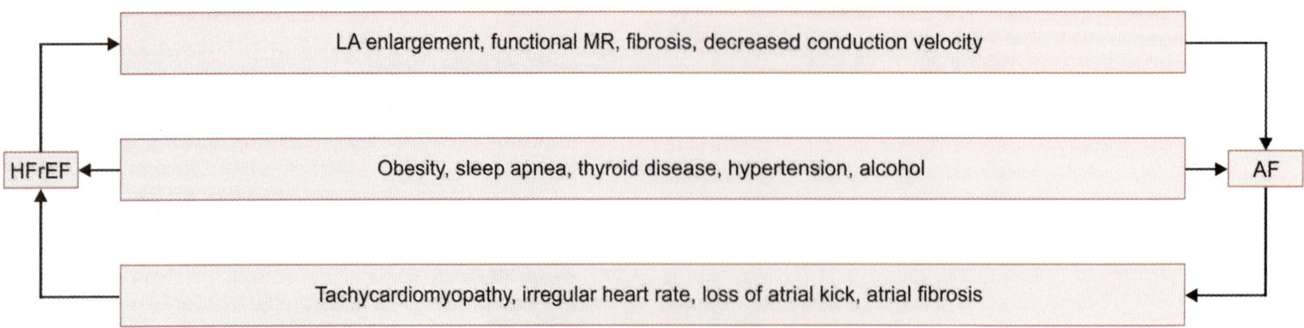

FLOWCHART 1: Mechanisms and pathways of progression of heart failure and atrial fibrillation.

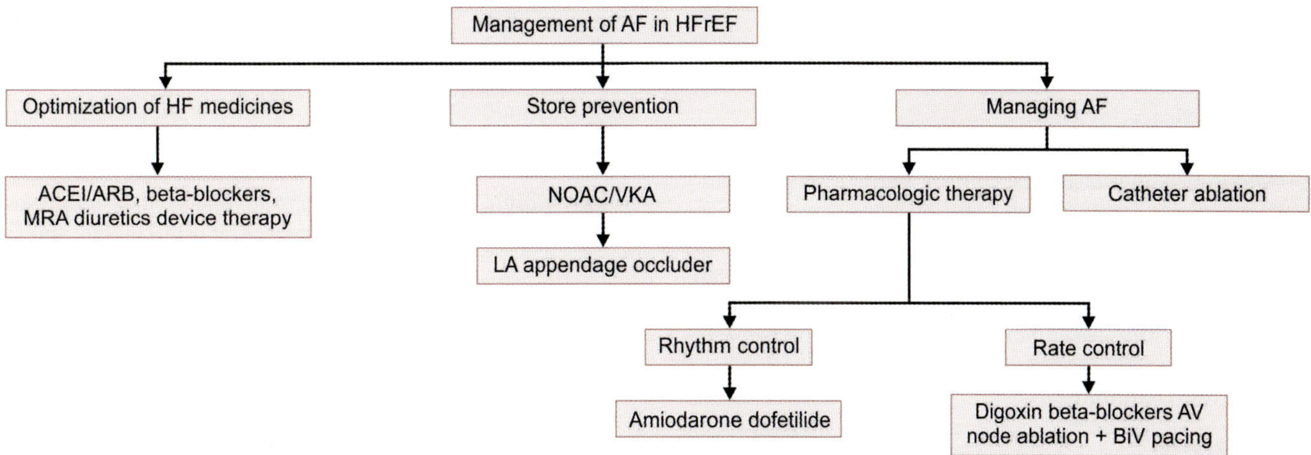

ACEI, angiotensin-converting enzyme inhibitor; ARB, angiotensin receptor blocker; AV, atrioventricular; AF, atrial fibrillation; BiV, biventricular; HFrEF, heart failure with reduced ejection fraction; LA, Left Atrium; MRA, mineralocorticoid receptor antagonist; VKA, vitamin K antagonist.

FLOWCHART 2: Management of atrial fibrillation in heart failure with reduced ejection fraction.

atrioventricular (AV) nodal blocking properties with positive inotropic action. There is no randomized controlled trial (RCT) evidence of benefit with Digoxin in the setting of AF.

All other AV nodal blocking agents have a potentially negative inotropic action. Calcium blockers like verapamil and diltiazem are relatively contraindicated in HF. Amiodarone, though a drug used to maintain sinus rhythm, is also used for rate control strategy in combination with other drugs. Appropriate anticoagulation is essential given the potential conversion to sinus rhythm with amiodarone. Patients on long-term amiodarone for rate or rhythm control in HFrEF who develop fast ventricular response should be screened for amiodarone-induced thyrotoxicosis.

Beta-blockers remain the mainstay of rate control in HFrEF. Various trials have proven efficacy of beta-blockers in HFrEF in terms of morbidity and mortality reduction. Hypotension remains a limiting factor in titrating dose of beta-blockers. Very frequently a combination therapy may be necessary.

In a meta-analysis of 11 trials of beta-blockers in HFrEF, Kotecha et al.[2] found that regardless of pretreatment heart rate, beta-blockers reduce mortality in patients with HF with reduced ejection fraction in sinus rhythm. However, lowering ventricular rate with beta-blockers did not appear to be a predictor of outcomes in patients with HF and AF. The mechanism of this is still unclear. Therefore, although indicated and useful for rate control, beta-blockers have little prognostic impact as compared to patients of HF who are in sinus rhythm.

Patients presenting with decompensated HF and AF with fast ventricular rate should not be initiated on beta-blockers. Rate control can be achieved to reach a goal of 85 per minute at rest and 110 per minute during exercise.

Lenient Rate Control

Lenient rate control with target heart rate of less than 110 per minute at rest is much easier to achieve and in the Rate Control Efficacy in Permanent Atrial Fibrillation (RACE) 2 trial[3] has been found to have similar outcomes. However, RACE 2 patients were mostly in New York Health Association (NYHA) CL 1-2 and very few patients had HFrEF. Hence, these results may not apply to HFrEF patients.

Adequate rate control is even more important in HFrEF patients. Besides, fast ventricular response may lead to tachycardiomyopathy.

Nonpharmacological Rate Control: Pace and Ablate

Atrioventricular node ablation remains the last resort in patients who have failed drug therapy. Both European[4] and American[5] guidelines state that AV junction ablation and pacing is reasonable in patients with AF where rhythm control by drugs or ablation is not achievable and where rate control with drugs has failed. Choice of right ventricular pacing versus biventricular (BiV) pacing must be judiciously done ideally based on baseline left ventricular (LV) ejection fraction. His bundle pacing is now being considered increasingly in patients with AV block and LV dysfunction who will need long-term ventricular pacing.

Patients who have received a BiV device and now develop AF frequently leads to loss of BiV pacing. Achieving BiV pacing in excess of 90% is of paramount importance. This is achieved by uptitrating drugs that control ventricular rates. However, AV node ablation is now considered a superior strategy. In a systematic review, Ganesan et al.[6] found AV node ablation was associated with better overall and cardiovascular mortality and better functional class.

Rhythm Control

Whenever possible establishing and maintaining sinus rhythm remains the long-standing goal in patients with AF and HFrEF. This is accomplished by pharmacologic therapy, electrical cardioversion, and catheter ablation.

Pharmacology Therapy

Maintaining sinus rhythm is challenging in the setting of AF and HF due to limited availability of drugs that can be used and poor efficacy.

In multiple RCTs, rhythm control strategy has not been proven to be superior to rate control. In the atrial fibrillation and congestive heart failure (AF-CHF) trial[7], patients were randomized to aggressive rhythm control strategy using electrical cardioversion with amiodarone and if necessary, sotalol or dofetilide. Over a 3-year period, there was no difference in cardiovascular mortality between the two arms.

Therefore, rate control strategy was equally effective in terms of hard endpoints.

Amiodarone

It remains the mainstay in managing AF in patients with HFrEF. This is due to its almost no risk of proarrhythmia-like torsades. Two major drawbacks of amiodarone are relative lack of efficacy and significant systemic side effects often necessitating withdrawal. Intravenous amiodarone is known to have a conversion rate to sinus rhythm of around 30%. It does increase the chance of maintaining sinus rhythm when administered in long run. However, 30% of patients on long-term amiodarone do not tolerate and hence discontinue the medicine. Common systemic side effect is hypothyroidism; however, rarely hyperthyroidism is also known to occur. Besides liver and pulmonary toxicity also need monitoring. While administering amiodarone, close monitoring of international normalized ratio (INR) is necessary in patients anticoagulated with VKA due to its potentiation of VKA.

Sotalol

It is a class III antiarrhythmic drug that has been used in patients with coronary artery disease and AF. It should be used with caution in patients with severe LV dysfunction or with renal dysfunction. QT prolongation must be monitored as it is known to precipitate torsades. Implantable cardioverter defibrillator (ICD) implant is necessary before sotalol is used. Dofetilide: It is a class III antiarrhythmic drug. Patients are initiated on dofetilide as an inpatient with serial QT monitoring and doses are adjusted according to creatinine clearance. In the Danish Investigations of Arrhythmia and Mortality on Dofetilide in congestive heart failure (DIAMOND CHF)[8] and DIAMOND substudy[9] trials, patients with HFrEF and AF were administered dofetilide. Rate of conversion to sinus rhythm was significantly higher (57% vs. 34%) than placebo. Probability of maintaining sinus rhythm was greater with dofetilide (79% vs. 42%). There was no survival benefit with dofetilide. Torsades De pointes was the most important side effect that was observed in 3.3% patients most of them happening in first 3 days of initiation of dofetilide. Due to its proarrhythmic effect ICD implantation prior to administration of drug is useful. Dofetilide is currently unavailable in India.

Electrical Cardioversion

Hemodynamic instability in the setting of AF and HF warrants urgent electrical cardioversion. Before electrical or pharmacologic cardioversion, achieving optimal anticoagulation is necessary. If there is a necessity to cardiovert early, intracardiac clot must be ruled out with a transesophageal echocardiogram. Unless pretreated with antiarrhythmic drugs a high proportion of patients who undergo electrical cardioversion will revert to AF. Preferably, patient should be initiated on amiodarone or other antiarrhythmic drug prior to cardioversion that increases the likelihood of long-term success. Any intercurrent illness like pneumonia will make long-term maintenance of sinus rhythm unlikely. In such scenario, rate control strategy may be appropriate. Attempt to achieve and maintain sinus rhythm must be done for every patient with HFrEF and AF.

Catheter Ablation

Catheter ablation remains second line of management of AF in patients with normal heart. Current guidelines recommend catheter ablation in patients symptomatic despite drug therapy or those who decline drug therapy. However, AF in patients with HFrEF remains a challenge due to limited options of drug. In a landmark study, the CASTLE AF study,[10] patients with AF and HF were randomly assigned to catheter ablation or medical therapy. At 3 years, there was a significant reduction of the combined endpoint of death and hospitalization in patients undergoing catheter ablation (28.5% vs. 44.6%). At the end of 60 months, 66% of catheter ablation patients were in sinus rhythm as compared to only 22% in the medical therapy arm. LV ejection fraction improved by 8% in the ablation arm as compared to 0.2% in the medical therapy arm. In a meta-analysis[11] of 26 RCTs, significant improvement of LV ejection fraction was observed with catheter ablation.

In the recently presented catheter ablation vs. antiarrhythmic drug therapy in atrial fibrillation (CABANA)[12] trial, ablation was not superior to drug therapy for cardiovascular outcomes at 5 years among patients with new-onset or untreated AF that required therapy. However, this happened due to lot of crossover between the treatment arms. In those patients who did receive catheter ablation, there was significant reduction in the primary composite endpoint. About 15% of patients in CABANA had HF.

Stroke Prevention

Fundamentally all patients with AF and HFrEF need anticoagulation. Current guidelines have no role of Aspirin for stroke prevention in this setting. Other than patients with mechanical valves or moderate to severe mitral stenosis, all other patients can receive direct oral anticoagulant (DOAC) in preference to VKA.

Direct Oral Anticoagulant or Vitamin K Antagonist

Direct oral anticoagulants have been proven to be non-inferior to VKA in terms of preventing stroke. Some of them have been even superior to VKA. A large meta-analysis[13] of four RCTs found DOAC use to be as safe and effective as VKA in the setting of AF and HF. Use of DOAC was associated with a 41% lesser risk of intracranial bleed as compared to VKA.

Renal dysfunction is a frequent association with HFrEF. None of the DOAC has been tried with creatinine clearance less than 30 mL/min. They can be used safely with appropriate dose modification in the rest.

Role of Left Atrial Appendage Occluder

Long-term anticoagulation with VKA is associated with narrow therapeutic range as well as increased bleeding risk. Most of the cardioembolic strokes in AF arise from the left atrial appendage (LAA). Occluding or clamping the LAA has been tried in various studies. These devices are currently approved for use in patients who have relative contraindications to long-term anticoagulation. In the percutaneous left atrial appendage closure versus warfarin for atrial fibrillation (PROTECT-AF)[14] study, the WATCHMAN LAA occluder was found to reduce the composite endpoint of stroke, systemic embolism, and cardiovascular death by an absolute value of 1.5%. This was driven mainly by decreased incidence of hemorrhagic stroke in the device arm.

CHALLENGES IN DEVICE MANAGEMENT IN PATIENTS WITH ATRIAL FIBRILLATION AND HEART FAILURE

Device-detected Atrial Fibrillation

Device-detected atrial high rate episodes (AHRE) pose a new question of stroke risk associated with such episodes and whether such patients will benefit from anticoagulation. In a meta-analysis[15] of 11 trials, device-detected or subclinical AF was associated with more clinical AF. Such episodes were also associated with elevated stroke risk although it was lower than those with clinical AF. Studies are underway to define indications for anticoagulation in patients with device-detected AF. Currently, patients with AHRE on device logs undergo further testing with ambulatory ECG and external loop recorders to document AF.

Inappropriate Shocks

Atrial fibrillation and other supraventricular tachycardias are responsible for most of the inappropriate shocks. Appropriate device discriminators have to be programmed in such patients. Aggressive management of AF with pharmacologic therapy and if necessary catheter ablation is necessary.

CONCLUSION

Atrial fibrillation and HF frequently coexist and perpetuate each other. Onset of AF adds to challenges in the management of HF. AF, therefore, needs to be treated aggressively to prevent progression of HF as well as prevent development of structural changes that make AF permanent. Pharmacologic therapy whether aiming rate control or rhythm control is highly inadequate. Catheter ablation is an effective alternative that is now proven in RCT to reduce hard endpoints of HF hospitalizations and mortality. Catheter ablation is now being increasingly used in preference to pharmacologic therapy. DOAC have definite advantage over VKA both in terms of safety and efficacy. LAA occlusion with devices is an evolving therapy that is currently approved for use in patients where long-term use of anticoagulation is contraindicated. Managing comorbidities by lifestyle changes and risk factor modification are of paramount importance. Besides, optimization of HF with guideline-directed medical therapy is essential. A multidisciplinary approach with electrophysiologists and HF specialists will provide optimal patient care in this challenging situation.

REFERENCES

1. Bhatia S, Qazi M, Erande A, et al. Racial differences in the prevalence and outcomes of atrial fibrillation in patients hospitalized with heart failure. Am J Cardiol. 2016;117:1468-73.
2. Kotecha D, Flather MD, Altman DG, et al. Heart rate and rhythm and the benefit of beta-blockers in patients with heart failure. J Am Coll Cardiol. 2017;69:2885-96.
3. Mulder BA, Veldhuisen DJV, Crijns HJ, et al. Lenient vs. strict rate control in patients with atrial fibrillation and heart failure: a post-hoc analysis of the RACE II study. Eur J Heart Fail. 2013;15:1311-8.
4. Kirchhof P, Benussi S, Kotecha D, et al. 2016 ESC Guidelines for the management of atrial fibrillation developed in collaboration with EACTS. Eur Heart J. 2016;37:2893-62.
5. January CT, Wann LS, Alpert JS, et al. 2014 AHA/ACC/HRS guideline for the management of patients with atrial fibrillation. J Am Coll Cardiol. 2014;64.
6. Ganesan AN, Brooks AG, Roberts-Thomson KC, et al. Role of AV nodal ablation in cardiac resynchronization in patients with coexistent atrial fibrillation and heart failure. J Am Coll Cardiol. 2012;59:719-26.
7. Roy D, Talajic M, Nattel S, et al. Rhythm control versus rate control for atrial fibrillation and heart failure. N Engl J Med. 2008;358:2667-77.
8. Torp-Pedersen C, Møller M, Bloch-Thomsen PE, et al. Dofetilide in patients with congestive heart failure and left ventricular dysfunction. N Engl J Med. 1999;341:857-65.
9. Pedersen OD, Bagger H, Keller N, et al. Efficacy of dofetilide in the treatment of atrial fibrillation-flutter in patients with reduced left ventricular function. Circulation. 2001;104:292-6.
10. Marrouche NF, Brachmann J, Andresen D, et al. Catheter ablation for atrial fibrillation with heart failure. N Engl J Med. 2018;378(5):417-27.
11. Anselmino M, Matta M, D'Ascenzo F, et al. Catheter ablation of atrial fibrillation in patients with left ventricular systolic dysfunction: a systematic review and meta-analysis. Circ Arrhythm Electrophysiol. 2014;7:1011.
12. Packer DL. Catheter ablation vs antiarrhythmic drug therapy in atrial fibrillation: the results of the CABANA multicenter international randomized clinical trial. Presented at: HRS 2018. May 10, 2018. Boston, MA: HRS 2018; 2018.
13. Xiong Q, Lau YC, Senoo K, et al. Non-vitamin K antagonist oral anticoagulants (DOACs) in patients with concomitant atrial fibrillation and heart failure: a systemic review and meta-analysis of randomized trials. Eur J Heart Fail. 2015;17(11):1192-200.
14. Reddy VY, Sievert H, Halperin J, et al. Percutaneous left atrial appendage closure vs warfarin for atrial fibrillation: a randomized clinical trial. JAMA. 2014;312(19):1988-98.
15. Mahajan R, Perera T, Adrian D. Subclinical device-detected atrial fibrillation and stroke risk: a systematic review and meta-analysis. Eur Heart J. 2018;39(16):1407-15.

CHAPTER 110

Managing Atrial Fibrillation in Acute Myocardial Infarction

Jayagopal P Balagopalan, Sarjun Basha

INTRODUCTION

Atrial fibrillation (AF) often complicates acute myocardial infarction (AMI) with an incidence between 6% and 21%. AF may be pre-existing, first time detected, or of new onset. ST-segment elevation myocardial infarction (STEMI) patients with documented AF have worse short and long-term prognosis when compared with patients in sinus rhythm.[1] Presence of AF is associated with a higher reinfarction rate, higher stroke rate, higher risk for heart failure, and increased risk for sudden cardiac death.[2-4]

PREDICTORS OF ATRIAL FIBRILLATION IN ACUTE MYOCARDIAL INFARCTION

Increased age, presence of heart failure symptoms, high heart rates at admission, and left ventricular dysfunction are the major predictors.

MANAGEMENT OF ATRIAL FIBRILLATION IN ACUTE MYOCARDIAL INFARCTION

Management includes:

- Rate control
- Rhythm control
- Prevention of thromboembolism.

Rate Control

High ventricular rates associated with AF may further impair hemodynamics in patients with AMI by increasing myocardial oxygen demand. Thus adequate rate control represents the first therapeutic approach. In patients with AF and rapid ventricular rate, acute heart rate (HR) control is usually achieved with intravenous (IV) medication namely IV beta-blocker, IV amiodarone, and IV digoxin (Table 1). IV beta-blocker is indicated when there are no clinical signs of acute heart failure or hypotension.[2,5] IV amiodarone is indicated in the presence of concomitant acute heart failure without hypotension.[6] IV digitalis is indicated in the presence of acute heart failure and hypotension.[7] When coadministering IV digoxin and amiodarone, close monitoring for digoxin toxicity is necessary as digoxin serum concentration may rise.

TABLE 1: Atrial fibrillation acute rate control—common medication dosage.

Beta-blockers	Intravenous administration	Usual oral maintenance dose
Metoprolol tartrate	2.5–5.0 mg IV bolus over 2 minutes: up to 3 doses	25–100 mg bid
Esmolol	500 μg/kg IV bolus over 1 minute, then 50–300 μg/kg/min IV	N/A
Digoxin	0.25 mg IV with repeat dosing to a maximum of 1.5 mg over 24 hours	0.125–0.25 mg od
Amiodarone	300 mg IV over 1 hour, then 10–50 mg/h over 24 hours	100–200 mg od

bid, twice daily; IV, intravenous; N/A, not applicable; od, once daily.

However, electrical cardioversion is considered when adequate rate control is not achieved with pharmacological agents, there is ongoing ischemia, severe hemodynamic compromise or heart failure. Even though electrical cardioversion effectively reverts AF, early recurrence is frequent after successful cardioversion particularly in patients who need catecholamine therapy for circulatory support. IV amiodarone promotes electrical cardioversion and also decreases risk for early recurrence, more so in recent onset AF.

Rhythm Control

There is scarce information indicating preferences for rate control over rhythm control for AF in AMI situation.[8] According to European Society of Cardiology (ESC) 2016 guidelines on AF, IV amiodarone is indicated for conversion to sinus rhythm in stable patients with recent onset AF and structural heart disease. Digoxin, calcium channel blockers, and beta-blockers, including sotalol are ineffective in converting recent onset AF to sinus rhythm.[9,10]

Prevention of Thromboembolism

Prevention of thromboembolism stroke is the most important aspect of management of AF. Reversion of AF to sinus rhythm does not eliminate the stroke risk in patients who do not have a pre-existing left atrial thrombus, as the atria remain stunned for several weeks after cardioversion. The risk of thromboembolism is evaluated by CHA2DS2-VASc score. The risk of bleeding should always be assessed before initiation of anticoagulation. This assessment is done using the HAS-BLED (Hypertension, Abnormal renal and liver function, Stroke, Bleeding Labile INR, Elderly, Drugs or alcohol) score.

Postcardioversion Anticoagulation

In patient with AF less than 48 hours from a definite onset, a bolus of UFH (5,000 units) or low-molecular-weight heparin (1 mg/kg IV) is given. If AF has occurred for more than 48 hours transesophageal echocardiography is necessary to exclude left atrial thrombus. Following cardioversion, further anticoagulation may be needed depending on underlying risk factor assessed by CHA2DS2-VASc score. For patients with CHA2DS2-VASc score 0 for males (or) 1 for female, no oral anticoagulation (OAC) is needed after cardioversion. In patient with AF more than 48 hours (or) risk factors for thromboembolism, heparin is continued together with warfarin targeting a lower international normalized ratio (INR) 2–2.5. Thereafter, anticoagulation is continued for 4 weeks and then further anticoagulation depends on the presence of risk factors. When AF cannot be cardioverted or cardioversion is contraindicated (presence of left atrial thrombus) acute rate control by IV medication alone is used.

Anticoagulation and Antiplatelets in Acute Myocardial Infarction

According to ESC 2017 guidelines on STEMI, in patients with clear indication for OAC that is AF with CHA2DS2-VACs score more than 2, and OAC is used is addition to antiplatelet therapy (Class IC).

For Patients Treated with Fibrinolysis

Consider triple therapy (aspirin, clopidogrel, and vitamin K antagonist to keep INR 2–2.5) for 14 days followed by a vitamin K antagonist plus a single antiplatelet agent (2013 ACC/AHA guidelines for management of STEMI).

For Patients Treated with Primary Percutaneous Coronary Intervention

After an ACS in patients with AF with stent implantation combination triple therapy with aspirin, clopidogrel and an OAC is recommended for 1–6 months (ACC/AHA 2013 guidelines on STEMI and 2016 update on duration of dual antiplatelet therapy). However without stent implantation dual treatment with an OAC and aspirin or clopidogrel is advised for up to 12 months.[11] If patient requires triple antithrombotic therapy combining dual antiplatelet therapy (DAPT) and OAC, duration of DAPT should be minimized to reduce bleeding risk (class IB). Triple therapy is required for at least 1 month. There is new data showing efficacy and safety of novel oral anticoagulants in this scenario. Dabigatran along with newer antiplatelets have been shown to be safe and efficacious in the recently published RE-DUAL study.[12] PIONEER-AF data[13] showed in selected patients who receive aspirin and clopidogrel, low-dose rivaroxaban (2.5 mg twice daily) can be used if the patient is at low bleeding risk. Gastric protection with a proton pump inhibitor is used for the duration of DAPT therapy in patients at high risk of bleeding (Class IC).

CONCLUSION

Atrial fibrillation is a common arrhythmia that complicates myocardial infarction early in the disease. AF in AMI is an independent predictor of short- and long-term unfavorable outcome irrespective of reperfusion strategy. A comprehensive approach which includes rate and rhythm control and TE episode prevention are the main aspects of management. Treatment of underlying cardiovascular causes and heart failure, the most common mode of death post-AMI, should be targeted as a priority.

REFERENCES

1. Zafari AM, Zarter SK, Heggen V, et al. A program encouraging early defibrillation results in improved in-hospital resuscitation efficacy. J Am Coll Cardiol. 2004;44(4):846-52.
2. Schmitt J, Duray G, Gersh BJ, et al. Atrial fibrillation in acute myocardial infarction: a systematic review of the incidence, clinical features and prognostic implications. Eur Heart J 2009;30(9):1038-45.
3. Batra G, Svennblad B, Held C, et al. All types of atrial fibrillation in the setting of myocardial infarction are associated with impaired outcome. Heart. 2016;102(12):926-33.
4. Siu CW, Jim MH, Ho HH, et al. Transient atrial fibrillation complicating acute inferior myocardial infarction: implications for future risk of ischemic stroke. Chest. 2007;132(1):44-9.
5. Segal JB, McNamara RL, Miller MR, et al. The evidence regarding the drugs used for ventricular rate control. J Fam Pract. 2000;49(1):47-59.
6. Hou ZY, Chang MS, Chen CY, et al. Acute treatment of recent-onset atrial fibrillation and flutter with a tailored dosing regimen of intravenous amiodarone. A randomized, digoxin-controlled study. Eur Heart J. 1995;16(4):521-8.
7. Metawee M, Charnigo R, Morales G, et al. Digoxin and short term mortality after acute STEMI: results from the MAGIC trial. Int J Cardiol. 2016;218:176-80.
8. Nilsson KR, Al-Khatib SM, Zhou Y, et al. Atrial Fibrillation management strategies and early mortality after myocardial infarction: results from the Valsartan in Acute Myocardial Infarction (VALIANT) Trial. Heart. 2010;96(11):838-42.
9. Jordaens L, Trouerbach J, Calle P, et al. Conversion of atrial fibrillation to sinus rhythm and rate control by digoxin in comparison to placebo. Eur Heart J. 1997;18(4):643-8.
10. Thomas SP, Guy D, Wallace E, et al. Rapid loading of sotalol or amiodarone for management of recent onset symptomatic atrial fibrillation: a randomized, digoxin-controlled trial. Am Heart J. 2004;147(1):E3.
11. Kirchhof P, Benussi S, Kotecha D, et al. Dual therapy with any OAC plus clopidogrel 75mg/day may be considered as an alternative to initial triple therapy. Eur Heart J. 2016;37:2893-962.
12. Cannon CP, Bhatt DL, Oldgren J, et al. Dual Antithrombotic Therapy with Dabigatran after PCI in Atrial Fibrillation. NEJM. 2017;377:1513-24.
13. Gibson CM, Mehran R, Bode C, et al. Prevention of Bleeding in Patients with Atrial Fibrillation Undergoing PCI. NEJM. 2016;375:2423-34.

SECTION 16

Ventricular Arrhythmias

CHAPTER 111

Ventricular Arrhythmias in Acute Myocardial Infarction

Rajesh A Dhopeshwarkar, Rakesh Yadav, Kewal C Goswami

INTRODUCTION

Sustained ventricular arrhythmias (VA) in the setting of acute myocardial infarction (AMI) remains a predominant cause of mortality both early and late after myocardial infarction (MI). A dynamic and changing cellular and intercellular milieu is responsible for the genesis of these arrhythmias. The true incidence of these arrhythmias in AMI occurring in the community is not clearly known as many sudden deaths that happen before the patient reaches the hospital are due to serious VA. Underlying genetic predisposition also contributes to this risk for VA. The incidence of VA is higher in patients with ST segment elevation MI (STEMI) than in patients with a non-ST elevation AMI. Management of VA in this setting is often challenging with limited effectiveness of current pharmacological therapy and frequently needing adjuvant treatment such as autonomic modulation, hemodynamics support, and rarely ablation.

TYPES OF VENTRICULAR ARRHYTHMIAS

Isolated ventricular premature beats (VPBs) is the most common arrhythmia seen in the setting of AMI with a reported frequency of 10–93%. More serious VAs are seen less frequently. Among patients with STEMI incidence of ventricular fibrillation (VF) is 3.7–6.7%.[1] In the GUSTO-1 trial,[2] the incidence of sustained ventricular tachycardia (VT) or VF was 10.2% with majority of these occurring in the first 48 hours of MI. In the current era of primary percutaneous coronary intervention (PCI) and pharmacotherapy using β-blockers and angiotensin-converting enzyme (ACE) inhibitors, the incidence of VA is markedly reduced.

MECHANISM AND PATHOGENESIS OF VENTRICULAR ARRHYTHMIAS AFTER ACUTE MYOCARDIAL INFARCTION

Acute myocardial infarction is an evolving dynamic state where multiple mechanisms are responsible for genesis of VA that are time-dependent. Various mechanisms are summarized in flowchart 1. Temporal distributions of VA during AMI are conventionally classified as early (<48 h) and late (>48 h). Patients with early (<48 h) VAs are classified as very early (Phase 1) within 30 minutes of occlusion of infarct-related artery (IRA) and (Phase 2) 1.5–72 hours of occlusion of IRA.

Phase 1 is a reversible phase where reperfusion can lead to complete salvage of myocardium. Phase 2 starts at 1.5 hours where there could be onset of irreversible myocardial injury.

Accompanying the loss of mechanical function with the occlusion of IRA are significant biochemical changes. These biochemical changes and associated myocyte edema and altered electrophysiologic properties of infarcting myocardium giving rise to areas of slow conduction, altered refractoriness, and altered excitability. Purkinje fibers are relatively resistant to ischemia and surviving Purkinje fibers exhibit shortened action potentials with depolarized membrane potential. These surviving and irritable Purkinje fibers have been proposed as the main cause for generating VA during Phase 2.

A multitude of biochemical and electrophysiological changes contribute to genesis of VA and are responsible for sudden cardiac death in AMI rather than an isolated mechanism or event. Particular interest is genetic predisposition that increases susceptibility to VA as identified in recent studies.

PREDICTORS OF SUSTAINED VENTRICULAR TACHYCARDIA AND VENTRICULAR FIBRILLATION

There are some factors that predispose a patient for VA after AMI. Patients with larger infarcts, low-ejection fraction, late presenters, or inability to achieve adequate perfusion all endow increased risk for VA, especially sustained VA. In addition, large peri-infarct border zone and extensive scar on magnetic resonance imaging (MRI) are potential risk factors.

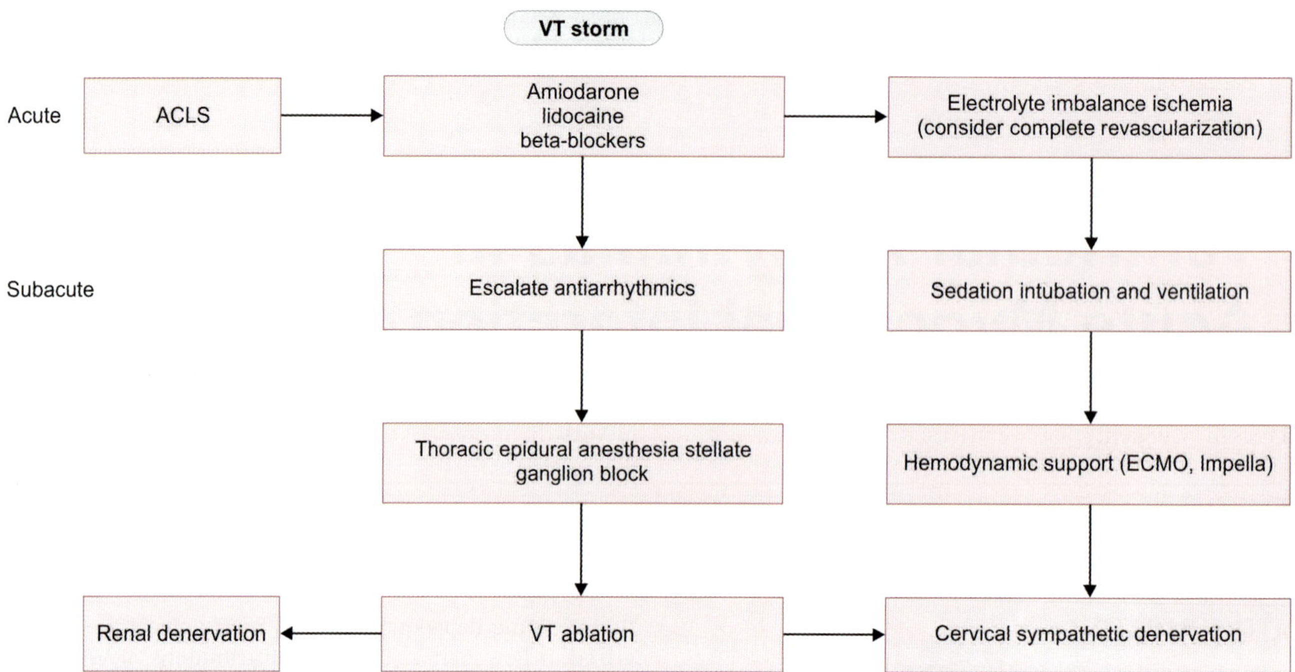

ACLS, advanced cardiac life support; ECMO, extracorporeal membrane oxygenator, VF, ventricular fibrillation; VT, ventricular tachycardia.

FLOWCHART 1: Algorithm for management of VT storm.

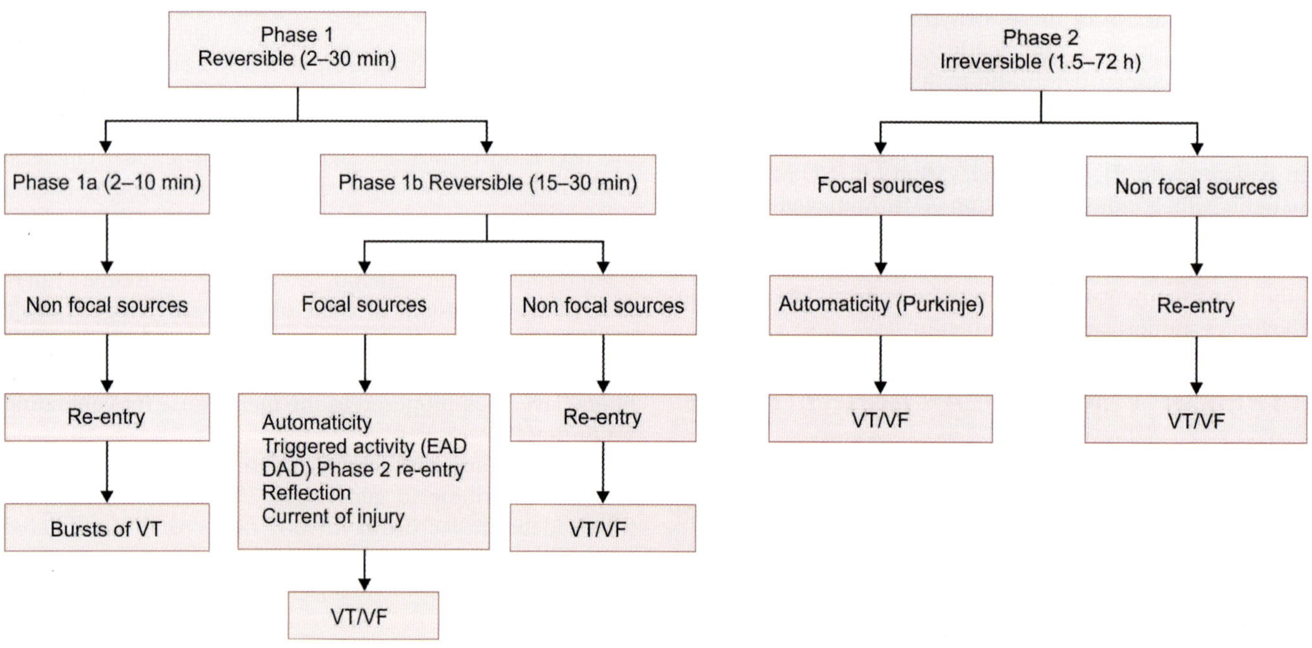

VF, ventricular fibrillation; VT, ventricular tachycardia; EAD, Early Afterdepolarization; DAD Delayed after depolarization.

FLOWCHART 2: Mechanisms of VT/VF in acute myocardial infarction.

DETERMINE[3] is a current large randomized trial looking into prophylactic implantable cardioverter defibrillator (ICD) therapy based on MRI-determined scar burden.

Programmed electrical stimulation has been used to assess the benefits of ICD therapy in patients late after AMI in the MADIT study. However, inducibility of sustained VT has low sensitivity in predicting future arrhythmic events. Other repolarization abnormalities, such as QT variability and dispersion, T-wave alternans, and measures of autonomic tone, such as heart rate variability and heart rate turbulence as well as baroreflex sensitivity, have been assessed as predictors.

However, they have not been proven to be beneficial. Higher prevalence of early repolarization has been observed in patients with VA and AMI in small studies.[4]

MANAGEMENT OF VENTRICULAR ARRHYTHMIAS

Ventricular Premature Beats

Isolated VPBs do not adversely affect prognosis after AMI. However, patients having complex ectopy, couplets, and multiform ectopics have a 3-fold increase in sudden deaths and 2-fold increase in all-cause mortalities.[5] In the GISSI-2 trial,[6] patients receiving thrombolytic therapy and having increased frequency of ventricular ectopy had higher mortality rate. In the CAMI study,[7] cardiac mortality was increased with increase in frequency of VPBs, but VPBs did not have an independent predictive value in multivariate analysis. With the advent of primary PCI, the absolute burden on VPBs in patients after AMI has been reduced. There is no evidence to support antiarrhythmic therapy to suppress VPBs. In fact there is evidence that drugs such as Encainide and Flecainide may increase mortality.[8]

Nonsustained Ventricular Tachycardia

With mechanism similar to sustained VT, nonsustained ventricular tachycardia (NSVT) is also seen in 12.7% patients following AMI. There is no evidence to treat asymptomatic episodes of NSVT with antiarrhythmic therapy other than β-blockers. However, frequent and hemodynamically unstable NSVT may need treatment with amiodarone.

Accelerated Idioventricular Rhythm

Accelerated idioventricular rhythm (AIVR) or slow VT is a ventricular rhythm with the heart rate between 50 and 100 beats/minute. Either an escape rhythm or an abnormal ectopic focus may be responsible for AIVR. AIVR is seen in up to 50% patients with AMI. Although seen post reperfusion, it is neither a sensitive nor a specific marker for successful reperfusion. AIVR is usually transient and needs no treatment.

Sustained Monomorphic Ventricular Tachycardia

Sustained monomorphic VT (SMVT) is observed in 2–3% of patients with STEMI and less than 1% of patients with non-ST elevation myocardial infarction (NSTEMI).[2] SMVT is less common than VF in the first few hours after AMI as the reentrant circuit needed for a SMVT is not established by then. SMVT occurring in the first 48 hours is generally due to enhanced automaticity or due to a prior infarct. SMVT occurring beyond 48 hours is usually due to structural changes leading to reentrant circuits. Scar from an old infarct may also be responsible for SMVT. While late SMVT is associated with a higher chance of recurrence of clinical VA, the clinical significance of early SMVT is still unclear as it may reflect presence of substrate for recurrence of VT. Available clinical data seems to suggest that patients who have SMVT in the post-MI period have a worse outcome than patients who have NSVT or VF.

Polymorphic Ventricular Tachycardia

Polymorphic VT is a rare arrhythmia following AMI (0.3%).[9] Coronary ischemia is the most common trigger for this arrhythmia. SMVT, within 48 hours of AMI, is associated with higher in-hospital mortality. However, its impact on long-term outcomes is unclear.[2] In a study[10] of 9,015 patients who had undergone PCI for AMI, sustained VT/VF was seen in 5.2% of the population and was associated with 4-fold increase in in-hospital mortality.

Late VT beyond 48 hours in the absence of ongoing ischemia is often due to arrhythmogenic substrate during healing of infarct. Patients with SMVT occurring beyond 48 hours have a worse in-hospital and 1-year mortality.[2]

Ventricular Fibrillation

The incidence of VF in the fibrinolytic era has ranged from 3% to 7% in various studies. Most of the episodes of VF are seen in the first 48–72 hours. They are usually due to ischemia and lack of perfusion.[2] VF is classified as primary when there is no ischemia or heart failure precipitating. VF due to recurrent ischemia or due to heart failure is classified as nonprimary VF.

Management of Sustained Ventricular Tachycardia/Ventricular Fibrillation[11]

Acute management of hemodynamically unstable sustained VT or VF is done as per ACLS guidelines. Prompt defibrillation is extremely important. Recurrent sustained VA could be due to residual ischemia or recurrence of acute ischemia. Prompt revascularization is important in eliminating it. This is especially true for polymorphic VT and VF. Patients with hemodynamically tolerated SMVT are treated with intravenous amiodarone. Use of other antiarrhythmic drugs in acute coronary syndrome such as Procainamide or Flecainide is not recommended.

Correction of acid-base balance and electrolytes are important adjuncts to the management. Patients with recurrent VT/VF should be promptly sedated and, if necessary, ventilated. SMVT that is recurrent and refractory to therapy is a challenging subset. Overdrive pacing can be used in these patients. Catheter ablation is a challenging but useful therapy in this subset of patients. Hemodynamic support with percutaneous left ventricular assist device (LVAD)[12] and extracorporeal membrane oxygenator (ECMO)-assisted primary PCI are extremely useful therapies in patients with refractory VA and cardiogenic shock.

In a study[13] comparing ECMO and intra-aortic balloon pump (IABP), 69.23% of patients on ECMO could be weaned as against only 12.5% with IABP. IABP is therefore not recommended.

Pharmacologic Therapy

Beta-blockers

Beta-blocker therapy remains the crux of management of patients with AMI. Multiple trials have proven reduction in sudden death and total mortality with β-blocker use in AMI.

Amiodarone

Amiodarone remains the drug of choice for managing sustained VT/VF after AMI. Amiodarone was found superior to lidocaine in patients with out-of-hospital cardiac arrest. However, amiodarone use has not been found to be associated with any long-term survival benefit. Lidocaine, mexiletine, and phenytoin have also been used in patients with incessant VA in the setting of AMI.

Catheter Ablation of Recurrent Sustained Ventricular Tachycardia and Electrical Storm

Three or more distinct episodes of VT or VF occurring within 24 hours of AMI is defined as electrical storm. Incessant VT and VF after AMI carries high mortality. It is often difficult to control with antiarrhythmic treatment alone. Recurrent VT or VF arise frequently from Purkinje fiber irritability in the infarct border zones. When it persists despite revascularization and adequate pharmacologic treatment, catheter ablation should be considered. These incessant VT and VF are due to macroreentrant circuits that develop early in the infarct border zone and due to triggering premature ventricular beats from irritable Purkinje fibers. Both can be targeted by ablation. Three-dimensional mapping and ablation using irrigated catheters is performed in this setting. Identifying and targeting late potentials, fragmented electrograms, channel ablation, and scar homogenization has been described in context to substrate-based ablation.[14] Activation mapping of VPBs that trigger VT and VF can be done provided they are frequent enough. Purkinje potentials before the VPBs are also identified in the infarct border zone.[15]

Noninducibility of VT/VF is a good marker for long-term success and survival.[16] Periprocedural mortality of up to 3% due to intractable VT and long-term mortality of 18% due to both VT and heart failure have been reported.[17]

Implantable Cardioverter Defibrillator

Patients who develop VT/VF within 48 hours of AMI have not been evaluated systematically. Current guidelines do not recommend ICD implantation in these patients. Patients developing sustained VT/VF beyond 48 hours without a correctable cause are candidates for ICD therapy.

Wearable Cardiac Defibrillator

Substantial mortality exists early after AMI. Two trials, DINAMIT and IRIS, have found the futility of primary prevention ICD within 40 days of AMI. To address this early period, VEST prevention of early sudden death trial, the VEST trial[18] was designed. Contrary to expectations wearable cardiac defibrillator (WCD) did not reduce sudden cardiac death (SCD) for up to 90 days after AMI. Surprisingly, all-cause mortality was significantly less in the WCD arm. Current ESC guidelines[11] recommend WCD (Cl IIb LOE C) in patients who are at high-risk for SCD for a limited time. They are likely to be modified in the setting of AMI after the VEST trial.

Autonomic Modulation for Management of Refractory Ventricular Tachycardia/Ventricular Fibrillation in the Setting of Electrical Storm[19]

Autonomic nervous system plays an important role in the genesis of VT and VF. AMI is frequently associated with sympathetic activation. Electrical storm with multiple ICD shocks is associated with high mortality. Thoracic epidural anesthesia (TEA) and percutaneous stellate ganglion block are two promising bedside interventions. Cervical sympathetic denervation (CSD), especially bilateral CSD, has been tried in patients with structural heart disease and electrical storm. In a small group of patients with refractory VA,[20] TEA was associated with 80% reduction and CSD with 50% reduction in arrhythmia burden. In an international multicenter study, CSD, especially bilateral CSD, was associated with 88% reduction in ICD shocks and 50% freedom from ICD shocks, transplant, or death.[21] Other neuromodulatory therapies, such as spinal cord stimulation, percutaneous stellate ganglion block, and renal denervation are also being evaluated for managing refractory VA.

CONCLUSION

Ventricular arrhythmias have been reported after STEMI and NSTEMI with varying frequency and severity. Setting of STEMI is dynamic and evolving with changing arrhythmia substrate and mechanisms responsible for arrhythmogenesis. Both early and late VAs, especially sustained VAs, are associated with worse prognosis after STEMI. Management of VA, especially refractory VA, after STEMI, remains challenging and involves drugs, hemodynamic and ventilatory support, as well as autonomic modulation and ablation.

Ventricular arrhythmias, especially sustained VT/VF, impart a substantial increase in mortality in patients after AMI. Prompt revascularization is of utmost importance not only in limiting the myocardial damage but also in reducing the incidence of VA. Management of VA in this setting is confounded by limited pharmacologic therapy at disposal. Management of associated electrolyte abnormalities and hemodynamic support is of use in patients with low cardiac output and cardiogenic shock. Heightened sympathetic tone and autonomic imbalance also contribute. Newer investigational therapies are being tried to address this. Catheter ablation is challenging and of high risk but offers reasonable options in an otherwise hopeless situation of drug refractory and incessant VT/VF.

REFERENCES

1. Volpi A, Cavalli A, Santoro L, et al. Incidence and prognosis of early primary ventricular fibrillation in acute myocardial infarction–results of the Gruppo Italiano per lo Studio della Sopravvivenza nell'Infarto Miocardico (GISSI-2) database. Am J Cardiol. 1998;82:265.

2. Newby KH, Thompson T, Stebbins A, et al. Sustained ventricular arrhythmias in patients receiving thrombolytic therapy: incidence and outcomes. The GUSTO investigators. Circulation. 1998;98(23):2567-73.
3. Kadish AH, Bello D, Finn JP, et al. Rationale and design for the Defibrillators to Reduce Risk by Magnetic Resonance Imaging Evaluation (DETERMINE) trial. J Cardiovasc Electrophysiol. 2009;20(9):982-7.
4. Tikkanen JT, Wichmann V, Junttila MJ, et al. Association of early repolarization and sudden cardiac death during an acute coronary event. Circ Arrhythm Electrophysiol. 2012;5:714-8.
5. Ruberman W, Weinblatt E, Goldberg JD, et al. Ventricular premature complexes and sudden death after myocardial infarction. Circulation. 1981;64:297-305.
6. Maggioni AP, Zuanetti G, Franzosi MG, et al. Prevalence and prognostic significance of ventricular arrhythmias after acute myocardial infarction in the fibrinolytic era. GISSI-2 results. Circulation. 1993;87:312-22.
7. Rouleau JL, Talajic M, Sussex B, et al. Myocardial infarction patients in the 1990s–their risk factors, stratification and survival in Canada: the Canadian assessment of myocardial infarction (CAMI) study. J Am Coll Cardiol. 1996;27:1119-27.
8. Echt DS, Liebson PR, Mitchell LB, et al. Mortality and morbidity in patients receiving Encainide, Flecainide, or Placebo. N Engl J Med. 1991;324:781-88.
9. Wolfe CL, Nibley C, Bhandari A, et al. Polymorphous ventricular tachycardia associated with acute myocardial infarction. Circulation. 1991;84:1543-51.
10. Piccini JP, Berger JS, Brown DL. Early sustained ventricular arrhythmias complicating acute myocardial infarction. Am J Med. 2008;121:797-804.
11. Priori SG, Blomström-Lundqvist C, Mazzanti A, et al. ESC guidelines for the management of patients with ventricular arrhythmias and the prevention of sudden cardiac death. Eur Heart J. 2015;36:2793-867.
12. O'neill WW, Schreiber T, Wohns DHW, et al. The current use of Impella 2.5 in acute myocardial infarction complicated by cardiogenic shock: results from the USpella registry. J Interv Cardiol. 2013;27:1-11.
13. Kim H, Lim SH, Hong J, et al. Efficacy of veno-arterial extracorporeal membrane oxygenation in acute myocardial infarction with cardiogenic shock. Resuscitation. 2012;83:971-5.
14. Tilz RR, Makimoto H, Lin T, et al. Electrical isolation of a substrate after myocardial infarction: a novel ablation strategy for unmappable ventricular tachycardias–feasibility and clinical outcome. Europace. 2014;16(7):1040-52.
15. Tan VH, Yap J, Hsu LF, et al. Catheter ablation of ventricular fibrillation triggers and electrical storm. Europace. 2012;14:1687-95.
16. Carbucicchio C, Santamaria M, Trevisi N, et al. Catheter ablation for the treatment of electrical storm in patients with implantable cardioverter-defibrillators: short- and long-term outcomes in a prospective single-center study. Circulation. 2008;117:462-9.
17. Stevenson WG, Wilber DJ, Natale A, et al. Irrigated radiofrequency catheter ablation guided by electroanatomic mapping for recurrent ventricular tachycardia after myocardial infarction: the multicenter thermocool ventricular tachycardia ablation trial. Circulation. 2008;118:2773-82.
18. Vest prevention of early sudden death trial (VEST) (Olgin J). [online] Available from http://www.clinicaltrialresults.org/Slides/ACC2018/VEST_Olgin.pdf [accessed March, 2018].
19. Bradfield JS, Ajijola OA, Vaseghi M, et al. Mechanisms and management of refractory ventricular arrhythmias in the age of autonomic modulation. Heart Rhythm. 2018;15(8):1252-60.
20. Bourke T, Vaseghi M, Michowitz Y, et al. Neuraxial modulation for refractory ventricular arrhythmias: value of thoracic epidural anesthesia and surgical left cardiac sympathetic denervation. Circulation. 2010;121:2255-62.
21. Vaseghi M, Barwad P, Corrales FJM, et al. Cardiac sympathetic denervation for refractory ventricular arrhythmias. J Am Coll Cardiol. 2017;69:3070-80.

CHAPTER 112

Ventricular Arrhythmias and Sudden Death: Problems and Opportunities in Clinical Practice

Kapil Kumawat

INTRODUCTION

Sudden cardiac death (SCD) accounts for 50% of all cardiovascular deaths,[1] and approximately 50% of cardiac disorders are first clinically recognized when patient unfortunately presents with SCD.[2] Ventricular arrhythmias (VAs) constitute the major underlying mechanism in SCD, especially in older age group. In out-of-hospital cardiac arrest, VAs constitute 30–70% of the initially observed rhythm,[3,4] though the exact rhythm would depend upon the time from actual event to evaluation of rhythm, with early observation leading to more VAs being observed and later evaluation leading to more asystole and pulseless electrical activity. Not all VAs lead to sudden death. VAs can range from being completely asymptomatic, as in ventricular premature beats (VPBs) to the most devastating ventricular fibrillation (VF) leading to sudden cardiac arrest (SCA) and SCD. Vast majority of sudden death by VA is seen in patients with underlying structural heart disease, especially coronary artery disease (CAD). Monomorphic ventricular tachycardia (VT) occurring in absence of underlying heart disease is called idiopathic VT and usually does not lead to SCD. The structural heart disease is either known before the SCD or is discovered after the event as postmortem analysis or in the clinical evaluation of the lucky few who are successfully resuscitated from SCA.

MECHANISMS OF VENTRICULAR ARRHYTHMIAS AND SUDDEN CARDIAC DEATH

Mechanisms of VA include: (1) enhanced normal automaticity or abnormal automaticity; (2) triggered activity induced by early or late afterdepolarizations; and (3) reentry. The initiation and progression of VA involves a complex interplay between substrate, triggers, and modifiers. The substrate may be structural changes secondary to an underlying disease process, and often includes a scar caused by prior myocardial infarction (MI) or surgical repair, or patchy fibrosis in the setting of cardiomyopathy or hypertrophy. With advancement in imaging like cardiac magnetic resonance (CMR), underlying structural changes are being elucidated in more and more diseases. Changes in ion channels, transporter proteins and other cell membrane proteins, cell-to-cell connections and coupling protein may be the underlying substrate in patients with so called structurally normal heart as these cannot be picked up by any clinical imaging modality.

The electrophysiological substrate is dynamically influenced by a variety of factors including electrolytes, cardiac metabolism, mechanical stretch, signaling pathways, and autonomic effects. Cardiac innervation and autonomic inputs (parasympathetic and sympathetic) are increasingly being recognized as significant modifying (sometimes initiating) factors in VAs and SCD and various new therapeutic modalities affecting cardiac nervous system are being developed and tested to prevent and treat VA and decrease SCD.

Most sustained VAs in the presence of structural heart disease are caused by reentry as underlying mechanism.[5] Reentry may occur around a fixed anatomical obstacle, such as scar after an MI or surgically repaired congenital heart disease. Reentry can also be functional reentry around areas of functional block without anatomical obstacles. There are two main proposed complex models of functional reentry to explain mechanism of VF.[6,7] The "leading circle model" has a functionally refractory core and no excitable gap. "Spiral wave reentry" is driven by a rotor with a curved wavefront and wavetail pivoting around an excitable but unexcited core. Phase 2 reentry can occur due to heterogeneity of repolarization between various areas of heart (e.g., between endocardium and epicardium). Phase 2 reentry may be one of the mechanisms of VT or VF in Brugada syndrome and during acute ischemia.[7]

Abnormal automaticity is one of the causes of VAs in acute ischemia and is caused by decreased transmembrane potential (due to increased extracellular potassium) nearing the activation potential of calcium channels.[5-7] Enhanced normal automaticity in Purkinje cells in ischemic zone may also trigger VA during acute coronary syndrome (ACS). Early afterdepolarizations (during late phase 2 or early phase 3 of action potential) are the trigger for torsades de pointes VT associated with QT prolongation (acquired or genetic channelopathies). Delayed afterdepolarizations occur after complete membrane repolarization, and develop under conditions of intracellular calcium overload caused by tachycardia, catecholamines, hypokalemia, digoxin toxicity, cardiac hypertrophy, and heart failure (HF).[8,9] Increased sarcoplasmic calcium and ryanodine receptor over activity can lead to activation of calcium-sodium currents leading to triggered action potential. Delayed afterdepolarizations are the underlying mechanism for VT in the setting of digoxin toxicity, catecholaminergic polymorphic VT, and idiopathic outflow tract VA, VAs in HF and some Purkinje fiber mediated VAs.

EPIDEMIOLOGY

By far the most common underlying disease in patient dying because of VA is CAD. The incidence of CAD in patients with SCD is pegged to be about 80% in patients above 35 years of age in western world.[10] The next most common cause of VA and SCD is cardiomyopathies [including dilated cardiomyopathy and hypertrophic cardiomyopathy (HCM)] accounting for 10–20% of SCD cases. Less than 5% of VA and SCD are caused by miscellaneous disorders like valvular heart disease, inflammatory and infiltrative heart disease. The infiltrative heart diseases like sarcoidosis are more and more being recognized as cause of VAs, but they still account for small numbers of SCD in general population. The genetic arrhythmia syndromes like channelopathies play a minor role numerically in general population above 35 years of age but are important cause of VAs and SCD. In younger age group of adolescents and young adults, myocarditis and congenital structural heart disease are responsible for majority of cases of VA and SCD. The age group 25–35 years is transition zone where CAD and cardiomyopathy increase as cause of SCD.[10] More men than women have SCD, especially with advancing age, due to increasing prevalence of CAD.[11]

It is a major exercise to determine in cause or mechanism of SCD, and the required tools like molecular autopsy and genetic analysis may not be readily available, especially in country like India. Even after autopsy and extensive postmortem evaluation up to 50% SCD may remain unexplained.[12]

THERAPIES FOR VENTRICULAR ARRHYTHMIAS AND SUDDEN CARDIAC DEATH

Treatment of VAs (and prevention of SCD) begins with management of underlying diseases and comorbidities to prevent formation or progression of substrate, and to prevent triggers leading to VA and SCD. The therapies involve medications, nonpharmacological medical management, and use of devices especially defibrillators (in various forms), catheter ablation and surgery. A lot of progress has been made in management of underlying disorders since the seminal trials of drugs and implantable cardioverter defibrillators (ICDs) were done and it is unlikely that any such new trials would be done. So we need to extrapolate the findings of these trials to the modern context.[13] An important aspect of treatment is discontinuation of proarrhythmic medications like those causing prolonged QT.

Antiarrhythmic Drugs

Of all the available antiarrhythmic medications, only β-blockers have shown to improve survival in randomized trials in VAs. A few trials have shown benefits with amiodarone.[14,15] All drugs have a significant potential for causing adverse events, including proarrhythmia. However, the use of these medications is essential in some patients to control arrhythmias and improve symptoms. Drugs can induce sinus bradycardia and atrioventricular (AV) block, impair His-Purkinje conduction and produce AV or bundle branch block, or prolong ventricular repolarization and the QT interval.

Beta-Blockers

Beta-blockers act by decreasing sympathetic activity by competitively blocking beta-adrenoceptors, decreasing sinus rate and by decreasing calcium release by ryanodine receptor channel.[16] They are usually the first line of therapy in a large spectrum of disorders with or without HF.[17,18] Beta-blockers reduce all-cause mortality and SCD in patients with HF with reduced ejection fraction (HFrEF).[19-21] In the setting of polymorphic VT after MI, β-blockers reduce mortality.[22] Beta-blockers (e.g., nadolol, propranolol) are also first-line therapy for some cardiac channelopathies [e.g., long QT syndrome (LQTS), catecholaminergic polymorphic VT].

Amiodarone

Amiodarone is multichannel blocker and blocks adrenergic receptors and sodium, potassium, and calcium channels. Effect of amiodarone on SCD is controversial. A few studies and a meta-analysis of several large studies have shown a reduction in SCD using amiodarone in patients with left ventricular (LV) dysfunction due to prior MI and nonischemic cardiomyopathy (NICM).[23-25] The SCD in Heart Failure Trial (SCD-HeFT) did not show any survival benefit with amiodarone versus placebo in patients with left ventricular ejection fraction (LVEF) less than 35%.[26] In fact, a secondary analysis of the SCD-HeFT showed increased risk of mortality with amiodarone in patients with New York Heart Association (NYHA) class III symptoms.[27] A meta-analysis in high-risk patients (LVEF <40%, with or without coronary disease), concluded that, for primary prevention, amiodarone decreased the risk of SCD [risk ratio 0.76; 95% confidence interval (CI) 0.66–0.88] and all-cause mortality (risk ratio: 0.88; 95% CI 0.78–1.00). The same systematic review suggested no significant benefit or harm in secondary prevention.[28] Intravenous amiodarone is used to reduce recurrent VT or VF during resuscitation.[29] Long-term administration of amiodarone has adverse effects on multiple systems including thyroid, lungs, liver, eyes, skin, and nerves.

These adverse effects are dependent on dose and duration of use and require discontinuation in significant number of patients. Hence, chronic treatment of young patients with amiodarone should be reserved as a bridge to more definitive treatment options such as catheter ablation.[30]

Sotalol

Sotalol is a blocker of delayed rectifier potassium channels with β-blocker properties. It has some efficacy in suppressing VA, but it has significant proarrhythmic effects and has not been shown to improve survival in a study of 146 patients with CAD and ICD.[31] D-sotalol was shown in the SWORD (Survival with Oral D-Sotalol) trial to increase the risk of death in patients with HF.[32] Sotalol may lead to HF decompensation, and so its use in patients with an LVEF less than 20% is generally avoided. Sotalol can be used safely in patients with CAD who do not have decompensated HF. The use of sotalol requires careful monitoring using electrocardiogram (ECG, QTc), especially in patients with a low body mass index or impaired renal function.

Sodium Channel Blockers

Class IA (e.g., quinidine, disopyramide) antiarrhythmic drugs that block the sodium current also block the rapid component of the delayed rectifier potassium current and may therefore prolong the QT interval. The CAST (Cardiac Arrhythmia Suppression Trial),[33] showed an increased mortality or nonfatal cardiac arrest rate (7.7%) among post-MI patients treated with encainide or flecainide. Hence, the use of class IC sodium channel blockers after MI has been contraindicated. The contraindication has been extended to other class I antiarrhythmic agents, because even if they do not increase mortality in post-MI patients they fail to reduce mortality.

Intravenous lidocaine can be used in cases of refractory VT or witnessed cardiac arrest[29] (most of the times along with amiodarone). Oral mexiletine is useful in congenital LQTS and quinidine is useful in Brugada syndrome patients.[34] Flecainide is used in catecholaminergic polymorphic VT patients not responding to β-blockers.[35]

Ranolazine, developed as antianginal agent, is a late sodium channel current blocking agent and has small blocking action on phase 3 repolarizing potassium current (Ikr). In small clinical studies, it has shown to decrease VTs, but not SCD.[36]

Others

In patients with HF with reduced EF (HFrEF), many HF medications have shown to decrease SCD. Angiotensin-converting enzyme inhibitors reduce mortality and SCD[37] in HFrEF patients. Mineralocorticoid-receptor antagonists, spironolactone, and eplerenone also reduce SCD along with overall mortality in this group of patients.[38,39] Recently published studies with the angiotensin receptor neprilysin inhibitor (sacubitril or valsartan) have shown a reduction in SCD along with cardiac mortality.[40]

Intravenous magnesium is first-line therapy in torsades de pointes VT.[41] It is recommended to keep the potassium level between 4.5 mmol/L and 5 mmol/L to prevent VA,[42,43] especially in high-risk conditions like acute myocardial infarction (AMI).

Combination Therapy

This should be reserved for patient with refractory VAs as it can be highly proarrhythmic. Combinations of sodium channel blockers and potassium channel blockers (e.g., amiodarone and flecainide/propafenone or mexiletine and sotalol) have been used in patients with frequent VT recurrences who have a defibrillator in place. Combination of β-blockers and amiodarone reduces the number of ICD shocks, however, side effects result in drug discontinuation in a significant number of patients.[44] Ranolazine has recently been tried in combined with other antiarrhythmic agents in cases of refractory VT, and has shown mixed results.[45]

DEVICES FOR TREATMENT OF VENTRICULAR ARRHYTHMIAS AND SUDDEN CARDIAC DEATH

Defibrillation is highly effective in terminating life-threatening VA. There are various forms of defibrillators: transvenous ICD; a subcutaneous ICD; a wearable cardioverter-defibrillator (WCD); or an external defibrillator.

Implantable Cardioverter Defibrillator

Implantable defibrillators have now been in use for last 30 years. Many high-quality randomized controlled trials (RCTs) support its use in various patient populations including survivors of cardiac arrest, patients with VT and structural heart disease, and patients with significant LV dysfunction. ICD therapy has been shown to prevent SCD and prolong life in patients at high-risk of sudden arrhythmic death, and is recommended in high-risk patients if the patient does not suffer from other conditions that limit life expectancy to less than 1–2 years.[46] However, ICD use may be associated with complications like infection and inappropriate shocks, which are especially frequent in children.[47] A retrospective analyses of 3,000 patients with ICD or cardiac resynchronization therapy defibrillator (CRT-D) showed a significant incidence of adverse events over a 12-year period: 20% inappropriate shocks, 6% device-related infections, and 17% lead failures.[48] Hence, careful selection of patients for ICD is very important. In spite of compelling evidence in favor of ICD, its utilization lags significantly in many countries like India. The major limiting factor being the high cost of ICDs.

A meta-analysis of the three major secondary prophylaxis ICD trials [Antiarrhythmics Versus Implantable Defibrillators (AVID), Cardiac Arrest Study Hamburg (CASH) and Canadian Implantable defibrillator study (CIDS)] demonstrated that ICD therapy was associated with a 50% ($p = 0.0001$) reduction in mortality by arrhythmia and a 28% ($p = 0.006$) reduction in total mortality in patients who have survived a cardiac arrest or life-threatening VA (hemodynamically unstable VA or VT with syncope) compared to antiarrhythmic drugs (predominantly amiodarone).[49]

Subcutaneous Cardioverter Defibrillator

The subcutaneous implantable cardioverter defibrillator does not require venous access and hence avoid complications of transvenous lead implantation including pneumothorax, hemothorax, and cardiac tamponade. Studies (mostly nonrandomized) have shown that the subcutaneous implantable cardioverter defibrillator can reliably detect and treat VF during defibrillation threshold testing at time of implantation and successfully terminate spontaneous clinical sustained VT and VF occurring during follow-up.[50] They are especially useful in patients who do not require anti-tachycardia pacing (or pacing in general) and patients with no venous access.

Wearable Cardioverter Defibrillator

The wearable cardioverter defibrillator is a vest to be worn under clothing, in contact with chest. The electrodes in this vest continuously monitor the heart rhythm and automatically deliver defibrillation shock when VF or VT is detected. The WCD has been approved in the United States by the US Food and Drug Administration for patients who are "at risk for SCA and are not candidates for or refuse an implantable defibrillator", e.g., patients having an LVEF of 35% or less within 40 days from MI or revascularization within the past 90 days (hence not yet a candidate for ICD), patients awaiting cardiac transplant, or patients with newly diagnosed NICM, myocarditis or secondary cardiomyopathy. A recently presented trial (Vest Prevention of Early Sudden Death Trial—VEST)[51] surprisingly showed that WCD does not reduce SCD (but reduces all-cause mortality) among patients with moderate-to-severe LV dysfunction immediately post-MI up to 90 days.

Automated Cardioverter Defibrillator

External defibrillation reduces mortality when delivered within minutes of onset of life-threatening VA including VF. The automated cardioverter defibrillator (AED) can be safely used by first responders including lay persons to deliver defibrillation to patients having out-of-hospital cardiac arrest.[52] Efforts should be made to popularize placement and use of AEDs at public places like airports, railway and bus stations, schools, sports facilities, etc.

Catheter Ablation

Catheter ablation is an important treatment option for patients with VA when antiarrhythmic medications are ineffective, not tolerated, or not desired by the patient. Whether catheter ablation can replace ICD therapy in well-tolerated sustained monomorphic VT in patients with an LVEF less than 40% requires further evaluation. Till then, ICD implantation is recommended in survivors of MI and other disorders with structural and molecular heart diseases suffering from sustained VT or VF, even if they undergo successful catheter ablation.[14] At present, there is no evidence that catheter ablation reduces mortality. It plays very useful role in decreasing ICD shocks, which have been shown to increase mortality.[53]

PREVENTION, PREDICTION, AND TREATMENT OF VAS AND SCD IN SPECIFIC DISORDERS

Coronary Artery Disease

Ischemic heart disease (IHD) due to CAD, recognized or unrecognized, remains the overwhelmingly largest underlying cause of VA and SCD. When VF is the first identified rhythm in a patient of out-of-hospital cardiac arrest, AMI is discovered in about half the patients and significant coronary stenosis was found in more than 50% patient of out-of-hospital cardiac arrest when they were subjected to coronary angiography immediately after resuscitation.[54] The mechanism of VA differs in the acute and chronic phases of IHD. In chronic phase it is the macroreentry around the scar which leads to VT which can then degenerate into VF leading to SCD. The mechanisms of VAs in acute phase of IHD are less well understood, but include heterogeneity of depolarization and repolarization due to ischemic damage to cell membranes, and abnormal or enhanced automaticity in Purkinje fibers. VA in acute phase is usually polymorphic VT or VF.

A large number of SCD events occur in patients of ACS even before they reach hospital. Hence, to reduce incidence of SCD in general population it is important to screen for patients at high risk of SCD. The incidence of VA in ACS undergoing treatment in hospital has declined in recent years, mainly due to early and intense revascularization, including primary angioplasty and also due to availability and adequate use of specific pharmacological treatment. However, in spite of adequate modern management in ACS, up to 6% of patients develop VT or VF within the first 48 hours after the onset of symptoms, most often before or during reperfusion.[13]

Acute Coronary Syndrome

Beta-blockers reduce VT or VF in ACS and are therefore recommended to be used early in ACS in patients who are hemodynamically stable.[55] Intravenous amiodarone should be considered only if episodes of VT or VF are frequent and cannot be controlled by repeated electrical cardioversion or defibrillation.[13] Intravenous lidocaine can be used in resistant cases of recurrent sustained VT or VF not responding to β-blockers and/or amiodarone. Some patients with recurrent VT or VF which is shown to be triggered by premature ventricular complex (PVC) arising from partially injured Purkinje fibers can be successfully treated by catheter ablation of initiating ventricular premature contraction.[13]

Immediate Post ACS

Sudden cardiac death is an important cause of death after AMI and is often due to recurrent infarction and not just because of VAs. Early ICD implantation after ACS has not been shown to improve prognosis, probably due to prevalence of nonarrhythmic causes of death, like reinfarction and cardiac rupture. Hence, it is recommended that LVEF be reassessed 6–12 weeks after MI in stable patients on optimized HF medications to assess for a primary preventive ICD implantation.[13,30]

Risk Stratification Post ACS

The LVEF is the most commonly used marker for the assessment of risk of SCD in IHD, and many studies have conclusively proved that ICDs reduce risk of SCD in patients with low LVEF. An LVEF of less than 30–35% is widely used as cut-off for ICD implantation. However, LVEF is not a very robust parameter to assess risk of SCD. When a LVEF of less than 35% is used as cut-off, 80% of cases of SCD will be missed. In the primary prevention population, only 5% of patients with ICDs for LVEF less than 35% will experience VT or VF per year.[26] In secondary prevention population, up to 50% of patients received ICD therapy in 1 year. SCD risk is highest in the immediate post-MI phase; however, the ICDs in Acute Myocardial Infarction Trial (DINAMIT) showed no mortality benefit with early placement of ICDs (at 6–40 days after MI).

In patients' history of MI and preserved LVEF, none of noninvasive risk stratification techniques were found to have sufficient specificity and sensitivity for clinical use. Many markers have been evaluated: microvolt T-wave alternans; QRS duration; signal-averaged ECG; ventricular ectopy; indicators of autonomic tone, such as heart rate variability, heart rate turbulence and baroreflex sensitivity.[56] However, in spite of initial promise, none of these were found to be superior to LVEF for SCD risk stratification and selection of patients for ICD implantation. QRS fragmentation seen in 12-lead ECG is due to conduction delays in different portions of heart. Some studies have shown usefulness of QRS fragmentation for prediction of VAs. However, assessment of this parameter is highly subjective and it can be seen as a normal variant. Hence, QRS fragmentation was never found to be sensitive or specific enough to predict SCD. More studies are needed to more accurately define relevant ECG morphologies to make it part of clinical decision making.[57-61]

More recently, late gadolinium enhancement cardiac magnetic resonance (LGE-CMR) has gained acceptance as gold standard for assessing myocardial fibrosis. The extent of myocardial fibrosis, especially in peri-infarct zone, as assessed by LGE-CMR appears to correlate with risk of SCD. However, routine use of LGE-CMR is limited in many centers due to its high cost, lack of expert radiologists, duration of study, and the need for potentially toxic contrast.[62-64]

Reduced right ventricular ejection fraction (RVEF) has also emerged as a useful parameter for assessing SCD risk: a strong correlation between RVEF less than 45% and SCD was documented in patients with LVEF greater than 35%.[65] Myocardial iodine-123 meta-iodobenzylguanidine imaging and (11)C-meta-hydroxyephedrine positron emission tomography (PET) have been used to demonstrate reduced sympathetic innervation of the heart and can predict an increased risk of SCD.[66,67]

Nonischemic Cardiomyopathy

Patients with NICM should be on adequate guidelines based medical treatment for HF for at least 3 months before a primary prevention ICD is considered.[30] LVEF is still the most robust measure for stratifying risk of SCD in NICM. Doubts have been raised about usefulness of ICD in primary prevention of SCD in NICM patients. A meta-analysis of the five primary prevention ICD trials (1,854 patients with nonischemic dilated cardiomyopathy) showed that in NICM, ICD reduce all-cause mortality by a significant 31% relative to medical therapy (risk ratio: 0.69; 95% CI 0.55–0.87, p = 0.002).[68] Recently published DANISH (the Danish Study to Assess the Efficiency of ICDs in Patients with Non-ischemic Systolic Heart Failure on Mortality) trial has stoked the controversy again.[69] DANISH trial showed that prophylactic ICD implantation in symptomatic NICM led to 50% reduction in SCD at 8 years compared with "usual clinical care". However, all-cause mortality was not significantly lowered. In DANISH study, CRT (either ICD or pacemaker) was used in 58% of patients in both the ICD and medical therapy arms. Therefore, the results of DANISH cannot be generalized to patients with NICM who are ineligible for CRT.[30]

Syncope in patients of NICM has shown to be associated with high mortality and appropriate ICD shocks in non-randomized studies and hence ICD was recommended in such patients.[70-72] However conflicting data has emerged, which challenges the assumption that syncope in NICM is due to malignant VAs. In a subgroup analysis of SCD-HeFT patients with NICM and syncope, ICD did not lead to decreased mortality.[73] Similarly, in a subgroup analysis of the MADIT-RIT (Multicenter Automatic Defibrillator Implantation Trial-Reduce Inappropriate Therapy) trial, syncope was found to be due to VAs in only 39% of patients.[74]

A meta-analysis of 29 studies regarding the use of LGE-CMR for risk stratification in NICM, suggested that it could be a significant predictor of SCD risk.[75] The distribution of fibrosis in LGE-CMR is of incremental value, mid-wall fibrosis appears to be associated with increased risk of VAs and SCD.[76,77]

Hypertrophic Cardiomyopathy

Hypertrophic cardiomyopathy is considered to be the most common identifiable cause of SCD in individuals less than 40 years of age.[78] HCM patients who have survived SCA, VF, or sustained VT resulting in syncope or hemodynamic compromise are indicated to have ICD implantation.[30] Risk of SCD in HCM is estimated to be 1% per year. Decision regarding ICD implantation in patients apart from the above group of patients can be very difficult and requires substantial workup. ICD risk stratification needs to be performed every 1–3 years even when initial workup denotes low-risk. Box 1 gives the risk factors associated with SCD in HCM.[30]

Late gadolinium enhancement CMR is fast emerging as an important and reliable marker for assessing SCD risk in HCM. However, studies of LGE-CMR in HCM have not been conclusive so far. One study found LGE to be an independent risk factor for SCD on univariate analysis, but the effect was lost on multivariate analysis.[79] T1 mapping in CMR appears to be promising in future evaluation of HCM, because it

BOX 1 Risk factors associated with increased sudden cardiac death in patients with hypertrophic cardiomyopathy

Established risk factors:

- Survival from a cardiac arrest due to VT or VF
- Spontaneous sustained VT causing syncope or hemodynamic compromise
- Family history of SCD associated with HCM
- LV wall thickness ≥30 mm
- Unexplained syncope within 6 months
- NSVT ≥3 beats
- Abnormal blood pressure response during exercise

Potential risk modifiers:

- Age <30 years
- LGE on cardiac MRI
- Severe LVOT obstruction
- Syncope >5 years ago

High-risk subsets:

- LV apical aneurysm
- LVEF <50%

HCM, hypertrophic cardiomyopathy; LGE, late gadolinium enhancement; LV, left ventricle; LVEF, left ventricular ejection fraction; LVOT, left ventricular outflow tract; MRI, magnetic resonance imaging; NSVT, nonsustained ventricular tachycardia; SCD, sudden cardiac death; VF, ventricular fibrillation; VT, ventricular tachycardia.

assesses general expansion of the extracellular space, and hence better in detecting diffuse myocardial fibrosis.[80]

Syncope in HCM poses significant clinical dilemma. Syncope in HCM can be neurally mediated (vasovagal), medication related, due to LV outflow obstruction, as well as due to VA. Hence, cause of syncope should be carefully evaluated before considering it to be associated with increased SCD risk. In one study, syncope that was unexplained or thought not to be neurally mediated was associated with SCD risk only when it occurred within previous 6 months but not if most episodes occurred more than 5 years previously.[81]

Nonsustained ventricular tachycardia (NSVT) is not considered to be an independent risk factor for SCD in patients with HCM if present alone. However, the risk of SCD increases if risk modifiers are present along with NSVT, especially in patients less than 30 years of age.[82] Electrophysiology study (EPS) and programed ventricular stimulation is not recommended in patients with HCM as it has low predictive value.[30]

Arrhythmogenic Right Ventricular Cardiomyopathy

Arrhythmogenic right ventricular cardiomyopathy (ARVC) is a genetically determined heritable disorder associated with replacement of right ventricular (and sometimes LV) myocardium by fibro-fatty tissue. ARVC is an important cause of SCD in young people and athletes. ARVC was found in 5–20% cases of undiagnosed SCD in patients of less than 35 years age.[83,84] A recent observational study of 301 ARVC patients suggested that rate of life-threatening VAs is ranging between 1.5 and 4.0 per 100 person-years; with the risk distributed from adolescence to later life and peaking at the ages of 21–40 years.[85]

BOX 2 Risk factors for sudden cardiac death in arrhythmogenic right ventricular cardiomyopathy

Major risk factors:

- Prior cardiac arrest or of sustained VT
- Unexplained syncope
- Nonsustained VT
- Severe ventricular dysfunction (RV or LVEF <35%)

Minor risk factors:

- Amount and distribution of scarring on MRI
- Frequent PVCs
- T-wave inversions beyond right precordial leads
- Presence of multiple desmosomal gene mutations

LVEF, left ventricular ejection fraction; PVCs, premature ventricular complex; RV, right ventricular; VT, ventricular tachycardia.

Competitive sports increase the risk for VT or SCD in patients with ARVC and hence they are advised to limit exercise intensity and duration to less than 650 metabolic equivalents hours (MET-Hr) per year, or 12.5 MET-Hr per week.[32] Asymptomatic patients of ARVC (usually diagnosed by family screening) with no VA or ventricular dysfunction are generally observed without antiarrhythmic therapy other than β-blockers. Periodic reassessment is recommended in these patients to look for development of arrhythmias or ventricular dysfunction.[30] Atenolol was shown in one study to reduce VA in ARVC patients.[86]

There is no clear value of electrophysiological study in asymptomatic ARVC patients (a small subgroup) with preserved ventricular function in predicting SCD risk and hence is not recommended.[87] In experienced centers, use of epicardial and endocardial mapping and ablation is associated with decrease in VA incidence in ARVC. However, successful VT ablation does not eliminate the need for an ICD in appropriate candidates. Box 2 enumerates the major and minor risk factors for SCD in ARVC.

Cardiac Channelopathies

Brugada Syndrome

Brugada syndrome is a genetically mediated heritable ion channel disorder resulting in an increased risk of SCD, despite an apparently structurally normal heart. It is characterized by coved ST elevation in leads V1 or V2 (positioned in the second, third, or fourth intercostal space) either spontaneously or induced by a sodium channel blocking drug, in the absence of other causes of ST elevation. Brugada syndrome is associated with syncope or SCA due to VF, seen predominantly in young males, although it can occur in all age groups. In Brugada syndrome-related SCD, short-coupled VPBs evolve into polymorphic VT and finally degenerate to VF.

Recently, imaging studies, specifically cardiac magnetic resonance imaging (MRI), have pointed toward potential anatomic substrate for arrhythmogenesis in Brugada syndrome.

Right ventricular outflow tract (RVOT) and upper RV anterior wall have been shown to be involved in the generation of VF and sudden death in Brugada syndrome, and studies have detected structural abnormalities like epicardial fibrosis in these regions.[88-92] Ablation of abnormal areas of late activation in the epicardial RVOT has been shown to suppress or eliminate VAs in small group of patients.[92] In these studies, the spontaneous type 1 Brugada pattern on ECG was eliminated in more than 75% of patients and recurrences of VT or VF were significantly reduced.[88,92-94]

After initial presentation, the SCD risk in Brugada syndrome is approximately 10% in first 4 years. Risk of arrhythmia is much lower in asymptomatic Brugada syndrome "patients", about 0.5% per year.[95,96] The only treatment which can reduce the risk of SCD in Brugada syndrome is the ICD implantation, therefore, the device is recommended in patients with documented VT or VF and in patients presenting with a spontaneous type 1 ECG and a history of syncope.[13] Inducibility of VT or VF on EPS has been debated to be of any value as a risk marker and most clinical studies have been inconclusive.[13] Certain ECG changes like QRS fragmentation and presence of a wide or large S-wave in lead I in spontaneous type I pattern patients (suggestive of RVOT conduction delay), appear to be associated with increased SCD risk.[97,98] Family history of SCD is not considered to increase risk of SCD in index patient.

Quinidine can suppress VF storm and suppress arrhythmia in Brugada patients. Some anesthetic agents, certain psychotropic medicines, cocaine, excessive alcohol intake, heavy meals, and fever (www.brugadadrugs.org) have been shown to trigger VF and SCA in Brugada syndrome. These agents and conditions should be avoided and fever should be aggressively treated to reduce temperature.[30] SCD in Brugada syndrome mostly occurs at rest or during sleep.

Long QT Syndrome

Long QT syndrome is characterized by a prolonged QT interval at some or all the times in patient (Table 1)[99] and is associated with VAs, usually triggered by increased sympathetic stimulation. LQTS presents at a young age with mean age of presentation being 14 years. Rate of SCD in untreated LQTS is estimated to be between 0.33 and 0.9% per annum, whereas rate for syncope is estimated to be about 5% per annum.[100,101] Assessment of SCD risk in an individual of LQTS requires evaluation of genetic parameters along with clinical and ECG features. Cardiac arrest survivors have a high risk of recurrence of malignant VAs, even when receiving β-blockers (14% within 5 years on therapy) and hence, ICD is indicated in all survivors of cardiac arrest with LQTS.[13] Left cardiac sympathetic denervation has been shown to reduce number of appropriate ICD shocks and VA burden in LQTS. In LQTS type 3, ranolazine, mexiletine, and flecainide can be used as they have been shown to shorten the QTc and can reduce recurrent arrhythmias.[102-104]

Implantable cardioverter defibrillator for primary prophylaxis may be considered in certain high-risk patients

TABLE 1: Scoring system for diagnosis of LQTS

Criteria			Points
ECG			
QTc (Bazett's formula)	≥480 ms		3
	460–479 ms		2
	450–459 ms (males)		1
	≥480 ms during 4th minute of recovery from exercise stress test		1
Torsade de pointes (mutually exclusive of syncope)			2
T-wave alternans			1
Notched T wave in 3 leads			1
Low heart rate for age (<2nd percentile for age at rest)			0.5
Clinical History			
Syncope (mutually exclusive of Torsades)		With stress	2
		Without stress	1
Family History (one family member to be counted once)			
Family member(s) with definite LQTS			1
Unexplained SCD at age <30 years in immediate family			0.5

Scoring:
≤1.0 point = low probability of LQTS
1.5–3.0 points = intermediate probability of LQTS
≥3.5 points = high probability of LQTS

ECG, electrocardiogram; LQTS, long QT syndrome; SCD: sudden cardiac death.

such as women with LQTS type 2 and QTc more than 500 ms, patients with QTc more than 500 ms and signs of electrical instability and in patients with high-risk genetic profiles (carriers of two mutations, including Jervell and Lange-Nielsen syndrome or Timothy syndrome). Invasive EPS in patients with LQTS for risk stratification is of no use.

Beta-blockers consistently reduce adverse cardiac events in patients of LQTS type 1 (>95%), type 2 (>75%), and females with LQTS type 3 by more than 60%. However, efficacy of β-blockers in males with LQTS type 3 is not very well proven.[30] There is some difference in efficacy of individual β-blockers and propranolol, atenolol, and nadolol have been found to be more effective than metoprolol.[105]

Medications which prolong QT (www.crediblemeds.org) should not be used in patients with LQTS unless there is no suitable alternative. Normal potassium and magnesium balance should be maintained in all LQTS patients to prevent VAs.

REFERENCES

1. Goldberger JJ, Buxton AE, Cain M, et al. Risk stratification for arrhythmic sudden cardiac death: identifying the roadblocks. Circulation. 2011;123(21):2423-30.
2. Fishman GI, Chugh SS, Dimarco JP, et al. Sudden cardiac death prediction and prevention: report from a National Heart, Lung, and Blood Institute and Heart Rhythm Society Workshop. Circulation. 2010;122(22):2335-48.
3. Bayés de Luna A, Coumel P, Leclerq JF. Ambulatory sudden cardiac death: mechanisms of production of fatal arrhythmia on the basis of data from 157 cases. Am Heart J. 1989;117(1):151-9.
4. Girotra S, Nallamothu BK, Sepertus JA, et al. Trends in survival after in-hospital cardiac arrest. N Engl J Med. 2012;367(20):1912-20.
5. Cherry EM, Fenton FH, Gilmour RF Jr. Mechanisms of ventricular arrhythmias: a dynamical systems-based perspective. Am J Physiol Heart Circ Physiol. 2012;302(12):H2451-63.
6. Pandit SV, Jalife J. Rotors and the dynamics of cardiac fibrillation. Circ Res. 2013;112(5):849-62.
7. Tsuji Y, Heijman J, Nattel S, et al. Electrical storm: recent pathophysiological insights and therapeutic consequences. Basic Res Cardiol. 2013;108:336.
8. Lerman BB. Mechanism, diagnosis, and treatment of outflow tract tachycardia. Nat Rev Cardiol. 2015;12(10):597-608.
9. Priori SG, Chen SR. Inherited dysfunction of sarcoplasmic reticulum Ca2+ handling and arrhythmogenesis. Circ Res. 2011;108(7): 871-3.
10. Myerburg RJ, Castellanos A. Cardiac arrest and sudden cardiac death. In: Mann DL, Zipes DP, Libby P, et al (Eds). Braunwald's Heart Disease: A Textbook Of Cardiovascular Medicine, 10th edition. Oxford (United Kingdom): Elsevier; 2015. pp. 821-60.
11. Eckart RE, Shry EA, Burke AP, et al. Sudden death in young adults: an autopsy-based series of a population undergoing active surveillance. J Am Coll Cardiol. 2011;58(12):1254-61.
12. Mazzanti A, O'Rourke S, Ng K, et al. The usual suspects in sudden cardiac death of the young: a focus on inherited arrhythmogenic diseases. Expert Rev Cardiovasc Ther. 2014;12(4):499-519.
13. Priori SG, Blomstrom-Lundqvist C, Mazzanti A, et al. 2015 ESC guidelines for the management of patients with ventricular arrhythmias and the prevention of sudden cardiac death. The Task Force for the Management of Patients with Ventricular Arrhythmias and the Prevention of Sudden Cardiac Death of the European Society of Cardiology. G Ital Cardiol (Rome). 2016;17(2):108-70.
14. Amiodarone Trials Meta-Analysis Investigators. Effect of prophylactic amiodarone on mortality after acute myocardial infarction and in congestive heart failure: meta-analysis of individual data from 6500 patients in randomised trials. Lancet. 1997;350(9089):1417-24.
15. Boutitie F, Boissel JP, Connolly SJ, et al. Amiodarone interaction with beta-blockers: analysis of the merged EMIAT (European Myocardial Infarct Amiodarone Trial) and CAMIAT (Canadian Amiodarone Myocardial Infarction Trial) databases. The EMIAT and CAMIAT Investigators. Circulation. 1999;99(17):2268-75.
16. Reiken S, Wehrens XH, Vest JA, et al. Beta-blockers restore calcium release channel function and improve cardiac muscle performance in human heart failure. Circulation. 2003;107(19):2459-66.
17. Reiter MJ, Reiffel JA. Importance of beta blockade in the therapy of serious ventricular arrhythmias. Am J Cardiol. 1998;82(4A):9I-19I.
18. Ellison KE, Hafley GE, Hickey K, et al. Effect of beta-blocking therapy on outcome in the Multicenter Unsustained Tachycardia Trial (MUSTT). Circulation. 2002;106(21):2694-9.
19. MERIT-HF Group. Effect of metoprolol CR/XL in chronic heart failure: Metoprolol CR/XL Randomised Intervention Trial in Congestive Heart Failure (MERIT-HF). Lancet. 1999;353(9169):2001-7.
20. Packer M, Bristow MR, Cohn JN, et al. The effect of carvedilol on morbidity and mortality in patients with chronic heart failure. U.S. Carvedilol Heart Failure Study Group. N Engl J Med. 1996;334(21):1349-55.
21. Committees of the Cardiac Insufficiency Bisoprolol Study II. The cardiac insufficiency Bisoprolol Study II (CIBIS-II): a randomised trial. Lancet. 1999;353(9146):9-13.
22. Nademanee K, Taylor R, Bailey WE, et al. Treating electrical storm: sympathetic blockade versus advanced cardiac life support-guided therapy. Circulation. 2000;102(7):742-7.
23. Connolly SJ. Meta-analysis of antiarrhythmic drug trials. Am J Cardiol. 1999;84(9A):90R-3R.
24. Steinberg JS, Martins J, Sadanandan S, et al. Antiarrhythmic drug use in the implantable defibrillator arm of the Antiarrhythmics Versus Implantable Defibrillators (AVID) Study. Am Heart J. 2001;142(3):520-9.
25. Farré J, Romero J, Rubio JM, et al. Amiodarone and "primary" prevention of sudden death: critical review of a decade of clinical trials. Am J Cardiol. 1999;83(5B):55D-63D.
26. Bardy GH, Lee KL, Mark DB, et al. Amiodarone or an implantable cardioverter-defibrillator for congestive heart failure. N Engl J Med. 2005;352(3):225-37.
27. Thomas KL, Al-Khatib SM, Lokhnygina Y, et al. Amiodarone use after acute myocardial infarction complicated by heart failure and/or left ventricular dysfunction may be associated with excess mortality. Am Heart J. 2008;155(1):87-93.
28. Claro JC, Candia R, Rada G, et al. Amiodarone versus other pharmacological interventions for prevention of sudden cardiac death. Cochrane Database Syst Rev. 2015;(12):CD008093.
29. Kudenchuk PJ, Brown SP, Daya M, et al. Amiodarone, lidocaine, or placebo in out-of-hospital cardiac arrest. N Engl J Med. 2016;374(18):1711-22.
30. Al-Khatib SM, Stevenson WG, Ackerman MJ, et al. 2017 AHA/ACC/HRS guideline for management of patients with ventricular arrhythmias and the prevention of sudden cardiac death: A report of the American College of Cardiology/American Heart Association Task Force on clinical practices guidelines and the Heart Rhythm Society. Circulation. 2017;pii:S1547-5271(17)31249-3..
31. Kuhlkamp V, Mewis C, Mermi J, et al. Suppression of sustained ventricular tachyarrhythmias: a comparison of d-sotalol with no antiarrhythmic drug treatment. J Am Coll Cardiol. 1999;33(1):46-52.
32. Waldo AL, Camm AJ, deRuyter H, et al. Survival with oral d-sotalol in patients with left ventricular dysfunction after myocardial infarction: rationale, design, and methods (the SWORD trial). Am J Cardiol. 1995;75(15):1023-7.
33. Cardiac Arrhythmia Suppression Trial (CAST) Investigators. Preliminary report: effect of encainide and flecainide on mortality in a randomized trial of arrhythmia suppression after myocardial infarction. N Engl J Med. 1989;321(6):406-12.
34. Mazzanti A, Maragna R, Faragli A, et al. Gene-specific therapy with mexiletine reduces arrhythmic events in patients with long QT syndrome type 3. J Am Coll Cardiol. 2016;67(9):1053-8.
35. Watanabe H, Chopra N, Laver D, et al. Flecainide prevents catecholaminergic polymorphic ventricular tachycardia in mice and humans. Nat Med. 2009;15(4):380-3.
36. Gupta T, Khera S, Kolte D, et al. Antiarrhythmic properties of ranolazine: a review of the current evidence. Int J Cardiol. 2015;187:66-74.
37. Cohn JN, Johnson G, Ziesche S, et al. A comparison of enalapril with hydralazine-isosorbide dinitrate in the treatment of chronic congestive heart failure. N Engl J Med. 1991;325(5):303-10.
38. Pitt B, Zannad F, Remme WJ, et al. The effect of spironolactone on morbidity and mortality in patients with severe heart failure. Randomized Aldactone Evaluation Study Investigators. N Engl J Med. 1999;341(10):709-17.
39. Zannad F, McMurray JJ, Krum H, et al. Eplerenone in patients with systolic heart failure and mild symptoms. N Engl J Med. 2011;364(1):11-21.
40. Desai AS, McMurray JJ, Packer M, et al. Effect of the angiotensin-receptor-neprilysin inhibitor LCZ696 compared with enalapril on mode of death in heart failure patients. Eur Heart J. 2015;36(30):1990-7.
41. Tzivoni D, Banai S, Schuger C, et al. Treatment of torsade de pointes with magnesium sulfate. Circulation. 1988;77(2):392-7.
42. Cohn JN, Kowey PR, Whelton PK, et al. New guidelines for potassium replacement in clinical practice: a contemporary review by the National Council on Potassium in Clinical Practice. Arch Intern Med. 2000;160(16):2429-36.
43. Macdonald JE, Struthers AD. What is the optimal serum potassium level in cardiovascular patients? J Am Coll Cardiol. 2004;43(2):155-61.
44. Hohnloser SH, Dorian P, Roberts R, et al. Effect of amiodarone and sotalol on ventricular defibrillation threshold: the optimal pharmacological therapy in cardioverter defibrillator patients (OPTIC) trial. Circulation. 2006;114(2):104-9.
45. Bunch TJ, Mahapatra S, Murdock D, et al. Ranolazine reduces ventricular tachycardia burden and ICD shocks in patients with drug-refractory ICD shocks. Pacing Clin Electrophysiol. 2011;34(12):1600-6.
46. Smith T, Jordaens L, Theuns DA, et al. The cost effectiveness of primary prophylactic implantable defibrillator therapy in patients with ischaemic or non-ischaemic heart disease: a European analysis. Eur Heart J. 2013;34(3):211-9.

47. Garnreiter JM, Pilcher TA, Etheridge SP, et al. Inappropriate ICD shocks in pediatrics and congenital heart disease patients: risk factors and programming strategies. Heart Rhythm. 2015;12(5):937-42.
48. van der Heijden AC, Borleffs CJ, Buiten MS, et al. The clinical course of patients with implantable defibrillators: extended experience on clinical outcome, device replacements, and device-related complications. Heart Rhythm. 2015;12(6):1169-76.
49. Connolly SJ, Hallstrom AP, Cappato R, et al. Meta-analysis of the implantable cardioverter defibrillator secondary prevention trials. AVID, CASH and CIDS studies. Antiarrhythmics vs Implantable Defibrillator study. Cardiac Arrest Study Hamburg. Canadian Implantable Defibrillator Study. Eur Heart J. 2000;21(24):2071-8.
50. Olde Nordkamp LR, Knops RE, Bardy GH, et al. Rationale and design of the PRAETORIAN trial: a prospective, randomized comparison of subcutaneous and transvenous implantable cardioverter-defibrillator therapy. Am Heart J. 2012;163(5):753-60.
51. Vest Prevention of Early Sudden Death Trial—VEST. Presented by Dr Jeffrey E Olgin at the American College of Cardiology Annual Scientific Session (ACC 2018), Orlando, FL, March 10, 2018.
52. Blom MT, Beesems SG, Homma PC, et al. Improved survival after out-of-hospital cardiac arrest and use of automated external defibrillators. Circulation. 2014;130(21):1868-75.
53. Poole JE, Johnson GW, Hellkamp AS, et al. Prognostic importance of defibrillator shocks in patients with heart failure. N Engl J Med. 2008;359(10):1009-17.
54. Dumas F, Cariou A, Manzo-Silberman S, et al. Immediate percutaneous coronary intervention is associated with better survival after out-of-hospital cardiac arrest: insights from the PROCAT (Parisian Region Out of hospital Cardiac Arrest) registry. Circ Cardiovasc Interv. 2010;3(3):200-7.
55. Piccini JP, Hranitzky PM, Kilaru R, et al. Relation of mortality to failure to prescribe beta blockers acutely in patients with sustained ventricular tachycardia and ventricular fibrillation following acute myocardial infarction [from the Valsartan in Acute myocardial Infarction trial (VALIANT) Registry]. Am J Cardiol. 2008;102(11):1427-32.
56. Dagres N, Hindricks G. Risk stratification after myocardial infarction: is left ventricular ejection fraction enough to prevent sudden cardiac death? Eur Heart J. 2013;34(26):1964-71
57. Das MK, Saha C, El Masry H, et al. Fragmented QRS on a 12-lead ECG: a predictor of mortality and cardiac events in patients with coronary artery disease. Heart Rhythm. 2007;4(11):1385-92.
58. Das MK, Maskoun W, Shen C, et al. Fragmented QRS on twelve-lead electrocardiogram predicts arrhythmic events in patients with ischemic and nonischemic cardiomyopathy. Heart Rhythm. 2010;7(1):74-80.
59. Das MK, Khan B, Jacob S, et al. Significance of a fragmented QRS complex versus a Q wave in patients with coronary artery disease. Circulation. 2006;113(21):2495-501.
60. Terho HK, Tikkanen JT, Junttila JM, et al. Prevalence and prognostic significance of fragmented QRS complex in middle-aged subjects with and without clinical or electrocardiographic evidence of cardiac disease. Am J Cardiol. 2014;114(1):141-7.
61. Wang DD, Buerkel DM, Corbett JR, et al. Fragmented QRS complex has poor sensitivity in detecting myocardial scar. Ann Noninvasive Electrocardiol. 2010;15(4):308-14.
62. Watanabe E, Abbasi SA, Heydari B, et al. Infarct tissue heterogeneity by contrast-enhanced magnetic resonance imaging is a novel predictor of mortality in patients with chronic coronary artery disease and left ventricular dysfunction. Circ Cardiovasc Imaging. 2014;7(6):887-94.
63. Yang Y, Connelly KA, Zeidan-Shwiri T, et al. Multicontrast late enhancement CMR determined gray zone and papillary muscle involvement predict appropriate ICD therapy in patients with ischemic heart disease. J Cardiovasc Magn Reson. 2013;15(1):57.
64. Ng AC, Bertini M, Borleffs CJ, et al. Predictors of death and occurrence of appropriate implantable defibrillator therapies in patients with ischemic cardiomyopathy. Am J Cardiol. 2010;106(11):1566-73.
65. Mikami Y, Jolly U, Heydari B, et al. Right ventricular ejection fraction is incremental to left ventricular ejection fraction for the prediction of future arrhythmic events in patients with systolic dysfunction. Circ Arrhythm Electrophysiol. 2017;10(1).
66. Fallavollita JA, Heavey BM, Luisi AJ Jr, et al. Regional myocardial sympathetic denervation predicts the risk of sudden cardiac arrest in ischemic cardiomyopathy. J Am Coll Cardiol. 2014;63(2):141-9.
67. Jacobson AF, Senior R, Cerqueira MD, et al. Myocardial iodine-123 meta-iodobenzylguanidine imaging and cardiac events in heart failure. Results of the prospective ADMIRE-HF (AdreView Myocardial Imaging for Risk Evaluation in Heart Failure) study. J Am Coll Cardiol. 2010;55(20):2212-21.
68. Desai AS, Fang JC, Maisel WH, et al. Implantable defibrillators for the prevention of mortality in patients with nonischemic cardiomyopathy: a meta-analysis of randomized controlled trials. JAMA. 2004;292(23):2874-9.
69. Kober L, Thune JJ, Nielsen JC, et al. Defibrillator implantation in patients with nonischemic systolic heart failure. N Engl J Med. 2016;375(13):1221-30.
70. Fonarow GC, Feliciano Z, Boyle NG, et al. Improved survival in patients with nonischemic advanced heart failure and syncope treated with an implantable cardioverter-defibrillator. Am J Cardiol. 2000;85(8):981-5.
71. Knight BP, Goyal R, Pelosi F, et al. Outcome of patients with nonischemic dilated cardiomyopathy and unexplained syncope treated with an implantable defibrillator. J Am Coll Cardiol. 1999;33(7):1964-70.
72. Middlekauff HR, Stevenson WG, Stevenson LW, et al. Syncope in advanced heart failure: high risk of sudden death regardless of origin of syncope. J Am Coll Cardiol. 1993;21(1):110-6.
73. Olshansky B, Poole JE, Johnson G, et al. Syncope predicts the outcome of cardiomyopathy patients: analysis of the SCD-HeFT study. J Am Coll Cardiol. 2008;51(13):1277-82.
74. Ruwald MH, Okumura K, Kimura T, et al. Syncope in high-risk cardiomyopathy patients with implantable defibrillators: frequency, risk factors, mechanisms, and association with mortality: results from the multicenter automatic defibrillator implantation trial-reduce inappropriate therapy (MADIT-RIT) study. Circulation. 2014;129(5):545-52.
75. Di Marco A, Anguera I, Schmitt M, et al. Late gadolinium enhancement and the risk for ventricular arrhythmias or sudden death in dilated cardiomyopathy: systematic review and meta-analysis. JACC Heart Fail. 2017;5(1):28-38.
76. Assomull RG, Prasad SK, Lyne J, et al. Cardiovascular magnetic resonance, fibrosis, and prognosis in dilated cardiomyopathy. J Am Coll Cardiol. 2006;48(10):1977-85.
77. Gulati A, Jabbour A, Ismail TF, et al. Association of fibrosis with mortality and sudden cardiac death in patients with nonischemic dilated cardiomyopathy. JAMA 2013;309(9):896-908.
78. Maron BJ, Shen WK, Link MS, et al. Efficacy of implantable cardioverter-defibrillators for the prevention of sudden death in patients with hypertrophic cardiomyopathy. N Engl J Med. 2000;342(6):365-73.
79. Ismail TF, Jabbour A, Gulati A, et al. Role of late gadolinium enhancement cardiovascular magnetic resonance in the risk stratification of hypertrophic cardiomyopathy. Heart. 2014;100(23):1851-8.
80. Moon JC, Messroghli DR, Kellman P, et al. Myocardial T1 mapping and extracellular volume quantification: a Society for Cardiovascular Magnetic Resonance (SMCR) and CMR working group of the European Society of Cardiology consensus statement. J Cardiovasc Magn Reson. 2013;15:92.
81. Spirito P, Autore C, Rapezzi C, et al. Syncope and risk of sudden death in hypertrophic cardiomyopathy. Circulation. 2009;119(13):1703-10.
82. Monserrat L, Elliott PM, Gimeno JR, et al. Non-sustained ventricular tachycardia in hypertrophic cardiomyopathy: an independent marker of sudden death risk in young patients. J Am Coll Cardiol. 2003;42(5):873-9.
83. Thiene G, Nava A, Corrado D, et al. Right ventricular cardiomyopathy and sudden death in young people. N Engl J Med. 1988;318(3):129-33.
84. Winkel BG, Holst AG, Theilade J, et al. Nationwide study of sudden cardiac death in persons aged 1-35 years. Eur Heart J. 2011;32(8):983-90.
85. Mazzanti A, Ng K, Faragli A, et al. Arrhythmogenic right ventricular cardiomyopathy: clinical course and predictors of arrhythmic risk. J Am Coll Cardiol. 2016;68(23):2540-50.
86. Marcus GM, Glidden DV, Polonsky B, et al. Efficacy of antiarrhythmic drugs in arrhythmogenic right ventricular cardiomyopathy: a report from the North American ARVC Registry. J Am Coll Cardiol. 2009;54(7):609-15.
87. Piccini JP, Dalal D, Roguin A, et al. Predictors of appropriate implantable defibrillator therapies in patients with arrhythmogenic right ventricular dysplasia. Heart Rhythm. 2005;2(11):1188-94.

88. Nademanee K, Veerakul G, Chandanamattha P, et al. Prevention of ventricular fibrillation episodes in Brugada syndrome by catheter ablation over the anterior right ventricular outflow tract epicardium. Circulation. 2011;123(12):1270-9.
89. Haissaguerre M, Extramiana F, Hocini M, et al. Mapping and ablation of ventricular fibrillation associated with long-QT and Brugada syndromes. Circulation. 2003;108(8):925-8.
90. Morita H, Fukushima-Kusano K, Nagase S, et al. Site-specific arrhythmogenesis in patients with Brugada syndrome. J Cardiovasc Electrophysiol. 2003;14(4):373-9.
91. Nademanee K, Raju H, de Noronha SV, et al. Fibrosis, connexin-43, and conduction abnormalities in the brugada syndrome. J Am Coll Cardiol. 2015;66(18):1976-86.
92. Brugada J, Pappone C, Berruezo A, et al. Brugada syndrome phenotype elimination by epicardial substrate ablation. Circ Arrhythm Electrophysiol. 2015;8(6):1373-81.
93. Sunsaneewitayakul B, Yao Y, Thamaree S, et al. Endocardial mapping and catheter ablation for ventricular fibrillation prevention in Brugada syndrome. J Cardiovasc Electrophysiol. 2012;23(suppl 1):S10-6.
94. Zhang P, Tung R, Zhang Z, et al. Characterization of the epicardial substrate for catheter ablation of Brugada syndrome. Heart Rhythm. 2016;13(11):2151-8.
95. Priori SG, Gasparini M, Napolitano C, et al. Risk stratification in Brugada syndrome: results of the PRELUDE (Programmed Electrical stimulation Predictive Value) registry. J Am Coll Cardiol. 2012;59(1):37-45.
96. Probst V, Veltmann C, Eckardt L, et al. Long-term prognosis of patients diagnosed with Brugada syndrome: results from the FINGER Brugada Syndrome Registry. Circulation. 2010;121(5):635-43.
97. Morita H, Kusano KF, Miura D, et al. Fragmented QRS as a marker of conduction abnormality and a predictor of prognosis of Brugada syndrome. Circulation. 2008;118(17):1697-704.
98. Calo L, Giustetto C, Martino A, et al. A new electrocardiographic marker of sudden death in Brugada syndrome: the S-wave in lead I. J Am Coll Cardiol. 2016;67(12):1427-40.
99. Schwartz PJ, Crotti L. QTc behavior during exercise and genetic testing for the long-QT syndrome. Circulation. 2011;124(20):2181-4.
100. Priori SG, Schwartz PJ, Napolitano C, et al. Risk stratification in the long-QT syndrome. N Engl J Med. 2003;348(19):1866-74.
101. Moss AJ, Schwartz PJ, Crampton RS, et al. The long QT syndrome. Prospective longitudinal study of 328 families. Circulation. 1991;84(3):1136-44.
102. Chorin E, Hu D, Antzelevitch C, et al. Ranolazine for congenital long-QT syndrome type III: experimental and long-term clinical data. Circ Arrhythm Electrophysiol. 2016;9(10):e004370.
103. Chorin E, Taub R, Medina A, et al. Long-term flecainide therapy in type 3 long QT syndrome. Europace. 2017;20(2):370-6.
104. Mazzanti A, Maragna R, Faragli A, et al. Gene-specific therapy with mexiletine reduces arrhythmic events in patients with long QT syndrome type 3. J Am Coll Cardiol. 2016;67(9):1053-8.
105. Chockalingam P, Crotti L, Girardengo G, et al. Not all beta-blockers are equal in the management of long QT syndrome types 1 and 2: higher recurrence of events under metoprolol. J Am Coll Cardiol. 2012;60(20):2092-9.

CHAPTER 113

Electrocardiography Clues in a Sudden Cardiac Death Survivor

Ranjan Modi, Aparna Jaswal

INTRODUCTION

There have been numerous papers published on electrocardiography (ECG) and cardiac diseases. The literature has established the profound correlation between ECG and sudden cardiac death (SCD) with most SCD attributed to cardiac diseases. Studies on SCD survivors indicate that 5–10% of cases occur in the absence of any apparent cardiac disease.[1] Primary electrical disorders resulting from channelopathies are believed to play a role in such patients. ECG provides important clues to the differential diagnosis of these entities. The ECG clues in these conditions may be broadly classified in table 1.

In a study in Korea for distribution of underlying cardiac diseases in SCD survivors, ECG abnormalities in structural heart disease and nonstructural heart disease were identified and respective underlying diseases prevalence noted (Fig. 1).

TABLE 1: Electrocardiography in sudden cardiac death

Structural	Nonstructural
• Hypertrophic obstructive cardiomyopathy • Arrhythmogenic right ventricular dysplasia • Ischemic heart disease	• Inherited • Noninherited

Underlying discases	Percent
Long QT syndrome (LQTS)	3.2
Brugada syndrome (BS)	9.4
Early repolarization syndrome (ERS)	5.2
J wave-related VF in the absence of structural heart diseases (IVF-J)1	6.1
Idiopathic ventricular fibrillation (IVF)	8.4
Myocardial infraction or coronary artery disease	25.6
Variant angina	3.2
Dilated cardiomyopathy	10.7
Hypertrophic cardiomyopathy	14.6
Arrhythmogenic right ventricular cardiomyopathy	4.2
Others (Sarcoidosis, valve, congenital disease, etc.)	9.4
Total	100.0

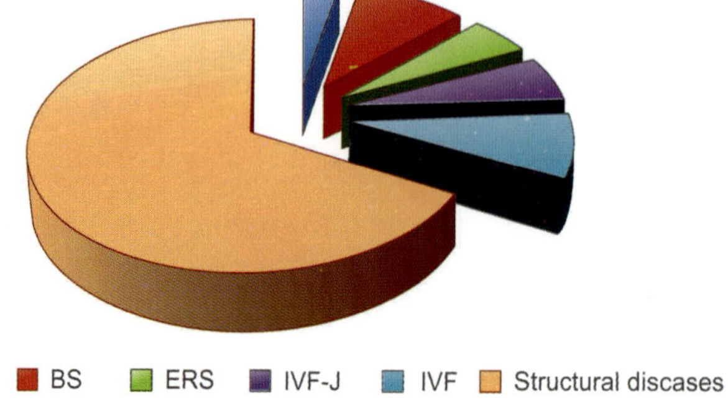

FIG. 1: Prevalence of underlying cardiac diseases in sudden cardiac death.

Recently various clinical entities such as Brugada syndrome (BS), long QT syndrome (LQTS), short QT syndrome (SQTS), arrhythmogenic right ventricular dysplasia (ARVD) and early repolarization syndrome (ERS) have gained importance in SCD survivors.

STRUCTURAL HEART DISEASE

Hypertrophic Cardiomyopathy

- Hypertrophic cardiomyopathy (HCM) is one of the most common inherited cardiac disorders; it affects almost 1 in 500 people and is the number one cause of SCD in young athletes
- The mortality in HCM is estimated at 1–2% annually
- It is produced by mutations in multiple genes coding for sarcomeric proteins (e.g., beta-myosin heavy chain, troponin T)
- It is an autosomal dominant disease.
- The chief abnormality is left ventricular hypertrophy (LVH), occurring in the absence of any stimulus such as hypertension or aortic stenosis
- The most common pattern is asymmetrical thickening of the anterior interventricular septum. It is associated with systolic anterior motion (SAM) of the mitral valve and dynamic left ventricular outflow tract (LVOT) obstruction. In the majority of cases almost 75%, HCM is not associated with LVOT obstruction
- Other patterns of LVH include concentric hypertrophy (20% of cases) and apical hypertrophy (10%), which are less common.

Electrocardiographic Features of Hypertrophic Cardiomyopathy

- Left atrial enlargement
- Left ventricular hypertrophy with associated ST/T abnormalities
- Deep, narrow ("dagger-like") Q waves in the lateral more than the inferior leads
- Giant precordial T-wave inversions which are mainly seen in apical HCM
- Short PR and delta wave which are signs suggestive of Wolff-Parkinson-White syndrome
- It is estimated that 5–10% of patient with HCM have ventricular pre-excitation[2]
- *Dysrhythmias*: Atrial fibrillation, supraventricular tachycardia (Fig. 2).

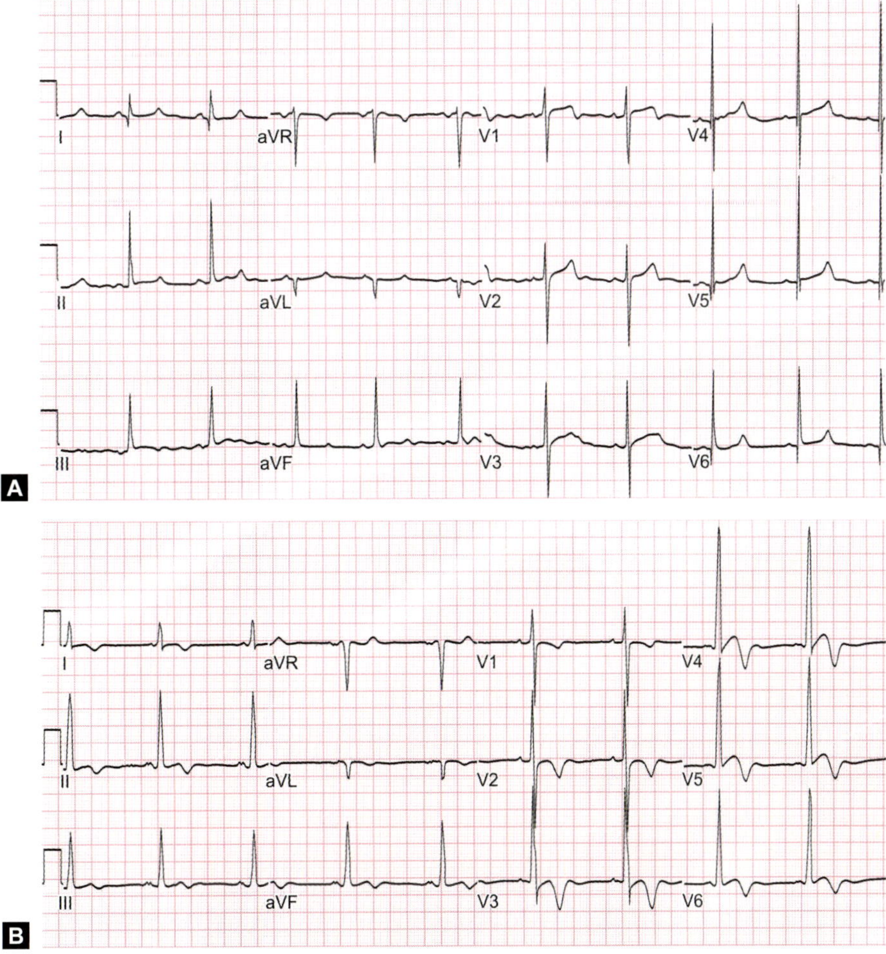

aVF, augmented vector foot; aVL, augmented vector left; aVR, augmented vector right.

FIG. 2: Electrocardiography features of hypertrophic cardiomyopathy.

Classic HCM pattern with asymmetrical septal hypertrophy (Fig. 2A):

- Voltage criteria for LVH.
- Deep narrow Q waves less than or equal to 40 ms wide in the lateral leads I, augmented vector left, and V5-6.

Figure 2B ECG shows the typical pattern of apical HCM:

- Large precordial voltages
- Giant T wave inversions in the precordial leads
- Inverted T waves are also seen in the inferior and lateral leads.

Arrhythmogenic Right Ventricular Dysplasia

- It is an autosomal dominant inherited myocardial disease
- It is characterized by fibro-fatty replacement of the right ventricular myocardium on pathology
- It is second most common cause of SCD in the young (after HCM)
- It is reported to cause 20% of SCDs in patients less than 35 years of age
- More common in men than women (3:1)
- It approximately affects 1 in 5,000.

Electrocardiographic Features

Arrhythmogenic right ventricular dysplasia is associated with characteristic ECG abnormalities:

- Epsilon wave (most specific finding, seen in 30% of patients)
- T-wave inversions in V_1–V_3 seen in 85% of patients.
- Prolonged S-wave upstroke of 55 ms in V_1–V_3 (95% of patients)
- Localized QRS widening of 110 ms in V_1–V_3
- Paroxysmal episodes of ventricular tachycardia with left bundle branch block (LBBB) morphology (Fig. 3).

ISCHEMIC HEART DISEASE

Ischemic heart disease (IHD) accounts for majority of cases of SCD. Presence of q waves in the ECG suggest old evolved myocardial infarction, such patients may have scarred myocardium resulting in scar ventricular tachycardia (VT)/ventricular fibrillation (VF). These patients may also have severe left ventricular dysfunction which may lead to predisposition of VT/VF and may result in SCD. Many articles and numerous literatures' have discussed the diagnosis, management, and complications of IHD (Fig. 4).[3]

NONSTRUCTURAL HEART DISEASE: INHERITED

Brugada Syndrome

Brugada syndrome is an autosomal dominant inherited arrhythmic disorder characterized by ST elevation with successive negative T wave in the right precordial leads without structural cardiac abnormalities.[4-6] Patients are at risk for VF which may lead to SCD. The ECG pattern similar to coved-type ST-segment elevation was reported as a normal variant in the healthy population or related to VF with structural abnormality,[7,8] but as a distinct entity, Brugada and Brugada[5] were the first to report eight patients with VF, right bundle branch block (BBB), and ST-segment elevation on 12-lead ECG.[9] Later, structural changes were reported.[10-12]

Genetic Background

The first causal mutations were found in *SCNSA* in 1998, which encodes for the α-subunit of the sodium channel.[13] Ever since, more than 100 *SCNSA* mutations have been reported in BS and currently represent the most common genotype, which is inherited as an autosomal-dominant trait with incomplete penetrance. The other mutations reported are missense mutation, nonsense mutation, nucleotide insertion/deletion, and splice site mutation.[14]

The *SCNSA* mutations not only may cause BS, but also may lead to other diseases. *SCNSA* mutations can also be seen in LQTS type 3, progressive cardiac conduction disease, sick sinus syndrome, or combinations of these,[15-17] congenital atrial standstill; or dilated cardiomyopathy (Fig. 5).[18-21]

Brugada syndrome is more common in males and has a variable penetrance.[22,23] Symptoms include syncope and seizures. ECG remains the cornerstone of diagnosis of BS24.

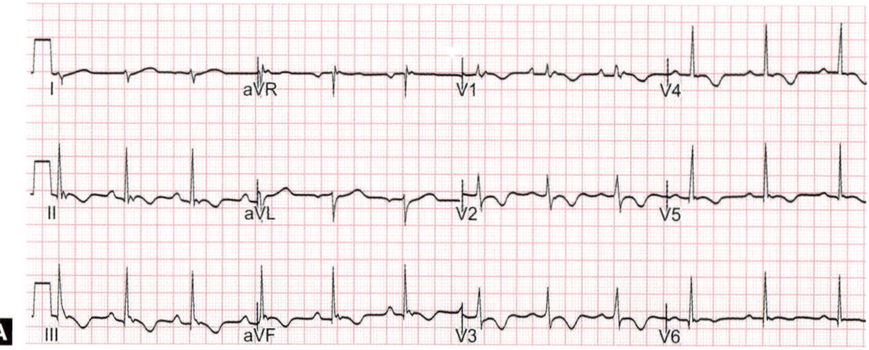

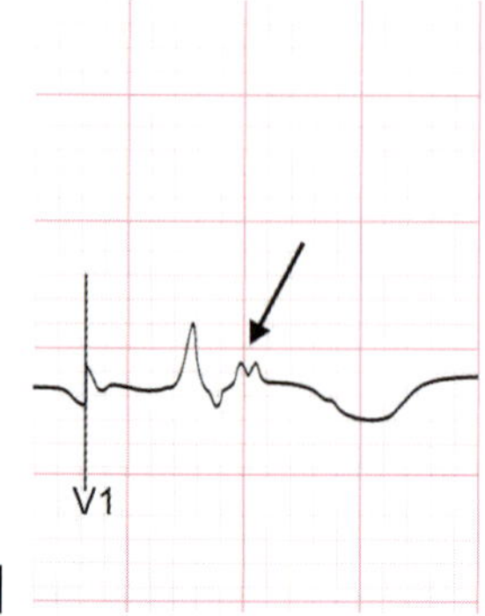

aVF, augmented vector foot; aVL, augmented vector left; aVR, augmented vector right.

FIG. 3: Electrocardiography of arrhythmogenic right ventricular dysplasia with Epsilon wave.

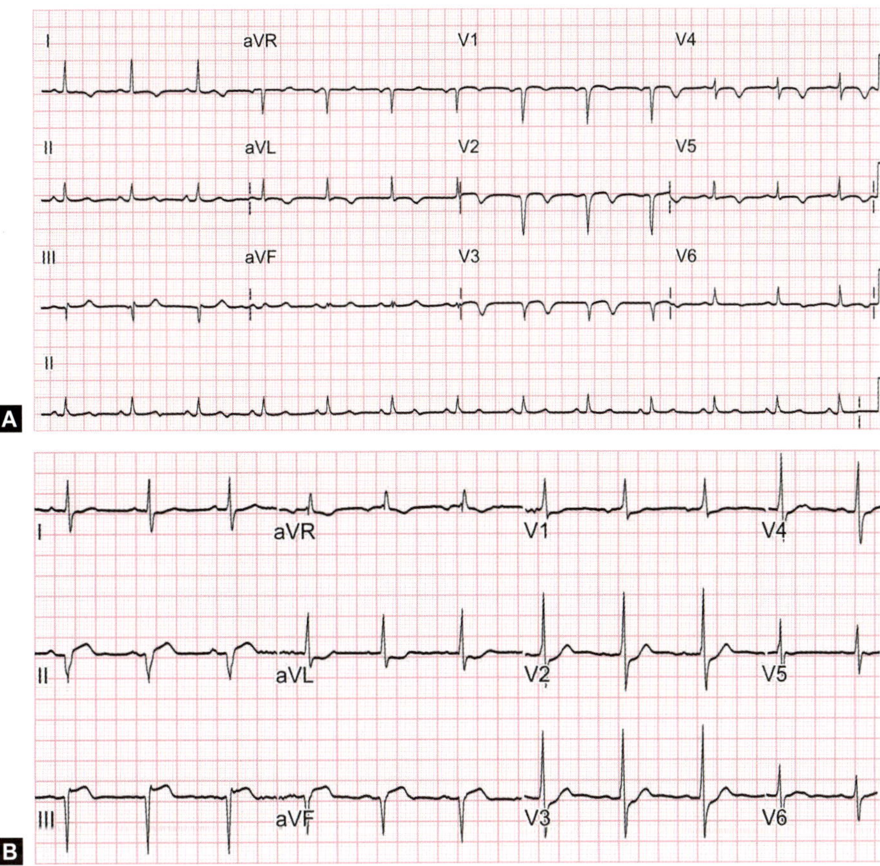

aVF, augmented vector foot; aVL, augmented vector left; aVR, augmented vector right.

FIG. 4: Electrocardiography of ischemic heart disease.

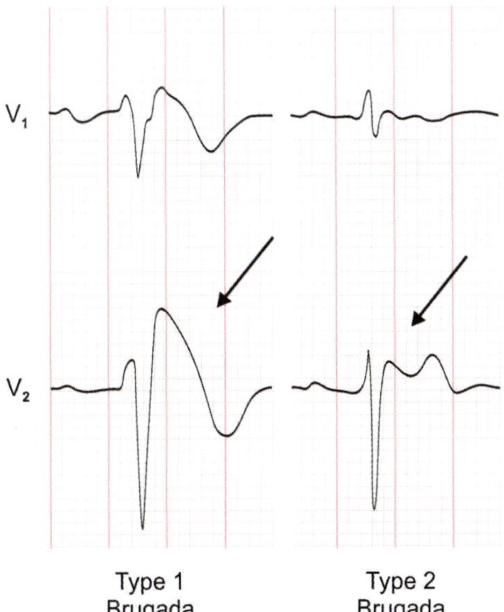

FIG. 5: Electrocardiography of Brugada syndrome.

Provocation of Brugada ECG feature by sodium-channel blocker is a specific marker for BS and the J-point is augmented by sodium-channel blockers in the right precordial leads in patients with a Brugada ECG.

A pitfall in the ECG diagnosis of BS is the so-called "masked" BS. In patients with BBB, the BS-type ST changes may be buried within the wide QRS complex, being unmasked only when the BBB is relieved. Therefore, in patients with cardiac arrest and right BBB, the possibility of masked BS should be considered in the differential diagnosis.[24-27]

The consensus for the management of BS is mentioned in figure 6.

Early Repolarization Syndrome

Early repolarization (ER), also recognized as "J-waves" or "f-point elevation", is an electrocardiographic abnormality consistent with elevation of the junction at the end of the QRS complex and the beginning of the ST segment in two contiguous leads.[28,29] Grant et al.[30] are considered to be the first who used the term ER to describe ST-segment deviations and related T-wave inversion. It was assumed that premature repolarization was the underlying etiology. The so-called "ERS" was regarded as "normal", a "normal variant", or a "benign ER" until 2000.[31] However, numerous reports have suggested a relationship between ER and an increased risk of death from cardiac arrhythmias.[32,33] ERS is an ECG finding which is characterized by J-point elevation manifested as either QRS slurring or notching, ST-segment elevation with upper concavity and prominent T waves in at least two contiguous leads (Fig. 7).[34]

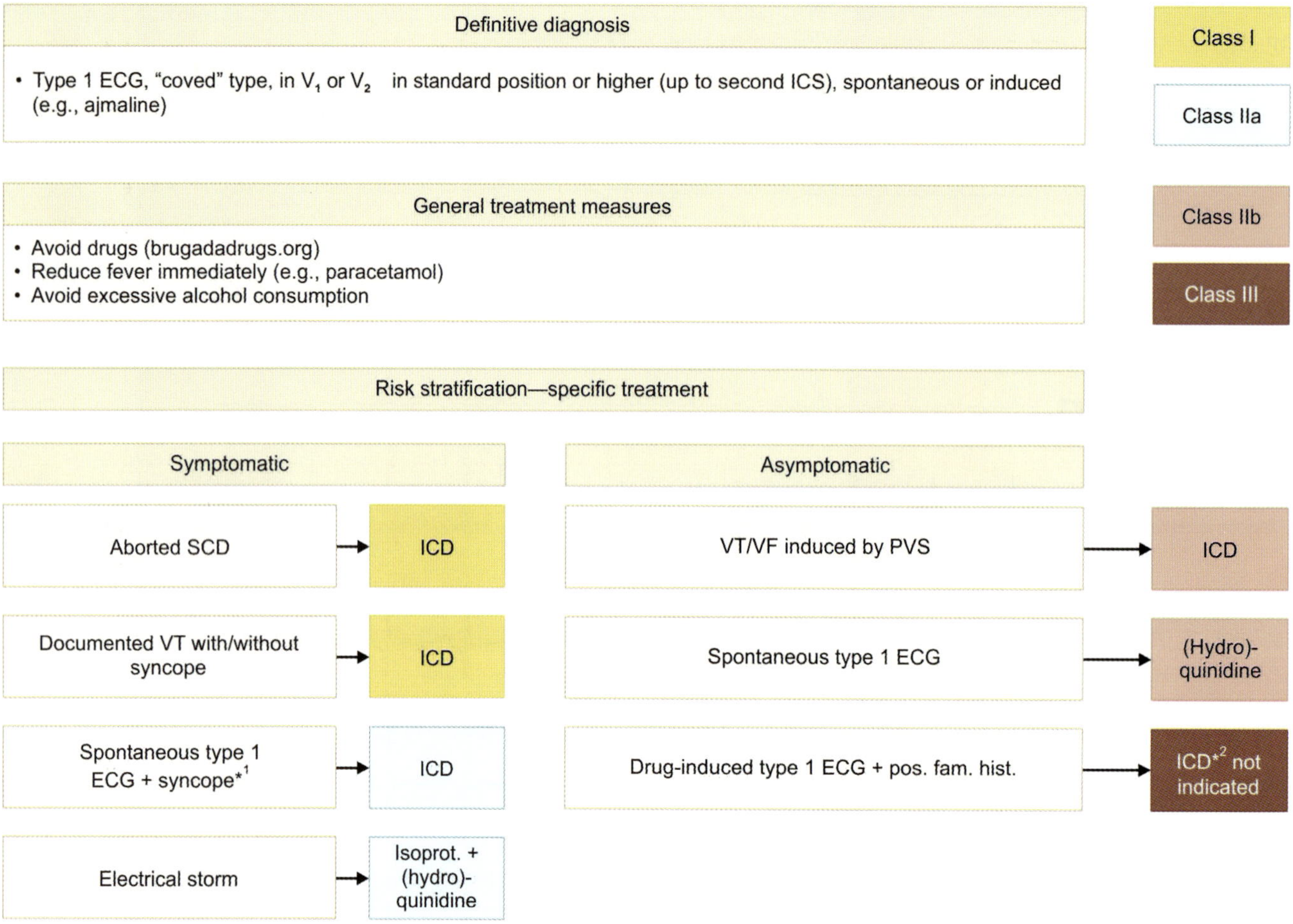

Definitive diagnosis

- Type 1 ECG, "coved" type, in V_1 or V_2 in standard position or higher (up to second ICS), spontaneous or induced (e.g., ajmaline)

Class I | Class IIa | Class IIb | Class III

General treatment measures

- Avoid drugs (brugadadrugs.org)
- Reduce fever immediately (e.g., paracetamol)
- Avoid excessive alcohol consumption

Risk stratification—specific treatment

Symptomatic

- Aborted SCD → ICD
- Documented VT with/without syncope → ICD
- Spontaneous type 1 ECG + syncope*[1] → ICD
- Electrical storm → Isoprot. + (hydro)-quinidine

Asymptomatic

- VT/VF induced by PVS → ICD
- Spontaneous type 1 ECG → (Hydro)-quinidine
- Drug-induced type 1 ECG + pos. fam. hist. → ICD*[2] not indicated

ICD, implantable cardioverter defibrillator; SCD, sudden cardiac death; VT, ventricular tachycardia; VF, ventricular fibrillation.

FIG. 6: The Heart Rhythm Society/European Heart Rhythm Association/Asia Pacific Heart Rhythm Society (HRS/EHRA/APHRS) Expert consensus statement on the diagnosis and management of patients with inherited primary arrhythmia syndromes of Brugada syndrome.

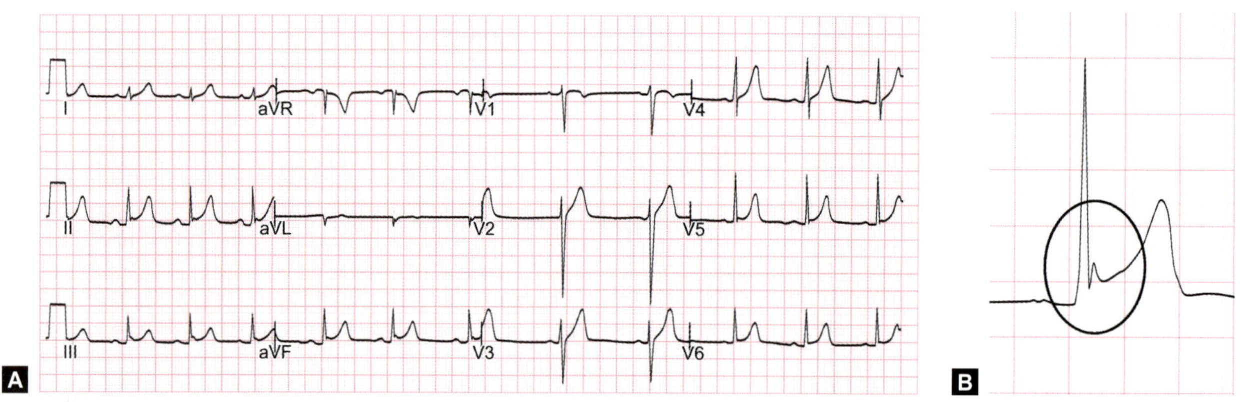

aVF, augmented vector foot; aVL, augmented vector left; aVR, augmented vector right.

FIG. 7: Electrocardiography of early repolarization syndrome.

The ERS is usually seen in athletes, cocaine users, hypertrophic obstructive cardiomyopathy and defects, and/or hypertrophy of interventricular septal defects.[35,36] ERS have a prevalence of 3–24% in the general population. Young individuals, males, African Americans, and athletes are known to have a higher prevalence of ERS.[34-37]

The pathophysiologic basis of the ER, the most common hypothesis, says that this may be related to either an increased susceptibility or vulnerability to cardiac arrest in critical ischemic conditions such as acute coronary syndromes, or to subtle changes in the cardiac action potential (AP).[38,39] ER occurs in early phase of the cardiac AP. It is caused by the

TABLE 2: The Heart Rhythm Society/European Heart Rhythm Association/Asia Pacific Heart Rhythm Society (HRS/EHRA/APHRS) consensus statement on the diagnosis and management of primary inherited arrhythmia syndromes recommendation for therapeutic intervention in early repolarization syndrome[44]: Expert consensus recommendations on early repolarization therapeutic interventions

Class I	1	ICD implementation is recommended in patients with a diagnosis of ER syndrome who have survived a cardiac arrest
Class IIa	2	Isoproterenol infusion can be useful in suppressing electrical storms in patients with a diagnosis of ER syndrome
	3	Quinidine in addition to an ICD can be useful for secondary prevention of VF in patients with a diagnosis of ER syndrome.
Class IIb	4	ICD implantation may be considered in symptomatic family members of ER syndrome patients with a history of syncope in the presence of ST-segment elevation >1 mm in 2 or more inferior or lateral leads
	5	ICD implantation may be considered in asymptomatic individuals who demonstrate a high-risk ER ECG pattern (high J-wave amplitude. horizontal/descending ST-segment) in the presence of a strong family history of juvenile unexplained sudden death with or without a pathogenic mutation
Class III	6	ICD implantation is not recommended ill asymptomatic patients with an isolated BR BCG pattern

ER, early repolarization; ICD, implantable cardioverter defibrillator; VF, ventricular fibrillation.

cardiac transient outward potassium current (I_{to}). In some situations the density of the I channels in endocardium is reduced compared to myocardium and epicardium.[40] At such situations a large I_{to} current can occur that results in ECG ER and large voltage gradients that may generate J-wave elevation (Fig. 6). These have the propensity to initiate life-threatening arrhythmias.[39,40] Another hypothesis regarding the mechanism causing ER suggests an association of localized depolarization abnormalities with repolarization anomalies, as it happens in type1 BS.[41]

The gene mutations involved in the syndrome include the *KCNJ8* gene (responsible for the ATP sensitive potassium channel K_{ir}6.1-IKATP current), *CACNAIC, CACNB2, CACNA2D1* genes (responsible for the cardiac L-type calcium channel I_{CaL} current), and the *SCNSA* gene (responsible for the sodium channel-I_{Na} current).[42] All these genes increase the imbalance between the underlying inward-outward currents and are responsible for accelerated epicardial repolarization.[43]

Electrocardiography Diagnosis

The ECG hallmark of ERS is elevation (>1 mm above baseline) of the QRS–ST junction manifested as either QRS slurring or notching, ST-segment elevation with upper concavity, and prominent T-waves in two or more contiguous inferior and/or lateral leads in a patient resuscitated from otherwise unexplained ventricular arrhythmia.[34] Recent studies have omitted ST-segment elevation from the definition of ERS, and say that the J point changes are sufficient to diagnose ERS. Although, the inclusion or exclusion of right precordial leads is also an area for debate.

Antzelevitch et al.[41] described three subtypes of ERS, and highlighted the risk profile.

Type 1: It shows ER in the lateral precordial leads that is seen in healthy male athletes and has the lowest risk of malignant arrhythmias.

Type 2: It shows ER in the inferior and inferolateral leads and is associated with a greater risk of malignant arrhythmias.

Type 3: It shows ER pattern in all ECG leads and has the highest risk of malignant arrhythmias and electrical storms.

The Heart Rhythm Society/European Heart Rhythm Association/Asia Pacific Heart Rhythm Society (HRS/EHRA/APHRS) consensus statement on the diagnosis and management of primary inherited arrhythmia syndromes recommended criteria for the diagnosis of ER is shown in table 2.[44]

Tikkanen et al. again identified a subgroup of patients with ER who show a benign long-term prognosis.[45] If the ST segment after the J wave is ascending, the long-term mortality is not significantly different from the general population, whereas subjects with a J wave and horizontal or descending ST segment changes are at higher risk of arrhythmic death.[45-47]

Long QT Syndrome

The congenital LQTS is a cardiac arrhythmia syndrome that represents one of the most leading causes of sudden death in the young. LQTS is typically characterized by a prolongation of the QT interval on the ECG and by the occurrence of syncope or cardiac arrest, mainly precipitated by emotional or physical stress.

Since ages,[46] hereditary variants, the Romano-Ward (RW) syndrome[47,48] and the extremely severe Jervell and Lange-Nielsen (JLN) syndrome,[49,50] which are associated with congenital deafness, have been included under the comprehensive name of LQTS. The usual mode of inheritance for RW is autosomal dominant, whereas JLN shows autosomal recessive inheritance.

Several reasons make LQTS an important disease. Symptomatic patients left without therapy are known to have a high mortality rate, 21% within 1 year from the first syncope.[51] However, with proper treatment, mortality is now almost 1% during a 15-year follow-up.[52]

Genetics of Long QT Syndrome

The QT interval represents the depolarization and repolarization phases of the cardiac AP. The combined interaction of these several ion channels determine the AP duration. A decrease in repolarizing outward K^+ current or increase in depolarizing inward sodium or calcium current can lead to prolongation of the QT interval, thus representing a pathophysiological substrate for LQTS.

The *KCNQ1* (LQT1), *KCNH2* (LQT2), and *SCNSA* (LQT3) are mostly 90% of the times the common genes accounted for in LQTS.[53,54]

Electrocardiography Presentation

The ventricular tachyarrhythmia that potentiates the cardiac events of LQTS is torsades de pointes (TdP), a type of ventricular tachycardia that may be self-limiting, produces transient syncope but can also lead into VF causing cardiac arrest or sudden death.[55]

Short QT Syndrome

Introduction

Short QT (SQT) refers to the ECG manifestation of accelerated cardiac repolarization. Its association with atrial and VF was suggested by Gussak et al.[56] Various articles have confirmed the familial nature and arrhythmogenic potential of SQT.[57] The most common cause is the acquired disease which results from electrolyte disturbances or drugs, in addition to hypercalcemia, hyperkalemia, and acidosis; SQT also manifests with drugs like digoxin, androgen use, increased vagal tone, and after VF.[58-60] SQTS is autosomal dominant and can manifests with atrial and ventricular arrhythmias leading to SCD.[61] Cardiac arrest can be the presenting symptom in up to 40% of the cases.[62]

Molecular Basis and Genetics

The manifestation can be attributed to mutations in potassium (KCNH2, KCNQ1, KCNJ2) and calcium (CACNA1C, CACNB2, CACNA2D1) channels (Table 3). Calcium-channel mutations also lead to a correlation with diseases, such as BS or ERS. Recently carnitine deficiency has also been linked to ECG manifestations of SQT.[63,64]

Gain of function mutations in the potassium channels have been shown to hasten earlier repolarizing currents, this decreases the AP causing lower threshold for arrhythmias. Calcium channel mutations cause loss of function in the slow inward calcium channel or L-type channel.[65,66] Mouse models of carnitine deficiency showed response to carnitine supplementation with reduction in ventricular arrhythmias, linking indirect effect of long-chain fatty acid on the regulation of the potassium channels.

Diagnosis

According to the HRS/EHRA/APHRS expert consensus statement on the diagnosis and management of patients with inherited primary arrhythmia syndromes, SQTS is diagnosed in the presence of a QTc less than or equal to 330 ms. It can also be diagnosed in combination with the presence of a QTc less than 360 ms and one of the following: a pathogenic mutation, family history of SQTS, family history of sudden death at age less than or equal to 40, or survival of a VT/VF episode in the absence of heart disease (Fig. 8).[67]

TABLE 3: Diagnostic criteria of long QT syndrome[55]

Electrocardiographic findings*		Points
A	QTc.	
	≥480 ms	3
	460–479	2
	450–459 (men)	1
B	QTc. t 4th minute of recovery from exercise stress test ≥480 ms	1
C	Torsades de pointes	2
D	T-wave alternans	1
	Notched T wave in 3 leads	1
	Low heart rate for age	0.5
Clinic history		
A	Syncope	
	With stress	2
	Without stress	1
B	Congenital deafness	0.5
Family history		
A	Family members with definite LQT	1
B	Unexplained sudden cardiac death younger than age 30 among immediate family members	0.5

In 2011, A diagnostic criteria was proposed for the assessment of patients with suspected SQTS[68] (Table 4). The criteria included ECG findings as well a family history, clinical history, and genotyping.[69] An overall score of 4 or more was considered to indicate a high probability diagnosis of SQTS.

The QTc generally is fixed and short in relation to changing heart rate (HR) of patients with SQTS.[69] This failure of adaptation to a faster HR has allowed more specific identification of subjects with QTc intervals between 340 ms and 360 ms, and a QT/HR slope under –0.9 ms/beat/min.[70,71]

Another ECG finding noted in SQTS is the high prevalence of early repolarization patterns (ERP). A study depicted that the presence of ERP in patients with SQTS is associated with higher arrhythmic events. The study looked at the uncorrected J point-T peak interval (JTp) and found that patients with symptomatic SQTS had shorter uncorrected JTp (<150 ms), shorter uncorrected J point-T end interval (JTe; <230 ms), and a high rate-corrected Tpeak-Tend c/QTc ratio.

J Wave Syndromes

Brugada syndrome and ERS share many ECG and clinical features, and have been collectively grouped as J wave syndrome (JWS). The concept has now expanded to include other structural heart diseases such as acute myocardial infarction, variant angina, and even some forms of cardiomyopathy.[3,4] This emphasizes the possibility that J waves may be even more important than previously recognized and may serve as a common mechanism of VF in various clinical settings (Box 1).

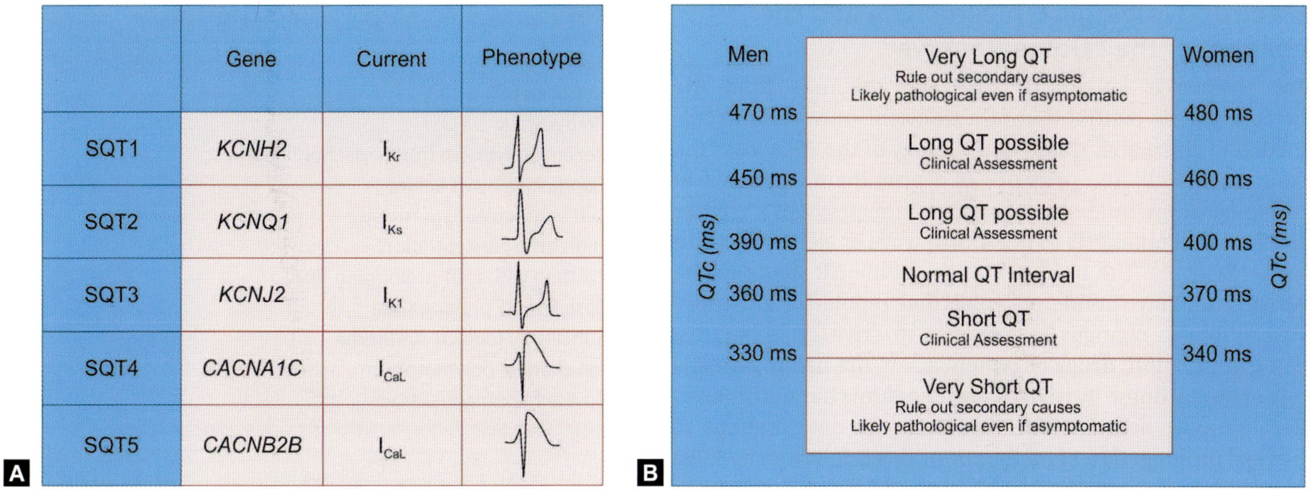

A

	Gene	Current	Phenotype
SQT1	*KCNH2*	I_{Kr}	
SQT2	*KCNQ1*	I_{Ks}	
SQT3	*KCNJ2*	I_{K1}	
SQT4	*CACNA1C*	I_{CaL}	
SQT5	*CACNB2B*	I_{CaL}	

B

Men	QTc (ms)	Women
	Very Long QT Rule out secondary causes Likely pathological even if asymptomatic	
470 ms		480 ms
	Long QT possible Clinical Assessment	
450 ms		460 ms
	Long QT possible Clinical Assessment	
390 ms		400 ms
	Normal QT Interval	
360 ms		370 ms
	Short QT Clinical Assessment	
330 ms		340 ms
	Very Short QT Rule out secondary causes Likely pathological even if asymptomatic	

LQTS, long QT syndrome; SQT, short QT; SQTS, short QT syndrome.

FIG. 8: Diagnosis and management of short QT syndrome.

TABLE 4: The short QT syndrome diagnostic scoring scheme[67]

Short QT syndrome	Points
QTc, ms	
<370	1
<350	2
<330	3
J point-T peak interval <120 ms	1
Clinical history	
History of sudden cardiac arrest	2
Document polymorphic ventricular tachycardia or ventricular fibrillation	2
Unexplained syncope	1
Atrial fibrillation	1
Family history	
First- or second-degree relative with high-probability short QT syndrome	2
First- or second-degree relative with autopsy-negative sudden cardiac death	1
Sudden infant death syndrome	1
Genotype	
Genotype positive	2
Mutation of undetermined significance in a culprit gene	1

J Wave-related Syndrome in Patients with Structural Heart Disease or Other Conditions

The J wave phenomenon can be observed both in structurally normal hearts and in patients with structural heart diseases. The pathogenic role of the epicardial notch and phase 2 re-entry in the early stages of acute myocardial ischemia was demonstrated by Yan et al.[72] who showed that acute regional myocardial ischemia results in heterogeneous loss of the epicardial AP dome across the ischemic border zone, leading to phase 2 re-entry and R-on-T extra-systoles inducing VFs. Although direct evidence is lacking, as the J wave is an electrocardiographic marker of vulnerability to phase 2 re-entry, its presence in the setting of acute myocardial ischemia is presumed to cause a higher likelihood of VF and SCD (Table 5).

BOX 1 Conditions with J waves

Conditions with predominant J waves

- Hypothermia
- Hypercalcemia
- Hyperkalemia
- Vasospastic angina
- Brugada syndrome
- Early repolarization syndrome
- Short QT syndrome
- Hypoxia
- Acidosis
- Pulmonary embolism
- Arrhythmogenic right ventricular cardiomyopathy
- Subarachnoid hemorrhage

TABLE 5: Risk factors for ventricular arrhythmias in long QT syndrome and J wave-related ventricular fibrillation syndromes

Risk factors for Torsades de pointes in LQTS (markers of reduced "repolarization reserve")	Risk factors for polymorphic VT/VF in J-wave syndrome (markers of reduced dome reserve")
Female	Male
Congestive heart failure, acute ischemia	Acute ischemia
Hypokalemia, hypomagnesemia	Hypocalcemia
K-channel blocker, psychotropic drugs, antibiotics, antifungals, antihistamine	Na-channel blocker, Ca-channel blocker, K-channel opener, psychotropic drugs, cocaine intoxication
Fever	Hypothermia (ERS), fever (some patients with BS)
Bradycardia, pause	Bradycardia, pause
QT prolongation	Prominent J wave

BS, Brugada syndrome; ERS, early repolarization syndrome; LOTS, long QT syndrome; VF, ventricular fibrillation; VT, ventricular tachycardia.

Electrophysiological mechanism and the concept of the "Dome Reserve"

The J wave is known to arise and originate from the heterogeneous distribution of a transient outward current-mediated spike and, dome morphology of the AP across the ventricular wall. The presence of a prominent AP notch in the epicardium, but not the endocardium, provides a voltage gradient that manifests as J (Osborn) wave or elevated J point in the ECG.[73,74] The unique features of the AP shape in the epicardium have rendered epicardial repolarization more susceptible to changes in response to drive cycle lengths, extra stimulation, drugs or ischemia.[75,76] The heterogeneous loss of the AP dome by ischemia, the sodium channel blocker, flecainide, or acetylcholine results in the development of marked prolongation of AP duration. This is followed by local re-excitation (phase 2 re-entry) due to AP propagating from sites where it was maintained to ones where it was abolished. Thus, the ECG J wave, a clinical marker of the AP notch, represents the vulnerability of the epicardial AP to an all-or-none repolarization, and susceptibility to fatal ventricular tachyarrhythmias. It is presumed that individuals with prominent J waves are thought to have the potential to lose their AP dome by extrinsic factors such as vagal stimulation, sodium channel blocker or ischemia. This ability of the ventricular myocardium to preserve this AP dome may be called "dome reserve", and the lack of this reserve may simply be expressed by the electrocardiographic J waves. A study proposed the concept of a "repolarization reserve" in which normal hearts have multiple repolarization currents during the physiologic repolarization process.[77,78] Defects in one of these multiple mechanisms may not produce the full-blown electrocardiographic features of LQTS. When multiple subclinical lesions are already present in the repolarization process that superimposition of an I_{Kr}-blocking drug can produce marked AP prolongation, resulting in TdP.

NONSTRUCTURAL HEART DISEASE: NONINHERITED

Acquired Long QT Syndrome

Acquired LQTS is defined as a disorder of cardiac repolarization mostly due to specific drugs, hypokalemia, or hypomagnesemia that may precipitate TdP and cause SCD. Selzer and Wray first reported QT prolongation and VF as a response to a drug which was quinidine in 1964 (Box 2).[79]

The QT interval on the surface electrocardiogram represents the summation of AP. QT prolongation entails AP prolongation, which results from an increase in inward current (through sodium or calcium channels) or a decrease in outward current (through potassium channels). Myocardial repolarization is primarily mediated by efflux of potassium ions. The two subtypes of the delayed rectifier I_{to}, I_{Kr} (rapid) and I_{Ks} (slow), are predominantly responsible for repolarization. These two currents have different activation, inactivation, and deactivation characteristics, different sensitivities to blocking drugs,[80-82] different rate, and catecholamine sensitivity[83,84] and are also result of expression of different genes.[85,86]

BOX 2 Risk factors for drug-induced torsade de pointes

- Female sex
- Hypokalemia
- Bradycardia
- Recent conversion from atrial fibrillation
- Congestive heart failure
- Left ventricular hypertrophy
- High drug concentration
- Infusion with a QT prolonging drug
- Base line QT prolongation
- Subclinical long QT syndrome
- Ion channel polymorphism
- Severe hypomagnesemia

TABLE 6: Drugs implicated in torsade de pointes

Antiarrhythmic medications • Class 1A (quinidine, procainamide, and disopyramide) • Class III (dofetilide, ibutilide, sotalol, and amiodarone) • Class III (dofetilide, ibutilide, sotalol, and amiodarone) • Class IV (Verapamil)	**Pentamidine**
Promotility medications • Cisapride	**Antimalarial**
Antimicrobial medications • Macrolides • Erythromycin • Clarithromycin • Fluoroquinolones • Antiprotozoals	**Chloroquine**
Antipsychotic medications • Phenothiazine neuroleptics • Thioridazine • Chlorpromazine • Butyrophenone neuroleptics • Haloperidol	**Arsenic trioxide**
Miscellaneous medications	**Methadone**

The hallmark mechanism of acquired LQTS and TdP is the blockade of I_{Kr} by specific drugs.[87] I_{Kr} current proteins are encoded by the *HERG* gene (now termed *KCNH2*) (Table 6).[88]

The I_{Kr} blockade results in a delay in phase 3 rapid repolarization of the AP, which is reflected by QT prolongation. Prolonged repolarization can cause early after depolarization (EADs) due to activation of inward depolarizing currents (L-type calcium channels or sodium-calcium exchange current.[89] These EADs that reach threshold voltage can result in a ventricular extrasystole preceded by a long QT interval on the surface ECG.

ELECTROCARDIOGRAPHY-BASED TESTS

The 12-lead electrocardiogram (ECG) is a widely available, inexpensive, noninvasive tool, used and familiar to all clinicians. As a time tested modality reflecting the electrical activity of the heart, it seems to be the one to contribute significantly to identifying risk of SCD, which may be the result of electrical disturbances in the heart (Table 7).

COMMON FORMS OF SUDDEN CARDIAC DEATH

Most SCD in the general population is associated with coronary artery disease (CAD),[90] while a smaller proportion is due to other cardiomyopathies. Assessment of SCD risk is complex since it represents a combination of multiple processes acting together.[91]

TABLE 7: Electrocardiography-based tests

ECC-based test	Advantages	Disadvantages/Limitations	Practical value for risk stratification
12-lead ECG	Cheap, quick and easy to perform; can be obtained serially at each follow-up visit to reassess risk; large databases can be generated and analyzed retrospectively/ prospectively	Many abnormal parameters are markers of increased mortality, rather than specifically SCD; low positive predictive and negative predictive accuracies; subject to interobserver variability (unless automated software is used); considerable overlap in some parameters between healthy subjects and patients	Remains a standard investigation in patients with CAD; low positive and negative predictive accuracies for SCD limit its practical use in (risk stratification and selection of ICD candidates
Signal-averaged ECG	Easy and quick to perform; high negative predictive accuracy; can be used in patients with AF	Low positive predictive accuracy; numerous negative studies, especially in current era of interventional cardiology; better at predicting risk of VT than VF; normal standards for patients with bundle branch block or paced rhythm have not been established	Improved risk stratification when used in combination with other tests: probably more useful In identifying low-risk patients; not useful alone for risk stratification
Standard 24-hour Holter	Provides information on other arrhythmias in patients with CAD (e.g., AF, heart block); standard test, easy to perform; can be used in patients in AF or paced rhythms	Low sensitivity and specificity	Most promising use is in combination with other parameters (e.g., HRV and HRD obtained from Holter recordings; not useful alone for risk stratification
Heart rate variability	Can be automatically recorded with standard Holter (using additional software); short (2–30 min) and longer (24 h) measurements are possible	Cannot be reliably assessed in patients with AF or frequent PVCS Influenced by a number of factors (e.g., age, medication); may be affected by functional state of sinus node; short-term measurements in risk prediction have not been well tested; no consensus on which parameters of HRV or method of assessment is best	Current practical use for risk stratification is limited as a consensus opinion on which parameters of HRV to record and which method of assessing HRV is required
Heart rate turbulence	Value in risk prediction post-AMI supported by several recent large-scale prospective studies; provides prognostic information in patients with normal and impaired IVEF	Optimal time post-AMI to perform the test has not been established; can only be performed in patients in SR with a significant number of PVCs: use in patients with CAD and no history of AMI not well established	A promising test for risk prediction that can be used with other Holter-based measurements; limited practical use at present in the absence of clear guidelines for risk stratification
T-wave alternans	Easy to perform; can use existing equipment or modification of equipment; high negative predictive accuracy	Can only be used in patients in SR; "clean" ECG trace required (difficult to obtain during exercise); indeterminate result if target heart rate not achieved during exercise; low positive predictive accuracy	Useful in risk stratifying patients with impaired and preserved LVEF; useful role in determining which patients are unlikely to benefit from ICD insertion; improved risk stratification when used in combination with other tests: dear guidelines awaited for practical use for risk stratification

AF, atrial fibrillation; AMI, acute myocardial infarction; CAD, coronary artery disease; HRD, heart rate detection; HRV, heart rate variability; ICD, implantable cardioverter defibrillators; LVEF, left ventricular ejection fraction; PVC, premature ventricular contraction; SCD, sudden cardiac death; VF, ventricular fibrillation; VT, ventricular tachycardia; ECG, electrocardiography.

Resting Heart Rate

A higher resting HR has been linked to SCD risk in several studies. In the Paris Prospective Study, subjects with an HR more than 75 beats/min had an almost 4-fold risk of SCD compared with those with a HR less than 65.[92,93] HR is linked to autonomic tone which influences the risk of arrhythmia.[94] However, there has been some concern that HR may be a nonspecific marker;[95] furthermore, it is influenced by several factors of which drugs are the most common.

Abnormalities of Depolarization

Various abnormalities related to the QRS complex, which reflects ventricular depolarization, can help evaluate SCD risk. Q waves, representing loss of myocardium and possibly LV dysfunction and scar, have been associated with an increased risk.[96] Various QRS scores have been calculated and shown to correlate with ventricular arrhythmic events.[97-99]

A longer QRS duration (QRSD) has been shown to be associated with the risk of SCD irrespective of the presence of BBB.[100,101] A study showed a 27% increase in SCD risk for every 10 ms increase in the QRSD.[102] Also dynamic prolongation of QRSD has been shown to occur in acute myocardial ischemia.[103] While prolonged QRSD has been well studied as a risk factor for SCD, there is very less data on the relevance of QRS morphologies. A large population-based study reported that intraventricular conduction delay was associated with arrhythmic death, it may also be weakly associated with LBBB, while right BBB has not been correlated.[104] Fragmentation of the QRS (fQRS) is defined as the presence of various RSR patterns. This results from disrupted electrical conduction in areas of diseased or fibrosed myocardium;[105] thus, it can be related to re-entrant arrhythmias. A study[106] demonstrated that fQRS was better than Q waves in detecting myocardial scar. Subsequent studies have shown that fQRS is related to SCD as well as implantable cardioverter defibrillator (ICD) shocks.[107,108] The evidence for fQRS as a prognostic marker in patients with beyond CAD, such as in arrhythmogenic right ventricular cardiomyopathy[109] and cardiac amyloidosis,[110] suggests that it may be a useful risk marker for SCD risk.[111] Another often overlooked risk factor in the context of SCD is the presence of LVH on the ECG. While ECG-LVH has been shown to be associated with SCD risk,[112] it has been associated as an indicator of increased LV mass.[113,114] A subsequent study demonstrated diagnoses of LVH with respect to the risk of developing new atrial fibrillation.[115] These reports suggest that increased myocardial voltage may reflect adverse electrical' remodeling, leading to a risk higher than just anatomic LV hypertrophy.

Abnormalities of Repolarization

Prolongation of the QT interval has long been associated with an increased risk of ventricular arrhythmias (like LQTS). However, multiple findings suggest that this may also be an important risk factor for SCD.

Oregon-Sudden Unexpected Death study suggested that though diabetes and QT-affecting drugs contributed to SCD risk, idiopathic QT prolongation unrelated to either of these factors was the strongest predictor of SCD in CAD, conferring up to a 5-fold increased risk.[116] Kinoshita et al.[117] found a QTc of more than or equal to 450 ms in men and more than or equal to 470 ms in women to be an independent predictor of SCD in subjects undergoing cardiac surgery. A recent meta-analysis incorporating 23 studies confirmed an increased risk of SCD in subjects in the highest versus lowest categories of QTc; thus, relative variations even within the traditionally defined normal limits for the QTc may be relevant in terms of risk.[118] The measurement of JT interval may be a more useful measure in patients of prolonged QT.[119]

Another new novel ECG marker recently is the T-peak to T-end interval (Tpe). This has been thought to be a measurement of the transmural dispersion of repolarization.[120] A prolonged Tpe may reflect a period where the epicardium has fully repolarized, but the subendocardium is still recovering. This could create an electrical disturbance for after depolarization driven re-entrant ventricular arrhythmias.[121,122] A recent study showed the Tpe to be significantly prolonged in cases of SCD. Also, Tpe was significantly associated with SCD in patients with prolonged QRSD, where measurement of QTc is challenging.[123] Thus, Tpe may be a useful addition to the QTc in assessing abnormal repolarization.

Studies have also shown the Tpe or the Tpe/QT ratio to be a predictor of arrhythmic events in inherited conditions such as BS[124] and HCM.[125] The ER pattern or J point elevation, previously was considered to be a benign finding, but recently has been reported to have a link with idiopathic VF.[126-127]

A new parameter that involves both depolarization and repolarization is the QRS-T angle, which can be assumed as the difference between the net directions of depolarization and repolarization in the heart. Recently in studies, this increased QRS-T angle has been associated with an increased SCD risk.[128,129]

MULTIPLE RISK MARKERS: CUMULATIVE RISK

While several of the markers indicated in the article from a pathological aspect have the potential to lead to SCD, it is unlikely that a single marker would have adequate discriminative power to be noted as a singular potential risk predictor.[130] As SCD represents the combination of multiple risk processes, the use of multiple risk markers, which reflect the different facets of the heart's electrical activity, would help to convey more information than a single marker. The validation of these multiple markers in large population-based studies would be needed to finally be able to develop an "electrical" risk score based on ECG which could be by a primary physician to target potential at-risk individuals. This early concept for a cumulative risk approach using a combination of variables has been noted in various analyses from all the defibrillator trials.[131]

Though ECG represents only one arm of the approach to SCD risk prediction, ECG with cumulative risk markers can be useful combined with clinical markers, genetics, biomarkers, and imaging.[132]

IMPORTANCE OF DYNAMIC MONITORING

One study suggested that the total magnitude of ST elevation in all leads can predict VF in patients with ST elevation MI.[133] Moreover, continuous monitoring may help identify dynamic changes immediately before the onset of VF which may give insights into pathophysiology and etiology of the arrhythmia. Implantable loop recorders may help yield dynamic information as well. Dynamic monitoring approaches may aid SCD risk assessment. It can be assumed that parameters from an ECG at one point in time can help attain information about long-term risk of susceptibility to arrhythmia which may be the static risk of the patient, wherever the dynamic monitoring in the acute setting, including ECG in the field at the time of an ACS and various forms of ambulatory ECG monitoring can help understand changes preceding arrhythmia[134,135] which could help identify the markers for triggers of arrhythmia.

CONCLUSION AND FUTURE DIRECTIONS

The 12-lead ECG continues to be a simple and useful tool for identification of individuals at increased risk of SCD. At present, the utility of this modality is unquestionable for making a diagnosis and assessing at risk patients with primary and inherited arrhythmia syndromes; and even the acquired forms of drug-induced LQTS. As clinicians we should be able to put this widely available and inexpensive tool to use in decision making for who may be in need to receive a primary prevention defibrillator. It is likely that these ECG variables will not be the individual predictors of increased SCD risk but will rather be utilized to predict risk as cumulative markers.

REFERENCES

1. Chugh SS, Kelly KL, Titus JL. Sudden cardiac death with apparently normal heart. Circulation. 2000;102:649-54.
2. Marian AJ, Roberts R. The molecular genetic basis for hypertrophic cardiomyopathy. J Mol Cell Cardiol. 2001;33(4):655-70.
3. Henkel DM, Witt BJ, Gersh BJ. Ventricular arrhythmias after acute myocardial infarction: A 20-year community study. Am Heart J. 2006;151:806-12.
4. Naruse Y, Tada H, Harimura Y, et al. Early repolarization is an independent predictor of occurrences of ventricular fibrillation in the very early phase of acute myocardial infarction. Circ Arrhythm Electrophysiol. 2012;5:506-13.
5. Brugada P, Brugada J. Right bundle branch block, persistent ST segment elevation and sudden cardiac death: A distinct clinical and electrocardiographic syndrome. A multicenter report. J Am Coll Cardiol. 1992;20:1391-6.
6. Wilde AA, Antzelevitch C, Borggrefe M, et al. Proposed diagnostic criteria for the Brugada syndrome: Consensus report. Circulation. 2002;106:2514-9.
7. Osher HL, Wolff L. Electrocardiographic pattern simulating acute myocardial injury. Am J Med Sci. 1953;226:541-5.
8. Edeiken J. Elevation of the RS-T segment, apparent or real, in the right precordial leads as a probable normal variant. Am Heart J. 1954;48:331-9.
9. Martini B, Nava A, Thiene G, et al. Ventricular fibrillation without apparent heart disease: Description of six cases. Am Heart J. 1989;118:1203-9.
10. Coronel R, Casini S, Koopmann TT, et al. Right ventricular fibrosis and conduction delay in a patient with clinical signs of Brugada syndrome: A combined electrophysiological, genetic, histopathologic, and computational study. Circulation. 2005;112:2769-77.
11. Frustaci A, Priori SG, Pieroni M, et al. Cardiac histological substrate in patients with clinical phenotype of Brugada syndrome. Circulation. 2005;112:3680-7.
12. Martini B, Nava A. A long lasting electrocardiographic history. Heart Rhythm. 2010;7:1521.
13. Chen Q, Kirsch GE, Zhang D, et al. Genetic basis and molecular mechanism for idiopathic ventricular fibrillation. Nature. 1998;392:293-6.
14. Priori SG, Napolitano C, Giordano U, et al. Brugada syndrome and sudden cardiac death in children. Lancet. 2000;355:808-9.
15. Wang DW, Yazawa K, George AL Jr, et al. Characterization of human cardiac Na+ channel mutations in the congenital long QT syndrome. Proc Natl Acad Sci USA. 1996;93:132005.
16. Schott JJ, Alshinawi C, Kyndt F, et al. Cardiac conduction defects associate with mutations in SCN5A. Nat Genet. 1999;23:20-21.
17. Smits JP, Koopmann TT, Wilders R, et al. A mutation in the human cardiac sodium channel (E161K) contributes to sick sinus syndrome, conduction disease and Brugada syndrome in two families. J Mol Cell Cardiol. 2005;38:969-81.
18. Makita N, Sasaki K, Groenewegen WA, et al. Congenital atrial standstill associated with coinheritance of a novel SCN5A mutation and connexin 40 polymorphisms. Heart Rhythm. 2005;2:1128-34.
19. Bezzina CR, Rook MB, Groenewegen WA, et al. Compound heterozygosity for mutations (W156X and R225W) in SCN5A associated with severe cardiac conduction disturbances and degenerative changes in the conduction system. Circ Res. 2003;92:159-68.
20. McNair WP, Ku L, Taylor MR, et al. SCN5A mutation associated with dilated cardiomyopathy, conduction disorder, and arrhythmia. Circulation. 2004;110:2163-7.
21. Olson TM, Michels VV, Ballew JD, et al. Sodium channel mutations and susceptibility to heart failure and atrial fibrillation. JAMA. 2005;293:44754.
22. Survivors of out-of-hospital cardiac arrest with apparently normal heart. Need for definition and standardized clinical evaluation. Consensus statement of the Joint Steering Committees of the Unexplained Cardiac Arrest Registry of Europe and of the Idiopathic Ventricular Fibrillation Registry of the United States. Circulation. 1997;95:265-72.
23. Tan HL, Hofman N, van Langen IM, et al. Sudden unexplained death: heritability and diagnostic yield of cardiological and genetic examination in surviving relatives. Circulation. 2005;112:207-13.
24. Behr ER, Camm AJ. Letter by Behr and Camm regarding article, "Induced Brugada-type electrocardiogram, a sign for imminent malignant arrhythmias." Circulation. 2008;118:e701.
25. Matsuo K, Akahoshi M, Nakashima E, et al. The prevalence, incidence and prognostic value of the Brugada type electrocardiogram: a population-based study of four decades. J Am Coll Cardiol. 2001;38:765-70.
26. Rolf S, Haverkamp W, Eckardt L. True right bundle branch block masking the typical ECG in Brugada syndrome. Pacing Clin Electrophysiol. 2005;28:258-9.
27. Priori SG, Wilde AA, Horie M, et al. HRS/EHRA/APHRS Expert consensus statement on the diagnosis and management of patients with inherited primary arrhythmia syndromes: Document endorsed by HRS, EHRA, and APHRS in May 2013 and by ACCF, AHA, PACES, and AEPC in June 2013. Heart Rhythm. 2013;10:1932-63.
28. Klatsky AL, Oehm R, Cooper RA, et al. The early repolarization normal variant electrocardiogram: Correlates and consequences. Am J Med. 2003;115:171-7.
29. Mehta M, Jain AC, Mehta A. Early repolarization. Clin Cardiol. 1999;22:59-65.
30. Grant RP, Estes EH, Doyle JT. Spatial vector electrocardiography; the clinical characteristics of S-T and T vectors. Circulation. 1951;3:182-97.
31. Gussak I, Antzelevitch C. Early repolarization syndrome: Clinical characteristics and possible cellular and ionic mechanisms. J Electrocardiol. 2000;33:299-309.
32. Tikkanen JT, Anttonen O, Junttila MJ, et al. Long-term outcome associated with early repolarization on electrocardiography. N Engl J Med. 2009;361:2529-37.
33. Rosso R, Kogan E, Belhassen B, et al. J-point elevation in survivors of primary ventricular fibrillation and matched control subjects: incidence and clinical significance. J Am Coll Cardiol. 2008;52:1231-8.
34. Miyazaki S, Shah AJ, Haïssaguerre M. Early repolarization syndrome—a new electrical disorder associated with sudden cardiac death. Circ J. 2010;74:2039-44.

35. Serra-Grima R, Doñate M, Álvarez-García J, et al. Long-term follow-up of early repolarization pattern in elite athletes. Am J Med. 2015;128:192.e1-192.e9.
36. Barbosa EC, Bomfim Ade S, Benchimol-Barbosa PR, et al. Ionic mechanisms and vectorial model of early repolarization pattern in the surface electrocardiogram of the athlete. Ann Noninvasive Electrocardiol. 2008;13:301-7.
37. Nam GB, Ko KH, Kim J, et al. Mode of onset of ventricular fibrillation in patients with early repolarization pattern vs. Brugada syndrome. Eur Heart J. 2010;31:330-9.
38. Tikkanen JT, Wichmann V, Junttila MJ, et al. Association of early repolarization and sudden cardiac death during an acute coronary event. Circ Arrhythm Electrophysiol. 2012;5:714-8.
39. Benito B, Guasch E, Rivard L, et al. Clinical and mechanistic issues in early repolarization of normal variants and lethal arrhythmia syndromes. J Am Coll Cardiol. 2010;56:1177-86.
40. Li GR, Lau CP, Ducharme A, et al. Transmural action potential and ionic current remodeling in ventricles of failing canine hearts. Am J Physiol Heart Circ Physiol. 2002;283:H1031-41.
41. Antzelevitch C, Yan GX. J wave syndromes. Heart Rhythm. 2010;7:549-58.
42. Haïssaguerre M, Chatel S, Sacher F, et al. Ventricular fibrillation with prominent early repolarization associated with a rare variant of KCNJ8/KATP channel. J Cardiovasc Electrophysiol. 2009;20:93-98.
43. Perez MV, Friday K, Froelicher V. Semantic confusion: The case of early repolarization and the J point. Am J Med. 2012;125:843-4.
44. Tikkanen JT, Junttila MJ, Anttonen O, et al. Early repolarization: Electrocardiographic phenotypes associated with favorable long-term outcome. Circulation. 2011;123:2666-73.
45. Rollin A, Maury P, Bongard V, et al. Prevalence, prognosis, and identification of the malignant form of early repolarization pattern in a population-based study. Am J Cardiol. 2012;110:1302-8.
46. Sshwartz PJ, Periti M, Malliani A. The long QT syndrome. Am Heart J. 1975;89:378-90.
47. Romano C, Gemme G, Pongiglione R. Rare cardiac arrhythmias of the pediatric age, syncopal attacks due to paroxysmal ventricular fibrillation. (Presentation of 1st case in Italian pediatric literature). Clin Pediatr (Bologna). 1963;45:656-83.
48. Ward OC. A new familial cardiac syndrome in children. J Ir Med Assoc. 1964;54:103-6.
49. Jervell A, Lange-Nielsen F. Congenital deaf mutism, functional heart disease with prolongation of the QT interval and sudden death. Am Heart J. 1957;54: 59-68.
50. Schwartz PJ, Spazzolini C, Crotti L, et al. The Jervell and Lange-Neilsen syndrome: Natural history, molecular basis and clinical outcome. Circulation. 2006;113:783-90.
51. Schwartz PJ. Idiopathic long QT syndrome: Progress and questions. Am Heart J. 1985;109:399-411.
52. Schwartz PJ, Crotti L. Long QT and short QT syndrome. Zipes DP, Jalife J (eds). Cardiac Electrophysiology: From Cell to Bedside. Philadelphia, PA: Elsevier/ Saunders; 2009. pp. 731-44.
53. Kapplinger JD, Tester DJ, Salisbury BA, et al. Spectrum and prevalence of mutations from the first 2500 consecutive unrelated patients referred for the FAMILION long QT syndrome genetic test. Heart Rhytm. 2009;6:1297-303.
54. Tester DJ, Will ML, Haglund CM, et al. Compendium of cardiac channel mutations in 541 consecutive unrelated patients referred for long QT syndrome genetic testing. Heart Rhytm. 2005;2:507-17.
55. Schwartz PJ, Crotti L. QTc behavior during exercise and genetic counseling for the long QT syndrome. Circulation. 2011;124:2181-4.
56. Gussak I, Brugada P, Brugada J, et al. Idiopathic short QT interval: A new clinical syndrome? Cardiology. 2000;94:99-102.
57. Gaita F, Giustetto C, Bianchi F, et al. Short QT syndrome: A familial cause of sudden death. Circulation. 2003;108:965-70.
58. Cheng TO. Digitalis administration: An underappreciated but common cause of short QT interval. Circulation. 2004;109:E152.
59. Hancox JC, Choisy SC, James AF. Short QT interval linked to androgen misuse: Wider significance and possible basis. Ann Noninvasive Electrocardiol. 2009;14:311-2.
60. Ramakrishna H, O'Hare M, Mookadam F, et al. Sudden cardiac death and disorders of the QT interval: Anesthetic implications and focus on perioperative management. J Cardiothorac Vasc Anesth. 2015;29:1723-33.
61. Brugada R, Hong K, Dumaine R, et al. Sudden death associated with short-QT syndrome linked to mutations in HERG. Circulation. 2004;109:30-5.
62. Mazzanti A, Kanthan A, Monteforte N, et al. Novel insight into the natural history of short QT syndrome. J Am Coll Cardiol. 2014;63:1300-8.
63. Roussel J, Labarthe F, Thireau J. Carnitine deficiency induces a short QT syndrome. Heart Rhythm. 2016;13:165-74.
64. Giustetto C, Schimpf R, Mazzanti A, et al. Long-term follow-up of patients with short QT syndrome. J Am Coll Cardiol. 2011;58:587-95.
65. Antzelevitch C, Pollevick GD, Cordeiro JM, et al. Loss-of-function mutations in the cardiac calcium channel underlie a new clinical entity characterized by ST-segment elevation, short QT intervals, and sudden cardiac death. Circulation. 2007;115:442-9.
66. Templin C, Ghadri JR, Rougier JS, et al. Identification of a novel loss-of-function calcium channel gene mutation in short QT syndrome (SQTS6). Eur Heart J. 2011;32:1077-88.
67. Giudicessi JR, Ackerman MJ. Determinants of incomplete penetrance and variable expressivity in heritable cardiac arrhythmia syndromes. Trans Res. 2013;161:1-14.
68. Gollob MH, Redpath CJ, Roberts JD. The short QT syndrome: Proposed diagnostic criteria. J Am Coll Cardiol. 2011;57:802-12.
69. Redpath CF, Green, MS, Birnie DH, et al. Rapid genetic testing facilitating the diagnosis of short QT syndrome. Can J Cardiol. 2009;25:e133-5.
70. Giustetto C, Scrocco C, Schimpf R, et al. Usefulness of exercise test in the diagnosis of short QT syndrome. Europace. 2015;17:628-34.
71. Bellocq C, van Ginneken AC, Bezzina CR, et al. Mutation in the *KCNQ1* gene leading to the short QT-interval syndrome. Circulation. 2004;109:2394-7.
72. Yan GX, Joshi A, Guo D, et al. Phase 2 reentry as a trigger to initiate ventricular fibrillation during early acute myocardial ischemia. Circulation. 2004;110: 1036-41.
73. Yan GX, Antzelevitch C. Cellular basis for the electrocardiographic J wave. Circulation. 1996;93:372-9.
74. Yan GX, Antzelevitch C. Cellular basis for the Brugada syndrome and other mechanisms of arrhythmogenesis associated with ST-segment elevation. Circulation. 1999;100:1660-6.
75. Litovsky SH, Antzelevitch C. Differences in the electrophysiologic response of canine ventricular subendocardium and subepicardium to acetylcholine and isoproterenol: A direct effect of acetylcholine in ventricular myocardium. Circ Res. 1990;67:615-27.
76. Krishnan SC, Antzelevitch C. Sodium channel blockade produces opposite electrophysiologic effects in canine ventricular epicardium and endocardium. Circ Res. 1991;69:277-91.
77. Roden DM. Taking the "idio" out of "idiosyncratic": Predicting torsades de pointes. Pacing Clin Electrophysiol. 1998;21:1029-34.
78. Roden DM. Long QT syndrome: Reduced repolarization reserve and the genetic link. J Intern Med. 2006;259:59-69.
79. Selzer A, Wray HW. Quinidine syncope. Paroxysmal ventricular fibrillation occurring during treatment of chronic atrial arrhythmias. Circulation.1964;30:17-26.
80. Sanguinetti MC, Jurkiewicz NK. Two components of cardiac delayed rectifier K+ current: Differential sensitivity to block by class III antiarrhythmic agent. J Gen Physiol. 1990;96(1):195-215.
81. Sanguinetti MC, Jurkiewicz NK. Delayed rectifier outward K+ current is composed of two currents in guinea pig atrial cells. Am J Physiol—Heart Circ Physiol. 1991;260(2):H3939.
82. Gintant GA. Two components of delayed rectifier current in canine atrium and ventricle: Does IKs play a role in the reverse rate dependence of class III agents? Circ Res. 1996;78(1):26-37.
83. Sanguinetti MC, Kurkiewicz NK, Scott A, et al. Isoproterenol antagonizes prolongation of refractory period by the class III antiarrhythmic agent E-4031 in guinea pig myocytes: Mechanism of action. Circ Res. 1991;68(1):77-84.
84. Jurkiewicz NK, Sanguinetti MC. Rate-dependent prolongation of cardiac action potentials by a methanesulfonanilide class III antiarrhythmic agent: Specific block of rapidly activating delayed rectifier K+ current by dofetilide. Circ. Res. 1993;72(1):7583
85. Sanguinetti MC, Curran ME, Zou A, et al. Coassembly of K(V)LQT1 and minK (IsK) proteins to form cardiac I(Ks) potassium channel. Nature. 1996;384(6604): 80-3.

86. Barhanin J, Lesage F, Guillemare E, et al. K(V)LQT1 and IsK (minK) proteins associate to form the I(Ks) cardiac potassium current. Nature. 1996;384(6604):78-80.
87. Roden DM, Viswanathan PC. Genetics of acquired long QT syndrome. J Clin Invest. 2005;115:2025-32. comprehensive review of molecular and cellular mechanisms underlying acquired LQTS.
88. Curran ME, Splawski I, Timothy KW, et al. A molecular basis for cardiac arrhythmia: HERG mutations cause long QT syndrome. Cell. 1995;80(5): 795-803.
89. Roden DM, Lazzara R, Rosen M, et al. Multiple mechanisms in the long-QT syndrome: Current knowledge, gaps, and future directions. Circulation. 1996;94(8):1996-2012.
90. Adabag AS, Peterson G, Apple FS, et al. Etiology of sudden death in the community: Results of anatomical, metabolic, and genetic evaluation. Am Heart J. 2010;159:33-9.
91. Chugh SS, Reinier K, Teodorescu C, et al. Epidemiology of sudden cardiac death: Clinical and research implications. Prog Cardiovasc Dis. 2008;51:213-28.
92. Jouven X, Zureik M, Desnos M, et al. Resting heart rate as a predictive risk factor for sudden death in middle-aged men. Cardiovasc Res. 2001;50:373-8.
93. Cale R, Mendes M, Brito J, et al. Resting heart rate is a powerful predictor of arrhythmic events in patients with dilated cardiomyopathy and implantable cardioverter-defibrillator. Rev Port Cardiol. 2011;30:199-212.
94. Hohnloser SH, Klingenheben T, van de Loo A, et al. Reflex versus tonic vagal activity as a prognostic parameter in patients with sustained ventricular tachycardia or ventricular fibrillation. Circulation. 1994;89:1068-73.
95. Jouven X, Escolano S, Celermajer D, et al. Heart rate and risk of cancer death in healthy men. PLoS One. 2011;6:e21310.
96. Smith WC, Kenicer MB, Tunstall-Pedoe H, et al. Prevalence of coronary heart disease in Scotland: Scottish Heart Health Study. Br Heart J. 1990;64:295-8.
97. Strauss DG, Selvester RH, Lima JA, et al. ECG quantification of myocardial scar in cardiomyopathy patients with or without conduction defects: Correlation with cardiac magnetic resonance and arrhythmogenesis. Circ Arrhythm Electrophysiol. 2008;1:327-36.
98. Strauss DG, Poole JE, Wagner GS, et al. An ECG index of myocardial scar enhances prediction of defibrillator shocks: An analysis of the sudden cardiac death in heart failure trial. Heart Rhythm. 2011;8:38-45.
99. Loring Z, Zareba W, McNitt S, et al. ECG quantification of myocardial scar and risk stratification in MADIT-II. Ann Noninvasive Electrocardiol. 2013;18:427-35.
100. Morin DP, Oikarinen L, Viitasalo M, et al. QRS duration predicts sudden cardiac death in hypertensive patients undergoing intensive medical therapy: The LIFE study. Eur Heart J. 2009;30:2908-14.
101. Teodorescu C, Reinier K, Uy-Evanado A, et al. Prolonged QRS duration on the resting ECG is associated with sudden death risk in coronary disease, independent of prolonged ventricular repolarization. Heart Rhythm. 2011;8:1562-7.
102. Kurl S, Makikallio TH, Rautaharju P, et al. Duration of QRS complex in resting electrocardiogram is a predictor of sudden cardiac death in men. Circulation. 2012;125:2588-94.
103. Wiegerinck RF, Galvez-Monton C, Jorge E, et al. Changes in QRS duration and R-wave amplitude in electrocardiogram leads with ST segment elevation differentiate epicardial and transmural myocardial injury. Heart Rhythm. 2010;7:1667-73.
104. Aro AL, Anttonen O, Tikkanen JT, et al. Intraventricular conduction delay in a standard 12-lead electrocardiogram as a predictor of mortality in the general population. Circ Arrhythm Electrophysiol. 2011;4:704-10.
105. Das MK, Saha C, El Masry H, et al. Fragmented QRS on a 12-lead ECG: a predictor of mortality and cardiac events in patients with coronary artery disease. Heart Rhythm. 2007;4:1385-92.
106. Das MK, Khan B, Jacob S, et al. Significance of a fragmented QRS complex versus a Q wave in patients with coronary artery disease. Circulation. 2006;113:2495-501.
107. Brenyo A, Pietrasik G, Barsheshet A, et al. QRS fragmentation and the risk of sudden cardiac death in MADIT II. J Cardiovasc Electrophysiol. 2012;23: 1343-8.
108. Terho HK, Tikkanen JT, Junttila JM, et al. Prevalence and prognostic significance of fragmented QRS complex in middle-aged subjects with and without clinical or electrocardiographic evidence of cardiac disease. Am J Cardiol. 2014;114: 141-7.
109. Pei J, Li N, Gao Y, et al. The J wave and fragmented QRS complexes in inferior leads associated with sudden cardiac death in patients with chronic heart failure. Europace. 2012;14:1180-7.
110. Canpolat U, Kabakci G, Aytemir K, et al. Fragmented QRS complex predicts the arrhythmic events in patients with arrhythmogenic right ventricular cardiomyopathy/dysplasia. J Cardiovasc Electrophysiol. 2013;24:1260-6.
111. Perlini S, Salinaro F, Cappelli F, et al. Prognostic value of fragmented QRS in cardiac AL amyloidosis. Int J Cardiol. 2013;167:2156-61.
112. Rosengarten JA, Scott PA, Morgan JM. Fragmented QRS for the prediction of sudden cardiac death: A meta-analysis. Europace. 2015;17:969-77.
113. Wachtell K, Okin PM, Olsen MH, et al. Regression of electrocardiographic left ventricular hypertrophy during antihypertensive therapy and reduction in sudden cardiac death: The LIFE study. Circulation. 2007;116:700-5.
114. Devereux RB, Casale PN, Wallerson DC, et al. Cost-effectiveness of echocardiography and electrocardiography for detection of left ventricular hypertrophy in patients with systemic hypertension. Hypertension. 1987;9 (2 Pt 2):II69-76.
115. Narayanan K, Reinier K, Teodorescu C, et al. Electrocardiographic versus echocardiographic left ventricular hypertrophy and sudden cardiac arrest in the community. Heart Rhythm. 2014;11:1040-6.
116. Chrispin J, Jain A, Soliman EZ, et al. Association of electrocardiographic and imaging surrogates of left ventricular hypertrophy with incident atrial fibrillation: MESA (Multi-Ethnic Study of Atherosclerosis). J Am Coll Cardiol. 2014;63: 2007-13.
117. Chugh SS, Reinier K, Singh T, et al. Determinants of prolonged QT interval and their contribution to sudden death risk in coronary artery disease: The Oregon Sudden Unexpected Death Study. Circulation. 2009;119:663-70.
118. Kinoshita T, Asai T, Suzuki T, et al. Time course and prognostic implications of QT interval in patients with coronary artery disease undergoing coronary bypass surgery. J Cardiovasc Electrophysiol. 2012;23:645-9.
119. Zhang Y, Post WS, Blasco-Colmenares E, et al. Electrocardiographic QT interval and mortality: A meta-analysis. Epidemiology. 2011;22:660-70.
120. Crow RS, Hannan PJ, Folsom AR. Prognostic significance of corrected QT and corrected JT interval for incident coronary heart disease in a general population sample stratified by presence or absence of wide QRS complex: the ARIC Study with 13 years of follow-up. Circulation. 2003;108:1985-9.
121. Opthof T, Coronel R, Wilms-Schopman FJ, et al. Dispersion of repolarization in canine ventricle and the electrocardiographic T wave: Tp-e interval does not reflect transmural dispersion. Heart Rhythm. 2007;4:341-8.
122. Gupta P, Patel C, Patel H, et al. T(p-e)/QT ratio as an index of arrhythmogenesis. J Electrocardiol. 2008;41:567-74.
123. Liu T, Brown BS, Wu Y, et al. Blinded validation of the isolated arterially perfused rabbit ventricular wedge in preclinical assessment of drug-induced proarrhythmias. Heart Rhythm. 2006;3:948-56.
124. Panikkath R, Reinier K, Uy-Evanado A, et al. Prolonged Tpeak-to-tend interval on the resting ECG is associated with increased risk of sudden cardiac death. Circ Arrhythm Electrophysiol. 2011;4:441-7.
125. Letsas KP, Weber R, Astheimer K, et al. Tpeak-Tend interval and Tpeak-Tend/QT ratio as markers of ventricular tachycardia inducibility in subjects with Brugada ECG phenotype. Europace. 2010;12:271-4.
126. Shimizu M, Ino H, Okeie K, et al. T-peak to T-end interval may be a better predictor of high-risk patients with hypertrophic cardiomyopathy associated with a cardiac troponin 1 mutation than QT dispersion. Clin Cardiol. 2002;25: 335-9.
127. Haissaguerre M, Derval N, Sacher F, et al. Sudden cardiac arrest associated with early repolarization. N Engl J Med. 2008;358:2016-23.
128. Barra S, Providência R, Paiva L, et al. Early repolarization patterns and the role of additional proarrhythmic triggers. Europace. 2013;15:482-5.
129. Kardys I, Kors JA, van der Meer IM, et al. Spatial QRS-T angle predicts cardiac death in a general population. Eur Heart J. 2003;24:1357-64.
130. Aro AL, Huikuri HV, Tikkanen JT, et al. QRS-T angle as a predictor of sudden cardiac death in a middle-aged general population. Europace. 2012;14: 872-6.

131. Pepe MS, Janes H, Longton G, et al. Limitations of the odds ratio in gauging the performance of a diagnostic, prognostic, or screening marker. Am J Epidemiol. 2004;159:882-90.
132. Goldenberg I, Vyas AK, Hall WJ, et al. Risk stratification for primary implantation of a cardioverter-defibrillator in patients with ischemic left ventricular dysfunction. J Am Coll Cardiol. 2008;51:288-96.
133. Chugh SS. Early identification of risk factors for sudden cardiac death. Nat Rev Cardiol. 2010;7:318-26.
134. Demidova MM, Carlson J, Erlinge D, et al. Predictors of ventricular fibrillation at reperfusion in patients with acute ST-elevation myocardial infarction treated by primary percutaneous coronary intervention. Am J Cardiol. 2015;115:417-22.
135. Shenthar J, Deora S, Rai M, et al. Prolonged Tpeak-end and Tpeak-end/QT ratio as predictors of malignant ventricular arrhythmias in the acute phase of ST-segment elevation myocardial infarction: A prospective case control study. Heart Rhythm. 2015;12:484-9.

CHAPTER 114

Premature Ventricular Complex: When and How to Ablate?

Joseph Theodore, Raja Selvaraj

INTRODUCTION

Premature ventricular complexes (PVCs) are fairly common in the general population. They are more frequently seen in the elderly and in patients with hypertension, obesity, sleep apnea, and structural heart disease. PVCs can arise from anywhere in the heart but have a predilection for specific sites. The most common sites of origin are in the ventricular outflow tracts (right > left).[1] Other sites for PVCs include the His-Purkinje system, especially the left posterior fascicle, endocavitary structures including the papillary muscles, moderator band, and false tendons.

The mechanisms of PVCs are varied. Outflow tract PVCs are caused by delayed afterdepolarizations or triggered automaticity, and are provoked by catecholamines, exercise, and menstrual cycles. Extensions around fibrous valvular annuli have also been hypothesized to allow conduction slowing and unidirectional block, which can lead to reentrant PVCs. Delayed afterdepolarizations also cause pathologic PVCs, frequently in a bigeminal pattern, in channelopathies such as Andersen–Tawil syndrome or catecholaminergic polymorphic ventricular tachycardia (VT), and in digoxin toxicity. On the other hand, early afterdepolarizations may cause PVCs that are precursors for torsades de pointes in long QT syndromes and drug-related QT prolongation. Reentry is the likely mechanism for PVCs originating from regions of fibrosis or infiltration in cardiomyopathies such as ischemic heart disease, arrhythmogenic right ventricular (RV) cardiomyopathy, sarcoidosis, hypertrophic cardiomyopathies, dilated cardiomyopathies, valvular cardiomyopathy, and postsurgical cardiac patients.

WHEN DO PREMATURE VENTRICULAR COMPLEXES NEED TO BE TREATED?

In most patients, PVCs in the structurally normal heart are considered benign and do not need treatment especially when asymptomatic. A few patients may complain of palpitations, while some may complain of fatigue due to decreased cardiac output caused by high frequency of PVCs. Presence of any significant symptoms provides a justification to treat PVCs to provide symptom relief to the patient.

In patients with ventricular dysfunction and frequent PVCs, the possibility that ventricular dysfunction is caused by the PVCs and may be reversible with abolition of the PVCs has to be considered. In the presence of such a possibility, consideration should be given to treat the PVCs. Even in patients with coronary artery disease (CAD) or other causes of ventricular dysfunction, the presence of a large number of PVCs may contribute to further worsening of left ventricular (LV) function. In these patients, partial improvement of LV function may be seen with treatment of the PVCs.

In patients with a normal LV function, frequent PVCs may be associated with a small risk of developing PVC-induced cardiomyopathy in the future. The number or proportion of PVCs associated with this risk varies in different reports and probably reflects the fact that the risk is linear without a single threshold. Commonly, more than 15–20% PVC burden per day[1] is considered to be associated with a risk of developing cardiomyopathy, but the burden may be as low as 10% and the risk may depend on the duration, coupling interval, and other characteristics of the PVC apart from only the burden. Presence of even 1,000 PVCs per day (<1%) for 4–8 years may sometimes be significant.[2]

Other rare indications for treating PVCs include PVCs triggering sustained tachycardia and PVCs that interfere with optimal delivery of resynchronization therapy.

TO TREAT OR NOT TO TREAT A PREMATURE VENTRICULAR COMPLEX

In summary, the situations in which treatment of PVCs may be considered include:

- Symptoms
- Likely presence of PVC-induced cardiomyopathy

- Risk of developing PVC-induced cardiomyopathy [asymptomatic burden >15%, left bundle branch block (BBB) morphology, wide QRS, large variability in the coupling interval, interpolated PVCs][1]
- Premature ventricular complex observed to induce VT/VF (ventricular fibrillation)
- Premature ventricular complex interference with cardiac resynchronization therapy (CRT) function.

Use of electrocardiogram (ECG), echocardiography, and long-term ECG monitoring [Holter, pocket ECG, implantable loop recorder (ILR)] is required to evaluate the patients and helps to make a decision regarding treating PVC. The management of several forms of structural heart disease associated with PVCs may be guided by magnetic resonance imaging (MRI), including dilated cardiomyopathy, hypertrophic cardiomyopathy (HCM), sarcoidosis, amyloidosis, and arrhythmogenic right ventricular cardiomyopathy (ARVC).

HOW TO TREAT?

Reversible factors causing PVCs are uncommon, but should be looked for and treated. Electrolyte abnormalities (potassium, magnesium) should be corrected. Treat contributing diseases like hypertension, sleep apnea, and obesity. Although some continue to recommend reducing or stopping caffeine intake, there is no evidence that this is required.[3]

Beta-blockers and calcium channel blockers [nondihydropyridine (non-DHP)] are the first-line pharmacologic agent to suppress PVCs. Antiarrhythmic drugs like flecainide [caution in reduced ejection fraction (EF), CAD], sotalol (QTc, structural heart disease) can be used as second line drugs. Even though amiodarone can be effective in selected patients, long-term use is avoided because of toxicity, especially in patients with a structurally normal heart. Medical therapy is, however, limited by lack of efficacy for many patients. Additionally, beta-blockers, calcium channel blockers, and sodium channel blockers might cause unacceptable adverse effects such as fatigue or reduced inotropy and are difficult to take regularly on a long-term basis.

Catheter ablation of PVC is considered when treatment of PVCs is considered necessary, but drug therapy is ineffective, not tolerated or not preferred.

TECHNIQUE OF PREMATURE VENTRICULAR COMPLEX ABLATION

Prior to ablation, a careful assessment of justification, risks, and success of ablation is essential. Infrequent PVCs might make mapping impossible and all drugs-suppressing PVC are to be stopped prior to the procedure depending on their half-lives. Triggered PVCs (outflow) are catecholamine sensitive and can be completely inhibited with anesthesia. Therefore, general anesthesia and even sedation should be avoided if possible. Sympathomimetic agents (isoproterenol) or awakening the patient on the table may provoke PVCs. Rapid atrial or ventricular pacing causes an increase in triggered PVCs. Atrial or ventricular extrastimulation can provoke reentrant PVCs.

Localization from 12-lead Electrocardiogram

First step in ablating PVC is to get an idea of approximate origin of PVC from surface ECG and decide about the chamber to be mapped (Table 1). Clues to mapping, regarding the chamber of interest, endocardial or epicardial mapping (coronary

TABLE 1: Electrocardiographic features that suggest particular region as site of origin or exit of PVC

ECG finding	PVC localization
Inferior axis with tall positive leads II, III, aVF, and QS complex in aVR, aVL	**Outflow tract**
LBBB morphology in lead V1 with late precordial transition (after lead V3)	Right ventricular outflow tract (RVOT)
Early precordial transition	Left ventricular outflow tract
Lead V1	
QS	RVOT free wall
rS	Posterior RVOT, pulmonary valve, right (or left) coronary cusp (RCC/LCC)
qR	Aortomitral continuity
R	Mitral annulus
Left-sided leads (I and aVL)	
Positive lead I	RCC, rightward parts of RVOT
Negative lead I	Leftward portions of outflow tracts including pulmonary valve, LCC and mitral valve annulus
Positive aVL and I	Para-Hisian region
Pseudo delta wave (34 ms) or maximum deflection index >0.55	Epicardial or coronary sinus
RBBB morphology with R (slurred) in V1 and transition to rS in V4-6	**Papillary muscle or fascicular system**
Axis	
Left/superior	Posteromedial papillary muscle/left posterior fascicle
Right/inferior	Anterolateral papillary muscle/left anterior fascicle
Tall positive precordial leads	**Valve annuli**
LBBB morphology in V1	Tricuspid annulus
Negative aVR, positive aVL	Anterior tricuspid annulus
RBBB morphology in V1	Mitral annulus
Positive aVR, negative aVL	Anterolateral mitral annulus
Superiorly directed frontal plane axis	Posterior annulus

ECG, electrocardiograms; LBBB, left bundle branch block; PVC, premature ventricular complex; RBBB, right bundle branch block; aVR, augmented vector right; aVL, augmented vector left; aVF, augmented vector foot.

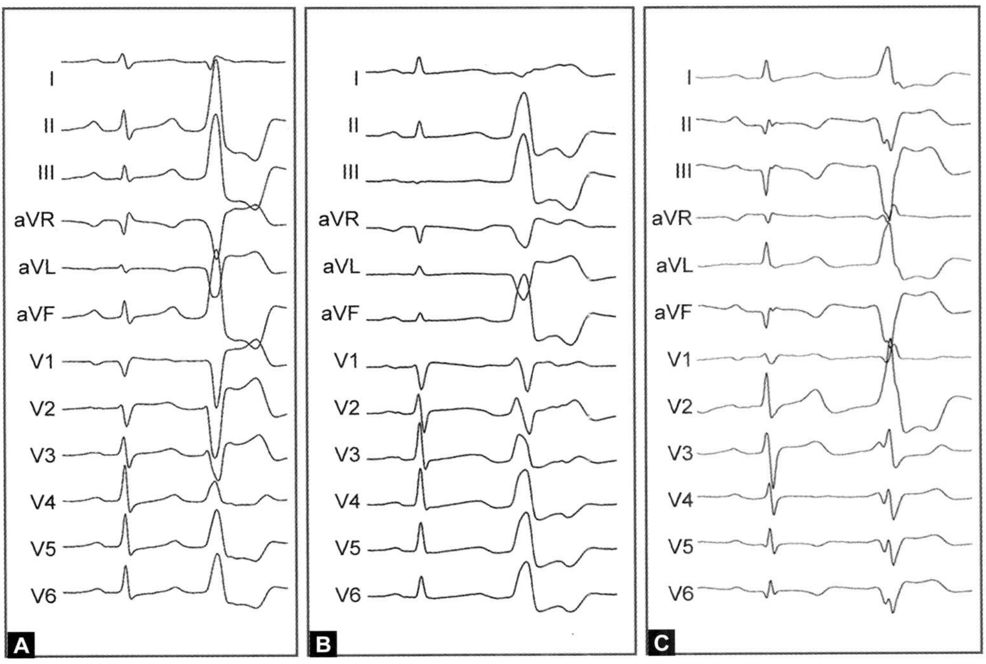

PVC, premature ventricular complexes; RBBB, right bundle branch block; aVR, augmented vector right; aVL, augmented vector left; aVF, augmented vector foot.

FIG. 1: Identifying site of origin from PVC morphology. A sinus beat and a PVC are shown from three different patients. **In panels A and B,** tall upright QRS complexes in the inferior leads with a QS morphology in aVR and aVL are suggestive of PVC arising from the outflow tract. The precordial transition is at V4 in panel A, consistent with origin from the right ventricular outflow tract. Whereas, a transition earlier than V3 in panel B suggests origin in the left ventricular outflow tract. **Panel C** shows a PVC with a totally different frontal plane axis. There is left axis deviation and right bundle branch block like morphology in lead V1 with negative QRS complexes in the inferior leads suggests origin from the inferior wall of the left ventricle. In the sinus beat, deep Q-waves are seen in the inferior leads, suggesting an old inferior wall myocardial infarction with PVCs arising from the scar.

sinus may be used in appropriate PVC) would be suggested by 12-lead ECG.

Figure 1 shows representative PVCs to illustrate identification of site of origin from the PVC morphology.

Activation Mapping

Activation mapping is the principal modality for mapping PVCs as it helps in precise localization of PVC origin. As opposed to sustained VT, entrainment of single PVCs is not possible, and mapping of both focal and reentrant PVCs is largely dependent on activation mapping. Local ventricular activation is assessed in different regions in the chamber of interest and the earliest local ventricular signal with respect to the QRS onset of the clinical PVC is mapped. For assessment of local activation time, the first sharp deflection in the bipolar signal is used. Recording of unipolar signals can be very useful and a completely negative unipolar signal is typically seen at the origin of the PVC. Figure 2 shows illustrative bipolar and unipolar signals at the site of successful ablation of a PVC. Activation mapping can be done using a three-dimensional (3D) electroanatomical system where a 3D map of the ventricle is created and colored according to the local activation time at each site. To maximize success, care is needed to ensure only the relevant PVC morphology is being mapped and to exclude fused beats different morphologies, or catheter ectopy.

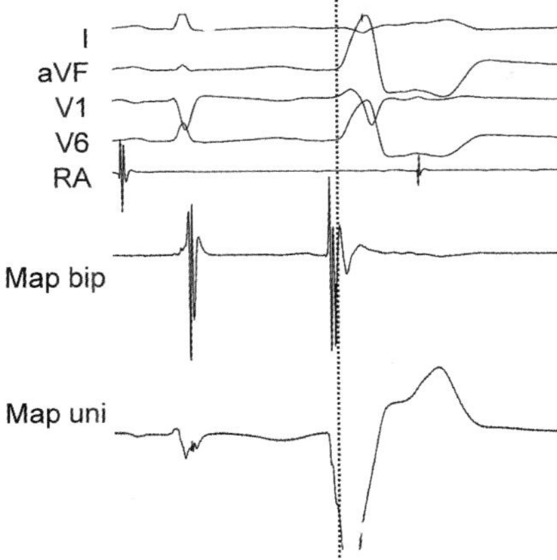

FIG. 2: Signals at the site of successful ablation in the right ventricular outflow tract in a patient with frequent premature ventricular complexes (PVCs). Shown are a sinus beat and a PVC. A dotted line is drawn at the onset of the QRS. The bipolar signal (map bip) shows local activation 30 ms ahead of the QRS onset. The unipolar signal shows a QS morphology with the local activation (steep negative deflection) occurring before the QRS onset.

Pace Mapping

In certain situations, e.g., in the case of infrequent PVCs, pace mapping is an alternative method that may be useful. The mapping catheter is positioned at a possible site of interest and pacing is performed from this catheter. Comparing the morphology of the paced QRS to the clinical PVC will help in assessing the proximity to the origin of the PVC. At the origin of a focal PVC, a 12/12 match (good match of morphology in all 12 surface ECG leads) will be observed. The disadvantage is that pace mapping is not very accurate and pacing from a reasonably large surrounding area may also result in an exact pace map. Therefore, activation mapping is always to be preferred when possible.

ABLATION OF PREMATURE VENTRICULAR COMPLEXES

During mapping and while preparing for ablation, careful attention is needed to prevent a mechanical bump to the PVC focus with the catheter that will suppress PVCs temporarily. Confirming catheter contact and integrating information from the bipolar and the unipolar recordings can facilitate correct annotation of the breakout site at the tip of ablation catheter. Radiofrequency (RF) energy is delivered at the origin of the PVC using a nonirrigated or irrigated catheter depending on the situation. Common outflow tract PVCs will require 20–30 watts energy.[4] Anterior or free wall locations will require lesser energy than septal location or a transmural lesion targeting an epicardial focus. Cryoablation (not available in India) can be used safely in areas closer to conduction tissue or coronary artery where RF ablation might pose danger.

OUTCOMES

The success rate of ablation of outflow tract or fascicular PVCs is 80–100%.[5]

In 60% of patients undergoing PVC ablation due to PVC-mediated cardiomyopathy, LV function improves to normal within 4 months, although it may take more than a year in a few patients.[5] Recurrence after successful ablation is possible due to remodeling of the arrhythmogenic substrate. The risk of collateral injury with ablation of PVCs close to critical structures needs to be considered. Coronary artery injury can occur when ablating in the coronary veins, epicardial space, above the coronary cusps close to coronary ostia, and in posterior right ventricular outflow tract (RVOT) near the pulmonary valve. Ablation at noncoronary aortic cusp (NCC), midseptum, and parahisian region can cause AV blocks. Thromboembolic complications can be minimized with therapeutic heparin anticoagulation during and following procedure. Cardiac tamponade or valve perforation is rare but catastrophic complications for which the operator has to be watchful.

CONCLUSION

Premature ventricular complexes are generally benign and are only occasionally symptomatic. In patients showing a clear association between PVCs and symptoms, PVC-induced ventricular tachyarrhythmia, PVC-mediated cardiomyopathy, or with a high PVC burden with future risk of developing cardiomyopathy, catheter ablation is safe and feasible alternative to long-term medical therapy. Localizing with 12-lead ECG, approximation with pace mapping and precise localization with activation mapping, using an electroanatomical mapping system when required, will improve procedural success.

REFERENCES

1. Del Carpio Munoz F, Syed FF, Noheria A, et al. Characteristics of premature ventricular complexes as correlates of reduced left ventricular systolic function: Study of the burden, duration, coupling interval, morphology and site of origin of PVCs. J Cardiovasc Electrophysiol. 2011;22:791-8.
2. Yokokawa M, Kim HM, Good E, et al. Relation of symptoms and symptom duration to premature ventricular complex-induced cardiomyopathy. Heart Rhythm. 2012;9(1):92-5.
3. Dixit S, Stein PK, Dewland TA, et al. Consumption of caffeinated products and cardiac ectopy. J Am Heart Assoc Cardiovasc Cerebrovasc Dis. 2016;5(1): e002503.
4. Suleiman M, Asirvatham SJ. Ablation above the semilunar valves: When, why, and how? Part I. Heart Rhythm. 2008;5(10):1485-92.
5. Noheria A, Deshmukh A, Asirvatham SJ. Ablating premature ventricular complexes: Justification, techniques, and outcomes. Methodist Debakey Cardiovascular J. 2015;(2):109-20.

CHAPTER 115

Epicardial Ventricular Tachycardia: Recognition and Approach

Maki Ono, Walid I Saliba, Oussama Wazni, Mandeep Bhargava

INTRODUCTION

Failure of endocardial radiofrequency catheter ablation for ventricular tachycardia (VT) has often been thought to be due to subepicardial or midmyocardial circuits, where the ability of delivering energy epicardially can greatly enhance the efficacy of the ablation procedure. In 1996, Sosa et al. demonstrated the efficacy of an epicardial ablation by subxiphoid approach in Chagas disease and since then the utility of gaining access into the normal pericardial sac has been described with increasing enthusiasm.[1-3] We are now in an era where epicardial ablation has been shown to be useful not only for structural heart disease such as nonischemic cardiomyopathy (NICM), arrhythmogenic right ventricular cardiomyopathy (ARVC), and hypertrophic cardiomyopathy (HCM) but also for channelopathies like Brugada syndrome.

PREOPERATIVE ASSESSMENT AND RECOGNITION

Epicardial ablation has potential risks of both cardiac and noncardiac complications while obtaining access, during ablation and that of postprocedural adhesions and inflammation, which make it difficult to perform a second epicardial ablation in the future. Hence, the decision to obtain epicardial access should be made carefully and limited to the patients who have higher likelihood of having an epicardial origin of the arrhythmia. Electrocardiographic criteria, imaging features, and other clinical characteristics like activation and voltage mapping information from previous ablation attempts should be considered while determining the indication for the same. Many algorithms for making such decisions have been suggested by various authors.[4-8] It can often be the access of choice for patients where retrograde and trans-septal routes are not an option at all, as in patients with a left ventricular thrombus or in patients with a metallic valve in both the aortic and mitral position.

If a 12-lead electrocardiography (ECG) of the VT is available and the QRS onset is easy to identify, evaluating certain "interval criteria" and "morphology criteria" can be helpful to differentiate an epicardial origin.[5,6,9] Sometimes, the onset of QRS or deflection points can be difficult to determine or the 12-lead ECG may not be available until the VT is induced at the electrophysiological study as the only diagnosis of the VT may have been from the intracardiac electrograms on an implantable cardioverter-defibrillator (ICD). Berruezo et al.[5] initially evaluated and described important QRS intervals which could be used to predict an epicardial origin of the VT. They described four important intervals as follows:

1. *Pseudo-delta wave (PDW):* Interval from the earliest ventricular activation to the onset of rapid deflection in any precordial lead
2. *Intrinsicoid deflection time (IDT):* Interval from the earliest ventricular activation to the peak of the R wave in V2
3. *Shortest RS complex (SRS):* Interval from the earliest ventricular activation to the nadir of the first S wave in any precordial lead
4. QRS duration.

Using these criteria, they showed that a PDW of more than or equal to 34 ms had a sensitivity of 83% and a specificity of 95%, an IDT of more than or equal to 85 ms had a sensitivity of 87% and specificity of 90%, and an SRS of more than or equal to 121 ms had a sensitivity of 76% and specificity of 85%, respectively for identifying an epicardial origin for the VT. Most patients had coronary artery disease and the study was based on pace mapping which were realized as limitations over a period of time but the study clearly showed that epicardial breakout is associated with wider QRS and slower initial forces as it engages the His-Purkinje system later when compared to endocardial breakouts from similar areas.

Patients with ischemic cardiomyopathy often have endocardial circuits as these scars are "inside out". A fair number of these patients may have epicardial circuits, but many such circuits may have a critical endocardial isthmus or may be approachable by deep endocardial lesions. Later studies have shown that ECG criteria are less useful to predict epicardial origin in patients with ischemic cardiomyopathy and patients on antiarrhythmic drugs.[10] Additionally, prior open heart surgery, bypass grafts and adhesions may make epicardial access difficult in these patients. Hence, in these patients, we usually reserve access for patients with failed endocardial ablation, patients with left ventricular thrombus or rarely in the primary procedure when the conviction for an epicardial circuit is very high.

Nonischemic cardiomyopathy patients have a higher chance of having an epicardial circuit as their scars can often be epicardial. Figure 1 shows a patient with nonischemic cardiomyopathy who has a relatively small scar on the endocardial map which can be deceptive as the epicardial access and mapping showed that the patient had a large epicardial scar as shown and was harboring the circuit for the culprit VT. Different types of ECG criteria have been proposed to especially look at the VT from the basal anterolateral walls but Valles et al. proposed a four-step algorithm.[6] The criteria include first looking for "Q" waves in the inferior leads and their presence for VTs in that region high up would suggest initial forces going away from the inferior leads and would suggest an endocardial origin. One would then look for a PDW of more than or equal to 75 ms or a maximal deflection index (ratio of onset to peak to that of the total QRS duration in the mid-precordial leads) and the presence of either of these would favor an epicardial origin. If neither of these helps, they recommend looking for "Q" waves in leads I and the presence of that would also favor an epicardial origin. The four-step algorithm claims to have a sensitivity of 96% and specificity of 93% for predicting an epicardial origin in patients with nonischemic cardiomyopathy. Figure 2 shows

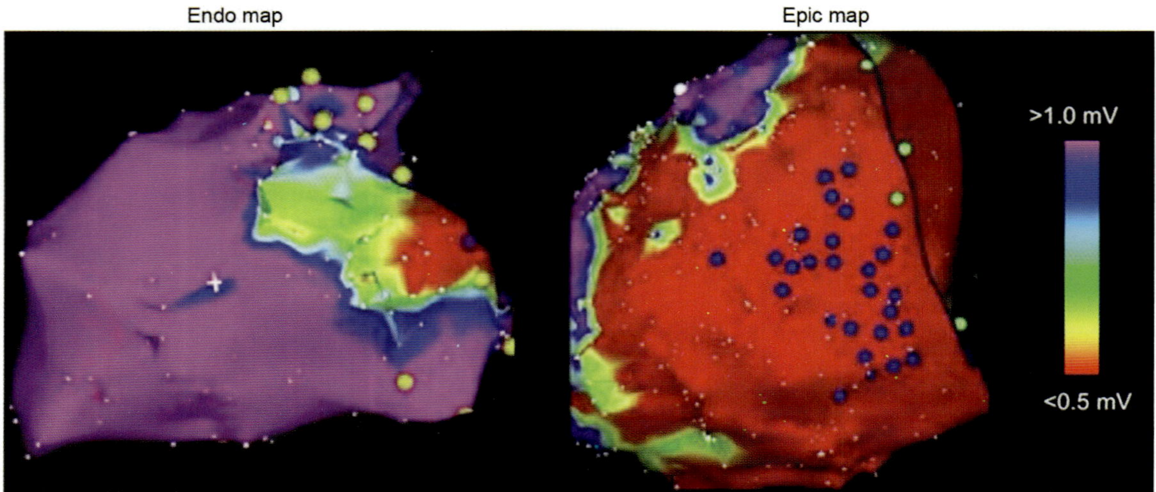

FIG. 1: A left lateral view of a voltage map of the endocardium and the epicardium in a patient with nonischemic cardiomyopathy. The endocardial map on the left panel shows a small scar along the basal lateral wall close to the mitral annulus. The voltage map on the right shows that the scar is much larger and predominantly epicardial and spans the basal and mid-anterolateral, lateral and inferolateral walls of the left ventricle.

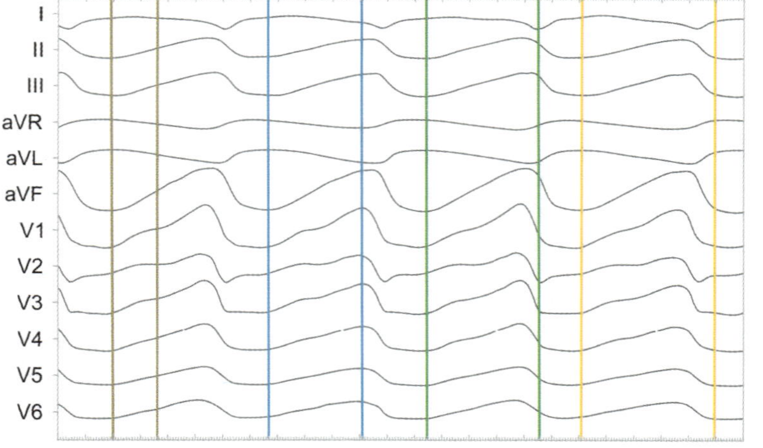

IDT, intrinsicoid deflection time; MDI, maximum deflection index; PDW, pseudo-delta wave; SRS: shortest RS complex; aVF, augmented vector foot; aVL, augmented vector right; aVR, augmented vector right.

FIG. 2: The various "interval criteria" on an electrocardiography measured in a patient with ventricular tachycardia originating from an epicardial focus from the basal lateral wall in a patient with nonischemic cardiomyopathy. The "morphology criteria" also show a Q-wave in leads I and augmented vector left.

one of our patients with a VT with right bundle branch block like pattern with a right inferior axis. The VT was originating from an epicardial focus along the basal lateral wall and the surface ECG shows a pattern consistent with an epicardial focus as per the various "interval criteria" and "morphology criteria" noted.

There are also ECG criteria for predicting epicardial origin for patients with VT from an ARVC but we feel that this decision is less stressful because patients with ARVC do not usually need anticoagulation during mapping and ablation for VT and epicardial access can be obtained anytime without concerns for reversing anticoagulation if not obtained at the beginning of the procedure. Similar to patients with NICM, patients with ARVC also can have a fair percentage of patients with epicardial circuits as both these disease states can be associated with scars which are epicardial or "outside in".

Imaging has been shown to be useful to identify the arrhythmogenic substrate of VT and to plan an appropriate mapping and ablation strategy. Bogun et al. showed the utility of delayed-enhancement magnetic resonance imaging (DE-MRI) in 29 nonischemic cardiomyopathy patients.[7] Scar was identified in 14 of 29 patients. Five patients with predominant endocardial scar were successfully ablated from the endocardium, two patients with predominant epicardial scar were successfully ablated from the epicardium, and no effect on VT could be achieved in five patients with predominant intramural scar. Intracardiac echo has also been described to look for epicardial scars but we do not use it often as a predictive tool. Recent studies have also shown that preserved endocardial bipolar voltages on electroanatomical maps with reduced unipolar voltages are also predictive of epicardial scars and may be a "far-field reflection" of low voltages in the epicardium.

Hence, the patient's clinical background is important to assess the probability of an epicardial focus given the cardiac substrate.[8] Assessing ECG, imaging, and probability before procedure is important to plan a safe and effective ablation. Other important assessment and preparation before procedure includes discontinuation of anticoagulants and antiplatelet agents and the availability of surgical backup in the event of a complication.

APPROACH TO ACCESS THE PERICARDIAL SPACE

It is critical to understand relevant anatomy to prevent complications while obtaining subxiphoid access. The normal pericardium[11] is a double-layered flask-shaped sac with an outer fibrous envelope and an inner serous sac, i.e., invaginated by the heart. The serous pericardium is divided into the visceral pericardium which surrounds the myocardium and the great vessels also called the epicardium and the outer parietal layer which is the inner serous layer of the fibrous pericardium. The pericardial space is the virtual space in between these two serous linings and by separating it from the heart and its surrounding structures, in normal conditions, it provides a smooth lubricated space for free motion around the heart. The pericardial space contains about 20–25 mL of fluid in the physiological state and in the supine position this is largely seen in the posterior network of sinuses and recesses of the pericardium.

A blunt tipped epidural Tuohy needle (17G, 90 mm, BD, Medical Franklin Lakes, NJ, or 17G, 152 mm, Hakko Co, Ltd., Tokyo, Japan) is used with a spring guidewire. Hydrophilic wires cannot be used with metal Tuohy needle. Recently a "needle-in-needle" method using two needles (21G micropuncture needle in 18G needle) was reported[12,13] and the new methods using pressure sensor lines[14] have also been described.

For most averagely built patients, it is best to start about an inch below the line between the xiphoid process and the costal margin but adjustments may need to be made in accordance with the patient's size and depth that need to be negotiated. Given the relatively blunt and angulated nature of the Tuohy needle, it may often be helpful, especially in patients with thicker skin, to give a skin incision. This could also allow the operator to have a better tactile sensation of the structures encountered and their pulsatility. This also makes it easier to feel the give-away sensation on entering the pericardial space or to appreciate the contractile nature of the myocardium. The Tuohy needle is gently aimed at an angle toward the left scapula with the patient in the supine position. Under fluoroscopic guidance, the needle is gently moved toward the cardiac border. There are two approaches—an anterior versus posterior approach—and the angle of the needle is guided by the intent to achieve access for one or the other approach. Table 1 shows comparable differences between the two approaches.

The anterior approach requires a shallower angle of the needle. The guidance by a catheter placed at the right ventricular (RV) apex or pre-existing lead of an implantable cardiac rhythm device can be of additional help. Fluoroscopically, a shallow left anterior oblique (LAO) view may help to show the anterior and posterior relationship and a slight right anterior oblique (RAO) view to stay midway between the apex and the annulus can be extremely helpful. A left lateral projection[15] has also been described to address the needle angle posterior to the sternum and to help to avoid the diaphragm. In the posterior approach, a steeper

TABLE 1: Comparison of anterior versus posterior approach for epicardial access

	Anterior approach	Posterior approach
Angle of the needle	Shallow, <30°	Steep, >30–45°
Direction of the needle edge and wire	Anterior	Posterior
Marker of the direction	RV apex catheter or lead	RV apex catheter or lead, and coronary sinus catheter or lead
Useful fluoroscopic angle	RAO, LAO, and left lateral	LAO and RAO
Intra-abdominal bleeding	Rare	Possible

LAO, left anterior oblique; RAO, right anterior oblique; RV, right ventricle.

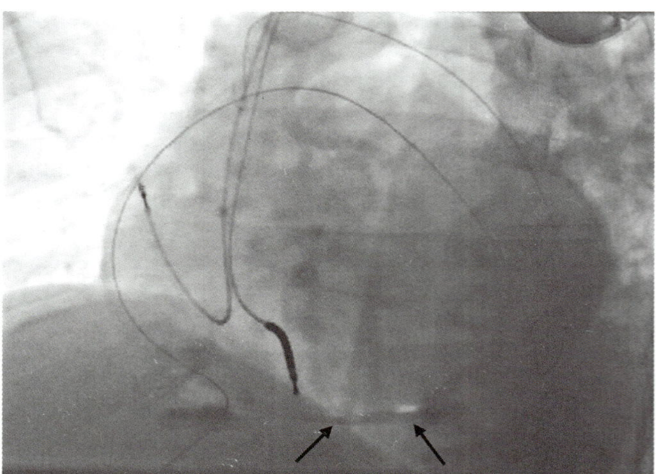

FIG. 3: A fluoroscopic left anterior oblique view of a patient with a relatively anterior approach to access the pericardial space. The tip of the implantable cardioverter defibrillator lead is close to the right ventricular apex. The wire is seen to span the complete heart border from the anterior portion on the left of the screen to the posterior portions on the right of the screen confirming that it is in the pericardial space and not in one of the chambers. The arrows show the layering of contrast at the bottom.

angle of the needle is required and both catheters or leads at RV apex and in coronary sinus are helpful. Intra-abdominal hemorrhage by diaphragmatic and hepatic puncture is higher with posterior approach. We like to make sure that the site of entry is preferably close to the midpoint between the annulus (as seen by the coronary sinus catheter or lead) and the RV apex (as assessed by an RV apical catheter/lead) in a RAO projection.

As the needle comes in close proximity to the cardiac border, small puffs of contrast are injected to visualize tenting of the parietal pericardium or entry into the pericardial space. The latter is most often identified by layering of contrast into the pericardial space (Fig. 3). With experience, this is usually preceded by a sensation of the pericardium "giving away" but this may not be appreciated all the time. A common mistake by inexperienced operators is a combination of minimal advancement of the needle with injection of too much contrast. This tends to cloud the fluoroscopic view and should be avoided.

As soon as the sensation of the parietal pericardium "giving away" is achieved or contrast layering is seen in the pericardium, it is crucial to stabilize the needle with one hand and gently pass a guidewire into the pericardial space with the other. Some operators prefer using a Y connector with the Tuohy needle, so that they can inject contrast from the side port and insert a wire from the main port at the same time. Under usual circumstances, this wire should pass and move freely into the pericardial space. Our preference is to visualize the wire in LAO position (Fig. 3). It is important to see that the wire crosses over on both, the right and left sides of the cardiac border and hence seen anterior and posterior in this view as this would further confirm that the wire is in the pericardium. It is also best if the wire can be seen along the posterior and anterior border of the heart. Any contact with the myocardium with the needle or the wire is likely to produce ventricular ectopy and should be watched for. It is of absolute importance to confirm that the wire is in the pericardial space and not in a cardiac chamber prior to insertion of a dilator or a sheath over the wire. If there is doubt that the needle or wire is in the cardiac chamber, it should be gently withdrawn and attempts to slowly retract and stay in the pericardial space are often successful. However, if a dilator or sheath is passed over the wire and then a realization is made that it is in one of the cardiac chambers, surgical help should be sought before pulling this back any further. Most often, gentle invasion of the ventricle with the needle or wire per se is usually forgiving but injuries to the epicardial vessels, diaphragmatic vessels or the liver can be much more serious.

Once access has been achieved with a guidewire, it is reasonable to exchange that with a stiffer sheath and in procedures needing more stability, we may often use a steerable or a metallic sheath to have better navigation within the pericardial space. Through this, one may pass catheters or wires at will but it is important to try and minimize the time where the sheath is left without a catheter as the sharp and stiff edges of a sheath can often cause damage to the fragile blood vessels on the epicardial surface of the heart which can lead to incessant bleeding.

Epicardial access for the patient with prior cardiac surgery has been reported to be feasible;[16,17] but, in our experience, it may be limited to about 15–40% patients at best. It is suggested that a more inferior approach is helpful in these patients. Such patients are likely to have more adhesions and scarring even after successful access. Care should also be taken to protect the bypass grafts coursing through this space. Gentle disruption of adhesions with catheters and guidewires has been reported when presents, but this should be cautiously ventured into. Soejima et al. first reported the feasibility of surgical subxiphoid epicardial approach in the electrophysiology laboratory in six patients with prior cardiac surgery or failed percutaneous epicardial access.[18] Michowits et al. did detailed analysis of the relationship of surgical window and accessibility.[19] While limited anterior thoracotomy enabled access to the apex, anterior, and mid to apical anterolateral walls, subxiphoid surgical window provided access to the inferior and diaphragmatic surface of the heart extending posteriorly to the basal lateral wall.

MAPPING AND ABLATION

Mapping by epicardial approach creates less premature ventricular complexes (PVCs) and is relatively smooth in handling ablation catheter if there are no adhesions. We find the short steerable sheath very useful to obtain better stability and navigation for the catheter. Three-dimensional mapping systems such as CARTO (Biosense Webster, Diamond Bar, CA), Ensite (St Jude Medical/Abbott, St Paul, MN), and Rhythmia (Boston Scientific, Marlborough, MA) can be used with multielectrode catheter such as Pentarray (Biosense Webster, Diamond Bar, CA) and Intellamap Orion (Boston Scientific, Marlborough, MA). Orion should be used without full expansion, and small amount of normal saline (10–20 mL) can be added into the epicardial space if the noise is significant. If an irrigated-tip ablation catheter is chosen for the mapping, irrigation during mapping can be stopped but care should be taken to regularly aspirate the epicardial space if irrigation is used during mapping and ablation.

Mapping approaches to epicardial VT could include substrate mapping during sinus rhythm, activation mapping during VT, or pace mapping. Low voltage has been reported as 0.5–1.5 mV[20] or less than 0.94 mV[21] but these criteria obtained by mapping with conventional ablation catheters need to be reassessed in the era of high-density mapping.

It is important to understand the distribution of fat in relation to the pericardium during mapping. The presence of epicardial fat is seen in relation to the sulcus, the interventricular grooves, and the coronary vasculature and can vary from 0–14 mm in thickness. The thickness is often related to age and may not necessarily have a relationship to the body habitus of an individual but has two important implications. The fat could act as a layer of electrical disturbance and could falsely give low amplitude signals in an area of viable tissue by causing a layer of inertness electrically or increase pacing thresholds and could also act as a layer of insulation which prevents the delivery of radiofrequency energy in the most optimal manner. In animal studies, scar from healed myocardial infarction exhibits more fractionation and longer EGM duration when compared to fat and late potentials are highly specific for locating infarct scars.[22]

An irrigated-tip ablation catheter that can show the contact force and vector orientation is most useful for ablation. It is most important to make the catheter tip vector toward heart muscle, not toward lung or pleura to obtain effective ablation and to avoid collateral damage.[23] Caution should also be exercised along the lateral and posterolateral walls of the left ventricle as these areas could be in close proximity to the left phrenic nerve. Appropriate energy is unknown but we usually use 20–40 Watts of power with irrigated tip catheters and occasionally up to 50 Watts while keeping a very close watch on the impedance and temperature.

Coronary angiography can sometimes be necessary before ablation to define the proximity of coronary arteries (Fig. 4). High-output pacing may be required on the left anterior and lateral border to determine the location of the left phrenic nerve. While ablating with irrigated catheters, intermittent or continuous pericardial aspiration from the sheath is necessary to avoid fluid accumulation and cardiac tamponade.

After the ablation, evaluate and aspirate pericardial effusion before removing the sheath. It may be safe to use transthoracic echocardiography or intracardiac echocardiography to see the remaining pericardial effusion before withdrawing the sheath to avoid the situation that epicardial sheath is obstructed with blood clot and fluid cannot be aspirated or that epicardial access has been lost in the face of a significant effusion or tamponade. Prophylaxis of inflammation and adhesions is important and intrapericardial steroid injection using pig-tail before

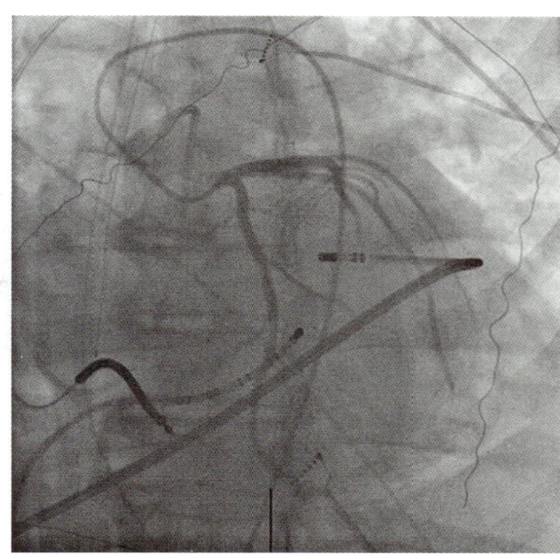

FIG. 4: A left anterior oblique caudal view of a coronary angiogram done in a patient just prior to ablation. The mapping or ablation catheter can be seen close to the left circumflex artery and its branches but at a fair distance where ablation can be deemed safe in this area.

removing sheath reduces postprocedure pain and we tend to use 1–2 mg/kg of triamcinolone on a routine basis.

Although epicardial access is most commonly required for patients with nonischemic cardiomyopathy and arrhythmogenic RV dysplasia, it can often be a useful bailout strategy in patients with normal hearts or ischemic cardiomyopathy. Figure 5 shows a patient with a focal tachycardia in a patient with a normal heart where the VT shows a right bundle branch like pattern with an inferior axis. The morphology of the QRS in lead V1 would change with lead position and mapping of the right and left ventricular endocardium did not show any great sites of early activation or pace matching. The activation pattern was focal with a centrifugal spread suggesting a non-reentrant mechanism. Epicardial mapping showed sites which were more than 80 ms earlier than the endocardial sites and ablation in those areas resulted in prompt termination and noninducibility of the tachycardia. In contrast, Figure 6 shows a re-entrant tachycardia along the apical anterior wall on an aneurysm in a patient with ischemic cardiomyopathy, old anterior wall myocardial infarction, and a left ventricular thrombus. The arrhythmia had a critical isthmus within the scar (noted on the left panel in the voltage map) and ablation in this area resulted in a successful outcome.

COMPLICATIONS

It is important to be aware of the possible complications during percutaneous epicardial access and ablation and only then can we focus on the prevention and management of these complications.[24] An RV puncture can happen in 4–5% of the cases but usually safe if observed with just the needle but without advancement of the sheath. RV puncture can be detected at the time of puncture with contrast. The needle should gently be withdrawn and the pericardial space should be cannulated with the wire. We must carefully monitor for

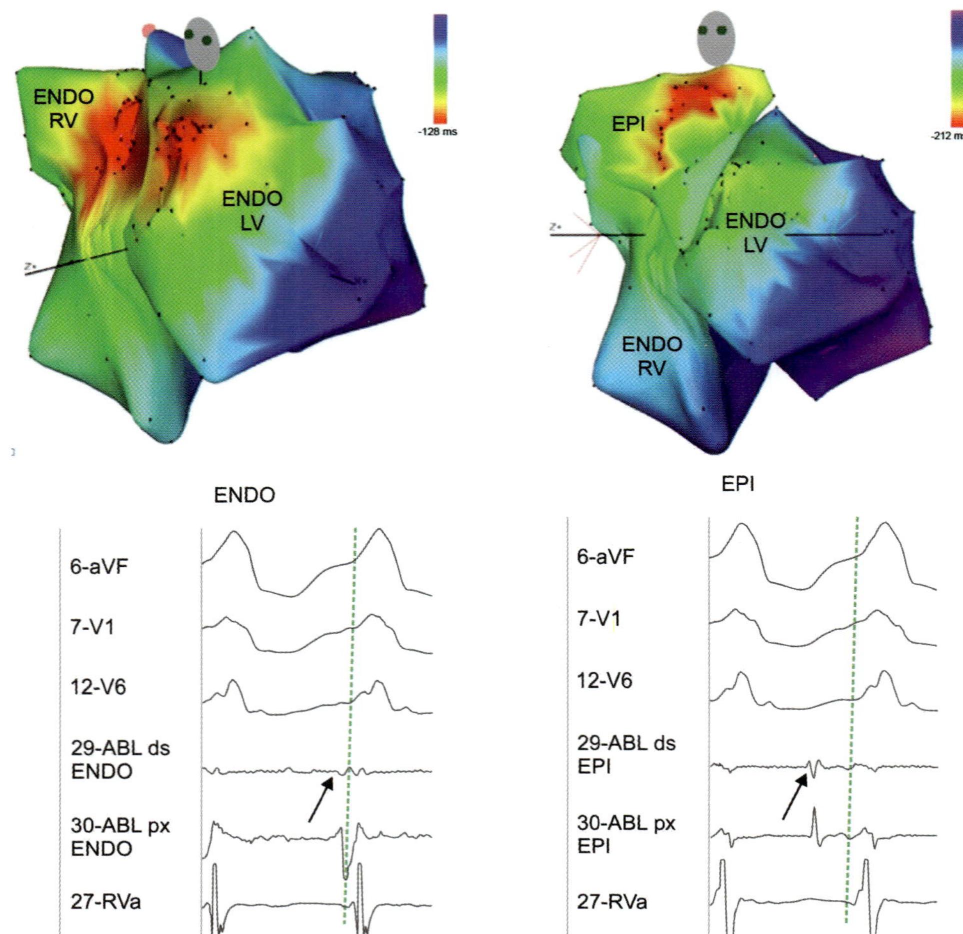

aVF, augmented vector foot; RV, right ventricular.

FIG. 5: An activation map of a focal ventricular tachycardia in a patient with a normal heart. The left panel shows activation map of the right and left ventricular outflow tract respectively in this patient with a ventricular tachycardia showing a right bundle branch block pattern with an inferior axis. Both show large areas of early activation and even the earliest point of activation shows that it is just at best at the onset of the rapid deflection of the QRS but not earlier than the pseudo-delta wave. Epicardial access was obtained and it showed a much earlier site of activation at the basal anterior portion of the left ventricle with a near-field electrogram and ablation was successful at this site.

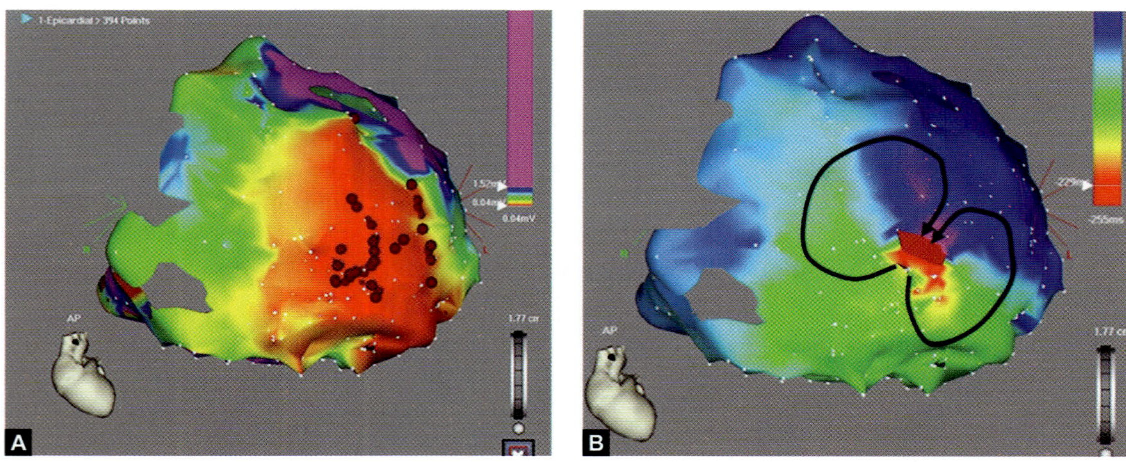

AP, anteroposterior.

FIG. 6: The voltage and activation map of a patient with ventricular tachycardia involving the apical aneurysm in the patient with an old anterior wall myocardial infarction. **A,** Right anterior oblique view of a bipolar voltage map shows a large apical scar; **B,** An activation map with a circular activation pattern with a figure of 8 appearance. The narrow critical isthmus is the area highlighted as the one where "early meets late" as highlighted by the bold red band. Ablation along this critical isthmus resulted in prolongation, termination and non-inducibility of the tachycardia. Epicardial ablation was performed as the patient had a left ventricular thrombus.

pericardial effusion not only at the time of puncture but also after the procedure. To prevent RV puncture, it is important to advance needle slowly with using contrast and with appropriate needle direction, and to carefully observe for PVCs. Intrapericardial bleeding can happen at 4–5% of the cases anytime from puncture to the time after the procedure. Discontinuation of anticoagulant agents before the procedure and careful handling of both sheath and mapping and ablation catheters are warranted. The sheath should not be left in the epicardial space without a catheter because of the possible damage by its sharp edges. Intra-abdominal bleeding and diaphragmatic injury are rare but can occur in 0.5% of patients and may require careful assessment for diagnosis. Anatomical evaluation with imaging before the procedure may be critical to assess the appropriate approach. Anterior approach reduces the risk of intra-abdominal bleeding. Any bleeding can be observed if it stops spontaneously but may require surgery if it shows no signs of settling on its own.

Damage to the coronary artery and coronary veins can happen in about 0.6% patients but can happen anytime from puncture to ablation. Access very septally increases the risk of damage to the posterior descending artery or middle cardiac vein injury. Expert consensus recommends at least 5 mm distance from coronary artery by assessing coronary angiography even during ablation.[25] Before ablating in the lateral left ventricular area, evaluation of left phrenic nerve should be assessed by high output pacing to avoid the rare complication of phrenic nerve injury. Fan et al. reported the utility of high output pacing more than 10 mA to determine the pathway of phrenic nerve.[26] A fertile substrate for ventricular arrhythmias is often observed around the basal to mid-lateral and basal to mid-anterolateral left ventricle in patients with nonischemic cardiomyopathy which increases the risk of phrenic nerve injury. If the nerve is in close proximity to ablation targets, injection of normal saline or insertion of balloon into epicardial space has been reported[27,28] to protect the same.

Mild pericarditis occurs in almost all patients after the procedure, and clinically important pericarditis happens in 30%, but severe pericarditis is rare at 0.6%. Dyrda et al. reported on the incidence of pericarditis in 85 consecutive patients after epicardial VT ablation.[29] Intrapericardial steroids (triamcinolone 2 mg/kg) significantly reduced the incidence of pericardial pain (58% vs. 21%; $p = 0.006$) compared to no steroid, but the difference was not significant with systemic steroids alone (58% vs. 43%; $p = 0.31$).

CONCLUSION

Epicardial VT ablation is a relatively novel approach which can significantly enhance the efficacy of catheter ablation for arrhythmias, especially in patients with VT. This requires invasive electrophysiologists to understand anatomy for areas other than the heart itself. The rate of any complications goes higher by adding this approach to an endocardial ablation and we should take all precautions to avoid the same.

REFERENCES

1. Sosa E, Scanavacca M, d'Avila A, et al. A new technique to perform epicardial mapping in the electrophysiology laboratory. J Cardiovasc Electrophysiol. 1996;7(6):531-6.
2. Sosa E, Scanavacca M, D'Avila A, et al. Endocardial and epicardial ablation guided by nonsurgical transthoracic epicardial mapping to treat recurrent ventricular tachycardia. J Cardiovasc Electrophysiol. 1998;9(3):229-39.
3. Sosa E, Scanavacca M, d'Avila A, et al. Nonsurgical transthoracic epicardial catheter ablation to treat recurrent ventricular tachycardia occurring late after myocardial infarction. J Am Coll Cardiol. 2000;35(6):1442-9.
4. Boyle NG, Shivkumar K. Epicardial interventions in electrophysiology. Circulation. 2012;126(14):1752-69.
5. Berruezo A, Mont L, Nava S, et al. Electrocardiographic recognition of the epicardial origin of ventricular tachycardias. Circulation. 2004;109(15):1842-7.
6. Valles E, Bazan V, Marchlinski FE. EKG criteria to identify epicardial ventricular tachycardia in nonischemic cardiomyopathy. Circ Arrhythm Electrophysiol. 2010;3(1):63-71.
7. Bogun FM, Desjardins B, Good E, et al. Delayed-enhanced magnetic resonance imaging in nonischemic cardiomyopathy: utility for identifying the ventricular arrhythmia substrate. J Am Coll Cardiol. 2009;53(13):1138-45.
8. Sacher F, Roberts-Thomson K, Maury P, et al. Epicardial ventricular tachycardia ablation a multicenter safety study. J Am Coll Cardiol. 2010;55(21):2366-72.
9. Bazan V, Gerstenfeld EP, Garcia FC, et al. Site-specific twelve-lead EKG features to identify an epicardial origin for left ventricular tachycardia in the absence of myocardial infarction. Heart Rhythm. 2007;4(11):1403-10.
10. Martinek M, Stevenson WG, Inada K, et al. QRS characteristics fail to reliably identify ventricular tachycardias that require epicardial ablation in ischemic heart disease. J Cardiovasc Electrophysiol. 2012;23(2):188-93.
11. D'Avila A, Scanavacca M, Sosa E, et al. Pericardial anatomy for the interventional electrophysiologist. J Cardiovasc Electrophysiol. 2003;14(4):422-30.
12. Kumar S, Bazaz R, Barbhaiya CR, et al. "Needle-in-needle" epicardial access: Preliminary observations with a modified technique for facilitating epicardial interventional procedures. Heart Rhythm. 2015;12(7):1691-7.
13. Gunda S, Reddy M, Pillarisetti J, et al. Differences in complication rates between large bore needle and a long micropuncture needle during epicardial access: time to change clinical practice? Circ Arrhythm Electrophysiol. 2015;8(4):890-5.
14. Di Biase L, Burkhardt JD, Reddy V, et al. Initial international multicenter human experience with a novel epicardial access needle embedded with a real-time pressure/frequency monitoring to facilitate epicardial access: Feasibility and safety. Heart Rhythm. 2017;14(7):981-8.
15. Weerasooriya R, Jais P, Sacher F, et al. Utility of the lateral fluoroscopic view for subxiphoid pericardial access. Circ Arrhythm Electrophysiol. 2009;2(4):e15-7.
16. Killu AM, Ebrille E, Asirvatham SJ, et al. Percutaneous epicardial access for mapping and ablation is feasible in patients with prior cardiac surgery, including coronary bypass surgery. Circ Arrhythm Electrophysiol. 2015;8(1):94-101.
17. Sosa E, Scanavacca M, D'Avila A, et al. Nonsurgical transthoracic epicardial approach in patients with ventricular tachycardia and previous cardiac surgery. J Interv Card Electrophysiol. 2004;10(3):281-8.
18. Soejima K, Couper G, Cooper JM, et al. Subxiphoid surgical approach for epicardial catheter-based mapping and ablation in patients with prior cardiac surgery or difficult pericardial access. Circulation. 2004;110(10):1197-201.
19. Michowitz Y, Mathuria N, Tung R, et al. Hybrid procedures for epicardial catheter ablation of ventricular tachycardia: Value of surgical access. Heart Rhythm. 2010;7(11):1635-43.
20. Desjardins B, Morady F, Bogun F. Effect of epicardial fat on electroanatomical mapping and epicardial catheter ablation. J Am Coll Cardiol. 2010;56(16):1320-7.
21. Cano O, Hutchinson M, Lin D, et al. Electroanatomic substrate and ablation outcome for suspected epicardial ventricular tachycardia in left ventricular nonischemic cardiomyopathy. J Am Coll Cardiol. 2009;54(9):799-808.
22. Tung R, Nakahara S, Ramirez R, et al. Distinguishing epicardial fat from scar: analysis of electrograms using high-density electroanatomic mapping in a novel porcine infarct model. Heart Rhythm. 2010;7(3):389-95.
23. Jesel L, Sacher F, Komatsu Y, et al. Characterization of contact force during endocardial and epicardial ventricular mapping. Circ Arrhythm Electrophysiol. 2014;7(6):1168-73.
24. Lim HS, Sacher F, Cochet H, et al. Safety and prevention of complications during percutaneous epicardial access for the ablation of cardiac arrhythmias. Heart Rhythm. 2014;11(9):1658-65.

25. Aliot EM, Stevenson WG, Almendral-Garrote JM, et al. EHRA/HRS Expert Consensus on Catheter Ablation of Ventricular Arrhythmias: developed in a partnership with the European Heart Rhythm Association (EHRA), a Registered Branch of the European Society of Cardiology (ESC), and the Heart Rhythm Society (HRS); in collaboration with the American College of Cardiology (ACC) and the American Heart Association (AHA). Heart Rhythm. 2009;6(6):886-933.
26. Fan R, Cano O, Ho SY, et al. Characterization of the phrenic nerve course within the epicardial substrate of patients with nonischemic cardiomyopathy and ventricular tachycardia. Heart Rhythm. 2009;6(1):59-64.
27. Di Biase L, Burkhardt JD, Pelargonio G, et al. Prevention of phrenic nerve injury during epicardial ablation: Comparison of methods for separating the phrenic nerve from the epicardial surface. Heart Rhythm. 2009;6(7):957-61.
28. Buch E, Vaseghi M, Cesario DA, et al. A novel method for preventing phrenic nerve injury during catheter ablation. Heart Rhythm. 2007;4(1):95-8.
29. Dyrda K, Piers SR, van Huls van Taxis CF, et al. Influence of steroid therapy on the incidence of pericarditis and atrial fibrillation after percutaneous epicardial mapping and ablation for ventricular tachycardia. Circ Arrhythm Electrophysiol. 2014;7(4):671-6.

CHAPTER 116

Cardiopulmonary Resuscitation: What's New?

Nitin Modi, Sunil Sharma

INTRODUCTION

The practice of cardiopulmonary resuscitation (CPR) has a long history dating back to 1740 when the Paris Academy of Sciences recommended mouth-to-mouth resuscitation for rescue of drowning victims. The first documented chest compression for resuscitation was performed by Dr Friedrich Maass in 1891. However, mouth-to-mouth resuscitation remained the mainstay of resuscitative efforts with Dr Peter Safar and Dr James Elam promoting respiratory support for resuscitation. It was only in 1960s that a program on CPR was initiated in the US. In 1947 Dr Claude Beck reported first successful ventricular defibrillation of a 14-year-old boy using open chest massage and internal defibrillation with alternating current.

The CPR guidelines have been periodically published every 5 years and were last revised in 2015 when they were published as the 2015 American Heart Association Guideline Update for Cardiopulmonary Resuscitation and Emergency Cardiovascular Care jointly by the American Heart Association (AHA), the European Resuscitation Council (ERC) and the International Liaison Committee on Resuscitation (ILCOR). These bodies reviewed the evidence published since 2010 and published these guidelines as an update to the 2010 Guidelines. Though an update, it is interesting to note that only 1% of all recommendations put forward in 2015 guidelines have the highest level of scientific evidence (Level of Evidence A) and only 25% have a class I recommendation. Majority of these guideline updates have a low level of scientific evidence (either evidence ids based on expert opinion guided by clinical experience or based on studies that have limitations in study design or execution (including meta-analysis) or are based on physiologic or mechanistic studies involving human subjects. As a result most of the recommendations in these guidelines carry only a Class IIb recommendation. Yet, there are major implications for clinical practice and are hence reviewed in this chapter.

2015 AMERICAN HEART ASSOCIATION GUIDELINE UPDATE FOR CARDIO-PULMONARY RESUSCITATION AND EMERGENCY CARDIOVASCULAR CARE

The updated guidelines have revisited the entire process of CPR and have come up with major changes in the entire steps of CPR. Hence, important changes in these new guidelines will be discussed in connection with the revised changes.

Chain of Survival

The revised 2015 AHA guidelines have suggested separate chain of survival for out-of-hospital versus in-hospital cardiac arrest, emphasizing the importance of surveillance and prevention of cardiac arrest in in-hospital patients by paying adequate importance to clinical symptoms and signs that may predict occurrence of cardiac arrest (Fig. 1). The guidelines have paid emphasis to the formation of rapid response teams (RRT) to improve survival of cardiac arrest victims especially in general care wards in both adult and pediatric patients. In additions hospital are encouraged to initiate quality improvement programs to assess and improve upon existing systems of care in their hospitals. Recognizing the importance of primary percutaneous coronary intervention (PCI) in patients with cardiac arrest, communities are encouraged to develop regional centers that have expertise in cardiac resuscitation. The use of mobile phones and social media to initiate the call for help has been recognized and added to the 2015 guidelines.

Chest Compression, Depth, and Rate

The 2015 guidelines have emphasized the lay rescuers may perform chest compression only CPR for adult victims. If the lay rescuer is trained and willing to perform rescue breaths then he should deliver rescue breaths in a ratio of 30 compressions to 2 rescue breaths (for both single and 2 rescuer CPR). In infants and children, the rescuer should

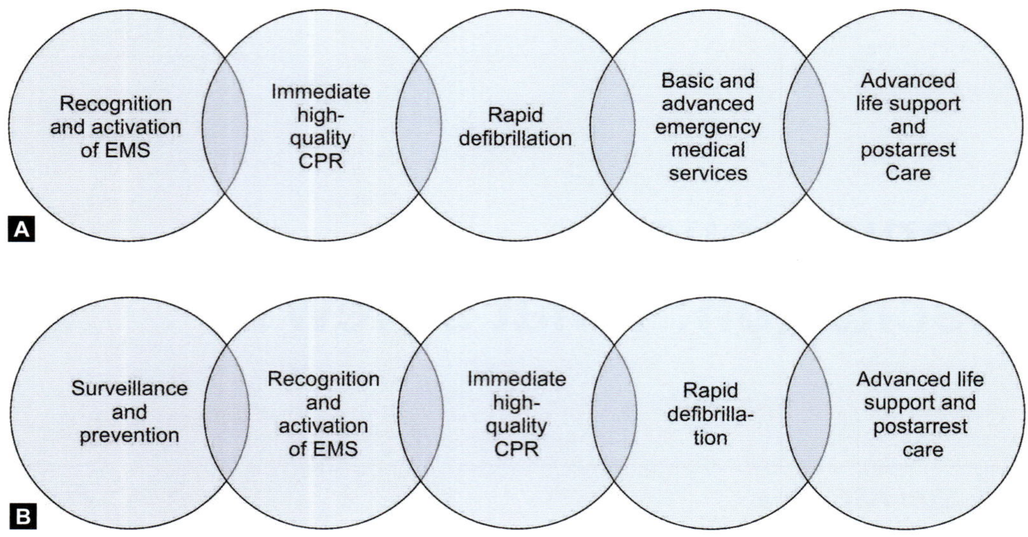

CPR, cardiopulmonary resuscitation; EMS, emergency medical services.

FIG. 1: Chain of survival for cardiac arrest victims in **A,** out-of-hospital; **B,** in-hospital conditions.

maintain the 30:2 ratio for a single rescuer situation while in a two-rescuer situation this should be augmented to 15:2. The rate of chest compression has been changed from at least 100 per minute in 2010 to a rate of 100–120 per minute in the current guidelines. This range has been defined as chest compression i.e., either too fast or too slow can limit cardiac output during CPR and variations beyond this range have been associated with a lower rate of return of spontaneous circulation (ROSC). In addition, the extent of chest compression has also been defined—chest compression in an adult should be at least 5 cm (2 inches) and not more than 6 cm (2.4 inches). In children, the appropriate depth is about one-third of the anteroposterior diameter of the chest (usually about 2 inches); in infants chest compression should be about one-third of the anteroposterior diameter of the chest (usually about one and a half inches). To achieve these criteria rescuers are encouraged to use CPR feedback devices. Many new defibrillators now incorporate these guidelines with voice prompts to ensure high-quality CPR. To ensure high-quality CPR the 2015 guidelines have reemphasized that there should be no interruptions in chest compression of more than 10 seconds. Guidelines have therefore been accordingly simplified—e.g., if a patient has an advanced airway in position then ventilation should be provided in a ratio of 1 breath every 6 seconds (10 breaths/min).

An important update is in victims who have had a witnessed out of hospital cardiac arrest. In these victims ventilation may be delayed by using a strategy of 3 cycles on 200 chest compressions with passive oxygen insufflation using airway adjuncts. In addition, patients who have had a witnessed cardiac arrest and an automated external defibrillator (AED) is immediately available then it is reasonable to use the AED as soon as possible. Previous guidelines had suggested that a brief period of chest compression (1.5–3 min) before defibrillation maybe useful. Though scientific evidence has not shown any difference in clinical outcomes, current guidelines recommend that chest compression should be continued even as the AED is being applied and the AED should be used as early as possible.

Use of Mechanical Devices for Chest Compression

The 2015 guidelines have suggested that when available mechanical compression devices may be used to provide high-quality CPR when performing manual CPR is difficult or impossible (e.g., in a moving ambulance, during PCI, limited rescuers, hypothermic cardiac arrest, prolonged CPR, etc.). However, it should be noted that piston-type devices have not been found to be superior to manual CPR in clinical studies.

Extracorporeal Techniques

Extracorporeal membrane oxygenator (ECMO) may be used as an alternative to conventional CPR in selected patients in whom the cause of cardiac arrest is deemed reversible and when this can be rapidly implemented. Available data is on a very select patient population from limited centers with this expertise. As there are no clinical trials of ECMO in patients with cardiac arrest and this decision needs to be individualized depending upon availability, center expertise, and clinical condition. ECMO allows time to reverse potentially treatable causes during cardiac arrest.

Advanced Cardiac Life Support Monitoring and Pharmacotherapy

Vasopressin

The use of vasopressin (40 units IV or intraosseous) in conjunction with epinephrine in cardiac resuscitation has been dispensed with in the 2015 guidelines as there is no evidence of benefit in cardiac arrest victims. As the two drugs have equal efficacy, vasopressin has been removed to simplify cardiac arrest care.

Epinephrine

The new guidelines have suggested that epinephrine may be administered as soon as possible after cardiac arrest due to an initial nonshockable rhythm. This is because the results of a clinical study reported improved outcomes in patients who were administered epinephrine at 1 minute and 3 minutes in cardiac arrest due to a nonshockable rhythm.

Lidocaine

Routine use of lidocaine during cardiac arrest due to pulseless ventricular tachycardia or ventricular fibrillation has been removed. However, use of lidocaine in postcardiac arrest care after ROSC remains.

Beta-blockers

An observational study had reported improved outcomes in patients with cardiac arrest due to pulseless VT/VF (ventricular tachycardia/ventricular fibrillation) who were administered beta-blockers. However, at present current guidelines do not recommend routine use of beta-blockers in such cardiac arrest victims. They may however be considered after ROSC in appropriate clinical conditions.

End-Tidal Carbon Dioxide Level

Monitoring of end-tidal carbon dioxide level ($ETCO_2$) to assess ROSC in intubated patients; conversely failure to achieve $ETCO_2$ of more than 10 mm Hg in intubated patients even 20 minutes after CPR is considered a poor prognostic marker and may be useful in association with other clinical markers to assess termination of ventilation. It however should not be used in isolation to determine when to terminate resuscitative efforts.

Postcardiac Arrest Care

Coronary Angiography and Acute Coronary Syndrome Assessment

An important change in the 2015 guidelines is the early use of coronary angiography in select patients with cardiac arrest. Patients with electrocardiogram (ECG) evidence of ST elevation on the ECG after cardiac arrest as well as those patients who are electrically unstable but without ST elevation on the ECG in whom cardiovascular disease is suspected should be considered for emergency coronary angiography to rule out acute coronary syndrome as a cause of cardiac arrest.

Targeted Temperature Management

Current guidelines recommend that all comatose adult patients after ROSC following cardiac arrest should be considered for targeted temperature management with a goal to achieve temperatures between 32 and 36°C for at least 24 hours. However, a recent high-quality study did not report superior outcomes in patients who received temperature management during postcardiac arrest care. Current guidelines are still based on previous studies that found superior outcomes in patients who received targeted temperature management during the postcardiac arrest care.

However, there is no evidence that prehospital cooling of patients after ROSC with IV fluids does not improve outcomes and is not recommended.

Prognostication

Neurologic prognostication of patients who have had poor neurologic outcomes after ROSC is best done 72 hours after cardiac arrest. This is because various drugs used during cardiac arrest including sedatives and neuromuscular blockers may take a prolonged time to clear from the body. Multiple modalities should be used to arrive at a clinical decision as no single method is accurate in predicting clinical outcomes. Poor prognostic markers include absence of pupillary reflex 72 hours after cardiac arrest, status myoclonus in the first 72 hours, marked reduction in gray-white ratio on CT brain within 2 hours of cardiac arrest, absence of electroencephalogram (EEG) reactivity to external stimuli at 72 hours after cardiac arrest, and extensive restriction of diffusion on brain MRI 72 hours after cardiac arrest.

Cardiopulmonary Resuscitation in Special Situations

Pregnancy

The 2015 guidelines have made a significant change in the recommendations on how to perform CPR in pregnancy. These guidelines have recommended just manual left uterine displacement in pregnant women with cardiac arrest if the fundal height is above the umbilicus. This prevents aortocaval compression which may impede venous return during chest compression. The previous guidelines had suggested that a wedge maybe used to tilt the patient to an angle of up to 30° to prevent uterine effect on venous return.

Opioid Overdose

Current guidelines suggest empiric intramuscular or intratracheal administration of naloxone in suspected opioid overdose in patients who are unresponsive and have a definite pulse, but are not breathing or are gasping. These measures should not in any way delay standard resuscitative measures. In patients who have no definite pulse focus should be on standard resuscitation. It may be that some of these patients are in respiratory arrest and not in cardiac arrest with a weak and slow pulse—it may be reasonable to administer naloxone based on clinical suspicion.

Prone Cardiopulmonary Resuscitation

Though not specifically addressed in the 2015 guidelines, when patient have cardiac arrest in prone position, e.g., as in neurosurgical procedures, in road traffic accident victims when it is impossible to switch to a supine position, the only viable option is to perform CPR in prone position. In the prone position, heart area is maximum behind 1–2 vertebral segments below the inferior angle of scapula. Delivering compression at this location gives adequate hemodynamic results. Defibrillation maybe performed in prone position by placing one of the pads in the left fifth intercostal space in the midaxillary line and the other between the tip of right scapula and the spine.

Ineffectual Therapies

Many therapies during CPR have noted to be ineffective yet continued to be practiced at times. These include the following described here.

Sodium Bicarbonate

Use of sodium bicarbonate during CPR is widely prevalent despite ample evidence to suggest that it does not but may rather impair outcomes in patients with cardiac arrest. Though, it is clinically logical to counteract metabolic acidosis during cardiac arrest with sodium bicarbonate, use of this drug may lead to intracellular acidosis, hypernatremia, and even metabolic alkalosis on recovery from cardiac arrest. The only indication for use of sodium bicarbonate is in patients with cardiac arrest due to hyperkalemia or that occurring due to drug toxicity like tricyclic antidepressants or antiarrhythmic drugs such as flecainide. Many clinicians still support the use of sodium bicarbonate in cardiac arrest especially in those with pre-existing metabolic acidosis (pH <7.10), clinical outcomes do not support its use.

Magnesium Sulfate

Magnesium sulfate should not be used routinely in patients with VT/VF unless these rhythms result from QT prolongation (acquired or congenital).

Cardiac Pacing

Temporary pacemakers are often inserted during cardiac arrest presenting as asystole. However, pacing is not a recommended technique for CPR as it does not improve outcomes. The only indication for temporary cardiac pacemaker is in cardiac arrest resulting from complete heart block.

Fibrinolysis

Although both myocardial infarction and pulmonary embolism account for a large number of cardiac arrest episodes, fibrinolysis in cardiac arrest has not been shown to improve outcomes. A number of studies including randomized controlled trials have failed to demonstrate any benefit of fibrinolysis. However, it may be useful in some selected patients with suspected pulmonary embolism.

"Cough" Cardiopulmonary Resuscitation

Coughing increases intrathoracic pressure which increases peripheral perfusion pressure. In a monitored condition such as in the cardiac catheterization laboratory a patient with a nonperfusing cardiac rhythm offers a few seconds before he or she losses consciousness. In this period, vigorous coughing can maintain consciousness for a few seconds and can give time for reversal of cardiac arrhythmia. However, it is not recommended as a method for CPR.

Precordial Thump

A precordial thump is ineffective in majority of cases of malignant ventricular arrhythmias though there are occasional occasions when these arrhythmias may convert to sinus rhythm with thump version. However, it may result in sternal fracture and strokes have been reported as well.

Active Compression–Decompression Cardiopulmonary Resuscitation

This is method of chest compression in which a suction device is used over the chest to convert passive chest recoil into an active mode in order to improve venous return. Preliminary studies in both animals and humans evoked some interest with improvement in some cardiac parameters. However, clinical trials have not found any major advantage of this method in improving patient outcomes. As a result current guidelines have neither supported nor rejected this method of CPR.

REFERENCES

1. Kronick SL, Kurz MC, Lin S, et al. Part 4: Systems of Care and Continuous Quality Improvement: 2015 American Heart Association Guidelines Update for Cardiopulmonary Resuscitation and Emergency Cardiovascular Care. Circulation. 2015;132(18 Suppl 2):S397-413.
2. Adams JG. Emergency Medicine: Clinical Essentials (Expert Consult – Online). Elsevier Health Sciences. 2012;1771. ISBN 1455733946.
3. Who Is at Risk for Sudden Cardiac Arrest? NHLBI. 2016.
4. Hasselqvist-Ax I, Riva G, Herlitz J, et al. Early cardiopulmonary resuscitation in out-of-hospital cardiac arrest. N Engl J Med. 2015;372:2307-15.
5. Lenzer J. Peter Josef Safar. BMJ. 2003;327(7415):624.
6. Beck CS, Pritchard WH, Feil HS. Ventricular fibrillation of long duration abolished by electric shock. JAMA. 1947;135:1230-33.
7. Part1: Executive Summary 2010 American Heart Association Guidelines for Cardiopulmonary Resuscitation and Emergency Cardiovascular Care; 2010. [online] Available from circ.ahajournals.org/content/122/18_suppl_3.
8. 2017 American Heart Association Focused Update on Adult Basic Life Support and CPR. Available from circ.ahajournals.org/content/circulationaha/Nov 6, 2017.
9. 2012 National Utstein Report. CARES Cardiac Arrest Registry to Enhance Survival.
10. Huang Y, He Q, Yang LJ, et al. Cardiopulmonary resuscitation (CPR) plus delayed defibrillation versus immediate defibrillation for out-of-hospital cardiac arrest. The Cochrane Database Syst Rev. 2014;9.
11. Assar D, Chamberlain D, Colquhoun M, et al. Randomized controlled trials of staged teaching for basic life support. 1. Skill acquisition at bronze stage. Resuscitation. 2000;45:7-15.
12. Heidenreich JW, Higdon TA, Kern KB, et al. Single rescuer cardiopulmonary resuscitation: 'two quick breaths'–an oxymoron. Resuscitation. 2004;62:283-9.
13. Alwan AA, Ehlenbach WJ, Menon PR, et al. Cardiopulmonary resuscitation among mechanically ventilated patients. Intensive Care Med. 2014;40(4):55663.
14. Lee IH, How CK, Lu WH, et al. Improved survival outcome with continuous chest compressions with ventilation compared to 5:1 compressions-to-ventilations mechanical cardiopulmonary resuscitation in out-of-hospital cardiac arrest. J Chin Med Assoc. 2013;76:158-63.
15. Chen YS, Lin JW, Yu HY, et al. Cardiopulmonary resuscitation with assisted extracorporeal life support versus conventional cardiopulmonary resuscitation in adults with in hospital cardiac arrest: An observational study and propensity analysis. Lancet. 2008;372:554-61.

16. Shih CL, Lu TC, Jerng JS, et al. A web-based Utstein style registry system of in-hospital cardiopulmonary resuscitation in Taiwan. Resuscitation. 2007;72:394-403.
17. LeGuen M, Nicolas Robin A, Carreira S, et al. Extracorporeal life support following out of hospital refractory cardiac arrest. Crit Care. 2011;15:R29.
18. International Liaison Committee on Resuscitation: 2005 International Consensus on Cardiopulmonary Resuscitation and Emergency Cardiovascular Care Science with Treatment Recommendations. Part 2: Adult basic life support. Resuscitation. 2005;67(2-3):187-201.
19. Riou B, Adnet F, Baud F, et al. Guidelines for indications for the use of extracorporeal life support in refractory cardiac arrest. Ann Fr Anesth Reanim. 2009;28:182-90.
20. Wei J, Tung D, Sue SH, et al. Cardiopulmonary resuscitation in prone position: A simplified method for outpatients. J Chin Med Assoc. 2006;69:202-6.
21. Kwon MJ, Kim EH, Song IK, et al. Optimizing prone cardiopulmonary resuscitation: Identifying the vertebral level correlating with the largest left ventricle cross-sectional area via computed tomography scan. Anesth Analg. 2017;124:520-3.
22. Miller B, Cohen A, Serio A, et al. Hemodynamics of cough cardiopulmonary resuscitation in a patient with sustained torsades de pointes/ventricular flutter. J Emerg Med. 1994;12:62732.
23. Keeble W, Tymchak WJ. Triggering of the Bezold Jarisch Reflex by reperfusion during primary PCI with maintenance of consciousness by cough CPR: A case report and review of pathophysiology. J Invasive Cardiol. 2008;20:E239-42.
24. Niemann JT, Rosborough J, Hausknecht M, et al. Cough-CPR: Documentation of systemic perfusion in man and in an experimental model: A "window" to the mechanism of blood flow in external CPR. Crit Care Med. 1980;8:14 -6.
25. Saba SE, David SW. Sustained consciousness during ventricular fibrillation: case report of cough cardiopulmonary resuscitation. Cathet Cardiovasc Diagn. 1996;37:47-8.
26. Pellis T, Kette F, Lovisa D, et al. Utility of pre-cordial thump for treatment of out of hospital cardiac arrest: A prospective study. Resuscitation. 2009;80:17-23.
27. Pennington JE, Taylor J, Lown B. Chest thump for reverting ventricular tachycardia. N Engl J Med. 1970;283:1192-5.
28. Amir O, Schliamser JE, Nemer S, et al. Ineffectiveness of precordial thump for cardioversion of malignant ventricular tachyarrhythmias. Pacing Clin Electrophysiol. 2007;30:153-6.
29. Ahmar W, Morley P, Marasco S, et al. Sternal fracture and osteomyelitis: An unusual complication of a precordial thump. Resuscitation. 2007;75:540-2.
30. American Heart Association Guidelines for Cardiopulmonary Resuscitation and Emergency Cardiovascular Care. Part 4. 2010

SECTION 17

Cardiac Implantable Electronic Devices

CHAPTER 117

Improving Outcomes in Patients with Cardiac Resynchronization Therapy

Rohit Malhotra

INTRODUCTION

As patient survival has improved postmyocardial infarction, congestive heart failure (CHF) has become increasingly prevalent. Cardiac resynchronization therapy (CRT) reduces morbidity and mortality in these patients but optimizing therapies in these patients can be challenging. There are well-established guidelines for patients who qualify for CRT and derive the most benefit (Table 1). It is estimated that up to 30% of patients do not respond to therapy.[1] There are a number of approaches to improving outcomes in these patients.

PATIENT SELECTION

Requirements for medical therapy prior to implantation suggest benefits to patients who have taken optimal guideline directed therapy for at least 3 months as medical therapy is the cornerstone for heart failure management in these patients. The first trials examining CRT (COMPANION and CARE-HF)[2,3] included 1,502 and 813 patients, respectively. In each of these trials, angiotensin-converting enzyme inhibitors (ACEIs) and angiotensin receptor blockers (ARBs) were utilized in roughly 90% of patients. Beta-blockade therapy was utilized in approximately 70% of patients, and spironolactone in about 50%. More recent data, from the DANISH[4] trial, indicated that 90% of patients received both beta-blockers and ACEI or ARB therapy with 60% receiving mineralocorticoid receptor antagonists. While this trial did not demonstrate a benefit to implantable cardioverter-defibrillator (ICD) therapy, and the impact of CRT was not clear and was not studied, it does demonstrate the increased utilization of medical therapy in patients eligible for these medications. In addition, with the impact of valsartan or sacubitril on patient outcomes, the definition of optimal medical therapy becomes more nebulous. In summary, optimal medical therapy is defined by the implanting physician and not specifically by medications being utilized.

The QRS duration is a large determinant of patient responsiveness to CRT. Recent American[5,6] and European[7] guidelines differ from prior guidelines, changing the class I indication for CRT implantation from more than or equal to 120 ms[8] to more than or equal to 150 ms (Table 2). While QRS duration is the cornerstone of guidelines for CRT therapy, there is a lot of controversy regarding response to therapy in left bundle branch block (LBBB) and non-LBBB patients.

The predominance of these data arises from differences in outcomes in patients with LBBB and non-LBBB. Mechanistically, earliest electrical activation of the left ventricle in non-LBBB patients is at the septum[9] with the free wall of the right ventricle (RV) contracting last. However, if there are issues with conduction in the left ventricle, such as fascicular blocks, patients may have some benefit from left ventricular (LV) lead implantation, though these data are less clear. For example, Chandra et al.[10] demonstrated that patients with RBBB and fascicular block had better outcomes as assessed by New York Heart Association (NYHA) class or an improvement of more than or equal to 5% in ejection fraction. Varma[11] demonstrated that the initiation of QRS deflection and time to basal lateral LV depolarization correlated with QRS duration, suggesting that those patients with significantly prolonged QRS duration may have more benefit from CRT. While these studies suggest that patients with non-LBBB may benefit from CRT, other data are contradictory. However, analysis of MADIT-CRT indicates that while patients with left anterior hemiblock on ECG may have improvement in echocardiographic parameters such as LV end systolic volume, end diastolic volume, and left atrial volume, survival did not differ.[12]

Furthermore, this change is based upon the data from multiple studies, including analysis of echocardiographic dyssynchrony in patients with prolonged QRS durations.[13] This study indicates that QRS duration does not correlate with the area of mechanical dyssynchrony. Analysis of large population post-CRT implantation with non-LBBB indicates that outcomes did not improve post-CRT implantation and were actually worse.[14] Thus, while echocardiographic

TABLE 1: United States guidelines for the year 2012

United States guidelines	2012
Class I indications	CRT indicated for patients with normal sinus rhythm and EF ≤35% with LBBB and QRS duration of ≥150 ms with NYHA class II, III, or ambulatory class IV symptoms on guideline-directed medical therapy (GDMT)
Class IIa indications	CRT useful for: • Normal sinus rhythm with EF ≤35% with QRS duration between 120 and 149 ms with LBBB with NYHA class II, III, or ambulatory class IV symptoms on GDMT • Normal sinus rhythm with EF ≤35% with QRS duration ≥150 ms with non-LBBB with NYHA class III or ambulatory class IV symptoms on GDMT • Patients with atrial fibrillation with EF ≤35% if pacing is required or AV nodal ablation or pharmacologic therapy will allow near 100% pacing • Patients on GDMT with EF ≤35% and ventricular pacing is anticipated to be 40% or greater
Class IIb	CRT considered for patients: • EF ≤30% due to ischemia, normal sinus rhythm, and LBBB with QRS ≥150 ms with NYHA class I symptoms • EF ≤35% with normal sinus rhythm with non-LBBB pattern and QRS between 120 and 149 ms with class III or ambulatory class IV symptoms on GDMT • EF ≤35%, normal sinus rhythm with non-LBBB pattern with QRS duration ≥150 ms and class II symptoms on GDMT
Class III	CRT not recommended for patients: • Class I or II symptoms and non-LBBB pattern with QRS duration <150 ms • With comorbidities that limit life expectancy to less than 1 year

AV, atrioventricular; CRT, cardiac resynchronization therapy; EF, ejection fraction; LBBB, left bundle branch block; NYHA, New York Heart Association.

TABLE 2: European guidelines for the year 2016

European guidelines	2016
Class I with evidence level A	CRT indicated for: • Symptomatic patients with EF ≤35% and CHF in normal sinus rhythm with QRS duration ≥150 ms and LBBB morphology despite optimal medical therapy (OMT) • CRT rather than RV pacing recommended for patients with heart failure with reduced EF and indication for ventricular pacing
Class I with evidence level B	CRT considered for patients: • Symptomatic patients with EF ≤35% and CHF in normal sinus rhythm with QRS duration between 130 and 149 ms and LBBB morphology despite OMT
Class IIa evidence level B	CRT should be considered: • Symptomatic patients with CHF in sinus rhythm with QRS ≥150 ms and non-LBBB pattern with EF ≤35% • Symptomatic patients with CHF in sinus rhythm with QRS between 130 and 149 ms and non-LBBB pattern with EF ≤35% • EF ≤35% with NYHA class III or IV CHF despite OMT if they have atrial fibrillation and QRS duration ≥130 ms with a strategy to induce pacing or restoration of sinus rhythm is anticipated
Class IIB evidence level B	CRT may be considered for: • Patients symptomatic with CHF with QRS between 130 and149 ms and non-LBBB pattern with EF ≤35% despite OMT • Patients with existing pacemaker or ICD with worsening CHF despite OMT and have a high-proportion of RV pacing may be considered for upgrade to CRT
Class III	CRT contraindicated in patients with QRS duration <130 ms

CRT, cardiac resynchronization therapy; CHF, congestive heart failure; EF, ejection fraction; ICD, implantable cardioverter-defibrillator; LBBB, left bundle branch block; NYHA, New York heart association; RV, right ventricular.

or electrocardiographic parameters may improve post-CRT implantation, survival may not improve. As a result, indications for CRT implantation have changed (Fig. 1). While non-LBBB patients are not excluded, these patients are most likely to benefit if the QRS duration is long.

Studies of CRT implantation[15] in patients with echocardiographic dyssynchrony but with QRS duration less than 130 ms do not demonstrate benefit. In this study, which terminated early due to futility of therapy, 809 patients with class III or IV CHF and ejection fraction of 35% or less with LV

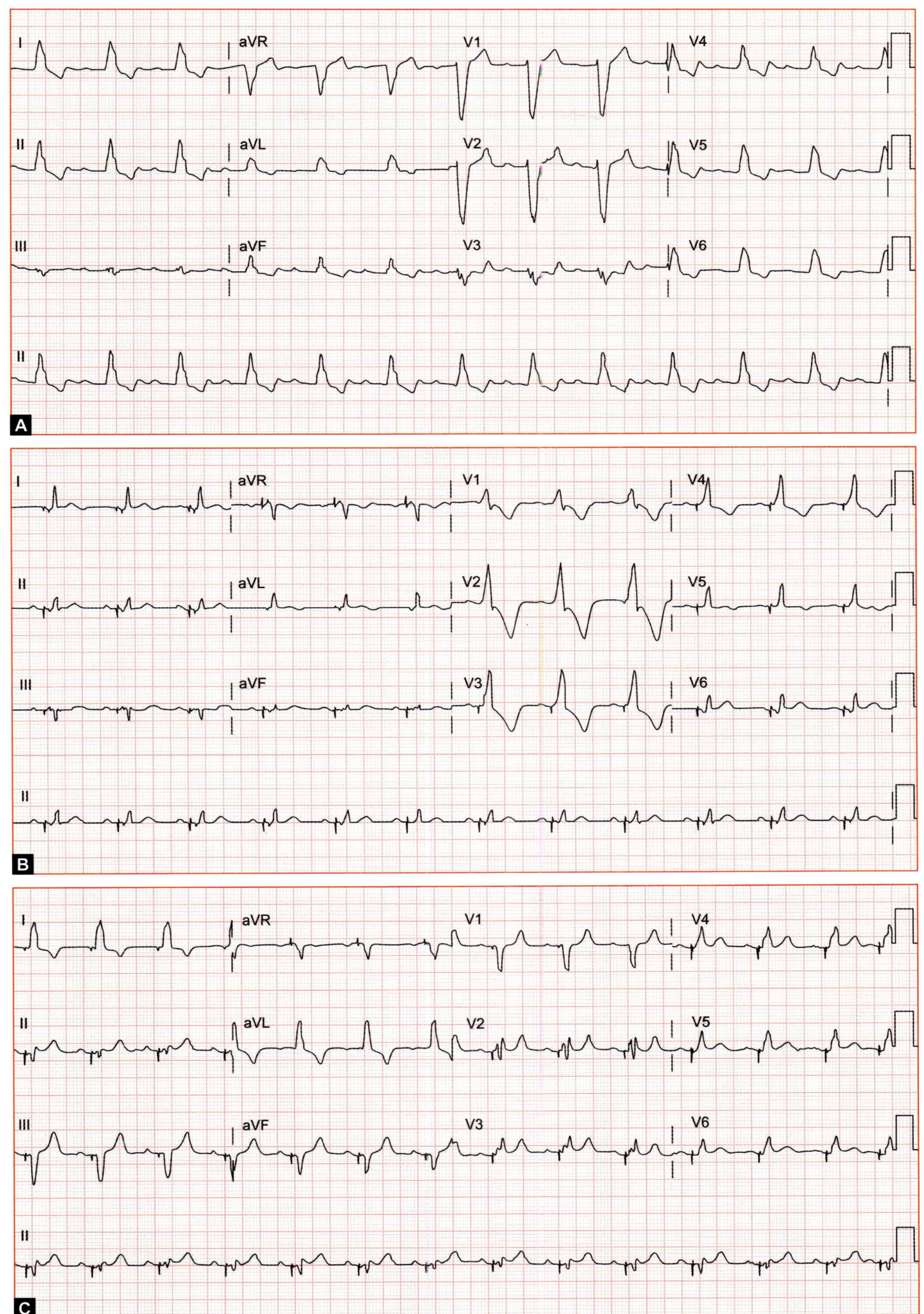

aVR, augmented vector right; aVL, augmented vector left; aVF, augmented vector foot.

FIG. 1: A, Preimplantation ECG; **B,** Post-cardiac resynchronization therapy (CRT) implantation ECG; **C,** Post CRT implantation ECG with altered left ventricular and right ventricular timing.

dyssynchrony demonstrated by echocardiography underwent CRT implantation with a 1:1 randomization to either CRT therapy or no CRT therapy, if the LV lead was successfully implanted. Dyssynchrony was defined by tissue Doppler with opposing wall delay of 80 ms or more in apical four-chamber view or apical long-axis views or by speckle tracking analysis of radial strain of the anteroseptal to posteroseptal walls of 130 ms or more in the short-axis view. Patients were followed every 3 months. The primary outcome was death or first CHF hospitalization. Unfortunately, the study was stopped early due to a potential for harm. In total, 1,680 patients were consented, but due to lack of echocardiographic dyssynchrony, 602 were excluded. There was no difference in death from any cause or first CHF hospitalization between groups.

Some studies do indicate that QRS duration may not alone predict a favorable response. A number of studies have analyzed QRS duration relative to body surface area, body mass index, or LV mass and have demonstrated CRT benefit even in patients with QRS durations less than 150 ms.[16-18] These studies suggest that smaller patients, particularly women, may benefit from CRT at shorter QRS durations. However, these studies have not been sufficient to alter current guidelines for CRT.

PREPROCEDURE PLANNING

In clinical practice, QRS duration is the predominant predictor of benefit from CRT implantation, though calculators do exist that may predict outcomes postimplantation.[19] However, in trying to determine factors that may contribute to response to therapy, a number of approaches have been undertaken, including echocardiographic and magnetic resonance imaging (MRI)-based evaluation.

Echocardiography is a widely available and inexpensive method to assess baseline ejection fraction. For example, analysis of echocardiography pre- and postimplantation demonstrated that patients who responded to therapy had improvement in lateral and anteroseptal activation while nonresponders did not (Auger). Unfortunately, this analysis does not help with prediction of response to CRT implantation. However, it may provide insight into where to implant leads.

More advanced echocardiographic techniques, such as speckle tracking, have been utilized to assess response to therapy. Prior trials have attempted to predict response to therapy, and they have not demonstrated power to predict response based upon one echocardiographic parameter.[20] This trial evaluated regional strain and was unable to identify a predictor of response, which was in part attributed to variability in interpretation. In order to predict responses to therapy, Park et al.[21] developed a score using a combination of LV global longitudinal strain (LVGLS), end diastolic dimension, left atrial area, RV end diastolic area, right ventricular fractional area change (defined as the percentage change in right ventricular end diastolic and end-systolic areas), and right atrial area that predicted response to therapy. The higher the score, the better the outcome, independent of clinical factors such as age, gender, baseline functional class, and heart failure etiology. However, performing this difficult analysis is not often undertaken in clinical practice given the complexity.

Another study[22] examining speckle tracking suggests that strain offers prediction of clinical outcome as defined by time to death, LV assist device implantation, or transplant. However, this single center study does note that performing a portion of the analysis (global circumferential strain) is more dependent upon the skills of the sonography and the interpretation, complicating the generalizability of this approach.

Additionally, speckle tracking has been utilized to aid in LV lead implantation at the time of the procedure.[23] In this study, a double-blinded approach to echocardiographic LV lead implantation was performed over the course of 6 years, from 2005–2011 in 187 total patients, with 110 undergoing echocardiographic guidance. Speckle tracking echocardiography was performed prior to the procedure, and the areas of latest activation designated. LV leads were implanted in areas closest to the area of latest activation based upon the left anterior oblique fluoroscopic view in echocardiographically-guided patients and placed routinely in a lateral or posterior position in control patients, regardless of activation site. Patients with leads implanted at the site of latest activation had significantly better outcomes with fewer hospitalizations in the echocardiogram-guided implant group and an overall 26% reduction in events in the intervention group. However, while outcomes were better in this group, the intervention is cumbersome and expensive, particularly, since 66% of patients in the control group had LV lead placement in the site of latest mechanical activation, suggesting that performing speckle echocardiography prior to implantation would likely be costly to perform in all patients. Cost analysis was not performed in this study, but this practice has not become a part of routine clinical care.

Finally, MRI has been utilized to assess scar, mechanical, and electrical properties at the site of LV lead placement.[24] Using displacement encoding with stimulated echoes (DENSE), a technique that allows for strain assessment without the potentially subjective and operator dependent aspects of echocardiographic speckle tracking coupled with an algorithm to evaluate the time to regional peak strain, analysis of patients who underwent CRT implantation was performed to determine CRT response. Of the parameters compared, including lead not in scar, stretch at the LV lead position, and time from QRS onset to the electrogram at the lead position, the time to regional peak strain was most predictive of response to therapy. However, much like speckle tracking, this technique involves a costly test prior to device implantation.

A final approach to optimal placement of LV leads is to seek out longest time from onset of QRS to the electrogram at the site of the LV lead, also called QLV. A substudy of the SMART-AV trial, which examined atrioventricular (AV) optimization techniques in patients with CHF undergoing CRT implantation, evaluated the effect of QLV on outcomes. In this study, Gold et al. compared the QRS and the RV and

LV lead electrograms, allowing measurement of the QLV. A total of 426 patients were analyzed. Those patients with a QLV longer than the median had better outcomes overall as assessed by LV end systolic volume, end diastolic volume, ejection fraction, and quality of life. However, QRS duration did not correlate with QLV.

While preprocedural imaging with MRI or echocardiography can identify areas of dyssynchrony, incorporating this testing into routine clinical practice can be costly and potentially not helpful. Examination of QLV can be helpful in predicting a favorable response and can potential direct implanting physicians to the ideal location for lead placement and pacing. This technique can be used at the time of the procedure, unlike the preprocedural imaging.

Lead Implantation

Coronary sinus leads are placed via a guiding sheath that allows for implantation of the lead. Commonly, the left anterior oblique cinefluoroscopy is utilized to identify coronary sinus branches and their locations (anterior or posterior/inferior).[25] Unfortunately, endovascular lead implantation is limited to the available anatomy, which may lead to implantation of LV leads in areas of scar, and thus, poor response and high thresholds. In addition, pacing energy can lead to stimulation of the phrenic nerve, resulting in significant patient discomfort. Furthermore, LV leads do not have any support and sit in a large pool of blood in the coronary sinus vein. As a result, some areas of the lead may be close to ventricular myocardium and others far away, potentially impacting the amount of energy required to pace the left ventricle. The quadripolar LV lead was designed to combat these issues.

Prior generation LV leads were capable of unipolar or bipolar pacing, exposing patients to the noted risks. Quadripolar leads have four pacing electrodes with variable spacing, depending upon manufacturer. In addition to allowing for variable pacing vectors which may reduce pacing threshold and help reduce the risk of phrenic nerve capture, these leads allow for changes in pacing vector over the duration of device implant. If there is a small movement in the lead, lead repositioning can be avoided in many cases. In addition, if the heart configuration changes, such as due to response to LV pacing and reduction in LV volume, pacing poles can be altered to help maintain battery longevity and to avoid phrenic nerve stimulation if this should become an issue. Furthermore, given the data on QLV, current devices can give automated read-outs on the timing differential between RV and LV electrogram timing, potentially allowing for pacing at the longest QLV.

Additionally, quadripolar leads allow for multipoint pacing (MPP). When utilized in this configuration, pacing can occur at two different LV sites. There may be benefits to this type of pacing configuration, if there are areas of scar that lead to delay in signal conduction through the left ventricle.[26] To maximize the possibility of simultaneous LV depolarization despite areas of slowed conduction that may limit response to CRT, these devices can be programed to pace at different points. Niazi et al.[27] demonstrated safety and efficacy of this technology in 2017. In this Investigation Device Exemption (IDE) trial, indicated patients underwent implantation of CRT devices. At 3 months postimplant, patients underwent echocardiographic analysis, with particular emphasis on velocity-time integral of the transmitral flow (EA VTI) as this parameter most closely replicates dP/dt_{max}, which has been documented to best assess hemodynamic response to CRT, and those patients who had the best response to MPP in various configurations were randomized to biventricular pacing or MPP. MPP was programed per investigator discretion. Subsequently, analysis was performed on which programing performed best in terms of clinical response, and those patients who were programed to pace at points of maximal anatomic separation with short pacing delay between electrodes had significantly better clinical outcomes than those programed to other configurations. Furthermore, patients who were nonresponders to CRT had a significant improvement with MPP activated. This technology holds promise for improving outcomes in nonresponders. Integration of imaging techniques such as MRI and speckle tracking may further improve response to therapy.

Noncoronary Sinus Left Ventricular Pacing

Unfortunately, while successful implantation rates of LV leads has increased overtime, there is up to a 20% rate of LV lead implantation failure.[28] There are a number of reasons that coronary sinus leads cannot be implanted, such as poor venous targets, lack of coronary sinus access, and scar in areas near the coronary sinus. As a result, alternative approaches to LV pacing have been developed.

First, for patients with poor vascular targets in the coronary sinus, venoplasty, and snares have been used to improve lead delivery. For example, Worley et al.[29] described a technique where the coronary sinus is cannulated. A long wire is delivered to the vein, and the end of the wire snared. This loop of wire, with both ends controlled outside the body, allows the lead to be advanced to targeted vessels, even when they are small. In addition, techniques to venoplasty small veins to facilitate lead implantation have been utilized. Hesselson et al. describe a single center experience of this technique in 47 patients over 12 years. Using the guiding sheath size as a gauge for measurement of angioplasty balloon, veins were dilated to allow lead passage beyond valves, to small vessels, and past focal stenoses. In this series, there was a 77% success rate though others have described 88–99% success rates. Unfortunately, Worley et al. have also describe coronary sinus vein rupture related to venoplasty, so this technique must be used with appropriate caution. The patient described was able to have the LV lead implanted. These techniques have been used in combination to assist in LV lead delivery.

For patients in whom the coronary sinus is not identified, surgical LV lead implantation has also been utilized to surmount issues with coronary sinus lead implantation. There are a number of different approaches to surgical LV lead implantation,[30] including left thoracotomy and thoracoscopic approaches, both with video assistance or without. There are data that suggest that patients did not do as well with surgically placed leads, predominantly due to anterior LV implantation. However, more recent data indicate that patients post epicardial lead implantation have similar outcomes to endovascularly placed leads, though the initial recovery period has higher morbidity.[31] Recovery in these patients can be prolonged, and due to poor LV function, the surgical risk is high.

Recent advances in His bundle pacing tools have led to an increased usage of His bundle pacing, and this approach may become an option for management of patients with unsuitable anatomy for LV lead implantation. Pacing from the His bundle position can lead to QRS narrowing, even in patients with underlying bundle branch block. Placing leads in this position is technically challenging, with higher outputs required to maintain His bundle capture, and is thus not performed standardly. Lustgarten et al.[32] implanted standard CRT devices with both a LV lead and a lead in the His bundle position. Patients who had narrowing of QRS due to His bundle pacing were then randomized to undergo either biventricular pacing or His bundle pacing for 6 months. After 6 months, patients were crossed-over to the alternate therapy. Ultimately, 12 patients completed the protocol. In both groups, there was an improvement in quality of life, ejection fraction, and NYHA class. Echocardiographic parameters were not significantly different from baseline in either group. This approach allows for alternative pacing sites in patients where coronary sinus leads cannot be implanted due to anatomy, high pacing thresholds due to LV scar, or phrenic nerve stimulation.

Finally, there are data to suggest that endocardial pacing of the left ventricle may have more benefit than epicardial pacing.[33,34] As a result, and in the setting of poor coronary sinus options, an endocardial approach has been attempted in some patients. These leads have been placed in the left ventricle via either transatrial septal, transventricular septal, or trans-ventricular apical techniques. Response rates to these approaches are not as high as with conventionally placed LV leads. However, due to surgical risk and the difficulty of placing surgical LV leads on the posterior aspect of the heart, these patients underwent these types of procedures. There is also an increased rate of stroke and transient ischemic attacks in these patients due to the need for anticoagulation related to endovascular leads in the arterial circulation. There is limited experience with these types of leads, and refinements of both implant techniques and ventricular locations will develop, with likely improvements in outcomes. In fact, new technologies using an endovascular pacing approach are in development and have been recently tested in a trial intended to assess feasibility and safety.[35] In this nonrandomized trial, 34 of 35 patients had a novel endocardial LV pacing system implanted. In this system, an ultrasound receiving electrode is placed endocardially in the LV via a retrograde aortic approach and a transmitter that emits focused ultrasound to the receiver to induce pacing is placed subcutaneously in the 4th to 6th intercostal space lateral to the parasternal border. The transmitter requires a direct line of site view to the receiver, without lung or bone intervening. This transmitter is attached to a battery supply that may be placed up to 30 cm away. The transmitter senses pacing signals from an existing RV pacing device (either a pacemaker or ICD) that prompts LV pacing that will occur 3–5 ms post RV pacing. Endpoints in the study included demonstrated biventricular pacing at 1 and 6 months. This endpoint was achieved in 33 out of 34 patients at 1 month and 31 out of 33 at 6 months with the absence of biventricular pacing in 2 patients due to transmitter failure that improved with transmitter replacement. Approximately, 66% of patients had improvement in clinical parameters (improvement in NYHA class ≥1 and improved quality of life scores. Unfortunately, 3 patients had complications related to implantation, with one dying 4 days postimplantation after suffering ventricular fibrillation during endocardial receiver implant and the other two having arterial issues. With the potential freedom to place the endovascular pacing element in very targeted locations, the data gleaned from the speckle-tracking or MRI-based methods discussed may provide insight on exactly where to pace the left ventricle for maximal patient benefit.

Postimplant Programing

Postimplantation, device programing can impact response to therapy. In 2010, Ellenbogen et al. examined 3 approaches to AV timing intervals. The 980 patients enrolled were randomized to either a fixed AV delay of 120 ms, echocardiographically optimized AV delays, or an algorithm designed to optimize AV delays based upon the initial AV interval and QRS duration. The primary end point of this trial was LV end systolic volume with secondary end points of NYHA class, Quality of life based upon survey analysis, 6 minute walk distance, LV end-diastolic volume, and ejection fraction. Patients enrolled in the trial had class III to IV CHF based upon NYHA classification, ejection fraction less than or equal to 35%, and QRS duration of more than or equal to 120 ms. Patients in the algorithmic arm had programing performed at randomization (1–14 days postimplantation) and then again at 3 months post reprograming. Unfortunately, this trial demonstrated that there was no difference in setting a fixed AV timing delay of 120 ms, echocardiographic timing of AV-delays, or the algorithmic approach.

While this trial demonstrated no difference in the algorithm based approach with reprograming performed again 3 months postimplantation of the device, the FREEDOM trial was intended to analyze more frequent reprograming of AV delays. This trial, presented only in abstract form, did not demonstrate significant improvements in LV ejection fraction, quality of life, or other echocardiographic parameters. In addition, a number of trials have examined RV and LV timing, and no significant clinical differences have been noted in outcomes. Thus, interest in avoiding RV pacing has evolved.

More recently, attention has been directed to pacing the left ventricle rather than pacing both the right and left ventricle, thus relying on intrinsic depolarization of the RV. Small scale studies have demonstrated that RV function is improved in patients if intrinsic RV conduction is relied upon[36] rather than RV pacing. Furthermore, LV pacing has been demonstrated to have a positive effect on ejection fraction.[37] These data were integrated and applied to a larger population as described by Martin et al.[38] In this study, 522 patients were randomized to conventional echocardiographic optimization of biventricular pacing versus pacing using an algorithm designed to paced the left ventricle when the AV interval is normal, and to pace both ventricles if the AV interval is prolonged. This algorithm periodically assesses conduction and alters pacing based upon the sensed results. Patients enrolled had NYHA Class III or IV symptoms, ejection fraction more than or equal to 35%, and QRS duration more than or equal to 120 ms. There were three primary endpoints. The first was a commonly utilized clinical composite score where patients can be defined as worse, unchanged, or better depending upon death, hospitalization, NYHA class, and other clinical parameters. The second was that the aortic velocity time integral (AoVTI) was greater than 0.82 in both the echo-optimization group and the algorithm group. The third endpoint was to evaluate the safety of dynamic programing adjustment. Patients who had changes in either the AV delay or the ventricle to ventricle delay of greater than 60 ms in a 28 day period were reviewed in an unblinded fashion. The adaptive algorithm was deemed noninferior to echocardiographic programing in terms of clinical composite score. AoVTI in each group was not significantly different in each group, and the programing changes did not exceed 60 ms in the adaptive group in any patient in any month, suggesting safety of this algorithm.

CONCLUSION

Cardiac resynchronization therapy has evolved significantly in the time since this approach to management of patients with heart failure was devised. Approaches to LV pacing, from interventional approaches to coronary sinus lead implantation, endocardial pacing, and His bundle pacing provide physicians and patients with a number of different options to help with resynchronization. Furthermore, for leads that are successfully implanted in the coronary sinus, quadripolar LV leads offer options to lower pacing thresholds and prolong battery life. In nonresponders, MPP provides options for pacing that may help improve symptoms. Imaging techniques that are being pioneered now may help with future approaches to providing synchronization by helping to direct placement of endocardial pacing electrodes.

REFERENCES

1. Curtis AB, Lopera G. CRT Optimization. Don't Forget the Atrium! 2011;4(7) 699-701.
2. Bristow MR, Saxon LA, Boehmer J, et al. Cardiac-Resynchronization Therapy with or without an Implantable Defibrillator in Advanced Chronic Heart Failure. New England J Med. 2004;350(21):2140-50.
3. Cleland JGF, Daubert JC, Erdmann E, et al. The Effect of Cardiac Resynchronization on Morbidity and Mortality in Heart Failure. New England J Med. 2005;352(15):1539-49.
4. Køber L, Thune JJ, Nielsen JC, et al. Defibrillator implantation in patients with nonischemic systolic heart failure. New Engl J Med. 2016;375(13):1221-30.
5. Epstein AE, DiMarco JP, Ellenbogen KA, et al. 2012 ACCF/AHA/HRS Focused Update Incorporated Into the ACCF/AHA/HRS 2008 Guidelines for device-based therapy of cardiac rhythm abnormalities. A Report of the American College of Cardiology Foundation/American Heart Association Task Force on Practice Guidelines and the Heart Rhythm Society. 2013;127(3):e283-352.
6. Russo AM, Stainback RF, Bailey SR, et al. ACCF/HRS/AHA/ASE/HFSA/SCAI/SCCT/SCMR 2013 Appropriate Use Criteria for Implantable Cardioverter-Defibrillators and Cardiac Resynchronization Therapy. A Report of the American College of Cardiology Foundation appropriate use criteria task force, Heart Rhythm Society, American Heart Association, American Society of Echocardiography, Heart Failure Society of America, Society for Cardiovascular Angiography and Interventions, Society of Cardiovascular Computed Tomography, and Society for Cardiovascular Magnetic Resonance. 2013;61(12):1318-68.
7. Ponikowski P, Voors AA, Anker SD, et al. 2016 ESC Guidelines for the diagnosis and treatment of acute and chronic heart failureThe Task Force for the diagnosis and treatment of acute and chronic heart failure of the European Society of Cardiology (ESC)Developed with the special contribution of the Heart Failure Association (HFA) of the ESC. European Heart J. 2016;37(27):2129-200.
8. Epstein AE, DiMarco JP, Ellenbogen KA, et al. ACC/AHA/HRS 2008 Guidelines for Device-Based Therapy of Cardiac Rhythm Abnormalities. A Report of the American College of Cardiology/American Heart Association Task Force on Practice Guidelines (Writing Committee to Revise the ACC/AHA/NASPE 2002 Guideline Update for Implantation of Cardiac Pacemakers and Antiarrhythmia Devices): Developed in Collaboration With the American Association for Thoracic Surgery and Society of Thoracic Surgeons. 2008;117(21):e350-408.
9. Cecilia F, Mihoko K, Raimondo M, et al. Right and left ventricular activation sequence in patients with heart failure and right bundle branch block: A detailed analysis using three-dimensional non-fluoroscopic electroanatomic mapping system. J Cardiovascular Electrophysiol. 2005;16(2):112-9.
10. Chandra R, Zolty R, Palma E. A left hemiblock improves cardiac resynchronization therapy outcomes in patients with a right bundle branch block. Clin Cardiol. 2010;33(2):89-93.
11. Varma N. Left ventricular conduction delays and relation to QRS configuration in patients with left ventricular dysfunction. Am J Cardiol. 2009;103(11):1578-85.
12. Tompkins C, Kutyifa V, McNitt S, et al. Effect on cardiac function of cardiac resynchronization therapy in patients with right bundle branch block (from the Multicenter Automatic Defibrillator Implantation Trial with Cardiac Resynchronization Therapy [MADIT-CRT] trial). Am J Cardiol. 2013;112(4):525-9.
13. Haghjoo M, Bagherzadeh A, Fazelifar AF, et al. Prevalence of mechanical dyssynchrony in heart failure patients with different QRS durations. Pacing Clin Electrophysiol. 2007;30(5):616-22.
14. Bilchick KC, Kamath S, DiMarco JP, et al. Bundle-branch block morphology and other predictors of outcome after cardiac resynchronization therapy in medicare patients. Circulation. 2010;122(20):2022-30.
15. Ruschitzka F, Abraham WT, Singh JP, et al. Cardiac-Resynchronization Therapy in Heart Failure with a Narrow QRS Complex. New Engl J Med. 2013;369(15):1395-405.
16. Varma N, Lappe J, He J, et al. Sex-Specific Response to Cardiac Resynchronization Therapy: Effect of Left Ventricular Size and QRS Duration in Left Bundle Branch Block. JACC: Clin Electrophysiol. 2017;3(8):844-53.
17. Oguz K, Om O, Beytullah C, et al. Adjusting the QRS duration by body mass index for prediction of response to cardiac resynchronization therapy: Does one QRS size fit all? Annals of Noninvasive Electrocardiol. 2016;21(5):450-9.
18. De Pooter J, Kamoen V, El Haddad M, et al. Gender differences in electro-mechanical characteristics of left bundle branch block: Potential implications for selection and response of cardiac resynchronization therapy. Int J Cardiol. 2018;257:84-91.
19. Hcke U, Mertens B, Khidir MJH, et al. Usefulness of the CRT-SCORE for shared decision making in cardiac resynchronization therapy in patients with a left ventricular ejection fraction of ≤35. Am J Cardiol. 2017;120(11):2008-16.
20. Chung ES, Leon AR, Tavazzi L, et al. Results of the predictors of response to CRT (PROSPECT) Trial. Circulation. 2008;117(20):2608-16.
21. Park JH, Negishi K, Grimm RA, P et al. Echocardiographic Predictors of reverse remodeling after cardiac resynchronization therapy and subsequent events. Circulation: Cardiovascular Imaging. 2013;6(6):864-72.
22. Delgado-Montero A, Tayal B, Goda A, et al. Additive Prognostic value of echocardiographic global longitudinal and global circumferential strain to

electrocardiographic criteria in patients with heart failure undergoing cardiac resynchronization therapy. Circ Cardiovasc Imaging. 2016;9(6).

23. Saba S, Marek J, Schwartzman D, et al. Echocardiography-guided left ventricular lead placement for cardiac resynchronization therapy. Circulation: Heart Failure. 2013;6(3):427.
24. Bilchick KC, Kuruvilla S, Hamirani YS, et al. Impact of mechanical activation, scar, and electrical timing on cardiac resynchronization therapy response and clinical outcomes. J Am Col Cardiol. 2014;63(16):1657-66.
25. Eie AA, Cosedis NJ, Kirstein PA, et al. Left ventricular lead performance in cardiac resynchronization therapy: Impact of lead localization and complications. Pac Clin Electrophysiol. 2005;28(6):483-8.
26. van Everdingen WM, Cramer MJ, Doevendans PA, et al. Quadripolar leads in cardiac resynchronization therapy. JACC: Clinical Electrophysiol. 2015;1(4):225-37.
27. Niazi I, Baker J, 2nd, Corbisiero R, et al. Safety and efficacy of multipoint pacing in cardiac resynchronization therapy: The Multi Point Pacing Trial. JACC Clin Electrophysiol. 2017;3(13):1510-8.
28. Gamble JHP, Herring N, Ginks M, et al. Procedural Success of Left ventricular lead placement for cardiac resynchronization therapy: A meta-analysis. JACC: Clin Electrophysiol. 2016;2(1):69-77.
29. Worley SJ, Gohn DC, Pulliam RW. Goose neck snare for LV lead placement in difficult venous anatomy. Pac Clin Electrophysiol. 2009;32(12):1577-81.
30. Shah RV, Lewis EF, Givertz MM. Epicardial left ventricular lead placement for cardiac resynchronization therapy following failed coronary sinus approach. Congestive Heart Fail. 2006;12(6):312-6.
31. Miller AL, Kramer DB, Lewis EF, et al. Event free survival following CRT with surgically implanted LV leads versus standard transvenous approach. Pacing Clin Electrophysiol. 2011;34(4):490-500.
32. Lustgarten DL, Crespo EM, Arkhipova-Jenkins I, et al. His-bundle pacing versus biventricular pacing in cardiac resynchronization therapy patients: A crossover design comparison. Heart Rhythm. 2015;12(7):1548-57.
33. Gamble JHP, Herring N, Ginks M, et al. Endocardial left ventricular pacing for cardiac resynchronization: systematic review and meta-analysis. EP Europace. 2018;20(1):73-81.
34. Strik M, Rademakers LM, van Deursen CJM, et al. Endocardial left ventricular pacing improves cardiac resynchronization therapy in chronic asynchronous infarction and heart failure models. Circulation: Arrhythmia and Electrophysiol. 2012;5(1):191-200.
35. Reddy VY, Miller MA, Neuzil P, et al. Cardiac resynchronization therapy with wireless left ventricular endocardial pacing: The SELECT-LV Study. J Am Coll Cardiol. 2017;69(17):2119-29.
36. Lee KL, Burnes JE, Thomas MJ, et al. Avoidance of right ventricular pacing in Cardiac resynchronization therapy improves right ventricular hemodynamics in heart failure patients. J Cardiovascular Electrophysiol. 2007;18(5):497-504.
37. Thibault B, Ducharme A, Harel F, et al. Left ventricular versus simultaneous biventricular pacing in patients with heart failure and a QRS Complex ≥120 milliseconds. Circulation. 2011;124(25):2874-81.
38. Martin DO, Lemke B, Birnie D, et al. Investigation of a novel algorithm for synchronized left-ventricular pacing and ambulatory optimization of cardiac resynchronization therapy: results of the adaptive CRT trial. Heart Rhythm. 2012;9(11):1807-14.

CRT-D versus CRT-P—What should be the Standard of Care in Nonischemic Cardiomyopathy?

TS Kler, Avinash Verma

INTRODUCTION

There are two ways to interpret the new data that has emerged from the recent trials of patients of cardiac resynchronization in heart failure (HF) due to nonischemic dilated cardiomyopathy (NICM). One and more direct way to look, it will be as further evidence in the series of evidence that addition of implantable cardioverter defibrillator (ICD) therapy in HF patients due to NICM is of little value. However, as with most things in medical research, the result should be interpreted for and hence applied to the specific subset of patient population. That is the second, and the correct way of looking the results of DANISH trial.[1] DANISH trial asked a specific question, i.e., Does adding ICD therapy over and above of Guideline Directed Medical Therapy (GDMT), including cardiac resynchronization therapy (CRT) provide any incremental benefit? The answer was "No". This result cannot, and should not, be generalized to include NICM patients not receiving CRT therapy.

As we can see there are two separate questions about usefulness of ICD in NICM patients.

1. Does ICD therapy provide survival benefit in patients of NICM in current medical era?
2. Does addition of ICD therapy to CRT provide additional survival advantage?

The DANISH investigators wanted answers for the first question. However, by trial design 323 out of 560 (57 7%) patients in control group and 322 out of 556 (57.9%) patients in the ICD group had CRT device implanted. Therefore, by trial design the DANISH study answers the second question.

Hence, one thing should be clear, DANISH study did not provide any evidence to withhold ICD therapy in patients of NICM with narrow QRS. They still qualify for ICD therapy for prevention of sudden cardiac death (SCD). As per current guidelines, ICD should be prescribed to the NICM patients [class 1 recommendation Level of Evidence A as per American College of Cardiology (ACC) and Level of Evidence B as per European Society of Cardiology (ESC)].

Now the question which remains is whether in patients with NICM who are eligible for CRT, does addition of ICD provide any incremental benefit? Let's examine the available body of data.

BURDEN OF SUDDEN CARDIAC DEATH IN NICM

To date, no single randomized trial has demonstrated that ICD implantation for primary prevention has a significant effect on overall mortality in patients with NICM (Table 1), and only the Sudden Cardiac Death in Heart Failure (SCD-HeFT) trial demonstrated a mortality benefit in a group that included both ICM and NICM patients.[2] However, many meta-analysis (Table 2), many of which included the recent DANISH study, have shown that all the studies combined to give an evidence base that ICD is beneficial for primary prevention of SCD in NICM and HF.[2]

Burden of Sudden Cardiac Death in Presence of CRT

Drug therapy, ICD, and CRT are all available modalities to treat HF in present era and to reduce HF symptoms and risk of SCD. Each treatment given according to GDMT reduces all-cause mortality by approximately 15–35%. However, the mortality reduction, by guideline-directed medical therapy (GDMT) and HF devices, varies for different modes of death. ICD is a very specific therapy which provides protection only against SCD in HF patients. Unlike CRT, it does nothing to the disease progression, symptoms, and deaths related to pump failure.

Cardiac resynchronization therapy on the other hand has more profound effect on HF disease progression. It works by remodeling the heart and in effect it can potentially lift the patient out of high-risk with low ejection fraction (EF) bracket to the low risk with higher EF category. It has been postulated that by this disease modifying and remodeling effects, CRT

TABLE 1: Randomized control trials on primary prevention implantable cardioverter defibrillator in nonischemic dilated cardiomyopathy patients

Study year published	Total no. of patients, N (ICD/MT)	Follow-up period (years)	Inclusion criteria	Design of the study	Death from any cause with event rate
CAT 2002[3]	104 (50/54)	1.9	NICM EF ≤30% NYHA II–III	ICD vs. medical therapy	Early termination of the study
AMIOVIRT 2003[4]	103 (51/52)	2	NICM EF ≤35% NYHA I–III NSVT	ICD vs. medical therapy	Early termination of the study
DEFINITE 2004[5]	458 (229/229)	2.4	NICM EF <36% NYHA I–III PVCs or NSVT	ICD vs. medical therapy	• ICD: 12.2% • Medical therapy: 17.4% • HR, 0.65 • 95% CI, 0.40–1.06 • p = 0.08
SCD-HeFT 2005[6]	1211 (398/394/419) (NICM subgroup)	3.8 (median)	ICM or NICM EF ≤35% NYHA II–III	ICD vs. amiodarone vs. medical therapy	• ICD: 21.4% • Medical therapy: 27.9% • HR, 0.73 • 95% CI, 0.50–1.07 • p = 0.06
COMPANION 2004[7]	397 (270/127) (NICM subgroup)	1.3 (median)	ICM or NICM	CRT-ICD vs. CRT vs. medical therapy	• HR, 0.50 in favor if CRT-ICD group in NICM patients • 95% CI: 0.29–0.88 • p = 0.015 • CRT-ICD vs. CRT only: • p = 0.12
DANISH 2016[1]	1116 (556/560)	5.6 (median)	NICM EF ≤35% NYHA II–III NYHA IV if CRT NT-pro-BNP >200	ICD vs. medical therapy including CRT	• ICD: 21.6% • Medical therapy: 23.4% • HR, 0.87 • 95% CI, 0.68–1.12 • p = 0.28

CI, confidence interval; CRT, cardiac resynchronization therapy; EF, ejection fraction; HR, hazard ratio; ICD, implantable cardioverter defibrillator; MT, medical therapy; NICM, nonischemic dilated cardiomyopathy; ICM, ischemic cardiomyopathy; NT-proBNP, N-terminal prohormone of brain natriuretic peptide; NVST, nonsustained ventricular tachycardia; NYHA, New York Heart Association; PVCs, premature ventricular contractions.

may also reduce risk of malignant ventricular arrhythmias. At 12-month follow-up in MADIT-CRT, 85% of the patients with CRT had left ventricular ejection fraction (LVEF) greater than 35% with significantly lower risk of ventricular arrhythmias compared to those with EF less than 35%.[17]

The CARE-HF (Cardiac Resynchronization-Heart Failure) extension phase study also suggested that CRT pacing, without an ICD function, could reduce the rate of sudden death [54 vs. 32 or 4.3% vs. 2.5% per annum; hazard ratio (HR) 0.54, 95% confidence interval (CI): 0.35–0.84, p = 0.005].[18] Similarly in the COMPANION study, the mortality with CRT alone vs a CRT defibrillator was similar after 2 years of follow-up.[7]

It can thus be inferred that the ability of CRT to reduce sudden death is probably delayed and possibly dependent on improvements in cardiac function and positive ventricular remodeling. Therefore, the inclusion of CRT patients in a study evaluating the impact of ICDs on mortality and SCD may impact the potential benefit of ICD therapy.

CRT-D IN NICM—LACK OF BENEFIT IS CONSISTENT

In an observational study by Martens et al, during a mean follow-up of 38 ± 22 months, five patients with cardiac resynchronization therapy pacemaker (CRT-P) (1.4%) experienced an episode of ventricular tachycardia with syncope whereas in patients with primary prevention cardiac resynchronization therapy defibrillator (CRT-D) with a nonischemic etiology the rate of appropriate therapy was 3.5% per patient year.[19] In comparison in the same study, the patient's primary prevention CRT-D with an ischemic etiology the rate of appropriate therapy was 6.7% per patient year.[19]

This observation of less arrhythmia burden in NICM as compared to ICM in equally diseased heart is very important and is a consistent observation. In an interesting study, Shadman et al. found a higher risk for SCD in patients with ICM in their proportional hazards model.[20]

TABLE 2: Recent systematic reviews and meta-analysis of implantable cardioverter defibrillator for primary prevention in nonischemic dilated cardiomyopathy

Study year	No. of trials	Total no. of patients (ICD/MT)	Primary end-point all-cause mortality (in favor of ICD arm)	Sudden death	Summary
Al-Khatib et al. 2017[8]	4 (CAT, DEFINITE, SCD-HeFT, DANISH)	1874(937/937)	HR, 0.75 95% CI 0.61–0.93 p = 0.008	N/A	Primary prevention ICDs are efficacious in reducing all-cause mortality in NICM
Narayanan et al. 2017[9]	6 (CAT, AMIOVIRT, DEFINITE, SCD-HeFT, COMPANION, DANISH)	2347(962/1385)	RR, 0.76 95% CI 0.63–0.91; p = 0.003	RR, 0.27 95% CI 0.15–0.50 p <0.001	ICDs associated with 24% reduction in all-cause mortality and 73% reduction in SCD in non- CRT patients
Golwala et al. 2017[10]	6 (CAT, AMIOVIRT, DEFINITE, SCD- HeFT, COMPANION, DANISH)	2970	HR, 0.77 95% CI 0.64–91	N/A	Meta-analysis of all published RCTs to date shows significant clinical benefit on primary prevention ICDs on all-cause mortality in patients with NICM
Kołodziejczak et al. 2017[11]	5 (CAT, AMIOVIRT, DEFINITE, SCD- HeFT, DANISH)	2992(1284/1708)	HR, 0.81 95% CI 0.72–0.91 p = 0.006	HR, 0.44 95% CI, 0.17–1.12 p = 0.064	ICD therapy associated with statistically significant reduction in all-cause mortality along with numerical trend in the same direction in case of sudden death
Barakat et al. 2017[12]	5 (CAT, AMIOVIRT, DEFINITE, SCD-HeFT, DANISH)	2573(1284/1289)	HR, 0.79 95% CI 0.64–0.93 p <0.001	RR, 0.47% 95% CI, 0.30–0.73 p = 0.001	Primary prevention ICD is associated with significant reduction in all-cause mortality in NICM patients
Stavrakis et al. 2017[13]	6 (CAT, AMIOVIRT, DEFINITE, SCD-HeFT, COMPANION, DANISH)	2967 (1553/1414)	HR, 0.78 95% CI, 0.66–0.92 p = 0.003	N/A	Primary prevention ICD is associated with 22% significant reduction in all-cause mortality in NICM patients
Romero et al. 2017[14]	5 (CAT, AMIOVIRT, DEFINITE, SCD-HeFT, DANISH)	2573	RR, 0.84 95% CI, 0.71–0.99 p = 0.03	RR, 0.47 95% CI, 0.30–0.73 p <0.001	Primary prevention ICD significantly reduced all-cause mortality and SCD in patients with NICM
Akel et al. 2017[15]	5 (CAT, AMIOVIRT, DEFINITE, SCD-HeFT, DANISH)	2573	HR, 0.80 95% CI, 0.67–0.96 p = 0.02	HR, 0.51 95% CI, 0.34–0.76 p = 0.001	ICD therapy beneficial in terms of all-cause mortality in certain subgroups of patients with NICM
Masri et al. 2017[16]	5 (CAT, DEFINITE, SCD-HeFT, COMPANION, DANISH)	2867 (1503/1364)	HR, 0.76 95% CI, 0.64–0.91 p = 0.002	RR, 0.40 95% CI, 0.18–0.90 p = 0.03	ICD therapy reduces all-cause mortality and SCD in patients with NICM

CI, confidence interval; HR, hazard ratio; ICD, implantable cardioverter defibrillator; RCT, randomized controlled trials; SCD, sudden cardiac death ; MT, medical therapy; NICM, nonischemic dilated cardiomyopathy RR, relative risk.

Source: Adapted from Ganga HV, Maan A, Kevin Heist E. Should Primary Prevention ICDs Still Be Placed in Patients with Non-ischemic Cardiomyopathy? A Review of the Evidence. Curr Cardiol Rep. 2018;20(5):31.

In a 2017 large observational study in Europe Barra et al.[21] after a mean follow-up period of 41.4 ± 29.0 months, in patients with NICM no difference in survival was observed when receiving CRT with a defibrillator compared with those who received CRT without a defibrillator (HR for mortality adjusted on propensity score and all mortality predictors: 0.92; 95% CI: 0.73–1.16; p = 0.49). Compared with recipients of defibrillators, the excess mortality in patients who did not receive defibrillators was related to SCD in 8.0% among those with ICM but in only 0.4% of those with NICM.[21] Similarly, in a study of 1,122 patients Kutyifa et al. reported there was no mortality benefit of CRT-D over CRT-P in NICM patients (HR 0.98; 95% CI: 0.73–1.32; p = 0.894, interaction p value = 0.15).[22]

Other putative reason for lack of benefit of CRT-D over CRT-P in NICM as compared to ICM may be that NICM are better responders to CRT than ICM. MADIT-CRT and CARE-HF both showed that NICM were more favorable responders to CRT.[23] In their review article Yokoshiki et al. have shown

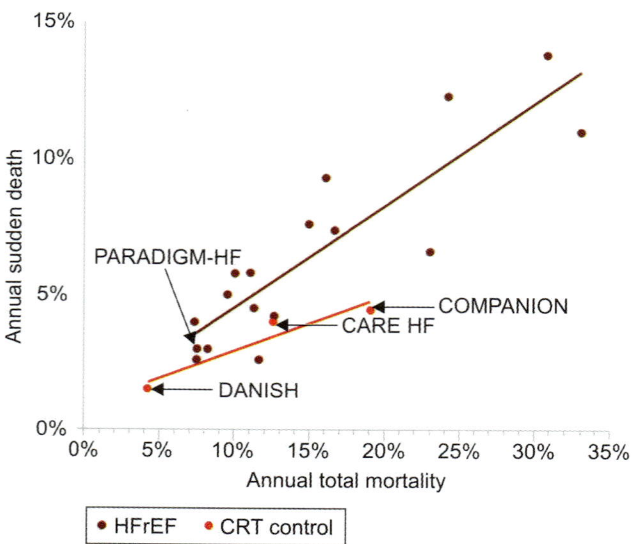

CRT, cardiac resynchronization therapy; HF, heart failure; HRrEF, heart failure with preserved ejection fraction.

FIG. 1: Annual sudden cardiac death rate versus total annual mortality in large heart failure trials.

Source: Adapted from Levy WC. Should Nonischemic CRT Candidates Receive CRT-P or CRT-D? J Am Coll Cardiol. 2017;69(13):1679-82.

that magnitude of favorable response in reverse remodeling was inversely correlated with the additional benefit which a patient will derive from addition of an ICD.[23] As the reverse remodeling is more with NICM patients, hence additional benefit of ICD is difficult to prove.

IS THE TRAIL DESIGN AT FAULT?

Wayne Levy in his editorial proposed that the differential response of ICD in the trials may be due to the proportion of sudden death; the ICD has a greater benefit when the proportion of sudden death is high (>50%), and CRT has greater benefit when the proportion of sudden death is low (<50%).[24] If large HF trials are examined, approximately 40% of all deaths are sudden, and approximately 50–60% of these may be preventable with the addition of an ICD. However, in CRT-P trials, sudden death is only 23–32% in the control subjects, and it was only 35% of all deaths in the DANISH trial. This lower proportion of sudden death diminishes the ICD benefit, because the residual sudden death rate approaches the 20% residual proportion of sudden death seen in patients with CRT-Ds and ICDs.[24]

Similarly, DANISH trail by design included 58% CRT patients in both control and ICD arm. Presence of CRT in both arms combined with lower proportional event rate of SCD in both the arms may have led to the lack of expected benefit of ICD in the study.

SO WHICH NICM PATIENT NEEDS ICD OR CRT-D?

That might be a more pertinent question to ask. It has been shown that not all NICM are same and that their risk for malignant arrhythmias are different, and possibly can be risk stratified accordingly for the need of ICD.

Most of the clinical outcome studies of ICDs in NICM, including DANISH,[1,3-5] have defined NICM based on findings from echocardiography, and had no imaging modalities, to provide tissue characterization. LV midwall fibrosis (MWF) is a type of myocardial scar found in approximately 30% of patients with NICM.[25] Gulati et al. in their study reported a death rate of 26.8% in patients with MWF versus death rate of 10.6% in patients without fibrosis [HR 2.96 (95% CI, 1.87–4.69); absolute risk difference, 16.2% (95% CI, 8.2%–24.2%); p < 0.001] during a median follow-up of 5.3 years (2,557 patient-years of follow-up).[26] The arrhythmic composite was reached by 42 patients with fibrosis (29.6%) and 23 patients without fibrosis (7.0%) [HR, 5.24; (95% CI, 3.15–8.72); absolute risk difference, 22.6% (95% CI, 14.6%–30.6%); p < .001].[26]

The association between late gadolinium enhancement (LGE) on CMR (suggestive of MWF) and ventricular arrhythmias or SCD in patients with NICM was studied in a systemic review and meta-analysis by Andrea Di Marco et al.[27] 29 studies were included, accounting for 2,948 patients. LGE was significantly associated with the arrhythmic endpoint both in the overall population (odds ratio: 4.3; p <0.001). The association between LGE and the arrhythmic endpoint remained significant among studies with mean LVEF more than 35% (odds ratio: 5.2; p <0.001) and was maximal in studies that included only patients with primary prevention ICDs (odds ratio: 7.8; p = 0.008).[27]

It can thus be inferred that presence of ICD with CRT will affect the clinical outcomes if case selection was done by screening for MWF. This hypothesis was tested in a study by Levya et al.[25] The study showed that in the +MWF and –MWF groups CRT-D was associated with lower total mortality (HR: 0.23; 95% CI: 0.07–0.75), than CRT-P in +MWF, but not in –MWF. Also compared with –MWF, +MWF was associated with a 3.75-fold higher risk for SCD and a 2.6-fold higher risk for the combined endpoint of SCD or hospitalization for ventricular arrhythmias.

Apart from the arrhythmic substrate, patient demographics and disease progression also play a vital role in susceptibility to ventricular arrhythmias and SCD. Wayne C Levy[24] has given an elegant metric for favorable response to ICD. ICDs (CRT-Ds vs. CRT-Ps) provide the greatest benefit in patients with the following:[24]

- High proportion of sudden death (>35%)
- Sudden death rate ≥1.2%/year (≥6% over 5 years), and
- Annual mortality of ≤25% (3-year mean survival).

Age does matter: A study of survival benefit of the primary prevention ICD among older patients (including ICM patients) by Hess et al. reported that the survival benefit of the ICD exists but is attenuated with increasing age.[28] Similar trend was reported by the DANISH trial where the investigators found that in the subgroup of patients who were younger than 68 years of age, the rate of death from any cause was significantly lower in the ICD group than in the control group (HR, 0.64; 95% CI, 0.45–0.90; p = 0.01).[1]

CONCLUSION

Based on all the above evidence we can come to a reasonable conclusion about whom to give CRT-D in NICM. Routine use of CRT-D for primary prevention of SCD in elderly NICM patient with low expected survivability has not been proven effective and should not be done. Younger patients of NICM, particularly those having LV midwall fibrosis should be given benefit of SCD prevention by ICD or CRT-D.

REFERENCES

1. Kober L, Thune JJ, Nielsen JC, et al. Defibrillator Implantation in Patients with Nonischemic Systolic Heart Failure. N Engl J Med. 2016;375(13):1221-30.
2. Ganga HV, Maan A, Kevin Heist E. Should Primary Prevention ICDs Still Be Placed in Patients with Non-ischemic Cardiomyopathy? A Review of the Evidence. Curr Cardiol Rep. 2018;20(5):31.
3. Bansch D, Antz M, Boczor S, et al. Primary prevention of sudden cardiac death in idiopathic dilated cardiomyopathy: the Cardiomyopathy Trial (CAT). Circulation. 2002;105(12):1453-8.
4. Strickberger SA, Hummel JD, Bartlett TG, et al. Amiodarone versus implantable cardioverter-defibrillator:randomized trial in patients with nonischemic dilated cardiomyopathy and asymptomatic nonsustained ventricular tachycardia--AMIOVIRT. J Am Coll Cardiol. 2003;41(10):1707-12.
5. Kadish A, Dyer A, Daubert JP, et al. Prophylactic defibrillator implantation in patients with nonischemic dilated cardiomyopathy. N Engl J Med. 2004;350(21):2151-8.
6. Bardy GH, Lee KL, Mark DB, et al. Amiodarone or an implantable cardioverter-defibrillator for congestive heart failure. N Engl J Med. 2005;352(3):225-37.
7. Bristow MR, Saxon LA, Boehmer J, et al. Cardiac-resynchronization therapy with or without an implantable defibrillator in advanced chronic heart failure. N Engl J Med. 2004;350(21):2140-50.
8. Al-Khatib SM, Fonarow GC, Joglar JA, et al. Primary prevention implantable cardioverter defibrillators in patients with nonischemic cardiomyopathy: A Meta-analysis. JAMA Cardiol. 2017;2(6):685-8.
9. Anantha Narayanan M, Vakil K, Reddy YN, et al. Efficacy of Implantable cardioverter-defibrillator therapy in patients with nonischemic cardiomyopathy: A systematic review and meta-analysis of randomized controlled trials. JACC Clin Electrophysiol. 2017;3(9):962-70.
10. Golwala H, Bajaj NS, Arora G, et al. Implantable cardioverter-defibrillator for nonischemic cardiomyopathy: An updated meta-analysis. Circulation. 2017;135(2):201-3.
11. Kolodziejczak M, Andreotti F, Kowalewski M, et al. Implantable cardioverter-defibrillators for primary prevention in patients with ischemic or nonischemic cardiomyopathy: A systematic review and meta-analysis. Ann Intern Med. 2017;167(2):103-11.
12. Barakat AF, Saad M, Elgendy AY, et al. Primary prevention implantable cardioverter defibrillator in patients with non-ischaemic cardiomyopathy: a meta-analysis of randomised controlled trials. BMJ Open. 2017;7(6):e016352.
13. Stavrakis S, Asad Z, Reynolds D. Implantable cardioverter defibrillators for primary prevention of mortality in patients with nonischemic cardiomyopathy: A Meta-Analysis of Randomized Controlled Trials. J Cardiovasc Electrophysiol. 2017;28(6):659-65.
14. Romero J, Chaudhary R, Garg J, et al. Role of implantable cardioverter defibrillator in non-ischemic cardiomyopathy: a systematic review and meta-analysis of prospective randomized clinical trials. J Interv Card Electrophysiol. 2017;49(3):263-70.
15. Akel T, Lafferty J. Implantable cardioverter defibrillators for primary prevention in patients with nonischemic cardiomyopathy: A systematic review and meta-analysis. Cardiovasc Ther. 2017;35(3).
16. Masri A, Hammadah M, Adelstein E, et al. Implantable cardioverter defibrillator in non-ischemic cardiomyopathy: a meta-analysis of randomized controlled trials. Cardiovasc Diagn Ther. 2017;7(4):397-404.
17. Breithardt G. MADIT-CRT (Multicenter Automatic Defibrillator Implantation Trial-Cardiac Resynchronization Therapy): cardiac resynchronization therapy towards early management of heart failure. Eur Heart J. 2009;30(21):2551-3.
18. Cleland JG, Daubert JC, Erdmann E, et al. Longer-term effects of cardiac resynchronization therapy on mortality in heart failure [the CArdiac REsynchronization-Heart Failure (CARE-HF) trial extension phase]. Eur Heart J. 2006;27(16):1928-32.
19. Martens P, Verbrugge FH, Nijst P, et al. Incremental benefit of cardiac resynchronisation therapy with versus without a defibrillator. Heart. 2017;103(24):1977-84.
20. Shadman R, Poole JE, Dardas TF, et al. A novel method to predict the proportional risk of sudden cardiac death in heart failure: Derivation of the Seattle Proportional Risk Model. Heart Rhythm. 2015;12(10):2069-77.
21. Barra S, Boveda S, Providencia R, et al. Adding defibrillation therapy to cardiac resynchronization on the basis of the myocardial substrate. J Am Coll Cardiol. 2017;69(13):1669-78.
22. Kutyifa V, Geller L, Bogyi P, et al. Effect of cardiac resynchronization therapy with implantable cardioverter defibrillator versus cardiac resynchronization therapy with pacemaker on mortality in heart failure patients: results of a high-volume, single-centre experience. Eur J Heart Fail. 2014;16(12):1323-30.
23. Yokoshiki H, Mitsuyama H, Watanabe M, et al. Cardiac resynchronization therapy in ischemic and non-ischemic cardiomyopathy. J Arrhythm. 2017;33(5):410-6.
24. Levy WC. Should Nonischemic CRT Candidates Receive CRT-P or CRT-D? J Am Coll Cardiol. 2017;69(13):1679-82.
25. Leyva F, Zegard A, Acquaye E, et al. Outcomes of cardiac resynchronization therapy with or without defibrillation in patients with nonischemic cardiomyopathy. J Am Coll Cardiol. 2017;70(10):1216-27.
26. Gulati A, Jabbour A, Ismail TF, et al. Association of fibrosis with mortality and sudden cardiac death in patients with nonischemic dilated cardiomyopathy. JAMA. 2013;309(9):896-908.
27. Di Marco A, Anguera I, Schmitt M, et al. Late Gadolinium Enhancement and the Risk for Ventricular Arrhythmias or Sudden Death in Dilated Cardiomyopathy: Systematic Review and Meta-Analysis. JACC Heart Fail. 2017;5(1):28-38.
28. Hess PL, Al-Khatib SM, Han JY, et al. Survival benefit of the primary prevention implantable cardioverter-defibrillator among older patients: does age matter? An analysis of pooled data from 5 clinical trials. Circ Cardiovasc Qual Outcomes. 2015;8(2):179-86.

CHAPTER 119

ICD in HFrEF—When are They not Needed?

Rajnish Sardana, Praloy Chakraborty

INTRODUCTION

In the initial era, automatic implantable cardioverter defibrillator (AICD) implantation was primarily considered for secondary prevention of sudden cardiac arrest or hemodynamically unstable ventricular arrhythmias. With time, the concept of primary prevention evolved. Patients with heart failure and reduced ejection fraction (HFrEF, both ischemic and nonischemic) carries substantial risk of sudden cardiac death. Eight large randomized trials have evaluated the use of implantable cardioverter defibrillators (ICDs) in patients at risk of sudden cardiac death due to heart failure (HF) or left ventricular (LV) dysfunction (Table 1). Based on results of these trials, current guidelines (both American[1] and European[2]) consider AICD implantation, in large subset of HFrEF patients, as Class I indication for primary prevention. However, that does not justify AICD implantation in all patients in this group. In certain subsets in this group of patients, AICD implantation is not justified on the basis of evidence-based practice.

EARLY AFTER MYOCARDIAL INFARCTION

The risk of sudden cardiac death (SCD) is highest immediately after acute myocardial infarction (AMI). In the Valsartan in Acute Myocardial Infarction Trial (VALIANT), risk of sudden death was highest in the first 30 days after a myocardial infarction (MI).[3] Multicenter Automatic Defibrillator Implantation Trial II (MADIT-II) trial clearly demonstrated mortality benefit with AICD in patients after acute MI[4] [The study population included patients with an MI >1-month from study entry and an left ventricular ejection fraction (LVEF) ≤0.30]. Looking at the highest risk of SCD in early post MI and benefits of ICD therapy in post-AMI LV dysfunction, it seems that ICD implantation will be beneficial to prevent SCD in immediate post-MI period. However, Defibrillator in Acute Myocardial Infarction Trial (DINAMIT) and IRIS trial failed to demonstrate benefit of ICD implantation within 30–40 days after MI. DINAMIT trial included patients within 6–40 days of AMI. AICD implantation in this group reduced the incidence of arrhythmic death [95% confidence interval (CI) 0.22–0.83; p = 0.009] but the benefit was offset by an increased incidence of nonarrhythmic death; thus, overall survival was not improved.[5] IRIS trial enrolled patients within 1-month of MI and once again there was a 45% lower risk of sudden arrhythmic death in the ICD group. However, this lower risk was offset by a significantly increased risk of nonarrhythmic death (p = 0.001).[6] Evaluation of autopsy records demonstrated that in the 1st month after AMI, 80% of sudden deaths were due to mechanical complications like myocardial rupture and only 20% were attributed due to arrhythmic death.[7] By 1 year, the proportions of sudden deaths due to nonarrhythmia versus arrhythmia causes were equal and over time there appeared to be a very gradual increase in the proportion of sudden deaths due to arrhythmia (approximately 60% at 30 months). Recurrent ICD shocks can result in injury to the myocardium, and that ventricular function can be further impaired as a consequence of backup ventricular pacing, thus increases the nonarrhythmic mortality due to pump failure and cardiogenic shock.[5,6] Analysis of 16,793 patients[8] who were referred to the cardiac catheterization laboratory for acute management of MI, found that a 90-day cardiovascular mortality rate of 9%, out of which 75% of the deaths were due to coronary artery disease (CAD) related nonsudden death, 9% CAD-related sudden death, and 4% due to sudden death not related to CAD.

Aggressive therapy to reduce the risk of sudden cardiac death in the early period after MI directed toward revascularization and improvement in LV function and clinical HF can be a more prudent and effective strategy as compared with early ICD implantation. As per current guidelines implantation of an ICD is not recommended within the first 40 days after the MI. However, ICD implantation in patients within 40 days of AMI is justified in any of following conditions.[11]

TABLE 1: Major randomized controlled trials of AICD in primary prevention in heart failure with reduced ejection fraction

Name of trial	Etiology of heart failure	Early after AMI	Early after revascu-larization	Early after diagnosis of NICM	Specific inclusion criteria	Result
Multicenter Automatic Defibrillator Implantation Trial (MADIT)[10]	Ischemic	No	No	N/A	LVEF <35%, NSVT, inducible nonsuppressible sustained VT/VF at EPS	Mortality benefit with ICD
Coronary Artery Bypass Graft (CABG) Patch Trial[11]	Ischemic	No	Yes	N/A	LVEF ≤0.35, abnormal SAECG, undergoing CABG	No mortality benefit with ICD
Multicenter Unsustained Tachycardia Trial[12]	Ischemic	Yes	Yes	N/A	EF ≤0.40 • NSVT within the last 6 months • ≥4 days post-MI or revascularization	Risk of sudden death reduced in patients with ICDs
Multicenter Automatic Defibrillator Implantation Trial-II (MADIT-II)[4]	ischemic	No	No	N/A	EF ≤0.30 • >1-month after MI • >3 months after revascularization	Mortality benefit with ICD
Defibrillators in Nonischemic Cardiomyopathy Treatment Evaluation (DEFINITE)[13]	Nonischemic	N/A	NA	Yes	EF <36% due to NICM • NYHA Class I–III • NSVT or PVCs	Trend to mortality reduction with ICD (both in recently diagnosed and remote diagnosed patients)
Sudden Cardiac Death in Heart Failure Trial (SCD-HeFT)[14]	Both ischemic and nonischemic	Yes (33 patients)	No	No	EF <35% • NYHA Class II or III	Mortality benefit with ICD
Defibrillator in Acute Myocardial Infarction Trial (DINAMIT)[5]	Acute CAD	Yes	No	N/A	MI past 6–40 days • EF <0.35 • Abnormal HRV	No mortality benefit with ICD (decrease in arrhythmic death but increase in nonarrhythmic death)
Immediate Risk-stratification Improves Survival (IRIS) Study[6]	Acute CAD	Yes	No	N/A	MI in the past 5–31 days and either: • EF ≤40% and initial HR >90 beats/min • NSVT >150 beats/min	No mortality benefit with ICD (decrease in arrhythmic death but increase in nonarrhythmic death)

AICD, automatic implantable cardioverter defibrillator; AMI, acute myocardial infarction; CAD, coronary artery disease; EF, ejection fraction; HRV, heart rate variability; ICD, implantable cardioverter defibrillator; LVEF, left ventricular ejection fraction; MI, myocardial infarction; NICM, nonischemic cardiomyopathy; NSVT, nonsustained ventricular tachycardia; NYHA, New York Heart Association; SAECG, signal-averaged electrocardiography; N/A, not applicable.

1. Presence of sustained (or hemodynamically significant) ventricular tachyarrhythmia more than 48 hours after an MI and in the absence of ongoing ischemia
2. In patients who require nonelective permanent pacing, who also would meet primary prevention criteria for implantation of an ICD, and recovery of LV function is uncertain or not expected
3. Patients presenting with syncope that is thought to be due to ventricular tachyarrhythmia [by clinical history, documented nonsustained ventricular tachycardia (NSVT) or electrophysiological study]
4. In patients who have an ICD that requires elective replacement due to battery depletion (after careful assessment of comorbidities and the current clinical situation).

EARLY AFTER MYOCARDIAL REVASCULARIZATION

Pathophysiological consequences of coronary ischemia is formation of nonviable (dead or scar) as well as ischemic but viable myocardium. The second category is of immense electrophysiological and mechanical importance. This partially damaged myocardium has electrophysiological properties (conduction velocities and refractory periods) different from healthy myocardium and the electrical heterogeneity creates the milieu for generation of reentrant ventricular tachycardia (VT), the commonest cause of SCD in this subset. This ischemic but viable myocardium is dysfunctional at rest contributing to ventricular dysfunction. Contrary to dead myocardium, the physiological derangement of the second group is reversible. Revascularization can lead to complete normalization of electrophysiological as well as mechanical properties of ischemic but viable myocardium although the normalization process is not instant after revascularization and the exact time period is not known. The rationale for waiting after revascularization to implant an ICD is based upon the hypothesis that LV function can improve. As a result of improvement in perfusion in ischemic but viable myocardium, it leads to reduction in life threatening ventricular arrhythmia events. It remains a major challenge to predict those patients who will or will not significantly improve their LV function. Although imaging studies like magnetic resonance imaging (MRI) and positron emission tomography (PET) are supposed to identify the viable myocardium, in a large study, preoperative imaging failed to identify the group of patients who will show benefits after revascularization.[15] None of the primary prevention trial analyzed the benefit of AICD in early period after revascularization. Both multicenter automatic defibrillator implantation trial (MADIT) and MADIT-II trial excluded patients after revascularization. Sudden cardiac death in heart failure trial (SCD-HeFT) made no specific exclusion with respect to the timing of revascularization. However, in SCD-HeFT, the median time from coronary artery bypass graft (CABG) to enrollment was 3.1 years and from percutaneous coronary intervention (PCI) to enrollment was 2.3 years.[14] Early revascularization was permitted in multicenter unsustained tachycardia trial (MUSTT) and CABG Patch trial. CABG Patch trial which randomized patients to ICD therapy or no ICD at the time of CABG, failed to demonstrate any survival benefit with ICD.[11] Although, it is clear that patients with LVEF less than 35% are at high-risk for revascularization procedure (both PCI and CABG)[16,17] and early mortality after revascularization is high in this group, the proportion of arrhythmic death is not clear. In a substudy of MUSTT, patients enrolled within 30 days of CABG had significantly lower rates of arrhythmic events despite other high risk characteristics, than patients not enrolled within 30 days after CABG. Few nonrandomized, retrospective studies, however, have suggested a benefit of ICD implant early after coronary revascularization.[18,19] Based on evidences from primary prevention studies, current guidelines recommend waiting for 90 days after revascularization for implantation of AICD for primary prevention. However, a limitation of these studies was that they analyzed patients several months to years from revascularization and not within 90 days from revascularization. However AICD implantation is justified within 90 days of revascularization in following conditions.[9]

- If secondary prevention criteria is fulfilled (in patient with cardiac arrest or hemodynamically unstable or sustained VT before or after revascularization where the arrhythmia is not related to ischemia
- Patient of nonelective permanent pacing, who would also meet primary prevention criteria for implantation of an ICD, and in whom recovery of LV function is uncertain or not expected
- Patient with syncope that is thought to be due to VT [by clinical history or documented NSVT, or electrophysiologic (EP) study]
- Patient who have been listed for heart transplant or implanted with a ventricular assist device, and who are not within 40 days of an AMI
- In patients who have an ICD that requires elective replacement due to battery depletion (after careful assessment of comorbidities and the current clinical situation).

RECENT ONSET NONISCHEMIC CARDIOMYOPATHY

Natural history of nonischemic cardiomyopathy (NICM) is unpredictable. Before the widespread usage of optimal medical therapy (OMT), 5 years mortality was estimated to be 50%, of which 30% were due to sudden death. However, in the last few decades, remarkable progress took place in the field of pharmacotherapy in HF. Introduction of disease modifying drugs like angiotensin-converting enzyme inhibitor (ACEi), angiotensin receptor blockers (ARBs), β-blocker, mineralocorticoid receptor antagonists (MRA) and angiotensin receptor–neprilysin inhibitors (ARNI) has made a change in the natural history of NICM. The primary challenge is to decide whether to advise ICD implantation in newly diagnosed patient or to try OMT for a specific period. Long term follow-up with OMT was found to reduce mortality and significant improvement in LVEF was documented in more than 50% patients. In 4 year follow-up, 25% of the cohort achieved near normalization of LVEF (>50%) with OMT.[20] In patients with NICM, LVEF has been found to be significant independent risk factor for major arrhythmic events, with each 10% decrease in ejection fraction associated with a 2.3-fold increase in risk.[21] Subgroup analysis in Defibrillators in Nonischemic Cardiomyopathy Treatment Evaluation (DEFINITE) study found similar benefit in AICD implantation regardless of the duration of NICM.[13] It is important to note that patients with potentially reversible causes of cardiomyopathy such as peripartum cardiomyopathy, myocarditis or acute drug-induced cardiomyopathy were excluded from the study. Although studies have included different electrocardiography (ECG), biopsy,[20] and MRI criteria,[22] it is difficult to separate patients who will have improvement in LVEF on initial OMT, from those patients with irreversible or progressive LV dysfunction. Genetic testing can also play a role in risk stratification of patients with NICM. Preliminary studies suggest that NICM due to LMNA, TNNT2, SGCD, RBM20, and CHRM2 mutations can be at higher risk of sudden cardiac death.[23-25] Patients with cardiac sarcoidosis and LVEF less than 0.30 are unlikely to improve with medical therapy.[26] Giant cell myocarditis is a rare cause of myocarditis characterized by large multinucleated cells, has an extremely virulent course that does not respond to therapy.[27]

Taken together, the published literature suggests that significant number of newly diagnosed NICM patients will have improvement in LVEF with OMT. The current guideline supports that for all patients with NICM, it is imperative that patients be on OMT for HF for at least 3 months before a primary prevention ICD is offered. The clinician must carefully evaluate those patients with relatively recent onset NICM and early AICD implantation can be useful in selected patients with NICM who are unlikely to have recovery of LV function. An early AICD (between 3 and 9 months of diagnosis of NICM) will also be useful for primary prevention in patients with sarcoidosis, giant cell myocarditis or familial cardiomyopathy with a family history of sudden death.[9]

Incessant Ventricular Tachycardia

Automatic implantable cardioverter defibrillator is considered as double-edge sword in patients of HFrEF. An infrequent, appropriate ICD shock aborts sudden cardiac death and is life saving and at the same time repeated shocks (appropriate or inappropriate) is detrimental for the patients. The repeated shocks are painful and increase the psychogenic stress of the patient. At the same time each shock causes myocardial injury and increase in serum troponin level.[28] This transient postshock myocardial dysfunction,[29] complicated by dyssynchrony due to backup pacing is detrimental in patients with already compromised LV function. Shocks, both inappropriate and appropriate, have been associated with increased HF and mortality in this group of patients.[30,31] Keeping in mind the detrimental effect of repeated shocks, AICD should not be implanted in patients with incessant VT. If a patient with AICD has incessant VT, the ICD should be switched-off and appropriate pharmacological or interventional strategy (like catheter ablation) should be taken for the refractory VT.

New York Heart Association Class IV Patients

Mode of death in HF depends on stage of HF. Contrary to early stage, where sudden death is common, in advanced stage the pump failure death is common. On the other hand, shock can increase the HF and mortality in advanced HF. Most of randomized controlled trials (RCTs) in AICD did not include New York Heart Association (NYHA) class IV patients. Ambulatory class IV patients with HF were included in the COMPANION (Comparison of Medical Therapy, Pacing, and Defibrillation in Heart Failure) trial, which showed an overall improved functional status and survival with a cardiac resynchronization therapy (CRT) defibrillator.[32] Unless such a patient is a candidate for CRT or advanced HF therapies such as heart transplantation or a left ventricular assist device (LVAD), an ICD is not expected to meaningfully prolong survival.

Patient with Life Expectancy More Than 1 Year

Economic outcomes of ICD implantation for primary prevention of SCD were assessed in MADIT-I,[10] MADIT-II,[4] and SCD-HeFT.[14] All studies reported increased survival and life expectancy and higher lifetime costs of medical care with an ICD than without an ICD. The incremental cost-effectiveness ratios were generally less than $50,000 per year of life added by an ICD, which provides high value according to the benchmarks adopted for the current guideline.[30] The value provided by an ICD was consistently high when life expectancy was projected to increase by more than 1.4 years.[31]

On the other hand the survival benefit with ICD is not instant. In MADIT II[4] trial, the benefit did not become evident until approximately 9 months after device implantation. Similarly, separation of the survival curves in SCD-HeFT was also observed 12–15 months after device implantation.[14] Considering the economic outcomes and survival benefit curve, patients with serious comorbidities associated with a survival of less than 1-year are generally not considered ICD candidates. Since, its introduction before more than 30 years ago, the ICD has evolved to a widely accepted and important treatment for patients with cardiovascular disease who are at risk of life threatening ventricular arrhythmias. However, the device is not free of complications and is expensive. Cardiologists must continue to refine their understanding of who benefits from ICD implantation and how to optimally implement ICD therapy in these patients.

CONCLUSION

Since its introduction before more than 40 years ago, the ICD has evolved to a widely accepted and important treatment for patients with cardiovascular disease who are at risk of life threatening ventricular arrhythmias. However, the device is not free of complications and is expensive. Cardiologists must continue to refine their understanding of who benefits from ICD implantation and how to optimally implement ICD therapy in these patients.

REFERENCES

1. Al-khatib SM, Stevenson WG, Ackerman MJ, et al. 2017 AHA/ACC/HRS Guideline for management of patients with ventricular arrhythmias and the prevention of sudden cardiac death: Executive summary: A report of the American College of Cardiology/American Heart Association Task Force on Clinical Practice Guidelines and the Heart Rhythm Society. Heart Rhythm. 2017.
2. Priori SG, Blomström-Lundqvist C, Mazzanti A, et al. 2015 ESC Guidelines for the management of patients with ventricular arrhythmias and the prevention of sudden cardiac death: The Task Force for the Management of Patients with Ventricular Arrhythmias and the Prevention of Sudden Cardiac Death of the European Society of Cardiology (ESC).Endorsed by: Association for European Paediatric and Congenital Cardiology(AEPC). Eur Heart J. 2015;36(41):2793-867.
3. Solomon SD, Zelenkofske S, McMurray JJ, et al. for the Valsartan in Acute Myocardial Infarction Trial (VALIANT) Investigators. Sudden death in patients with myocardial infarction and left ventricular dysfunction, heart failure, or both. N Engl J Med. 2005;352:2581-8.
4. Moss AJ, Zareba W, Hall WJ, et al. Prophylactic implantation of a defibrillator in patients with myocardial infarction and reduced ejection fraction. N Engl J Med. 2002;346:877-83.
5. Hohnloser SH, Kuck KH, Dorian P, et al. for the DINAMIT Investigators. Prophylactic use of an implantable cardioverter-defbrillator after acute myocardial infarction. N Engl J Med. 2004;351:2481-8.
6. Steinbeck G, Andresen D, Seidl K, et al. for the IRIS Investigators. Defbrillator implantation early after myocardial infarction. N Engl J Med. 2009;361:1427-36.
7. Pouleur AC, Barkoudah E, Uno H, et al. for the VALIANT Investigators. Pathogenesis of sudden unexpected death in a clinical trial of patients with

myocardial infarction and left ventricular dysfunction, heart failure, or both. Circulation. 2010;122:597-602.
8. Bunch TJ, May HT, Bair TL, et al. Trends in early and late mortality in patients undergoing coronary catheterization for myocardial infarction: implications on observation periods and risk factors to determine ICD candidacy. Heart Rhythm. 2011;8:1460-6.
9. Kusumoto FM, Calkins H, Boehmer J, et al. HRS/ACC/AHA expert consensus statement on the use of implantable cardioverter-defibrillator therapy in patients who are not included or not well represented in clinical trials. Circulation. 2014;130(1):94-125.
10. Moss AJ, Hall WJ, Cannom DS, et al. Improved survival with an implanted defibrillator in patients with coronary disease at high risk for ventricular arrhythmia. Multicenter Automatic Defbrillator Implantation Trial Investigators. N Engl J Med. 1996;335:1933-40.
11. Bigger JT, Jr. Prophylactic use of implanted cardiac defbrillators in patients at high risk for ventricular arrhythmias after coronary-artery bypass graft surgery. Coronary Artery Bypass Graft (CABG) Patch Trial Investigators. N Engl J Med. 1997;337:1569-75.
12. Buxton AE, Lee KL, Fisher JD, et al. A randomized study of the prevention of sudden death in patients with coronary artery disease. Multicenter Unsustained Tachycardia Trial Investigators. N Engl J Med. 1999;341:1882-90.
13. Kadish A, Dyer A, Daubert JP, et al. for the Defbrillators in Non-Ischemic Cardiomyopathy Treatment Evaluation (DEFINITE) Investigators. Prophylactic defbrillator implantation in patients with nonischemic dilated cardiomyopathy. N Engl J Med. 2004;350:215-8.
14. Bardy GH, Lee KL, Mark DB, et al. for the Sudden Cardiac Death in Heart Failure Trial (SCD-HeFT) Investigators. Amiodarone or an implantable cardioverter-defbrillator for congestive heart failure. N Engl J Med. 2005;352:225-37.
15. Bonow RO, Maurer G, Lee KL, et al. Myocardial viability and survival in ischemic left ventricular dysfunction. N Engl J Med. 2011;364:1617-25.
16. Shahian DM, O'Brien SM, Sheng S, et al. Predictors of long-term survival after coronary artery bypass grafting surgery: results from the society of thoracic surgeons adult cardiac surgery database (the ASCERT study). Circulation. 2012;125:1491-500.
17. Weintraub WS, Grau-Sepulveda MV, Weiss JM, et al. Prediction of long-term mortality after percutaneous coronary intervention in older adults: results from the national cardiovascular data registry. Circulation. 2012;125:1501-10.
18. Bolad I, MacLellan C, Karanam S, et al. Effectiveness of early implantation of cardioverter defbrillator for postoperative ventricular tachyarrhythmia. Am J Cardiol. 2004;94:376-8.
19. John JM, Hussein A, Imran N, et al. Underutilization of implantable cardioverter defbrillators post coronary artery bypass grafting in patients with systolic dysfunction. Pacing Clin Electrophysiol. 2010;33:727-33.
20. McNamara DM, Starling RC, Cooper LT, et al. for the IMAC Investigators. Clinical and demographic predictors of outcomes in recent onset dilated cardiomyopathy: results of the IMAC (Intervention in Myocarditis and Acute Cardiomyopathy)-2 study. J Am Coll Cardiol. 2011;58:1112-8.
21. Grimm W, Christ M, Bach J, et al. Noninvasive arrhythmia risk stratification in idiopathic dilated cardiomyopathy: results of the Marburg Cardiomyopathy Study. Circulation. 2003;108:2883-91.
22. Gulati A, Jabbour A, Ismail TF, et al. Association of fibrosis with mortality and sudden cardiac death in patients with nonischemic dilated cardiomyopathy. JAMA. 2013;309:896-908.
23. Ackerman MJ, Priori SG, Willems S, et al. HRS/EHRA expert consensus statement on the state of genetic testing for the channelopathies and cardiomyopathies: this document was developed as a partnership between the Heart Rhythm Society (HRS) and the European Heart Rhythm Association (EHRA). Heart Rhythm. 2011;8:1308-39.
24. Meune C, Van Berlo JH, Anselme F, et al. Primary prevention of sudden death in patients with lamin A/C gene mutations. N Engl J Med. 2006;354:209-10.
25. Brauch KM, Karst ML, Herron KJ, et al. Mutations in ribonucleic acid binding protein gene cause familial dilated cardiomyopathy. J Am Coll Cardiol. 2009;54:930-41.
26. Yazaki Y, Isobe M, Hiramitsu S, et al. Comparison of clinical features and prognosis of cardiac sarcoidosis and idiopathic dilated cardiomyopathy. Am J Cardiol. 1998;82:537-40.
27. Kandolin R, Lehtonen J, Kupari M. Cardiac sarcoidosis and giant cell myocarditis as causes of atrioventricular block in young and middle-aged adults. Circ Arrhythm Electrophysiol. 2011;4:303-9.
28. Hasdemir C, Shah N, Rao AP, et al. Analysis of troponin I levels after spontaneous implantable cardioverter defibrillator shocks. J Cardiovasc Electrophysiol. 2002;13(2):144-50.
29. Xie J, Weil MH, Sun S, et al. High-energy defibrillation increases the severity of postresuscitation myocardial dysfunction. Circulation. 1997;96(2):683-8.
30. Anderson JL, Heidenreich PA, Barnett PG, et al. ACC/AHA statement on cost/value methodology in clinical practice guidelines and performance measures: a report of the American College of Cardiology/American Heart Association Task Force on Performance Measures and Task Force on Practice Guidelines. Circulation. 2014;129:2329-45.
31. Sanders GD, Hlatky MA, Owens DK. Cost-effectiveness of implantable cardioverter-defibrillators. N Engl J Med. 2005;353(14):1471-80.
32. Bristow MR, Saxon LA, Boehmer J, et al. Cardiac-resynchronization therapy with or without an implantable defibrillator in advanced chronic heart failure. N Engl J Med. 2004;350:2140-50

CHAPTER **120**

Leadless Pacemakers: Current Review and Future Directions

Vanita Arora

INTRODUCTION

Bradyarrhythmia with symptoms is a clinical condition which affects millions of people worldwide. Patients with symptomatic bradycardia are eligible to get a pacemaker implanted but an estimated 1.5 million pacemakers are implanted annually worldwide.[1] The increasing usage of these novel devices has led to proper diagnosis and improvement in the quality of lives of bradycardia patients.[2] In addition, the latest technological achievements in the field of pacing, which are related to battery longevity and miniaturization, device software and programming, lead performance, remote monitoring systems, and implantation techniques, have transformed pacing into an extremely reliable and safe therapy.

POTENTIAL COMPLICATIONS WITH CONVENTIONAL PACING SYSTEM

Although conventional pacemakers with leads improve the clinical status of patients, the pacing leads have long been considered their Achilles' heel.[3] Some of the early postprocedural complications include micro- or complete dislodgement of lead, perforation of right ventricular (RV) or right atrial (RA) wall, pneumothorax and tamponade. However, chronic lead problems affect in around 10% of cases. These are but not limited to conditions such as thrombosis in the venous access, superior vena cava (SVC) block, severe tricuspid regurgitation (TR), and infections which occur at a rate of 1–2% and often require a lead extraction procedure which is technically demanding.[5] Overall, the rate of periprocedural and early postprocedural complications in cardiac pacing therapy is estimated, approximately, to be 10%. Adoption of strict sterile techniques in electrophysiology (EP) laboratories are not sufficient to contain pacemaker related infections especially pocket infections. The occurrence of the same is a dreaded situation for the patient and the doctor alike. This leads to removal of pulse generator or sometimes the entire assembly which increases the morbidity. The incidence of pacemaker lead fracture is about 1–4%,[5] phenomenon happening due to subclavian crush.

Insulation breach can also be a cause for potential lead failure which leads to pace or sense error and battery longevity (Fig. 1). Leadless cardiac pacemakers (LCPs) can overcome these issues due to absence of leads and no requirement for a surgical pocket. Spickler et al. in 1970 were the first to introduce the concept of LCP.[6] The LCP is an innovative concept which involves the placement of a completely self-contained intracardiac device. Like other innovations usage of LCP also were thought to be possible in humans only when they were successfully studied in animals.[6] In this article, we would review the progress made in the leadless space and analyze the potential use of the same in various arrhythmic disorders.

ANIMAL STUDIES AND TECHNOLOGICAL ADVANCEMENTS

Various animal studies have been conducted to understand the technological advancements.[7-11] Spickler et al. tried implanting the nuclear-powered device in the dog way back in the early 90's but the concept was not commercialized due to battery longevity and safety. Vardas et al. in 1991 tried to pace dog heart (8 dogs) asynchronously with an LCP powered by three 1.5 V battery in 1991; the commercial introduction of this was also not possible.

Spickler et al. and Vardas et al.'s research was ahead of its time, and it was not until 1999 that Goto et al., explored the concept of using an automatic power-generating system (AGS) to power the LCP. The AGS worked on the principle of conversion of kinetic energy into electrical energy like quartz watches. The investigators successfully paced a mongrel dog's heart at 140 beats/min for 60 minutes with a fully charged AGS system.[12] Ultrasound as a power source was later used by Echt et al. in 2006.[13] This later became a viable power source and was accepted in multiple studies.

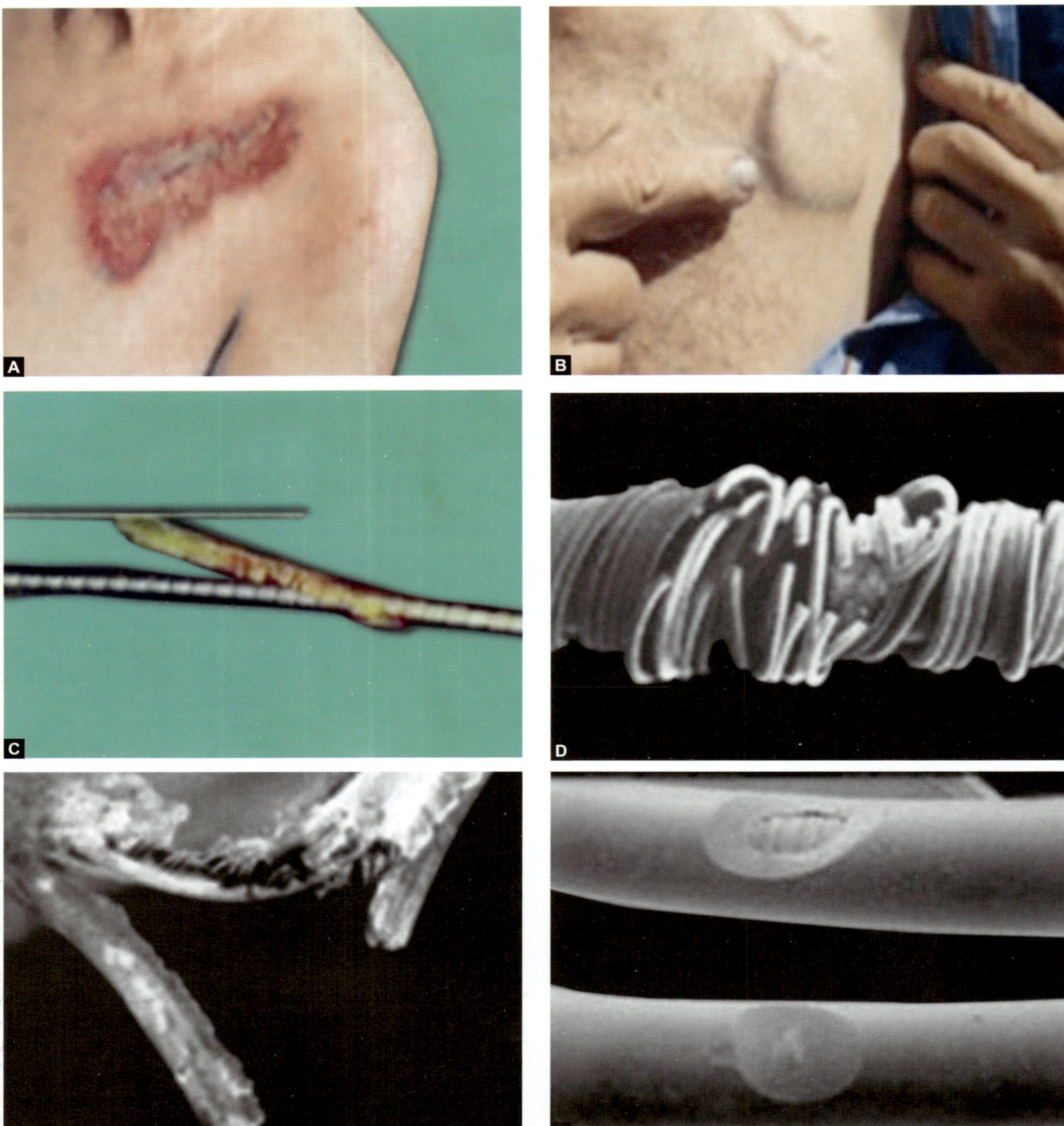

FIG. 1: Postimplant complications affecting transvenous pacing components: (Clockwise from L to R: Pocket infection, Twiddler's Syndrome, insulation Break. Lead Fracture).

CURRENT LEADLESS CARDIAC PACEMAKERS

The new era of miniaturization started with leadless devices and currently there are three companies which are into leadless pacing devices (Table 1). The first is the device called Micra Transcatheter Pacing System (TPS), made by Medtronic Inc., which is the "world's smallest pacemaker" (93% smaller than a conventional pacemaker) with dimensions of just 7 mm in width, 26 mm long and 2 g in weight (Fig. 2). In a postapproval registry, the device was successfully implanted in 792 of 795 patients (99.6%) by

TABLE 1: Comparison of different leadless pacemaker characteristics

	Nanostim wireless pacer	Micra Transcatheter Pacing System	Wireless Cardiac Stimulation system (WCS)
Parent company	Abbott Inc.	Medtronic PLC	EBR Systems
Pacing mode	VVI/VVIR	VVI/VVIR	CRT when used with conventional right ventricle pacer
Battery	Lithium carbon monofluoride	Lithium silver vanadium oxide/ carbon monofluoride (C3H)	Ultrasound transmitter in chest wall with receiver electrode in left ventricle
Device retrieval	Yes	Possible although, rationale is to put another device with coexisting one	Not studied yet
Fixation mechanism	Screw in helix	Self-expanding nitinol tines	Anchor barbs
Human studies	Yes	Yes	Yes
Estimated battery life (company reported)	9–10 years	7–15 years	Not reported

EBR, electronic batch record; VVI, indication for ventricular demand; VVIR, ventricular single-chamber rate-modulated; CRT, cardiac resynchronization therapy.

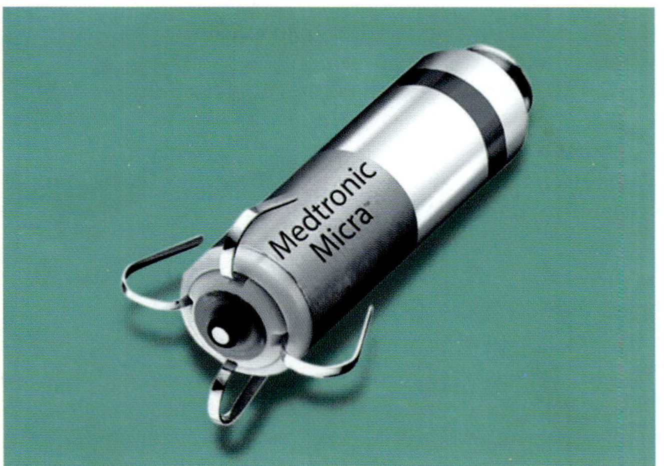

FIG 2: Micra device.

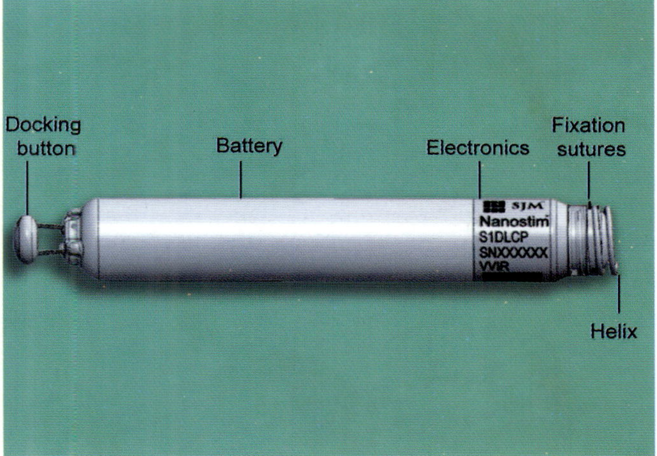

FIG 3: Nanostim device.

149 implanters at 96 centers in 20 countries. Through 30 days post implant, a total of 13 major complications occurred in 12 patients, for a major complication rate of 1.51% (confidence interval, 0.78–2.62%). Major complications included cardiac effusion or perforation (1, 0.13%), device dislodgement (1, 0.13%), and sepsis (1, 0.13%). The rate of major complications in the registry was lower than that of the Investigational Device Exemption (IDE) but after the baseline differences were adjusted (odds ratio, 0.58, 95% confidence interval, 0.27–1.25). The TPS is delivered through a 27-French (Fr) outer diameter catheter the inner diameter of which is 25 Fr through the femoral route. the pacemaker could be repositioned as many number of times as possible. The pacing capture thresholds were low during the study period. The estimated battery life was around 10–12 years. The TPS uses self-expanding nitinol tines to fixate in the trabeculae. At the end of battery life of Micra and other Micra can be implanted in the ventricle, in fact three Micra devices can be accommodated in the ventricle.[14]

Nanostim device is manufactured by Abbott Inc. The device is smaller than a AAA battery and can be directly placed inside the heart through the femoral route approach.

Implantation technique: Nanostim LPS has a screw-in helix. A steroid-eluting disk is located at the center of the helix acts as the cathode, whereas the anode is the uncoated ring of the titanium case (Fig. 3). The Nanostim LPs uses conductive communication via a dedicated programmer, which uses skin leads to apply subliminal 250 kHz pulses for signal transmission and programming. The Nanostim LPs uses a temperature-based sensor for rate control. This LCP which is 4 cm long, 6 mm wide and just 2 g in weight is delivered by an 18 Fr catheter attached to a docking button on the end of the device, which introduces it into the body via the femoral vein and subsequently into the right ventricle. In order to tug on the device after implantation, a tether mode is used. If positioning has to be changed or if it has not been completely fixed the LCP can be unscrewed during the operation. The device has a long battery life of 9–10 years as it uses electrical impulses to communicate rather than the standard antenna and coil system leading to a need for fewer replacements.[15]

After the LEADLESS trial, this LCP was given the CE mark. A Wireless Cardiac Stimulation system for the left ventricle (WiCS-LV) is also being developed by electronic batch record (EBR systems) (Sunnyvale, CA, USA). The system utilizes ultrasound emitted from a transmitter implanted subcutaneously in the left chest and a receiver implanted in the ventricle which converts ultrasound energy to electrical energy that can be used to pace the heart (Fig. 4). In contrast to the aforementioned devices, the WiCS-LV system has been used in cardiac resynchronization therapy (CRT) when used with conventional RV pacers. This results in both ventricles contracting almost simultaneously thus allowing resynchronization. Another added advantage of the EBR system (WiCS-LV) is its capability of endocardial pacing which runs contrary to epicardial pacing seen with conventional CRT devices.

Endocardial pacing may be more physiological and theoretically could improve patients' clinical response to CRT therapy. This hypothesis clearly requires study.

Figure 5 shows evolution of leadless pacemakers from animal studies to past and currently ongoing human studies.[16]

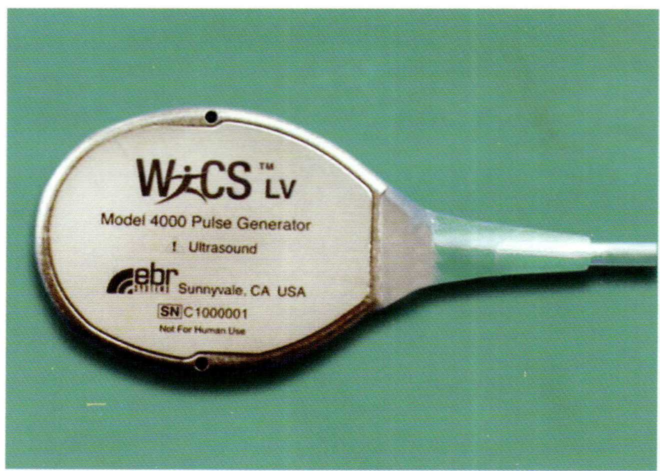

FIG 4: Wireless Cardiac Stimulation system for the left ventricle.

It should be noted that Nanostim from St Jude Medical (now Abbott) is not available commercially while WiCS-LV is not commercially launched in many countries worldwide.

Clinical indications where ventricular single-chamber rate-modulated (VVIR) leadless pacemaker is recommended:

- Symptomatic intermittent or permanent high-grade atrioventricular (AV) block in the presence of atrial fibrillation (AF)
- Symptomatic intermittent or permanent high-grade AV block (AVB) in the absence of AF as an alternative to dual chamber pacing when atrial lead placement is considered difficult, high risk, or not deemed necessary for effective therapy
- Symptomatic tachy-brady syndrome or sinus node dysfunction (SND) (sinus bradycardia or sinus pauses), as an alternative to atrial or dual chamber pacing when atrial lead placement is considered difficult, high risk, or not deemed necessary for effective therapy.

Unique indications for leadless pacemaker:

- Prior device and lead infection
- Vascular access issue (dialysis, subclavian thrombosis)
- Potential Twiddler's syndrome
- Renal failure
- Tricuspid regurgitation probably because of conventional lead implantation.

Comparative Review of Micra IDE Study and Micra Postapproval Registry

In comparison to IDE study patients, significantly fewer patients in the postapproval registry had congestive heart failure, coronary artery disease, hypertension, chronic obstructive pulmonary disease, or AF. A couple of more characteristics at enrolment in patients of the registry were: the mean left ventricular ejection fraction (LVEF) was significantly lower, patients had a cardiac device previously implanted and or did not have any venous access as the

1970: Spickler et al. tested his nuclear powered device in dogs

1991: Vardas et al. used a battery powered leadless pacemaker in dogs

1999: Goto et al, successfully used an automatic power' generating system in his leadless cardiac pacemaker

2006: Echt et al, used ultrasound to power his device

2009: Wieneke et al. used induction technology to power his device

2011: WiSE-CRT trial started using the wireless cardiac stimulation system

2013: Sperzel et al. used his device in sheep successfully to show case of retrieval

2013: Nanostim device received CM mark approval

2013: Medtronic Micra system completed first its first in-man implantation

2014: Reddy et al, published the results of the LEADLESS trials (first human trials)

2015: Ritter et al. published early results from the Micra Transcatheter eter Pacing Study

FIG 5: Evolution timeline diagram.

TABLE 2: Comparative analysis of Micra postapproval and investigational studies

	Micra Transcatheter Pacing System Postapproval	Micra Investigational Device Exemption Study	
Success rate (%)(n/N)	99.6 (792/795)	99.2 (719/725)	–
Procedure duration (min)	–	35 ± 24	–
30-day event rate			
Major complication criterion	**Postapproval (n = 795) no. (patients, %)**	**Investigational (n =726) no. (patients, %)**	**Odds ratio (postapproval vs. investigational) (95% CI)**
Total Major Complications	13 (12, 1.51%)	24 (21, 2.89%)	0.58 (0.27, 1.25)*
Death	1 (1, 0.13%)	1 (1, 0.14%)	0.91 (0.06–14.66)
Hospitalization	4 (4, 0.50%)	9 (8, 1.10%)	0.45 (0.14–1.51)
Prolonged hospitalization	9 (8, 1.01%)	16 (14, 1.93%)	0.52 (0.22–1.24)
System revision	2 (2, 0.25%)	3 (3, 0.41%)	0.61 (0.10–3.65)
Loss of device function	0 (0, 0%)	2 (2, 0.28%)	NE

*Adjusted analyses for baseline characteristics (p <0.16). Unadjusted results were similar (0.52, 95% CI: 0.25–1.05).
CI, confidence interval; NE, not estimable.

later was an exclusion criterion in the IDE study. The major complication rate trended lower in the registry compared with that of the IDE study (1.51% vs. 2.89%; odds ratio, 0.515, 95% CI, 0.251 1.053; p 0.0691), although this did not reach statistical difference. (Table 2). Among the 795 patients in the registry, there were fewer cardiac effusion or perforation major complications, compared with the 726 patients from the IDE study (1 patient, 0.13% vs. 10 patients, 1.38%). The number of major complications related to the groin puncture site was similar in both studies (6 events, 0.75% for the registry vs. 5 events, 0.69% for the IDE study). Though the patient demographics were slightly different between the groups, the implant success rate was similar (99.6%) with a low level of major complications (1.51%). The registry population had less congestive heart failure, coronary artery disease, hypertension, chronic obstructive pulmonary disease, and AF, but a higher percentage of patients had no venous access for a transvenous pacemaker. The outstanding electrical performance of Micra TPS has also been maintained within the registry population, with a 97% implant threshold of 2 V, and 87.2% had a pacing capture threshold 1 V, like what was reported for the IDE study.[17] The average impedance was 721 Ω at implant, and the mean R-wave amplitude was 11.4 mV. Longer term follow-up in the IDE study has shown a trend to improvement of these parameters with time.

Current Challenges

Leadless pacemakers eventually would become the first-choice for treatment of symptomatic bradycardia, but this novel technique offers its own challenges like:

- Learning curve associated to implantation techniques, interpretation of data diagnostics is different for different manufacturers.

The current devices are capable of single chamber pacing and not dual-chamber (DDD) pacing or[1] CRT pacing. The WiCS-LV system is capable of CRT pacing but unfortunately doesn't have a defibrillator.

Although, the promising technology of leadless pacemakers might minimize the lead associated complications, the possibility of new complications such as device dislodgement, late perforation or tamponade, early battery depletion and mechanically induced arrhythmia has yet to be clinically explored.

Optimal management of patients who develop gram-positive bacteremia late after LCP implantation (which represents a class I indication for transvenous lead extraction) remains unknown.[2]

Transfemoral explantation of the device when dense adhesions form at the interface with the endocardium may also prove difficult.

Future Perspectives

The use of single-chamber pacemakers is limited to 14% of pacemaker implantations only.[19] This is largely due to the potential benefits of atrial pacing in patients with SND as well as the recognized benefits of AV synchrony (AVS) in decreasing the incidence of pacemaker syndrome, improving stroke volume, and positively influencing functional status and quality of life in patients with AVB.[20-22] Three clinical trials were conducted to develop and evaluate the performance of a novel downloadable algorithm for the Micra single-chamber ventricular leadless pacemaker, based on intracardiac accelerometer data. The development and performance of this algorithm in successfully achieving AVS in a large proportion of patients with high grade AVB and an implanted Micra device is reported.

HOW THE ALGORITHM FUNCTIONS[3]

Accelerometer signals collected from MASS/MASS 2 (Micra Accelerometer Sensor Sub-Study) patients demonstrated that four distinct segments of cardiac activity were seen in the accelerometer signal. These segments corresponded to isovolumic Q2 contraction and mitral or tricuspid valve closure (A1), aortic or pulmonic valve closure (A2), passive ventricular filling (A3), and atrial contraction (A4). Accelerometer segments corresponding to passive filling and atrial contraction was associated with mitral valve flow E- and A-wave measurements.[3]

Based on these signals, an AV synchronous algorithm was developed to provide a VDD pacing mode. Blanking periods must be manually set to reject signals in the accelerometer originating from the ventricular region as the accelerometer can also sense mitral and aortic valves closure movements. Atrial contraction was detected when the filtered and rectified accelerometer signal exceeded one of two programmable thresholds. There is a high probability that at high sinus rates of >80 bpm, the two ventricular signals can fuse creating a large accelerometer signal hence two programming thresholds should be looked into—a larger passive ventricular filling threshold to detect fused passive ventricular filling or atrial contraction threshold and a lower atrial contraction threshold for detecting the same signal later in diastole. If atrial contraction was detected, an atrial marker (AS) was[3] output via telemetry, and a programmable AV interval was initiated. Because of the electromechanical delay between the electrical p wave and the atrial signal, the accelerometer, the A4 VP was typically programmed to 10 msec. The algorithm incorporated a rate smoothing feature designed to maintain AVS during intermittent atrial under sensing. If an atrial contraction was not detected, a ventricular pace was delivered a programmable rate smoothed interval (typically 100 m) longer than the median Q3 R-R interval.[3]

Clinical Evidence

The purpose of the (MASS/MASS 2) was to characterize the intracardiac accelerometer signals during various patients' activities and to assess the feasibility of sensing atrial contraction through the sensor and these studies were conducted in prospective patients in multiple centers and was nonrandomized. The Micra implanted patients were followed up in an office setting at the end of 12 months from implant. The software was incorporated in these devices and accelerometer signal was collected from all three vectors. The primary endpoint of interest was to measure the atrial contraction amplitude by the accelerometer signal during each cardiac cycle. The mean atrial contraction amplitude which varied across postures and vectors were analyzed for 75 patients. The findings from the MASS/MASS 2 studies were used to develop an AV synchronous pacing algorithm.[3]

The Micra Atrial TRacking Using A Ventricular AccELerometer (MARVEL) study was an acute, prospective, nonrandomized, multicenter clinical feasibility study. The primary aim of MARVEL was to test the feasibility of providing AVS pacing in patients with AVB using the algorithm developed from MASS and MASS 2 studies. Usable Holter recordings from 64 patients enrolled in the MARVEL study were evaluated. Majority of these patients had a second or third degree AVB while 48% had an intrinsic conduction. The AVS percentage was 87%. The AVS percentage age was noticed mostly at rest when the AV algorithm mode was put on (Table 3).

TABLE 3: Baseline and medical history of patients in Micra Atrial TRacking Using a Ventricular AccELerometer

Characteristics	Enrolled (n = 70)	Usable Holter (n = 64)
Age (years):		
Mean ± SD	71.3 ± 15.1	72.0 ± 14.4
Range	24–92	30–92
Female	24 (34)	20 (31)
Months from Micra implant:		
Mean ± SD	11.6 ± 12.3	11.5 ± 12.4
Range	0–41.4	0–41.4
Comorbidities:		
Hypertension	41 (59)	38 (59)
Paroxysmal atrial fibrillation	14 (20)	11 (17)
Diabetes	17 (24)	16 (25)
Coronary artery disease	16 (23)	15 (23)
Chronic obstructive pulmonary disease	5 (7)	5 (8)
Device location:		
Apex	19 (27)	16 (25)
Septum	47 (67)	46 (72)
Right ventricular outflow tract	2 (3)	2 (3)
Not reported	2 (3)	0 (0)
Predominant rhythm during Holter recording:		
Second-/third-degree AVB	NA	33 (52)
Intrinsic AV conduction	–	32 (48)

AVB, atrioventricular block; AV, atrioventricular.

Importance of these Studies

The MARVEL study demonstrated the feasibility of tracking atrial contractions and providing AVS using a mechanical accelerometer-based sensor in the Micra[3] ventricular pacemaker. Specifically, the average AVS percentage at rest was 87%.[3] In patients with high-grade AVB, AVS improved from 37.5 to 80% when comparing VVI versus AV algorithm mode.[3] The presence of the algorithm had no detrimental impact on AVS in patients with intrinsic AV conduction. The achievement of AVS had a significant effect on stroke volume as measured by velocity time integral (VTI)[3] on echocardiography. It was very natural that, SND, premature ventricular complexes and low-amplitude signals contributed to a lack of synchrony,[3] although this was evident in a relatively small number of patients. The study demonstrated that AVS with this algorithm was impacted by activity. With increase in heart rate, the atrial and ventricular signals superimposed on the accelerometer resulting in loss of AVS. The AVS was not impacted by changes in posture while at rest. In this circumstance, it is important to consider that the loss of atrial synchrony is compensated for by an increase in heart rate and ejection fraction during exercise, particularly in patients with preserved left ventricular systolic function.[23] When sensing atrial contraction was difficult a rate smoothing feature takes over so that AVS is maintained; this increased the AVS by 9%.[3] There were no instances of pacemaker-mediated tachycardia or significant interruption in ventricular pacing resulting in symptomatic pauses.[3] The literature and published guidelines support use of single-chamber pacemakers in patients with AVB under certain circumstances.[24] These include infrequent need for pacing, vascular access issues, sedentary patients, and comorbidities likely to impact clinical outcomes.[6] However, this does not preclude the benefit of AVS, if it can be achieved safely in this population of patients.[6] This provides the opportunity for this patient population to benefit from AVS and increased stroke volume, reduction in pacemaker syndrome incidence, and improvement in functional status and quality of life; however, this would require long-term evaluation.[25-27] A limitation of the algorithm could be the loss of AVS with increased levels of activity. However, this may be mitigated by the fact that cardiac output at higher rates has been shown to be more dependent on heart rate than AVS.[27] Thus, rate responsive pacing (i.e., VVIR) may be an adequate option for patients when active. Patients with lower AVS tended to have SND (manifesting primarily as sinus arrhythmia, sinus bradycardia, and sinus tachycardia) or had low-amplitude A4 signals.[3] It is clear that implantation of these devices would not benefit those patients with persisting or permanent atrial arrhythmias; furthermore, the A4 signal during AF will likely be low and not detected, resulting in pacing near the lower rate.[3] Loss of AVS also occurred because of low-amplitude signals measured by the accelerometer.[3] The accelerometer signals can be complex and setting up the algorithm will require knowledge of the cardiac components of the accelerometer signal.

CONCLUSION

There is a paradigm shift in pacing. It is a little early to know if leadless pacing is the future of pacing but it looks very promising from the results.

Curious thoughts:

- Will all pacemakers be leadless soon? Is that what we want?
- VDD will be a programmable option soon and what about DDD version?
- Dual chamber and triple chamber devices, how will they communicate with each other?
- What will be the ideal battery longevity?
- What will be the role of LCP with S/C ICD for postshock pacing and ATP?

The early results from clinical evaluations suggest that leadless pacing could gain wider adoption.Whether leadless systems expand beyond a small niche to replace traditional transvenous pacing systems remains to be determined and will likely depend in large part on the evolution of feasibility and ease of multichamber headless stimulation. Long-term follow-up will need to verify device performance, including the projected battery longevity, stable stimulation thresholds, adequate sensing, and the safety of extraction, if needed.

REFERENCES

1. Statista. Estimated global cardiac pacemaker sales from 2015 to 2021 (in million units). [Online] Available from https://www.statista.com/statistics/731763/cardiac-pacemaker-units-sales-worldwide/ [Accessed October, 2018].
2. Greenspon AJ, Patel JD, Lau E, et al. Trends in permanent pacemaker implantation in the United States from 1993 to 2009: increasing complexity of patients and procedures. J Am Coll Cardiol. 2012;60(16):1540-5.
3. Reddy VY, Knops RE, Sperzel J, et al. Permanent leadless cardiac pacing: results of the LEADLESS trial. Circulation. 2014;129(14):1466-71.
4. Fanourgiakis J, Simantirakis E, Maniadakis N, et al. Complications related to cardiac rhythm management device therapy and their financial implication: a prospective Single-Center Two-year Survey. Hellenic J Cardiol. 2016;57(1):33e38.
5. Birgersdotter-Green UM, Pretorius VG. Lead extractions: indications, procedural aspects, and outcomes. Cardiol Clin. 2014;32(2):201-10.
6. Spickler JW, Rasor NS, Kezdi P, et al. Totally self-contained intracardiac pacemaker. J Electrocardiol. 1970;3(3-4):325-31.
7. Sperzel J, Khairkhahan A, Ligon D, et al. Feasibility efficacy and safety of percutaneous retrieval of a leadless cardiac pacemaker in an in vivo ovine model. Europace. 2013;15(Suppl. 2).ii112-3.
8. Vardas PE, Politopoulos C, Manios E, et al. A miniature pacemaker introduced intravenously and implanted endocardially. Preliminary findings from an experimental study. Eur J CPE. 1991;1:27-30.
9. Koruth JS, Rippy MK, Khairkhahan A, et al. Feasibility and efficacy of percutaneously delivered leadless cardiac pacing in an in vivo ovine model. J Cardiovasc Electrophysiol. 2015;26(3):322-8.
10. Wieneke H, Konorza T, Erbel R, et al. Leadless pacing of the heart using induction technology: a feasibility study. Pacing Clin Electrophysiol. 2009;32(2):177-83.
11. Wieneke H, Rickers S, Velleuer J, et al. Leadless pacing using induction technology: impact of pulse shape and geometric factors on pacing efficiency. Europace. 2013;15(3):453-9.
12. Goto H, Sugiura T, Harada Y, et al. Feasibility of using the automatic generating system for quartz watches as a leadless pacemaker power source. Med Biol Eng Comput. 1999;37(3):377-80.
13. Echt DS, Cowan MW, Riley RE, et al. Feasibility and safety of a novel technology for pacing without leads. Heart Rhythm. 2006;3(10):1202-6.
14. Omdahl P, Eggen MD, Bonner MD, et al. Right Ventricular Anatomy Can Accommodate Multiple Micra Transcatheter Pacemakers. Pacing Clin Electrophysiol. 2016;39(4):393-7.
15. Mountfort K, Knops R, Sperzel J, et al. The promise of leadless pacing. Arrhythm Electrophysiol Rev. 2014;3(1):51-5.
16. Duray GZ, Ritter P, El-Chami M, et al. Micra Transcatheter Pacing Study Group. Long-term performance of a transcatheter pacing system: 12-month results from the Micra Transcatheter Pacing Study. Heart Rhythm. 2017;14(5):702-9.
17. Piccini JP, Stromberg K, Jackson KP, et al. Micra Transcatheter Pacing Study Group. Long-term outcomes in leadless Micra transcatheter pacemakers with elevated thresholds at implantation: results from the Micra Transcatheter Pacing System Global Clinical Trial. Heart Rhythm. 2017;14(5):685-91.
18. Medtronic. Micra: Transcatheter Pacing System. [online] Available from http://www.medtronic.com/us-en/healthcare-professionals/products/cardiac-rhythm/pacemakers/micra-pacing-system/indications-safety-warnings.html/ [Accessed October, 2018].
19. Lamas GA, Ellenbogen KA. Evidence base for pacemaker mode selection: from physiology to randomized trials. Circulation. 2004;109(4):443-51.
20. Lamas GA, Orav EJ, Stambler BS, et al. Quality of life and clinical outcomes in elderly patients treated with ventricular pacing as compared with dual-chamber pacing. Pacemaker Selection in the Elderly Investigators. N Engl J Med. 1998;338(16):1097-104.
21. Nielsen JC, Andersen HR, Thomsen PE, et al. Heart failure and echocardiographic changes during long-term follow-up of patients 368 with sick sinus syndrome randomized to single-chamber atrial or ventricular pacing. Circulation. 1998;97:987-95.
22. Ausubel K, Steingart RM, Shimshi M, et al. Maintenance of exercise stroke volume during ventricular versus atrial synchronous pacing: role of contractility. Circulation. 1985;72(5):1037-43.

23. Gillis AM, Russo AM, Ellenbogen KA, et al. HRS/ACCF expert consensus statement on pacemaker device and mode selection. Developed in partnership between the Heart Rhythm Society (HRS) and the American College of Cardiology Foundation (ACCF) and in collaboration with the Society of Thoracic Surgeons. Heart Rhythm. 2012;9(8):1344-65.
24. Masuyama T, Kodama K, Uematsu M, et al. Beneficial effects of atrioventricular sequential pacing on cardiac output and left ventricular filling assessed with pulsed Doppler echocardiography. JPN Circ J. 1986;50(9):799-807.
25. Ouali S, Neffeti E, Ghoul K, et al. DDD versus VVIR pacing in patients, ages 70 and over, with complete heart block. Pacing Clin Electrophysiol. 2010;33(5): 583-9.
26. Toff WD, Camm AJ, Skehan JD, et al. Single-chamber versus dual-chamber pacing for high-grade atrioventricular block. N Engl J Med. 2005;353(2):145-55.
27. Benditt DG, Milstein S, Buetikofer J, et al. Sensor-triggered, rate-variable cardiac pacing. Current technologies and clinical implications. Ann Intern Med. 1987;107(5):714-24.

SECTION 18

Cardiac Surgery

CHAPTER 121

Time to Embrace Total Arterial Revascularization

Ramakanta Panda, Sunil Vanzara

INTRODUCTION

The left internal mammary artery (LIMA) to the left anterior descending artery (LAD) graft, unanimously considered the gold standard of coronary revascularization and conduits, has not only shown to improve survival but also decrease the rate of reoperation compared to the use of only vein grafts.[1] However, the conventional surgery of one internal mammary artery (IMA) and vein grafts do not reduce the incidence of recurrence of angina and late myocardial infarction (MI) because of the high occlusion rates of vein grafts of 12%, 25%, 50%, and 75% within 1 , 5, 12, and 15 years, respectively, after coronary artery bypass grafting (CABG).[2-4] Conceptually arterial grafts with higher patency rate should reduce above adverse events if grafted to circumflex (Cx) and right coronary artery (RCA). This has been corroborated by numerous retrospective analyses documenting an incremental survival benefit by increasing the number of arterial grafts.[5-9] Two independent meta-analyses have corroborated the long-term benefit.[5],[10] A large retrospective study (8,622 patients),[11] which involved a large cohort of multivessel coronary artery disease (MVCAD) patients, has shown that in isolated CABG performed more than 15 years ago with the use of LIMA to the LAD, bypassing the non-LAD targets with at least one additional arterial graft, was an independent predictor of survival during the succeeding 15 years. The improved survival was seen among both sexes, all ages, patients with preserved as well as impaired left ventricular function, those with pre-existing diabetes, chronic lung disease, or renal failure, and those without those risk factors. Patients with clinically significant left main coronary artery disease (CAD), double- and triple-vessel disease patients, operated electively or emergently also had improved survival. Despite this compelling evidence in the published literature, multiple arterial grafting is currently performed in <13% of CABG operations,[12] bilateral internal thoracic artery (ITA) in 4.1%, and radial artery (RA) in 10.8% patients.[13]

REASON FOR LOW ATHEROSCLEROSIS IN ARTERIAL CONDUITS

The superiority of IMAs over saphenous vein grafts (SVGs) can be attributed to its striking resistance to the development of atherosclerosis. Structurally its endothelial layer shows fewer fenestrations, lower intercellular junction permeability, greater antithrombotic molecules such as heparin sulfate and tissue plasminogen activator, and higher endothelial nitric oxide production, which are some of the unique ways that make the IMA impervious to the transfer of lipoproteins, which are responsible for the development of atherosclerosis. The IMA, an elastic artery, is dominated by a media with discrete lamellae of wavy collagen and smooth muscle, aligned nearly circumferentially. The SVG, in contrast, is more variable in its size and structure, characteristically with a narrow circumferential media comprised mostly of collagen, which is straightened and highly aligned at arterial pressures contributing to high mechanical stiffness of this vessel when exposed to arterial pressure. The high fraction of longitudinal muscle, in addition to the circumferential muscle cells in the SVG, makes it vulnerable to any pre-implant surgical preparation, and to the cyclical luminal pressures and longitudinal strains characteristic for epicardial arteries.[14]

Radial artery has a significantly greater prevalence of intimal hyperplasia, atherosclerosis, and medial calcification than the IMA. However, all severity indices are fairly low in both the RA and the IMA. Age, smoking, diabetes, and peripheral vascular disease (PVD) are correlated with intimal hyperplasia and atherosclerosis in the RA and the IMA. The left IMA is used almost exclusively as a graft to the LAD coronary artery; however, the choice of the second graft varies widely among surgeons. A caution should be exercised in selecting the RA in favor of the right IMA as a bypass conduit in patients who are elderly, diabetic, smoker, or have PVD, especially in patients with a combination of any of the above. Doppler ultrasonography may be useful in evaluating these patients before surgery to select only disease-free RAs and to avoid an unnecessary incision.[15]

TYPES OF ARTERIAL CONDUITS

Left Internal Thoracic Artery

Since the landmark publication by Loop et al. in 1986[1] demonstrating the significant survival benefit of LIMA-to-LAD over SVG-to-LAD, LIMA is universally accepted as the best conduit for CABG, and LIMA-LAD graft is the gold standard as well as the single most important component of any coronary revascularization.

The Right Internal Mammary Artery

The right internal mammary artery (RIMA) is biologically identical to the LIMA.[16-18] The RIMA is usually of greater diameter than the LIMA in right-handed people, easier to dissect and because of larger diameter easier to use.

Radial Artery (Unilateral and Bilateral)

Over the past 20 years RA has proven to be an important conduit, and for those not experienced with using bilateral IMA (BIMA), it is the second best conduit after LIMA. It is easy to harvest, has excellent length up to 22 cm to reach most distal coronary arteries, has appropriate size match for coronaries, and is very comfortable for surgeons to use.

Gastroepiploic Artery

The gastroepiploic artery (GEA) is the largest terminal branch of the gastroduodenal artery and is a muscular artery. The diameter of the right GEA (RGEA) is approximately 3 mm or more at its origin and is 1.5–2.0 mm in the middle of the greater curvature and length up to 24 cm can be harvested.[19]

Inferior Epigastric Artery

Like GEA, the inferior epigastric artery (IEA) is a muscular artery and originates from the external iliac artery. Though proximal diameter is between 3.0 and 4.0 mm, the short length (in between 6 and 10 cm) and smaller distal size of 1.0–2.0 mm limit its use.

INDICATIONS AND CONTRAINDICATIONS TO USE TOTAL ARTERIAL REVASCULARIZATION

While total arterial revascularization (TAR) is not necessarily indicated in all patients, it should be the primary objective in any coronary bypass surgery with BIMA grafting forming the foundation and RA as the third conduit when needed. Patients with a body mass index (BMI) of over 35, diabetes or severe airway disease, or who had or are undergoing radiotherapy or immunosuppression are only relatively contraindicated for BIMA use.[20] If more conduits are required, the RA can be harvested at the same time as the LIMA, and its harvesting is associated with favorable early and late outcomes.[21] Prior to harvesting RA, a modified Allen test, duplex examination, and pulse oximetry can also be used to preoperatively evaluate the RA and ulnar artery. Moreover, the RA should be avoided when cardiac catheterization has been recently performed through RA thereby injuring the vessel (RA) and when the RA might be used for future fistulae in patients with significant renal impairment.[22] RAs <2 mm in diameter are also avoided due to the possibility of vasospasm. In 5–10% cases it cannot be used because of RA dominance, calcification, prior trauma, especially if a recent coronary angiogram is performed through the RA route, and collagen disease.[23] Another absolute contraindication is hypoplasia of ulnar artery or inadequate accentuation in ulnar artery (<20%) in response to compression of ipsilateral radial on Doppler study.

With greater acceptance of RA, GEA use has been restricted to limited centers or when there is a paucity of arterial conduits especially in coronary reoperations. It is usually used to graft RCA or its branches mostly as *in situ* graft and occasionally as free graft from aorta or composite from LIMA to proximal vessels such as diagonal (Dg), intermediate, or obtuse marginal (OM).

Inferior epigastric artery is extremely infrequently used but can be considered in situations of non-availability of other arterial conduits in redo CABG situations. Because of its limited length, it can be used to anastomose proximal coronary branches such as Dg or intermediate and OM1 from aorta or as composite conduit as Y from LIMA to Dg, intermediate or OM, or to RIMA as Y graft or extension to graft PDA or OM.

Finally, the extent of stenosis of the target coronary vessel with stenosis of <70% in the left coronary bed and <90% in a dominant RCA may also constitute a contraindication for arterial conduit use due to competitive flow causing graft attrition.[20]

Commonly raised concerns regarding the use of BIMA that discourages many surgeons are:

- Surgeons not trained in RIMA harvest: Technique of harvesting RIMA is same as LIMA and there is no additional learning curve
- Not comfortable with the actual use of the RIMA to perform coronary grafting: The RIMA is usually larger than the LIMA in most right-handed individual and the wall is identical or sometimes slightly thicker than that of the LIMA. Technically, it is not more difficult to use RIMA for anastomosis
- Prolonging the operation: Though the operation time is prolonged approximately by 30–60 minutes, the benefits of using RIMA outweigh the additional operating time
- *Uncertainty as to how best to deploy the RIMA*: The common concerns are:
  - Whether to use *in situ*, free, or Y graft,
  - Whether to graft to single coronary artery or sequential to multiple coronary arteries, and
  - Whether to route the RIMA anterior or posterior to the aorta to reach the Cx, the RCA, or posterior descending artery (PDA).

Regardless of all of the above concerns, the patency of *in situ* RIMA is identical to free RIMA to the same vessel and should not be a concern.[24]

- Concern regarding sternal infection, necrosis, and non-union: Though BIMA harvest is associated with increased incidence of sternal wound infection, it is so when the IMA is harvested in a pedicle manner. The sternal wound infection is minimized by skeletonized harvesting of the RIMA,[25,26] appropriate prophylactic antibiotic regimens, and meticulous perioperative glucose management.[16,27-29] A subgroup analysis of the ART trial showed that the risk of sternal wound infection is same with pedicled single IMA (SIMA) versus skeletonized BIMA. Though the risk of skeletonized SIMA was the lowest, the difference when compared with skeletonized BIMA was negligible.[30] However, there is no doubt that BIMA should be avoided in morbidly obese (BMI >40), insulin-dependent diabetes patients, female patients with diabetes, and those with severe chronic obstructive airways disease (COAD).[16] At authors' institution, since the introduction of skeletonized IMA in 2006, we have been able to increase the use of BIMA from 17% in 2004 to more than 60% today, without any significant increase in wound infection.
- Concern regarding RIMA patency: Despite multiple angiographic studies showing higher patency of RIMA as both *in situ* and free grafts, there are still concerns among surgeons about the superior patency of RIMA over SVG.[16] Patency of conduits depends on multiple factors including the degree of proximal stenosis of the grafted vessel, surgical team experience, and harvesting technique. Many of the studies comparing patency of RIMA to vein grafts are intermediate-term follow-up studies and we know that while IMA attrition rate is highest in the first 5 years,[31] the vein graft attrition is highest after 5 years. Short- and intermediate-term angiographic studies will not show the difference between RIMA and SVG. Only long-term angiographic studies (preferably >10 years) will show superior patency of RIMA or any other arterial grafts over SVG
- Concern regarding lack of additional survival benefit: Adding even one arterial graft to LIMA-to-LAD has shown to reduce late cardiac events such as recurrence of angina or MI, but short-term follow-up studies including ART trial 5-year midterm outcome have failed to show additional survival benefit of BIMA over single internal mammary artery (SIMA).[32] That is because firstly, the significant survival benefit of LIMA-to-LAD accrues from LAD mostly supplying the largest area of myocardium among the three coronary arteries and anatomic location of LIMA in relation to LAD providing the best patency rate among all conduits grafted to any other coronary arteries. To show additional survival benefit of multiple or total arterial grafting over only LIMA-to-LAD plus SVG, an equivalent or large area of myocardium needs to be revascularized using arterial conduits, presuming the patency rate of other arterial conduits will be as good as LIMA-to-LAD. Secondly, as mentioned earlier, many of these studies are short- to medium-term follow-up[32] and we know that while IMA attrition rate is highest in the first 5 years,[31] the vein graft attrition is highest after 5 years. In fact, most follow-up observational studies of beyond 10 years have shown the additional survival benefit and protection from late cardiac events of multiple arterial grafting.[7,33]
- Lack of randomized trials: Numerous single and multi-institutional observational, propensity-matched reports, and meta-analyses support survival benefit of BIMA over SIMA[6,33-36] However, this issue is being addressed by randomized trials as well. Five-year results of arterial revascularization trial (ART), a multi-institutional randomized study, did not show any benefit between SIMA and BIMA, though close to statistical significance was observed in favor of BIMA in patients under 70 years.[32,37,38] Recently, the 10-year ART results presented in the European Society of Cardiology meeting in August, 2018, though did not show difference in mortality or MI, surgeon's experience appeared to play a crucial factor for outcomes with BIMA graft. Again the follow-up duration of 5–10 years is short to show beneficial effect because while arterial graft attrition is maximum in first 5 years, the SVG attrition is more after 5 years and especially after 10 years. Also, the study suffered from high crossover: 14% of BIMA group received SIMA and a large number of single SIMA group received an additional RA graft. We know that RA grafts have nearly similar patency as that of RIMA.

While the above listed issues are real dilemmas, none of them justify not using BIMA.

TECHNIQUES OF HARVESTING

Basic Principles

- Proper exposure using appropriate specialized IMA retractor
- No touch technique of dissection without handling the arterial conduit
- Avoid injury to IMA - most dissections must be done with no touch and minimal handling
- Using harmonic scalpel or cautery at a very low setting
- If not using harmonic scalpel, using clips on either side of IMA branches and cutting with a sharp 45° angle Castroviejo scissors
- Irrigating the surface of IMA with dilute papaverine solution intermittently to avoid spasm
- Identifying occasional large pericardiophrenic and highest intercostal branch and clipping to prevent competitive flow
- Routing the IMA: If preserving pleura (to reduce pulmonary complications), create a space between mediastinal and parietal pleura and making an incision on extrapleural dissected area of pericardium and directing IMA behind lung to avoid stretching of IMA by lungs.

If pleura is opened, making an incision in the pericardium to direct the IMA behind lung as above.

Skeletonized Harvesting

- Internal mammary artery is dissected by ligating IMA branches close to it without removing the accompanying vein and surrounding tissues, so that collateral circulation to the sternum is maintained[39]
- Avoid using electrocautery to divide branches to prevent thermal injury to IMA
- Minimal use of electrocautery at low thermal setting
- Divide branches using harmonic scalper or cutting them with a fine scissor in between metal clips
- Cover the mammary bed, after IMA dissection, with the endothoracic fascia.

As discussed earlier, skeletonization of IMA not only reduces superficial and deep sternal wound infection[25,26] but also increases the length of IMA reaching out *in situ* to distal coronary branches such as PDA or OM and also increases diameter of IMA thus increasing flow.[40] Because of higher flow a skeletonized IMA, especially *in situ* IMA, can be used to graft a less critically stenosed coronary artery or stenosed vein graft,[41] a relative contraindication for using pedicled IMA.

Prevention of Arterial Graft Spasm

The commonest cause of spasm of arterial conduits is due to injury to vessel wall or endothelium from rough handling during harvesting. The basic principles enumerated earlier, i.e., no touch harvest, with minimal conduit handling, low electrocautery setting, etc. must be adhered to. Spraying diluted papaverine during dissection is the most common method used. Other pharmacological agents used are:

- Intraluminal use of 2–3 mL solution of milrinone buffered in warm heparinized blood into lumen of harvested arterial conduit using a catheter with bulbous tip (milrinone mix = 10 mL milrinone + 18 mL heparinized blood + 2 mL – 2,000 IU – heparin)
- Storing harvested arterial conduits in buffered blood containing phenoxybenzamine or verapamil.[23]

The above is supplemented in the postoperative period for 24–48 hours with intravenous nitroglycerine or/and IV diltiazem for 24 hours and amlodipine 5 mg daily for 6–36 months.[23]

FACTORS INFLUENCING GRAFT PATENCY

Patency of arterial grafts depends on multitude of factors not intrinsic to arterial conduits, be it IMA or RA or RGEA or IEA. Extrinsic modifiable factors influencing graft patency include:

- Harvesting technique
- Graft ischemia
- Degree of stenosis in coronary artery (competitive flow)
- Coronary artery grafted
- Lie and length of the conduit
- Experience of surgical team.

Harvesting Technique

Importance of technique cannot be overemphasized. Many of the events that lead to an arterial graft failure occur early in the operation. Careful dissection, vasodilatation, storage, etc. as discussed earlier can avoid graft injury and ischemia leading to reduction in graft closure. While dissecting conduits, any direct, thermal, electrical injury, kinking, hematoma in arterial wall, branch avulsion, drying of blood vessel over distension should be avoided.

Graft Ischemia

Reducing graft ischemia, i.e., time between interruption of blood supply to the conduit (disconnection of arterial graft) and re-establishing circulation (i.e., by completing one anastomosis), is important in preventing damage to endothelium and vessel wall. Thatte et al.[42] had reported that in veins, within 60 minutes of storing autologous heparinized blood, exhibited markedly diminished calcium mobilization and nitric oxide generation, as well as non-viability of 90% of endothelial cells. The ischemic period of a conduit should be kept minimum by careful planning of grafting order and disconnecting the arterial conduit at the last moment just before the particular anastomosis.

Degree of Stenosis in Coronary Artery

Unlike SVG, which are not affected by native coronary artery stenosis (NCAS) or competitive flow, all arterial grafts' (especially free grafts) patency are affected by NCAS.[23,43,44] When the block in coronary artery is not critical (<70%), there is still significant flow in the native vessel which competes with the constructed graft. IMAs are less sensitive to this and their graft patency rate reduces if the NCAS is <60%. RA and RGEA are extremely vulnerable. The best patency rate of these conduits are achieved only when the NCAS is more than 80%, more so if NCAS is more than 90% especially for RCA. Unfortunately, assessment of NCAS is subjective and flow through a 80% stenosed 4 mm RCA will be far more than through 80% stenosis in a 2 mm Cx. Residual coronary artery diameter is probably a more objective indicator, with 1 mm or less residual diameter a threshold for significant influence on arterial graft patency.[45]

Coronary Artery Grafted

Patency of arterial grafts depends on the coronary artery grafted, with highest patency of arterial grafts achieved when grafted to LAD, followed by Cx and grafts to RCA has the lowest patency rate.[17]

Lie and Length of the Conduit

The length, lie, and rotation of the conduit are important technical points affecting a graft's patency. A long graft may get kinked or a short graft may get stretched, especially if routed in front of the lung instead of behind it risking its patency. Skeletonized IMA are prone to 180–360° rotation of conduit in long axis, which can lead to graft closure.

Experience of Surgical Team

The relationship between center or operator (surgeon) experience and outcome has been extensively described in medicine and surgery.[46] Construction of coronary anastomosis using arterial conduits, especially BIMA or RGEA, is technically complex and surgical volume and experience plays a very important role. Grandjean et al.[47] have reported an RGEA patency of 77% in their first year of experience, which increased to 95% at the end of their learning curve by the fourth year. The results of 10-year ART data (unpublished) presented at the European Society of Cardiology meeting in August, 2018, suggest surgeon experience to be a crucial factor for outcomes with arterial grafts.

COMPARATIVE PATENCY DATA OF ARTERIAL GRAFTS

Graft Patency

Since the publication by Loop et al. in 1986[1] (and other publications around that time), it is universally accepted that LIMA is the best coronary graft, and LIMA-to-LAD is the single most important component of any coronary revascularization in reducing recurrent cardiac events and enhancing survival[48] It is often described as "gold standard" or "benchmark". LIMA–LAD improves perioperative mortality and can be used, and is strongly recommended, in all situations including emergency revascularization, older age, and in patients with comorbid states (diabetes, obesity, renal dysfunction, and COAD).[49] The only situations where it may not be usable are if it is damaged, is of insufficient size, and has inadequate flow to sustain the dependent vessel and myocardium. In our experience, it is extremely rare to find an IMA which is small for grafting to a coronary artery, and the low flow is usually due to improper harvesting techniques. As many as 80% of IMA conduits have been shown to be free from failure in the third decade after CABG.[19] RIMA-to-LAD has the same patency as that of LIMA-to-LAD.[50] Tatoulis et al.[17] reported similar patency between RIMA and LIMA when grafted to the same target vessel. When grafted to LAD, it was 98% versus 98% at 5 years and 95% versus 96% at 10 years. When grafted to Cx, it was 96% versus 96% at 5 years and 91% versus 89% at 10 years. Several angiographic studies from 6.7 to 12 years following surgery have reported similar RIMA patency rates (ranges from 86 to 97%) as compared to LIMA[4,51] (Fig. 1).

The patency rates of the RA range from 83 to 91% at 5–7 years postoperatively, thus demonstrating a superior patency of the RA versus SVG.[52-54] A meta-analysis of 35 studies showed a significantly lower RA graft failure compared to SV grafts (9.6% vs. 18.8%).[44] The graft patency of RAs of 88.6% was superior to that of the SVGs of 75.8%. Similar findings have been reported by a recent single-institution study involving 1,851 patients showing a superiority of the RA compared to the SV in terms of graft patency and graft failure.[55] When grafted to largest non-LAD artery, the free RIMA patency is not significantly different from that of RA.[18,55]

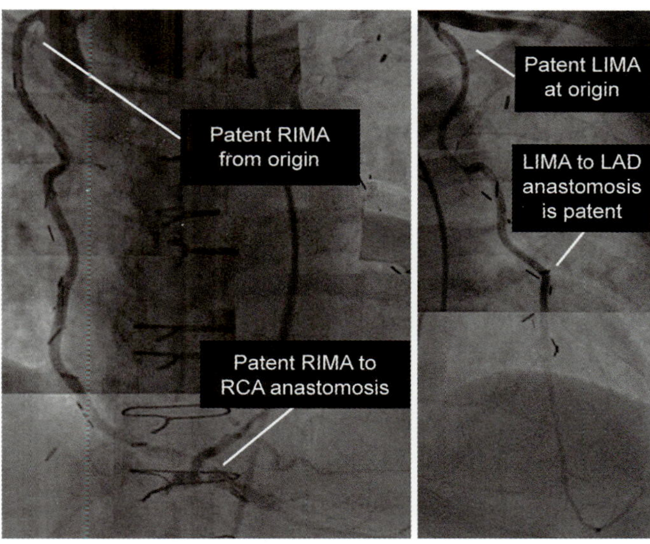

LIMA, left internal mammary artery; RIMA, right internal mammary artery; RCA, right coronary artery; LAD, left anterior descending artery.

FIG. 1: Patent bilateral internal mammary artery at 22 years postoperatively.

Patency of GEA grafts is dependent on tight stenosis and if grafted to RCA, must be done to one with a stenosis of >90%. Suma et al.[56] reported a graft patency of 85.5% at 5 years and 66.4% at 10 years in 172 angiographic studies among 1,352 patients receiving a GEA. However, most of these were grafted to an RCA with <90% stenosis. This poor long-term result has been improved to 94.7% at 5 years and 90.2% at 8 years by skeletonizing of GEA and grafting to >90% stenosed vessel[57] (Fig. 2).

Very few studies published about the use and patency of IEA. Buche et al.[58] reported a patency rate of 92% at 8.5 months, 86% at 2 years, and all the five grafts studied at 5 years were patent. Of the grafts occluded, most were anastomosed to a non-critically blocked artery.

Multiarterial CABG, including bilateral ITA grafts, has been consistently associated with better arterial graft patencies (better than 90% at 10 years) and long-term survival in diabetic patients, those with renal dysfunction, women, and older patients.[21]

In summary, most of the arterial grafts have a good long-term patency, with RIMA equivalent or slightly superior to RA, which in turn is superior to GEA. The huge disparity in literature among the arterial conduit patency is because analysis of most studies has not included other factors affecting graft patency, mainly noncritical stenosis and the coronary artery grafted, i.e., Cx versus RCA. Table 1 summarizes some of the long-term patency rates of arterial grafts versus SVG published in literature.[59,60]

SURVIVAL BENEFIT

Adding even one arterial graft to LIMA-to-LAD has shown to improve survival and reduce late cardiac events such as recurrence of angina or MI[6,7] but some studies have failed

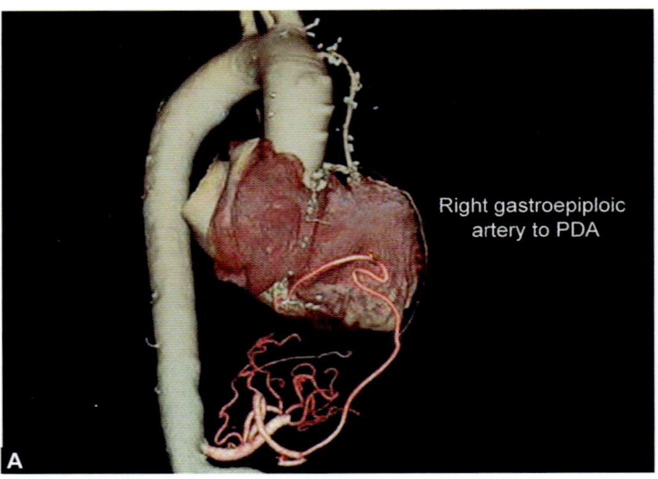

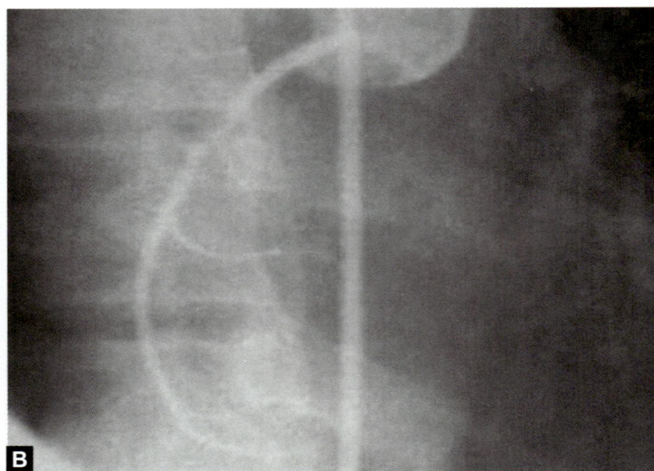

PDA, posterior descending artery.

FIG. 2: **A,** Computed tomography angiogram of right gastroepiploic artery to posterior descending artery; **B,** Inferior epigastric artery 10 years postoperative angiogram.

TABLE 1: Patency of coronary artery bypass conduits

Conduit	Author	Year	Follow-up (years)	Patency (%)
LIMA	Tatoulis[17]	2011	15	91
IMA	Sabik[59]	2005	15	92
RIMA	Tatoulis[17]	2011	15	79
RA	Tranbaugh[44]	2012	8.1	82
RA	Achouh[60]	2012	7	82.8
RA	Tatoulis[17]	2011	10	78
RA	Possati[52]	2003	9	90
RGEA-pedicled	Suma[56]	2007	10	66
RGEA-skeletonized	Suzuki[57]	2013	8	90
IEA	Buche[58]	1995	2	86
SVG	Tatoulis[17]	2011	15	50.7
SVG	Sabik[59]	2005	15	53
SVG	Possati[52]	2003	9	67

LIMA, left internal mammary artery; IMA, internal mammary artery right or left; RA, radial artery; RGEA, right gastroepiploic artery; SVG, saphenous venous graft.

to show additional survival benefit.[32] This is because the significant survival benefit of LIMA-to-LAD derives from high patency rate of the graft supplying to the largest area of myocardium. An equivalent area of myocardium needs to be supplied by additional arterial conduits to show benefit. Grafting the second or third arterial conduit to a small Dg or OM or small PDA will not show survival benefit. Secondly, many of these studies are short- to medium-term follow-up and we know while arterial graft attrition is maximum in the first decade that the vein graft attrition increases after 5 years and more so after 10 years. In fact most follow-up studies of more than 10 years have shown the additional survival benefit and protection from late cardiac events of multiple arterial grafting.[6,7]

There is no significant differences between BIMA and LIMA use with regard to perioperative complications and postoperative length of stay, deep sternal wound infection in non-diabetic or diabetic (if IMA is skeletonized), although more BIMA patients required blood transfusions and reoperation for bleeding.[36,61] The in-hospital and 30-day mortality rates were not significantly different between BIMA and LIMA groups.

Multiple observational long-term follow-up studies have shown advantages of BIMA/TAR in terms of long-term survival, reoperation, and the need for angioplasty.[6,7] A clear benefit is seen in the first postoperative decade and its advantage becomes even more apparent during the second postoperative decade as vein graft attrition increases. A retrospective study by Lytle et al.[62] demonstrated survival in the BIMA group of 94%, 84%, and 67% versus 92%, 79%, and 64% in the LIMA group at 5, 10, and 15 years postoperatively, respectively ($p < 0.001$). Similar superiority of BIMA grafting over LIMA with regard to long-term survival throughout the follow-up period (96% vs. 91% at 5 years, 89% vs. 79% at 10 years, and 79% vs. 61% at 15 years) was reported by Grau et al.[36] The survival benefit of BIMA over SIMA has been reported to be from 8 years throughout the study period[63] to >10% for BIMA grafting at 20 postoperative years.[6,7,62] Similar survival benefit of 10% at 10 years and 18% at 18 years was reported by Grau et al.[36] among patients receiving BIMA compared to LIMA use only.

Bilateral internal mammary artery grafting showed similar survival benefit over SIMA in diabetic patients too. In a large meta-analysis that compared 19,277 BIMA to 59,786 LIMA patients,[64] diabetic patients who underwent BIMA harvesting had an increased 10-year survival rate and a lower perioperative mortality rate compared to the LIMA group.[65]

Although no freedom from adverse events such as angina recurrence, new MI is observed during the first 4 years, a clear benefit is gained from the use of BIMA after 10 years,[66] and a 9% decrease in angina recurrence at 15 years.[67] BIMA is also associated with an additional 7 years of freedom

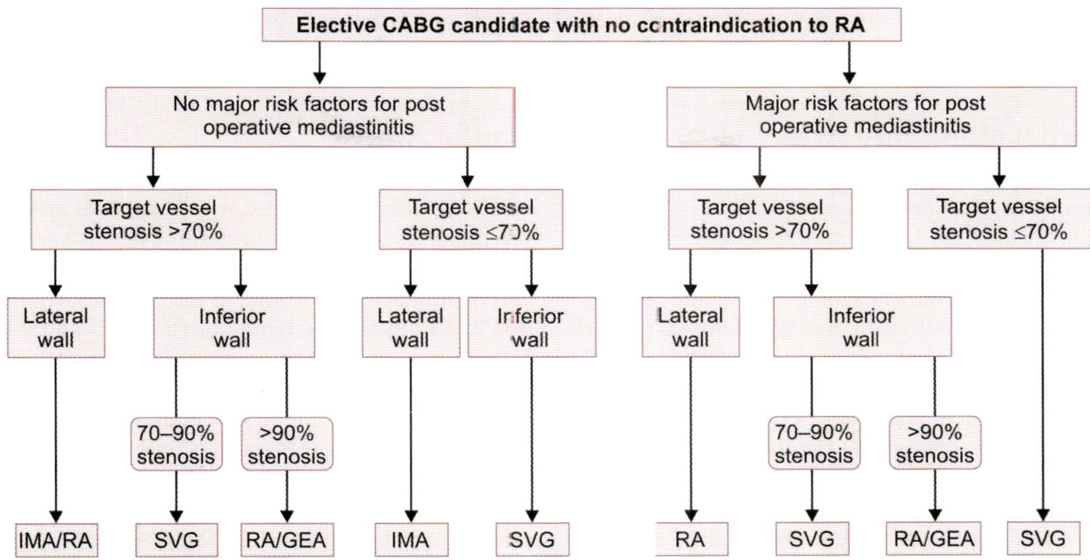

CABG, coronary artery bypass grafting; GEA, gastroepiploic artery; IMA, internal mammary artery; RA, radial artery; SVG, saphenous vein graft.

FLOWCHART 1: Algorithm for total arterial revascularization, while considering that left internal mammary artery is always grafted to left anterior descending artery.

from reoperation as a result of better graft patency rates.[63] Incremental benefit of BIMA grafting has been shown in elderly though the data is not as convincing. Kurlansky et al.[68] have reported an enhanced long-term survival in patients older than 75 years receiving BIMA. There is evidence that RA and LIMA grafting has a strong protective effect against native CAD in previously grafted vessels, whereas SVG does not have such protective effect, again emphasizing the advantage of total arterial grafting.[69]

Gastroepiploic Artery and Survival

Right gastroepiploic artery has poor long-term prognosis and patency when grafted to LAD[70] and should be avoided. Suzuki et al.[71] in a comparative study of GEA versus SVG as a complement third conduit to left-sided BIMA graft reported superior freedom from death from all causes (96% GEA vs. 82.2% SVG) and freedom from cardiac events (cardiac death, MI, angina pectoris, repeat intervention, and heart failure) of 89.3% for GEA versus 77.5% for SVG.

DISCUSSION

In spite of overwhelming evidence of superiority of multiple arterial grafts over use of SIMA with vein grafts, hardly 5% patients receive BIMA whereas RA is used between 5 and 40% patients worldwide. Between 2004 and 2014, only one arterial graft was used in over 95.9% of all CABG in the United States (Society of Thoracic Surgeons (STS) database) and in 95.7% in the Australia and New Zealand (ANZ) patients.[72] This trend is no different from usage of BIMA in earlier decade among STS participating institutions.[13] Single arterial coronary bypass rate increased both in STS from 85.2 to 91.7% and in ANZ patients from 17.3 to 51.4%. BIMA use was very low (STS: 4.1%, ANZ: 4.3%), unchanged in STS, and decreased in ANZ patients. RA graft use decreased among STS patients from 10.5 to 3.7% and ANZ patients from 65.8 to 39%. Total arterial/multiple arterial bypass grafting was an abysmal 0.5% among STS patients and a little better but still very low of 5.9% among ANZ patients. The reason for low use of arterial conduits is complex and multifactorial. The perceived concerns as mentioned earlier (technical difficulties, enhanced postoperative complications, lack of randomized trials, etc.) and focus on short-term "quality metrics" such as longer operating time and avoidance of deep sternal wound infection by hospital administrators contribute significantly to this low use. In many countries, insurance does not reimburse cost of treatment of deep sternal wound infection.

Though long-term conduit patency is the key factor for success of CABG, no precise guideline exists and the choice of revascularization strategy by most surgeons is more of an art than science. LIMA-to-LAD is the gold standard and forms the cornerstone of CABG. As discussed earlier, there is robust evidence to suggest that an additional arterial graft (RIMA or RA), rather than a vein, is associated with improved late survival and reduced cardiac event.[6,7,36,63] The benefits of second arterial grafts also apply to those with unstable angina or reduced ventricular function.[73,74] The location of second arterial conduit does not modify the extent of survival advantage.[75] In patients with risk of mediastinitis, the use of RA instead of RIMA can safely increase the use of second arterial conduit.[76] All the available evidence in literature points to the use of multiple arterial graft/total arterial graft except where contraindicated (Flowchart 1). Lack of proper protocol for BIMA grafting contributes to the variation of its use among the surgeons which can be mitigated by developing guidelines for BIMA usage taking into variables such as age, diabetes, obesity, LV function, and a scoring system taking into consideration the SYNTAX and EuroSCORE can help standardize BIMA usage.[77]

Right Internal Mammary Artery

After LAD territory, Cx territory revascularization is more important than RCA except in patients with a large tightly stenosed RCA.[9] RIMA can be used as *in situ* graft to intermediate or OM across midline behind thymus, either in front of aorta or behind through transverse sinus. Alternately, it can be used as free graft, with proximal anastomosis on aorta over hood of a vein graft, over vein patch, or directly to it. To reach the inferolateral and RCA branches, it can be attached as Y or T graft to the side of LIMA. RIMA preferably be grafted to a critically stenosed (>90%)[4,17] large RCA, especially to its distal PDA and posterior left ventricular branches. It is better to avoid grafting to main RCA as either there is nonocclusive disease at crux at the time of grafting or crux develops occlusive disease over the next 5–10 years.[4,17] If the length of RIMA does not reach distal RCA branches, it is better to use as free graft. Skeletonization of RIMA helps getting additional length to reach distal RCA or Cx branches.

Radial Artery

The length and size of RA allows it to reach most distal coronary arteries and perform sequential anastomosis. The proximal anastomosis is preferably done to aorta over a vein graft hood, or vein patch or directly on aorta. Alternately, it can be attached to the side of LIMA or occasionally to RIMA as a T or Y graft to reach out both distal Cx and RCA branches. RA is more sensitive to competitive flow compared to IMA. While IMAs are resistant to competitive flow in coronary stenosis >70% and can be grafted to any coronary artery with >70% stenosis, RA preferably should only be grafted to an artery with stenosis of >90%.[20,23]

In summary, BIMA (Flowchart 1), especially an *in situ* IMA, should be grafted to LAD and Cx with stenosis of >60% and RA-to-Cx with >70% stenosis, preferably >80% stenosis.

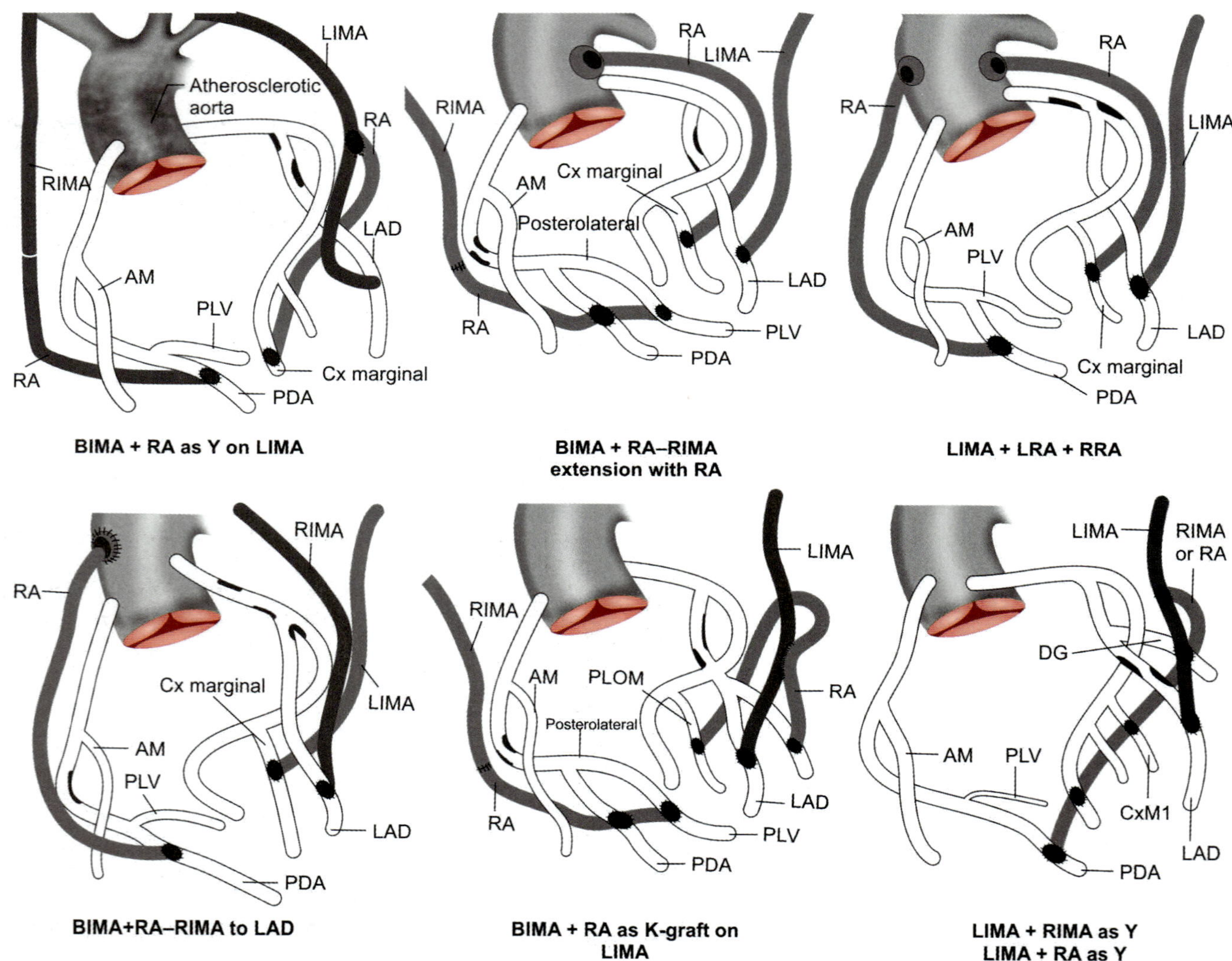

BIMA, bilateral internal mammary artery; LIMA, left internal mammary artery; RIMA, right internal mammary artery; RA, radial artery; LAD, left anterior descending artery; DG, diagonal artery; Cx, circumflex; PDA, posterior descending artery; AM, acute marginal artery; PLV, posterior left ventricular; PLOM, posterolateral obtuse marginal; CxM, circumflex marginal.

FIG. 3: A few suggested arterial graft configurations.

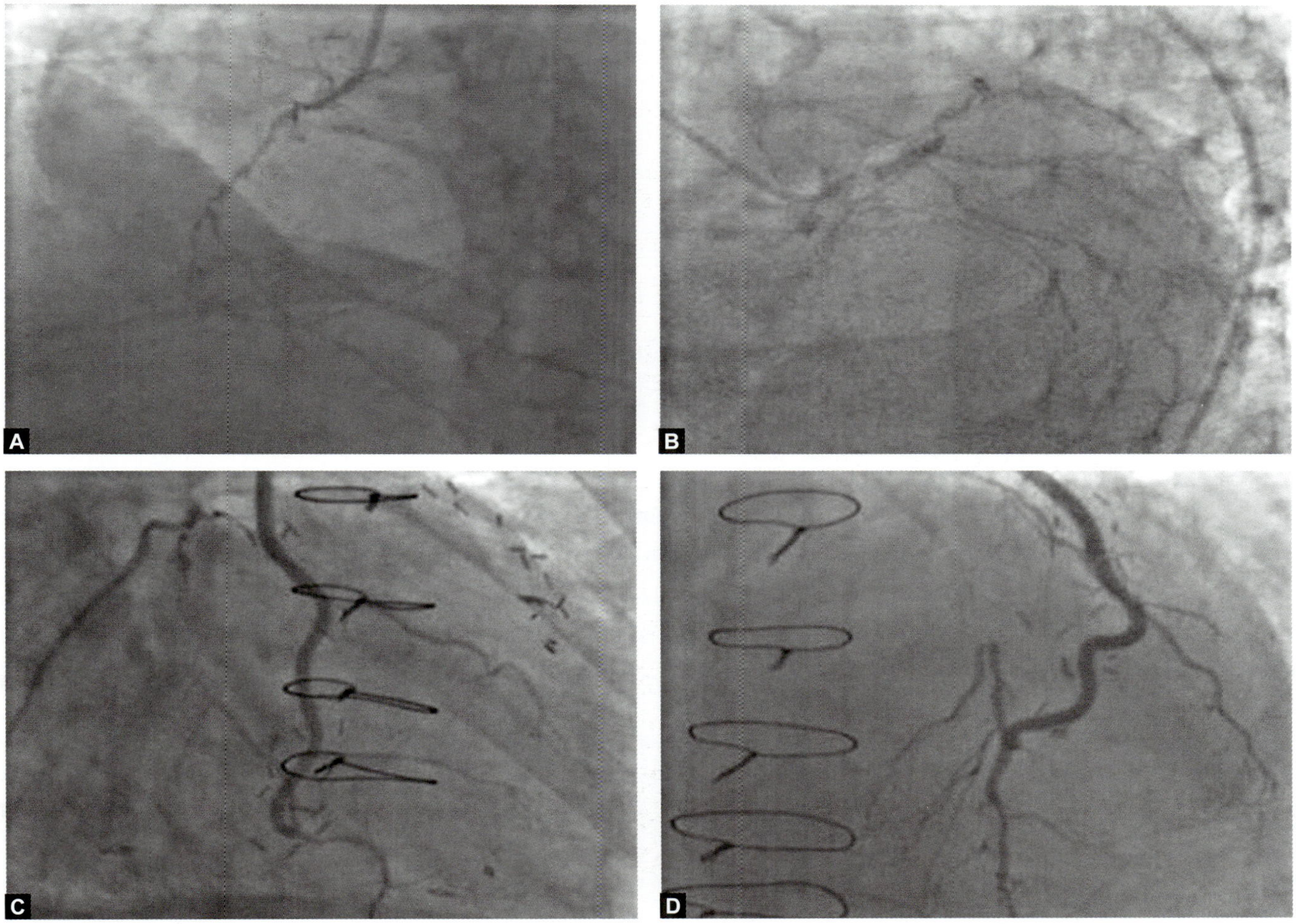

FIG. 4: Preoperative and 7 years postoperative angiogram of a patient with diffuse coronary artery disease. (**A and B**) Preoperative angiogram; (**C and D**) Postoperative angiogram.

Arterial conduits should only be grafted to RCA with >90% stenosis. SVG should be used in RCA stenosis of <90% and Cx stenosis of <60%. The choice of coronaries grafted by arterial conduits are BIMA to left system (preferably LIMA-to-LAD and RIMA-to-Cx) with RA to RCA if stenosis is >90% or SVG if <90%.

Graft Configurations

Left internal mammary artery, RIMA, and RA can be used in innumerable combinations depending on needs (Fig. 3).

Internal mammary artery can be *in situ*, LIMA–RIMA "Y," RIMA can be brought across midline to LAD territory, and LIMA can go to Cx and PDA territory (both *in situ*). RITA can be used *in situ* for proximal Cx territory across transverse sinus. RA can be used as "Y" on any ITA or can be attached to aorta for proximal anastomosis. Any conduit length saved from one territory may be used to extend other conduit. Our preference is to use BIMA with RA when needed. In patients with high risk of deep sternal infection, we use LIMA with RA.

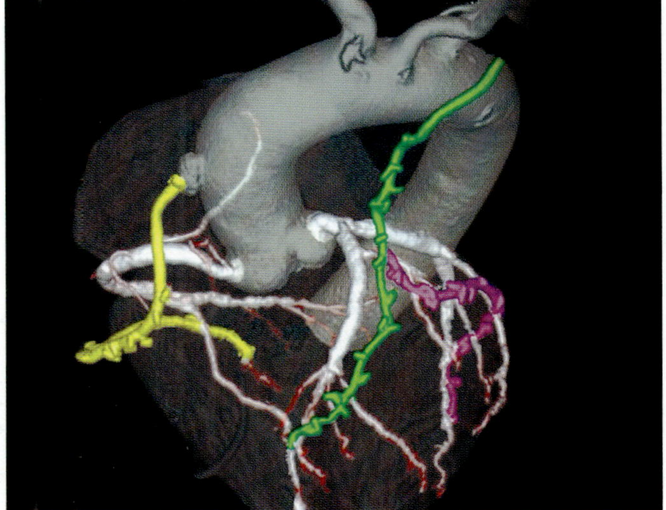

FIG. 5: First 1-year follow-up computed tomography angiogram of a patient with 12 grafts.

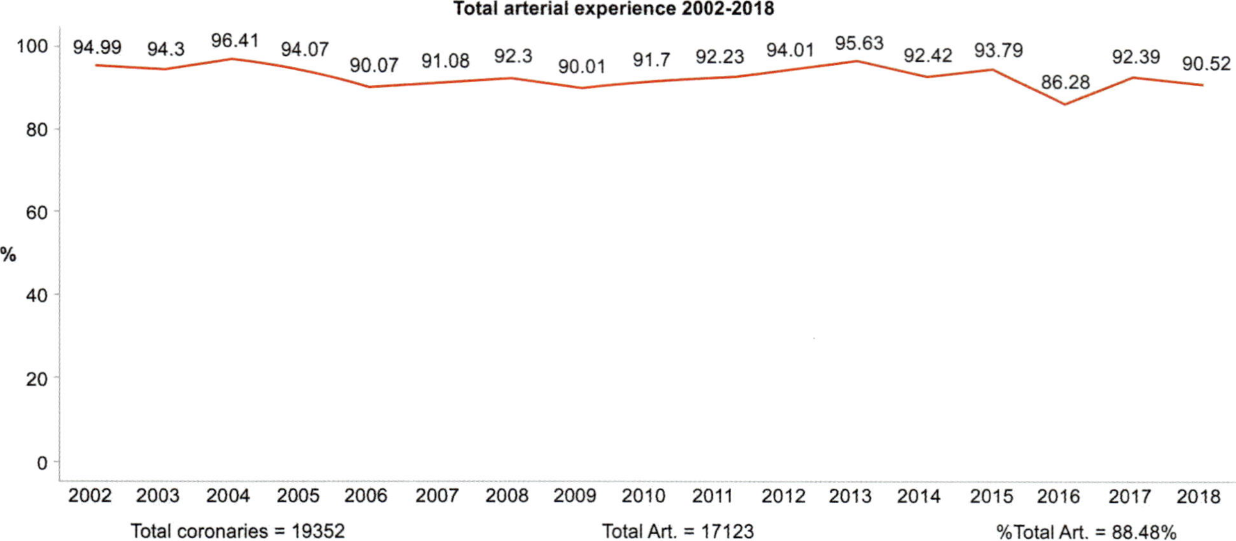

FIG. 6: Total arterial grafting—author's institution experience between 2002 and 2018.

Young Patients with Coronary Artery Disease

Though there is a paucity of information in literature, the few reports available in literature on short- and long-term results of young patients (a significant number of Indian patients fall into this category) with CAD undergoing conventional CABG of one IMA and SVG portray a very bleak outcome in this subcategory of patients. Lytle et al.[78] in a follow-up study of younger patients had reported an overall vein graft patency of 56% at mean interval of 47 months compared to 80% in older patients. Compared to this, IMA had a better overall graft patency of 93% in younger patients compared to 98% in older patients. A 20-year follow-up of young patients (below 40 years) undergoing predominant SVGs showed 27% mortality at 10 years and an estimated mortality of 69% in the second decade, while all these patients were still <60 years age.[79] Only 31% of patients who were operated when they were below 40 years were alive at 60 years. These horrendous results in young patient undergoing conventional CABG with one IMA and SVG grafts emphasizes the need for total arterial grafting in these subset of patients (Fig. 4).

Diffuse Coronary Atherosclerosis

Subgroup of patients with diffuse distal coronary athero-sclerosis and small coronary arteries pose a difficult decision-making dilemma. This is more so in Indian scenario, where because of small body surface area resulting in smaller coronary arteries and high incidence of diabetes, more patients undergoing CABG have diffuse CAD with small coronary arteries. In our experience and that of Kasliwal et al.,[80] close to 50% patients undergoing CABG in India have diabetes compared to 40% among Western counterpart.[13] As discussed earlier, most of these patients are younger and the short- and long-term vein grafts patency rate in these patients are extremely poor[77] and long-term survival is abysmal.[79] We strongly believe that extending the principles of multiple arterial grafting, to revascularize all coronary branches above 1 mm, in symptomatic patients especially with a strongly positive exercise scintigraphy is the best option. We quite often perform more than five arterial grafts (Fig. 5), and our incidence of patients needing more than five grafts has increased from 23% patients in 2003 to 50% today (unpublished data).

CONCLUSION

Most patients with MVCAD, except those with non-critically blocked coronary artery, can and should receive total arterial grafting. Skeletonization of both IMAs reduces sternal infection, increases available length reaching out to distal coronary arteries, and improves flow thus increasing the number of patients who will benefit. BIMA grafting can be safely performed and increasing evidence points to fewer perioperative complications, higher graft patency rates, excellent long-term survival rate, reduced adverse cardiac events resulting in reoperation, and lower CAD progression in grafted arteries in patients undergoing TAR. Total arterial coronary revascularization (TACR) should be done in all patients except where contraindicated and is possible to achieve in over 80% patients (Fig. 6). Since 2003, we have been able to achieve TACR in close to 90% patients undergoing CABG at our institution.

REFERENCES

1. Loop FD, Lytle BW, Cosgrove DM, et al. Influence of the internal-mammary-artery graft on 10-year survival and other cardiac events. N Engl J Med. 1986;314:1-6.
2. FitzGibbon GM, Kafka HP, Leach AJ, et al. Interventions for coronary stenosis—a Canadian experience of 30 revolutionary years. Can J Cardiol. 1996;12:893-900.

3. Bourassa MG. Long-term vein graft patency. Curr Opin Cardiol. 1994;9:685-91.
4. Tatoulis J, Buxton BF, Fuller JA, et al. Patencies of 2127 arterial to coronary conduits over 15 years. Ann Thorac Surg. 2004;77(1):93-101.
5. Pick AW, Orszulak TA, Anderson BJ, et al. Single versus bilateral internal mammary artery grafts: 10-year outcome analysis. Ann Thorac Surg. 1997;64: 599-605.
6. Taggart DP, D'Amico R, Altman DG. Effect of arterial revascularisation on survival: a systematic review of studies comparing bilateral and single internal mammary arteries. Lancet. 2001;358(9285):870-5.
7. Lytle BW, Blackstone EH, Sabik JF, et al. The effect of bilateral internal thoracic artery grafting on survival during 20 postoperative years. Ann Thorac Surg. 2004;78:[2005-12; discussion 2012-4].
8. Zacharias A, Habib RH, Schwann TA, et al. Improved survival with radial artery versus vein conduits in coronary bypass surgery with left internal thoracic artery to left anterior descending artery grafting. Circulation. 2004;109:1489-96.
9. Rankin JS, Tuttle RH, Wechsler AS, et al. Techniques and benefits of multiple internal mammary artery bypass at 20 years of follow-up. Ann Thorac Surg. 2007;83:1008-14; [discussion 1014-5].
10. Rizzoli G, Shiavon L, Bellini P. Does the use of bilateral internal mammary artery (IMA) grafts provide incremental benefit relative to the use of a single IMA graft? A meta-analysis approach. Eur J Cardiothorac Surg. 2002;22:781-6.
11. Locker C, Schaff HV, Dearani JA, et al. Multiple arterial grafts improve late survival of patients undergoing CABG: analysis of 8,622 patients with multivessel disease. Circulation. 2012;126:1023-30.
12. Ruttmann E, Fischler N, Sakic A, et al. Second internal thoracic artery versus radial artery in coronary artery bypass grafting: a long term, propensity score-matched follow-up study. Circulation. 2011;124:1321-29.
13. ElBardissi A, Aranki S, Sheng S, et al. Trends in isolated coronary artery bypass grafting: an analysis of the Society of Thoracic Surgeons Database. J Thorac Cardiovasc Surg. 2012;143:273-81.
14. Canham PB, Finlay HM, Boughner DR. Contrasting structure of the saphenous vein and internal mammary artery used as coronary bypass vessels. Cardiovasc Res. 1997;34(3):557-67.
15. Ruengsakulrach P, Sinclair R, Komeda M, et al. Comparative histopathology of radial artery versus internal thoracic artery and risk factors for development of intimal hyperplasia and atherosclerosis. Circulation. 1999;100(19 Suppl.):II139-44.
16. Tatoulis J, Buxton BF, Fuller JA. The right internal thoracic artery: is it underutilized? Curr Opin Cardiol. 2011;26:528-35.
17. Tatoulis J, Buxton BF, Fuller JA. The right internal thoracic artery: the forgotten conduit—5,766 patients and 991 angiograms. Ann Thorac Surg. 2011;92:9-15; [discussion 15-7].
18. Buxton BF, Ruengsakulrach P, Fuller J, et al. The right internal thoracic artery graft—benefits of grafting the left coronary system and native vessels with a high grade stenosis. Eur J Cardiothorac Surg. 2000;18:255-61.
19. Suma H. Gastroepiploic artery graft in coronary artery bypass grafting. Ann Cardiothorac Surg. 2013;2(4)493-8.
20. Buxton BF, Hayward PA. The art of arterial revascularization and total arterial revascularization in patients with triple vessel coronary artery disease. Ann Cardiothorac Surg. 2013;2:543-51.
21. Tatoulis J, Wynne R, Skillington PD, et al. Total arterial revascularization: achievable and prognostically effective—a multicenter analysis. Ann Thorac Surg. 2015:100(4),1268-75.
22. Blitz A, Osterday RM, Brodman RF. Harvesting the radial artery. Ann Cardiothorac Surg. 2013;2:533-42.
23. Tatoulis J, Buxton BF, Fuller JA, et al. Long-term patency of 1108 radial arterial-coronary angiograms over 10 years. Ann Thorac Surg. 2009; 88:23-9; [discussion 29-30].
24. Tatoulis J. Total arterial coronary revascularization—patient selection, stenoses, conduits, targets. Ann Cardiothorac Surg. 2013;2(4):499-506.
25. Peterson MD, Borger MA, Rao V, et al. Skeletonization of bilateral internal thoracic artery grafts lowers the risk of sternal infection in patients with diabetes. J Thorac Cardiovasc Surg. 2003;126:1314-9.
26. De Paulis R, de Notaris S, Scaffa R, et al. The effect of bilateral internal thoracic artery harvesting on superficial and deep sternal infection: the role of skeletonisation. J Thorac Cardiovasc Surg. 2005;129:536-43.
27. Dion R, Etienne PY, Verhelst R, et al. Bilateral mammary grafting. Clinical, functional and angiographic assessment in 400 consecutive patients. Eur J Cardiothorac Surg. 1993;7:287-93; [discussion 294].
28. Baskett RJ, Cafferty FH, Powell SJ, et al. Total arterial revascularization is safe: multicenter ten-year analysis of 71,470 coronary procedures. Ann Thorac Surg. 2006;81:1243-8.
29. Puskas JD, Sadiq A, Vassiliades TA, et al. Bilateral internal thoracic artery grafting is associated with significantly improved long-term survival, even among diabetic patients. Ann Thorac Surg. 2012;94:710-5; [discussion 715-6].
30. Benedetto U, Altman DG, Gerry S, et al. Pedicled and skeletonized single and bilateral internal thoracic artery grafts and the incidence of sternal wound complications: Insights from the arterial revascularization trial. J Thorac Cardiovasc Surg. 2016;152:270-6.
31. Robinson BM, Paterson HS, Naidoo R, et al. Bilateral Internal thoracic artery composite Y grafts: analysis of 464 angiogram in 296 patients. Ann Thorac Surg. 2016;101:974-80.
32. Taggart DP, Altman DG, Gray AM, et al. Randomised trial of bilateral versus single internal-thoracic-artery grafts. N Engl J Med. 2016;375:2540-9.
33. Buxton BF, Komeda M, Fuller JA, et al. Bilateral internal thoracic artery grafting may improve outcome of coronary artery surgery. Risk-adjusted survival. Circulation. 1998;98 (Suppl. 19):II1-6.
34. Dorman MJ, Kutaggarlansky PA, Traad EA, et al. Bilateral internal mammary artery grafting enhances survival in diabetic patients: a 30-year follow-up of propensity score-matched cohorts. Circulation. 2012;126(25):2935-42.
35. Buttar SN, Yan TD, Taggart DP, et al. Long-term and short-term outcomes of using bilateral internal mammary artery grafting versus left internal mammary artery grafting: a meta-analysis. Heart. 2017;103:1419-26.
36. Grau JB, Ferrari G, Mak AW, et al. Propensity matched analysis of bilateral internal mammary artery versus single left internal mammary artery grafting at 17-year follow-up: validation of a contemporary surgical experience. Eur J Cardiothorac Surg. 2012;41(4):770-5; [discussion 776].
37. Taggart DP, Altman DG, Gray AM, et al. Randomized trial to compare bilateral vs. single internal mammary coronary artery bypass grafting: 1-year results of the Arterial Revascularisation Trial (ART). Eur Heart J. 2010;31:2470-81.
38. Damgaard S, Lund JT, Lilleør NB, et al. Comparably improved health-related quality of life after total arterial revascularization versus conventional coronary surgery—Copenhagen arterial revascularization randomized patency and outcome trial. Eur J Cardiothorac Surg. 2011;39:478-83.
39. Berdajs D, Zund G, Turina MI, et al. Blood supply of the sternum and its importance in internal thoracic artery harvesting. Ann Thorac Surg. 2006;81: 2155-9.
40. Wendler O, Tscholl D, Huang Q, et al. Free flow capacity of skeletonized versus pedicled internal thoracic artery grafts in coronary artery bypass grafts. Eur J Cardiothorac Surg. 1999;15:247-50.
41. Yaku H, Doi K. Redo coronary artery bypass grafting. Gen Thorac Cardiovasc Surg. 2014;62:453-60.
42. Thatte HS, Biswas KS, Najjar SF, et al. Multi-photon microscopic evaluation of saphenous vein endothelium and its preservation with a new solution, GALA. Ann Thorac Surg. 2003;75:1145-52.
43. Zacharias A, Schwann TA, Riordan CJ, et al. Late results of conventional versus all-arterial revascularization based on internal thoracic and radial artery grafting. Ann Thorac Surg. 2009;87:19-26.
44. Tranbaugh RF, Dimitrova KR, Friedmann P, et al. Coronary artery bypass grafting using the radial artery: clinical outcomes, patency, and need for reintervention. Circulation. 2012;126:S170-5.
45. Glineur D, D'Hoore W, de Kerchove L, et al. Angiographic predictors of 3 year patency of bypass grafts implanted on the right coronary artery system: a prospective randomized comparison of gastroepiploic, saphenous vein, and right internal thoracic artery grafts. J Thorac Cardiovasc Surg. 2011;142: 980-8.
46. Birkmeyer JD, Siewers AE, Finlayson EV, et al. Hospital volume and surgical mortality in the United States. N Engl J Med. 2002;346:1128-37.
47. Grandjean JG, Boonstra PW, den Heyer P, et al. Arterial revascularization with the right gastroepiploic artery and internal mammary arteries in 300 patients J Thorac Cardiovasc Surg. 1994;1309-15.

48. Barner HB, Swartz MT, Mudd JG, et al. Late patency of the internal mammary artery as a coronary bypass conduit. Ann Thorac Surg. 1982;34:408-12.
49. Leavitt BJ, O'Connor GT, Olmstead EM, et al. Use of the internal mammary artery graft and in-hospital mortality and other adverse outcomes associated with coronary artery bypass surgery. Circulation. 2001;103:507-12.
50. Shah PJ, Durairaj M, Gordon I, et al. Factors affecting patency of internal thoracic artery graft: clinical and angiographic study in 1,434 symptomatic patients operated between 1982 and 2002. Eur J Cardiothorac Surg. 2004;26:118-24.
51. Chow MS, Sim E, Orszulak TA, et al. Patency of internal thoracic artery grafts: comparison of right versus left and importance of vessel grafted. Circulation. 1994;90(5 Pt 2):II129-32.
52. Possati G, Gaudino M, Prati F, et al. Long term results of the radial artery used for myocardial revascularization. Circulation. 2003;108(11):1350-4.
53. Cao C, Manganas C, Horton M, et al. Angiographic outcomes of radial artery versus saphenous vein in coronary artery bypass graft surgery: a meta-analysis of randomized controlled trials. J Thorac Cardiovasc Surg. 2013;146(2):255-61.
54. Athanasiou T, Saso S, Rao C, et al. Radial artery versus saphenous vein conduits for coronary artery bypass surgery: forty years of competition which conduit offers better patency? A systematic review and meta-analysis. Eur J Cardiothorac Surg. 2011;40(1):208-20.
55. Hayward PAR, Hare DL, Gordon I, et al. Which arterial conduit? Radial artery versus free right internal thoracic artery: six-year clinical results of a randomized controlled trial. Ann Thor Surg. 2007;84(2):493-7;[discussion 497].
56. Suma H, Tanabe H, Takahashi A, et al. Twenty years experience with the gastroepiploic artery graft for CABG. Circulation. 2007;116(11 Suppl.):I188-91.
57. Suzuki T, Asai T, Nota H, et al. Early and long-term patency of in situ skeletonized gastroepiploic artery after off-pump coronary artery bypass graft surgery. Ann Thorac Surg. 2013;96(1):90-5.
58. Buche M, Schroeder E, Gurné O, et al. Coronary artery bypass grafting with the inferior epigastric artery. Midterm clinical and angiographic results. J Thorac Cardiovasc Surg. 1995;109(3):553.
59. Sabik JF, Lytle BW, Blackstone EH, et al. Comparison of saphenous vein and internal thoracic artery graft patency by coronary system. Ann Thorac Surg. 2005;79(2):544-51; [discussion 544-51].
60. Achouh P, Isselmou KO, Boutekadjirt RD, et al. Reappraisal of a 20-year experience with the radial artery as a conduit for coronary bypass grafting. Eur J Cardio-Thorac Surg. 2011;41(1):87-92.
61. Momin AU, Deshpande R, Potts J, et al. Incidence of sternal infection in diabetic patients undergoing bilateral internal thoracic artery grafting. Ann Thorac Surg. 2005;80(5):1765-72.
62. Lytle BW, Blackstone EH, Loop FD, et al. Two internal thoracic arteries are better than one. J Thorac Cardiovasc Surg. 1999;117(5):855-72.
63. Endo M, Nishida H, Tomizawa Y, et al. Benefit of bilateral IMA grafts over single IMA graft for multiple coronary artery bypass grafting. Circulation. 2001;104(18):2164-70.
64. Weiss AJ, Zhao S, Tian DH, et al. A meta-analysis comparing bilateral internal mammary artery with left internal mammary artery for coronary artery bypass grafting. Ann Cardiothorac Surg. 2013;2(4):390-400.
65. Savage EB, Grab JD, O'Brien SM, et al. Use of bilateral internal thoracic arteries in diabetic patients increases deep sternal wound infection. Ann Thorac Surg. 2007;83(3):1002-6.
66. Berreklouw E, Rademakers PPC, Koster JM, et al. Better ischemic event-free survival after two internal thoracic artery grafts: 13 years of follow-up. Ann Thorac Surg. 2001;72(5):1535-41.
67. Naunheim KS, Barner HB, Fiore AC. 1990: Results of internal thoracic artery grafting over 15 years: single versus double grafts. 1992 update. Ann Thorac Surg. 1992;53(4):716-8.
68. Kurlansky PA, Traad EA, Dorman MJ, et al. Thirty-year follow-up defines survival benefit for second internal mammary artery in propensity-matched groups. Ann Thorac Surg. 2010;90:101-8.
69. Dimitrova KR, Hoffman DM, Geller CM, et al. Arterial grafts protect the native coronary vessels from atherosclerotic disease progression. Ann Thorac Surg. 2012;94(2),475-81.
70. Takahashi K, Daitoku K, Nakata S, et al. Early and mid-term outcome of anastomosis of gastroepiploic artery to left coronary artery. Ann Thorac Surg. 2004;78(6):2033-6; [discussion 2036].
71. Suzuki T, Asai T, Matsubayashi K, et al. In off-pump surgery, skeletonized gastroepiploic artery is superior to saphenous vein in patients with bilateral internal thoracic arterial grafts. Ann Thorac Surg. 2011;91(4):1159-64.
72. Schwann TA, Tatoulis J, Puskas J, et al. Worldwide trends in multi-arterial coronary artery bypass grafting surgery 2004-2014: A tale of 2 continents. Semin Thorac Cardiovasc Surg. 2017;29(3):273-80.
73. Hayward PA, Yap CH, Shi WY, et al. Does the addition of a radial artery graft improve survival after higher risk coronary artery bypass grafting? A propensity-score analysis of a multicenter database. Eur J Cardiothorac Surg. 2013;44(3):497-504, [discussion 504-5].
74. Galbut DL, Kurlansky PA, Traad EA, et al. Bilateral internal thoracic artery grafting improves long-term survival in patients with reduced ejection fraction: a propensity-matched study with 30-year follow-up. J Thorac Cardiovasc Surg. 2012;143(4):844-53.
75. Sabik III JF, Stockins A, Nowicki ER, et al. Does location of the second internal thoracic artery graft influence outcome of coronary artery bypass grafting? Circulation. 2008;118(14 Suppl.):S210-5.
76. Tranbaugh RF, Dimitrova KR, Lucido DJ, et al. The second best arterial graft: a propensity analysis of the radial artery versus the free right internal thoracic artery to bypass the circumflex coronary artery. J Thorac Cardiovasc Surg. 2014;147(1):133-40.
77. Parissis H, Soo AW, Al-Alao B. Is there any further advantage of using more than one internal mammary artery? Literature review and analysis. Asian Cardiovasc Thorac Ann. 2013;21(1):101-13.
78. Lytle BW, Kramer JR, Golding LA, et al. Young adults with coronary atherosclerosis: ten year results of surgical myocardial revascularization. J Am Coll Cardiol. 1984;4(3):445-53.
79. Ng WK, Vedder M, Whitlock RM, et al. Coronary revascularisation in young adults. Eur J Card Thorac Surg. 1997;11(4):732-8.
80. Kasliwal RR, Kulshreshtha A, Agrawal S, et al. Prevalence of cardiovascular risk factors in Indian patients undergoing coronary artery bypass surgery. J Assoc Physicians India. 2006;54:371-5.

CHAPTER 122

Surgery in Acute Myocardial Infarction

Ganesh K Mani, Pramod K Sharma, Manju Mani

INTRODUCTION

The most serious consequence of coronary artery disease is acute coronary syndrome (ACS) which can lead to long-term disability and death. Mortality rates for men and women older than 40 years of age are 18% and 23%, respectively and account for nearly 1.5 million hospital admissions annually in the United States of America.[1]

Prompt restoration of myocardial blood flow is essential to optimize myocardial salvage and decrease mortality in the first few hours after acute myocardial infarction (AMI). About 20–30% of patients with AMI come forward for coronary artery bypass grafting (CABG) as they are considered ineligible for percutaneous coronary intervention (PCI). The optimal timing of CABG in AMI setting has remained a matter of discussion and debate, making "myocardial salvage", the combined responsibility of both the cardiologist and cardiac surgeons.[2]

Both the American College of Cardiology/American Heart Association (ACC/AHA) and European Society of Cardiology/European Association for Cardio-Thoracic Surgery (ESC/EACTS) *guidelines* provide guidance on the use of CABG as an emergency procedure.[3]

- *Class I*: Indication for CABG in the context of ST-segment elevation myocardial infarction (STEMI) if PCI has been impossible to perform or has failed and the patient has persistent pain and ischemia threatening a significant area of myocardium despite medical therapy
- *Class I:* Indication for emergency surgery:
  - Ventricular septal defect (VSD) (post MI)
  - Papillary muscle rupture resulting in acute and severe mitral regurgitation (MR)
  - Free wall rupture
  - Ventricular pseudoaneurysm
  - Life-threatening ventricular arrhythmias
  - Cardiogenic shock (CS).

However, emergency CABG is not recommended:

- Persistent angina, but only a small area of myocardium at jeopardy and patient is hemodynamically stable
- No reflow state (unsuccessful microvascular reperfusion)
- Ventricular tachycardia with scar and no evidence of ischemia.

CORONARY ARTERY BYPASS SURGERY AFTER FAILED PCI

Recommendations for emergency CABG after failed PCI include the following:

- Ongoing ischemia or threatened occlusion with myocardium at risk (class I)
- Hemodynamic compromise with impairment of coagulation and without previous sternotomy (class IIa)
- Hemodynamic compromise in a previous sternotomy (class IIb)
- Retrieval of foreign body (e.g., fractured guidewire or stent) in a critical location (class IIa).

Over the past decade, PCI has become primary treatment not only for STEMI but also non-STEMI (NSTEMI) (or unstable angina). CABG is reserved for multivessel disease or left main disease (LMD) and is most often performed as an elective or semiacute procedure after stabilization of acute ischemic symptoms.[3,4]

Advancements in PCI have altered the need for emergency CABG.[5] The unpredictable outcomes after emergency CABG triggered the strategy of allowing a "cooling off" period after AMI. However, mortality in patients undergoing emergency CABG could be reduced substantially[6] by using a prospective treatment protocol.

A predictive formula was proposed on the basis of regression analysis (30-day mortality) (Table 1).[7]

When patients were taken up for CABG immediately (1–6 hours), mortality rate for NSTEMI was 2% and STEMI was 15%.[8] Because of the relatively low mortality in NSTEMI, Caceres et al. concluded that in general, delaying CABG especially in hemodynamically stable patients cannot be considered "standard of care" any longer, especially in NSTEMI! The question however remains as to what is the

TABLE 1: Regression analysis (30-day mortality)[7]

Factor	p	p (logistic regression)
Cardiogenic shock	0.043	–
IABP preoperative	0.064	–
LVEF	0.002	–
STEMI	0.014	–
CK-MB >100 (U/L) 6-h	<0.001	–
CK-MB >100 (U/L) 24-h	0.054	–
EUROSCORE	0.04	p <0.001 HR 1.216 95% confidence interval 1.082–1.366

CKMB, creatine kinase-MB; HR, hazard ratio; IABP, intra-aortic balloon pump; LVEF, left ventricular ejection fraction; STEMI, ST-segment elevation myocardial infarction.

Source: Khaladj N, Bobylev D, Peterss S, et al. Immediate surgical coronary revascularisation in patients presenting with acute myocardial infarction. J Cardiothorac Surg. 2013;8:167.

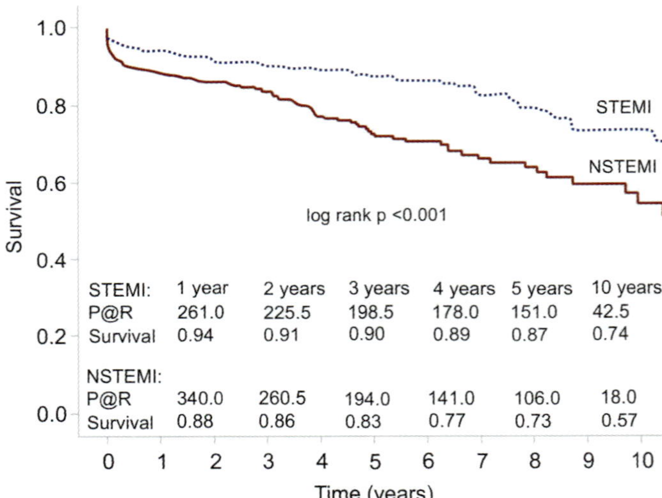

STEMI, ST-segment elevation myocardial infarction; NSTEMI, non-ST-segment elevation myocardial infarction; P@R, patients at risk.

FIG. 1: Ten-year survival after acute myocardial infarction and coronary artery bypass. Kaplan–Meier survival curves for STEMI and NSTEMI patients showed significant survival differences.

Source: Grothusen C, Friedrich C, Loehr J, et al. Outcome of Stable Patients With Acute Myocardial Infarction and Coronary Artery Bypass Surgery Within 48 Hours: A Single-Center, Retrospective Experience. J Am Heart Assoc. 2017;6(10). pii: e005498.

optimal timing for CABG, especially in the era of clopidogrel, ticagrelor or prasugrel.

Timing of CABG in ACS appears a critical factor in predicting outcomes after emergency CABG. Caceres et al.[6] surmised that CABG had relatively similar outcomes in NSTEMI and STEMI though they maintained STEMI as a risk factor for CABG.[6]

But in 2017, quite a contrary view was noted by workers in Germany.

In the absence of CS, Grothusen et al. (2017)[2] found superior short- and long-term outcomes for STEMI patients vis-a-vis NSTEMI patients. STEMI patients were significantly younger with lower risk profiles and shorter referral times. The NSTEMI patients were older, had diabetes, hypertension, renal dysfunction, and multivessel involvement and were referred later in the course of their hospital stay.

OUTCOME OF SURGERY WITHIN 6 HOURS

Grothusen et al. noted that 56% patients of STEMI were operated within 6 hours whereas only 20% of NSTEMI underwent CABG within 6 hours.

Presumably, the NSTEMI patients were sicker as evidenced by higher lactate levels, the higher incidence of preoperative balloon pump insertions. They observed that increased lactate level in excess of 2 mmol/L was associated with higher morbidity and mortality.

Some previous studies indicated that delayed surgery may improve outcomes because of the "proinflammatory" state of these patients causing a "shock"-like state.

Until recently, majority of surgical data indicated that it was indeed worthwhile to wait after AMI for the proinflammatory state to cool off.

Caceras et al. in 2013 was one of the first authors to differentiate between STEMI and NSTEMI as outcomes appeared different.[6] STEMI was considered an incremental risk factor (because of thrombolytics or other antiplatelet drugs on board). However, subsequent data from Grothusen et al. in 2017 indicate that hemodynamically stable STEMI patients can safely undergo early revascularization. In contrast, the surgical NSTEMI population described in this study consisted of older and sicker patients with consequently higher preoperative risk! The ACC/AHA guidelines advice seem to be in line with this experience in NSTEMI.

However, contrary to expectations, Grothusen observed that the CABG after STEMI fared better in the short-term as well as long-term! Survival of STEMI and NSTEMI at 1-year was 94% versus 88% (p <0.001), 87% versus73% after 5 years (p <0.001), and 74% versus 57% after 10 years (p <0.001). Thus they concluded that STEMI patients (not in CS) fared better than NSTEMI patients when subjected to CABG within 48 hours. This observation of outcome in STEMI patients after CABG somewhat challenges the guidelines which have hitherto recommended surgery only after the cooling off of the proinflammatory state (Fig. 1).

OPTIMAL TIMING OF CORONARY ARTERY BYPASS SURGERY IN ACUTE MYOCARDIAL INFARCTION

Nichols et al. 2017[9] found that crude in-hospitality mortality was higher for those whose MI to CABG time was less than 24 hours (5.1%) compared to 1–2 days (1.6%) or 6–7 days (1.6%). These results were similar to those of Parikh et al. 2010[10] whose analysis showed no difference in mortality rates between patients undergoing CABG less than 48 hours or more than 48 hours.

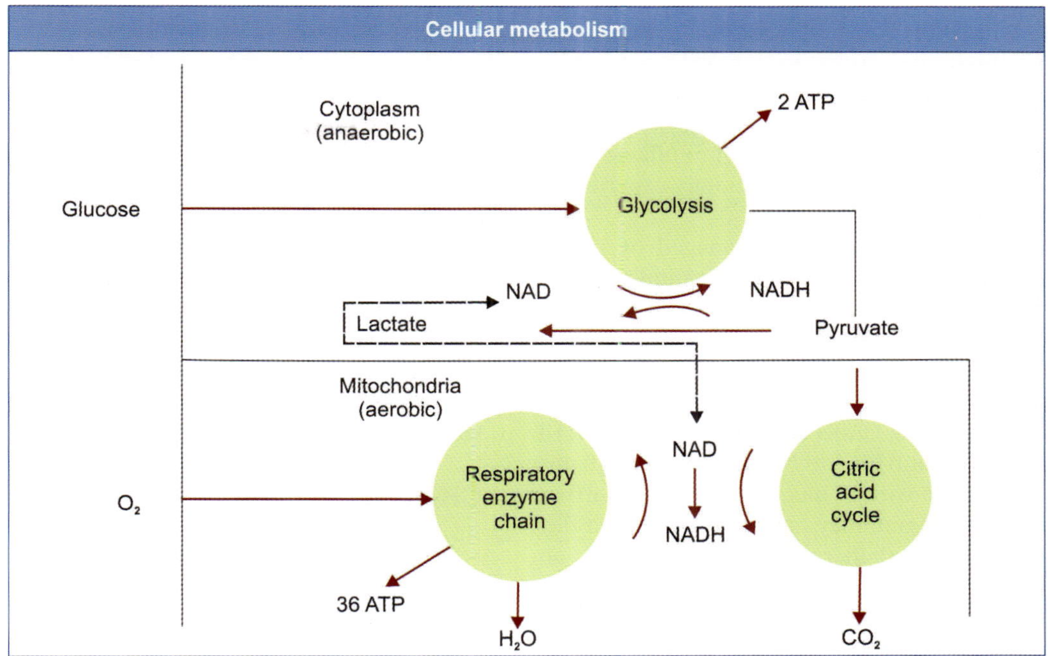

NAD, nicotinamide adenine dinucleotide.

FIG. 2: Beating heart techniques maintain the myocardium in an aerobic state and there by preserve 18 times more adenosine triphosphate (ATP) than the arrested heart which maintain the myocardium in an anaerobic state.

OPERATIVE STRATEGY (ARRESTED OR BEATING HEART?)

Chikara Ueki et al. 2016[11] postulated that on-pump beating heart CABG (On-BH-CABG) is associated with significantly lower morbidity and mortality (45%) as a result of lesser incidence of perioperative myocardial infarction ($p < 0.001$), lesser renal failure ($p < 0.001$) and lesser low output syndromes ($p < 0.001$).

The On-BH-CABG could be an attractive planned alternative to conventional cardioplegic arrest CABG in this high-risk patient population.

However, they observed that it was important to maintain a high arterial pressure during perfusion as it ensured better results.

The myocardial metabolism is maintained in an aerobic state during both off-pump coronary artery bypass graft (OPCABG) as well as On-BH-CABG which is essentially a nonischemic surgery. The preservation of mitochondrial adenosine triphosphate (ATP) could be the reason for less myocardial stunning and thereby better outcomes (Fig. 2).

PERSONAL EXPERIENCE

Though we have had a vast experience of over 15,000 CABGs (1985 to date), we concede that suboptimal record-keeping has precluded the publishing of our results! About 600 CABGs would have been done so far by us within 48 hours after AMI in the last 33 years. Of these, over 300 would have been done by beating heart technique (on- pump or off- pump). The unit policies have changed over the last three decades and so have clinical strategies.

The recent unified "Heart Team" strategy is offering the best option to the ischemic myocardium in AMI. It has been our current policy that CABG is first option in left main stem disease. However, in severe triple vessel disease, stabilizing hemodynamics with plain old balloon angioplasty (POBA) to restore some flow in the culprit artery and wheeling the patient at the earliest to the operating room possibly preserves myocardium better. Intra-aortic balloon pump (IABP) support is particularly valuable if the operation is planned on a beating heart. However, we have readily put the patient on cardiopulmonary bypass whenever hemodynamics were compromised. Before 2000, almost all these operations were done with anoxia and cardioplegia. But since 2000 onwards, all emergency CABGs whether done "off- pump" or "on- pump" were done on beating heart.

Excessive bleeding consequent to the recent use of reteplase and ticagrelor have been managed with cell saver assisted autotransfusion, fractionated blood products, and pharmacological agents like tranexamic acid.

However, a more detailed study comparing surgical outcomes in urgent and delayed CABG in AMI and those of CABG in STEMI and NSTEMI is warranted before we establish that both PCI or CABG emerge to have the same therapeutic value in AMI.

CONCLUSION

Surgery in AMI (excluding postinfarction VSD, acute MR, impending cardiac rupture) is an area where cardiac surgery was not routinely envisaged due to former erroneous attitudes of permitting "cooling off" of a proinflammatory clinical condition following AMI. Contemporary experiences of authors have busted this myth!

The presence of CS (if effectively managed by timely institution of IABP) is no longer a contraindication to CABG and has infarct become an indication.

Though earlier cancers in 2013 had observed that NSTEMI patients fared better[6] after CABG, more recently Grothusen in 2017 has shown that STEMI without CS actually fared better![2]

If logistics are favorable, CABG should be undertaken (if necessary with IABP support) as early as possible, though this subset needs specialized care of blood pressure and arrhythmia. However, usually, one may have to wait till next day for logistic reasons. As per all literature reviewed there is no further advantage by waiting further to "cool" the patient as perceived earlier.

Though most of the Western literature pertains to CABG on the arrested heart, there have been some recent reports favoring off- pump.[8] On-pump beating heart CABG,[11] our own personal experience supports the view that nonischemic technique (avoiding cardioplegic arrest) is a safer option in an already ischemic heart.

RECOMMENDED GUIDELINES

In India, in the middle of 2018, the possible recommended guidelines for revascularization in AMI would be:

- Percutaneous coronary intervention of culprit artery whenever possible
- Heart team to decide early for CABG whenever PCI is not possible
- In the presence of ongoing ischemia in triple vessel disease, culprit artery dilatation (POBA) and insertion of IABP could be done in cath laboratory as "bridge to CABG".
- Early CABG can safely be undertaken in both STEMI and NSTEMI
- Avoiding ischemic cardioplegic arrest may be an advantage in this subset
- Ventricular septal defect repair or mitral valve replacement is necessarily done by on-pump cardioplegic strategies only and has not been addressed in this chapter.

Patients with biochemical values of creatine phosphokinase MB >100, and lactate level >2 mmol are higher risk patients and appropriate consents are advisable. Intra-aortic balloon pump is valuable adjunct and preferable to catecholamines and facilitates OPCABG. Though CABG on arrested heart is the prevalent therapeutic modality in the West, OPCABG (maintaining a higher mean arterial pressure during perfusion) seems to have superior outcomes.

EPILOGUE

The last word is yet to be written and that may alter the ACC/AHA and ESC/EACTS guidelines of the future.[12,13] However as of the June 2018, CABG is indicated in AMI whenever PCI cannot be done. Beating heart surgery on IABP support and adjunctive cell saver support offers an equally safe option be it STEMI or NSTEMI. If ventricular arrhythmia or extremely unstable hemodynamics prevail despite IABP counterpulsation, off-pump or on-pump beating heart CABG should be the "standard of care" for revascularizing the ischemic or infarcting myocardium.

In any case, in LMD or severe triple vessel disease, present day strategies tend to equalize the outcomes of emergency CABG to elective CABG (and PCI)!

ACKNOWLEDGMENTS

- Rajiv Agarwal, DM (senior cardiologist)
- Ripen Gupta, DM (senior cardiologist)
- Prasanta Borthakur, MD (senior anesthesiologist)
- Subhashish Bhowmik, DA (senior anesthesiologist)

REFERENCES

1. Schumer EM, Chaney JH, Trivedi JR, et al. Emergency Coronary Artery Bypass Grafting: Indications and Outcomes from 2003 through 2013.
2. Grothusen C, Friedrich C, Loehr J, et al. Outcome of Stable Patients With Acute Myocardial Infarction and Coronary Artery Bypass Surgery Within 48 Hours: A Single-Center, Retrospective Experience. J Am Heart Assoc. 2017;6(10). pii: e005498.
3. Kolh P, Windecker S, Alfonso F, et al. 2014 ESC/EACTS Guidelines on myocardial revascularization: the Talk Force on Myocardial Revascularization of the European Society of Cardiology (ESC) and the European Association for Cardio-Thoracic surgery (EACTS). Developed with the special contribution of the European Association of Percutaneous Cardiovascular Interventions (EAPCI). Eur J Cardiothorac Surg. 2014;46:517-92.
4. Fox KA, Clayton TC, Damman P, et al. Long term outcome of a routine versus selective invasive strategy in patients with non-ST segment elevation acute coronary syndrome a meta-analysis of individual patient data. J Am Coll Cardiol. 2010;55:2435-45.
5. Axelsson TA, Mennander A, Malmberg M, et al. Is emergency and salvage coronary artery bypass grafting justified? The Nordic Emergency/Salvage coronary artery bypass grafting study. Eur J Cardiothorac Surg. 2016;49(2016):1451-6.
6. Caceres M, Weiman DS. Optimal timing of coronary artery bypass grafting in acute myocardial infarction. Ann Thorac Surg. 2013;95:365-72.
7. Khaladj N, Bobylev D, Peterss S, et al. Immediate surgical coronary revascularisation in patients presenting with acute myocardial infarction. J Cardiothorac Surg. 2013;8:167.
8. Bárta J, Brát R, Gaj J, et al. Immediate coronary artery bypass graft surgery for acute coronary syndrome – Outcomes and trends over the past eight years. Cor et Vasa. 2015;57(2):e63.
9. Nichols EL, McCullough JN, Ross CS, et al.; for the Northern New England Cardiovascular Disease Study Group. Optimal Timing From Myocardial Infarction to Coronary Artery Bypass Grafting on Hospital Mortality. Ann Thorac Surg. 2017;103(1):162-71.
10. Parikh SV, de Lemos JA, Jessen ME, et al. Timing of in-hospital coronary artery bypass graft surgery for non-ST-segment elevation myocardial infarction patients results from the National Cardiovascular Data Registry

ACTION Registry-GWTG (Acute Coronary Treatment and Intervention Outcomes Network Registry-Get With The Guidelines). JACC Cardiovasc Interv. 2010;3:419-27.

11. Ueki C, Sakaguchi G, Akimoto T, et al.; Department of Cardiovascular Surgery, Shizuoka General Hospital, Shizuoka, Japan. On-pump beating-heart technique is associated with lower morbidity and mortality following coronary artery bypass grafting: a meta-analysis. Eur J Cardiothorac Surg. 2016;50(5):813-21.
12. Steg PG, James SK, Atar D, et al. ESC Guidelines for the management of acute myocardial infarction in patients presenting with ST-segment elevation. Eur Heart J. 2012;33:2569-619.
13. Roffi M, Patrono C, Collet JP, et al. 2015 ESC Guidelines for the management of acute coronary syndromes in patients presenting without persistent ST-segment elevation: task Force for the Management of Acute Coronary Syndromes in Patients Presenting without Persistent ST-Segment Elevation of the European Society of Cardiology (ESC). Eur Heart J. 2016;37:267-315.

CHAPTER 123

Recent Advances in Coronary Artery Bypass Graft

OP Yadava

INTRODUCTION

1965 was a revolutionary year the in the field of coronary artery disease (CAD) when sutured anastomosis for coronary artery bypass graft (CABG) surgery was first performed by Kolessov and Potashov. Such was the impact of CABG that it surpassed any other cardiac surgery in numbers. Basking in the glory of the initial success, cardiac surgeons developed a kind of inertia and coronary surgery remained static in the 1970s and 1980s. However, challenged and egged on by the advances in percutaneous coronary interventions (PCI), surgeons too started innovating both as means of improving patient outcomes and experiences as also to protect their turf and advances came fast and furious in 1990s and thereafter in the millennium (Fig. 1).

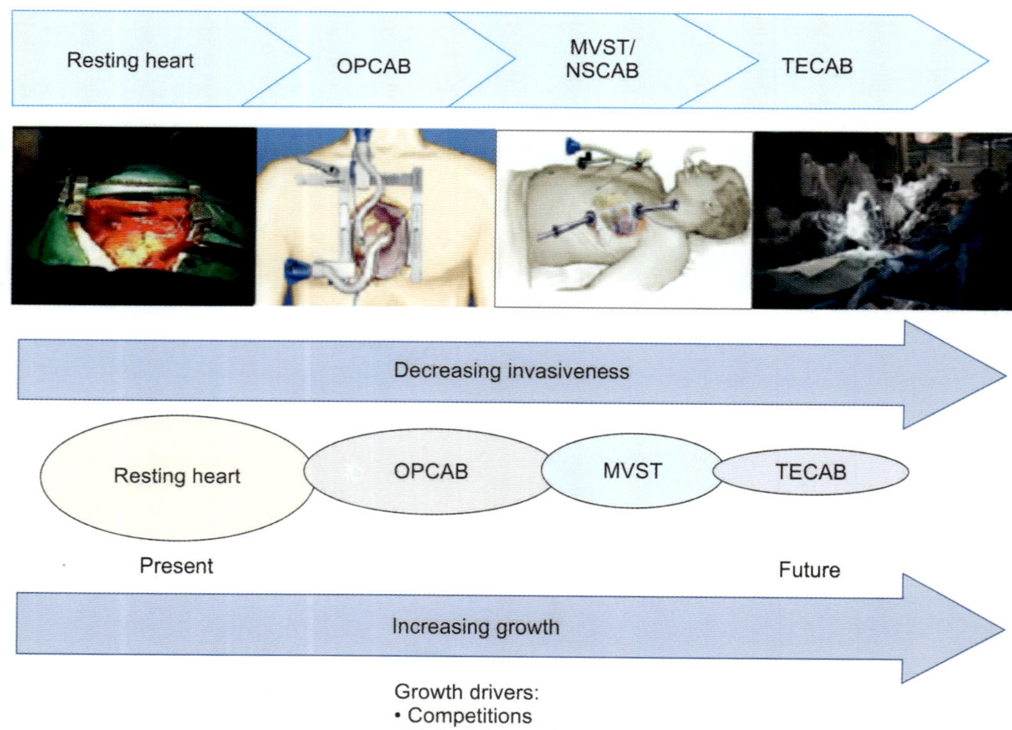

OPCAB, off-pump coronary artery bypass; MVST, Multivessel sternotomy NSCAB, Non sternotomy coronary artery bypass; TECAB, total endoscopic coronary artery bypass.

FIG. 1: Evolution of coronary artery bypass surgery.

MINIMALLY INVASIVE CABG

Minimally invasive cardiac surgery (MICS) envisages avoidance of both the cardiopulmonary bypass (CPB) and the sternotomy as its primary objective and reduction in the size of the incision as its secondary objective. Another advantage of MICS is avoidance of aortic manipulation thereby leading to a reduction of the stroke rates.[1] By avoiding sternotomy, respiratory functions are maintained better and the dreaded complication of mediastinitis can be eliminated. Avoidance of CPB prevents the whole body inflammatory response and its attendant side effects.[2] All this leads to fast tracking of the patients, besides improved cosmesis, as a small anterior or lateral thoracotomy is used for MICS.[3] Left internal mammary artery (LIMA) can be harvested endoscopically, but is now being replaced with robotically assisted LIMA harvest. Simple LIMA to left anterior descending (LAD) coronary artery through an anterior thoracotomy (Figs. 2A and B) has been labeled minimally invasive direct coronary artery bypass (MIDCAB) but even multiple bypasses can be performed with use of nonsternotomy stabilizer and positioner.[4] Excellent results have been demonstrated in skilled hands,[5] with reduced need for blood transfusion, reduced atrial fibrillation, and postoperative strokes. MICS-CABG has been validated against PCI[6] and conventional CABG.[7] However, Rabindranauth et al. found less number of grafts being performed with a MICS-CABG than with sternotomy off-pump coronary artery bypass (OPCAB)—(2.1 vs. 3.2%, respectively)[8] and graft patency too has been a matter of concern in some studies.[9]

Future is likely to witness increased penetration of MICS-CABG in the surgical fraternity as the surgical instrumentation and techniques improve. Robotically assisted CABG is another new development which is likely to see more traction going forwards. In fact Ishikawa et al.[10] performed robotically assisted awake CABG—ultra MICS, under epidural anesthesia and even day care MICS—CABG have been reported. Though currently, robotically assisted total endoscopic CABG (TECAB) may be inferior to MIDCAB,[11] but this may change as more and more experience is gained. As it stands today, MICS-CABG is a niche area meant for a limited few but with new anastomotic automated devices,[12,13] these techniques are going to percolate widely as they have mass appeal to the patients too. Coronary-conduit coupling devices, magnetic couplers, and even glues and laser welding are being evaluated and may fructify in the future.

Simulation-based learning in the skills labs too would help matters going forward. Even bilateral internal mammary artery (IMA) can be harvested through a left mini thoracotomy using direct vision.[14] In a limited survey carried out in India, 69% of the cardiac surgeons confirmed undertaking minimally invasive work, with a majority carrying 5–20% of their cardiac procedures using MICS techniques. However, only one-third of surgeons doing minimally invasive work were undertaking MICS-CABG.[3] Future is going to witness personalized medicine and customized operations with "one size fit all" operations—a paradigm of the gone by era.

CONDUITS—IMPROVING PATENCY

Though arterial grafts have superior patency and total arterial revascularization (TAR) improves long-term survival rates (10 years survival 85.4% for TAR and 81.2% for non-TAR—p <0.001),[15] almost 80% of all conduits used in CABG are saphenous vein (SV) grafts. Newer molecular targets involved in smooth muscle proliferation are being targeted to enhance SV patency.[16] Even external vein graft support stents[17] are being developed and gene and cell-based therapies too are being tried.[18] Alternative conduits in form of nonautologous umbilical vein grafts, long SV homografts, treated bovine IMA, 3D printing of conduits, and tissue engineered conduits, available off the shelf, are on the horizon.

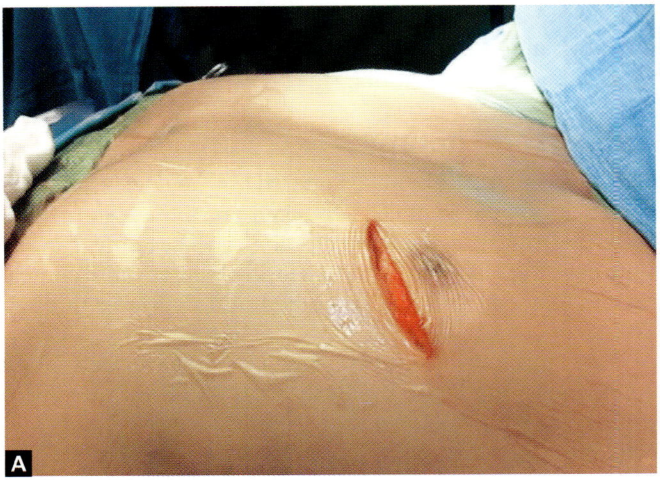

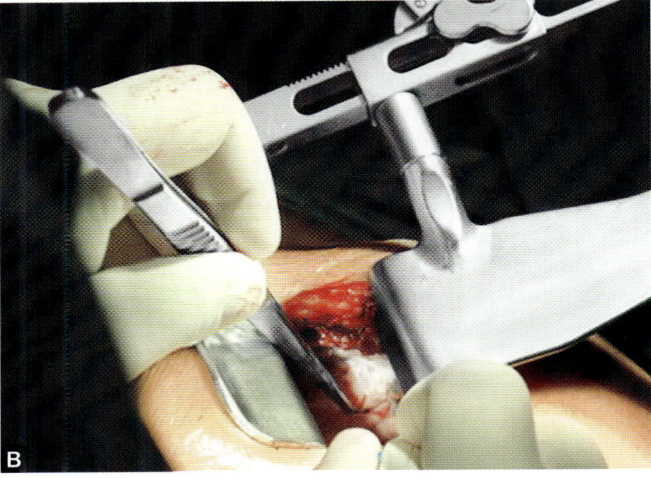

FIG. 2: Minimally invasive direct coronary artery bypass grafting through a small anterior thoracotomy. **A,** Submammary small incision; **B,** LIMA - LAD anastomosis.

Source: From Yadava OP, Lokeswara S. Cardiac Surgery in India: Coronary: At Par with the Rest of the World. CSI Textbook of Cardiology; 2017.

ON VERSUS OFF-PUMP CABG

Like any new technology, off-pump CABG came into vogue in 1990s with a lot of promise[19] with the hope that avoidance of CPB will ameliorate all the systemic inflammatory ill effects of conventional CABG.[2] However, ROOBY (Randomized On/Off Bypass) trial[20] challenged it and even 5 years results showed higher mortality, myocardial infarction (MI), and lower graft patency with off-pump vs. on-pump CABG [relative risk (RR) 1.14; $p = 0.046$].[21]

However, the CORONARY (CABG Off- or On-Pump Revascularization Study) trial[22] and Afilalo's meta-analysis[23] could not demonstrate any difference in the mortality, stroke, MI or quality of life measures between the two techniques. Even the patency rates[24] and survival up to 6–8 years[25] were same in the BHACAS I and II trials. Recent meta-analysis by Deppe et al.[26] and Luo et al.[27] too failed to demonstrate any difference in early mortality at 30 days and 6 months, respectively, between the two techniques.

Off-pump CABG may be associated with incomplete myocardial revascularization as suggested by the CORONARY trial.[22] To the contrary, Palmer et al.[28] found that the ratio of anastomosis to lesions was same, thereby implicating patient selection for less number of grafts off-pump, i.e., probably patients needing less number of grafts were chosen for off-pump CABG.

With the use of anaortic, off-pump techniques, the perioperative stroke rates is likely to come down[29] and high-risk patients tend to benefit more from off-pump CABG[30] with less postoperative renal dysfunction, less bleeding and use of blood products, and early mobilization and discharge from hospital.

This raging controversy therefore seems to be surreal and those committed to off-pump ideology are likely to continue performing this procedure. In our experience of 3500 CABGs, off-pump CABG reduced mortality, specially in women, from 4.5% on-pump to 1.4% off-pump ($p = 0.01$).[31]

HYBRID MYOCARDIAL REVASCULARIZATION

Though a noble intent, of harnessing the survival benefits of the gold standard surgical LIMA to LAD anastomosis, and the use of PCI with drug-eluting stents for non-LAD vessels, with a view to lowering periprocedural complications, hybrid myocardial revascularization (HMR) has till date not lived up to the hype generated. HMR may be performed sequentially, with either CABG first, or PCI first, or it can be performed simultaneously in a hybrid theater. Though the safety and the feasibility of HMR is fully established, the POL-MIDES study[32] failed to demonstrate any hard end-point advantage of HMR over CABG (all-cause mortality—CABG 2.9% vs. HMR 2% and 1 year survival CABG 92.2% vs. HMR 89.8%). Similarly, the HREVS (Hybrid Revascularization Versus Standards) study[33] found that residual myocardial ischemia and major adverse cardiac and cerebrovascular event (MACCE) were the same in the three study arms, viz. CABG, PCI, and HMR. Multicenter observational study by John Puskas et al.[34] again failed to demonstrate any advantage of HMR over multivessel PCI. Even in a meta-analysis by Zhu et al.,[35] feasibility and safety of HMR was demonstrated along with reduced need for transfusion of blood products and faster recovery, but there was no difference with regards to in-hospital mortality or 1 year survival. To the contrary, Kahn et al.[36] found HMR superior in terms of only 1 stent failure in the HMR group vs. 7 SV graft failures in the CABG group with MACE occurring in 7% of HMR patients versus 23% in the CABG group ($p = 0.05$). Excellent results using fractional flow results-guided HMR have been demonstrated by Davidavicius et al.[37]

The costs and the logistics of hybrid operating theater may be a barrier for its use, specially in a developing country like India. However, randomized controlled trials for diligent scientific scrutiny of the hard end-points are called for and likely to be launched in the future. HMR with robotically assisted LIMA harvest seems a promising prospect.[38]

NO OPTION CORONARY ARTERY DISEASE

Transmyocardial Laser Revascularization

For patients with diffused coronary atherosclerosis and sub-optimum targets for conventional myocardial revascularization in form of CABG or PCI, transmyocardial laser revascularization (TMLR) is an approved form of therapy. Two kinds of laser systems, the holmium "yttrium-aluminum-garnet" and the carbon dioxide laser systems have been approved by the United States FDA. TMLR can be performed either as a standalone procedure (Sole Therapy) or in conjunction with CABG.[39] In these patients, TMLR has been shown to improve symptoms, reduce hospitalization, and increase event-free survival,[40,41] which sustained over long term.[42] In fact even in a very recent study, improved survival was demonstrated in these patients (65% vs. 52% $p = 0.05$).[43] The mechanism of action of TMLR is debatable and the postulations are that it works through either laser-induced sympathetic regional denervation, angiogenesis, and neovascularization or increased blood flow through patent channels.[44] It may even be a placebo effect. Probably the effects are multifactorial.

Cell-based Therapies

Cell therapies, till now, have flattered only to deceive, but the use of embryonic stem cells, induced pluripotent stem cells, bone marrow mononuclear cells and most recently, cardiac stem cells[45] are likely to bring this form of therapy into clinical realm. They can even be combined and delivered through TMLR.

Bone marrow laser revascularization involves delivery of autologous bone marrow cells through TMLR with a view to using their paracrine effects of secreting growth factors and cytokines and thereby potentiating the neoangiogenesis of TMLR.[46] However, the results are equivocal.

Besides TMLR, coronary venous bypass grafting in form of arterialization of the great and middle cardiac veins using a

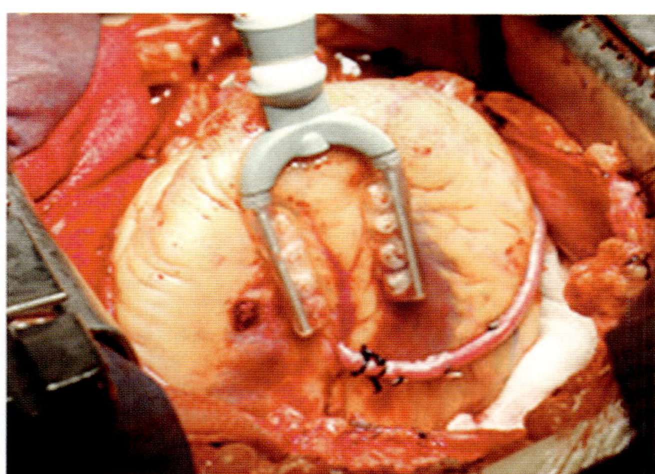

FIG. 3: Flow limiting coronary venous bypass graft.[47]

pedicled IMA and its various iterations, including flow limited coronary venous bypass graft, are being explored[47] (Fig. 3).

QUALITY INITIATIVES

Contemporary CABG relies on qualitative cine coronary angiography for assessment of the coronary artery stenosis. However, the importance of looking at the physiological impact of an anatomical stenosis has been adequately demonstrated by the FAME (Fractional Flow Reserve Versus Angiography for Multivessel Evaluation) study. Though there were no mortality benefits, other clinical outcomes were superior with fractional flow reserve (FFR)-based revascularization as compared to conventional angiography based PCI.[48] Already some centers are using noninvasively assessed FFR measurements in CABG and GRAFFITI (Graft Patency After FFR-guided Versus Angio-guided CABG) trial is comparing angiographically driven CABG versus FFR driven CABG. Physiologically driven surgical myocardial revascularization is likely to become a routine and a normative quality matrix to avoid unnecessary grafting and to improve the outcomes of CABG.

In future, it is likely that intraoperative graft validation will become mandatory and in fact a norm for quality initiatives. Though cine angiography is the gold standard, however, in absence of free availability of hybrid operation theatres, noninvasive graft validation in form of either transit time flowmetry (TTFM) or indocyanine fluorescence imaging, thermal coronary angiography or high-resolution epicardial coronary ultrasonography (HR-ECUS) are likely to find greater application. In fact, DiGiammarco et al. recommend combining TTFM with HR-ECUS as it increases the positive predictive value of TTFM to virtually 100%.[49]

MISCELLANEOUS

Advancements in CPB technology in form of biocompatible and miniaturized circuits, as also better myocardial protection, will make the surgeries safer. Artificial intelligence may make the protocol-dictated delivery of intensive care safer and computers and mathematical modeling too will help in planning and execution of surgery.

Future is going to see increased cooperation between the interventional cardiologist and the cardiac surgeons to the point of may be amalgamation of the two, with the surgeons learning catheter-based skills.

A more holistic view is being taken currently with a realization that no single form of therapy is panacea to all the attendant ills of CAD. Therefore, heart-team concept assumes increasing importance and amalgamation of alternative forms of therapy—AYUSH with allopathy is likely to give better long-term outcomes. The development of the new specialty of "vascular psychiatry" with a view to bringing about behavioral change is again a futuristic well-intended trend. A "Heart Team", indeed a "Platonic illusion"[50] till date, is likely to see more traction and patient and his personal physicians will form an integral part of decision making, thereby making treatment of CAD more organic and socially relevant. With the launch of social insurance schemes like "AYUSHMAN BHARAT" as also with deeper penetration of other health insurance schemes, the availability and affordability of coronary interventions, both percutaneous and surgical, will improve.

CONCLUSION

Total arterial revascularization and miniaturization of incision using minimally invasive and robotically assisted techniques and off the shelf, tissue engineered or biological conduits will make the surgery customized to each patients' needs. There is a need for increased cooperation and collaboration between the family physician, interventional cardiologist, and the cardiac surgeon for an organic approach to the problem.

However, final answer to the woes of CAD will lie in molecular biology, genetics, and behavioral change with a view to preventing the disease rather than treating it.

REFERENCES

1. Misfeld M, Brereton RJ, Sweetman EA, et al. Neurologic complications after off-pump coronary artery bypass grafting with and without aortic manipulation: meta-analysis of 11,398 cases from 8 studies. J Thorac Cardiovasc Surg. 2011;142:e11-17.
2. Czerny M, Baumer H, Kilo J, et al. Inflammatory response and myocardial injury following coronary artery bypass grafting with or without cardiopulmonary bypass. Eur J Cardiothorac Surg. 2000;17:737-42.
3. Kayatta MO, Halkos ME, Narayan P. Minimally Invasive Coronary Artery Bypass Grafting. Ind J Cardiothorac Surg. 2018. In Press.
4. McGinn JT Jr, Usman S, Lapierre H, et al. Minimally invasive coronary artery bypass grafting: dual-center experience in 450 consecutive patients. Circulation. 2009;120:S78-84.
5. Kettering K, Dapunt O, Baer FM. Minimally invasive direct coronary artery bypass grafting: a systematic review. J Cardiovasc Surg (Torino). 2004;45:255-64.
6. Blazek S, Rossbach C, Borger MA, et al. Comparison of sirolimus-eluting stenting with minimally invasive bypass surgery for stenosis of the left anterior descending coronary artery: 7-year follow-up of a randomized trial. JACC Cardiovasc Interv. 2015;8:30-8.

7. Deppe AC, Liakopoulos OJ, Kuhn EW, et al. Minimally invasive direct coronary bypass grafting versus percutaneous coronary intervention for single-vessel disease: a meta-analysis of 2885 patients. Eur J Cardiothorac Surg. 2015;47:397-406.
8. Rabindranauth P, Burns JG, Vessey TT, et al. Minimally invasive coronary artery bypass grafting is associated with improved clinical outcomes. Innovations (Phila) 2014;9:421-6.
9. Vicol C, Nollert G, Mair H, et al. Midterm results of beating heart surgery in 1-vessel disease: minimally invasive direct coronary artery bypass versus off-pump coronary artery bypass with full sternotomy. Heart Surg Forum. 2003;6:341-4.
10. Ishikawa N, Watanabe G. Ultra-minimally invasive cardiac surgery: robotic surgery and awake CABG. Surg Today. 2015;45(1):1-7.
11. Jegaden O, Wautot F, Sassard T, et al. Is there an optimal minimally invasive technique for left anterior descending coronary artery bypass? J Cardiothorac Surg. 2011;6:37.
12. Cohn WE. Advances in surgical treatment of acute and chronic coronary artery disease. Tex Heart Inst J. 2010;37:328-33.
13. Soylu E, Harling L, Ashrafian H, et al. A systematic review of the safety and efficacy of distal coronary artery anastomotic devices. Eur J Cardiothorac Surg. 2016;49:732-45.
14. Nambiar P, Mittal C. Minimally invasive coronary bypass using internal thoracic arteries via a left minithoracotomy: "the Nambiar Technique". Innovations (Phila). 2013;8:420-6.
15. Tatoulis J, Wynne R, Skillington PD, et al. Total Arterial Revascularisation - Achievable and Prognostically effective. A multicenter analysis. Ann Thorac Surg. 2015;100:1268-75.
16. Walker T, Muller I, Raabe C, et al. Effective silencing of adhesion molecules on venous endothelial cells for protection of venous bypass grafts. Eur J Cardiothorac Surg. 2011;40:1241-47.
17. Taggart DP, Amin S, Djordjevic J, et al. A prospective study of external stenting of saphenous vein grafts to the right coronary artery: the VEST II study. Eur J Cardiothorac Surg. 2017;51(5):952-8.
18. Katz MG, Fargnoli AS, Kendle AP, et al. Gene Therapy in Cardiac Surgery: Clinical Trials, Challenges, and Perspectives. Ann Thorac Surg. 2016;101(6): 2407-16.
19. Benetti FJ, Naselli G, Wood M, et al. Direct myocardial revascularization without extracorporeal circulation; Experience in 700 patients. Chest. 1991;100(2):312-16.
20. Shroyer AL, Grover FL, Hattler B, et al. For the Veterans Affairs Randomized On/Off Bypass (ROOBY) Study Group. On-Pump versus Off-Pump Coronary Artery Bypass Surgery. New Engl J Med. 2009;361:1827-37.
21. Shroyer AL, Hattler B, Wagner TH, et al. for the Veterans Affairs ROOBY - FS Group. Five year outcomes after On Pump and Off-Pump Coronary Artery Bypass. New Engl J Med. 2017;377:623-32.
22. Lamy A, Devereaux PJ, Prabhakaran D, et al.; for the CORONARY Investigators. Five Year Outcomes after Off-Pump and On-Pump Coronary Artery Bypass Grafting. New Engl J Med. 2016;375:2359-68.
23. Afilalo A, Rasti M, Ohayon SM. Off-pump vs. on-pump coronary artery bypass surgery: an updated meta-analysis and meta-regression of randomized trials. Eur Heart J. 2012;33(10):1257-67.
24. Angelini GD, Taylor FC, Reeves BC, et al. Early and midterm outcome after off-pump and on-pump surgery in Beating Heart Against Cardioplegic Arrest Studies (BHACAS 1 and 2): a pooled analysis of two randomised controlled trials. Lancet. 2002;359(9313):1194-99.
25. Angelini GD, Culliford L, Smith DK, et al. Effects of on- and off-pump coronary artery surgery on graft patency, survival, and health-related quality of life: long-term follow-up of 2 randomized controlled trials. J Thorac Cardiovasc Surg. 2009;137:295-303.
26. Deppe AC, Arbash W, Kuhn EW, et al. Current evidence of coronary artery bypass grafting off-pump versus on-pump: a systematic review with meta-analysis of over 16,900 patients investigated in randomized controlled trials. Eur J Cardiothorac Surg. 2016;49:1031-41.
27. Luo T, Ni Y. Short-term and Long-term Postoperative Safety of Off-Pump versus On- Pump Coronary Artery Bypass Grafting for Coronary Heart Disease: A Meta-analysis for Randomized Controlled Trials. Thorac Cardiovasc Surg. 2015;63:319-27.
28. Palmer G, Herbert MA, Prince SL, et al. Coronary Artery Revascularization (CARE) registry: an observational study of on-pump and off-pump coronary artery revascularization. Ann Thorac Surg. 2007;83:986-91.
29. Yadava OP. An-aortic Total Arterial OPCAB - Panacea to all ills ? Indian Heart J. 2015;67:196-200.
30. Kuss O, von Salviati B, Börgermann J. Off-pump versus on-pump coronary artery bypass grafting: a systematic review and meta-analysis of propensity score analyses. J Thorac Cardiovasc Surg. 2010;140:829-35, 835.e1-13.
31. Yadava OP, Prakash A, Kundu A, et al. Coronary Artery Bypass Grafting in women - Is OPCAB mandatory? Ind Heart J. 2011;63:425-8.
32. Gasior M, Zembala MO, Tajstra M, et al. Hybrid revascularization for multivessel coronary artery disease. JACC Cardiovasc Interv. 2014;7:1277-83.
33. Ganyukov V, Kochergin N, Shilov A, et al. The Comparative Effectiveness of Hybrid Revascularization (MIDCAB Then PCI) With DES Versus Multivessel DES PCI or CABG (HREVS). [online] Available from https://clinicaltrials.gov/ct2/show/NCT01699048.
34. Puskas JD, Halkos ME, DeRose JJ, et al. Hybrid coronary revascularization for the treatment of multivessel coronary artery disease: A multicenter observational study. J Am Coll Cardiol. 2016;68:356-65.
35. Zhu P, Zhou P, Sun Y, et al. Hybrid coronary revascularization versus coronary artery bypass grafting for multivessel coronary artery disease: systematic review and meta-analysis. J Cardiothorac Surg. 2015;10:63.
36. Kon ZN, Kwon MH, Collins MJ, et al. Off-Pump coronary artery bypass leads to a regional hypercoagulable state not detectable using systemic markers. Innovations (Phila.). 2006;1:232-8.
37. Davidavicius G, Van Praet F, Mansour S, et al. Hybrid revascularization strategy: a pilot study on the association of robotically enhanced minimally invasive direct coronary artery bypass surgery and fractional-flow-reserve-guided percutaneous coronary intervention. Circulation. 2005;112: I317-22.
38. Kiaii B, McClure S, Stewart P, et al. Simultaneous integrated coronary artery revascularisation with long-term angiographic follow-up. J Thorac Cardiovasc Surg. 2008;136:702-8.
39. Allen KB, Dowling RD, Heimansohn DA, et al. Transmyocardial revascularization utilizing a holmium: YAG laser. Eur J Cardiothorac Surg. 1998;14:S100-4.
40. Burkhoff D, Schmidt S, Schulman SP, et al. Transmyocardial revascularization compared with continued medical therapy for treatment of refractory angina pectoris: a prospective randomized trial. Lancet. 1999;354:885-90.
41. Aaberge L, Norstrand K, Dragsund M, et al. Transmyocardial Revascularization with CO2 laser in patients with refractory angina pectoris: clinical results from the Norwegian randomized trial. J Am Coll Card. 2000;35:1170-77.
42. Horvath KA, Aranki SF, Cohn LC, et al. Sustained angina relief 5 years after transmyocardial laser revascularization with a CO2 laser. Circulation. 2001;I: 81-8.
43. Allen KB, Dowling RD, Angell W, et al. Transmyocardial revascularization: five-year follow-up of a prospective, randomized, multicenter trial. Ann Thorac Surg. 2004;77:1228-34.
44. Allen KB, Mahoney A, Aggarwal S, et al. Transmyocardial Revascularization (TMR): Current Status and Future Directions. Ind J Thorac Cardiovasc Surg. 2018. In Press.
45. Katz MG, Fargnoli AS, Kendle AP, et al. Gene Therapy in Cardiac Surgery: Clinical Trials, Challenges, and Perspectives. Ann Thorac Surg. 2016;101(6):2407-16.
46. Reyes G, Allen KB, Alegre A, et al. Bone marrow laser revascularization for treating angina due to diffuse CAD. Eur J Cardiovasc Thorac Surg. 2009;36: 192-4.
47. Gu C-X, Yu Y, Wang C. (2013). Surgical Treatment for Diffuse Coronary Artery Diseases. [online] Available from http://dx.doi.org/10.5772/54416 [Accessed August 2018].
48. van Nunen LX, Zimmermann FM, Tonino PA, et al. FAME Study Investigators. Fractional flow reserve versus angiography for guidance of PCI in patients with multivessel coronary artery disease (FAME): 5-year follow-up of a randomized controlled trial. Lancet. 2015;386:1853-60.
49. Di Giammarco G, Canosa C, Foschi M, et al. Intraoperative graft verification in coronary surgery: increased diagnostic accuracy adding high-resolution epicardial ultrasonography to transit-time flow measurement. Eur J Cardiothorac Surg. 2014;45:e41-5.
50. Yadava OP. 'Heart Team' Concept - A reality or a 'Platonic Illusion'. Ind Heart J. 2017;69(5):681-3.

CHAPTER 124

Redo Coronary Artery Bypass Grafting: Challenges and Outcomes

Ramakanta Panda, Muzil Munshi

INTRODUCTION

A patient needs redo coronary artery bypass grafting (CABG) when there is graft occlusion or progression of their native coronary artery disease (CAD) or a combination of both. Redo CABG is far more challenging than primary CABG because the patients are older, have more compromised ventricular function, more comorbid conditions, severe and diffuse native distal coronary atherosclerosis and frequently have more advanced atherosclerosis in aortic and noncardiac arteries. Moreover, adhesions from previous operations predisposing the patient to higher risk of injury to cardiac structures or a patent arterial graft as well as saphenous vein graft (SVG) atherosclerosis with its attendant higher risk of distal embolization of atherosclerotic material adds up to the higher risk to patient and technical challenge to the surgical team. The availability of conduits if both internal thoracic arteries (ITAs) and saphenous veins were used up in first operation adds up to the challenge.

INCIDENCE

Likelihood of patient needing reoperation depends on variables related to patient, variables related to first time surgery and strict control of risk factors postprimary surgery. Patient-related variables are young age at first operation, preserved left ventricular (LV) function, single or double vessel disease, class III or IV symptoms at primary operation. Variables related to first time surgery predicting reoperation are: not using an ITA especially to left anterior descending (LAD) coronary artery and incomplete revascularization.

Even though Cosgrove et al.[1] have reported a cumulative incidence of reoperation of 3% at 5 years, 10% by 10 years, and 25% by 20 years, over last three decades, there has been a gradual decline in the total number of patients undergoing isolated repeat CABG as well as frequency of redo CABG relative to total CABG performed. This is due partly to universal use of at least one ITA especially to LAD compared to earlier decades, more use of arterial conduits, improved surgical technique, possibly more effective risk factor control, optimal medical therapy with universal use of statins as well as antiplatelet therapy and more use of catheter interventions in patients with prior CABG.

Cleveland Clinic, one of the highest volume redo surgery centers, saw their numbers decline from 37% in 1990 to 30% in 2000[2] and more dramatically in current decade to 4.6% of all isolated CABG operations. This is similar to a decline from 6.0% in 2000 to 3.4% in 2009 from analysis of 72.322 isolated redo CABG patients from 1,035 institutions from Society of Thoracic Surgeons (STS) Adult Cardiac Surgery Database.[3] Spiliotopoulos et al.[4] from Toronto General Hospital, in a most recent largest single center study of changing pattern of redo CABG of 1,204 patients, among 25,347 patients undergoing isolated CABG procedure, reported a decline from 7.2% (1990–1994) to 2.2% (2005–2009). The Japanese Association for Thoracic Surgery (JATS) also reported[5] a significant decline of ratio of redo CABG to total number of CABG from 10% in 2001 to 2% in 2010. The prevalence of redo CABG among elderly patients who undergo CABG is very uncommon.[6] Fosbol et al. in a review of STS database of 723,134 patients older than 65 years who underwent isolated CABG between 1991 and 2007 found repeat revascularization incidence of 0.1, 0.6, 1.3, and 1.7% at 1, 5, 10 and 18 years, respectively. Mode of repeat revascularization among these patients was mostly percutaneous coronary intervention (PCI) (93%).

Emphasis on medical therapy over revascularization in patients with stable angina[7] and improved medical management with use of beta-blockers, statins, and angiotensin-converting enzyme (ACE) inhibitors that can slow the progression of coronary disease delays or obviates the need for surgical revascularization.[8] Among the patients in STS database, more patients were receiving statin and ACE inhibitors in 2009 than in 2004.[3] PCI on native arteries or the grafts of re-operated patients, before redo CABG significantly increased from 14.5% (1990 through 1994) to 26.6% (2005 through 2009).[4] Similar increase was reported by Riley et al.[9] who reported an increase of 31% among US Medicare population from 2001 to 2004 but decreased by 20% thereafter presumably from clinical trials demonstrating of lack of benefit of additional PCI (above optimal medical therapy) in stable CAD. Among the patients in the STS database of 72,431 patients undergoing reoperative CABG, incidence of patients treated with previous PCI had increased from 35% in 2000 to 53% in 2009.[3]

During past few decades, there has been universal use of a left internal thoracic artery (LITA) graft to LAD combined with an increase in use of arterial grafts during primary operation,[10] possibly contributing to higher graft patency of arterial grafts thus decreased need for reoperation.[3,11-14]

PATIENT RISK PROFILE

Patients undergoing coronary reoperation exhibit significantly worse risk profile. They are older, have more comorbidities, more unstable angina, higher New York Heart association (NYHA) class, worse LV function, previous myocardial infarction (MI), higher incidence of peripheral vascular disease.[2,15] In the study of STS database from 2000 to 2009, though there was no significant change in age or gender of reoperation patients, there were significant prevalence of comorbidities like diabetes (42.5% vs. 31.7%), hypertension (90.9% vs. 73.4%), hypercholesterolemia (93.0% vs. 71.8%), renal failure (2.2% vs. 0.7%), chronic obstructive pulmonary disease (25.5% vs. 16.6%), cerebrovascular disease (12.4% vs. 8.5%) in 2009 than 2000.[3] They had worse presentation like congestive failure (18.4 vs. 14.2%), left main disease (35.1% vs. 25.7%), MI (60.9% vs. 55.9%), renal failure (2.2% vs. 0.7%), and cerebrovascular disease (12.4% vs. 8.5%). They more likely needed an urgent procedure than a routine one. The study of risk profile from Toronto General Hospital[4] showed similar increase over the years from 1990 to 2009. The patients were significantly older, had higher incidence of diabetes, hypertension, dyslipidemia, left main disease, peripheral vascular disease, and cerebrovascular accidents. The mean interval between first operation and reoperation had increased.

INDICATIONS

Unlike the randomized trials of bypass surgeries versus medical management in the 1970s and subsequent studies that provided information that formed the basis of indication for first time bypass surgeries, no such information exists for decision making regarding redo CABG. The coronary pathology of patients with prior CABG especially with vein graft, that progresses more rapidly and erratically, are different from that of patients with native CAD. The natural history of both cannot be equated to behave similarly.

The pathology of SVG to coronary arteries is different at various time intervals after surgery.[16-20] Most vein grafts develop proliferative intimal fibroplasia within 2–3 months which evolves with time to a nonfriable fibrous lesion. This may or may not cause stenosis or occlusion. This is completely different from vein graft atherosclerosis which starts as early as 3–4 years after surgery and is due to lipid infiltration into areas of intimal hyperplasia. Vein graft atherosclerosis is a friable, diffuse, superficial lesion and is often associated with overlying mural thrombus. This is different from native coronary atherosclerosis which is segmental, and proximal, eccentric, encapsulated, and is usually not friable or associated with mural thrombus.

Because of above and greater surgical risk of redo CABG compared to primary CABG, indications for the former are stricter and based on careful assessment of risk benefit ratio. Patients with early (<5 years after operation) vein graft stenosis (mostly intimal hyperplasia and nonatherosclerotic) have approximately the same outcomes as those with no stenosis[19,20] and can be managed medically. However, patients with late (>5 years after operation) vein graft stenosis, especially to that of LAD has poor long-term prognosis.[19,20] Patients with late stenosis in SVG to LAD associated with other risk factors have an abysmal late survival. Patients with 50–99% stenosis in SVG-LAD who had additional impaired ventricular function or left main stenosis or triple vessel disease (TVD) had only 46% survival at 2 years. Patients with stenosis in SVG to LAD had far worse long-term survival than native LAD coronary atherosclerosis and should be treated with PCI or redo CABG.

Percutaneous Coronary Interventions Versus Redo Coronary Artery Bypass Grafting

Percutaneous coronary intervention of stenosed vein graft or native coronary artery is an alternative anatomical treatment for symptomatic post-CABG patients. PCI on native arteries or the grafts of operated patients, before redo CABG, significantly increased from 14.5% (1990 through 1994) to 26.6% (2005 through 2009).[4] Similar increase was reported by Riley et al.[9] who reported an increase of 31% among US Medicare population from 2001 to 2004 but decreased by 20% thereafter presumably from clinical trials demonstrating of lack of benefit of additional PCI (above optimal medical therapy) in stable CAD. Among the patients in the STS database of 72,431 patients undergoing reoperative CABG, incidence of patients treated with previous PCI had increased from 35% in 2000 to 53% in 2009.[3]

However, PCI for SVGs is associated with an increased risk of distal coronary embolization from more friable SVG atheroma, resulting in perioperative MI. Glycoprotein (GP) IIb/IIIa inhibitors are less effective in the intervention of SVG compared to native coronary artery.[21] Compared to occlusive devices, distal embolic protection devices using filters during SVG PCI seem to offer better protection.[22,23]

Symptomatic patients with prior CABG are a very heterogeneous group with a group at one end considered low-risk group who do not need any anatomic treatment (redo CABG or PCI) and a group at other end who are at high risk without the above therapy. Whether PCI or redo CABG is the most effective form of therapy must be based on multiple factors.

Some of the factors favoring PCI over redo CABG are listed in table 1.

TABLE 1: Indications of coronary artery bypass grafting versus percutaneous coronary intervention

Redo CABG	PCI
Late (>5 years) SVG stenosis	Early (<5 years) SVG stenosis
Diffusely atherosclerotic vein graft	Other patent non-stenotic vein grafts
Stenotic LAD vein graft especially diffuse disease	Focal stenotic LAD vein graft
Multiple stenotic vein graft	Single stenotic vein graft
No patent ITA graft especially to LAD	Patent ITA-LAD graft
Abnormal left ventricular function	Normal ventricular function

CABG, coronary artery bypass grafting; ITA, internal thoracic artery; LAD, left anterior descending; PCI, percutaneous coronary intervention; SVG, saphenous vein graft.

PREOPERATIVE EVALUATION AND PLANNING

As complete understanding of the patient's native coronary and bypass graft anatomy is very essential before undertaking redo CABG, preoperative planning (Table 2) is more important in coronary reoperations than it is in primary CABG. The patient's history and previous operation note must be reviewed thoroughly including any relevant procedures or comorbidities that may affect surgeon's approach to the reoperation. For example, a patient with history of mediastinitis following primary operations may be better to operate through lateral thoracotomy if coronary anatomy is favorable to this approach.

Preoperative Assessment

- *Review of available conduits*:
  - Physical examination
  - Inferior thoracic artery (ITA) shoot
  - Radial artery (RA) ultrasound and Doppler.
- X-ray posterior-anterior (PA) and left lateral view
- Vascular Doppler imaging of Carotid Arteries and lower extremities
- Dobutamine echocardiography/thallium scintigraphy
- Computed tomography of chest
- Coronary angiography
- Review of previous operation note
- Review old angiograms before previous operations
- Adequate blood arrangement.

Availability of Conduits for Bypass Grafting

The importance of preoperative physical examination and testing to assess the availability and quality of conduits cannot be overstated. ITA angiography during coronary angiography provides a more complete evaluation of these arteries and should be done whenever possible. Venous Doppler studies are often used to determine the size and quality of greater and lesser saphenous vein segments. Arterial Doppler studies of the radial arteries combined with modified Doppler Allen's test to assess adequacy of flow to digits should be done whenever RA harvesting is contemplated.

Chest X-ray and Computed Tomography

A posteroanterior and lateral chest X-ray can give an idea of the proximity of important cardiac structures to the sternum

TABLE 2: Indications for redo coronary artery bypass grafting from the European guidelines for revascularization

	Class of recommendation	Level of evidence
In early graft failure:		
Coronary angiography is indicated for highly symptomatic patients, or in the event of postoperative instability, or with abnormal biomarkers/ECG suggestive of perioperative MI	I	C
Decision of redo CABG or PCI should be made by the Heart Team	I	C
In late graft failure following CABG:		
PCI or redo CABG is indicated in patients with severe symptoms or extensive ischemia despite OMT	I	B
PCI is preferred over CABG If considered safe	I	C
Revascularization modalities:		
ITA is the conduit of choice for redo CABG when available/ Not used earlier	I	B
Redo CABG is considered for patients without patent ITA graft to LAD	IIa	B
Distal protection devices is considered for PCI of SVG lesions	IIa	B
PCI of the bypassed native artery should be considered over PCI of the bypass graft	IIa	C
In Stent Restenosis:		
In patients with recurrent events of diffuse in-stent restenosis, CABG should be considered by the Heart Team over a new PCI attempt	IIa	C

CABG, coronary artery bypass grafting; ECG, electrocardiography; ITA, internal thoracic artery; MI, myocardial infarction; OMT, optimal medical therapy; PCI, percutaneous coronary intervention; SVG, saphenous vein graft.

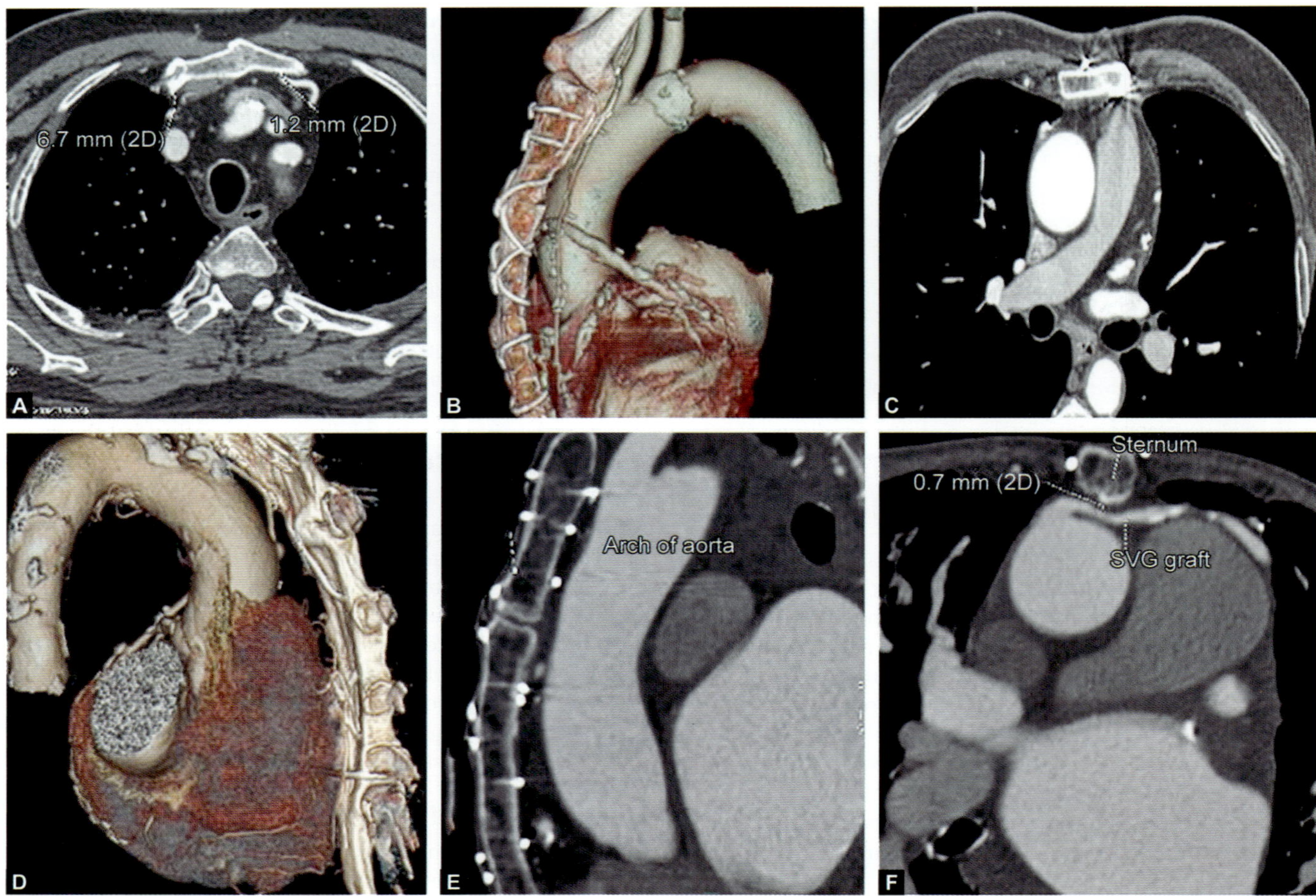

SVG, saphenous vein graft.

FIG. 1: Computed tomography (CT) angiogram. Preoperative CT angiogram to detect proximity of vascular structures and previous grafts to sternum. CT images showing proximity of cardiovascular structures to sternum: **A,** Left internal thoracic artery; **B,** Aorta; **C,** Brachiocephalic vein; **D,** Right ventricle; **E,** Aorta; **F,** Saphenous vein graft.

and helps the surgeon in evaluating the risk of sternal reentry. Steel clips, used in the harvest of ITA graft, visible on chest radiograph give information about risk of injury during sternotomy. Routine use of multi-detector computed tomographic angiography (CTA) (Fig. 1) is recommended in redo CABG to detect proximity of cardiovascular structures and conduits to the posterior surface of sternum, any patent grafts missed out during coronary angiography, ascending aorta calcification, and pseudoaneurysms. It is also helpful in assessing unused ITA if not demonstrated during conventional coronary angiography.

Coronary Angiography

A complete and well-performed angiography is a necessary step in the preoperative assessment of patients undergoing redo CABG. Review of previous angiogram and operation notes are invaluable tools for the surgeon as well as the interventional cardiologist performing angiogram to gain a better understanding of the patient's coronary anatomy. Multiple views, injecting all relevant branches and grafts as well as allowing enough time for filling of the coronaries by collaterals are critical to identify potential targets. Non-demonstration of bypass graft, venous or arterial, usually means that they are occluded but it is also possible that the angiogram had failed to demonstrate their location.

Assessment of Viable Myocardium

Because of the increased morbidity and mortality in patients undergoing coronary reoperations especially those with impaired ventricular function, it is important to be reasonably sure that there is a matchup between the patient's graftable arteries and viable myocardium to provide some long-term benefits. This is especially so in patients with patent LITA-to-LAD who have non-LAD territory disease. Because these patients derive no survival benefit from reintervention, viability assessment is important to verify a substantial non-LAD territory at jeopardy. The commonly used diagnostic tools are dobutamine echocardiography, thallium scintigraphy, positron-emission tomography (PET), and cardiac magnetic resonance imaging (cMRI).

TECHNICAL ASPECTS AND CHALLENGES ASSOCIATED WITH REDO CORONARY ARTERY BYPASS GRAFTING

Coronary reoperations are technically more difficult and challenging than primary CABG for various reasons,[24] and recognition of all pitfalls and a thorough planning is essential. They are:

- Sternotomy and dissection
- Myocardial protection
- Stenotic or patent vein or arterial graft
- Aortic atherosclerosis
- Availability of conduits for bypass
- Identification of coronary arteries.

Detailed preoperative evaluation as mentioned earlier and operative planning are key to minimizing complications and their importance cannot be overemphasized in achieving superior results.

Sternotomy and Dissection

Unlike primary CABG, opening the sternum during redo CABG is always risky because the pericardium has been opened in earlier operation and the heart, major vessels or bypass grafts may be close or adherent to under surface of sternum. The most common re-entry injury is to a patent bypass graft,[25] i.e., a patent graft to right coronary artery (RCA) or a patent LITA to left side artery close to sternum or a right ITA graft to left coronary artery. The sternotomy is performed with an oscillating saw. In high-risk cases, alternative access to go on emergency cardiopulmonary bypass like prior exposure of femoral vein and axillary artery or wire access of femoral artery and vein for percutaneous cannulation must be planned out before sternotomy. In extremely high-risk cases, prior cannulation (femoral vein and preferably axillary artery) may be required before commencing sternotomy. Axillary artery cannulation is preferred over femoral artery because of risk of retrograde atherosclerotic embolization from femoral artery. Sternal wires are divided anteriorly and not removed to protect the underlying structures. The sternotomy is performed till the posterior table, at which stage the ventilation is stopped temporarily. While the posterior table is cut, the assistant lifts up both ends of the cut wires thus elevating the posterior surface of sternum from cardiac structures (Fig. 2). Once the posterior table is divided, the wires are removed and the heart is carefully dissected away from under surface of sternum, first on right side and then left side. Once the heart is freed from the posterior table and chest wall, the dissection of heart starts from diaphragmatic surface of heart (where there is very little risk of injuring any critical structure) and carried cranially first dissecting out the right atrium and aorta for central aortic and venous cannulation if needed. The right ITA is dissected first followed by dissection of left side of heart. One must be extremely careful while dissecting patent ITA, especially near second and third rib. The risk of injury to a patent ITA can be reduced significantly if the ITA is routed posterior to the lung (Fig. 3) through a

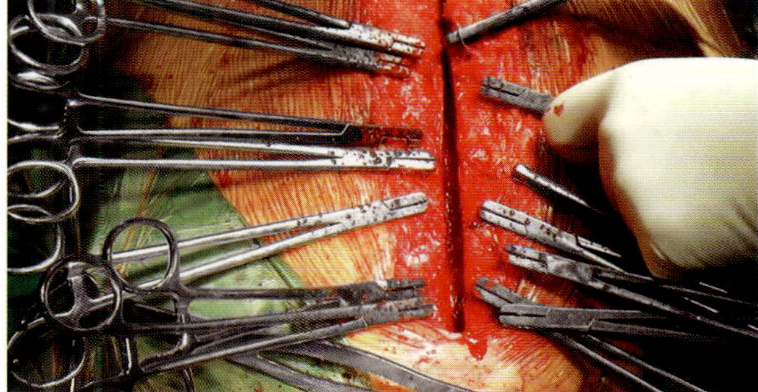

FIG. 2: Sternotomy lifting. Lifting of the anterior sternal wires during sternotomy reduces the risk of the injury to underlying structures.

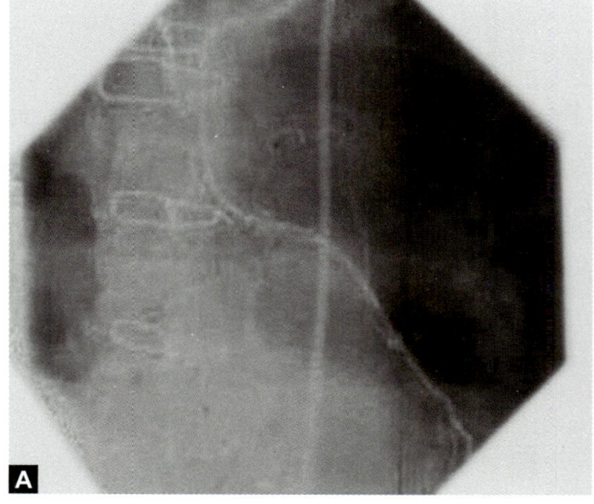

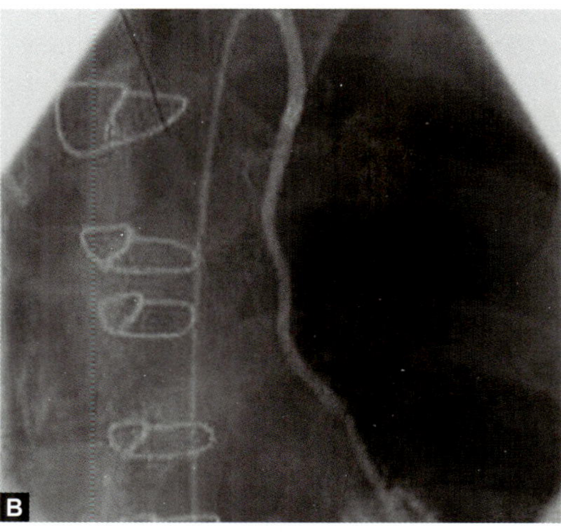

FIG. 3: Left internal thoracic artery (LITA) position. LITA position with **A,** closed pleura; **B,** pleura open.

cut in pericardium during primary CABG. One should do minimum dissection of atherosclerotic vein grafts just away from pericardium to prevent athero-embolism.

Myocardial Protection

Redo CABG patients with more diffuse distal atherosclerosis in coronary arteries, totally occluded vessels, patent arterial graft supplying an occluded coronary artery, friable vein graft atherosclerosis pose a more difficult myocardial protection challenge compared to primary operation, with perioperative MI being the most common cause of in-hospital death.[26,27] Conventional antegrade cardioplegia may not be effective in above situations and may be dangerous because of risk of embolization from atherosclerotic vein grafts. A combination of antegrade and retrograde cardioplegia seems to be a better option. Retrograde cardioplegia delivered through the coronary sinus is extremely useful not only in reaching areas not protected by antegrade cardioplegia like areas supplied by patent arterial grafts or occluded coronary arteries which significantly decreases hospital mortality[28] but, also can be helpful in removing embolized atherosclerotic debris from diseased vein grafts or air from coronary arteries. This can also be combined with cardioplegia through newly constructed vein graft, if any.

Choice of Conduits and Grafting Pattern (Fig. 4)

The basic concept of conduit selection for coronary reoperations is same as primary CABG and arterial conduits should be the first choice wherever possible, especially in younger patients or older patients with reasonable life expectancy. Vein grafts are less suitable in redo CABG

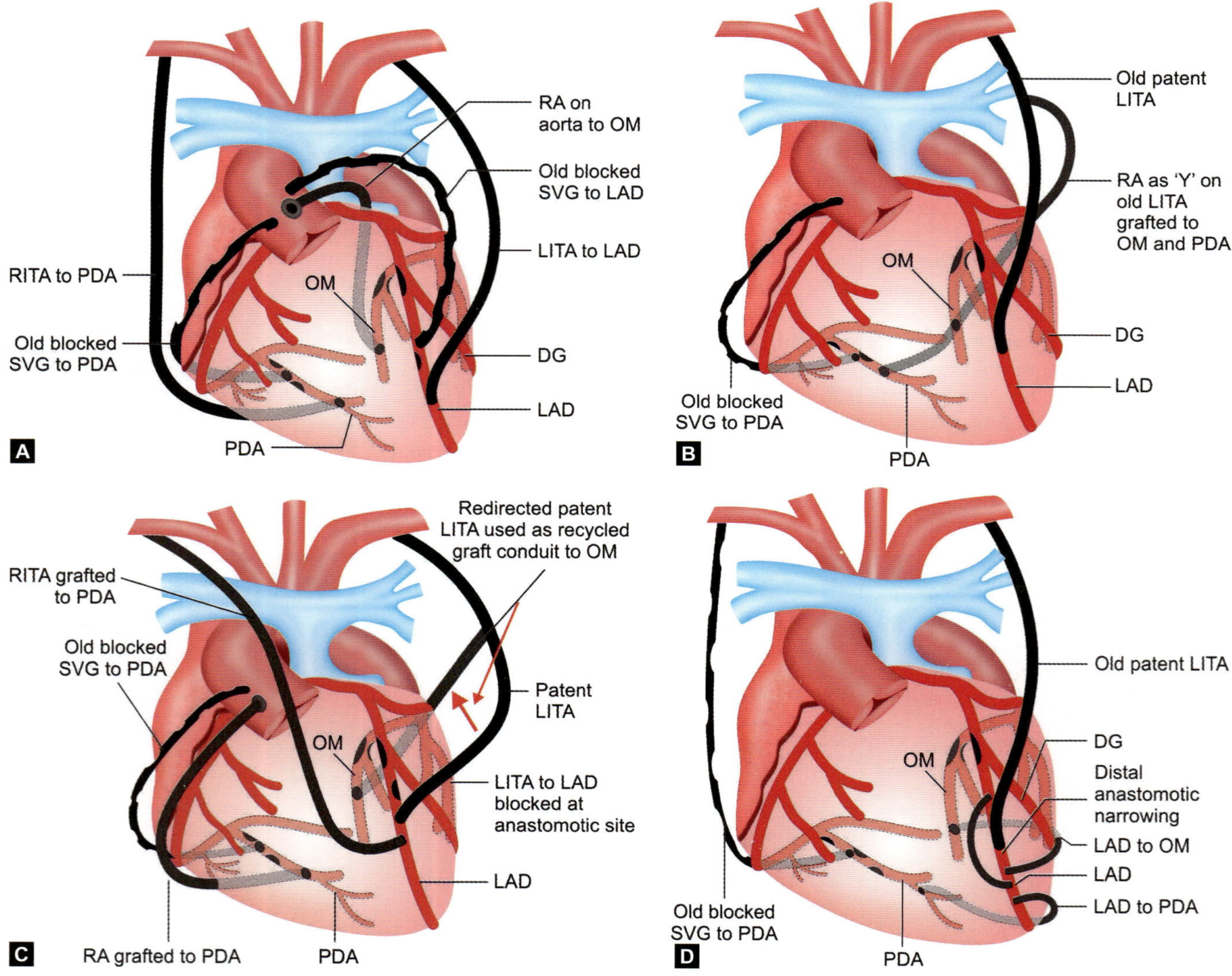

RITA, right internal thoracic artery; PDA, posterior descending artery; LITA, left internal thoracic artery; RA, radial artery; LAD, left anterior descending artery; DG, diagonal artery; SVG, saphenous vein graft; OM, obtuse marginal.

FIG. 4: Graft configurations. Examples of arterial conduit permutations in redo to achieve total arterial revascularization.

because patients have more diffuse and distal atherosclerosis and better quality vein grafts are utilized during primary operation leaving poor quality veins for reoperations. If only SVG was used in the primary CABG, then either one ITA or both ITAs should be the conduit of choice. Like primary operation, revascularization of LAD with LITA in reoperation is associated with increase in early and late survival compared to use of SVG to LAD.[29]

In patients with patent LITA-to-LAD and non-grafted or occluded grafts to circumflex and RCA, using the right internal thoracic artery (RITA) does not increase the risk of deep sternal wound infection.[30] The right ITA can be used as in situ or as a free graft anastomosed to the side of patent left ITA in a T or Y fashion to graft circumflex and RCA branches. Such graft arrangements using bilateral ITAs may have a survival benefit as in primary operations.[31] RA is a good alternative conduit that can be used in conjunction with right ITA or alone and is associated with improved outcomes,[32] but this should only be used in native vessels with severe stenosis to avoid competitive flow and graft attrition.[33]

The right gastroepiploic artery (RGEA) can be a good option to graft inferior wall especially to isolated RCA disease through a sternal-sparing transabdominal approach with good short-term and mid-term outcomes.[34] However, the RGEA has limited length, small diameter, vulnerable to spasm and is being infrequently used especially since the resurgence of RA as a conduit.

Handling Saphenous Vein Grafts

Whether a patent or stenotic vein graft be left alone or replaced and if replaced, should it be with a vein or arterial graft are difficult technical decisions that need to be taken during coronary reoperations. Vein grafts more than 5 years old are more likely to be atherosclerosed and need to be replaced. If using an arterial conduit to revascularize a coronary artery with a pre-existing patent SVG, the old venous graft flow must be interrupted (unless critically stenosed) to avoid competitive flow and possible graft closure. If the LAD was not grafted during primary operation or a SVG was used, every effort must be made to revascularize it with an ITA as there is evidence of increase in early and late survival when at reoperation, LAD is bypassed with an ITA compared to SVG-to-LAD.[29] However, when a patent vein graft is replaced with an arterial graft, especially supplying a large territory, patient may develop a hypoperfusion syndrome[35] resulting in myocardial ischemia or infarction because of lesser flow through a smaller diameter arterial graft compared to a vein graft, even if stenosed. RA may be more suitable in this situation because of larger diameter. A skeletonized ITA has better flow than pedicled ITA[36] and may be used to replace a diseased vein graft. Every effort must be made to use multiple arterial grafts at reoperation to improve long-term survival and event-free survival. However, if there is shortage of arterial conduits or available venous conduits are of poor quality, any existing SVG free of atherosclerosis (both angiographically and on inspection) especially if less than 5 years, old grafts should be left alone.

Lack of Conduits and Recycling Conduits

Poor quality of conduits or lack of conduit[24] is a common problem in redo CABG patient populations due to older age, obesity, calcification of RAs, use of ITAs or better quality veins in prior CABG leaving no or poor quality veins. When conduit shortage is an issue and anatomy is suitable, recycling arterial grafts previously used is a good adjunct to performing redo CABG. A distal stenosis in a LITA-to-LAD can be managed by dividing distally and anastomosing to a diagonal or early obtuse marginal and grafting RITA to LAD (Fig. 5).

A proximal stenosis in an in situ LITA can be managed by using as a free graft off the hood RA or an old vein graft. A free RITA can be used in Y or T fashion to the side of existing patent

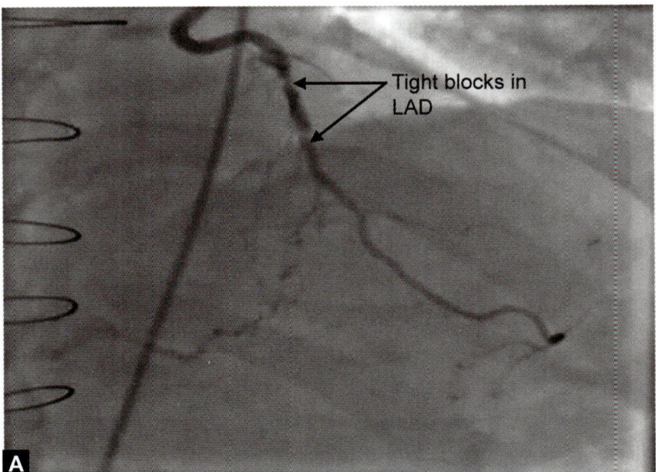

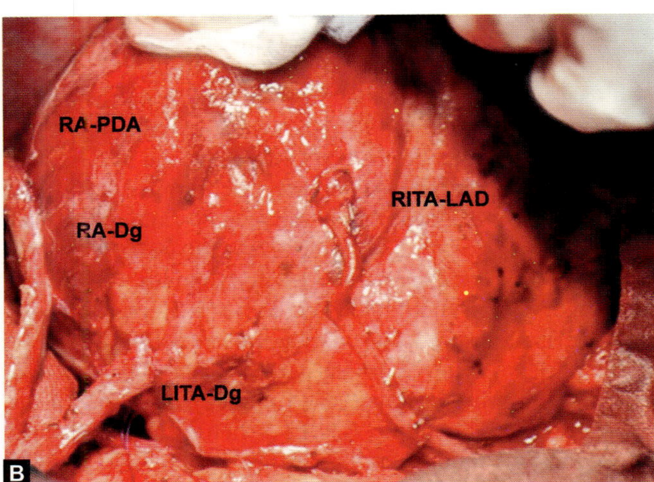

LAD, left anterior descending artery; LITA, left internal thoracic artery; PDA, posterior descending artery; RA, radial artery; RITA, right internal thoracic artery.

FIG. 5: Tight block in left anterior descending (LAD). Left internal transthoracic artery (LITA)–LAD artery anastomotic restenosis. Recycling of conduit with right internal thoracic artery to LAD and LITA to diagonal and sequential radial artery to intermediate (inter) and posterior descending artery.

LITA to revascularize rest of myocardium. Combination of arterial conduits to optimize usage in situations of limited availability of conduits is depicted in Fig. 4. The RGEA or inferior epigastric arteries (IEA) can be used in extreme situations of non-availability of conduits.

Off-pump Versus On-pump

Though there have been concerns related to perceived greater threat of atherosclerotic vein graft embolization, incomplete revascularization, and poor outcomes in patients converted to on pump, there is increasing evidence that off-pump coronary artery bypass (OPCAB) grafting may provide superior early results especially in high-risk patients and prospective randomized trials as well as large retrospective reviews have shown that compared to on pump CABG, OPCAB is associated with improved early risk adjusted morbidity and mortality.[37,38] A meta-analysis of 12 studies from Imperial College, London showed that in selected patients undergoing coronary reoperations off-pump technique significantly reduced early mortality.[39]

The advantages of off-pump technique in coronary reoperations are:

- Elimination of cardiopulmonary bypass-induced complications
- Reducing or eliminating aortic manipulation and attendant reduction in cerebrovascular accident by avoiding aortic cannulation or cross clamp and basing grafts off ITA inflow
- Elimination of concerns relating to effective protection of myocardium by cardioplegia.

In spite of evidence of superior early results of off-pump redo CABG, use of the technique for coronary reoperations varies widely between various centers. An analysis of STS database revealed an increase prevalence of off-pump reoperative CABG from 12% in 2000 to 18% in 2009 among 72,431 patients undergoing isolated coronary reoperations.[3] However, Maltais et al.[40] from Mayo Clinic, recently reported use of only cardiopulmonary bypass among 748 patients undergoing redo CABG with a 6% perioperative mortality. On the other hand, Dohi et al.[41] in an analysis of Japanese Cardiovascular Surgery Database reported 59% use of off-pump technique among 617 patients undergoing coronary reoperations. Whether to use OPCAB technique in coronary reoperations and success of off-pump technique depends on skill and experience of surgeon and anesthesiologist as well as number and location of target coronary arteries, aortic atherosclerosis, and patient's hemodynamics. However, the primary goal should always be to achieve complete revascularization with lowest perioperative morbidity.

In patients with hemodynamic instability, dilated heart with impaired ventricular function, insertion of an intra-aortic balloon pump (IABP) is helpful in improving hemodynamics and avoiding cardiopulmonary bypass. One should have a low threshold for its use. In patients undergoing on pump redo CABG, its use also helps ease perioperative hemodynamic instability and postoperative recovery and has been used as high as in 20% patients.[40] To avoid hemodynamic instability during dissection of lateral wall, it is important to graft LAD and RCA with minimal dissection and perform circumflex area dissection and anastomosis last. One should complete the proximal anastomosis first, as this has the advantage of supplying blood to ischemic myocardium immediately upon completion of distal grafting and stabilizing an unstable patient.

Alternative Approaches

Although vast majority of patients undergoing redo CABG need grafts to multiple vessels and the procedure is performed through a median sternotomy, alternative approaches may be useful especially if a limited target area revascularization is needed or if combined with PCI (hybrid approach). A thoracotomy[42] may be an alternative route to avoid injury to underlying structures especially if a patent graft is adherent to sternum or a patent ITA is crossing midline and has the additional advantage of less blood loss and wound complications. This is risky in patients who are obese, need grafts to multiple regions of the heart or cannot tolerate single lung ventilation. This is performed through a muscle-sparing lateral thoracotomy through the fourth, fifth or sixth interspace and provide good exposure of entire anterolateral wall and the LITA if not used previously. The proximal end of the conduit can be anastomosed to descending aorta or the subclavian artery, if the patient only needs grafts to LAD territory and/or intermediate, minimally invasive direct coronary artery bypass grafting (MIDCAB) approach with a small anterior thoracotomy may be a preferable approach. If the patient needs revascularization of RCA, a transabdominal approach may be preferable using RGEA[34] as described earlier. Hybrid procedure with robotic left thoracotomy LITA graft to LAD combined with PCI has been described,[43] although its usefulness is yet to be determined.

Early Results

Technically redo CABG operations are far more complex than primary operations and the patient populations are more vulnerable resulting in a higher operative mortality and morbidity than primary operations. The early mortality of redo CABG is reported to be 2–5 times higher than expected for primary CABG and associated with increased stroke, renal failure, reoperation for bleeding, and deep sternal wound infection.[3] However, over past few decades, there has been a steady improvement in early operative mortality despite an increase in risk profile of patient populations undergoing reoperations. Cleveland Clinic reported an operative mortality of 3.4%[26] between 1967 and 1994 which continued to decrease to 2.5% in 2002.[29] Similar results were reported by Ghanta et al.[3] in an analysis of STS database of 72,431 patients undergoing reoperations between 2000 and 2009, at 1,035 institutions. They reported a 23.7% reduction in the relative risk of redo CABG mortality during the period, despite increase in morbidity like more left main disease, MI, heart failure, renal failure, and cerebrovascular disease. The risk-adjusted mortality decreased from 6.0 to 4.7%. In 2013, the mortality had further reduced to 3.5% among the STS participants institutions. This is attributed to increase in surgical team experience resulting in better patient management pre- and postoperative, better myocardial protection, handling of atherosclerotic vein graft, avoiding injury to patent vein graft, frequent use of arterial (especially ITA graft). In high-volume centers, the risk of redo CABG approaches that of primary CABG.[2] However, hospital risks increase with number of previous operations. Sabik et al.[2] reported operative mortality of 4.3% for first reoperations, 5.1% for second reoperations, and 6.4% for three or more reoperations.

The two most important factors that determine the outcome of redo CABG are surgical team experience as mentioned earlier and patient risk profiles. While surgical experience especially in high-volume centers has neutralized the risk of operation due to technical difficulties, patient characteristics now has a greater influence on hospital mortality.[2]

The higher perioperative mortality in coronary reoperations is mostly because of an increased risk of perioperative MI. Causes of MI identified are incomplete revascularization from diffuse distal atherosclerosis, atherosclerotic emboli from old vein grafts, injury to bypass grafts including patent ITA and thrombosis of constructed vein graft. In Cleveland Clinic series, 85% of cause of perioperative death was cardiovascular, in contrast to mostly non-cardiac cause of death in primary CABG.[26,44] The early in-hospital mortality was associated with a new perioperative MI in 67% cases. The higher incidence of perioperative MI may be attributable to multiple factors unique to coronary reoperations like incomplete revascularization due to diffuse distal atherosclerotic CAD, vein graft thrombosis, atherosclerotic embolization from diseased vein grafts, injury to earlier bypass grafts, ITA graft failure, hypoperfusion from new arterial grafts, perioperative MI, and complications of percutaneous transluminal coronary angioplasty (PTCA).

Predictors of in-hospital mortality of coronary reoperations identified in multiple studies are increased age, female gender, and emergency operations.[27,45] Though by itself, advanced age does not increase the risk of operative mortality it does so when combined with other variables. Emergency operations are a strong predictor and the operative mortality is more than three times higher than that of elective coronary reoperations.[26,27,45,46] Anatomic conditions specific to reoperations like presence of an ITA graft or atherosclerotic vein grafts or patent graft attached to undersurface of sternum in midline can increase the risk of reoperation but with experience, these technical factors can be neutralized.

Late Results

Patients undergoing redo CABG are older and at a later stage in the natural history of CAD than those undergoing primary CABG resulting in more diffuse atherosclerosis, inferior quality coronary revascularization. So the long-term results after coronary reoperations are not as favorable as that of primary CABG, with more frequent recurrence of angina and inferior late survival. Weintraub et al.[27] have reported a 41% recurrence of angina at 4-year follow-up and 76% survival at 5-year and 55% at 10-year. This is similar to 89%, 77%, and 51% survival at 1-, 5-, and 10-year respectively reported from Mayo Clinic[40] recently (Fig. 6). LV dysfunction, advanced age, and diabetes have been the consistent predictors of late survival in most studies, though current cigarette smoking, hypertension, TVD have been identified as decreasing late survival in some studies.[47] Unlike primary CABG, the influence of ITA graft on late survival has been difficult to determine for reoperation, probably due to non-LAD coronary artery grafting by ITA. However, extrapolating the positive influence of ITA grafts at least partially contributing to the dramatic reduction in coronary reoperations among STS participating institutions[10] one could extrapolate a similar positive effect of ITA, especially multiple ITA, or arterial grafting on late survival.

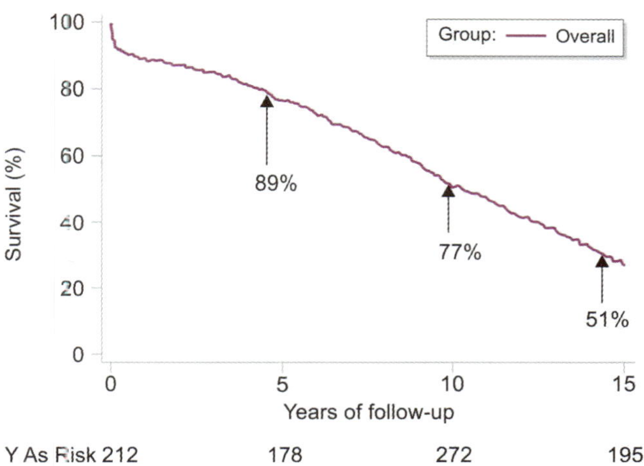

FIG. 6: Survival curve for redo. Kaplan–Meier survival curve for redo patients at 1, 5, and 10 years.

Multiple Reoperations

Patients needing more than one coronary reoperations represent a very small fraction of all redo CABG patients. Of the 4518 patients undergoing coronary reoperations at Cleveland Clinic between 1990 and 2003, 3919 had first, 552 second, 43 third, 3 fourth, and 1 fifth reoperations.[2] Similarly Maltais et al.[40] from Mayo Clinic reported an incidence of 8% second reoperation, and 1% third reoperation. The indications for additional reoperations remain the same as first time redo CABG especially in patients with disabling angina unresponsive to medical therapy. In addition to having more complex and diffuse CAD, availability of conduits is a limiting factor in these patients. Even though the risk of first reoperation in high-volume experienced centers approaches that of primary CABG, the hospital risk of multiple re-operations still remains high with reported operative mortality of 4.3% for first reoperations, 5.1% for second reoperations, and 6.4% for three or more reoperations.[2] Age greater than 65 years and LV dysfunction with ejection fraction less than 35% are predictors of early mortality, with 10% mortality in patients above 70 years.[2] Patients above 70 years who survived multiple reoperations have a poor late survival of 50% at 5 years.[2]

CONCLUSION

Redo CABG is a complicated procedure and far more technically challenging than primary CABG. The surgical team must recognize the challenges involved and careful preoperative planning as well as meticulous surgical technique is essential to successful outcomes. Surgical outcomes of redo CABG are improving in spite of increasing high-risk patients and in high-volume experienced centers the operative mortality is nearing that of primary CABG.

REFERENCES

1. Cosgrove DM, Loop FD, Lytle BW, et al. Predictors of reoperation after myocardial revascularization. J Thorac Cardiovasc Surg.1986;92(5):811-21.
2. Sabik JF, Blackstone EH, Houghtaling PL, et al. Is reoperation still a risk factor in coronary artery bypass surgery? Ann Thorac Sur. 2005;80(5):1719-27.
3. Ghanta RK, Kaneko T, Gammie JS, et al. Evolving trends of reoperative coronary artery bypass grafting: An analysis of the Society of Thoracic Surgeons Adult Cardiac Surgery Database. J Thorac Cardiovasc Surg. 2013;145(2):364-72.
4. Spiliotopoulos K, Maganti M, Brister S, et al. Changing pattern of reoperative coronary artery bypass grafting: A 20-year study. Ann Thorac Surg. 2011; 92:40-7.
5. Amano J, Kuwano H, Yokomise H. Thoracic and cardiovascular surgery in Japan during 2011. Annual report by The Japanese Association for Thoracic Surgery. Gen Thorac Cardiovasc Surg. 2013;61:578-607.
6. Fosbol EL, Zhao Y, Shahian DM, et al. Repeat coronary surgeon's national experience, 1991-2007. Circulation. 2013;127:1656-63.
7. Boden WE, O'Rourke RA, Teo KK, et al. The evolving pattern of symptomatic coronary artery disease in the United States and Canada: Baseline characteristics of the Clinical Outcomes Utilizing Revascularization and Aggressive Drug Evaluation (COURAGE) trial. Am J Cardiol. 2007;99:208-12.
8. LaRosa JC, He J, Vupputuri S. Effect of statins on risk of coronary disease: A meta-analysis of randomized controlled trials. JAMA. 1999;282:2340-6.
9. Riley RF, Don CW, Powell W, et al. Trends in coronary revascularization in the United States from 2001 to 2009: Recent decline in percutaneous coronary intervention volumes. Circ Cardiovasc Qual Outcomes. 2011;4:193-7.
10. ElBardissi A, Aranki S, Sheng S, et al. Trends in isolated coronary artery bypass grafting: An analysis of the Society of Thoracic Surgeons Database. J Thorac Cardiovasc Surg. 2012;143:273-81.
11. Loop FD, Lytle BW, Cosgrove DM, et al. Influence of the internal-mammary-artery graft on 10-year survival and other cardiac events. N Engl J Med. 1986;314:1-6.
12. Cameron A, Davis KB, Green G, et al. Coronary bypass surgery with internal-thoracic-artery grafts—effects on survival over a 15-year period. N Engl J Med. 1996;334:216-9.
13. Sabik JF III, Blackstone EH, Gillinov AM, et al. Influence of patient characteristics and arterial grafts on freedom from coronary reoperation. J Thorac Cardiovasc Surg. 2006;131:90-8.
14. Head SJ, Milojevic M, Taggart DP, et al. Current practice of state-of-the-art surgical coronary revascularization. Circulation. 2017;136:1331-45.
15. Yap CH, Sposato L, Akowuah E, et al. Contemporary results show repeat coronary artery bypass grafting remains a risk factor for operative mortality. Ann Thorac Surg. 2009;87:1386-91.
16. Neitzel GF, Barboriak JJ, Pintar K, et al. Atherosclerosis in aortocoronary bypass grafts: Morphologic study and risk factor analysis 6 to 12 years after surgery. Arteriosclerosis. 1986;6:594.
17. Ratliff NB, Myles JL. Rapidly progressive atherosclerosis in aortocoronary saphenous vein grafts: Possible immune-mediated disease. Arch Pathol Lab Med. 1989;113:772.
18. Solymoss BC, Leung TK, Pelletier LC, et al. Pathologic changes in coronary artery saphenous vein grafts and related etiologic factors. Cardiovasc Clin. 1991;21:45.
19. Lytle BW, Loop FD, Taylor PC, et al. Vein graft disease: The clinical impact of stenosis in saphenous vein bypass grafts to coronary arteries. .J Thorac Cardiovasc Surg. 1992;103:831.
20. Lytle BW, Loop FD, Taylor PC, et al. The effect of coronary reoperation on the survival of patients with stenosis in saphenous vein to coronary bypass grafts .J Thorac Cardiovasc Surg. 1993;105:605.
21. Roffi M, Mukherjee D, Chew DP, et al. Lack of benefit from intravenous platelet glycoprotein IIb/IIIa receptor inhibition as adjunctive treatment for percutaneous interventions of aortocoronary bypass grafts: A pooled analysis of five randomized clinical trials. Circulation. 2002;106(24):3063-7.
22. Stone GW, Rogers C, Hermiller J, et al. Randomized comparison of distal protection with a filter-based catherter and a balloon occlusion and aspiration system during percutaneous intervention of diseased saphenous vein aorto-coronary bypass grafts. Circulation. 2003;108(5):548-53.
23. Mauri L, Cox D, Hermiller J, et al. The PROXIMAL trial: Proximal protection during saphenous vein graft intervention using the Proxis Embolic Protection System: A randomized, prospective, multicenter clinical trial. J Am Coll Cardiol. 2007;50(15):1442-9.
24. Machiraju VR How to avoid problem in redo coronary artery bypass surgery. J Card Surg. 2004;19:284-90.
25. Solomon NW, Page US, Bigelow JC, et al. Reoperative coronary surgery: Comparative analysis of 6591 patients undergoing primary bypass and 508 patients undergoing reoperative coronary artery bypass. J Thorac Cardiovasc Surg. 1990;100:250-9.
26. Lytle BW, McElroy D, McCarthy P, et al. Influence of arterial coronary bypass grafts on the mortality in coronary reoperations. J Thorac Cardiovasc Surg. 1994;107(3):675-82.
27. Weintraub WS, Jones EL, Craver JM, et al. In-hospital and long-term outcome after reoperative coronary artery bypass graft surgery. Circulation. 1995;92(9 Suppl):II50-7.
28. Borger MA, Rao V, Weisel RD, et al. Reoperative coronary bypass surgery: effect of patent grafts and retrograde cardioplegia. J Thorac Cardiovasc Surg. 2001;121:83-90.
29. Sabik JF, Sajjad R, Blackstone EH, et al. Value of internal thoracic artery grafting to the left anterior descending coronary artery at coronary reoperation. J Am Coll Cardiol. 2013;61:302-10.
30. Svensson LG, Mumtaz MA, Blackstone EH, et al. Does use of a right internal thoracic artery increase deep wound infection and risk after previous use of a left internal thoracic artery? J Thorac Cardiovasc Surg. 2006;131:609-13.
31. Taggart DP, D'Amico R, Altman DG. Effect of arterial revascularization on survival: A systematic review of studies comparing bilateral and single internal mammary arteries. Lancet. 2001;358:870-5.
32. Zacharias A, Schwann TA, Riordan CJ, et al. Late outcomes after radial artery versus saphenous vein grafting during reoperative coronary artery bypass surgery. J Thorac Cardiovasc Surg. 2010;139:1511-8.
33. Aldea GS, Bakaeen FG, Pal J, et al. The Society of Thoracic Surgeons clinical practice guidelines on arterial conduits for coronary artery bypass grafting. Ann Thorac Surg. 2016;101:801-9.
34. Tavilla G, Bruggemans EF. Avoiding sternotomy in repeat coronary artery bypass grafting: Feasibility, safety, and mid-term outcome of the transabdominal off-pump technique using the right gastroepiploic artery. J Thorac Cardiovasc Surg. 2012;144:124-9.
35. Navia D, Cosgrove DM 3rd, Lytle BW, et al. Is the internal Thoracic artery the conduit of choice to replace a stenotic vein graft? Ann Thorac Surg. 1994;57(1):40-3.
36. Wendler O, Tscholl D, Huang Q, et al. Free flow capacity of skeletonized versus pedicled internal thoracic artery grafts in coronary artery bypass grafts. Eur J Cardiothorac Surg. 1999;15:247-50.
37. Puskas JD, Cheng D, Knight J, et al. Off-pump versus conventional coronary artery bypass grafting: A meta-analysis and consensus statement from the 2004 ISMICS Consensus Conference. Innovations Fall. 2005;1(1):3-27.
38. Puskas JD, Edwards FH, Pappas PA, et al. Off-pump techniques benefit men and women and narrow the disparity in mortality after coronary bypass grafting. Ann Thorac Surg. 2007;84(5):1447-54.

39. Sepehripour AH, Saso S, Harling L, et al. Does off-pump coronary revascularization reduce mortality in reoperative coronary artery bypass surgery? A meta-analysis of observational studies. Perfusion. 2013;28:340-9.
40. Maltais S, Widmer RJ, Bell MR, et al. Reoperation for coronary artery bypass grafting surgery: outcomes and considerations for expanding interventional procedures. Ann Thorac Surg. 2017;103:1886-92.
41. Dohi M, Miyati H, Doi K, et al. The off-pump technique in redo coronary artery bypass grafting reduces mortality and major morbidities; propensity score analysis of data from the Japan Cardiovascular Surgery Database. Eur J Cardiothorac Surg. 2015;47:299-307.
42. Takahashi K, Takeuchi S, Ito K, et al. Reoperative coronary artery bypass surgery: Avoiding repeat median sternotomy. Ann Thorac Surg. 2012;94(6):1914-9.
43. Ejiofor JI, Leacher M, Byrne JG. Robotic CABG and hybrid approaches: The current landscape. Prog Cardiovasc Dis. 2015;58:356-64.
44. Loop FD, Lytle BW, Cosgrove DM, et al. Influence of the internal-mammary-artery graft on 10-year survival and other cardiac events. N Engl J Med. 1986;314:1-6.
45. Akins CW, Buckley MJ, Daggett WM, et al. Reoperative coronary grafting: Changing patient profiles, operative indications, techniques, and results. Ann Thorac Surg. 1994;58:359.
46. He GW, Acuff TE, Ryan WH, et al. Determinants of operative mortality in reoperative coronary artery bypass grafting. J Thorac Cardiovasc Surg. 1995;110:971.
47. Loop FD, Lytle BW, Cosgrove DM, et al. Reoperation for coronary atherosclerosis. Changing practice in 2509 conservative patients. Ann Surg. 1990;212(3):378-85.

CHAPTER 125

LVAD—Should Indians Borrow to Afford Them?

Sachin Talwar, Harsha V Niraghatam

INTRODUCTION

Heart failure (HF) is a state characterized by reduced cardiac index, stroke volume, and mean arterial pressure with the heart unable to meet the circulatory demands of the body. Initially heart tries to meet the circulatory demands by various compensatory mechanisms. As one reaches the chronic phase due to remodeling the architecture of the ventricular musculature causes chamber dilatation causing the ventricle to attain spherical shape as a result of which, the cardiac myocytes are subjected to maximal stress leading to myocyte apoptosis which lead to progressive ventricular dysfunction and end-stage HF.[1]

EPIDEMIOLOGY

The incidence of HF in the Western population is 1–5/1,000/ year and it is 3–20/1,000 population.[2,3] HF affects an estimated 4.7 million Americans, with 550,000 new patients diagnosed annually.[4,5] The risk of HF in adults around 40 years of age in the US is 14–20%.[6]

Magnitude of Problem in Indian Scenario

Actual data and small studies suggest that the number of patients with HF in India is not less than 2–5 million patients with and at any point of time, 2–3/1,000 population suffers HF. In a study by Chaturvedi and Seth,[7] 1.2/1,000 patients in rural areas suffer from HF. Approximately, 0.1–0.16 million patients die from HF annually. As per the AFAR study the patients enrolled were middle aged (mean 50.8 years) with an in-hospital mortality estimated to be 30.8% with a post-discharge 6-month rehospitalization and mortality rates of 39.5% and 26.3%. The mean age was lower than Western cohorts (ranging from 65 to 73 years) described in Euro-HF Study, the Acute Decompensated HF National Registry, the organized program to initiate life-saving treatment in hospitalized patients with HF and the effects of oral tolvaptan in patients hospitalized for worsening HF (EVEREST). The reason for mortality in the hospital was progression of HF in 92% patients, majority of in-hospital deaths were due to progressive HF in 92%, refractory arrhythmias in 6% and/or renal failure in the remaining. One-month death rate in patients who were discharged from the hospital was 15.8% that approached 26.3% at 3 and 6 months.[8] HF was found to the cause of death in 2.4% of all deaths in around 50 villages in South India.[9] These figures represent those patients in whom all medical therapeutic options have been exhausted. Heart transplantation has been considered to the gold-standard in managing patients with end-stage HF and mechanical support using various devices is considered in the interim in patients awaiting heart transplant. In some patients these devices are used as the only final palliation. However, these devices come at a heavy cost to the patients, insurance companies and the health sector. In addition they are associated with many complications. In this chapter, we present the detailed indications, methods, complications of these devices and will attempt to perform a risk-benefit analysis of these devices and attempt to answer the question "Should Indians borrow to afford them?".

THE INDIAN SCENARIO

In another study of admitted patients of HF (as per Framingham criteria) from South India (Fig. 1),[7] 94 consecutive patients aged more than 60 years were studied between 2003 and 2005. Mean age of these patients was 69 years and just less than half were females. Coronary artery disease was responsible for majority of these cases (55%) and diseases affecting single or multiple heart valves was the next most common cause (13%). The other causes were dilated cardiomyopathy in 10% and hypertension in 6% patients. In 12% patients, no causes could be ascertained.[10]

Disease-wise Heart Failure

Rheumatic Heart Disease

A previous estimate has shown that close to 200,000 deaths that account for 1% of all deaths are due to rheumatic heart disease in southeast Asia,[11] majority of these being due to HF. According to project carried out by the World Health

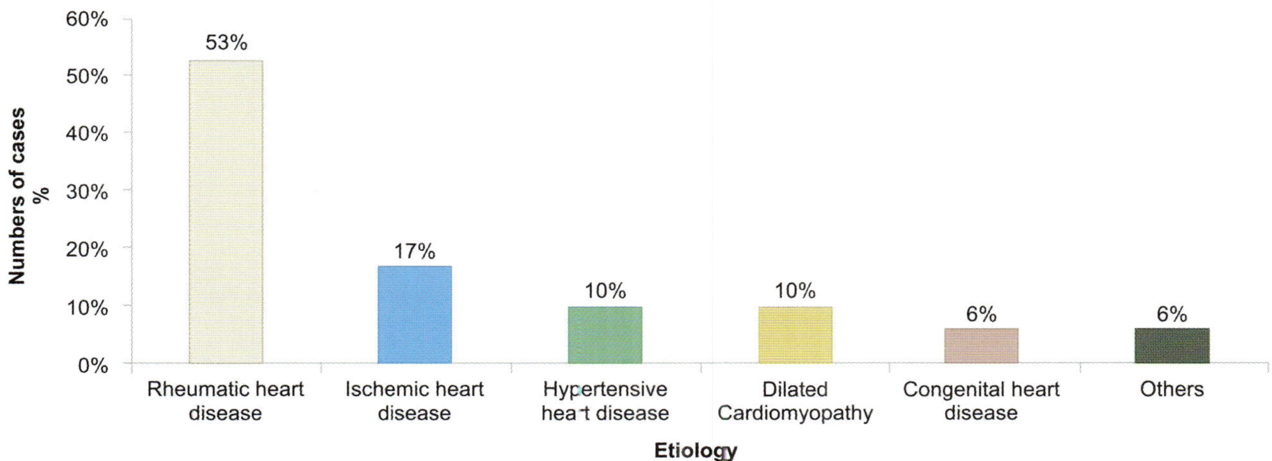

FIG. 1: Common etiologies of heart failure in India.

Source: Chaturvedi V, Parakh N, Seth S, et al. Heart failure in India: The Indus (India Ukieri Study) study. J Pract Cardiovasc Sci. 2016;2:28.

Organization in seven developing nations including India, approximately 19% patients with rheumatic heart disease had congestive heart failure (CHF).[12] In a study by Arora et al. in the 1980s, 20% of the patients with rheumatic heart disease needed multiple hospitalizations.[13] Grover et al. have estimated that 10% of patients with chronic rheumatic heart disease may die particularly in the presence of lesions that are not.[14] Therefore, it is easily inferred that 20–30% patients with rheumatic heart disease may develop HF and it can easily account for 3% yearly deaths.

Ischemic Heart Disease

Jose and Gupta have shown that 5% patients may develop HF within 30 days of an ST-segment elevation myocardial infarction (STEMI).[15] In the CREATE-ECLA study, 17% patients developed HF within 30 days and 10% died.[16] In the OASIS 2 registry, that studied the outcome following acute coronary syndromes, HF was prevalent in 7.2% patients.[17] In CREATE registry that was carried out in India, HF was documented in 1.6%.[18]

Hypertension and Heart Failure

As many as 90,000 patients per year are estimated die from consequences of hypertension in Southeast Asia and a large number of these have HF.[19] In the LIFE study, as many as 8.8% patients may have HF of new onset with abnormal features on an electrocardiogram (ECG).[20] In study that was carried out in Mumbai, significant hypertension was present in 13.1% of males and 16.7% of females. On a yearly basis, it was estimated these accounted for 0.2% annual deaths. Of all deaths related to hypertension, 14% deaths in males and 25% in females resulted from cardiac disease and consequences of hypertension.[21]

PROTOCOL FOR MANAGEMENT OF HEART FAILURE IN INDIA (FLOWCHART 1)[22]

Ventricular Assist Devices

A ventricular assist device (VAD) helps patients with HF by (A) arresting the remodeling process; (B) by reversing the remodeling process; (C) limiting or reducing dilatation of the heart due to HF. This is achieved by proving rest to the heart gradually helping improve its contractile function. The artificial heart program at the National Institute of Health (NIH) commenced in 1964 following which various mechanical devices were developed for use in patients with unresponsive and refractory HF. The Jarvik 7 artificial heart was first implanted in 1982 and the recipient survived for 112 days.[23] Domingo Liotta from Houston are credited with the development of the first left ventricular assist device (LVAD) in the early sixties.[24] These devices were approved as a bridge to heart transplantation in 1994 in the United States.

Heart transplantation is considered to be the final and desired management options for patients with refractory and unresponsive HF. However, the numbers of these procedures has remained stationary worldwide. The number of heart transplants performed annually in the United States has remained fairly constant at approximately 2,100 for many years (2001 heart and stroke update). The total number of heart transplants performed in India has not grown beyond 500 (number since 3rd August 1994) and only a few centers are equipped for this purpose. Due to these limitations there was a need to explore for alternative means of hemodynamic support and VADs play an important role as a "Bridge to transplant" because there is a shortfall of a sufficient number of donors. In about 5–15 % of transplant candidates the native ventricular function is restored by VAD support. Bridging to heart transplantation occurs in 300–400 patients annually in USA.[25] Transplantation is performed after VAD implantation in about 20% of patients.[26] The published total number of VAD implanted in India is approximately 25,[27] although current data suggests the number to be around 60 (data collected by means of telephonic conservation from Dr KR Balakrishnan, Chief Cardiothoracic, Fortis Malar Hospital, Adyar, Chennai, India). VADs also have a place in providing circulatory support in patients who have end stage HF who are ineligible for transplant (old age >65 years, renal dysfunction, pulmonary hypertension and high body mass index) as "Destination Therapy".[28] VADs have also been used in patients with

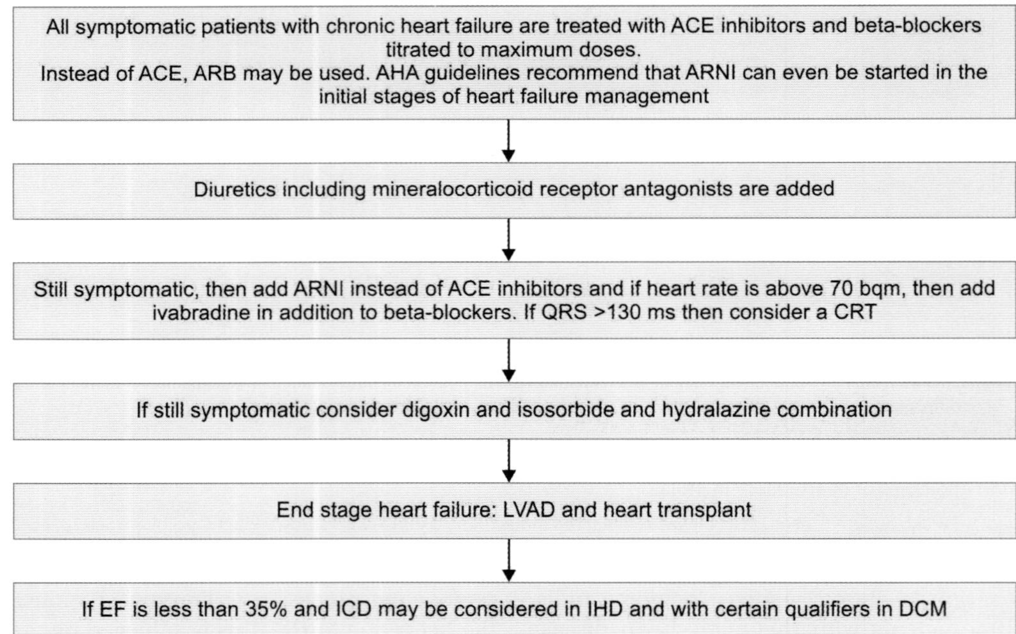

ACE, angiotensin-converting enzyme; ARB, angiotensin receptor blocker; AHA, American Heart Association; ARNI, angiotensin receptor-neprilysin inhibitor; CRT, cardiac resynchronization therapy; LVAD, left ventricular assist device; EF, ejection fraction; ICD, implantable cardioverter-defibrillator; IHD, ischemic heart disease; DCM, dilated cardiomyopathy.

FLOWCHART 1: Algorithm for heart failure management as per the 2017 guidelines ESC/AHA 2017.

Source: Chaturvedi V, Parakh N, Seth S, et al. Heart failure in India: The INDUS (India Ukieri Study) study. J Pract Cardiovasc Sci 2016;2:28-35.

potentially reversible cardiomyopathy and in whom the candidacy for heart transplantation cannot be determined immediately and in order to buy time to make a judicious decision as "Bridge to Recovery or Decision".[29]

Classification of Ventricular Assist Devices[1,30]

Left Ventricular Assist Devices

They reduce the left ventricular wall stress by 80% and decreases the myocardial oxygen demand by 40% by left ventricle decompression and provide systemic perfusion.

Indications:

- Presence of a cardiac index less than 1.8 L/min/m^2 with a systolic blood pressure (BP) less than 80 mm Hg
- Pulmonary capillary wedge pressure (PCWP) or left atrial pressure (LAP) more than 20 mm Hg on maximal medical support
- An intra-aortic balloon pump, systemic vascular resistance (SVR) more than 2100 dyne-s/cm,[5] urine output less than 20 mL/hour.

Technique

Drainage is provided from the left atrium or left ventricular apex with return of blood to the aorta and a left atrial catheter is inserted for accurate monitoring of left-sided filling pressures.

Evolution of Left Ventricular Assist Devices[1,31]

First Generation

They are also known as pulsatile and volume displacement pumps. They are powered by pneumatic or electrical drive systems. Examples are Abiomed BVS 5000, Thoratec IVAD, Novacor II, Worldheart Heart Saver, Arrow LionHeart are designed for long term support. Thoratec IVAD and Novacor II are para corporeal while Worldheart HeartSaver and Arrow LionHeart are totally implantable. Lion Heart is a totally implantable VAD without the need for a percutaneous drive line or external catheter but instead uses a transcutaneous energy transmission (TET) system. The LionHeart also has the potential for permanent use in patients not listed for transplantation, such as those with a history of cancer and advanced age. It has the advantage of preventing infection and improving patients' quality of life.

Second Generation

These are also known as continuous flow LVADs which are further classified as:

- *Axial flow pumps*: Nimbus HeartMate II/TCI, Jarvik 2000, (Fig. 2)[32] DeBakey/Micromed VAD (Fig. 3),[32] and Impella pump system
- *Centrifugal pumps*: AB 180, HeartMate II (Fig. 4),[32] Cor Aide, Tandem Heart (PTVA), Heartware (HVAD) system (Fig. 5).[32]

Third Generation

These are continuous flow devices which are being developed with an aim search for better material, longer battery life, and smaller size of the device. Examples are VentrAssist, DuraHeart, and HeartMate III LVAD (Fig. 6).[32]

Volume unloading is better with pulsatile pumps EVAHEART 2, (Fig. 7),[32] but left ventricular pressure unloading is similar with both pulsatile and non-pulsatile pumps.[33,34]

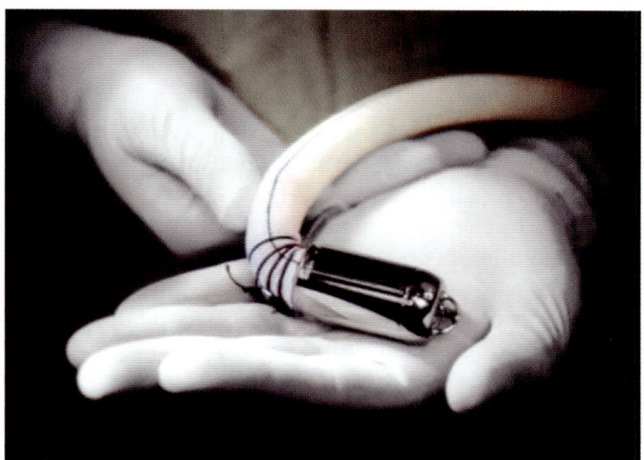

FIG. 2: Jarvik 2000 left ventricular assist device.

Source: Reproduced with permission from Imamura T, Chung B, Nguyen A, et al. Clinical implications of hemodynamic assessment during left ventricular assist device therapy. J Cardiol. 2017.

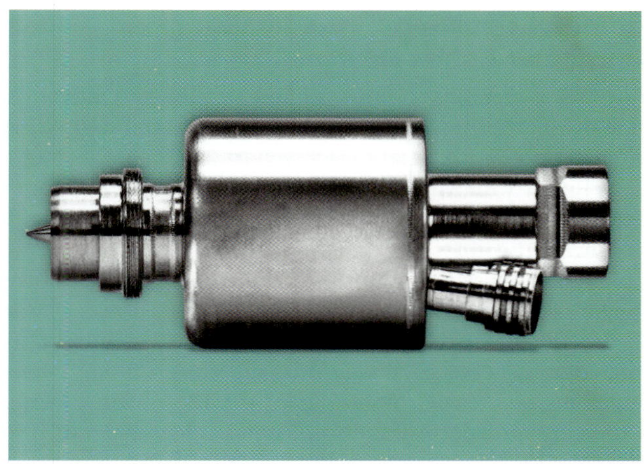

FIG. 3: The DeBakey Heart Assist device.

Source: Reproduced with permission from Imamura T, Chung B, Nguyen A, et al. Clinical implications of hemodynamic assessment during left ventricular assist device therapy. J Cardiol. 2017.

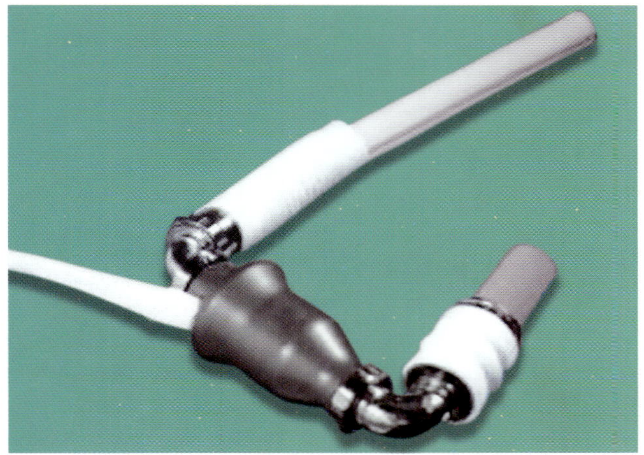

FIG. 4: HeartMate II left ventricular assist device.

Source: Reproduced with permission from Imamura T, Chung B, Nguyen A, et al. Clinical implications of hemodynamic assessment during left ventricular assist device therapy. J Cardiol. 2017.

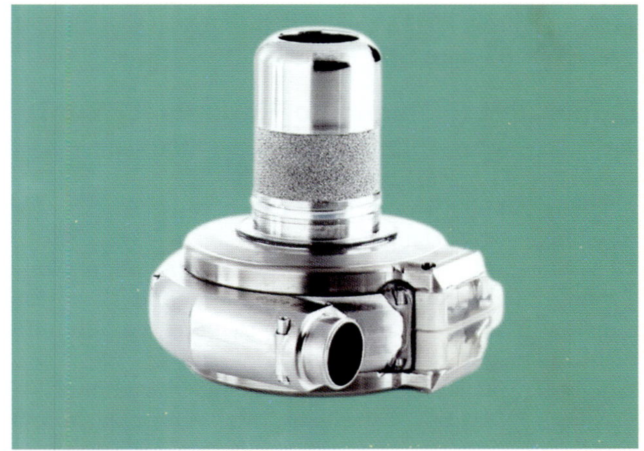

FIG. 5: Heartware (HVAD) system.

Source: Reproduced with permission from Imamura T, Chung B, Nguyen A, et al. Clinical implications of hemodynamic assessment during left ventricular assist device therapy. J Cardiol. 2017.

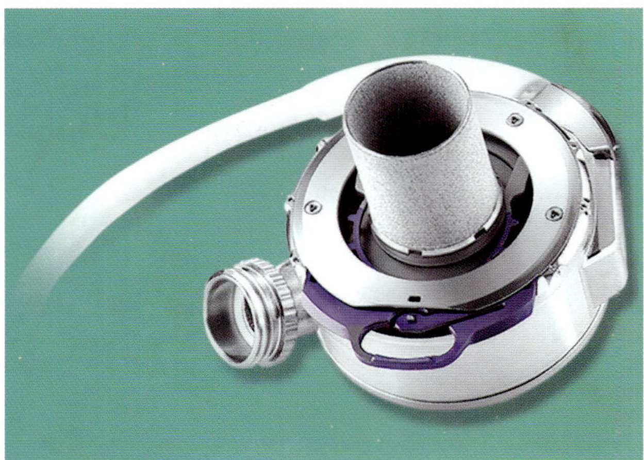

FIG. 6: HeartMate III left ventricular assist device.

Source: Reproduced with permission from Imamura T, Chung B, Nguyen A, et al. Clinical implications of hemodynamic assessment during left ventricular assist device therapy. J Cardiol. 2017.

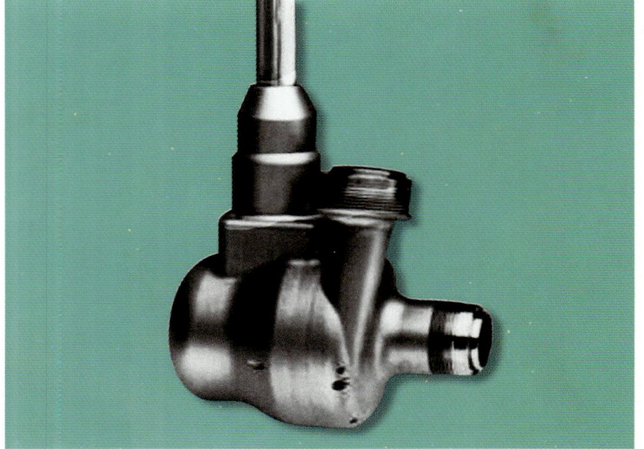

FIG. 7: EVAHEART 2 pulsatile flow device.

Source: Reproduced with permission from Imamura T, Chung B, Nguyen A, et al. Clinical implications of hemodynamic assessment during left ventricular assist device therapy. J Cardiol. 2017.

Timing of Decision Strategies for Ventricular Assist Devices

With the worsening hemodynamic profile and advanced stage of HF, traditional New York Heart Association (NYHA) classification is not reliable (Flowchart 2). Thus, the Interagency Registry for Mechanically Assisted Circulatory Support (INTERMACS) profile system assigns a level depending on how severe the illness is (Figs. 8 and 9).[28,35,36]

Patients classified under INTERMACS level 2 and 3 constitute about 66% of all LVAD patients. These classes HF are the ideal patients for durable LVAD implantation which could serve in the interim till they undergo heart transplant or for the remainder of the life of the patients. In the randomized evaluation of mechanical assistance for the treatment of congestive HF (REMATCH) trial out of 129 nontransplant patients of HF randomized into two arms one with ongoing medical therapy and in the other arm patients receiving HeartMate XVE implantation, those receiving circulatory device support showed 53% survival versus 25% survival in medical therapy arm at the end of 1 year.[35] Thus, LVAD implantation confers a definite survival benefit in the presence of end stage HF.

Preoperative Evaluation of Patients for LVAD[27]

Issues that can jeopardize functioning of LVAD which needs to be assessed prior to implantation are:

- Patent foramen ovale (PFO) which cause severe hypoxemia post-LVAD implantation
- Presence of significant aortic regurgitation which increases further post-LVAD implantation as a result increases LVAD preload leading to increased pump flow and fall in systemic blood flow
- Right ventricular function and tricuspid regurgitation (TR) as high LVAD flow can distort inter ventricular septum and cause tethering of tricuspid valve and exacerbate preexisting TR.

Post Ventricular Assist Device Implantation Management[31]

Left Ventricular Assist Device

- Flows are initiated to achieve a systemic flow of 2.2 L/min/m^2 with a LAP maintained at 10–15 mm Hg
- Maintain mean BP of 75 mm Hg
- As LVAD patients manifest commonly with vasodilatory shock alpha agents and vasopressin infusions may be started
- Heparinization should be done to maintain activated partial thromboplastin time (aPTT) 2–2.5 times normal and activated clotting time (ACT) 185–200 s.

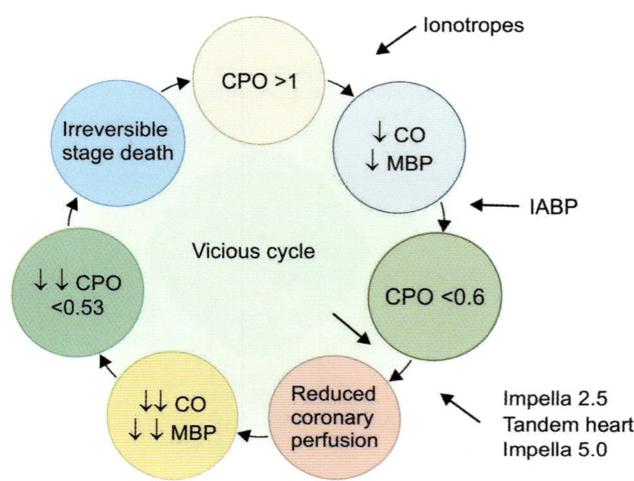

CPO, cardiac power output; CO, cardiac output; MBP, mean blood pressure.

FIG. 8: Timing of strategies providing hemodynamic support.

Source: Reproduced with permission from Mishra S. Upscaling cardiac assist devices in decompensated heart failure: Choice of device and its timing. Indian Heart J. 2016:S1-4.

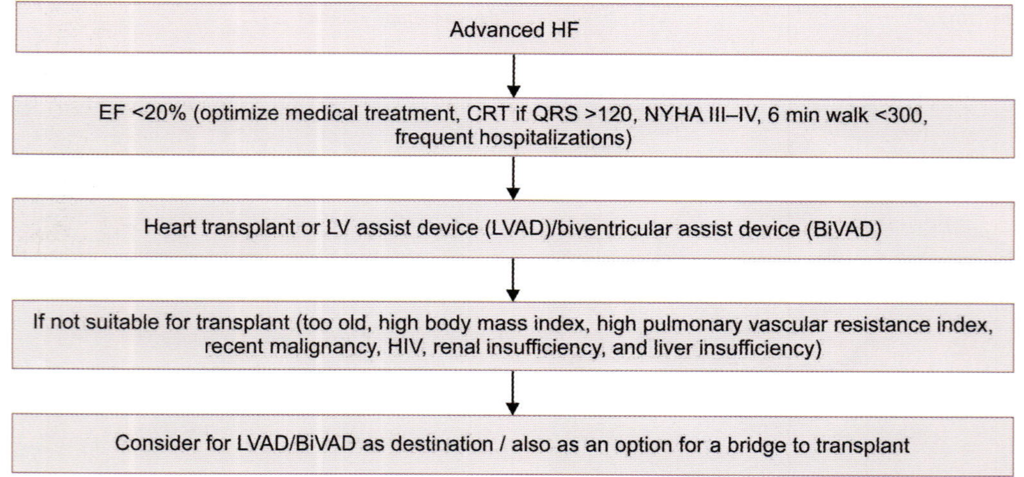

CRT, cardiac resynchronization therapy; HF, heart failure; LV, left ventricular; NYHA, New York Heart Association; EF, ejection fraction; HIV, human immunodeficiency virus.

FLOWCHART 2: Decision process for ventricular assist devices.

Source: Reproduced with permission from Seth S, Bhargava B, Maulik SK, et al. Consensus statement on management of chronic heart failure in India. J Pract Cardiovasc Sci. 2015;1:105-12.

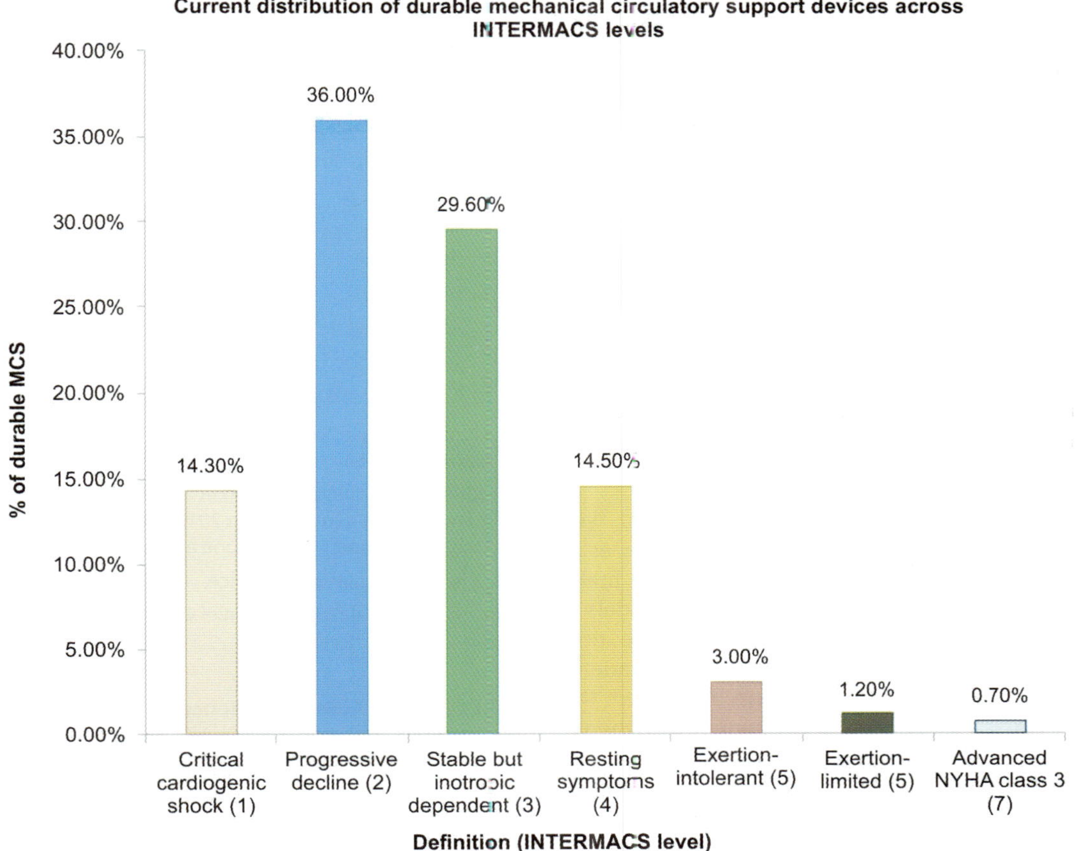

INTERMACS, Interagency Registry For Mechanical Circulatory Support; MCS, mechanical circulatory support; NHYA, New York Heart Association.

FIG. 9: Distribution of durable mechanical circulatory support devices across INTERMACS level.

Source: Shah SP, Mehra MR. Durable left ventricular assist device therapy in advanced heart failure: Patient selection and clinical outcomes. Indian Heart J. 2016;68:S45-51.

Problems with LVAD: Post-LVAD Implantation Complications[30,37]

A discussion of these is important as the frequent occurrence of these complications mandates that the patients either remain in the hospital for extended duration or live in close proximity or manage to return for follow-up at short intervals or in times of need. This is not difficult in the Western world because of wide awareness and because of multiple set-ups that are available within close distance of the patient's place of residence. However, this is practically impossible in countries like India where there are less than 10 setups for the entire country, which means that these patients have to be in the hospital for extended periods of time, significantly increasing the costs of health care.[38,39]

Bleeding

As a result of anticoagulation with warfarin, shear stress from pump induced platelet dysfunction causes bleeding mostly from gastro intestinal tract at the rate of 8–23%[40] Heyde's syndrome [a gastrointestinal (GI) bleeding initially described in patients with severe calcific aortic stenosis from angiodysplasias] is seen in candidates with continuous flow LVADs which results due to low pulsatility on micro circulation and increased oxidative stress.[41]

Up to 60% of patients require re-exploration for evacuation of mediastinal clots as a result of mediastinal bleeding that causes tamponade which manifests as improper drainage of the device.[42]

Pump Thrombosis

This complication carries a high risk of death and may also lead to postoperative neurological events. Incidence rate of pump thrombosis is 6–12%.[43,44] From the time of confirmed pump thrombosis, there is a two-fold increase in mortality at 30 days, 90 days, and 6 month.[45] Patients with suspected LVAD thrombosis who do not undergo LVAD exchange or cardiac transplantation have 48.2% mortality within 6 months.

Infection

Incidence of infection in post-VAD implantation patients is about 20% which manifests as sepsis, mediastinitis or a drive-line infection.[40] This data is from the Western world and the incidence of infectious complications is expected to be much higher in India. The most common organisms are *Staphylococcus aureus*, coagulase-negative staphylococci, *Candida* and *Pseudomonas aeruginosa*. Infection should be treated aggressively which may require long term antibiotics, antifungal agents unless the device is exchanged or the patient is considered for cardiac transplantation.

Cerebrovascular Complications

Thromboembolic events like stroke occur at a rate of 6%. Patients with mechanical aortic valves should have them covered with tissue or sewn shut to prevent thromboembolism.

Malignant Ventricular Arrhythmias

Ventricular arrhythmias occur as a result of myocardial ischemia, infarction, or the use of catecholamines. Fibrillation may lead to thrombus formation in the ventricle and it should be treated aggressively by early cardioversion to prevent RV injury from prolonged fibrillation.[46] Chest compressions can be used for percutaneous and continuous flow devices but are contraindicated for pulsatile devices.[47]

Case Series on Ventricular Assist Device Implantation from India

A case series comprising of 11 patients implanted with LVAD as destination therapy was reported by Kumar et al. in 2015 from Fortis Malar Hospital Chennai[48] in 8 males and 3 females with a mean age of 47 years. Two models of LVADs HEARTMATE-II for patients weighing more than 70 kg in 3 patients and HeartWare (HVAD) for patients weighing less than 70 kg in 8 patients were implanted. Out of 11 patients primary diagnoses for 4 patients was ischemic cardiomyopathy, 3 had dilated cardiomyopathy, one patient had recent anterior wall myocardial infarction (AWMI) with recurrent VT and LV dysfunction and one had severe valvular aortic stenosis with severe LV dysfunction. Seven patients were classified as INTERMACS level 2, 3 patients in INTERMACS level 3 and one patient in INTERMACS level 4. Two patients were on prior ECMO and 8 patients were on inotropic support. In postoperative period 9 patients were successfully discharged. Two patients had in hospital mortality: one due to sepsis and intracerebral hemorrhage and other due to severe right heart and liver failure. There was one late mortality 18 months postoperatively due to fulminant hepatic failure. Remaining 7 patients are doing well with no signs of HF after a maximum of 3 years follow-up. Current Fortis experience is listed in table 1.

A case series of 3 patients of LVAD implantation was reported by Jayanth Kumar et al. in 2013 from Narayana Hrudayalaya Institute of Medical Sciences, Bangalore.[45] The average age was 42.3 years. Etiology of HF in 2 cases was ischemic cardiomyopathy and 1 was idiopathic cardiomyopathy. All 3 patients under went LVAD implantation with VentrAssist model. All 3 patients underwent a cardiac rehabilitation program prior to discharge. All of them were in NYHA class I cardiac status at the time of discharge.

A case report was described by Singh et al. from AIIMS New Delhi[48] of a 35-year-old male with primary diagnoses of dilated cardiomyopathy who underwent LVAD implantation with HeartWare (HVAD). During the postoperative period patient developed hematuria on second postoperative day and acute kidney injury in the first postoperative week. This patient underwent mediastinal exploration on day 11 and bilateral pleural drains were placed for pleural effusion which did not subside by repeated tapping during the first week.

TABLE 1: LVAD: The Chennai experience

Variable	Values
• Duration	2012–2018
• Number of cases	55
• Type of LVAD	
○ HeartMate III	20
○ Heartware	25
○ HeartMateII	10
• Cost per case	80–90 lakh rupees
• Survival rates	
○ At 1 year	>80%
○ At the end of 5 years	<40%
• Number of cases who ended in transplantation	4

In addition, Centrimag was used in 28 patients in 2016, 55 patients in 2017 and in 50 patients so far in 2018. Majority of these patients were postcardiotomy and 10 were done as bridge to transplant.

LVAD, left ventricular assist device.

Courtesy: Dr KR Balakrishnan, Chief Cardiothoracic, Fortis Malar Hospital, Adyar, Chennai.

TABLE 2: LVAD AIIMS experience

Variable	Value
Number of cases	8
Median age	41.5 (range 34–49) years
Etiology of heart failure	DCM (N = T), Post-transplant: 1

Planned as bridge to transplant in all patients except one, with only one patient receiving the transplant.

LVAD, left ventricular assist device; AIIMS, All India Institute of Medical Sciences; DCM, dilated cardiomyopathy.

Patient also developed depression due to prolonged ICU stay. Mean hospital stay was 45 days. Postdischarge patient developed driveline site infection leading to formation of granulation tissue. During follow-up visit 6 months postoperative, patient developed severe RV dysfunction and hepatomegaly. Current AIIMS experience is listed in table 2.

HEART TRANSPLANTATION VERSUS VAD'S FOR END STAGE HEART FAILURE

Cardiac transplantation is the desired optimal management for patients with end stage HF, but compatible donor availability is a major limiting factor.[49] Optimal patient selection determines is important to get good results. Heart transplantation is contraindicated in the presence of significant pulmonary hypertension; however mechanical support is considered in these patients.[50] Patients with end-stage right-sided HF are suitable for mechanical LV assist. In these patients cardiac transplantation is useful.[51-53] Mechanical assist of the left ventricle improves renal function.[54] Contraindications are infection, older age, and significant aortic insufficiency.[55-58] Mechanical LV assist may however lead to ventricular arrhythmias.[59] In addition, many patients on LV assist may not remain suitable candidates or may never undergo cardiac transplantation due to scarcity of a suitable donor.[52]

Theochari et al.,[60] conducted a meta-analysis of eight multi-centric studies involving close to 8,000 patients. Almost 5,000 of these received a cardiac transplant whereas a LV assist device was implanted in 92 as the final palliation. In more than 2,500 patients, the mechanical assist was used while these patients awaited a transplant. The follow-up in patients undergoing transplant was 12–50 months and for those on assist, awaiting transplant, it was 9.4–30 months. The average LVEF was 14–24% in the transplant group, 15.6–20.4% in the bridge to transplant group and 13–20% in the destination group 1-year death rates in all groups were similar. Stroke rate was 0–4.3% in those undergoing cardiac transplantation, 0– 6.1% those undergoing mechanical assist as a bridge to transplant and 4.3–6.1% in patients where the mechanical assist was used as a destination therapy. Infection occurred in 0.5–25.5% undergoing transplant, 21.1–26.5% with destination mechanical assist and 0–32% with bridge mechanical assist. The total cost per-patient for the transplantation group was 128,474–230,009 US Dollars, for the mechanical assist as a bridge, it was 95,428–166,415 US Dollars and in patients where mechanical LV assist was the final palliation, it was 152,931–174,165 US Dollars. On comparing 1-year survival following heart transplantation after a period of mechanical circulatory assist with mechanical assist as a final therapy, both strategies carried similar results.

Retrospective Study by Mishra et al.[61] showed that 1- and 5-year survival rates were 96% and 83% in the bridging to HTx (LVADHTx group), 92% and 81% in heart transplant (HTx group), 48% and 36% in those who were treated by LVAD alone (LVAD group). Total hospital cost at 1 year was \$151,685 ± 86,892 for HTx, \$427,337 ± 365,154 for LVAD, and \$600,897 ± 198,109 for LVADHTx. The study concluded that LVADHTx and HTx groups showed excellent 1- and 5-year survival rates and the expenses per patient was almost four times in LVADHTx group. However, as these devices are not indigenous, it is apparent that these costs are prohibitive and not within reach of even 0.5% of the population. The average per capita income in India was \$1,410 in 2011, in some states it was as low as \$ 294–436 ("India Country Overview 2013". World Bank. 2014. Retrieved 28 July 2014.)—World Bank: India Country Overview 2013.

India is a developing mixed economy.[62] It is the world's sixth largest economy by nominal gross domestic product (GDP) and the third largest by purchasing power parity (PPP). The country ranks 139th in per capita GDP (nominal) with \$2,134 and 122nd in per capita GDP (PPP) with \$7,783 as of 2018.[62]

A study by Garbade J et al.[63] compared the two therapeutic options VAD versus heart transplantation for end stage HF (Table 3).[63]

TABLE 3: Comparing questions and challenges between the two end-stage heart failure treatment modalities

Feature	Ventricular assist devices	Heart transplantation
Availability	Immediately	Unmet needs with waiting list
2 years survival benefit	80%	80%
5 years survival benefit	40%	70%
QoL and functional capacity	Proven up to 2 years	Proven
Showering and bathing	Very limited	Unrestricted
Long-term stability	Proven	Proven
Complications	• Thrombo embolic events • Bleedings • Drive-line infections	• Drug toxicities • Allograft vasculopathy • Malignancies
Drug monitoring	Required, anticoagulation, different protocols	Required, immunosuppression, multiple protocols
Myocardial biopsy	No	Yes, different protocols
Infrastructure, outstanding, and hospital care	Under construction and development	Available
Team and coordinator	Yes	Yes
Remote monitoring	Under development	Not available
Organ supply	–	Limited, despite newer conservation technique and organ care systems
VAD development and new technique, peripherals	Stringent development	–
Reimbursement	Unclear	Defined
Public policy	Insurance & costs	Insurance and costs
Ethical aspects	Undefined, decision making: device selection for individual patients not defined clearly (e.g., considering age, comorbidities, palliative care)	Regulated by different societies

VAD, ventricular assist device; QoL, quality of life.

A retrospective single center study by Marasco SF et al.[64] comparing costs of 35 post-heart transplantation patients with 33 post-LVAD implantation patients, demonstrated the significantly increased costs of VAD implantation compared to HTx over the first 12 months of care. The total costs of care during the index admission, procurement, blood products, and subsequent admissions were approximately $411.414 per patient in the VAD group which is almost double versus $189.988 per patient in the heart transplant group. Procurement costs for the current generation VAD in our country are approximately 27 times higher than for a donor heart as they are not indigenously manufactured. Emergency admissions for duration of several days in the subsequent periods are also high for VAD implantation group culminating in very high postoperative management expenditures.

Patel et al.[65] compared costs over 12 months of LVAD treatment versus heart transplantation including follow-up with immunosuppressive drugs and surveillance biopsies, it was found that the index admission and postoperative management costs for 1 year were higher in LVAD implantation by approximately 15%, but the overall costs were almost similar in both the groups balanced by the higher outpatient costs in the transplant group.

In a study by Mulloy et al.,[66] in-hospital deaths following mechanical LV assist occurred in 17% compared to 6.5% following cardiac transplant. The mean cost per patient increased for both orthotopic heart transplantation and LV assist device placement which were 40% and 17%, respectively. With the observed increase in both device usage and cost per patient, the cumulative LV assist device cost increased 232% within 5 years from $143 million to $479 million.

PROS AND CONS OF LVADS IN INDIA (TABLE 4)

Made in India Ventricular Assist Device[67]

On May 23rd 2016, Cherian from Frontier Lifeline, Chennai signed entered into collaboration with Russian scientists to manufacture a low-cost VAD which potentially fulfil the objectives of LV assist. This is proposed to be manufactured in India and may cost only around Rs 30 lakh, one-third of the market prices of other devices. The device called Sputnik, in envisaged to be manufactured in in a facility near Chennai. India will be the first Asian country and the third in the world to manufacture VADs, after US and Germany. Currently this device is still in the testing phase in various preclinical animal studies.

TABLE 4: Pros and cons of ventricular assist devices in India

Pros	Cons
Off the shelf availability	Prohibitive costs
Size not an issue	Risk of complications: bleeding, infection, thromboembolism
Blood group not an issue	Need and risks of anticoagulation
No need to wait for donors	May unmask right ventricular failure with need of ventricular assist
No need for immunosuppressants	Technical issues with implantation
Can be used as bridge to transplant/destination therapy	Patient mobility (flexibility with newer modules)

CONCLUSION

The cost of VAD implant is approx. US$ 100,000 and in India Rs. 9,000,000.[27,67,68] The cost of implant is obviously a factor in slow growth of VADs assistance programs for patients. VAD costs as well as perioperative care need to reduce substantially in order to make this treatment option a more available alternative for larger groups of the severe HF patients. It is likely that this will happen, as results improve and complications reduce. Favorable reimbursement policies even in developing countries like India are expected to trigger the entry of these devices penetration into the health care in the near future. However, at the moment this remains a costly treatment option despite an expanding pool of recipients and probably does not justify the need to borrow to afford them.[69,70]

REFERENCES

1. Ghosh P. Surgery for heart failure. Ind J Thorac Cardiovasc Surg. 2002;18(3): 125-36.
2. McMurray JJ, Stewart S. Epidemiology, aetiology, and prognosis of heart failure. Heart. 2000;83:596-602.
3. Cowie MR, Mosterd A, Wood DA, et al. The epidemiology of heart failure. Eur Heart J. 1997;18:208-25.
4. American Heart Association. 2001 Heart and stroke statistical update. Dallas: Texas. American Heart Association, 2000.
5. O'Connell JB, Birstow MR. Economic impact of heart failure in the United States: Time for a different approach. J Heart Lung Transplant. 1994;13:S107-12.
6. Lloyd-Jones DM, Larson MG, Leip EP, et al. Lifetime risk for developing congestive heart failure: The Framingham heart study. Circulation. 2002;106:3068-72.
7. Chaturvedi V, Parakh N, Seth S, et al. Heart failure in India: The Indus (India Ukieri Study) study. J Pract Cardiovasc Sci. 2016;2:28.
8. Seth S, Khanal S, Ramakrishnan S, et al. Epidemiology of acute decompensated heart failure in India: The AFAR study (Acute failure registry study). J Pract Cardiovasc Sci. 2015;1:35.
9. Joshi R, Chow CK, Raju PK, et al. Fatal and nonfatal cardiovascular disease and the use of therapies for secondary prevention in a rural region of India. Circulation. 2009;119:1950-5.
10. Docherla M, Hande MH, Kavitha S, et al. Comparative study of systolic and diastolic cardiac failure in elderly hospitalized patients in a tertiary care hospital in Southwest India. J Clin Diagn Res. 2009;3:1529-36.
11. Lopez AD, Mathers CD, Ezzati M, et al. Global and regional burden of disease and risk factors, 2001: Systematic analysis of population health data. Lancet. 2006;367:1747-57.
12. Strasser T, Dondog N, El Kholy A, et al. The community control of rheumatic fever and rheumatic heart disease: Report of a WHO international cooperative project. Bull World Health Organ. 1981;59:285-94.
13. Arora R, Subramanyam G, Khalilullah M, et al. Clinical profile of rheumatic fever and rheumatic heart disease: A study of 2,500 cases. Indian Heart J. 1981;33:264-9.
14. Grover A, Dhawan A, Iyengar SD, et al. Epidemiology of rheumatic fever and rheumatic heart disease in a rural community in Northern India. Bull World Health Organ. 1993;71:59-66.
15. Jose VJ, Gupta SN. Mortality and morbidity of acute ST segment elevation myocardial infarction in the current era. Indian Heart J. 2004;56:210-4.

16. Mehta SR, Yusuf S, Díaz R, et al. Effect of glucose-insulin-potassium infusion on mortality in patients with acute ST-segment elevation myocardial infarction: The CREATE-ECLA randomized controlled trial. JAMA. 2005;293:437-46.
17. Prabhakaran D, Yusuf S, Mehta S, et al. Two-year outcomes in patients admitted with non-ST elevation acute coronary syndrome: Results of the OASIS registry 1 and 2. Indian Heart J. 2005;57:217-25.
18. Xavier D, Pais P, Devereaux PJ, et al. Treatment and outcomes of acute coronary syndromes in India (CREATE): A prospective analysis of registry data. Lancet. 2008;371:1435-42.
19. Lawes CM, Vander Hoorn S, Rodgers A. International Society of Hypertension. Global burden of blood-pressure-related disease, 2001. Lancet. 2008;371:1513-8.
20. Okin PM, Devereux RB, Nieminen MS, et al. Electrocardiographic strain pattern and prediction of new-onset congestive heart failure in hypertensive patients: The Losartan Intervention for Endpoint Reduction in Hypertension (LIFE) study. Circulation. 2006;113:67-73.
21. Pednekar MS, Gupta R, Gupta PC. Association of blood pressure and cardiovascular mortality in India: Mumbai cohort study. Am J Hypertens. 2009;22:1076-84.
22. Seth S, Ramakrishnan S, Parekh N, et al. Heart failure guidelines for India: Update 2017. J Pract Cardiovasc Sci. 2017;3:133-8.
23. Barron H (2007). The 25th Anniversary of Barney Clark's Artificial Heart. Celebrity Health, 2007. [online] Available from: http://www.HealthDiaries.com [Accessed on September 2018].
24. Liotta D, Descotes JP, Cooley DA, et al. L'assistance circulatoire prolongee par pompe intrathoracique, realisant un bypass partiel du ventricule gauche: etude experimentale. Ann Chir Thorac Cardiovasc. 1963;2:3-7.
25. Stevenson LW, kormos RL, Mechanical Cardiac Support 2000. Current applications and future trial design. Consensus conference report. J Am Coll Cardiol. 2001;37:340-70.
26. Hamdan MH, Zagrodzky JD, Joglar JA, et al. Biventricular pacing decreases sympathetic activity compared with right ventricular pacing in patients with depressed ejection fraction. Circulation. 2000;102:1027-32.
27. Neema PK. Heart failure: Advances and Issues. Ann Card Anaesth. 2013;16:235-7.
28. Seth S, Bhargava B, Maulik SK, et al. Consensus statement on management of chronic heart failure in India. J Pract Cardiovasc Sci. 2015;1:105-12.
29. The artificial heart program: Current status and history. In: Hogness JR, VanAntwerp M (Eds). The artificial heart: Prototypes, policies, and patients. Washington, D.C.: National Academy Press, 1991. pp. 14-25.
30. Bojar RM. Cardiovascular management. Manual of Perioperative Care in Adult Cardiac Surgery, Fifth Edition. 2005; pp. 439-580.
31. Klotz S, Deng MC, Stypmann J, et al. Left ventricular pressure and volume unloading during pulsatile versus nonpulsatile left ventricular assist device support. Ann Thorac Surg. 2004;77:14-9.
32. Imamura T, Chung B, Nguyen A, et al. Clinical implications of hemodynamic assessment during left ventricular assist device therapy. J Cardiol. 2017.
33. Garcia S, Kandar F, Boyle A, et al. Effects of pulsatile- and continuous-flow left ventricular assist devices on left ventricular unloading. J Heart Lung Transplant. 2008;27:261-7.
34. Marquez TT, D'Cunha J, John R, et al. Mechanical support for acute right ventricular failure: evolving survival paradigms. J Thorac Cardiovasc Surg. 2009;137:e39-40.
35. Mishra S. Upscaling cardiac assist devices in decompensated heart failure: Choice of device and its timing. 2016:S1-4.
36. Shah SP, Mehra MR. Durable left ventricular assist device therapy in advanced heart failure: Patient selection and clinical outcomes. Indian Heart J. 2016;68: S45-51.
37. Rose EA, Gelijns AC, Moskowitz AJ, et al. Long-term use of a left ventricular assist device for end-stage heart failure. New Eng J Med. 2001;345(20): 1435-43.
38. Klodell CT Jr, Morey TE, Lobato EB, et al. Effect of sildenafil on pulmonary artery pressure, systemic pressure, and nitric oxide utilization in patients with left ventricular assist devices. Ann Thorac Surg. 2007;83:68-71.
39. McIlvennan CK, Magid KH, Ambardekar AV, et al. Clinical outcomes after continuous-flow left ventricular assist device CLINICAL PERSPECTIVE: A Systematic Review. Circulation: Heart Failure. 2014;7(6):1003-13.
40. Suarez J, Patel CG, Felker M, et al. Mechanisms of bleeding and approach to patients with axial-flow left ventricular assist devices. Circ Heart Fail. 2011;4:779-84.
41. Goldstein DJ, Beauford RB. Left ventricular assist devices and bleeding: adding insult to injury. Ann Thorac Surg. 2003;75(6 suppl):S42-7.
42. Kirklin JK, Naftel DC, Kormos RL, et al. Interagency Registry for Mechanically Assisted Circulatory Support (INTERMACS) analysis of pump thrombosis in the HeartMate II left ventricular assist device. J Heart Lung Transplant. 2014;33(1):12-22.
43. Starling RC, Moazami N, Silvestry SC, et al. Unexpected abrupt increase in left ventricular assist device thrombosis. New Eng J Med. 2014;370(1):33-40.
44. Najjar SS, Slaughter MS, Pagani FD, et al. An analysis of pump thrombus events in patients in the HeartWare ADVANCE bridge to transplant and continued access protocol trial. J Heart Lung Transplant. 2014;33(1):23-34.
45. Singh SP, Seth S, Sahu MK, et al. HeartWare HVAD: Postoperative issues in our first patient. J Pract Cardiovasc Sci. 2017;3:63-6.
46. Rao GS, Balakrishnan KR. Left ventricular assist device (LVAD) as destination therapy in end stage heart failure–First Indian report. Indian Heart J. 2015;67:S105-6.
47. Jayanthkumar HS, Murugesan C, Rajkumar J, et al. Our experience with implantation of VentrAssist left ventricular assist device. Indian J Anaesth. 2013;57:56-61.
48. Wiedemann D, Haberl T, Angleitner P, et al. Minimally invasive approaches for implantation of left ventricular assist devices. Ind J Thorac Cardiovasc Surg. 2018;1:1-6.
49. Blanche C, Kamlot A, Blanche DA, et al. Heart transplantation with donors fifty years of age and older. J Thorac Cardiovasc Surg. 2002;123(4):810-5.
50. Murali S, Uretsky BF, Reddy PS, et al. Reversibility of pulmonary hypertension in congestive heart failure patients evaluated for cardiac transplantation: comparative effects of various pharmacologic agents. Am Heart J. 1991;122(5):1375-81.
51. Cordtz J, Nilsson JC, Hansen PB, et al. Right ventricular failure after implantation of a continuous-flow left ventricular assist device: early haemodynamic predictors. Eur J Cardio-Thorac Surg. 2013;45(5):847-53.
52. Drakos SG, Janicki L, Horne BD, et al. Risk factors predictive of right ventricular failure after left ventricular assist device implantation. Am J Cardiol. 2010;105(7):1030-5.
53. Atluri P, Goldstone AB, Fairman AS, et al. Predicting right ventricular failure in the modern, continuous flow left ventricular assist device era. Ann Thorac Surg. 2013;96(3):857-64.
54. Hasin T, Topilsky Y, Schirger JA, et al. Changes in renal function after implantation of continuous-flow left ventricular assist devices. J Am Col Cardiol. 2012;59(1):26-36.
55. Kirklin JK, Naftel DC, Pagani FD, et al. Seventh INTERMACS annual report: 15 000 patients and counting. J Heart Lung Transplant. 2015;34(12):1495-504.
56. Cotts WG, McGee Jr EC, Myers SL, et al. Predictors of hospital length of stay after implantation of a left ventricular assist device: An analysis of the INTERMACS registry. J Heart Lung Transplant. 2014;33(7):682-8.
57. Holley CT, Fitzpatrick M, Roy SS, et al. Aortic insufficiency in continuous-flow left ventricular assist device support patients is common but does not impact long-term mortality. J Heart Lung Transplant. 2017;36(1):91-6.
58. Pal JD, Klodell CT, John R, et al. Low operative mortality with implantation of a continuous-flow left ventricular assist device and impact of concurrent cardiac procedures. Circulation. 2005;120(11 suppl 1):S215-9.
59. Sims DB, Uriel N, González-Costello J, et al. Human immunodeficiency virus infection and left ventricular assist devices: a case series. J Heart Lung Transplant. 2011;30(9):1060-4.
60. Theochari CA, Michalopoulos G, Oikonomou EK, et al. Heart transplantation versus left ventricular assist devices as destination therapy or bridge to transplantation for 1-year mortality: a systematic review and meta-analysis. Ann Cardiothorac Surg. 2018;7(1):3.
61. Mishra V, Fiane AE, Winsnes BA, et al. Cardiac replacement therapies: outcomes and costs for heart transplantation versus circulatory assist. Scand Cardiovasc J. 2017;51(1):1-7.
62. Wikipedia (2018). Economy of India [online]. Available from https://en.wikipedia.org/wiki/Economy_of_India [Accessed September 2018]

63. Garbade J, Barten MJ, Bittner HB, et al. Heart transplantation and left ventricular assist device therapy: two comparable options in end-stage heart failure? Clin Cardiol. 2013;36(7):378-82.
64. Marasco SF, Summerhayes R, Quayle M, et al. Cost comparison of heart transplant vs. left ventricular assist device therapy at one year. Clinical Transplant. 2016;30(5):598-605.
65. Patel SR, Sileo A, Bello R, et al. Heart transplantation versus continuous-flow left ventricular assist device: comprehensive cost at 1 year. J Cardiac Fail. 2015;1;21(2):160-6.
66. Mulloy DP, Bhamidipati CM, Stone ML, et al. Orthotopic heart transplant versus left ventricular assist device: a national comparison of cost and survival. J Thorac Cardiovasc Surg. 2013;145(2):566-74.
67. Times of India (2016). India-made-heart-pump-at-1/3rd-cost. [Online]. Available from https://timesofindia.indiatimes.com/life-style/health-fitness/health-news/India-made-heart-pump-at-1/3rd-cost/articleshow/52667592.cms [Accessed September 2018].
68. Stehlik J, Edwards LB, Kucheryavaya AY, et al. The Registry of the International Society for Heart and Lung Transplantation: 29th official adult heart transplant report—2012. J Heart Lung Transplant. 2012;31(10):1052-64.
69. Kirklin JK, Naftel DC, Kormos RL, et al. Third INTERMACS Annual Report: the evolution of destination therapy in the United States. J Heart Lung Transplant. 2011;30(2):115-23
70. Matthews JC, Koelling TM, Pagani FD, et al. The right ventricular failure risk score. A preoperative tool for assessing the risk of right ventricular failure in left ventricular assist device candidates. J Am Coll Cardiol. 2008;51:2163-72.
71. Fitzpatrick JR 3rd, Frederick JR, Hsu VM, et al. Risk score derived from preoperative data analysis predicts the need for biventricular mechanical circulatory support. J Heart Lung Transplant. 2008;27:1286-92.

CHAPTER **126**

Heart Transplantation in India: Successes and Challenges

Balram Airan, Milind Hote

INTRODUCTION

The events that led to the first human heart transplant and the relevant history of this phenomenal surgical feat is fascinating. Cardiac surgery progressed from the days of Stephen Paget in 1890s who condemned any contemplation of surgery on a human heart as being beyond the "limit set by nature" to controlled cross-circulation and first-oxygenator based open-heart surgeries in 1950s.[1] The next big leap in this field came from a teaching hospital near Devil's peak in Cape Town, South Africa when a young surgeon named Christiaan Barnard captured public imagination all over the world by doing the first human heart transplant in 1967.[2] Many thought this was flattery only to deceive, when several successive attempts at heart transplantation failed worldwide. Essentially the field went into hibernation and only very few determined pioneers at Stanford University persisted with this daring undertaking.[3]

There have been significant advances in medical and device therapies for heart failure (HF) in the last two decades. However, for patients in stage D HF (established end-stage HF), heart transplantation is the gold standard option for suitable candidates.[4]

This chapter is an attempt to look back into the journey of the heart transplant procedure in India, its successes and the challenges to be faced in the road ahead.

SUCCESSES

Overcoming Difficulties in Performing the First Heart Transplant in India

While major experimental work was going on at Stanford, Indian efforts were also on at King Edward Memorial (KEM) hospital in Mumbai, in early 1960s. Professor PK Sen was actively harvesting and transplanting canine hearts (dogs) in his laboratory, worth reasonable success.[5] Having gained strong insight into surgical technique required and donor organ function after transplant, Professor Sen awaited permission from the Maharashtra state medical board to carry out the first human heart transplant since 1965. However, the permission did not come until the first such operation was done in South Africa. In February 1968 (the sixth heart transplant operation in the world) and then again in September 1968, Dr Sen performed two human heart transplants, in both, hearts were retrieved from severe head injury patients.[5] Both the patients succumbed within the first 24 hours of their surgery; first one due to graft dysfunction and the other due to severe pulmonary hypertension in recipient. It is interesting to note here that even in South Africa, in 1967, there had been no set guidelines for diagnosis of death in beating heart potential donors.

These initial failures and the lack of a robust medicolegal document (act pertaining to human organ transplantation) put a mental block in the minds of other surgeons about performing this procedure. By early 1990s All India Institute of Medical Sciences (AIIMS), New Delhi and Madras Medical Mission (MMM), Chennai were ready to perform their own cases of heart transplantation. However, even up to this time, the laws defining organ donation in India were not crystal clear. Major efforts to convince the governmental bodies about the feasibility of this procedure, need for the organ donation, and examples of successful systems in the west, were finally sufficient to convince the regulatory bodies of that time, to come up with a set of rules [THOA (Transplantation of Human Organs Act, 1994)]. The act defined for the first time, the concept of brain stem death (BSD), organ donation, and set forth the regulations governing such organ donation and transplantation for the various hospital setups in India. This was a major breakthrough which kick started the program of solid organ transplant in 1990s. With this major roadblock gone, Professor Venugopal did the first successful heart transplant in India on 3rd August 1994.[6] This was soon followed by several heart transplants both at AIIMS and at MMM, Chennai (Dr KM Cherian). Dr Cherian is credited with our country's first pediatric heart transplant and also the first heart-lung transplant operation.[7] At KEM, where this operation was first attempted in 1968, no further heart transplant operation was done until 2015.

Number of Heart Transplant Centers in Our Country

For almost 14 years since 1994, there were only three to four active centers doing heart transplants in the country. However, since 2008, there has been a rapid increase in the number of centers certified to do heart transplant operation. This increase has been mostly in the metro and large tier-II cities. With a continuous increase in the number of qualified surgeons with more than 2,000 cases surgical experience of open-heart surgery and also the establishment of various multidisciplinary facilities in both government and private sector hospitals, the requirements of certification of an applying center are usually met with and hence the increase in the number of certified centers has materialized. The concern here remains that of the 87 odd centers now certified (Fig. 1),[8] only about 10 are actively doing heart transplants frequently (>5 cases a year), and the other centers have yet to cross a cumulative figure of five.

Number of Operations[8]

Paralleling the increase in the number of centers, there has been an encouraging increase in the number of operations also year-wise, as can be seen in fig. 2. With increase in the experience of transplant teams, the initial teething problems of a successful program are frequently over after the third or fourth operation and subsequent limitation to number is only related to the availability of donor heart. There are three centers which have experience of more than 50 transplants (AIIMS, New Delhi >60, Fortis Malar, Chennai >200 and Fortis Mulund, Mumbai >50). The number of organ donations is increasing especially in some states in our country and more and more surgical teams are geared up to utilize the available donor hearts. The evolution of HF teams (especially cardiologists, cardiac surgeons) enables increasing referrals of end-stage HF patients to heart transplant registries. In addition, there are increasing numbers of pediatric heart transplants also which is very encouraging.

Availability of Standard Immunosuppressive Drugs

Cyclosporin was introduced to the world in early 1980s and the success of solid organ transplants increased exponentially thereafter. There is standard immunosuppression protocol followed across heart transplant centers in India, and there is no dearth of the availability of common drugs used including cyclosporine, tacrolimus, mycophenolate mofetil, and OKT 3. The spectrum of Indian patients varies widely compared to the west in terms of our patients' nutrition, pre-existing latent infections and external environmental hygiene. This has mandated the titration of dosages of steroids and immunosuppressive drugs in Indian patients, these doses being different from western heart transplant recipients. It is a tightrope walk between achieving adequate immune suppression versus inviting infection in Indian setup. With increasing experience in our country, these long-term immunosuppressive drug dosage regimes also have been standardized, as different from Western dosages.

Good Survival and Heart Transplant Outcomes

The standard 1-year survival in busy centers in our country is more than 80%. This compares very favorably with the International Society for Heart and Lung Transplantation (ISHLT) Western data (88%).[9] The main losses previously have been due to flaring up of latent infections or patients who were in extremis preoperatively (on extracorporeal membrane oxygenation, etc.). The problem of flaring up of subclinical infection has been minimized due to aggressive tapering of steroid therapy administered postoperatively, to the minimum required dosage. In terms of long-term recovery, patients are becoming more aware about the possibilities after this major surgery and they are able to actively participate in their cardiac rehabilitation program which enables their return to routine work and lifestyle. Many long-term survivors (>10 years) are inspiring motivators to preoperative HF patients. Good long-term survival also depends significantly on the regular and routine follow-up of these recipients in specialized heart transplant clinics managed mainly by intensivists and cardiologists with important support from radiologists, nephrologists, pathologists and physiotherapists, and counselors.

Increase in Organ Donation, Heart Utilization[8]

Till 2008, the number of organ donations overall in India was abysmally low. If we compare the organ donation rates (number per million population) following 2008, there has been a significant increase. The leading state in terms of organ donation has been Tamil Nadu and the regions of Maharashtra, Chandigarh, Indore, and Kerala also have picked up encouragingly (Fig. 3). Primary cause of increased donation is the increased awareness amongst people about the benefits of organ donation and removal of taboos from their minds (about possible deficiencies in future lives following organ donation), etc. The states starting with Tamil Nadu have taken good corrective action in minimizing red tapes related to organ donation following accident (medicolegal case) deaths, in the sense that no further postmortem is necessary. The forensic team arrives in the operation theatre itself whilst organ harvesting process is underway. In addition, some of the states have taken commendable action toward promoting organ donation by giving ethical soft incentives like government job to one member of a donor family, health insurance to all close family members of a donor family for 5 years, special recognition and thanksgiving functions organized periodically to honor the family of organ donors, and special status to family member of a donor if he/she needs any organ donation. Various states adopt these various measures and the response has definitely been encouraging.

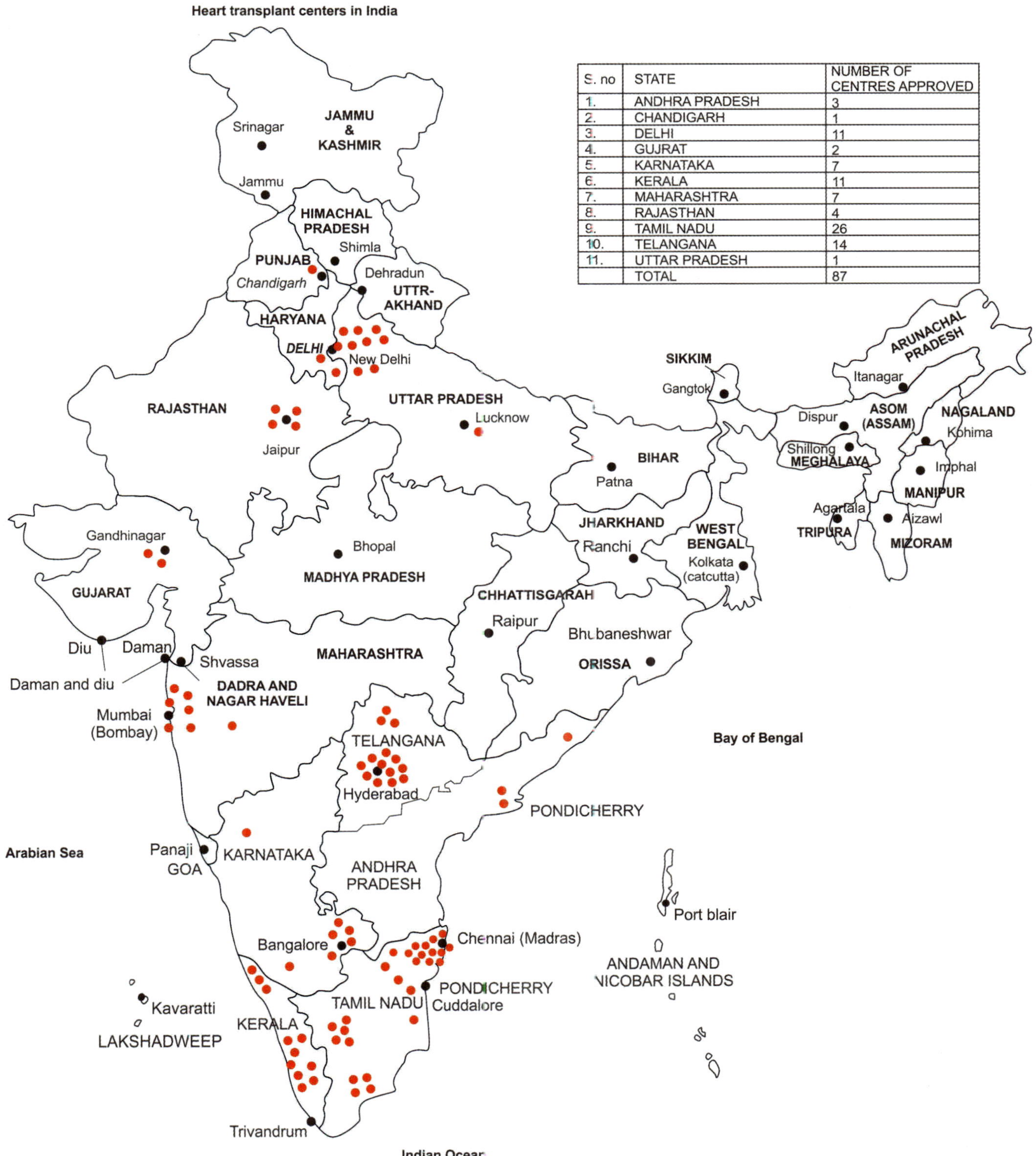

S. no	STATE	NUMBER OF CENTRES APPROVED
1.	ANDHRA PRADESH	3
2.	CHANDIGARH	1
3.	DELHI	11
4.	GUJRAT	2
5.	KARNATAKA	7
6.	KERALA	11
7.	MAHARASHTRA	7
8.	RAJASTHAN	4
9.	TAMIL NADU	26
10.	TELANGANA	14
11.	UTTAR PRADESH	1
	TOTAL	87

FIG. 1: Red dots on map show the cities with hospitals licensed to perform heart transplants.

Recipient Characteristics and Pediatric Heart Transplant

In recent years and in experienced centers, the patient profile is visibly changing. All patients on waiting list for heart transplant are New York Heart Association Class IV, but in addition, several patients are now being taken up whilst being on heavy inotropic support with additional mechanical support (intra-aortic balloon pump or left ventricular assist device) frequently. It becomes a real emergency to offer a

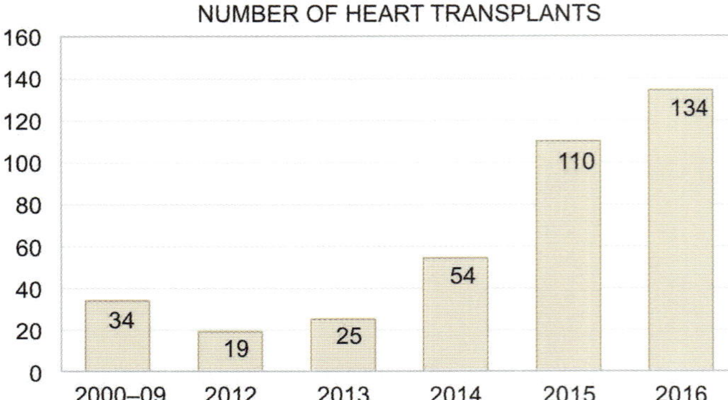

FIG. 2: Yearwise figures - number of heart transplants in India.

donor heart to such patients who are in extremis and are not expected to survive for more than a week in the absence of a donor heart. In these patients, even borderline donor hearts have been transplanted as a desperate measure. Centers are also taking up transplant in the pediatric age group (<14 years). Pediatric age group patients usually belong to the subset having late ventricular failures following some primary operation (usually Fontan operation). There are a very large number of patients in our country who have undergone a Fontan procedure and many of them are gradually returning back with increasing HF. The complexity of surgery increases many times in both the above subsets but outcomes have been gratifying.

National Organ and Tissue Transplant Organization Coordination and Outstation Harvests

With a limited pool of recipients registered in a city, it is a frequent happening that a donor available in a city has no takers for the heart in that city. In the initial years (1995–2008), there was no central organization in the field of coordinating organ donation. Important regional players were nongovernmental organizations (NGOs) like Mohan foundation in South India, Organ Retrieval Banking Organization (ORBO) in AIIMS, New Delhi, and others. Later there was formation of Tamil Nadu Network for Organ Sharing (TNOS) and Transplant Authority of Tamil Nadu (TRANSTAN), and the organ donation rates were significantly increased. Recently, a robust central coordination system is being gradually put into place by National Organ and Tissue Transplant Organization (NOTTO) and it has been instrumental in judicious utilization of available donor hearts nationwide. Nowadays, most of the transplants are happening with donor heart harvesting being done in some other city. NOTTO informs various transplant teams across the country about the availability of a donor heart with all the details. The allocated recipient hospital then makes arrangement to retrieve the donor heart from another city. Use of both chartered flights (air ambulances, cost 6–10 lakh rupees) and routine commercial flights (Indigo, Jet airways, Air India, etc.) has been done to procure the precious donor hearts. The cooperation extended by the flight staff, airport security officials, and traffic police in creating a green corridor in both cities has always been magnanimous, and this concept of outstation harvests is primarily responsible for the recent spurt in the number of heart transplants being done in India.

Experienced Transplant Teams

Surgical technique for heart transplantation is simple. Essentially it involves good myocardial protection while harvesting the heart (give cardioplegia, pack it properly in cold cardioplegia solution—ice), ensure transport of donor heart back to recipient OT within 4 hours, and perform five structural anastomoses—left atrial cuff, inferior vena cava (IVC), superior vena cava (SVC), pulmonary artery and aorta. Any cardiac surgeon with an open-heart surgery experience of more than 1,000 cases can perform the above steps without difficulty. The real challenge comes in the postoperative management in the intensive care unit (ICU) and ward. Many patients go into low renal output and a good all-around team care—from the cardiologist, intensivist, anesthesiologist, nephrologist, physiotherapist, transplant nurses, pathologist, psychologist and others—is mandatory for a successful outcome following this major surgery. This close model of care needs to be followed up even after discharge and late after transplant. Having a successful transplant program essentially depends on having a competent, cohesive, committed core team comprising the above. These are now available in many hospitals and many cities in India, that is, an important factor in the success of the transplant program in India.

CHALLENGES

In India, there still are several challenges faced by the specialty of heart transplantation. We are still not performing as many number of transplants as needed and the factors determining postoperative outcome here are slightly different from what is seen in the western data. Herein we briefly look at the factors that cause still a suboptimal heart transplant program in India.

Low Donation Rate[8]

The bar graph (Fig. 4) shows the organ donation rate per million population in various countries. It is amply clear that India stands way far behind in terms of national average donation rate.

About 10 states and two union territories only are reasonably active in the field of organ donation. Many states are large states like UP, Bihar, Chhattisgarh, Himachal Pradesh (Fig. 5), etc. but have not yet seen a single organ donation. If we see the road traffic figures, we had 1% (of the world) road vehicles and 6% of road traffic accidents (in the world). By 2006, these accident figures have swelled to 10%. In absolute numbers, 137,572 people died on Indian roads due to accidents (1.1% of world's total death figure). If even 5–10% of these deaths are converted into organ donating individuals,[10] it will largely suffice the need for donors for heart and lung transplants in our country. We need to have more number and enthusiastic transplant coordinators

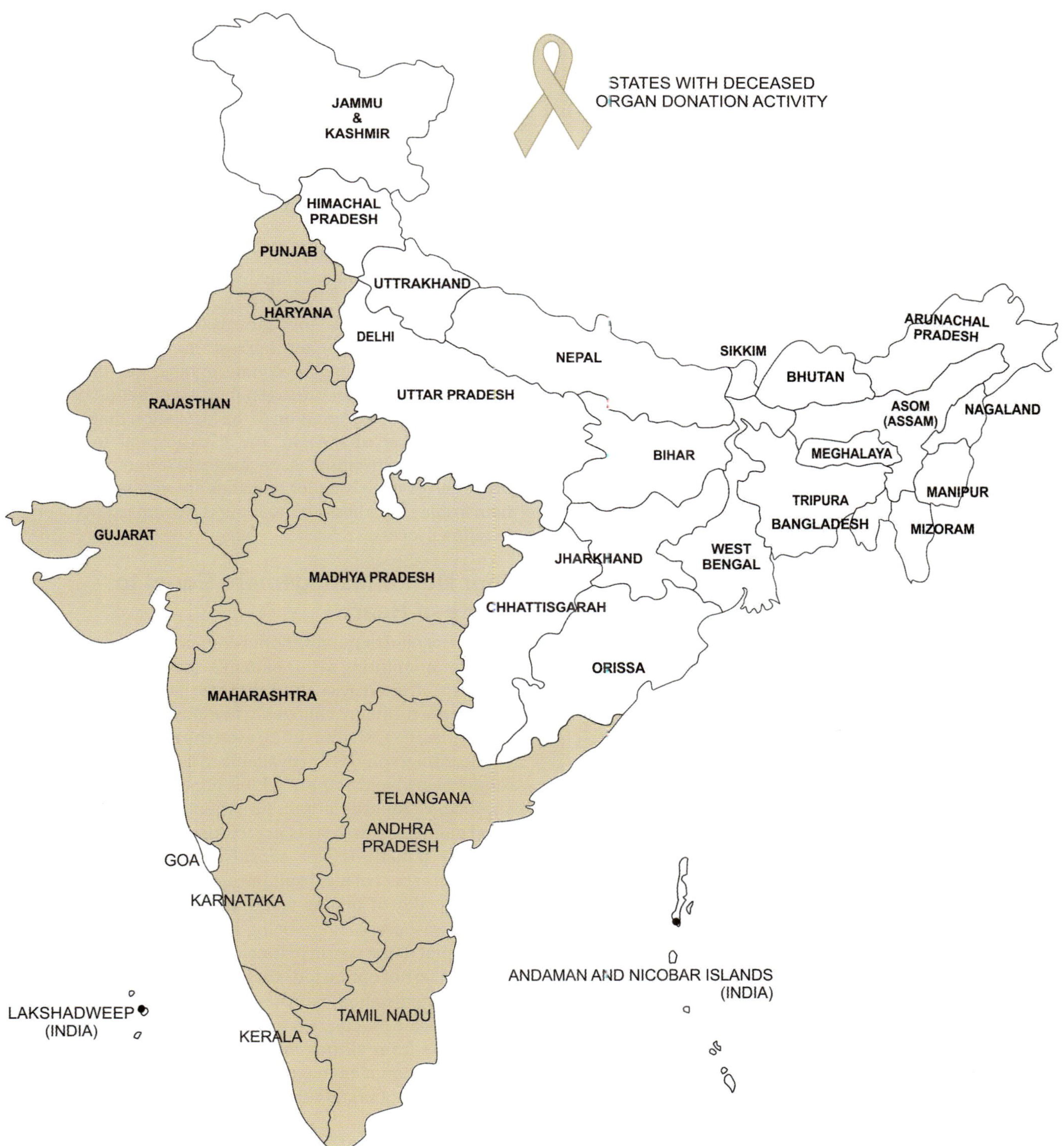

FIG. 3: States active in organ donation.

who can empathize with such road traffic accident victims' families and can coordinate with the treating neurosurgeons or intensivists to motivate the families for organ donation.

The reasons for low convincing rate for donation in donor's family are manifold: cultural beliefs amongst people of various religions about incomplete next-birth form; multiplicity of family people involved in decision-making process; fear of mutilation of body; delay in cremation process, etc. Several recent attempts by religious leaders and prominent sports and political personalities (including Prime Minister himself) to convince the people about organ donation are working to reduce this sociocultural factor.

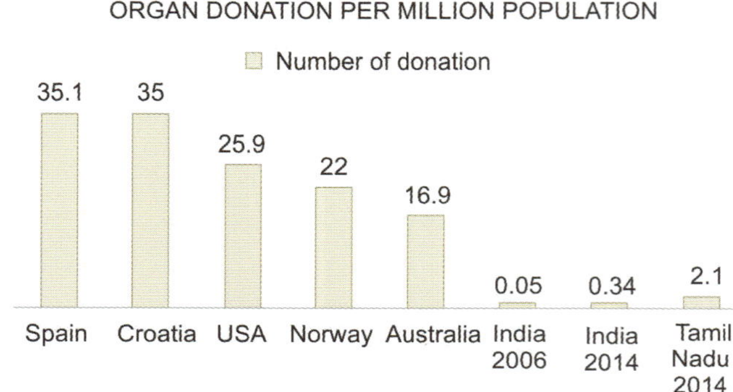

FIG. 4: Abysmally low levels of donation in India.

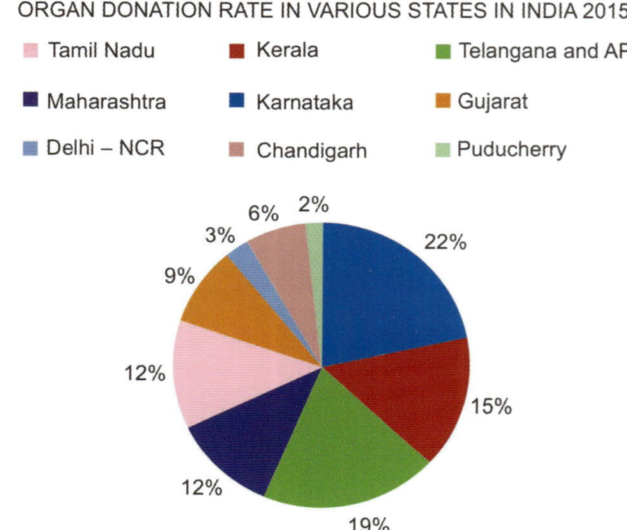

FIG. 5: States where most donors have come from.[8]

Recipient Attrition

Sometimes, the patients on the waiting list get "used to" their class IV status and relegate themselves to this bedridden life. Their motivation levels are low. Many patients when offered the option of heart transplantation refuse because the high costs involve. At AIIMS, New Delhi, most of the heart transplants were done at a very nominal cost of 1 lakh rupees, but recently, the commitment toward lifelong immunosuppression has made it necessary to give higher estimate for this surgery (Rs 10 lakhs). In most corporate hospitals, the package rates for heart transplant are between 15 and 22 lakhs. In addition, sometimes the recipients refuse when informed about availability of a donor heart by giving reasons as upcoming festival or family event scheduled shortly, etc. Several others die while in the waiting list.

Not Identifying or Notifying Brain Stem Death

Many centers in metro cities and especially in tier-II cities are inexperienced in handling all aspects of BSD. Even if they have identified a patient of head injury or spontaneous subarachnoid hemorrhage with Glasgow Coma Scale (GCS) of 3 and absent brain stem reflexes, they are hesitant to declare BSD. The common reasons for not identifying BSD include:

- They do not have the BSD certification panel
- It is cumbersome for them to arrange the logistics for organ donation
- They are not clear about who will bear the costs of "maintaining" a BSD patient in ICU who is willing for organ donation
- They are not having forensic medicine backup and hence unable to tackle the medicolegal aspects of organ donation
- They do not have the advanced surgical facilities for facilitating multiorgan harvest. In several cases the families are willing to donate organs, but the hospital lacks the infrastructure to enable this donation of organs.

Stronger implementation of the legislation that mandates the notification of BSD in any ICU/hospital to the state transplant organization is necessary. Donor management programs for these smaller hospitals are necessary to enable them to allay their hesitations about the complexities of organ donation process.

Poor Donor Management Equal to Waste of Heart

A small hospital or nursing home does not have good facilities either for monitoring a BSD patient's hemodynamics, nor the expertise of intensivist or anesthetist available to expertly manage the turbulent changes in hemodynamics of a possible donor after BSD. Many a times, even the most basic screening (echocardiography) is not available to assess the suitability of a donor heart. Neither the machine, nor an echocardiographer is available. No arterial pressure monitoring line or arterial blood gas (ABG) analysis is in records. The person managing the BSD patient is not sensitive to understanding the protective aspect of ideal volume and inotropic management for the health of organs to be harvested. Often very high doses of vasopressors are being administered which can be detrimental to the sensitive function of the heart. The volume status is also not optimized. There is a tussle between the lung and liver teams about sufficiency of volume infusion. These points indicate that there is a need to adequately train at least two people from all possible donor centers in the country about ideal donor management. In our country with acute scarcity of donor organs, these precious organs should not be wasted.

Inconstant Transplant Teams

Due to various reasons, the faculty at institutes or corporate hospitals performing heart transplant operations is not constant. As mentioned above, the postoperative care of a recipient is the real Achilles' heel over which the final outcome critically depends. Loss of even one member of the team can seriously compromise the results of a transplant program at any institute unless very standard protocols are set in and uniformly followed all over the country. However, since there is no database in the country of the transplants done and their final outcome, development and vetting of such a protocol is not even in a nascent stage. The transplant teams need to get their act together on this issue about the database so that their own success can be replicated elsewhere and the chain reaction of one transplant leading to at least three more by other teams will materialize.

Lack of Flights

Many a times there is a call from a center far away from the recipient center. In the absence of affordable air ambulance flights, commercial flights have to be utilized for this critical transfer. The whole harvesting process has to be coordinated between three to four teams and appropriate harvest time decided. Many a times, the flight distance or timings preclude harvesting of the available organ and these precious hearts are lost.[10] The government needs to eke out a policy wherein a special status is made available to chartered flights for the purpose of organ transplantation. This is routine in European and other western countries where all donor organ transfers are done through chartered flights. There is a pleasant collaboration between the private aircraft owners who perform these "transfer helps" as a part of their corporate social responsibility.

Postoperative Problems in Indian Scenario

The results of heart transplantation have been uniformly encouraging. There is however scope for improvement. We need to bring further down the 1 year mortality of 1–25%. This mortality is due to the fact that ours is a developing country, usually people are from middle to poor socioeconomic backgrounds, average education, minimum sense about hygiene, poor self-discipline, dry dusty climate that throws up a battery of environmental pathogens attacking the immunocompromised steroid-dependent heart transplant recipient. The 1 year results range between 70 and 90% survival across the country. There are many more than 5 years and more than 10 years survival too. The common complications seen in the Indian scenario include infections (fungal and bacterial pulmonary infections, cytomegalovirus—neurological infection), early prosthetic graft dysfunction, reversible renal compromise, psychological disturbances, and rarely cardiac allograft vasculopathy. Common cause of death in the Indian scenario has been infection and not rejection as is prevalent in the western literature. At any individual center, with more experience, the complications reduce and overall recoveries are faster.

ROADMAP FOR THE FUTURE

Some important steps which may help to make the heart transplant program more robust in our country include:

- Stronger legislation making notification of brain death mandatory in all hospitals. It must be ensured and documented that reasonable efforts were made to counsel the family of a BSD patient for organ donation before the final certification of death
- Gradual shift of THOA laws to "opt out" policy. This is consistent with the standards of organ donation in many Western countries
- Hiring of trained and enthusiastic transplant coordinators who can strongly educate and motivate families to donate organs in the setting of BSD. They should be continuously upgraded with continuing medical education and periodic seminars
- Ensuring ideal donor management and facilitation of organ harvesting by NOTTO or regional coordinating authority
- Cost support to any hospital enabling the organ donation process
- Increasing the awareness amongst public that heart transplant is a good viable option with excellent quality of life after surgery
- Covering the heart (and other solid organ) transplant surgery under the proposed national healthcare insurance scheme. Majority of our citizens cannot afford the operation costs and hence, it is high time the government took up financing this program under its mantle. Similarly, cost subsidy to post-transplant recipients for lifelong immunosuppression
- Robust national, regional and state organ and tissue transplant organizations (NOTTO, ROTTO, and SOTTO). The coordination activity should be efficient, organ allocation process should be fair and transparent and there should be no wastage of any available donor heart
- A continuous and comprehensive pool of end-stage HF patients should be available waitlisted with all hospitals who are licensed to do heart transplants. The active participation of cardiologists here is important to ensure the same
- Initiating special and ethical incentives for donor families to encourage organ donation
- Audit of centers dealing with BSD patients to ensure they are encouraging organ donation. Audit of centers performing heart transplants to ensure that centers of transplant excellence are there, at least one per state so that the overall results continually improve
- All above measures should seek to improve the annual transplant rate to at least 1,000 operations per year, distributed equally in all geographical regions of our country.

CONCLUSION

The progress made in the field of heart transplantation in India has been slow & steady but is now seeing robust growth. There still are many challenges to be overcome , but as India makes a transition towards a more developed country, it is only to be expected that over the next two decades, the advances in science and the combined efforts of the state, medical personnel and the society will make the option of heart transplantation for our large end-stage heart failure population a very feasible and viable choice.

REFERENCES

1. Larry WS. History of Cardiac Surgery. Surgery. 2008;7:1471-9.
2. Barnard CN. The operation. A human cardiac transplant: An interim report of a successful operation performed at Groote Schuur Hospital, Cape Town. S Afr Med J. 1967;41:1271-4.
3. EB Stinson, E Dong Jr, J Schroeder, et al. Initial clinical experience with cardiac transplantation. Am J Cardiol. 1968;22:791-803.
4. Rodriguez Cetina Biefer H, Sündermann SH, Emmert MY, et al. Surviving 20 years after heart transplantation: a success story. Ann Thorac Surg. 2014;97:499-504.
5. Jones DS, Sivaramakrishnan K. Transplant Buccaneers: P.K. Sen and India's First Heart Transplant, February 1968. J Hist Med Allied Sci. 2018;73(3):303-32.
6. Venugopal P. The first successful heart transplant in India. Natl Med J India. 1994;7(5):213-5.
7. Madhu Sankar N, Kurian VM, Rajan S, et al. Heart-lung transplantation in India: initial experience. Indian Heart J. 2003;55(2):185-7.
8. Transplant centres in India Retrieved on 05/20/2018 from http://www.mohanfoundation.org/transplant-centres/index.asp.
9. Lund LH, Khush KK, Cherikh WS, et al. The Registry of the International Society for Heart and Lung Transplantation: Thirty-fourth Adult Heart Transplantation Report—2017; Focus Theme: Allograft ischemic time. J Heart Lung Transplant. 2017;36(10):1037-46.
10. Singh NP, Anish K. Kidney transplantation in India: Challenges and future recommendation. MAMC J Med Sci. 2016;2(1);12-7.

SECTION 19

Stroke

CHAPTER 127

Atrial Fibrillation and Stroke: An Update

Rohit Bhatia, Rimpy Joseph

INTRODUCTION

Atrial fibrillation (AF), the most prevalent sustained disorder of cardiac rhythm, has in recent times emerged as a major global public health concern, in terms of substantial morbidity and mortality.[1] Global estimates indicate 20–25% of all strokes to be cardio embolic in origin; of these, nearly one-half cases are caused by nonvalvular AF, one-fourth by valvular heart disease, and one-third by left ventricular (LV) thrombi.[2] Thus, worldwide, AF contributes to almost 80% of cardioembolic strokes and approximately 33% of all ischemic strokes.[2,3] While the risk of stroke is increased by 4–5 fold, the mortality is almost doubled compared to age-matched controls in the presence of AF.[4-6] Although, the annual risk of stroke related to AF alone is 0.2%, it rises exponentially to more than 10% in the presence of additional risk factors.[7] Significantly, in as many as 25% of AF-related strokes, stroke is the presenting manifestation of a hitherto undetected AF. Regardless to say, AF-related strokes are significantly more disabling and fatal. Fortunately, AF is an eminently preventable and treatable cause of stroke. There has been a surge in the evidence available with newer avenues for tackling several issues concerning concomitant AF and stroke management. This chapter envisages to provide a lucid and comprehensive overview on AF and stroke, with particular emphasis on thromboprophylactic and therapeutic strategies.

EPIDEMIOLOGY AND GLOBAL BURDEN

Data suggest that globally nearly 33 million individuals are affected with AF. This figure is a gross underestimation of sorts, as evidenced by the fact that majority of AF patients (1 in 12 paroxysms) remain asymptomatic. The lifetime risk of developing AF stands at 25%. Available data indicate 1–2% AF prevalence in the general population.[8] The prevalence of AF rises with age steadily, affecting 2% patients less than 65 years of age and nearly 9% of patients more than 65 years of age. The risk of stroke in AF is also age-dependent, rising exponentially from 1.5% in the fifth decade to 23.5% in the eighth decade.[9] This translates to a 1.5-fold increase in the risk of AF-related stroke for every decade of life. In the western world, the median age of patients with AF is 75 years, with nearly 70% being in 65–75 years age group.[10] It is estimated that by 2050, nearly 50% of those affected in US will be aged 80 years and above.[11] As regards the Asian population which is rapidly aging, estimates suggest a staggering 72 million AF-afflicted patients by 2050, of which nearly 2.9 million would have AF-related stroke.[12] Valvular AF confers a 17-fold higher risk of stroke compared to 5-fold higher risk with nonvalvular AF.[13] Available data also suggest that AF-related stroke translates to a high mortality (20%) and substantial morbidity (60%).

There remains paucity of epidemiological data pertaining to AF from India. Regional population based registries from India have estimated AF prevalence of 8–10%.[14,15] Recent data from the Indian population indicate AF to be associated with 15% of all strokes.[16] Indian Heart Rhythm Society (IHRS-AF) registry – till date, the single largest epidemiological study of its kind from the Indian subcontinent, was a prospective, multicenter observational study conducted over 24 centers across India, enrolling 1,537 AF patients during the time period 2011–2012. The salient observations were that the annual stroke rate was 1%; mean age of AF in the Indian population was 54.7 years, which is at least a decade lesser than the western counterparts and females constituted 51.5% while males were 48.5%. In contrast to the west, rheumatic heart disease (RHD)-related AF constituted a significant proportion (47.6%) in the Indian population. The younger age of onset of RHD AF is attributed to higher prevalence of RHD, hypertension, diabetes, and coronary artery disease among the young population of India.[17] Regional registries such as Ludhiana-based urban population stroke registry, which found an AF-related stroke prevalence of 10% (203/1,942 patients) have corroborated the findings of IHRS-AF registry except that nonvalvular AF constituted 97% of cases.[15] However, most of the Indian studies, albeit done on small scale, have found RHD-related valvular AF to be the most common cause of AF related stroke in our

Indian population.[18,19] In addition, AF-related strokes are more common in women (F:M 1.2 to 1.38:1) in contrast to western studies (F:M = 1:1.5). This again is speculated to be due to larger proportion of causative RHD cases in India which in turn are more common in women. Also in deviation to the global trends, only one-third cases of AF in India are constituted by paroxysmal AF.

UPDATED MODEL FOR STROKE MECHANISM IN ATRIAL FIBRILLATION AND CONCEPT OF ATRIAL CARDIOPATHY

Atrial cardiopathy refers to structural remodeling of the heart resulting in changes in the atrial tissue properties (chiefly fibrosis), size [left atrial (LA) enlargement and cellular ultrastructure (alterations in sarcoplasmic reticulum, nuclear chromatin, redistribution of mitochondria, glycogen accumulation, myolysis, proteolysis due to calcium dependent calpain activation, etc.)]. This leads to reduced and ineffective atrial contractility underlying AF, which further contributes to atrial dilatation and the vicious cycle continues. Atrial fibrosis with resultant conduction slowing, could either be reactive interstitial fibrosis where the individual muscle bundles are separated by fibrous tissue or reparative fibrosis wherein, there is replacement of the dead cardiac myocytes. The resultant increased fibroblast coupling to the cardiac myocytes promotes re-entry and focal ectopic firing. Since, atrial fibrosis predicts progression to permanent AF, it has become a potential target for suppression of arrhythmogenesis as well as predicting response to treatment.[20-22] It is interesting to note that, atrial cardiopathy can occur independent of AF. In fact, the surrogate markers of atrial dysfunction such as premature atrial contractions, paroxysmal supraventricular tachycardia, LA size, and ECG-defined LA enlargement, etc. can result in stroke (embolic/cryptogenic), independent of AF.[23-26]

Kamel et al. proposed the updated model for stroke in AF which highlights the causative role of systemic and atrial abnormal substrates, in addition to abnormal rhythm in AF-related strokes. They proposed that atrial cardiopathy or abnormal atrial tissue substrate which underlies both AF and thromboembolism is predisposed to by ageing and other systemic vascular risk factors; either of which can also predispose to stroke independently via nonatrial stroke mechanisms (such as large artery atherosclerosis, small vessel occlusion, ventricular dysfunction, etc.). Conversely, AF per se, by causing reduced atrial contractility resulting in atrial stretch, dilatation and remodeling, also contributes to atrial cardiopathy over a period of weeks which further increases the risk of stroke and thromboembolism. Moreover, AF also leads to ventricular dysfunction due to fast ventricular rate with irregular rhythm, loss of atrial kick, and reduced coronary flow reserve. This model could explain the fact that nearly 25% cases of AF and stroke manifest AF only after stroke occurrence and brief AF periods could result in strokes several months later. In addition, the occurrence of nonembolic strokes in AF patients is also explained by this model which suggests that AF acts as a marker for upstream vascular risk factors. It also provides plausible explanation to the fact that rhythm controlling therapies (including catheter ablation of AF) alone cannot by itself eliminate stroke risk. In particular, among the systemic vascular risk factors, obesity needs special mention as concurrent local epicardial fat accumulation leads to local atrial inflammation and also by increasing propensity to obstructive sleep apnea (OSA), elevates intra-arterial pressures resulting in atrial cardiopathy. A major therapeutic implication of this model is that strategies aimed at reversing atrial cardiopathy are essential for reducing thromboembolic risk. Future trials are anticipated to specifically address this issue. Not all strokes in AF are due to left atrial appendage (LAA) thromboembolism. While two-thirds of stroke in AF patients are postulated to be due to embolism arising from thrombi lodged within the LAA; a significant one-third cases are due to alternative stroke mechanisms such as carotid atherosclerosis, complex aortic arch plaque, small vessel disease, LV origin thrombi, etc.[27,28]

The need of the hour is thus concomitant global risk factor reduction rather than tunneled focus on anticoagulation alone.

ATRIAL FIBRILLATION DETECTION IN STROKE

Atrial Fibrillation Detected after Stroke and Transient Ischemic Attack

Cerasuolo et al. coined the term AFDAS [AF diagnosed or detected after stroke and transient ischemic attack (TIA)] in 2017. The term encompasses all forms of AF (paroxysmal/persistent/permanent) detected by any ECG monitoring technology and could either be prestroke AF which was hitherto undiagnosed/asymptomatic and detected only after stroke (cardiogenic origin) or incident AF which has developed after stroke/TIA (neurogenic origin)–new onset AF. It is estimated that AFDAS constitutes nearly 25% of AF cases and approximately 50% of AFDAS are asymptomatic.[29]

Till date, whether poststroke AF is a cause or consequence of stroke remains unclear. A plausible hypothesis for AFDAS suggests an interplay of autonomic dysregulation and systemic inflammation. Normally, the extrinsic or cerebral autonomic nervous system (ANS) (comprising of cerebral cortex, especially insula, cingulate, and prefrontal regions with projections to the hypothalamus, limbic, and brainstem nuclei) exerts control over the intrinsic ANS constituted by the ganglionated plexi within the pulmonary vein (PV) endings and pericardium. In acute ischemic strokes affecting the aforesaid regions, the central modulation is lost, with consequent activation of intrinsic ANS resulting in ectopic firing from PV and non-PV foci, and paroxysmal AF ensues. Following acute cardioembolic strokes, there also exists a brief lasting inflammatory response with release of cytokines [interleukin (IL)-6, tumor necrosis factor (TNF) alpha, IL-1 antagonists)], chemokines (CXCL16), and adhesion molecules [intercellular adhesion molecule (ICAM) 1, E/P selectins)] which can trigger AF either by focal ectopic firing via the autonomic cascade or re-entry circuits located in the atrial myocardium. Other contributing factors in AFDAS include sleep-disordered breathing (SDB) which confers 4 times higher risk of AF and AF per se, doubles the risk of developing SDB in the poststroke period.[29,30]

Compared to known AF patients, those with poststroke AF are younger (median age 72 vs. 79 years, p = 0.058); have significantly lesser proportion of LA enlargement (60.9 vs. 91.2, p = 0.001), and overall 4 cm^2 lesser median LA area.[31] A study identified 3 positive clinical predictors of poststroke paroxysmal AF which would warrant intensive work up including 7 days prolonged Holter. These included advanced age [74 ± 10.5 vs. 67 ± 13, p <0.001; odds ratio (OR) 1.05: 95% confidence interval (CI) 1.01–1.08], clinical symptoms more than 24 hours (OR 5.17, 95% CI 1.73–15.48), and a history of coronary artery disease (OR 3.14, 95% CI 1.35–7.28).[32] Since, the peaks of inflammation and autonomic dysfunction occur in the initial few days of stroke onset, majority of neurogenic poststroke AF is manifest in the initial few days (71% in first 3 days; 75% in 1–2 weeks)—emphasizing the need for early Holter monitoring to get better diagnostic yield. Targeted strategies to reduce myocardial inflammation and thus reduce poststroke AF recurrence are being extensively studied.

Occult Atrial Fibrillation Detection in Stroke

The commonly available tools for detection of AF include ECG, continuous ECG monitoring with Holter recording (both routine short term: 24 hours and long-term recording using efficient memory Holter and patch monitors), intermittent long-term monitoring using loop recorders (external and implantable), and event monitors; and telemetry systems (inpatient and outpatient). Digital innovations including apps for easy detection of AF have also entered into the foray.

The 2016 European Society of Cardiology (ESC) guidelines for management of AF has placed class I recommendation for AF screening by short-term ECG followed by at least 72-hour Holter monitoring for all patients with ischemic stroke and TIA.[33]

Find-AF is a recently published open label randomized control trial (RCT), based on the premise that enhanced and prolonged Holter recording would increase the odds of AF detection in poststroke patients. The study which was conducted on 398 patients of acute ischemic stroke (AIS) (within 7 days of onset and aged ≥60 years) across four German centers, found a significantly higher AF detection rate of 14% in the enhanced and prolonged monitoring group (10 days Holter monitoring at 0, 3, and 6 months) compared to 5% in control group (95% CI 3.4–14.5, p = 0.002).[34]

Cryptogenic stroke and underlying AF (Crystal AF study) was a RCT done on 441 patients with stroke aged more than or equal to 40 years, without pre-enrolment evidence of AF during 24 hours of ECG monitoring, who were then randomized to insertable cardiac monitor (ICM) group (221 patients) and control group (220 patients). The results indicated a higher AF (>30 s duration) detection rate in the ICM group at 6 months [8.9% vs. 1.4%; hazard ratio (HR): 6.4; 95% CI 1.9–21.7; p <0.001]. Also, ICM group registered a significantly higher AF detection rate at 12 months (12.4% vs. 2%; HR 7.3; 95% CI 2.6–20.8; p <0.001) and 36 months, 30% (ICM group vs. 3%; HR 8.8, 95% CI 3.5–22.2, p <0.001).[35]

Event Monitoring Belt for Recording Atrial fibrillation after a Cerebral ischemic Event (EMBRACE)-AF trial observed that 30-day event triggered loop recorder (intervention group) was superior than conventional 24-hour Holter recording: control group (AF detection rates 16.1% vs. 3.2%; 95% CI 1–17.6; p <0.001, number needed to screen 8); also AF with duration more than or equal to 2.5 minutes was detected more in the intervention group (9.9% vs. 2.5%; 95% CI 3.4–11.3; p <0.001) and the rate of anticoagulant treatment nearly doubled in the intervention arm.[36]

Importantly, brief subclinical AF acts as an important predictor of AF recurrence and subsequent stroke, as corroborated by the ASSERT study (ASymptomatic atrial fibrillation and Stroke Evaluation in pacemaker patients and the atrial fibrillation Reduction atrial pacing Trial); subclinical atrial tachyarrhythmia more than 6 minutes predicts clinical AF (HR 5.56; 95% CI 3.78–8.17, p <0.001) and MOST (MOde Selection Trial) trial (atrial high rate episode) more than 5 minutes predicted clinical AF (HR 5.9).[37,38]

However, the minimum duration or frequency of AF that necessitates anticoagulation remains controversial. Nevertheless, the frequency of atrial premature beats (APBs) detected on routine 24-hour Holter monitoring serves as a marker for subclinical AF, especially among older cryptogenic stroke and TIA patients, as evidenced by the EMBRACE-AF[36] trial, which suggested a cutoff of more than 500 APBs or 24 hours for defining frequent APBs.[39] This study also proposed a minimum of 2 weeks of targeted noninvasive ECG monitoring with mobile outpatient telemetry or autodetect loop recorder for patients with infrequent APBs less than 500 or 24 hours; 4 weeks for frequent APBs more than 500 or 24 hours and longer monitoring with implantable loop recorders for those with excessive APBs more than 1,000 or 24 hours.[39]

Another AF prediction score is STAF score (Score for the Targeting of Atrial Fibrillation) which takes into account 4 factors—age more than 62 years (2 points), NIHSS (The National Institutes of Health Stroke Scale) more than or equal to 8 (1 point), LA dilatation (2 points), absence of symptomatic intracranial or extracranial stenosis more than or equal to 50% or clinical radiological lacunar syndrome (3 points). The STAF score more than or equal to 5 had a high sensitivity (89%) and specificity (88%) of having underlying AF.[40]

Recently, Yoshioka et al. developed the iPAB score [acronym for—Identified by Past history of arrhythmia or antiarrhythmic agent use, Atrial (left) dilatation and Brain natriuretic peptide (BNP) elevation] to predict the presence of AF in acute stroke patients. In this scoring system, a score of 3 is given if there is a past history of arrhythmia or antiarrhythmic agent use; LA dilatation more than or equal to 40 mm gets a score of 1 while BNP elevation (pg/mL) is sub classified into 3 groups—levels more than or equal to 50 are scored 1, levels more than or equal to 90 are given a score of 2, and levels more than or equal to 150 get a score of 3. Score of more than or equal to 2 was found to have a sensitivity of 93% and specificity of 71% while scores of more than or equal to 4 had sensitivity of 60% and specificity of 95% in predicting paroxysmal AF in acute stroke patients.[41]

Other ongoing RCTs in this direction include SAFFO trial[42] (Silent AF detection aFter ischemic strOke) in patients more than or equal to 65 years, with first ever atherothrombotic or lacunar stroke, using implantable loop recorders at first diagnosis and MonDAFIS trial (Impact of standardized MONitoring for Detection of AF in Ischemic Stroke), largest of its kind RCT, which aims to evaluate whether initial prolonged 7-day Holter recording has impact on secondary stroke prevention.[43]

STROKE RISK STRATIFICATION SCORES

Over the past few decades, several scores for prediction of stroke risk in AF have been devised, aimed at aiding in decision making regarding initiation of antithrombotic strategies.[44-49] The major scores used for stroke risk stratification are outlined in table 1.

ARE TYPE OF ATRIAL FIBRILLATION AND DURATION OF EPISODES PREDICTIVE OF STROKE RISK?

Published data provide conflicting results on the association between type of AF and stroke risk prediction, although

TABLE 1: Stroke risk stratification scores among patients with atrial fibrillation

CHADS$_2$ score* (2001)	CHA$_2$DS$_2$VASc score** (2010)	Modified CHA$_2$DS$_2$VASc score (mCHA$_2$DS$_2$VASc score) (2016)	Delta CHA$_2$DS$_2$VASc (follow-up CHA$_2$DS$_2$VASc score—Baseline CHA$_2$DS$_2$VASc score): 2018	ATRIA score (AnTicoagulation and Risk factors In Atrial fibrillation): 2013
Congestive cardiac failure 1	Congestive cardiac failure 1	Congestive cardiac failure 1	Congestive cardiac failure 1	Age Prior stroke - + ≥85 6 9 75–84 5 7 65–74 3 7 <65 0 8
Hypertension 1	Hypertension 1	Hypertension 1	Hypertension 1	Female 1 1
Age ≥75 1	Age ≥75 2 Age 65–74 1	Age ≥75 2 Age 50–74 1	Age ≥75 2 Age 65–74 1	Diabetes 1 1
Diabetes 1	Diabetes 1	Diabetes 1	Diabetes 1	Hypertension 1 1
Prior stroke or TIA 2	Prior stroke or TIA 2	Prior stroke or TIA 2	Prior stroke or TIA 2	CHF 1 1
	Vascular disease (prior MI, peripheral arterial disease or aortic plaque) 1	Vascular disease (prior MI, peripheral arterial disease or aortic plaque) 1	Vascular disease (prior MI, peripheral arterial disease or aortic plaque) 1	Proteinuria 1 1
	Sex category Female 1	Sex category Female 1	Sex category Female 1	ESRD or eGFR 1 <45 mL/min/1.73m^2
	Annual stroke rate Score 0 0% Score 1 1.3% Score 2 2.2% Score 3 3.2% Score 4 4.0% Score 5 6.7% Score 6 9.8% Score 7 9.6% Score 8 6.7% Score 9 15.2%	Annual stroke risk Score 0 males 0.46% Score 1 females 0.63% Score 1(males) 2.44% Score 2 3.24% Score 3 4.27% Score 4 5.21% Score 5 5.27% Score 6 5.43% Score 7 5.87% Score 8 6.87% Score 9 10.72%	Annual stroke risk Delta CHA$_2$DS$_2$VASc Score 0: 0.92 % Score 1: 2.04% Score ≥4: 4.99%	Annual stroke risk Low-risk (0–5 points; annual event rate <1%) Moderate-risk (6 points; annual event rate 1–2%) High-risk (7–15 points; annual event rate ≥2%)

*CHADS$_2$—acronym for *C*ongestive cardiac failure, *H*ypertension, *A*ge ≥75 years, *D*iabetes and prior *S*troke/transient ischemic attack (TIA).

**CHA$_2$DS$_2$VASc score—acronym for *C*ongestive cardiac failure, *H*ypertension, *A*ge (≥75 years and 65–74 years) , *D*iabetes, prior *S*troke/TIA, *V*ascular disease [prior myocardial infarction (MI), peripheral arterial disease or aortic plaque] and *S*ex category (female).

CHF, congestive heart failure; ESRD, end stage renal disease; eGFR, estimated glomerular filtration rate; MI, myocardial infarction; TIA, transient ischemic attack.

the odds of thromboembolism are more in favor toward permanent or persistent AF vis-a-vis paroxysmal AF. The ACTIVE-W trial (Atrial Fibrillation Clopidogrel Trial with Irbesartan for Prevention of Vascular Events) was equipoised as regards the risk of stroke or systemic embolism in paroxysmal AF versus persistent AF [relative risk (RR) 0.7; 95% CI 0.59–1.30].[50] However, the recent evidence obtained from ENGAGE-AF (Edoxaban versus warfarin in patients with Atrial Fibrillation) trial, *ROCKET-AF (Rivaroxaban-Once-daily, oral, direct Factor Xa inhibition Compared with vitamin K antagonism for prevention of stroke and Embolism Trial in Atrial Fibrillation) trial*, and meta-analysis by Ganesan et al. proves that the risk of thromboembolism is much higher in nonparoxysmal forms of AF.[51-53]

The establishment of correlation, if any, between duration of AF episodes and stroke risk has been the focus of numerous studies. The ASSERT study (ASymptomatic atrial fibrillation and Stroke Evaluation in pacemaker patients and the atrial fibrillation Reduction atrial pacing Trial) was conducted on 2,580 elderly hypertensive patients (≥65 years), without previous AF history, who had undergone pacemaker or defibrillator implantation recently. It was found that during the initial 3 months postprocedure, 10% patients developed subclinical tachyarrhythmias lasting at least 6 minutes, and this was associated with 2.5-fold higher risk of stroke or systemic embolism in the 2.5 years follow-up period (HR 2.49; 95% CI 1.28–4.85; p = 0.007).[37] These findings were corroborated by the SOS-AF study (Stroke PreventiOn Strategies based on Atrial Fibrillation information from implanted devices) which found a statistically significant association between AF episodes more than or equal to 5 minutes and stroke (HR 1.76; 95% CI 1.02–3.02); the highest HR was observed for more than or equal to 1 hour duration AF burden (HR 2.11, 95% CI 1.22–3.64, p = 0.008); also there was a 3% increase in the relative risk for stroke for every additional hour in the daily maximum AF burden.[54] The RATE study (RAte control Therapy Evaluation in permanent atrial fibrillation) observed that the risk of stroke or TIA in brief lasting AF episodes less than 20 seconds is similar to that in non-AF patients while episodes more than or equal to 20 seconds have 1.5 times higher risk of developing stroke or TIA (HR 1.51, 95% CI 1.03–2.21).[55]

SERUM BIOMARKERS AS PREDICTORS OF STROKE RISK IN ATRIAL FIBRILLATION?

Current evidence suggests high sensitivity cardiac troponins and NT-proBNP as positive predictors of stroke risk in AF patients. The RE-LY trial[56] (Randomized Evaluation of Long-term Anticoagulation Therapy) observed that Trop I levels more than or equal to 0.040 were associated with highest annual stroke risk rate of 2.09% (HR 1.99, 95% CI 1.17–3.39; p = 0.0040) and elevated NT-proBNP levels more than 1,402 ng/L were associated with 2.3% annual stroke risk rate (HR 2.40, 95% CI 1.41–4.07; p = 0.0014) while levels between 801 ng/L and 1,402 ng/L had HR of 1.31 (95% CI 0.76–2.27, p = 0.0014) and for levels 387–800 ng/L, HR was 1.35 (95% CI 0.80–2.27, p = 0.0014).[56] The results of ARISTOTLE trial add impetus to the value of elevated high sensitivity troponin (≥24 ng/L) and NT-proBNP in predicting stroke and systemic embolism (HR 1.98; 95% CI 1.42–2.78).[57,58] The role of inflammatory biomarkers such as C-reactive protein (CRP) and IL-6 in stroke prediction remain controversial.[59-61] The ABC stroke risk score (acronym for Age, Biomarkers–high sensitivity troponin and NT-proBNP and Clinical history, i.e., prior stroke/TIA) is a recent biomarker-based score for 1 year and 3 years stroke risk prediction in AF which has demonstrated benefit over all clinical stroke risk scores recommended by current guidelines.[62] Modifications of ABC score like ABC death risk score (additionally incorporates GDF-15, i.e., growth differentiation factor 15 and congestive heart failure as variables) and ABC bleeding risk scores have also been proposed recently and validated.[63,64]

STRUCTURAL AND FUNCTIONAL MARKERS OF LEFT ATRIAL AND LEFT ATRIAL APPENDAGE AS STROKE PREDICTORS IN ATRIAL FIBRILLATION

Available evidence suggests moderate-to-severe LA enlargement as predictor of recurrent embolic or cryptogenic stroke, irrespective of AF.[65] Studies on AF patients have shown convincing evidence on association between LA enlargement and stroke; in addition to correlating strongly with surrogate markers of stroke risk such as LAA thrombus and spontaneous echocardiographic contrasts (SECs).[66,67] Also, LA function markers such as decreased myocardial strain rate, MRI evidence of atrial fibrosis, higher $CHADS_2$ (*C*ongestive cardiac failure, *H*ypertension, *A*ge ≥75 years, *D*iabetes and prior *S*troke/TIA) score, presence of persistent or permanent AF, mitral valve inflow, and atrial electromechanical delay also serve as markers of thromboembolic risk.[67]

Left atrial appendage is a major source of thrombus formation in AF and has been the focus of continuing research. Echocardiographic evidence of reduced LAA antegrade flow velocities is taken as marker of stasis within LAA; a cross-sectional study on nonvalvular AF showed that LAA velocities less than 36 cm/sec had significant association with prior stroke than those without stroke who had LAA velocity of 55 cm/sec (p <0.001).[68] Also, post-hoc analysis of 721 patients from SPAF (the Stroke Prevention in Atrial Fibrillation) III trial showed LAA velocities less than 20 cm/sec as independent predictor of LAA thrombus (RR 2.6, p = 0.02).[69]

Spontaneous echocardiographic contrasts are also taken as markers of stroke risk, these refer to the echocardiographic dynamic smoke-like appearance, secondary to stasis, hypercoagulability and RBC aggregation, and is strongly associated with LAA thrombus and thromboembolic risk.[67,70] Morphological appearance of LAA serves as a structural marker of stroke risk. Amongst the four morphologies of LAA (chicken wing-48%, windsock-19%, cactus-30%, and cauliflower-3%), most studies suggest nonchicken wing morphologies to have higher odds of stroke risk. This is attributed to lower LAA flow velocities in nonchicken wing LAA morphologies and extensive trabeculation specifically in the cauliflower morphology. Other structural LAA markers include larger LAA orifice size and greater number of lobes.[71-73]

ASSESSMENT OF BLEEDING RISK (TABLE 2)

Although bleeding risk in AF is much less than the thromboembolic risk, assessment of bleeding risk assumes significance as it decides the net clinical benefit of anticoagulation. Several bleeding risk prediction scores exist for AF patients such as HEMORR$_2$AGES [*H*epatic or Renal disease, *E*thanol abuse, *M*alignancy, *O*lder age (>75 years), *R*educed platelet number/function, *R*ebleeding, *A*nemia, *G*enetic factors, *E*xcessive fall risk and *S*troke][74], HAS-BLED [*H*ypertension, *A*bnormal renal and liver function, *S*troke, *B*leeding, *L*abile international normalized ratio (INR), *E*lderly (>65 years) and *D*rugs (antiplatelets or NSAIDs or Alcohol)],[75] ATRIA (*An*T*i*coagulation and *R*isk factors *I*n *A*trial fibrillation)[76], ORBIT (Outcomes Registry for Better Informed Treatment of AF)[77] and ABC-bleeding risk score, which is biomarker based.[64] The major scores are summarized in table 2. In the universally recommended HAS-BLED score, the annual bleeding rate steadily increased from 1.13% for 0 score, to 1.88% for score 2, 3.74% for score 3, 8.7% for score 4, and 12.5% for score 5.[75] The HAS-BLED score more than or equal to 3 predicts major bleeding during bridging of chronic anticoagulant therapy. The AMADEUS trial of 2012, which compared the performances of HEMORR$_2$AGES, ATRIA, and HAS-BLED scores, concluded that HAS-BLED score has better predictive value for intracranial haemorrhage.[78] While validation studies have proven superiority of ORBIT score over HAS-BLED for predicting major bleeding, it is the recent ABC-bleeding risk score which has outperformed all previous bleeding scores.[64]

MANAGEMENT STRATEGIES

The management of AF primarily revolves around a three pronged strategy of rate control, rhythm control (which includes both acute rhythm restoration strategies in the form of pharmacological cardioversion, electrical cardioversion and pill in the pocket cardioversion using self-administered

TABLE 2: Bleeding risk prediction scores for patients with atrial fibrillation

HEMORR$_2$AGES*		HAS-BLED**		ATRIA***		ORBIT****	ABC-bleeding risk score #
Hepatic/renal disease	1	Hypertension	1	Anemia	3	Older ≥75	Age
Ethanol abuse	1	Abnormal renal and liver function	1+1	Severe renal disease	3	Reduced hemoglobin (<13 mg/dL males; <12 mg/dL females) or Hct <40% in males and <36% in females or H/O anemia	Biomarkers: • High sensitivity cardiac troponin T • GDF-15 • Hemoglobin
Malignancy	1	Stroke	1	Age ≥75	2	Bleeding history	Clinical history • Prior bleeding
Older age(>75)	1	Bleeding	1	Any prior hemorrhage	1	Insufficient renal function (eGFR <60 mg/dL/1.73 m^2)	–
Reduced platelet no./function	1	Labile INR	1	Hypertension	1	Treatment with antiplatelet	–
Rebleeding	2	Elderly (>65)	1	–		–	–
Anemia	1	Drugs (antiplatelets or NSAIDs/alcohol)	1+1	–		–	–
Genetic factors	1	–		–		–	–
Excessive fall risk	1	–		–		–	–
Stroke	1	–		–		–	–

*HEMORR$_2$AGES: acronym for *H*epatic or Renal disease, *E*thanol abuse, *M*alignancy, *O*lder age (>75 years), *R*educed platelet number/function, *R*ebleeding, *A*nemia, *G*enetic factors, *E*xcessive fall risk and *S*troke.

**HAS-BLED: acronym for *H*ypertension, *A*bnormal renal and liver function, *S*troke, *B*leeding, *L*abile INR, *E*lderly (>65 years) and *D*rugs (antiplatelets or NSAIDs or Alcohol).

***ATRIA: acronym for *An*T*i*coagulation and *R*isk factors *I*n *A*trial fibrillation.

****ORBIT: acronym for *O*lder (≥75), *R*educed hemoglobin, *B*leeding history, *I*nsufficient renal function and *T*reatment with antiplatelet.

ABC-bleeding risk score: acronym for *A*ge, *B*iomarkers and *C*linical history.

Hct, hematocrit; GDF-15, growth differentiation factor 15; eGFR, growth differentiation factor 15; INR, international normalized ratio; NSAIDs, nonsteroidal anti-inflammatory drugs.

oral flecainide 200–300 mg or propafenone 400–600 mg and long-term antiarrhythmic measures), and prevention of thromboembolism; alongside prompt management of vascular risk factors implicated in atrial cardiopathy which can beget AF. We shall focus on thrombophylactic strategies in AF, which are core to prevention of AF-related stroke and its recurrence.

Primary Prevention of Stroke in Atrial Fibrillation

Oral Anticoagulation Therapy

The best form of stroke prevention and avoidance of consequent stroke-related disability is primary prevention. Oral anticoagulation therapy comprising vitamin K antagonists (VKA), and non-vitamin K newer or directly acting oral anticoagulants (NOACs or DOACs) is currently the standard of care for thromboprophylaxis in AF. Irrespective of the stroke risk, antiplatelets are not recommended for stroke prevention in AF.

While VKAs form the sole thromboprophylactic option in valvular AF (mechanical heart valves or rheumatic moderate and severe mitral stenosis), nonvalvular AF offers a choice between VKAs and NOACs. High-bleeding risk is one of the reasons cited for deferring oral anticoagulants (OACs). However, there is concrete evidence to suggest that while bleeding risk of OACs is similar to antiplatelets, it is only the OACs which are effective in stroke prevention.[79-82]

Recently, in 2017, a functional EHRA classification (Evaluated Heart valves, Rheumatic or Artificial) was proposed based on the type of OAC use in patients with AF. The EHRA Type *I* refers to valvular heart disease patient, especially rheumatic moderate; severe MS and mechanical prosthetic valves who need VKA therapy while EHRA Type 2 refers to all other native valvular disease along with mitral valve repair, bioprosthetic valves, and transaortic valve interventions, where either VKAs or NOACs would suffice.[83] All current guidelines advocate a thromboembolic risk-based antithrombotic strategy for stroke prevention in nonvalvular AF. Flowchart 1 summarizes the current guidelines-based recommendations for primary prevention of stroke in AF.[33,46,84]

Vitamin K Antagonists

There is sufficient evidence to prove that VKAs reduce stroke risk by 64% while reducing mortality by 26%, when compared to either aspirin or no treatment, provided the INR is within therapeutic range (2.0–3.0).[85] The clinical superiority of warfarin over aspirin, with similar risk of intracranial hemorrhage was also corroborated by the BAFTA (Birmingham Atrial Fibrillation Treatment of the Aged) study which showed a 52% risk reduction with warfarin.[86] VKA therapy is associated with a 0.2% increase in absolute risk of intracranial hemorrhage (ICH). Notable among the various limitations of VKA therapy include a narrow therapeutic window (with resultant frequent monitoring and adjustments in dose), varied drug and food interactions, unpredictable response, slow onset and offset of action, warfarin resistance, and increased baseline ICH risk. However, if administered with adequate time in therapeutic range (TTR >70%), they provide effective and cheaper thromboprophylaxis in AF. In 2013, using the AFFIRM trial (Atrial Fibrillation Follow Up Investigation of Rhythm Management) data, authors put forth a simple predictive score, *SAMe-TT$_2$R$_2$* [acronym for *S*ex, female; *A*ge <60 years; *Me*dical history (atleast 2 of the following – hypertension/diabetes/CAD/peripheral arterial disease/CCF/previous stroke /pulmonary disease/hepatic or renal disease); *T*reatment (warfarin interacting drugs, e.g., amiodarone); current *T*obacco use (within 2 years) and *R*ace, noncaucasians] for likelihood of INR control. Except for current tobacco use and race which are scored 2, all others

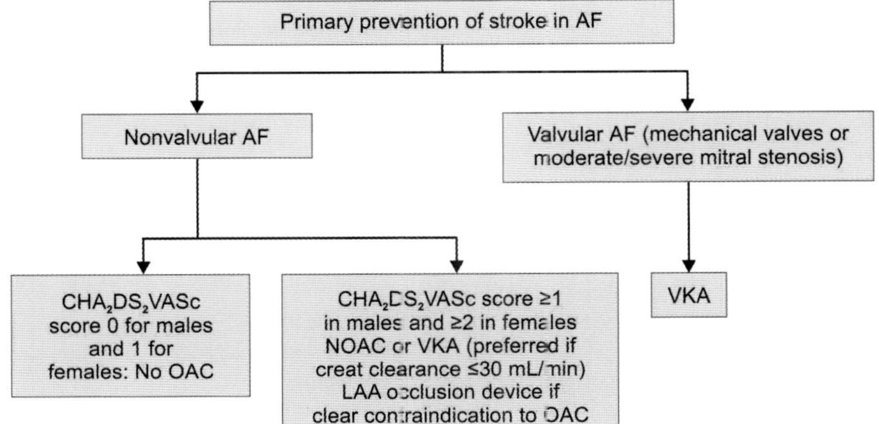

AF, atrial fibrillation; CHA2DS2VASC score, Congestive Heart Failure, Hypertension, Age ≥75 (Doubled), Diabetes Mellitus, Prior Stroke or Transient Ischemic Attack (Doubled), Vascular Disease, Age 65–74, Female; LAA, left atrial appendage; NOAC, newer oral anticoagulants; OAC, oral anticoagulants; VKA, vitamin K antagonists.

FLOWCHART 1: Summary of primary prevention of stroke in atrial fibrillation.

are scored 1. Higher the SAMe-TT_2R_2 score, poorer will be the INR control and more will be the rationale to choose NOACs over VKA.[87] A SAMe-TT_2R_2 score of less than or equal to 2 (which translates to an adequate time in therapeutic range, i.e., >70%) may be used as a reasonable cutoff to choose between either NOACs or VKAs as stroke thrombophylactic strategies in nonvalvular AF with CHA_2DS_2VASC scores more than or equal to 1 in males or more than or equal to 2 in females. However, the presence of SAMe-TT_2R_2 score of more than or equal to 3 precludes the use of VKAs and necessitates exclusive NOAC usage.[46]

Nevertheless, VKAs are the only thromboprophylactic strategy available for valvular AF (rheumatic disease and mechanical heart valves) and stage V chronic kidney disease (CKD) (creatinine clearance ≤15 mL/min).

Novel Oral Anticoagulants

These have emerged in recent years as an effective and safer alternative to VKAs in the field of stroke prevention in nonvalvular AF. In all AF patients who are otherwise eligible for NOACs, ESC 2016 guidelines places class Ia recommendation for choosing NOACs over VKAs.[33] As of

TABLE 3: Novel anticoagulants used in clinical practice for primary and secondary stroke prevention

	Dabigatran	Apixaban	Rivaroxaban	Edoxaban
Prodrug	+	–	–	–
Bioavailability	3–7% (not affected by food)	60% (not affected by food)	66% (in fasting state and higher with food, up to 100%)	50% (6–22% more absorption with food)
Time to peak plasma concentration	0.5–2 hours	1–4 h	2–4 h	1–2 h
Renal clearance	80%	27%	35%	50%
Half-life	12–14 h (in normal renal function) 18 h, creatinine clearance 30–50 mL/min >24 h, creatinine clearance <30 mL/min	12 h	7–11 h	8–10 h
Drug interactions	P-glycoprotein inhibitors (e.g., ketoconazole)	P-glycoprotein and CYP3A4 inhibitors	P-glycoprotein and CYP3A4 inhibitors	P-glycoprotein inhibitors and CYP3A4 inhibitors (<4%)
Adverse effect other than bleeding	Dyspepsia (due to acidic coating on capsule)	Nil	Nil	Nil
Dosing frequency	Twice daily	Twice daily	Once daily	Once daily
Intake with food	No interaction	No interaction	Mandatory	No guidelines
Administration through Ryle's tube	Cannot be given*	Yes	Cannot be given**	Yes
NOAC	**Standard dose**		**Dose modification**	
Apixaban	5 mg bd		2.5 mg bd if two out of the following three criteria present: • Serum creatinine ≥1.5 mg/dL (or creatinine clearance 15–29 mL/min) • Weight <60 kg • Age >80 years	
Dabigatran	150 mg bd/110 mg bd		110 mg bd >80 years and high-risk of bleeding; not recommended if creatinine clearance <30 mL/min	
Rivaroxaban	20 mg od		15 mg od if creatinine clearance 15–50 mL/min	
Edoxaban	60 mg od (creatinine clearance 50–95 mL/min)		30 mg od if: • Creatinine clearance 15– 50 mL/min • Weight ≤60 kg • Concomitant treatment with strong P-glycoprotein inhibitor (e.g., verapamil, quinidine, dronedarone) Not recommended when creatinine clearance >95 mL/min or <15 mL/min	

*Dabigatran capsules should not be crushed or chewed or administered through Ryles tube since removal of intact capsule shell increases bioavailability of the drug by 75%.

**Edoxaban administration through Ryles tube is not recommended, pending trial results.[97]

NOAC, newer oral anticoagulants.

now, the approved NOACs ensemble includes 4 drugs--dabigatran (direct thrombin inhibitor), apixaban, edoxaban, and rivaroxaban (factor Xa inhibitors). The major landmark trials for NOACs include RELY[88] for dabigatran, ARISTOTLE[89] and AVERROES[90] trials (Apixaban Versus ASA to Prevent Stroke In AF Patients Who Have Failed or Are Unsuitable for Vitamin K Antagonist Treatment) for apixaban, ROCKET-AF[91] trial for rivaroxaban and ENGAGE-AF TIMI (Effective Anticoagulation with factor Xa Next Generation in Atrial Fibrillation-Thrombolysis In Myocardial Infarction 48)[92] trial for edoxaban. The advantages of NOACs include a predictable pharmacokinetic profile, offsetting the need for frequent anticoagulation, better compliance, considerably less drug and food interactions, faster onset of action, and lower risk of systemic and intracranial hemorrhage. Potential limitations include high cost, absence of readily available antidote, difficulty in coagulation monitoring, and possible drug toxicity in the presence of renal failure.[88] Table 3 provides a concise summary of (1) pharmacokinetic profile and (2) the approved dose recommendations for NOACs for stroke prevention in nonvalvular AF.[93-96]

Choice of Specific Newer Oral Anticoagulants

Current evidence remains inadequate as regards the choice of individual NOACs. Once daily dosage NOACs such as rivaroxaban and edoxaban may be preferred in patients with compliance issues. Similarly, apixaban is a viable option in patients prone to gastrointestinal (GI) bleeding as it is the only NOAC associated with lower GI bleeding risk compared to warfarin. In patients with renal dysfunction and dyspepsia, rivaroxaban and apixaban are preferred over dabigatran in view of predominant nonrenal modes of drug clearance and absence of dyspepsia as an adverse effect. Dabigatran 150 mg bd is preferred in patients with high stroke risk (CHA_2DS_2VaSc) while reduced dosage (110 mg bd) or apixaban 5 mg bd is preferred in patients with bleeding risk or past history of life-threatening bleeds. In the very elderly patients, more than or equal to 80 years with impaired renal function and low weight, apixaban 2.5 mg bd is preferred.[95]

Newer oral anticoagulant usage in presence of renal dysfunction is guided by the differences in renal clearance. As warfarin has the lowest renal clearance of <1%, it is undoubtedly, the safest OAC option in severe CKD, especially end stage renal disease (ESRD) (creatinine clearance ≤15 mL/min). Among the NOACs, dabigatran has the highest renal clearance (80%) followed by edoxaban (50%), rivaroxaban (35%), and apixaban (27%). Meta-analysis of NOACs in CKD by Sardar et al. (10 RCTs) and Nielsen et al. (5 RCTs) has shown that when compared to warfarin, NOACs significantly reduce the risk of stroke or systemic embolism in mild-to-moderate CKD (creatinine clearance 30–79 mL/min) and risk of major bleeding is comparable to warfarin in moderate CKD (creatinine clearance 30–49 mL/min) but significantly reduced in mild CKD (creatinine clearance 50–79 mL/min).[98,99] As per majority of recent guidelines, low-dose NOACs (except dabigatran) can be used in severe CKD (creatinine clearance 15–30 mL/min) with regular renal function monitoring.[46] Though dabigatran 75 mg bd has been approved by United States Food and Drug Administration (US FDA) in patients with creatinine clearance 15–30 mL/min (not approved in Europe). All NOACs are contraindicated in ESRD. RCTs regarding OAC use in hemodialysis patients are lacking There are conflicting data on efficacy of warfarin in ESRD with majority of studies indicating reduced stroke or systemic embolism risk but with increased risk of bleeding. The 2018 EHRA guidelines have suggested that NOACs are better avoided in patients with ESRD and those on dialysis in concordance with available evidence.[100]

Available evidence indicates that all NOACs are contraindicated in the presence of Child-Turcotte-Pugh C cirrhosis and in liver disease with coagulopathy and resultant increased bleeding risk. Additionally, rivaroxaban is also contraindicated in Child-Pugh B cirrhosis.[100]

Role of Left Atrial Appendage Occlusion Strategies in Primary Prevention of Stroke in Atrial Fibrillation

As stasis and thrombi formation within the LAA are harbingers of stroke and systemic thromboembolism in AF patients, it seems reasonable that occlusion or exclusion of LAA by interventional or surgical measures would aid thromboprophylaxis. Some of the devices available for LAA occlusion include WATCHMAN, PLAATO, Amulet, ACP, LAmbre, WaveCrest, Sideris patch, and ultrasept. The percutaneous left atrial cardioversion closure vs warfarin for atrial fibrillation (PROTECT-AF) and PREVAIL trials (Evaluation of the WATCHMAN LAA Closure Device in Patients With Atrial Fibrillation Versus Long Term Warfarin Therapy) compared long-term VKA treatment to LAA occlusion in AF patients. Both studies revealed that LAA occlusion using WATCHMAN device was noninferior to VKA treatment in moderate stroke risk patients of AF, with reduced risk of bleeding on prolonged follow-up.[101,102] These findings were corroborated in a meta-analysis on LAA occlusion, as an alternative to VKA therapy, for stroke prevention in AF.[103]

Surgical occlusion or exclusion of LAA is an alternative to interventional procedures for LAA closure; these can be done either as an isolated thoracoscopic procedure or with surgical AF foci ablation or open-heart surgery. A recent trial did not demonstrate definite benefit of surgical LAA occlusion in preventing strokes.[104] The LAAOS III (Left atrial appendage occlusion study), a large ongoing RCT on surgical LAA removal during concomitant open heart surgery in AF patients, estimates to enroll 4,700 patients from July 2012 to November 2020. The results of this trial would provide answers to the speculated beneficial role of LAA surgical removal.[105]

Secondary Stroke Prevention in Atrial Fibrillation

Appropriate and timely initiation of optimum therapeutic strategies is core to the precept of secondary stroke prevention among patients with AF. It is imperative to initiate the patient on lifelong anticoagulation therapy after the occurrence of ischemic stroke in the presence of AF. While valvular AF is an exclusive indication for VKA therapy, nonvalvular AF offers a broader therapeutic choice between NOACs and VKAs.

The core principles of drug choices, details, adverse effects, bleeding risk stratification are already outlined in the section above in detail.

Timing of Initiation of Anticoagulation after Ischemic Stroke/Transient Ischemic Attack

The optimum and safest time for initiating anticoagulation in AF-related stroke/TIA remains a matter of debate. Published data suggest 1–10% early stroke recurrence rate following a cardioembolic stroke within 2 weeks. Hence, it is prudent to initiate anticoagulation at an apt time without increasing the risk of ICH. Paciaroni et al. in their meta-analysis (Stroke, 2007) concluded that administration of parenteral anticoagulation within 48 hours of stroke onset, only resulted in more ICH without causing any reduction in recurrent stroke risk.[106] However, Abdul-Rahim et al. in their recent analysis of VISTA trial concluded that early initiation of OAC within 2–3 days of AIS, resulted in significant reduction in stroke recurrence, without causing increased risk of ICH.[107] Another study, observed that early NOAC initiation within 7 days did not prove beneficial in reducing stroke or ICH risk.[108]

The Dieners rule (1-3-7-14) or the EHRA proposed 1-3-6-12 rule is an easy aid which is practically used for selecting the timing of anticoagulation initiation. According to this rule, anticoagulation may be started 1 day after a TIA, 3 days after a mild stroke (NIHSS <8), 6 days after a moderate stroke (NIHSS 8–16), and 12 days after a severe stroke (NIHSS >16); after excluding hemorrhagic transformation on noncontrast computed tomography (NCCT). Clinical points, which would favor early initiation of anticoagulation, include a low NIHSS (<8), presence of small infarct on imaging, spontaneous echo contrast, LA thrombi, younger age, and absence of hemorrhagic transformation.[33] Two large ongoing RCTs namely, TIMING study and START study, have been designed to specifically address the issue of optimum timing of NOAC initiation.[109]

Atrial Fibrillation Patients on Oral Anticoagulants with Acute Ischemic Stroke Presenting within the Window Period

In general, as a standard of care, in all eligible AIS patients, current guidelines recommend intravenous thrombolysis in all patients with AIS presenting within 4.5 hours of onset and in the presence of large vessel occlusion (LVO), mechanical thrombectomy is recommended (standard thrombectomy window period of 6 hours or even within the delayed thrombectomy period of 6–24 hours, based on strict selection criteria).

However, patients who are already on OAC therapy and especially on NOAC's pose a special challenge in the management of AIS. Intravenous thrombolysis is NOT permissible until details of medication use, INR status, laboratory parameters like activated partial thromboplastin time (aPTT), INR, platelet count, ecarin clotting time, thrombin time, or appropriate direct factor Xa activity assays, and dosing details are known. "Strict individualized risk benefit assessment will be required to make a decision on treating such patients in view of bleeding risk concerns".

In the presence of current OAC usage–either VKA or NOAC (with unknown or subtherapaeutic coagulation parameters), direct endovascular mechanical thrombectomy is preferred over intravenous thrombolysis as the initial reperfusion strategy, in the presence of LVO.[33,110,111] Bridging using thrombolysis and mechanical thrombectomy could be undertaken among patients with definite subtherapeutic coagulation parameters as discussed above, if available rapidly.

For patients without any proximal major vessel occlusion on computed tomographic angiography (CTA)/magnetic resonance angiography (MRA); severity of stroke, history of OAC intake details (dose, last dose timing), rapid availability of coagulation assays, and risk benefit assessment need to be done before proceeding for thrombolysis. Flowchart 2 provides an algorithmic representation of the practical management options of known AF patients on OACs presenting with AIS.

Resuming Anticoagulation after Intracerebral Hemorrhage—Timing?

Restarting OACs after an ICH is a difficult decision which merits serious risk benefit consideration. Current guidelines recommend OAC to be restarted 4–8 weeks after ICH in AF patients, provided the benefits of stroke risk reduction outweigh the harms of recurrent ICH. In a study on 2,619 ICH patients with AF, maximum benefit was obtained when OACs were restarted after 7–8 weeks.[112] In a meta-analysis of eight trials, authors observed that restarting of anticoagulation after ICH was associated with reduced risk of ischemic stroke, and there was no increase in recurrence of ICH.[113] While the need for long-term anticoagulation after lobar bleed is controversial, published evidence indicate cerebral amyloid angiopathy as a contraindication to OAC.[33,95]

CONCLUSION

The past few years have borne witness to tremendous advancements in the field of AF and stroke. The advent of NOACs is a major milestone and has revolutionized the thromboprophylactic arena of AF and stroke. The growing research in this field is anticipated to open up a plethora of high quality, patient-friendly treatment approaches. The development of antidotes to NOACs has further added to the armamentarium of management of AF-related strokes in the acute period. Ongoing research in the fields of occult AF detection, with better understanding of AF-related stroke pathophysiology and newer markers of stroke prediction also portend a brighter future with better pragmatic approaches in the thromboprophylactic and therapeutic realm.

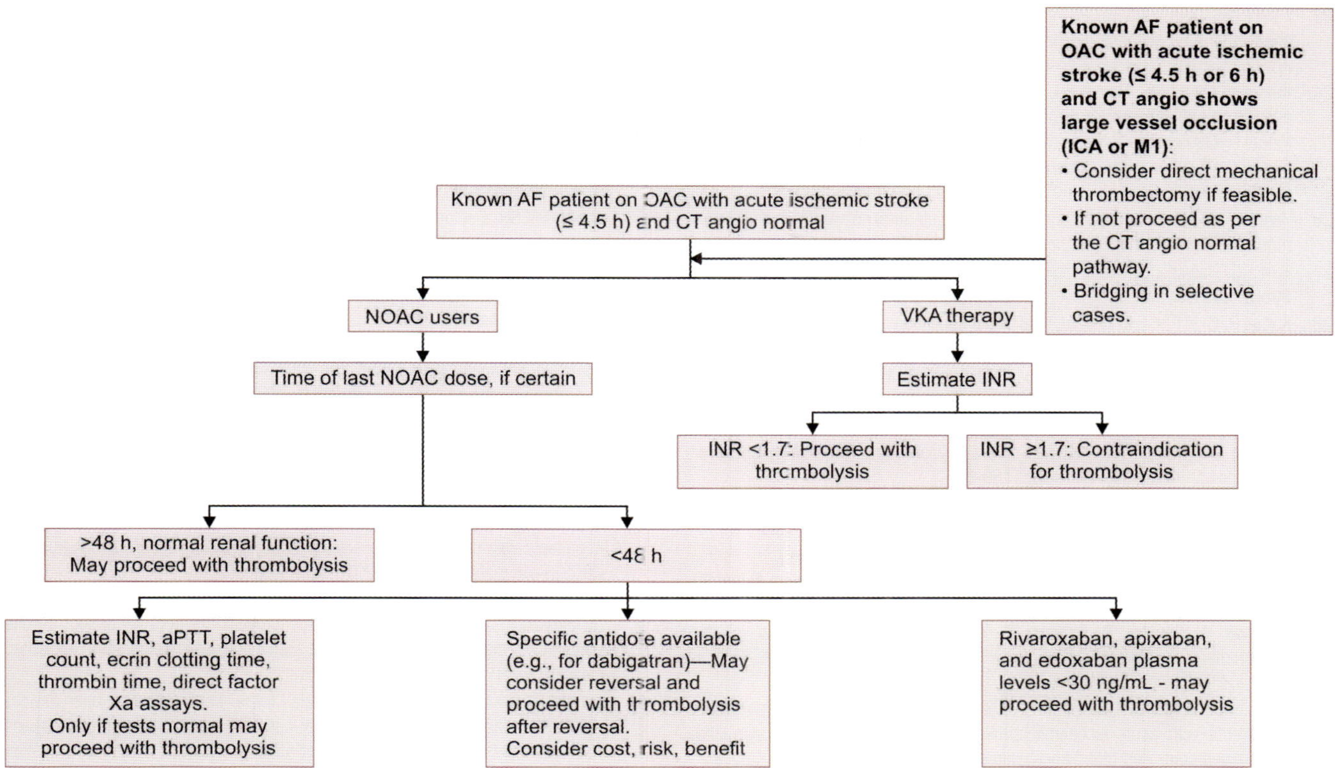

AF, atrial fibrillation; aPTT, activated partial thromboplastin time; CT, computed tomography; ICA, internal carotid artery; INR, international normalized ratio; NOAC, newer oral anticoagulants; OAC, oral anticoagulant; VKA, vitamin K antagonists.

FLOWCHART 2: An outline for the practical management of AF patients on OAC who present within the stroke window period. Please see the text for detailed discussion and concerns.

REFERENCES

1. Chugh SS, Havmoeller R, Narayanan K, et al. Worldwide Epidemiology of Atrial Fibrillation: a Global Burden of Disease 2010 study. Circulation. 2014;129:837-47.
2. Leary MC, Caplan LR. Cardioembolic stroke: An update on aetiology, diagnosis and management. Ann Indian Acad Neuro. 2008;11:S52-S63.
3. Freedman B, Potpara TS, Lip GYH. Stroke prevention in atrial fibrillation. Lancet. 2016;388:806-17.
4. Phillips SJ. Is atrial fibrillation an independent risk factor for stroke? Can J Neurol Sci. 1990;17:163-8.
5. Go AS, Hylek EM, Phillips KA, et al. Prevalence of diagnosed atrial fibrillation in adults: National implications for rhythm management and stroke prevention: The AnTicoagulation and Risk factors in Atrial Fibrillation (ATRIA) Study. JAMA. 2001;285:2370-5.
6. Miyasaka Y, Bames ME, Bailey KR, et al. Mortality trends in patients diagnosed with first atrial fibrillation: A 21 year community based study. J Am Coll Cardiol. 2007;49:986-92.
7. Bungard TJ, Shuaib A, Tsuyuki RT. Stroke prophylaxis in nonvalvular atrial fibrillation. Curr Opin Neurol. 2001;14:59-65.
8. Andrade J, Khairy P, Dobrev D, et al. The clinical profile and pathophysiology of atrial fibrillation relationships among clinical features, epidemiology, and mechanisms. Circ Res. 2014;114:1453-68.
9. Wolf PA, Abbott RD, Kannel WB. Atrial fibrillation as an independent risk factor for stroke: The Framingham study. Stroke. 1991;22:983-8.
10. Feinberg WM, Blackshear JL, Laupacis A, et al. Prevalence, age distribution, and gender of patients with atrial fibrillation .Analysis and implications. Arch Intern Med. 1995;155(5):469-73.
11. Deiner HC, Weber Ralph, Lip GYH, et al. Stroke prevention in atrial fibrillation: Do we still need warfarin? Curr Opin Neurol. 2012;25:27-35.
12. Chiang CE, Wang KL, Lip GY. Stroke prevention in atrial fibrillation: An Asian perspective. Thromb Haemost. 2014;111:789-97.
13. Wolf PA, Benjamin EJ, Belanger AJ, et al. Secular trends in the prevalence of atrial fibrillation: the Framingham study. Am Heart J. 1996;131:790-5.
14. Sridharan SE, Unnikrishnan JP, Sukumaran S, et al. Incidence, types, risk factors, and outcome of stroke in a developing country: The Trivandrum stroke registry. Stroke. 2009;40:1212-8.
15. Akarsha GW, Paramdeep K, Gagandeep S, et al. Clinical features, risk factors, and short-term outcome of ischemic stroke, in patients with atrial fibrillation: Data from a population based study. Ann Indian Acad Neurol. 2017;20:289-93.
16. Deore R, Vora A. Epidemiology and risk factor for AF in India. J Prev Cardiol. 2013;3:505-7.
17. Vora A, Kapoor A, Nair M, et al. Clinical presentation, management, and outcomes in the Indian Heart Rhythm Society-Atrial Fibrillation (IHRS-AF) registry. Indian Heart J. 2017;69:43-47.
18. Bhardwaj R. Atrial fibrillation in a tertiary care institute – A prospective study. Indian Heart J. 2012;64:476-8.
19. Narasimhan C, Verma JS, Ravi Kishore AG, et al. An International, observational cross sectional survey evaluating AF Management and Cardiovascular Risk profile of AF patients, Indian subset data presented at the ISE Meeting Jaipur; 2012.
20. Yue L, Xie J, Nattel S. Molecular determinants of cardiac fibroblast electrical function and therapeutic implications for atrial fibrillation. Cardiovasc Res. 2011;89:744-53.
21. Burstein B, Nattel S. Atrial fibrosis: Mechanisms and clinical relevance in atrial fibrillation. J Am Coll Cardiol. 2008;51:802-9.
22. Akoum N, Daccarett M, McGann C, et al. Atrial fibrosis helps select the appropriate patient and strategy in catheter ablation of atrial fibrillation: A DE-MRI guided approach. J Cardiovasc Electrophysiol. 2011;22:16-22.

23. Larsen BS, Kumarathurai P, Falkenberg J, et al. Excessive atrial ectopy and short atrial runs increase the risk of stroke beyond incident atrial fibrillation. J Am Coll Cardiol. 2015;66:232-41.
24. Kamel H, Elkind MS, Bhave PD, et al. Paroxysmal supraventricular tachycardia and the risk of ischemic stroke. Stroke. 2013;44:1550-4.
25. Kamel H, O'Neal WT, Okin PM, et al. Electrocardiographic left atrial abnormality and stroke subtype in the atherosclerosis risk in communities study. Ann Neurol. 2015;78:670-8.
26. Yaghi S, Moon YP, Mora-McLaughlin C, et al. Left atrial enlargement and stroke recurrence: the Northern Manhattan Stroke Study. Stroke. 2015;46:1488-93.
27. Hart RG, Halperin JL. Atrial fibrillation and stroke concepts and controversies. Stroke. 2001;32:803-8.
28. Kamel H, Okin PM, Elkind MSV, et al. Atrial fibrillation and mechanisms of stroke – time for a new model. Stroke. 2016;47:895-900.
29. Cerasuolo JO, Cipriano LE, Sposato LA. The complexity of atrial fibrillation newly diagnosed after ischemic stroke and transient ischemic attack: advances and uncertainties. Curr Opin Neurol. 2017;30:28-37.
30. Sposato LA, Riccio PM, Hachinski V. Post stroke atrial fibrillation: Cause or consequence. Neurology. 2014;82:1180-6.
31. González Toledo ME, Klein FR, Riccio PM, et al. Atrial fibrillation detected after acute ischemic stroke: Evidence supporting the neurogenic hypothesis. J Stroke Cerebrovasc Dis. 2013;22:e486-91.
32. Wohlfahrt J, Stahrenberg R, Weber-Kruger M, et al. Clinical predictors to identify paroxysmal atrial fibrillation after ischaemic stroke. Eur J Neurol. 2014;21:21-7.
33. Kirchhoff P, Benussi S, Kotecha D, et al. 2016 ESC guidelines for the management of atrial fibrillation developed in collaboration with EACTS. Eur Heart J. 2016;37:2893-962.
34. Wachter R, Groschel K, Gelbrich G, et al. Holter-electrocardiogram-monitoring in patients with acute ischaemic stroke (Find-AF $_{\text{RANDOMISED}}$): An open-label randomised controlled trial. Lancet Neurol. 2017;S1474-4422(17):30002-9.
35. Sanna T, Diener HC, Passman RS, et al. Cryptogenic stroke and underlying atrial fibrillation. N Engl J Med. 2014;370:2478-86.
36. Gladstone DJ, Spring M, Dorian P, et al. Atrial fibrillation in patients with cryptogenic stroke. N Engl J Med. 2014;370:2467-77.
37. Healey JS, Connolly SJ, Gold MR, et al. Subclinical atrial fibrillation and the risk of stroke. N Engl J Med. 2012;366:120-9.
38. Glotzer TV, Hellkamp AS, Zimmerman J, et al. Atrial high rate episodes detected by pacemaker diagnostics predict death and stroke: Report of the atrial diagnostics ancillary study of the Mode Selection Trial (MOST). Circulation. 2003;107:1614-9.
39. Gladstone DJ, Dorien P, Spring M, et al. Atrial premature beats predict atrial fibrillation in subclinical stroke – Results from the EMBRACE trial. Stroke. 2016;46:936-41.
40. Suissa L, Bertora D, Lachaud S, et al. Score for the Targeting of Atrial Fibrillation (STAF) – A new approach for the detection of atrial fibrillation in the secondary prevention of stroke. Stroke. 2009;40:2866-8.
41. Yoshioka K, Watanabe K, Zeniya S, et al. A score for predicting paroxysmal atrial fibrillation in acute stroke patients: iPAB score. J Stroke Cerebrovas Dis. 2015;24:2263-9.
42. Toni D, Lorenzano S, Strano S, et al. Detection of Silent Atrial Fibrillation aFter Ischemic StrOke (SAFFO) guided by implantable loop recorder: multicentre Italian trial based on stroke unit network with paired cardio-arrhythmology units. Int J Stroke. 2016;11(3):361-7.
43. Haeusler KG, Kirchhof P, Heuschmann PU, et al. Impact of standardized MONitoring for Detection of Atrial Fibrillation in Ischemic Stroke (MonDAFIS): rationale and design of a prospective randomized multicenter study. Am Heart J. 2016;172:19-25.
44. Gage BF, Waterman AD, Shannon W, et al. Validation of clinical classification schemes for predicting stroke: Results from the national registry of atrial fibrillation. JAMA. 2001;285:2864-70.
45. Lip GY, Nieuwlaat R, Pisters R, et al. Refining clinical risk stratification for predicting stroke and thromboembolism in atrial fibrillation using a novel risk factor-based approach: the euro heart survey on atrial fibrillation. Chest. 2010;137:263-72.
46. Chiang CE, Okumura K, Zhang S, et al. 2017 consensus of the Asia- Pacific Heart Rhythm society on stroke prevention in atrial fibrillation. J Arrhythmia. 2017;33:345-67.
47. Chao TF, Lip GYH, Liu CJ, et al. Validation of a modified CHA2DS2-VASc score for stroke risk stratification in Asian patients with atrial fibrillation: A nationwide cohort study. Stroke. 2016;47:2462-9.
48. Singer DE, Chang Y, Borowsky LH, et al. A new risk scheme to predict ischemic stroke and other thromboembolism in atrial fibrillation: The ATRIA study stroke risk score. J Am Heart Assoc. 2013;2:e000250.
49. Chao TF, Lip GYH, Liu CJ, et al. Relationship of aging and incident comorbidities to stroke risk in patients with atrial fibrillation. J Am Coll Cardiol. 2018;71:122-32.
50. Hohnloser SH, Pajitnev D, Pogue J, et al. Incidence of stroke in paroxysmal versus sustained atrial fibrillation in patients taking oral anticoagulation or combined antiplatelet therapy: An ACTIVE W substudy. J Am Coll Cardiol. 2007;50:2156-61.
51. Link MS, Giugliano RP, Ruff CT, et al. Stroke and mortality risk in patients with various patterns of atrial fibrillation: Results from the ENGAGE AF-TIMI 48 trial (effective anticoagulation with factor Xa next generation in atrial fibrillation-thrombolysis in myocardial infarction 48). Circ Arrhythm Electrophysiol. 2017;10:e004267.
52. Ganesan AN, Chew DP, Hartshorne T, et al. The impact of atrial fibrillation type on the risk of thromboembolism, mortality, and bleeding: A systematic review and meta-analysis. Eur Heart J. 2016;37:1591-602.
53. Steinberg BA, Hellkamp AS, Lokhnygina Y, et al. Higher risk of death and stroke in patients with persistent versus paroxysmal atrial fibrillation: Results from the ROCKET-AF trial. Eur heart J. 2015;36(5):288-96.
54. Boriani G, Glotzer TV, Santini M, et al. Device-detected atrial fibrillation and risk for stroke: An analysis of >10000 patients from the SOS AF project (Stroke preventiOn Strategies based on Atrial Fibrillation information from implanted devices). Eur Heart J. 2014;35:508-16.
55. Swiryn S, Orlov MV, Benditt DG, et al. Clinical implications of brief device-detected atrial tachyarrhythmias in a cardiac rhythm management device population: Results from the registry of atrial tachycardia and atrial fibrillation episodes. Circulation. 2016;134:1130-40.
56. Hijazi Z, Oldgren J, Andersson U, et al. Cardiac biomarkers are associated with an increased risk of stroke and death in patients with atrial fibrillation: a randomized evaluation of long-term anticoagulation therapy (RE-LY) substudy. Circulation. 2012;125:1605-16.
57. Hijazi Z, Siegbahn A, Andersson U, et al. High-sensitivity troponin I for risk assessment in patients with atrial fibrillation: insights from the Apixaban for Reduction in Stroke and other Thromboembolic Events in Atrial Fibrillation (ARISTOTLE) trial. Circulation. 2014;129:625-34.
58. Hijazi Z, Wallentin L, Siegbahn A, et al. N-terminal pro-B-type natriuretic peptide for risk assessment in patients with atrial fibrillation: insights from the ARISTOTLE trial (apixaban for the prevention of stroke in subjects with atrial fibrillation). J Am Coll Cardiol. 2013;61:2274-84.
59. Lip GY, Patel JV, Hughes E, et al. High-sensitivity C-reactive protein and soluble CD40 ligand as indices of inflammation and platelet activation in 880 patients with nonvalvular atrial fibrillation: relationship to stroke risk factors, stroke risk stratification schema, and prognosis. Stroke. 2007;38:1229-37.
60. Aulin J, Siegbahn A, Hijazi Z, et al. Interleukin-6 and C-reactive protein and risk for death and cardiovascular events in patients with atrial fibrillation. Am Heart J. 2015;170:1151-60.
61. Hijazi Z, Aulin J, Andersson U, et al. Biomarkers of inflammation and risk of cardiovascular events in anticoagulated patients with atrial fibrillation. Heart. 2016;102:508-17.
62. Hijazi Z, Lindback J, Alexander JH, et al. The ABC (age, biomarkers, clinical history) stroke risk score: A biomarker based risk score for predicting stroke in atrial fibrillation. Eur Heart J. 2016;37:1582-90.
63. Hijazi Z, Oldgren J, Lindback J, et al. A biomarker-based risk score to predict death in patients with atrial fibrillation: the ABC (age, biomarkers, clinical history) death risk score. Eur Heart J. 2018;39:477-85.
64. Hijazi Z, Oldgren J, Lindback J, et al. The novel biomarker-based ABC (age, biomarkers, clinical history)-bleeding risk score for patients with atrial fibrillation: A derivation and validation study. Lancet. 2016;387:2302-11.
65. Yaghi S, Moon YP, Mora-McLaughlin C, et al. Left atrial enlargement and stroke recurrence: The Northern Manhattan stroke study. Stroke. 2015;46:1488-93.
66. Hamatani Y, Ogawa H, Takabayashi K, et al. Left atrial enlargement is an independent predictor of stroke and systemic embolism in patients with non-valvular atrial fibrillation. Sci Rep. 2016;6:31042.

67. Calenda BW, Fuster V, Halperin JL, et al. Stroke risk assessment in atrial fibrillation: Risk factors and markers of atrial myopathy. Natur Rev Cardiol. 2016;13(9):549-59.
68. Lee JM, Shim J, Uhm JS, et al. Impact of increased orifice size and decreased flow velocity of left atrial appendage on stroke in nonvalvular atrial fibrillation. Am J Cardiol. 2014;113:963-9.
69. Goldman ME, Pearce LA, Hart RG, et al. Pathophysiologic correlates of thromboembolism in nonvalvular atrial fibrillation: I. Reduced flow velocity in the left atrial appendage (the stroke prevention in atrial fibrillation [SPAF-III] study). J Am Soc Echocardiogr. 1999;12:1080-7.
70. Yaghi S, Kamel H. Stratifying stroke risk in atrial fibrillation beyond clinical risk scores. Stroke. 2017;48:2665-70.
71. Yaghi S, Song C, Gray WA, et al. Left atrial appendage function and stroke risk. Stroke. 2015;46:3554-9.
72. Khurram IM, Dewire J, Mager M, et al. Relationship between left atrial appendage: Morphology and stroke in patients with atrial fibrillation. Heart Rhythm. 2013;10:1843-9.
73. Yamamoto M, Seo Y, Kawamatsu N, et al. Complex left atrial appendage morphology and left atrial appendage thrombus formation in patients with atrial fibrillation. Circ Cardiovasc Imaging. 2014;7:337-43.
74. Gage BF, Yan Y, Milligan PE, et al. Clinical classification schemes for predicting haemorrhage: Results from the National Registry of Atrial Fibrillation (NRAF). Am Heart J. 2006;151(3):713-9.
75. Pisters R, Lane DA, Nieuwlaat R, et al. A novel user-friendly score (HAS-BLED) to assess 1 year risk of major bleeding in patients with atrial fibrillation: The Euro Heart Survey. Chest. 2010;138(5):1093-100.
76. Fang MC, Go AS, Chang Y, et al. A new risk scheme to predict Warfarin-associated haemorrhage: The ATRIA (Anticoagulation and risk factors in atrial fibrillation) study. J Am Coll Cardiol. 2011;58:395-401.
77. O'Brien EC, Simon DN, Thomas LE, et al. The ORBIT bleeding score: A simple bedside score to assess bleeding risk in atrial fibrillation. Eur Heart J. 2015;36:3258-64.
78. Apostolakis S, Lane DA, Guo Y, et al. Performance of the $HEMORR_2HAGES$, ATRIA and HAS-BLED bleeding risk-prediction scores in patients with atrial fibrillation undergoing anticoagulation: The AMADEUS (Evaluating the Use of SR34006 Compared to Warfarin or Acenocoumarol in Patients With Atrial Fibrillation) study. J Am Coll Cardiol. 2012;60:861-7.
79. Culebras A, Messe SR, Chaturvedi S, et al. Summary of evidence-based guideline update: Prevention of stroke in nonvalvular atrial fibrillation: Report of the Guideline Development Subcommittee of the American Academy of Neurology. Neurology. 2014;82:716-24.
80. Connolly SJ, Eikelboom J, Joyner C, et al. AVERROES Steering Committee Investigators. Apixaban in patients with atrial fibrillation. N Engl J Med. 2011;364:806-17.
81. Mant J, Hobbs FD, Fletcher K, et al. Warfarin versus aspirin for stroke prevention in an elderly community population with atrial fibrillation (the Birmingham Atrial Fibrillation Treatment of the Aged Study, BAFTA): A randomised controlled trial. Lancet. 2007;370:493-503.
82. Diener HC, Eikelboom J, Connolly SJ, et al. Apixaban versus aspirin in patients with atrial fibrillation and previous stroke or transient ischaemic attack: A predefined subgroup analysis from AVERROES, a randomised trial. Lancet Neurol. 2012;11:225-31.
83. Lip GYH, Collet JP, Caterina R, et al. Antithrombotic therapy in atrial fibrillation associated with valvular heart disease: a joint consensus document from the European Heart Rhythm Association (EHRA) and European Society of Cardiology Working Group on Thrombosis, endorsed by the ESC Working Group on Valvular Heart Disease, Cardiac Arrhythmia Society of Southern Africa (CASSA), Heart Rhythm Society (HRS), Asia Pacific Heart Rhythm Society (APHRS), South African Heart (SA Heart) Association and Sociedad Latinoamericana de Estimulacion Cardiaca y Electrofisiologia (SOLEACE). Europace. 2017;19:1757-8.
84. January CT, Wann LS, Alpert JS, et al. AHA/ACC/HRS guideline for the management of patients with atrial fibrillation: Executive summary: A report of the American College of Cardiology/American Heart Association Task Force on Practice Guidelines and the Heart Rhythm Society. J Am Coll Cardiol. 2014;64:2246-80.
85. Hart RG, Pearce LA, Aguilar MI. Meta-analysis: Antithrombotic therapy to prevent stroke in patients who have nonvalvular atrial fibrillation. Ann Intern Med. 2007;146:857-67.
86. Mant J, Hobbs FD, Fletcher K, et al. Warfarin versus aspirin for stroke prevention in an elderly community population with atrial fibrillation (the Birmingham Atrial Fibrillation Treatment of the Aged Study, BAFTA): A randomised controlled trial. Lancet. 2007;370:493-503.
87. Apostolakis S, Sullivan RM, Olshansky B, et al. Factors affecting quality of anticoagulation control among patients with atrial fibrillation on warfarin. Chest. 2013;144(5):1555-63.
88. Connolly SJ, Ezekowitz MD, Yusuf S, et al. Dabigatran versus warfarin in patients with atrial fibrillation. N Engl J Med. 2009;361:1139-51.
89. Granger CB, Alexander JH, McMurray JJV, et al. Apixiban versus warfarin in patients with atrial fibrillation. N Engl J Med. 2011;365:981-92.
90. Connolly SJ, Eikelboom J, Joyner C, et al. Apixaban in patients with atrial fibrillation. N Engl J Med. 2011;364:806-17.
91. Patel MR, Mahaffey KW, Garg J, et al. Rivaroxaban versus warfarin in nonvalvular atrial fibrillation. N Engl J Med. 2011;365:883-91.
92. Giugliano RP, Ruff CT, Braunwald E, et al. Edoxaban versus warfarin in patients with atrial fibrillation. N Engl J Med. 2013;369:2093-104.
93. Alberts MJ, Eikelboom JW, Hankey GJ. Antithrombotic therapy for stroke prevention in nonvalvular atrial fibrillation. Lancet. 2012;11:1066-81.
94. Aguilar MR, Kuo RS, Freeman WD. New anticoagulants (dabigatran, apixiban, rivaroxaban) for stroke prevention in AF. Neurol Clin. 2013;31:659-75.
95. Dalal J, Bhave A, Oomman A, et al. The Indian Consensus guidance on stroke prevention in atrial fibrillation: A practical view on the use of non-Vitamin K antagonist oral anticoagulants. JAPI. 2018;66(suppl):S6-26.
96. Hinojar R, Jimenez-Natcher JJ, Fernandez-Golfin C, et al. New oral anticoagulants: A practical guide for physicians. Eur Heart J Cardiovasc Pharamacother. 2015;1:134-45.
97. Petersen JJ, Hoehns JD. Administration of direct oral anticoagulants through enteral feeding tubes. J Pharm Tech. 2016;32(5)196-200.
98. Sardar P, Chatterjee S, Herzog E, et al. Novel oral anticoagulants in patients with renal insufficiency: A meta-analysis of randomized trials. Can J Cardiol. 2014;30:888-97.
99. Nielsen PB, Lane DA, Rasmussen LH, et al. Renal function and nonvitamin K oral anticoagulants in comparison with warfarin on safety and efficacy outcomes in atrial fibrillation patients: A systemic review and meta-regression analysis. Clin Res Cardiol. 2015;104:418-29.
100. Steffel J, Verhamme P, Potpara TS, et al. The 2018 European heart rhythm Association practical guide on the use of nonVitamin K antagonist oral anticoagulants in patients with atrial fibrillation. Eur Heart J. 2018;39:1330-93.
101. Reddy VY, Sievert H, Halperin J, et al. Percutaneous left atrial appendage closure vs warfarin for atrial fibrillation: A randomized controlled trial. JAMA. 2014;312(19):1988-98.
102. Holmes DR Jr, Kar S, Price MJ, et al. Prospective randomized evaluation of the Watchman left atrial appendage closure device in patients with atrial fibrillation versus long-term warfarin therapy: The PREVAIL trial. J Am Coll Cardiol. 2014;64(1):1-12.
103. Holmes DR Jr, Doshi SK, Kar S, et al. Left atrial appendage closure as an alternative to warfarin for stroke prevention in atrial fibrillation: A patient-level meta-analysis. J Am Coll Cardiol. 2015;65:2614-23.
104. Gillinov AM, Gelijns AC, Parides MK, et al. Surgical ablation of atrial fibrillation during mitral-valve surgery. N Engl J Med. 2015;372:1399-409.
105. Whitlock R, Healey J, Vincent J, et al. Rationale and design of the Left Atrial Appendage Occlusion Study (LAAOS) III. Ann Cardiothorac Surg. 2014;3:45-54.
106. Paciaroni M, Agnelli G, Micheli S, et al. Efficacy and safety of anticoagulant treatment in acute cardio embolic stroke: A meta-analysis of randomized controlled trials. Stroke. 2007;38:423-43.
107. Abdul-Rahim AH, Fulton RL, Frank B, et al. Association of improved outcome in acute ischaemic stroke patients with atrial fibrillation who receive early antithrombotic therapy: Analysis from VISTA. Eur J Neurol. 2015;22:1048-55.
108. Seiffge DJ, Traenka C, Polymeris A, et al. Early start of DOAC after ischemic stroke: Risk of intracranial hemorrhage and recurrent events. Neurology. 2016;87:1856-62.
109. Asberg S, Hijazi Z, Norrving B, et al. Timing of oral anticoagulant therapy in acute ischemic stroke with atrial fibrillation: Study protocol for a registry-based randomised controlled trial. Trials. 2017;18:581.

110. Powers WJ, Rabinstein AA, Ackerson T, et al. 2018 guidelines for the early management of patients with acute ischemic stroke. Stroke. 2018;49(3):e46-110.

111. Kernan WN, Ovbiagele B, Black HR, et al. Guidelines for the prevention of stroke in patients with stroke and transient ischemic attack. A guideline for healthcare professionals from the American Heart Association/American Stroke Association. Stroke. 2014;45:2160-236.

112. Pennlert J, Overholser R, Asplund K, et al. Optimal timing of anticoagulant treatment after intracranial haemorrhage in patients with atrial fibrillation. Stroke. 2017;48:314-20.

113. Murthy SB, Gupta A, Merkler AE, et al. Restarting anticoagulant therapy after intracranial haemorrhage: a systematic review and meta-analysis. Stroke. 2017;48:1594-600.

CHAPTER 128

Current Reperfusion Strategy in Acute Ischemic Stroke

MV Padma Srivastava, Vishnu VY

INTRODUCTION

The primary aim in management of acute ischemic stroke (AIS) is reestablishment of blood flow to save brain tissue which has not yet infarcted. In the last three decades, the management strategies have evolved from nihilism to thrombolytic therapy followed by endovascular therapy and recently to next generation endovascular devices and thrombolytic agents. The eligibility criteria and the drugs or devices for these two approved therapies have further evolved over the last two decades. In this review, we will discuss briefly the evolution of reperfusion therapy followed by the current best available evidence on reperfusion strategies in AIS.

THROMBOLYSIS IN ACUTE ISCHEMIC STROKE: "TIME CLOCK"

Thrombolysis in AIS arrived as a game changer but much later compared to cardiology practice. The main concept in the initial evolution of stroke thrombolysis was "time is brain" and the thrombolytic drug should be administered as early as possible.

The thrombolytic agent activates plasminogen to plasmin which cleaves the cross-linkages between fibrins in blood clots.[1] The efficacy of these agents depends on the age of clot, size and location, since higher density of cross linking of fibrin makes clot harder, more compact and difficult to dissolve.[1] Unlike the initial thrombolytic agents like streptokinase and urokinase, the only Food and Drug Administration (FDA)-approved tissue plasminogen activator (tPA) in stroke, alteplase (recombinant rtPA), is a fibrin selective analogue with short half-life. The dose of intravenous alteplase is 0.9 mg/kg up to 90 mg; 10% as a bolus followed by 1 hour infusion. Several trials like National Institute of Neurological Disorders and Stroke (NINDS) and European Collaborative Acute Stroke Study (ECAS) had proven the benefit for rtPA in AIS within 3 hours.[2,3] Several prospective observational registries like Canadian Alteplase for Stroke Effectiveness Study (CASES) registry,[4] and Safe Implementation of Thrombolysis in Stroke-International Stroke Thrombolysis Register (SITS-ISTR) showed similar rates of mortality, symptomatic intracerebral hemorrhage (ICH) within 24 hours and functional independence.[5] An individual patient data (IPD) meta-analysis of randomized controlled trials (RCTs) showed that thrombolysis using alteplase within 3 hours of stroke onset led to a good outcome {33% vs. 23%, or 1.75 [confidence interval (CI) 1.35–2.27]}.[6]

European Collaborative Acute Stroke Study III trial showed benefit of thrombolysis with alteplase in patients with clearly defined symptom onset between 3–4.5 hours of stroke onset [modified ranking scale, mRS 0–1 at 3 months, 52.4% vs. 45.2%, odds ratio (OR) 1.34, CI 1.02–1.76]. Third International Stroke (IST-3) trial had 1,177 patients in the 3–4.5 hours window period and the primary outcome was mRS 0–2 at 6 months (adjusted OR 0.73; 99% CI, 0.5–1.07). In the IPD meta-analysis, thrombolysis with alteplase showed benefit for patients with stroke onset within 3–4.5 hours (mRS 0–1, 35.3% vs. 30.1%, adjusted OR 1.26; 95% CI, 1.05–1.51).[6] Thrombolysis with alteplase is approved from 3–4.5 hours in Europe, Australia, and many countries including all the leading guidelines. But US FDA has approved alteplase for thrombolysis only up to 3 hours. This may be due to the controversy in the evidence for thrombolysis using alteplase in 3–4.5 hours. In the ECAS III trial, there were baseline differences in the form of lower proportion of patients with previous stroke in alteplase group (7.7% vs. 14.1%, p = 0.003). When these patients were excluded and analyzed there was no significant difference in the primary outcome between alteplase and placebo (OR 1.19, 95% CI 0.89–1.59).[7] In the IST-3 trial, even though the statistical analysis plan mentioned subgroup analysis using 95% CI, in the final analysis the authors used 99% CI. BS Alper et al. had done an unadjusted analysis of this data using 95% CI and uncovered a significant reduction in functional outcome (OR 0.76, 95% CI 0.60–0.97, number needed to harm, NNH = 16).[8] Thrombolytic therapy beyond 4.5 hours was not found beneficial in three trials which used then existing conventional inclusion criteria

[Alteplase Thrombolysis for Acute Noninterventional Therapy in Ischemic Stroke-A (ATLANTIS-A), ATLANTIS-B and IST-3].[9-11]

RECENT ADVANCES IN STROKE THROMBOLYSIS

Risk of major intracranial hemorrhage, low recanalization rates for large vessel occlusion (LVO), requirement for continuous infusion, and narrow window period are the major limitations of the currently approved thrombolytic agent, alteplase. Stroke research in the last decade had tried to surpass these limitations.

Low-dose versus Standard-dose Alteplase

The popular belief that there is higher risk of bleeding in Asians had led to approval of lower dose alteplase (0.6 mg/kg) in Japan based on a single group, open-label study with 103 patients.[12,13] The Enhanced Control of Hypertension and Thrombolysis Stroke Study (ENCHANTED) trial assessed whether low-dose alteplase was as effective as usual dose in efficacy and risk for hemorrhage in a noninferiority hypothesis. It did not show noninferiority of low-dose alteplase in decreasing death or disability after AIS (mRS 2–6, 53.2% vs. 51.1%; OR 1.09; 95% CI, 0.95–1.25, p = 0.51 for noninferiority). But the rate of symptomatic ICH was significantly lower in low-dose alteplase (1.0% vs. 2.1%, OR 0.48; 95% CI, 0.27–0.86, p = 0.01). The secondary analysis of ENCHANTED trial found no clear differential benefit of low-dose alteplase in older, Asian, or severely affected patients with AIS compared to standard-dose alteplase.[14] Hence, the clinical equipoise remains regarding low-dose alteplase even though we now know that risk of symptomatic ICH is lesser.

Thrombolysis in Minor Nondisabling Stroke

The role of thrombolysis with alteplase in minor non-disabling stroke is ambiguous. The American Heart Association (AHA) 2018 guidelines states "within 3 hours from symptom onset, treatment of patients with mild ischemic stroke symptoms that are judged as nondisabling may be considered. Treatment risks should be weighed against possible benefits, however, more study is needed to further define the risk-to-benefit ratio [Class IIb; level of evidence C (LoE C)]". The first RCTs on thrombolysis in acute mild ischemic stroke with no disabling deficit (PRISMS: A Study of the Efficacy and Safety of Alteplase in Participants with Mild Stroke-NCT02072226) was stopped early recently due to slow recruitment (not published yet, abstract presented in International Stroke Conference, 2018). The trial had enrolled 313 patients (out of intended 948 patients) and hence was underpowered. An intention-to-treat (ITT) analysis was done for 156 patients in the alteplase group and 157 in the aspirin only group. The rate of symptomatic ICH (32% vs. 0) and any ICH (7.1% vs. 3.3%) was more in alteplase. Hence, among patients with low National Institute of Health Stroke Scale (NIHSS) scores and with no disabling deficits, alteplase may not provide benefit and increases the risk of intracranial hemorrhage.[15]

Thrombolysis in Wake-up Stroke

Role of thrombolytic agents in wake-up stroke was controversial since time of onset of stroke was unknown. WAKE-UP trial [Magnetic Resonance Imaging (MRI)-Guided Thrombolysis for Stroke with Unknown Time of Onset] was designed to answer this highly clinically relevant research question.[16] It was a multicenter, randomized double-blind placebo controlled trial which recruited stroke patients with unknown onset and coexisting diffusion-fluid-attenuated inversion recovery (FLAIR) mismatch in MRI. This mismatch (ischemic lesion visible in diffusion images but no lesion in FLAIR images) indicates that stroke might have occurred within 4.5 hours. They had excluded patients planned for thrombectomy. The trial was stopped early due to lack of funding after enrolling 500 patients of the estimated 800 patients. The primary outcome of mRS 0–1 was achieved significantly higher by alteplase group compared to placebo (53.3% vs. 41.8%; adjusted OR 1.61; 95% CI, 1.09–2.36, p = 0.02) with number needed to treat (NNT) of 8.7. There was no difference in rate of symptomatic hemorrhage (2% vs. 0.4%; OR 4.95; 95% CI, 0.57 to 42.87, p = 0.15). This gives hope to wake-up stroke patients without LVO and still have a salvageable ischemic penumbra.

NEXT GENERATION THROMBOLYTIC AGENT: TENECTEPLASE

An ideal thrombolytic agent should be efficacious, fast and long acting, with higher fibrin specificity, without pro-coagulant effect, lesser intracranial or systemic hemorrhages, active in platelet rich thrombi and finally also be cost-effective. Many "next generation" thrombolytic agents evolved over last decade and the most promising one is tenecteplase (TNK) which is a genetically modified tissue plasminogen activator with pharmacologic advantage over alteplase. TNK amino acid sequence differs from alteplase at three sites. TNK has similar mechanism of action but has 14-fold greater fibrin specificity, 80-fold greater resistance to inactivation by plasminogen activator inhibitor-1, no procoagulant action, longer half-life (18 min) and slower plasma clearance compared to alteplase (Table 1).[17,18] Hence, the availability of a thrombolytic agent which can be given as a single intravenous bolus in AIS was exciting.

Evidence for Tenecteplase in Acute Ischemic Stroke

Haley et al. showed safety of TNK in AIS in an open-labeled dose escalation study involving 88 patients using four doses of TNK (0.1, 0.2, 0.4, and 0.5 mg/kg). Symptomatic ICH occurred only in 0.5 mg/kg (2/13, 13% patients).[19] This was followed by four phase 2 trials which gave reasonable assurance regarding safety and efficacy of TNK. Parson et al. (2009) showed in a prospective non-randomized trial, greater

TABLE 1: Comparison of pharmacokinetic and pharmacodynamic properties of alteplase and tenecteplase

Properties	tPA	TNK
Fibrin specificity	++	+++
Thrombolytic potency	+	+++
PAI-1 resistance	–	++
Fibrinogen depletion	++	+
PRT activity	++	+++
Clearance (mL/kg/min)	16.1	1.9

PAI, plasminogen activator inhibitor; PRT, platelet-rich thrombus; tPA, tissue plasminogen activator; TNK, tenecteplase.

efficacy of intravenous TNK (0.1 mg/kg) in AIS patients with a defined ischemic-perfusion mismatch from a proximal vessel occlusion. Intravenous (IV) TNK arm had greater reperfusion, lesser infarct growth, and better early clinical improvement than patients who received IV tPA (0.9 mg/kg) in the 3 hours window. But the first randomized controlled trial comparing three doses of TNK with alteplase within the 3 hours window period was stopped early due to slow enrolment. But the 0.4 mg/kg TNK arm had an increased risk of hemorrhage. No definite conclusion on superiority or non-inferiority could be drawn from it. Parson et al. (2012) came up with their first phase 2 RCT on 75 AIS patients (perfusion mismatch with LVO, 0–6 h) with three arms (0.1 mg/kg TNK, 0.25 mg/kg TNK and 0.9 mg/kg tPA). Both the TNK arms had better reperfusion and clinical improvement at 24 hours compared to alteplase. The study had a selection bias for small cerebral infarctions affecting its generalizability.[20-23] Another phase 2 trial (ATTEST: Alteplase versus TNK for Thrombolysis after Ischemic Stroke) failed to show any significant difference between alteplase and TNK in AIS patients within 4.5 hours.[24] They used conventional eligibility criteria for inclusion in trial and then used computed tomography (CT) perfusion and CT angiography to find out the percentage of "initial territory-at-risk" on CT perfusion that did not ultimately developed into infarct on the follow-up non-contrast CT scan (primary outcome). Around 35% of patients were excluded from primary analysis since they did not have adequate imaging and also there were significant baseline differences which might have affected the results ultimately.[25]

The first phase 3 clinical trial with 1,100 patients was published in 2017 (NOR-TEST: Norwegian Tenecteplase Stroke Trial) which had a clinical primary outcome.[26] There was no difference in the primary outcome of mRS 0–1 at 3 months (64% vs. 63%, OR 1.08, CI 0.84–1.38, p = 0.52). In both the groups, the frequency of symptomatic ICH was similar. The major limitation of the trial was that more than 80% of patients had minor stroke or stroke mimic who were anyway more likely to have good prognosis.[27] EXTEND-TNK (Tenecteplase versus Alteplase before Endovascular Therapy for Ischemic Stroke) trial (2018) showed that in AIS patients (<4.5 h) with LVO eligible for thrombectomy, TNK caused better reperfusion (22% vs. 10%; OR 2.6; CI, 1.1–5.9) compared to alteplase. There was no difference in proportion of patients who had functionally independent outcome (mRS 0–2) or excellent outcome (mRS 0–1).

A meta-analysis of three phase 2 RCTs[21,23,24] and one phase 3 RCT[26] involving 1,334 patients did not show any significant difference in mRS at 90 days, mortality at 90 days or any ICH/symptomatic ICH.[28] The authors claimed that "TNK group compared to the alteplase group had significantly better early major neurological improvement (relative risk; RR = 1.56, 95% CI 1.00, 2.43, p = 0.05)". The authors have mentioned its grade evidence profile as critical outcome with moderate certainty. The meta-analysis did not include EXTEND-TNK trial. There is a compelling cost-effective argument favoring TNK over alteplase but we need cost-effective/benefit analysis studies to prove the advantage. Since, TNK can reperfuse 22% of LVO, it may be useful in settings where endovascular therapy is not available. We still need to await on-going clinical trials [Tenecteplase versus Alteplase for Stroke Thrombolysis Evaluation (TASTE), ATTEST-2, TNK-tPA for Minor Ischemic Stroke with Proven Acute Symptomatic Occlusion Trial 2 (TEMPO-2), Tenecteplase in Wake-up Ischemic Stroke (TWIST), Extending the Time for Thrombolysis in Emergency Neurological Deficits-Intra-arterial with Tenecteplase (EXTEND-IA TNK) Part 2] before having the final verdict on clinical superiority of TNK over alteplase.

ENDOVASCULAR THERAPY: "TISSUE CLOCK"

Early Window Endovascular Trials

Ever since the results of Multicenter Randomized Clinical Trial of Endovascular Treatment for Acute Ischemic Stroke in the Netherlands (MR CLEAN) trial and the following domino effect of multiple trials being stopped prematurely (Table 2), the standard of care for AIS (<6 h) with an anterior circulation LVO has been mechanical thrombectomy with stent retrievers.[29] The result of these six endovascular RCTs [MR CLEAN, Evaluation Study of Congestive Heart Failure and Pulmonary Artery Catheterization Effectiveness (ESCAPE), REVASCAT, Solitaire with the Intention for Thrombectomy as Primary Endovascular Treatment (SWIFT PRIME), EXTEND-1A, THRACE] contradicted the results of the three previous RCTs [Intervention Management of Stroke (IMS) III, SYNTHESIS and Mechanical Retrieval and Recanalization of Stroke Clots Using Embolectomy (MR RESCUE)]. The reasons for the success of these trials are many including newer (better) technology, better work flow, and patient selection (smaller baseline infarct volume with confirmed LVO). The IPD meta-analysis of five trials [Highly Effective Reperfusion Evaluated in Multiple Endovascular Stroke trials (HERMES) collaboration] with 1,287 patients showed precise superiority of mechanical thrombectomy (mRS 0–1 at 90 days, 26.9% vs. 12.9%; OR 2.49; 95% CI, 1.84–3.35; p <0.0001; mRS 0–2 at 90 days, 46% vs. 26.5%; OR 2.35; CI, 1.85–2.98, p <0.0001).[30] NNT to reduce one point in mRS was 2.6.

Late Window Endovascular Trials

The year 2018 witnessed two landmark trials [DAWN and Diffusion and Perfusion Imaging Evaluation for Understanding Stroke Evolution (DEFUSE) 3] which brought high-quality evidence to extend the window period for

TABLE 2: Comparison of endovascular trials with second generation devices[1]

RCT	MR CLEAN	ESCAPE	EXTEND-IA	SWIFT PRIME	REVASCAT	THERAPY	THRACE
No. of points	500 (267/233)	315 (150/165)	70 (35/35)	196 (98/98)	206 (103/103)	108 (54/54)	412 (208/204)
Baseline NIHSS (median)	18 (14–22) vs. 17 (14–21)	17 (12–20) vs. 16 (13–20)	13 (9–19) vs. 17 (13–20)	17 (13–19) vs. 17 (13–20)	17 (12–19) vs. 17 (14–20)	NR	17 (13–20) vs. 18 (15–21)
Median stroke onset to groin puncture (min)	260	241	210	224	269	226	255
mRS (0–2) at 90 days %	19.1 vs. 32.6	29.3 vs. 53	40 vs. 70	35.5 vs. 60.2	28.2 vs. 43.7	30.4 vs. 38	42.1 vs. 54.2
NNT	7.1	4.2	3.2	4.0	6.3	13.2	8.3

ESCAPE, Evaluation Study of Congestive Heart Failure and Pulmonary Artery Catheterization Effectiveness; EXTEND-IA, Extending the Time for Thrombolysis in Emergency Neurological Deficits-Intra-arterial; MR CLEAN, Multicenter Randomized Clinical Trial of Endovascular Treatment for Acute Ischemic Stroke in the Netherlands; NNT, number needed to treat; NIHSS, National Institute of Health Stroke Scale; RCT, randomized controlled trials; SWIFT PRIME, Solitaire with the Intention for Thrombectomy as Primary Endovascular Treatment; REVASCAT, Randomized trial of revascularization with Solitaire FR device versus best medical therapy in teh treatment of acute stroke due to anterior circulation large vessel occlusion presenting with in eight hours of symptom onset; THERAPY, The randomized concurrent controlled trial to assess the Penumbra systems safety and effectiveness in the treatment of acute stroke; THRACE, Mechanical thrombectomy after intravenous alteplase versus alteplase alone after stroke.

endovascular intervention up to 24 hours by careful selection of patients.[31,32] DAWN (DWI or CTP Assessment with Clinical Mismatch in the Triage of Wake-Up and Late Presenting Strokes Undergoing Neurointervention with Trevo) trial was the first RCT to compare endovascular therapy with standard of care in AIS patients who were last known to be well 6–24 hours earlier.[31] Similar to RCTs with second generation devices, DAWN trial carefully selected patients with small established infarct and a LVO in the anterior circulation. The trial used the concept of "clinical-core mismatch" which was significant clinical deficit disproportionately severe compared to the already established infarct. The infarct volume was measured by automated software on CT perfusion or MRI DWI imaging. The eligibility criteria were one of the following: "group A: age ≥80 years, NIHSS ≥10, core infarct <21 mL; group B: age <80 years, NIHSS ≥10, infarct <31 mL; group C: age <80 years, NIHSS ≥20, infarct 31–<51 mL". DAWN trial enrolled 206 patients (EVT 107 vs. medical 99). The enrolment was stopped early after prespecified interim analysis which showed a high probability of success. Around 60% of patients had wake-up stroke (unknown stroke onset). Compared to medical arm, thrombectomy arm had significant benefit on the 90-day utility-weighted mRS (5.5 vs. 3.4) and rate of functional independence (mRS 0–2, 49% vs. 13%). This benefit was consistent across stroke severity, age, site of vessel involvement and stroke presentation (witnessed vs. unwitnessed vs. wake-up). The patients selected by "tissue window" in DAWN trial had similar rate of functional independence (mRS 0–2) when compared to "time window" in HERMES meta-analysis (DAWN, mRS 0–2 49% vs. HERMES mRS 0–2 46%).

Endovascular Therapy Following Imaging Evaluation for Ischemic Stroke (DEFUSE 3) trial reinforced the shift in paradigm created by DAWN trial. It enrolled 182 AIS patients (6–16 h after the time last known well) and also was stopped early for efficacy.[32] The inclusion criteria were presence of proximal LVO, initial infarct volume less than 70 mL and ratio of volume of ischemic tissue on perfusion imaging to infarct volume of 1.8 or more and an absolute volume of penumbra 15 mL or more assessed by CT perfusion or MR diffusion. Thrombectomy arm had a favorable shift in mRS at 90 days (OR, 2.77; $p < 0.001$) and a higher percentage of patients who were functionally independent (mRS 0–2, 45% vs. 17%, $p < 0.001$). There was lesser 90-day mortality in the endovascular arm and there were no difference in symptomatic ICH or serious adverse events. Thus, both DAWN and DEFUSE 3 have brought class I evidence for mechanical thrombectomy for selected patients satisfying their inclusion criteria.

Both these trials were stopped early which could have led to over estimation of effect of mechanical thrombectomy.[33,34] Majority of patients in both the trials were wake-up strokes, which tend to occur close to awakening. Hence, many of these patients might be biologically within the established window period of 6 hours and the control group in these trials might have been at disadvantage. Even then these trials have shown the wake-up strokes with small core and large penumbra with LVO, mechanical thrombectomy can significantly change the outcome.

Late Window Paradox

Both DAWN and DEFUSE trials have shown us the concept of "late window paradox".[35] Since "time is brain", interventions done more than 6 hours of stroke onset should be less beneficial than those done within 6 hours. But results of DEFUSE and DAWN were better than those endovascular trials done within 6 hours. In fact, DAWN had the largest absolute increase (35.5%) in functional independence across any stroke therapy trial even after median time from stroke onset being 12.5 hours. DEFUSE 3 had 28% increase in functional independence and had the largest reduction in mortality/severe morbidity (20%) ever achieved. Even HERMES (pooled analysis of five early window endovascular RCTs) had only 19.5% absolute increase in functional independence and 11% decrease in mortality. All these trials had similar patients, stroke severity, thrombectomy devices and reperfusion achievement. These better results in late window endovascular trials are called "late window paradox". Various factors affect this phenomenon. A significant number of stroke patients with LVO have very protracted growth of the ischemic core for 12 hours or even longer. It is the good collateral circulation which keeps the ischemic core size small for this long period and eventually fails to increase the size of infarct. So, DAWN and DEFUSE had enrolled patients with very small ischemic core, very slow growth rate of infarct and large penumbra. The medical arm of these trials would have poor outcomes as most of them would not receive IV tPA as they are out of window period of 4.5 hours and their collateral circulation will eventually fail causing large infarct.

CONCLUSION

The recent advances in the reperfusion strategies have added "tissue window" to the existing "time window" and many patients with small ischemic core, large penumbra, good collaterals may benefit from mechanical thrombectomy if they have a proximal LVO even if they arrive within 6–24 hours of stroke onset. Wake-up stroke patients with unknown stroke onset may also benefit from thrombolysis with alteplase if they have diffusion-FLAIR mismatch. The next generation thrombolytic agent, TNK has shown huge promise and we eagerly wait for the on-going trials to provide definite evidence for its clinical superiority over alteplase.

REFERENCES

1. Bhaskar S, Stanwell P, Cordato D, et al. Reperfusion therapy in acute ischemic stroke: dawn of a new era? BMC Neurol. 2018;18(1):8.
2. National Institute of Neurological Disorders and Stroke rt-PA Stroke Study Group. Tissue plasminogen activator for acute ischemic stroke. N Engl J Med. 1995;333(24):1581-7.
3. Hacke W, Kaste M, Fieschi C, et al. Intravenous thrombolysis with recombinant tissue plasminogen activator for acute hemispheric stroke. The European Cooperative Acute Stroke Study (ECASS). JAMA. 1995;274(13):1017-25.
4. Shobha N, Buchan AM, Hill MD, et al. Thrombolysis at 3-4.5 hours after acute ischemic stroke onset—evidence from the Canadian Alteplase for Stroke Effectiveness Study (CASES) registry. Cerebrovasc Dis. 2011;31(3):223-8.
5. Ahmed N, Wahlgren N, Grond M, et al. Implementation and outcome of thrombolysis with alteplase 3–4.5 h after an acute stroke: an updated analysis from SITS-ISTR. Lancet Neurol. 2010;9(9):866-74.
6. Emberson J, Lees KR, Lyden P, et al. Effect of treatment delay, age, and stroke severity on the effects of intravenous thrombolysis with alteplase for acute ischaemic stroke: a meta-analysis of individual patient data from randomised trials. Lancet Lond Engl. 2014;384(9958):1929-35.
7. Shy BD. Implications of ECASS III error on emergency department treatment of ischemic stroke. J Emerg Med. 2014;46(3):385-6.
8. Alper BS, Malone-Moses M, McLellan JS, et al. Thrombolysis in acute ischaemic stroke: time for a rethink? BMJ. 2015;350:h1075.
9. Clark WM, Albers GW, Madden KP, et al. The rtPA (alteplase) 0- to 6-hour acute stroke trial, part A (A0276g) : results of a double-blind, placebo-controlled, multicenter study. Thrombolytic therapy in acute ischemic stroke study investigators. Stroke. 2000;31(4):811-6.
10. Clark WM, Wissman S, Albers GW, et al. Recombinant tissue-type plasminogen activator (Alteplase) for ischemic stroke 3 to 5 hours after symptom onset. The ATLANTIS Study: a randomized controlled trial. Alteplase Thrombolysis for Acute Noninterventional Therapy in Ischemic Stroke. JAMA. 1999;282(21):2019-26.
11. Sandercock P, Wardlaw JM, Lindley RI, et al. The benefits and harms of intravenous thrombolysis with recombinant tissue plasminogen activator within 6 h of acute ischaemic stroke (the third international stroke trial [IST-3]): a randomised controlled trial. Lancet Lond Engl. 2012;379(9834):2352-63.
12. Anderson CS, Robinson T, Lindley RI, et al. Low-dose versus standard-dose intravenous alteplase in acute ischemic stroke. N Engl J Med. 2016;374(24):2313-23.
13. Sila C. Finding the right t-PA dose for Asians with acute ischemic stroke. N Engl J Med. 2016;374(24):2389-90.
14. Wang X, Robinson TG, Lee T-H, et al. Low-dose vs standard-dose alteplase for patients with acute ischemic stroke: secondary analysis of the ENCHANTED randomized clinical trial. JAMA Neurol. 2017;74(11):1328-35.
15. Ellis F. (2018). Treating tPA in mild strokes found not protective. [online] Available from https://journals.lww.com/neurotodayonline/blog/NeurologyTodayConferenceReporterInternationalStrokeConference/pages/post.aspx?PostID=23. [Accessed August 2018].
16. Thomalla G, Simonsen CZ, Boutitie F, et al. MRI-guided thrombolysis for stroke with unknown time of onset. N Engl J Med. 2018;379(7):611-22.
17. Keyt BA, Paoni NF, Refino CJ, et al. A faster-acting and more potent form of tissue plasminogen activator. Proc Natl Acad Sci U S A. 1994;91(9):3670-4.
18. Behrouz R. Intravenous tenecteplase in acute ischemic stroke: an updated review. J Neurol. 2014;261(6):1069-72.
19. Haley EC, Lyden PD, Johnston KC, et al. A pilot dose-escalation safety study of tenecteplase in acute ischemic stroke. Stroke. 2005;36(3):607-12.
20. Parsons MW, Miteff F, Bateman GA, et al. Acute ischemic stroke: imaging-guided tenecteplase treatment in an extended time window. Neurology. 2009;72(10):915-21.
21. Haley EC, Thompson JLP, Grotta JC, et al. Phase IIB/III trial of tenecteplase in acute ischemic stroke: results of a prematurely terminated randomized clinical trial. Stroke. 2010;41(4):707-11.
22. Molina CA. Reperfusion therapies for acute ischemic stroke: current pharmacological and mechanical approaches. Stroke. 2011;42(1 Suppl):S16-9.
23. Parsons M, Spratt N, Bivard A, et al. A randomized trial of tenecteplase versus alteplase for acute ischemic stroke. N Engl J Med. 2012;366(12):1099-107.
24. Huang X, Cheripelli BK, Lloyd SM, et al. Alteplase versus tenecteplase for thrombolysis after ischaemic stroke (ATTEST): a phase 2, randomised, open-label, blinded endpoint study. Lancet Neurol. 2015;14(4):368-76.
25. González RG. Tenecteplase versus alteplase for acute ischemic stroke. N Engl J Med. 2012;367(3):275-6.
26. Logallo N, Novotny V, Assmus J, et al. Tenecteplase versus alteplase for management of acute ischaemic stroke (NOR-TEST): a phase 3, randomised, open-label, blinded endpoint trial. Lancet Neurol. 2017;16(10):781-8.
27. Anderson CS. NOR-TEST-ing tenecteplase in acute ischaemic stroke. Lancet Neurol. 2017;16(10):762-3.
28. Thelengana A, Radhakrishnan DM, Prasad M, et al. Tenecteplase versus alteplase in acute ischemic stroke: systematic review and meta-analysis. Acta Neurol Belg. 2018. [Epub ahead of print]
29. Powers WJ, Derdeyn CP, Biller J, et al. 2015 American Heart Association/American Stroke Association Focused Update of the 2013 Guidelines for the Early Management of Patients With Acute Ischemic Stroke Regarding Endovascular Treatment: A Guideline for Healthcare Professionals From the American Heart Association/American Stroke Association. Stroke. 2015;46(10):3020-35.
30. Goyal M, Menon BK, van Zwam WH, et al. Endovascular thrombectomy after large-vessel ischaemic stroke: a meta-analysis of individual patient data from five randomised trials. Lancet Lond Engl. 2016;387(10029):1723-31.
31. Nogueira RG, Jadhav AP, Haussen DC, et al. Thrombectomy 6 to 24 Hours after Stroke with a Mismatch between Deficit and Infarct. N Engl J Med. 2018;378(1):11-21.
32. Albers GW, Marks MP, Kemp S, et al. Thrombectomy for Stroke at 6 to 16 Hours with Selection by Perfusion Imaging. N Engl J Med. 2018;378(8):708-18.
33. Vinny PW, Vishnu VY, Padma Srivastava MV. Thrombectomy 6 to 24 Hours after Stroke. N Engl J Med. 2018;378(12):1161.
34. Vinny PW, Vishnu VY, Srivastava MVP. Thrombectomy for Stroke with Selection by Perfusion Imaging. N Engl J Med. 2018;378(19):1849.
35. Albers GW. Late Window Paradox. Stroke. 2018;49(3):768-71.

CHAPTER 129

Prevention of Stroke in Cardiac Patients

Harsh Wardhan, Nitin Aggarwal

INTRODUCTION

Stroke remains a major global health problem, and due to the ongoing demographic changes, including aging and health transitions observed in developing countries its impact is likely to increase in the future. The increasing global stroke burden strongly suggests that currently implemented primary stroke prevention strategies are not sufficiently effective, and new primary prevention strategies with larger effect sizes are needed. For the prevention of early recurrent ischemic stroke, the advantages of aspirin are greater than previously recognized. Direct oral anticoagulants (OACs) as an alternative to warfarin for atrial fibrillation (AF), and carotid stenting as an alternative to endarterectomy for symptomatic carotid stenosis are the other strategies used nowadays to prevent recurrent stroke. Despite stable incidence rates and declining mortality rates over the past two decades, the number of incident strokes, prevalent stroke survivors, disability-adjusted life years (DALYs) lost due to stroke, and stroke-related deaths are increasing. This review highlights recent developments in prevention of stroke in cardiac patients.

DEFINITION OF STROKE AND TRANSIENT ISCHEMIC ATTACK

Stroke is distinguished from transient ischemic attack (TIA), if the symptoms persist longer than 24 hours (or lead to earlier death). An updated definition of stroke is an acute episode of focal dysfunction of the brain, retina, or spinal cord lasting longer than 24 hours, or of any duration if imaging [computed tomography (CT) or magnetic resonance imaging (MRI)] or autopsy shows focal infarction or hemorrhage relevant to the symptoms.[1] This definition includes subarachnoid hemorrhage.[1] A TIA has been redefined as focal dysfunction of less than 24 hours duration and with no imaging evidence of infarction.[1]

CARDIAC EMBOLISM AND STROKE

Cardioembolic stroke accounts for 25% of all ischemic strokes[2] and due the advancement in cardiac imaging, its frequency has increased over time.[2] Various cardiac disorders may be the cause of cardioembolic stroke; however, it occurs most commonly as a result of AF in adults (50%) (Fig. 1).[3,4] Other important causes include ventricular thrombus (20%), structural heart defects or tumors (15%), and valvular heart disease (15%) (Box 1).[5] Although the aortic arch is not a cardiac structure, it is usually considered under sources of cardiac embolism.

Cardioembolic stroke is therefore a syndrome with diverse causes and not a single disease entity. A systematic approach, including a detailed history, physical examination, and review of neuroimaging, electrocardiogram, and echocardiographic

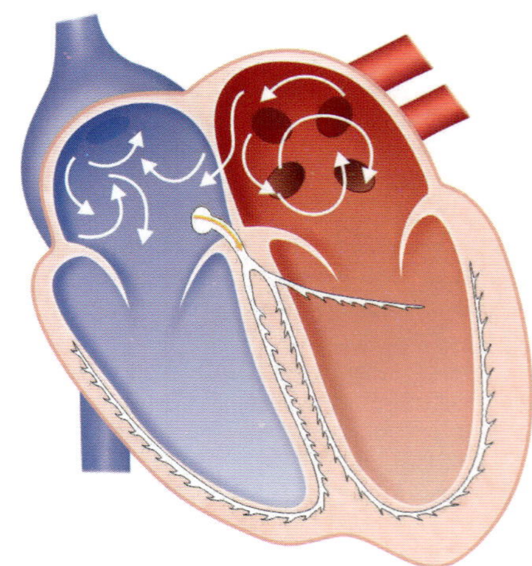

FIG. 1: Atrial fibrillation. Diagram depicts the abnormal electrical activity within the atria, which may lead to uncoordinated contraction of the atria, stagnant blood, and thrombus formation, and an irregular heart rhythm.

BOX 1 Major causes of cardioembolic stroke

Etiology of cardioembolism

- Atrial fibrillation
- Valvular heart disease
- Ventricular thrombus
- Structural heart defects or tumors
- Myocardial infarction
- Congestive heart failure
- Patent foramen ovale
- Infective endocarditis
- Prosthetic valves

data, may be helpful to know the cause of cardioembolic stroke. Echocardiography, especially transesophageal echocardiography (TEE), remains the diagnostic standard to evaluate for cardioembolic sources of stroke.[6] TEE is superior to transthoracic echocardiography (TTE) for the detection of cardioembolic sources.[7] Overall, cardiac embolism as the cause of stroke is diagnosed in the absence of a large artery stenosis or occlusion, a clinical syndrome or radiographic appearance of a lacunar stroke, and unusual causes of stroke (e.g., vasculitis and drug abuse). However, approximately 15% of patients who have lacunar syndromes would also have risk factors for cardioembolism.[8]

STROKE PREVENTION IN ATRIAL FIBRILLATION

Atrial fibrillation is the most common cardiac arrhythmia and the incidence and prevalence of this disease are rising. It is estimated that by the year 2050 there will be over 7.5 million patients with AF in the USA alone.[9] This disease carries a significant risk of morbidity and mortality driven in large part by the development of heart failure and thromboembolism.[10] Oral anticoagulation therapy is effective in reducing risk of stroke and systemic embolism and is the standard of care for patients undergoing either a rhythm or rate control strategy.

Systemic embolization is a potential complication of any form of AF, and it can occur in patients with acute AF lasting as little as 72 hours. The forms of AF proposed by the American College of Cardiology or American Heart Association (AHA) or European Society of Cardiology are as follows:[11,12]

- *Paroxysmal*: Self-terminating AF, in which episodes generally last less than 7 days and usually less than 24 hours; it may be recurrent
- *Persistent*: Fails to self-terminate and lasts longer than 7 days
- *Permanent*: Lasts for more than 1 year
- *Lone*: Paroxysmal, persistent, or permanent AF in the absence of structural heart disease
- *Nonvalvular*: Cases without rheumatic mitral valve disease, prosthetic heart valve, or valve repair.

However, the stroke risk is increased fivefold in AF; it is not homogeneous and is associated with the presence of various stroke risk factors.[13] The more commonly encountered risk factors have been used to formulate stroke risk stratification scores, such as the CHA_2DS_2-VASc score.[14] The latter was designed to be simple, extending the older CHADS2 score by recognizing that age is an important driver of stroke risk (with the risk increasing above 65 years of age, although in Asians, this risk may rise from age 50 upwards, hence requiring a recalibration of the CHA_2DS_2-VASc score),[15,16] and that other commonly encountered risk factors such as "complicated" vascular disease (e.g., myocardial infarction and peripheral artery disease) would also increase risks. CHA_2DS_2-VASc is consistently good at identifying "low risk" patients and if an AF patient is defined as low risk using CHA_2DS_2-VASc (i.e., 0 in males and 1 in females), event rates (whether stroke or death) are usually less than 1% per year.

Treatment thresholds for stroke prevention with a stroke event rate of 1% per year is generally regarded as the threshold for thromboprophylaxis, given that AF-related strokes are more likely to be fatal or severely disabling.[17] Even a single stroke risk factor confers an excess risk of stroke or mortality,[18] and the net clinical benefit is positive for OAC compared to aspirin or leaving such patients untreated.[19]

The "Birmingham 3-step" management pathway to streamline decision-making for stroke prevention in patients with AF is shown in the flowchart 1.[20] The first step is to identify and offer stroke prevention to AF patients with low or even more than 1 stroke risk factors. At second step, a practical stroke score is meant to be reductionist, so that it does not matter whether the CHA_2DS_2-VASc score is 2 or 9 points, or whether biomarkers are positive or negative—that AF patient needs stroke prevention, which is OAC. For the latter or the third step, decision making between a vitamin K antagonist (VKA) or new oral anticoagulant (NOAC) can be helped by using the SAMe-TT_2R_2 score,[21] [sex, age (<60 years); medical history (at least two of the following—hypertension, diabetes, coronary artery disease or myocardial infarction, peripheral arterial disease, congestive heart failure, previous stroke, pulmonary disease, and hepatic or renal disease); treatment (interacting drugs, e.g., amiodarone for rhythm control) (all 1 point); and the current tobacco use (2 points) and race (non-Caucasian; 2 points)] where patients with a score 0–2 are likely to do well on VKA with a good time in therapeutic range (TTR), whilst those with a score more than 2 are less likely to achieve a good TTR and additional measures such as regular follow-up [with international normalized ratio (INR) checks] and counseling, or a NOAC could be considered.[21] Persistence and adherence with OAC are additional considerations, with some evidence for better compliance with NOACs compared to VKA.

Bleeding risk assessment has also been subjected to much misinformation and bleeding risk scores have been misused by the ill-informed.[22] Many of the potentially reversible bleeding risk factors are contained within the HAS-BLED (Hypertension, Abnormal renal or liver function, Stroke, Bleeding, Labile INR, Elderly, Drugs or alcohol) score,[22] which is a simple and well-validated score that has been tested in AF and non-AF patients, and is also predictive of bleeding risks in a patient not on antithrombotic therapy, aspirin, and on anticoagulation (whether with a VKA or a non-VKA anticoagulant); thus, the HAS-BLED score is applicable throughout the patient pathway. A high HAS-BLED score more than or equal to 3 is not an excuse to withhold OAC, and has been shown to be predictive of intracranial hemorrhage, the most feared complication of OAC.

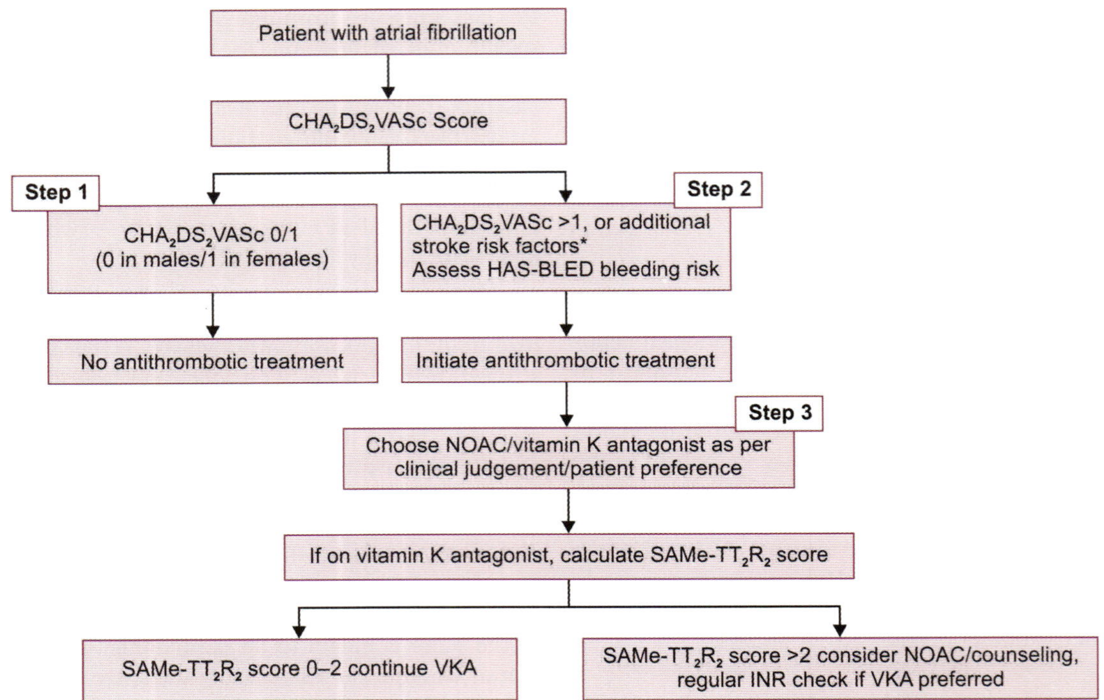

*Also calculate the HAS-BLED score. If HAS-BLED ≥3, address the modifiable bleeding risk factors and plan a closer clinical follow-up.

HAS-BLED, Hypertension, Abnormal renal or liver function, Stroke, Bleeding, Labile international normalized ratio, Elderly, Drugs or alcohol; NOAC, new oral anticoagulant; VKA, vitamin K antagonist; INR, international normalized ratio.

FLOWCHART 1: The Birmingham 3 step management pathway to streamline decision making for stroke prevention in patients with atrial fibrillation.

ORAL ANTICOAGULANTS

Vitamin K antagonists have been the main drugs for the antithrombotic prevention in AF for 60 years. Despite its unquestionable impact to prevent strokes, medical community has to deal with significant limitations, such as common drug or food interactions, and the necessity of regular monitoring to adjust doses and inter alia. In the last 10 years, OAC therapy is now witnessing a revolution after the completion of large phase III clinical trials on the commonly termed NOACs. Advantage of the new agents is the use of fixed-dosing with no need for monitoring, few interactions, and a wider therapeutic window counteract their current disadvantages. The lack of an effective antidote, cost, or reservations in patients with kidney disease may explain their slow rate of expansion.

Two classes of NOACs are currently available, (1) the oral direct thrombin inhibitors (DTIs; e.g., dabigatran) and (2) oral direct factor Xa inhibitors (e.g., rivaroxaban, apixaban, and edoxaban). These drugs block only a single step in coagulation, unlike VKAs, which block the formation of multiple active vitamin K-dependent coagulation factors (factors II, VII, IX, and X). Recent data from seven European countries show a much better adherence to evidence and recommendations for oral anticoagulation.[23]

Dabigatran

Dabigatran etexilate was the first NOACs studied and Food and Drug Administration (FDA) approved, is a highly specific and competitive DTI, based on the results of the RE-LY (Randomized Evaluation of Long-term anticoagulant therapY with dabigatran etexilate) trial.[24] The RE-LY trial comparing two blinded doses of dabigatran etexilate (110 or 150 mg BID) with warfarin in 18,113 patients with AF and at least one additional risk factor (a mean CHADS score of 2.1). Dabigatran 150 mg BID was superior to warfarin with no significant differences in major bleedings. Gastrointestinal (GI) bleeding was more frequent with dabigatran 150 mg BD. Dabigatran 110 mg BD was noninferior to warfarin for the primary efficacy endpoint of stroke and systemic embolism, with a reduction of 20% in major bleedings. RELY-ABLE (The subsequent Long-term Multicenter Extension of Dabigatran Treatment in Patients with Atrial Fibrillation) study threw light on the long-term effects of two doses of dabigatran in patients completing RE-LY by extending the follow-up of patients on dabigatran from a mean of 2 years at the end of RE-LY by an additional 2.3 years.[25] Patients on warfarin were not enrolled in this study. RELY-ABLE confirmed the results reported in RE-LY.

Rivaroxaban

Rivaroxaban, a competitive and dose-dependent direct inhibitor of factor Xa and the second NOAC approved by the FDA and European Medicines Agency (EMA) based on the ROCKET AF (Rivaroxaban-Once Daily Oral Direct Factor Xa Inhibition Compared with Vitamin K Antagonism for Prevention of Stroke and Embolism Trial in Atrial

Fibrillation).[26] The ROCKET AF was a double-blinded study, which included 14,264 patients with nonvalvular AF and CHADS2 scores more than or equal to 2 (mean 3.5). The subjects were randomly assigned to rivaroxaban 20 mg once daily or dose adjusted warfarin. Patients with creatinine clearance (CrCl) of 30–49 mL/min received 15 mg of rivaroxaban. After a median follow-up of 1.93 years, Rivaroxaban was noninferior to warfarin for the prevention of stroke or systemic embolism; however, rivaroxaban failed to show superiority over warfarin in the intention-to-treat analysis (p <0.12). There were no differences in the risk of major bleeding, although intracranial and fatal bleeding occurred less frequently in the rivaroxaban group.

Apixaban

Apixaban, a direct, reversible, competitive, and selective inhibitor of factor Xa and the last NOAC approved by the FDA and EMA for the prevention of stroke and embolism in nonvalvular AF. The ARISTOTLE[27] (Apixaban for Reduction In STroke and Other ThromboemboLic Events in AF) was a randomized, double-blinded, double-dummy, and phase III trial comparing apixaban (5 mg BID) with dose-adjusted warfarin in 18,201 patients with nonvalvular AF (a mean CHADS2 score of 2.1). After a mean follow-up of 1.8 years, apixaban was found to be superior than warfarin, with fewer primary outcomes (overall strokes—both ischemic and hemorrhagic—and systemic emboli); however, there was no significant difference in the rate of ischemic strokes. Patients treated with apixaban had significantly fewer intracranial bleeds, but GI bleedings were similar between both groups. All-cause mortality was found to be significantly lower in the apixaban group. Similar results were found in the AVERROES study[28] when compared with aspirin alone.

Edoxaban

Edoxaban is another reversible factor Xa inhibitor, recently approved by the FDA but not yet by the EMA. The ENGAGE AF-TIMI 48 (Effective Anticoagulation with Factor Xa Next Generation in Atrial Fibrillation-Thrombolysis in Myocardial Infarction 48)[29] was a three-group, randomized, double-blinded, and double-dummy phase III trial, which compared the two dose regimens of edoxaban (30 mg once daily and 60 mg once daily) with warfarin in a total of 21,026 patients with nonvalvular AF. After a follow-up of 2.8 years, Both the regimens of edoxaban were noninferior to warfarin with respect to the prevention of stroke or systemic embolism, after a follow-up of 2.8 years; however, the lower dose trended toward inferiority, with a hazard ratio of 1.13 versus warfarin, and was inferior to specifically prevent ischemic stroke. Edoxaban was associated with lower, dose-related rates of bleeding, including major bleeding, intracranial bleeding, and life-threatening bleeding. An exception was GI bleeding, which occurred more frequently with high-dose edoxaban, but less frequently with low-dose edoxaban compared with warfarin.

Comparison between New Oral Anticoagulants

For the time being, no direct head-to-head comparisons between NOACs have been made in randomized controlled trials. The choice of one or another NOAC for a given patient is influenced by individual patient characteristics, including risk of stroke or venous thromboembolism (VTE), risk of bleeding, and comorbidity such us the presence of impaired renal function. Figure 2 show the comparative efficacy of high-dose of NOACs and warfarin.[30] Comparative analysis of the four NOACs confirmed that NOACs significantly reduced the composite of stroke or systemic embolic events by 19% compared with warfarin, which very much depended on large reduction in hemorrhagic strokes. Table 1 summarizes general recommendations based on patient characteristics, drug compliance, and tolerability. All NOACs except apixaban were associated with more GI bleeding than warfarin. However, it is important to highlight that at present all NOACs are clinically indicated in nonvalvular AF regardless of the estimated risk of stroke or bleeding. Finally, VKAs remain the first-line anticoagulant for patients with mechanical heart valves or rheumatic heart disease and for those with severe renal insufficiency, in whom NOACs are contraindicated.

PATENT FORAMEN OVALE

Patent foramen ovale (PFO) is a flap-like defect in the interatrial septum (Fig. 2) and a common finding (25%) in the general population, but in 40% of adults with cryptogenic stroke. The relationship of PFO and ischemic stroke remains an area of considerable debate. The mechanism through which PFO causes ischemic stroke remains speculative. The

TABLE 1: Suggested use of new oral anticoagulants according to patient characteristics

Patients characteristics	NOAC	Dose regimen
High risk of stroke	Dabigatran	150 mg BID (high CHADS-VASC score)
Previous stroke	Rivaroxaban	20 mg QD
High risk of bleeding or	Dabigatran	110 mg BID
Previous life-threatening bleedings	Apixaban	5 mg BID
Dyspepsia	Rivaroxaban	20 mg QD
	Apixaban	5 mg BID
GI bleeding	Apixaban	5 mg BID
Medication compliance problems	Rivaroxaban	20 mg QD
Elderly (≥80 years) and impaired renal function	Apixaban	2.5 mg BID

BID, twice daily; GI, gastrointestinal; NOAC, new oral anticoagulants; QD, once daily.

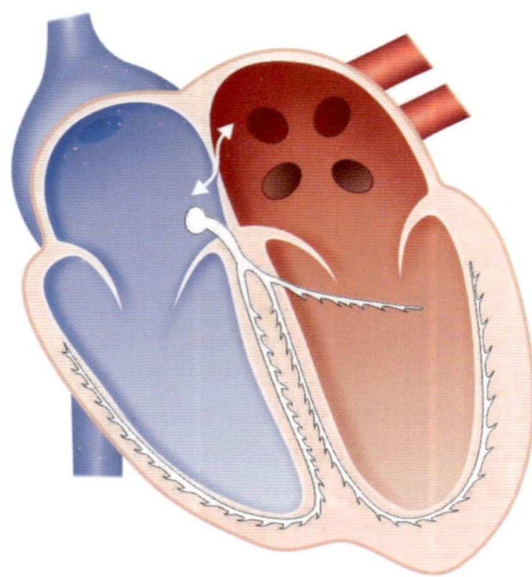

FIG. 2: Right to left shunting through patent foramen ovale.

prevailing hypothesis is that PFO-mediated stroke results from "paradoxical" (right to left) embolism caused by clots originating in the right side of the venous circulation proximal to the PFO that then traveling to the left atrium and the systemic circulation. Clinical examination of patients with PFO, documented deep vein thrombosis (DVT) and simultaneous pulmonary embolism (PE), and ischemic stroke support a right-sided to left-sided, or "paradoxical," circulatory mechanism for stroke. Another hypothesis regarding PFO-mediated stroke is that vasoactive substances (e.g., serotonin) usually deactivated in the pulmonary circulation cross into the systemic circulation and lead to ischemic stroke. The latter hypothesis is weakly supported by the finding of patients with PFO and experience migraines who improve after PFO closure. Some studies suggest that the size of the PFO defect is important, with a large PFO (≥2 mm) more likely to be associated with an embolic stroke than a small PFO (<2 mm).[31]

Medical Therapy versus Closure for Patent Foramen Ovale

Despite the association between PFO and cryptogenic stroke, three early randomized clinical trials [CLOSURE I (Evaluation of the STARFlex Septal Closure System in Patients with a Stroke and/or Transient Ischemic Attack due to Presumed Paradoxical Embolism through a Patent Foramen Ovale),[32] PC (Percutaneous Closure of Patent Foramen Ovale in Cryptogenic Embolism) trial,[33] and RESPECT (Randomized Evaluation of Recurrent Stroke Comparing PFO Closure to Established Current Standard of Care Treatment)[34] short-term] did not show a clear benefit of PFO closure for secondary stroke prevention. However, after FDA approval of the Amplatzer PFO occluder device and the results of two new randomized controlled trials,[35,36] PFO closure seems to be have better results in comparison to medical therapy, in CLOSE (Patent Foramen Ovale Closure or Anticoagulants Versus Antiplatelet Therapy to Prevent Stroke Recurrence),[35] after a mean follow-up of 5.3 years, subjects who underwent PFO closure had a lower risk of recurrent stroke than those maintained on antiplatelet therapy (0% vs. 6%). In REDUCE (Patent Foramen Ovale Closure or Antiplatelet Therapy for Cryptogenic Stroke),[36] after a median follow-up of 3.2 years, subjects who underwent PFO closure had a lower risk of recurrent stroke than those maintained on antiplatelet therapy (1.4% vs. 5.4%). In both these trials, PFO closure was associated with a higher risk of AF, which was believed to be primarily due to the closure procedure itself (i.e., self-limited). Therefore, PFO closure is of moderate benefit compared to antiplatelet therapy alone in the prevention of recurrent ischemic stroke in adults up to 60 years of age. It remains unknown how PFO closure compares to systemic anticoagulation (e.g., with novel OACs) for the prevention of recurrent ischemic stroke.

AORTIC ARCH DISEASE

An overlooked but a potentially serious source of embolic stroke is the aortic arch, especially when proximal aortic atheromatous disease is present. Large (>4 mm) and mobile plaques have a definite embolic potential. The stroke mechanism in patients with large or complex aortic plaques is believed to be predominantly thromboembolic. Aortic embolic disease manifests in different forms, including mobile and ulcerated plaques, aortic dissection, and aneurysms. Patients who have ascending aorta or proximal arch plaques of 4 mm thickness are up to seven times more likely to have cerebral infarction than controls (14.4% vs. 2%; $p < 0.001$).[37] For nonmobile aortic plaque, statin therapy may be protective in preventing stroke,[38] whereas uncertainty remains about whether aspirin or warfarin is the optimal antithrombotic therapy for mobile plaques. Recently published ARCH trial[39] results suggest that in general, patients with stroke or TIA with aortic arch atherosclerosis should be treated with antiplatelet therapy rather than warfarin.

MYOCARDIAL INFARCTION, LEFT VENTRICULAR DYSFUNCTION, AND HEART FAILURE

Myocardial infarction and associated ventricular wall immobility lead to cardiomyopathy resulting in left ventricular thrombus formation and subsequent cardioembolic stroke. Cardioembolic strokes may occur within 1 day of myocardial infarction, and approximately half occur within the first week, although stroke risk remains high up to 3 months and then decreases gradually.[40,41] Anterior wall myocardial infarction bears a higher risk for stroke than inferior wall myocardial infarction (25% vs. 5%). Management of patients who have experienced myocardial infarction with heparin for coronary disease helps decrease the risk for ventricular wall thrombus formation. TEE is the preferred test for detecting left ventricular wall and apical thrombi. Patients who experience anterior wall myocardial infarction and are found to have ventricular wall thrombus should be prescribed warfarin, with the goal of attaining an INR of 2.0–3.0 for up to 6 months, thereafter, aspirin therapy may be given. Prolonged anticoagulation decreased stroke risk up to 40% over 3 years in the ASPECT (Anticoagulants in the Secondary Prevention of Events in Coronary Thrombosis) trial,[41] although major bleeding complications were increased. If AF develops after myocardial infarction, anticoagulation may be considered indefinitely depending on other ischemic stroke risk factors, such as age more than 70 years, hypertension, heart failure, diabetes, and stroke, as per the CHADS-VASc Score.[10-12,17]

DILATED CARDIOMYOPATHY

Dilated cardiomyopathy is associated with different causes (ischemic and nonischemic, infectious, and infiltrative). The Study of Left Ventricular Dysfunction (SOLVD)[42] elucidated the relation between risk of embolic stroke and worsening ventricular function. In this study, warfarin and aspirin were associated with a lower rate of death or hospitalization due to heart failure than aspirin; however, only warfarin reduced death from worsening heart failure. Although, embolic stroke risk doubles when left ventricular ejection fraction (LVEF) declines below 28% compared with 35%, patients also benefit from aspirin alone (56% relative risk reduction in Survival and Ventricular Enlargement (SAVE),[43] without the bleeding complications. The Warfarin and Aspirin Therapy in Chronic Heart Failure trial (WATCH)[44] compares aspirin 160 mg/day, clopidogrel 75 mg/day, and warfarin (INR, 2.5–3.0) in 4,500 patients who had poor left ventricular function. Results showed that warfarin reduced nonfatal stroke compared with aspirin and clopidogrel ($p < 0.05$), but the combined end point of nonfatal myocardial infarction or stroke and death did not reach statistical significance ($p < 0.21$). The WARCEF trial (Warfarin Versus Aspirin in Patients With Reduced Cardiac Ejection Fraction)[45] compares the efficacy of warfarin (INR, 2.5–3.0; target, 2.75) versus aspirin (325 mg/day) on all-cause mortality and stroke (both ischemic and hemorrhagic) in patients who have LVEF of 35% or less. However, there was no significant overall difference in the primary outcome between treatment with warfarin and treatment with aspirin. A reduced risk of ischemic stroke with warfarin was offset by an increased risk of major hemorrhage. Therefore, as per the available data, warfarin did not provide an overall benefit and was associated with an increased risk of bleeding, there is no compelling reason to use warfarin rather than aspirin in patients with a reduced LVEF who are in sinus rhythm.

VALVULAR HEART DISEASE[46,47]

Aortic Stenosis

In calcific aortic valve disease, clinically symptomatic cerebral embolic events are less common, unless concomitant AF, reduced LVEF, or mitral valve disease is present. Calcific emboli to the retina (i.e., asymptomatic emboli) or after valvuloplasty are reported. Antiplatelet therapy may be initiated in patients with TIA and bicuspid calcific aortic stenosis, but anticoagulation is generally not recommended.

Mitral Valve Stenosis

Mitral valve stenosis due to rheumatic heart disease with or without AF is an indication for warfarin anticoagulation, with INR ranging between 2.0 and 3.0, to prevent thromboembolic events (cerebral and systemic). Anticoagulation is recommended in some patients with mitral valve stenosis without AF and evidence of spontaneous echo contrast (SEC) ("smoke") within a large left atrium (>5.5 cm). In these patients, valvuloplasty may be attempted after a sufficient duration of anticoagulation.

Mitral Annular Calcification

Mitral annular calcification (MAC) not only denotes simply calcification of the mitral annulus, but also a syndrome characterized in elderly patients by a calcified mitral annulus, mitral stenosis or regurgitation, aortic stenosis, conduction disturbances, embolic phenomenon, and even endocarditis. Antiplatelet agents are reasonable first-line therapy but if recurrent embolic events occur or AF develops, anticoagulation or valvular repair should be considered.

Mitral Valve Prolapse

Mitral valve prolapse (MVP) is the most common echocardiographic finding in normal individuals (4–6%). Palpitations or chest pain may be observed in symptomatic individuals. MVP is typically a benign echocardiographic finding and not associated with increased stroke risk unless it occurs in combination with MAC, mitral regurgitation, or AF. Antiplatelet agents remain first-line therapy, but anticoagulation is considered for recurrent cerebral ischemic events or MVP associated with AF or another embolic risk factor.

Prosthetic Cardiac Valves

Antithrombotic therapy depends on the type and location of the prosthetic valve and the presence of AF. For metallic valves, warfarin anticoagulation is typically recommended to attain a target INR ranging from 2.5 to 3.5. Prosthetic valves in the mitral position are associated with a higher thrombotic risk than those in the aortic position. Patients who have a bileaflet aortic valve without AF or left ventricular dysfunction should be prescribed warfarin to achieve a target INR ranging from 2.0 to 3.0. In patients with higher risk, aortic bileaflet valves, mitral bileaflet, or caged disc location in association with AF, warfarin with INR intensity of 2.5–3.5 and aspirin, 81–100 mg/day, may be given. Bioprosthetic valves complicated by thrombus formation, AF, or thromboembolism failing antiplatelet therapy may require warfarin anticoagulation with an INR ranging from 2.0–3.0.

Nonbacterial Thrombotic Endocarditis

Nonbacterial thrombotic endocarditis (NBTE), or marantic endocarditis, is a noninfectious process affecting normal or degenerative cardiac valves caused by fibrin thrombi deposits in patients with hypercoagulable states associated with adenocarcinomas of the lung, colon, or pancreas that produce mucin.[48] Patients with NBTE may present with arterial and VTE and disseminated intravascular coagulation. Heparin, but not warfarin, has provided benefit[48] and helped treat the underlying neoplastic disorder. Libman-Sacks endocarditis is a noninfectious valvular abnormality associated with autoimmune disorders, such as systemic lupus erythematosus and the antiphospholipid antibody syndrome. No large-scale randomized trials exist to provide evidence-based data; however, some experts recommend anticoagulation with warfarin as primary treatment to prevent stroke.[49]

Infectious Endocarditis

Before the advent of antibiotics, infectious seeding of heart valves or endocarditis was associated with a very high rate of cerebral embolism (70–90%), which decreased (12–40%) with the advent of antibiotics.[7,50] Based on the blood culture results, specific antibiotic therapy for endocarditis remains the first-line treatment, whereas anticoagulation remains controversial or contraindicated[48] given the early rates of cerebral hemorrhage and the fact that anticoagulation does not decrease the incidence of embolism in native valve endocarditis. However, patients who have mechanical prosthetic valves may be at higher risk if anticoagulation is discontinued. Prosthetic valve endocarditis may be considered an anticoagulation dilemma, because patients have equal risks for ischemic stroke and cerebral hemorrhage, considering the patient's valve type, location, and presence of AF in weighing the ischemic and hemorrhagic risks.

Infective endocarditis of a prosthetic heart valve warrants early surgical consultation. Surgical replacement of an infected prosthetic valve presents a high risk for morbidity and mortality, especially for mitral position valves. Surgical removal or repair is considered for patients who have congestive heart failure, cardiac abscess, or persistently positive blood cultures despite antibiotic treatment. Early surgery is also warranted in fungal endocarditis.

Cardiac Tumors[51-53]

Primary cardiac tumors are rare (<0.2% in unselected autopsy series), and most are benign (50% myxomas and papillary fibroelastoma) but associated with a high frequency of embolic events. Myxomas commonly occur in the left atrium and arise from the interatrial septum. They may embolize to the systemic circulation, particularly to the brain when tumor pieces break off or secondary thrombus formation occurs. TEE is invaluable in defining tumor location, size, and morphology. To prevent embolization, surgical resection of the tumor is recommended in all cases of myxomas. Papillary fibroelastomas are benign tumors that tend to originate on cardiac valves as single or multiple masses. Embolic events are typically the first clinical manifestation, because they are present on highly mobile valve leaflets. The embolic mechanism is the same as myxomas, caused by tumor fragmentation or secondary thrombus generation. Surgical resection is also indicated for fibroelastomas. Metastatic tumors to the heart are 20–40 times more frequent than primary cardiac tumors, which are rare (e.g., angiosarcoma and rhabdomyosarcoma). Cerebral embolization can also occur from these tumors. Surgical treatment can be offered but depends on the underlying tumor type and prognosis.

Left Atrial Thrombus and Spontaneous Echo Contrast ("Smoke")[46,47,54,55]

Risk factors for left atrial appendage thrombus formation include AF, mitral stenosis, severe left ventricular dysfunction, left atrial dilatation, or presence of a prosthetic mitral valve. Demonstration of a left atrial appendage thrombus on TEE is associated with a threefold increase in the risk for stroke. SEC is defined as a smoke-like echo density moving within the cardiac chamber, typically the left atrium or left ventricle in LV dysfunction, indicating stagnant blood flow. TEE best visualizes SEC in the left atrium. The presence of SEC is a predisposing factor to thrombus formation and risk for ischemic stroke by three-to-fourfold. Oral anticoagulation decreases the stroke risk associated with SEC. Therefore, prophylactic anticoagulation is recommended for at least 3 weeks before electrical cardioversion for AF.

CONCLUSION

The past decade has seen extraordinary advances in the treatment and prevention of stroke. The magnitude and nature of the early benefits of immediate aspirin for TIA and ischemic stroke are recognized. AF is so common, and the default should be to offer stroke prevention to all AF patients unless deemed to be at low risk. Risk stratification is also not a "one off" assessment but a dynamic process, reflecting the elderly AF population with a high rate of hospitalizations, comorbidities, and polypharmacy. The advent of direct OACs has increased the uptake of effective anticoagulant thromboprophylaxis among patients with AF at high risk of recurrent cardioembolic stroke. The key to preventing recurrent stroke is to identify the cause of the initial event so that therapy can be individualized to the patient. While the vascular risk factors should be treated in all patients, anticoagulation and PFO closure would be appropriate in only some patients. Modification of risk factors is the main resource for effective prevention of stroke. Many therapeutic options are available at present, and continued research efforts are expanding the available options. A multidisciplinary approach with organized continued education will likely improve the efficacy of these measures. In the near future, studies embarking on the evaluation of the genetic determinants of cerebrovascular risk factors and outcomes will increase our understanding of cerebrovascular disease and will likely result in new therapies, with individualized programs for stroke prevention.

REFERENCES

1. Sacco RL, Kasner SE, Broderick JP, et al. An updated definition of stroke for the 21st century: a statement for healthcare professionals from the American Heart Association /American Stroke Association. Stroke. 2013;44:2064-89.

2. Asinger RW, Dyken ML, Fisher M, et al. Cardiogenic brain embolism: the second report of Cerebral Embolism Task Force. Arch Neurol. 1989;46:723.
3. Bogousslavsky J, Cachin C, Regli F, et al. Cardiac sources of embolism and cerebral infarction–clinical consequences and vascular concomitants: the Lausanne Stroke Registry. Neurology. 1991;41:855-9.
4. Gage BF, Waterman AD, Shannon W, et al. Validation of clinical classification schemes for predicting stroke: results from the National Registry of Atrial Fibrillation. JAMA. 2001;285:2864-70.
5. Sila CA. Neurological therapeutics: principles and practice. In: Noseworthy JH (Ed). Cardioembolic Stroke. London: Martin Dunitz; 2003. pp. 450-7.
6. Adams HP Jr, del Zoppo G, Alberts MJ, et al. Guidelines for the early management of adults with ischemic stroke: a guideline from the American Heart Association/American Stroke Association Stroke Council, Clinical Cardiology Council, Cardiovascular Radiology and Intervention Council, and the Atherosclerotic Peripheral Vascular Disease and Quality of Care Outcomes in Research Interdisciplinary Working Groups: the American Academy of Neurology affirms the value of this guideline as an educational tool for neurologists. Circulation. 2007;115:e478.
7. Douglas PS, Khandheria B, Stainback RF, et al. ACCF/ASE/ACEP/ASNC/SCAI/SCCT/ SCMR 2007 appropriateness criteria for transthoracic and transesophageal echocardiography: are port of the American College of Cardiology Foundation Quality Strategic Directions Committee Appropriateness Criteria Working Group, American Society of Echocardiography, American College of Emergency Physicians, American Society of Nuclear Cardiology, Society for Cardiovascular Angiography and Interventions, Society of Cardiovascular Computed Tomography, and the Society for Cardiovascular Magnetic Resonance endorsed by the American College of Chest Physicians and the Society of Critical Care Medicine. J Am Coll Cardiol. 2007;50:187.
8. Horowitz DR, Tuhrim S, Weinberger JM, et al. Mechanisms in lacunar infarction. Stroke. 1992;23:325-7.
9. Naccarelli GV, Varker H, Lin J, et al. Increasing prevalence of atrial fibrillation and flutter in the United States. Am J Cardiol. 2009;104:1534-9.
10. January CT, Wann LS, Alpert JS, et al. 2014 AHA/ACC/HRS guideline for the management of patients with atrial fibrillation: a report of the American College of Cardiology/American Heart Association Task Force on Practice Guidelines and the Heart Rhythm Society. J Am Coll Cardiol. 2014;64.
11. Fuster V, Rydén LE, Cannom DS, et al. European Heart Rhythm Association. ACC/AHA/ESC 2006 guidelines for the management of patients with atrial fibrillation–executive summary: a report of the American College of Cardiology/ American Heart Association Task Force on Practice Guidelines and the European Society of Cardiology Committee for Practice Guidelines. J Am Coll Cardiol. 2006;48:854-906.
12. Fuster V, Rydén LE, Cannom DS, et al. ACC/AHA/ESC 2006 guidelines for the management of patients with atrial fibrillation: a report of the American College of Cardiology/ American Heart Association Task Force on Practice Guidelines and the European Society of Cardiology Committee for Practice Guidelines. Circulation. 2006;114:e257-354.
13. Guo Y, Wang H, Tian Y, et al. Multiple risk factors and ischaemic stroke in the elderly Asian population with and without atrial fibrillation. An analysis of 425,600 Chinese individuals without prior stroke. Thromb Haemost. 2016;115(1):184-92.
14. Pisters R, Lane DA, Nieuwlaat R, et.al. A novel user- friendly score (HAS-BLED) to assess 1-year risk of major bleeding in patients with atrial fibrillation. Chest. 2010;138(5):1093-100.
15. Chao TF, Wang KL, Liu CJ, et.al. Age Threshold for Increased Stroke Risk Among Patients With Atrial Fibrillation: A Nationwide Cohort Study From Taiwan. J Am Coll Cardiol. 2015;66(12):1339-47.
16. Chao TF, Lip GY, Liu CJ, et al. Validation of a Modified CHA2DS2-VASc Score for Stroke Risk Stratification in Asian Patients With Atrial Fibrillation: A Nationwide Cohort Study. Stroke. 2016;47(10):2462-9.
17. Overvad TF, Nielsen PB, Lip GY. Treatment thresholds for stroke prevention in atrial fibrillation: observations on the CHA2DS2-VASc score. Eur Heart J Cardiovasc Pharmacother. 2016;3(1):37-41.
18. Olesen JB, Torp-Pedersen C. Stroke risk in atrial fibrillation: Do we anticoagulate CHADS2 or CHA2DS2-VASc >/=1, or higher? Thromb Haemost. 2015;113(6):1165-9.
19. Lip GY, Skjøth F, Nielsen PB, et al. Non-valvular atrial fibrillation patients with none or one additional risk factor of the CHA2DS2-VASc score. A comprehensive net clinical benefit analysis for warfarin, aspirin, or no therapy. Thromb Haemost. 2015;114(4):826-34.
20. Lip GYH. Stroke prevention in atrial fibrillation. Eur Heart J. 2017;38(1):4-5.
21. Esteve-Pastor MA, Roldan V, Valdes M, et al. The SAMe-TT2R2 score and decision-making between a vitamin K antagonist or a non-vitamin K antagonist oral anticoagulant in patients with atrial fibrillation. Expert Rev Cardiovasc Ther. 2016;14(2):177-87.
22. Lip GY, Lane DA. Bleeding risk assessment in atrial fibrillation: observations on the use and misuse of bleeding risk scores. J Thromb Haemost. 2016;14(9):1711-4.
23. Kirchhof P, Ammentorp B, Darius H, et al. Management of atrial fibrillation in seven European countries after the publication of the 2010 ESC Guidelines on atrial fibrillation: primary results of the PREvention oF thromboemolic events--European Registry in Atrial Fibrillation (PREFER in AF). Europace. 2014;16:6-14.
24. Connolly SJ, Ezekowitz MD, Yusuf S, et al. RE-LY Steering Committee and Investigators. Dabigatran vs. warfarin in patients with atrial fibrillation. N Engl J Med. 2009;361:1139-51.
25. Connolly SJ, Wallentin L, Ezekowitz MD, et al. The Long-Term Multicenter Observational Study of Dabigatran Treatment in Patients with Atrial Fibrillation (RELY-ABLE) study. Circulation. 2013;128:237-43.
26. Patel MR, Mahaffey KW, Garg J, et al. Rivaroxaban versus warfarin in nonvalvular atrial fibrillation. N Engl J Med. 2011;365:883-91.
27. Granger CB, Alexander JH, McMurray JJ, et.al; ARISTOTL Committees and Investigators. Apixaban vs. warfarin in patients with atrial fibrillation. N Engl J Med. 2011;365:981-92.
28. Connolly SJ, Eikelboom J, Joyner C, et al. Apixaban in patients with atrial fibrillation. N Engl J Med. 2011;364:806-17.
29. Giugliano RP, Ruff CT, Braunwald E, et al. Edoxaban versus warfarin in patients with atrial fibrillation. N Engl J Med. 2013;369:2093-104.
30. Ruff CT, Giugliano RP, Braunwald E, et al. Comparison of the efficacy and safety of new oral anticoagulants with warfarin in patients with atrial fibrillation: a meta-analysis of randomised trials. Lancet. 2014;383:955-62.
31. Schwedt TJ, Demaerschalk BM, Dodick DW. Patent foramen ovale and migraine: a quantitative systematic review. Cephalalgia. 2008;28:531-40.
32. Furlan AJ, Reisman M, Massaro J, et al., CLOSURE I Investigators. Closure or medical therapy for cryptogenic stroke with patent foramen ovale. N Engl J Med. 2012;366:991-9.
33. Meier B, Kalesan B, Mattle HP, et al. PC Trial Investigators. Percutaneous closure of patent foramen ovale in cryptogenic embolism. N Engl J Med. 2013;368:1083-91.
34. Carroll JD, Saver JL, Thaler DE, et al. RESPECT Investigators. Closure of patent foramen ovale versus medical therapy after cryptogenic stroke. N Engl J Med. 2013;368:1092-100.
35. Mas JL, Derumeaux G, Guillon B, et al. CLOSE Investigators. Patent foramen ovale closure or anticoagulation vs. antiplatelets after stroke. N Engl J Med. 2017;377:1011-21.
36. Søndergaard L, Kasner SE, Rhodes JF, et al. Gore REDUCE Clinical Study Investigators. Patent foramen ovale closure or antiplatelet therapy for cryptogenic stroke. N Engl J Med. 2017;377:1033-42.
37. Amarenco P, Cohen A, Tzourio C, et al. Atherosclerotic disease of the aortic arch and the risk of ischemic stroke. N Engl J Med. 1994;331:1474-9.
38. Tunick PA, Nayar AC, Goodkin GM, et al. Effect of treatment on the incidence of stroke and other emboli in 519 patients with severe thoracic aortic plaque. Am J Cardiol. 2002;90:1320-5.
39. Amarenco P, Davis S, Jones E, et al. Clopidogrel plus aspirin versus warfarin in patients with stroke and aortic arch plaques. Stroke. 2014;45:1-10.
40. Medical Research Council. Assessment of short-term anticoagulant administration after myocardial infarction. BMJ. 1969;1:335-42.
41. Effect of long-term oral anticoagulant treatment on mortality and cardiovascular morbidity after myocardial infarction. Anticoagulants in the Secondary Prevention of Events in Coronary Thrombosis (ASPECT) Research Group. Lancet. 1994; 343 499-503.
42. Dries DL, Rosenberg YD, Waclawiw MA, et al. Ejection fraction and risk of thromboembolic events in patients with systolic dysfunction and sinus rhythm: evidence for gender differences in the studies of left ventricular dysfunction trials. J Am Coll Cardiol. 1997;29:1074-80.

43. Loh E, Sutton MS, Wun CC, et al. Ventricular dysfunction and the risk of stroke after myocardial infarction. N Engl J Med. 1997;336:251-7.
44. Massie BM, Krol WF, Ammon SE, et al. The Warfarin and Antiplatelet Therapy in Heart Failure trial (WATCH): rationale, design, and baseline patient characteristics. J Card Fail. 2004;10:101-12.
45. Homma S, Thompson LP, et al. Warfarin versus aspirin in patients with reduced cardiac ejection fraction (WARCEF) trial. N Engl J Med. 2012; 366:1859-69.
46. Baumgartner H, Falk V, Bax JJ, et al. 2017 ESC/EACTS Guidelines for the management of valvular heart disease The Task Force for the Management of Valvular Heart Disease of the European Society of Cardiology (ESC) and the European Association for Cardio-Thoracic Surgery (EACTS). Eur Heart J. 2017;38(36):2739-91.
47. Nishimura RA, Otto CM, Bonow RO, et al. 2017 AHA/ACC Focused Update of the 2014 AHA/ACC Guideline for the Management of Patients With Valvular Heart Disease A Report of the American College of Cardiology/American Heart Association Task Force on Clinical Practice Guidelines. Circulation. 2017;135(25):e1159-95.
48. Salem DN, Levine HJ, Pauker SG, et al. Antithrombotic therapy in valvular heart disease. Chest. 1998;114:590S-601S.
49. Sila CA. Neurological therapeutics: principles and practice. In: Noseworthy JH (Ed). Cardioembolic Stroke. London: Martin Dunitz; 2003. pp. 450-7.
50. Prabhakaran S. Neurologic complications of endocarditis. Continuum Lifelong Learning in Neurology. 2008;14(1):53-73.
51. Castelman B. Roth S. Tumors of the cardiovascular system, 1st edition. Washington DC: Armed Forces Institute of Pathology; 1978.
52. Reynen K. Frequency of primary tumors of the heart. Am J Cardiol. 1996;77:107.
53. Reynen K. Cardiac myxomas. N Engl J Med. 1995;333:1610-17.
54. Di Tullio MR, Homma S. Mechanisms of cardioembolic stroke. Curr Cardiol Rep. 2002;4:141-8.
55. Transesophageal echocardiographic correlates of thromboembolism in high risk patients with nonvalvular atrial fibrillation. The stroke prevention in atrial fibrillation investigators committee on echocardiography. Ann Intern Med. 1998;128:639-47.

CHAPTER 130

Stroke in Cath Lab

Neeraj Parakh, Kewal C Goswami

INTRODUCTION

Stroke is an uncommon complication in modern cardiac catheterization laboratories (Cath lab). To a large extent this is an avoidable complication, if basic diktats of catheterization are strictly followed. However, it is one of the most debilitating complication resulting in high incidence of mortality and morbidity.

INCIDENCE

Incidence of stroke in cath lab within 36 hours is <0.01% for diagnostic procedures and 0.1–0.4% for therapeutic procedures. As per Euro Heart Survey, incidence of stroke in cath lab for elective percutaneous coronary intervention (PCI) is 0.3% and the same is 0.6% for PCI in acute coronary syndrome. Higher incidence of stroke has been reported for valve interventions and for atrial fibrillation ablation. Asymptomatic embolism has been reported in 2–22% of cases in various studies. Thirty-day mortality for stroke in cath lab is up to 19% for ischemic stroke and up to 50% for hemorrhagic stroke.[1]

MECHANISM AND RISK FACTORS

Embolization of clot/thrombus is the commonest cause for ischemic stroke in cath lab. Thrombus may form over wires, catheters, etc., especially if anticoagulation is not appropriate. Plaque or atherosclerotic material may get dislodged from aorta or arch vessels during catheter or wire manipulation.[2] Embolization of valve tissue or other material may rarely cause stroke.[3] Various reasons for ischemic stroke in catheterization laboratory are as follows:

- Thrombus
- Calcific material
- Plaque/cholesterol particles
- Clot dislodgement from left ventricle (LV)/left atrium (LA)
- Air embolism
- Broken hardware
- Periprocedural hypotension
- Arterial dissection
- Valve tissue

Hemorrhagic stroke is usually attributed to the use of thrombolytics, anticoagulation, Gp IIb/IIIa inhibitors, and antiplatelets. Risk factors for stroke are mentioned in table 1 and box 1.

TABLE 1: Risk factor for ischemic stroke

Patient-related factors	Procedure-related factors
Older age >75 years	Emergent procedure
Diabetes	Prolonged procedure
Hypertension	Greater contrast use
Previous stroke	Retrograde catheterization of left ventricle in aortic stenosis
Renal failure	Bypass graft intervention
Heart failure	Intra-aortic balloon pump
Atherosclerotic burden such as triple-vessel disease	Coronary artery thrombus

BOX 1 Risk factor for hemorrhagic stroke

Risk factors

- Thrombolytics, Gp IIb/IIIa, anticoagulants, antiplatelets
- Age >75 years
- Female gender
- Low-body weight
- Systolic blood pressure (BP) >160 mm Hg
- Black race
- Acute coronary syndrome

PRESENTATION

Clinically, most of the strokes present either during the procedure or within 24 hours of the procedure. Common presenting complaints are visual disturbance, aphasia, dysarthria, hemiparesis, and altered mental status. Ischemic strokes present with maximal deficit at the onset and a fluctuating course thereafter, while hemorrhagic stroke presents with gradual worsening and raised intracranial pressure. Clinical features and focal deficit corresponds to the affected vascular territory. Nonfocal encephalopathy as presenting feature indicates diffuse bilateral infarcts.

EVALUATION

An immediate evaluation by a neurologist or stroke team for a focused history and examination should be the first step. Basic ABC (airway, breathing, circulation) for the management of critically ill patients should be followed. Hypoglycemia remains an important differential diagnosis, especially in diabetic patients. Determination of symptom onset is very important in planning for thrombolysis or mechanical intervention in case of ischemic stroke. Noncontrast computed tomography (CT)/magnetic resonance (MR) and concurrent neurovascular imaging should be performed immediately after the basic neurological examination for determining the type and localization of the lesion. CT or MR perfusion imaging is required only for uncertain diagnosis.

Differential Diagnosis

The differential diagnosis of stroke in cath lab includes transient ischemic attack, seizure disorder, migraine, encephalopathy, and hypoglycemia. Use of sedatives during the procedure or comorbid medical or neurologic conditions may confound the accurate diagnosis of stroke. Contrast-induced transient cortical blindness is another rare occurrence with use of contrast media.[4] Blurring of vision starts within minutes of the procedure and rapidly progresses to complete blindness, usually associated with headache. Vomiting, confusion, aphasia, memory impairment, and limb weakness may also be present. A CT scan done immediately after the symptom onset shows extravasation of the dye into the subarachnoid space and brain tissue in the posterior third of the brain. This at times is mistaken for subarachnoid hemorrhage. In nearly all cases, the neurologic impairments and neuroimaging abnormalities gradually resolve over days. Postulated mechanisms include direct neurotoxic effect, idiosyncratic reaction, microembolization, hypoxia, edema, and endothelin release (large volumes of radiocontrast is associated with elevated endothelin levels and endothelins have been implicated in posterior leukoencephalopathy).

TREATMENT

Hemorrhagic Stroke

Basic principle of treatment of hemorrhagic stroke is the reversal of anticoagulation, blood pressure control, treatment of raised intracranial pressure, and supportive treatment.

Ischemic Stroke

Given the rarity of stroke in cath lab, there are no randomized studies regarding revascularization in these patients. Usually, the guidelines for stroke in general population are also followed in case of stroke in cath lab (Boxes 2 and 3). Specific therapy for ischemic stroke includes the following:

BOX 2 rtPA in stroke—NINDS inclusion criteria

Inclusion criteria

- Clinical diagnosis of ischemic stroke causing measurable neurologic deficit
- Onset of symptoms <4.5 hours before beginning treatment; if the exact time of stroke onset is not known, it is defined as the last time the patient was known to be normal
- Age ≥18 years

rTPA, recombinant tissue plasminogen activator; NINDS, National Institute of Neurological Disorders and Stroke.

BOX 3 rTPA in stroke—NINDS exclusion criteria

Exclusion criteria

- Historical
  - Stroke or head trauma in the previous 3 months
  - History of intracranial hemorrhage
  - Intracranial tumor, arteriovenous malformation, or aneurysm
  - Recent neurosurgery
  - Noncompressible arterial puncture in the previous week
- Clinical
  - Symptoms suggestive of subarachnoid hemorrhage
  - Persistent blood pressure elevation (systolic ≥185 mm Hg or diastolic ≥110 mm Hg)
  - Hypoglycemia (serum glucose <50 mg/dL)
  - Active internal bleeding
  - Acute bleeding diathesis
- Hematologic
  - Platelet count <100,000 mm^{-3}
  - Current anticoagulant use with an international normalized ratio (INR) >1.7 or prothrombin time (PT) >15 seconds
  - Heparin use within 48 hours and an abnormally elevated activated partial thromboplastin time (aPTT)
  - Current use of a direct thrombin inhibitor or direct factor Xa inhibitor
- Head CT scan
  - Evidence of hemorrhage
  - Irreversible injury
- Relative exclusion criteria
  - Only minor and isolated neurologic signs
  - Rapidly improving stroke symptoms
  - Major surgery or serious trauma in the previous 14 days
  - Gastrointestinal or urinary tract bleeding in the previous 21 days
  - Myocardial infarction in the previous 3 months
  - Seizure at the onset of stroke with postictal neurologic impairments
  - Pregnancy
- Additional relative exclusion criteria for treatment from 3 hours to 4.5 hours from onset
  - Age >80 years
  - Oral anticoagulant use regardless of INR
  - Severe stroke (NIHSS score >25)
  - Combination of both previous ischemic stroke and diabetes mellitus

CT, computed tomography; NIHSS, National Institutes of Health Stroke Scale, rTPA, recombinant tissue plasminogen activator; NINDS, National Institute of Neurological Disorders and Stroke.

- Intravenous thrombolysis—within 4.5 hours
- Intra-arterial thrombolysis
- Intra-arterial mechanical thrombectomy—within 6 hours

Treatment of acute stroke after cardiac catheterization (TASCC) registry included 66 cases of ischemic strokes from seven major North American academic centers. Twelve (18%) of these patients were treated with thrombolysis by recombinant tissue plasminogen activator (rTPA) (seven intravenous and five intra-arterial).

Thrombolysed patients had better National Institutes of Health Stroke Scale (NIHSS) score from baseline to 24 hours as compared to nontreated cases (p <0.001). There was no significant difference in bleeding events and mortality rates were also similar. This data suggests that emergent cerebral revascularization should be a routine consideration.[5]

Thrombolysis in Stroke (Flowchart 1)

Intravenous tissue plasminogen activator (tPA) is initiated within 4.5 hours of clearly defined symptom onset (at a dose of 0.9 mg/kg, not exceeding 90 mg, given as a 10% bolus followed by continuous infusion of the remaining 90% over 60 minutes), followed by adjunctive endovascular therapy in patients with large vessel occlusions. In case of ischemic stroke due to large artery occlusion in the proximal anterior circulation, intra-arterial mechanical thrombectomy using a second-generation stent retriever device should be initiated within 6 hours of symptom onset. Intra-arterial tPA (20–40 mg) should be initiated in the 4.5- to 6-hour time window in patients otherwise eligible for tPA (but not eligible for mechanical thrombectomy). Intra-arterial tPA requires infrastructure and expertise. Doses of tPA required in intra-arterial thrombolysis are much lower than intravenous tPA. Before starting thrombolysis, normal activated partial thromboplastin time (aPTT) should be documented if heparin was administered within 48 hours. Protamine can be used to reverse the effect of heparin. For patients with a prolonged aPTT, endovascular therapies with intra-arterial tPA and/or mechanical embolectomy are treatment options. Gp IIb/IIIa inhibitor therapy may increase the risk of hemorrhagic complications with intravenous tPA. In such cases, endovascular interventions are treatment options. Antiplatelet therapy is not a contraindication to intravenous tPA.[6]

Stroke during Transcatheter Aortic Valve Replacement

Transcatheter aortic valve replacement (TAVR) has become the latest treatment option for high-risk patients with aortic stenosis (AS). Incidence of stroke has been one of the main

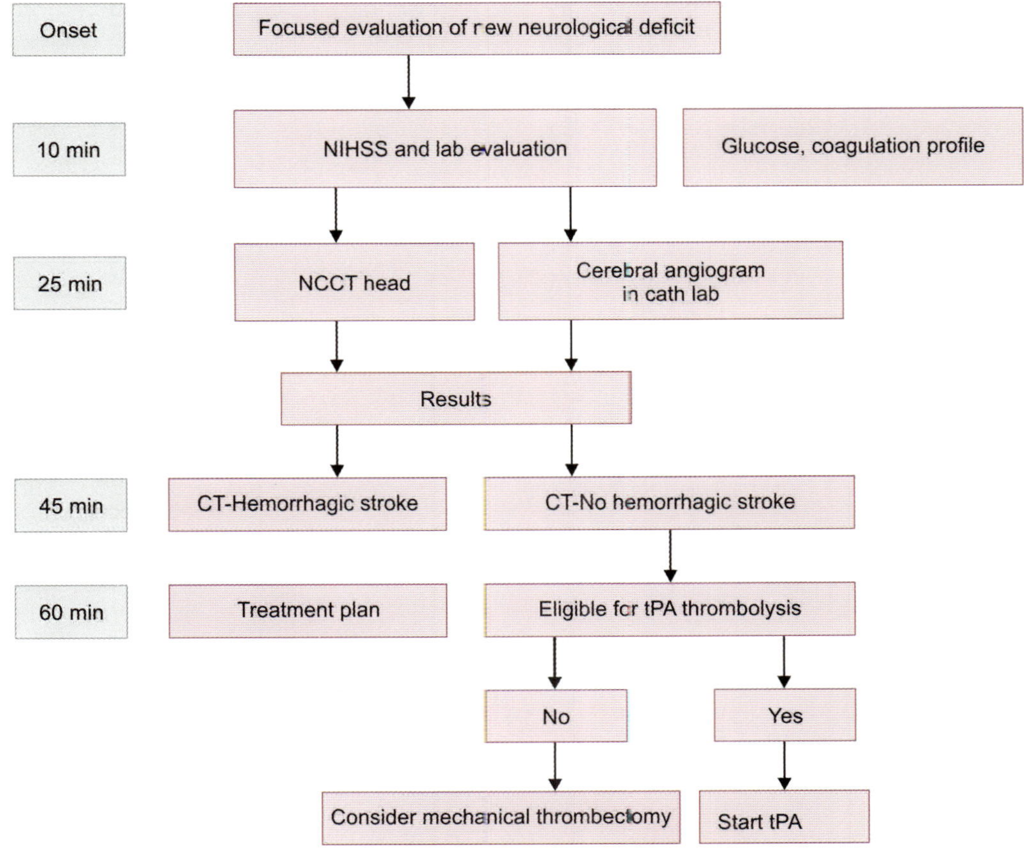

NIHSS, National Institutes of Health Stroke Scale; tPA, tissue plasminogen activator; CT, computed tomography; NCCT,Non Contrast Computed Tomography

FLOWCHART 1: Stroke algorithm.

concerns associated with TAVR. In the PARTNER I trial comparing TAVR and surgical valve replacement, stroke rates were higher after TAVR.[7] Periprocedural stroke leads to a five times higher incidence of death after TAVR.[8] Transcatheter aortic valve registry reported overall stroke rate of 2% during hospital stay. Up to 50% of all strokes during TAVR happen during first 24 hours after the procedure.[9] Embolic protection devices (EPDs) are emerging as a promising approach to decrease the incidence of stroke during TAVR. A reduction in the frequency of ischemic lesions has been seen; however, more research and trial data are required before their routine clinical use is established. At least three EPDs (Sentinel, Embrella, TriGuard) are under evaluation and preliminary results are encouraging.[10]

CONCLUSION

Each cath lab should set up a stroke protocol. Time is brain, so this inevitable complication should be handled expeditiously in cath lab.[11] Prevention strategy, such as adequate flushing of lumened catheters and balloons is a must, to keep the system air-free. Adequate heparinization and frequent neuro-checks should reduce the stroke incidence to a minimum. Routine intra-arterial thrombolysis is not recommended over intravenous therapy, but the judgment should be left to the consulting stroke team depending upon the need, infrastructure, and expertise. Stroke in cath lab remains the most treatable neurological conditions, and expeditious use of the stroke protocol is the fastest, safest, and most effective way to manage such patients.

REFERENCES

1. Korn-Lubetzki I, Farkash R, Pachino RM, et al. Incidence and risk factors of cerebrovascular events following cardiac catheterization. J Am Heart Assoc. 2013;2(6):e000413.
2. Eggebrecht H, Oldenburg O, Dirsch O, et al. Potential embolization by atherosclerotic debris dislodged from aortic wall during cardiac catheterization: histological and clinical findings in 7,621 patients. Catheter Cardiovasc Interv. 2000;49:389.
3. Shetkar SS, Parakh N, Singh B, et al. Cardio-embolic stroke due to valve tissue embolization during percutaneous transseptal mitral commissurotomy (PTMC). Indian Heart J. 2014;66(5):546-9.
4. Math RS, Singh S, Bahl V. An uncommon complication after a common procedure. J Invasive Cardiol. 2008;20(10):E301-3.
5. Khatri P, Taylor RA, Palumbo V, et al. Treatment of acute stroke after cardiac catheterization (TASCC) study group. The safety and efficacy of thrombolysis for strokes after cardiac catheterization. J Am Coll Cardiol. 2008;51(9):906-11.
6. Powers WJ, Rabinstein AA, Ackerson T, et al. Guidelines for the early management of patients with acute ischemic stroke: a guideline for healthcare professionals from the American Heart Association/American Stroke Association. Stroke. 2018;49:e46.
7. Smith CR, Leon MB, Mack MJ, et al. PARTNER trial investigators. Transcatheter versus surgical aortic-valve replacement in high-risk patients. N Engl J Med. 2011;364:2187-98
8. Werner N, Zeymer U, Schneider S, et al.. Incidence and clinical impact of stroke complicating transcatheter aortic valve implantation: results from the German TAVI registry. Catheter Cardiovasc Interv. 2016;88:644-53.
9. Mack MJ, Brennan J, Brindis R, et al. STS/ACC TVT registry. Outcomes following transcatheter aortic valve replacement in the United States. JAMA. 2013;310:2069-77.
10. Haussig S, Mangner N, Dwyer MG, et al. Effect of a cerebral protection device on brain lesions following transcatheter aortic valve implantation in patients with severe aortic stenosis: the CLEAN-TAVI randomized clinical trial. JAMA. 2016;316:592-601.
11. Lyden PD. Code stroke in the cath lab. J Am Coll Cardiol. 2008;51(9):912.

SECTION 20

Peripheral Vascular Disease

CHAPTER 131

Varicose Veins: Interventional Approach

Sanjeev Kumar, Vineeta Ojha

INTRODUCTION

Chronic venous insufficiency (CVI) is characterized by insufficient venous return to the heart, is related primarily to retrograde flow in lower extremity veins (venous reflux). Chronic venous insufficiency and reflux are usually caused by valvular incompetence, which may or may not be associated with venous obstruction. Patients may present with symptoms ranging from spider veins or telangiectasias to varicose veins, lipodermatosclerosis or venous ulcers. Fifteen percent of the men and 25% of the women suffer from varicose veins and in most of them, it appears by 30 years of age.[1,2] The current challenge in front of us is to provide the patients an effective treatment strategy for symptoms related to venous reflux that is associated with low recurrence rates, lesser recovery time, less morbidity, and visibly better outcomes. The past two decades have witnessed the development of some minimally invasive strategies that achieve these goals.

ANATOMY AND PATHOPHYSIOLOGY

The major superficial veins of the legs are the short saphenous vein (SSV), which runs in the posterior compartment and the great saphenous vein (GSV), which runs from ankle to groin in medial compartment. Superficial veins communicate with deep veins of the leg via multiple perforating veins which pass through openings in the deep fascia. The main deep vein of the leg is the popliteal vein until it courses upward into the thigh and becomes the femoral vein (FV) (Fig. 1). The veins have valves which are one way and prevent retrograde flow. When these valves start malfunctioning, there is backward flow of blood into these veins. Major valves whose dysfunctions cause varicose veins are saphenofemoral junction (SFJ) and saphenopopliteal junction (SPJ). The major risk factors for causation of varicose veins are: female hormones, family history, gravitational forces (more in pregnant patients), and hydrostatic forces in the muscular compartments of the legs.[1]

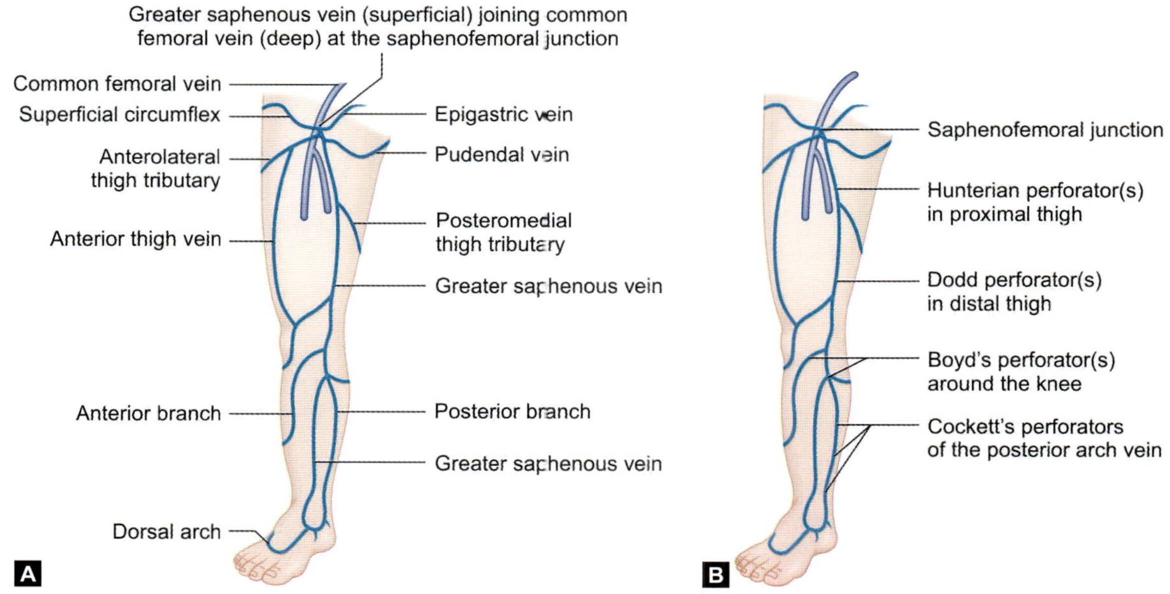

FIG. 1: Anatomy of superficial venous system. **A,** Superficial veins of the leg; **B,** Perforators.

NATURAL HISTORY

Literature on the natural history of lower extremity varicosities show that, at a mean follow-up of 19 months, 73% of limbs remain stable, 11% develop worsening clinical stage, and a few percent more develop worsening reflux on duplex ultrasound without associated symptomatic progression.[3] In normal individuals, the progression of chronic venous disease (CVD) is slow. Poor prognostic factors for progressive CVD include the combination of both reflux and obstruction, recurrent deep venous thrombosis (DVT), and multisegmental disease.[4]

CLASSIFICATION

To standardize the treatment and reporting of the chronic venous disorders, a dedicated classification (CEAP) has been proposed to help in diagnosis and comparison of varied manifestations of CVD. It was developed by a committee of the American Venous Forum in 1994 and it was subsequently accepted as a standard for classifying CVD. The basic CEAP classification gives a brief description of the clinical class of the CVD (C) based upon the symptoms, the etiology (E), the anatomical (A) distribution, and the underlying pathophysiology (P), whether reflux or obstruction. Clinical classification is shown in table 1.

INDICATIONS FOR TREATMENT

Indications for treatment include symptoms from uncomplicated varicose veins and complications from varicose vein disease. Uncomplicated varicose veins are associated with a variety of symptoms: pain/aching, fatigue/heaviness, itching/burning sensation, leg cramps, calf/ankle swelling, restless legs, and leg warmth.[5] Complications include blood stasis in the varicosities with subsequent superficial phlebitis, progression of disease, and rarely, variceal bleeding. The CEAP class C3 to C6 are actively treated and sometimes C2 class is also treated because of esthetic reasons. Decision to treat is based on four major concerns: symptoms, reflux, concerns for future worsening and complications, and lastly, unesthetic appearance of varices.

TREATMENT OPTIONS FOR VARICOSE VEINS

The approach is determined by anatomy and the clinical status of the patient. Therapy needs to be targeted to the veins that are actually the source of the problem whether it is the GSV, SSV, perforators, or accessory veins. The therapeutic approach will also be determined in large part by the size and morphology of the specific veins to be treated. The traditional

TABLE 1: Clinical classification of chronic venous disorders

CEAP classification	
C—Clinical	Description
C0	No visible or palpable signs of venous disease
C1	• Spider veins ("telangiectasias") (<1 mm in diameter) • Reticular veins ("venulectasias") (1 to <3 mm in diameter)
C2	Varicose veins (3 mm or larger in standing position)
C3	Venous edema; corona phlebectatica ("ankle flare")
C4	• Skin changes ascribed to venous disease • C4a: Eczema ("stasis dermatitis") or brownish hyperpigmentation • C4b: Lipodermatosclerosis or atrophie blanche
C5	Healed ulcer (and skin changes as described above)
C6	Active ulcer (and skin changes as described above)
E—Etiological	
Ec	Congenital
Ep	Primary
Es	Secondary (post-thrombotic)
En	No venous cause identified
A—Anatomical	
As	Superficial veins
Ap	Perforator veins
Ad	Deep veins
An	No venous location identified
P—Pathophysiological	
Pr	Reflux
Po	Obstruction
Pr, o	Reflux and obstruction
Pn	No venous pathophysiology identifiable

gold standard is a flush ligation of GSV at SFJ, followed by stripping of the GSV. Surgery of varicose veins is usually performed under anesthesia and might cause neurological damage (7–40%), scars, hematoma, and postoperative pain.[6-8] Though surgery is very effective in short term, 5-year recurrence rates are approximately 30% for GSV and 50% for SSV.[9] There are multiple minimally invasive therapies that can be applied to venous reflux disease as discussed subsequently.

Evaluation before Treatment

- *Clinical*: A thorough history should include duration and types of symptoms and history of DVT, any prothrombotic condition and prior treatments. Treatment should not be done in the setting of acute DVT. Physical examination should include the evaluation of the arterial system, signs of CVD, and size and location of patient's varicosities. The CEAP score is determined for each patient
- *USG Doppler*: Doppler evaluation of venous system should be done in details. Points to be evaluated are SFJ, SPJ incompetence or reflux or transient reflux (criteria to intervene), diameter of SFJ or SPJ [more than 3 mm are usually amenable to endovenous laser ablation (EVLA) or radiofrequency ablation (RFA)], superficial dilated varicosities in the legs, sites of incompetent perforators, presence of DVT (contraindication to thermal-based therapy), etc. In addition to the superficial, deep and perforator veins, attention should be paid to accessory veins too, like anterior accessory vein, vein of Giacomini, etc. which also serve as a source of venous reflux
- *Preprocedure steps*: After medical history and clinical as well as Doppler evaluation, informed consent needs to be taken. Patients must be told about the likely complications and the likely need for more than one session. Adequate hydration needs to be ensured. Intravenous (IV) cannula should be in place for all the patients, if need arises, premedication in the form of injection Emeset and IV Tramadol can be administered to the apprehensive patients.

INTERVENTIONAL APPROACH TO MANAGEMENT OF VARICOSE VEINS

Minimally Invasive Options

To increase the effectiveness and patients' health-related quality of life (HRQOL) and to reduce postoperative time, therapy-related complications and costs, newer minimally invasive methods such as ultrasound-guided foam sclerotherapy (UGFS), EVLA, and RFA are now widely used in the treatment of lower extremity varicosities. Venous ablation using n-butyl cyanoacrylate (NBCA) is a newer technique that does not require tumescent anesthesia (TA) or compression.

USG-guided Foam Sclerotherapy

Sclerotherapy is the method using the biological, physical, and chemical properties of an agent used to damage the target vessel. First described in 1939, foam sclerotherapy has recently increased in popularity.[10]

Mechanism of Action

Sclerotherapy causes endothelial damage by selective intravascular delivery of a sclerosant into an intravascular space that exerts its injury by direct contact with endothelium in a dose-dependent way. Other than fibrosis, agents might produce other effects like denaturation of proteins, thrombosis, cell dehydration, osmosis, and physical obstruction due to polymerization. Therapeutic effect of sclerotherapy is dependent on the choice of agent, the sclerosant concentration *in vivo*, and the duration for which the sclerosant is in contact with endothelium, also called "dwell-time".

Sclerosing Agents

The salient features of various sclerosing agents are summarized in table 2.[11] Sodium tetradecyl sulfate (STS) and polidocanol are the most widely used sclerosants. Allergy to the sclerosant, infection, DVT, and severe arterial disease are the major contraindications to sclerotherapy.

Procedure

It is performed in an angiography suite with USG facility. No sedation is required in most cases, however, if patient is apprehensive, conscious sedation or local nerve block is recommended. A tourniquet may be tied proximally for proper distension. Percutaneous introduction of butterfly needle into the varicosity is done under ultrasound guidance till free backflow of blood is observed. Further, venography is performed during gentle contrast injection and stopped as soon as deep vein is seen to fill and contrast amount is noted. Same amount of sclerosant foam is injected slowly into the vein. There are two main techniques of foam preparation: Tessari, and Monfreux. The Tessari method has become the more popular technique (Fig. 2). The foam, thus formed, displaces blood from the vein to be treated and persists in the vein to maximize its sclerosant effect (Fig. 3). Some authors also advocate aspirating the contrast before introducing the sclerosant to prevent more dilution. If there are signs of extravasation, in the form of induration or skin blanching, injection of sclerosant is stopped immediately. Compression at the SFJ during the procedure can be done to prevent passage of sclerosant into deep venous system. Local compression for 5–10 minutes is applied after injection. Staged sclerotherapy can be done 6–8 weeks apart.[11-13] Parsi et al. recommended a novel approach for saphenous vein ablation, i.e., catheter-directed sclerotherapy, in which access to GSV can be gained at knee or ankle, and catheter is advanced till 5 cm proximal to SFJ. Tumescent anesthesia is applied in perivenous plane. Foam is injected while catheter is withdrawn.[14]

Complications

Minor local complications are pain, swelling, reddish discoloration, hyperpigmentation, and telangiectatic matting (~16%). Other complications are juxtalesional skin necrosis, thrombophlebitis, neuropathy, DVT (0–0.2%), compartment

TABLE 2: Sclerosing agents and their salient features

Agent	Salient features
Ethanol	• Most efficacious, lowest recurrence • Denudation and destruction of intima • Inexpensive • Highest complication rate (7.5–27.9%) very toxic, procedure always under general anesthesia • Skin necrosis—major complication • Other complications—adjacent nerve palsy, hemoglobinuria, acute pulmonary hypertension • Maximum dose—1 mL/kg (however, limited to 10 mL/session)
Sodium tetradecyl sulfate	• Thrombosis and obliteration of the vessel • Safer than ethanol—lower rates of skin and nerve damage • Maximum dose—3 mL of 3% solution
Polidocanol	• Anesthetic properties—painless procedure • Less degree of endothelial damage • Hemolysis and elevation of D-dimers—at high dose • Maximum dose—10 mL of 3% solution
Ethanolamine oleate	• Causes fibrosis and sclerosis in delayed manner • Less penetrative effect—less adjacent nerve injury • Maximum dose—1 mL of 5% ethanolamine solution
Bleomycin	• Indications—painful bleeding, ulcerated lesions • Maximum 15 mg per session
Doxycycline	• Cellular reaction with deposition of fibrin • Dose range 100–1,000 mg per session

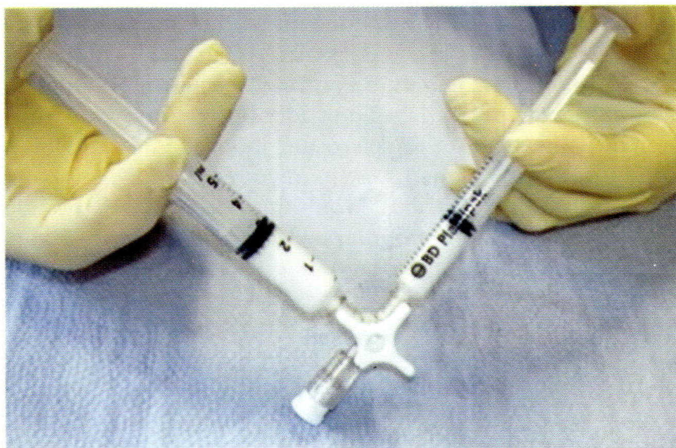

FIG. 2: Tessari technique: A syringe containing 1–2 mL of sclerosant is connected to a syringe containing 2 mL air via three-way stopcock. Twenty rapid passages are made.

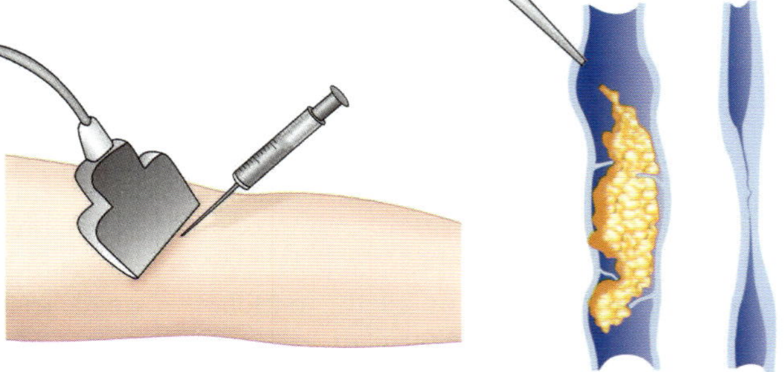

FIG. 3: Sclerotherapy technique.

syndrome, hemoglobinuria, pulmonary embolism, cardiopulmonary collapse, etc. A complication specific to intravascular administration of ethanol is precapillary pulmonary arterial spasm with increase in the pulmonary arterial pressure and right heart failure rarely. Sustained pulmonary hypertension has been described in 30% of patients per ethanol administration, but does not have a long-lasting effect, and it does not correlate with the total dose given.[15]

Success Rates or Efficacy of Sclerotherapy

Success rates for sclerotherapy alone as in literature vary from 31 to 100%. O'Hare et al. published the results of UGFS for varicose veins. After 2 weeks, 93% of the major veins were totally occluded on Doppler examination. After 6 months, in 74% of the patients, the major veins remained occluded. No patient had DVT.[16] In another study which included 453 patients with a follow up period of 3 years, sclerotherapy was done using the Monfreux and Tessari methods, immediate success rates were 88.1% and 93.3%, respectively.[17]

Thermal or Heat-based Therapies—RFA and EVLA

Radiofrequency Ablation

Radiofrequency ablation was approved by the United States Food and Drug Administration (US FDA) in 1999 (VNUS

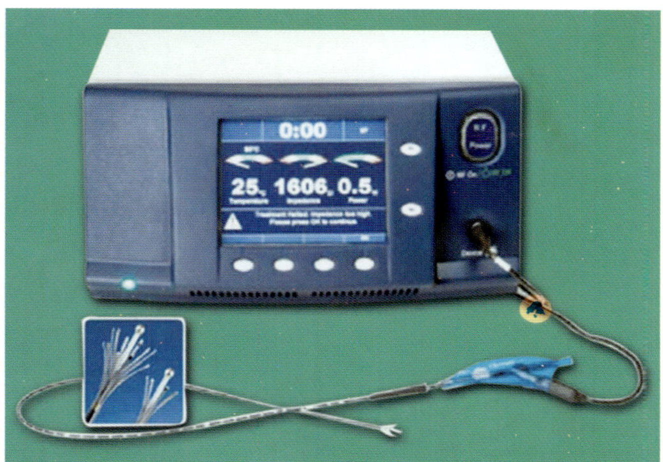

FIG. 4: VNUS Medical Technologies, Inc. device components for radiofrequency ablation. The ClosurePlus catheter possesses a microthermocouple that continuously measures vein wall temperature and provides feedback to the VNUS radiofrequency generator. Delivery of radiofrequency energy via the Closure electrodes (inset) causes resistive heating of the vein wall resulting in vein shrinkage and occlusion.

Closure; VNUS Medical Technologies, CA), as a minimally invasive method to obliterate superficial veins with reflux. Later, ClosurePlus and ClosureFast devices have also been developed.

Mechanism of Action

With RFA, high-frequency alternating current is applied to the vein wall by direct contact of the prongs of the RFA catheter with the venous endothelial layer. This causes disruption of vessel wall architecture and carbonization of the vessel. Very little thrombus is formed and precise tissue destruction is achieved.[12] Since there is a need for the direct contact of the catheter prongs with the endothelium, the application of RFA may be limited to veins smaller than 12 mm (Fig. 4).

Technique

The target vein is accessed using USG guidance, generally at the knee for GSV, and above the ankle for SSV. Further, the RFA catheter advanced to approximately 2–3 cm below the SFJ under USG guidance, immediately below the superficial epigastric vein. Tumescent anesthesia (a combination of 30 mL 0.1% lidocaine, 2 ampoules of epinephrine, and 10 mL bicarbonate with 200 mL cold saline) is injected perivenously along the vein. Tumescent anesthesia serves multiple purposes: analgesia, prevention of heat injuries to skin and also, compression of the vein to improve contact between the catheter prongs and the endothelium. Electrodes are available in two sizes—6Fr and 8Fr. The 6Fr probe treats vessels up to 8 mm and the 8Fr probe can be used for vessels measuring 8–12 mm in diameter. Larger vessels can be treated using additional strategies like extreme Trendelenburg position, increased TA volume, applying Esmarch bandage, etc. Radiofrequency ablation is performed with an intraluminally introduced ClosureFast catheter with a heating element measuring 7 cm. Segmental energy is delivered in 20-second cycles at a temperature of 120°C. In older RFA systems like VNUS, the temperature of probe was 85°C, and pullback rate was low (2.5–3 cm/min). During catheter withdrawal, impedance, temperature, and generator output should be monitored, to adjust the rate of withdrawal accordingly.[18] After completing catheter withdrawal, ultrasonography is performed to assess the patency of deep veins and for success of closure. It is recommended that after the procedure, patients should use compression stockings for 2 weeks, and resume normal daily activities immediately. Follow-up USG at 24–48 hours postprocedure is performed to confirm the occlusion of treated vein and absence of DVT.

Complication

Endovenous heat-induced thrombosis (extension of thrombus in common FV) is considered a major complication of thermal treatment of varicose veins and its incidence varies from 0 to 5.7% in literature. Minor side effects are pain, bruising, ecchymoses, paresthesias, etc.[19]

Outcomes

In a prospective multicenter study, review of 1,078 limbs in 890 patients was done at 1 week, 6 months, and 1, 2, 3, and 4 years. The vein closure rates were 91%, 88.8%, 86.2%, 84.2%, and 88.8%, respectively.[20] In a prospective, randomized controlled trial (RCT) comparing RFA and ligation with stripping (EVOLVeS Study), 2-year results showed RFA to be at least equivalent to surgery for GSV occlusion and that QOL scores were higher in RFA group at 2 years.[21] The RECOVERY Study (RFA vs. Laser) established that RFA was superior to EVLA by a significant margin as measured by multiple parameters like postprocedure recovery duration and QOL parameters. All scores like that of pain, tenderness, and ecchymosis were statistically lower in the ClosureFast (RFA) group.[22]

Endovenous Laser Ablation

Application of laser energy intraluminally to treat superficial venous reflux disease started to rise in popularity in the 1990s. It was approved by FDA in 2002 (Fig. 5).

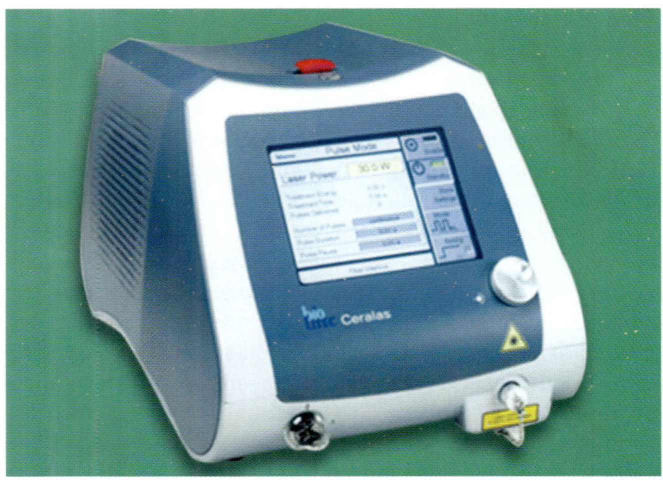

FIG. 5: Endovenous laser ablation machine.

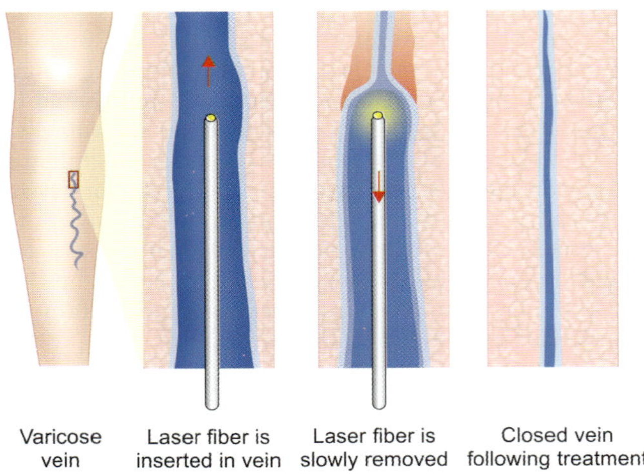

FIG. 6: Mechanism of action of endovenous laser ablation.

Mechanism of Action

Endovenous laser ablation applies laser energy directly inside the vein which causes boiling of the blood inside the vein, and there is spread of these steam bubbles up to the vein wall which disrupts the vessel wall architecture.[23] Some authors argue that the heat produced by the steam is not sufficient to destroy the wall of the vein, and that it needs direct contact of the venous wall with the laser energy itself. Whichever theory is accepted, the final mechanism is that heating the vein wall leads to contraction of the collagen and endothelial destruction. The final result is the fibrosis of the vein (Fig. 6).[24]

Technique

The patient is asked to lie down and is placed in reverse Trendelenburg position and GSV is accessed at the knee under USG guidance. A 5Fr sheath is introduced inside the vein over a guidewire. A laser fiber is then introduced through the sheath so that the tip lies approximately 2 cm below the SFJ. The location of the tip is confirmed on USG and the visible red beam through the skin. Laser fibers emitting energies at variety of wavelengths are available for, e.g., 810/940/980/1,320/1,470/1,560 nm. The one most commonly used at our institution is 1,470 nm fiber. After applying the TA in perivenous sheath, the GSV is treated in the pulsed mode or continuous mode at 6–12 watts of power. Pulsed mode has been shown to have a higher risk of adverse events than continuous mode Doppler. Hence, continuous mode is more commonly used. Radial endovenous energy density of 60–80 J/cm^2 is applied with simultaneous and gradual withdrawal of the catheter (Figs. 7 to 9). Higher wavelengths are associated with less postoperative pain and ecchymosis. Postprocedure patients wear compression stocking for 2 weeks, undergo follow-up USG at 48 hours, and resume normal daily activities almost immediately.[12,23] A covered tip design of the laser fiber, which has been recently developed, prevents the bare tip to directly come in contact with the venous wall, which prevents perforation of the vein wall and subsequently reduces pain and bruising, but failure rate of this design is quite high. Deep venous thrombosis, an inability to move, target vein thrombus, severe arterial disease, and pregnancy are contraindications to EVLA.

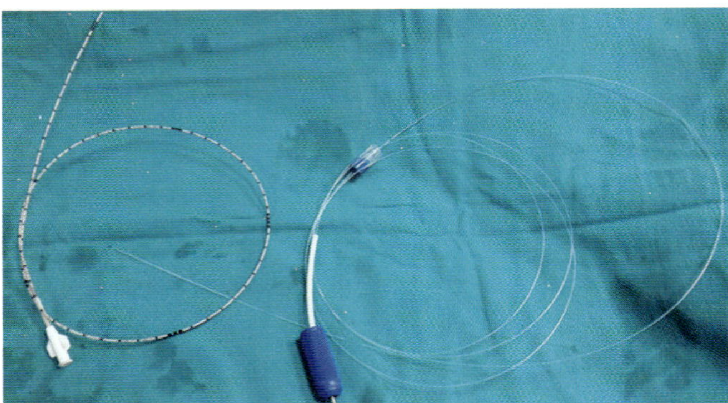

FIG. 7: Endovenous laser ablation catheter and laser fiber.

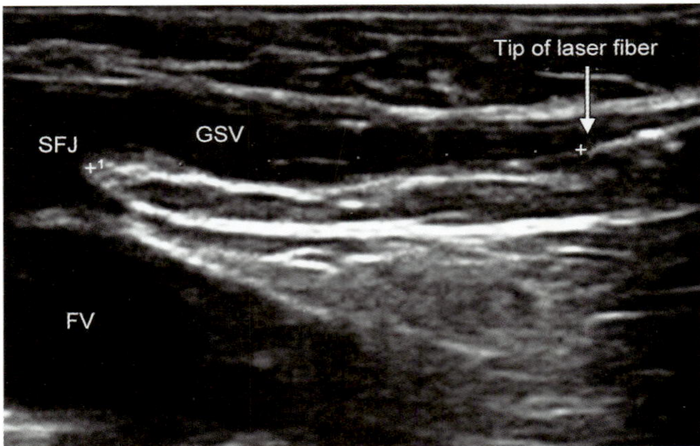

FV, femoral vein; GSV, great saphenous vein; SFJ, saphenofemoral junction.

FIG. 8: The tip of the laser is visualized by ultrasonography imaging and is kept at least 2 cm away from saphenofemoral junction.

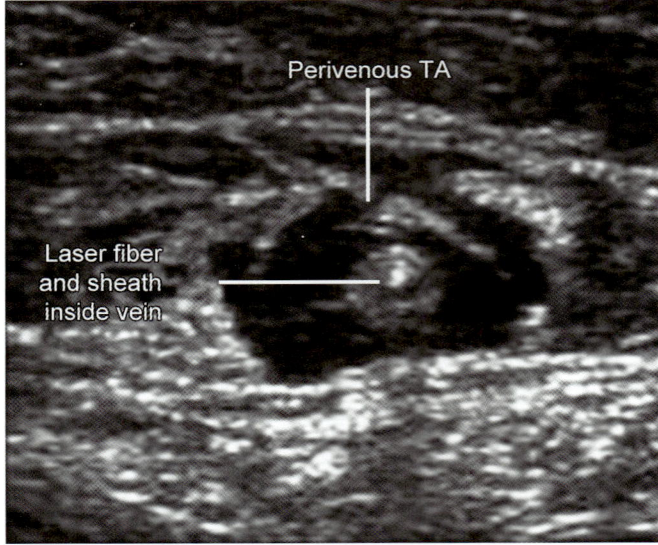

FIG. 9: Perivenous tumescent anesthesia (TA).

Outcomes

Endovenous laser treatment (EVLT) has shown excellent results in early obliteration of GSV. A retrospective review of 130 limbs in 92 patients at Mayo Clinic demonstrated an immediate occlusion rate in GSV to be 100% and reintervention rate of 0% in EVLT (vs. 17% in RFA).[25] A bigger trial evaluating 499 limbs demonstrated immediate obliteration rates of 98.2% in GSV and a 2-year success rate to be about 93.4%.[23] A meta-analysis also showed that results of EVLA are more effective than surgery, UGFS, and RFA.[26]

Complications

Similar to RFA. Pain, bruising, and induration of the thigh are common adverse effects of EVLA as compared to RFA which may be due to laser-induced perforation of the venous wall and extravasation of blood into adjacent tissue.

Comparative outcomes of different modalities are summarized in table 3.

Glue

Endovenous cyanoacrylate closure (CAC) is a newer technique approved by the US FDA (2015). It is a nontumescent, nonthermal, nonsclerosant procedure which is used endovenously to permanently close the vein [VenaSeal; Sapheon, VariClose Vein Sealing System (VVSS); Biolas]. The glue used is NBCA.

Trials and Outcomes

Early evidence from two studies does support the efficacy and safety of CAC for treatment of refluxing GSV.[22,29] Koramaz et al. published a retrospective study comparing CAC (VariClose) with EVLA for incompetent GSVs. The average procedure time and 1 year closure rates in the CAC and EVLA groups were 7 and 18 minutes and 98.6% and 97.3%, respectively. There was lesser incidence of adverse events after CAC (pigmentation and phlebitis).[30] First major randomized control trial evaluating CAC for varicose veins is VenaSeal Sapheon Closure System Study (VeClose Trial), a comparison of CAC versus RFA. Radiofrequency ablation was done with ClosureFast catheter. Out of 222 subjects, a 12-monthly follow-up was done for 192 subjects. At month 1, there was complete occlusion of vein in 100% of CAC patients and 87% of RFA patients. At month 12, both the groups showed nearly similar complete occlusion rates (97.2% in the CAC, 97 % in the RFA). Hence, occlusion is fast with CAC compared with RFA. Likelihood to recanalize was more in RFA group than the CAC group.[31]

TABLE 3: Intermediate and long-term success rates of endovenous therapies[20,21,23,27,28]

Reference, year	Sample size	Therapy	Follow-up in years	Occlusion (%)
Cabrera et al., 2000	500	Foam	3	95
Min et al., 2003	499	EVLA	2	93
Merchant et al., 2005	1,078	RFA	4	88
Lurie et al., 2005	65	RFA	2	96
Christenson et al., 2010	100	EVLA	2	93
Zuniga et al., 2012	355	RFA	1	98

EVLA, endovenous laser ablation; RFA, radiofrequency ablation.

Technique

After taking venous access using a 7Fr introducer sheath, a 5Fr delivery catheter is taken 5 cm inferior to the SFJ. Compressing the proximal GSV with the USG probe, two 0.1 mL drops of glue are administered 1 cm apart and additionally the treated segment is compressed with hand for 3 minutes. Subsequently serial 0.1 mL aliquots are administered at 3 cm distances along the target vein, and each treated segment is compressed for 30 seconds. Perivenous TA is not needed.

Complications

Complications are usually mild, with phlebitis being the most common as glue is an irritant. Mean intraprocedural pain ratings, paresthesias, and incidence ecchymoses are low. Burn marks and pigmentation which are common with thermal therapies are not observed.

Cryosclerosis

It was introduced by Milleret et al. in 1981. A cryoprobe which is quite flexible, is introduced inside the vessel with its tip refrigerated to –89°C after local anesthesia. The process causes thrombosis with very little inflammatory reaction and almost no pain. Then there is progressive fibrosis of the vein and recanalization almost never happens.[32]

There have been very few RCTs to support this therapy; however, Balint et al. published the results of a prospective trial in the year 2016. Out of 96 patients, 48 patients were administered cryosclerosis and the others were treated with conventional stripping. The occlusion rate was 81%. Recurrent varicosities were observed in 35% and 42% of the patients who received cryosclerosis and surgery, respectively. There was no significant difference between the groups ($p = 0.391$). Yet, cryosclerosis seems to be effective in the occlusion of the GSV.[33]

Mechanochemical Ablation

The ClariVein mechanochemical ablation (MOCA) system is the first ablation technique which employs a hybrid method in a single system. The tip of the catheters rotating wire causes endomechanical abrasion; and there is simultaneous injection of sclerosing agent over the rotating wire which causes chemical destruction.[34]

The device is composed of a catheter and a motor handle (to rotate the bent tip of abrasion wire). Catheter lumen is also connected to sclerosant syringe via side port. It is recommended to let the wire rotate for 3 seconds and withdraw simultaneously for about 0.5 cm to cause a venospasm at the proximal site, which is then followed by continuous rotation and withdrawal along with sclerosant delivery.[34] Occlusion rates are high (~97%) in the limited number of trials that have demonstrated its use.[35]

Endovenous Steam Ablation

All access steps are similar to EVLA. After TA and placement of catheter, pulses of steam at 120°C are released via generator. Catheter is withdrawn stepwise. About 3 cm below the SFJ or SPJ, four steam puffs are delivered with gentle manual

TABLE 4: Advantages and disadvantages of endovenous therapies for varicose veins

Therapy	Advantages	Disadvantages
Foam sclerotherapy	• Technical ease • Low cost • Less complications	• Microemboli • Skin necrosis
RFA	• Short- and long-term safety and efficacy is high • Superior to EVLA for postoperative ecchymosis and pain[38]	• Slow pull back time • Frequent need for a second catheter pass • High rate of additional treatments needed • Relative difficulty in treating larger veins
EVLA	• Very-high immediate success rate • Fast pull-back rate	• More minor complications, such as pain, edema, and bruising • Vein perforation with high energy
Glue	• TA is not required, fast • Early closure • Lower recanalization • Less ecchymosis • Compression stockings not required postprocedurally • Nonthermal—absence of paresthesias, burn, pigmentation, nerve injury • Due to viscosity and rapid polymerization, less incidence of deep venous thrombosis or pulmonary embolism[39]	• Phlebitis more common
ClariVein MOCA	• TA not required • Mechanical + chemical ablation • No risk of thermal injury to skin, nerves, and muscle	• Not Food and Drug Administration approved for varicose veins • Noise or vibration form catheter

EVLA, endovenous laser ablation; MOCA, mechanochemical ablation; RFA, radiofrequency ablation; TA: tumescent anesthesia.

pressure on the SFJ or SPJ. Subsequently, two to three puffs are delivered at 1 cm intervals depending on vein diameter. For the proximal segment during treatment, junction is compressed manually since the steam can reach some distance beyond the catheter tip. Postprocedure, patients should be advised to wear compression stockings for 2 weeks and to mobilize immediately after the treatment. The reported occlusion rates vary between 65 and 96%.[36] However, more RCTs are required to establish the use of this technique (Table 4).[37]

CONCLUSION

Chronic venous disease or varicose veins are important health issues with large loss in quality of life to the patient. Early recognition and management is important. With the introduction of endovenous strategies for superficial venous reflux, conventional surgical therapies are now rarely performed because endovenous therapies are minimally invasive, less morbid, done in outpatient basis with equal long-term efficacy as surgery. Ideally, treatment selection is according to individual patients' needs. The thermal-based techniques have widely been used in last decade. The newer nonthermal methods like glue and MOCA have multiple advantages and hold promise in future.

REFERENCES

1. Callam MJ. Epidemiology of varicose veins. Br J Surg. 1994;81:167-73.
2. Bergan JJ. Excision of varicose veins. In: Ernst CB, Stanley JC (Eds). Current Therapy in Vascular Surgery, 4th edition. St Louis, MO: Mosby; 2001. pp. 838-40.
3. Labropoulos N, Leon L, Kwon S, et al. Study of the venous reflux progression. J Vasc Surg. 2005;41:291-5.
4. Labropoulos N, Gasparis AP, Pefanis D, et al. Secondary chronic venous disease progresses faster than primary. J Vasc Surg. 2009;49:704-10.
5. Walters AS, LeBrocq C, Dhar A, et al. Validation of the International Restless Legs Syndrome Study Group rating scale for restless legs syndrome. Sleep Med. 2003;4:121-32.
6. Ramon RJP, van Eekeren, Boersma D, et al. Update of endovenous treatment modalities for insufficient saphenous veins—a review of literature. Semin Vasc Surg. 2014;27(2):118-36.
7. Morrison C, Dalsing MC. Signs and symptoms of saphenous nerve injury after greater saphenous vein stripping: prevalence, severity, and relevance for modern practice. J Vasc Surg. 2003;38:886-90.
8. Rautio T, Ohinmaa A, Perala J, et al. Endovenous obliteration versus conventional stripping operation in the treatment of primary varicose veins: A randomized controlled trial with comparison of the costs. J Vasc Surg. 2002;35:958-65.
9. Hartmann K, Klode J, Pfister R, et al. Recurrent varicose veins: sonography-based re-examination of 210 patients 14 years after ligation and saphenous vein stripping. Vasa. 2006;35:21-6.
10. Barrett JM, Allen B, Ockelford A, et al. Microfoam ultrasound-guided sclerotherapy of varicose veins in 100 legs. Dermatol Surg. 2004;30:6-12.
11. Legiehn GM, Heran MK. Venous malformations: classification, development, diagnosis, and interventional radiologic management. Radiol Clin North Am. 2008;46(3):545-97.
12. Sadick NS. Advances in the treatment of varicose veins: Ambulatory phlebectomy, foam sclerotherapy, laser and radiofrequency Closure. Dermatol Clin. 2005;23:443-55.
13. Hsu T. Foam sclerotherapy: A new era. Arch Dermatol. 2003;139:1494-6.
14. Parsi K. Catheter directed sclerotherapy. Phlebology. 2009;24:98-107.
15. Shin BS, Do YS, Lee BB, et al. Multistage ethanol sclerotherapy of soft-tissue arteriovenous malformations: effect on pulmonary arterial pressure. Radiology. 2005;235(3):1072-7.
16. O'Hare JL, Parkin D, Vandenbroeck CP, et al. Mid Term Results of Ultrasound Guided Foam Sclerotherapy for Complicated and Uncomplicated Varicose Veins. Eur J Vasc Endovasc Surg. 2008;36:109-13.

17. Frullini A, Cavezzi A. Sclerosing foam in treatment of varicose veins and telangiectases: History and analysis of safety and complications. Dermatol Surg. 2002;28:11-5.
18. Teruya TH, Ballard JL. New approaches for the treatment of varicose veins Surg Clin North Am. 2004;84:1397-417.
19. Stirling M, Shortell C. Endovascular Treatment of Varicose Veins. Semin Vasc Surg. 2006;19:109-15.
20. Merchant RF, Pichot O, Myers KA. Four-year follow-up on endovascular radiofrequency obliteration of great saphenous reflux. Dermatol Surg. 2005;31: 129-34.
21. Lurie F, Creton D, Eklof B, et al. Prospective randomised study of endovenous radiofrequency obliteration (closure) versus ligation and vein stripping (EVOLVeS): Two-year follow-up. Eur J Vasc Endovasc Surg. 2005;29:67-73.
22. Almeida JI, Kaufman J, Göckeritz O, et al. Radiofrequency endovenous ClosureFAST versus laser ablation for the treatment of great saphenous reflux: a multicenter, single-blinded, randomized study (RECOVERY study). J Vasc Interv Radiol. 2009;20(6):752-9.
23. Min RJ, Khilnani N, Zimmet SE. Endovenous laser treatment of saphenous vein reflux: Long-term results. J Vasc Interv Radiol. 2003;14:991-6.
24. Perrin M. Endoluminal treatment of lower limb varicose veins by endovenous laser and radiofrequency techniques. Phlebology. 2004;19:170-8.
25. Puggioni A, Kalra M, Carmo M, et al. Endovenous laser therapy and radiofrequency ablation of the great saphenous vein: Analysis of early efficacy and complications. J Vasc Surg. 2005;42:488-93.
26. Van den Bos R, Arends L, Kockaert M, et al. Endovenous therapies of lower extremity varicosities: A meta-analysis. J Vasc Surg. 2009;49:230-9.
27. Cabrera J, Cabrera J Jr, Garcia-Olmedo A. Treatment of varicose long saphenous veins with sclerosant in microfoam form: Long-term outcomes. Phlebology. 2000;15:19-23.
28. Christenson JT, Gueddi S, Gemayel G, et al. Prospective randomized trial comparing endovenous laser ablation and surgery for treatment of primary great saphenous varicose veins with a 2-year follow-up. J Vasc Surg. 2010;52(5):1234-41.
29. Almeida JI, Javier JJ, Mackay E, et al. First human use of cyanoacrylate adhesive for treatment of saphenous vein incompetence. J Vasc Surg Venous Lymphat Disord. 2013;1:174-80.
30. Koramaz I, El Kılıç H, Gökalp F, et al. Ablation of the great saphenous vein with nontumescent n-butyl cyanoacrylate versus endovenous laser therapy. J Vasc Surg. Venous and Lym Dis. 2017;5:210-5.
31. Morrison N, Gibson K, Vasquez M, et al. VeClose trial 12-month outcomes of cyanoacrylate closure versus radiofrequency ablation for incompetent great saphenous veins. J Vasc Surg Venous and Lym Dis. 2017;5:321-30.
32. Milleret R, Le Pivert P. Cryosclerosis of the saphenous veins in varicose reflux in the obese and elderly. Phlebologie. 1981;34(4):601-5.
33. Balint IB, Farics Á, Vizsy L, et al. [Cryosclerosis. The forgotten endovenous cryoablation of the great saphenous vein. Mid-term results of a prospective comparative trial]. Orv. Hetil. 2016;157(50):1994-2001.
34. Mueller RL, Raines JK. ClariVein mechanochemical ablation: background and procedural details. Vasc Endovascular Surg. 2013;47(3):195-206.
35. Elias S, Raines J. Mechanochemical tumescentless endovenous ablation: final results of the initial clinical trial. Phlebology. 2012;27:67-7.
36. Van den Bos RR, Malskat WS, De Maeseneer MG, et al. Randomized clinical trial of endovenous laser ablation versus steam ablation (LAST trial) for great saphenous varicose veins. Br J Surg. 2014;101(9):1077-83.
37. Proebstle TM, Lehr HA, Kargle A, et al. Endovenous treatment of the greater saphenous vein with a 940-nm diode laser: Thrombotic occlusion after endoluminal thermal damage by laser-generated steam bubbles. J Vasc Surg. 2002;45:729-36.
38. Anastasie B, Celerier A, Cohen-Solal G, et al. Laser endoveineux. Phlebologie. 2003;56:369-82.
39. Proebstle TM, Alm J, Dimitri S, et al. Twelve-month follow-up of the European multicenter study on cyanoacrylate embolization of incompetent great saphenous veins. J Vasc Surg Venous and Lym Dis. 2014;2:105-6.

CHAPTER 132

Deep Vein Thrombosis: Controversies and Consensus

Surender Deora, Kewal C Goswami

INTRODUCTION

Venous thromboembolism (VTE) is a thrombotic disorder manifesting as deep vein thrombosis (DVT) and pulmonary embolism (PE). Almost two-third cases of VTE are of DVT with involvement of proximal veins of legs but may also affect upper limb, splanchnic veins, and cerebral veins.[1] It is the third leading cause of vascular disease after myocardial infarction and stroke.[2] The incidence of DVT is 1:1000 per year and it increases with age with females more commonly affected in younger age group and males in elderly age group.[3-5] It is more common in African Americans as compared to Native Americans and Asians. The lifetime risk of VTE increases by 8% after the age of 45 years.[6] There are mainly three contributing factors as suggested by Virchow (Virchow's triad) for the formation of thrombus: stasis, vascular injury, and hypercoagulability (Flowchart 1). In 30–50% of the clinical cases, the cause of DVT is unknown and is unprovoked but it may also be secondary to provoking factors such as prolonged immobilization, cancer, oral contraceptives, trauma, and thrombophilia.[7] Proximal DVT is mainly due to chronic conditions whereas distal DVT in calf veins is mostly transient. It is high after orthopedic surgery with approximately 1% of patients developing DVT even after prophylactic anticoagulation.[8] Overall, the most common provoking factor is cancer in 19% of the patients followed by surgery and immobilization contributing to 15%.[9,10]

EVALUATION AND MANAGEMENT OF DEEP VEIN THROMBOSIS

There is significant morbidity and mortality in patients of VTE with mortality reaching up to 20% with PE and 2–5% with DVT mainly in those with proximal vein involvement.[11] The DVT itself can also impair the quality of life (QoL) with 20–50% of patients developing post-thrombotic syndrome (PTS) within 2 years after proximal DVT.[12] There is high recurrence risk in initial 3–6 months and therefore anticoagulation is needed in this period.[13] Therefore, the diagnosis of DVT should be made at the earliest and managed to prevent PE.

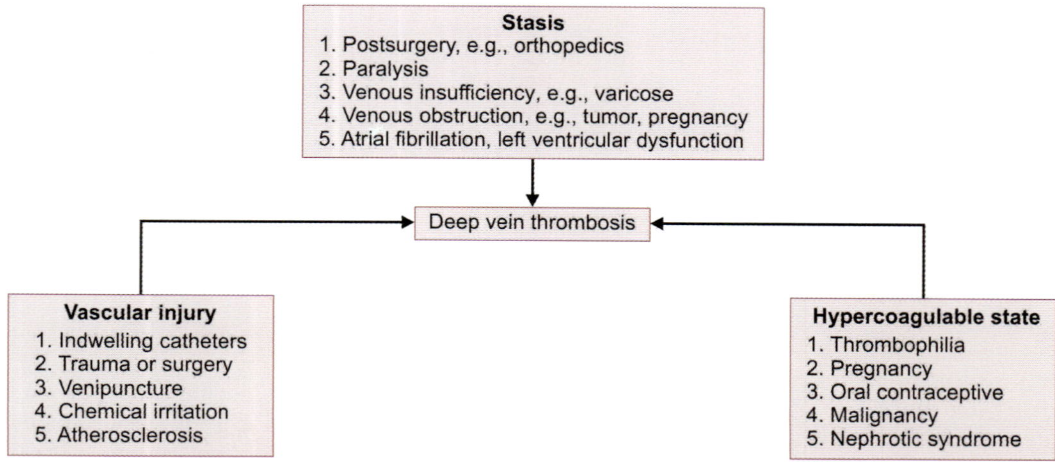

FLOWCHART 1: Clinical conditions associated with Virchow's triad leading to deep vein thrombosis.

TABLE 1: Therapeutic options available for the treatment of deep vein thrombosis

Duration treatment	Acute (5–10 days)	Short-term (3–6 months)	Long-term (>6 months)
IV heparin	Yes	No	No
SQ LMWH	Yes	Yes (cancer)	Yes (cancer)
SQ FONADAPARINUX	Yes	No	No
WARF	No	Yes	Yes
NOACs	Yes	Yes	Yes
	Rivaroxaban, apixaban—start day 1, no overlap heparin		
	Dabigatran, edoxaban—heparin overlap 5–10 days		
Aspirin	No	No	Yes

LMWH, low-molecular-weight heparin; NOACs, non-VKA oral anticoagulants; IV, intravenous.

Various practice guidelines have been published for the diagnosis and management of DVT patients. Many recommendations are based on strong clinical evidence and there is no controversy in applying those in clinical practice (Table 1). However, many recommendations are still based only on expert opinion and thus lead to significant practice variations across the regions and therefore need a consensus. This review will concentrate on these gray zones in the evaluation and management of DVT.

Imaging of Contralateral Asymptomatic Leg

The diagnosis of DVT is mainly based on clinical symptoms and imaging. Although venography is the gold standard, venous ultrasound (VUS) is most commonly practiced in clinical setting. VUS includes direct imaging of thrombus, compression ultrasonography, and abnormal spectral and color-Doppler flow. The sensitivity and specificity of VUS in diagnosing proximal DVT is 94.2% and 93.8%, respectively. The sensitivity increases with color Doppler although with reduced specificity.[14] After the diagnosis of DVT in the affected leg, it is debatable whether the contralateral leg should be scanned or not. The studies conducted for evaluation of prevalence of DVT in asymptomatic contralateral leg had inconsistent findings. Some studies have shown frequent association whereas some has shown no DVT in contralateral leg.[15,16] Le Gal et al. reported in their retrospective cohort study that for the diagnosis of unilateral clinically suspected DVT, the whole limb VUS is sufficient.[17] The study included 2,804 patients with clinically suspected DVT in which 21.8% had positive VUS. Out of these only 0.8% of patients had thrombus in both affected leg and contralateral leg and 0.2% had thrombus in only contralateral leg. The authors concluded that VUS of contralateral leg in clinically suspected DVT has very low yield and needs large number of scanning to diagnose one case of contralateral DVT. On the other hand, data from the OPTIMEV study had different results. This was a large multicenter, prospective, observational French study in patients with suspected DVT. Galanaud et al. performed the data analysis in the subgroup of patients who underwent bilateral VUS for unilateral DVT.[18] The study included 5,206 patients with clinical DVT, with 27% having positive VUS. In 5% of these patients contralateral DVT was diagnosed along with affected limb and 4.2% had positive VUS in only contralateral leg. The study finally concluded that bilateral VUS is necessary in certain groups of patients presenting with unilateral clinical DVT. However, the consensus is that the patients with active cancer, those with PE and normal ipsilateral VUS, and admitted elderly patients of >75 years of age are mostly benefitted with bilateral VUS. In conclusion, the VUS for contralateral leg is needed only in specific subgroup of patients at high risk of recurrent DVT.

Management of Isolated Distal Deep Vein Thrombosis

There is uncertainty regarding benefits of anticoagulation in patients with isolated distal DVT. The CACTUS study evaluated acute calf DVT in low-risk patients from 23 centers in Canada, France, and Switzerland.[19] In this randomized, double-blind placebo-controlled trial, patients were randomized to either low-molecular-weight heparin (LMWH) nadroparin (171 UI/kg, subcutaneously, once a day) or placebo (saline 0.9%, subcutaneously, once a day) for 6 weeks. There was no difference in rate of proximal extension or VTE between LMWH and placebo but there was an increased risk of clinically relevant nonmajor bleeding. At least 15% of untreated patients with isolated distal DVT may have either extension of thrombus to popliteal vein or may cause PE.[20] Therefore, these patients either need anticoagulation or VUS surveillance. These patients are to be risk stratified so that the anticoagulation can be started in high-risk distal DVT only (Table 2). After risk stratification, high-risk patients should be managed with full-dose anticoagulation for at least 3 months and low-risk patients may be either given anticoagulation for short time (4–6 weeks) or may have a VUS surveillance. The role non-VKA oral anticoagulants (NOACs) are not well

TABLE 2: Risk factors associated with increased risk of progression to proximal veins or venous thromboembolism in patients with isolated distal deep vein thrombosis

Risk factors for increased complication after distal DVT	
High-risk conditions	**Low-risk conditions**
• Male • Age >50 years • Unprovoked DVT • History of VTE • Extensive thrombosis (>5 cm length, >7 mm maximum diameter, multiple veins) • Cancer • Positive D-dimer • Isolated DVT involving popliteal trifurcation	• Transient risk factors e.g., OCP, hormone replacement therapy • Transient clinical conditions which are completely resolved e.g., fracture, long travel

DVT, deep vein thrombosis; VTE, venous thromboembolism; OCP, oral contraceptive.

established in isolated distal DVT but all patients are advised for compression stockings.

Thrombolysis versus Anticoagulation in Acute Proximal Deep Vein Thrombosis

Current standard treatment of DVT is anticoagulation and compression stockings. The main aim of anticoagulation is to prevent thrombus extension, reduce the incidence of VTE and recurrent DVT. Anticoagulation with heparin and oral therapy has reduced the thrombosis-related complications and mortality in DVT patients and is in the range of 2.5–5% with comparable risk of bleeding.[21] Despite the use of adequate anticoagulation, almost half of the patients with DVT develop PTS.[12,22] It is mainly caused by valvular and vascular injuries due to chronic DVT leading to raised venous pressure. This results in chronic tissue edema, subcutaneous fibrosis, and sometimes venous ulcers. The patients with PTS complain of heaviness in legs especially after prolonged standing and in evening hours, chronic mild pain in legs, and in severe cases venous ulcers. The QoL in these patients with PTS is significantly hampered and therefore the need was felt for revascularization of the affected veins as early as possible leading to the concept of "open vein hypothesis." The updated Cochrane review of 17 randomized controlled trials assessed the effects of thrombolytic therapy and anticoagulation versus anticoagulation in the management of patients with acute DVT of the lower limb.[23] Results of early and intermediate follow-up of 1,103 patients showed complete clot lysis and improved venous patency in the treatment group. Also the PTS and leg ulcerations were significantly less in patients that received thrombolysis but with complications. Patients receiving thrombolysis had more stroke and data on recurrent DVT and PE were inconclusive. There was also no significant effect on mortality and the incidence of severe PTS was not reduced. Thus, the authors concluded that the thrombolysis increases venous patency and reduces the risk of PTS by one-third but at the cost of increased risk of bleeding. Therefore, the usefulness of this strategy is limited to select patients only.

The use of catheter-directed thrombolysis (CDT) by directly infusing the drug into the clot is safer probably due to lower drug dose and was equally effective as systemic thrombolysis. The 5-year result of CAVENT trial studying 209 patients of acute proximal DVT treated with alteplase and anticoagulation versus anticoagulation alone found no significant difference in the QoL.[24] Similar results were also shown in ATTRACT trial where pharmacomechanical CDT did not reduce the risk of PTS but caused increased bleeding.[25] Therefore, in conclusion, any thrombolysis, either systemic or catheter-directed, in patients presenting with acute DVT, has not proven any long-term clinical benefits in terms of recurrent DVT, severe PTS, or mortality and hence is not recommended in patients with high proximal DVT.

Role of Compression Stockings for Post-thrombotic Syndrome

Post-thrombotic syndrome may occur in half of the patients with DVT with latency period extending up to 10 years. The cumulative frequency has been estimated to be 23% at 2 years and 28% at 5 years.[26] Treatment of PTS is difficult once it is established and only limited modalities are available. The cornerstone of PTS prevention was use of elastic compression stockings. This was based on two small randomized trials which have shown benefits in prevention of PTS by half after 2 years in DVT patients.[27,28] The effectiveness of compression stocking was recently challenged by findings from the SOX trial.[29] This was multicenter, randomized, placebo-controlled trial that enrolled patients from 24 centers in USA and Canada. A total of 806 patients having first proximal DVT diagnosed by VUS were randomized to either compression stocking (ankle pressure 30–40 mm Hg) or placebo (ankle pressure <5 mm Hg). There was no significant difference observed in the PTS with the incidence of 14.2% in the active stocking group and 12.7% in the placebo group using the Ginsberg criteria and was 52.3% in the active group and 52.3% in the placebo group using Villalta criteria. However, the major limitation of SOX trial was insufficient adherence to compression therapy and compliance definition (stockings wearing for ≥3 days/week) was significantly lower than in previous studies (56% vs. 90%).[27] The main reason cited for poor adherence was local irritation and cosmetic look. This result had affected the practice of routine use

TABLE 3: Indication of inferior vena cava filter according to various societies

Status of various guidelines for the indications for inferior vena cava filter insertion		
Indications	**Supporting societies**	**Opposing societies**
Acute VTE and contraindication for anticoagulation	ACCP, AHA, SIR, ACR	–
Anticoagulation failure	AHA, SIR, ACR	–
Hemodynamically unstable patients with VTE	ACCP, AHA, SIR, ACR	–
Massive PE treated with thrombolysis or mechanical thrombectomy	ACCP, SIR, ACR	AHA
Prophylaxis in high-risk population (polytrauma, spinal cord injury)	SIR, ACR	ACCP
Iliocaval DVT, mobile thrombus	SIR, ACR	–

ACCP, American College of Chest Physicians; AHA, American Heart Association; ACR, American College of Radiology; DVT, deep vein thrombosis; PE, pulmonary embolism; SIR, Society for Interventional Radiology; VTE, venous thromboembolism.

of compression stocking in DVT patients and also gave rise to changes in some guidelines. The incidence of PTS and adherence to compression stocking decreases with time, and therefore the exact duration of the compression needed to be defined. Till the publication of the SOX trial the usual duration for compression stocking was 24 months, but because of the adherence issue, shorter durations of compression stocking were studied. The OCTAVIA trial evaluated the duration of compression stocking 24 months versus 12 months on the occurrence of PTS and QoL.[30] The study concluded that strict adherence to the compression stocking decreases the incidence of PTS but is not noninferior to 24 months of therapy. The IDEAL DVT was multicenter, randomized, single-blind, noninferiority trial at 14 centers in the Netherlands and Italy, and compared the effectiveness of individualized duration of elastic compression therapy, with standard duration of therapy of 24 months for the prevention of PTS.[31] The participants were given the compression stockings for first 6 months and then individualized according to the Villalta scores to extended duration. The study concluded individualized tailored approach to be highly efficient as treatment could be stopped in 55% of patients at 6 months, and in an additional 11% of patients at 12 months, and is cost effective. Therefore, based on the available evidence the consensus is that the compression stocking is helpful in reducing the incidence of PTS but each patient needs individualized approach for the duration of the compression stocking.

Role of Inferior Vena Cava Filter

Acute PE is a dreaded complication of DVT and the 1-month mortality is twice that of DVT, although DVT is diagnosed twice as often as PE.[1] Anticoagulation is the cornerstone in the management of acute VTE patients. Current recommendation for inferior vena cava (IVC) filter is in patients with acute VTE and contraindications for anticoagulation or with any complication related to anticoagulation. There is a paucity of high-quality data for the use of IVC filter in patients with acute VTE. In spite of that the use of IVC filter is increasing in clinical practice especially with the introduction of retrievable filter. The PREPIC (Prevention du Risque d'Embolie Pulmonaire par Interruption Cave) trial randomized 400 patients with proximal DVT to receive anticoagulation with a permanent IVC filter versus anticoagulation alone.[32] After 2 years of follow-up, the patients in IVC filter had twice as common nonsignificant symptomatic PE but significantly more symptomatic DVT. At 8 years follow-up, there were significantly fewer symptomatic PEs in the filter group, but more symptomatic DVTs in the filter group with no difference in mortality.[33] The PREPIC 2 was open-label, randomized trial with 6 months of follow-up to evaluate the efficacy and safety of retrievable vena cava filters plus anticoagulation versus anticoagulation alone for preventing PE recurrence in patients presenting with acute PE and a high-risk of recurrence.[34] The study results at 3 months did not reduce the risk of recurrent PE and hence concluded no role of IVC filter in patients who can be anticoagulated. The meta-analysis by Bikdeli et al. in patients with DVT and at risk of PE has shown insignificant decrease in risk of PE, increased risk of DVT, and no change in all-cause mortality.[35] This meta-analysis included 11 studies of which six were randomized-controlled trials, but all of these randomized trials were considered low-to-moderate quality and none of them included the patients with contraindications to anticoagulation. Therefore, the routine use of IVC filter in patients with proximal DVT is not indicated and even its use in patients with contraindication to anticoagulation is purely based on expert consensus (Table 3).

Management in Cancer Patients with Deep Vein Thrombosis

Venous thromboembolism is a frequent complication in cancer patients and is the second leading cause of death after cancer progression. The annual incidence is as high as 20% depending on the type and site of tumor and associated risk factors.[36] It is associated with 2–6-fold increased risk of mortality and significantly affects the management of these patients.[37] Various practice guidelines have been published for the management of cancer-associated thrombosis but still many challenging clinical scenario persists where controversy prevails.

Type and Duration of Anticoagulation

All international practice guidelines recommend the use of LMWH for initial 3–6 months of diagnosis of DVT in cancer patients. It has many added advantages as compared to oral vitamin K antagonist (VKA). LMWH does not need frequent monitoring and is absorbed even if the patient is having nausea and vomiting. It has less drug-to-drug interactions. It also appears to have antiinflammatory properties and may have effect on cancer progression.[38,39] The role of VKA is restricted only as an alternative to LMWH. The safety and efficacy of NOACs in cancer patients is still unclear. There are systematic reviews and meta-analysis comparing the NOACs and VKA in cancer patients and has shown nonsignificant lower risk of recurrent VTE and major bleeding episodes as compared to VKA.[40] However, the quality of evidence is low as the trials were underpowered to show noninferiority or superiority of NOACs to VKA in cancer patients and included lower risk patients. Therefore, the use of NOACs is not recommended in the acute and long-term management of cancer-related VTE until large, well-conducted, high-quality randomized control trials are ensured.

There is limited data available for anticoagulation beyond 6 months of treatment, which is still debatable. These patients need risk stratification based on type of tumor, disease stage, and comorbid conditions of the patients.[41] Any randomized clinical trial in this subset of cancer patients is not feasible. Also the type and dose of anticoagulation beyond 6 months is uncertain. LMWH is preferable because of its strong data in acute management and in recurrent VTE. The use of VKA or NOACs is still unclear because of lack of clinical data. These cases are to be managed according to individual, case-by-case approach and tailored according to patient's clinical status.

Recurrent Venous Thromboembolism Despite Anticoagulation

Patients with cancer and VTE have high risk of recurrent VTE despite adequate anticoagulation. The incidence of recurrent VTE at 6 month is 7–9% and 10–17% in patients receiving VKA and LMWH, respectively.[42,43] There is lack of randomized clinical trials to guide management in such patients and potential therapeutic options available either change the anticoagulant or dose escalation of the given anticoagulant. These patients may also be offered IVC filter to prevent PE. Based on retrospective cohort studies and International Society on Thrombosis and Haemostasis (ISTH) registry, many professional societies recommend full therapeutic doses of LMWH in patients with recurrent VTE despite anticoagulation with VKA or NOACs.[44] Similarly, based on two cohort studies, it is recommended to escalate the dose of LMWH by 20–33% in patients with recurrent VTE despite treatment with LMWH.[45] Patients developing recurrent VTE despite dose escalation are very challenging and need to be managed on a case-by-case basis. IVC filters are used only in those patients who have absolute contraindications to anticoagulation and have been shown to have no net benefit in preventing recurrent VTE and no impact on survival. Therefore, the American College of Chest Physicians panel recommends IVC filter as last resort in such patients.[44]

Anticoagulation in Thrombocytopenia

Management of cancer patients on anticoagulation and thrombocytopenia is very challenging. The approach to these patients is on a case-to-case basis and depends upon the cause of thrombocytopenia, its severity, and expected duration. Thrombocytopenia may be due to chemotherapy-induced or by direct bone-marrow infiltration of cancer. There is general consensus that platelet count of 50×10^9/L is safe for initiation of therapeutic doses of anticoagulation. Those patients with moderate ($30–50 \times 10^9$/L) and severe ($<30 \times 10^9$/L) thrombocytopenia need special risk stratification in terms of bleeding risk and chances of recurrent VTE. The first month after VTE is the highest risk period for recurring events and therefore the management also differs depending upon the time since diagnosis of VTE (Flowchart 2).

Treatment of Incidental Cancer-related Pulmonary Embolism

There is an increase in the rate of diagnosis of cancer-related PE with use of multiple-detector computed tomography (MDCT) and up to 50% are incidentally detected.[46] There is limited available literature on the management of incidental PE in cancer patients. The prognosis of cancer patients with incidental detection of PE is similar to patients with symptomatic PE and therefore needs the same management. For the first 6 months, LMWH is the recommended

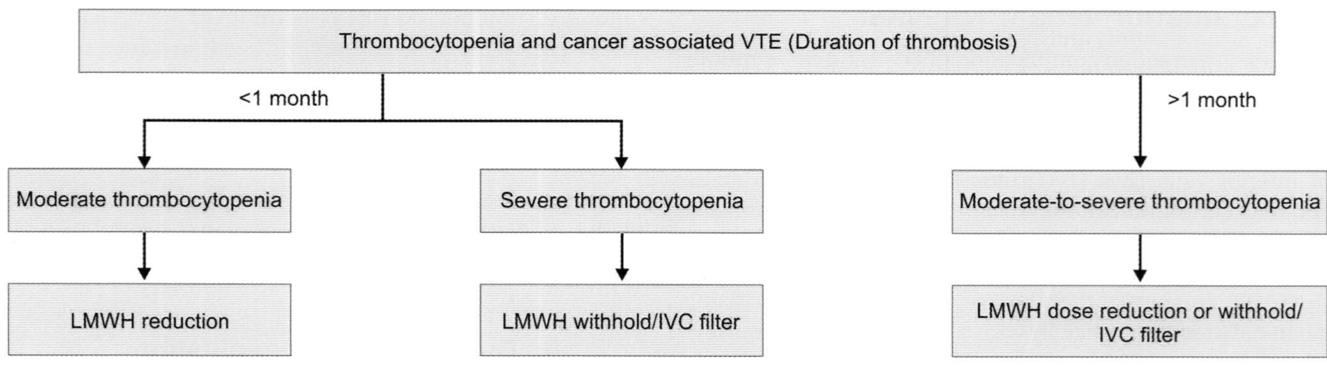

VTE, venous thromboembolism; LMWH, low-molecular-weight heparin; IVC, inferior vena cava.

FLOWCHART 2: Management strategy in cancer patients with venous thromboembolism and thrombocytopenia.

therapy and after that individual case-based approach is needed after risk stratification. For patients detected with isolated subsegmental PE (SSPE) and without DVT can be managed conservatively without anticoagulation. In patients with multiple SSPE, consensus suggests of anticoagulation therapy.[47]

Screening for Cancer in Unprovoked Deep Vein Thrombosis

Cancer is one of the important risk factor for VTE and the risk increases by 4.1-fold as compared to noncancer patients.[48] There is a complex interaction between tumor cells releasing cytokines, the hemostatic system causing platelet activation, and characteristics of the individual patient.[49] VTE may be the presenting manifestation of cancer in some patients, especially if DVT is unprovoked. The SOMIT trial randomized 201 patients with unprovoked VTE to extensive screening for cancer or no screening within 4 weeks of diagnosis.[50] The extensive screening strategy identified malignancies at an earlier stage and almost 93% of the malignancies were detected. However, there was no difference in mortality between the two groups. Similarly, the study was performed between 2002 and 2008 of 630 patients having objectively confirmed unprovoked VTE, who underwent extensive screening versus standard screening.[51] The extensive screening led to a diagnosis of cancer in 5.5% of patients at baseline and 3.7% during a median 2.5-year follow-up period as compared to 2.5% at baseline and 5.0% during a median 2.6-year follow-up period in standard screening group. Again there was no benefit in overall or cancer-related mortality in extensive screening group. Therefore, both these trials have concluded that extensive screening for cancer in patients with unprovoked VTE leads to more diagnosis of cancer with less time delay without having any effect on mortality. Also extensive screening is not cost-effective and may have procedure-related complications. The sensitivity of detecting cancer is also 50–70% and 30–50% of patients still remain undetected. Therefore, in conclusion, extensive screening for detection of cancer in patients with unprovoked VTE is not indicated.

CONCLUSION

Deep vein thrombosis is a commonly encountered clinical problem in community and hospitals. Despite advances in the diagnosis and management of DVT there are controversies in many clinical settings because of the insufficient available data. Mostly the consensus on these controversies is based on expert reviews and needs a case-by-case approach.

REFERENCES

1. White RH. The epidemiology of venous thromboembolism. Circulation. 2003; 107(23Suppl 1):I4-8.
2. Raskob GE, Angchaisuksiri P, Blanco AN, et al. Thrombosis: a major contributor to global disease burden. Arterioscler Thromb Vasc Biol. 2014;34:2363-71.
3. Silverstein MD, Heit JA, Mohr DN, et al. Trends in the incidence of deep vein thrombosis and pulmonary embolism: a 25-year population-based study. Arch Intern Med. 1998;158:585-93.
4. Heit JA. The epidemiology of venous thromboembolism in the community. Arterioscler Thromb Vasc Biol. 2008;28:370-2.
5. White RH, Zhou H, Romano PS. Incidence of idiopathic deep venous thrombosis and secondary thromboembolism among ethnic groups in California. Ann Intern Med. 1998;128:737-40.
6. Bell EJ, Lutsey PL, Basu S, et al. Lifetime risk of venous thromboembolism in two cohort studies. Am J Med. 2016;129:339. e19-26.
7. Goldhaber SZ. Risk factors for venous thromboembolism. J Am Coll Cardiol. 2010;56(1):1-7.
8. Januel JM, Chen G, Ruffieux C, et al. Symptomatic in-hospital deep vein thrombosis and pulmonary embolism following hip and knee arthroplasty among patients receiving recommended prophylaxis: a systematic review. JAMA. 2012;307:294-303.
9. Timp JF, Braekkan SK, Versteeg HH, et al. Epidemiology of cancer-associated venous thrombosis. Blood. 2013;122:1712-23.
10. Jensvoll H, Severinsen MT, Hammerstrøm J, et al. Existing data sources in clinical epidemiology: the Scandinavian Thrombosis and Cancer Cohort. Clin Epidemiol. 2015;7:401-10.
11. Galanaud JP, Kahn SR, Khau Van Kien A, et al. [Epidemiology and management of isolated distal deep venous thrombosis]. Rev Med Interne. 2012;33:678-85.
12. Kahn SR, Comerota AJ, Cushman M, et al. The postthrombotic syndrome: evidence-based prevention, diagnosis, and treatment strategies: a scientific statement from the American Heart Association. Circulation. 2014;130:1636-61.
13. Mearns ES, Coleman CI, Patel D, et al. Index clinical manifestation of venous thromboembolism predicts early recurrence type and frequency: a meta-analysis of randomized controlled trials. J Thromb Haemost. 2015;13:1043-52.
14. Goodacre S, Sampson F, Thomas S, et al. Systematic review and meta-analysis of the diagnostic accuracy of ultrasonography for deep vein thrombosis. BMC Med Imaging. 2005;5:6.
15. Naidich JB, Torre JR, Pellerito JS, et al. Suspected deep venous thrombosis: is US of both legs necessary? Radiology. 1996;200:429-31.
16. Sheiman RG, McArdle CR. Bilateral lower extremity US in the patient with unilateral symptoms of deep venous thrombosis: assessment of need. Radiology. 1995;194:171-3.
17. Le Gal G, Robert-Ebadi H, Carrier M, et al. Is it useful to also image the asymptomatic leg in patients with suspected deep vein thrombosis? J Thromb Haemost. 2015;13:563-6.
18. Galanaud JP, Sevestre MA, Genty C, et al. Is it useful to also image the asymptomatic leg in patients with suspected deep vein thrombosis? J Thromb Haemost. 2015;13:2127-30.
19. Righini M, Galanaud JP, Guenneguez H, et al. Anticoagulant therapy for symptomatic calf deep vein thrombosis (CACTUS): a randomised, double-blind, placebo-controlled trial. Lancet Haematol. 2016;3:e556-62.
20. Masuda EM, Kistner RL, Musikasinthorn C, et al. The controversy of managing calf vein thrombosis. J Vasc Surg. 2012;55(2):550-61.
21. Wells PS, Forgie MA, Rodger MA. Treatment of venous thromboembolism. JAMA. 2014;311:717-28.
22. Baldwin MJ, Moore HM, Rudarakanchana N, et al. Postthrombotic syndrome: a clinical review. J Thromb Haemost. 2013;11:795-805.
23. Watson L, Broderick C, Armon MP. Thrombolysis for acute deep vein thrombosis. Cochrane Database Syst Rev. 2014;1:CD002783.
24. Haig Y, Enden T, Grotta O, et al. Post-thrombotic syndrome after catheter-directed thrombolysis for deep vein thrombosis (CaVenT): 5-year follow-up results of an open-label, randomized controlled trial. Lancet Haematol. 2016;3:e64-71.
25. Vedantham S, Goldhaber SZ, Julian JA, et al. ATTRACT trial investigators. Pharmacomechanical catheter-directed thrombolysis for deep-vein thrombosis. N Engl J Med. 2017;377(23):2240-52.
26. Prandoni P, Lensing A, Cogo A, et al. The long term clinical course of acute deep venous thrombosis. Ann Intern Med. 1996;125:1-7.
27. Brandjes DP, Buller HR, Heijboer H, et al. Randomised trial of effect of compression stockings in patients with symptomatic proximal-vein thrombosis. Lancet. 1997;349:759-62.
28. Prandoni P, Lensing AW, Prins MH, et al. Below-knee elastic compression stockings to prevent the post-thrombotic syndrome: a randomized, controlled trial. Ann Intern Med. 2004;141:249-56.

29. Kahn SR, Shapiro S, Wells PS, et al. Compression stockings to prevent post-thrombotic syndrome: a randomized placebo controlled trial. Lancet. 2014;383:880-8.
30. Mol GC, van de Ree MA, Klok FA, et al. One versus two years of elastic compression stockings for prevention of post-thrombotic syndrome (OCTAVIA study): randomised controlled trial. BMJ. 2016;353:i2691.
31. Ten Cate-Hoek AJ, Amin EE, Bouman AC, et al. Individualised versus standard duration of elastic compression therapy for prevention of post-thrombotic syndrome (IDEAL DVT): a multicentre, randomised, single-blind, allocation-concealed, non-inferiority trial. Lancet Haematol. 2018;5(1):e25-33.
32. Decousus H, Leizorovicz A, Parent F, et al. A clinical trial of vena caval filters in the prevention of pulmonary embolism in patients with proximal deep-vein thrombosis. N Engl J Med. 1998;338(7):409-15.
33. PREPIC Study Group. Eight-year follow-up of patients with permanent vena cava filters in the prevention of pulmonary embolism: the PREPIC (Prevention du Risque d'Embolie Pulmonaire par Interruption Cave) randomized study. Circulation. 2005;112(3):416-22.
34. Mismetti P, Laporte S, Pellerin O, et al. Effect of a retrievable inferior vena cava filter plus anticoagulation vs anticoagulation alone on risk of recurrent pulmonary embolism: a randomized clinical trial. JAMA. 2015;313(16): 1627-35.
35. Bikdeli B, Chatterjee S, Desai NR, et al. Inferior vena cava filters to prevent pulmonary embolism: systematic review and meta-analysis. J Am Coll Cardiol. 2017;70(13):1587-97.
36. Khorana AA. Venous thromboembolism and prognosis in cancer. Thromb Res. 2010;125:490-3.
37. Elting LS, Escalante CP, Cooksley C, et al. Outcomes and cost of deep venous thrombosis among patients with cancer. Arch Intern Med. 2004;164:1653-61.
38. Mousavi S, Moradi M, Khorshidahmad T, et al. Anti-inflammatory effects of heparin and its derivatives: a systematic review. Adv Pharmacol Sci. 2015;2015:507151.
39. Tieken C, Versteeg HH. Anticoagulants versus cancer. Thromb Res. 2016; 140(Suppl 1):S148-53.
40. Carrier M, Cameron C, Delluc A, et al. Efficacy and safety of anticoagulant therapy for the treatment of acute cancer-associated thrombosis: a systematic review and network meta-analysis. Thromb Res. 2014;134:1214-9.
41. Carrier M, Lazo-Langner A, Shivakumar S, et al. Clinical challenges in patients with cancer-associated thrombosis: Canadian expert consensus recommendations. Curr Oncol. 2015;22:49-59.
42. Lee AY, Levine MN, Baker RI, et al. Low-molecular-weight heparin versus a coumadin for the prevention of recurrent venous thromboembolism in patients with cancer. N Engl J Med. 2003;349:146-53.
43. Lee AY, Kamphuisen PW, Meyer G, et al. Tinzaparin vs warfarin for treatment of acute venous thromboembolism in patients with active cancer: a randomized clinical trial. JAMA. 2015;314:677-86.
44. Kearon C, Akl EA, Ornelas J, et al. Antithrombotic therapy for VTE disease: CHEST guideline and expert panel report. Chest. 2016;149:315-52.
45. Ihaddadene R, Le GG, Delluc A, et al. Dose escalation of low molecular weight heparin in patients with recurrent cancer-associated thrombosis. Thromb Res. 2014;134:93-5.
46. Van EN, Bleker SM, Di NM. Cancer-associated unsuspected pulmonary embolism. Thromb Res. 2014;133(Suppl 2):S172-8.
47. Di Nisio M, Lee AY, Carrier M, et al. Diagnosis and treatment of incidental venous thromboembolism in cancer patients: guidance from the SSC of the ISTH. J Thromb Haemost. 2015;13:880-3.
48. Heit JA, Silverstein MD, Mohr DN, et al. Risk factors for deep vein thrombosis and pulmonary embolism: a population-based case-control study. Arch Intern Med. 2000;160:809-15.
49. Bick RL Cancer-associated thrombosis. N Engl J Med. 2003;349:109-11.
50. Piccioli A, Lensing AWA, Prins MH, et al. Extensive screening for occult malignant disease in idiopathic venous thromboembolism: a prospective randomized clinical trial. J Thromb Haemost. 2004;2:884-9.
51. Van Doormaal FF, Terpstra W, Van Der Griend R, et al. Is extensive screening for cancer in idiopathic venous thromboembolism warranted? J Thromb Haemost. 2011;9:79-84.

CHAPTER 133

Renal Artery Stenosis: When and How to Intervene?

George Joseph

INTRODUCTION

Renal artery stenosis (RAS) is a common cause of secondary hypertension. The etiology in more than 90% of cases of RAS is atherosclerotic renal artery stenosis (ARAS), with fibromuscular dysplasia (FMD) coming a distant second.[1] In India and other tropical/subtropical countries, RAS with secondary hypertension is not uncommonly caused by Takayasu arteritis (TA). This chapter will focus on these three etiologies of RAS, though several others such as aortorenal dissection, trauma, extrinsic compression, and posttransplant RAS may be occasionally encountered.

ATHEROSCLEROTIC RENAL ARTERY STENOSIS

Atherosclerotic renal artery stenosis produces a spectrum of clinical syndromes ranging from asymptomatic incidentally detected lesions to renovascular hypertension, ischemic nephropathy, and accelerated cardiovascular disease.[2] The underlying pathophysiology begins with RAS-induced reduction in renal blood flow resulting in activation of the renin–angiotensin–aldosterone axis, which in turn causes vasoconstriction, sodium retention, aldosterone secretion, vascular remodeling, sympathetic activation, and myocardial effects including left ventricular hypertrophy.[2] Later these processes, transition to alternate vascular mechanisms mediated by signals such as oxidative stress, endothelin, and vasoconstrictor prostaglandins that are not entirely dependent on the renin–angiotensin system.[2] Kidney injury in ARAS is produced by complex interactions between factors such as vascular rarefaction, oxidative stress injury, and recruitment of inflammatory cellular elements that ultimately produce fibrosis.[3] ARAS has profoundly adverse effects on the cardiovascular system and the kidney, i.e., in excess of what can be explained simply on the basis of hypertension or degree of renal impairment.[4] Patients with ARAS have more cardiovascular comorbidity and a greater prevalence of left ventricular hypertrophy and diastolic dysfunction than those without ARAS with the same level of blood pressure and degree of renal dysfunction.[5] Another important consideration is that ARAS is a progressive disorder; in one study,[6] progression of ARAS occurred in 53% of affected arteries, and total occlusion developed in 9%, all of which had a high-grade stenosis at baseline. In another study,[7] renal atrophy occurred in 21% of ARAS cases with high-grade stenosis and in nearly 6% of those with less than 60% stenosis.

Detection of Renal Artery Stenosis

Apart from the occasional abdominal bruit radiating to the flank, physical examination provides no specific clues to the presence of hemodynamically significant RAS.[1] Clinical suspicion of its presence may arise in certain situations (Box 1) and should initiate appropriate diagnostic evaluation.[1,8]

Noninvasive Diagnostic Evaluation

The 2017 European Society of Cardiology (ESC) guidelines[8] and the 2013 American College of Cardiology Foundation/American Heart Association (ACCF/AHA) guidelines[9] recommend duplex ultrasonography (DUS) as the first-line imaging modality to screen for significant RAS [class I, level of evidence (LOE) B]. Peak systolic velocity (PSV) in the main renal artery has 85% sensitivity and 92% specificity to identify angiographically significant RAS.[8] PSV and end-diastolic velocity (EDV) obtained using DUS can be used to determine the renal resistive index, calculated as (PSV-EDV)/PSV. Renal resistive index correlates closely with pressure gradient across the stenosis in patients with unilateral RAS[10] and may help to identify more severe RAS.[8] DUS has advantages such as being inexpensive, noninvasive, and easily repeatable to assess disease progression; however, it requires experience, may be difficult in overweight subjects, may fail to visualize portions of the renal artery, and may miss the highest PSV tracing and accessory renal arteries.[8] Computed tomography angiography (CTA) and magnetic resonance angiography (MRA) show

BOX 1 Clinical situations suggesting presence of renal artery stenosis*

- Onset of hypertension before age of 30 years
- Onset of severe hypertension after the age of 55 years, when associated with chronic kidney disease or heart failure
- Hypertension and abdominal bruit
- Rapid and persistent worsening of previously controlled hypertension
- Resistant hypertension (other secondary cause unlikely and target not achieved despite four drug classes including a diuretic and a mineralocorticoid-receptor antagonist in appropriate doses)
- Hypertensive crisis (acute renal failure, acute heart failure, hypertensive encephalopathy, or grades 3–4 retinopathy)
- New azotemia or worsening of renal function after treatment with renin–angiotensin–aldosterone system blockers
- Unexplained atrophic kidney or discrepancy in kidney size, or unexplained renal failure
- Flash pulmonary edema
- Multivessel coronary artery disease or peripheral artery disease
- Unexplained congestive heart failure or refractory angina

Source: *Adapted from Parikh SA, Shishehbor MH, Gray BH, et al. SCAI expert consensus statement for renal artery stenting appropriate use. Catheter Cardiovasc Interv. 2014;84:1163-71; Aboyans V, Ricco JB, Bartelink ME, et al. 2017 ESC Guidelines on the Diagnosis and Treatment of Peripheral Arterial Diseases, in collaboration with the European Society for Vascular Surgery (ESVS): Document covering atherosclerotic disease of extracranial carotid and vertebral, mesenteric, renal, upper and lower extremity arteries. Endorsed by: The European Stroke Organization (ESO), The Task Force for the Diagnosis and Treatment of Peripheral Arterial Diseases of the European Society of Cardiology (ESC) and of the European Society for Vascular Surgery (ESVS). Eur Heart J. 2018;39:763-816.

equally high sensitivities and specificities for the detection of RAS, but are more costly than DUS.[1,8] CTA has higher spatial resolution, but involves exposure to radiation and iodinated contrast.[8,9] Gadolinium-enhanced MRA provides excellent characterization of the renal arteries and kidney, but tends to overestimate stenosis severity and produces artifacts in patients with renal artery stents.[8] CTA and MRA are recommended as screening tests to establish the diagnosis of RAS in both the ACCF/AHA and the ESC guidelines (class I, LOE B).[8,9]

Invasive Diagnostic Evaluation

Invasive diagnostic angiography remains the gold standard for the diagnosis of RAS and should be considered for patients with inconclusive noninvasive testing and a high clinical suspicion of RAS and for patients at high risk for RAS and who require invasive angiography for other indications (ACCF/AHA and ESC class IIb, LOE B/C).[1,8,9] The 2014 Society for Cardiovascular Angiography and Interventions (SCAI) expert consensus statement classifies visually estimated angiographic RAS severity of less than 50%, 50–70%, and more than 70% as being mild, indeterminate, and significant, respectively. However, the correlation between degree of stenosis and hemodynamic impact is poor and so a variety of physiological parameters have been studied to guide treatment.[4] Pressures proximal (Pa) and distal (Pd) to the

TABLE 1: Invasive physiologic parameters used in renal artery stenosis evaluation*

Parameters	Acronym	Condition	Calculation
Mean resting pressure gradient	MPG	Rest	Pa – Pd (mean)
Mean hyperemic pressure gradient	MHG	Hyperemia	Pa – Pd (mean)
Peak resting systolic pressure gradient	RSG	Rest	Pa – Pd (peak)
Peak hyperemic systolic pressure gradient	HSG	Hyperemia	Pa – Pd (peak)
Resting pressure ratio	RPR	Rest	Pd/Pa (mean)
Renal fractional flow reserve	rFFR	Hyperemia	Pd/Pa (mean)
Renal flow reserve	RFR	Both	APVh – APVr

APVh, average peak intrarenal flow velocity during hyperemia; APVr, average peak intrarenal flow velocity at rest; *Pa, pressure proximal to renal artery stenosis; Pd, pressure distal to renal artery stenosis.

Source: Adapted from van Brussel PM, van de Hoef TP, de Winter RJ, et al. Hemodynamic measurements for the selection of patients with renal artery stenosis: a systematic review. JACC Cardiovasc Interv. 2017;10:973-85.

RAS using a 014-inch pressure wire or peak flow velocities using a Doppler wire are studied under resting and hyperemic conditions and various parameters are calculated (Table 1).

Using these parameters, the SCAI guidelines reclassify 50–70% RAS as significant if physiologic testing reveals mean resting pressure gradient (MPG) >10 mm Hg, or peak hyperemic systolic pressure gradient (HSG) >20 mm Hg (induced with intra-renal bolus of papaverine 30 mg or dopamine 50 μg/kg), or renal fractional flow reserve (rFFR) ≤0.8.[1] The ESC guidelines classify ≥60% stenosis by DUS as significant; however, an invasively determined peak resting systolic pressure gradient (RSG) >20mmHg or a resting pressure ratio (RPR) <0.90 is considered necessary to confirm significant stenosis in symptomatic patients.[8] Van Brussel et al. recently reviewed 15 studies concerning basal and hyperemic hemodynamic measurements in patients with RAS as a guide to treatment and concluded that the correlation between angiographic stenosis severity and hemodynamic data was relatively poor, and the predictive value of intrarenal functional data for outcome is still insufficient; this may be at least partly related to the heterogeneity in methodology and subjects' characteristics.[11] Myocardial and renal physiologies have distinct differences, because of which physiological indexes successful in coronary artery interventions may not be fully transferable to the setting of RAS.[11] Currently, adequate tools to reliably establish the hemodynamic significance of any degree of ARAS in humans do not as yet exist.[4]

Medical Management of Atherosclerotic Renal Artery Stenosis

The ESC and ACCF/AHA guidelines recommend medical therapy as the first-line treatment for ARAS.[8,9] Both recommend angiotensin-converting enzyme inhibitors (ACEIs), angiotensin receptor blockers (ARBs), calcium channel blockers, and beta-blockers (class I), but the ESC guidelines recommend diuretics as well (class I), and caution that ACEI/ARB therapy in patients with bilateral severe RAS or RAS in a single functional kidney must be done only if well-tolerated and under close monitoring (class IIb). The ESC also considers statins and antiplatelet therapy as part of best medical therapy.[8]

Revascularization in Atherosclerotic Renal Artery Stenosis

The potential benefit of renal revascularization in ARAS seems intuitive. Indeed, several nonrandomized studies of percutaneous transluminal renal angioplasty (PTRA) and renal artery stenting (RASt) in ARAS showed clinical benefit.[12-17] Early randomized trials comparing PTRA with medical therapy in patients with moderate to severe ARAS showed modest but significant effect on blood pressure.[18] However, three recent major randomized controlled trials (Table 2) showed no difference between endovascular therapy and best medical therapy.[19-21] Apart from having design flaws, these trials have been criticized for excluding categories of patient who might have benefited from revascularization and for not defining the length of kidney disease in their patient population making it impossible to determine if the duration of renal dysfunction had any impact on outcome after intervention.[22] Another criticism is that data was not provided on different subgroups of patients, some of whom might have benefited from renal revascularization.[22] However, a later subgroup analysis on the Cardiovascular Outcomes with Renal Atherosclerotic Lesion (CORAL) trial data did not support a benefit of stenting based on the degree of stenosis, hemodynamic significance of the lesion, or higher pretreatment blood pressure.[23] In 2016, an expert panel systematically reviewed all data from randomized and nonrandomized studies concerning the comparative effectiveness and safety of RASt, surgical revascularization, and medical therapy to treat ARAS with regard to clinically important outcomes; they concluded that the strength of the evidence, that there is no or only a minimal clinically relevant difference between these treatments with regard to outcome or blood pressure control, is low.[24] In other words, it remains uncertain whether mechanical treatment of ARAS is beneficial or not.[4]

Current Indications for Percutaneous Revascularization in Atherosclerotic Renal Artery Stenosis

Given the prevailing uncertainty whether mechanical treatment of ARAS is beneficial or not and the negative results of recent randomized trials, it is unsurprising that the 2017 ESC guidelines state that routine revascularization is not

TABLE 2: Major randomized clinical trials comparing renal artery stenting to medical therapy*

Trials (reference)	STAR[19]	ASTRAL[20]	CORAL[21]
Year of publication	2009	2009	2014
Follow-up duration	2 years	5 years	5 years
Centers	10	57	109
RASt + MT group (N)	64	403	467
MT only group (N)	76	403	480
Inclusion criteria	• eGFR <80 mL/min/1.73 m² • Ostial ARAS ≥50% • Stable BP <140/90 mm Hg	ARAS >50% with clinician unsure of best treatment	ARAS >60% + HTN on ≥ two drugs or CKD with eGFR <60 mL/min/1.73 m²
Primary endpoint	≥20% eGFR decrease	1/Cr slope over time	Major CV or renal event
Main outcome	GFR decline similar	Favored RASt + MT but p = 0.06 (NS)	No difference
Renal outcome	GFR decline similar	Renal events same	No difference
BP outcome	No difference	No difference	Favored RASt + MT
Procedure-related complications N(%)	• Two early/one late death (5%) • Hematoma 11 (17%) • Others seven (11%)	Serious complications in 23 (6%) including two deaths (0.5%)	26 (5.5%)
Limitations	• Underpowered for estimating efficacy • 28% of stent group not stented as ARAS <50%	Considerable crossover between groups	<20% reached 5-year endpoint. Significant heterogeneity of technique

ARAS, atherosclerotic renal artery stenosis; ASTRAL, Angioplasty and Stenting for Renal Artery Lesion; BP, blood pressure; Cr, creatinine; CV, cardiovascular; CKD, chronic kidney disease; CORAL, Cardiovascular Outcomes with Renal Atherosclerotic Lesion; eGFR, estimated glomerular filtration rate; HTN, hypertension; MT, medical therapy; N, number; RASt, renal artery stenting; STAR, Stenosis and Impaired Renal Function.

Source: *Adapted from Aboyans V, Ricco JB, Bartelink ME, et al. 2017 ESC Guidelines on the Diagnosis and Treatment of Peripheral Arterial Diseases, in collaboration with the European Society for Vascular Surgery (ESVS): Document covering atherosclerotic disease of extracranial carotid and vertebral, mesenteric, renal, upper and lower extremity arteries. Endorsed by: the European Stroke Organization (ESO), The Task Force for the Diagnosis and Treatment of Peripheral Arterial Diseases of the European Society of Cardiology (ESC) and of the European Society for Vascular Surgery (ESVS). Eur Heart J. 2018;39:763-816.

recommended in ARAS (class III, LOE A) and make a class IIb LOE C recommendation for RAS with unexplained recurrent congestive heart failure or sudden pulmonary edema (cardiac destabilization syndromes).[8]

The pre-CORAL[21] 2013 ACCF/AHA guidelines accord class IIb, LOE C recommendation to percutaneous revascularization in asymptomatic ARAS, whether unilateral, bilateral, or in a solitary kidney.[9] In three specific situations class IIA, LOE B recommendation is made by the ACCF/AHA: (1) one is hemodynamically significant RAS and accelerated hypertension, resistant hypertension, malignant hypertension, hypertension with an unexplained unilateral small kidney, and hypertension with intolerance to medication; (2) the second is RAS and progressive chronic kidney disease (CKD) with bilateral RAS or a RAS to a solitary functioning kidney; and (3) the third is significant RAS with unstable angina.[9] A class I, LOE B recommendation is made for hemodynamically significant RAS and cardiac destabilization syndromes.[9]

Based on an expert panel review of available data,[1] the SCAI concluded that revascularization of significant (>70%) RAS may be considered appropriate care in the following situations:

- Cardiac destabilization syndromes (flash pulmonary edema or acute coronary syndrome with severe hypertension)
- Resistant hypertension (uncontrolled hypertension with failure of maximally tolerated doses of at least three antihypertensive agents, one of which is a diuretic, or intolerance to medications)
- Ischemic nephropathy with CKD with estimated glomerular filtration rate (eGFR) less than 45 mL/min/1.73 m^2 and global renal ischemia (unilateral significant RAS with a solitary kidney or bilateral significant RAS) without other explanation.

Current Indications for Surgical Revascularization in Atherosclerotic Renal Artery Stenosis

The ESC guidelines state that in case an indication for revascularization of ARAS exists, then surgical revascularization should be considered for patients with complex anatomy of the renal arteries, after a failed endovascular procedure or during open aortic surgery (class IIa, LOE B).[8] The ACCF/AHA gives class I, LOE B/C recommendations to surgical revascularization in ARAS with multiple small renal arteries or early primary branching of the main renal artery, and in combination with pararenal aortic reconstruction.[9]

Revascularization Modality

With the exception of a few situations discussed earlier, open surgical renal revascularization has been largely replaced by percutaneous intervention (PI) for ARAS because of the increased morbidity and mortality associated with surgery.[25] Of the two percutaneous renal revascularization techniques available, RASt is significantly better than PTRA. Van de Ven et al.[26] performed a randomized trial comparing PTRA with RASt for ARAS. About 42 patients in each arm were followed up for 6 months. Complications were similar. However, primary success rate (<50% residual stenosis) was worse with PTRA compared to RASt (57% vs. 88%), as were primary patency rate at 6 months (29% vs. 75%) and restenosis after a successful primary procedure (48% vs. 14%). Secondary RASt (performed in 12 patients) for primary or late failure of PTRA was as successful as primary RASt. Intention to treat analysis showed no difference in clinical results at 6 months between PTRA and RASt. The authors concluded that RASt was a better technique than BA to achieve vessel patency in ostial ARAS. Primary RASt and primary PTRA plus rescue RASt have similar outcomes, but the burden of reintervention after PTRA outweighs the potential saving in stents. The ACCF/AHA guidelines recommend renal stent placement for ostial ARAS lesions that meet the clinical criteria for intervention (class I, LOE B).[9]

Vascular Access

Conventionally, femoral arterial access has been used for renal interventions and offers several advantages such as the large caliber of the access vessel and proximity to the renals. However, radial artery access is being increasingly used to reduce access site complications and improve patient comfort. However, the operator needs specific technical skills as well as knowledge of device compatibility. Both radial arteries are suitable for renal intervention. Generally, the left radial access allows a shorter distance to renal arteries, but the right radial approach is ergonomically more comfortable with lower radiation exposure for the operator. Extra-long guiding catheters and balloons may be required in taller patients or with excessive aortic arch tortuosity.[27] The brachial artery may also be used, but is associated with a higher local complication rate.

Embolic Protection Device and "No-touch" Technique

Atheroembolization during stenting for ARAS occurs in virtually every patient[28] and could be responsible for deterioration of renal function postprocedure. Embolic protection devices (EPDs) have, therefore, been used during RASt for ARAS. Khosla et al.[29] retrospectively studied 18 patients who underwent RASt for ARAS using EPDs and compared them with matched controls. At 12-month follow-up, stage-4 CKD patients treated with EPD had significantly higher eGFR than controls. Use of EPDs adds to the procedure cost and is technically challenging in renal arteries that bifurcate early. Generally, use of EPDs is confined to RASt procedures in patients with impaired renal function.[25] Another technique used to limit atheroembolization and prevent potential ostial renal artery injury during RASt for ARAS is the "no-touch" technique (Fig. 1).[30] In this technique, two guidewires are used, the first is placed in the aorta to prevent contact between the guiding catheter and the renal artery ostium, and the second is placed in the renal artery and serves as a rail over which the balloon and stent are passed.

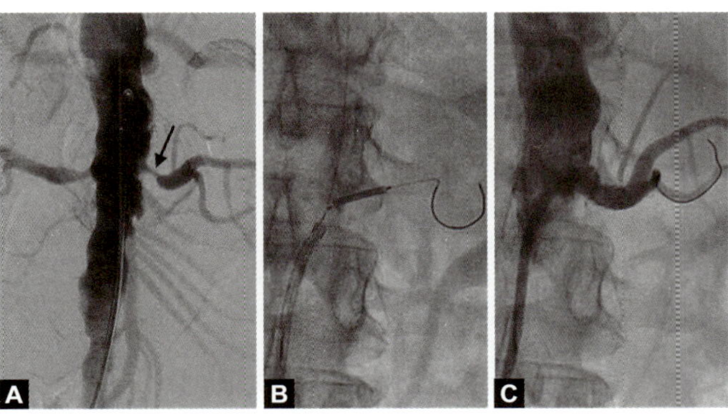

FIG. 1: "No touch" technique of renal artery stenting. **A,** Severe atherosclerotic ostioproximal stenosis of the left renal artery with extensive atheromatous aortic plaques in the vicinity; **B,** Two 014-inch guidewires are introduced through a 7-F guiding catheter, one is passed up the abdominal aorta and the other enters the left renal artery. A balloon-expandable stent is ready for deployment in the left renal artery; **C,** Poststenting selective left renal angiogram showing a good angiographic result.

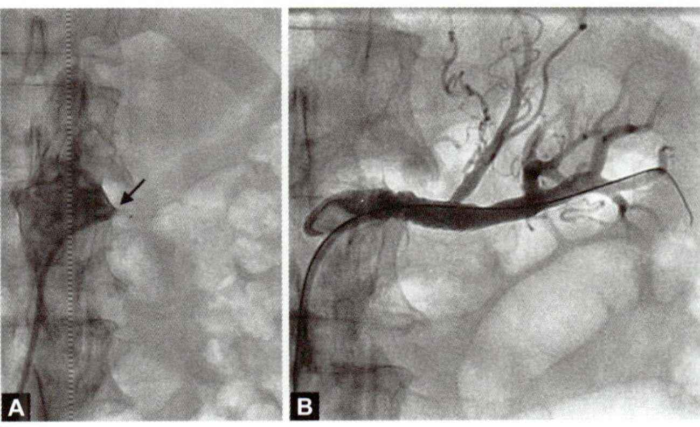

FIG. 2: Recanalization and stenting of a recently occluded renal artery in a patient presenting with pulmonary edema. **A,** Atherosclerotic ostial occlusion of the left renal artery; **B,** Postintervention selective left renal angiogram showing a good angiographic result.

Hardware

Renal interventions are performed using either a guiding catheter (such as a 7-F Renal Double Curve) and 014 or 018-inch guidewires, or long sheaths (such as the 6-F Ansel 55 cm) and 035-inch guidewires. Predilatation is usually reserved for severe lesions. Stents used in ARAS should be balloon expandable for accurate positioning and better radial strength. Bare-metal stents (BMSs) are almost always used, though drug-eluting stents have been tried in an effort to reduce restenosis. Zahringer et al.,[31] in a prospective multicenter nonrandomized trial (GREAT Trial), compared 52 patients undergoing RASt for ARAS using BMSs with 53 using sirolimus-eluting stents (SESs). Both stents significantly improved blood pressure, but angiographic outcome at 6 months did not show any significant difference (binary restenosis rate 6.7% for SES vs. 14.6% for BMS, $p = 0.30$).

Renal Artery Occlusions

The SCAI consensus document[1] considers revascularization of unilateral, solitary, or bilateral renal artery chronic total occlusion as rarely appropriate care probably because such kidneys are atrophic and revascularization is unlikely to restore any significant function. However, atrophic kidneys can be hormonally active and, therefore, contribute to significant hypertension and pulmonary edema;[32] also, not all kidneys with occluded arteries are atrophic, as the occlusion may be recent (Fig. 2) and viability may be preserved by collateral blood flow. Torsello et al.[33] surgically revascularized 52 kidneys with occluded arteries; they found that postoperatively blood pressure normalized or became easier to control in 89% of patients and mean plasma creatinine levels reduced significantly, enabling two severely uremic patients to discontinue hemodialysis; these benefits have to be weighed against an operative mortality of 5.7%. Percutaneous recanalization techniques in general have improved significantly of late and carry much lower risks. Very recently, Petrov et al.[34] reported successful recanalization of occluded renal arteries in six of seven hypertensive patients with elevated plasma renin levels; in the six patients with successful recanalization, blood pressure reduced significantly and plasma renin levels normalized at 6 months and 12 months follow-up.

Restenosis

The incidence of restenosis after RASt with BMS was 17% in a meta-analysis of 14 studies involving 678 patients.[35] The optimal treatment of in-stent restenosis is unclear. Zeller et al.[36] used four different treatment modalities in 31 patients with 33 second-time (reoccurring) in-stent restenotic lesions. Primary success rate was 100% with all modalities. During follow-up, repeat in-stent restenosis was seen in 71% with balloon angioplasty, 43% with drug-eluting stents, 17% with covered stents, and 100% with cutting balloon angioplasty.

Follow-up

Atherosclerotic renal artery stenosis patients undergoing RASt should be followed at 1 month, 6 months, 1 year, and annually thereafter.[25] Parameters to be assessed are blood pressure control, renal functions, and DUS imaging. DUS is the recommended imaging technique to screen for in-stent restenosis. DUS should take into account that a stented artery is less compliant than a native artery and that PSV and renal/aortic velocity ratio obtained by DUS are higher for any given degree of arterial narrowing within the stent, and hence obtaining a postprocedure DUS is reasonable to establish a new baseline PSV.[37]

FIBROMUSCULAR DYSPLASIA

Fibromuscular dysplasia is a nonatherosclerotic, noninflammatory vascular disease that most commonly affects the renal and internal carotid arteries, but can involve other arterial territories as well.[38]

Pathology

The pathological classification scheme of renal artery FMD is based on the arterial layer in which the lesion predominates.[38] Medial fibroplasia is the most common type, involves the middle to distal portion of the artery and is characterized by the classic "string of beads" appearance with the beading being larger than the normal caliber of the artery; only the arterial media is involved, the intima and adventitia being spared. Perimedial fibroplasia is another type of FMD that spares the intima and adventitia, characterized by a homogeneous collar of elastic tissue at the junction of the media and the adventitia; it is diagnosed when focal stenoses or multiple constrictions are observed, often with a robust collateral network; the "beads" are usually less numerous than in medial fibroplasia and are typically smaller in diameter than the normal caliber of the artery. Intimal fibroplasia occurs in less than 10% of FMD cases and appears angiographically as: (1) focal concentric stenosis, (2) long smooth narrowing, or (3) redundancy of the artery. Adventitial hyperplasia is the rarest type of FMD featuring sharply localized, tubular areas of stenosis.

Clinical Features and Imaging

Women, 15–50 years of age, are most commonly affected by renovascular FMD.[38] In most cases, it is detected incidentally, though evaluation for systemic hypertension may also reveal this condition. Angiographic progression of disease occurs in up to 37% of cases of renovascular FMD. DUS is an important diagnostic modality; elevated flow velocities in the distal portion of the renal arteries are suggestive of renovascular FMD; a renal resistive index less than 0.8 in the cortical vessels suggests a favorable response to revascularization. CTA and MRA are useful in detecting renovascular FMD, though the spatial resolution of the latter may be inadequate. Conventional angiography remains the most accurate method for diagnosing FMD.

Therapy

Medical treatment for systemic hypertension in FMD should follow standard guidelines. According to the 2017 ESC guidelines,[8] revascularization using balloon angioplasty with bail-out stenting is recommended (class IIa, LOE B) in cases of hypertension and/or signs of renal impairment related to renovascular FMD. The 2013 ACCF/AHA criteria also recommend balloon angioplasty with bail-out stenting (class I, LOE B) for FMD lesions that meet the clinical criteria for intervention; vascular surgical intervention is also recommended at the same level, especially for those exhibiting complex disease that extends into the segmental arteries and those having macroaneurysms. Although, there is a paucity of prospective data suggesting superiority of one treatment modality over the other, the percutaneous approach is increasingly favored in view of lower cost, invasiveness, and morbidity.[38] Successful angioplasty often results in substantial and rapid reduction in blood pressure (Fig. 3). Restenosis is seen in 7–27% of cases. Follow-up using periodic DUS imaging is important to detect progression of disease, restenosis, or loss of kidney volume.[38]

TAKAYASU ARTERITIS

Takayasu arteritis is a rare large-vessel vasculitis affecting the aorta and its primary branches producing stenotic or aneurysmal lesions. The renal artery is frequently stenosed or occluded in TA, resulting in secondary systemic hypertension, kidney atrophy, and renal insufficiency. Over the last three decades, there have been numerous reports of surgical[39-42] and endovascular[43-49] treatment of RAS in TA. These have fuelled two debates: (1) one is whether surgical treatment is superior to PI, and (2) the second is that if PI is performed, whether balloon angioplasty is better than stenting.[49,50] Surgical revascularization preceded PI historically, and is better established in the existing guidelines,[51,52] which

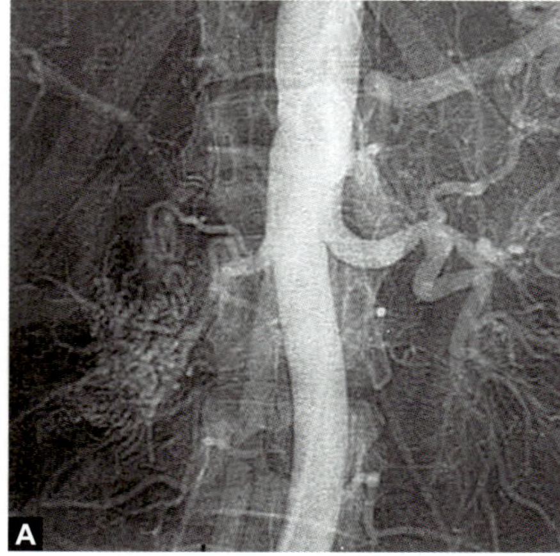

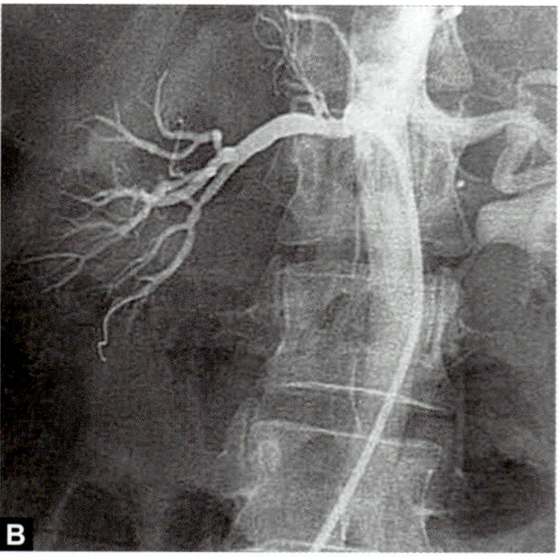

FIG. 3: Renal angioplasty in fibromuscular dysplasia. **A,** Abdominal aortogram in a young hypertensive woman showing perimedial fibroplasia type of fibromuscular dysplasia affecting the right renal artery; the involvement is nonostial, with multiple constrictions and a robust collateral network; "beading", typical of medial fibroplasia, is not seen; **B,** Angiogram, performed after balloon angioplasty of the main and first-order branches of the right renal artery, showing a good result. The patient had a rapid and substantial reduction in blood pressure.

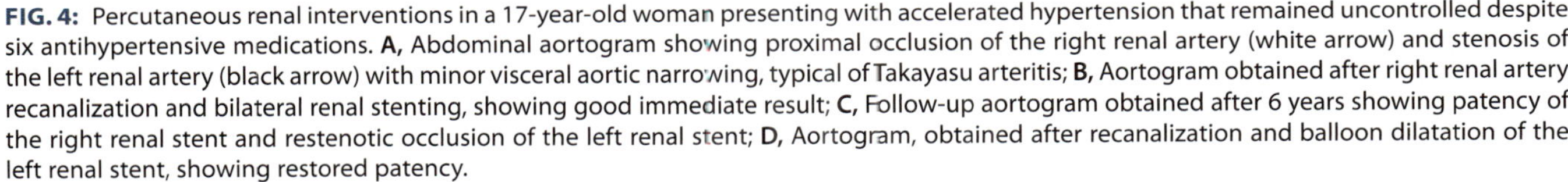

FIG. 4: Percutaneous renal interventions in a 17-year-old woman presenting with accelerated hypertension that remained uncontrolled despite six antihypertensive medications. **A,** Abdominal aortogram showing proximal occlusion of the right renal artery (white arrow) and stenosis of the left renal artery (black arrow) with minor visceral aortic narrowing, typical of Takayasu arteritis; **B,** Aortogram obtained after right renal artery recanalization and bilateral renal stenting, showing good immediate result; **C,** Follow-up aortogram obtained after 6 years showing patency of the right renal stent and restenotic occlusion of the left renal stent; **D,** Aortogram, obtained after recanalization and balloon dilatation of the left renal stent, showing restored patency.

do not consider PI in TA as standard therapy, and recommend restriction of its use to discrete lesions in high-risk patients during disease remission with the caveat that restenosis frequently occurs after PI in TA. However, these recommendations were based on small case series that used PI techniques developed largely for atherosclerotic vascular disease.[53] The relative rarity of TA, small numbers of patients in most TA case series, and wide variation in treatment strategies have retarded elucidation of the best way to treat vascular lesions in TA.[53] Arterial lesions in TA pose several distinctive impediments to obtaining successful PI outcomes and mandate development of disease-specific PI techniques to overcome these hurdles.

CHRISTIAN MEDICAL COLLEGE, VELLORE INTERVENTIONAL EXPERIENCE IN TAKAYASU ARTERITIS RENAL ARTERY STENOSIS

A total of 717 TA patients (mean age 29.6 years, 74.9% female) underwent 2,932 PIs to treat 1,893 arterial lesions in all vascular territories over 23 years (1996–2018) at Christian Medical College (CMC), Vellore, India. Of these patients, 315 of these patients underwent 676 renal artery PI procedures to treat 436 RAS lesions (214 left-sided and 222 right-sided). In 105 patients 2 renal arteries were treated, while in 9 patients 3 renal arteries were treated. Baseline serum creatinine was above 1.4 mg/dL during the first PI (PI-1) in 45 (10%) lesions, and inflammatory markers were elevated in 48%. 96% of the lesions were in hypertensive TA patients. Of the 436 renal lesions, 56 (12.8%) were occlusions, of which 48 (86%) were successfully recanalized (Fig. 4) with eight failures to cross. PTRA alone was done in 56 lesions during PI-1, using a mean balloon diameter of 4.8 mm and mean pressure of 8.8 atm; early successful outcome (residual <50%) was obtained in 52 (92.8%). RASt was done in 372 lesions during PI-1, either electively or to overcome suboptimal PTRA results, using a mean balloon diameter of 5.7 mm and mean pressure of 17 atm; early successful outcome was obtained in 359 (96.5%). Follow-up was obtained in 336/436 (77%) of all lesions at a mean of 31.8 months after PI-1. Follow-up obtained in 41/56 (73%) of lesions treated with PTRA during PI-1 revealed successful outcome (stenosis <50%) in 19 (46%) and suboptimal outcome/failure (stenosis >50%) in 22 (54%); 20 lesions in the latter subgroup were subjected to PI-2 (stenting in 14, repeat PTRA in 6). Follow-up obtained in 294/372 (79%) of lesions treated with RASt during PI-1 revealed successful outcome in 170 (58%) and suboptimal outcome/failure in 124 (42%); 117 lesions in the latter subgroup were subjected to PI-2 (balloon dilatation in 93, second stent in 24). Further

PIs (mostly simple balloon dilatation only) were performed at subsequent follow-up visits if required (average number of PIs per lesion was 1.55, range 1–8), leading to progressive increase in the cumulative success rate. At the final follow-up obtained after a mean of 40.6 months after the last performed PI, successful outcome was obtained in 223/269 (87%) of lesions. In the 386 lesions that were stented, BMSs alone were used in 236 and covered stents with or without BMS in 150; use of covered stents was associated with reduction in the number of PIs required (1.39 vs. 1.55) and time required (10.1 months vs. 61.9 months) to achieve sustained success. There were no in-hospital deaths. Complications included arterial dissection 16, rupture three, perforation one, distal embolization two, stent thrombosis six, inadequate stent expansion nine, stent displacement/distortion nine, and groin complications five; given that these occurred in 676 renal PI procedures, their absolute rate is low. Thus, PI used to treat RAS in TA yields a high level of mid- to long-term success with acceptably low morbidity; the key factors to achieve this are aggressive immunosuppressive therapy to control disease activity, use of high-pressure noncompliant balloons and covered stents, and repeated PIs till sustained success is obtained.

REFERENCES

1. Parikh SA, Shishehbor MH, Gray BH, et al. SCAI expert consensus statement for renal artery stenting appropriate use. Catheter Cardiovasc Interv. 2014;84:1163-71.
2. Garovic VD, Textor SC. Renovascular hypertension and ischemic nephropathy. Circulation. 2005;112:1362-74.
3. Textor SC, Lerman LO. Paradigm shifts in atherosclerotic renovascular disease: where are we now? J Am Soc Nephrol. 2015;26:2074-80.
4. de Leeuw PW, Postma CT, Spiering W, et al. Atherosclerotic renal artery stenosis: Should we intervene earlier? Curr Hypertens Rep. 2018;20:35.
5. Wright JR, Shurrab AE, Cooper A, et al. Left ventricular morphology and function in patients with atherosclerotic renovascular disease. J Am Soc Nephrol. 2005;16:2746-53.
6. Tollefson DF, Ernst CB. Natural history of atherosclerotic renal artery stenosis associated with aortic disease. J Vasc Surg. 1991;14:327-31.
7. Caps MT, Zierler RE, Polissar NL, et al. Risk of atrophy in kidneys with atherosclerotic renal artery stenosis. Kidney Int. 1998;53:735-42.
8. Aboyans V, Ricco JB, Bartelink ME, et al. 2017 ESC Guidelines on the Diagnosis and Treatment of Peripheral Arterial Diseases, in collaboration with the European Society for Vascular Surgery (ESVS): Document covering atherosclerotic disease of extracranial carotid and vertebral, mesenteric, renal, upper and lower extremity arteries. Endorsed by: the European Stroke Organization (ESO), The Task Force for the Diagnosis and Treatment of Peripheral Arterial Diseases of the European Society of Cardiology (ESC) and of the European Society for Vascular Surgery (ESVS). Eur Heart J. 2018;39:763-816.
9. Anderson JL, Halperin JL, Albert NM, et al. Management of patients with peripheral artery disease (compilation of 2005 and 2011 ACCF/AHA guideline recommendations): a report of the American College of Cardiology Foundation/ American Heart Association Task Force on Practice Guidelines. Circulation. 2013;127:1425-43.
10. Noory E, Rastan A, Beschorner U, et al. Duplex derived intrarenal resistance index correlates with invasive pressure gradient measurements in detecting relevant unilateral renal artery stenosis. Vasa. 2016;45:175-80.
11. van Brussel PM, van de Hoef TP, de Winter RJ, et al. Hemodynamic measurements for the selection of patients with renal artery stenosis: a systematic review. JACC Cardiovasc Interv. 2017;10:973-85.
12. Gray BH, Olin JW, Childs MB, et al. Clinical benefit of renal artery angioplasty with stenting for the control of recurrent and refractory congestive heart failure. Vasc Med. 2002;7:275-9.
13. Zeller T, Frank U, Müller C, et al. Stent-supported angioplasty of severe atherosclerotic renal artery stenosis preserves renal function and improves blood pressure control: long-term results from a prospective registry of 456 lesions. J Endovasc Ther. 2004;11:95-106.
14. Kashyap VS, Sepulveda RN, Bena JF, et al. The management of renal artery atherosclerosis for renal salvage: does stenting help? J Vasc Surg. 2007;45:101-8.
15. Laird JR, Rundback J, Zierler RE, et al. Safety and efficacy of renal artery stenting following suboptimal renal angioplasty for de novo and restenotic ostial lesions: results from a nonrandomized, prospective multicenter registry. J Vasc Interv Radiol. 2010;21:627-37.
16. Mannarino A, Spatoliatore G, Caselli GM, et al. Different outcomes of atherosclerotic renal artery stenosis managed with stenting: results from a cohort study. Ren Fail. 2012;34:142-8.
17. Jaff MR, Bates M, Sullivan T, et al. Significant reduction in systolic blood pressure following renal artery stenting in patients with uncontrolled hypertension: Results from the HERCULES trial. Catheter Cardiovasc Interv. 2012;80:343-50.
18. Nordmann AJ, Woo K, Parkes R, et al. Balloon angioplasty or medical therapy for hypertensive patients with atherosclerotic renal artery stenosis? A meta-analysis of randomized controlled trials. Am J Med. 2003;114:44-50.
19. Bax L, Woittiez AJ, Kouwenberg HJ, et al. Stent placement in patients with atherosclerotic renal artery stenosis and impaired renal function: A randomized trial. Ann Intern Med. 2009;150:840-8.
20. Wheatley K, Ives N, Gray R, et al. Revascularization versus medical therapy for renal-artery stenosis. N Engl J Med. 2009;361:1953-62.
21. Cooper CJ, Murphy TP, Cutlip DE, et al. Stenting and medical therapy for atherosclerotic renal-artery stenosis. N Engl J Med. 2014;370:13-22.
22. Mousa AY, Bates MC, Broce M, et al. Issues related to renal artery angioplasty and stenting. Vascular. 2017;25:618-28.
23. Murphy TP, Cooper CJ, Matsumoto AH, et al. Renal artery stent outcomes: effect of baseline blood pressure, stenosis severity, and translesion pressure gradient. J Am Coll Cardiol. 2015;66:2487-94.
24. Balk EM, Raman G, Adam GP, et al. Renal Artery Stenosis Management Strategies: An Updated Comparative Effectiveness Review [Internet]. Rockville (MD): Agency for Healthcare Research and Quality (US); 2016.
25. Tafur JD, White CJ. Renal Artery Stenosis: When to Revascularize in 2017. Curr Probl Cardiol. 2017;42:110-35.
26. van de Ven PJ, Kaatee R, Beutler JJ, et al. Arterial stenting and balloon angioplasty in ostial atherosclerotic renovascular disease: a randomised trial. Lancet. 1999;353:282-6.
27. Trani C, Tommasino A, Burzotta F. Transradial renal stenting: why and how. Catheter Cardiovasc Interv. 2009;74:951-6.
28. Olin JW. Atheroembolic renal disease: underdiagnosed and misunderstood. Catheter Cardiovasc Interv. 2007;70:789-90.
29. Khosla A, Misra S, Greene EL, et al. Clinical outcomes in patients with renal artery stenosis treated with stent placement with embolic protection compared with those treated with stent alone. Vasc Endovascular Surg. 2012;46:447-54.
30. Funaki B. Renal Ostial Angioplasty and Stenting. Part 1: The Routine Procedure. Semin Interv Radiol. 2009;26:74-81.
31. Zähringer M, Sapoval M, Pattynama PM, et al. Sirolimus-eluting versus bare-metal low-profile stent for renal artery treatment (GREAT Trial): angiographic follow-up after 6 months and clinical outcome up to 2 years. J Endovasc Ther. 2007;14:460-8.
32. Wykrzykowska JJ, Williams M, Laham RJ. Stabilization of renal function, improvement in blood pressure control and pulmonary edema symptoms after opening a totally occluded renal artery. J Invasive Cardiol. 2008;20:E26-9.
33. Torsello G, Szabo Z, Kutkuhn B, et al. Ten years experience with reconstruction of the chronic totally occluded renal artery. Eur J Vasc Surg. 1987;1:327-33.
34. Petrov I, Tasheva I, Garvanski I, et al. Recanalization and stenting of total occlusions of the renal arteries for blood pressure control in resistant to treatment hypertension. Cardiovasc Revasc Med. 2018:S1553-8389(18)30275-6.
35. Leertouwer TC, Gussenhoven EJ, Bosch JL, et al. Stent placement for renal arterial stenosis: where do we stand? A meta-analysis. Radiology. 2000;216:78-85.
36. Zeller T, Sixt S, Rastan A, et al. Treatment of reoccurring in stent restenosis following reintervention after stent-supported renal artery angioplasty. Catheter Cardiovasc Interv. 2007;70:296-300.

37. Chi YW, White CJ, Thornton S, et al. Ultrasound velocity criteria for renal in-stent restenosis. J Vasc Surg. 2009;50:119-23.
38. Slovut DP, Olin JW. Fibromuscular dysplasia. N Engl J Med. 2004;350:1862-71.
39. Teoh MK. Takayasu's arteritis with renovascular hypertension: results of surgical treatment. Cardiovasc Surg. 1999;7:626-32.
40. Chiche L, Kieffer E, Sabatier J, et al. Renal autotransplantation for vascular disease: late outcome according to etiology. J Vasc Surg. 2003;37:353-61.
41. Weaver FA, Kumar SR, Yellin AE, et al. Renal revascularization in Takayasu arteritis-induced renal artery stenosis. J Vasc Surg. 2004;39:749-57.
42. Ladapo TA, Gajjar P, McCulloch M, et al. Impact of revascularization on hypertension in children with Takayasu's arteritis-induced renal artery stenosis: a 21-year review. Pediatr Nephrol. 2015;30:1289-95.
43. Tyagi S, Singh B, Kaul UA, et al. Balloon angioplasty for renovascular hypertension in Takayasu's arteritis. Am Heart J. 1993;125:1386-93.
44. Sharma S, Gupta H, Saxena A, et al. Results of renal angioplasty in nonspecific aortoarteritis (Takayasu disease). J Vasc Interv Radiol. 1998;9:429-35.
45. Bayrak AH, Numan F, Cantasdemir M, et al. Percutaneous balloon angioplasty of renovascular hypertension in pediatric cases. Acta Chir Belg. 2008;108:708-14.
46. Park HS, Do YS, Park KB, et al. Long term results of endovascular treatment in renal arterial stenosis from Takayasu arteritis: angioplasty versus stent placement. Eur J Radiol. 2013;82:1913-8.
47. Zhu G, He F, Gu Y, et al. Angioplasty for pediatric renovascular hypertension: a 13-year experience. Diagn Interv Radiol. 2014;20:285-92.
48. Kinjo H, Kafa A. The results of treatment in renal artery stenosis due to Takayasu disease: comparison between surgery, angioplasty, and stenting. A monocentrique retrospective study. G Chir. 2015;36:161-7.
49. Peng M, Ji W, Jiang X, et al. Selective stent placement versus balloon angioplasty for renovascular hypertension caused by Takayasu arteritis: Two-year results. Int J Cardiol. 2016;205:117-23.
50. Jeong HS, Jung JH, Song GG, et al. Endovascular balloon angioplasty versus stenting in patients with Takayasu arteritis: A meta-analysis. Medicine (Baltimore). 2017;96:e7558.
51. JCS Joint Working Group. Guideline for management of vasculitis syndrome (JCS 2008). Japanese Circulation Society. Circ J. 2011;75:474-503.
52. Mukhtyar C, Guillevin L, Cid MC, et al. EULAR recommendations for the management of large vessel vasculitis. Ann Rheum Dis. 2009;68:318-23.
53. Joseph G. Percutaneous interventions in Takayasu arteritis. La Presse Medicale Quarterly Med Rev. 2013;42:635-37.

CHAPTER 134

Carotid Artery Stenting in 2018

Vivudh P Singh, Ranjan Modi, Atul Mathur

INTRODUCTION

Stroke is a major global health problem accounting for the second most common cause of death.[1] India being in midst of epidemiological and economical transition is particularly affected.[2] Besides being most populous we are also facing brunt of an increasing aging population. Approximately 20% of cases are due to extracranial carotid artery stenosis. Unlike coronary artery disease symptoms are due to embolization, rather than thrombosis. Symptomatic patient have much higher rate of embolism than asymptomatic patients although asymptomatic patients outweigh symptomatic patient by 4:1. Principally the source is internal carotid artery (ICA, 25%); however, intracranial small vessel disease (25%) cardiac embolism (20%), and idiopathic (25%) are other significant contributors.

In order to prevent stroke, carotid endarterectomy (CEA) has been used extensively as a primary option to eliminate both hemodynamic instability as well as the source of cerebral atheroembolism. Its efficacy was evaluated in four well-designed randomized controlled trials: North American Symptomatic Carotid Endarterectomy Trial (NASCET) the European Carotid Surgery Trial (ECST), Asymptomatic Carotid Atherosclerosis Study (ACAS), and Asymptomatic Carotid Surgery Trial (ACST). These studies have established a class Ia indication for CEA.

Carotid artery stenting (CAS) has been evaluated by multiple large randomized clinical trials (RCTs) that recognize CAS as an alternative to CEA for stroke prevention[1] in surgical-risk symptomatic patients when the anticipated risk of periprocedural stroke or mortality is less than 6% [(class I, level of evidence (LOE) B]. They also preferred CAS to CEA when carotid lesions were anatomically unfavorable (i.e., in cases of restenosis, high cervical or intrathoracic lesions, or following radiation therapy) (class IIa, LOE B). Finally, they have also recommended that CAS may be considered in highly selected asymptomatic patients with more than or equal to 60% angiographic stenosis (class IIb, LOE B).

Primary prevention is defined as aims to prevent carotid disease from ever developing. Secondary prevention is defined as aims at reducing the clinical impact of asymptomatic carotid stenosis [i.e., stenosis are present and the aim is to prevent them from causing a transient ischemic attack (TIA) or stroke]. The goal of tertiary prevention is to reduce the risk of recurrent TIA or stroke in patients who present with a TIA or stroke secondary to carotid stenosis. Decisions regarding carotid interventions should involve a multidisciplinary team (MDT) including neurologists or stroke physicians, vascular surgeons, and interventional radiologists at every hospital.

MANAGEMENT OF CAROTID ARTERY DISEASE

Definition of Stroke and Transient Ischemic Attack

Stroke diagnosis has been based on the World Health Organization (WHO) definition of a focal, occasionally global, loss of neurological function lasting more than 24 hours (or leading to death) and which has a vascular etiology. A TIA was defined in a similar manner, but the duration was less than 24 hours.[3] Imaging has shown that many TIA patients have evidence of acute infarction (particularly when symptoms lasted several hours) and this led to proposals that the classical definitions of stroke or TIA should be revised. One revised definition of TIA proposed by the American Heart Association (AHA) is "a brief episode of neurologic dysfunction resulting from focal temporary cerebral ischemia, which is not associated with acute cerebral infarction". Ischemic stroke is defined as "an episode of neurologic dysfunction caused by focal cerebral or retinal infarction, where infarction is defined as brain or retinal cell death, attributable to ischemia, based on neuropathology, neuroimaging, and/or clinical evidence of permanent injury".

Silent infarction is defined as "imaging or neuropathological evidence of cerebral/retinal infarction without a history of acute neurological dysfunction attributable to the lesion".[4]

Methods for Measuring Carotid Artery Stenosis Severity

The ECST and the NASCET trials used different methods for measuring stenosis severity.

- A 50% NASCET stenosis is equivalent to a 75% ECST stenosis
- A 70% NASCET stenosis equates to an 85% ECST stenosis.[5]

The ECST measurement method has important advantages over NASCET. The NASCET method does not permit reliable measurement of stenosis severity in patients with large volume plaques within dilated carotid bulbs. Here, the residual luminal diameter may be only slightly less than that of the distal ICA. In this situation, the NASCET measurement method will record a less than 50% stenosis, whereas the ECST method will measure this as being more than 70%. In this rare situation, recently symptomatic patients with large volume plaques consistent with an ECST more than 70% stenosis should be considered for revascularization.

Imaging Strategies in Carotid Artery Disease

Angiography has now been abandoned because of angiography-related stroke. In the ACAS, the 30-day deathor stroke rate was 2.3% after CEA, but about half of these strokes (1.2%) were angiographic related.[6]

Duplex ultrasound (DUS) is usually the first-line imaging modality because of its low cost and accessibility.

The advantage of computed tomographic angiography (CTA) and magnetic resonance angiography (MRA) is the ability to simultaneously image the aortic arch, supra-aortic trunks, carotid bifurcation, distal ICA, and the intracranial circulation, which is mandatory if a patient is being considered for CAS.

Contrast-enhanced MRA (CEMRA) has a higher accuracy than noncontrast MRA techniques but requires administration of a paramagnetic contrast agent such as gadolinium.[7] Catheter angiography is now rarely required, unless there are discrepancies on noninvasive imaging.

SECONDARY PREVENTION IN ASYMPTOMATIC PATIENTS

Medical Therapy

Control of Risk Factors

In a pooled analysis smoking was associated with a significant increase in the prevalence of a more than 50% ICA stenosis.[8] About 5% of males aged more than 65 years who are current smokers have a more than 50% ICA stenosis on DUS screening[9] and smoking was shown to increase plaque progression.[10] In a meta-analysis of 32 studies, smoking was associated with a significant increase in late ischemic stroke.[11] In a meta-analysis, moderate physical activity was associated with a 25% relative risk reduction (RRR) in ischemic stroke.[12]

Antiplatelet Therapy

There is conflicting opinion regarding antiplatelet therapy in asymptomatic patients because of concerns of increase in bleeding events. In the Asymptomatic Cervical Bruit study, patients with more than 50% asymptomatic ICA stenoses were randomized to 325 mg aspirin versus placebo, at follow-up, there was no difference in ischemic events or death.[13] By contrast, the Asymptomatic Carotid Emboli Study (ACES) reported that antiplatelet therapy was an independent predictor of lower rates of ipsilateral stroke or TIA in patients with asymptomatic 70–99% stenoses.[14]

In the Clopidogrel for High Atherothrombotic Risk and Ischemic Stabilization Management and Avoidance (CHARISMA) study, where 7% had asymptomatic 50–99% ICA stenosis, there was no evidence that dual antiplatelet therapy (DAPT) conferred any benefit over single antiplatelet therapy.[15] The net effect on stroke was not significant.[16]

Presently monotherapy with aspirin remains the antiplatelet agent in asymptomatic carotid artery stenosis patients, with clopidogrel reserved for patients who are aspirin intolerant.

Lipid-lowering Therapy

In ACST-1 patient who were on lipid-lowering therapy, the 10-year risk of stroke was 13.4% in medical therapy patients and 7.6% after CEA. However, in patients not on statins, the 10-year stroke risk was 24.1% in Optimal medical treatment (OMT) patients, versus 17.9% after CEA, suggesting that statins reduce long-term stroke in patients with asymptomatic stenoses.[17] With regard to dosage of statin therapy in these asymptomatic patients there are insufficient data available.

Management of Hypertension

Hypertension is associated with an increased risk of carotid disease.[18] Treatment of hypertension reduces stenosis progression (14% vs. 31%) and promotes regression (32% vs. 0%) compared with placebo.[19] Regression of carotid intima-media thickness (IMT) has been shown with patients with reductions in carotid pulse pressure.[20] The European Lacidipine Study on Atherosclerosis, compared lacidipine with atenolol, and concluded that lacidipine was associated with greater reductions in carotid IMT progression and fewer atherosclerotic plaques, despite smaller falls in blood pressure (BP), suggesting an independent, antiatherosclerotic action.[21] Similar results have been obtained for angiotensin-converting enzyme (ACE) inhibitors; however, calcium channel blockers (CCBs) reduce IMT progression more than diuretics, beta-blockers, or ACE inhibitors in many studies.[22]

None of the studies or RCTs has evaluated the effect of antihypertensive therapy on stroke prevention in patients

TABLE 1: Recommendations for management of asymptomatic carotid artery disease (European Society of Cardiology Guidelines 2017)

Recommendations	Class	Level
In "average surgical risk" patients with an asymptomatic 60–99% stenosis, CEA should be considered in the presence of clinical and/or more imaging characteristics that may be associated with an increased risk of late ipsilateral stroke, provided documented perioperative stroke/death rates are <3% and the patient's life expectancy is >5 years	IIa	B
In asymptomatic patients who have been deemed "high-risk for CEA" and who have an asymptomatic 66–99% stenosis in the presence of clinical and/or imaging characteristics that may be associated with an increased risk of late ipsilateral stroke, CAS should be considered, provided documented perioperative strike death rates are <3% and the patient's life expectancy is >5 years	IIa	B
In "average surgical risk" patients with an asymptomatic 60–99% stenosis in the presence of clinical and/or imaging characteristics that may be associated with an increased risk of late ipsilateral stroke, CAS may be an alternative to CEA provided documented perioperative stroke/death rates are <3% and patient's life expectancy is >5 years	IIb	B

CAS, carotid artery stenting; CEA, carotid endarterectomy.

with asymptomatic carotid stenoses (ACS). In practice, BP should be maintained less than 140/90 mm Hg in patients with carotid artery stenosis and ACS.[23]

Management of Diabetes

Diabetes is associated with a twofold increased risk of ACS,[24] as well as stroke.[25,26] In various meta-analyses, it has been shown that there is no evidence that tight glycemic control reduces stroke risk,[27] the UK Prospective Diabetes Study observed that tight BP control, mean BP 144/82 mm Hg, in patients with diabetes was associated with a 44% relative RRR in stroke, compared with patients with mean BP 154/87 mm Hg (Table 1).[28,29]

TERTIARY PREVENTION IN RECENTLY SYMPTOMATIC PATIENTS

The term "symptomatic" refers to any patient who has suffered a carotid territory symptom within the preceding 6 months. Carotid territory symptoms include (1) hemisensory impairment, (2) hemimotor deficits, and (3) higher cortical dysfunction.

"Crescendo TIAs" involve multiple TIAs within a short time period, with full recovery in between.

"Stroke-in evolution" refers to a fluctuating deficit (never fully back to normal) or a progressively worsening neurological deficit.[30]

Medical Therapy

Control of Risk Factors

The control of modifiable risk factors including smoking, exercise, diet, and obesity is an important aspect of tertiary prevention in patients of carotid stenosis.

Antiplatelet Therapy

The importance of starting antiplatelet therapy at an earlier time was documented in various meta-analysis which compared aspirin started in the first few days after symptoms onset, compared to control. Early aspirin therapy reduced the 6-week risk of recurrent stroke by 60% as well as disabling or fatal stroke by 70%.[31,32]

Antiplatelet Therapy during Carotid Artery Stenting

All guidelines recommend that patients of CAS should receive DAPT. However, this is mainly based on the coronary literature, with no data from large RCTs in CAS patients.

Meta-analyses of the various RCTs suggested aspirin plus clopidogrel therapy after coronary artery stenting;[33] however, the only RCT in CAS patients, aspirin plus heparin was associated with significantly higher perioperative neurological events and a nonsignificantly higher risk of bleeding complications compared with aspirin plus clopidogrel.[34]

Presently, most guidelines advise at least 4 weeks of treatment with aspirin and clopidogrel after CAS.[34] Literature shows long-term DAPT confers no additional benefit over single antiplatelet, unless indicated for cardiac reasons.[35,36]

Statins during Carotid Artery Stenting

Various studies have reported that statin therapy started prior to CAS are associated with significant reductions in 30-day risk.[37-39] Studies reported that 30-day death/stroke/myocardial infarction (MI) risk was significantly lower in CAS patients who were pretreated with statins (4%), versus 15% who were not.[37] A similar study reported that preoperative statin therapy was associated with significant reductions in perioperative death/stroke/MI (6.8%) versus 13.9% in those not taking statins pre-CAS.[39,38] Statin usage has not been evaluated in RCTs, but the evidence from these various studies suggest that pretreatment with statins in patients undergoing CAS is advocated.

Treatment of Hypertension

No RCT has evaluated the role of antihypertensives in patients with symptomatic carotid stenoses. However, a meta-analysis of 13 BP treatment trials in patients with history of stroke reported a significant RRR in stroke on antihypertensive therapy.[40]

TABLE 2: European Society of Cardiology recommendations: features associated with high risk of carotid endarterectomy

Recommendations	Class	Level
CEA is recommended in symptomatic patients with 70–99% carotid stenoses, provided the documented procedural seath/stroke rate is <6%	I	A
CEA should be considered in symptomatic patients with 70–99% carotid stenoses, provided the documented procedural death/stroke rate is <6%	IIa	A
In recently symptomatic patients with a 50–99% stenosis who present with adverse anatomical features or medical comorbidities that are considered to make them "high-risk for CEA", CAS should be considered, provided the documented procedural death/stroke rate is <6%	IIa	B
When revascularization is indicated in "average surgical risk" patients with symptomatic carotid disease, CAS may be considered as an alternative to surgery, provided the documented procedural death/stroke rate is <5%	IIb	B
When decided,it is recommended to perform revascularization of symptomatic 50–99% carotid stenoses as soon as possible, preferably with in 14 days of symptom onset	I	A
Revascularization is not recommended in patients with a <50% carotid stenosis	III	A

CAS, carotid artery stenting; CEA, carotid endarterectomy.

Though in symptomatic patients with severe bilateral ICA stenoses, aggressive BP lowering before revascularization may not be advisable.[41]

CAROTID ARTERY STENOSIS VERSUS CAROTID ENDARTERECTOMY

There has been a large section of literature published regarding choice of procedure for carotid artery stenosis (CAS vs. CEA).

Carotid artery stenting is the procedure of choice for high-risk patients compared to CEA. Features associated with high risk of CEA (Tables 2 and 3) (ESC recommendations) and predictors of high perioperative risk of CEA (Table 4) are independent variables for the choice of treatment. These factors can predict CAS as the choice of treatment for CAS (Table 5).

TABLE 3: Features associated with high risk of carotid endarterectomy

Medical comorbidity	Anatomic criteria
Elderly >75 years	Surgically inaccessible lesions
Congestive heart failure (NYHA class III/IV)	At or below C2
Unstable angina	Below the clavicle
CAD with >2 vessels >70%stenosis	Ipsilateral neck irradiation
Recent myocardial infarction <30 days	Spinal immobility of the neck
Planned open heart surgery (<30 days)	Contralateral carotid artery occlusion
Ejection fraction <30%	Laryngeal palsy
Severe pulmonary disease (COPD)	Tracheostoma
Severe renal disease	Previous ipsilateral CEA or neck surgery

CAD, coronary artery disease; CEA, carotid endarterectomy; COPD, chronic obstructive pulmonary disease; NYHA, New York Heart Association.

TABLE 4: Predictors of perioperative risk in carotid endarterectomy

Neurologic
- Deficit within past 24 h Stroke within past 7 days Crescendo TIA
- Global cerebral ischemia
- CT evidence of stroke

Angiographic
- Ulcerated plaque on stenosis
- >3 cm distal carotid stenosis
- >5 cm proximal carotid stenosis High bifurcation (at C2) Intraluminal thrombus

Medical
- Age >50 years
- Hypertension, COPD, severe obesity, DM

DM, diabetes mellitus; TIA, transient ischemic attack; COPD, chronic obstructive pulmonary disease.

TIMING OF INTERVENTIONS AFTER ONSET OF SYMPTOMS

The following are the definitions of "first event", "index event", and "most recent event".[42]

- The "first event" is the first symptom to affect the patient
- The "index event" is the symptom that led the patient to seek medical advice
- The "most recent event" is the symptom that occurred most recently.[42]

Timing of Carotid Artery Stenting

The time of performing CAS after symptom onset is controversial. A pooled series from four registries reported higher 30-day stroke rates (8.8%) when CAS was performed early less than 14 days, compared with 5.9% when CAS was performed later than 14 days.[43,44]

Timing of Carotid Interventions after Intracranial Endovascular Therapies

A meta-analysis of randomized trials reported that emergency endovascular treatment of acute ischemic stroke

TABLE 5: Indication associated with carotid endarterectomy

Indication	Recommendation	LOE
• Symptomatic high surgical risk • Among patients with symptomatic severe stenosis (>70%) in whom the stenosis is difficult to access surgically, medical conditions are present that greatly increase the risk of surgery , or when other specific circumstances exist, such as radiation-induced stenosis or restenosis after CEA, CAS may be considered when performed by an experienced operator	Class IIa	B
It is reasonable to choose CAS over CEA when revascularization is indicated in patients with neck anatomy unfavorable for arterial surgery	Class IIa	B
• Symptomatic average surgical risk • CAS is indicated as an alternative to CEA for symptomatic patients at average or low risk of complications associated with endovascular intervention when the diameter of the lumen of the internal carotid artery is reduced by >70% as documented by noninvasive imaging or >50% as documented by catheter angiography and the anticipated rate of periprocedural stroke or mortality is <6%	Class I	B
CAS is indicated as an alternative to CEA for symptomatic patients at average or low risk of complications associated with endovascular intervention when the diameter of the lumen of the internal carotid artery is reduced by >70% by noninvasive imaging or >50% by catheter angiography	Class I	B
• Asymptomatic high surgical risk patients • Selection of asymptomatic patient for carotid revascularization should be guided by an assessment of comorbid conditions, life expectancy and other individual factors and should include a thorough discussion of the risks and benefits of the procedure with an understanding of patient preferences	Class I	C
It is reasonable to choose CAS over CEA when revascularization is indicated in patients with neck anatomy unfavorable for arterial surgery	Class IIa	B
• Asymptomatic average surgical risk patients • Prophylactic CAS might be considered in highly selected patients with asymptomatic carotid stenosis (minimum 60% by angiography, 70% by validated Doppler ultrasound), but its effectiveness compared with medical therapy alone in this situation is not well established	Class IIb	B

CAS, carotid artery stenting; CEA, carotid endarterectomy; LOE, level of evidence.

was associated with a twofold improvement in functional outcome, compared with patients on medical therapy. Presently, there is no data to whether adjuvant CEA or CAS should be performed as a synchronous or staged intervention in these patients, but ESCAPE (The Evaluation Study of Congestive Heart Failure and Pulmonary Artery Catheterization Effectiveness) trial advised not to routinely perform CAS at the time of endovascular therapy.[45]

Benefit of Revascularization in Less than 50% Stenosis

In patients with less than 50% stenoses who report recurrent symptoms, it is important to ensure that optimal medical treatment should be initiated. If symptoms persist, despite optimal medical therapy, it may be reasonable to consider CEA or CAS.

CAROTID ARTERY STENTING OVER CAROTID ENDARTERECTOMY

Carotid artery stenting can be considered as an alternative to CEA in high-risk patients.

STAGED OR SYNCHRONOUS BILATERAL CAROTID INTERVENTIONS

Few patients can present with bilateral 70–99% stenoses. Either they will be totally asymptomatic, or have one stenosis symptomatic. It is extremely rare for bilateral severe ICA stenoses to be symptomatic simultaneously. The question is whether synchronous bilateral CEAs should be considered. While it is feasible to undertake bilateral synchronous CEAs,[46] the most dangerous complication is injury to both recurrent laryngeal and/or hypoglossal nerves. Accordingly, if bilateral (synchronous) revascularization is absolutely necessary, it may be better to consider bilateral CAS. However, in most patients, staged bilateral CEAs is appropriate, especially in the patient with a symptomatic 50–99% stenosis on one side and an asymptomatic 70–99% stenosis on the other.

CAROTID ARTERY STENTING TECHNIQUE

Adjuvant medical therapy has been a cornerstone of our intervention advances. It is now in guidance to start dual antiplatelet with aspirin and clopidogrel, if patient is not on any drug. Aspirin 300 mg loading should be done.

Postprocedure dual antiplatelet should be continued for at least 1 month followed by clopidogrel. It is now recommended to routinely administered 0.6–1.2 mg of atropine in view of anticipated hypotension and bradycardia (Table 6). Femoral is choice of access for most operators although radial may be preferred in aortoiliac tortuosity or occlusion or hostile aortic arch anatomy. The choice of sheath or guide catheter approach depends on the perceived technical difficulty of the procedure. Guide catheters have better torque control and are preferred for more challenging cases, such as steep aortic arch (types II or III), tortuous carotid artery, or extremely stenotic or calcified carotid lesions. Traditionally, Judkins Right and Amplatz 1, multipurpose have been used. In sheath approach a 6 Fr 90-cm Shuttle sheath is typically used. Either a 5 Fr diagnostic JR4 or VTK catheter can be used to engage the innominate or left common carotid artery. Following arterial access, intravenous (IV) heparin (50–100 U/kg) is given to achieve an optimal activated clotting time between 250 and 300 seconds (Table 7).

There has been lot of ongoing debate over stent cell design. Self-expanding tapered stents (nitinol or stainless steel) are preferred as they enable easy and accurate one-handed deployment. They are designed for low profile and rapid exchange. There are two types of cell designs. Open cell design enhances deliverability while remaining conformable and gentle on the vessel. Closed cell design secures the lesion and holds plaque in place. Hybrid cell design (See figure 1) ensure combination of better trackability and protection.

The International Carotid Stenting Study (ICSS)[47] reported 5.1 % risk of death or stroke at 30 days with closed cell design versus 9.5% with open cell (p = 0.024) there is no guideline recommendation for dual stent reducing procedural risk. Routine predilatation which predisposes to higher stroke risk is only advisable when there is anticipated difficulty is passing stent or filter protection devices.

Cerebral protection device (CPD): They are has now been relegated to class IIa (level II) as there has been conflicting evidence supporting their use. A meta-analytics comprising of 11,655 patient favored CPD as it reduced perioperative stroke death. Proximal protection device which work without crossing the stenotic lesion are an attractive option in prevention of embolic drug all stage of CAS. In a systematic review there has been reduction in periprocedural stroke 0.62 [RRR 95% (1.054–0.72)].

TABLE 6: Carotid artery stenting technique

Guiding catheter	Long sheath system
*Better torque control	Less torque control
*More rigid better support	Less rigid less support
*Better for tortuosity	–
7F/8F sheath size	*6F sheath size
Uneven transition with inner catheter	*Dilator provides smooth transition

*Comparison of choice of hardware, advantage of either technique marked as green.

TABLE 7: Recommendations for carotid artery stenting

Recommendation	Class	Level
The use to embolic protection devices should be considered in patient undergoing CAS	IIa	B
Proximal protection devices are not recommended in patients with advanced common carotid disease, or those with external carotid artery disease (where an occlusion balloon is to be positioned in the external carotid artery) or in patients with contralateral occlusion and insufficient collateralization	III	C

CAS, carotid artery stenting.

COMPLICATIONS

Perioperative Stroke

Stroke because of aortic arch manipulation is the most common intraprocedural cause. Protection device filters are also not full proof as they may be malapposed or incompetently deployed. Even if they are completely deployed it is worthwhile to remember that smallest pore size is 80 µm even in latest filter, so small particle can escape through then (Table 8).

If stroke do occurs, dedicated neurological devices can be used for cleaning of embolic material from main branch of ICA that gives to M2 segment. Thrombosuction can also be tried. Thrombolysis is not beneficial as embolism comprises of plaque rather than fibrin clot. However, if needed the agent studied are urokinase (500,000 two unit) at half as bolus or rTPA can be given as a 5-mg bolus, followed by slow infusion (maximum dose 20 mg). Selective glycoprotein (Gp) IIb/IIIa inhibitor (abciximab) has been tried in treatment of stroke.[48] Delphi et al. have enumerated predictor of periprocedural stroke (1) Type II aortic arch, (1) Bovine arch, (3) arch atheroma, (4) external carotid artery disease, (5) markedly angulated distal ICA, (6) long stenosis, and (7), pinhole stenosis (Table 9).[49]

Poststenting hypotension is generally a self-limiting event. To prevent it is important to hold antihypertensive

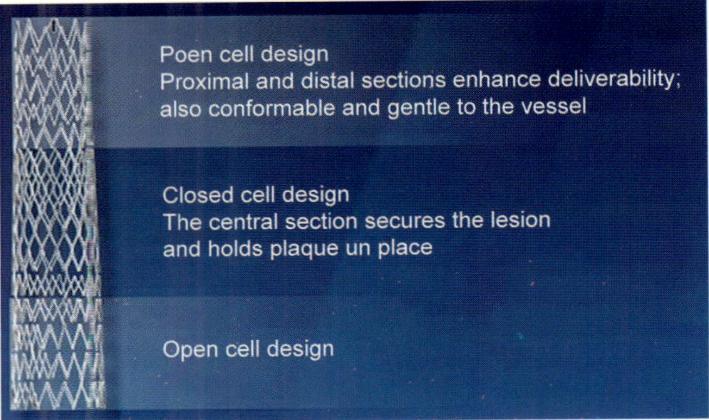

FIG 1: Hybrid cell design.

TABLE 8: Carotid artery stenting: Procedural factors likely to be associated with adverse procedural outcomes

Medical comorbidity	Anatomical criteria	Procedural factor
Elderly (>75/82 years)	Type III aortic arch	Inexperienced operator/center
Symptom status	Vessel tortuosity	EPD not used
Bleeding risk/ hypercoagulable state	Heavy calcification	Lack of femoral access
Severe aortic stenosis	Lesion-related thrombus	Time delay to perform procedure from onset of symptoms
Chronic kidney disease	Echolucent plaque	–
Decreased cerebral reserve	Aortic arch atheroma	–

EPD, embolic protection device.

TABLE 9: Complication related to carotid endarterectomy or carotid artery stenting

Recommendation	CLASS	LEVEL
Patients suffering a late ipsilateral stroke or transient ischemic attack (TIA) in the presence of an ipsilateral 50–90% restenosis should undergo redo carotid endarterectomy or carotid artery stenting	I	A
It is recommended that patients suffering a late ipsilateral stroke or TIA in the presence of an ipsilateral <50% restenosis should be treated medically	I	A
Reintervention may be considered in carotid endarterectomy patients with an asymptomatic 70–90% restenosis, following multidisciplinary team review	IIb	B
It is recommended that carotid stent patients who develop an asymptomatic restenosis >70% are treated medically	I	A

medicine on morning of procedure, having venous access and adequate hydration (N crystalloid plus volume expands) problem with IV expander is post-CAS in a state of decrease peripheral vascular resistance and hence IV vasopressor are more beneficial (preferably norepinephrine).

Restenosis

Symptomatic ipsilateral carotid territory symptom should undergo repeat CAS within 14 days. Regarding asymptomatic restenosis data is uncertain Kumar's meta-analysis suggested little or no benefit of intervention (0.8% over 4 year).[50]

Carotid Stenosis Patients Undergoing Major Cardiac Surgery

Routine screening in view of low prevalence of perioperative stroke cannot be supported. It should only be done in patient who are elderly, presence of carotid, prior stroke or staged left main triple vessel disease (TVD).[51] Etiology of perioperative stroke can be multifactorial however intervention is indicated in patient with prior history of stroke or TIA[52] or bilateral asymptomatic 70–99% stenosis.[53] However, evidence is less supportive in asymptomatic significant unilateral stenosis where risk of strokes is 20%.[53] Choice of strategy CAS versus CEA will depend on urgency of performing surgery, choice of antiplatelet (Table 10).

TABLE 10: Screening of cardiac stenosis patients for cardiac surgery

Recommendation	CLASS	LEVEL
Routine screening for carotid disease prior to open heart surgery is not recommended	III	C
Ultrasound screening for carotid disease prior to coronary bypass should be considered in patients aged >70 years, those with a history of transient ischemic attack or stroke, a carotid bruit or left mainstream disease so that the patient can be better informed of the increased risk associated with coronary artery bypass surgery in patients with concurrent carotid disease	IIa	C
Staged or synchronous carotid intervention should be considered in coronary artery bypass surgery patients with a history of stroke or transient ischemic attack in the preceding 6 months and a 50–90% carotid stenosis	IIa	B
Staged or synchronous carotid endarterectomy should be considered, instead of stenting plus coronary bypass in patients with a history of stroke or transient ischemic attack in the preceding 6 months and a 50–90% carotid stenosis	IIa	B
A staged or synchronous carotid intervention is not recommended in coronary artery bypass patients with an asymptomatic unilateral 70–90% carotid stenosis for the prevention of stroke after coronary bypass	III	B
A staged or synchronous carotid intervention may be considered in coronary artery bypass patients with bilateral asymptomatic 70–99% carotid stenosis, or a 70–99% stenosis with contralateral occlusion	IIb	C
The choice between carotid endarterectomy and carotid stenting in asymptomatic patients in whom a carotid intervention is deemed necessary prior to coronary artery bypass should be based on the urgency of performing surgery, choice of antiplatelet strategy during coronary bypass, individual patient characteristics, symptom status and local expertise	IIa	C

Carotid Artery Disease and Major Noncardiac Surgeries

Patient undergoing elective noncardiac surgery with history of stroke within last 6 months should undergo carotid artery imaging (class I), if possible surgery should be deferred for 6 months (class 1) and patient who come out with ipsilateral 50–99% carotid stenosis should undergo CAS before elective non cardiac surgery. In patient of known asymptomatic carotid artery disease statin and antiplatelet should not be stopped. Prophylactic CAS is not recommended in this subject.

NEW ASPECTS OF 2017 GUIDELINES ADDED TO THE 2009 GUIDELINES

- Evidence supporting the prevention of stroke in patients with asymptomatic and symptomatic carotid disease
- Evidence supporting rapid interventions in recently symptomatic patients and the timing of interventions after thrombolysis
- Evidence supporting various CAS techniques including adjuvant medical therapy, wires, catheters, and stents, and CPDs
- Management of concurrent carotid and cardiac disease
- Management of patients with ACS undergoing major noncardiac surgical procedures.

REFERENCES

1. Murray C, Lopez A. Global health statistics: A compendium of incidence, prevalence and mortality estimates for over 200 conditions. Cambridge, MA. Harvard University Press; 1996.
2. Strong K, Mathers C, Bonita R. Preventing stroke: Saving lives around the world. Lancet Neurol. 2007;6:182-7.
3. Aho K, Harmsen P, Hatano S, et al. Cerebrovascular disease in the community: Results of a WHO collaborative study. Bull World Health Organ. 1980;58:113-30.
4. Sacco RL, Kasner SE, Broderick JP, et al. An updated definition of stroke for the 21st century. A statement for healthcare professionals from the American Heart Association/American Stroke Association. Stroke. 2013;44:2064-89.
5. Rothwell PM, Gibson RJ, Slattery J, et al. On behalf of the ECST Collaborative Group. Equivalence of measurements of carotid stenosis: a comparison of three methods on 1001 angiograms. Stroke. 1994;25:2435-9.
6. Executive Committee for the Asymptomatic Carotid Atherosclerosis Study. Endarterectomy for asymptomatic carotid artery stenosis. JAMA. 1995;273: 1421-8.
7. Wardlaw JM, Chappell FM, Stevenson M, et al. Accurate, practical and cost-effective assessment of carotid stenosis in the UK. Health Technol Assess. 2006;10:1-182.
8. de Weerd M, Greving JP, Hedblad B, et al. Prediction of asymptomatic carotid artery stenosis in the general population identification of high-risk groups. Stroke. 2014;45:2366-71.
9. Hogberg D, Kragsterman B, Bjorck M, et al. Carotid artery atherosclerosis among 65-year-old Swedish men: A population-based screening study. Eur J Vasc Endovasc Surg. 2014;48:5-10.
10. Herder M, Johnsen SH, Arntzen KA, et al. Risk factors for progression of carotid intima-media thickness and total plaque area: A 13-year follow-up study: the Tromso Study. Stroke. 2012;43:1818-23.
11. Shinton R, Beevers G. Meta-analysis of relation between cigarette smoking and stroke. BMJ. 1989;298:789-94.
12. Lee CD, Folsom AR, Blair SN. Physical activity and stroke risk: A meta-analysis. Stroke. 2003;34:2475-81.
13. Cote R, Battista R, Abrahamowicz M, et al. Lack of effect of aspirin in asymptomatic patients with carotid bruits and substantial carotid narrowing. The Asymptomatic Cervical Bruit Study Group. Ann Intern Med. 1995;123:649-55.
14. King A, Shipley M, Markus H.. The effect of medical treatments on stroke risk in asymptomatic carotid stenosis. Stroke. 2013;44:542-6.
15. Bhatt DL, Flather MD, Hacke W, et al. Patients with prior myocardial infarction, stroke, or symptomatic peripheral arterial disease in the CHARISMA trial. J Am Coll Cardiol. 2007;49:1982-8.
16. Baigent C, Blackwell L, Collins R, et al. Aspirin in the primary and secondary prevention of vascular disease: collaborative meta-analysis of individual participant data from randomised trials. Lancet. 2009;373:1849-60.
17. Halliday A, Harrison M, Hayter E, et al. 10-year stroke prevention after successful carotid endarterectomy for asymptomatic stenosis (ACST-1): A multicentre randomised trial. Lancet. 2010;376:1074-84.
18. Mathiesen EB, Joakimsen O, Bonaa KH. Prevalence of and risk factors associated with carotid artery stenosis: the Tromso Study. Cerebrovasc Dis. 2001;12:44-51.
19. Sutton-Tyrrell K,Wolfson Jr SK, Kuller LH. Blood pressure treatment slows the progression of carotid stenosis in patients with isolated systolic hypertension. Stroke. 1994;25:44-50.
20. Boutouyrie P, Bussy C, Hayoz D, et al. Local pulse pressure and regression of arterial wall hypertrophy during long-term antihypertensive treatment. Circulation. 2000;101:2601-6.
21. Zanchetti A, Bond MG, Hennig M, et al. On behalf of the ELSA investigators. Calcium antagonist lacidipine slows down progression of asymptomatic carotid atherosclerosis: principal results of the European Lacidipine Study on Atherosclerosis (ELSA), a randomized, double-blind, long-term trial. Circulation. 2002;106:2422-7.
22. Wang JG, Staessen JA, Li Y, et al. Carotid intima-media thickness and antihypertensive treatment: A meta-analysis of randomized controlled trials. Stroke. 2006;37:1933-40.
23. Neal B, MacMahon S, Chapman N. Blood Pressure Lowering Treatment Trialists' Collaboration. Effects of ACE inhibitors, calcium antagonists, and other blood-pressure-lowering drugs: Results of prospectively designed overviews of randomized trials. Lancet. 2000;356:1955-64.
24. de Weerd M, Greving JP, Hedblad B, et al. Prediction of asymptomatic carotid artery stenosis in the general population identification of high-risk groups. Stroke. 2014;45:2366-71.
25. Schoites VP, Peeters W, van Lammeren GW, et al. Type 2 diabetes is not associated with an altered plaque phenotype among patients undergoing carotid revascularization. A histological analysis of 1455 carotid plaques. Atherosclerosis. 2014;235:418-23.
26. Banerjee C, Moon YP, Paik MC, et al. Duration of diabetes and risk of ischemic stroke: The Northern Manhattan Study. Stroke. 2012;43:1212-7.
27. Zhang C, Zhou YH, Xu CL, et al. Efficacy of intensive control of glucose in stroke prevention: A meta-analysis of data from 59197 participants in 9 randomized controlled trials. PLoS One. 2013;8:e54465.
28. UK Prospective Diabetes Study Group. Tight blood pressure control and risk of macrovascular and microvascular complications in type 2 diabetes: UKPDS. BMJ. 1998;317:703-13.
29. ESH/ESC Task Force for the Management of Arterial Hypertension. 2013 ESH/ESC Guidelines for the management of arterial hypertension: The Task Force for the management of arterial hypertension of the European Society of Hypertension (ESH) and of the European Society of Cardiology (ESC). J Hypertens. 2013;31:1281-357.
30. Mendrinos E, Machinis TG, Pournaras CJ. Ocular ischemic syndrome. Surv Ophthalmol. 2010;55:2-34.
31. Rothwell PM, Algra A, Chen Z, et al. Effects of aspirin on risk and severity of early recurrent stroke after transient ischaemic attack and ischaemic stroke: Time-course analysis of randomised trials. Lancet. 2016;388:365-75.
32. Markus HS, King A, Shipley M, et al. Asymptomatic embolisation for prediction of stroke in the asymptomatic carotid emboli study: a prospective observational study. Lancet Neurol. 2010;9:663-71.
33. Bhatt DL, Bertrand ME, Berger PB, et al. Meta-analysis of randomized and registry comparisons of ticlopidine with clopidogrel after stenting. J Am Coll Cardiol. 2002;39:9-14.
34. McKevitt FM, Ranbdall MS, Cleveland TJ, et al. The benefits of combined anti-platelet treatment in carotid artery stenting. Eur J Vasc Endovasc Surg. 2005;29:522-7.
35. Navarese EP, Andreotti F, Schulze V, et al. Optimal duration of dual antiplatelet therapy after percutaneous coronary interventions with drug eluting stents: Meta-analysis of randomised trials. BMJ. 2015;350:L1618.
36. Diener HC, Bogousslavsky J, Brass LM, et al. Aspirin and clopisogrel compared with clopidogrel alone after recent ischaemic stroke or transient ischaemic attack in high-risk patients (MATCH): Randomised, double-blind, placebo-controlled trial. Lancet. 2004;364(9431):331-7.

37. Groschel K, Ernemann U, Schulz JB, et al. Statin therapy at carotid angioplasty and stent placement: effect on procedure related stroke, myocardial infarction and death. Radiology. 2006;240:145-51.
38. Verzini F, De Rango P, Parlani G, et al. Effects of statins on early and late results of carotid stenting. J Vasc Surg. 2011;53:71-9.
39. Reiff T, Amiri H, Rohde S, et al. Statins reduce periprocedural complications in carotid stenting. Eur J Vasc Endovasc Surg. 2014;48:626-32.
40. Law MR, Morris JK,Wald NJ. Use of blood pressure lowering drugs in the prevention of cardiovascular disease: meta-analysis of 147 randomised trials in the context of expectations from prospective epidemiological studies. BMJ. 2009;338:b1665.
41. Rothwell PM, Howard SC, Spence JD. Relationship between blood pressure and stroke risk in patients with symptomatic carotid occlusive disease. Stroke. 2003;34:2583-90.
42. den Hartog AG, Moll FL, van der Worp HB, et al. Delay to carotid endarterectomy in patients with symptomatic carotid artery stenosis. Eur J Vasc Endovasc Surg. 2014;47:233-9.
43. Aronow HD, Gray WA, Ramee SR, et al. Predictors of neurological events associated with carotid artery stenting in high surgical risk patients: insights from the Cordis Carotid Stent Collaborative. Circ Cardiovasc Interv. 2010;3:577-84.
44. Gray WA, Yadav JS, Verta P, et al. The CAPTURE Registry: Predictors of outcomes in carotid artery stenting with embolic protection for high surgical risk patients in the early post-approval setting. Catheter Cardiovasc Interv. 2007;70:1025-33.
45. Goyal M, Demchuk AM, Menon BK, et al. on behalf of the ESCAPE Trial Investigators. Randomised assessment of rapid endovascular treatment of ischemic stroke. N Engl J Med. 2015;372(11):1019-30.
46. Kumar ID, Singh S, Williams G, et al. Bilateral one-stage carotid endarterectomy: Is there an indication? Eur J Vasc Endovasc Surg. 2001;21:575-6.
47. Gupta R, Horowitz M, Jovin TG. Hemodynamic instability after carotid artery angioplasty and stent placement: a review of the literature. Neurosurg Focus. 2005;18:e6.
48. van den Berg JC. Neuro-rescue during carotid stenting. Eur J Vasc Endovasc Surg. 2008;36:627-36.
49. Nandalur MR, Cooper H, Satler LF, et al. Vasopressor use in the critical care unit for treatment of persistent post-carotid artery stent induced hypotension. Neurocrit Care. 2007;7:232-7.
50. Kumar R, Batchelder A, Saratzis A, et al. Restenosis after carotid interventions and its relationship with recurrent ipsilateral stroke: a systematic review and meta-analysis. Eur J vasc Endovasc Surg. 2017;53:766-75.
51. Naylor AR, Mehta Z, Rothwell PM, et al. Carotid artery disease and stroke during coronary artery bypass: A critical review of the literature. Eur J Vasc Endovasc Surg. 2002;23:283-94.
52. D'Agostino RS, Svensson LG, Neurmann DJ, et al. Screening carotid ultrasonography and risk factors for stroke in coronary artery surgery patients. Ann Thorac Surg. 1996;62:1714-23.
53. Naylor AR, Bown MJ. Stroke after cardiac surgery and its association with asymptomatic carotid disease: An updated systematic review and meta-analysis. Eur J Vasc Endovasc Surg. 2011;41:607-24.

CHAPTER 135

Critical Limb Ischemia: Current Management

Narendra N Khanna, Chukwudi Nwagbara, Suparna Rao

INTRODUCTION

Clinically, critical limb ischemia (CLI) is defined as ischemic rest pain, tissue loss or gangrene in the presence of peripheral artery disease (PAD) and hypoperfusion of the lower extremity.[1] This definition is recommended by the Trans-Atlantic Inter-Society Consensus on management of PAD.[2] CLI is a severe manifestation of PAD and it is usually as a result of a combination of atherosclerotic and atherothrombotic disease process.[3]

The term CLI implies chronicity and it is reserved for patients with ischemic symptoms of more than 2 weeks.[4] It differs from acute limb ischemia, which is a sudden loss of limb perfusion (defined as within 2 weeks) and typically caused by embolus or thrombus. Significance of CLI is the fact that it is associated with not only a high degree of loss to limb but also to life. Total 25% of patients with CLI die within 1-year following presentation and 30% undergo amputation during the same period.[5]

CLI is characterized by:

- Rest pain of more than 2 weeks duration
- Impending loss of tissue or ulceration because of severe multisegmental arterial disease
- Associated high-risk of loss of limb and life.

The goal of treatment is relieving pain, prevention or minimizing tissue or limb loss, healing of ulcers, and improving quality of life and survival. These goals are usually achieved by a combination of aggressive medical therapy, endovascular or surgical revascularization, and sometimes amputation. Treatment such as stem cell therapy, gene therapy, hyperbaric oxygen therapy, intermittent pneumatic compression, and spinal cord stimulation may also be of some benefit in relieving pain and promoting wound healing among those who are either unfit or unwilling to undergo revascularization or amputation.[3] Other therapies include control of infection, local wound care, offloading and pressure relief, good analgesics and optimal therapy to modify atherosclerotic risk factors, and treatment of other comorbidities.[3]

EPIDEMIOLOGY AND RISK FACTORS

The incidence of CLI is approximately 22% per 100,000 per year, affecting 1–2% of patients with PAD.[6] However with increasing life expectancy and the prevalence of diabetes, obesity, sedentary lifestyles, these estimates are likely to increase.[7] A national survey by the Vascular Surgery Society of Great Britain and Ireland showed an annual incidence of 400 per million per year.[8] In a Finnish study, 39% of patients presenting with CLI experienced symptoms of previous claudication, out of which 54% were diabetic and 89% had ulcers as the initial feature of CLI.[9] About 10% of the patients with symptomatic PAD and another 5–10% of patients with asymptomatic PAD progress to CLI over a period of 5 years.[10] In the PREVENT trial, more than 40% of patients with CLI had advanced coronary artery disease.[11]

The major risk factors for the development of CLI are smoking, diabetes mellitus, age, and dyslipidemia. Studies have shown that diabetic PAD patients are more likely to need a major amputation than nondiabetic PAD patients.[12] A Danish national discharge survey showed that in 1980, the incidence of lower limb major amputations increased from 0.3 per 100,000 per year in those younger than 40 years to 226 per 100,000 per year in those older than 80 years.[13] Also nondiabetic heavy smokers undergo major amputation more frequently among PAD patients.[14]

PATHOPHYSIOLOGY OF CRITICAL LIMB ISCHEMIA

The etiology of CLI is multifactorial; however, the common factor is impaired blood flow to the lower extremities due to occlusive lesions. As a result of this, there is reduced oxygen and nutrient supply to the affected region leading to ischemic pain. Patients with CLI usually have multilevel vessel disease such that even the resting blood supply cannot meet the nutritional requirements of the limbs leading to rest pain and ulcer formation.[15] The cause of ulcer may be related to pressure, trauma, venous insufficiency or poor hygiene.[16] However, an increased level of blood supply is usually required when skin ulcers are present to successfully complete the healing process.[17] Impaired blood supply can lead to cell death, endothelial dysfunction, inflammation, and an inability to provide proper local immunologic response to the infection.[18] This leads to autonomic dysregulation, altered blood viscosity, and decreased erythrocyte fluidity.[19]

Abnormalities in the microcirculation is another contributory factor to the pathophysiology of CLI. Individuals with CLI have a reduced number of perfused skin capillaries. Other factors that contribute to the decreased capillary perfusion in CLI patients include platelet aggregation, reduced red blood cell deformability, increased leukocyte adhesiveness, fibrinogen, microvascular thrombosis, excessive vasoconstriction, and interstitial edema.[20]

CLINICAL FEATURES

Symptoms

The classical symptom of CLI is pain which usually occurs at the lower extremity of the limb. The pain occurs usually at rest and worst at night. It is usually wakes the patient up and it is exacerbated by elevation of the limb and exercise. The pain is temporary relieved by cold and also by keeping the leg at dependent position. The pain of CLI should be carefully distinguished from other related disease conditions that causes limb pain like venous disease (the pain occurs usually at rest and increases in the evening which often disappears with some form of muscle activity), osteoarthritis (pain on walking but not relieved by rest), neuropathic pain (usually characterized by instability while walking and pain not relieved by rest), and complex regional pain syndrome (previously known as reflex sympathetic dystrophy). In addition to pain, CLI patients also have paresthesia.

Physical Findings

Clinical examination demonstrates features of poor tissue perfusion: hair loss, muscle atrophy, subcutaneous tissue and skin atrophy, skin fissures, thickened and brittle toe nail, discoloration of the skin of the affected tissue, weak or absent peripheral pulses, poor capillary refilling, loss of temperature, nonhealing ulcer, pallor, and gangrene.

CLASSIFICATION

Categorization of patients with CLI depends on the severity of the disease. The Rutherford classification has classically defined CLI as rest pain (class IV), tissue loss (class V), and gangrene (class VI) (Table 1).[21]

Alternatively, the Fontaine classification put rest pain as class III and tissue loss or gangrene as class IV (Table 2).[22]

These classifications did not address the wound size, perfusion assessment, or infection. The Society for Vascular Surgery Lower Extremity Guidelines Committee came up with Threatened Limb Classification System: Risk stratification based on wound, ischemia, foot infection (WIfI).[23]

TABLE 1: Modified Rutherford classification of peripheral artery disease

Grade	Category	Clinical presentation
	0	Asymptomatic
I	1 2 3	Mild claudication Moderate claudication Severe claudication
II	4 5	Ischemic rest pain Minor tissue loss: Nonhealing ulcer, focal gangrene with diffuse pedal ulcer
III	6	Major tissue loss extending above the transmetatarsal level, functional foot no longer salvageable

Source: Modified from Rutherford RB, Baker JD, Ernst C, et al. Recommended standard for reports dealing with lower extremity ischemia: revised version. J Vasc Surg. 1997;26:517-13.13.

TABLE 2: Fontaine classification of peripheral artery disease

Stage	Symptoms
I	Asymptomatic
II	Intermittent claudication
IIa	Pain free, claudication walking >200 m
IIb	Pain free, claudication walking <200 m
III	Rest and nocturnal pain
IV	Necrosis, gangrene

DIFFERENTIAL DIAGNOSIS OF LEG PAIN ON EXERTION

Vascular causes:
- Atherosclerosis
- Embolism
- Thrombosis
- Vasculitis:
  - Thromboangiitis obliterans
  - Takayasu arteritis
  - Giant cell arteritis.
- Aortic coarctation
- Fibromuscular dysplasia
- Irradiation
- Endofibrosis of the external iliac artery
- Extravascular compression:
  - Arterial entrapment (e.g., popliteal artery entrapment)
- Adventitial cysts

Nonvascular causes:
- Venous insufficiency
- Osteoarthritis; hip and knee
- Myositis
- Glycogen storage disease
- Lumbosacral radiculopathy:
  - Degenerative arthritis
  - Spinal stenosis.

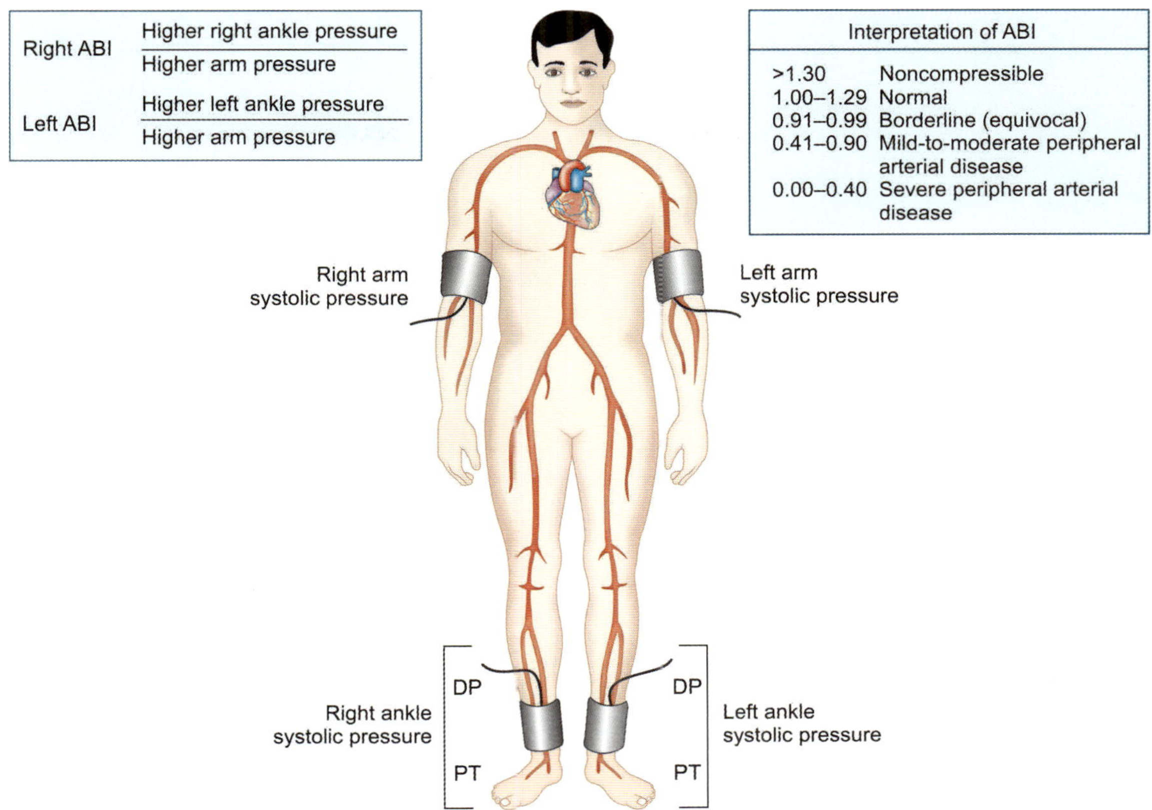

FIG. 1: Assessment of ankle brachial index.

EVALUATION OF CRITICAL LIMB ISCHEMIA

Ankle Brachial Index

Ankle brachial index (ABI) is the primary noninvasive test for the diagnosis of CLI. Determination of the ABI is a simple procedure and it can be done at the bedside. It is a ratio of systolic blood pressure (SBP) in the ankle and SBP in the arm. A pneumatic cuff placed just above the ankle is inflated to a value just above the systolic pressure and it then gradually deflated to obtain the onset of flow with a hand held Doppler instrument (5–10 MHz) place over the posterior tibial and anterior tibial arteries of each foot, the value obtained represents the ankle SBP (Fig. 1). The highest ankle systolic pressure is divided by the highest brachial systolic pressure, resulting in an ABI per leg. Measuring ABI after exercise increases the sensitivity of the test. For this, the patient is asked to exercise on a treadmill at 3.2 km/h at 10–20% slope until claudication occurs.

The normal ABI range is 1.00–1.40. ABI less than 0.4 is strongly suggestive of CLI. In patients with ischemic ulcers, the ankle systolic pressure is usually 50–70 mm Hg and 30–50 mm Hg among patients with ischemic rest pain. In patients with calcified vessels as seen among diabetics, end-stage renal disease patients and elderly, leg BP measurement are not reliable because the pneumatic cuff cannot compress the calcified vessels. ABI higher than 1.40 suggests a non-compressible artery and a toe-brachial index (TBI) or toe pressure measurement is indicated for such patients. TBI with a ratio of 0.70 or toe pressure less than 30 mm Hg is suggestive of CLI (Table 3).

TABLE 3: Features of critical limb ischemia (CLI)

Noninvasive vascular laboratory test for CLI	Value
Ankle-brachial Index	≤0.4
Ankle systolic pressure	≤50 mm Hg
Toe systolic pressure	≤30 mm Hg
Measures of skin microcirculation	
Capillary density	≤20/mm^2
Absent reactive hyperemia on capillary microscopy	
TcPO$_2$	≤10 mm Hg

TcPO$_2$, transcutaneous oxygen pressure.

Duplex Ultrasound

Duplex ultrasound provides a direct, noninvasive means of assessing the anatomic characteristics of the peripheral arteries, morphology of the plaques and to monitor bypass grafts. It is a popular procedure due to its noninvasive nature, use of no contrast, and freedom from exposure to radiation.[24,25] The lesions are identified by two dimensional ultrasonography and color Doppler mapping, while the degree of stenosis is estimated by Doppler waveform analysis,

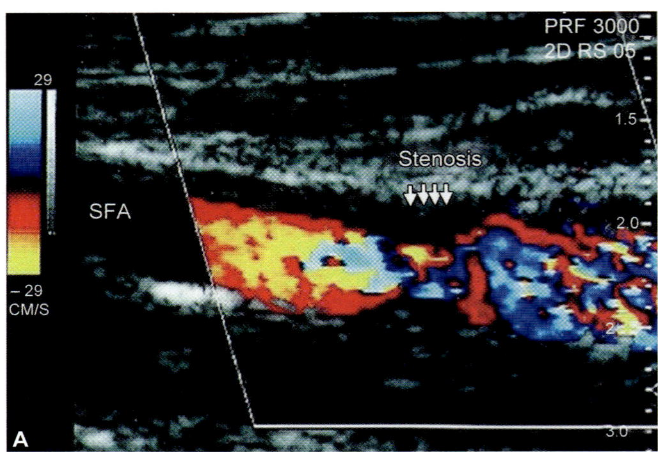

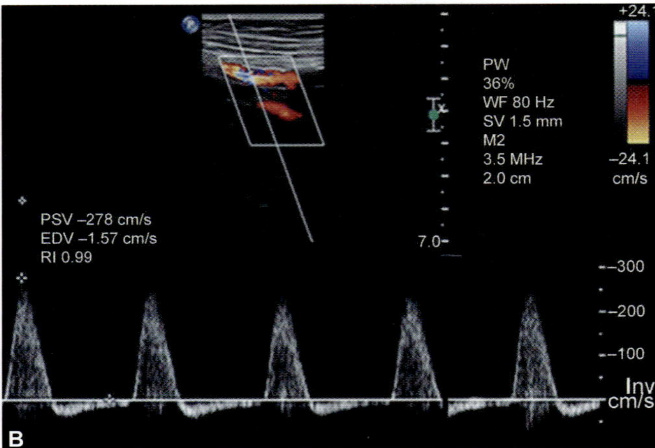

FIG. 2: Duplex ultrasound assessment showing stenosis of superficial femoral artery.

peak systolic velocities, and ratios (Fig. 2). The major pitfall of duplex ultrasound is its difficulty in assessment of the lumen in deeply calcified arteries as seen among diabetics, and also those with open ulcers or severe scarring. Another significant setback of duplex ultrasound when compared with other imaging modalities like digital subtraction angiography (DSA), computed tomography angiography (CTA), or magnetic resonance angiography (MRA) is its difficulty in providing full arterial road map.

Computed Tomography Angiography

Computed tomography angiography using multidetector CT technology allows imaging with high resolution. The advantage of CT is its ability to visualize calcifications, clips, stents, and bypasses (Fig. 3). CTA has some disadvantages which include ionizing radiation exposure, use of nephrotoxic contrast materials, and the visualization of artifacts due to blooming effect.

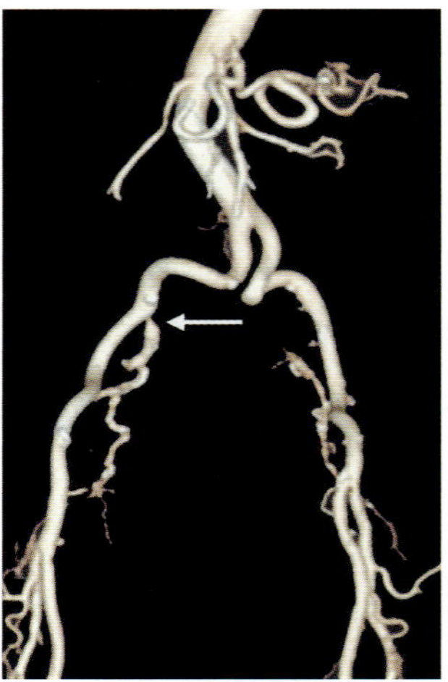

FIG. 3: Computed tomography angiography showing stenosis of right ostial internal iliac artery.

Magnetic Resonance Angiography

Magnetic resonance angiography is one of the most non-invasive sensitive imaging modality that is used for visualization of the lower limb vessels[26] (Fig. 4). MRA however cannot be used in the presence of pacemaker or metallic implants and also among patients with claustrophobia. MRA cannot visualize arterial calcifications, which may be a limitation for the selection of the anastomotic site for a surgical bypass. Another significant disadvantage is the occurrence of nephrogenic fibrosing dermopathy with gadolinium contrast agents.

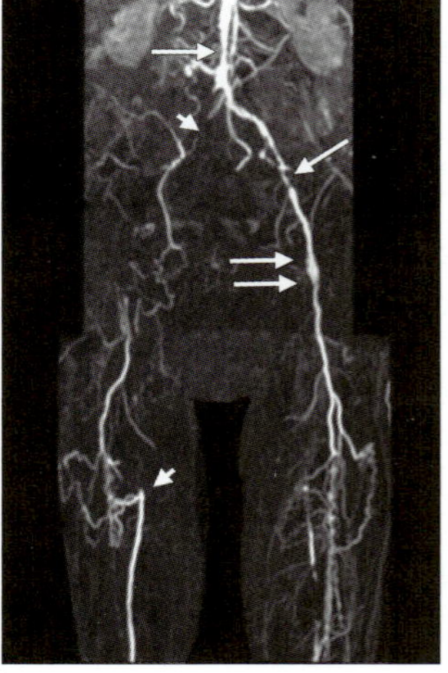

FIG. 4: Magnetic resonance angiography showing diffuse arterial disease.

Peripheral Angiography

Conventional peripheral angiography is essential in evaluation of arterial anatomy before endovascular revascularization procedure (Fig. 5). This is considered as the gold standard but it is now reserved only for patients undergoing endovascular intervention and also used when the diagnosis

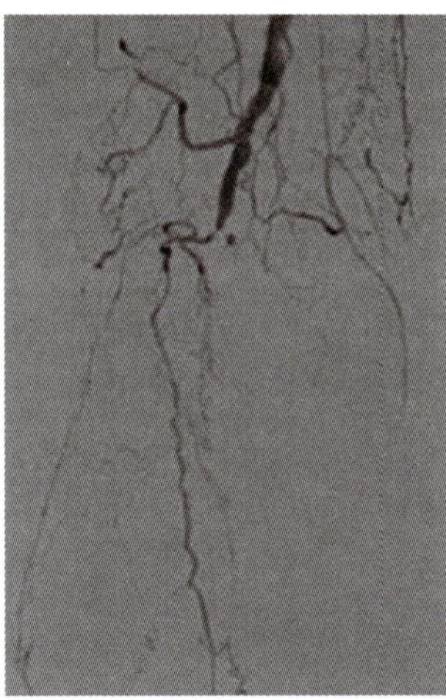

FIG. 5: Peripheral angiography showing long segment total occlusion.

is not clear. It has an advantage of using digital subtraction technique to enhance resolution of the lesion.

TREATMENT OF CRITICAL LIMB ISCHEMIA

Critical limb ischemia treatment requires a multidisciplinary team approach that may be responsible to address all the contributory factors.

The goal of treatment includes the following:

- Risk factors modification
- Optimal medical treatment
- Wound care
- Revascularization.

Risk Factors Modification

Smoking Cessation

Smoking is one of the major risk factors for the development of CLI. In general population, smoking increases the risk of developing CLI by twofold to 6-fold. Smokers with CLI have an increased risk of amputation, higher morbidity, and mortality rate. Smoking cessation is a class 1 recommendation for smokers with CLI.

Blood Pressure Control

Blood pressure control reduces the risk of coronary artery disease and stroke among CLI patients. Studies have shown that intensive blood pressure control reduces cardiovascular events in diabetic patient with PAD.[27] In the Heart Outcome Prevention Evaluation study, the risk of heart attack, stroke, and death from vascular causes decreased by 22% for patients who received angiotensin-converting enzyme inhibitor.[28]

Dyslipidemia

The presence of PAD is considered a coronary artery risk equivalent. Intensive statin (HMG-CoA reductase inhibitors) therapy consistently lowers cardiovascular events in patients with PAD than those are not on statin or low intensity statin. The mechanism by which statin reduces cardiovascular events and mortality is through plaque stabilization and improvement of endothelial function.[29]

Diabetes Mellitus

Intensive treatment of diabetes mellitus reduces the risk of microangiopathies. However, such benefits have not been observed in macrovascular complications.[30] The United Kingdom Prospective Diabetes Study has shown that a 1% increase in hemoglobin A1C was associated with a 28% increase in risk of incident of PAD.[31]

Optimal Medical Therapy

The definitive treatment of CLI is revascularization; however, the optimal medical treatment is targeted at symptoms (claudication), delay in progression of the disease, and reduction of cardiovascular events.

The drugs used are as follows:

- *Cilostazol*: It is a quinolinone derivative that inhibits phosphodiesterase 3, thereby decreasing the degradation of cyclic adenosine monophosphate and increasing its concentration in platelets and blood vessels.[15] In a meta-analysis by Momsen, the maximal walking distance increased on an average by 70 m with 100 mg dose of cilostazol.[32] Cilostazol is contraindicated in heart failure patients
- *Pentoxifylline*: It, also known as oxpentifylline, is a xanthine derivative. It improves tissue oxygenation by its ability to decrease blood viscosity and to improve erythrocyte flexibility
- *Naftidrofuryl*: It, also known as nafronyl, is a vasodilator which inhibits 5-hydroxytryptamine type 2 (5-HT2) thereby reducing erythrocyte and platelet aggregation. It is effective in treating muscle pain and cramps thereby improving walking distance[33]
- *Statins*: Statin is a HMG-CoA inhibitor. In addition to cardiovascular risk reduction, it may improve symptoms of claudication and also reduce the risk of tissue loss.[34] This occurs through plaque stabilization and improvement of endothelial function[29]
- *Antiplatelets*: These are used for the treatment of CLI mostly to prevent the risk of cardiovascular events, stroke, and vascular death. However, after revascularization, antiplatelets improve the stent patency rate.

Wound Care

The principles of wound care include improving perfusion to the limb, treatment of the infection, avoiding pressure on the wound by off-loading the foot, debridement, and good nutrition.

The local temperature of the limb can be increased using sheepskin boots and this may improve tissue perfusion.[35] Biosurgery with sterile maggots has been shown to have some beneficial effects in increasing vascularity and promoting wound healing.[36]

Some adjuvant therapies include hyperbaric oxygen, intermittent pneumatic compressions, spinal cord stimulation, ultrasound therapy, noncontact low-intensity frequency, topical therapy of platelet-derived growth factor (stem cell therapy), and low-dose diode laser therapy at the wound margins.

Hyperbaric Oxygen Therapy

Hyperbaric oxygen therapy is one of the adjuvant management modalities for the treatment of nonhealing wound among patients with CLI.[37] During hyperbaric oxygen therapy, patients are usually placed in the hyperbaric chamber and exposed to 100% oxygen at 2–3 times greater pressure than ambient atmosphere. Protocols usually vary depending on the indication. Hyperbaric oxygen therapy enhances collagen synthesis and maturation, fibroblast proliferation, epithelialization, increases leukocyte bacterial killing capacity, and induces angiogenesis. Hyperbaric oxygen therapy also exhibits some antibacterial effects on selected microorganisms thereby enhancing wound healing. Hyperbaric oxygen therapy should always be initiated along with other conventional treatment.

Stem Cell Therapy

Stem cell therapy involves the use of various cell-stimulating factors that promote angiogenesis and bone marrow-derived pluripotent cells in the management of CLI. These factors include fibroblast growth factor-1, vascular endothelial growth factor, and hepatocyte growth factor. Angiogenesis is defined as the expansion of the vasculature through the formation of new capillary network from the pre-existing vessels. In pilot studies, these therapies have demonstrated efficacy in improving outcome of CLI.[38]

Revascularization

Revascularization is the gold standard for treatment of CLI and it is a class 1 recommendation for CLI treatment.[5] Without revascularization, about 40% of patients with CLI will require lower limb amputation by 1-year. Adequate inflow and outflow are required in order to keep the revascularized vessel patent and functional.

The options of revascularization for patients with CLI include endovascular revascularization, surgical revascularization or hybrid procedure. Several factors influence the choice of revascularization strategy, including anatomical factors, comorbidities, available level of expertise, and patient preference.

One randomized controlled trial, BASIL (Bypass versus Angioplasty in Severe Ischemia of Leg), compared surgery versus balloon angioplasty among 452 patients with CLI; after 5 years of follow-up, both therapies had similar rates of amputation-free survival and mortality.[39] Recently, a review by the Agency for Healthcare Research and Quality that included the BASIL trial, in addition to 19 other observational studies, found no differences in all-cause mortality, amputation, and amputation-free survival between surgical and endovascular revascularization.[40]

Despite the increasing nationwide numbers of endovascular revascularization for CLI, a personalized approach in selecting the best revascularization option is advocated.[41,42] Several factors which influence the choice of revascularization strategy include anatomical factors (such as availability of venous conduit, distal target, runoff, calcifications, previous procedures), patients age, comorbidities, life expectancy, kidney function, risk associated with anesthesia, and compliance.

Lesion Classification According to the Trans-Atlantic Inter-Society Consensus for the Management of Peripheral Artery Disease (TASC II)

Lesion classification according to the Trans-Atlantic Inter-Society Consensus for the Management of Peripheral Artery Disease has been shown in figure 6.

Endovascular Revascularization

Endovascular revascularization is a minimally invasive procedure. Majority of patients prefer endovascular procedure for the treatment of CLI because of its minimally invasive nature and reduced duration of hospital stay, lower health care cost, lower morbidity, and mortality rate. TASC recommends that in a situation where endovascular revascularization and open repair or bypass of a specific lesion causing symptoms of peripheral arterial disease give equivalent short-term and long-term symptomatic improvement, endovascular technique should be used first. In the United States of America, the rate of surgical revascularization has reduced from 13.9% in 2003 to 8.8% in 2011 while rate of endovascular revascularization have increased from 5.1 to 11% during the same period.[43] Table 4 shows personal experience of 196 cases of CLI treated by endovascular revascularization.

Angiosome Concept

A new concept of defining vascular territories by means of angiosomes is currently under review. An angiosome is an anatomic unit of tissue (consisting of skin, subcutaneous tissue, fascia, muscle, and bone) supplied by specific source of arteries and drained by specific vein (Fig. 7). There are five angiosomes in the leg and six angiosomes in the foot and ankle area as described by Taylor and Palmer in 1987. Utilizing the particular source of artery has shown promising results in terms of complete wound healing and limb salvage. Hence, they should be considered in planning the revascularization strategy.

Vascular Access Approach for Endovascular Revascularization

The choice of vascular access approach for endovascular revascularization depends on the site and type of the lesion. Retrograde vascular access and crossover is good for iliac-femoral lesions. Antegrade femoral vascular access is good for tibia-popliteal stenotic lesions. For tibia-popliteal occlusion lesions, retrograde pedal-tibial approach is a good option (Fig. 8).

Techniques for Endovascular Revascularization

Several techniques are now available for endovascular revascularization, which include the following:

- Percutaneous transluminal balloon angioplasty (PTA):

Type A lesions
- Unilateral or bilateral stenoses of CIA
- Unilateral or bilateral single, short (≤3 cm) stenosis of EIA

Type B lesions
- Short (≤3 cm) stenosis of infrarenal aorta
- Unilateral CIA occlusion
- Single or multiple stenosis totaling 3–10 cm involving the EIA, not extending into the CFA
- Unilateral EIA occlusion not involving the origins of internal iliac or CFA

Type C lesions
- Bilateral CIA occlusions
- Bilateral EIA stenoses 3–10 cm long, not extending into the CFA
- Unilateral EIA stenosis extending into the CFA
- Unilateral EIA occlusion that involves the origins of internal iliac and/or CFA
- Heavily calcified unilateral EIA occlusion with or without involvement of origins of internal iliac and/or CFA

Type D lesions
- Infrarenal aortoiliac occlusion
- Diffuse disease involving the aorta and both iliac arteries, requiring treatment
- Diffuse multiple stenoses involving the unilateral CIA, EIA, and CFA
- Unilateral occlusions of both CIA and EIA
- Bilateral occlusions of EIA
- Iliac stenoses in patients with AAA requiring treatment and not amenable to endograft placement or other lesions requiring open aortic or iliac surgery

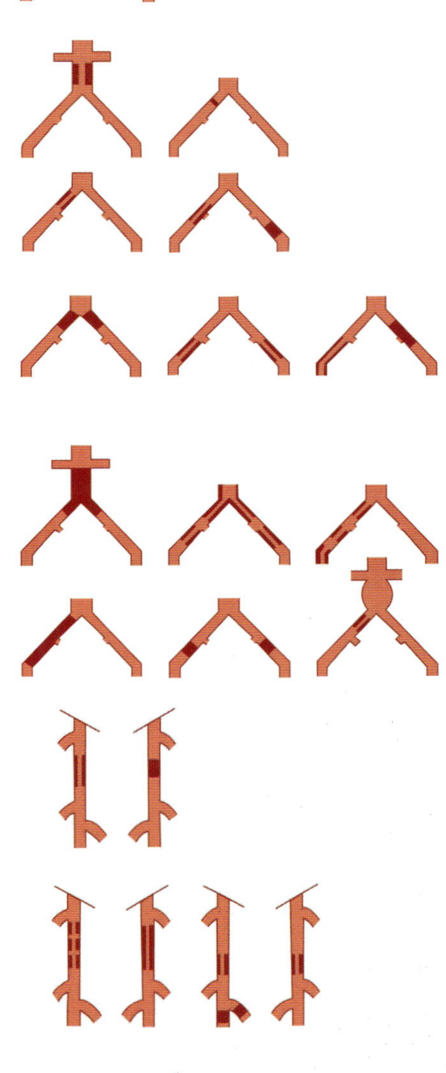

Type A lesions
- Single stenosis ≤10 cm long
- Single occlusion ≤5 cm long

Type B lesions
- Multiple lesions (stenoses or occlusions), each ≤5 cm
- Single stenosis or occlusion ≤5 cm, not involving the infrageniculate popliteal artery
- Single or multiple lesions in the absence of continuous tibial vessels to improve inflow for a distal bypass
- Heavily calcified occlusion ≤5 cm long
- Single popliteal stenosis

Type C lesions
- Multiple stenoses or occlusions totaling >15 cm with or without heavy calcification
- Recurrent stenoses or occlusions that need treatment after two endovascular interventions

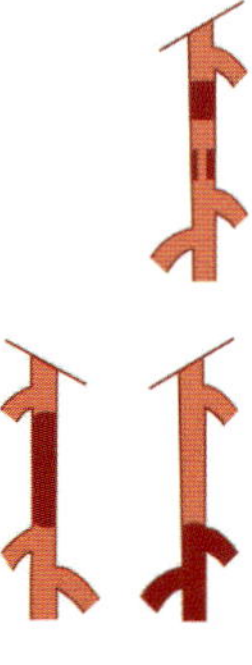

Type D lesions
- Chronic total occlusions of CFA or SFA (>20 cm, involving the popliteal artery)
- Chronic total occlusion of popliteal artery and proximal trifurcation vessels

AAA, abdominal aortic aneurysm; CIA, common iliac artery; CFA, common femoral artery; EIA, external iliac artery; SFA, superficial femoral artery.

FIG. 6: Lesion classification according to the Trans-Atlantic Inter-Society Consensus for the Management of Peripheral Artery Disease.

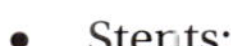

- Plain balloon angioplasty
- Cutting balloon angioplasty
- Scoring balloons
- Drug-coated balloons (DCBs).

- Stents:
  - Bare metal stents
  - Self-expandable stents: Stainless steel and nitinol
  - Covered stents

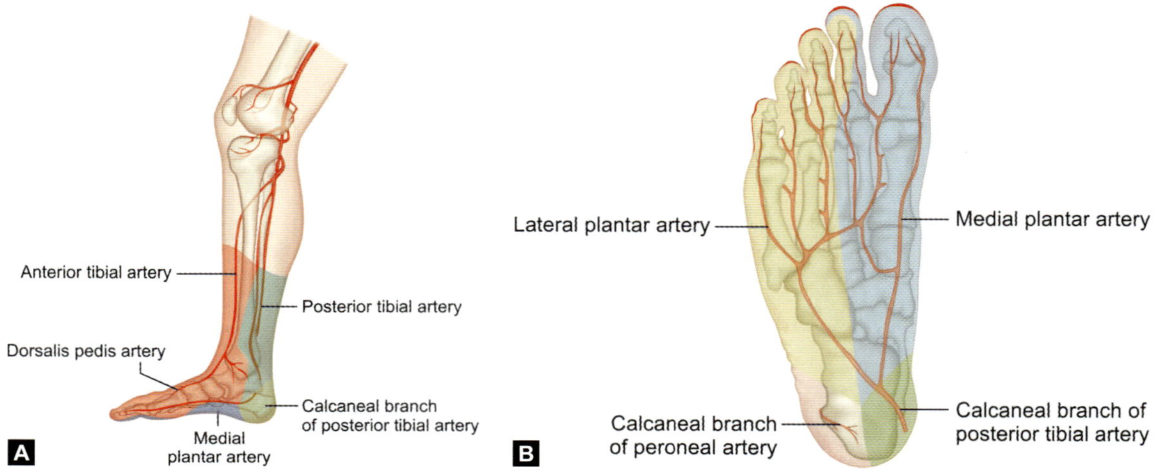

FIG. 7: **A,** Angiosome concept in lower limb; **B,** Angiosome concept in foot.

TABLE 4: Personal experience on endovascular revascularization

Endovascular treatment of CLI—personal experience of 196 cases	Number	Percentage
Total number = 196		
Femoral	107	54%
Below the knee	89	45%
Percutaneous transluminal balloon angioplasty	113	58%
Stents	83	42%
Drug-coated balloon	17	8%
Drug-eluting stents	27	14%
Adjuvant stem cell therapy	04	2%
Technical success	176	96%
Amputation free survival at 6 months	146	76%
Ulcer healing	147	75%

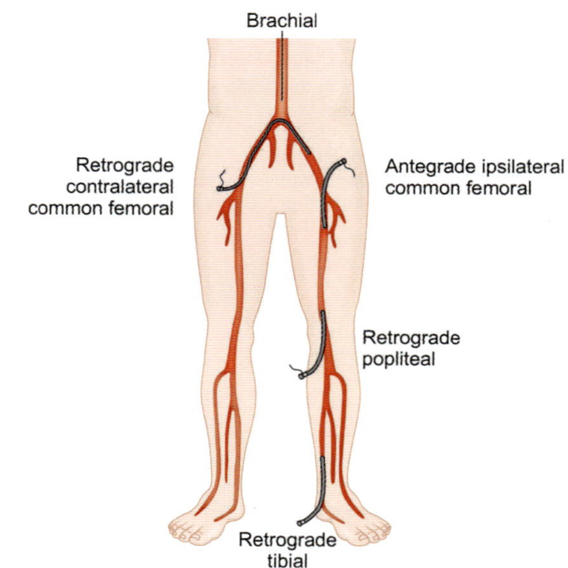

FIG. 8: Types of vascular access approach for endovascular revascularization.

 - Drug-eluting stents (DESs)
 - Bioresorbable vascular scaffolds.
- Debulking devices:
 - Rotablation
 - Atherectomy devices: Directional atherectomy, Silver hawk, and orbital atherectomy device
 - Laser
 - Re-entry devices: Pioneer, outback catheter, and front runner.
- Other modalities:
 - Cryoplasty
 - Photodynamic therapy
 - Gene therapy
 - Autologous stem cell implantation.

Percutaneous transluminal balloon angioplasty

Percutaneous transluminal balloon angioplasty is found to be better than optimal medical therapy for CLI. The development of DCB is an important milestone in endovascular revascularization. In the above knee lesions, DCBs have shown to be superior to PTA as shown in the 2015 IN.PACT SFA Trial.[44] In the below knee lesions, DCB is preferred to PTA in the 2012 ACHILLES trial.[45] DCBs have been widely adopted in the femoral and popliteal arteries lesion and found to be superior than plain balloon angioplasty. DCBs are also favored over stenting in situations in which significant dissection or vessel recoil is absent.

Drug-coated balloons

The PACIFIER, LEVANT-1, FEM-PAC, and THUNDER trials were some of the first randomized controlled trials for treating SFA disease by paclitaxel coated balloons. In all of these trials, DCBs were found to have higher patency rates and lower incidence of target lesion revascularization (TLR) (Table 5). In the IN.PACT trial, DCBs were used to treat in-stent restenosis (ISR) in SFA lesions. 12-month

TABLE 5: Comparison of various trials of drug-coated balloon and drug-eluting stent

	Absolute	Resilient	Sirocco	Strides
Lesion length (cm)	~10	~6.7	~8.4	9.0
Diabetes mellitus	~38%	38%	~47%	39%
Ca^{++} (moderate/ severe)	~82%	~35%	~77%	78%
Occlusion	~18	~18	~57%	47%
Restenosis	N/A	~3%	~7%	10%
12-month patency	63%	81%	82% (18 months)	63%
	Zilver PTX	**Thunder**	**Fem-PAC**	**Levant**
Lesion length (cm)	5.4	7.5	4.5	8.1%
Diabetes mellitus	46%	50%	47%	47%
Ca^{++} (mod/ severe)	72%	46% (site)	52%	N/A
Occlusion	25%	50%	13%	41%
Restenosis	6%	22% (14% ISR)	27% (7% ISR)	11%
12-month patency	76%	75%	18% (6 months)	72% (6 months)

ISR, in-stent restenosis.

TLR and restenosis rates were 7.8%. Two types of coatings-crystalline or amorphous are done on DCBs. Amorphous coatings have higher update and lower retention. Sirolimus-based nanocrystal balloon coating technology is also in the pipeline.

Debulking devices

Debulking devices include laser, rotablation, and atherectomy devices; directional atherectomy, silver hawk, and orbital atherectomy device. Laser involves the delivery of a burst of ultraviolent energy in a short pulse that ablates tissue directly in contact with the catheter. There is usually a minor thermal injury following laser procedure. Rotablation uses the mechanism of concentrically rotating burr to debulk the plaque. Atherectomy devices are very beneficial in crossing heavily calcified lesions that are resistant to balloon and stent dilatation (Fig. 9).

Chronic total occlusions

Chronic total occlusions (CTOs) are commonly encountered in CLI and occur in about 40% of cases of symptomatic PAD.[46] It is usually a big challenge to some operators. Usually, the lesions are long and calcified and are accompanied by diffuse and extensive disease in the outflow tracts. The technical challenge is the difficulty in crossing the wire. However this difficulty can be overcome by using wire escalation, in which wires of increasing diameter, tip loads, and hydrophobicity are used to cross the lesion. Retrograde vascular access through the pedal-tibial approach is also beneficial in a situation of inability to cross the wire through femoral antegrade approach. Debulking devices are of great benefit in CTOs.

Subintimal angioplasty

Subintimal angioplasty is a minimally invasive procedure in which a guidewire is passed between the intima and the media to create a new track along the vessel wall thereby by passing the atherosclerotic occlusion and angioplasty is done using an appropriate balloon along the new tract (Fig. 10). This technique of angioplasty was first reported by Bolia et al.[47] This technique is reserved when there is difficulty in crossing a lesion with 100% occlusion after all available options fail.

Procedural Specifications

All procedures are done under locoregional anesthesia, which has a number of advantages: accurate digital imaging by eliminating any artifacts due to limb movement on DSA, reduced arterial spasm, and also permits concomitant ulcer debridement.

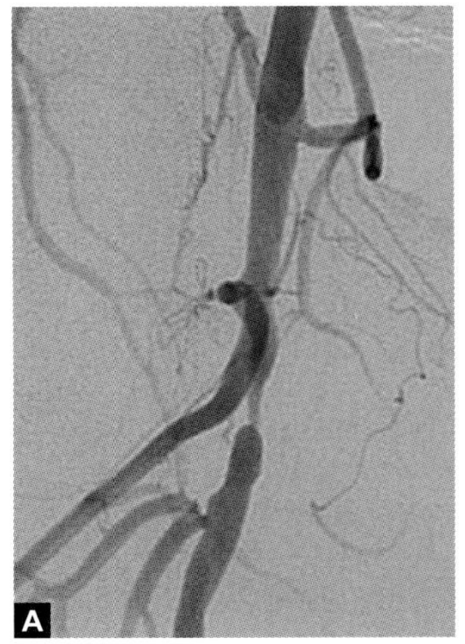

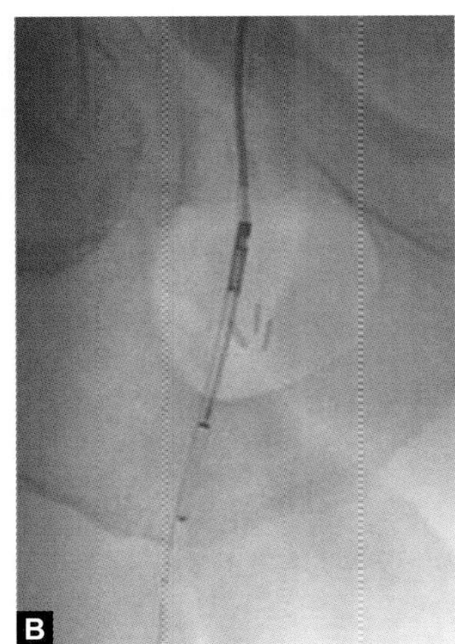

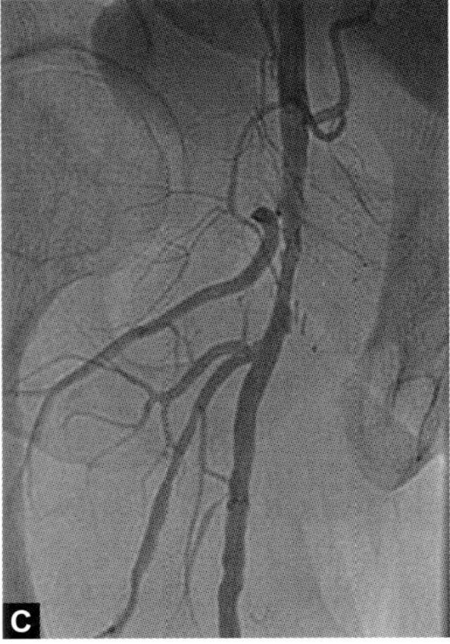

FIG. 9: A, Lesion at the ostial superficial femoral artery; **B,** been treated with atherectomy device; **C,** final result.

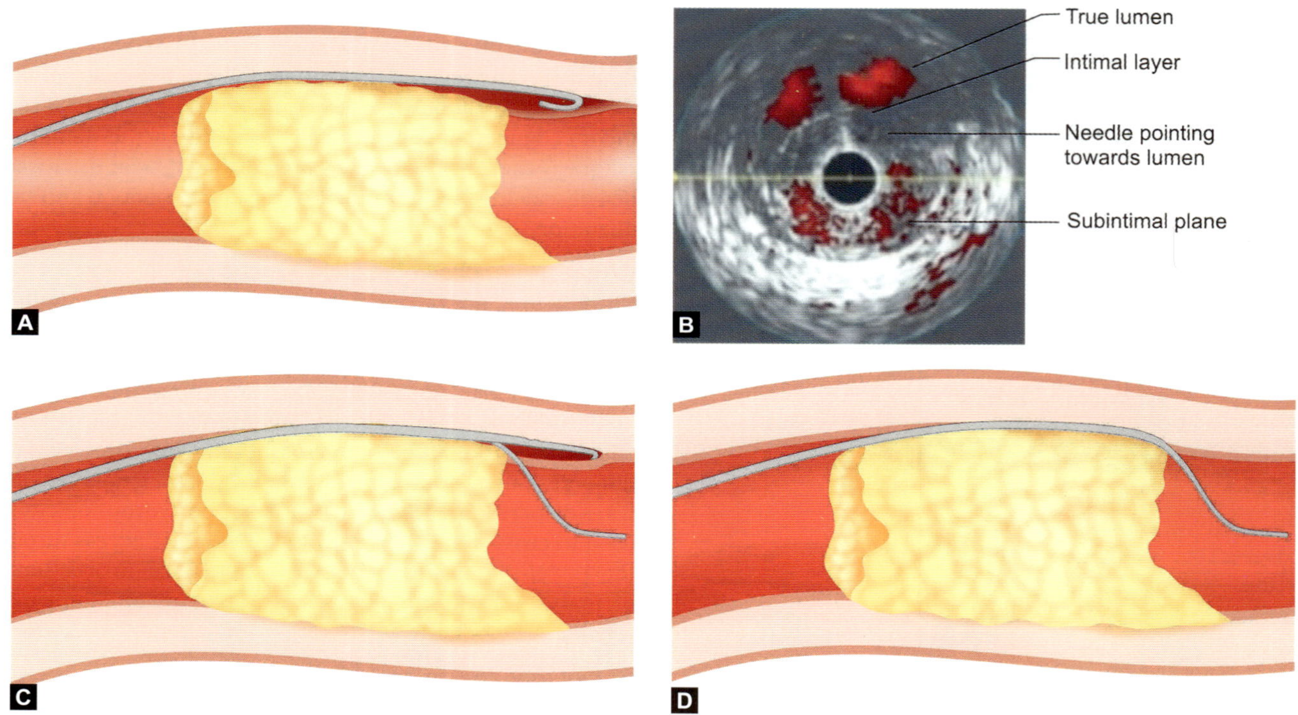

FIG. 10: Subintimal entry of device.

Technique for Femoropopliteal Segment Endovascular Revascularization

The procedure is done under strict aseptic and antiseptic procedure. Femoropopliteal disease can be approach by retrograde contralateral common femoral artery or antegrade ipsilateral common femoral artery route, the region is sterilized and locoregional anesthesia is given. The common femoral artery is accessed with a micropuncture needle and then 6-F introducer sheath is introduced. The sheath provides access for the guidewire. An appropriate-sized guidewire, 0.035'', 0.025'' or 0.018, is used to intubate the lesion under angiographic guidance. After crossing the lesion, the appropriate-sized catheter and percutaneous transluminal balloon is used to treat the lesion (Figs. 11 and 12).

Surgical Revascularization

Surgical revascularization is one of the modalities of revascularization in the treatment of CLI. There is preservation of limb viability and improvement of symptoms of CLI following surgical revascularization. The anatomical location of the lesion and other comorbidities should be considered before taking patient up for surgical revascularization. Preoperative preparation of the patient involves imaging to locate the exact anatomy of the lesion and access for the arterial inflow and outflow. Surgical revascularization has become more significant in complex and calcified lesions that are not adequate for endovascular revascularization and also in younger age groups because of its higher patency rate.

Hybrid Procedures

Hybrid procedure involves the use of both endovascular and surgical revascularization in the treatment of CLI. Hybrid procedures, due to their short procedure time and relatively lesser risk of intra- and postoperative complications represent an attractive option in patients who are older, frail or have limited autologous conduit for bypass. Multilevel disease is often treated with hybrid revascularization using endovascular techniques to treat inflow disease (e.g., iliac stenting) and surgical revascularization for femoral or infrainguinal disease (e.g., common femoral endarterectomy and femoral popliteal bypass).[48]

In a hybrid procedure of 125 patients analyzed by Dougherty, the perioperative mortality was less than 1% and the primary patency was 39.6% over a mean follow-up of 27.6 months.[49] Similar results were seen by other authors when this technique was analyzed for freedom from amputation and event-free survival.[50,51]

Amputation

Amputation is what every interventionist wants to prevent in the course of management of CLI. However, it is inevitable in some occasions.

Indications of amputation in CLI patients:

- Failed revascularization
- Patients with tissue loss or infection
- Potential nonambulating patients
- Patients unfit for surgical or endovascular revascularization.

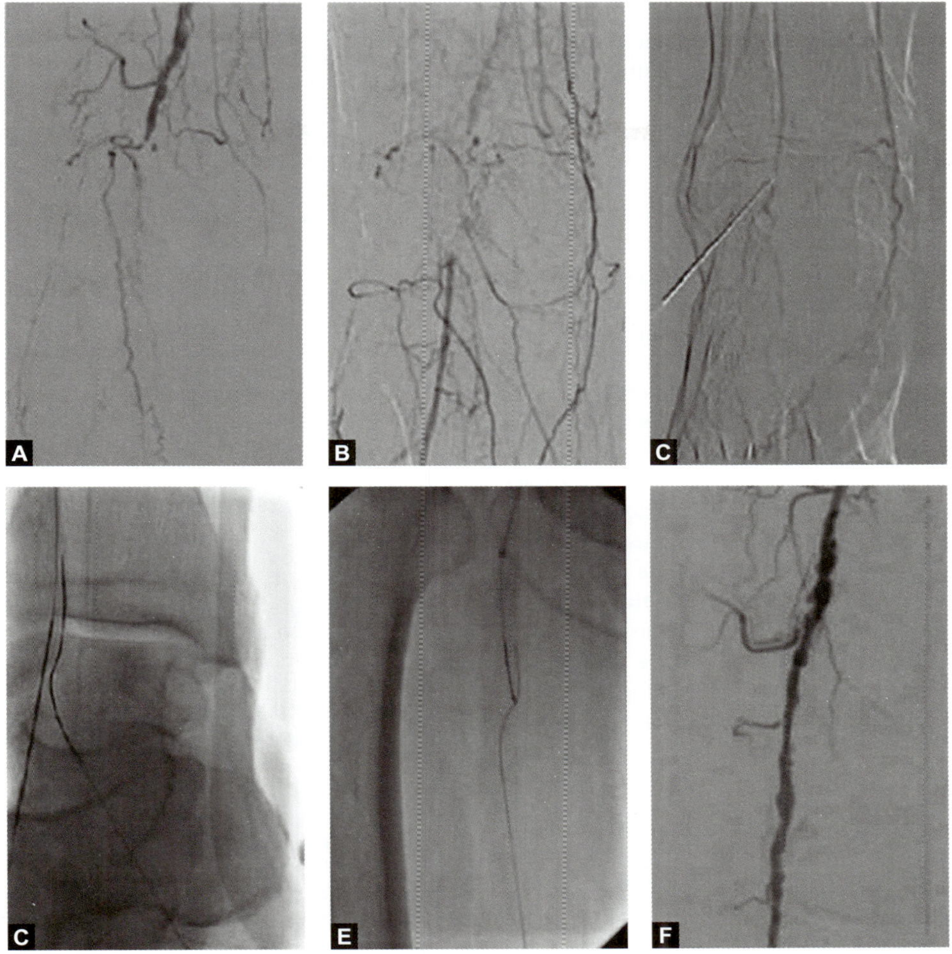

FIG. 11: **A and B**, Long segment total occlusion; **C**, Access through the dorsalis pedis artery; **D**, Retrograde entry of the wire; **E**, Wire snared through the antegrade puncture; **F**, Final result.

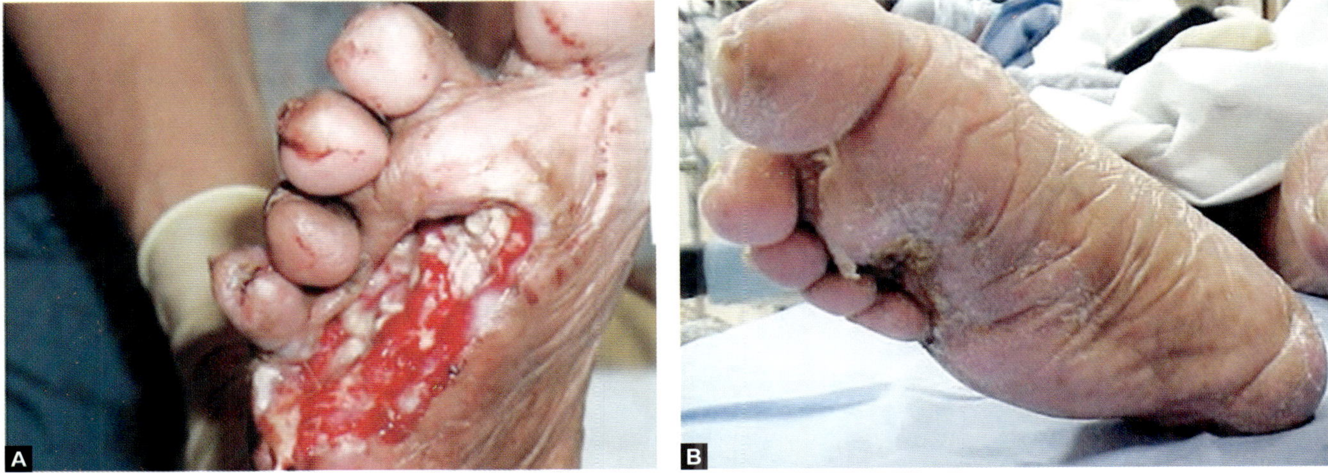

FIG. 12: **A**, Before revascularization; **B**, After revascularization.

Usually, adequate blood supply is required for proper wound healing following amputation. Minor amputations which include disarticulation of the toe or metatarsals do not limit functional independence of the patient or require prosthesis. Major amputations (below knee or above knee amputation) are usually a great concern to patients and usually require prosthesis. There are some factors which limits the use of prosthesis which include dementia, old age, bilateral or above knee amputation, and poor function before the amputation.[52]

CONCLUSION

Critical limb ischemia represents an advanced stage of PAD. It is a significant cause of morbidity and mortality among patients with PAD. Patients with CLI have high risk of limb loss and increase risk of cardiovascular events. Multidisciplinary approach remains the key factor in the treatment of CLI. Intensive medical therapy is very important in reducing the cardiovascular events that is associated with CLI. Revascularization is the gold standard of the treatment of CLI. Selection of the revascularization strategy should be based on individual patient basis and factors such as patient age, anatomy of the arterial lesion, comorbidities, life expectancy, kidney function, risk associated with anesthesia, and compliance should be considered. All patients who present with rest pain, tissue loss or gangrene should be offered hemodynamic assessment followed by revascularization. Newer drug-eluting balloons offer better long term results after some endovascular procedure. Close postoperative care monitoring is essential in order to prevent recurrent disease.

REFERENCES

1. Patel MR, Conte MS, Cutip DE, et al. Evaluation and treatment of patients with lower extremity peripheral artery disease. Consensus definition from peripheral Academic Research Consortium (PARC). J Am Cardiol. 2015;65:931-41.
2. Management of peripheral arterial disease (PAD). Transatlantic Inter-Society Consensus (TASC). J Vasc Surg. 2000;31:SI-21.
3. Khanna NN, Henry M (Eds). Handbook of Interventions for Structural Heart and Peripheral Vascular disease, 1st edition. New Delhi: Jaypee Brothers Medical Publishers Pvt. Ltd.; 2016. pp. 171-93.
4. Second European Consensus Documentation on chronic critical leg ischemia. Circulation. 1991;84(4 Suppl):1-26.
5. Norgren L, Hiatt WR, Dormandy JA, et al. Inter-Society Consensus for the Management of peripheral arterial disease (TACS II). J Vasc Surg. 2007;45 (suppls):S5-67.
6. Howard DP, Banerjee A, Fairhead JF, et al. Oxford Vascular Study: population-based study of incidence, risk factors, outcome, and prognosis of ischemic peripheral arterial events: implications for prevention. Circulation. 2015;132:1805-15.
7. Fowkes FG, Rudan D, Aboyans V, et al. Comparison of global estimates of prevalence and risk factors for peripheral artery in 2000 and 2010: a systematic review and analysis. Lancet. 2013;382(9901):1329-40.
8. The Vascular Surgical Society of Great Britain and Ireland. Critical limb ischemia: Management and outcome. Report of a National Survey. Eur J Vasc Endovasc Surg. 1995;10:108-13.
9. Matzke S, Lepantalo M. Claudication does not always precede critical limb ischemia. Vasc Med. 2001;6:77-80.
10. Farber A, Eberhardt RT. The current state of critical limb ischemia: A systematic review. JAMA Surg. 2016;151(11):1070-7.
11. Schanzer A, Mega J, Meadows J, et al. Conte Risk stratification in critical limb ischemia: Derivation and validation of a model to predict amputation-free survival using multicenter surgical outcomes data. J Vasc Surg. 2008;48:1464-71.
12. Da Silva A, Widmer LK, Ziegler HW, et al. The Basle longitudinal study; report on the relationship of initial glucose level to baseline ECG abnormalities, peripheral artery disease and subsequent mortality. J Chorn Dis. 1979;32:797-803.
13. Erikhoff JH, Hansen HJ, Lorentzen JE. The effects of arterial reconstruction on lower limb amputation rate. An epidemiological survey based on reports from Danish hospitals. Acta Chir Scand Suppl. 1980;502:181-7.
14. McGrath MA, Graham AR, Hill DA, et al. The natural history of chronic leg ischemia. World J Surg. 1983;7:314-8.
15. Zipes D, Libby P, Bonow R, et al. Braunwald's Heart Disease, 11th edition. Elsevier; 2018.
16. Bumpus K, Maier MA. The ABC's of wound care. Curr Cardiol Rep. 2013;15:346.
17. Singer AJ, Clark RA. Cutaneous wound healing. N Engl J Med. 1999;341:738-46.
18. Sumpio BE. Foot ulcers. N Engl J Med. 2000;343:787-93.
19. Rossi M, Carpi A. A skin microcirculation in peripheral arterial obliterative disease. Biomed Pharmacother. 2004;58:427-31.
20. Hiatt WR, Armstrong EJ, Larson CJ, et al. Pathogenesis of the limb manifestation and exercise limitations in peripheral artery disease. Circ Res. 2015;116:1527-39.
21. Rutherford RB, Baker JD, Ernst C, et al. Recommended standard for reports dealing with lower extremity ischemia: revised version. J Vasc Surg. 1997;26:517-13.
22. Fontain R, KIM M, Kieny R. Surgical treatment of peripheral circulation disorders (article in German). Helv Chir Acta. 1954;21:499-533.
23. Mills JL Sr, Conte MS, Armstrong DG, et al. Society for Vascular Surgery Lower Extremity Guidelines Committee. The Society for Vascular Surgery Lower Extremity Threatened Limb Classification System: risk stratification based on wound, ischemia and foot infection (WIFI). J Vasc Surg. 2014; 59:220-34.
24. Bandy DF, Chauvapun JP. Duplex ultrasound surveillance can be worth-while after arterial intervention. Perspect Vasc Surg Endovasc Ther. 2007; 19:354-9;discussion 360-51.
25. Ferris BL, Mills JL Sr, Hughes JD, et al. Is early postoperative duplex scan surveillance of leg bypass graft clinically important? J Vasc Surg. 2003;37:495-500.
26. Koelemay MJ, Lijmer JG, Stroker J, et al. Magnetic resonance angiography for the evaluation of lower extremity arterial disease: a meta-analysis. JAMA. 2001;285:1338-45.
27. Beckman JA, Paneni F, Cosentino F, et al. Diabetes and vascular disease: pathophysiology, clinical consequences, and medical therapy. Part II. Eur Heart J. 2013;34:2444-52.
28. Yusuf S, Sleight P, Pogue J, et al. effects of an angiotensin converting-enzyme inhibitor, ramipril, on cardiovascular events in high risk patients. N Engl J Med. 2000;342:145-53.
29. Heart Protection Study Collaborative Group. MRC/BHF Heart Protection Study of cholesterol lowering with simvastatin 20,536 high-risk individual: a randomized placebo-controlled trial. Lancet. 2002;360:7-22.
30. The Diabetes Control and Complications Trial Research Group. The effect of intensive treatment of diabetes on the development and progression of long-term complication in insulin-dependent diabetes mellitus. N Engl J Med. 1993;329:977-86.
31. Alder AI, Stevens RJ, Neil A, et al. UKPDS 59: hyperglycemic and other potential modifiable risk factors for peripheral vascular disease in type 2 diabetes. Diabetes Care. 2002;25:894-9.
32. Momsen AH, Jensen MB, Norager CB, et al. Drug therapy for improving walking distance in intermittent claudication: a systematic review and meta-analysis of robust randomized controlled studies. Eur J Vasc Endovasc Surg. 2009;38:463-74.
33. Katzberg HD, Khan AH, So YT. "Assessment: Symptomatic treatment for muscle cramps (an evidenced based review): Report of the Therapeutics and Technology Assessment Subcommittee of American Academy of Neurology". Neurology. 2010;74(8):691-6.
34. Kumbhani DJ, Steg PG, Cannon CP, et al. REACH Registry Investigators. Statin therapy and long-term adverse limb outcomes in patients with peripheral artery disease: insights from the REACH registry. Eur Heart J. 2014;35:2864-72.
35. Rooke TW, Hollier LH, Osmundson PJ. The influence of sympathetic nerves on transcutaneous oxygen tension in normal and ischemic lower extremities. Angiology. 1987;38:400-10.
36. Enoch S, Grey JE, Harding KG. ABC of wound healing. Nonsurgical and drug treatment. BMJ. 2006;332:900-3.

37. Gunalp U, Senol Y, Samil A. Hyperbaric oxygen therapy in the management of nonhealing wounds in patients with critical limb ischemia: future medicine part of future science group. Therapy. 2008;5(1):99-108.
38. KO SH, Bandyk DF. Therapeutic angiogenesis in critical limb ischemia. Semin Vasc Surg. 2014;27:23-31.
39. Adam DJ, Beard JD, Cleveland T, et al. BASIL Trial Participants. Bypass versus angioplasty in severe ischemia of the leg (BASIL): Multicentre randomized controlled trial. Lancet. 2005;366:1925-34.
40. Jones WS, Dalor RJ, Hasselblad V, et al. Comparative effectiveness of endovascular and surgical revascularization in patients with peripheral artery disease and critical limb ischemia: systematic review of revascularization in critical limb ischemia. Am Heart J. 2014; 167:489-98.
41. Shishehbor MH. Acute and critical limb ischemia: when time is limb. Cleve Clin J Med. 2014;81:209-16.
42. Stegman BM, Shishehbor MH. Commentary: optimal revascularization for critical limb ischemia: one approach does not always fit all. J Endovasc Ther. 2015;22:482-4.
43. Agarwal S, Sud K, Shishehbor MH. Nationwide trends of hospital admission and outcomes among critical limb ischemia patients: From 2003-2011. J AM Coll Cardio. 2016;67:1901-13.
44. Tepe G, Laird J, Schneider P, et al. Drug coated balloon versus standard percutaneous transluminal angioplasty for the treatment of superficial femoral and popliteal peripheral artery disease: 12-months results from the IN.Pact SFA randomized trial. Circulation. 2015;131:495-502.
45. Scheinert D, Katsanos K, Zeller T, et al. A prospective randomized multicenter comparison of balloon angioplasty and infrapopliteal stenting with the sirolimus-eluting stents in patients with ischemic peripheral artery disease. 1-year result from ACHILLES trial. J Am Coll Cardiol. 2012;60:2290-5.
46. Boguszewski AN, Torey JA, Pai R, et al. Intraluminal recanalization of SFA CTOs. Endovasc Today. 2010;9:33-8.
47. Bolia A, Miles KA, Brennan J, et al. Percutaneous transluminal angioplasty of occlusions of the femoral and popliteal arteries by subintimal dissection. Cardiovasc Intervent Radiol. 1990;13:357-63.
48. Slovut DP, Lipsitz EC. Surgical technique and peripheral artery disease. Circulation. 2012;126:1127-38.
49. Dougherty MJ, Young LP, Calligaro KD. One hundred twenty five concomitant endovascular and open procedures for lower extremity arterial disease. J Vasc Surg. 2003;37:316-22.
50. Melliere D, Cron J, Allaire E, et al. Indications and benefits of simultaneous endoluminal balloon angioplasty and open surgery during elective lower limb revascularization. Cardiovasc Surg. 1999;7:242-6.
51. Miyahara T, Miyata T, Shigematsu H, et al. Long-term results of combined iliac endovascular intervention and infrainguinal surgical revascularization for the treatment of multilevel arterial occlusive disease. Int Angiol. 2005;24: 340-8.
52. Taylor SM, Kalbaugh CA, Blackhurst DW, et al. Preoperative clinical factors predict postoperative functional outcomes after major lower limb amputation: an analysis of 553 consecutive patients. J Vasc Surg. 2005;42:227-35.

SECTION 21

Women and Heart Disease

CHAPTER 136

Coronary Artery Disease in Women: Unfair Assessment and Outcomes

Roopa Salwan

"The learning and knowledge that we have, is, at the most, but little compared with that of which we are ignorant."

–Plato

INTRODUCTION

Cardiovascular disease (CVD) is the world's leading and arguably the most preventable cause of death and disability among women. Cardiovascular disease kills more women than lung cancer and breast cancer combined.[1] The incidence of coronary artery disease (CAD) in women is lower than in men during the fourth and fifth decade of life, it rises sharply after menopause and equals that of men by the sixth and seventh decade. Once CAD is clinically manifest, women experience similar, if not worse outcomes than men.

India has a population of 1,252 million, 48.5% are women, the life expectancy at birth is 65 years for men and 68 years for women. India is undergoing a rapid health transition with rising burden of coronary heart disease (CHD). As the lifespan is increasing, so is the prevalence of heart disease. In India, more than 10.5 million deaths occur annually, 20.3% of deaths in men and 16.9% of deaths in women are caused by CVD.[2] Increase in deaths from CVD is driven by a 55% increase in mortality due to the aging of populations and a 25% increase due to population growth.[3] In a recent study from Kerala, the prevalence of any CAD was 14.3% in women and 9.8% in men, and the prevalence of definite CAD was 2.6% in women, 3.5% in men.[4] An improved understanding of disease that could affect half the population is essential to be able to improve health and outcomes.

Women and men differ in their genetic complement by a single chromosome that affects the mechanism and expression of disease (biological differences related to X chromosome) as well as the psychosocial and behavioral characteristics and environment of the individual (gender bias), which may protect from or enhance the susceptibility to CVD. Medical research in women has traditionally focused on diseases of breast and reproductive system, i.e., bikini boundaries and neglected sex and gender differences in the spectrum of CVDs.[5] Women live longer than men, but the quality of life, of those added years, is burdened by chronic disease that is preventable and treatable.

Bernadine Healy described bias in treatment of women with CAD as "Yentl Syndrome". "Yentl" was a young lady, in a Jewish community in the 19th century, who had to dress and act like a boy to be able to get education.[6] Two studies published in the New England Journal of Medicine in 1991 showed that women were significantly less likely to undergo coronary angiography or revascularization when admitted with unstable or stable angina, acute myocardial infarction (MI) or chest pain when women who underwent coronary angiography were studied, there was no difference between the sexes in treatment. Once a woman showed she was like a man by having severe CAD or MI then she was treated as a man would be.[7,8] This led to an awareness that women have not been studied as thoroughly as men—the results from studies in men have been generalized to women, which may not be appropriate. These publications were followed by sex and gender-specific research in the last three decades that has improved understanding of the pathophysiology and management of coronary disease in women.

Loss of hormones with menopause contributing to CVD is oversimplification of a complex issue. The HERS (Heart and Estrogen Replacement Study) and WHI (Women's Health Initiative) were large hormone trials, which documented that hormone replacement therapy had no role in primary or secondary prevention of heart disease in postmenopausal women, in fact they did more harm. Estrogen and progestin therapy was associated with an increased risk of breast cancer, stroke, pulmonary embolism, and coronary events, estrogen alone increased the risk of stroke with no benefit for CAD.[9-11]

RISK FACTORS FOR CORONARY ARTERY DISEASE

Traditional risk factors are similar to men; however, there is an increased prevalence and clustering of risk factors with age in women. The impact of risk factors is more adverse and placing them at a higher risk.

Established Risk Factors

Age

The prevalence of CVD increases with age, one in eight women 45–64 years have CHD while one in three women older than 65 have CHD. The highest mortality is seen in younger- and middle-aged women.[12] Women less than 50-year old have twice the likelihood of dying in hospital compared with age matched men. Why young premenopausal women who are protected by estrogens and are considered to be low-risk have worse outcomes is not known.

Hypertension

Women older than 60 years have a higher prevalence and poorer control of hypertension than men. It increases the prevalence of stroke and congestive heart failure in women. Hypertension rises 2- to 3-fold in women taking oral contraceptives. Hypertension is predictive of a higher risk in premenopausal women.

Diabetes

It confers greater cardiovascular risk for women than men. The risk of fatal CHD is three times compared to nondiabetic women. Impaired glucose tolerance may be more detrimental in women. Gestational diabetes increases the risk of diabetes later in life. Diabetic women have more complications and higher mortality following ST-elevation myocardial infarction (STEMI) and surgical revascularization.[13-16] In the INTERHEART study, hypertension and diabetes were more strongly associated with MI in women than men.[17]

Smoking

It is one of the strongest risk factors for CAD, more so in women on oral contraceptives, there is a significant increase in risk of venous thromboembolism, stroke, and MI.[18-20] It is of concern that smoking is increasing in women in India. The INTERHEART has documented increased risk with all forms of tobacco use including chewing tobacco or smoking beedies.[21]

Dyslipidemia

Adverse changes in lipids accompany menopause, with increase in low-density lipoprotein (LDL) cholesterol, triglycerides (TGs), and decrease in high-density lipoprotein (HDL). Low-density lipoprotein is the main atherogenic lipoprotein in the development of atherosclerosis. At any level of LDL, the risk depends on the level of HDL and TG. High-density lipoprotein cholesterol less than 30 mg/dL is strongly associated with increased cardiovascular mortality in women. Secondary prevention to reduce cardiac events and mortality is equally effective in women and men.[22,23]

Family History of Premature Coronary Heart Disease

Family history of premature CHD in a first-degree female relative is a relatively more potent family history risk factor than in male relative. A family history of premature CAD is seen more frequently in women with CAD.

Physical Activity and Fitness

Physical inactivity is more common in women, as they get older and is associated with higher blood pressure, worse cholesterol levels, poorer glucose metabolism, poor mental health, and obesity. Those with higher physical activity have lower rates of CVD. Physically fit obese women are at lower risk than lean women who are not physically fit.[24,25]

Emerging Risk Factors

Metabolic Syndrome

It is more prevalent in women and increases the risk of developing CVD 2.6-fold. Obesity, a body mass index (BMI) more than 30 kg/m^2 increases the risk of diabetes, CVD and is a powerful predictor of mortality in women. High BMI in adolescents has been linked with early menarche; and later in life, obesity, insulin resistance, dyslipidemia, and metabolic syndrome.

Autoimmune Disease

Rheumatoid arthritis and systemic lupus erythematosus (SLE) are more prevalent in women and lead to accelerated atherosclerosis with 2- to 3-fold increase in risk of acute MI, congestive cardiac failure and stroke.[26-28]

Gestational Hypertension

Pregnancy is like a stress test for future cardiovascular events—gestational hypertension and preeclampsia increase the risk of CVD, later in life, 2-fold.[29]

Polycystic Ovarian Disease

Estrogen deficiency causing irregular menstrual cycles from polycystic ovarian disease (PCOD) or hypothalamic dysfunction in premenopausal women is associated with an increased risk of coronary atherosclerosis, diabetes mellitus, and adverse CVD events.[30-33]

Breast Cancer

Women surviving breast cancer have an elevated risk of developing CVD. Radiotherapy exposes the heart to ionizing radiation that increases the risk of developing ischemic heart disease (IHD) within a few years after exposure that continues up to 20 years. The risk is proportionate to the mean dose of radiation to the heart and the presence of other CVD risk factors.[34-36] There are similarities in predisposing risk factors—obesity, sedentary lifestyle, tobacco use, diet, and age. Modification of risk factors during cancer treatment is not given its due attention.

Hysterectomy

Increased risk of CVD has been reported in observational studies after hysterectomy with or without bilateral salpingo-oophorectomy (BSO). Compromised ovarian function after hysterectomy has been reported even when the ovaries have been preserved is likely related to reduced ovarian blood flow. However, there is no independent association between hysterectomy and CVD after controlling for other major risk factors. Hysterectomy does not change CVD risk factors such as blood pressure and lipid profile. Women who have had a hysterectomy tend to have worse CVD risk profile.[37]

In the Swedish registry, data on 184,441 women who underwent hysterectomy between 1973 and 2003 has shown that hysterectomy in women less than 50 years age substantially increases the risk for CVD later in life. Oophorectomy further adds to the risk of both CHD and stroke. In women older than 50 years, there was no significant association between hysterectomy and incident CVD.[38]

There are no published guidelines specifically for the management of BRCA mutation carriers after prophylactic BSO.

Psychosocial Factors

Psychological factors and emotional stress can influence the onset and clinical course of IHD in women. Depression is twice as common and is a consistent predictor of CHD events in women.[39,40] Psychological factors associated with increased risk are hostility, work stress, and anger suppression. Increased attention to emotional regulation may give a better understanding of role of negative emotions in CAD in women.[41,42] Strain of multiple roles and lack of supportive relationships, low level of social integration is associated with increased risk of recurrent events and mortality.[43-45] Optimism has been found to be associated with reduced risk of MI and mortality in WHI.

PATHOPHYSIOLOGY OF IHD IN WOMEN

Ischemic Heart Disease

Ischemic heart disease comprehensively describes the spectrum of disease in women. Besides CAD, i.e., atherosclerotic disease of the epicardial vessels, it includes—ischemia related to endothelial dysfunction, coronary microvascular dysfunction (CMD), coronary spasm, supply-demand mismatch, spontaneous coronary dissection, and stress-related cardiomyopathy.

Atherosclerotic Coronary Artery Disease

Plaque rupture with disrupted fibrous cap, large necrotic core with macrophages is more prevalent in men and older women.[46] Plaque erosion is seen in younger women, the underlying lesion is fibroatheroma or intimal thickening characterized by smooth muscle cells in a proteoglycan and collagen-rich matrix with absence of surface endothelium and increased frequency of distal microembolization from platelet-rich debris. Plaque erosion is associated with less thrombus burden, less calcification, less percentage vessel stenosis, less overall plaque burden, minimal inflammation, and negative arterial remodeling.[47] Infrequently, coronary event is from a calcified nodule, that represents fibrocalcific plaques with little or no underlying necrotic core but there is disruption of the luminal surface, i.e., absence of collagen and endothelium with luminal thrombosis overlying the eruptive dense calcified nodules.[48]

Endothelial Dysfunction

Endothelium is responsible for the vasomotor tone of coronary vessels, platelet aggregation, leukocyte migration, and thrombogenicity. Patients with coronary endothelium dysfunction have an increased vasoconstrictor response to autonomic system leading to increased resistance in arterioles.

Coronary Microvascular Dysfunction

It is known that women have smaller coronary arteries per 100 g of left ventricular (LV) mass and their arteries have increased stiffness. The epicardial arteries are 500 microns to 5 mm in size, the prearterioles 100–500 microns, intramural arterioles 100 microns, and capillaries 5–10 microns—the coronary microcirculation regulates coronary blood flow and adapts to metabolic demands of the body. Coronary microvascular dysfunction may occur in the presence or absence of obstructive CAD, myocardial disease or may be iatrogenic. Intrinsic genetic factors also contribute to coronary smooth muscle reactivity.[49]

Young patients with acute MI have been classified into five phenotypes in the VIRGO (Variation in Recovery: Role of Gender on Outcomes of Young Acute MI Patients) study: Class I patients with plaque-mediated obstructive culprit lesions (94.9% in men and 82.5% in women); Class II obstructive CAD (>50% stenosis) without evidence of plaque rupture or thrombosis (2% in men and 3.8% in women); Class III nonobstructive CAD (<50% stenosis, 2.7% in men and 11.35 in women); Class IV nonplaque mechanism of ischemia including vasospasm, dissection, and embolism (0.2% in men and 1.5% in women); Class V indeterminate (0.2% in men and 0.8% in women).

Further Class II and II are divided into "a" and "b" on the presence or absence of supply-demand mismatch: increased myocardial oxygen demand, defined as systolic blood pressure more than or equal to 180 mmHg; diastolic blood pressure more than or equal to 100 mmHg; heart rate more than or equal to 120 bpm; atrial fibrillation or flutter regardless of heart rate; ventricular tachycardia or fibrillation; acute life-threatening comorbid illness on presentation (e.g., severe pneumonia or exacerbation of chronic obstructive pulmonary disease; trauma; acute renal failure; stroke; sepsis; surgical complication; any fracture; diabetes ketoacidosis/hyperosmolar hyperglycemia syndrome/hypoglycemia; seizure; acute liver failure; and other acute and severe infections), or decreased myocardial oxygen supply, defined as systolic blood pressure less than 90 mmHg, hemoglobin less than 10 mg/dL, hypoxia, gastrointestinal bleed, and other major bleeding.[50]

ASSESSMENT OF ISCHEMIC HEART DISEASE IN WOMEN

Women have more symptoms, are older with higher risk factor burden, but paradoxically have less severe obstructive CAD. The relatively low prevalence of obstructive CAD in women produces a higher ratio of false-positive to true-positive results. Physicians underestimate women's cardiovascular risk and underutilize noninvasive diagnostic modalities for concern on the diagnostic accuracy of these tests.

Exercise Stress Testing

Exercise stress test is the initial diagnostic test for symptomatic women who can exercise more than 5 metabolic equivalents (METs), the negative predictive value of the test is comparable to men (78% vs. 81%). Integrating the Duke Treadmill score improves the accuracy. In women, resting electrocardiography (ECG) frequently has ST-T changes related to hormonal factors that leads to higher false-positive rate of exercise stress test. The positive predictive value of ST depression with exercise testing in women is significantly lower than men (47% vs. 77%). Stress imaging should be limited to women with indeterminate or abnormal ECG findings—ECG test leads to nuclear scan or stress echocardiography (ECHO) in one in five women.[51,52]

Stress Echocardiography

Stress ECHO with exercise or dobutamine stress has high-diagnostic accuracy in women, sensitivity 79%, and specificity 83%. In institutions with high volume and expertise, stress ECHO has comparable accuracy to nuclear imaging. Echocardiography can also be helpful in assessing noncoronary etiologies for symptoms such as diastolic dysfunction, abnormal filling pressures, abnormal myocardial mechanics using tissue Doppler or speckle tracking.[53,54]

Stress Myocardial Perfusion Single-photon Emission Computed Tomography

Stress myocardial perfusion single-photon emission computed tomography (SPECT) has sensitivity of 81% and specificity of 78%. While traditional imaging has been done with thallium, it was associated with lower accuracy due to breast tissue artifact in women. Use of Technetium 99m sestamibi and technetium 99m tetrofosmin has decreased incidence of false-positive results. The high energy results in less tissue attenuation, and simultaneous ECG gating has been shown to significantly improve the specificity over nuclear imaging for women. The overall radiation burden is higher with the use of stress myocardial perfusion SPECT than for cardiac computed tomography angiography (CCTA) or positron emission tomography (PET) imaging. To limit radiation, stress imaging should be performed first and if findings are normal, elimination of resting scan can reduce radiation exposure considerably. In patients with left bundle branch block, dobutamine SPECT is more accurate than exercise perfusion imaging.[55]

Stress Myocardial Perfusion Positron Emission Tomography

Stress myocardial perfusion PET has improved spatial resolution and increased diagnostic accuracy for detecting obstructive CAD in obese women when compared to SPECT (88% vs. 78%). Conventional cardiac PET using rubidium-82 or N ammonia has markedly reduces radiation exposure 2–3 mSv. It also allows measurement of coronary blood flow and coronary flow reserve (CFR) less than 2 indicated microvascular dysfunction in patients with nonobstructive disease on angiography.[56,57]

Stress Cardiovascular Magnetic Resonance

Stress cardiovascular magnetic resonance (CMR) has comparable sensitivity to SPECT and ECHO. Cardiovascular magnetic resonance measures myocardial flow reserve on vasodilator stress, which may improve detection of CMD in symptomatic women. Stress MR demonstrates diffuse subendocardial perfusion defects in patients with microvascular dysfunction. Late gadolinium enhancement CMR imaging to improve detection of scarred or infarcted myocardium in women with previous undocumented MI.[58-60]

Noninvasive Imaging of Atherosclerosis

Coronary Artery Calcium

Coronary artery calcium (CAC) is a marker of subclinical atherosclerosis, is highly predictive of CVD risk, and potentially identifies patients for more intensive risk factor modification. In the Multiethnic Study of Atherosclerosis (MESA) trial, increased severity of CAC is associated with higher mortality rates. Women with a CAC score more than or equal to 300 had an annual IHD event rate of 2.2%.[61] The IHD event risk for women with a high-risk CAC score and multiple risk factors is 10% greater in women than men, comorbidity disproportionately accelerates risk in women. It has a sensitivity of 96–100% and specificity of 40–60% in detecting obstructive CAD in women.[62]

Computed Tomography Coronary Angiography

The diagnostic accuracy of CCTA is similar in men and women, sensitivity of 85–99% and specificity of 64–90%, and is useful for evaluation of women with indeterminate stress test. In the PROMISE trial, CT Angiography as an initial evaluation approach does not improve clinical outcomes when compared to a functional test for CAD evaluation, however, is associated with fewer invasive angiographies.[63] In the ROMICAT II trial, women undergoing CCTA in emergency department for evaluation of chest pain suggestive of acute coronary syndrome (ACS) had a greater reduction in length of hospital stay and lower hospital admission rate. CCTA-detected CAD in a third of patients, 58% had normal coronaries and 5% had obstructive disease. CCTA is able to visualize nonobstructive CAD, which is not detected during stress tests, that enables patients to be on better preventive therapy when indicated.[64] In the CRESCENT trial, with CCTA, in women, diagnosis was established earlier with lesser additional downstream testing and patients were more likely to have resolution of chest pain at 1 year.[65]

Invasive Testing for Ischemic Heart Diseas

In women with a high-risk on noninvasive testing, symptomatic on optimal medical therapy or with evidence of ACS, coronary angiography is indicated for diagnosis with revascularization when appropriate. Women are more likely to experience severe bleeding and access site complications, use of radial access substantially reduces these complications. Women have smaller arteries and a higher incidence of spasm, they are more likely to cross over to femoral access than men (11.1% vs. 6.3%).[66] Dose adjusting of antithrombotic/antiplatelet therapies to weight and creatinine clearance reduces bleeding complications. Despite worse symptoms, women usually have less obstructive disease and greater microvascular dysfunction.

Invasive Coronary Vasomotor

Invasive coronary vasomotor testing is a safe method for definitive diagnosis and assessment of CMD. Nitroglycerin (NTG) is an endothelium-independent vasodilator that acts directly on the smooth muscles and dilates coronary vessels greater than 200 mcm. Lack of response to NTG suggests endothelium-independent epicardial vessel dysfunction. Adenosine acts on smooth muscle cells of coronary vessels less than 150 mcm in diameter CFR ratio more than 2.5 is normal, abnormal response is seen with microvascular dysfunction. Acetylcholine produces a uniform endothelium-dependent dilation of both micro- and macrovasculature leads to more than 50% increase in coronary blood flow. Lack of response to acetylcholine reflects endothelial disease.

CLINICAL SPECTRUM OF ISCHEMIC HEART DISEASE

Although the Framingham study previously suggested that development of CAD in women lags approximately 10 years behind men, it is now believed, this lag is substantially less and women are susceptible to CAD at a much younger age. The mean age of women in the Kerala ACS registry was 64.4 ± 11.7 years, was older than men by 5 years (mean age in men 59.3 ± 11.9 years, p <0.001).[67] Chest pain is the most frequent symptom, women are more likely to be overwhelmed with by a multiplicity of associated symptoms—back, neck and jaw pain, dyspnea, paroxysmal nocturnal dyspnea, nausea, indigestion, and weakness or fatigue. Thirty seven percent of women present without chest pain (as compared to 27% men). Women were more likely to delay seeking care had more diabetes, hypertension, and heart failure with preserved ventricular systolic function. Women more commonly present with non-ST-elevation myocardial infarction (NSTEMI) than STEMI. Women are also more likely to have spontaneous coronary artery dissection (SCAD) or coronary artery spasm (CAS).[68,69] Compared with men, women with ACS and those after coronary revascularization have longer hospitalizations, more bleeding complications, higher in-hospital mortality, and up to 30% more readmissions within 30 days after the index hospitalization. In the setting of ACS, normal coronary arteries do not have a benign prognosis. Worse prognosis of women has been attributed to advanced age, comorbidities, underutilization of life-saving therapies.

Young women with AMI had higher rates of cardiovascular risk factors and comorbidities than men, including diabetes, morbid obesity, congestive heart failure, and renal failure. They also have higher levels of depression, stress, poorer physical health, and lower quality of life at baseline. They are more likely to present with atypical chest pain or no symptoms (16% vs. 10%; p = 0.008) and more likely to present more than 6 hours after symptom onset (35% vs. 23%; p = 0.002).[70]

The GLOW meta-analysis of gender-based outcomes in 731,990 patients (32% women), women with STEMI had more risk factors, longer door to balloon times, and with a greater than 2-fold higher in-hospital mortality. They were more likely to have more in hospital complications such as shock, heart failure, mechanical complications, reinfarction, recurrent ischemia, bleeding, and stroke as compared with men. Adjustments for comorbidities suggest that modifiable risk factors account primarily for the difference in mortality.[71] With primary percutaneous coronary intervention (PCI), women have a lower 30-day mortality, 7.7% versus 9.6% for those presenting within 2 hours of symptom onset and 8.5% versus 14.4% for those presenting later than 2 hours.[72,73] Thrombolytic therapy is indicated in patients presenting within 12 hours of symptoms, with no contraindications, who have an anticipated delay more than 120 minutes to a PCI-capable facility. Women often have multiple relative contraindications (advanced age, hypertension, and small body size) to thrombolysis and female sex is an independent predictor of intracranial bleeding.[74]

Among patients undergoing coronary artery bypass grafting (CABG), however, women have a higher risk of morbidity and mortality and they experience less relief from angina than do men after CABG, when off-pump surgery is performed, women have a lower mortality rate.[75,76]

Guideline-directed medical therapy is the same for all patients, women are less likely to receive optimal therapy. Lifestyle changes are pivotal. Statins in intermediate to high-risk women besides controlling lipids, have a pleiotropic effect, improve endothelial dysfunction, along with angiotensin-converting enzyme (ACE) inhibitors, and improve coronary flow reserve. Aspirin has no role in primary prevention in women less than 65 years; and for others, it should be given on long-term basis.

INDIAN DATA

In the CREATE Registry, 23.5% patients were women, in 47% of women, the presentation of ACS was STEMI. The mean age of the entire group was 57.5 (SD 12.1) years. The mean time to presentation was significantly longer for women 410 versus 340 minutes (p <0.0001), 30.9% women were treated with thrombolysis (vs. 44.9% men, p <0.0001), 5.6% underwent primary PCI (vs. 6.9% men p <0.0001). The 30-day mortality was 8.9% in women versus 6.5% in men (p <0.0001).[77]

The Detection and Management of Coronary Heart Disease (DEMAT) Registry was specifically evaluated gender differences in ACS patients (334 women; 1,231 men). Women were less likely to present with STEMI (38% vs. 55%). Women were also more likely than men to have a history of hypertension (62% vs. 42%; p = 0.001) and diabetes (46% vs. 38%; p = 0.01) but were less likely to be tobacco users (2% vs. 33%; p = 0.001).[78] There was no gender difference in the in-hospital management, discharge treatment and 30 day mortality and major adverse CV event (MACE) (13.5% vs. 12.5%).

MYOCARDIAL INFARCTION WITH NONOBSTRUCTIVE CORONARY ARTERIES

Myocardial infarction with non obstructive coronary arteries (MINOCA) refers to patients with coronary-related ischemia in the absence of coronary artery obstruction (<50% disease) or from nonplaque-mediated mechanisms (coronary spasm, spontaneous coronary dissection, coronary embolism or unidentified mechanisms). The MINOCA represents 6–14% of all acute MIs—two-thirds cases are NSTEMI. In the VIRGO trial, 11.1% of patients had MINOCA, the presentation was STEMI in 21.4%. Young premenopausal women are five times more likely to have MINOCA (14.9% vs. 3.5%).[79] Hypertension is frequently associated, while hyperlipidemia and diabetes are less frequent. Hypercoagulable state is more frequent (3% vs. 1.3%). Autoimmune disease, cocaine or illicit drug use, and psychosocial factors did not differ by type of MI. Those with obstructive CAD are more likely to have history of gestational diabetes and early menarche.

The MINOCA is not benign—all-cause in-hospital mortality is 0.9%, with a 2% risk of death or reinfarction over 6 months, and 1-year mortality of 4.7% is reported. These patients tend to have a 15% readmission rate within 6 months because of persistent disabling symptoms. At 10 years, CVD death or MI occurred in 6.7% of those with no evident angiographic CAD and in 12.8% among those with nonobstructive CAD.[80] In the VIRGO trial, the 1-month mortality was 1.1% and 12-month mortality was 0.6%.

In the absence of obstructive CAD, postulated pathophysiologic mechanism includes atherosclerosis with plaque disruption, distal embolization, and endothelial and microvascular dysfunction that would amplify the consequences of an upstream spastic or thrombotic event.

Coronary Artery Spasm

Coronary artery spasm can cause recurrent chest pain episodes at rest with associated transient ST-segment elevation, infrequently causes AMI. It is caused by autonomic imbalance, vascular smooth muscle hyperactivity, and endothelial dysfunction. Cigarette smoking, cocaine and other drug abuse may lead to coronary spasm. Studies of patients with stable CHD have reported higher rates of mental stress-induced ischemia in women.

Takotsubo Cardiomyopathy

Takotsubo cardiomyopathy (TTC) is characterized by acute and rapidly reversible systolic and diastolic LV dysfunction, triggered by profound psychological or physical stress. Signs and symptoms of myocardial ischemia occur in the absence of obstructive CAD. A distinctive abnormality of LV contraction consists of akinesia or dyskinesia of the apical and/or midventricular segments of the left ventricle (apical ballooning), together with hypercontractility of the base that usually recovers on follow-up.

Myocardial biopsy in patients with stress cardiomyopathy shows interstitial infiltrates consisting primarily of mononuclear lymphocytes, leukocytes, and macrophages; myocardial fibrosis; and contraction band necrosis.

Prevalence

Takotsubo cardiomyopathy accounts for 1.7–2.2% of all patients admitted with a presumed diagnosis of ACS; this rate increases up to 6–7%, if only females are considered. In the HORIZONS-AMI trial, TTC was diagnosed with a frequency of 0.5% of all patients and 2.1% of the female patients.

The cause of TTC remains unknown, the role of brain-heart axis, exaggerated sympathetic stimulation and the negative inotropic effect of high-dose epinephrine on the LV myocardium have been postulated. The LV apex contains a higher density of β-adrenoceptors, making it more susceptible to catecholamine-induced cell injury. The density of sympathetic nerve endings approximately 40% higher in the basal myocardium than in the apical myocardium, the heart is dependent on neuronal uptake for inactivating catecholamines in the extracellular fluid. Supraphysiological catecholamines induce a β2-adrenoceptor stimulation that leads to a Gi-mediated negative inotropy—which is more pronounced at the apex and completely reversible on removal of the catecholamine stimulus. The coronary microcirculation is innervated by neurons that originate in the brainstem and mediate vasoconstriction leading to myocardial stunning.

The International Takotsubo Registry is the largest data base of 1,750 patients.[81] Takotsubo cardiomyopathy is predominantly a disease of postmenopausal women (89.8%), mean age—66.8 ± 13 years, and 79.1% were women older than 50 years of age. Symptoms at presentation are chest pain (75.9%), dyspnea (46.9%), and syncope (7.7%). It may be triggered by physical (36%) or emotional (27.7%) strain, 55.8% patients had a previous neurological or psychiatric illness.

Takotsubo cardiomyopathy is a heart failure syndrome associated with significant elevation of brain natriuretic peptide and lesser elevation of troponin I. Apical TTC is the most common form (81.7%), the other being midventricular form (14.6%), basal (2.2%), and focal forms (1.5%). Early angiography is necessary to rule out ACS. In hospital, major adverse events were seen in 21.8% of patients, 9.9% developed cardiogenic shock, 17.3% required ventilatory support, 3% had ventricular tachycardia and a mortality of 4.1%. On long-term follow-up, the death rate from any cause was 5.6% per patient per year, the rate of stroke or transient ischemic attack was 1.7% per patient per year and the rate of recurrence of TTC was 1.8% per patient per year.

Spontaneous Coronary Artery Dissection

Spontaneous coronary artery dissection is a coronary artery dissection that is not atherosclerotic, traumatic, or iatrogenic. Spontaneous coronary artery dissection accounts for 1–4% of ACS, 80% of patients are female, average age is 42 years, 20–25% of cases occur in the peripartum period. The classic presentation is of a young healthy woman, without risk factors, and sudden onset of ACS. It results from an intimal tear, which allows blood from the true lumen to enter media and generate a false lumen or from spontaneous hemorrhage in the vasa vasorum within the vessel wall—formation of an intramural hematoma that compresses the true lumen leading to coronary insufficiency and MI. Histopathology is characterized by a periadventitial inflammatory infiltrate with predominant eosinophils. Fibromuscular dysplasia in extracoronary vascular beds is frequently seen, most common involved are the renal arteries (79.7%) and extracranial carotids (74.3%). Intracranial aneurysm is seen in 14–23%. The left anterior descending artery is the most commonly affected (32–46% of cases), left main is involved in 4%. In the majority of cases, the mid to distal segments of coronary arteries are affected; multivessel SCAD occurs in 9–23% of cases. Spontaneous healing of SCAD lesion is seen in majority of patients, angiography done more than 35 days after diagnosis, spontaneous healing seen in 88.5%. Recurrent MI is seen in 7–10% within the 1st week due to extension of dissection. In-hospital mortality is low, 2.6–8% require revascularization for ongoing ischemia, left main dissection, or hemodynamic instability. Angiographic three patterns are described: (1) type I multiple radiolucent lumens or arterial wall contrast staining (29.1%); (2) type II diffuse stenosis that can be of varying severity and length usually more than 20 mm (67.5%); and (3) type III Focal or tubular stenosis less than 20 mm in length that mimics atherosclerosis (3.4%). Percutaneous coronary intervention for SCAD has been associated with lower technical success and higher complications, the affected arteries are inherently weak and susceptible to iatrogenic dissection and extension of dissection. Recommended therapy includes a single antiplatelet, avoidance of statin, use of beta-blockade, avoidance of systemic hormones including oral contraceptives. Statins were associated with recurrent SCAD, therefore, these are recommended only when hyperlipidemia is documented. The largest series of SCAD from Mayo Clinic has reported a high MACE (death, recurrent SCAD, MI, and HF) rate of 47.4%, recurrence rate of 17% (occurring solely in women), and a 10-year mortality rate of 7.7%.[82,83]

CONCLUSION

The CVD is a leading cause of death in women. Synergistic effect of multiple risk factors contributes to the disease burden. Unique aspects of risk factors and manifestation of heart disease in women are better understood today. Aggressive risk factor control by physicians early in life with optimal use of guideline-directed therapy is essential to improve cardiovascular outcomes in women. Women must be educated that they are vulnerable to heart disease, and risk factors need to be prevented and controlled. Physicians need to be aware of the entire spectrum of disease in women, and be sensitive in their approach to diagnosis and treatment.

REFERENCES

1. Benjamin EJ, Blaha MJ, Chiuve SE, et al. Heart disease and stroke statistics 2017 update a report from the American Heart Association. Circulation. 2017;135:e146-e603.
2. Gupta R. Burden of Coronary Heart Disease in India. Indian Heart J. 2005;57:632-8.
3. Roth GA, Forouzanfar MH, Moran AE, et al. Demographic and Epidemiologic Drivers of Global Cardiovascular Mortality. N Engl J Med. 2015;372:1333-41.
4. McSweeney JC, Rosenfeld AG, Abel WM, et al. Preventing and experiencing Ischemic Heart Disease as a woman: State of the Science. A scientific statement from the American Heart Association. Circulation. 2016;133:1302-31.
5. Krishnan MN, Zachariah G, Venugopal K, et al. Prevalence of coronary artery disease and its risk factors in Kerala, South India: a community-based cross-sectional study. BMC Cardiovasc Disord. 2016;16:12.
6. Healy B. The Yentl Syndrome. N Engl J Med. 1991;325:274-6.
7. Ayanian JZ, Epstein AM. Differences in the use of procedures between women and men hospitalised for coronary heart disease. N Engl J Med. 1991;325:221-5.
8. Steingart RM, Packer M, Hamm P, et al. Sex Differences in the management of Coronary Artery Disease. N Engl J Med. 1991;325:226-30.
9. Bairey Merz CN, Shaw LJ, Reis SE, et al.; Insights from the NHLBI—Writing Group for the Women's Health Initiative Investigators. Risks and benefits of estrogen plus progestin in healthy postmenopausal women: principal results from the Women's Health Initiative randomized controlled trial. JAMA. 2002;288:321-33.
10. Grady D, Herrington D, Bittner V, et al. Cardiovascular disease outcomes during 6.8 years of hormone therapy: Heart and Estrogen/progestin Replacement Study Follow-up (HERS II). JAMA. 2002;288:49-57.
11. Hulley S, Grady D, Bush T, et al. Randomized trial of estrogen plus progestin for secondary prevention of coronary heart disease in postmenopausal women: Heart and Estrogen/progestin Replacement Study (HERS) Research Group. JAMA. 1998;280:605-13.
12. Lerner DJ, Kannel WB. Patterns of coronary heart disease morbidity and mortality in the sexes: a 26-year follow-up of the Framingham population. Am Heart J. 1986;111:383-90.
13. Barrett-Connor EL, Cohn BA, Wingard DL, et al. Why is diabetes mellitus a stronger risk factor for fatal ischemic heart disease in women than in men? The Rancho Bernardo Study. JAMA. 1991;265:627-631.
14. Manson JE, Colditz GA, Stampfer MJ, et al. A prospective study of maturity onset diabetes mellitus and risk of coronary heart disease and stroke in women. Arch Intern Med. 1991;151:1141-7.
15. Juutilainen A, Kortelainen S, Lehto S, et al. Gender difference in the impact of type 2 diabetes on coronary heart disease risk. Diabetes Care. 2004;27:2898-904.

16. Huxley R, Barzi F, Woodward M. Excess risk of fatal coronary heart disease associated with diabetes in men and women: meta-analysis of 37 prospective cohort studies. BMJ. 2006;332:73-8.
17. Anand SS, Islam S, Rosengren A, et al. Risk factors for myocardial infarction in women and men: insights from the INTERHEART study. Eur Heart J. 2008;29:932-40.
18. Huxley RR, Woodward M. Cigarette smoking as a risk factor for coronary heart disease in women compared with men: a systematic review and meta-analysis of prospective cohort studies. Lancet. 2011;378:1297-305.
19. Lidegaard O. Smoking and use of oral contraceptives: impact on thrombotic diseases. Am J Obstet Gynecol. 1999;180:S357-63.
20. Pomp ER, Rosendaal FR, Doggen CJ. Smoking increases the risk of venous thrombosis and acts synergistically with oral contraceptive use. Am J Hematol. 2008;83:97-102.
21. Goyal A, Yusuf S. The burden of cardiovascular disease in the Indian subcontinent. Indian J Med Res. 2006;124:235-44.
22. Langendorfer A, Stein EA, Kruyer W, et al. Primary prevention of acute coronary events with lovastatin in men and women with average cholesterol levels: results of AFCAPS/TexCAPS. Air Force/Texas Coronary Atherosclerosis Prevention Study. JAMA. 1998;279:1615-22.
23. Pedersen TR, Kjekshus J, Berg K, et al.; Scandinavian Simvastatin Survival Study Group. Randomised trial of cholesterol lowering in 4444 patients with coronary heart disease: the Scandinavian Simvastatin Survival Study (4S). 1994. Atheroscler Suppl. 2004;5:81-7.
24. Wilson PW, D'Agostino RB, Sullivan L, et al. Overweight and obesity as determinants of cardiovascular risk: the Framingham experience. Arch Intern Med. 2002;162:1867-72.
25. Wilson PW, Kannel WB, Silbershatz H, et al. Clustering of metabolic factors and coronary heart disease. Arch Intern Med. 1999;159:1104-9.
26. del Rincón I, Polak JF, O'Leary DH, et al. Systemic inflammation and cardiovascular risk factors predict rapid progression of atherosclerosis in rheumatoid arthritis. Ann Rheum Dis. 2015;74:1118-23.
27. Gianturco L, Bodini BD, Atzeni F, et al. Cardiovascular and autoimmune diseases in females: The role of microvasculature and dysfunctional endothelium. Atherosclerosis. 2015;241:259-63.
28. Esdaile JM, Abrahamowicz M, Grodzicky T, et al. Traditional Framingham risk factors fail to fully account for accelerated atherosclerosis in systemic lupus erythematosus. Arthritis Rheum. 2001;44:2331-7.
29. Bellamy L, Casas JP, Hingorani AD, et al. Pre-eclampsia and risk of cardiovascular disease and cancer in later life: systematic review and meta-analysis. BMJ. 2007;335:974.
30. Bairey Merz CN, Johnson BD, Sharaf BL, et al. Hypoestrogenemia of hypothalamic origin and coronary artery disease in premenopausal women: a report from the NHLBI-sponsored WISE study. J Am Coll Cardiol. 2003;41:413-9.
31. Tannenbaum C, Barrett-Connor E, Laughlin GA, et al. A longitudinal study of dehydroepiandrosterone sulphate (DHEAS) change in older men and women: the Rancho Bernardo Study. Eur J Endocrinol. 2004;151:717-25.
32. Ding EL, Song Y, Malik VS, et al. Sex differences of endogenous sex hormones & risk of type 2 diabetes. JAMA. 2006;295:1288-99.
33. Shaw LJ, Bairey Merz CN, Azziz R, et al. Postmenopausal women with a history of irregular menses and elevated androgen measurements at high risk for worsening cardiovascular event-free survival: results from the National Institutes of Health-National Heart, Lung, and Blood Institute sponsored Women's Ischemia Syndrome Evaluation. J Clin Endocrinol Metab. 2008;93:1276-84.
34. Darby SC, Ewertz M, McGale P, et al. Risk of ischemic heart disease in women after radiotherapy for breast cancer. N Engl J Med. 2013;368:987-98.
35. Herrmann J, Lerman A, Sandhu NP, et al. Evaluation and management of patients with heart disease and cancer: cardio-oncology. Mayo Clin Proc. 2014;89:1287-306.
36. Lancellotti P, Nkomo VT, Badano LP, et al. Expert consensus for multi-modality imaging evaluation of cardiovascular complications of radiotherapy in adults: a report from the European Association of Cardiovascular Imaging and the American Society of Echocardiography. J Am Soc Echocardiogr. 2013;26:1013-32.
37. Colditz GA, Willett WC, Stampfer MJ, et al. Menopause and the risk of coronary heart disease in women. N Engl J Med. 1987;316:1105-10.
38. Ingelsson E, Lundholm C, Johansson ALV, et al. Hysterectomy and risk of cardiovascular disease a population based cohort study. Eur Heart J. 2011;32:745-50.
39. Musselman DL, Evans DL, Nemeroff CB. The relationship of depression to cardiovascular disease: epidemiology, biology, and treatment. Arch Gen Psychiatry. 1998;55:580-92.
40. Xu X, Bao H, Strait K, et al. Sex differences in perceived stress and early recovery in young and middle-aged patients with acute myocardial infarction. Circulation. 2015;131:614-23.
41. Rutledge T, Reis SE, Olson MB, et al. Depression symptom severity and reported treatment history in the prediction of cardiac risk in women with suspected myocardial ischemia: the NHLBI-sponsored WISE study. Arch Gen Psychiatry. 2006;63:874-80.
42. Frasure-Smith N, Lespérance F, Juneau M, et al. Gender, depression, and one-year prognosis after myocardial infarction. Psychosom Med. 1999;61:26-37.
43. Orth-Gomér K, Wamala SP, Horsten M, et al. Marital stress worsens prognosis in women with coronary heart disease: the Stockholm Female Coronary Risk Study. JAMA. 2000;284:3008-14.
44. Wang HX, Leineweber C, Kirkeeide R, et al. Psychosocial stress and atherosclerosis: family and work stress accelerate progression of coronary disease in women; the Stockholm Female Coronary Angiography Study. J Intern Med. 2007;261:245-54.
45. Bucholz EM, Strait KM, Dreyer RP, et al. Effect of low perceived social support on health outcomes in young patients with acute myocardial infarction: results from the VIRGO (Variation in Recovery: Role of Gender on Outcomes of Young AMI Patients) study. J Am Heart Assoc. 2014;3:e001252.
46. Falk E. Plaque rupture with severe pre-existing stenosis precipitating coronary thrombosis: characteristics of coronary atherosclerotic plaques underlying fatal occlusive thrombi. Br Heart J. 1983;50:127-34.
47. van der Wal AC, Becker AE, van der Loos CM, et al. Site of intimal rupture or erosion of thrombosed coronary atherosclerotic plaques is characterized by an inflammatory process irrespective of the dominant plaque morphology. Circulation. 1994;89:36-44.
48. Virmani R, Burke AP, Farb A, et al. Pathology of the vulnerable plaque. J Am Coll Cardiol. 2006;47(suppl):C13-8.
49. Kothawade K, Merz CNB. Microvascular dysfunction in women—pathophysiology, diagnosis and management. Curr Probl Cardiol. 2011;36:291-318.
50. Spatz ES, Curry LA, Masoudi FA, et al. The Variation in recovery: role of gender on outcomes of young AMI patients (VIRGO) classification system: a taxonomy for young women with acute myocardial infarction. Circulation. 2015;132:1717-8.
51. Mieres JH, Gulati M, Merz BN, et al. Role of noninvasive testing in the clinical evaluation of women with suspected ischemic heart disease: a consensus statement from the American Heart Association. Circulation. 2014;130:350-79.
52. Shaw LJ, Mieres JH, Hendel RH, et al. Comparative effectiveness of exercise electrocardiography with or without myocardial perfusion single photon emission computed tomography in women with suspected coronary artery disease: Results from What is the Optimal Method of Ischemia Evaluation in Women (WOMEN) trial. Circulation. 2011;124:1239-49.
53. Shaw LJ, Vasey C, Sawada S, et al. Impact of gender on risk stratification by exercise and dobutamine stress echocardiography: long-term mortality in 4,234 women and 6,898 men. Eur Heart J. 2005;26:447-56.
54. Metz LD, Beattie M, Hom R, et al. The prognostic value of normal exercise myocardial perfusion imaging and exercise echocardiography: a meta-analysis. J Am Coll Cardiol. 2007;49:227-37.
55. Shaw LJ, Iskandrian AE. Prognostic value of stress gated SPECT in patients with known or suspected coronary artery disease. J Nucl Cardiol. 2004;11:171-85.
56. Yoshinaga K, Chow BJ, Williams K, et al. What is the prognostic value of myocardial perfusion imaging using rubidium-82 positron emission tomography? J Am Coll Cardiol. 2006;48:1029-39.
57. Lertsburapa K, Ahlberg AW, Bateman TM, et al. Independent and incremental prognostic value of left ventricular ejection fraction determined by stress gated rubidium 82 PET imaging in patients with known or suspected coronary artery disease. J Nucl Cardiol. 2008;15:745-53.
58. Panting JR, Gatehouse PD, Yang GZ, et al. Abnormal subendocardial perfusion in cardiac syndrome × detected by cardiovascular magnetic resonance imaging. N Eng J Med. 2002;346:1948-53.

59. Pilz G, Klos M, Ali E, et al. Angiographic correlations of patients with small vessel disease diagnosed by adenosine-stress cardiac magnetic resonance imaging. J Cardiovasc Magn Reson. 2008;10:8.
60. Vermeltfoort IA, Bondarenko O, Raijmakers PG, et al. Is subendocardial ischaemia present in patients with chest pain and normal coronary angiograms? A cardiovascular MR study. Eur Heart J. 2007;28:1554-8.
61. Lakoski SG, Greenland P, Wong ND, et al. Coronary artery calcium scores and risk for cardiovascular events in women classified as "low risk" based on Framingham risk score: the Multi-Ethnic Study of Atherosclerosis (MESA). Arch Intern Med. 2007;167:2437-42.
62. Greenland P, Bonow RO, Brundage BH, et al. ACCF/AHA 2007 clinical expert consensus document on coronary artery calcium scoring by computed tomography in global cardiovascular risk assessment and in evaluation of patients with chest pain: a report of the American College of Cardiology Foundation Clinical Expert Consensus Task Force (ACCF/AHA Writing Committee to Update the 2000 Expert Consensus Document on Electron Beam Computed Tomography) developed in collaboration with the Society of Atherosclerosis Imaging and Prevention and the Society of Cardiovascular Computed Tomography. J Am Coll Cardiol. 2007;49:378-402.
63. Douglas PS, Hoffmann U, Patel MR, et al.; PROMISE Investigators. Outcomes of anatomical versus functional testing for coronary artery disease. N Engl J Med. 2015;372:1291-300.
64. Truong QA, Hayden D, Woodard PK, et al. Sex differences in the effectiveness of early coronary computed tomographic angiography compared with standard emergency department evaluation for acute chest pain: the rule-out myocardial infarction with Computer-Assisted Tomography (ROMICAT)-II Trial. Circulation. 2013;127:2494-502.
65. Lubbers M, Dedic A, Coenen A, et al. Calcium Imaging and selective computed tomography in comparison to functional testing for suspected coronary artery disease: the multicentre randomised CRESCENT trial. Eur Heart J. 2016;37:1232-43.
66. Pandie S, Mehta SR, Cantor WJ, et al. Radial versus femoral access for coronary angiography/intervention in women with acute coronary syndrome: insights from RIVAL trial (Radial vs Femoral access for coronary interventions). JACC Cardiovasc Interv. 2015;8:505-12.
67. Mohanan PP, Mathew R, Harikrishnan S, et al.; Kerala ACS Registry Investigators. Presentation, management, and outcomes of 25748 acute coronary syndrome admissions in Kerala, India: results from the Kerala ACS Registry. Eur Heart J. 2013;34(2):121-9.
68. Canto JG, Goldberg RJ, Hand MM, et al. Symptom presentation of women with acute coronary syndromes myth vs reality. Arch Intern Med. 2007;167:2405-13.
69. Khan NA, Daskalopoulou SS, Karp I, et al. Sex differences in acute coronary syndromes presentation in young patients. JAMA Intern Med. 2013;173:1863-71.
70. D'Onofrio G, Safdar B, Lichtman JH, et al. Sex differences in reperfusion in young patients with ST-segment-elevation myocardial infarction: results from the VIRGO study. Circulation. 2015;131:1324-32.
71. Lee HJ, Haimi I, Mehta S, et al. Gender Disparities in ST-Elevation Myocardial Infarction Care and Outcomes in Emerging Countries: A Systematic Meta-Analysis of 731,990 patients: GLOW. J Am Coll Cardiol. 2016;67(13):2356.
72. Vaccarino V, Rathore SS, Wenger NK, et al.; National Registry of Myocardial Infarction Investigators. Sex and racial differences in the management of acute myocardial infarction, 1994 through 2002. N Engl J Med. 2005;353:671-82.
73. Pancholy SB, Shantha GP, Patel T, et al. Sex differences in short term and long-term all-cause mortality among patients with ST-segment elevation myocardial infarction treated by primary percutaneous intervention: a meta-analysis. JAMA Intern Med. 2014;174:1822-30.
74. Brass LM, Lichtman JH, Wang Y, et al. Intracranial hemorrhage associated with thrombolytic therapy for elderly patients with acute myocardial infarction: results from the Cooperative Cardiovascular Project. Stroke. 2000;31:1802-11.
75. Edward FH, Carey JS, Grover FL, et al. Impact of gender on coronary bypass mortality. Ann Thorac Surg. 1998;66:125-31.
76. Pushas JD, Kilgo PD, Lutner M, et al. Off pump technique disproportionately benefit women and narrows the gender disparity in outcomes after coronary artery bypass surgery. Circulaltion. 2007;116:1192-9.
77. Xavier D, Pais P, Devereaux PJ, et al.; CREATE Registry Investigators. Treatment and outcomes of acute coronary syndromes in India (CREATE): a prospective analysis of registry data. Lancet. 2008;371:1435-42.
78. Pagidipati NJ, Huffman MD, Jeemon P, et al. Association between gender, process of care measures and outcomes in ACS in India: results from the Detection and Management of Coronary Heart Disease (DEMAT) Registry. PLoS One. 2013;8(4):e62061.
79. Safdar B, Spatz ES, Dreyer RP, et al. Presentation, clinical profile and prognosis of young patients with myocardial infarction with nonobstructive coronary arteries (MINOCA): results from VIRGO study. J Am Heart Assoc. 2018;7:e009174.
80. Claudio CP, Quesada O, Pepine CJ, et al. Why names matter for women MINOCA/INOCA (myocardial infarction/ischemia and no obstructive CAD). Clin Cardiol. 2018;41:185-93.
81. Templin C, Ghadri JR, Diekmann J, et al. Clinical features and outcomes of Takotsubo (Stress) cardiomyopathy. N Engl J Med. 2015;373:929-38.
82. Tweet MS, Hayes SN, Pitta SR, et al. Clinical features, management, and prognosis of spontaneous coronary artery dissection. Circulation. 2012;126: 579-88.
83. Hayes SN, Kim ESH, Saw J, et al. Spontaneous Coronary Artery Dissection: current state of the science: a scientific statement from American Heart Association. Circulation. 2018;137(19):e523-57.

CHAPTER 137

Hypertension in Pregnancy—A Stepwise Approach

Cherian Koshy, K Venugopal

INTRODUCTION

Hypertensive disorders of pregnancy, including preeclampsia, complicate up to 10% of pregnancies,[1] constituting a leading cause of maternal morbidity and mortality.[1] It is estimated that 50,000–60,000 deaths per year occur worldwide due to preeclampsia itself.[2]

CLASSIFICATION OF HYPERTENSIVE DISORDERS IN PREGNANCY

Chronic Hypertension

Chronic hypertension is defined as a systolic blood pressure (SBP) of 140 mm Hg or more or a diastolic blood pressure (DBP) of 90 mm Hg or more on two separate occasions at least 2 hours apart occurring before pregnancy or developing less than 20 weeks during pregnancy.[3]

Gestational Hypertension

Detection of hypertension after 20 weeks of gestation and BP falls back to normal within 12 weeks of delivery. Approximately, 15–25% of women with gestational hypertension will develop preeclampsia.

Preeclampsia

Hypertension after 20 weeks of pregnancy with proteinuria more than or equal to 300 mg in a 24-hour urine collection or a urinary protein/creatinine ratio more than or equal to 0.3.[3] Thrombocytopenia, renal insufficiency, impaired liver function, pulmonary edema, and cerebral or visual symptoms can occur with severe preeclampsia.[3]

Chronic Hypertension with Superimposed Preeclampsia (ACOG 2013)

Patients with pre-existing chronic hypertension can develop features of pre-eclampsia as per the recommendations of the American College of Obstetrics and Gynecology. Any one criteria is enough for the diagnosis of preeclampsia in patients with chronic hypertension.

Postpartum Hypertension

In addition preeclampsia can develop for the first time in the postpartum period and is called postpartum hypertension.

GRADING OF HYPERTENSION (NICE GUIDELINES)[4]

The grading of hypertension as per the National Institute for Health and Care Excellence (NICE) guidelines is described as:

- Mild hypertension: SBP 140–149 mm Hg or DBP 90–99 mm Hg
- Moderate hypertension: SBP 150–159 mm Hg or DBP 100–109 mm Hg
- Severe hypertension: SBP 160 mm Hg or DBP 110 mm Hg or higher.

MANAGEMENT

Gestational Hypertension

Control of hypertension in pregnancy has been a matter of debate regarding the nature of control, tight control versus less tight control.[5] The NICE guidelines on hypertension in pregnancy advocate starting antihypertensive treatment in patients with systolic pressures 150 mm Hg or more. A systolic pressure more than 160 is an emergency and requires quick control of BP to prevent hemorrhagic stroke.

Drugs used in the Treatment of Gestational Hypertension

Alpha-Methyldopa

Most widely used drug in the treatment of hypertension in pregnancy. It is a centrally acting drug affecting the sympathetic outflow from the brain stem. It is safe to use in pregnancy and has been the preferred agent in the national high blood pressure education program guidelines.

Labetalol

Labetalol is an alpha beta-blocker (combined). It is now being increasingly used in hypertensive situations in pregnancy, both for chronic hypertension as well as acute reduction of BP (parenteral).

Nifedipine

Among the calcium channel blockers, nifedipine has the maximum experience. It has also been used in emergency situations by rapidly acting oral preparations. Sublingual use has also been tried but caution has to be used to avoid precipitous fall in blood pressure in some patients.

In uncomplicated cases bed rest or inpatient management is not required. All patients need close monitoring of BP. Fetal growth and fetoplacental well-being assessment with ultrasonography (USG) and umbilical artery Doppler studies may be required.

Preeclampsia

Etiopathogenesis of preeclampsia is still not clearly understood. There is a genetic predisposition and usually seen more in primigravidas. There is abnormal immunological response of maternal tissue to trophoblasts, deficient trophoblast invasion, and hypoperfusion of placenta and increased circulating levels of interleukin and tumor necrosis factor (TNF) alpha. There is vascular endothelial activation leading to clinical symptoms of preeclampsia (Table 1).

INVESTIGATIONS

Urinary protein or urine protein/creatinine ratio, should be done in every antenatal visit in mild cases. Urinary protein or urine protein/creatinine ratio should be done daily in severe cases. Full blood counts, renal function tests, transaminases, bilirubin, lactate dehydrogenase (LDH), electrolytes, and peripheral smear are to be done in severe cases and repeated three times a week. Ultrasonography for fetal biophysical profile and Doppler velocimetry of the umbilical artery should also be done to optimize the timing of delivery.

TABLE 1: Risk factors for preeclampsia

Risk factor	Unadjusted relative risk (95% confidence interval)[4]
Age >40 years, primigravida	1.68 (1.23–2.29)
Age >40 years, multipara	1.96 (1.34–2.87)
Family history	2.90 (1.70–4.93)
Nulliparity	2.91 (1.28–6.61)
Multiple pregnancy	2.93 (2.04–4.21)
Preexisting diabetes	3.56 (2.54–4.99)
Prepregnancy body mass index	4.29 (3.52–5.49)
Previous preeclampsia	7.19 (5.85–8.83)
Antiphospholipid syndrome	9.72 (4.34–21.75)

TABLE 2: The NICE identifies high- and moderate-risk factors for developing preeclampsia

High-risk factors	Moderate-risk factors
• Hypertension in previous pregnancy • Chronic kidney disease • Autoimmune disease, e.g., SLE, antiphospholipid • Type 1 or type 2 diabetes • Chronic hypertension	• First pregnancy • Age 40 or older • Pregnancy interval >10 years • BMI >35 at first visit • Family history of pre-eclampsia

Advise women with one high-risk factor or 2 or more moderate-risk factors to take 75 mg aspirin daily from 12 weeks until the baby is born *(this is an unlicensed indication and should be discussed and documented appropriately)*

BMI, body mass index; NICE, National Institute for Health and Care Excellence; SLE, systemic lupus erythematous.

Prevention of Preeclampsia

High-risk women stand to gain maximum with low dose aspirin 75 mg to prevent development of preeclampsia [number needed to treat (NNT) of 19 to prevent one episode of preeclampsia]. One recent trial showed that a higher dose of aspirin 150 mg versus placebo from 11 to 34 weeks of gestation showed an absolute reduction of preeclampsia of 2.7% (1.6% vs. 4.3% p = 0.004).[6]

Table 2 guides the initial care provider in managing uncomplicated gestational hypertension and referring those with preeclampsia or severe hypertension to fully equipped centers.

Management of Severe Preeclampsia

Standardized, evidence-based clinical guidelines for the management of preeclampsia and eclampsia have been demonstrated to reduce incidence of adverse maternal outcomes. Treatment with first-line agents should be instituted as soon as possible, within 30–60 minutes of confirmed severe hypertension (BP greater than 160/110 mm Hg and persistent for 15 minutes) to reduce the risk of maternal stroke. Appropriate measurement of BP is of paramount importance (mercury sphygmomanometer or appropriately validated equivalent automated equipment, use of correct cuff size, positioning in sitting or semi reclining position with back support).

Intravenous (IV) labetalol and hydralazine have long been considered first-line medications. Immediate release oral nifedipine is also considered as first-line therapy, particularly when IV access is not available. Immediate release of oral nifedipine capsules should be administered orally and not punctured or otherwise administered sublingually (because of risk of hypotension).

Boxes 1–3 outline standardized order sets for the use of oral nifedipine, IV hydralazine, and IV labetalol in initial management of acute severe hypertension. Administration of above drugs does not require cardiac monitoring or other monitoring more than what is mentioned in boxes 1–3. In addition, personnel in all hospital settings, should be able to provide these initial medications without transferring to another unit (JNC 7 recommendations).

BOX 1 Suggested algorithm for management of severe intrapartum hypertension using immediate release Nifedipine

- Monitor BP and treat if systolic blood pressure (SBP) ≥160 or diastolic (DBP) ≥110 mm Hg
- Monitor fetal well being
- If SBP or DBP remain persistently elevated for ≥ 15 min, administer 10 mg nifedipine orally
- Short acting nifedipine should not be used
- Monitor BP every 15–20 min, if still above range then administer additional dose
- Maximal total dose of nifedipine is 30 mg
- Use nifedipine with caution in patients on magnesium sulfate as it can marked fall in BP. Please note that the use of Nifedipine in treatment of hypertension in pregnancy is still controversial and is not generally preferred
- If BP still above range, administer labetalol (40 mg IV over 2 min)
- Assess fetal well being and consult obstetrician
- Additional antihypertensive drugs may be administered as per need
- Once BP returns to acceptable range, monitor BP periodically (repeat BP measurement every 10 min for 1 h, then every 15 min for 1 h, then every 30 min for 1 h, and then every hour for 4 h)

BOX 2 Suggested algorithm for management of severe intrapartum hypertension using hydralazine

- Monitor BP and treat if systolic blood pressure (SBP) ≥160 or diastolic (DBP) ≥110 mm Hg
- Monitor fetal well being
- If SBP or DBP remain persistently elevated for ≥15 min, administer Hydralazine (5 mg IV)
- Monitor BP every 15–20 min, if still above range then administer additional dose (10 mg IV)
- Maximal total dose of hydralazine is 25 mg
- If BP still above range, administer labetalol (40 mg IV over 2 min)
- Assess fetal wellbeing and consult obstetrician
- Additional antihypertensive drugs may be administered as per need
- Once BP returns to acceptable range, monitor BP periodically (repeat BP measurement every 10 min for 1 h, then every 15 min for 1 h, then every 30 min for 1 h, and then every hour for 4 h)

Second-line Alternatives

In rare circumstances, when above-mentioned drugs fail, second-line drugs are recommended. They include nicardipine or esmolol infusion. Sodium nitroprusside is reserved for extreme emergencies. It should be used only for the shortest time in view of concerns regarding cyanide or thiocyanate toxicity and increase in intracranial pressure with worsening cerebral edema in the mother.

Magnesium sulfate is not recommended as an antihypertensive agent, but still remains the drug of choice for seizure prophylaxis in preeclampsia with severe features and for controlling seizures in eclampsia.

BOX 3 Suggested algorithm for management of severe intrapartum hypertension using Labetalol

- Monitor BP and treat if systolic blood pressure (SBP) ≥160 or diastolic (DBP) ≥110 mm Hg
- Monitor fetal well being
- If SBP or DBP remain persistently elevated for ≥15 min, administer labetalol 20 mg IV
- Monitor BP every 15–20 min, if still above range then administer additional dose (20–40 mg IV)
- If BP still above range, administer labetalol (40–80 mg IV over 2 min)
- Maximal total dose of labetalol is 220 mg
- Assess fetal well being and consult obstetrician
- Additional antihypertensive drugs may be administered as per need
- Once BP returns to acceptable range, monitor BP periodically (repeat BP measurement every 10 min for 1 h, then every 15 min for 1 h, then every 30 min for 1 h, and then every hour for 4 h)

CHRONIC HYPERTENSION

Hypertension which predates pregnancy is associated with adverse pregnancy outcomes. These patients require preconception counseling regarding antihypertensive use, reducing obesity, and stopping smoking and getting pregnant at an earlier age. Angiotensin-converting enzyme inhibitors (ACEIs), angiotensin receptor blocker (ARB), and chlorothiazide increase the risk of congenital anomalies and should stopped before conception. It is also advisable to stop direct renin inhibitors and spironolactone. There is no known risk for other antihypertensive. Antihypertensive treatment, if BP is more than 150/100 mm Hg, will reduce the risk of severe hypertension, but there is no effect on perinatal outcomes. Low-dose aspirin is also advisable to reduce the chance of development of superadded preeclampsia. Increased surveillance during pregnancy like more frequent antenatal visits, ultrasound monitoring of fetal growth, and consideration of home BP monitoring is required.

TIMING OF TERMINATION OF PREGNANCY

Termination of pregnancy is the definitive treatment for preeclampsia. Factors which decide timing of termination of pregnancy include the severity of preeclampsia, and the period of gestation and fetal maturity. In severe cases where the patient has reached 34 weeks pregnancy should be terminated either by vaginal delivery or by cesarean section. In mild cases of preeclampsia pregnancy can be continued till term with frequent assessment of maternal and fetal conditions and judicious decisions can be taken. The HYPITAT (Hypertension and Preeclampsia Intervention) trial advocated delivery by 37 weeks of gestation to reduce adverse maternal outcomes.[7] HELLP syndrome is a severe manifestation of preeclampsia characterized by hemolysis, elevation of hepatic enzymes, and platelet abnormalities associated with grave maternal outcomes and requires urgent termination of pregnancy. In cases of severe preeclampsia, pregnancy should be terminated before 34 weeks in the setting of HELLP syndrome, renal failure, pulmonary edema, placental abruption, intracerebral bleed, and abnormal fetal biophysical profile.[8]

POSTPARTUM HYPERTENSION

Postpartum hypertension and preeclampsia is the cause for 0.3% of all visits to emergency department in the postpartum period. In women with preeclampsia or superimposed preeclampsia, BP starts decreasing within 48 hours of delivery, but increases again within 3–6 days. So, all women should be educated regarding symptoms of severe hypertension and report if needed as preeclampsia and eclampsia can develop up to 4 weeks postpartum. BP should be measured at 72 hours and 7–10 days postdelivery in all with gestational hypertension, preeclampsia, or superimposed preeclampsia. Antihypertensive therapy to be instituted, if BP is more than 150/100 mm Hg on two occasions at least 4–6 hours apart. Magnesium sulfate has to be given for features of impending eclampsia.

INDIAN DATA

The National Eclampsia Registry 2011[9] indicates a prevalence of 9% of hypertensive disorders and preeclampsia of 5%.

KEY MESSAGES

- Hypertension during pregnancy is the second most common cause of maternal morbidity and mortality
- Careful measurement of BP as per guidelines should be done during each antenatal visit
- Once pregnancy is suspected ACEI, ARBs, mineralocorticoid antagonists should be stopped and replaced by appropriate antihypertensive treatment
- Patients with BP 150/100 mm Hg or more should be admitted for proper monitoring and appropriate management. Severe BP elevation 160/110 mm Hg needs urgent control of BP
- Labetalol, alpha-methyldopa, and nifedipine are three key drugs in the management of hypertension during pregnancy. In severe cases parenteral labetalol, hydralazine, and rapid acting oral nifedipine should be used. Sublingual nifedipine is contraindicated because of severe hypotension which may ensue
- Timing of termination of pregnancy in preeclampsia depends on severity of preeclampsia and the fetal biophysical profile and should be decided judiciously
- Postpartum hypertension with preeclampsia can occur in the immediate postnatal period and can result in complications. This entity should be considered in postpartum periods and appropriate treatment should be instituted.

REFERENCES

1. Amro FH, Moussa HN, Ashimi OA, et al. Treatment options for hypertension in pregnancy and puerperium. Expert Opin Drug Saf. 2016;15:1635-42.
2. Hypertensive Disorders in pregnancy. (2014) ICOG guidelines [online]. Available from https://fogsi.org/wp-content/uploads2015/11/hdp.pdf [Accessed August 2018].
3. Roberts JM, August PA, Bakris G, et al. Hypertension in pregnancy. Report of the American College of Obstetricians and Gynecologists' Task Force on Hypertension in Pregnancy. Obstet Gynecol. 2013;122:1122-31.
4. NICE Guidelines (2010). Hypertension in Pregnancy: Diagnosis and management. Clinical guideline (CG107) [online]. Available from http://www.nice.org.uk/guidance/cg107 [Accessed August 2018].
5. Ryan RM, McCarthy FP. Hypertension in pregnancy, Obstetrics gynecology and Reproductive Medicine. 2018.
6. Rolnik DL, Wright D, Poon LC, et al. Aspirin vs placebo in pregnancy at high risk for preterm preeclampsia. New England J Med. 2017;377:613-22.
7. Magee LA, von Dadelszen P, Rey E, et al. Less tight versus tight control of hypertension in pregnancy. New England J Med. 2015;372:407-17.
8. Koopmans CM, Bijlenga D, Groen H, et al. Induction of labour versus expectant monitoring for gestational hypertension or mild pre-eclampsia after 36 weeks' gestation (HYPITAT): a multicentre, open-label randomised controlled trial. Lancet. 2009;374(9694):979-88.
9. Gole S. (2015). Report of the National Eclampsia Registry [online]. Available from http://www.fogsi.org/the-national-eclampsia-registry/ [Accessed August 2018].

CHAPTER 138

Peripartum Cardiomyopathy

Abhishek Roy, Debabrata Roy

INTRODUCTION

Occasionally, peripartum cardiomyopathy (PPCM) can be a serious pregnancy complication, often occurring in pregnant women who were earlier quite healthy. Women with this disorder usually have an infant to take care of, along with a frequently disabling heart condition, and a higher mortality risk.

The definition of PPCM is based on the following criteria:

- Symptomatic heart failure (HF) in the last month of pregnancy or within 5 months ofdelivery
- Absence of an identifiable cause of HF
- Absence of pre-existing heart disease prior to the last month of pregnancy, and
- Left ventricular (LV) systolic dysfunction [left ventricular ejection fraction (LVEF) <45% and/or fractional shortening <30% on echocardiogram.][1]

The diagnosis of PPCM is thus made when no other etiology of HF can be readily identified.

Peripartum cardiomyopathy is not a very common condition. Estimations of the population incidence of PPCM are scarce due to several reasons. These include an inability to correctly diagnose the condition, as well as the absence of a reliable reporting system. In the United States, the incidence is estimated to be 1 in 1,000 to 1 in 4,000 pregnancies.[2,3] On the other hand, Nigeria and Haiti appear to be global hotspots, where high incidence rates of almost 1 in every 100 to 1 in every 300 are reported.[4,5] Why the incidence rates of PPCM have such extreme global variations is yet to be fully understood. However, it is encountered more often and portends a graver prognosis in women with an African ancestry.[2,6-8]

The exact incidence of PPCM in the Indian subcontinent has not yet been properly elucidated. Reported incidence from a tertiary care hospital from southern India was 1 in 1374 live births.[9] Apart from ethnic and racial differences, multiparous women, women with multifetal pregnancies, advanced maternal age, pregnancy-induced hypertension, and preeclampsia are classically associated with a higher risk of PPCM.[1,10-15]

PHYSIOLOGY OF NORMAL PREGNANCY

Starting with the first trimester of pregnancy, maternal systemic vascular resistance decreases along with a proportional increase in the cardiac output.[16] The renin–angiotensin–aldosterone system is activated, thereby retaining salt and water and thus helping to maintain the blood pressure. Estrogen, progesterone, and relaxin, the pregnancy hormones, promote vascular relaxation at the same time.[17,18] There is also a significant increase in LV mass via physiological cardiac remodeling. Since coagulation factors increase throughout gestation,[19] the risk for thrombosis during pregnancy is 4–10 times higher and reaches the maximum at term. The amount of oxidative stress is raised in pregnancy, and this is accompanied by an increase in antioxidant capability, though slightly delayed.[20] Hence, profound system-wide hemodynamic, metabolic, and hormonal adaptations are noted during pregnancy.

The dilemma in the diagnosis of PPCM lies in the fact that several of the presenting symptoms such as ankle, foot and abdominal swelling, easy fatigability, weakness, and a reduced exercise capacity maybe interpreted erroneously as the consequences of pregnancy rather than a failing heart.[21]

ETIOPATHOGENESIS OF PERIPARTUM CARDIOMYOPATHY

Through the decades, there has been wide speculation regarding the cause of PPCM. Several theories have been considered in the past, including myocarditis, fetal antigen autoimmunity, fetal microchimerism, selenium deficiency or excess salt consumption. Research carried out in recent times, however, suggests that PPCM is likely a vascular disease, triggered by placental and pituitary secretion of strong antiangiogenic agents late in gestation.

Prolactin

That apoptosis has an important role in PPCM has been suggested by several clinical observations and analyses of plasma in affected women,[22,23] but the cause of this apoptosis was not quite clear.

Denise Hilfiker-Kleiner and Helmut Drexler first provided experimental support for the hypothesis that PPCM was a vascular disease that was initiated by late gestational hormonal changes.[24] On deletion of transcription factor STAT3 (signal transducer and activator of transcription 3) in cardiomyocytes of pregnant mice, they developed PPCM. Protection of the heart against reactive oxygen species (ROS) is conferred by STAT3, and is essentially regulated by the expression of the gene for superoxide dismutase 2 (SOD2). SOD2 counteracts superoxides generated by the activity of mitochondria in cardiac myocytes. Hence, an increase in ROS was observed after the deletion of STAT3, which in turn led to the inappropriate secretion of peptidases, particularly cathepsin D, from the cardiomyocytes (Fig. 1). Prolactin is then cleaved into a 16-kD fragment by extracellular cathepsin D. This 16-kD prolactin fragment has potent vasculotoxic properties and causes endothelial cell apoptosis. Using bromocriptine to treat STAT3 cardiac knockout (KO) mice blocked the production of prolactin and dramatically reversed the clinical features of PPCM.

More recently, deeper assessment of the mechanism of vascular damage by 16-kD prolactin showed that there is increased endothelial expression of microRNA-146a on exposure to it.[25,26] Ultimately target genes, especially the neuregulin/ErbB pathway, are suppressed in the cardiomyocytes via microRNA action. This is known to be vital in the prevention of cardiomyocyte apoptosis. There is a profound increase in the levels of microRNA-146a in PPCM, and treatment with bromocriptine significantly reduces these levels. Micro-RNA146a could thus potentially be used as a PPCM biomarker or alternatively, be targeted therapeutically.

Soluble Fms-like Tyrosine Kinase-1 and Preeclampsia

A potent transcriptional regulator, PGC-1α (peroxisome proliferatoractivated receptor gamma coactivator 1α) is known to have important effects on various angiogenic and metabolic pathways. Similar to the STAT3 cardiac KO mice, those mice with absent PGC-1α in cardiac myocytes developed PPCM.[27] Like STAT3, SOD2 expression is controlled by PGC-1α, thus giving rise to increased ROS levels in PGC-1α cardiac KO mice. However, only bromocriptine use was unable to revert the PPCM in these mice. The reason for this is because transcriptional induction of vascular endothelial growth factor (VEGF) is influenced by PGC-1α, thereby directly regulating the health of the vasculature.[28] Thus, vasculotoxicity is caused by two different pathways in a PGC-1α deficient heart: stimulation of a vasculotoxic 16-kD mediated pathway, and inhibition of a VEGF-mediated provascular pathway (Fig. 1). Consequently, these mice with PPCM could be successfully rescued only with dual therapy combining bromocriptine as well as VEGF.

The hormonal milieu of pregnancy is predominantly regulated by the pituitary and the placenta. Toward the end

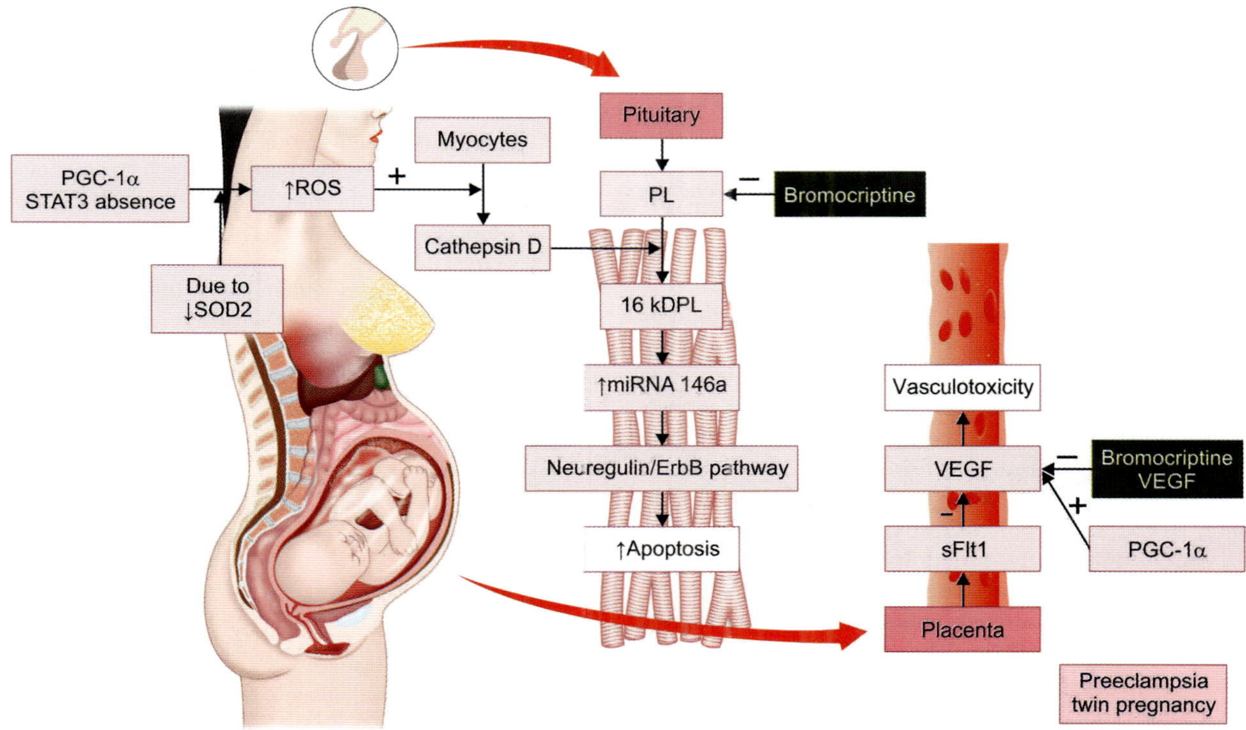

PL, prolactin; PPCM, peripartum cardiomyopathy; ROS, reactive oxygen species; sFlt-1, soluble Fms-like tyrosine kinase 1; SOD2, superoxide dismutase 2; VEGF, vascular endothelial growth factor; PGC-1α, peroxisome proliferator-activated receptor gamma coactivator 1-alpha; STAT3, signal transducer and activator of transcription 3.

FIG. 1: Mechanisms in peripartum cardiomyopathy.

of gestation, several compounds are secreted into the circulation by the placenta. This particularly includes a soluble VEGF receptor 1 or soluble fms-like tyrosine kinase 1 (sFlt-1). Members of the VEGF family present in the circulation are bound to and neutralized by this sFlt-1, leading to the neutralization of most of the circulating VEGF by the end of gestation.[29] Placental secretion of additional sFlt-1 during the later part of gestation establishes further hormonal damage to the cardiac vasculature. In defense, there is strong secretion of VEGF locally in the heart. This local secretion of VEGF is reduced in the absence of PGC-1α, and this coupled with a high gestational sFlt-1, gives rise to vasculotoxicity. Accordingly, when nulliparous mice were administered sFlt-1, PGC-1α cardiac KO mice started exhibiting signs of cardiomyopathy.

In preeclampsia, a disease of pregnancy characterized by hypertension and proteinuria, secretion of sFlt-1 by the placenta is profoundly increased.[29] This is in accordance with the fact that preeclampsia is one of the strongest risk factors associated with PPCM.[30] About 25% of PPCM patients are concomitantly diagnosed with preeclampsia. Twin pregnancies have higher sFlt-1 levels, probably due to increased mass of the placenta,[31] and similarly are associated with 10–16% of PPCM occurrences.[32-34] Collectively, these observations argue strongly in favor of the fact that placental sFlt-1, secreted toward the end of gestation, poses a formidable noxious challenge to the heart. When adequate defensive mechanisms are unavailable, PPCM is quick to develop.

A "Two-Hit" Hypothesis

When the available recent evidence is collectively considered, it appears that PPCM develops in the presence of two simultaneous "hits": the first hit being the vasculotoxic hormonal milieu, involving prolactin and sFlt-1, late in gestation, and the second one is the incapability of certain women to counter this vasculotoxicity. Unfortunately, at this point, there is only speculation about the true nature of this susceptibility toward PPCM (the second "hit").

One of the possibilities is that cardiac defenses might be weakened by an acute insult such as viral myocarditis. Even though such a rationalization would be consistent with earlier hypotheses about PPCM, evidence for it is scarce. Genetic predisposition could be another possible second hit. This notion is favored by a few studies. In a genome-wide association study (GWAS), an association was found between PPCM and a polymorphism close to the *PTHLH* gene, which apparently functions as an angiogenesis inhibitor.[35,36] It is also interesting to note that mutations, especially titin, which are associated with familial dilated cardiomyopathy (DCM), have been identified in certain families with both PPCM and DCM.[37,38] However, predisposition to PPCM in familial DCM is still unable to explain most cases of PPCM. This likely represents the heterogeneity of the disease.

CLINICAL FEATURES

Clinical features of PPCM are no different than in nonpregnant patients with systolic dysfunction. New or rapid onset of dyspnea, cough, paroxysmal nocturnal dyspnea, orthopnea, fatigue, palpitations, chest pain, and unexplained weight gain should always be promptly evaluated. Tachycardia, tachypnea, a subnormal SPO_2 and evidence of cardiomegaly are often found on physical examination. The jugular venous pressure is usually raised, blood pressure may however be normal, S3 is often auscultable and the P2 component of the second heart sound might be loud. Mitral regurgitation, tricuspid regurgitation, and bibasal fine crepitations are often found. Dependent edema may worsen and ascites along with congestive hepatomegaly are quite common. Arrhythmias are not infrequent and may give rise to cardioembolic phenomenon. Occasionally mild-to-moderate pericardial effusions are noted. Preeclampsia is suspected on detection of raised blood pressures and evidence of proteinuria. The hemodynamic alterations and overall clinical picture of PPCM cannot be reliably distinguished from other forms of DCM.[39] There are also few reported instances of PPCM with high output cardiac failure.[40]

DIAGNOSIS

As there are no clearly defined specific symptoms of PPCM, especially during the last trimester of pregnancy, the diagnosis of PPCM is delayed many times. One should keep in mind the possibility of PPCM in all pregnant women presenting with symptoms of cardiac failure or in postpartum women who have a slower recovery to the pregestational state. In such cases, an in-depth family history should be taken to find out any familial trends of cardiomyopathy Diagnostic testing that may be performed in suspected cases of PPCM are enumerated in box 1.[41]

- *X-ray chest*: An increased cardiothoracic ratio or evidence of pulmonary edema may be seen. Pleural effusion may also be occasionally noted. However, the routine use of X-ray chest during pregnancy should be discouraged as it is nonessential for the diagnosis of PPCM. It should only

BOX 1 Diagnostic testing for peripartum cardiomyopathy

- Blood test
  - Complete blood cell count
  - Urea, creatinine, electrolytes
  - Cardiac enzymes, including troponin
  - BNP or N-terminal pro-BNP
  - Liver function test
  - Thyroid-stimulating hormone
- Chest radiograph
- Electrocardiogram
- Transthoracic echocardiogram
- Cardiac magnetic resonance imaging (if needed)

BNP, brain-type natriuretic peptide.

be performed if absolutely necessary using abdominal shielding

- *Electrocardiography (ECG):* A normal ECG does not rule out PPCM. Sinus tachycardia is the most common abnormality, though atrial fibrillation, abnormalities of conduction and other types of arrhythmias along with nonspecific ST-T changes are occasionally encountered.
- *Echocardiography*: Echocardiography is one of the most important modalities for the initial evaluation and subsequent monitoring of women with PPCM. Evidence of LV systolic dysfunction (LV ejection fraction <45% and/or fractional shortening <30%) is quintessential for the diagnosis of PPCM. Frequently, the left ventricle is also dilated, especially in patients who present late. Compensatory hypertrophy of the left ventricle may be present to a mild extent, however, pronounced LV wall hypertrophy might be suggestive of a primary hypertrophic cardiomyopathy. Small pericardial effusions are not infrequent in the immediate postpartum period. Morphologically, valves are generally normal. However, when extensive LV dilatation sets in, mitral regurgitation as a consequence of annular dilatation may be seen. On occasion, tricuspid regurgitation and pulmonary regurgitation may also be seen. Overall PPCM is indistinguishable from primary idiopathic DCM on the basis of echocardiography alone[42]
- *Endomyocardial biopsy*: Features of myocarditis may be seen on endomyocardial biopsy since quite a few cases of PPCM appear to be related to myocarditis. The best time to perform endomyocardial biopsies in these patients is early after symptom onset. However, sufficient data about this diagnostic modality in the context of PPCM is lacking
- *Viral and bacterial assays*: Antibody titers for Coxsackie B virus may be estimated in carefully selected cases. However, the implications of such titers are currently more research related rather than diagnostic
- *Magnetic resonance imaging (MRI)*: MRI is the gold standard in the evaluation of cardiac volumes and ventricular systolic functions, and may complementarily be used in the workup of a patient with PPCM. Patterns of late gadolinium enhancement can often aid in making a definitive diagnosis. A cardiac MRI can also guide biopsy from an affected area, thereby increasing the yield and diagnostic accuracy
- *Right heart catheterization*: Right heart catheterization can assess filling pressures and reliably estimate the cardiac output in patients with refractory HF, unstable hemodynamics or target organ damage. Dilatation of all cardiac chambers, especially the left ventricle can also be readily established
- *Biochemical evaluation*: Creatine kinase or cardiac troponins are usually not raised. Evaluation of renal and liver function may provide valuable information about organ perfusion in patients with cardiac failure and compromised hemodynamics.

DIFFERENTIAL DIAGNOSIS

Diagnosis of PPCM should be made when all other probable causes of HF have been ruled out. Box 2 enumerates the differential diagnosis of PPCM.

The various causes of cardiomyopathy should be evaluated before making a diagnosis of PPCM. The closest in clinical manifestation is DCM, the possibility of which should be carefully looked into. PPCM is more common in the young and has a better prognosis, mostly occurring after delivery (78–93%) unlike DCM, which occurs by second trimester. Unlike DCM, PPCM can cause faster deterioration of clinical symptoms leading to poorer consequences. Clinical history, physical examination, and investigations should be done in order to exclude other probable causes of cardiac failure like coronary artery disease, diseases of the cardiac valves, pulmonary thromboembolism, pneumonia, and severe eclampsia.

Transthoracic echocardiography can rule out the most probable differential diagnosis which happens to be previously undetected valvular heart disease. The presence of normal systolic function can rule out PPCM and should point toward further probing into causes of high output HF like thyrotoxicosis and anemia. Even though this population is at low risk for ischemic heart diseases, women with known and important risk factors like type I diabetes mellitus should be evaluated by noninvasive methods for coronary ischemia, and if required angiography should be done. In women with persistent cardiac failure, unstable hemodynamics or in cases of organ dysfunction, catheterization of the right heart can be done to determine the filling pressures and cardiac output.

Fett et al. have devised an easy to use, efficacious, self-administered test to differentiate early clinical features of cardiac failure from healthy term pregnancy (Table 1).

MANAGEMENT

Insufficient evidence-based data on management of cardiac failure in pregnancy poses challenges in the treatment of PPCM.

Presently, it is treated as per the protocol of management of cardiac failure keeping in mind the pregnant condition

BOX 2 Differential diagnoses of peripartum cardiomyopathy

- Pre-existing dilated cardiomyopathy
- Pre-existing other forms of cardiomyopathy
- Pre-existing valvular heart disease, particularly valvular stenosis
- Pre-existing congenital heart disease
- Hypertensive heart disease including preeclampsia and eclampsia
- Acute myocarditis
- Acute pulmonary embolism
- Acute coronary spasm, coronary dissection, coronary thrombosis, and acute myocardial infarction
- Thyrotoxicosis
- Maternal sepsis

TABLE 1: Probability scores for peripartum cardiomyopathy proposed by Fett et al.[43]

Symptom/Sign	0 point	1 point	1 point
Dyspnea	None	When climb >8 steps	Walking
Orthopnea	None	Elevate head only	Elevate boy >45°
Unexplained cough	None	Night-time	Day and night
Pitting edema	None	Below Knee	Above knee
Weight gain 9th month	<1 kg/week	1–2 kg/week	>2 kg/week
Palpitations	None	Night-time	Day and night

0–2 : low risk, continue observation
3–4 : mild risk, consider blood BNP
5 or > : high risk, blood BNP and echo
BNP, brain-type natriuretic peptide.

of the women. Therapy in late pregnancy should take into consideration both the mother's as well as the fetus' health (Table 2).[41] Drugs like beta-blockers, thiazide diuretics or furosemide may be mandatory in few patients of PPCM before delivery of the fetus. In this regard, it is imperative to use lowest recommended dose of diuretics as they can cause impairment in perfusion of the placenta posing a threat to the fetus.

In patients of PPCM postdelivery, the therapeutic management is like that of HF which includes use of beta-blockers, mineralocorticoid receptor antagonists (MRAs), diuretics and angiotensin converting enzyme inhibitors (ACEIs)/angiotensin receptor blockers (ARBs). Due to lack of data on inotrope usage in PPCM patients and the fact that myocardial damage may be aggravated by the use of catecholamines, use of inotropes should be done only in cases of severe hypotension with or without evidence of cardiogenic shock. Once the patient becomes hemodynamically stable,

TABLE 2: Peripartum cardiomyopathy medications

Classification	Medication	Dose	Remark
ACEIs	Captopril	Starting dose 6.25 mg TDS	Contraindicated in pregnancy
		Increase upto 25–50 mg TDS	
	Enalapril	Starting dose 1.25 mg BD	Contraindicated in pregnancy
		Increase upto 10 mg BD	
	Ramipril	Starting dose 1.25 mg BD	Lack of data in pregnancy
		Increase upto 5 mg BD	
ARBs	Candesartan	Starting dose 2 mg OD	Contraindicated in pregnancy and lactation
		Increase upto 32 mg OD	
	Valsartan	Starting dose 40 mg BD	Contraindicated in pregnancy and lactation
		Increase upto 160 mg BD	
MRAs	Spironolactone	Starting dose 12.5 mg OD	Contraindicated in pregnancy and lactation
		Increase upto 50 mg OD	
β-Blockers	Extended-release Metoprolol	Starting dose 12.5 mg OD Increase upto 50 mg OD	Rare risk of bradycardia or respiratory distress in newborn
	Carvedilol	Starting dose 3.125 mg BD	Same as metoprolol
		Increase upto 25 mg BD	–
Vasodilators	Hydralazine	Starting dose 10 mg TDS	–
		Increase upto 40 mg TDS	–
	Nitroglycerin	Starting dose 10–20 μg/min IV	Risk of hypotension
		Increase according to BP	
Diuretic	Hydrochlorothiazide	12.5–50 mg OD	Risk of insufficient uteroplacental circulation
	Furosemide	20–80 mg OD-BD (oral/IV)	Risk of insufficient uteroplacental circulation
Inotropes	Digoxin	0.125–0.25 mg OD	Risk of toxicity to drug
	Dobutamine	2.5–10 μg/kg/min	–
	Milrinone	0.125–0.5 μg/kg/min	–
Prolactin inhibition	Bromocriptine	2.5 mg OD for 1 week (short-term)	Thrombotic risk
		5 mg for 2 weeks, followed by 2.5 mg for 6 weeks (long-term)	

ACEIs, angiotensin-converting enzyme inhibitors; ARBs, angiotensin receptor blockers; BD, twice daily; BP, blood pressure; IV, intravenous; MRAs, mineralocorticoid receptor antagonists; OD, once daily; TDS, thrice daily.

tapering of the inotropes should be done and the treatment protocol for pregnant patients with HF should be adopted. In patients who have severely compromised ejection fraction, initiation of beta-blockers at very low doses appears to have a protective effect. Ivabradine may alternatively be used in patients of persistent sinus tachycardia where increase in beta-blocker dose is not recommended for fear of cardiac failure or hypotension.

In South Africa, a pilot study showed beneficial effect of bromocriptine in addition to drugs used for cardiac failure, in patients of PPCM where the onset was acute in nature.[44,45] Similarly, a German registry of PPCM patients also showed that the above therapy gave better results in most of the patients (96%).[46] Another randomized multicenter trial in Germany explored the efficacy of bromocriptine. Treatment with bromocriptine had higher rates of full recovery of the left ventricle, along with reduced mortality and morbidity, in patients with PPCM, when compared with other cohorts of PPCM who were not administered bromocriptine.[47] However, considering use of bromocriptine suppresses lactation, how this data relates to other parts of the world where the survival of infants is affected by lack of availability of breast milk is yet to be fully ascertained.

The risk of sudden death is more in patients with PPCM and the outcome can be improved by the use of implantable cardioverter defibrillators (ICDs) and cardiac resynchronization therapy (CRT).[48-50] For the purpose of primary prevention, a wearable cardioverter-defibrillator can be considered as many of the PPCM patients show significant improvement of systolic function of the left ventricle and some may even show complete recovery. Wearable cardioverter-defibrillators can be recommended for 3–6 months as interim management. The LV function should be assessed by echocardiography at regular intervals during this period. Another observational study conducted on a small group of PPCM patients who had severely compromised cardiac function with/without ventricular arrhythmias also showed the usage of wearable cardioverter-defibrillators to be valuable in such patients.[51] The use of LV assist device may be done in patients who are critically ill; who do not show any signs of recovery over a period of many weeks. Cardiac transplantation should be considered as the last option as there is quite an improvement in the condition of most PPCM patients in the first 6–12 months.

PROGNOSIS AND FOLLOW-UP

The disease prognosis may range from full recovery to even death of the patient. In most of the cases, the LV function recovers either fully or partially. It has been seen that about 23–72% of patients have had full recovery of systolic function of left ventricle (i.e., LVEF > 50%).[23,52,53] The recovery can be seen within 2–6 months after diagnosis of the disease, but in some cases, it may take upto 5 years.[4] Those patients of PPCM who had LVEF less than 35% or had severe remodeling of the left ventricle [left ventricular end-diastolic diameter (LVEDD) ≥60 mm] are the ones who are at risk of slow recovery or nonrecovery.[54]

The treatment for cardiac failure which includes beta-blockers, ARBs, and ACEIs should be done in patients with systolic dysfunction of the left ventricle for at least 12 months. This is because some patients may have late recovery.[55,56] Also, in patients with normal function of left ventricle the therapy should be continued for at least 6 months. This is because normal ejection fraction or return of left ventricle size to normal does not mean stability in the long run.[56]

Even after maximally tolerated therapy, 20–25% patients develop end-stage cardiac failure in later years. The requirement of heart transplantation or LV assist device is seen in 4–11% of patients with PPCM.[55] Most of the deaths occur within 3–6 months of diagnosis of the disease.[57] Recently, due to early diagnosis and better management of cardiac failure, there has been a decrease in mortality rates. Nonetheless, mortality due to PPCM is still quite high in young women who were previously healthy. Thromboembolism, progression to refractory cardiac failure and ventricular arrhythmias are some of the important causes of death. The factors which can predict the long-term prognosis are yet not clear. However, it has been seen that women with poor functional reserve, LVEDD more than or equal to 60 mm, LVEF less than or equal to 25–35% and women of non-European descent have poorer prognosis.[52,53,55]

COUNSELING FOR FUTURE PREGNANCIES

Once a patient has suffered from PPCM, there is 30–50% chance of it occurring in subsequent pregnancies.[58,59] In those women who have persistent LV dysfunction, risk of PPCM occurring recurrently is higher. Also, women with severe LV dysfunction have higher mortality and morbidity rates.[58,60] Even a normal LVEF does not mean that the subsequent pregnancy will have a normal outcome. Hence, all women who have had PPCM should be cautioned regarding risk of PPCM in future pregnancies which can even lead to death. All relevant information regarding choice of contraceptive methods should be given to the patient.

In case a woman is already pregnant, her and her family's decision regarding continuation of the pregnancy should be of primary importance. This is because many pregnant women may remain healthy even if they have had a history of PPCM during previous pregnancies. This is particularly true in cases where the LV systolic function was not compromised. Hence, termination of pregnancy in all cases of recurrent PPCM is not warranted.[61] A tailor-made plan can be adopted if the woman wishes to continue her pregnancy.

During the last trimester echocardiography should be done every 1–2 weeks for monitoring the status of the patient. Also, therapeutic management of cardiac failure can prevent serious unwanted complications.

CONCLUSION

Healthy pregnancy is jeopardized by PPCM. Having a clinical foresight is very important for diagnosing the condition early. The investigation of prime importance is echocardiography which is required for screening, diagnosis, and even follow-up of the patient. Treatment for PPCM is the same as that of cardiac failure, although the treatment should be modified keeping in mind the safety of the fetus. In future, more studies are required in order to fully understand the pathophysiology of the disease, determine specific biomarkers and better treatment protocols. Studies are also needed to explore various measures for prevention of PPCM.

REFERENCES

1. Pearson GD, Veille J, Rahimtoola S, et al. Peripartum cardiomyopathy: National heart, lung, and blood institute and office of rare diseases (National Institutes of Health) workshop recommendations and review. J Am Med Assoc. 2000;283:1183-8.
2. Brar SS, Khan SS, Sandhu GK, et al. Incidence, mortality, and racial differences in peripartum cardiomyopathy. Am J Cardiol. 2007;100:302-4.
3. Deneux-Tharaux C, Berg C, Bouvier-Colle MH, et al. Underreporting of pregnancy-related mortality in the United States and Europe. Obstet Gynecol. 2005;106:684-92.
4. Fett JD, Christie LG, Carraway RD, et al. Five-year prospective study of the incidence and prognosis of peripartum cardiomyopathy at a single institution. Mayo Clinic Proc. 2005;80:1602-6.
5. Isezuo SA, Abubakar SA. Epidemiologic profile of peripartum cardiomyopathy in a tertiary care hospital. Ethn Dis. 2007;17:228-33.
6. Goland SMK, Hatamizadeh P, Elkayam U. Differences in clinical profile of African-American women with peripartum cardiomyopathy in the United States. J Card Fail. 2013;19:214-8.
7. Fett JD, Murphy JG. Infant survival in Haiti after maternal death from peripartum cardiomyopathy. Int J Gynaecol Obstet. 2006;94:135-6.
8. Gentry MB, Dias JK, Luis A, et al. African-American women have a higher risk for developing peripartum cardiomyopathy. J Am Coll Cardiol. 2010;55:654-9.
9. Pandit V, Shety S, Kumar A, et al. Incidence and outcome of peripartum cardiomyopathy from a tertiary hospital in South India. Trop Doct. 2009;39:168-9.
10. Abboud J, Murad Y, Chen-Scarabelli C, et al. Peripartum cardiomyopathy: A comprehensive review. Int J Cardiol. 2007;118:295-303.
11. Brown CS, Bertolet BD. Peripartum cardiomyopathy: A comprehensive review. Am J Obstet Gynecol. 1998;178:409-14.
12. Desai P. Peripartum cardiomyopathy. A review. J Obstet Gynecol India. 2010;60:25-32.
13. Johnson-Coyle L, Jensen L, Sobey A. Peripartum cardiomyopathy: Review and practice guidelines. Am J Crit Care. 2012;21:89-99.
14. Karaye KM, Henein MY. Peripartum cardiomyopathy: A review article. Int J Cardiol. 2011;164:333-8.
15. Ntusi NBA, Mayosi BM. Aetiology and risk factors of peripartum cardiomyopathy: A systematic review. Int J Cardiol. 2009;131:168-79.
16. Chung E, Leinwand LA. Pregnancy as a cardiac stress model. Cardiovasc Res. 2014;101(4):561-70.
17. Sanghavi M, Rutherford JD. Cardiovascular physiology of pregnancy.Circulation. 2014;130:1003-8.
18. Conrad KP, Davison JM. The renal circulation in normal pregnancy and preeclampsia: Is there a place for relaxin? Am J Physiol Renal Physiol. 2014;306:F1121-35.
19. Brenner B. Haemostatic changes in pregnancy. Thromb Res. 2004;114:409-14.
20. Toescu V, Nuttall SL, Martin U, et al. Oxidative stress and normal pregnancy. Clin Endocrinol (Oxf). 2002;57:609-13.
21. Hunt SA, Abraham WT, Chin MH, et al. 2009 focused update incorporated into the ACC/AHA 2005 Guidelines for the Diagnosis and Management of Heart Failure in Adults: a report of the American College of Cardiology Foundation/ American Heart Association Task Force on Practice Guidelines developed in collaboration with the International Society for Heart and Lung Transplantation. J Am Coll Cardiol. 2009;53:e1-90.
22. Sliwa K, Forster O, Libhaber E, et al. Peripartum cardiomyopathy: Inflammatory markers as predictors of outcome in 100 prospectively studied patients. Eur Heart J. 2006;27:441-6.
23. Sliwa K, Skudicky D, Bergemann A, et al. Peripartum cardiomyopathy: Analysis of clinical outcome, left ventricular function, plasma levels of cytokines and Fas/ APO-1. J Am Coll Cardiol. 2000;35:701-5.
24. Hilfiker-Kleiner D, Sliwa K, Drexler H. Peripartum cardiomyopathy: Recent insights in its pathophysiology. Trends Cardiovasc Med. 2008;18:173-9.
25. Halkein J, Tabruyn SP, Ricke-Hoch M, et al. MicroRNA-146a is a therapeutic target and biomarker for peripartum cardiomyopathy. J Clin Invest. 2013;123:2143-54.
26. Bajou K, Herkenne S, Thijssen VL, et al. PAI-1 mediates the antiangiogenic and profibrinolytic effects of 16k prolactin. Nat Med. 2014;20:741-7.
27. Patten IS, Rana S, Shahul S, et al. Cardiac angiogenic imbalance leads to peripartum cardiomyopathy. Nature. 2012;485:333-8.
28. Arany Z, Foo SY, Ma Y, et al. HIF-independent regulation of VEGF and angiogenesis by the transcriptional coactivator PGC-1 . Nature. 2008;451:1008-12.
29. Powe CE, Levine RJ, Karumanchi SA. Preeclampsia, a disease of the maternal endothelium: The role of antiangiogenic factors and implications for later cardiovascular disease. Circulation. 2011;123:2856- 69.
30. Bello N, Rendon IS, Arany Z. The relationship between pre-eclampsia and peripartum cardiomyopathy: A systematic review and meta-analysis. J Am Coll Cardiol. 2013;62:1715-23.
31. Bdolah Y, Lam C, Rajakumar A, et al. Twin pregnancy and the risk of preeclampsia: bigger placenta or relative ischemia? Am J Obstet Gynecol. 2008;198:428.e1-6.
32. Kamiya CA, Kitakaze M, Ishibashi-Ueda H, et al. Different characteristics of peripartum cardiomyopathy between patients complicated with and without hypertensive disorders. Results from the Japanese Nationwide survey of peripartum cardiomyopathy. Circ J. 2011;75:1975-81.
33. Kao DP, Hsich E, Lindenfeld J. Characteristics, adverse events, and racial differences among delivering mothers with peripartum cardiomyopathy. JACC Heart Fail. 2013;1:409-16.
34. Elkayam U, Akhter MW, Singh H, et al. Pregnancy-associated cardiomyopathy: Clinical characteristics and a comparison between early and late presentation. Circulation. 2005;111:2050-5.
35. Horne BD, Rasmusson KD, Alharethi R, et al. Genome-wide significance and replication of the chromosome 12p11. 22 locus near the PTHLH gene for peripartum cardiomyopathy. Circ Cardiovasc Genet. 2011;4:359-66.
36. Bakre MM, Zhu Y, Yin H, et al. Parathyroid hormone related peptide is a naturally occurring, protein kinase A-dependent angiogenesis inhibitor. Nat Med. 2002;8:995-1003.
37. van Spaendonck-Zwarts KY, van Tintelen JP, van Veldhuisen DJ, et al. Peripartum cardiomyopathy as a part of familial dilated cardiomyopathy. Circulation. 2010;121:2169-75.
38. van Spaendonck-Zwarts KY, Posafalvi A, van den Berg MP, et al. Titin gene mutations are common in families with both peripartum cardiomyopathy and dilated cardiomyopathy. Eur Heart J. 2014;35:2165-73.
39. Van Hoevan KH, Kitsis RN, Kat SD, et al. Peripartum versus idiopathic dilated cardiomyopathy in young women: A comparisons of clinical pathological and prognostic features. Int J Cardiol. 1993;40:57.
40. Martin Neto JA, Maciel BC, Teran Urbanet LL, et al. High output failure in patients with peripartum cardiomyopathy. A comparative study with dilated cardiomyopathy. Am Heart J. 1990;121:134.
41. Kim M-J, Shin M-S. Practical management of peripartum cardiomyopathy. The Korean Journal of Internal Medicine. 2017;32(3):393-403. doi:10.3904/ kjim.2016.360.
42. Braunwald Zl. Heart Diseases: A Textbook of Cardiovascular Medicine. HIE Saunders, 8th edition, 65;2179-81.
43. Fett JD. Validation of a self-test for early diagnosis of heart failure in peripartum cardiomyopathy. Crit Pathw Cardiol. 2011;10:44-45.
44. Sliwa K, Fett J, Elkayam U. Peripartum cardiomyopathy. Lancet. 2006;368: 687-93.
45. Sliwa K, Blauwet L, Tibazarwa K, et al. Evaluation of bromocriptine in the treatment of acute severe peripartum cardiomyopathy: A proof-of-concept pilot study. Circulation. 2010;121:1465-73.
46. Haghikia A, Podewski E, Libhaber E, et al. Phenotyping and outcome on contemporary management in a German cohort of patients with peripartum cardiomyopathy. Basic Res Cardiol. 2013;108:366.

47. Hilfiker-Kleiner D, Haghikia A, Berliner D, et al. Bromocriptine for the treatment of peripartum cardiomyopathy: A multicentre randomized study. Eur Heart J. 2017;38(35):2671-9.
48. Forster O, Hilfiker-Kleiner D, Ansari AA, et al. Reversal of IFN-gamma, oxLDL and prolactin serum levels correlate with clinical improvement in patients with peripartum cardiomyopathy. Eur J Heart Fail. 2008;10:861-8.
49. Sliwa K, Forster O, Tibazarwa K, et al. Long-term outcome of peripartum cardiomyopathy in a population with high seropositivity for human immunodeficiency virus. Int J Cardiol. 2011;147:202-8.
50. Mouquet F, Mostefa Kara M, Lamblin N, et al. Unexpected and rapid recovery of left ventricular function in patients with peripartum cardiomyopathy: Impact of cardiac resynchronization therapy. Eur J Heart Fail. 2012;14:526-9.
51. Duncker D, Haghikia A, Konig T, et al. Risk for ventricular fibrillation in peripartum cardiomyopathy with severely reduced left ventricular function-value of the wearable cardioverter/defibrillator. Eur J Heart Fail. 2014;16:1331-6.
52. Goland S, Modi K, Bitar F, et al. Clinical profile and predictors of complications in peripartum cardiomyopathy. J Card Fail. 2009;15:645-50.
53. McNamara DM, Elkayam U, Alharethi R, et al. Clinical outcomes for peripartum cardiomyopathy in North America: Results of the IPAC study (Investigations of Pregnancy-Associated Cardiomyopathy). J Am Coll Cardiol. 2015;66:905-14.
54. Fett JD. Peripartum cardiomyopathy: A puzzle closer to solution. World J Cardiol. 2014:6:87-99.
55. Sliwa K, Hilfker-Kleiner D, Petrie MC, et al. Current state of knowledge on aetiology, diagnosis, management, and therapy of peripartum cardiomyopathy: A position statement from the Heart Failure Association of the European Society of Cardiology Working Group on peripartum cardiomyopathy. Eur J Heart Fail. 2010;12:767-78.
56. Hilfker-Kleiner D, Haghikia A, Nonho J, et al. Peripartum cardiomyopathy: Current management and future perspectives. Eur Heart J. 2015;36:1090-7.
57. Whitehead SJ, Berg CJ, Chang J. Pregnancy-related mortality due to cardiomyopathy: United States, 1991-1997. Obstet Gynecol. 2003;102:1326-31.
58. Elkayam U, Tummala PP, Rao K, et al. Maternal and fetal outcomes of subsequent pregnancies in women with peripartum cardiomyopathy. N Engl J Med. 2001;344:1567-71.
59. Fett JD, Sannon H, Thelisma E, et al. Recovery from severe heart failure following peripartum cardiomyopathy. Int J Gynaecol Obstet. 2009;104:125-7.
60. Elkayam U. Risk of subsequent pregnancy in women with a history of peripartum cardiomyopathy. J Am Coll Cardiol. 2014;64:1629-36.
61. Habli M, O'Brien T, Nowack E, et al. Peripartum cardiomyopathy: Prognostic factors for long-term maternal outcome. Am J Obstet Gynecol. 2008;199:415.e1-415.e5.

CHAPTER 139

Mitral Stenosis in Pregnancy: The Last Straw on the Camel's Back!

AJ Swamy, Deepak Saha, Sarat Chandra

INTRODUCTION AND EPIDEMIOLOGY

Mitral stenosis (MS) is the most common manifestation of chronic rheumatic heart disease, and its age of occurrence, natural history, and hemodynamic load imposed on the circulatory system ensure that it will always be an important consideration if present in a pregnant patient. The earliest description was in the last quarter of the 19th century by James Mackenzie, a Scottish physician who observed a young woman with MS and pregnancy.[1] The patient had severe pulmonary congestion in the second trimester and succumbed during labor.

PREVALENCE AND INCIDENCE IN INDIA

In one large study, rheumatic MS formed 88% of the heart diseases complicating pregnancy in a tertiary referral center in India.[2] Significant MS causes maternal complications (pulmonary edema, atrial fibrillation, thromboembolic complications) and fetal complications (premature birth, intrauterine growth retardation, and still birth).[3] Severe MS is particularly malignant: in one study of pregnant patients with severe MS, 67% developed a maternal cardiac event, and 44% of infants were born prematurely or died.[4] These events can be prevented and outcomes improved by proper management during pregnancy and better perinatal care.[5]

HEMODYNAMIC CHANGES IN PREGNANCY

Pregnancy brings about significant changes in hemodynamics throughout gestation. The blood volume progressively increases throughout pregnancy starting at 6 weeks of gestation. It reaches peak at 32 weeks of gestation (at this time blood volume reaches 45% more than the prepregnancy level). Maternal heart rate gradually increases from fifth week of gestation till 32 weeks of gestation after which it plateaus. An increase of 15–20 beats/min is usual. Cardiac output (which is a product of stroke volume and heart rate) gradually increases from sixth week of gestation and usually peaks at 32 weeks. A 50% increase of cardiac output is seen at peak level compared to prepregnancy measurements. Cardiac output fluctuates significantly with changes in maternal position in the latter half of pregnancy. The enlarged gravid uterus compresses the inferior vena cava (IVC) in the supine position leading to decreased venous return to the heart and thus decreased cardiac output.

Systemic vascular resistance (SVR) decreases significantly during pregnancy starting from fifth week reaching nadir at about 20 weeks of gestation, during which it decreases by approximately 35% compared to baseline levels. It remains constant till 32 weeks beyond which a mild increase in SVR is noted till term. Blood pressure starts decreasing from seventh week of gestation reaching nadir at 20 weeks wherein, an average fall by 5–10% is observed. Thereafter blood pressure gradually increases returning to base line level (sometimes exceeds by 5–10%) by term.[6]

The hemodynamic burden during pregnancy may unmask previously unrecognized asymptomatic heart disease which sometimes results in significant morbidity and mortality. Other disorders of the heart like peripartum cardiomyopathy, aortic dissection or spontaneous coronary dissection may be precipitated by hormonal and hemodynamic alterations during pregnancy.[7]

HEMODYNAMICS DURING LABOR AND DELIVERY

Women with heart disease require close monitoring during labor and delivery. Uterine contractions at the time of labor transfer approximately 400 mL of blood from the uterus to the general circulation. The cardiac output may further increase in the second stage owing to the maternal pushing efforts, pain and anxiety causing increased sympathetic tone leading to increased heart rate and systolic blood pressure (SBP). Additionally, cardiac output may increase up to 70% immediately after delivery with increase in venous return caused by relief of vena caval compression and transfer of blood from the placental circulation.[8]

PATHOPHYSIOLOGY OF MITRAL STENOSIS DURING PREGNANCY

Pregnancy burdens significantly the maternal heart suffering from MS. The increased blood volume, increased filling pressure, and increased heart rate all contribute to the rise in left atrial (LA) mean pressure and thus pulmonary edema. Additionally, due to decreased diastolic time due to tachycardia, there is significant underfilling of left ventricular (LV) leading to low-stroke volume and low cardiac output state. This is the major contributor to uteroplacental insufficiency and cause of fetal morbidity.[8,9]

Natural History

Mitral stenosis causes significant maternal adverse events that are related to New York Heart Association (NYHA) class and severity of MS. Symptoms depend upon the severity of MS prior to conception. In a study of a Cohort of 80 patients with pregnancy and rheumatic MS by Silverside CK et al., the rate of cardiac complications (pulmonary edema/arrhythmia), was 26% in mild MS [mitral valve area (MVA) >1.5 cm^2], 38% in moderate MS (MVA 1–1.5 cm^2), and 67% in severe MS (MVA <1 cm^2).[4] Symptoms correlate closely with NYHA class with regard to maternal and fetal outcomes. Mortality rates for class I and II amount to less than 1%, whereas they range between 5 and 15% for class III and IV. The perinatal mortality rate for class III and IV may be high as 20–30%. In another 2001 study that reported the effect of valvular heart disease on maternal and fetal outcome in 46 pregnancies in 44 patients with MS, a high incidence of maternal morbidity but no mortality was found. Hospitalization due to heart failure was reported in 61% of moderate MS patients (MVA 1–1.5 cm^2) and 78% of women with severe stenosis. In those with moderate or severe stenosis, deterioration in functional status was noted in 82% of class I and 61% of class II patients. Outcomes in patients with mild MS were not statistically different from controls.[10]

The major adverse events related to pregnancy are acute pulmonary edema, arrhythmia (atrial fibrillation), and thromboembolic phenomena. Maternal death is rare in pregnancy. The risk of maternal death is greatest during labor and during the immediate postpartum period. The sudden increase in the preload immediately after delivery, due to autotransfusion from the uterus, may flood the central circulation, resulting in severe pulmonary edema. In addition, there continues to be autotransfusion of blood for 24–72 hours after delivery. Thus, the risk of pulmonary edema extends for several days after delivery.[7,8] Other studies have described additional markers of adverse outcomes in heart disease with pregnancy. These include prior heart failure, arrhythmia, transient ischemic attack or stroke, a baseline NYHA III class or more or cyanosis, systemic ventricular dysfunction (ejection fraction <40%) pulmonary hypertension (pulmonary arterial systolic pressure 50% of systemic pressure), left heart obstruction, severe aortic stenosis (valve area less than or equal to 1 cm^2, Doppler jet velocity 4 m/s) symptomatic or severe MS, and severe aortic or mitral regurgitation with NYHA class III or IV symptoms.[11]

Adverse fetal outcomes are also related to severity of MS and NYHA class, occurring almost exclusively in symptomatic patients. Fetal and neonatal mortality up to 30% has been reported in patients with severe MS.[12] This is caused by uteroplacental insufficiency due to low cardiac output and includes preterm delivery, intrauterine growth retardation, low birth weight, and fetal or neonatal death.[8,10] A large multicenter study in 2001 identified five predictors of neonatal events including NYHA class, maternal left heart obstruction, smoking during pregnancy, multiple gestations, and use of anticoagulants during pregnancy. Thus, women with poor functional class are at maximum risk for adverse neonatal outcomes.[9,13]

Diagnosis

The symptoms due to MS are due to pulmonary or systemic congestion or low cardiac output. Common presentation is with progressive breathlessness, fatigue and/or pedal edema, which may be sometimes confused with the physiological effect of pregnancy. In women without known diagnosis of MS, a high suspicion of underlying heart disease is the key for early detection and timely management.[8]

Good clinical examination will give a clue to the diagnosis. Electrocardiogram (ECG) may show LA enlargement, atrial fibrillation or features of right ventricular hypertrophy (RVH) due to pulmonary hypertension. Chest X-ray (CXR) is usually avoided in pregnancy. The cornerstone of diagnosis is an echocardiographic evaluation that will reveal the severity of MS, the gradient across the valve, degree of subvalvular disease, the presence of pulmonary hypertension, the LV function, the presence of any additional valve involvement, pericardial effusion, or rheumatic activity. The 2D derived valve area may be more reliable than that derived by pressure half time.[7,14]

Management

The functional class of patient prior to conception usually governs the prognosis of maternal and fetal outcome. In general, worsening by one NYHA Functional Class is anticipated during pregnancy usually at second and third trimester. Patients with moderate or severe MS do not tolerate hemodynamic burden of pregnancy well. Women with symptomatic MS, MS with significant pulmonary hypertension or valve area less than 1.5 cm^2 must be advised intervention, ideally, before pregnancy.[7,8]

In all patients, medical therapy is initiated to relieve the pulmonary congestion. Restricted physical activity, salt restriction, and iron supplements should be routinely advised.[7,8]

Beta-blockers: Cardioselective beta-blockers, usually short acting, are ideal. Atenolol has been shown to be associated with intrauterine growth restriction (IUGR) and so metoprolol is preferred.[15,16] Maternal heart rate is slowed, thus reducing LA pressure and increasing cardiac output by increased LV filling. It may be used along with diuretics. Beta-blockade has been shown to improve NYHA Functional Class. It has been shown to decrease maternal adverse events without adverse events on the fetus.[17] Digoxin may be added for control of heart rate in cases with atrial fibrillation.[7,10]

Diuretics: Loop diuretics are preferred but need careful monitoring under obstetric care so that placental insufficiency in avoided.[7,8,18]

Anticoagulants: Since, pregnancy is a hypercoagulable state, anticoagulation [with vitamin K antagonist (VKA)] must be considered to prevent stroke and systemic embolism even if the patient is in sinus rhythm. In patients with mild MS, anticoagulants are better avoided. In moderate-to-severe MS, the risk to benefit ratio favors the use of anticoagulation if the LA dimensions exceeds 55 mm, however, there is a lack of evidence in this subset.

Patients who have established or intermittent atrial fibrillation should be treated with anticoagulation. VKAs are associated with fetal anomalies if used in the first trimester, especially if warfarin dose exceeds 5 mg/day. Ideally, warfarin should be used between 12 and 36 weeks. The consensus is to use low-molecular-weight heparin (LMWH) in weight adjusted doses for the first and third trimester, warfarin between 12 and 36 weeks and switch to unfractionated heparin 24 hours before delivery or lower (uterine) segment cesarean section (LSCS).[19] In patients on heparin, the drug should be withdrawn 4 hours before cesarean section or at the onset of labor and resumed 6–12 hours after either surgical or vaginal delivery.[20]

PERCUTANEOUS BALLOON MITRAL VALVULOPLASTY

Percutaneous balloon mitral valvuloplasty (PBMV) is the treatment of choice for isolated, noncalcified MS in symptomatic, moderate (or more) MS. Ideally, this should be performed preconception. It should also be considered in patients with echocardiographically severe MS even if asymptomatic. Contraindications include LA thrombi, more than 2+ mitral regurgitation, and severe subvalvular stenosis. The procedure may electively be performed in second trimester of pregnancy in patients who are at high-risk of developing pulmonary edema in late stage of pregnancy. If feasible, the procedure may be postponed beyond 28 weeks to ensure viability of the issue.[8] In an emergency, it should be performed, irrespective of the timing of pregnancy.

Steps of balloon mitral valvuloplasty (BMV) are similar to conventional procedure. However, prolonged compression of the IVC in supine position due to a long procedure or prolonged balloon inflation may cause adverse hemodynamic effects especially on uteroplacental circulation resulting in fetal distress and higher incidence of cesarean section.[21] All patients need abdominal shielding with lead shields from diaphragm to pubic symphysis. Two lead shields may be placed for the patient to lie on and a light shield over the anterior abdominal wall so as not to compress the gravid uterus. Fluoroscopy should be monitored and minimum. Right heart catheterization is thus usually avoided. The risk due to radiation exposure to the fetus is considerably less than the adverse effect of hemodynamic instability in later phase of pregnancy.

Percutaneous balloon mitral valvuloplasty must be performed at high-volume centers with appropriate shielding and where the speed of procedure can be minimized with optimum care both to mother and fetus. Short- and long-term outcomes have been reported after BMV in pregnancy. Immediate short-term success approaches 100%.[22,23] In one series with 71 women with Class III or IV who underwent PBMV in Brazil, mean MVA increased from 0.9 to 2.0 cm^2. A total of 98% were in NYHA Class I or II at conclusion of pregnancy.[23] In another study of PBMV in pregnancy, 49 pregnant women were included. The mean gestational age was 23.5 ± 5.2 weeks (range: 12–36 weeks). The mean 2D area increased from 0.93 to 1.75 cm^2 with a procedural success of 95.9%. One patient had a major complication with tamponade and another aborted 2 days after the procedure.[24] Other studies have reported similar results.[25,26] Long-term outcomes have also been reported after BMV.[27,28] A 17-year outcomes following BMV have been reported; subsequent pregnancies were normal with children exhibiting normal physical and mental development.

Echocardiographically guided PBMV has been reported[29] as has intracardiac echocardiography (ICE)-assisted BMV.[30]

SURGICAL MITRAL VALVOPLASTY/ MITRAL REPLACEMENT

Closed mitral valvotomy has been largely replaced by PBMV in most centers. Although the surgical risk to the mother has been quite low (1–5% mortality), the fetal mortality due to surgery has been high (up to 30% of cases).[31] Open valvotomy carries a higher risk than closed valvotomy especially with regard to fetal mortality (15–30% vs. 5–15%).[26] But both have been replaced by PBMV for the last two decades with evidence from registries and comparative studies. PBMV resulted in lesser fetal morbidity and mortality in a nonrandomized study.[32]

In patients with mixed stenosis and regurgitation, mitral valve replacement is the treatment of choice, but due to higher maternal and fetal morbidity and mortality, it should be reserved for symptomatic patients who have failed aggressive medical therapy.[8] Cardiopulmonary bypass should be done at normal temperature and high flow and pressure for as brief a time period as possible. Important principles include use of high-flow, high-pressure, normothermic bypass during the procedure, fetal heart and uterine monitoring to allow adjustments to the blood flow and pharmacological manipulations to ensure adequate placental perfusion, and if the fetus is more than 28 weeks of gestational age, to opt for cesarean section concurrently just prior to the cardiac operation.[7]

Management during Delivery or Labor

Tachycardia, secondary to labor pain, increases flow across the mitral valve, producing sudden rises in LA pressure, leading to acute pulmonary edema.[33] Good analgesia is of paramount importance during labor. Epidural anesthesia is ideal with vaginal delivery unless contraindicated. Cesarean section is recommended for obstetric indications only. In one study, only 29–31% of the 522 women with heart disease required caesarean section and nearly 70% of them underwent vaginal delivery under epidural analgesia.[34] Invasive monitoring with radial artery cannulation and pulmonary catheter are of use in real-time assessment of cardiac output and pulmonary artery pressure and to guide fluid and drug therapy and are often used in NYHA III and IV patients.[35]

During the second stage of labor, maternal expulsive effort, i.e., always associated with the Valsalva maneuver should not be permitted and only uterine expulsive force should be allowed. Thus, the second stage should be cut short by instrumentation. Supplementary analgesia for instrumentation may be required.[36]

Fetal heart rate monitoring should be carried out during all stages of labor. Supplemental oxygen administration and supplementary epidural anesthesia can be maintained throughout the immediate postpartum period. The epidural catheter may be left in situ to provide anesthesia for immediate or postpartum tubal sterilization if advised.[35] The goals of anesthetic management of a patient with MS are maintain slow heart rate, immediate cardioversion of acute atrial fibrillation, avoid aortocaval compression, maintain adequate SVR, and prevention of pain, hypoxia, acidosis and hypercarbia.

There is a lack of evidence regarding ideal anesthetic protocol during LSCS for patients with significant MS. Thus, the technique with which the treating team has maximum experience and safety in the available resources and expertise are recommended. Regional anesthesia is a safe technique for anesthesia for LSCS in patients with cardiac disease. Epidural and continuous spinal anesthetic techniques are favored. General anesthesia is associated with increased pulmonary arterial pressure and tachycardia during intubation. However, if general anesthesia is contemplated, drugs-associated tachycardia (atropine, ketamine, pancuronium and meperidine) should be totally avoided. A beta-blocker and an opioid are recommended during the induction of general anesthesia.

Whatever be the mode of delivery and anesthetic technique, autotransfusion of blood from the uterus adds significant hemodynamic stress. Therefore, intensive monitoring needs to be performed till all parameters return to normal.[36]

CONCLUSION

Mitral stenosis is the commonest rheumatic valvular manifestation and occurrence of significant MS coincides with child-bearing age in women. The additional cardiac stresses imposed by pregnancy can be life-threatening to mother and baby in severe MS. This high-risk pregnancy needs careful management by a team with cardiology, obstetrics, critical care, and neonatology elements working together. However, with close monitoring and coordination, this dangerous combination can be controlled and a gratifying result ensured in the vast majority of cases.

REFERENCES

1. Mackenzie J. Mitral stenosis; In. Heart disease and Pregnancy. Henry Froude and Hodder and Stoughton. London. Oxford Medical Publications. 1921; pp 78-87.
2. Bhatla N, Lal S, Behera G, et al. Cardiac disease in pregnancy. Int J Gynaecol Obstet. 2003;82:153-9.
3. Norrad SN, Salehian O. Management of severe mitral stenosis during pregnancy. Circulation. 2011;124:2756-60.
4. Siversides C, Colman J, Sermer M, et al. Cardiac risk in pregnant women with rheumatic mitral stenosis. Am J Cardiol. 2003;91:1382-5.
5. Malhotra M, Sharma JB, Tripathii R, et al. Maternal and fetal outcome in valvular heart disease. Int J Gynaecol Obstet. 2004;84:11-16.
6. Soma-Pillay P, Catherine NP, Tolppanen H, et al. Physiological changes in pregnancy. Cardiovasc J Africa. 2016;27(2):89-94.
7. Anandaraja S, Kothari SS, Bahl VK. Management of valvular heart disease during pregnancy. Indian Heart J. 2005;57:101-8.
8. Tsairass S, Poppas A. Mitral valve disease in pregnancy. Obstet Med. 2009;2: 6-10.
9. Siu SC, Sermer M, Colman JM, et al. Prospective multicenter study of pregnancy outcomes in women with heart disease. Circulation. 2001;104:515-21.
10. Hameed A, Karaalp IS, Tummala PP, et al. The effect of valvular heart disease on maternal and fetal outcome of pregnancy. J Am Coll Cardiol. 2001;37:893-9.
11. Siu SC, Sermer M, Harrison DA, et al. Risk and predictors for pregnancy-related complications in women with heart disease. Circulation. 1997;96:2789-94.
12. Brady K, Duff P. Rheumatic heart disease in pregnancy. Clin Obstet Gynecol. 1989;32:21-40.
13. Siu SC, Colman JM, Sorensen S, et al. Adverse neonatal and cardiac outcomes are more common in pregnant women with cardiac disease. Circulation. 2002;105:2179-84.
14. Fokey R, Hsu HW, Moise KJJ, et al. Inaccurate noninvasive mitral valve area calculation during pregnancy. Obstet Gynecol. 1994;84:950-5.
15. Lydakis C, Lip GY, Beevers M, et al. Atenolol and fetal growth in pregnancies complicated by hypertension. Am J Hypertens. 1999;12:541-7.
16. Easterling TR, Brateng D, Schmucker B, et al. Prevention of preeclampsia: A randomized trial of atenolol in hyperdynamic patients before onset of hypertension. Obstet Gynecol. 1999;93:725-33.
17. Al Kasab SM, Sabag T, al Zaibag M, et al. Beta-adrenergic blockade in the management of pregnant women with mitral stenosis. Am J Obstet Gynecol. 1990;165:37-40.
18. Norrad RS, Salehian O. Management of severe mitral stenosis during pregnancy. Circulation. 2011;124:2756-60.
19. Toyoda K. Antithrombotic therapy for pregnant women. Neurol Med Chir (Tokyo). 2013.53(8):526-30.
20. Siu SC, Colman JM. Heart disease and pregnancy. Heart. 2000;85:710-5.
21. Sananes S, Iung B, Vahanian A, et al. Fetal and obstetrical impact of percutaneous balloon mitral commissurotomy during pregnancy. Fetal Diagn Ther. 1994;9(4);218-25.
22. Aggarwal N, Suri V, Goyal A, et al. Closed mitral valvotomy in pregnancy and labor. Int J Gynaecol Obstet. 2005;88:118-21.
23. Routray SN, Mishra TK, Swain S, et al. Balloon mitral valvuloplasty during pregnancy. Int J Gynaecol Obstet. 2004;85:18-23.
24. Vinayakumar D, Vinod GV, Madhavan S, et al. Maternal and fetal outcomes in pregnant women undergoing balloon mitral valvotomy for rheumatic mitral stenosis. Indian Heart J. 2016;68:780-2.
25. Mishra S, Narang R, Sharma M, et al. Percutaneous transseptal mitral commissurotomy in pregnant women with critical mitral stenosis. Indian Heart J. 2001;53:192-6.

26. Singh Y, Manjunath C Nanjappa. Immediate and intermediate-term outcomes of percutaneous transvenous mitral commissurotomy during pregnancy: our experience with Accura balloon at a high-volume center. Indian Heart J. 2013;65:S333.
27. Gulraze A, Kurdi W, Niaz F, et al. Mitral balloon valvuloplasty during pregnancy: The long-term up to 17 years obstetric outcome and childhood development. Pak J Med Sci. 2014;30(1);86-90.
28. Esteves CA, Munoz JS, Braga S, et al. Immediate and long-term follow-up of percutaneous balloon mitral valvuloplasty in pregnant patients with rheumatic mitral stenosis. Am J Cardiol. 2006;98:812-6.
29. Trehan V, Mukhopadhyay S, Nigam A, et al. Mitral valvuloplasty by inoue balloon under transthoracic echocardiographic guidance. J Am Soc Echocardiogr. 2005;18:964-9.
30. Ahmari SA, Amro A, Otabi MA, et al. Initial experience of using intracardiac echocardiography (ICE) for guiding balloon mitral valvuloplasty (BMV). J Saudi Heart Assoc. 2012;24(1):23-27.
31. Weiss BM, von Segesser LK, Alon E, et al. Outcome of cardiovascular surgery and pregnancy: A systematic review of the period 1984–1996. Am J Obstet Gynecol. 1998;179:1643-53.
32. de Souza JA, Martinez EEJ, Ambrose JA, et al. Percutaneous balloon mitral valvuloplasty in comparison with open mitral valve commissurotomy for mitral stenosis during pregnancy. J Am Coll Cardiol. 2001;37:900-3.
33. Sharma SK, Gambling DR, Gajraj NM, et al. Anesthetic management of a parturient with mixed mitral valve disease and uncontrolled atrial fibrillation. Int J Obstet Anesth. 1994;3:157-62.
34. Gomar C, Errando CL. Neuroaxial anaesthesia in obstetrical patients with cardiac disease. Curr Opin Anaesthesiol. 2005;18:507-12.
35. Kannan M, Vijayanand G. Mitral stenosis and pregnancy: Current concepts in anaesthetic practice. Indian J Anaesth. 2010;54:439-44.
36. Ngan Kee WD, Shen J, Chiu AT, et al. Combined spinal-epidural analgesia in the management of labouring parturients with mitral stenosis. Anaesth Intensive Care. 1999;27:523-6.

CHAPTER 140

Heart Failure in Pregnancy

Kajal Ganguly, Anindya Mukherjee, Malay Acharya, Auriom Kar

INTRODUCTION

Pregnancy is a physiological stress test. In normal subjects as well as known patients of cardiac ailments, pregnancy and peripartum period with all its physiological changes poses as a challenge. There is 30–50% increase in cardiac output close to term.[1] Labor induces more hemodynamic stress and newly developed cardiovascular disease (CVD) during pregnancy and the effects of pregnancy on them continue even after delivery over several months.[2]

EPIDEMIOLOGY

Cardiac disease is not related to any complication of pregnancy itself. Hence, it is termed as an "indirect" cause of maternal mortality when it complicates pregnancy.[3] In the article by Mulubrhan F Mogos et al. among the 50,995,050 pregnancy-related hospitalizations between January 1, 2001, and December 31, 2011, there were 7,542 antepartum, 15,620 delivery, and 34,110 postpartum hospitalizations with a diagnostic indication of hearf failure (HF). Across the pregnancy continuum, the overall prevalence of HF among the study population was 112 cases per 100,000 pregnancy-related hospital discharges [95% confidence interval (CI), 107–118]. Although the postpartum period represented only 1.5% of pregnancy-related hospitalizations, this period saw the occurrence of 60% of the HFs related to pregnancy, followed by the delivery (27%), and antepartum (13%) periods.[4] Incidence of HF due to peripartum cardiomyopathy varies in cosmopolitan societies. Genetic and social variations within individual communities give rise to these disparities. One out of 1,421 African-Americans develops HF in pregnancy in the United States of America compared with an incidence of 1:2,675 in Asians, 1:4,075 in Caucasians and 1:9,861 in people of Hispanic origin.[5] Prevalence of cardiac disease in pregnancy differs from one country to another, but in various countries across various socioeconomic strata, it is a common cause of maternal death. HF is usually the most common mechanism of death.[6]

PHYSIOLOGY

The uterine enlargement and increased activity along with the increased blood flow into the choriodecidual space accounts for 12% of the total cardiac output in a pregnancy.[7] Hyperaldosteronism leads to increased blood volume and thus leads to an increase in cardiac output. The cardiac output starts to rise from the first trimester and it peaks toward the end of the second trimester. The peak cardiac output during pregnancy is between 3.5 L/min and 6 L/min, which is 30–50% higher than nonpregnant values.[8,9] From the first trimester, the peripheral vasculature is dilated with a progressive fall of systemic vascular resistance and it receives the progressively increasing cardiac output. There is increase in left and right ventricular mass and end diastolic volume as pregnancy progresses which is a reflection of the rising cardiac output and intravascular volume. These changes reverse in postpartum period.[10] The summary of these adaptations are given in figure 1.[6]

ETIOLOGY AND PATHOPHYSIOLOGY

Preeclampsia, peripartum cardiomyopathy, and amniotic fluid embolism are the three causes of HF which are specific to pregnancy. Apart from these are the other causes of HF which are not related to pregnancy but may complicate pregnancy.[6]

Preeclampsia

Pulmonary edema is a common occurrence in preeclampsia. A South African confidential enquiry has found that pulmonary edema and cerebrovascular bleeding are the dominant causes of maternal mortality due to hypertension.[3] Diastolic dysfunction directly and increased systemic vascular resistance indirectly, contributes to this pulmonary edema.[6,11] Transient systolic dysfunction may occasionally occur in severe preeclampsia.[6]

Hypertension

Around 17–25% of preeclampsia develops in known hypertensive subjects, compared to 3–5% occurring in the general

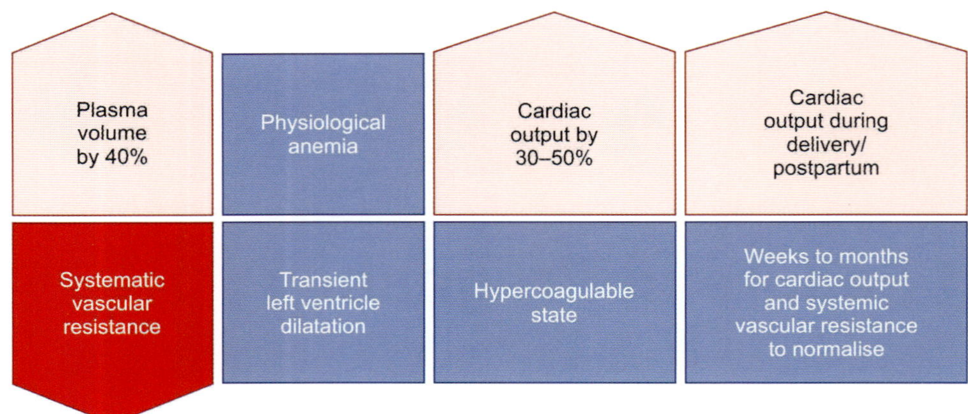

FIG. 1: Summary of physiological changes occurring during pregnancy.

population. Placental abruption, fetal growth restriction, and preterm birth are also more common in hypertensive patients.[12] At 32–34 weeks of gestation plasma volume expansion peaks. This increase in preload together with hypertension induced diastolic dysfunction predisposes some patients to develop mild pulmonary edema.[13,14]

Pulmonary Hypertension and Right Heart Failure

Pulmonary hypertension has been classified in a consensus statement.[15] Acute right-sided HF may occur in pregnant patients with primary pulmonary hypertension after delivery. These patients are at risk of sudden cardiac death.[16]

Diseases Affecting the Aortic Root

Takayasu's disease predominantly presents with hypertension and sometimes with HF.[17] Patients of Marfan's syndrome with aortic root dilatation commonly present with arterial dissection and acute aortic regurgitation during pregnancy.[18]

Peripartum Cardiomyopathy

The most common cause of mortality developing during or after pregnancy is peripartum cardiomyopathy.[19,20] Previously well women develop left ventricular (LV) systolic dysfunction with an ejection fraction of less than 45% during the last month of pregnancy or 6 months postpartum.[21] A 16 kDa cathepsin cleavage product of prolactin has been proposed as a possible mechanism of peripartum cardiomyopathy. This mechanism is based upon the induction of myocyte apoptosis.[21,22] Other proposed mechanisms include inflammation, oxidative stress, and autoimmunity to cardiac proteins.[23] Imbalance between angiogenic and antiangiogenic factors has been linked to association of peripartum cardiomyopathy with preeclampsia and multiple pregnancy.[24]

Hereditary Cardiomyopathies

Symptom-free hypertrophic cardiomyopathy is tolerated well during pregnancy.[25,26] In patients of dilated cardiomyopathy, pregnancy outcome depends on the severity of symptoms before developing pregnancy.[6] Risk of sudden cardiac death is always associated with arrhythmogenic right ventricular dysplasia and it is not altered by pregnancy or its complications.[27]

Drugs

Drug abuse is rarely associated with HF during pregnancy.[6]

Autoimmune Diseases and Infections

Infective carditis or autoimmune disease-related myocarditis may result in dilated cardiomyopathy. Chronic HF can ensue in these cases of dilated cardiomyopathies.[6]

Amniotic Fluid Embolism

Large amounts of amniotic fluid may get released into the maternal circulation and results in acute pulmonary hypertension. This leads to left HF and associated arrhythmias.[6]

Ischemic Heart Disease

Heart failure rarely occurs during pregnancy in patients having myocardial ischemia.[6]

Valvular Lesions

Time for LV filling diminish during pregnancy due to tachycardia, which is further aggravated during labor. Thus in patients with mitral inflow obstruction, HF ensues.[6] Mitral and aortic regurgitation are well tolerated in pregnancy.[28]

Congenital Diseases

Congenital diseases can be classified as high-risk, moderate-risk and low-risk in pregnancy. Greatest risk of mortality lies with Marfan syndrome with aortic root dilatation and Eisenmenger syndrome. Moderate-risk lesions for HF are congenitally stenosed valves, cyanotic heart disease without pulmonary hypertension, a systemic right ventricle or Fontan circulation. The septal defects and repaired coarctation are the low-risk lesions for HF.[29]

CLINICAL PRESENTATION

Normal subjects with pregnancy experience some breathlessness on exertion. Exertional dyspnea together with orthopnea, paroxysmal nocturnal dyspnea, syncope, and palpitations, signifies the presence of associated heart ailment and warrants for further investigations.

Pregnancy does mimic certain signs of heart disease.[30] A clinician must look for any cyanosis, clubbing, resting tachycardia, presence of any arrhythmia, a water hammer pulse, hypertension or hypotension, any signs of respiratory distress, an abnormal jugular venous pressure (JVP), any diastolic or pansystolic murmur, any thrill or murmur radiation beyond left sternal border or signs of pulmonary venous hypertension.[6]

INVESTIGATIONS

Normal pregnancy may be associated with ST-T abnormalities in electrocardiogram and supraventricular arrhythmias.[30] Echocardiography is a routine procedure nowadays to rule out cardiac diseases in pregnancy if the patient is symptomatic.

Assigning Severity of Risk

The morbidity and mortality of adverse events in pregnant women has been defined by Modified World Health Organization classification.[29,31] Class I cardiac disease includes mild pulmonary stenosis, patent ductus arteriosus, mitral valve prolapse, repaired septal defects, and isolated supraventricular, and ventricular ectopics. These are not associated with any risk. Class II diseases are associated with a small increase in risk. All other arrhythmias apart from isolated supra-ventricular and ventricular ectopics, repaired tetralogy of Fallot and operated septal defects are included in class II. Category III include all forms of cardiomyopathy, prosthetic heart valves, Marfan syndrome with dilated aortic root, cyanotic heart disease, Fontan circulation, and a systemic right ventricle. In these diseases there is a significantly increased risk of morbidity and mortality. Class IV includes pulmonary hypertension, severe symptomatic LV inflow or outflow tract obstruction, previous peripartum cardiomyopathy with residual disease, severe LV failure (ejection fraction <30%) and aortic coarctation or Marfan's syndrome with dilated aortic root of more than 45 mm. Pregnancy is contraindicated in the class IV conditions.

DIFFERENTIAL DIAGNOSIS

In the patients developing pulmonary edema, all possible cardiac causes must be ruled out before a diagnosis of non-cardiogenic pulmonary edema is made. Even all the clinical and radiological armamentarium may sometimes fail to distinguish infection from pulmonary edema. Pulmonary thromboembolism is also an important differential diagnosis demanding special investigations, more so because pregnancy is a procoagulant condition.[32] Diabetic ketoacidosis and lactic acidosis both may mimic breathlessness due to acidotic breathing pattern. Subdiaphragmatic pathology may hinder respiration and cause rapid shallow breathing, which may appear as breathlessness.

MANAGEMENT PRINCIPLES

Diuretics

Diuretics form the first-line of treatment for HF in pregnancy.[33] Though there is a theoretical concern that diuretics limit the necessary increase in uterine and placental perfusion but there is no evidence that diuretics are an independent risk factor for fetal growth restriction. The use of diuretics reduces the increased preload, thus have positive effects on LV function as well as symptoms and this justifies the use of diuretic therapy as first-line treatment.

Elevated vascular resistance and LV diastolic dysfunction is the rule in preeclampsia presenting as acute severe disease.[34] Parenteral vasodilators reduce afterload and the fall of vascular resistance leads to increase in LV stroke volume and cardiac output which ultimately leads to reduction of left-sided filling pressures.[35] Diuretic therapy leads to depletion of an already contracted intravascular volume whereas there is no reduction in systemic vascular resistance.

Nitroglycerine is a combined arterial and venous vasodilator. It is used in pregnant patients with HF who are acutely ill and not responding to diuretics alone.

Angiotensin-converting Enzyme Inhibitors

These drugs are relatively contraindicated in pregnancy, pregnancy being a state of physiological hyperreninism.[30] Neonatal renal failure may develop in babies delivered by mothers who were treated with angiotensin-converting enzyme (ACE) inhibitors during pregnancy.[36] ACE inhibitors have sufficient data as a safe drug while breastfeeding.

Beta-blockers

Use of β-blockers as antihypertensive has been associated with intrauterine growth restriction and increased perinatal mortality.[37] When adverse perinatal outcome may result from either underlying maternal disease or its treatment, but there is risk of maternal mortality, β-blockers can be used in pregnancy with HF.

Spironolactone

Spironolactone is a mineralocorticoid receptor antagonist. Its antiandrogenic actions and teratogenic potentials contraindicate its use during pregnancy. This drug can be used after the delivery of the fetus. Less than 1% of the drug passes from mother to child in the breastmilk.[6]

Digoxin

Digoxin is the safest antiarrhythmic drug to be used during pregnancy. It is Food and Drug Administration category C drug which is permeable though placenta and expressed in breastmilk.[29]

Angiotensin Receptor-Neprilysin Inhibitor

These drugs should be discontinued as soon as pregnancy is detected. During the second and third trimesters of pregnancy these drugs cause oligohydramnios which may cause fetal injury (e.g., hypotension, neonatal skull hypoplasia, anuria, reversible, and irreversible renal failure) and death. It is unknown if angiotensin receptor-neprilysin inhibitor (ARNi) is distributed in human breast milk, hence use is not recommended during lactation.

Hydralazine-Isosorbide Dinitrate

This combination can be considered for afterload reduction in pregnancy, instead of ACE inhibitors or angiotensin receptor blockers, though definite recommendations and robust studies are lacking.[29]

Ivabradine

Ivabradine is contraindicated in pregnancy and lactation due to lack of human data and animal studies showing adverse intrauterine and postnatal outcomes.

Bromocriptine

As discussed previously, a 16 kDa cathepsin-cleavage product of prolactin is incriminated for the pathophysiology of peripartum cardiomyopathy.[38] Bromocriptine suppresses lactation and is a reasonable treatment for this condition, though data is limited and needs further research.

Arrhythmias

Atrial fibrillation is the common arrhythmia in pregnancy. Beta-blockers are the drugs of choice and digoxin can be used if necessary. Implantable devices used for continuous monitoring may help to diagnose serious ventricular arrhythmias. Amiodarone is commonly used for treating sustained ventricular tachycardia. Implantable cardioverter defibrillators can be planned if indicated.[39]

Assist Devices and Inotropic Support

Inotropic support is a necessity in managing patients with acute HF in pregnancy. Treatment and dosage depend on the clinical situation and physician discretion as there is no randomized data guiding the same. Assist devices may act as a bridge between the initial presentation of the patient and access to cardiac transplantation services. Inspite of limited evidence these are potential adjuncts in the management of intractable HF.[39]

TREATING REVERSIBLE FACTORS

Structural heart diseases, like inflow or outflow tract obstructions, lead to HF during pregnancy. Second trimester balloon valvotomy of mitral, pulmonary and aortic valves in these patient subsets have been reported to be beneficial in multiple studies. Anemia, infections, and hyperthyroidism lead to increase of heart rate and aggravate HF. Subclinical thyroiditis affects up to 5% of women in the first postpartum year.[6] Urinary tract infection may frequently lead to genital tract sepsis during or after pregnancy and thus needs to be identified and managed properly.

SUPPORTIVE MEASURES

In HF patients during pregnancy thromboprophylaxis with once daily dosage of low molecular weight heparin is advocated.[40] If preeclamptic mothers develop pulmonary edema, the risk of maternal mortality is very high and thus medical termination of pregnancy is indicated.[6] Other treatable causes of pulmonary edema must be searched for and treated before considering termination of pregnancy.

THE MODE OF DELIVERY

The onset of labor leads to acute increase in LV workload and intravascular blood volume. There is also pain-mediated increase in catecholamine secretion. These changes are compensated to some extent by blood loss during delivery. The mother may need to do valsalva maneuver during second stage of labor. Assisted vaginal delivery using forceps limit the duration of second stage of labor and also the CV effects of valsalva. Induced labor is unpredictable and the possibility of emergency cesarean section always remains. The risks of anesthesia, hemorrhage, and postoperative complications must be kept in mind while performing a cesarean delivery, either elective or emergency. The decision to allow either vaginal delivery or to perform an elective cesarean delivery is peculiar to the individual case with multiple factors to be considered including the parity of the mother, any other. Though there is no justification for routine cesarean delivery in pregnant females with HF, a case-specific approach is necessary considering the parity, obstetric comorbidities, and the severity of the cardiac lesion. European Society of Cardiology Guidelines on the management of CVD during pregnancy provide individualized recommendations.[29]

THE PUERPERIUM AND LONG-TERM MANAGEMENT

Fluid overload must be avoided in the immediate postpartum period. The placental delivery and associated uterine contraction leads to expulsion of blood from this vascular organ and resultant fluid overload in the systemic circulation. Herein lies the benefit of IV diuretic therapy at the time of delivery in patients of HF and severe cardiac valvular stenosis. In general, ergometrine is avoided and low-dose oxytocin is advocated for the active management of the third stage of labor. Prophylactic antibiotics are necessary to prevent infections and to limit the risk of bacterial endocarditis.[41] Breastfeeding and its effects in patients of pregnancy with HF requires attention and further research.

HEART FAILURE WITH PRESERVED EJECTION FRACTION

No separate guideline exists for this group of patients in pregnancy till date. In the article titled Heart failure with preserved ejection fraction in women—the Dutch Queen of Hearts program, H. den Ruijter et al. have mentioned about preeclampsia as an important cause of HF with preserved ejection fraction (HFpEf) besides other known cardiac and systemic diseases. Diastolic dysfunction can develop in the patients of preeclampsia even 1 year after pregnancy. Management revolves around treatment of the cause and symptomatic relief with diuretics.

CONCLUSION

Women at increased risk of developing HF must be identified early and this would likely lead to proper monitoring and early intervention. Usual discharge from the hospital is planned within 2–3 days of delivery and next postdischarge visit is planned at around 6 weeks postpartum. Multidisciplinary team including cardiologists must keep proper surveillance on at-risk mothers during this period. This leads to better outcomes and fewer readmissions.[42,43] In addition, information, education, and counseling of the pregnant patients with HF regarding their condition can help them seek timely medical attention. These women can spread awareness and support among their social network after delivery and discharge from hospital.[44] HF-related maternal morbidity and mortality are disproportionately more among poor, advanced maternal age, and black population. Increased awareness and public health measures are needed to address the problems and search for management strategies among these high-risk population subgroups.

REFERENCES

1. Hunter S, Robson SC. Adaptation of the maternal heart in pregnancy. Br Heart J. 1992;68:540-3.
2. Clapp JF III, Capeless E. Cardiovascular function before, during, and after the first and subsequent pregnancies. Am J Cardiol. 1997;80:1469-73.
3. Saving Mothers 2011-2013: Sixth report on confidential enquiries into maternal deaths in South Africa. Short report, Republic of South Africa Department of Health, 2015.
4. Mogos MF, Piano MR, McFarlin BL, et al. Heart failure in pregnant women: A concern across the pregnancy continuum. Circ Heart Fail. 2018;11:e004005.
5. Brar SS, Khan SS, Sandhu G, et al. Incidence, mortality, and racial differences in peripartum cardiomyopathy. Am J Cardiol. 2007;100:302-4.
6. Anthony J, Sliwa K. Decompensated heart failure in pregnancy. Cardiac Fail Rev. 2016;2(1):20-6.
7. Thaler I, Manor D, Itskovitz J, et al. Changes in uterine blood flow during human pregnancy. Am J Obstet Gynecol. 1990;162:121-5.
8. Nolten WE, Ehrlich EN. Sodium and mineralocorticoids in normal pregnancy. Kidney Int. 1980;18:162-72.
9. Carlin A, Alfirevic Z. Physiological changes of pregnancy and monitoring. Best Pract Res Clin Obstet Gynaecol. 2008;22:801-23.
10. Dorn GW. The fuzzy logic of physiological cardiac hypertrophy. Hypertension. 2007;49:962-70.
11. Young P, Johanson R. Haemodynamic, invasive and echocardiographic monitoring in the hypertensive parturient. Best Pract Res Clin Obstet Gynaecol. 2001;15:605-22.
12. Seely EW, Ecker J. Chronic hypertension in pregnancy. N Engl J Med. 2011;365:439-46.
13. Vazquez Blanco M, Roisinblit J, Grosso O, et al. Left ventricular function impairment in pregnancy-induced hypertension. Am J Hypertens. 2001;14: 271-5.
14. Lindheimer MD, Taler SJ, Cunningham FG, et al. ASH position paper: Hypertension in pregnancy. J Clin Hypertens (Greenwich). 2009;11:214-25.
15. Simonneau G, Robbins IM, Beghetti M, et al. Updated clinical classification of pulmonary hypertension. J Am Coll Cardiol. 2009;54:S43-54.
16. Weiss BM, Zemp L, Seifert B, et al. Outcome of pulmonary vascular disease in pregnancy: a systematic overview from 1978 through 1996. J Am Coll Cardiol. 1998;31:1650-7.
17. Sharma BK, Jain S, Vasishta K. Outcome of pregnancy in Takayasu arteritis. Int J Cardiol. 2000;75:S159-62.
18. Milewicz DM, Dietz HC, Miller DC. Treatment of aortic disease in patients with Marfan syndrome. Circulation. 2005;111:e150-7.
19. Roos-Hesselink JW, Ruys TP, Stein JI, et al. Outcome of pregnancy in patients with structural or ischaemic heart disease: Results of a registry of the European Society of Cardiology. Eur Heart J. 2013;34:657-65.
20. Sliwa K, Libhaber E, Elliott C, et al. Spectrum of cardiac disease in maternity in a low-resource cohort in South Africa. Heart. 2014;100:1967-74.
21. Hilfiker-Kleiner D, Sliwa K. Pathophysiology and epidemiology of peripartum cardiomyopathy. Nat Rev Cardiol. 2014;11:364-70.
22. Sliwa K, Fett J, Elkayam U. Peripartum cardiomyopathy. Lancet. 2006;368: 687-93.
23. Ansari AA, Fett JD, Carraway RE, et al. Autoimmune mechanisms as the basis for human peripartum cardiomyopathy. Clin Rev Allergy Immunol. 2002;23:301-24.
24. Patten IS, Rana S, Shahul S, et al. Cardiac angiogenic imbalance leads to peripartum cardiomyopathy. Nature. 2012;485:333-8.
25. Autore C, Conte MR, Piccininno M, et al. Risk associated with pregnancy in hypertrophic cardiomyopathy. J Am Coll Cardiol. 2002;40:1864-9.
26. Krul SP, van der Smagt JJ, van den Berg MP, et al. Systematic review of pregnancy in women with inherited cardiomyopathies. Eur J Heart Fail. 2011;13:584-94.
27. Basso C, Corrado D, Marcus FI, et al. Arrhythmogenic right ventricular cardiomyopathy. Lancet. 2009;373:1289-300.
28. Sliwa K, Johnson MR, Zilla P, et al. Management of valvular disease in pregnancy: A global perspective. Eur Heart J. 2015;36:1078-89.
29. European Society of Gynecology (ESG), Association for European Paediatric Cardiology (AEPC), German Society for Gender Medicine (DGesGM), et al. ESC Guidelines on the management of cardiovascular diseases during pregnancy. Eur Heart J. 2011;32:3147-97.30. Hytten F, Chamberlain G. Clinical physiology in obstetrics. Boston, MA: Blackwell Scientific Publications, 1980.
31. Thorne S, Nelson-Piercy C, MacGregor A, et al. Pregnancy and contraception in heart disease and pulmonary arterial hypertension. J Fam Plann Reprod Health Care. 2006;32:75.
32. Soubra SH, Guntupalli KK. Critical illness in pregnancy: An overview. Crit Care Med. 2005;33:S248-55.
33. ter Maaten JM, Dunning AM, Valente MA, et al. Diuretic response in acute heart failure—an analysis from ASCENDHF. Am Heart J. 2015;170:313-21.
34. Belfort M, Anthony J, Kirshon B. Respiratory function in severe gestational proteinuric hypertension: The effects of rapid volume expansion and subsequent vasodilatation with verapamil. BJOG. 1991;98:964-72.
35. Belfort M, Akovic K, Anthony J, et al. The effect of acute volume expansion and vasodilatation with verapamil on uterine and umbilical artery Doppler indices in severe preeclampsia. J Clin Ultrasound. 1994;22:317-25.
36. Shotan A, Widerhorn J, Hurst A, et al. Risks of angiotensin-converting enzyme inhibition during pregnancy: Experimental and clinical evidence, potential mechanisms, and recommendations for use. Am J Med. 1994;96:451-6.
37. Swan L, Lupton M, Anthony J, et al. Controversies in pregnancy and congenital heart disease. Congenit Heart Dis. 2006;1:27-34.
38. Sliwa K, Fett J, Elkayam U. Peripartum cardiomyopathy. Lancet. 2006;368: 687-93.

39. Dickstein K, Cohen-Solal A, Filippatos G, et al. ESC Guidelines for the diagnosis and treatment of acute and chronic heart failure 2008. Eur J Heart Fail. 2008;10:933-89.
40. Ageno W, Squizzato A, Garcia D, et al. Epidemiology and risk factors of venous thromboembolism. Semin Thromb Hemost. 2006;32:651-8.
41. Dayer MJ, Jones S, Prendergast B, et al. Incidence of infective endocarditis in England, 2000–13: A secular trend, interrupted time-series analysis. Lancet. 2015;385:1219-28.
42. Rich MW, Beckham V, Wittenberg C, et al. A multidisciplinary intervention to prevent the readmission of elderly patients with congestive heart failure. N Engl J Med. 1995;333:1190-5.
43. Hanumanthu S, Butler J, Chomsky D, et al. Effect of a heart failure program on hospitalization frequency and exercise tolerance. Circulation. 1997;96:2842-8.
44. Weiss ME, Lokken L. Predictors and outcomes of postpartum mothers' perceptions of readiness for discharge after birth. J Obstet Gynecol Neonatal Nurs. 2009;38:406-17.

SECTION 22

Systemic Diseases and Heart

CHAPTER 141

Hypothyroidism and Heart

Niteen V Deshpande

INTRODUCTION

Thyroid hormones have a profound effect on the functioning of cardiovascular system and thus the common signs and symptoms of thyroid dysfunction are those arising from its effects on the heart and vascular system.[1] The relationship goes beyond the risk of atherosclerosis in hypothyroidism and atrial fibrillation in hyperthyroidism. Thyroid hormones modulate function of every component of cardiovascular system—the heart, blood vessels, and blood and thus alterations in cardiac contractility, myocardial oxygen consumption, systemic vascular resistance (SVR), cardiac output and blood pressure are observed in thyroid dysfunction. It is interesting to note that in almost all cases the cardiovascular abnormalities are reversible once thyroid dysfunction is recognized and treated.

Hypothyroidism affects between 4 and 10% of the population and has higher prevalence in women and patients over 60 years of age. Subclinical hypothyroidism is seen in around 10% population in various studies.[2-4] Diagnosis of hypothyroidism rests on demonstration of low levels of thyroid hormones (levothyroxine—T4 and triiodothyronine—T3) coupled with elevated levels of thyroid-stimulating hormone (TSH). Subclinical hypothyroidism is diagnosed when TSH levels are elevated with normal values of thyroid hormones. Overt hypothyroidism is diagnosed when TSH levels are more than 20 mIU/L with suppressed levels of T4 and T3 while TSH levels between 3 mIU/L and 20 mIU/L with normal T4 and T3 constitute subclinical hypothyroidism.[5-7] Estimation of TSH is thus appropriate initial test to evaluate thyroid dysfunction.

EFFECTS OF THYROID HORMONE ON CARDIOVASCULAR SYSTEM

The cardiovascular effects of thyroid hormone are mediated by T3. Heart relies mainly on serum T3 as the myocytes do not have significant deiodinase activity. Cellular actions of T3 are mediated through its binding with thyroid receptors (TRs). These receptor proteins induce transcription by binding to thyroid hormone response elements (TREs) in the promoter regions of positively regulated genes (Fig. 1).[8-10] Regulation of the key structural and regulatory genes by thyroid hormones thus modulates cardiac structure and function.[2] Thyroid hormone responsive cardiac genes include sarcoplasmic reticulum Ca^+ adenosine triphosphatase (SERCA) and its inhibitor phospholamban which regulate calcium uptake in sarcoplasmic reticulum in diastole, α-myosin heavy chain and β-myosin heavy chain and a number of ion channels which regulate electromechanical response of the myocardium.[1,8,11] Nongenomic effects of thyroid hormones include changes in various membrane ion channels for sodium, potassium, and calcium, effects on actin polymerization, adenine nucleotide translocator I in the mitochondrial membrane and a number of intracellular signaling pathways in the myocytes and vascular smooth muscle cells.[12-14] As a result of these effects, thyroid hormones affect the action potential and repolarization currents in cardiac myocytes.[15]

Hemodynamic effects of thyroid hormones include decreased SVR, increased resting heart rate (HR), left ventricular contractility and blood volume (Fig. 2). Direct effect of thyroid hormone on vascular smooth muscle cells of the peripheral arterioles reduces SVR causing reduction in the mean arterial pressure. This reduction of MAP is sensed by kidney activating the renin-angiotensin-aldosterone system leading to sodium resorption. T3 also increases erythropoietin synthesis which increases red cell mass. Blood volume is increased as a result of these changes and preload increases. In hypothyroidism the effects of thyroid deficiency are diametrically opposite and cardiac output decreases by 30–50%.[16] T3 also alters endothelial function and increased nitric oxide production may result as result of genomic and nongenomic mechanisms. In hypothyroidism, thus the arterial compliance is reduced leading to increase in SVR. In fact impaired endothelium dependent vasodilatation

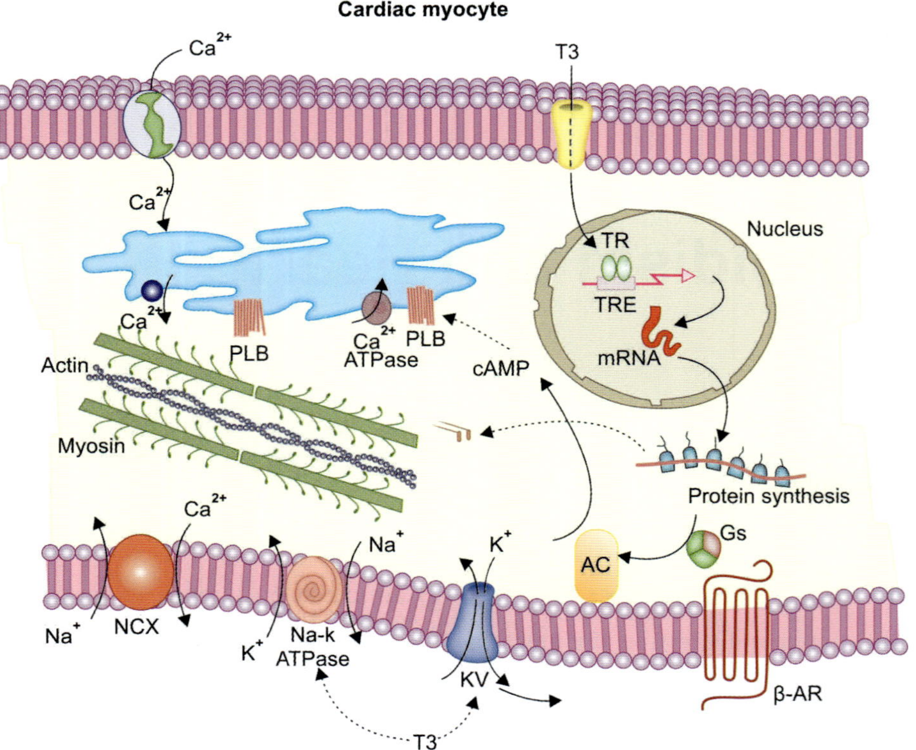

FIG. 1: Effects of T3 in the cardiac myocyte.
Source: Adapted from Klein I, Danzi S. Thyroid disease and the heart. Circulation. 2007;116:1725-35.

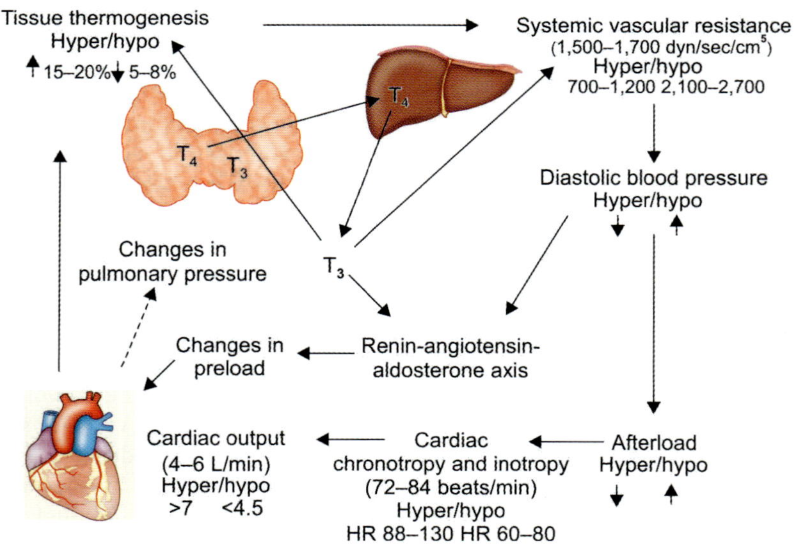

FIG. 2: Hemodynamic effects of thyroid hormone.
Source: Adapted from Klein I, Danzi S. Thyroid disease and the heart. Circulation. 2007;116:1725-35.

due to reduction in nitric oxide availability is demonstrated even in subclinical hypothyroidism.[17] Hypothyroidism is often associated with increase in diastolic pressure and its combination with reduced cardiac output results in narrowed pulse pressure. This diastolic hypertension in hypothyroidism occurs with low renin levels and is sodium sensitive.[18,19] Levels of serum erythropoietin are depressed in hypothyroidism resulting in normochromic, normocytic anemia in almost one-third patients.

Thyroid hormones also exert significant effect on lipid metabolism and it is well known fact that hypothyroid patients have elevated lipid levels with significant increase in low-density lipoprotein (LDL) cholesterol levels and apolipoprotein B.[20] The mechanism responsible for LDL-cholesterol elevation is reduction in the LDL receptor in liver and reduction in their activity.[20-22] Cholesterol metabolism is also altered by multiple mechanisms including biliary excretion leading to elevated cholesterol levels in hypothyroidism. This concept is supported by a recent study which showed that a liver specific thyroid hormone agonist—eprotirome had additive effect in statin treated patients in lowering total cholesterol.[23] A significant elevation in serum homocysteine levels and levels of C-reactive proteins are also common in patients with hypothyroidism.[2,24]

CARDIOVASCULAR MANIFESTATIONS

The most frequent cardiovascular signs and symptoms of hypothyroidism include bradycardia, mild diastolic hypertension, narrowed pulse pressure, and fatigue. Hypothyroidism is associated with reduced cardiac contractility, decreased cardiac output, accelerated atherosclerosis, and coronary artery disease.[25-27] Increased risk of stroke is also reported in hypothyroidism.[28,29] Acceleration of atherosclerosis is due to dyslipidemia, hypertension and hyperhomocysteinemia which develops in patients with hypothyroidism. Increase in cardiovascular morbidity and mortality was observed in a study in untreated subclinical hypothyroidism.[30] Some studies have also shown increased abdominal aortic atherosclerosis and increased carotid intima-media thickness and decreased myocardial perfusion which resolves with thyroid replacement therapy.[31] Small to moderate pericardial effusions occur in about 30% patients with hypothyroidism due increased volume of distribution of albumin and decrease in lymphatic clearance. The pericardial fluid may be golden in color due to presence of cholesterol crystals.[32] Pericardial effusions resolve in period of weeks to months following institution of thyroid replacement therapy[33] and rarely cause cardiac tamponade. Approximately 4% of the patients develop pericarditis. These patients need observation for development of pericardial effusion or cardiac tamponade although pericardial effusions can occur without pericarditis. Thus it is important to check serum TSH levels in patients with nontraumatic pericarditis where no other obvious cause is detected.[31] The electrocardiogram shows sinus bradycardia, low voltage complexes and prolongation of QT interval and rarely atrioventricular blocks. QT prolongation predisposes these patients to ventricular arrhythmias.[34] Echocardiography shows impaired relaxation in patients with overt as well as subclinical hypothyroidism. Early impairment can be demonstrated by prolongation of isovolumic relaxation time and reduction in E/A ratio.[35] More obvious findings include pericardial effusions and features suggestive of coronary artery disease with demonstration of regional wall motion abnormalities.

HYPOTHYROIDISM AND HEART FAILURE

Relationship of hypothyroidism and heart failure (HF) is recognized for long time. An early study by Schwimmer et al. showed improvement in HF and myxedema during therapy with desiccated thyroid extract.[36] Cases of hypothyroidism and reversible dilated cardiomyopathy have also been reported more recently.[37,38] Heart is a principle target of thyroid hormones and the transition from fetal to adult cardiac phenotype depends on the increase in thyroid hormones during the perinatal period.[39] In the adult life, normal thyroid hormone levels are required to maintain cardiovascular function. A number of attributes like inotropic and lusitropic properties of myocardium, cardiac growth, myocardial contractility, and vascular function are controlled by thyroid hormones. Hypothyroidism—overt or subclinical, has been shown to result in important changes in cardiac structure and function with their severity depending on the degree of deficiency.[40-44] Hypothyroidism results in decreased cardiac output due to bradycardia and low-stroke volume[40,41] and both systolic and diastolic functions are reduced at rest and during exercise. Impaired diastolic function and reduced blood volume lead to decreased preload and vascular function is also deranged.[43] Additionally, lower renal perfusion leads to impaired free water clearance and hyponatremia.[40] Experimental studies have demonstrated structural cardiac changes as well. Myocardial atrophy is seen in hypothyroidism due to decreased expression of α-myosin heavy chain genes and increased expression of β-myosin heavy chain genes. Dilatation of cardiac chambers and impaired myocardial blood flow are also observed in hypothyroidism.[45-47] Subclinical hypothyroidism is increasingly being recognized to be associated with HF. A recent meta-analysis of six prospective cohort studies which included more than 2,000 patients with subclinical hypothyroidism[48] confirmed that patients with serum TSH more than 10 mU/L are at increased risk of developing HF. Other way round, in patients with chronic HF, subclinical hypothyroidism is a risk factor for cardiac death.[49-51] Data on thyroid function in patients with HF from the Sudden Cardiac Death in Heart Failure Trial (SCD-HeFT) showed that HF patients who had abnormal thyroid function had higher risk of death even after adjustment for other factor associated with mortality.[52] Similar findings on HF patients discharged from hospital and followed for 3 years were reported by Sato et al.[53] The definition of subclinical hypothyroidism used in this study was serum TSH more than 4 mIU/L with normal T4 levels. The prevalence of subclinical hypothyroidism was 12% in this study and patients had worse outcomes as compared to those with normal thyroid function. Thyroid hormone metabolism is altered in patients with HF. The conversion of T4 to T3 is impaired leading to development of low T3 syndrome.[39,54-57] Low T3 syndrome is a strong predictor of mortality in patients with severe heart disease. Observed development of alteration in gene expression in failing heart is similar to that in experimental hypothyroidism indicating that thyroid dysfunction may play an important role in progression of HF.[58] More recently studies in rodent models have identified increased activity of cardiac type III deiodinase as a possible cause of diminished levels and action of thyroid hormones in HF.[59]

As thyroid hormone has such profound impact on HF and heart can develop in patients with hypothyroidism it is important to assess thyroid function in patients with HF. The American College of Cardiology guidelines for HF recommend a screening TSH test for all cases of newly diagnosed HF.[60]

EFFECT OF HEART DISEASE ON THYROID FUNCTION

Alterations in thyroid hormones metabolism accompany a number of disease states like sepsis, starvation and cardiac diseases. The primary abnormality in such conditions is reduced levels of serum T3 which has multifactorial origin. Reduction in hepatic 5'-monoiododinization is one of the important mechanism or reduced serum T3 levels.[25] Low serum T3 levels have been shown to correlate with increased all-cause and cardiovascular mortality in a population-based study.[57] Levels of T3 decline by almost 20% following uncomplicated myocardial infarction and thyroid replacement in experimental models may increase left ventricular function.[25] Serum T3 levels decrease predictably following cardiac surgery in the perioperative period in children and adults. However, intravenous T3 replacement in these situations has not resulted in mortality benefit although incidence of atrial fibrillation was reduced by 50%.[61] The decline in serum T3 levels is even greater in neonate following cardiac surgery and intravenous replacement of T3 in neonates has been shown reduce need of postoperative inotropic agents.[62] In patients with HF up to 30% patients have low serum T3 levels and this reduction in serum T3 levels correlate with function al class (NYHA).[63]

TREATMENT OF HYPOTHYROIDISM AND HEART

Thyroid replacement therapy with levothyroxine improves lipid profile, diastolic dysfunction, HR and delays progression of atherosclerosis.[11] However, treatment with levothyroxine in the setting of established or suspected cardiac disease poses a challenge of precipitating myocardial ischemia or arrhythmias. In older patients with heart disease it is recommended to start low (25–50 μg/day) and go slow (increase the dose gradually no sooner than 6–8 weeks) with thyroid replacement therapy. A predictable improvement in thyroid parameters and cardiac function is expected if these simple rules are followed.[26] Concerns about the euthyroid state achieved following treatment adversely affecting the cardiac status are largely unfounded. In fact, patients with atherosclerotic cardiovascular disease often improve, rather than worsening after levothyroxine therapy as observed by Keating et al.[64]

Treatment of subclinical hypothyroidism with levothyroxine has not shown to impact cholesterol levels or diastolic blood pressure in cohort studies.[65] A 18-month study of levothyroxine treatment in women with subclinical hypothyroidism however showed normalization of systolic and diastolic blood pressure, reduction in total cholesterol and LDL and decrease in carotid intima media thickness.[66] In patients with subclinical hypothyroidism and coronary artery disease levothyroxine treatment did not show any significant change while placebo treated patients had echocardiographic evidence of progression of diastolic dysfunction.[67] The elevated risk of cardiovascular disease in patients with subclinical hypothyroidism may be reduced with levothyroxine treatment as observed by a population-based study which found higher risk of cardiovascular events despite treatment in patients with TSH more than 4 mIU/L.[68] Interestingly the United Kingdom General Practitioner Research Database noted that treatment of subclinical hypothyroidism was associated with fewer ischemic heart disease events in patients younger than 70 years but not in patients older than 70 years. Based on the current evidence the European Thyroid Association guidelines recommend levothyroxine therapy for patients younger than 65 years of age and TSH levels above 10 mIU/L. Treatment for patients older than 80 years with TSH less than 10 is discouraged.[69] Treatment of subclinical hypothyroidism in patients with HF has shown to result in improvement of cardiovascular function.[70-72] Thyroid replacement therapy in these patients improves diastolic dysfunction, vascular function, and coronary flow reserve when euthyroid state is restored. In the cardiovascular health study risk of HF was significantly lower in T4 treated patients and patients with TSH more than 10 mIU/L had an increased risk of HF during periods of levothyroxine withdrawal than during its use.[73] Thus it appears that thyroid replacement therapy in patients with TSH more than 10 mIU/L should be considered to prevent HF events.[70] It is important to monitor these patients on replacement therapy for development of drug-induced hyperthyroidism, especially the elderly patients.

Amiodarone and Hypothyroidism

Amiodarone is a commonly used antiarrhythmic agent for treatment of tachyarrhythmia. It has very high iodine content (37% by weight) which exposes the patient to very high iodine load, almost 300 times the daily recommended allowance.[74,75] Due to its high iodine content, amiodarone can lead to thyroid dysfunction either hypothyroidism (5–25% of treated patients) or hyperthyroidism (2–10% of the treated patients).[76,77] Conversion of T4 to T3 is inhibited as a result of inhibition of 5'deiodinase activity. Also iodine released can directly inhibit thyroid gland function leading to hypothyroidism. Pre-existent thyroid disease and Hashimoto's thyroiditis, both are risk factor for amiodarone-induced thyroid dysfunction. A periodic evaluation is therefore recommended for patients being treated with amiodarone and thyroid replacement is advocated if TSH is persistently elevated. The antiarrhythmic effect of amiodarone is not affected by thyroid replacement therapy and is independent of the effect of the drug on thyroid hormone metabolism.[1] Amiodarone effect on thyroid hormone is not dose dependent and can occur anytime during the therapy and due to high lipid solubility of amiodarone the effect may be seen up to 1 year after discontinuation of the therapy.[78]

CONCLUSION

Thyroid hormones have profound effects on cardiovascular system through genomic as well as nongenomic mechanisms. Acceleration of atherosclerotic process leading to overt coronary artery disease occurs in hypothyroidism due to development of dyslipidemia, hypertension, and increased levels of homocysteine. Similarly, increased incidence of stroke is also associated with hypothyroidism. Subtle changes in cardiac structure and function are well documented in subclinical hypothyroidism. Association of clinical or subclinical hypothyroidism and HF is another area of current research and treatment. Population studies have shown a higher risk of developing HF in people with TSH levels exceeding 10 mIU/L. In HF patients hypothyroidism or low T3 syndrome is linked to higher morbidity and mortality. Thus recognition of these abnormalities and timely correction with thyroid replacement therapy can improve outcomes in patients with HF. However, correction of hypothyroidism is done gradually following the dictum "start low and go slow" to avoid precipitation of myocardial ischemia and arrhythmia.

REFERENCES

1. Klein I, Ojamaa K. Thyroid hormone and the cardiovascular system. N Engl J Med. 2001;344:501-9.
2. Klein I, Danzi S. Thyroid disease and the heart. Circulation. 2007;116:1725-35.
3. Ochs N, Auer R, Bauer DC, et al. Meta-analysis: subclinical thyroid dysfunction and the risk for coronary heart disease and mortality. Ann Intern Med. 2008;148:832-45.
4. Razvi S, Shakoor A, Vanderpump M, et al. The influence of age on the relationship between subclinical hypothyroidism and ischemic heart disease: a meta-analysis. J Clin Endocrinol Metab. 2008;93:2998-3007.
5. Demers LM, Spencer CA. Laboratory medicine practice guidelines: laboratory support for the diagnosis and monitoring of thyroid disease. Thyroid. 2003;13:3-126.
6. Levey GS, Klein I. Disorders of the thyroid. In: Stein DJ, Hollander E, Rothbaum BO (Eds). Stein's Textbook of Medicine, 2nd edition. Boston, Mass: Little Brown & Co.; 1994. p. 1383.
7. Surks MI, Ortiz E, Daniels GH, et al. Subclinical thyroid disease: scientific review and guidelines for diagnosis and management. JAMA. 2004;291:228-38
8. Kahaly GJ, Dillmann WH. Thyroid hormone action in the heart. Endocrine Rev. 2005;26:704-28.
9. Brent G. The molecular basis of thyroid hormone action. N Engl J Med. 1994;331:847-53.
10. Lazar MA, Chin WW. Nuclear thyroid hormone receptors. J Clin Invest. 1990;86:1777-82.
11. Napoli R, Biondi B, Guardasole V, et al. Impact of hyperthyroidism and its correction on vascular reactivity in humans. Circulation. 2001;104:3076-80.
12. Davis PJ, Davis FB. Nongenomic actions of thyroid hormone on the heart. Thyroid. 2002;12:459-466.
13. Hiroi Y, Kim HH, Ying H, et al. Rapid nongenomic actions of thyroid hormone. Proc Natl Acad Sci USA. 2006;103:14104-9.
14. Park K, Dai H, Ojamaa K, et al. Direct vasomotor effect of thyroid hormones on rat skeletal muscle resistance arteries. Anesth Analg. 1997;85:734-8.
15. Sun Z, Ojamaa K, Coetzee WA, et al. Effects of thyroid hormone on action potential and repolarization currents in rat ventricular myocytes. Am J Physiol Endocrinol Metab. 2000;278:E302-7.
16. Danzi S, Klein I. Thyroid hormone and the cardiovascular system. Minerva Endocrinologica. 2004;29:139-50.
17. Taddei S, Caraccio N, Virdis A, et al. Impaired endothelium-dependent vasodilatation in subclinical hypothyroidism: beneficial effect of levothyroxine therapy. J Clin Endocrinol Metab. 2003;88:3731-7.
18. Laragh JH, Sealey JE. Relevance of the plasma renin hormonal control system that regulates blood pressure and sodium balance for correctly treating hypertension and for evaluating ALLHAT. Am J Hypertens. 2003;16:407-15.
19. Marcisz C, Jonderko G, Kucharz EJ. Influence of short-time application of a low sodium diet on blood pressure in patients with hyperthyroidism or hypothyroidism during therapy. Am J Hypertens. 2001;14:995-1002.
20. Duntas LH. Thyroid disease and lipids. Thyroid. 2002;12:287-93.
21. Thompson GR, Soutar AK, Spengel FA, et al. Defects of receptor-mediated low-density lipoprotein catabolism in homozygous familial hypercholesterolemia and hypothyroidism in vivo. Proc Natl Acad Sci USA. 1981;78:2591-5.
22. Rush J, Danzi S, Klein I. Role of thyroid disease in the development of statin-induced myopathy. The Endocrinologist. 2006;16:279-85.
23. Ladenson PW, Kristensen JD, Ridgway EC, et al. Use of the thyroid hormone analogue eprotirome in statin treated dyslipidemia. N Engl J Med. 2010;362:906-16.
24. Vargas-Uricoechea H, Bonelo-Perdomo A, Sierra-Torres CH. Effects of thyroid hormones on the heart. Clin Investig Arterioscler. 2014;26:296-309.
25. Klein I. Endocrine disorders and cardiovascular disease. In: Zipes DP, Libby P Bonow R, Braunwald E (Eds). Braunwald's Heart Disease: A Textbook of Cardiovascular Medicine, 7th edition. Philadelphia, Pa: WB Saunders; 2005. pp. 2051-65.
26. Crowley WF Jr, Ridgway EC, Bough EW, et al. Noninvasive evaluation of cardiac function in hypothyroidism. Response to gradual thyroxine replacement. N Engl J Med. 1977;296:1-6.
27. Steinberg AD. Myxedema and coronary artery disease: a comparative autopsy study. Ann Intern Med. 1968;68:338-44.
28. Danzi S, Klein I. Thyroid hormone and blood pressure regulation. Curr Hypertens Rep. 2003;5:513-20.
29. Qureshi AI, Suri FK, Nasar A, et al. Free thyroxine index and risk of stroke: results from the National Health and Nutrition Examination Survey Follow-up Study. Med Sci Monit. 2006;12:CR501-6.
30. Walsh JP, Bremmer AP, Bulsara MK, et al. Subclinical thyroid dysfunction as a risk factor for cardiovascular disease. Arch Intern Med. 2005;165:2467-72.
31. Grais IM, Sowers JR. Thyroid and Heart. The Am J Med. 2014;127:691-8.
32. Alexander JS. A pericardial effusion of "Gold Paint" appearance due to presence of cholesterin. Br Med J. 1919;2:463.
33. Khaleeli AA, Memon N. Factors affecting resolution of pericardial effusions in primary hypothyroidism: a clinical biochemical and echocardiographic study. Postgrad Med J. 1982;58:473-6.
34. Fredlund BO, Olsson SB. Long QT interval and ventricular tachycardia of "torsade de pointe" type in hypothyroidism. Acta Med Scand. 1983;213:231-5.
35. Rodondi N, Bauer DC, Cappola AR, et al. Subclinical thyroid dysfunction, cardiac function, and the risk of heart failure. The Cardiovascular Health study. J Am Coll Cardiol. 2008;52:1152-9.
36. Schwimmer D, Vogel M, McGavack TH. Clinical manifestations in forty cases of myxedema. J Clin Endocrinol Metab. 1947;7:468.
37. Khochtali I, Hamza N, Harzallah O, et al. Reversible dilated cardiomyopathy caused by hypothyroidism. Int Arch Med. 2011;21:4-20.
38. Ladenson PW, Sherman SI, Baughman KL, et al. Reversible alterations in myocardial gene expression in a young man with dilated cardiomyopathy and hypothyroidism. PNAS. 1992;89:5251-5.
39. Gerdes AM, Iervasi G. Thyroid replacement therapy and heart failure. Circulation. 2010;122:385-93.
40. Fazio S, Palmieri EA, Lombardi G et al. Effects of thyroid hormone on the cardiovascular system. Recent Prog Horm Res. 2004;59:31-50.
41. Biondi B, Palmieri EA, Lombardi G, et al. Subclinical hypothyroidism and cardiac function. Thyroid. 2002;12:505-10.
42. Biondi B, Klein I. Hypothyroidism as a risk factor for cardiovascular disease. Endocrine. 2004;24:1-13.
43. Ripoli A, Pingitore A, Favilli B, et al. Does subclinical hypothyroidism affect cardiac pump performance? Evidence from a magnetic resonance imaging study. J Am Coll Cardiol. 2005;45:439-45.
44. Biondi B. Cardiovascular effects of mild hypothyroidism. Thyroid. 2007;17:625-30.
45. Liu Y, Redetzke RA, Said S, et al. Serum thyroid hormone levels may not accurately reflect thyroid tissue levels and cardiac function in mild hypothyroidism. Am J Physio. Heart Circ Physiol. 2008;294:H2137-43.

46. Liu Z, Gerdes AM. Influence of hypothyroidism and the reversal of hypothyroidism on hemodynamics and cell size in the adult rat heart. J Mol Cell Cardiol. 1990;22:1339-48.
47. Tang YD, Kuzman JA, Said S, et al. Low thyroid function leads to cardiac atrophy with chamber dilatation, impaired myocardial blood flow, loss of arterioles, and severe systolic dysfunction. Circulation. 2005;112:3122-30.
48. Gencer B, Collet TH, Virgini V, et al. Subclinical thyroid dysfunction and the risk of heart failure events: an individual participant data analysis from six prospective cohorts. Circulation. 2012;126:1040-9.
49. Nanchen D, Gussekloo J, Westendorp RG, et al. Subclinical thyroid dysfunction and the risk of heart failure in older persons at high cardiovascular risk. J Clin Endocrinol Metab. 2012;97:852-61.
50. Iacoviello M, Guida P, Guastamacchia E, et al. Prognostic role of sub-clinical hypothyroidism in chronic heart failure outpatients. Curr Pharm Design. 2008;14:2686-92.
51. Silva-Tinoco R, Castillo-Martı̀nez L, Orea-Tejeda A, et al. Developing thyroid disorders is associated with poor prognosis factors in patient with stable chronic heart failure. Int J Cardiol. 2011;147:e24-5.
52. Mitchell JE, Hellkamp AS, Mark DB, et al. Thyroid function in heart failure and impact on mortality. J Am Coll Cardiol. 2013;1:48-55.
53. Sato Y, Yoshihisa A, Kimishima Y, et al. Subclinical hypothyroidism is associated with adverse prognosis in heart failure patients. Can J Cardiol. 2018;34:80-7.
54. Khalife WI, Tang YD, Kuzman JA, et al. Treatment of subclinical hypothyroidism reverses ischemia and prevents myocyte loss and progressive LV dysfunction in hamsters with dilated cardiomyopathy. Am J Physio Heart Circ Physiol. 2005;289:H2409-H2415.
55. Mourouzis I, Forini F, Pantos C, et al. Thyroid hormone and cardiac disease: from basic concepts to clinical application. J Thyroid Res. 2011;2011:958626.
56. Pingitore A, Landi P, Taddei MC, et al. Triiodothyronine levels for risk stratification of patients with chronic heart failure. Am J Med. 2005;118:132-6.
57. Lervasi G, Pingitore A, Landi P, et al. Low-T3 syndrome: a strong prognostic predictor of death in patients with heart disease. Circulation. 2003;107:708-13.
58. Kinugawa K, Minobe WA, Wood WM, et al. Signaling pathways responsible for fetal gene induction in the failing human heart: evidence for altered thyroid hormone receptor gene expression. Circulation. 2001;103:1089-94.
59. Janssen R, Muller A, Simonides WS. Cardiac thyroid hormone metabolism and heart failure. Eur Thyroid J. 2017;6:130-7.
60. Jessup M, Abraham WT, Casey DE, et al. Focused update: ACCF/AHA guidelines for the diagnosis and management of heart failure in adults: a report of the American College of Cardiology Foundation/American Heart Association Task Force on Practice Guidelines: developed in collaboration with the International Society for Heart and Lung Transplantation. Circulation. 2009;119:1977-2016.
61. Klemperer JD, Klein I, Ojamaa K, et al. Triiodothyronine therapy lowers the incidence of atrial fibrillation after cardiac operations. Ann Thorac Surg. 1996;61:1323-7.
62. Chowdhury D, Parnell V, Ojamaa K, et al. Usefulness of triiodothyronine (T3) treatment after surgery for complex congenital heart disease in infants and children. Am J Cardiol. 1999;84:1107-9.
63. Pingitore A, Galli E, Barison A, et al. Acute effects of triiodothyronine (T3) replacement therapy in patients with chronic heart failure and low-T3 syndrome: A randomized placebo controlled study. J Clin Endocrinol Metab. 2008;93:1351-8.
64. Keating FR Jr, Parkin TW, Selby JB, et al. Treatment of heart disease associated with myxedema. Prog Cardiovasc Dis. 1961;3:364-81.
65. Uvodcic M, Pena RH, Patham B, et al. Hypothyroidism and the heart. Methodist Debakey Cardiovasc J. 2017;13:55-9.
66. Adrees M, Gibney J, El-Saeity N, et al. Effects of 18 months of L-T4 replacement in women with subclinical hypothyroidism. Clin Endocrinol. 2009;71:298-303.
67. Fadeyev VV, Sytch J, Kalashnikov V, et al. Levothyroxine replacement therapy in patients with subclinical hypothyroidism and coronary artery disease. Endocr Pract. 2006;12:5-17.
68. Flynn RW, Bonellie SR, Jung RT, et al. Serum thyroid-stimulating hormone concentration and morbidity from cardiovascular disease and fractures in patients on long-term thyroxine therapy. J Clin Endocrinol Metab. 2010;95:186-93.
69. Pearce SH, Brabant G, Duntas L, et al. 2013 ETA Guideline: Management of Subclinical Hypothyroidism. Eur Thyroid J. 2013;2:215-28.
70. Biondi B, Cooper DS. Subclinical thyroid disease. Lancet. 2012;379:1142-54.
71. Razvi S, Ingoe L, Keeka G, et al. The beneficial effect of L-thyroxine on cardiovascular risk factors, endothelial function and quality of life in subclinical hypothyroidism: randomized, crossover trial. J Clin Endocrinol Metab. 2007;92:1715-23.
72. Biondi B, Galderisi M, Pagano L, et al. Endothelial-mediated coronary flow reserve in patients with mild thyroid hormone deficiency. Eur J Endocrinol. 2009;161:323-9.
73. Klein I, Ojamaa K. Thyroid hormone and the cardiovascular system. N Engl J Med. 2001;344:501-9.
74. Batcher EL, Tang XC, Singh BN, et al. Thyroid function abnormalities during amiodarone therapy for persistent atrial fibrillation. Am J Med. 2007;120:880-5.
75. Cohen-Lehman J, Dahl P, Danzi S, et al. Effects of amiodarone therapy on thyroid function. Nat Rev Endocrinol. 2010;6:34-41.
76. Amico JA, Richardson V, Alpert B, et al. Clinical and chemical assessment of thyroid function during therapy with amiodarone. Arch Intern Med. 1984;144:487-90.
77. Martino E, Bartalena L, Bogazzi F, et al. The effects of amiodarone on the thyroid. Endocr Rev. 2001;22:240-54.
78. US Food and Drug Administration. (2009). Multaq (Dronederone): Briefing document. Advisory committee meeting of the cardiovascular and renal drug division of the US Food and Drug Administration. [online]. Available from http://www.fda.gov/downloads/AdvisoryCommittees/CommitteesMeetingMaterials/Drugs/CardiovascularandRenalDrugsAdvisoryCommittee/UCM134981.pdf [Accessed August, 2018].

CHAPTER 142

Cardiorenal Syndrome: Current Update

Dipak Sarma, Ritesh Kalwar

INTRODUCTION

Recent advances in medical sciences, both basic and clinical, have improved our understanding of organ crosslink in pathophysiological processes of disease conditions. The cardiorenal syndrome (CRS) is one example in this regard.

DEFINITION

Cardiorenal syndrome has been defined as "disorders of heart and the kidneys when acute or chronic dysfunction in one organ may induce acute or chronic dysfunction of the other".[1]

Brook et al. thus defined CRS as each dysfunctioning organ has the ability to initiate and participate disease in the other organ through common hemodynamic, neurohumoral, immunological, and/or biochemical feedback pathways.

CLASSIFICATION

Cardiorenal syndrome has been classified by Ronco et al. into five subtypes:[1]

- *Type I—acute cardiorenal syndrome*: Acute worsening of cardiac function leading to renal dysfunction. For example, acute cardiogenic shock and acute decompensated heart failure (ADHF)
- *Type II—chronic cardiorenal syndrome*: Chronic abnormalities in cardiac function leading to renal dysfunction. For example, congestive heart failure (CHF)
- *Type III—acute renocardiac syndrome*: Acute worsening of kidney function causing acute cardiac dysfunction. For example, acute kidney injury (AKI) and glomerulonephritis
- *Type IV—chronic renocardiac syndrome*: Chronic kidney disease (CKD) causing decline in cardiac dysfunction. For example, chronic glomerulonephritis (CGN) and interstitial disease
- *Type V—secondary cardiorenal syndrome*: Systemic conditions both causing kidney and cardiac dysfunction. For example, sepsis and diabetes mellitus.

LINK AND PATHOPHYSIOLOGY

The kidney and the heart are both highly vascular organs and both are supplied by sympathetic nervous system (SNS) and parasympathetic nervous system. Both organs play prominent role in blood pressure regulation as well as in intravascular homeostasis. Both have roles in natriuresis, diuresis, and oxygenation. The heart secrets the vasodilator, natriuretic peptide. The kidney is the main organ involved in the renin-angiotensin-aldosterone system (RAAS)[2] with so much in common, it is hardly surprising that dysfunction of one organ leads to the dysfunction of the other.

With advances in experimental and clinical sciences, it is now realized that the crosslink between the kidney and the heart is quite complicated, much more than what was believed in the past.

Low-flow State Hypothesis

For a long time it was believed that in ADHF patients, the reduced cardiac output leads to reduced renal perfusion, which in turn leads to activation of the RAAS leading to sodium and water retention, increased preload thus worsening pump failure.[3] Decreased glomerular filtration from afferent arteriolar constriction and profibrotic neurohormonal increase leads to ventricular remodeling, and further worsening of pump failure.[4] However, the findings of the recent ESCAPE (Evaluation Study of CHF and Pulmonary Artery Catheterization Effectiveness) trial showed that there was no correlation between renal function and cardiac index and that improvement of cardiac function did not result improvement of renal function. These findings, therefore suggested that the pathophysiology of CRS is more complex than just the low-flow hypothesis.[5]

Renin–Angiotensin–Aldosterone System

The activation of RAAS by the reduced perfusion pressure in the kidneys is a protective phenomenon in the initial stage. But when chronically stimulated, as in both cardiac and renal failure, the pathophysiological effect becomes harmful and severe. Renin which is produced by Juxtaglomerular apparatus in the kidneys in response to hypoperfusion carries out the conversion of angiotensinogen to angiotensin I and it is converted to angiotensin II (Ang II) by angiotensin-converting enzyme (ACE). Ang II has several deleterious effects on cardiovascular system (CVS), especially in the heart failure (HF) patients—increasing both preload and afterload thus myocardial organ demand. Ang II also converts nicotinamide adenine dinucleotide phosphate (NADPH) oxidase in cells, vascular and cardiomyocytes, mostly endothelial cells, vascular smooth muscle cell, renal tubular cell, and cardiomyocytes which lead to formation of reactive oxygen species (ROS) mostly superoxide which is responsible for the process of inflammation and organ dysfunction.[6-9] Nitric oxide (NO) is responsible for vasodilation and assist in renal control of extracellular fluid volume (ECFV). Superoxide not only antagonize these effects but also reduces the bioavailability of NO.[10] Oxidation stress damages deoxyribonucleic acid (DNA), proteins, carbohydrates, lipids and also shift cytokine production toward proinflammatory mediators, e.g., interleukin (IL)-1, IL-6, and tumor necrosis factor alpha (TNF-α). IL-6 also stimulates fibroblasts leading to increased cardiorenal fibrosis.[11]

Sympathetic Nervous System

Like the RAAS activation the SNS stimulation is also initially a protective mechanism in CHF patients. The SNS stimulation helps to maintain cardiac output by positive chronotropic and inotropic effects on the myocardium, but sustains SNS overactivity has several negative effects. It causes reduction of β-adrenergic receptor density within the ventricular myocardium.[12] It also reduces adrenoceptor density in both renal and HF[13] with the progression of ventricular systolic failure, there is diminution of renal blood flow and the perfusion pressure. This lead to baroreceptor mediated renal vasoconstriction, activation of renal sympathetic, and release of catecholaminergic hormones.[14] Also there is reduced clearance of catecholamines by the kidneys in patients with HF with advanced renal failure.[15]

Sympathetic nervous system activation also increases the release of the vascular growth promoter neuropeptide Y, leading to neointimal proliferation leading to atherosclerosis and vasoconstriction. It also interferes with normal immune system function.[16]

Intra-abdominal Hypertension

Intra-abdominal pressure (IAP) is said to be elevated when the pressure is more than 8 mm Hg. Intra-abdominal hypertension (IAH) is defined as IAP more than 12 mm Hg. HF is marked by an elevated central venous pressure which reduces the pressure gradient across the renal capillary bed. Earlier studies shown rising venous pressure could reduce or even abolish urine production.[17]

Extrinsic compression of renal vein has also been shown to compromise renal function.[18] A study of 40 patients with ADHF found that 24 had an IAP of more than 8 mm Hg and none had abdominal symptoms. The degree of reduction of IAP with diuretic treatment correlated with an improvement in renal function.[19]

The ESCAPE trial found that the baseline right atrial pressure but not atrial blood flow correlates with baseline serum creatinine.[20]

Arginine Vasopressin

Arginine vasopressin (AVP) has deleterious effect on CRS by retaining fluid and potentiating Ang II and potentiating activity. AVP also stimulates myocardial hypertrophy.[21]

Endothelin

Endothelin stimulates and potentiates noradrenergic, Ang II, aldosterone, and induces vasoconstriction.[22]

Drugs

Some drugs have adverse effect in progression of CRS. High-dose diuretics produces hypovolemia, intravenous vasodilators may cause hypotension. Inotropic drugs enhance neurohormonal activation. All these factors need to be taken into consideration while formulating treatment of CRS.

Cardiorenal Anemia Syndrome

Hemoglobin is an antioxidant, anemia which is common in both HF and CKD may contribute to the abnormal renal oxidative state. Normally, anemia induces increased production of erythropoietin (EP). But in CRS there is decreased concentration of EP. There is evidence to believe that a combination of anemia and decreased EP may exacerbate the underlying factor causing CRS.[23,24]

BIOMARKER IN CARDIORENAL SYNDROME

Renal Biomarker

Creatinine

As standard indicators of renal function, serum creatinine level and glomerular filtration rate (GFR) are vital for effective identification of renal disease and prognostic prediction of patients with renal disease.

Microalbuminuria

It is not only related to HF and CKD development but also rehospitalization and mortality rates in general population.[25] Mechanism linking microalbuminuria to HF remains unclear.

Neutrophil Gelatinase-associated Lipocalin

Neutrophil gelatinase-associated lipocalin (NGAL) is released due to an inflammatory reaction. NGAL predicts worsening of renal function correlates with inflammatory reaction and mediates ventricular remodeling in acute heart failure (AHF).[26]

In intensive care unit (ICU) adult patients with AKI secondary to sepsis, ischemia, nephrotoxins, NGAL is significantly increased in the plasma and urine.[27]

Cystatin C

It is a better predictor of glomerular function than serum creatinine in patients with CKD. Cystatin C has outperformed serum creatinine and estimated GFR in risk prediction for events in patients with cardiovascular disease (CVD).[28]

Kidney Injury Molecule-1

It is a transmembrane glycoprotein which is not normally detectable in urine.[29] It is measurable in urine after ischemic or nephrotoxic insults to proximal tubular cells.[30]

Importantly, kidney injury molecule-1 (KIM-1) may be elevated before there is histological evidence of proximal tubular cell death.[31]

N-Acetyl D Glucosaminidase

It is not only found in elevated urinary concentration in AKI and CKD but also in diabetic patients, and patients with essential hypertension and HF.[32]

Cardiac Biomarkers

Cardiac Troponin

As the component of the contractile apparatus in cardiomyocytes cardiac troponin-T and cardiac troponin-I are specific biomarkers of myocardial injury and infarction.[33] Elevated troponin T and I are related to myocardial injury, ventricular hypertrophy, HF and CKD.[34]

B-Type Natriuretic Peptide

B-type natriuretic peptide (BNP) is released from cardiomyocytes and plays diuretic, natriuretic, vasodilative and other cardioprotective roles. Patient with HF have over activated RAAS and SNS and compensated release of BNP due to ventricular and pressure overloaded. BNP is still deficient, in its role and are resisted in these patients.[35]

Myeloperoxidase

It predicts prognosis in patients with AHF. It has also elevated levels in CHF and can identify patients with HF irrespective of diastolic-systolic/right or left HF. It's positivity level correlate with CHF progression and predicts CV event in patients of CHF.[36] It also predicts CKD severity and mortality rates in patients with CKD.[37]

Copeptin

Whether heart releases copeptin, it is controversial[38] but it is a liable biomarker of CVD as well as significant predictor of mortality.[39] It has regarded as a hallmark of activated hypothalamus pituitary adrenal axis and thus received attention as a marker of AHF and AKI.

Soluble Vascular Endothelial Growth Factor Receptor-1

Vascular endothelial growth factor (VEGF), platelet-derived growth factor (PDGF) and soluble vascular endothelial growth factor receptor-1 (sFLT-1) have elevated levels in patients with HF. PDGF reduces infarct size and improves cardiac dysfunction, whereas sFLT-1 inhibits these role of PDGF. sFLT-1 is a biomarker that predicts prognosis in patients with HF.[40] SFLT-1 also contributes to endothelial dysfunction in CKD and links microvascular disease with HF in CKD.[41]

Mid-regional Pro-adrenomedullin

Adrenomedullin (ADM) is a potent vasodilator synthesized in the adrenal medulla whereas vascular endothelial cells, heart and elsewhere in response to physical stretch and specific cystokines.[42] It is very difficult to remove plasma ADM levels due to its short half-life and existing binding proteins.

Midregional pro-adrenomedullin (MR-proADM) is more stable and manufactured in a 1:1 ratio with active ADM.[43] MR-proADM thus a biomarker identity global disease burden in HF.[44] It also correlates with development of CKD and predicts the decline in renal function.

MANAGEMENT

Type-I Cardiorenal Syndrome

It occurs in the setting of ADHF or cardiogenic shock for a number of reasons.[45] While hypotension and decreased cardiac output with neurohormonal activation has been the traditional explanations for worsening renal function, however, recent evidence has implicated high venous pressure and raised intra-abdominal pressure leading to renal venous congestion as important contributor to impairment of kidney function,[46] as indeed many patient with ADHF and type-I CRS have preserved left ventricular ejection fraction and normal or high blood pressure. Hence diuretics, ultrafiltration (UF) and vasodilation are important steps in management.

Diuretics: Infusion or Bolus

Infusion therapy of diuretics has a greater efficacy than intermittent dosing.[47] However, in diuretic optimization strategies evaluation (DOSE) trial found that both bolus and infusion therapy have the same efficacy and similar renal outcomes. If the kidney function continues to worsen despite diuretic therapy, first possibility is that diuretic resistance secondary to mucosal edema decreased in intestinal absorption or excessive salt intake or concurrent use of nonsteroidal anti-inflammatory drugs (NSAIDs). Second possibility may be due to continuous blockade of RAAS with the use of ACE inhibitor (ACEi) or angiotensin receptor blockers (ARB) necessitating with holding or delaying the introduction of the same.[48]

Vasodilator

It is a modality for patients with a preserved or elevated blood pressure, nitroglycerin (NTG) are often used.[49] Nesiritide-B type natriuretic peptide helps in relieving dyspnea in AHF by decreasing preload and pulmonary vascular resistance and increased cardiac output.[50]

Inotropes

Positive inotropes like dobutamine or phosphodiesterase (PDE) inhibitor may be required, levosimendan with calcium sensitizing activity can be used, have shown mixed results.[51]

Other Measures

As a bridging therapy for the recovery of cardiac function or transplantation, more invasive therapies like intra-aortic balloon pump (IABP), ventricular assist devices or artificial hearts may be required.

TYPE-II Cardiorenal Syndrome

- Interruption of RAAS is the primary goal in the management of type-II CRS. Aldosterone blockers, spironolactone and eplerenone, are important adjunct therapy. However, use of these drugs, i.e., ACEI or acetate-free biofiltration (AFB) increases the risk of hyperkalemia, so have to avoid using the agent with serum creatinine more than 2.5
- Use of β-blocker: Interruption of sympathetic tone using β-blocker is another important strategy for patients with CHF or ischemic heart disease. Carvedilol has been demonstrated to have favorable effect on kidney function in CRS patients.[52]

Both CHF and CKD are associated with anemia and treated with EP which also helps in reducing apoptosis, fibrosis and inflammation,[53] and another approach is to use parenteral iron. In FAIR-HF (Ferinject Assessment in Patients with Iron Deficiency and Chronic Heart Failure) study, the patients/subjects in the treatment group (ferric carboxy maltose) were randomized to ferric carboxymaltose or placebo and active treatment group experienced improvement in HF symptoms, 6-minute walk test, and quality of life.

Type-III Cardiorenal Syndrome

Many strategies including hydration, diuretic, natriuretic peptide, N-acetylcysteine, dopamine have been studied, however, most successful intervention is isotonic fluid, along with some controversy regarding N-acetylcysteine.[54] Use of low-osmolar nonionic monomer iopamide in the prevention of contrast nephropathy[55] has been studied.

Type-IV Cardiorenal Syndrome

The management focused on the reduction of CV risk factor and complications common to CKD patients which are anemia, hypertension, altered bone and mineral metabolism, dyslipidemia, albuminuria, and malnutrition.[56]

Treatment of anemia seems to lessen CV events; however, randomized control trials have shown that higher hemoglobin targets associated with worse outcomes.[57]

Observational studies have shown that elevated phosphate, parathyroid hormone, and inadequate vitamin D receptor activities are potential risk factor for type-IV CRS.[58] Phosphate-binding products, cinacalcet, a drug used for lowering parathyroid hormone, decreased hospitalization related to CVD.[59]

Study of Heart and Renal Protection (SHARP) trial has suggested the use of statins in prevention of major atherosclerotic events.[60]

Type-V Cardiorenal Syndrome

- It includes a heterogeneous group of disorders like sepsis, systemic lupus erythematosus (SLE), diabetes mellitus, and amyloidosis
- Treatment should be done according to cause
- De Backer and colleagues compared dopamine versus noradrenaline in septic shock patient where they found that there is a higher incidence of cardiac arrhythmia in dopamine group[61]
- Another study indicates that low-dose vasopressin was effective in limiting cardiac and kidney injury in sepsis.[62]

CONCLUSION

The ability to make diagnosis of CRS will allow making early introduction of management strategies which will further help in better clinical and biochemical outcome.

Prognosis is not uniform in all subtypes and depend upon the underlying causes, worst is however for those patients with chronic dysfunction of both organ system.

Patient resistant to diuretic therapy may get benefit from UF. Infusion therapy of frusemide can be used in patients of ADHF with CRS.

It is a cross connecting process and difficult to understand and manage, more studies and trials are required for a better outcome. It is a challenging disease which has come across many physicians, cardiologists, and nephrologists.

REFERENCES

1. Ronco C, McCullough PA, Anker SD, et al. Cardio-renal syndromes: report from the consensus conference of the acute dialysis quality initiative. Eur Heart J. 2010;31(6):703-11.
2. Bock JS, Gottlieb SS. Cardiorenal syndrome: new perspectives. Circulation. 2010;121(23):2592-600.
3. Cannon PJ. The kidney in heart failure. N Eng J Med. 1977;296(1):26-32.
4. Smith GL, Vaccarino V, Kosiborod M, et al. Worsening renal function: what is a clinically meaningful change in creatinine during hospitalization with heart failure? J Card Fail. 2003;9(1):13-25.
5. Nohria A, Hasselblad V, Stebbins A, et al. Cardiorenal interactions: insights from the ESCAPE trial. J Am Coll Cardiol. 2008;51(13):1268-74.
6. Ushio-Fukai M, Zafari AM, Fukui T, et al. p22phox is a critical component of the superoxide-generating NADH/NADPH oxidase system and regulates angiotensin II-induced hypertrophy in vascular smooth muscle cells. J Biol Chem. 1996;271(38):23317-21.
7. Chabrashvili T, Kitiyakara C, Blau J, et al. Effects of ANG II type 1 and 2 receptors on oxidative stress, renal NADPH oxidase, and SOD expression. Am J Physiol Regular Integr Comp Physiol. 2003;285(1):117-24.
8. Nakagami H, Takemoto M, Liao JK. NADPH oxidase-derived superoxide anion mediates angiotensin II-induced cardiac hypertrophy. J Mol Cell Cardial. 2003;35(7):851-9.
9. Bock JS, Gottlieb SS. Cardiorenal syndrome: new perspective. Circulation. 2010;121(23):2592-600.
10. Zou AP, Li N, Cowley AW Jr. Production and actions of superoxide in the renal medulla. Hypertension. 2001;37(2):547-53.
11. Wikto-Sarsat V, Friedlander M, Capeillère-Blandin C, et al. Advanced oxidation protein products as a novel marker of oxidative stress in uremia. Kidney Int. 1996;49(5):1304-13.
12. Bock JS, Gottlieb SS. Cardiorenal syndrome: new prospective. Circulation. 2010;121(23):2592-600.
13. Leineweber K, Heinroth-Hoffmann I, Ponicke K, et al. Cardiac -adrenoceptor desensitization due to increased -adrenoceptor kinase activity in chronic uremia. J Am Soc Nephrol. 2002;13(1):117-24.
14. Bristow MR, Ginsburg R, Minobe W, et al. Decreased catecholamine sensitivity and beta-adrenergic-receptor density in failing human hearts. N Engl J Med. 1982;307(4):205-11.
15. Laederach K, Weidmann P. Plasma and urinary catecholamines as related to renal function in man. Kidney Int. 1983;31:107-11.

16. Li L, Lee EW, Ji H, et al. Neuropeptide Y-induced acceleration of postangioplasty occlusion of rat carotid artery. Arterioscler Thromb Vasc Biol. 2003;23:1204-10.
17. Winton FR. The influence of venous pressure on the isolated mammalian kidney. J Physiol. 1931;72(1):49-61.
18. Bradley SE, Bradly GP. The effect of increase intra-abdominal pressure on renal function in men. J Clin invest. 1947;26:1010-5.
19. Mullens W, Abrahams Z, Skouri HN, et al. Elevated intra-abdominal pressure in acute decompensated heart failure: a potential contributor to worsening renal function? J Am Coll Cardiol. 2008;51(3):300-6.
20. Nohria A, Hasselblad V, Stebbins A, et al. Cardiorenal interactions: insights from the ESCAPE trail. J Am Coll Cardiol. 2008;51(13):1268-74.
21. Lee CR, Watkins ML, Patterson JH, et al. Vasopressin: A new target for the treatment of heart failure. Am Heart J. 2003;146(1):9-18.
22. Moe GW, Rouleau JL, Nguyen QT, et al. Role of endothelin in congestive heart failure. Can J Physiol Pharmacol. 2003;81:588-97.
23. Burger D, Lei M, Geoghegan-Morphet N, et al. Erythropoietin protects cardio-myocytes from apoptosis via up regulation of endothelial nitric oxide synthase cardio vascular research. 2006;72(1):51-9.
24. Mancini DM, Katz SD, Lang CC, et al. Effect of erythropoietin on exercise capacity in patients with moderate to severe chronic heart failure. Circulation. 2003;107(2):294-9.
25. Iacoviello M, Leone M, Antoncecchi V, et al. Evaluation of chronic kidney disease in chronic heart failure: From biomarkers to arterial renal resistances. World J Clin Cases. 2015;3(1):10-9.
26. Jungbauer CG, Birner C, Jung B, et al. Kidney injury molecule-1 and N-acetyl-β-D- glucosaminidase in chronic heart failure: possible biomarkers of cardiorenal syndrome. Eur J Heart Fail. 2011;13(10):1104-10.
27. Mori K, Nakao K. Neutrophil gelatinase-associated lipocalin as the real time indicator of active kidney damage. Kidney Int. 2007;71(10):967-70.
28. McMurrary MD, Trivax JE, McCullough PA. Serum cystatin-C, renal filtration function, and left ventricular remodeling. Circ Heart Fail. 2009;2:86-9.
29. Prozialeck WC, Edwards JR, Lamar PC, et al. Expression of kidney molecule-1 (Kim-1) in relation to necrosis and apoptosis during the early stage of Cd-induced proximal tubule injury. Toxicol Appl Pharmacol. 2009;238(3):306-14.
30. Vaidya VS, Ramirez V, Ichimura T, et al. Urinary kidney injury molecule-1: a sensitive quantitative biomarker for early detection of kidney tubular injury. Am J Physiol Renal Physiol. 2006;290(2):F517-29.
31. Kobayashi M, Hirawa N, Morita S, et al. Silent brain infarction and rapid decline of kidney function in patients with CKD: a prospective cohort study. Am J Kidney Dis. 2010;56(3):468-76.
32. Wellwood JM, Ellis BG, Price RG, et al. Urinary N-acetyl-beta-D-glucosaminidase activities in patients with renal disease. Br Med J. 1975;3(5980):408-11.
33. Expert Group on Biomarkers. Biomarkers in Cardiology-Part 2: In Coronary Heart Disease, Valve Disease and Special Situations. Arq Bras Cardiol. 2015;104(5):337-46.
34. Morawiec B, Fournier S, Tapponnier M, et al. Performance of highly sensitive cardiac troponin T assay to detect ischemia at PET-CT in low-risk patients with acute coronary syndrome: a prospective observational study. BMJ Open. 2017;7(7)e014655.
35. Franeková J, Hošsková L, Se nik P Jr, et al. The role of timely measurement of galectin-3, NT-proBNP, cystatin C and hsTnT in predicting prognosis and heart function after heart transplantation. Clin Chem Lab Med. 2016;54(2):339-44.
36. Gedikli O, Kiris A, Hosoglu Y, et al. Serum myeloperoxidase level is associated with heart-type fatty acid-binding protein but not troponin T in patients with chronic heart failure. Med Princ Pract. 2015;24(1):42-6.
37. Afshinnia F, Zeng L, Byun J, et al. Myeloperoxidase levels and its product 3-chlorotyrosine predict chronic kidney disease severity and associated coronary artery disease. Am J Nephrol. 2017;46(1):73-81.
38. Boeckel JN, Oppermann J, Anadol R, et al. Analyzing the release of copeptin from the heart in acute myocardial infarction using a transcoronary gradient model. Sci Rep. 2016;6.
39. Tasevska I, Enhörning S, Persson M, et al. Copeptin predicts coronary artery disease cardiovascular and total mortality. Heart. 2016;102(2):127-32.
40. Vorovich E, French B, Ky B, et al. Biomarker predictors of cardiac hospitalization in chronic heart failure: a recurrent event analysis. J Card Fail. 2014;20(8):569-76.
41. Hannan NJ, Brownfoot FC, Cannon P, et al. Resveratrol inhibits release of soluble fms-like tyrosine kinase (sFlt-1) and soluble endoglin and improves vascular dysfunction-implications as a preeclampsia treatment. Sci Rep. 2017;7(1):1819.
42. Jougasaki M, Burnett JC Jr. Adrenomedullin: potential in physiology and pathophysiology. Life Sci. 2000;66(10):855-72.
43. Morgenthaler NG, Struck J, Alonso C, et al. Measurement of midregional proadrenomedullin in plasma with an immunoluminometric assay. Clin Chem. 2005;51(10):1823-9.
44. Klip IT, Voors AA, Anker SD, et al. Prognostic value of mid-regional pro-adrenomedullin in patients with heart failure after an acute myocardial infarction. Heart. 2011;97(11):892-8.
45. Hunt SA, Abraham WT, Chin MH, et al. 2009 focused update incorporated into the ACC/AHA 2005 Guidelines for the Diagnosis and Management of Heart Failure in Adults: a report of the American College of Cardiology Foundation/American Heart Association Task Force of Practice Guidelines: development in collaboration with the International Society for heart and Lung Transplantation. Circulation. 2009;119(14):e391-479.
46. Dickstein K, Cohen-Solal A, Filippatos G, et al. ESC guidelines for the diagnosis and treatment of acute and chronic heart failure 2008: the Task Force for the diagnosis and treatment of acute and chronic heart failure 2008 of the European Society of Cardiology. Developed in collaboration with the Heart Failure Association of the ESC (HFA) endorsed by the European Society of Intensive Care Medicine (ESICM). Eur J Heart Fail. 2008;10(10):933-89.
47. Salvador DR, Rey NR, Ramos GC, et al. Continuous infusion versus bolus injection of loop diuretics in congestive heart failure. Cocharane Database Syst Rev. 2004;(1):CD003178.
48. Heywood JT. The cardiorenal syndrome: lessons from the ADHERE database and treatment options. Heart Fail Rev. 2005;9(3):195-201.
49. den Uil CA, Lagrand WK, Valk SD, et al. Management of cardiogenic shock: focus on tissue perfusion. Curr Probl Cardiol. 2009;34(8):330-49.
50. Reichert S, Ignaszewski A. Molecular and physiological effect of nesiritide. Can J Cardiol. 2008;24(Suppl B):15B-18B.
51. Yilmaz MB, Yalta K, Yontar C, et al. Levosimendan improves renal function in patients with acute decompensated heart failure: comparison with dobutamine. Cardiovasc Drugs Ther. 2007;21(6):431-5.
52. Bakris GL, Hart P, Ritz E. Beta blockers in the management of chronic kidney disease. Kidney Int. 2006;70(11):1905-13.
53. Fu P, Arcasoy MO. Erythropoietin protects cardiac myocytes against anthra-cycline-induced apoptosis. Biochem Biophys Res Commun. 2007;354(2):372-8.
54. Jasuja D, Mor MK, Hartwig KC, et al. Provider knowledge of contrast-induced acute kidney injury. Am J Med Sci. 2009;338(4):280-6.
55. Solomon RJ, Mehran R, Natarajanet MK, et al. Contrast-induced nephropathy and long-term adverse events: cause and effect? Clin J Am Soc Nephrol. 2009; 4(7):1162-9.
56. Manley HJ. Disease progression and the application of evidence-based treatment guidelines diagnose it early: a case for screening and appropriate management. J Manag Care Pharm. 2007;13(9 Suppl D):S6-12.
57. Singh AK, Szczech L, Tang KL, et al. Correction of anemia with epoetin alfa in chronic kidney disease. N Engl J Med. 2006;355(20):2085-98.
58. Mathew S, Davies M, Lund R, et al. Function and effect of bone morphogenetic protein-7 in kidney bone and the bone-vascular links in chronic kidney disease. Eur J Clin Invest. 2006;36 Suppl 2:43-50.
59. Garside R, Pitt M, Anderson R, et al. The effectiveness and cost-effectiveness of cinacalcet for secondary hyperparathyroidism in end-stage renal disease patients on dialysis: a systemic review and economic evaluation. Health Technol Assess. 2007;11(18):1-167.
60. Baigent C, Landry M. Study of Heart and Renal Protection (SHARP). American Society of Nephrology Renal Week, Denver, CO, USA. 2010.
61. De Backer D, Biston P, Devriendt J, et al. Comparison of dopamine and norepinephrine in the treatment of shock. N Eng J Med. 2010;362(9):779-89.
62. Simon F, Giudici R, Scheuerle A, et al. Comparison of cardiac, hepatic and renal effects of arginine vasopressin and noradrenaline during porcine fecal peritonitis: a randomized controlled trail. Crit Care. 2009;13(4):R113.

CHAPTER 143

Anemia in Heart Failure

Umesh C Samal, Harikrishnan S

INTRODUCTION

Anemia is a frequent comorbidity in patients with heart failure (HF) and it increases mortality, recurrent hospitalizations, and morbidity in terms of impaired exercise capacity and poor quality of life (QoL).[1]

The World Health Organization defines anemia as a hemoglobin (Hb) value less than 13 g/dL for men and 12 g/dL for women.[2] Iron deficiency (ID) with or without anemia has been commonly associated with HF and is of renewed interest recently with new data.[3]

The major cardiology physician communities have understood the importance of this risk factor and has come out with specific guidelines addressing this issue.[4,5]

Even though there is a clear cut evidence that ID is an important comorbidity, it is often ignored or considered clinically only in the context of anemia.[1]

EPIDEMIOLOGY OF ANEMIA AND IRON DEFICIENCY IN HEART FAILURE

Most of the studies on HF indicates that the prevalence of anemia is more than 20%.[6] In a large meta-analysis of 1,53,180 patients, the prevalence of anemia was 34%.[7] In various studies, anemia was found to be associated with an increased risk of mortality in both HF with reduced ejection fraction (HFrEF) and HF with preserved ejection fraction (HFpEF).[7,8]

The reported prevalence of anemia varies with different studies due to the variability in the definitions used, the proportion of male and female patients in the study or whether it was acute or chronic where dilutional anemia influences the values.[4] The prevalence of anemia is higher in patients with advanced age, low functional capacity, and lower renal function.[6]

Iron deficiency is much more prevalent than anemia. In an international pooled analysis the prevalence of ID in HF was 50%.[9] It was found in the analysis that, anemic patients were more often iron deficient than nonanemic patients (61.2% vs. 45.6%).[9]

In a small study of 150 patients from Rajasthan, India, ID was present in 76% patients with 48.7% patients having absolute and 27.3% patients having functional type of ID.[10] Females had significantly higher (91.6% vs. 68.6%) prevalence of ID than males.

About one-fourth of the patients were having ID without anemia, which as the authors highlight, signifying the importance of workup to identify ID, rather than testing Hb alone.[10]

PATHOGENESIS OF ANEMIA IN HEART FAILURE

In HF, the sensitivity of bone marrow to erythropoietin (EPO) is low. Renin–angiotensin–aldosteron system (RAAS) activation which happens in HF even though leads to stimulation of EPO, it will not produce the desired effect. Also reduced renal perfusion in HF leads to renal dysfunction and we know that chronic kidney disease (CKD) is associated with anemia. Also some drugs acting on the RAAS system like angiotensin-converting enzyme inhibitor or angiotensin receptor blocker (ACEI/ARB) reduce EPO secretion and contribute to anemia (Flowchart 1).

CONSEQUENCES OF ANEMIA AND IRON DEFICIENCY IN HEART FAILURE

Iron deficiency often appears before the onset of clinically recognizable anemia and can be diagnosed by biochemical investigations.

To understand how ID can be diagnosed and managed, we have to know the details of iron metabolism in the body. Two body proteins (transferrin and ferritin) and a receptor (transferrin receptor) play the key role in the storage and transport of iron in the body. Transferrin carries iron in blood and other body fluids. The transferrin receptor present on cell membranes, internalizes transferrin, to make it intracellular iron. The protein ferritin stores iron in tissues.

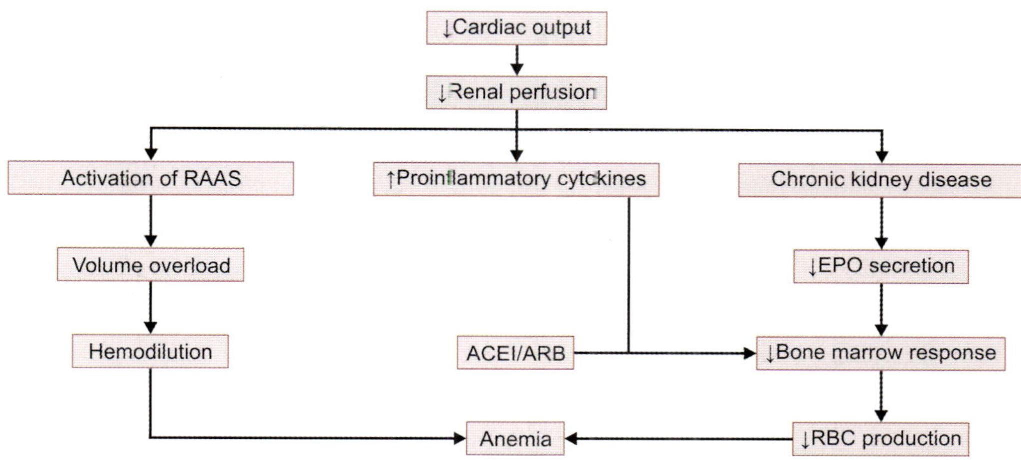

ACEI, angiotensin-converting enzyme inhibitor; ARB, angiotensin receptor blocker; EPO, erythropoietin; RAAS, renin–angiotensin–aldosterone system; RBC, red blood cell.

FLOWCHART 1: Mechanism of the development of anemia in heart failure.

Two important proteins are involved in iron metabolism—they are ferroportin and hepcidin. "Hepcidin is said to bind to ferroportin and induces its internalization, thus blocking iron export from intestinal cells and iron recycling in macrophages of the reticuloendothelial system (RES)".[1] So hepcidin is the main negative feedback component in the loop of iron metabolism. We know that hepcidin synthesis is induced by inflammatory states like HF and this contributes to ID.

HOW TO DIAGNOSE IRON DEFICIENCY?

Serum ferritin is the best indicator of iron stores, but ferritin is an acute phase reactant—its levels increase very rapidly in the presence of inflammatory states—HF is one such situation. Therefore, we cannot rely on low ferritin levels in HF to diagnose ID. Serum transferrin is less affected by changes in iron metabolism. A decrease of transferrin iron saturation indicates what is called the "functional ID".

In the 2016 European Society of Cardiology (ESC) guidelines[5] for the diagnosis and treatment of HF, systematic measurement of iron parameters [serum ferritin and transferrin saturation (TSAT)] is recommended in all patients suspected of having HF, as well as in the follow-up visits of HF patients. Transferrin saturation, measured as a percentage, is a medical laboratory value. It is the value of serum iron divided by the total iron-binding capacity (TIBC).

In the ESC guidelines 2016, ID is defined as follows:

- Serum ferritin less than 100 mg/L (absolute ID), or
- Serum ferritin 100–299 mg/L and TSAT less than 20% (functional iron deficiency). (TSAT = serum iron/TIBC).

TREATMENT OF ANEMIA AND IRON DEFICIENCY

European Society of Cardiology recommends detailed evaluation to find out the exact cause of anemia (e.g., occult blood loss, ID, B12 or folate deficiency, blood dyscrasias).

Iron therapy has proven to be effective in the treatment of ID and anemia. Erythropoiesis stimulating agents did not improve clinical outcomes in HFrEF patients.

Both oral and intravenous (IV) routes of iron have been tried in the treatment of ID. Because of intestinal edema which accompanies HF and also the high hepcidin levels which can impair absorption of oral iron, it is said that functional ID is more efficiently corrected by IV administration of iron because this can bypass the intestinal barrier and overcome the iron sequestration.[1]

But oral iron therapy is much cheaper than IV iron. There is a recently published study from North India which suggests that improvement in QoL and exercise tolerance might be achievable with use of oral iron supplementation (ferrous sulphate 100 mg, twice daily for 3 months).[11]

The Canadian HF recommendations[4] suggest that for patients with documented ID, oral or IV iron supplement be initiated to improve functional capacity.

But the ESC Guidelines recommend only IV iron for treatment of ID.

Intravenous iron was trialled in two randomized controlled trials (RCTs) in patients with HF and ID both with and without anemia. IV ferric carboxymaltose (FCM) has been shown to improve symptoms, QoL and New York Heart Association (NYHA) class in the Ferinject Assessment in Patients with Iron Deficiency and Chronic Heart Failure (FAIR-HF) trial[3] and in the CONFIRM-HF trial.[12]

In a meta-analysis of IV iron therapy in HFrEF patients with ID showed reduction in hospitalization rates and improved symptoms of HF, exercise capacity and QoL.[13] ESC recommendations say that the effect of treating ID in HFpEF or HF with midrange ejection fraction (HFmrEF) and the long-term safety of iron therapy in either HFrEF, HFmrEF or HFpEF is unknown.[5]

In a practical recommendation in British Medical Journal, Alain Cohen-Solal et al. recommends "oral iron should be prescribed for absolute ID for at least 3 months with assessment of iron replenishment after 1 month; in

TABLE 1: Dosage and administration of intravenous iron complexes[1]

Intravenous iron complexes	Dosage	Administration
Iron carboxymaltose (Ferinject 50 mg/mL)	Intravenous infusion at 15 mg/kg (for a total ≤1,000 mg) once/week Bolus intravenous injection of 200 mg/day (≤3 injections/week)	Intravenous infusion in normal saline (0.9%) with iron concentration >2 mg/mL: • From 100 to <200 mg: 50 mL of normal saline (0.9% NaCl) • From 200 to <500 mg: 100 mL of normal saline (0.9% NaCl, in ≥6 min) • From 500 to 1,000 mg: 250 mL of normal saline (0.9% NaCl, in ≥15 min) Bolus intravenous injection at a maximal dose of 200 mg
Iron hydroxide sucrose	100–300 mg/injection; 1–3 injections/week with a 48 h interval between each injection	Slow intravenous infusion (3.5 mL/min) with a duration ≥1.5 h; 1 ampoule diluted in ≤100 mL of normal saline (0.9% NaCl)
Iron hydroxide dextran	100–200 mg/injection (not exceeding 20 mg/kg); 1–3 injections/week with a 48 h interval between each injection	Intravenous infusion of 1 or 2 ampules (100 or 200 mg) in 100 mL of normal saline (0.9% NaCl) or 5% glucose Slow intravenous injection of 100–200 mg of iron (0.2 mL/min), preferably diluted in 10–20 mL of normal saline (0.9% NaCl) or 5% glucose

NaCl, sodium chloride.

case of inefficacy or intolerance, oral therapy is stopped and IV iron is administered. In case of functional ID, initial administration of IV iron is required since oral iron is ineffective in this clinical condition".[1]

All IV iron agents are colloids that mainly consist of iron-carbohydrate nanoparticles.[5] They are iron dextran, gluconate, sucrose, or FCM. Serious side effects, particularly anaphylactic reactions, have been reported with use of iron dextran, so it has become unpopular.

There are limited comparative data between the available IV iron preparations. Ferric hydroxide sucrose, ferric gluconate, and FCM are Food and Drug Administration (FDA)-approved for use in CKD patients. The recommended dose for FCM (750 mg) is higher than that for ferric sucrose (100–400 mg) or ferric gluconate (125 mg), so fewer injections of FCM may be needed to replenish the body iron stores (Table 1).

Serological iron profile should be performed 1 month after IV iron administration for evaluation of iron stores, and if necessary, repeat administration must be done.

CONCLUSION

Among patients with HF, one-third have anemia and half of the patients have ID. Anemia and ID have shown to affect the prognosis of patients with HF. The guidelines recommend the monitoring of iron parameters for all patients with HF. Iron supplementation, especially IV supplementation of iron, is shown to improve functional capacity and reduce hospitalizations.

REFERENCES

1. Cohen-Solal A, Leclercq C, Deray G, et al. Iron deficiency: an emerging therapeutic target in heart failure. Heart. 2014;100(18):1414-20.
2. World Health Organization. Vitamin and Mineral Nutrition Information System (VMNIS). Haemoglobin Concentrations for the Diagnosis of Anaemia and Assessment of Severity. Geneva: World Health Organization; 2011.
3. Anker SD, Comin Colet J, Filippatos G, et al. Ferric carboxymaltose in patients with heart failure and iron deficiency. N Engl J Med. 2009;361(25):2436-48.
4. Moe GW, Ezekowitz JA, O'Meara E, et al. The 2014 Canadian Cardiovascular Society Heart Failure Management Guidelines Focus Update: anemia, biomarkers, and recent therapeutic trial implications. Can J Cardiol. 2015;31(1):3-16.
5. Ponikowski P, Voors AA, Anker SD, et al. 2016 ESC Guidelines for the diagnosis and treatment of acute and chronic heart failure: The Task Force for the diagnosis and treatment of acute and chronic heart failure of the European Society of Cardiology (ESC) Developed with the special contribution of the Heart Failure Association (HFA) of the ESC. Eur Heart J. 2016;37(27):2129-200.
6. Tang YD, Katz SD. The prevalence of anemia in chronic heart failure and its impact on the clinical outcomes. Heart Fail Rev. 2008;13(4):387-92.
7. Groenveld HF, Januzzi JL, Damman K, et al. Anemia and mortality in heart failure patients a systematic review and meta-analysis. J Am Coll Cardiol. 2008;52(10):818-27.
8. Owan TE, Hodge DO, Herges RM, et al. Trends in prevalence and outcome of heart failure with preserved ejection fraction. N Engl J Med. 2006;355(3):251-9.
9. Klip IT, Comin-Colet J, Voors AA, et al. Iron deficiency in chronic heart failure: an international pooled analysis. Am Heart J. 2013;165(4):575-82.
10. Sharma SK, Agarwal SK, Bhargava K, et al. Prevalence and spectrum of iron deficiency in heart failure patients in south Rajasthan. Indian Heart J. 2016;68(4):493-7.
11. Sm M, Singh J, Laller K. Impact of oral iron therapy on quality of life in patients with heart failure. Int J Basic Clin Pharmacol. 2013;2(1):43.
12. Ponikowski P, van Veldhuisen DJ, Comin-Colet J, et al. Beneficial effects of long-term intravenous iron therapy with ferric carboxymaltose in patients with symptomatic heart failure and iron deficiency. Eur Heart J. 2015;36(11):657-68.
13. Jankowska EA, Tkaczyszyn M, Suchocki T, et al. Effects of intravenous iron therapy in iron-deficient patients with systolic heart failure: a meta-analysis of randomized controlled trials. Eur J Heart Fail. 2016;18(7):786-95.

CHAPTER 144

When to Screen and How to Manage OSA in Cardiology Practice

GC Khilnani, Pawan Tiwari

INTRODUCTION

Obstructive sleep apnea (OSA) is the most common sleep-related breathing disorder in adults worldwide. OSA is characterized by symptoms during sleep (excessive snoring, restlessness, or witnessed apneas) and daytime due to incomplete or disrupted sleep (morning headaches, excessive daytime somnolence, poor concentration); diagnosis is made by demonstrating obstructive events during sleep (apneas, hypopneas, or respiratory effort-related arousals) using polysomnography (PSG). Shakespeare described a character Sir Falstaff in his historic play Henry IV, who was found "fast asleep behind the arras, and snoring like a horse." The term "Pickwickian syndrome" originated with the obese character "Joe" in Charles Dickens novel. In 1965, Gastaut described the cardinal features of OSA, and first described use of polygraphy.[1] OSA was first successfully treated with tracheostomy in 1970s.[2] In 1981, Sullivan first described continuous positive airway therapy for treatment of OSA.[3] Wisconsin study by Young et al. examined the prevalence of OSA in general community and resulted in increased interest of medical community in this disease. OSA has been associated with increased risk of hypertension, coronary artery disease (CAD), stroke, heart failure (HF), and complex cardiac arrhythmias in various large prospective observational studies.[4-7] Due to ever increasing problem of obesity, and the fact that many patients may present with symptoms related to cardiovascular disease, a cardiologist is likely to be the first point of contact for patients with OSA. Thus, it is important for cardiologists to be proficient in management of OSA.

EXTENT OF THE PROBLEM

In a recent systematic review, the prevalence of OSA in adult population [defined as apnea-hypopnea index (AHI) >5 events per hour] ranges from 9 to 38%, with a higher prevalence in males (13–33%) as compared to females (6–19%); in advanced age groups, prevalence of OSA has been reported to be as high as 84%. Prevalence of moderate-to-severe OSA (AHI >15 events per hour) ranges from 6 to 17% in adults.[8] Prevalence of OSA in Asians has been reported to be similar to Western data, despite lower rates of obesity in this population.[9] Population prevalence of OSA and OSA syndrome (OSAS) has been reported to be 9.3% and 2.8%, respectively in a community-based observational study from Delhi.[10]

RISK FACTORS FOR OBSTRUCTIVE SLEEP APNEA

Increasing age,[5,11] male gender,[5,11,12] and obesity[5,13] are risk factors associated with increased prevalence of OSA. However, prevalence of OSA is increased in females postmenopause. Other risk factors include nasal congestion,[14] smoking,[15] positive family history,[16] and substance abuse (alcohol, sedative drugs, and narcotics).[17] Medical conditions that are associated with increased prevalence of OSA include pregnancy, chronic lung diseases (chronic obstructive pulmonary disease, asthma, and idiopathic interstitial fibrosis), congestive cardiac failure, acromegaly, hypothyroidism, polycystic ovarian syndrome, end-stage renal disease, and stroke.

Obesity remains the most consistent risk factor in development of sleep apnea. Incidence of OSA increased six times for each 10% increase in body weight in a prospective observational study.[18] Similarly, in a community-based study, there was progressive increase in prevalence of moderate-to-severe OSA with increasing body weight. Among subjects with normal body mass index (BMI), prevalence of OSA was 11% in males and 3% for females; among overweight subjects, prevalence increased to 21% in males and 9% in females; obese subjects had highest prevalence, i.e., 63% in males and 22% in females.[11]

Bony or soft tissue abnormalities of craniofacial region and upper airways are also associated with increased risk of OSA. This risk becomes more important in nonobese patients.[14,19] Recognition of these abnormalities is important as these may be amenable to surgical correction and potential cure for OSA.

CONSEQUENCES AND COMPLICATIONS OF OBSTRUCTIVE SLEEP APNEA

Obstructive sleep apnea is associated with higher all-cause mortality as compared to general population; positive dose-response relationship with higher mortality in moderate-to-severe OSA as compared to general population has been demonstrated, especially in middle-aged males.[20,21]

Obesity and OSA seem to be interlinked. Obesity is the most consistent risk factor for OSA, at the same time, OSA also independently contributes to development and worsening of obesity. This may be due to central dysregulation of appetite control,[22] leptin resistance,[23] increased ghrelin levels,[24] intermittent hypoxia, sleep disruption, arousals, increased inflammatory cytokines, and associated with OSA lead to obesity. Also, due to excessive daytime somnolence, there is decreased daily physical activity, aggravating weight gain. Both obesity and OSA are associated with similar comorbidities like hypertension and insulin resistance. Also, weight loss has been shown to improve severity of OSA in various studies.[25] Casual relationship between OSA and insulin resistance has been supported by large epidemiologic studies, with OSA conferring independent risk of diabetes mellitus.[26,27] Continuous positive airway pressure (CPAP) use in OSA has been shown to improve glycemic control.[28]

Association between OSA and hypertension has been reported in several large epidemiological studies.[7,29] In a recent meta-analysis of 20 studies, OSA was associated with increased risk of essential hypertension with pooled odds ratio of 1.18 [95% confidence interval (CI) 1.09–1.27] for mild OSA, 1.32 (95% CI 1.20–1.43) for moderate OSA and 1.56 (95% CI 1.29–1.84) for severe OSA.[30] OSA has been cited as the most common cause of resistant hypertension.[31] Use of CPAP for treating OSA has shown improvement in blood pressure control in various controlled trials and prospective studies[32,33] including refractory hypertension.[34,35] In a recent meta-analysis (30 studies, n = 1,900), CPAP use was associated with mean blood pressure reduction of 2.5 mm Hg, and was associated with significant reduction in cardiovascular events.[36] Recent guidelines also recommend screening for OSA in patients with refractory hypertension.[35]

Obstructive sleep apnea, apart from comorbid disorders like hypertension and CAD, may contribute independently to the development of HF by periodic increase in intrathoracic pressures during spells of apneas and hypopneas, intermittent hypoxemia, and increased sympathetic drive resulting in increased afterload. Though HF is usually associated with central apneas, OSA is being increasingly reported. In patients with HF, 12–53% were detected to have OSA in various studies.[37-40] In patients with OSA and low ejection fraction, fixed pressure CPAP reduces sympathetic activity and is associated with improvement in ejection fraction. However, advantages in HF with preserved ejection fraction are less clear.[40]

Premature contractions and atrial fibrillation (AF) are associated with OSA. OSA has been demonstrated to be an independent risk factor for complex arrhythmias in various observational studies.[41] The most common sustained arrhythmia associated with OSA is AF. Around 4.8% OSA patients had AF in sleep heart health study, as compared to 0.9% of controls.[6] Higher prevalence of OSA has also been reported in patients with AF.[41] Untreated OSA is associated with increased recurrence rates of AF; CPAP therapy is associated with decrease in AF recurrence.[42] Fatal arrhythmias due to recurrent sleep disruption and increased sympathetic drive are the likely cause of increased risk of sudden death during sleeping hours in OSA patients. Higher risk of sudden cardiac death has been reported in severe OSA as compared to mild-to-moderate disease.[43,44]

Coronary artery disease in OSA patients has been reported in up to 65% cases. Increased risk of myocardial infarction has been reported with history of snoring and severity of OSA.[45,46] Pre-existent OSA is an independent risk factor for cardiovascular death in patients with CAD[47,48] with decreased frequency and increased time to new cardiovascular events in patients treated with CPAP.[48] OSA has been associated with increased risk of stroke in various observational studies.[6] OSA was an independent predictor of stroke and all-cause mortality in another cohort study with a hazard ratio of 2.0.[49]

Other vascular complications of OSA include pulmonary hypertension. Usually, OSA causes only mild pulmonary arterial hypertension (PAH), unless there is associated cardiac or respiratory disease, or presence of obesity hypoventilation syndrome.[50] Postulated mechanisms for development of PAH include intermittent hypoxemia leading to pulmonary vasoconstriction with subsequent hypertrophy of smooth muscles and vascular remodeling.

Mood disorders including depression occur with increased frequency in patients with OSA, and can be presenting symptom of OSA in women.[51,52] Fibromyalgia and suicidal tendencies are other psychosomatic manifestations of OSA. OSA also contributes to significantly increased risk of cognitive impairment and road traffic accidents.[53]

SCREENING TOOLS FOR OBSTRUCTIVE SLEEP APNEA

As significant proportion of patients with OSA may present with cardiac symptoms, cardiologists should always evaluate patients for OSA. Patients presenting to cardiology services with hypertension, AF, coronary heart disease, HF, and PAH should be screened for OSA. Patients with comorbidities like obesity and diabetes mellitus should also be screened for OSA.

Screening tools for OSA include Berlin questionnaire (BQ), STOP-BANG questionnaire (SBQ), STOP questionnaire, and Epworth Sleepiness Scale (ESS). Commonly used scales are described in table 1. Modified Berlin scale is also available and has been validated for use in India. In a recent meta-analysis (108 studies, n = 47,989) comparing various screening tools (BQ, SBQ, STOP, and ESS) for the diagnosis of OSA, pooled sensitivity for mild OSA was 76%, 88%, 87%,

TABLE 1: Commonly used screening tools for identifying patients with obstructive sleep apnea

Modified Berlin Questionnaire*		Epworth Sleepiness Scale**	Score	STOP BANG***	Score
Category 1		Sitting and reading		Snoring (louder than talking/heard through closed doors)	
1. Do you snore?	Yes (1) No (0) Do not know (0)				
2. Your snoring is?	Slightly louder than breathing (0) As loud as talking (0) Louder than talking (1) Very loud—heard in adjacent rooms (1)	Watching TV		Tired/fatigued/sleepy during daytime	
3. How often do you snore?	Nearly every day (1) 3–4 times/week (1) 1–2 times/week (0) 1-2 times/month (0) Never/nearly never (0)	Sitting inactive in a public place		Observed stoppage of breathing during sleep	
4. Snoring bothering others?	Yes (1) No (0) Do not know (0)	Being passenger in motor vehicle for ≥1		Hypertension	
5. Has anyone noticed you quit breathing during sleep?	Nearly every day (2) 3–4 times a week (2) 1–2 times a week (0) 1–2 times a month (0) Never or nearly never (0)	Lying down in the afternoon		BMI >35 kg/m²	
Category 2		Sitting and talking to someone		Age >50 years	
6. Tired/ fatigued after sleep?	Nearly every day (1) 3–4 times a week (1) 1–2 times a week (0) 1–2 times a month (0) Never or nearly never (0)	Sitting quietly after lunch (no alcohol)		Neck circumference >40 cm	
7. Tired, fatigued or not up to par during waking time?	Nearly every day (1) 3–4 times a week (1) 1–2 times a week (0) 1–2 times a month (0) Never or nearly never (0)	Stopped for a few minutes in traffic while driving			
8. Nodded off or fallen asleep while driving a vehicle? If yes: 9. How often does this occur?	Yes (1) No (0) Nearly every day 3–4 times a week 1–2 times a week 1–2 times a month Never or nearly never			Male	
Category 3					
10. HTN	Yes/No/Do not know				
11. BMI	>30 kg/m² or ≤30 kg/m²				
Conclusion					

*Categories 1 and 2 are positive if score more than 2 points; Category 3 is positive if HTN present/BMI >30 kg/m².
Subject classified as high risk if score positive in 2 or more categories otherwise low risk for obstructive sleep apnea.
**Number for each situation: 0 = would never doze or sleep; 1 = slight chance of dozing or sleeping; 2 = moderate chance of dozing/sleeping; 3 = high chance of dozing or sleeping.
***To score 1 if answer is yes, 0 if answer is no.
BMI, body mass index; HTN, hypertension.

and 54%, respectively, whereas pooled specificity was 59%, 42%, 42%, and 65%. For severe OSA, pooled sensitivity was 84%, 93%, 90%, and 58%; pooled specificity was 38%, 35%, 28%, and 60%. The authors concluded that SBQ is best suited for screening for OSA in resource limited settings or when PSG is not available.[54] As stated above, the cardiologist should also be conscious of the varied presentations of OSA, and that all patients need not be obese or have excessive daytime somnolence. Refractory hypertension, recurrent arrhythmias, and ischemic events should prompt thorough history and polysomnographic evaluation to rule out OSA or concomitant sleep-related breathing disorders.

BARRIERS IN INTEGRATING OSA MANAGEMENT IN CARDIOLOGY PRACTICE AND SOLUTIONS

The barriers in integrating OSA diagnostics into cardiology practice stem from multiple factors. First and foremost barrier is the lack of awareness regarding OSA in cardiologists. Only visual screening of the patients for telltale signs of obesity or just relying on BMI may underdiagnose OSA, especially in high-risk patients. This can be taken care of by applying systematic screening tools as described above.

Second barrier or obstacle is referral of patient to a sleep physician. Though sleep medicine is rapidly expanding, certified, or experienced sleep physicians are few in number. Also, the patient may not understand the link between sleep and their cardiac disease, and may not make the effort to consult a sleep physician unless this is emphasized enough by the treating cardiologist. On the other hand, it may be difficult for cardiologists to provide sleep diagnostics and management adding more burden to already busy cardiology services. Also, due to limited number of quality PSG laboratories, full in-laboratory PSG may have a long waiting time. This can be sorted out by prior liaison with certified sleep physicians. Alternatively, cardiologists can improve their knowledge on sleep-related breathing disorders, to perform clinical evaluation on their own, and incorporate home-based sleep study as an initial method of diagnosis of OSA. Subsequently, patients can be managed in consultation with a sleep specialist. Patients with facial abnormalities or morbid obesity may be managed in consultation with surgical specialties.

Third obstacle is lack of connection with manufacturers of devices such as CPAP devices or mandibular advancement devices (MAD) for treatment of OSA. This is not a major problem and can be sorted out once cardiologist decides to incorporate sleep medicine in their practice.

DIAGNOSIS OF OBSTRUCTIVE SLEEP APNEA

Patients with OSA can primarily present with resistant hypertension, CAD, AF or pulmonary hypertension, without any overt manifestations of OSA. Patients should be asked for other symptoms of OSA including loud snoring, choking sensation, or gasping or witnessed choking spells during sleep, morning headaches, sore throat or dry mouth on getting up in morning, cognitive deficits, decreased vigilance, morning confusion, personality, or mood changes, erectile dysfunction, and gastroesophageal reflux. Excessive daytime somnolence is an important manifestation of OSA syndrome. On clinical examination, increased neck circumference, craniofacial abnormalities, nasal congestion, low soft palate, uvular hypertrophy, enlargement of palatine tonsils, and macroglossia should be looked for. BMI and waist-hip ratio should be assessed.

Polysomnography is the method of choice for diagnosis of OSA. Attended level 1 PSG is the gold standard for diagnosis of OSA. Level 1 PSG records comprehensive physiologic parameters during sleep which include electroencephalogram (EEG), electrooculogram, electromyogram, snoring frequency, thoracoabdominal movements, nasal airflow, and oximetry. Thus, it can provide accurate sleep staging along with type of apneas. It can be used for titration of optimal CPAP pressure to obviate apneas and hypopneas in a separate study or during a split night study. It can be used to assess complex sleep disorders. It can also be combined with percutaneous carbon dioxide (CO_2) monitoring to detect concomitant hypoventilation. Disadvantages include requirement of attendance of trained technical staff, limited availability of PSG laboratories, and higher cost.[55]

Home sleep apnea testing (HSAT) is an acceptable approach to diagnostic evaluation of suspected patients with OSA. These devices have been validated against in-laboratory PSG. As per American Academy of Sleep Medicine (AASM), minimum requirements of an HSAT device include sensors for nasal pressure monitoring, chest and abdominal respiratory inductance, and oximetry. Devices using peripheral arterial tonometry along with oximetry and actigraphy (e.g., WatchPAT) are also approved.

Advantages of HSAT devices for the patient include comfort of sleep testing at home, lesser waiting time, and lower cost. However, limitations include underestimation of AHI in mild-to-moderate OSA. Also, it is difficult to assess central and complex sleep apneas with HSAT devices. Therefore, these are not suitable for assessment of patients with comorbid disorders like chronic obstructive pulmonary disease (COPD), HF or other sleep disorders (hypersomnias, central sleep apnea, parasomnias, or periodic limb movement disorders). Also, CPAP titration using HSAT is not standardized, therefore, most patients diagnosed with OSA using HSAT devices may have to use auto titrating devices (auto CPAP) or retested with split night level 1 PSG.[55]

Diagnosis of OSA is based on symptoms along with respiratory events during sleep. Apneas are defined as diminished airflow by 90% of baseline for 10 seconds or more; definition of apnea does not include desaturation as a criteria. Hypopnea is defined as diminished airflow by 30% of baseline for 10 seconds or more, along with arousal on EEG or desaturation by more than or equal to 3% on oximetry. Apnea and hypopnea should be obstructive in character, i.e., associated with paradoxical thoracic and abdominal movements. Respiratory event-related arousals are defined as airflow limitation for 10 seconds or more along with EEG evidence of arousal, without satisfying criteria for apnea or hypopnea. The indices for defining severity of OSA can be AHI or respiratory disturbance index (RDI). AHI is defined as the sum of apneas and hypopneas per hour of sleep time. RDI comprises sum of apneas, hypopneas, and respiratory event related arousals per hour of sleep time.

Patients with 5–15 events per hour are classified as mild OSA, those with more than 15–30 events per hour are classified as moderate OSA. Patients with AHI more than 30 events per hour are classified as having severe OSA.[56]

OVERVIEW OF MANAGEMENT OF OBSTRUCTIVE SLEEP APNEA

Once diagnosis of OSA is achieved, multimodality treatment is required. General measures applicable to treatment of all patients with OSA include lifestyle modifications like weight reduction, aerobic exercises, and dietary modifications. Patients who have respiratory events only in particular postures, e.g., supine predominant OSA can be counseled to avoid those postures during sleep. Patients can also be counseled to avoid or refrain from substances and drugs that are known to worsen OSA like alcohol and benzodiazepines. Patients with treatable craniofacial abnormalities may be good candidates for surgery. Patients with morbid obesity or concomitant hypoventilation may be advised for weight reduction surgery.

Continuous positive airway pressure therapy is the mainstay of treatment for OSA. The AASM recommends CPAP for all patients with moderate or severe OSA. Patients with mild OSA along with comorbidities including cardiac diseases like CAD, HF or AF should also be treated with CPAP as per AASM guidelines.[57,58] CPAP works by splinting the upper airways and maintaining their patency during inspiration during sleep. CPAP therapy has been shown to reduce respiratory events during sleep, decrease daytime somnolence, improve alertness, improve systemic blood pressure, and improve glucose tolerance. CPAP has also been shown to reduce risk of nocturnal arrhythmias, recurrence of AF, and improve outcomes in patients with HF. Mortality benefit with CPAP has been shown in observational studies, but not in randomized trials.[59] Alternative to CPAP include MAD, however, they are less effective than CPAP,[28] and should only be offered as an alternatives in patients with mild-to-moderate OSA who are not willing or intolerant to CPAP. Hypoglossal nerve stimulation is another upcoming strategy for treatment of OSA.[60]

Various drugs like cannabinoids are being studied for efficacy in OSA, but are not currently recommended as pharmacologic therapy.[61] For residual sleepiness after CPAP therapy, modafinil or armodafinil have been used.

CONCLUSION

There have been great strides in management of HF, arrhythmias, and CAD. However, multiple factors lead to readmissions due to recurrence of these disorders. OSA has become increasingly prevalent, and is associated with increased risk of cardiovascular diseases. This association presents the cardiologist with a unique opportunity to be at the forefront of screening and diagnosis of OSA. Home-based sleep testing has come of age, is easy and cost-effective in carefully selected patients, and can be used for diagnosis of OSA. This can be incorporated easily into existing cardiology services. Also, cardiologists can be an important part of the team in management of OSA and related disorders. Practicing cardiologists have both this opportunity and obligation to become thoroughly educated on sleep-related breathing disorders, and incorporate management of sleep disordered breathing in their practice to deliver best quality care to their patients. Cardiology training programs should also emphasize on screening, diagnosis, and treatment of OSA. Future research should further explore the horizons of relationship between sleep and the heart.

REFERENCES

1. Gastaut H, Tassinari CA, Duron B. Polygraphic study of the episodic diurnal and nocturnal (hypnic and respiratory) manifestations of the Pickwick syndrome. Brain Res. 1966;1(2):167-86.
2. Lugaresi E, Coccagna G, Mantovani M, et al. Effects of tracheostomy in two cases of hypersomnia with periodic breathing. J Neurol Neurosurg Psychiatry. 1973;36(1):15-26.
3. Sullivan C, Berthon-Jones M, Issa F, et al. Reversal of obstructive sleep apnoea by continuous positive airway pressure applied through the nares. The Lancet. 1981;317(8225):862-5.
4. Lavie P. Incidence of sleep apnea in a presumably healthy working population: a significant relationship with excessive daytime sleepiness. Sleep. 1983;6(4):312-8.
5. Young T, Palta M, Dempsey J, et al. Burden of sleep apnea: Rationale, design, and major findings of the wisconsin sleep cohort study. WMJ Off Publ State Med Soc Wis. 2009;108(5):246-9.
6. Mehra R, Benjamin EJ, Shahar E, et al. Association of nocturnal arrhythmias with sleep-disordered breathing: The sleep heart health study. Am J Respir Crit Care Med. 2006;173(8):910-6.
7. Shahar E, Whitney CW, Redline S, et al. Sleep-disordered breathing and cardiovascular disease: cross-sectional results of the Sleep Heart Health Study. Am J Respir Crit Care Med. 2001;163(1):19-25.
8. Senaratna CV, Perret JL, Lodge CJ, et al. Prevalence of obstructive sleep apnea in the general population: A systematic review. Sleep Med Rev. 2017;34:70-81.
9. Redline S, Tishler PV, Hans MG, et al. Racial differences in sleep-disordered breathing in African-Americans and Caucasians. Am J Respir Crit Care Med. 1997;155(1):186-92.
10. Reddy EV, Kadhiravan T, Mishra HK, et al. Prevalence and risk factors of obstructive sleep apnea among middle-aged urban Indians: a community-based study. Sleep Med. 2009;10(8):913-8.
11. Tufik S, Santos-Silva R, Taddei JA, et al. A. Obstructive sleep apnea syndrome in the Sao Paulo Epidemiologic Sleep Study. Sleep Med. 2010;11(5):441-6.
12. Quintana-Gallego E, Carmona-Bernal C, Capote F, et al. Gender differences in obstructive sleep apnea syndrome: a clinical study of 1166 patients. Respir Med. 2004;98(10):984-9.
13. Peppard PE, Young T, Barnet JH, et al. Increased prevalence of sleep-disordered breathing in adults. Am J Epidemiol. 2013;177(9):1006-14.
14. Young T, Skatrud J, Peppard PE. Risk factors for obstructive sleep apnea in adults. JAMA. 2004;291(16):2013-6.
15. Wetter DW, Young TB, Bidwell TR, et al. Smoking as a risk factor for sleep-disordered breathing. Arch Intern Med. 1994;154(19):2219-24.
16. Redline S, Tishler PV. The genetics of sleep apnea. Sleep Med Rev. 2000;4(6):583-602.
17. Mason M, Cates CJ, Smith I. Effects of opioid, hypnotic and sedating medications on sleep-disordered breathing in adults with obstructive sleep apnoea. Cochrane Database Syst Rev. 2015;(7):CD011090.

18. Peppard PE, Young T, Palta M, et al. Longitudinal study of moderate weight change and sleep-disordered breathing. JAMA. 2000;284(23):3015-21.
19. Li KK, Kushida C, Powell NB, et al. Obstructive sleep apnea syndrome: a comparison between Far-East Asian and white men. The Laryngoscope. 2000;110(10 Pt 1):1689-93.
20. Lavie P, Lavie L, Herer P. All-cause mortality in males with sleep apnoea syndrome: declining mortality rates with age. Eur Respir J. 2005;25(3):514-20.
21. Marti S, Sampol G, Muñoz X, et al. Mortality in severe sleep apnoea/hypopnoea syndrome patients: impact of treatment. Eur Respir J. 2002;20(6):1511-8.
22. Grunstein RR. Metabolic aspects of sleep apnea. Sleep. 1996;19(suppl_10): S218-20.
23. Ip MS, Lam KS, Ho C, et al. Serum leptin and vascular risk factors in obstructive sleep apnea. Chest. 2000;118(3):580-6.
24. Spiegel K, Tasali E, Penev P, et al. Brief communication: Sleep curtailment in healthy young men is associated with decreased leptin levels, elevated ghrelin levels, and increased hunger and appetite. Ann Intern Med. 2004;141(11):846.
25. Harman EM, Wynne JW, Block AJ. The effect of weight loss on sleep-disordered breathing and oxygen desaturation in morbidly obese men. Chest. 1982;82(3):291-4.
26. Reichmuth KJ, Austin D, Skatrud JB, et al. Association of sleep apnea and type II diabetes: a population-based study. Am J Respir Crit Care Med. 2005;172(12):1590-5.
27. Al-Delaimy WK, Manson JE, Willett WC, et al. Snoring as a risk factor for type II diabetes mellitus: a prospective study. Am J Epidemiol. 2002;155(5):387-93.
28. Iftikhar IH, Khan MF, Das A, et al. Meta-analysis: Continuous positive airway pressure improves insulin resistance in patients with sleep apnea without diabetes. Ann Am Thorac Soc. 2013;10(2):115-20.
29. Peppard PE, Young T, Palta M, et al. Prospective study of the association between sleep-disordered breathing and hypertension. N Engl J Med. 2000;342(19):1378-84.
30. Hou H, Zhao Y, Yu W, et al. Association of obstructive sleep apnea with hypertension: A systematic review and meta-analysis. J Glob Health. 2013; 010405.
31. Parati G, Lombardi C, Hedner J, et al. European Respiratory Society. Position paper on the management of patients with obstructive sleep apnea and hypertension: joint recommendations by the European Society of Hypertension, by the European Respiratory Society and by the members of European COST (Cooperation in Scientific and Technological research) ACTION B26 on obstructive sleep apnea. J Hypertens. 2012;30(4):633-46.
32. Huang Z, Liu Z, Luo Q, et al. Long-Term effects of continuous positive airway pressure on blood pressure and prognosis in hypertensive patients with coronary heart disease and obstructive sleep apnea: A randomized controlled trial. Am J Hypertens. 2015;28(3):300-6.
33. Sanner BM, Tepel M, Markmann A, et al. Effect of continuous positive airway pressure therapy on 24-hour blood pressure in patients with obstructive sleep apnea syndrome. Am J Hypertens. 2002;15(3):251-7.
34. Logan AG, Perlikowski SM, Mente A, et al. High prevalence of unrecognized sleep apnoea in drug-resistant hypertension. J Hypertens. 2001;19(12):2271-7.
35. Whelton PK, Carey RM, Aronow WS, et al. 2017 ACC/AHA/AAPA/ABC/ACPM/AGS/APhA/ASH/ASPC/NMA/PCNA Guideline for the Prevention, Detection, Evaluation, and Management of High Blood Pressure in Adults: A Report of the American College of Cardiology/American Heart Association Task Force on Clinical Practice Guidelines. J Am Coll Cardiol. 2018;71(19):e127-248.
36. Blood Pressure Lowering Treatment Trialists' Collaboration. Blood pressure-lowering treatment based on cardiovascular risk: a meta-analysis of individual patient data. Lancet Lond Engl. 2014;384(9943):591-8.
37. Sezavar SH, Hajsadeghi S, Hejrati M, et al. Left ventricular mass index and pulmonary artery pressure in patients with the obstructive sleep apnea syndrome. J Tehran Univ Heart Cent. 2016;11(1):11-4.
38. Aslan K, Deniz A, Cayli M, et al. Early left ventricular functional alterations in patients with obstructive sleep apnea syndrome. Cardiol J. 2013;20(5):519-25.
39. Ferrier K, Campbell A, Yee B, et al. Sleep-disordered breathing occurs frequently in stable outpatients with congestive heart failure. Chest. 2005;128(4):2116-22.
40. Khattak HK, Hayat F, Pamboukian SV, et al. Obstructive sleep apnea in heart failure: review of prevalence, treatment with continuous positive airway pressure, and prognosis. Tex Heart Inst J. 2018;45(3):151-61.
41. Gami AS, Pressman G, Caples SM, et al. Association of atrial fibrillation and obstructive sleep apnea. Circulation. 2004;110(4):364-7.
42. Kirchhof P, Benussi S, Kotecha D, et al. 2016 ESC Guidelines for the management of atrial fibrillation developed in collaboration with EACTS. Eur Heart J. 2016;37(38):2893-962.
43. Gami AS, Howard DE, Olson EJ, et al. Day-night pattern of sudden death in obstructive sleep apnea. N Engl J Med. 2005;352(12):1206-14.
44. Sert Kuniyoshi FH, Garcia-Touchard A, Gami AS, et al. Day-night variation of acute myocardial infarction in obstructive sleep apnea. J Am Coll Cardiol. 2008;52(5):343-6.
45. Hung J, Whitford EG, Parsons RW, et al. Association of sleep apnoea with myocardial infarction in men. Lancet Lond Engl. 1990;336(8710):261-4.
46. Ben Ahmed H, Boussaid H, Hamdi I, et al. Prevalence and predictors of obstructive sleep apnea in patients admitted for acute myocardial infarction. Ann Cardiol Angeiol (Paris). 2014;63(2):65-70.
47. De Torres-Alba F, Gemma D, Armada-Romero E, et al. Obstructive sleep apnea and coronary artery disease: From pathophysiology to clinical implications. Pulm Med. 2013;2013:768064.
48. Milleron O, Pillière R, Foucher A, et al. Benefits of obstructive sleep apnoea treatment in coronary artery disease: a long-term follow-up study. Eur Heart J. 2004;25(9):728-34.
49. Yaggi HK, Concato J, Kernan WN, et al. Obstructive sleep apnea as a risk factor for stroke and death. N Engl J Med. 2005;353(19):2034-41.
50. Fletcher EC, Schaaf JW, Miller J, et al. Long-term cardiopulmonary sequelae in patients with sleep apnea and chronic lung disease. Am Rev Respir Dis. 1987;135(3):525-33.
51. Schröder CM, O'Hara R. Depression and obstructive sleep apnea (OSA). Ann Gen Psychiatry. 2005;4:13.
52. Shepertycky MR, Banno K, Kryger MH. Differences between men and women in the clinical presentation of patients diagnosed with obstructive sleep apnea syndrome. Sleep. 2005;28(3):309-14.
53. Sassani A, Findley LJ, Kryger M, et al. Reducing motor-vehicle collisions, costs, and fatalities by treating obstructive sleep apnea syndrome. Sleep. 2004;27(3):453-8.
54. Chiu HY, Chen PY, Chuang LP, et al. Diagnostic accuracy of the Berlin questionnaire, STOP-BANG, STOP, and Epworth sleepiness scale in detecting obstructive sleep apnea: A bivariate meta-analysis. Sleep Med Rev. 2017;36: 57-70.
55. Kapur VK, Auckley DH, Chowdhuri S, et al. Clinical practice guideline for diagnostic testing for adult obstructive sleep apnea: An American Academy of Sleep Medicine Clinical Practice Guideline. J Clin Sleep Med JCSM Off Publ Am Acad Sleep Med. 2017;13(3):479-504.
56. Sateia MJ. International classification of sleep disorders-third edition: highlights and modifications. Chest. 2014;146(5):1387-94.
57. Berry RB, Budhiraja R, Gottlieb DJ, et al. Rules for scoring respiratory events in sleep: update of the 2007 AASM Manual for the Scoring of Sleep and Associated Events. Deliberations of the Sleep Apnea Definitions Task Force of the American Academy of Sleep Medicine. J Clin Sleep Med JCSM Off Publ Am Acad Sleep Med. 201;8(5):597-619.
58. Epstein LJ, Kristo D, Strollo PJ, et al. Clinical guideline for the evaluation, management and long-term care of obstructive sleep apnea in adults. J Clin Sleep Med JCSM Off Publ Am Acad Sleep Med. 2009;5(3):263-76.
59. Jonas DE, Amick HR, Feltner C, et al. Screening for obstructive sleep apnea in adults: evidence report and systematic review for the US preventive services task force. JAMA. 2017;317(4):415-33.
60. Certal VF, Zaghi S, Riaz M, et al. Hypoglossal nerve stimulation in the treatment of obstructive sleep apnea: A systematic review and meta-analysis. The Laryngoscope. 2015;125(5):1254-64.
61. Ramar K, Rosen IM, Kirsch DB, et al. Medical Cannabis and the Treatment of Obstructive Sleep Apnea: An American Academy of Sleep Medicine Position Statement. J Clin Sleep Med JCSM Off Publ Am Acad Sleep Med. 2018;14(4):679-81.

SECTION 23

Emerging Issues in Cardiology

CHAPTER 145

mCardiology: mHealth in Cardiology

Ambuj Roy, Ajay S Vamadevan

INTRODUCTION

The term mHealth or mobile health refers to the use of integrated mobile telecommunication and multimedia technologies for wireless health care delivery systems. The first use of this term is widely attributed to Professor Robert Istepanian. He defined it as "mobile computing, medical sensor, and communications technologies for health care".[1] The footprints of mHealth has gradually expanded over the years and it has been used in collecting routine demographic and clinical health information from the community, delivery of health-related information to practitioners and patients, real-time monitoring of patient vital signs, provision of care via telemedicine and electronic clinical decision support system (e-DSS). The electronic decision support system (e-CDSS) is a way to support health personnel in providing evidence-based care using standard medical management protocol algorithms loaded on a mobile device (smartphones, tablets, etc.) that can be used by doctors and support staff.

NEED FOR TECHNOLOGY

India has seen a rapid transition in epidemiology of diseases over the past two decades. Noncommunicable diseases (NCDs) now constitute the leading cause of disease burden all over India. Cardiovascular diseases (CVDs) are the leading cause of mortality among NCDs.[2] The dominant reason for this is the high burden of the risk factors like diabetes, hypertension, tobacco use, dyslipidemia, and physical inactivity in the population.[3] The number of individuals with this conditions is mindboggling with over 175 million estimated to have hypertension and 73 million (2017) with diabetes in India. Given the dual burden of communicable and NCD, the primary focus of public health systems over the years being communicable diseases; and severe shortage of health care staff especially in rural India the health infrastructure is severely constrained in handling the NCD burden. In this context innovations and use of technology such as mHealth may assist in addressing these challenges.

The use of mHealth in India has been evaluated through multiple pilot research projects in India and is planned to be taken up by the Government of India as part of the National Program for the Prevention and Control of Cancer, Diabetes, Cardiovascular Diseases, and Stroke (NPCDCS) for implementation at different levels of primary and secondary care hospitals. The program also envisages mass screening by ancillary health care workers to screen for risk factors like diabetes, hypertension, and common cancers in the population. The screening activities in the communities, management at various levels of care will be supported through a mHealth-based android "App" that combine's electronic health record (EHR) and e-DSS capabilities. The App will connect all the levels of care by uploading patient data to central servers which would then facilitate seamless transmission of data across health centers. Screen detect patients from the communities could visit health facilities for confirmatory diagnosis, further treatment, referral care, and follow-up. The mHealth App thus will facilitate task sharing and avoid redundancy in human efforts and data collected. Some of the usage of mHealth in CV health is discussed below.

Electronic Decision Support System

mPOWER Heart Project

In 2012–2014, the All India Institute of Medical Sciences (AIIMS), New Delhi and the Centre for Chronic Disease Control (CCDC), New Delhi, in collaboration with the Himachal Pradesh Government implemented and evaluated a mHealth-enabled, nurse delivered NCD care delivery model in the Solan district. The project involved five Government community Health Centers (CHCs) and the District hospital. A copyrighted android-based smartphone App, *mPOWER Heart e-DSS,* was used in the NCD clinics primarily by nurses in helping the medical officers in screening, diagnosis, and computing clinical management of hypertension and diabetes. The e-DSS had the following features:

- Computing clinical risk score for detecting patients at risk of diabetes
- Generation of personalized management plan for diabetes and hypertension
- Suggestion for choosing optimal drugs, and contra-indications
- Storing patient data electronically to generate serial data to provide continuity of care during follow-up visits
- Utility to export data to statistical software packages for analyzing temporal trends.

A pre-post evaluation of the mHealth enabled care delivery model showed impressive results. A mean reduction of 14.6 mm Hg of systolic blood pressure (SBP), 7.6 mm Hg diastolic BP, and 50 mg/dL in fasting glucose level was observed among people with hypertension or diabetes during 18 months of follow-up.[4] This model has provided the basis for replication of mHealth enabled interventions for chronic disease care in India.

SimCard Trial

The SimCard trial in India and China evaluated a simplified cardiovascular management program (SimCard) delivered by community health workers (CHWs) in their communities, with the aid of a smartphone-based e-DSS.[5] People with high risk of CVDs, underwent the "2+2" SimCard intervention model: two lifestyle recommendations (dietary salt reduction and smoking cessation) and prescription of two accessible, effective, and low-cost drugs (aspirin and a diuretic or calcium channel blocker). The trial was conducted in 47 villages (27 in China and 20 in India) involving 2,086 "high CV risk" individuals (aged 40 years or older with self-reported history of coronary heart disease, stroke, diabetes, and/or measured SBP ≥160 mm Hg). Participants in the intervention villages were managed by CHWs through an Android e-DSS App on a monthly basis focusing on two medication use and two lifestyle modifications. Compared with the control group, the intervention group had a 25.5% ($p < 0.001$) higher net increase in the proportion of patient-reported antihypertensive medication use at 12 months of follow-up. There were also significant differences in certain secondary outcomes such as aspirin use (17.1%, $p < 0.001$) and SBP (–2.7 mm Hg, $p = 0.04$). The results from the trial indicated that the e-DSS facilitated simplified cardiovascular management program improved quality of primary care and clinical outcomes in resource-poor settings in China and India.

mWELLCARE Trial

This Wellcome trust funded trial expanded the e-DSS to include another important and undertreated NCD condition—mental health. This prospective, multicenter, open-label, cluster randomized controlled trial involving 40 CHCs in 20 districts of Haryana and Karnataka, evaluated the effect of mHealth system for the integrated management of five chronic conditions (high BP, diabetes, tobacco use, alcohol use disorder, and depression) versus enhanced usual care among patients with hypertension and diabetes.[6] The android-based App was again capable of e-DSS features along with storing health records, sending alerts and reminders for follow-up and adherence to medication. A total of 3,702 participants from 40 CHCs in the intervention and control (enhanced care) arms were recruited. The primary outcome was the difference in mean change (from baseline to 1 year) in SBP and glycated hemoglobin (HbA1c) between the two treatment arms. The secondary outcomes were the difference in mean change from baseline to 1 year in fasting plasma glucose, total cholesterol, predicted 10-year risk of CVD, depression, smoking behavior, body mass index (BMI), and alcohol use between the two treatment arms and cost-effectiveness of the intervention. The trial has been completed and the study results would be available soon.

Noncommunicable Disease Initiative, Tripura

This was a very important landmark for the mHealth in clinical hypertension and diabetes care, as it went from research to service mode, which is the ultimate goal for all translational research. The "NCD initiative in Tripura" was launched in May 2017 to address burden of CVDs. As part of the initiative, the *mPOWER Heart e-DSS* was used for management of diabetes, hypertension, and secondary prevention of CVD in health facilities all over the state of Tripura. A total of 40 NCD clinics running at governmental primary and secondary health care facilities rolled out the e-DSS. The nurses and medical officers manning these clinics were trained in use of the e-DSS. In addition, the doctors and nurses were oriented to evidence-based management of theses chronic conditions in separate orientation courses prior to launch of the NCD initiative. At the NCD clinic screening of all eligible subjects (30+ years) were done for diabetes and hypertension and the nurse records the clinical parameters into e-DSS on a tablet device that generated a personalized prescription, based on evidence-based algorithms. The prescription was subsequently vetted by the medical officer and changes made were recorded by the nurse in the App. She/he is also provided additional lifestyle counseling as per prompts of the e-DSS. The App served also as an EHR and was used for follow-up assessment of the patient. The initiative has screened more than 80,000 individuals and treated over 30,000 for hypertension, 8,000 for diabetes, and 4,500 for both. The program was monitored real-time, using big-data analytic tools, for informed decision-making. Data from e-DSS server (https://tripurancd.org/m-powerheartplus/login) are reliable source for health administrators to monitor real-time process or health outcomes in individual health facilities and overall in the state. Major challenges in implementing this initiative were making technology user-friendly, which we overcame through multiple iterations with the support of all stakeholders.

Text Messages for Behavior Change Support

Indian SMS Diabetes Prevention Study

The Indian SMS diabetes study in Southeast India investigated whether mobile phone messaging that encouraged lifestyle change could reduce incident type 2 diabetes (T2D) in Indian Asian men with impaired glucose tolerance, through a 2-year, prospective, parallel-group, randomized controlled trial.[7] Participants in the intervention group received frequent mobile phone messages compared with controls who received standard lifestyle modification advice at baseline only. At the end of the study, the cumulative incidence of T2D was lower (18% vs. 27%) in those who received mobile phone messages than in controls. Additional 3-year follow-up of these participants, even after withdrawal of the active intervention, also showed beneficial effects of intervention on diabetes prevention.[8]

Similar to these interventions, the Ministry of Health and Family Welfare (MoHFW), Government of India, in collaboration with the WHO country office for India and other partners, has launched a SMS-based initiatives for tobacco cessation (mCessation Program), and the prevention and care of diabetes (mDiabetes Program). Potential beneficiaries are encouraged to register their mobile numbers online (websites: https://www.nhp.gov.in/QUIT-tobacco & http://mdiabetes.nhp.gov.in/) to receive messages to support behavior change to effect quitting tobacco and prevention or self-management of diabetes, respectively. Reports on large scale evaluation of these efforts are yet to be available.

TEXTME Trial

This trial conducted in Australia assessed impact of a lifestyle-focused semipersonalized support program delivered by mobile phone text message on CV risk factors in patients with coronary artery disease.[9] It was a parallel-group, single-blind, randomized clinical trial that recruited 710 patients to two groups; those receiving text messages and control. Patients in the intervention group (n = 352) received four text messages per week for 6 months in addition to usual care. Text messages provided advice, motivational reminders, and support to change lifestyle behaviors. Messages for each participant were selected from a bank of messages based on baseline characteristics (e.g., smoking) and delivered through an automated computerized message management system. The program was not interactive. The primary end point was levels of low-density lipoprotein cholesterol (LDL-C) 6 months. Secondary end points included SBP, BMI, physical activity, and smoking status. At 6 months, levels of LDL-C were significantly lower in intervention participants and there were concurrent reductions in SBP and BMI, significant increase in physical activity and a significant reduction in smoking. The majority of participants reported the text-message program to be helpful (91%), easy to follow (97%), and optimum in frequency (86%). The groups have since developed text messages contextual to and in local language in North India.[10]

Evidence from Systematic Reviews

A Cochrane review of the impact of messaging in secondary prevention reports that overall there is improved adherence in the intervention arm. However, the studies are small and have not evaluated the impact of intervention on CV outcomes. It suggests sufficiently powered, high-quality randomized trials are needed, particularly in low- and middle-income countries.[11]

Another Cochrane review of similar studies for primary prevention reported mixed results. The quality of data was overall poor and results heterogeneous. The authors concluded that there was uncertainty around the effectiveness of these interventions at present. However, there are six ongoing trials being conducted in a range of contexts including in low-income settings with potential to generate more precise estimates of the effect of primary prevention medication adherence interventions delivered by mobile phone.[12]

Smoking Cessation Meta-analysis

A Cochrane meta-analysis of five studies with over 9,000 participants has shown that mobile phone interventions increase the long-term quit rates by 71% as compared with control programs, using a definition of abstinence of no smoking at 6 months since quit day but allowing up to three lapses or up to five cigarettes. Statistical heterogeneity was substantial as indicated by the I^2 statistic ($I^2 = 79\%$) among the studies. They suggest that more research is needed into other forms of mobile phone-based interventions for smoking cessation and that it should be studied in other contexts like in low income countries and the cost-effectiveness of the intervention should be assessed.

Systematic Review of mHealth-based Heart Failure Interventions

This review evaluated nine studies using mHealth technology as part of an heart failure (HF) monitoring system, which typically included a BP-measuring device, weighing scale, and an electrocardiogram recorder.[13] The impact of the mHealth interventions on all-cause mortality, CV mortality, HF-related hospitalizations, length of stay, New York Heart Association functional class, left ventricular ejection fraction, quality of life, and self-care were studied and they were inconsistent across these studies. The authors concluded that further research is needed to conclusively determine the impact of mHealth interventions on HF outcomes. The limitations of the studies were small sample size, quasi-experimental design, use of older mobile phone models, etc. This should be taken into consideration in planning larger trials as it may help improve dismal outcomes in HF patients especially in low resource settings like India.

CONCLUSION

The field of mHealth in cardiology is in its infancy but rapidly expanding. It provides a great opportunity to use technology to improve health care delivery. mHealth is not a substitute for conventional delivery of health delivery processes but it complements it to improve the efficiency of the system. It helps in task-sharing, evidence-based treatment, maintain records, and aid in follow-up even in resource poor setting. Mobile text messages have also shown promise in health promotion and improving medication adherence in various CVDs.

REFERENCES

1. Istepanian R, Jovanov E, Zhang YT. Introduction to the special section on M-Health: beyond seamless mobility and global wireless health-care connectivity. IEEE Trans Inf Technol Biomed. 2004;8(4):405-14.
2. Dandona L, Dandona R, Kumar GA, et al. Nations within nation variations in epidemiological transition across the states of India, 1990-2016 in the Global Burden of Disease Study. Lancet. 2017;390(10111):2437-60.
3. Prabhakaran D, Jeemon P, Roy A. Cardiovascular Diseases in India: Current Epidemiology and Future Directions. Circulation. 2016;133(16):1605-20.
4. Ajay VS, Jindal D, Roy A, et al. Development of a Smartphone-Enabled Hypertension and Diabetes Mellitus Management Package to Facilitate Evidence-Based Care Delivery in Primary Healthcare Facilities in India: The mPower Heart Project. J Am Heart Assoc. 2016;5(12). pii: e004343.
5. Tian M, Ajay VS, Dunzhu D, et al. A Cluster-randomized, controlled trial of a simplified multifaceted management program for individuals at high cardiovascular risk (SimCard Trial) in Rural Tibet, China, and Haryana, India. Circulation. 2015;132:815-24.
6. Jha D, Gupta P, Vamadevan SA, et al. Protocol for the mWellcare trial: a multicentre, cluster randomised, 12-month, controlled trial to compare the effectiveness of mWellcare, an mHealth system for an integrated management of patients with hypertension and diabetes, versus enhanced usual care in India. BMJ Open. 2017;7:e014851.
7. Ramachandran A, Snehalatha C, Ram J, et al. Effectiveness of mobile phone messaging in prevention of type 2 diabetes by lifestyle modification in men in India: a prospective, parallel-group, randomised controlled trial. Lancet Diabetes Endocrinol. 2013;1(3):191-8.
8. Nanditha A, Snehalatha C, Raghavan A, et al. The post-trial analysis of the Indian SMS diabetes prevention study shows persistent beneficial effects of lifestyle intervention. Diabetes Res Clin Pract. 2018;142:213-21
9. Chow CK, Redfern J, Hillis GS, et al. Effect of lifestyle-focused text messaging on risk factor modification in patients with coronary heart disease: A randomized clinical trial. JAMA. 2015;314(12):1255-63.
10. Thakkar J, Karthikeyan G, Purohit G, et al. Development of macaronic Hindi-English 'Hinglish' text message content for a coronary heart disease secondary prevention programme. Heart Asia. 2016;8(2):32-8.
11. Adler AJ, Martin N, Mariani J, et al. Mobile phone text messaging to improve medication adherence in secondary prevention of cardiovascular disease. Cochrane Database Syst Rev. 2017;4:CD011851.
12. Pamer Cochrane Database Syst Rev. 2018
13. Cajita MI, Gleason KT, Han HR. A systematic review of mHealth-based heart failure interventions. J Cardiovasc Nurs. 2016;31(3):E10-22.

CHAPTER 146

Telemonitoring in Cardiology

Pramod Sagar Arsikere, Aditya Kapoor

INTRODUCTION

Telehealthcare can be broadly defined as personalized healthcare delivered from a distance and represents an effective fusion of information and communication technologies with medical science. Among the range of medical specialties in which telemedicine has been successfully applied, cardiology is one of the most important. The usual components include—(1) acquiring patient data [e.g., blood pressure, pulse, weight, general well-being, symptoms, investigations like electrocardiography (ECG), echocardiography, etc.], (2) electronic transmission of patient data to a healthcare setup, (3) delivery of feedback tailored according to the individual patient need, which may range from ordering new investigation, drug titration or advising hospitalization.

The first recorded concept of telemedicine perhaps dates back to 1900s, when Willem Einthoven, a Dutch physiologist, developed the first electrocardiograph in his laboratory in Leiden and used a string galvanometer and telephone wires, recorded the ECG of patient in a hospital 1 km away.[1]

Data acquisition and transfer can be either real-time (synchronous), store-and-forward (asynchronous), or a combination (hybrid systems). While synchronous techniques mandate that patient and healthcare professional be available together at the same time with real-time data processing, store-and-forward techniques allow for flexibility. The key components utilized in telehealthcare comprise of portable data acquisition or imaging devices (e.g., blood pressure apparatus, ECG, echocardiography systems), computer/smart phones, and a stable wireless communication infrastructure that can transmit data. This data can viewed immediately or stored at the receiving station for later review. The following four generations of telehealthcare for remote management of patients have been practiced:[2]

1. Nonreactive data collection and analysis, with store-and-forward transmission of data (e.g., with ECG lop recorders)
2. Systems with real-time data transfer but nonimmediate decision-making structure. Therefore, although the healthcare provider can view data and recognize changes, delays can occur in analysis, especially if the system is only active during daytime
3. Systems with 24-hour ongoing, continuous, and consistent analytical, decision-making support, even outside office hours
4. Fully integrated telehealthcare where data from medical devices (invasive and noninvasive) are linked to telemedical platforms that are available for both the primary care provider and the telemedical center.

VARIOUS APPLICATIONS OF TELECARDIOLOGY

Various applications of telecardiology include:

- Teleauscultation
- Tele-ECG and its role in management of ST elevation myocardial infarction (STEMI)
- Remote monitoring for heart failure (HF)
- Remote monitoring for patients with implantable devices
- Others:
  - Patients with pulmonary hypertension
  - Tele-echocardiography services
  - Patients with prosthetic valves
  - Arrhythmia diagnosis
  - Radio Detection and Ranging (RADAR) systems.

Teleauscultation and Digital Stethoscope

Auscultation is an integral tool to establish diagnosis in cardiology and digital stethoscopes like ViScope offer high-resolution visual display combined with conventional auscultation (Fig. 1). Visual waveforms displayed in the format window of the phonocardiogram are transmitted to the cardiologist at the main server for analysis and interpretation. Using these tools for remote hearing has been shown to be more sensitive than traditional stethoscopes.[3]

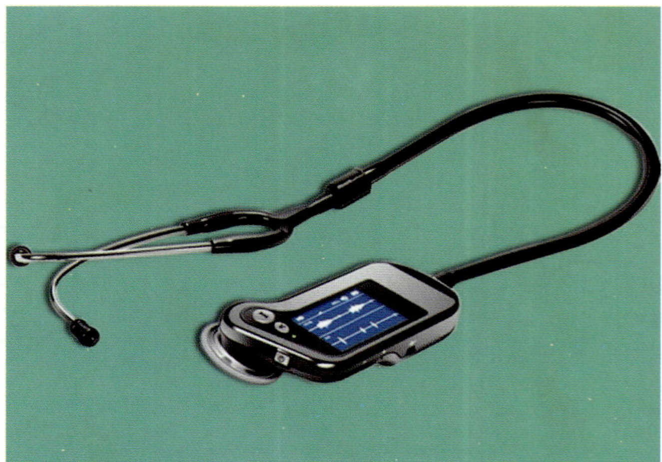

FIG. 1: Digital stethoscope.

Tele-electrocardiography

Although ECG equipment is widely available, and lack of interpretation skills at the primary care level is an important issue. This is especially true for the developing world where medical outreach to communities is low and getting accurate ECG reports with specialist input is challenging. In India, there is acute shortage of physicians to provide medical care in remote areas and the reported doctor patient ratio in 2016 was ~1:1,300 as opposed to the World Health Organization (WHO) recommended ratio of 1:1,000.[4]

Inability or errors in diagnosing cardiac arrhythmias, acute ischemic syndromes, channelopathies, etc. is common due to varying levels of skill in primary care physicians. Hence, it is important to have reliable ECG interpretation at the primary care level, so that correct diagnosis can be made especially in cases of atypical presentations and when needed, urgent referrals can be done. Advances in telecardiology have helped rapid and reliable remote ECG recording and interpretation, using hand-held ECG units, that encode the ECG into sound, play it telephonically to the telecardiology service where the audio input is decoded and displayed as a 12-lead ECG. Tele-ECG electronic devices can also record ECGs, display it on the phone via Bluetooth, and then send it to specialists via mobile cellular networks.

- Of all patients with chest pain and suspected acute coronary syndrome (ACS) or STEMI and referred to tertiary care centers only 25–50% turn out to have ACS/STEMI.[5] Hence, it is sensible to develop strategies to reduce such unnecessary referrals and limit the cost burden on health services
- Patients with STEMI are candidates for early reperfusion and primary percutaneous coronary intervention (PCI) remains the preferable strategy, if it can be performed in a timely manner and the patient can reach a PCI-enabled center. An early diagnosis is hence the cornerstone of managing such patients and can help in referring them to PCI centers in due time. Therefore prehospital diagnosis done via an ECG recorded in the field, interpreted by paramedics with field triage, followed by wireless transmission to emergency physicians or cardiologists at the tertiary care hospital has emerged as a successful method to help early diagnosis and appropriate management of STEMI patients[6-9]
- Techniques of prehospital (in-ambulance) ECG recording and transfer have evolved from the early days of single-lead telemetry (which primary helped to diagnose arrhythmias) followed by successful implementation of satisfactory quality 12-lead ECG transmission using error-correcting digital transmission via cellular phone links
- Telecardiology for such patients also facilitates prehospital continuous ECG surveillance that provides useful prognostic information (failed thrombolysis, ongoing ischemia, arrhythmias, etc.) which can potentially help to improve further triage with individualized treatment protocols
- Successful implementation of such programs has been reported to significantly shorten transfer times, decrease treatment delay, and is associated with a lower mortality.[10,11] While the early focus of most such studies was on prehospital fibrinolysis, Terkelsen et al. were one of the earliest to demonstrated the benefit of prehospital ECG diagnosis, field triage followed by transfer to a primary PCI center in patients with STEMI. The study reported that time from first medical contact to balloon was approximately 81 minutes shorter with prehospital diagnosis compared to patients diagnosed in the hospital. Even shorter (34 vs. 97 min, $p < 0.001$) door-to-PCI times have been reported in subsequent studies using better techniques and technology and studies from different countries have reported similar results, despite diverse geographic settings, healthcare structure, and prehospital logistics[12,13]
- *Body surface mapping*: A major limitation of the 12-lead ECG, whether in-hospital or prehospital phase, is the low sensitivity since the entire anatomic left ventricle is not completely covered by conventional leads. Hence, inferoposterior myocardial infarction (MI) could be missed on 12-lead ECG, a limitation, which can be overcome by using additional leads, like V7–V9. Body surface mapping using 80-lead ECG improves the ability to detect ischemia in all regions of the left ventricular (LV) including inferoposterior area, right ventricular (RV) MI, and can therefore improve sensitivity compared to conventional 12-lead ECG.[14,15] However, body surface mapping for evaluation of patients with chest pain has not gained widespread popularity because it is time consuming; development of newer, easy to apply technologies for this purpose could change this scenario in future
- *Development of new ECG lead systems*: Since recording ECGs in prehospital settings is fraught with technical issues including poor general condition of status and time is of essence, focus has been on developing novel ECG monitoring systems for easy and rapid electrode application. The EASI lead system, using only four leads

to extract a complete, diagnostic "12-lead" ECG, has been reported to be as effective as the conventional 12-lead ECG system. The 5-lead system tested in the synthesized 12-lead ST monitoring and real-time tele-ECG initiative was also shown to be effective.[16,17]

Remote Patient Management Systems for Heart Failure

Recurrent hospital admissions and episodes of cardiac decompensation are common in the first 6–12 months after the initial diagnosis as well as during the late phase of HF. Approximately, 50% of HF patients are rehospitalized within 6 months of hospital discharge. Follow-up of HF patients, even in the West, is inadequate at best, with suboptimal support at home and at the level of general or family physicians. Patients themselves have low adherence to drugs and fail to recognize early signs of cardiac decompensation. Telemonitoring of patients with chronic HF is now emerging as an innovative concept to detect early signs of acute decompensation, so that therapeutic measures can be instituted in time and recurrent hospitalizations are prevented. The use of telemonitoring for HF patients ensures "continuity of care" extending seamlessly from the hospitals to the patients' home.

- Although telemonitoring has been shown to be useful in detecting early warning signs of HF decompensation, the best monitoring room remains elusive. Simple tools like only monitoring body weight may be fraught with inconsistencies, and multiparametric monitoring of weight, heart rate, blood pressure, ECG, O_2 saturation, natriuretic peptide levels, symptoms, and drug intake may be more beneficial. Ideal systems provide for face-to-face two-way communication between patients and healthcare providers using telephone or satellite connection. Preferably, the patient's device should be portable with videoconferencing and data transmission ability, which can be managed by the healthcare professional using a remote control
- *Phone-based systems*: Use mobile phone-based telemonitoring equipment, a centralized center for automated data transfer and analysis, an internet-based graphical user interface with alert notifications for physicians-on-call. Patients measure their blood pressure, heart rate, body weight, etc. and enter this data along with daily dose of HF medications on the mobile phone. This data is then transferred to the central server via mobile networks
  - The Randomized Trial of Telephone Intervention in Chronic Heart Failure (DIAL) examined structured telephone support (STS) wherein nurses changed the diuretic dose and recommended nonscheduled medical consultations. This resulted in fewer HF readmissions (RR reduction 29%, p = 0.005) and better quality of life in the short term and even 1–3 years after stopping intervention[18]
  - The Trans-European Network-Home-Care Management System (TEN-HMS) study used twice daily home telemonitoring (HTM: self-measurement of weight, blood pressure, heart rate, and heart rhythm with automated devices linked to a cardiology center) or specialist nurses telephone support (NTS) or usual care. Although the number of admissions and mortality were similar among patients receiving NTS or HTM, the mean duration of admissions was lesser with HTM. Those receiving usual care had significantly higher 1-year mortality than patients getting HTM or NTS[19]
  - The Austrian Mobile Phone-based Telemonitoring for Heart Failure patients (MOBITEL) trial used an automatic algorithm to alert physicians, if the body weight gain exceeded a threshold of 2 kg within 2 days. Per-protocol analysis revealed that rate of reaching the primary endpoint (death and hospitalizations) was reduced by 54% (p = 0.04) and telemonitored patients who were hospitalized for worsening HF had a significantly shorter length of stay (6.5 vs. 10 days, p = 0.04)[20]
  - The Telemonitoring to Improve Heart Failure Outcomes (Tele-HF) study assessed the use of a telephone-based interactive voice response system in patients within 30 days of HF hospitalization. Readmissions, death, and number of days in the hospital were not reduced by telemonitoring. The study concluded that a thorough and independent evaluation of these strategies is important before their adoption in clinical practice[21]
- *Near-field communication (NFC) technology*: Difficulties in manual data entry via the mobile phone keypad often leads to inability to initiate data transmission. This is especially common for older patients or those from low socioeconomic and educational status. E-mail notifications about patient events also occasionally result in overloading the server due to inappropriately adjusted technical thresholds. Near-field communication technology, which supports a touch-based method for data acquisition and unlike Bluetooth, does not depend on device pairing and is likely to circumvent these problems.[22] This is a wireless connectivity-based technology that involves contactless identification based on magnetic inductive coupling, working in the frequency band of 13.56 MHz. Apart from ease of data acquisition, NFC also has the ability to provide access to data stored on radiofrequency identification (RFID) tags. This can facilitate acquisition of nonquantitative data, like medication intake and patient well-being stored on electronic barcodes. Specially designed blood pressure monitors (UA-767 plus NFC, AND, Japan) with integrated NFC module (AIT: Austrian Institute of Technology, Austria) to allow for wireless transmission of measurement values have been developed. In addition, body weight scales (UA-321, AND, Japan) with NFC extension have also been designed to help HF patients in acquiring data by just a touchscreen technology using NFC-enabled mobile phones. Patient identification on the central server is done using contactless smart cards (patient-specific ID cards)

- *Use of implantable electronic devices (IEDs) and implantable hemodynamic monitors (IHMs) in HF patients*: Although patients can be trained to recognize signs and symptoms of worsening HF and monitor body weight, the sensitivity of weight gain to detect decompensation is modest at best (<20%).[23] Implantable devices provide information about the filling pressures of the ventricles and help in guiding HF management optimally by measuring intrathoracic impedance, LV/RV filling pressures, RV oxygen saturation, pulmonary hypertension, etc. as surrogate markers of patient hemodynamics. Most devices (e.g., Chronicle® system) include a monitor, a passive fixation sensor lead, an external pressure reference along with data retrieval, and viewing components (Fig. 2). Studies have shown that the sensors function well over time, reliability is good, and the IHMs are usually well tolerated.[24,25] Many cardiac resynchronization therapy and implantable cardioverter defibrillators (CRT, ICDs) have the technology to monitor intrathoracic impedance and in-built algorithms alert patients by an audible alarm, if there is volume overload and incipient clinical worsening. Patients can then either increase drugs doses (e.g., diuretics) or instructed to get in touch with their home nurses/physicians
    - In the SENSE-HF study, OptiVol® (ICD/CRT-D) device measured intrathoracic impedance showed modest sensitivity for predicting recurrent hospitalizations[26]
    - In the MUSIC study, a noninvasive external device attached to the chest, measured bioimpedance, heart rate, respiratory rate, physical activity duration and intensity, and body posture. A multiparametric algorithm based on fluid index, breath index, and personalization parameters had a sensitivity of 65% and a specificity of 90% in predicting acute HF decompensations[27]
    - The Evolution of Management Strategies of Heart Failure Patients with Implantable Defibrillators (EVOLVO) study, randomized patients of HF to remote monitoring (ICD/CRT-D) of intrathoracic impedance, atrial arrhythmias and ICD-shocks versus usual care (scheduled visits every 4 months). A significant reduction of emergency visits by ~35% was reported in the remote monitoring group when compared to usual care[28]
    - In the Implant-based Multiparameter Telemonitoring of Patients with Heart Failure (IN-TIME) trial, daily multiparametric monitoring of data transmitted by devices was associated with benefit in clinical composite scores [all-cause death, hospital admission for HF, change in New York Heart Association (NYHA) class] in the telemonitoring group (risk reduction by 37%)[29]
    - However the OptiLink HF study, in patients of HF with ICD/CRT-Ds, reported that despite fluid status alerts, no significant effect was noted in the composite endpoint of all-cause death and hospitalizations.[30] The multicentric Remote Management of HF using IEDs (REM-HF) study, also reported no significant difference in death/hospitalizations between the remote monitoring group and usual care[31]
- Data on the effectiveness of STS telehealthcare in reducing hard endpoints like morbidity and mortality in HF has been conflicting. While some meta-analyses have reported that STS reduces all-cause mortality and HF hospitalizations, other studies did not confirm this.[21,32-34] Recent data confirm the benefit of telemonitoring in reducing death, emergency admission rates, and reduced duration of hospital stay in patients with HF and obstructive pulmonary disease[35]
- Telemonitoring of HF patients using invasive data (acquired from IHMs) has shown to be of greater benefit. In fact, intrathoracic impedance, LV-filling pressures, and pulmonary artery (PA) pressures monitoring have been reported to have greater sensitivity to predict worsening HF as compared to simple parameters like acute weight gain.[36] Use of wireless implantable hemodynamic monitoring systems to measure and monitor PA pressure has been reported to reduce rate of HF and duration of hospital stay.[37] Telemonitoring of left atrial pressure has also been reported to be associated with reduced risk of acute decompensation and HF death.[38] Trials with new generation telesystems that combine noninvasive and invasive parameters are required to further elaborate of the use of telehealthcare in HF
- The 2016 European Society of Cardiology Guidelines for HF recommend for the first time "remote patient monitoring" with a recommendation of grade IIb, LOE B.[39]

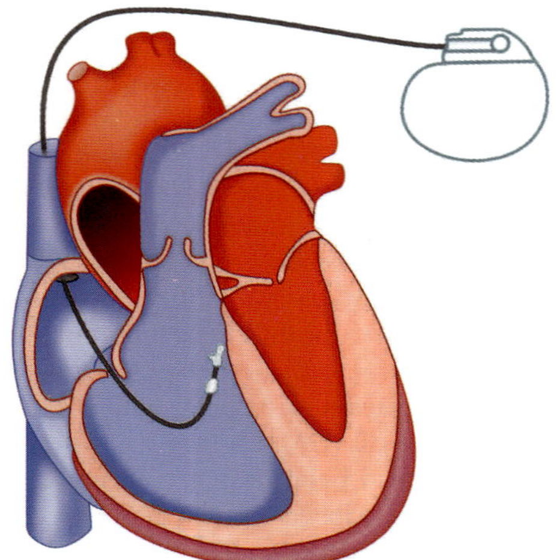

FIG. 2: An implantable hemodynamic monitoring device with lead placed near right ventricular outflow tract.

Remote Monitoring in Patients with Pacemakers and Implantable Cardioverter Defibrillators

The number of patients with implantable devices like pacemakers and ICDs is rising exponentially as indications of implant have widened to include more diverse patient groups. Generally, patients with devices need follow-up at 6 months to 1 year and sometimes more frequently depending on the clinical situation. These follow-up visits usually include evaluation of the device function (battery status, capture thresholds, and any events) and a general clinical examination. In most of these visits, no technical change is performed in device parameters rendering these hospital visits as clinically irrelevant. Studies have shown that only 5–15% of in-hospital visits for ICD checks are done for an unscheduled event (e.g., a shock, device alert).[40] Patients often travel from afar (with accompanying attendants) just to be told that everything is normal and these time-consuming visits mean long-waiting times and time off work leading to noncompliance. Hospital resources like physical space and manpower are also required to manage such visits; nurses, technical staff, and even doctors often compromise their time for attending to issues that are uneventful and only need reassurance.

- Recent technical innovations in devices have led to advancements in remote monitoring and data can be wirelessly transferred on a regular basis to servers that examine and analyze the data, so that remote follow-up can be performed. Information available from current devices can range from arrhythmia detection, battery and lead parameters, impedance, volume status, pulmonary and left atrial pressure, etc. Systems allow automatic transmission of data stored in the device to the outpatient clinic using wireless network for mobile communication network or via a landline. The alerts can be based on a change in device parameters (battery status and lead impedance), programming issues [sensing or capture margins, inadvertent disabling of ventricular fibrillation (VF) therapy] and clinical events (arrhythmias and lung fluid accumulation)
- Physicians in charge of the patients can be notified immediately, if any events or technical malfunctions are detected. Additional notification by E-mail, SMS, fax, or even phone messages can be sent, if critical data are available for consultation. This helps in earlier detection of relevant findings and conserves healthcare resources only for clinically important events. Depending on the clinical need and specific issues involved, follow-ups are still needed since due to safety issues systems do not yet allow routine remote device programming
- The technical reliability of such systems is in excellent and transmission of information is much faster than what would occur with face-to-face visits. Clinical benefit of telemonitoring in patients with implantable devices is well documented with nearly 50% reduction in follow-up visits without compromising patient safety.[40-42] It has been documented that telemonitoring to follow-up 100 ICD patients needed only 1.5 hours and 15 minutes per week nurse- and physician-time, respectively, and leading to significant reduction in unnecessary hospital visits.[43,44] In addition, unscheduled visits following ICD shocks can also be minimized, when after an event and patient upload of data, analysis reveals that the shock was inappropriate and a physical visit is not needed.

Others

Telemonitoring in Patients with Pulmonary Hypertension

The aim of pharmacological management of patients with primary/idiopathic pulmonary hypertension is alleviation of PA pressures. Although PA pressure can be measured by right heart catheterization or Doppler echocardiography, both provide only a single time snapshot of the hemodynamic status. Telemonitoring by devices like the Chronicle® system or CardioMEMS® system can help in continuous assessment of PA pressures and monitor long-term efficacy of new drug therapies.[45,46] Pressure sensors, in close contact with the PA, collect and store data of PA pressures and then transmit it to the central server.

Tele-echocardiography

Transmission of real-time echocardiography images between small peripheral hospitals and specialized tertiary care centers is especially important for diagnosing or excluding congenital heart disease (CHD) in newborns. In India nearly 180,000–210,000 children are born with CHD every year, and 30–50% of these have critical disease that requires early intervention. Nearest echocardiography machines and experienced pediatric cardiologists are often hundreds of kilometers away meaning that only a minority receives requisite therapy due to delay in diagnosis. Tele-echo services have been developed that involve training technicians or physicians to perform echocardiography on remote sites and then transferring images to the pediatric cardiologist via tele-echo links. This helps to make early diagnosis and ensure proper and early referrals when needed. Transmitting echocardiogram images needs efficient compression techniques without compromising image quality. After transmission, images are decompressed at the specialist making interpretation feasible and easy.

Patients with Prosthetic Valves

Patients with mechanical valvular heart prostheses can encounter life-threatening complications like endocarditis, valve thrombosis, pannus, and thromboembolism. Devices (the ThromboCheck device) can analyze and transmit the sound frequency spectra of valve motion. A baseline frequency spectrum is obtained immediately postoperatively. The device continuously monitors the sound frequency of the prosthetic valve motion and if the spectrum deviates from baseline, the signals are transmitted to the medical center via telephone or Internet.[47] If the nurse/physician in charge suspects prosthesis valve dysfunction, patients are instructed to come in and get an echocardiogram or fluoroscopy. The positive-predictive value (97%) and sensitivity (~100%) of ThromboCheck devices has been reported to be excellent. Patients living in remote or outreach areas, poorly compliant on anticoagulation or those with previous history of valve thrombosis are the optimal candidates for such monitoring.

Arrhythmia Diagnosis

Telecardiology is very useful for establishing diagnosis of paroxysmal arrhythmias, which are often missed by single time ECG/Holter recordings. Event and loop recorders record continuous ECGs (3–7 days) and transmit the data to physicians electronically, helping make remote diagnosis. In patients with paroxysmal atrial fibrillation, alerts can identify initiating episodes and identify triggers, which can call for unscheduled follow-up visits with tailoring of management (antiarrhythmic drugs, anticoagulation, external cardioversion, or device reprogramming).

RADAR Systems

Many currently available telemonitoring systems use sensors that need to be placed in close contact with the cardiac chamber and therefore require invasive techniques for insertion. RADAR systems using ultra-wideband (UWB) can potentially overcome these limitations and expand the use to a wider spectrum of population including sicker adults and even children without compromising patient mobility and comfort, and avoiding the complications of an invasive procedure. This technology can acquire and transmit large amount of digital data and high-resolution images. Although microwave radiation exposure was concern, the average emission level used (»1 μW) is much lower than international standards for continuous human exposure to microwaves, making these devices safe and useful. This technology has found application in monitoring cardiac volumes, respiration, early diagnosis of sudden infant death syndrome (SIDS) and in patients with obstructive sleep apnea.

CONCLUSION

An increasingly aging patient population, rising trends of coronary artery disease (CAD) and HF, and the widespread availability of new drugs and devices have highlighted the need for continuous and close contact between the patient and healthcare givers to ensure optimal care. Since there is a dearth of qualified healthcare professionals and medical resources, especially in developing countries like India, telehealthcare is a cost-effective way for evidence based care to be delivered at the doorstep of patients. It is mandatory that the remote monitoring system is organized comprehensively with seamless and rapid data transfer, fast reaction schemes with effective alert notifications and feedbacks systems for patient education and counseling. The system should be tiered to filter out only relevant events and hence not overburden the providers with unnecessary information.

Initiation into home follow-up telemonitoring systems should begin early after hospital discharge to help patients become familiar with these systems as early as possible. Physicians and para-medical staff should also be educated about the operational technicalities of the system. Keeping in mind cost and long-term sustainability issues, it is important to identify specific subgroups of patients that would maximally be benefited by such interventions. Although the cost of creating, operating, and monitoring such effective telemonitoring systems is a factor, this needs to be considered in light of the fact that only few (<10%) of routine hospital visits require subsequent physician evaluation as compared to more than 50% of those with unforeseen events. This large unmet clinical need of optimization of healthcare resources can help to make these systems cost-effective.

REFERENCES

1. Einthoven W. Le telecardiogramme. Arch Int de Physiol. 1906;4:132-64 [Translated into English Am Heart J. 1957;53:602-15].
2. Anker SD, Koehler F, Abraham WT. Telemedicine and remote management of patients with heart failure. Lancet. 2011;378:731-9.
3. Vörös K, Bonnevie A, Reiczgel J. Comparison of conventional and sensor-based electronic stethoscopes in detecting cardiac murmurs of dogs. Tierarzte Prax Ausg K Kleintiere Heimitiere. 2012;40(2):103-11.
4. WHO. (2018). Density of physicians (total number per 1000 population, latest available year). [online] Available from http://www.who.int/gho/health_workforce/physicians_density/en/. [Accessed July, 2018].
5. Capewell S, McMurray J. 'Chest pain—please admit': is there an alternative? A rapid cardiological assessment service may prevent unnecessary admissions. BMJ. 2000;320:951.
6. Terkelsen CJ, Nørgaard BL, Lassen JF, et al. Telemedicine used for remote prehospital diagnosing in patients suspected of acute myocardial infarction. J Intern Med. 2002;252:412-20.
7. Clemmensen P, Sejersten M, Sillesen M, et al. Diversion of ST-elevation myocardial infarction patients for primary angioplasty based on wireless prehospital 12-lead electrocardiographic transmission directly to the cardiologist's handheld computer: a progress report. J Electrocardiol. 2005;38 Suppl 4:194-8.
8. Adams GL, Campbell PT, Adams JM, et al. Effectiveness of prehospital wireless transmission of electrocardiograms to a cardiologist via hand-held device for patients with acute myocardial infarction (from the Timely Intervention in Myocardial Emergency. North East Experience [TIME-NE]). Am J Cardiol. 2006;98:1160-4.
9. Dieker HJ, Liem SS, El Aidi H, et al. Pre-hospital triage for primary angioplasty: direct referral to the intervention center versus interhospital transport. JACC Cardiovasc Interv. 2010;3:705-11.
10. Pedersen SH, Galatius S, Hansen PR, et al. Field triage reduces treatment delay and improves long-term clinical outcome in patients with acute ST-segment elevation myocardial infarction treated with primary percutaneous coronary intervention. J Am Coll Cardiol. 2009;54:2296-302.
11. Sørensen JT, Terkelsen CJ, Nørgaard BL, et al. Urban and rural implementation of pre-hospital diagnosis and direct referral for primary percutaneous coronary intervention in patients with acute ST-elevation myocardial infarction. Eur Heart J. 2011;32(4):430-6.
12. Terkelsen CJ, Lassen JF, Nørgaard BL, et al. Reduction of treatment delay in patients with ST-elevation myocardial infarction: impact of pre-hospital diagnosis and direct referral to primary percutaneous coronary intervention. Eur Heart J. 2005;26:770-7.
13. Atary JZ, De Visser M, Van den Dijk R, et al. Standardised pre-hospital care of acute myocardial infarction patients: MISSION! guidelines applied in practice. Neth Heart J. 2010;18(9):408-15.
14. Ornato JP, Menown IB, Peberdy MA, et al. Body surface mapping vs 12-lead electrocardiography to detect ST-elevation myocardial infarction. Am J Emerg Med. 2009;27:779-84.
15. Hoekstra JW, O'Neill BJ, Pride YB, et al. Acute detection of ST-elevation myocardial infarction missed on standard 12-Lead ECG with a novel 80-lead real-time digital body surface map: primary results from the multicenter OCCULT MI trial. Ann Emerg Med. 2009;54:779-88.e1.
16. Drew BJ, Dempsey ED, Joo TH, et al. Pre-hospital synthesized 12-lead ECG ischemia monitoring with transtelephonic transmission in acute coronary syndromes. Pilot study results of the ST SMART trial. J Electrocardiol. 2004;37 Suppl:214-21.
17. Drew BJ, Sommargren CE, Schindler DM, et al. A simple strategy improves prehospital electrocardiogram utilization and hospital treatment for patients with acute coronary syndrome (from the ST SMART Study). Am J Cardiol. 2011;107(3):347-52.

18. GESICA Investigators. Randomised trial of telephone intervention in chronic heart failure: DIAL trial. BMJ. 2005;331:425.
19. Cleland JG, Louis AA, Rigby AS, et al. Noninvasive home telemonitoring for patients with heart failure at high risk of recurrent admission and death: the Trans-European Network-Home-Care Management System (TEN-HMS) study. J Am Coll Cardiol 2005;45:1654-64.
20. Scherr D, Kastner P, Kollmann A, et al.; The MOBITEL investigators. Effect of home-based telemonitoring using mobile phone technology on the outcome of heart failure patients after an episode of acute decompensation: randomized controlled trial. J Med Internet Res. 2009;11(3):e34.
21. Chaudhry SI, Mattera JA, Curtis JP, et al. Telemonitoring in patients with heart failure. N Engl J Med. 2010;363:2301-9.
22. Morak J, Kollmann A, Schreier G. Feasibility and usability of a home monitoring concept based on mobile phones and near field communication (NFC) technology. Stud Health Technol Inform. 2007;12(Pt 1):112-6.
23. Chaudhry SI, Wang Y, Concato J, et al. Patterns of weight change preceding hospitalization for heart failure. Circulation. 2007;116:1549-54.
24. Pamboukian SV, Smallfield MC, Bourge RC. Implantable hemodynamic monitoring devices in heart failure. Curr Cardiol Rep. 2006;8(3):187-90.
25. Adamson PB. Ambulatory hemodynamics in patients with chronic heart failure: implications for volume management in elderly patients. Am J Geriatr Cardiol. 2005;14:236-41.
26. Conraads VM, Tavazzi L, Santini M, et al. Sensitivity and positive predictive value of implantable intrathoracic impedance monitoring as a predictor of heart failure hospitalizations: the SENSE-HF trial. Eur Heart J. 2011;32:2266-73.
27. Anand IS, Tang WH, Greenberg BH, et al. Design and performance of a multisensor heart failure monitoring algorithm: results from the Multisensor Monitoring in Congestive Heart Failure (MUSIC) study. J Card Fail. 2012;18(4):289-95.
28. Landolina M, Perego GB, Lunati M, et al. Remote monitoring reduces healthcare use and improves quality of care in heart failure patients with implantable defibrillators the Evolution of Management Strategies of Heart Failure Patients With Implantable Defibrillators (EVOLVO) study. Circulation. 2012;125:2985-92.
29. Hindricks G, Taborsky M, Glikson M, et al. Implant-based multiparameter telemonitoring of patients with heart failure (IN-TIME): a randomised controlled trial. Lancet. 2014;384(9943):583-90.
30. Böhm M, Drexler H, Oswald H, et al. Fluid status telemedicine alerts for heart failure: a randomized controlled trial. OptiLink HF study investigation. Eur Heart J. 2016;37:3154-63.
31. Morgan JM, Kitt S, Gill J, et al. Remote management of heart failure using implantable electronic devices. Eur Heart J. 2017;38(30):2352-60.
32. Inglis SC, Clark RA, McAlister FA, et al. Structured telephone support or telemonitoring programmes for patients with chronic heart failure. Cochrane Database Syst Rev. 2010;(8):CD007228.
33. Inglis SC, Clark RA, Dierckx R, et al. Structured telephone support or non invasive telemonitoring for patients with heart failure. Cochrane Database Syst Rev. 2015;(10):CD007228.
34. Koehler F, Winkler S, Schieber M, et al. Impact of remote telemedical management on mortality and hospitalizations in ambulatory patients with chronic heart failure: the telemedical interventional monitoring in heart failure study. Circulation. 2011;123:1873-80.
35. Steventon A, Bardsley M, Billings J, et al. Effect of telehealth on use of secondary care and mortality: findings from the Whole System Demonstrator cluster randomised trial. BMJ. 2012;344:e3874.
36. Abraham WT, Compton S, Haas G, et al. Intrathoracic impedance vs daily weight monitoring for predicting worsening heart failure events: results of the Fluid Accumulation Status Trial (FAST). Congest Heart Fail. 2011;17:51-5.
37. Abraham WT, Adamson PB, Bourge RC, et al. Wireless pulmonary artery haemodynamic monitoring in chronic heart failure: a randomised controlled trial. Lancet. 2011;377(9766):658-66.
38. Adamson PB, Magalski A, Braunschweig F, et al. Ongoing right ventricular hemodynamics in heart failure: clinical value of measurements derived from an implantable monitoring system. J Am Coll Cardiol. 2003;41:565-71.
39. Ponikowski P, Voors AA, Anchor SD, et al. Acute and chronic heart failure. ESC Clinical Practice Guidelines. EHJ. 2016;37:2129-200.
40. Heidbuchel H, Lioen P, Foulon S, et al. Potential role of remote monitoring for scheduled and unscheduled evaluations of patients with an implantable defibrillator. Europace. 2008;10(3):351-7.
41. Mabo P, Victor F, Bazin P, et al. A randomized trial of long-term remote monitoring of pacemaker recipients (the COMPAS trial). Eur Heart J. 2012;33:1105-11.
42. Brugada P. What evidence do we have to replace in-hospital implantable cardioverter defibrillator follow-up? Clin Res Cardiol. 2006;95 Suppl 3:3-9.
43. Ricci RP, Morichelli L, Santini M. Home monitoring remote control of pacemaker and implantable cardioverter defibrillator patients in clinical practice: impact on medical management and health-care resource utilization. Europace. 2008;10(2):164-70.
44. Varma N, Epstein AE, Irimpen A, et al. Evaluation of efficacy and safety of remote monitoring for ICD follow-up: the TRUST trial. Circulation (Abstract). 2008;118:2316.
45. Fruhwald FM, Kjellström B, Perthold W, et al. Continuous hemodynamic monitoring in pulmonary hypertensive patients treated with inhaled iloprost. Chest. 2003;124(1):351-9.
46. Karamanoglu M, McGoon M, Frantz RP, et al. Right ventricular pressure waveform and wave reflection analysis in patients with pulmonary arterial hypertension. Chest. 2007;132:37-43.
47. Fritzsche D, Schenk S, Eitz T, et al. Patient self-monitoring of prosthetic heart valve function. J Heart Valve Dis. 2007;16:558-66.

CHAPTER 147

Executive Cardiac Checkup: Is it Really Needed?

Brian Pinto, Neeraj A Desai

INTRODUCTION

Since independence, India has seen a drastic change in lifestyle and diet, moving from agrarian diets and hard physical labor to junk food, and sedentary lifestyles due to a capitalist economy ushered in, especially in the 80s and 90s. This has occurred in a much shorter duration compared to other nations. Hence, high mortalities related to cardiovascular diseases (CVDs), diabetes, and stroke have sky rocketed since then. In comparison with the Europeans, CVD affects Indians at least a decade earlier and in their most productive midlife years.[1,2] In the west, 23% of CVD deaths occur before the age of 70 years; while in India, this number is 52%.[3] Regarding case fatality related to CVD in developing countries like India, it is much higher compared to developed nations.[4,5] The World Health Organization (WHO) had reported that, due to burden of CVD, India had apparently lost $237 billion from the loss of productivity and spending on health care over a 10-year period (2005–2015).[6] The current and future forecasts is no different and shows continuing trend in the coming decades, where CVDs will lead to major loss of the human resource pool of the country. Slated to be one of the youngest nations in the world, India is set to give up this productive population to CVD morbidity and mortality which can hinder the economic growth in an otherwise beneficial phase of demographic transition.

In India, the preventive healthcare sector is growing. India's total preventive healthcare market now estimates over $800 million.[7] The current scenario in Indian markets offers a tremendous opportunity to bring in innovative technology solutions. Healthcare companies are moving in the upward direction empowering patients to engage more in health awareness. This has lead to people spending more time and resources on health which has given a boost to preventive healthcare at urban and to some extent semi-urban market.

It makes good sense for India Inc. to protect their top talent from the growing dearth of noncommunicable diseases which have reached a point of epidemic stature, irrespective of socioeconomic and cultural background. The healthcare industry in India is at a very important juncture. It is on the brink of a transformation, as it adopts new pathways, including latest innovative technology, to help executives manage their health in a better manner. Preventive healthcare is becoming an area of focus in most countries, and India is no different.

As the cost of healthcare increases in the corporate sector, there is an increasing interest in workplace for raising awareness about various diseases especially CVD and a need to practice prevention in healthcare. The ASSOCHAM (Associated Chambers of Commerce and Industry of India) report in January 2018 on preventive healthcare and its impact on corporate sector states that ₹1 spent on prevention saves ₹133 in absenteeism costs and ₹6.62 in healthcare costs. Hence, proper healthcare and wellness programs can change employees' perception about health and improve his risk profile and productivity.

Currently the executive cardiac health checkups in India offer a battery of test listed below:

- Routine blood and urine investigations [including lipid profile, apolipoprotein B (ApoB), lipoprotein(a), and serum homocysteine levels]
- Chest X-ray
- Electrocardiogram
- Two-dimensional echocardiography
- Treadmill test
- Cardiac consultation
- In some centers cardiac computed tomography (CT) (to assess calcium score).

Costs vary, but executive cardiac health programs can be cost-effective.[8] Considerable disparity exists among programs in terms of testing and other clinical services. Some executive checkups provide comprehensive, efficient, effective, and individualized patient-based care at a reasonable cost.

Although executive checkups have been around for 100 years, literature search has been futile and very few studies have documented the potential impact of a cardiac executive checkup on medical expenditure. In a study published in 2002, periodic executive cardiac checkup participants experienced an average 0.93 (or 2.78 for 3 years) short-term disability days absent per year in comparison with an average of 1.34 (or 4.02 for 3 years) short-term disability days absent for nonperiodic heath checkups. The net return on investment (ROI) for a worksite-based executive health examination which cost approximately $400 per executive whose total compensation (salary and benefits) is at least $125,000 is estimated to be 2.3:1, which compares favorably with other preventive health programs.[8]

The best available evidence suggests that patients benefit from cardiac executive health checks through its association with improved delivery of some important preventive clinical tests through reduction of patient worry. The available evidence does not reveal harms associated with the executive health checkup. Given that short- and long-term studies have shown that appropriate implementation of currently recommended preventive services improves health in short- and long-term studies.[9]

The main appeal of an executive health check stems partly from its variety. It usually includes a comprehensive exam, extensive blood work, and other checks for heart disease. The exclusive versions also call for a CT scan of the heart to asses for coronary artery calcium (CAC) scoring.

COMPUTED TOMOGRAPHY CORONARY CALCIUM SCORING

Several studies have shown how CAC can reclassify individuals previously stratified as per the atherosclerotic cardiovascular disease (ASCVD) risk factors.[10] Hence, preventive cardiac checkups in asymptomatic diabetic and age 40–75 years but with estimated ASCVD risk of 5% or higher or those in less than 5% 10 years risk group can definitely benefit from additional CAC scanning. The higher risk (>20% 10 years ASCVD risk) has little role except that it provides a persuasive confirmation of high-risk patients reluctant for statin therapy (Fig. 1). The 2013 American College of Cardiology/American Heart Association (ACC/AHA) prevention guidelines emphasized on absolute risk assessment of preventive therapy to determine maximum benefit.[11] CAC = 0 appears the strongest negative predictor of cardiovascular event when compared to other markers like ankle brachial index or carotid intimal thickness. There is strong evidence that CAC = 0 can downwardly classify risk when 10 years ASCVD risk is between 5 and 15% and a moderate evidence to reclassify risk in people between 15 and 20% ASCVD to a level where no statin is required. Those who have undergone CAC screening in the ASCVD 5–20% intermediate risk group statin therapy is initiated or not initiated as per the Society of Cardiovascular Computed Tomography recommendations (Fig. 2). In a few patients where a progression of CAC score is anticipated and would support intensifying the preventive management, repeat scanning at an interval of 5 years for 0 CAC and 3–5 years interval for patients with CAC more than 0.[12]

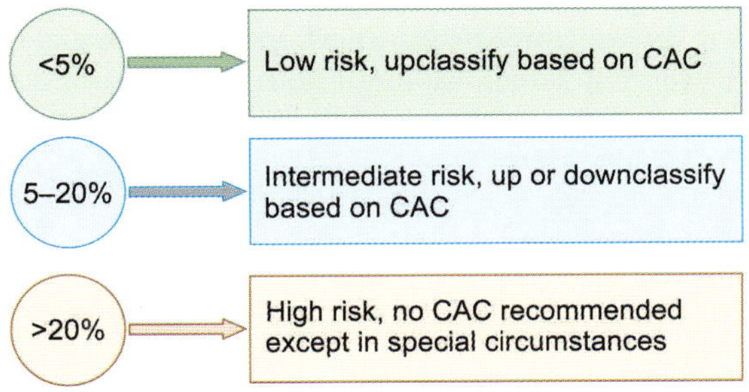

FIG. 1: The role of coronary artery calcium in reclassifying the 10-year atherosclerotic cardiovascular disease risk categories and guiding treatment.[13]

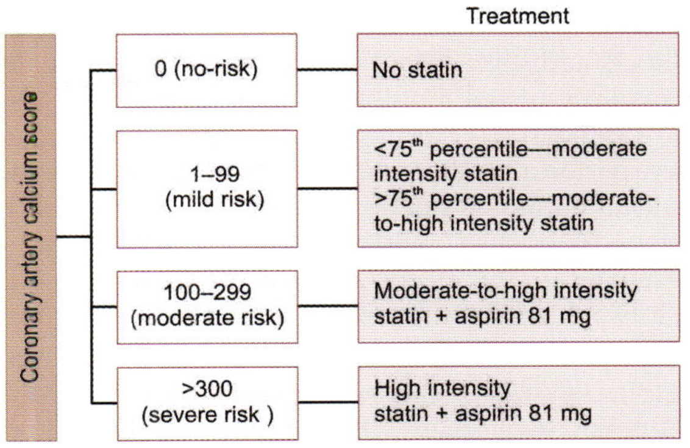

FIG. 2: Primary prevention based on coronary artery calcium score determined risks in the 5–20% atherosclerotic cardiovascular disease risk group.[13]

At first, you should think that an innovative medical technology can see a dormant disease lying with your body without so much as scratching the skin would be perfect. However, the monetary aspects with low circumstantial evidence deter most insurers to pay for them in a preventive context. And there are some drawbacks. Quite frequently these scans show false positives. They detect suspicious lesions that turnout to be harmless, raising needless worry, and frequently prompting invasive tests. Conversely they also can be falsely negative, that can create a false sense of security that leads the patient to ignore early warning signs. Even if a recent scan of an employee's coronary arteries indicates a low risk of heart disease, he/she should tell her doctor about angina and the mild nausea he/she has started to feel after a short time on the treadmill. Not doing so could prove fatal. As imaging technology continues to get better and safer, the day may come when the risk/benefit ratio justifies scans as screening tests for healthy people in a preventive care setup. Today, though, the feasibility in most situations would not see a return on their investment when they are included as part of the executive physical with the occasional exceptions.

Presumably, the employers believe that the extensive workup will help reveal hidden health issues while they are most treatable, through a process, i.e., both thorough and efficient. If there is nothing detected, at least the executive will feel cared for. However, more does not necessarily mean better.

However, today many executive cardiac checkups are conducted at distant corporate hospitals which have tie-ups with majority of the multinational companies. Ideally, the doctor talking to the executive and noting down his medical history, performing the general examination, and ordering investigations should not be someone the patient will never see again. He or she should be that person's primary doctor. Unfortunately in todays day and age time-pressured primary care, it is practically impossible to have sufficient time and opportunity during periodic executive health checkup exam for any type of detailed and personalized conversation necessary to create that meaningful doctor-patient relationship and to sustain it. The executive health check frequently becomes a rushed, impersonal, and largely bureaucratic activity which ends up being nothing more than a brief interview focused reviewing of health habits, medications, and allergies, with additional supplemented by a physical examination and ordering of recommended screening tests and procedures—in essence, checking all the requisite boxes for reimbursement. No wonder some observers question the value of the annual physical as it is currently implemented. Physician-ethicist-commentator Ezekiel Emanuel, for one, views it as an antiquated habit of little worth (and even of potential harm) that consumes scarce physician time; he has called for the public to skip it while acknowledging that the opportunity to "reaffirm the physician-patient relationship" is an important draw for patients.[13]

The talk of scrapping the executive health checkup should take into account factors that stall its implementation and limit its contributions to care, especially in terms of relationship building. Time and continuity are clearly in short supply in primary care, yet both are critical to establishing and maintaining a trusting doctor-patient relationship. Discussing a person's values and health care preferences are important addendums to that inquiry and help build a sense of caring, respect, mutuality, and trust. Trust is built by the relationships continuity and the availability, reliability, and safety of the care provided over time. When performed in a thorough, gentle, and considerate manner, the physical examination can communicate caring and help build trust. From this point of view, the executive health checkup becomes as much an act of relationship building and continuity as it is a means of searching for clinically significant findings. In the age of imaging and advanced medical technology, physicians scarcely rely on physical examination and lose appreciation for its therapeutic effect, not to mention the skills required to perform it.

Rather than completely eliminating such executive checkups, it should be improved. This requires time and a dedicated team effort on part of both the employer and primary caregiving institutions, to free the physician of a routinized aspect of screening, data collection, and examination. Instead of predetermining the investigations and concluding a health check with the physician consultation, the order should be reversed, where the primary physician gets to decide the course of the executive health check. This will lead to a more thorough evaluation in terms of physician-optimized value-added elements. For active medical problems, a problem-based review could be included, complemented by a careful evidence-based physical examination for relevant items. The visit could conclude with a summation of findings, recommendations for the coming year, and time for discussion. An hour-long visit could include about 30–40 minutes of physician time, making it practical and meaningful for both patient and physician. In this conceptualization, the executive health checkup would become the annual health review, just like an appraisal and managing your yearly health goals.

For low-risk patients (e.g., healthy young adults with health-conscious lifestyles), the interval between such visits might be longer than a year, but short enough to maintain the relationship and check on life events and stresses with health consequences. In places where primary care physicians are few and far between, this role, for patients without complex medical issues could very well be carried out by well-trained advanced-practice nurses or physician assistants with physician backup over communication.

CONCLUSION

To summarize, the mantra that "One size fits all" does not hold true for executive cardiac checkup as it does not have much value if too many tests are burdened on all asymptomatic individuals. However in my opinion, a basic cardiac checkup, comprising of routine blood investigations with lipid profile with high-risk lifestyles above the age of 30 years should be made a necessity in all corporate work places, not every year but once in 3 years. This can give the physician an idea about individual risk stratification and differentiate low-risk individuals from intermediate and high risk ones subjectively based on family history and physical examination. Those with a relatively higher risk can be subjected to further testing based on their subordinate features.

The health insurance, primary care providers and their affiliated organizations should create and maintain a well-oiled system for thorough and efficient preventive steps proven to be cost-effective and risk free. Executives get exactly what they want; they would get it from their own primary care physicians, which would save time and money for the employers. It seems reasonable for physicians to redouble their efforts to build meaningful relationships that can be trusted and sustained, particularly at a time when patients are experiencing problems at every step of healthcare delivery. Turning the executive health checkup into an annual health review will help create value for both patients and doctors, enabling the latter to serve as physicians rather than merely health care providers.

REFERENCES

1. Joshi P, Islam S, Pais P, et al. Risk factors for early myocardial infarction in South Asians compared with individuals in other countries. Jama. 2007;297(3):286-94.
2. Xavier D, Pais P, Devereaux PJ, et al. Treatment and outcomes of acute coronary syndromes in India (CREATE): a prospective analysis of registry data. Lancet. 2008;371(9622):1435-42.
3. Harikrishnan S, Leeder S, Huffman M, et al. A race against time: the challenge of cardiovascular disease in developing economies. New Delhi, India: Centre for Chronic Disease Control; 2014.

4. Yusuf S, Rangarajan S, Teo K, et al. Cardiovascular risk and events in 17 low-, middle-, and high-income countries. N Eng J Med. 2014;371(9):818-27.
5. Prabhakaran D, Yusuf S, Mehta S, et al. Two-year outcomes in patients admitted with non-ST elevation acute coronary syndrome: results of the OASIS registry 1 and 2. Indian Heart J. 2005;57(3):217-25.
6. Mendis S, Puska P, Norrving B, et al. Global atlas on cardiovascular disease prevention and control. Geneva: World Health Organization; 2011.
7. Naikawadi A. Preventive healthcare: The need of the hour for corporates. ETHealthWorld. 2017.
8. Burton WN, Chen CY, Conti DJ, et al. The value of the periodic executive health examination: experience at bank one and summary of the literature. J Occup Environ Med. 2002;44(8):737-44.
9. Sheridan S, Pignone M, Donahue K. Screening for high blood pressure: a review of the evidence for the US Preventive Services Task Force. Am J Prev Med. 2003;25(2):151-8.
10. Raggi P, Shaw LJ, Berman DS, et al. Prognostic value of coronary artery calcium screening in subjects with and without diabetes. J Am Coll Cardiol. 2004;43:1663-9.
11. Stone NJ, Robinson JG, Lichtenstein AH, et al. 2013 ACC/AHA guideline on the treatment of blood cholesterol to reduce atherosclerotic cardiovascular risk in adults: a report of the American College of cardiology/American heart association Task Force on practice guidelines. J Am Coll Cardiol. 2014;63(25 Pt B): 2889-934.
12. Hecht H, Blaha MJ, Berman DS, et al. Clinical indications for coronary artery calcium scoring in asymptomatic patients: Expert consensus statement from the Society of Cardiovascular Computed Tomography. J Cardiovasc Comput Tomogr. 2017;11(2):157-68.
13. Emanuel EJ. Skip your annual physical. New York Times; 2015.

CHAPTER 148

Cardiology and Ethics: Mission Impossible?

Raja Selvaraj, Jayaraman Balachander

INTRODUCTION

The practice of medicine is a unique blend of science and art and is exacting in its requirement of skills and qualities in its practitioners. Ethical issues have been interlinked with the practice of this discipline ever since the birth of modern medicine. Even today, taking the Hippocratic Oath continues as a rite of passage for medical trainees beginning practice and issues regarding ethics crop up each day while practicing.

An important reason why medical practice remains a minefield of ethical issues is that while providing medical care to a patient, the physician and patient enter into a contract which is inherently unbalanced. In this contract between unequal parties, the patient is always much more vulnerable than the physician, having less knowledge and understanding of the situation, usually less authority about deciding the course of action and always with more to lose. Being in a position of more power, the physician has to tread carefully and it is very easy to act in a manner that brings up questions of ethics. While this is common to all forms of medical practice, is there something unique about the field of cardiology, and especially about this time in history that makes it a challenge to practice ethical medicine in cardiology today?

CHALLENGES SPECIFIC TO CARDIOLOGY

At first glance, the odds appear to be stacked in favor of cardiologists. The heart is a vital organ and diseases of the heart remain one of the most common causes of death in the general population. Cardiologists who treat these diseases therefore have a large number of patients whom they can help and the potential change in the lives of these patients by good medical care is enormous. The most common heart disease, coronary artery disease, has an extensive evidence base for various treatment modalities with multiple large studies regarding the best treatment to offer. Guidelines are also provided and regularly updated by various national and international scientific bodies for various cardiac disorders. All these should help the cardiologist decide the correct course of action easily and advise the patient accordingly. Despite these, not many would argue with the fact that the practice of cardiology today is particularly enmeshed with ethical issues. There are a few specific reasons for this.

Cost-Benefit Ratio

The cost of many interventional treatments for heart diseases is high because of the specialized hardware required and the evolving treatment approaches with introduction of new technology which tends to be expensive. This makes the financial implications of choosing an interventional therapy over a noninterventional treatment huge. Therefore, avoiding bias while choosing therapies is challenging for the cardiologist. It is an even greater challenge to avoid the perception of bias from this financial gain in the mind of the patient when advising an interventional therapy.

This is not helped by the fact that the benefit of many interventions remains arguable, often small or limited to specific subsets of patients. As an example, the benefits of percutaneous coronary interventions in stable coronary artery disease are small and questionable and have to be balanced against the risks and disadvantages when compared with medical management[1] or coronary artery bypass surgery.[2] Use of an implantable cardioverter defibrillator for primary prevention is associated with a number needed to treat to save a life[3] which some consider acceptable, while others consider too large to justify for the cost. Communicating this uncertainty to the patient and taking a decision with their understanding is not an easy task.

Bias toward Interventions

Apart from financial gains, the technical aspects of a procedure may also prove very attractive for the cardiologist. This may be because of technical challenges presented by the procedure and the attendant satisfaction from completing it (e.g., percutaneous intervention for chronic total occlusion of coronaries) or being an initial adopter of a new procedure leading to adulation from industry and peers (e.g.,transcatheter aortic valve replacement). These can consciously or unconsciously introduce a bias in the mind of the cardiologist when taking a decision of doing a procedure.

The Uncertain Boundaries of Expertise

Cardiology continues to expand into a broad field of knowledge and skills where expertise in a specific area often is required to provide optimal treatment. Trained cardiologists are now available with specific expertise in fields like pediatric cardiology, interventional cardiology, or cardiac electrophysiology. At the same time, many specialized procedures continue to be performed by cardiologists who may not have special training in it. Especially in the absence of a strict certification system in our country, it becomes an ethical challenge for the practicing cardiologist to decide if he should do a certain procedure or refer it to a colleague who may have undergone specific training in that field.

Changing Doctor–Patient Relationship

The doctor–patient relationship is undergoing a sea change in our country which has led to a climate of distrust from both sides. From the traditional relationship of paternal beneficence wherein the physician was treated with reverence, equated with God and given a free hand to take all the important decisions, we are moving to a relationship of shared decision-making where the physician is seen as a caregiver with duties and responsibilities. In today's scenario, the physician is expected to act as mediator between the patient on one hand and medical science and technology on the other, providing the patient with adequate information in order to be able to participate in the decision-making process. In the field of cardiology especially, patient expectations run high because of the fear and awareness of heart disease and the implications of its treatment.

All these factors combine to make ethical issues a challenge in the practice of cardiology today. But is this a challenge that can be overcome with diligence or is it a mission impossible? We believe that it is the former, and that the challenge can be tackled with a concerted effort from the cardiologists and regulatory bodies of medicine and cardiology.

WHAT CAN THE CARDIOLOGIST DO?

The first step is for practicing cardiologists to recognize and understand that practice of cardiology is a challenge today and needs diligence from the practitioner to stick to an ethical path and avoid various biases. An acknowledgement of the challenge prepares him or her to consciously avoid these biases and practice ethical cardiology.

Evidence-based Medicine

It is important to zealously study the scientific literature, critically weighing the various studies and guidelines to decide on the scientifically correct treatment for various conditions. The vast body of literature and the often conflicting results in different studies takes a lot of effort from cardiologists to sift through the available information and separate the wheat from the chaff. But, it is important to follow the evidence and give it precedence over gut feeling and anecdotal evidence. A scientific approach forms the underlying basis for an ethical practice.

Avoiding Discrimination

Multiple studies have shown the existence of differences in diagnosis and treatment of heart disease based on gender, race, and financial status. While this is not a consciously practiced discrimination most of the time, it is an ethical responsibility of the cardiologist to be aware of the existence of this and consciously take steps to avoid it.

Shared Decision-Making

The decision-making practice for many conditions is complex. Often there is a choice to be made between various available therapies and sometimes, an option of no treatment. Each treatment choice is associated with its attendant risks and benefits and sometimes the difference between these might be small and may vary depending on individual perception. The cardiologist should consider the subtle individual differences in the assessment of such risks and benefits that may exist between patients. In the absence of a clear choice of treatment, an approach of shared decision-making should be followed. The role of the cardiologist should not be to make the decision for the patient, but to provide adequate information for the patient to make the decision himself or herself.

Shared decision-making involves not just the provision of the requisite information to the patient, but also time and space to take decisions. For example, *ad hoc* angioplasty has been criticized on this ground because it is difficult, if not impossible for a patient to take a decision when lying on the table after a coronary angiogram. Therefore, this approach should be restricted to specific situations, with preference for a deliberate, joint decision-making process at other times.

Team Approach

The assistance of colleagues is often required for an ideal, ethical practice and the cardiologist should not shy away from obtaining it. An opportunity to obtain a second opinion should be freely provided to patients when necessary. Such a second opinion should also be obtained by the cardiologist when a choice needs to be made among different treatment options to reduce the chance of individual bias. For example, in a situation where there is a choice between a surgical or medical therapy, a surgical colleague may be consulted on the patient. While a colleague from a different field may have a very different view of the situation and this may be initially be uncomfortable to confront, such a different look will ultimately be of benefit to the patient. Joint meetings between the cardiologist and cardiothoracic surgeon were common and played an important role in decision-making in patients with coronary artery disease. As percutaneous interventions have taken over a greater role in management of these patients, such meetings have become uncommon.

Performance Review

Periodic review of his or her own performance is important to do for every cardiologist. Clearly defined and objective key performance indicators may be used and provide an assessment of performance on an ongoing basis. Apart from this kind of self-audit, a periodic peer review process is also useful. In institutes and hospitals, this may take the form of group discussions where management of a patient is reviewed by multiple cardiologists.

Do No Financial Harm[4]

"Primum non nocere", do no harm, is the cardinal rule in medicine. Today, healthcare cost is considered one of the most important forms of financial harm to a person and family. Cardiologists have an important role and an ethical responsibility to mitigate this harm. This involves being aware of the financial status of the patient and tailoring treatment strategies according to this information.

WHAT SHOULD REGULATORY BODIES DO?

The regulatory bodies have an important role as a watchdog to ensure ethical practice of medicine. The American College of Cardiology has published a code of ethics[5] and similarly, code of ethics is published by the Medical Council of India.[6] Such a code of ethics specific to Cardiology can be published by the Cardiology Society of India (CSI).

The American Heart Association (AHA) runs advocacy campaigns among cardiologists and the general public to raise awareness of health disparities and create health equity. Health equity is the term that has been coined to indicate that every patient should have the same opportunity for accessing healthcare. This is achieved by eliminating bias by age, gender, ethnicity, or other differences. The AHA also runs a program called "Get With The Guidelines" to ensure that hospitals follow evidence-based management of heart disease. Such initiatives should also be undertaken by the CSI to improve cardiac care in our country.

Certification by the regulatory bodies as is in vogue in the west will guide cardiologists on the procedures they are allowed to do and the competency required to do them and to maintain proficiency to continue doing them.

Medical Council of India and CSI should also lobby for and guide the inclusion of medical ethics in the curriculum for undergraduates and postgraduates in medicine. Apart from medical ethics, a case has also been made to include medical humanities in teaching including the history of medicine, medicine in literature, patients' perception of illness, life as a doctor and the art of doctoring, subjects which are covered poorly or not at all at present.

CONCLUSION

Cardiology has seen major technological advances in the last few decades, expanding the horizon of what can be done. In contrast, less emphasis seems to be placed on what should be done. Ethical challenges are mostly centered on this conflict between can and should. Cardiology, especially in today's times, presents various challenges to ethical practice. However, with a conscientious and diligent approach from cardiologists and regulatory bodies, this is a challenge that can be overcome and should be overcome.

REFERENCES

1. Al-Lamee R, Thompson D, Dehbi HM, et al. Percutaneous coronary intervention in stable angina (ORBITA): A double-blind, randomised controlled trial. Lancet. 2018;391(10115):31-40.
2. Habib RH, Dimitrova KR, Badour SA, et al. CABG versus PCI: Greater benefit in long-term outcomes with multiple arterial bypass grafting. J Am Coll Cardiol. 2015;66(13):1417-27.
3. Betts TR, Sadarmin PP, Tomlinson DR, et al. Absolute risk reduction in total mortality with implantable cardioverter defibrillators: Analysis of primary and secondary prevention trial data to aid risk/benefit analysis. Europace. 2013; 15(6):813-9.
4. Moriates C, Shah NT, Arora VM. First, Do No (Financial) Harm. JAMA. 2013; 310(6):577-8.
5. American College of Cardiology code of ethics. [online] Available from https://www.acc.org/about-acc/our-bylaws-and-code-of-ethics/code-of-ethics [Accessed August 2018].
6. MCI code of ethics. [online] Available from https://www.mciindia.org/CMS/rules-regulations/code-of-medical-ethics-regulations-2002 [Accessed August 2018].

SECTION 24

Miscellaneous

CHAPTER 149

Development of Cardiology and Interventions in India—An Insider's Glimpse

M Khalilullah

INTRODUCTION

Cardiology was part of medicine until late 1950s when cardiology lectures, bedside clinics, and even cardiac patients were treated by faculty of medicine and physicians at large.

In early 1960s, clinical cardiology was pioneered by Prof JN Berry from Nagpur and Chandigarh, Dr KK Datey and Dr Rustom Jal Vakil from Mumbai, Dr CRR Pillai and Dr Rajagopalan from Chennai, Dr DP Basu and Dr JC Banerjee from Kolkata, but it was Prof Sujoy B Roy at the All India Institute of Medical Sciences (AIIMS), New Delhi and Dr Kamla Vytilingam of CMC Vellore who introduced invasive cardiology and established first catheterization laboratory and pioneered hemodynamic studies. Dr S Padmavati started a catheterization laboratory in Lady Hardinge Medical College at the same time. The superspecialized departments of Cardiology ushered in an era of structured and focused training of cardiology by starting DM cardiology program. This involved in-depth training of clinical cardiology, electrocardiography, hemodynamic studies, and cardiology research programs.

First batch of DM cardiology students passed from AIIMS in early 1960s and then from CMC Vellore in mid-1960s. These two institutions trained true and dedicated cardiologists, who in turn became eminent teachers and trained hundreds of students who fanned out all over the country. Department of Cardiology started getting separated from departments of Medicine with qualified faculties and DM Cardiology program started spreading all over the country.

Prof Rajendra Tandon at AIIMS and Prof IP Sukumar at CMC Vellore pioneered the training in pediatric cardiology. First pacemaker implantation was carried out at AIIMS in April 1966, and first indigenous pacemaker (Khalil Mendes pacemaker) was developed in the same department. Cardiac pacing spread to other parts of the country, especially in Kolkata, and became the large turnover center. Some of the pioneering research of acute mountain sickness, high-attitude pulmonary edema, and high-attitude pulmonary hypertension were carried out by Prof SB Roy. Dr Padmavati, who started her initial career at Lady Hardinge Medical College, became the Director Principal of Maulana Azad Medical College and GB Pant Hospital and soon started DM Cardiology program in 1970. Her pioneering work in rheumatic fever, school surveys of rheumatic heart disease, and prevention of rheumatic fever with establishment of All India Heart Foundation are huge contributionsto the medical field. Her farsightedness and resourcefulness soon made GB Pant Hospital as the center of excellence with about the best training facilities in the country. Students who have qualified from this institution have spread all over the country and abroad, and are the epitome of excellence. Soon the DM training program started in Bengaluru, Hyderabad, Chennai, Mumbai, Jaipur, Lucknow, Kanpur, Kolkata, Thiruvananthapuram, Chandigarh, and many more centers all over the country. Clinical cardiac electrophysiology was started on March 5, 1975, at GB Pant Hospital and became the only center for training in electrophysiology. Soon electrophysiology developed in other parts of country such as Hyderabad, Bangalore, Mumbai, Thiruvananthapuram, Kolkata, Chennai, Ahmedabad both in government and private sectors and became the area of deep interest for large number of young cardiologists.

First catheter ablation was carried out in June 1984 using direct current (DC) shock and improvised DC energy delivery system in GB Pant Hospital and ushered in an era of therapeutic and interventional electrophysiology. At the same time, arrhythmia surgery was established for the first time in GB Pant Hospital where more than 50 patients with Wolff–Parkinson-White syndrome were treated by epicardial mapping and surgical/cryoablation. Many cardiologists got trained abroad and infused new talent in the field of electrophysiology and ablation.

First international conference on Interventional Cardiology was organized on April 1–4, 1985, preceded by a workshop in Interventional Cardiology with assistance of Dr James E Locke and Prof John Keane from Boston Children's Hospital and the first balloon procedure was performed in

India on March 23, 1985, in a patient with severe valvular pulmonary stenosis with suprasystemic Right ventricular (RV) pressure. This deeply blue child became pink instantly after pulmonary valvuloplasty and RV systolic pressure dropped from 180 to 65. Between March 27 and 30, five patients with rheumatic mitral stenosis were subjected to transseptal mitral valvuloplasty - three with single balloon and two with double-balloon technique. Thus the practice of balloon mitral valvuloplasty (BMV) was born. This has changed the entire management of rheumatic mitral stenosis, not only in the Indian subcontinent but the world over, although now the Inoue balloon is used all over the world.

The first case of balloon aortoplasty of coarctation of aorta was performed at GB Pant Hospital in June 1985 and this opened up a new chapter in the management of coarctation of aorta. Soon balloon dilatation technique was attempted in aortic stenosis in operation theater and the balloon was introduced in the stenosed aortic valve and inflated. The aortic cusps got beautifully separated. This was followed by percutaneous balloon aortoplasty of valvular, membranous subaortic stenosis, and supravalvular aortic stenosis; renal artery stenosis was treated with balloon angioplasty along with iliofemoral arterial stenosis.

In December 1985, balloon dilatation of aortoarteritis was established and this pioneering work was published in Circulation in 1986. We had the largest experience of adult coarctation and aortoarteritis probably in the world. Patients with tricuspid stenosis were subjected to double-balloon valvuloplasty, at GB Pant Hospital again the first time in the history.

In 1987, a team from Texas Heart Institute, Houston arrived in GB Pant Hospital comprising Dr Mike Duncan, Cardiac Surgeon, Dr VS Mathur, Cardiologist, Dr Sabavala, Cardiac Anesthetist, and a senior OT nurse for a 2-week workshop on coronary angioplasty and coronary artery bypass grafting (CABG).

During this 2-week workshop, 15 cases of Percutaneous transluminal coronary angioplasty (PTCA) and ten patients were operated for CABG and thus began the era of coronary interventions in India. About the same time Dr Samuel Mathews did his first case of PTCA in Mumbai. Soon a group of cardiologists and cardiac surgeons got trained in PTCA and CABG and the country began to offer PTCA and CABG at many centers in Delhi, Mumbai, Hyderabad, Bangalore, Kolkata, Chennai, and others. In 1988, rotablation started and Dr Gary Ruben brought the rotablator technique to be started in GB Pant Hospital. Dr DS Gambhir was first to be trained in rotablation.

Having achieved a great success in balloon dilatation of valvular stenosis and peripheral arteries, the first neodymium-doped yttrium aluminum garnet (Nd:YAG) laser equipment arrived in GB Pant Hospital and Nd:YAG laser-assisted peripheral angioplasty in 1988, especially chronic total occlusion (CTO) of iliofemoral arteries, was successfully performed along with total occlusion of aorta in eight patients.

Prof John Keane of Boston's Children's Hospital arrived in GB Pant Hospital to start the program of percutaneous closure of patent ductus arteriosus (PDA) using Rashkind's umbrella device. Several cases were performed in GB Pant Hospital and I had the opportunity to demonstrate this technique in Sri Lanka, Peshawar, and in Jayadeva Institute of Cardiology in Bengaluru. I had overheard that a Greek doctor named Dr EA Sideris has developed a kite-shaped device for closure of atrial septal defect (ASD) secundum. He was invited to GB Pant Hospital in 1991 and 15 cases of ASD secundum were successfully closed in 5 days using this occluder and counter-occluder on a button device, and thus percutaneous closure of ASD started in India.

Sideris device of small size was also used to close large PDAs and even acquired ventricular septal defect (VSD) following anterior myocardial infarction. This is the first-ever device historically used to close ASDs. Subsequently, Amplatzer device for PDA and ASD closure was introduced which was easy to handle and retrievable and has been widely used all over the world. This also enabled submembranous VSD to be closed percutaneously. Devices are being used for closure of rupture of sinus of Valsalva, pulmonary arteriovenous (AV) fistula, and vascular plugs have been used to block AV malformations in liver, kidney, and large subcutaneous malformations.

Coronary stents emerged in the later part of 1990s and again Gary Ruben from Atlanta brought two stents to be implanted in GB Pant Hospital. Samuel Mathews was the first to popularize this technique and soon stenting became an addition to PTCA. Peripheral stents became available for peripheral angioplasty including renal artery stenosis, iliofemoral stenosis, coarctation of aorta, aortoarteritis of aorta, and peripheral arteries. Soon carotid artery stenting started in carotid stenosis.

Doctor Tejas Patel from Ahmedabad was the first to start radial artery approach to coronary angiography and angioplasty and complex CTO interventions with the help of Japanese cardiologists. Today the radial approach has become the route of choice for coronary angiography and interventions all over the country; credit of this revolution should entirely go to Dr Patel.

IMPLANTABLE VALVES

After Dr Alain Cribier implanted an aortic valve percutaneously in aortic stenosis, this technique has slowly grown in India. Although expensive, but in patients with serious comorbidities and inoperable patients, this has been a great relief in patients with aortic stenosis. Dr Ashok Seth from Escorts Heart Institute and Dr Praveen Chandra from Medanta Heart Institute have been pioneers in this area and this technique is now being performed in Kerala, Bangalore, and Tamil Nadu. First-ever pulmonary valve implantation has been carried out by Dr Radhakrishnan at the Pediatric Cardiology Department of Escorts Heart Institute this year.

LEFT ATRIAL APPENDAGE CLOSURE

Stroke prevention in atrial fibrillation (AF) in nonvalvular AF has been a cause of concern because of high morbidity and mortality. To prevent the cerebral embolization of thrombus from left atrial (LA) appendage, LA appendage closure has been started by Dr Balbir Singh at Medanta Heart Institute using Watchman's device and this is now being done in several centers in the country.

INTERVENTIONAL ELECTROPHYSIOLOGY

Even since the first DC ablation of paroxysmal supraventricular tachycardia was performed at GB Pant Hospital in 1984, interventional electrophysiology has grown extensively with the availability of variety of hardware, in-depth understanding of genesis and perpetuation of arrhythmias, and advances of imaging techniques with 3-D cardiac mapping, it is now possible to treat all types of SVT, atrial flutter, and AF. Pulmonary vein ablation has improved success rate of ablation of AF.

Ventricular ectopy and ventricular tachycardia can also be cured by ablation techniques. There are centers all over the country where enormous work has been done, which are also proving to be the advanced training centers for a young electrophysiologist.

The automatic implantable cardioverter-defibrillator (AICD) implantation started in 1980s and has been established all over the country. Lately, noninvasive ICD and implantable and leadless pacemakers have been added as newer therapeutic tools.

Interventional cardiology has been established in the country as an alternative to cardiac surgery in a large variety of cardiovascular diseases.

CHAPTER 150

Evidence-based Medicine: Are Randomized Controlled Trials the Gold Standard?

Vitull K Gupta, Meghna Gupta, Varun Gupta

HISTORY OF EVIDENCE-BASED MEDICINE

Medical progress and teachings through the centuries, since the time of Hippocrates, have been based on experiences and authority of eminent physicians, without any solid scientific basis, struggling to balance the uncontrolled experience of healers with scientifically trustworthy empirical evidence. So entrenched was eminence-based medicine that it took more than a millennia for Vesalius (1514–1564) to contradict successfully the teachings of Galen.[1] Since 11th century, testing medical interventions for efficacy has existed, but in 19th century, the systematic application of evidence to medical situations first occurred in the field of epidemiology. The idea of science in medicine was promoted by Rudolf Virchow, Claude Bernard, and Louis Pasteur in Europe and in early 20th century the Flexner report consolidated the concept of scientific inquiry in American medicine. Until recently, solid scientific evidence for many treatments did not exist and the principles governing such evidence did not even emerge until 1948 when the first randomized controlled trial (RCT) was performed. In 1962, US Food and Drug Administration Kefauver-Harris Act was passed in the USA, legally necessitating rigorous clinical trials in human beings to establish claims regarding drug efficacy.[2] David Sackett, David Eddy, and Archie Cochrane in 1970s and 1980s stressed on the need for strengthening the empirical practice of medicine and proposed initial evidentiary rules for guiding clinical decisions.[3-5] David Eddy first used the term "evidence-based" in 1990[6] and in 1992, the term "evidence-based medicine (EBM)" first appeared in the medical literature in a paper by Guyatt et al.[7] Evidence-based medicine focused on educating clinicians in assessing the credibility of medical research, understanding the results of clinical studies and determining how best to apply the results to their everyday practice.[8] Evidence-based medicine rapidly transformed into an energetic intellectual community committed for more scientific and empirically based clinical practice with an aim to achieve safer, consistent, and cost-effective care.[9] Evidence-based medicine caused shift in medical paradigms suggesting that clinical decision-making should be based on scientific evidence and not on intuition, clinical experience or unscientific pathophysiologic rationale. More and more, clinicians are moving away from using time honored but unproven practices in clinical decision-making to using the most valid and reliable scientific information available. The key words are validity and reliability.[10]

WHAT IS EVIDENCE-BASED MEDICINE?

Centre for Evidence-based Medicine defines EBM as, "Evidence-based medicine is the conscientious, explicit, and judicious use of current best evidence in making decisions about the care of individual patients".[11]

Best research evidence means clinically relevant research which is patient centric; it includes clinical examination, diagnostic tests, prognostic markers, the efficacy and safety of therapeutic, and rehabilitative and preventive regimens. New evidence generated by clinical research both invalidates and replaces old but accepted concepts in diagnostics and therapeutics with more accurate, safe, and powerful new ones.

Clinical expertise means the ability to utilize experience and clinical skills to identify patient's health status, diagnosis of the diseases, their individual risks and benefits of treatment according to their personal values and expectations.

Patient values mean consideration of patients concerns, preferences, and expectations integrated into clinical decisions.

With integration of these factors, a diagnostic and therapeutic alliance is formed between the clinicians and patients helping optimize clinical outcomes and quality of life (QoL).[12] Practice of EBM requires expertise in clinical sciences, expertise in collecting, retrieving, interpreting the data, and applying the results of scientific research in clinical practice and in communicating the patients about the risks and benefits of different courses of action.

"Half of what you are taught as medical students will in 10 years have been shown to be wrong. And the trouble is none of your teachers know which half."

Dr Sydney Burwell (1956),
Dean, Harvard Medical School

CLASSIFICATION OF EVIDENCE-BASED MEDICINE

Two types of EBM have been proposed:[13]

1. *Evidence-based guidelines*: At organizational or institutional level, EBM is practiced through evidence-based guidelines (EBG) or clinical practice guidelines (CPG) including the production, policy, and regulations of guidelines also known as evidence-based healthcare. In 1990, advisory committee of the Institute of Medicine issued a report which defined practice guidelines as: "Systematically developed statements to assist practitioner and patient decisions about appropriate health care for specific clinical circumstances"[14]
2. *Evidence-based individual decision-making*: When individual healthcare provider practices EBM, it is known as evidence-based individual decision (EBID) making and currently EBM focuses excessively on EBID.

QUALIFICATION OF EVIDENCE

A cornerstone of EBM is the hierarchical system of classifying evidence. This hierarchy is known as the levels of evidence (LoE) which is an important component of EBM. Different types of clinical evidence are categorized and ranked according to the strength of their freedom from the various biases that beset medical research. A system was developed by the US Preventive Services Task Force to classify the evidence based on quality and evidence was ranking according to the effectiveness of treatments or screening:

- *Level I*: Evidence generated by minimum of one properly designed RCT
- *Level II-1*: Evidence generated by nonrandomized well-designed controlled trials
- *Level II-2*: Evidence generated by preferably more than one research groups of centers which are case-control analytic studies or well-designed cohort studies
- *Level II-3*: Evidence generated from studies with or without intervention including multiple time series and uncontrolled trials expressing dramatic results
- *Level III*: Observations of learned authorities, based on expert committee reports, experience, or descriptive studies.

Similarly categories A, B, C, and D were developed by the UK National Health Service. Levels of evidence related to the design of the study and critical analysis of diagnosis, therapy, prevention, prognosis, and harm studies was developed by Oxford Centre for Evidence-based Medicine.[15] The levels are:

- *A Level*: Relates to cohort studies, clinical RCTs, all or none and validated clinical decision guidelines or rules in different populations
- *B Level*: Relates to evidence extrapolated from level A study or exploratory or retrospective cohort, outcome research studies, ecological study or case-control study
- *C Level*: Relates to evidence extrapolated from level B study or case series study
- *D Level*: Relates to first principles, expert opinion without explicit critical appraisal, or based on bench research or physiology.

Several other methods, categories or classifications for LoE are adopted by various organizations and journals. Research questions are divided into the categories: treatment, prognosis, diagnosis, and economic or decision analysis. Detailed discussion on LoE is not in the preview of this chapter.

STATISTICAL MEASURES IN EVIDENCE-BASED MEDICINE

Mathematical methods and tools used by practitioners of EBM to express various interventions, clinical benefits of tests, and treatments are:

- *Likelihood ratios*: Post-test probability is determined by likelihood ratio multiplied by the pretest probability of a specific diagnosis, which is reflecting the Bayes' theorem. Usefulness and priority of a clinical test in a clinical scenario is determined by the differences in likelihood ratio of those clinical tests
- Relationship between specificity and sensitivity of a test is determined by the area under the receiver operator characteristic curve (AUC-ROC) and it approaches one for high-quality tests and publications. Cutoff values for both negative and positive tests do not affect AUC-ROC, but can influence sensitivity and specificity.

Safety and affectivity of an intervention in a clinically meaningful way is expressed by number needed to harm or number needed to treat (NNT). Generally, NNT is used to analyze data in relation to study two treatments A and B, one of which is a drug and other is a placebo. A defined endpoint has to be specified. If the probabilities pA and pB of this endpoint under treatments A and B, respectively, are known, then the NNT is computed as 1/(pB-pA).

HOW DO WE ACTUALLY PRACTICE EVIDENCE-BASED MEDICINE?[16]

Five steps or Principles are important for practice of EBM:

- *Step 1*: Construct a well-built clinical question and classify it into one category (therapy, diagnosis, etiology or prognosis)
- *Step 2*: Find the evidence in healthcare literature
- *Step 3*: Critically appraise or formally evaluate for validity and usefulness.
- *Step 4*: Integrate the evidence with patient factors to carry out the decision.
- *Step 5*: Evaluate the whole process.

TYPES OF RESEARCH STUDY DESIGNS[17]

There are various types of study designs and some are superior to others in context of nature of the study and answering specific questions.

- *Randomized controlled trials*: (Quires related to prevention and treatment is answered by RCTs). Bias in selection is avoided by randomization
- *Cohort study*: (Quires related to etiology, prognosis, and prevention is answered by cohort studies). Cohorts are the research design to the subgroup characteristics in populations as a whole and over a specific period of time, two groups are compared and results analyzed
- *Case-control study*: (Quires related to etiology, prognosis, and prevention is answered by case-control studies) Research related to case-control studies are studies compare the patients with problem and controls without that problem and analyze the results
- *Case series and case reports*: (Quires related to etiology, prognosis, and prevention is answered by case series or reports). Research related to case series including several patients and case reports of a single patient.

Randomized Controlled Trial

It was initially introduced into clinical medicine for the evaluation of the efficacy of streptomycin for tuberculosis in 1948.[17] Further progress in understanding the strength of various study designs has resulted in RCT being the method of choice to assess the efficacy of interventions. Professor Archie Cochrane, a Scottish epidemiologist, through his book Effectiveness and Efficiency: Random Reflections on Health Services (1972) and subsequent advocacy caused increasing acceptance of the concepts behind evidence-based practice. The explicit methodologies used to determine "best evidence" were largely established by the McMaster University research group led by David Sackett and Gordon Guyatt.

LIMITATIONS OF EVIDENCE-BASED MEDICINE

Practice of EBM by clinicians has led to both negative as well as positive reactions. Universal limitations to science and medicine are: shortage of coherent, consistent scientific evidence, difficulties in applying any evidence to the care of individual patients, and barriers to any practice of high-quality medicine.

Practice of EBM specifically encounters unique limitations[6] like difficulty in developing new skills in searching and critical appraisal of scientific evidence, availability of little time for busy clinicians to master and apply these new skills and instant access to scientific evidence and information is often inadequate in clinical settings. The generation of data and scientific evidence on which EBM depends is a slow process. Biggest challenge faced by physicians today is related to application of EBM in solving multimorbidity problems faced by aging populations, which the current generalized EBM guidelines are unable to solve effectively.[18] Moreover generalized guidelines may not be good for patients with multiple morbidities because many conflicting therapies may be needed which may not fit the actual requirements of the patient. It is simply not possible or feasible to develop trials which may include all potential disease combinations.[19,20]

APPLICATION OF EVIDENCE-BASED MEDICINE IN DEVELOPING COUNTRIES LIKE INDIA

Foundation of EBM is based on systematically reviewed information generated from RCTs and meta-analysis and should be applied cautiously in the context of developing countries. Randomized controlled trials conducted in other countries like Europe or North America ignores well-documented issue of racial differences in therapeutic responses and survival rates and morbidity statistics are not directly applicable across races especially when geographical and cultural differences between continents are considered.

Based on their perceptions of health and illness, researchers of Europe or North America have developed QoL measures, which are used in some studies and their use in scientific research across continents and countries is questionable because these life measures are value-based and culturally sensitive.

CAN EVIDENCE-BASED MEDICINE BE INFLUENCED?

Many health professionals have expressed doubts about infiltration of medical research institutions and influence on peer-review process to promote drugs marketed by pharmaceutical companies undermining the validity and veracity of peer-reviewed research and so subverting the foundation of EBM.[21] Medical scientists believe that industry-influenced studies camouflage or eliminate unfavorable results, remodeling the data to present favorable results to create "hyped" medications.[22] It is believed by internists like John Abramson[23] that every aspect of health care, medical education, and basic research has been influenced by the pharmaceutical industry so much so that prominent and influential researchers are endorsing questionable studies and also influencing the mechanisms of evaluation of effective treatment for widely accepted illnesses.[24] Evidence-based medicine, a product of objective research, if conducted by disinterested medical researchers or under the influence of pharmaceutical industry or sponsored clinical trials, can have a corrosive impact both on physicians and the evidence itself. Results of all clinical trials are not published, particularly the pharma sponsored trials which do not show benefit of an agent.[25] In January 2006, an article was published in JAMA by imminent personalities sighting concerns about EBM being influenced and suggested a number of measures for protection of researchers and scientists from adverse influence of pharmaceutical industry on medical research.[26] Such a communication expressed increasing concerns of prominent medical researchers and faculty regarding growing risk of influence of pharmaceutical industry on EBM.

PHARMA INDUSTRY, RESEARCH, AND EVIDENCE-BASED MEDICINE

Funding of medical research by pharmaceuticals has been shown to have propharmaceutical results in several systematic reviews. Several causes like bias in trial protocols, results and publications have been documented expressing close relationship and influence of pharmaceuticals on medical research.[27] Statistically significant relationship was found between the study results and funding authority, like industry-selected drugs were likely to be proved more efficacious, in spite of the flawed study results, because scientists feared stoppage of funds in case of unfavorable results expressed by the study.[28] Influence of funding source on decision-making by the researcher has been documented in a number of research papers. Data analysis related to faculty of internal medicine at seven Midwest US teaching hospitals has shown that pharmaceutical support was an independent risk factor for making requests for formulary additions.[29]

ARE RANDOMIZED CONTROLLED TRIALS THE GOLD STANDARD?

What is "Gold Standard"?

The original gold standard was a monetary system where currency was based on a fixed quantity of gold. The gold standard allusion derives from international finance, in which the rates of exchange among national currencies were fixed to the value of gold. Actual gold standard is the technique of international finance that links the value of a nation's currency to a set amount of gold, facilitating exchange between different currencies. The gold standard system collapsed in 1971 following the United States' suspension of convertibility from dollars to gold and in 1976 US revised its definition of the dollar to remove all references to gold.

Randomized Controlled Trials as the "Gold Standard"

In 1747, James Lind conducted the first reported clinical trial in the history to identify treatment for scurvy.[30] In 1865, Claude Bernard published the general guidelines of modern experimental medicine[31] and in 1948 the paper entitled "Streptomycin Treatment of Pulmonary Tuberculosis" became the first published RCT in medicine.[18] After that, RCTs were increasingly being recognized as the standard method[32] providing the most rigorous test for preventive, diagnostic, and therapeutic interventions and generally referred to as the "gold standard" for clinical trials. Post World War II the importance of RCTs became critical especially in 1962 when the US Food and Drug Administration made well-controlled studies or RCTs mandatory before new drug approval as a proof of efficacy which lead to explosive increase in importance of RCTs throughout the world so much so that by 1990s most of the RCTs were funded by the pharma industry as compared to the government and academic bodies.[33] Over the past 70 years, RCTs have influenced medical research, knowledge, and clinical practice and since then researchers have introduced many different clinical trial methods and innovative statistical methods to eliminate bias.[34] Over time, international standards for clinical research were established in collaboration with the national bodies systematizing RCTs and RCTs were increasingly being promoted as the best means to achieve EBM with case reports at the bottom of methodological hierarchies and RCTs at the top.[35]

By early 1980s, government authorities and scientific associations responsible for methodological quality review and ranking of research studies gave RCTs the status of gold standard for therapeutics, medical research, and knowledge.[36] For the past two to three decades, medical and government organizations consider RCTs as a method for generating scientifically valid and reliable evidence about the usefulness of almost any type of therapy or for specific comparisons between treatments. Randomized controlled trials have achieved the status of gold standard of scientific evidence because RCTs employ randomization across study arms, eliminate patient-treatment selection bias, resulting in reliable causal inference. Randomized controlled trials challenged the popular beliefs of treatment like in Cardiac Arrhythmia Suppression Trial (CAST) conducted in 1989 in which the effect of antiarrhythmic drugs was tested versus a placebo in myocardial infarction patients. It was a known fact that ventricular arrhythmias were a poor prognostic factor in myocardial infarction and it was believed that suppressing ventricular arrhythmias will decrease the mortality rate. But the results of the trial showed about 3-fold increase in total mortality in patients on antiarrhythmic drugs. So, the use of antiarrhythmic drugs for treatment of ventricular arrhythmias in myocardial infarction became contraindicated.[32]

Limitations of Randomized Controlled Trials as Gold Standard

With increasing popularity of EBM, there was emergence of methodological hierarchies with RCTs at the top and case reports at the bottom. Despite being at the top of methodological hierarchies, RCTs have substantial limitations which challenge their "Gold Standard" status and RCTs have never been able to monopolize medical knowledge production especially now with the emergence of registries, electronic data bases, randomized registry trials, and other modes of production of knowledge and research in medicine. Major limitations of RCTs relate to scientific limitations, cost, and practicality. Scientific limitations relate to RCT patient population which may not represent the patient population in practical world. Tightly controlled environment, limited patient population, clearly defined inclusions and exclusions like age limits, the presence or absence of comorbidities, the concomitant use of drugs, a range of clinical and biochemical criteria, treatment of patients according to detailed protocols, making it impossible to follow the tight RCT criteria in clinical practice. The results of a single RCT may not be generalized to different populations and establishes only one data point. Moreover the outcome results of RCTs may be of interest to researchers and may not to the actual patients in real practice.

It may not be feasible to conduct an RCT in rare diseases as it may not be possible to recruit a sufficient number of patients to randomize across multiple treatment possibilities. Different approaches for clinical research have been experimented for the past several years and more flexible and acceptable new study designs have been developed to extract useful data from patient registries and electronic medical records which has erode the status of RCTs as a gold standard. Practice of personalized medicine focusing on several individual factors for determining the diagnostic and therapeutic strategies may not be influenced by the results of RCTs which analyze typical patients in a controlled environment.[37] Status of observational studies or nonrandomized trials in evaluating treatments is being debated and studies found greater effects of the same treatment comparisons in observational studies than in RCTs.[37,38] No difference was found in two studies comparing the treatment effects between RCTs and nonrandomized trials, but these findings were not confirmed by the two studies comparing individual RCTs with observational studies in 19 therapeutic areas[39] and meta-analyses of RCTs with meta-analyses of cohort and case–control studies in five therapeutic areas.[40]

No major differences were found between the estimates of treatment effects in the observational studies and RCTs. Previous systematic review estimating the effects of treatment in 22 areas, found no consistent difference between RCTs and observational studies. Evidence-based medicine popularly projecting that observational studies produce inferior results than that of RCTs may be misleading.[41] Greater effects in five of the nonrandomised trials were found in a systematic review, which compared same intervention in eight RCTs with nonrandomised trials.[42]

Comparison of different types of research modalities like RCTs, cross-sectional studies, cohort studies, and case–control studies shows that potential for external validity was more in cross-sectional studies, cohort studies, and case–control studies than RCTs, that is, the data can be extrapolated to a higher degree in general population. All the three study designs have the limitation of a lower internal validity, because the bias and confounding variables are difficult to eliminate and/or control.[43] Internal validity is more in a single well-done RCT as it is done for a specific intervention, for a specific sample, at a specific time and place producing valid results about that intervention only in that specific setting. For this reason most of the single RCTs lack external validity.[44] But other researchers suggest that strength of the instructional design and learning theory incorporated in the intervention can help guide which RCTs are carried out to establish external validity.[45] Registry studies are an important modality with several advantages for population-based case-control studies but are not free from bias.[46] The advantages of registry studies are large sample sizes, systematic data collection, faster studies, low costs, studies of rare effects and rare diseases is possible, informed consent is not required, and the analysis of long-term effects can be done easily. So, it is argued that relative importance of different research methodology is an unnecessary distraction and diverse approaches should be accepted for providing evidence basis for modern therapeutics replacing hierarchies of evidence.[47]

Randomized controlled trials were described by Feinstein and Horwitz as an elusive ideal research method in many circumstances and not as a gold standard, but supported other clinical epidemiological research designs and remarked, "epidemiological research has become increasingly important because it offers a substitute for the unattainable scientific gold standard of a randomized experimental trial". New methodology of observational research producing large comparative data from extensive databases of patients on different treatment outcomes in routine healthcare settings continued to emerge.[48] Intuitive logic of the techniques and angiography provided visual evidence to promote coronary angioplasty and stents and not the RCTs.[49]

Randomized controlled trials became standard modality in pharmaceutical research, but medical scientists struggled to apply them in other fields of medicine. Though numerous RCTs were conducted but were thought to be inappropriate and sometimes impossible to study highly individualized and long-term effects of psychotherapy and methodological concerns undermined major psychotherapy trials.[50] Disproportionately more robust data on psychotropic drugs than psychotherapy was generated because of easy to conduct RCTs on psychotropic drugs as compared to psychotherapy which benefited pharmaceuticals and lead to suboptimal use of comprehensive psychiatric care.[51] Similar limitations were faced by RCTs in surgery because pathological findings were different in different patients, surgical skills vary from surgeon-to-surgeon and numerous different choices existed for premedication, anesthesia, instrumentation, surgical approach, and postoperative care. All these different factors prevented standardization required for clinical trials.[52] Sham controls could not be used for major operations, which limited blinding of trials.

Large studies with benefits of RCTs in low-cost are possible with the data from patient registries and electronic health records like a study explored outcomes of treatment for type 2 diabetes showing that thiazolidinediones were much more effective in reducing hospitalization and death than sulfonylureas using the data from the Veterans Health Administration and Medicare. When RCTs are given undue importance, ignoring other rigorously generated evidences, misconceptions like whether tobacco has adverse health effects or soft drinks do not cause obesity crop up. Progressively, RCTs became costly requiring massive bureaucratic and corporate support for infrastructure, record keeping research design, ethical review, and statistical analysis. Presently, the cost estimate for a single phase three RCT could be 30 million dollars or more[53] which resulted in high cost of prescription drug without any price controls. Because of high-cost involved in conducting RCTs, a clinical trial industry came into being and contract research organizations (CROs) become a $25 billion industry.[54] Consequently the research was shifted from teaching and academic hospitals involving physicians and scientists to private sector employing nonacademic physicians on a contract basis.[55] With high cost involvement, much of the clinical research is focused on drugs with substantial marketing potential rather than drugs with limited impact on public health like tuberculosis and malaria. In present scenario, the global knowledge production is dependent on the industry which has raised public health and ethical questions regarding the role of RCTs in benefit of public health. Evidence suggests that the RCTs which are funded by the private industry are likely to produce favorable results as compared to public-funded trials[56] and industry has substantial interests in publishing positive results than negative conclusions which is extremely damaging to medical research and knowledge.

Randomized controlled trials sometime have practical difficulties as they can take many years to complete or not long enough to study long-term beneficial or adverse effects of an intervention such as vaccine immunity. Results of RCTs may be valid only for a specific population like trial results in high-risk population may not be applicable or relevant in low-risk population. Practical difficulties arise if RCTs are planned for population-wide interventions or urgent health issues such as infectious disease outbreaks, for which urgent public health decisions are required.

Patient's environment may influence many complex treatments making even cluster randomized trials impossible. No study design is perfect because different research requires different methodology and patients respond differently to different therapy in practice compared to therapy during trials and responses are influenced by age of the patient and presence of multiple diseases.[57] So, we suggest new and revolunatory innovation in EBM, like system dynamics and narrative, complementary research paradigms of complexity science, combination of research methodologies, and qualitative approaches to deliver meaningful evidence to help clinicians in daily practice.

CONCLUSION

Evidence-based medicine has been considered as the gold standard parameter in taking decisions and standard healthcare practice. Randomized controlled trails are generally considered as the basic research tool related to EBM. Randomized controlled trails are specifically useful in the diseases caused by single factor or acute diseases treated by single modality, but are not so useful in studies related to chronic and multimorbidity diseases especially in epidemiological context. Evidence-based medicine generally do not give importance to local conditions, social factors influencing health, and effect of various factors related to healthcare services. There is no single or best approach to obtain better information about health interventions. Evidence grading systems, policy makers, and researchers must embrace other study types in addition to RCTs. Review of literature suggests and supports a flexible approach in which RCTs, observational studies, and other type of research methodology have complementary roles. Glorifying RCTs above other approaches, even when these other approaches may either be superior or the only practical way to get an answer may force us to accept the evidence that is not based on best available evidence. An approach that uses all appropriate evidence types and builds on the existing evidence base using proven best practices is the one most likely to result in clinical and public health action that will save lives.

"Evidence-based practice", should be the valid ideal aimed to implement best proven clinical care and public policy interventions, but it is also important to develop "practice-based evidence", exploring and implementing programs in practice to generate data and document whether it is beneficial or not for the patients. Such interventions will help save lives and expand the data base.

REFERENCES

1. Reddy DS (Ed). History of Medicine: Prehistoric to Present, 1st edition. Hyderabad: Paras Medical Publisher; 2006.
2. Matthews JR. Quantification and quest for medical certainty. Princeton, NY: Princeton University Press; 1995.
3. Sackett DL. Rules of evidence and clinical recommendations on the use of antithrombotic agents. Chest. 1986;89(2 suppl):2S-3.
4. Eddy DM. Guidelines for the cancer-related checkup: recommendations and rationale. CA Cancer J Clin. 1980;30:193-240.
5. Cochrane A. Effectiveness and efficiency: random reflections on health services. London: Nuffield Provincial Hospitals Trust; 1972.
6. Eddy DM. "Practice policies: where do they come from?". JAMA. 1990;263(9):1265, 1269, 1272 passim.
7. Guyatt G, Cairns J, Churchill D, et al; Evidence-Based Medicine Working Group. Evidence-based medicine. A new approach to teaching the practice of medicine. JAMA. 1992;268:2420-5.
8. Evidence-based Medicine Working Group. Evidence-based medicine. A new approach to teaching the practice of medicine. JAMA. 1992;268:2420-5.
9. Pope C. Resisting evidence: the study of evidence-based medicine as a contemporary social movement. Health. 2003;7:267-82.
10. Kuhn TS. The Structure of Scientific Revolutions. Chicago: University of Chicago Press; 1970.
11. Sackett DL, Rosenberg WM, Gray JA, et al. "Evidence based medicine: what it is and what it isn't". BMJ. 1996;312(7023):71-2.
12. Sackett D. Evidence-based Medicine: How to Practice and Teach EBM, 2nd edition. Churchill Livingtone; 2000.
13. Eddy DM. Evidence-based medicine: a unified approach. Health Affairs (Project Hope). 2005;24(1):9-17.
14. Field MJ, Lohr KN (Eds). Clinical Practice Guidelines: Directions for a New Program. Washington DC: National Academy of Press; 1990.
15. CEBM. (2009). Oxford Centre for Evidence-based Medicine: Levels of Evidence and Grades of Recommendation. [online] Available from https://www.cebm.net/2009/06/oxford-centre-evidence-based-medicine-levels-evidence-march-2009/ [Accessed July 2018].
16. Evidence Based Medicine, Web based tutorials, Saab Memorial Medical Library. American University of Beirut. [online] Available from http://smlweb.aub.edu.lb/StaticContent.aspx?file=Tutorials/ EBM.htm [Accessed July 2018].
17. Streptomycin in Tuberculosis Trials Committee. "Streptomycin treatment of pulmonary tuberculosis. A Medical Research Council investigation". Br Med J. 1948;2(4582):769-82.
18. Farmer C, Fenu E, O'Flynn N, et al. Clinical assessment and management of multimorbidity: summary of NICE guidance. BMJ. 2016;354:i4843.
19. Boyd C, Darer J, Boult C, et al. Clinical practice guidelines and quality of care for older patients with multiple comorbid diseases. JAMA. 2005;216:716-24.
20. Upshur R. Looking for rules in a world of exceptions: reflections on evidence-based practice. Persp Biol Med. 2005;48:477-89.
21. Kushner HI. The other war on drugs: the pharmaceutical industry, evidence-based medicine, and clinical practice. J Policy History. 2007;19(1):49-70.
22. Moynihan R, Cassels A (Ed). Selling Sickness: How the World's Biggest Pharmaceutical Companies are Turning us all into Patients. New York: Nation Books; 2005.

23. Abramson J. Overdosed America: The Broken Promise of American Medicine. New York: Harper Collins; 2004. pp. 352.
24. Giacomini M. Theory-based medicine and the role of evidence: why the emperor needs new clothes, again. Perspect Biol Med. 2009;52(2):234-51.
25. Turner EH, Matthews AM, Linardatos E, et al. Selective publication of antidepressant trials and its influence on apparent efficacy. N Engl J Med. 2008;358(3):252-60.
26. Brennan TA, Rothman DJ, Blank L, et al. Health industry practices that create conflicts of interest: a policy proposal for academic medical centers. JAMA. 2006;295(4):429-33.
27. Sismondo S. How pharmaceutical industry funding affects trial outcomes: Causal structures and responses. Soc Sci Med. 2008;66(9):1909-14.
28. Davidson RA. Source of funding and outcome of clinical trials. J Gen Intern Med. 1986;1:155-8.
29. Chren MM, Landefeld CS. Does a doctor's interaction with a drug company influence that doctor's behavior? Evidence of company-specific behavior. Clin Res. 1992;40:302A.
30. Dunn PM. James Lind (1716-94) of Edinburgh and the treatment of scurvy. Arch Dis Child Fetal Neonatal Ed. 1997;76:F64-5.
31. Jaillon P. [Controlled randomized clinical trials]. Bull Acad Natl Med. 2007;191(4-5):739-56; discussion 756-8.
32. Meldrum ML. A brief history of the randomized controlled trial. From oranges and lemons to the gold standard. Hematol Oncol Clin North Am. 2000;14(4): 745-60.
33. Carpenter D. Reputation and power: organizational image and pharmaceutical regulation at the FDA. Princeton, NJ: Princeton University Press; 2010.
34. Opinel A, Tröhler U, Gluud C, et al. Commentary: the evolution of methods to assess the effects of treatments, illustrated by the development of treatments for diphtheria, 1825-1918. Int J Epidemiol. 2013;42:662-76.
35. Daly J. Evidence-based medicine and the search for a science of clinical care. Berkeley: University of California Press; 2005.
36. Jones DS, Podolsky SH. The history and fate of the gold standard. Lancet. 2015;385:1502-3.
37. Chalmers TC, Matta RJ, Smith H Jr, et al. Evidence favouring the use of anticoagulants in the hospital phase of acute myocardial infarction. N Engl J Med. 1977;297:1091-6.
38. Sacks H, Chalmers TC, Smith H Jr. Randomized versus historical controls for clinical trials. Am J Med. 1982;72:233-40.
39. Benson K, Hartz AJ. A comparison of observational and randomized controlled trials. N Engl J Med. 2000;342:1878-86.
40. Concato J, Shah N, Horwitz RI, et al. Randomized, controlled trials, observational studies and the hierarchy of research designs. N Engl J Med. 2000;342:1887-92.
41. Britton A, McKee M, Black N, et al. Choosing between randomised and non-randomised studies: a systematic review. Health Technol Assess. 1998;2(13).
42. Kunz R, Oxman AD. The unpredictability paradox: review of empirical comparisons of randomised and non-randomised clinical trials. BMJ. 1998;317:1185-90.
43. Carlson MD, Morrison RS. Study design, precision, and validity in observational studies. J Palliat Med. 2009;12(1):77-82.
44. Shadish WR, Cook TD, Campbell DT. Experimental and Quasi-Experimental Designs for Generalized Causal Inference. Boston: Houghton Mifflin; 2002.
45. Jaciw, Newman D. "External Validity in the Context of RCTs: Lessons from the Causal Explanatory Tradition", paper presented before the Society for Research on Educational Effectiveness; 2011.
46. Izquierdo JN, Schoenbach VJ. The potential and limitations of data from population-based state cancer registries. Am J Public Health. 2000;90:695-8.
47. Rawlins M. De testimonio: on the evidence for decisions about the use of therapeutic interventions. Lancet. 2008;372:2152-61.
48. Schneeweiss S, Avorn J. A review of uses of health care utilization databases for epidemiologic research on therapeutics. J Clin Epidemiol. 2005;58:323-37.
49. Gruntzig A. Transluminal dilatation of coronary-artery stenosis. Lancet. 1978;1:263.
50. Ablon JS, Jones EE. Validity of controlled clinical trials of psychotherapy: findings from the NIMH Treatment of Depression Collaborative Research Program. Am J Psychiatry. 2002;159:775-83.
51. Deacon BJ. The biomedical model of mental disorder: a critical analysis of its validity, utility, and effects on psychotherapy research. Clin Psychol Rev. 2013;33:846-61.
52. Love JW. Drugs and operations: some important differences. JAMA. 1975;232: 37-8.
53. Sertkaya A, Birkenbach A, Berlind A, et al. Examination of clinical trial costs and barriers for drug development: report to the Assistant Secretary of Planning and Evaluation (ASPE). Washington, DC: Department of Health and Human Services, July 25, 2014.
54. Bodenheimer T. Uneasy alliance—clinical investigators and the pharmaceutical industry. N Engl J Med. 2000;342(20):1539-44.
55. Fisher JA, Kalbaugh CA. United States private-sector physicians and pharmaceutical contract research: a qualitative study. PLoS Med. 2012;9(7):e1001271.
56. Bourgeois FT, Murthy S, Mandl KD. Outcome reporting among drug trials registered in ClinicalTrials.gov. Ann Intern Med. 2010;153:158-66.
57. Farmer C, Fenu E, O'Flynn N, et al. Clinical assessment and management of multimorbidity: summary of NICE guidance. BMJ. 2016;354:i4843.

CHAPTER 151

Erectile Dysfunction in a Cardiac Patient

Ranjit K Nath, Neil Bardoloi

INTRODUCTION

Erectile dysfunction (ED) is not very uncommon among cardiac patients and is linked with a lack of complete physical well-being. Its incidence is expected to increase significantly along with the increase in various lifestyle diseases. Indian men are known to be at a much higher risk of coronary artery disease than men in most other countries; a biological risk factor has been postulated. The increase in risk is found from fourth decade of life onwards, when most men are still sexually active. As coronary heart disease (CHD) and ED may share a common etiology of atherosclerosis, ED attributed to atherosclerosis may be commoner in India than elsewhere in the world.

Male sexual function is a complex phenomenon that includes libido, erection, and orgasm and impairment of any of these components may lead to impaired sexual health, which can be temporary or permanent, leading to impotence. ED is defined as a lack of ability to sustain or maintain penile erection for sufficient amount of time, which leads to unsatisfactory sexual intercourse. It affects almost 26 cases per 1,000 men-years, and annual incidence rate increases with each decade of age. Also the incidence increases gradually with increasing age, lower level of education, diabetes, heart disease, and hypertension.[1] India has been dubbed as the impotence capital of the world due to the high incidence of the lifestyle diseases and probably the largest population of males affected by impotence in the world. Lack of awareness about the problem and very low therapy utilization rates along with poor compliance make it difficult to treat.

Cardiovascular disease (CVD) remains a source of considerable morbidity and mortality despite advances in prevention, diagnosis, and treatment. ED and CVD are the result of common risk factors like increasing age, high blood pressure, diabetes, hypercholesterolemia, use of tobacco, obesity, metabolic syndrome, lack of physical activity, and depression.[2] CVD and ED are said to be the result of a same pathophysiological mechanism of causation and progression. Many studies have shown that ED is common in men who are already suffering from atherosclerotic CVD and so, it can be considered as an independent risk marker for CVD in future.[2]

ETIOLOGY

Erectile dysfunction can be the result of a broad spectrum of disorders, which interplays significantly among them and there are lot of overlaps. The causes can be simple, related to the sex organs or complex, related to the physiology of erection, where psychological factors play an important role and can be divided as:[3]

- Organic causes:
  - Vascular (endothelial dysfunction, atherosclerosis)
  - Hormonal (hypogonadism, hyperprolactinemia)
  - Neurogenic (Parkinson's disease, multiple sclerosis, spinal cord disorders, etc.)
  - Drug-induced
  - Local causes (carcinoma of prostate, disorders of the penis).
- Psychological causes:
  - Performance anxiety
  - Depression
  - Partner-related problems
  - Psychosocial stress.
- Mixed.

PATHOPHYSIOLOGIC BASIS OF ERECTILE DYSFUNCTION AND CARDIOVASCULAR DISEASE

The association between ED and CVD is said to be because of their similarity in pathophysiological and clinical features (Fig. 1). Vascular cause of ED is said to be the result of impaired of endothelial-dependent smooth muscle relaxation (functional ED of vascular cause), or due to narrowing or

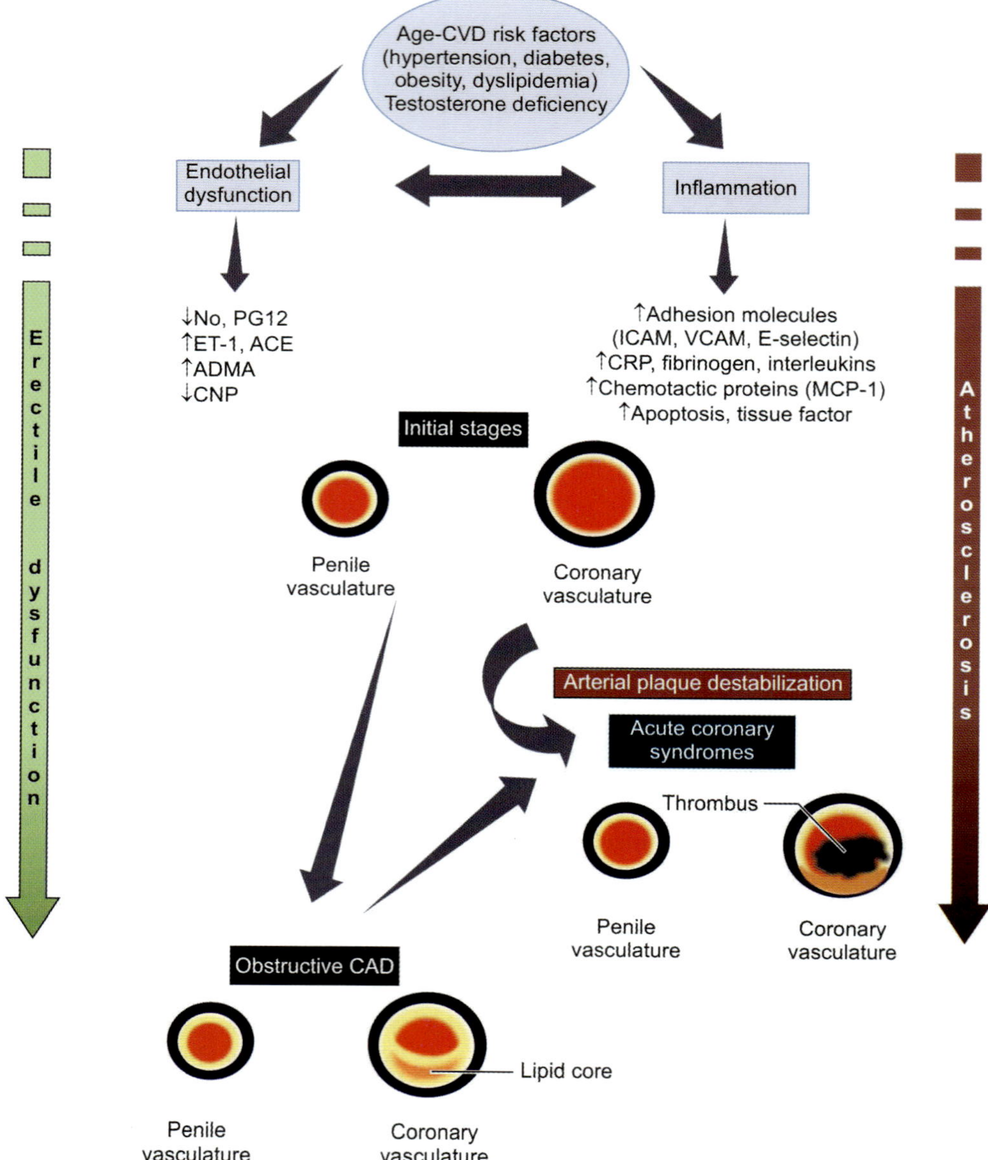

CVD, cardiovascular disease; CAD, coronary artery disease; NO, nitric oxide; PGI2, prostaglandin I2; ET, endothelin; ACE, angiotensin-converting enzyme; ADMA, asymmetrical dimethylarginine; CNP, C-type natriuretic peptide; CRP: C-reactive protein; MCP, monocyte chemoattractant protein; ICAM, intercellular adhesion molecule; VCAM, vascular cell adhesion molecule.

FIG. 1: Association and interplay between different risk factors, inflammatory markers, and pathophysiology of erectile dysfunction and coronary artery disease.

Source: Reprinted with permission from Vlachopoulos C, Jackson G, Stefanadis C, et al. Erectile dysfunction in the cardiovascular patient. Eur Heart J. 2013;34(27):2034-46.

occlusion of arteries of penis by the atherosclerotic process (structural ED of vascular cause) or a combined mechanism of both these causes. Patients with ED show increased inflammatory and endothelial-prothrombotic activation, which is thought to be responsible for altered activity of smooth muscle cells and endothelial lining of target organ arteries. This leads to endothelial dysfunction, which is observed in men with or without CAD.[4] Hence, endothelial dysfunction acts as the common pathophysiological similarity between ED and CVD. Endothelial dysfunction is said to be the initial stage of atherosclerosis and affects all arterial vascular tree including penile, coronary, and other vascular structures including peripheral vascular bed.

Montorsi et al.[5] postulated the artery size hypothesis, related to the involvement of the particular arteries of target organs, explaining that equal amount of atherosclerotic

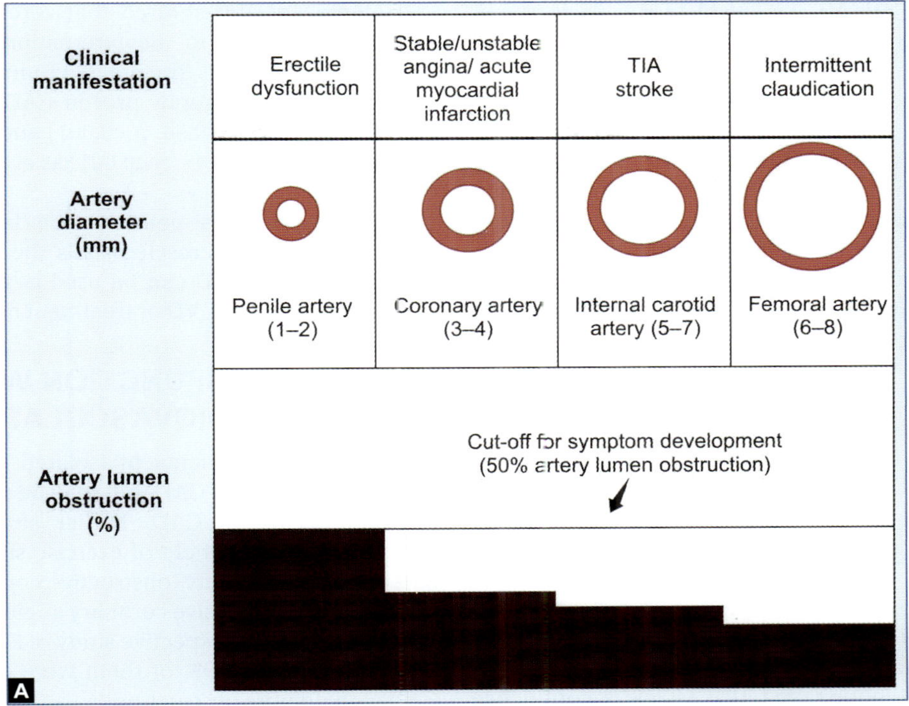

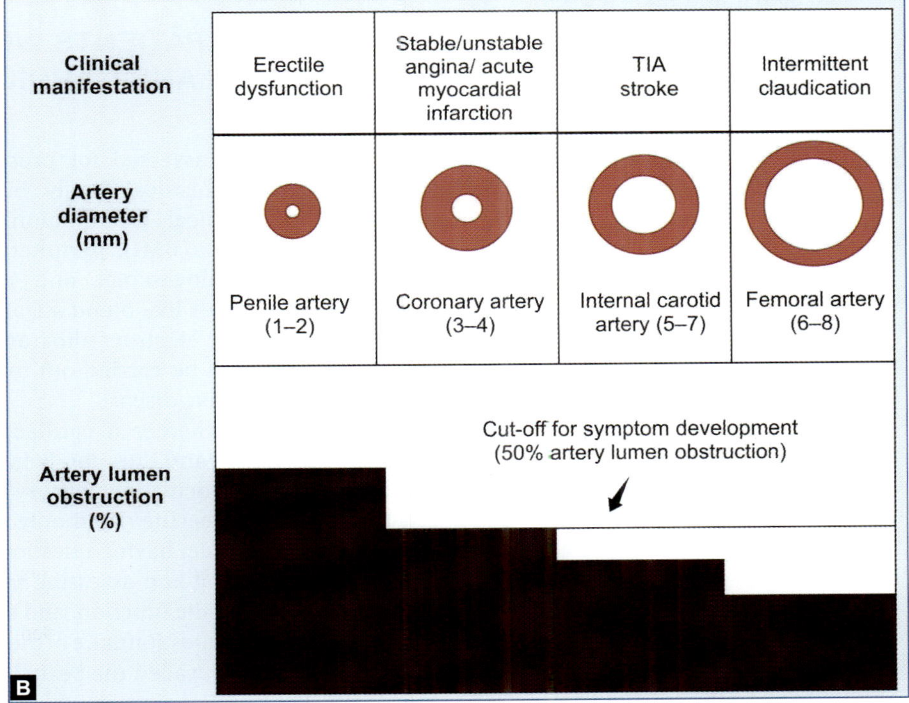

TIA, transient ischemic attack.

FIG. 2: The "artery size" hypothesis. Equal amount of atherosclerotic plaque burden may produce clinical features earlier; **A,** in small caliber cavernosal arteries than; **B,** in large lumen coronary arteries.

Source: Reprinted with permission from Vlachopoulos C, Jackson G, Stefanadis C, et al. Erectile dysfunction in the cardiovascular patient. Eur Heart J. 2013;34(27):2034-46.

burden may cause critical narrowing or occlusion of a small lumen artery like penile artery, whereas, it may not be sufficient to occlude or critically narrow a large lumen artery like the coronaries or other peripheral arteries (Fig. 2). So, when there is 50% narrowing of the lumen of an artery, large vessels may not develop symptoms due to large luminal size, but there will be significant reduction in lumen size in small caliber arteries like cavernosal arteries leading to symptoms.

ERECTILE DYSFUNCTION WITH ESTABLISHED CARDIOVASCULAR DISEASE

Erectile dysfunction is commonly detected in patients in whom other risk factors of endothelial dysfunction or atherosclerosis are prevalent, such as high blood pressure, diabetes, hypercholesterolemia, symptomatic CAD and chronic kidney disease (CKD).

Kloner et al.[6] administered a Sexual Health Inventory for Men Questionnaire for cardiac patients in the outpatient department to ascertain how often physicians treat ED in these patients with chronic CAD. The questionnaire took about 5 minutes to complete in the busy outpatient department. They found the prevalence of ED in 70% of CAD patients, suggesting an association between ED with stable CAD. Roumeguere et al.[7] compared 215 patients with ED and 100 patients without ED. CHD risk at 10 years were 56.6% in the ED group as compared to 32.6% in the group without ED ($p < 0.05$).

An epidemiological study from Japan[8] collected data from 6,112 male CAD patients from 447 clinics in 2003. The prevalence of ED was 81% in the cohort. ED was strongly associated with CVD [odds ratio (OR): 2.82; 95% confidence interval (CI): 1.95–4.23, $p < 0.0001$)] and diabetes (OR: 2.88; 95% CI: 2.26–3.70, $p < 0.0001$). Diabetes mellitus, CAD and high blood pressure showed significant associations with ED with ORs of 2.88, 2.82, and 1.79, respectively.

ERECTILE DYSFUNCTION AND FUTURE CARDIOVASCULAR EVENTS

Erectile dysfunction is regarded as a vascular marker for future CVD, as ED indicated initiation of endothelial dysfunction and atherosclerosis involving the vascular tree and can be used for screening and initiation of treatment for CVD risk reduction.

Uslu et al.[9] showed that flow-mediated dilatation (FMD) of the arteries decreases significantly in the group of patients having ED as compared to group without ED (4.1% ± 3.1% vs. 9.7% ± 3.5%; $p < 0.001$) and the relationship of suffering from ED and reduction of FMD was significant ($r = -0.66$, $p < 0.001$), concluding that aortic and brachial artery endothelial functions are impaired in men with ED without CVD.

Baumhakel et al.[10] tried to evaluate association of endothelial dysfunction and left ventricular ejection fraction (LVEF), and postulated that endothelial dysfunction is common in patients with reduced LVEF, and hence will have higher prevalence of ED in them. LVEF was measured by magnetic resonance imaging (MRI), contrast angiography and with the help of 2D echocardiography. Prevalence of ED was 80.6% among patients with moderate-to-severe reduction of LVEF ($p = 0.001$), and symptoms of ED were detected 3.04 ± 7.2 years before development of a cardiovascular event ($p = 0.005$). They concluded that reduced LVEF is a risk factor for ED in high CVD risk patients, probably caused by endothelial dysfunction.

Solomon et al.[11] showed that coronary plaque burden was well correlated to the International Index of Erectile Function (IIEF) score. The erectile function score of the 132 patients with angiography proven CAD correlated with the CVD risk factors ($r = 0.54$, $p < 0.001$) and with the severity of disease burden ($r = 0.44$, $p < 0.001$) as evaluated with the help of Gensini score.

All these studies point to the fact that endothelial dysfunction and atherosclerosis is the key for initiation of ED and CAD, and ED can be used as a clinical marker for prevention of future CVD or treatment of underlying CAD.

ERECTILE DYSFUNCTION WITH OCCULT CARDIOVASCULAR DISEASE

There are some patients of isolated ED not having any clinical symptoms of CAD, but may be suffering from asymptomatic or occult CAD. Earlier studies have reported prevalence with the help of exercise stress testing (EST) at 22%. More importantly, obstructive coronary artery disease was detected by invasive coronary angiography in 90% of the cases. In another prospective study of ED patients evaluated with angiography, 19% of them were suffering from silent CAD with definite obstruction.[12]

WORKUP FOR PATIENTS WITH ERECTILE DYSFUNCTION AND CARDIOVASCULAR DISEASE

Patients should be assessed for presence of risk factors through a proper history, family history of premature atherosclerosis, clinical examination to look especially for body mass index (BMI), peripheral pulsations, blood pressure, and cardiovascular and neurological examination. Investigations like blood sugar levels, lipid profile, renal function tests, electrocardiogram (ECG), and echocardiography should be carried out to identify risk factors and underlying cardiac disease.

Assessment of whether a cardiac patient is suffering from ED, its severity and duration is important aspects and can be obtained by meticulous history of sexual health and related questionnaires. The commonly used IIEF, a 15-item, self-evaluation module, having questionnaire as a validated method for evaluating and assessing male sexual functions including libido, erectile function, and satisfactory orgasm.[13] A shortened version questionnaire of the original 15-item IIEF is the 5-item module, called the Sexual Health Inventory for Men (SHIM) or IIEF-5 is given in table 1. The sum of the score of the responses to the questions can range from the worse (scoring 1) to the best (scoring 25); progressive decrease in score indicates gradual worsening of the erectile function, and a value of less than or equal to 21 is diagnostic of ED.

Exercise stress testing along with imaging or without imaging can be used to identify patients who are having underlying obstructive asymptomatic CAD, to identify patients with reversible ischemia, especially in detecting silent CAD in diabetic patients. Pharmacological stress evaluation methods

TABLE 1: The International Index of Erectile Function-5 (IIEF-5) scoring system used for screening and assessing severity of erectile dysfunction (ED). The total score is the sum of points scored to the five queries and overall score ranges from 1 to 25. ED is absent (score 22–25), mild (score 17–21), mild-to-moderate (score 12–16), moderate (score 8–11), and severe (score 1–7)

Questions	Score 0	Score 1	Score 2	Score 3	Score 4	Score 5
1. How do you rate your confidence over the past 6 months that you could get and keep an erection?	–	Very low	Low	Moderate	High	Very high
2. When you had erections with sexual stimulation over the past 6 months, how often were your erections hard enough for penetration (entering your partner)?	No sexual activity	Almost never or never	A few times (much less than half the time)	Sometimes (about half the time)	Most times (much more than half the time)	Almost always or always
3. During sexual intercourse in past 6 months, how often were you able to maintain your erection after you had penetrated (entered) your partner?	Did not attempt intercourse	Almost never or never	A few times (much less than half the time)	Sometimes (about half the time)	Most times (much more than half the time)	Almost always or always
4. During sexual intercourse in last 6 months, how difficult was it to maintain your erection to completion of intercourse?	Did not attempt intercourse	Extremely difficult	Very difficult	Difficult	Slightly difficult	Not difficult
5. When you attempted sexual intercourse during last 6 months, how often was it satisfactory for you?	Did not attempt intercourse	Almost never or never	A few times (much less than half the time)	Sometimes (about half the time)	Most times (much more than half the time)	Almost always or always

are more appropriate for those who are unable to perform EST due to physical limitations or with baseline significant ECG abnormalities. Patients with known CAD or diabetes are always considered to be at increased risk. So, patients with adequate exercise capacity or negative EST can restart or continue normal sexual activity along with proper treatment and lifestyle measures for ED. In patients with positive stress test results or in high-risk of repeat events, normal sexual activity is deferred until the condition of the patient is stabilized with adequate treatment. They need to be followed regularly with timely stress evaluation after treatment or interventions, before normal sexual activity can be advised.[2]

Measurement of serum testosterone level is strongly recommended in those with diagnosed organic ED especially if condition is not treated adequately with phosphodiesterase type 5 (PDE5) inhibitor agents. Low testosterone level can cause dyslipidemia by increasing total cholesterol and low-density lipoprotein cholesterol, and also to increased production of proinflammatory markers and mediators.[14] Endothelial dysfunction, progressive arterial wall thickening, gradual increase in arterial stiffness, and calcification also ensue in those with lower testosterone level. Hence, it is hypothesized that CVD risk is amplified by chronically reduced levels of testosterone.

MANAGEMENT OF ERECTILE DYSFUNCTION AND CARDIOVASCULAR DISEASE

As the basic mechanism and pathophysiology of CVD and ED are same, treatment of ED is mostly treatment of risk factors like treating high blood pressure, proper control of diabetes, treatment of dyslipidemia, cessation of all forms of tobacco use, maintaining a healthy body weight or loss of body weight in case of obesity, balanced diet, and regular physical exercise. Treatment of CAD may confer benefit in improving ED and conversely, treatment of ED may benefit patients with established CVD.

Lifestyle Measures

Lifestyle modifications is an important and integral part of treating patients of both CVD and ED. Regular physical exercise helps reducing CVD burden as well as control of the risk factors like hypertension, diabetes, hyperlipidemia, and obesity. Cessation of smoking or use of tobacco products, emphasis on proper diet with reduced salt intake, and weight control are necessary for treatment of ED.[15] Management of stress is another aspect of lifestyle measures necessary for treatment of ED.

Phosphodiesterase Type 5 Inhibitors for Erectile Dysfunction

Phosphodiesterase type 5 inhibitors are the main therapy for ED of nonfunctional etiology and they can be used safely if there is no contraindication for their use.[16] Mechanism of action include pulmonary artery and systemic arterial vasodilation, improvement in myocardial contractility, reduction in the stiffness of large arterial beds, improvement in the deteriorated endothelial function, and reduction in apoptosis, fibrosis and hypertrophy. Drug-to-drug interactions with other cardiac drugs are very minimal except nitrates and other nitric oxide (NO) donors (like nicorandil). Coadministration of these drugs may cause severe vasodilation, leading to hypotension. American Urological Association recent guidelines advise that cardiac patients who carry sublingual nitroglycerin for angina should be advised not to take nitrate within 24 hours of taking sildenafil and 48 hours of taking tadalafil. Transient systemic vasodilatation caused by these agents may be aggravated by coadministration of alpha-blocking agents. It is recommended that vardenafil and tadalafil, any dose, and sildenafil at 50 mg and 100 mg doses should be administered with caution in patients who are on alpha-blocker agents.[17]

All four agents of this group (sildenafil, tadalafil, vardenafil, and avanafil) have not shown to increase the risk of silent or overt myocardial ischemia, stroke, or cardiac death. These drugs also do not worsen ischemia or reduce exercise tolerance or exercise duration in patients with established CAD who are having good exercise capacity and are engaged in normal sexual activities.

Selection of Proper Cardiovascular Drugs in Erectile Dysfunction

Different cardiovascular drugs have been implicated by different investigators as to be having causal association with ED. Though all of them may not have been proven to have strong correlation other than thiazide diuretics that clearly lead to ED, they need to be remembered while treating a cardiac patient having ED. The drugs implicated are:

- *Sympathetic depressants*: Reserpine, alpha-methyldopa, and clonidine
- *Antihypertensive drugs*: Thiazide diuretic, some beta-blockers
- *Statin*: High-dose
- Spironolactone (antiandrogen side effect)
- *Cardiac glycosides*: Digoxin.

Some older beta-blockers are said to be responsible for causing ED, but this side effect was reported to be as low as 3% when the patients were blinded for the drug they were given. In fact, the newer vasodilator beta-blocker nebivolol is said to improve ED.[18] Botros SM et al.[19] studied hypertensive patients treated with beta-blockers atenolol, bisoprolol, carvedilol, and nebivolol. Pretreatment penile artery peak systolic and diastolic velocities were compared with 8–12 weeks post-treatment velocities. They found that blood flow was significantly reduced by atenolol, bisoprolol, and carvedilol but not by nebivolol.

Erectile dysfunction is frequently encountered in hypertensive population as a whole and sexual dysfunction is commonly encountered in treated than in untreated patients. Evidence suggests that older groups of drugs like diuretics, beta-blockers cause more ED as compared to the newer groups like nebivolol, angiotensin-converting enzyme inhibitors (ACEIs), angiotensin receptor blockers (ARBs), which are said to possess neutral or rather beneficial effect on erectile function in some studies.[20] However, they have not been studied extensively in large clinical trials from this angle.

Statins are helpful in improving endothelial dysfunction and preventing progression of atherosclerosis. So they should be helpful in ED prevention or treatment. Statins have mostly shown beneficial effect. However, higher statin doses may have a negative effect. In a clinical trial with patients of atherosclerosis on statin therapy, the baseline median IIEF score of 21 worsened to 6.5 after 6 months of statin therapy and baseline prevalence of ED of 57% increased to 79%. Difference in statin dose and type of the drugs prescribed showed no definite relation with the change in IIEF score.[21] Larger clinical trials with statin therapy need to be conducted to come to a conclusion in this regard as statin is the most essential drug in the treatment of atherosclerotic CVD.

Role of Testosterone and Prostaglandin Therapy

Testosterone replacement therapy (TRT) can be considered in patients who are symptomatic due to testosterone deficiency or who have laboratory documentation of low serum testosterone (TT <8 nmol/L or 2.3 ng/mL). Men with ED and/or with visceral obesity and metabolic diseases should be evaluated for testosterone deficiency.[22] TRT can be delivered by different routes like oral, injectable, gel, or transdermal. Bioavailability after oral administration is minimal, and hence, this route is not very effective. Gel applied regularly over skin or transdermal patches are effective alternatives of injectable therapy. Another option is prostaglandin E1 (PGE1), alprostadil that can be delivered by injection or by transurethral pallets.

While a PDE5 inhibitor is considered as first-line therapy, addition of TRT or PGE1 should be considered when the condition is not improved with PDE5 inhibitor alone. Improvement on TRT is dependent on the baseline testosterone levels and better results are expected at lower levels of testosterone.

CONCLUSION

Erectile dysfunction and coronary artery disease share the common platform of endothelial dysfunction and atherosclerosis, and associated with same risk factors like high blood pressure, diabetes, smoking, dyslipidemia, visceral obesity, and sedentary lifestyle, in its causation. Hence, ED can be an important risk marker of silent CVD. Assessment of sexual health should be a part of complete assessment of cardiovascular risk in men. A comprehensive approach of reducing cardiovascular risk with the help of both lifestyle measures and necessary pharmacological treatment improves overall vascular disease risk, including sexual function in persons suffering from this condition.

REFERENCES

1. Johannes CB, Araujo AB, Feldman HA, et al. Incidence of erectile dysfunction in men 40 to 69 years old: longitudinal results from the Massachusetts male aging study. J Urol. 2000;163(2):460-3.
2. Vlachopoulos C, Jackson G, Stefanadis C, et al. Erectile dysfunction in the cardiovascular patient. Eur Heart J. 2013;34(27):2034-46.
3. Solomon H, Man JW, Jackson G. Erectile dysfunction and the cardiovascular patient: endothelial dysfunction is the common denominator. Heart. 2003;89(3):251-4.
4. Vlachopoulos C, Aznaouridis K, Loakeimidis N, et al. Unfavourable endothelial and inflammatory state in erectile dysfunction patients with or without coronary artery disease. Eur Heart J. 2006;27(22):2640-8.

5. Montorsi P, Ravagnani PM, Galli S, et al. Common grounds for erectile dysfunction and coronary artery disease. Curr Opin Urol. 2004;14(6):361-5.
6. Kloner RA, Mullin SH, Shook T, et al. Erectile dysfunction in the cardiac patient: how common and should we treat? J Urol. 2003;170(2 Pt 2):S46-50.
7. Roumeguere T, Wespes E, Carpentier Y, et al. Erectile dysfunction is associated with a high prevalence of hyperlipidemia and coronary heart disease risk. Eur Urol. 2003;44(3):355-9.
8. Sasayama S, Ishii N, Ishikura F, et al. Men's health study: epidemiology of erectile dysfunction and cardiovascular disease. Circ J. 2003;67(8):656-9.
9. Uslu N, Gorgulu S, Alper AT, et al. Erectile dysfunction as a generalized vascular dysfunction. J Am Soc Echocardiogr. 2006;19(3):341-6.
10. Baumhakel M, Bohm M. Erectile dysfunction correlates with left ventricular function and precedes cardiovascular events in cardiovascular high risk patients. Int J Clin Pract. 2007;61(3):361-6.
11. Solomon H, Man JW, Wierzbicki AS, et al. Relation of erectile dysfunction and angiographic coronary artery disease. Am J Cardiol. 2003;91(2):230-1.
12. Vlachopoulos C, Rokkas K, Loakeimidis N, et al. Prevalence of asymptomatic coronary artery disease in men with vasculogenic erectile dysfunction: a prospective angiographic study. Eur Urol. 2005;48(6):996-1003.
13. Cappelleri JC, Rosen RC. The Sexual Health Inventory For Men (SHIM): a 5-year review of research and clinical experience. Int J Impot Res. 2005;17(4):307-19.
14. Carson CC 3rd, Rosano G. Exogenous testosterone, cardiovascular events, and cardiovascular risk factors in elderly men: a review of trial data. J Sex Med. 2012;9(1):54-67.
15. Gupta BP, Murad MH, Clifton MM, et al. The effect of lifestyle modification and cardiovascular risk factor reduction on erectile dysfunction: a systematic review and meta-analysis. Arch Intern Med. 2011;171(20):1797-803.
16. Giuliano F, Jackson G, Montorsi F, et al. Safety of sildenafil citrate: review of 67 double-blind placebo-controlled trials and the post-marketing safety database. Int J Clin Pract. 2010;64(2):240-55.
17. American Urological Association Guidelines. The management of erectile dysfunction: an update 2007. 2007. pp. 12-13.
18. Silvestri A, Galetta P, Cerquetani E, et al. Report of erectile dysfunction after therapy with beta-blockers is related to patient knowledge of side effects and is reversed by placebo. Eur Heart J. 2003;24(21):1928-32.
19. Boros SM, Hussein AM, Elserfy AS. Effect of different beta blockers on penile vascular velocities in hypertensive males. Egypt J Radiol Nucl Med. 2015;46:749-54.
20. Manolis A, Doumas M. Antihypertensive treatment and sexual dysfunction. Curr Hypertens Rep. 2012;14(4):285-92.
21. Solomon H, Samarasinghe YP, Feher MD, et al. Erectile dysfunction and statin treatment in high cardiovascular risk patients. Int J Clin Pract. 2006;60(2):141-5.
22. Buvat J, Maggi M, Guay A, et al. Testosterone deficiency in men: systematic review and standard operating procedures for diagnosis and treatment. J Sex Med. 2013;10(1):245-84.

CHAPTER 152

Noncardiac Surgery: How to "Clear" a Patient?

PC Manoria, Pankaj Manoria, Sharad Kumar Parashar

INTRODUCTION

Worldwide, it is estimated that around 20 million people undergo noncardiac surgery annually.[1] One-third of surgeries are performed in geriatric population. The overall mortality is 1–5%, in individual less than 65 years the average mortality is 1% whereas in individuals above 65 years the morality is higher about 5%. Cardiovascular (CV) complications are the most common cause of death.[2,3] All deaths in the first 48 hours are due to cardiac causes like heart failure (HF), acute coronary syndrome (ACS). The deaths from 48 hours to 6 weeks are usually due to a noncardiac cause like pneumonia, sepsis, pulmonary embolism, renal failure, etc.

Preoperative evaluation is of paramount importance as appropriate preventive and therapeutic strategies may decrease CV morbidity and mortality and shorten the hospital stay.

The main purpose of perioperative evolution is to get familiar with the following basic questions:

1. What are the underlying risk factors which the patient is having prior to noncardiac surgery?
2. What is the anticipated patient-related risk?
3. What is the proper preoperative treatment to reduce the anticipated risk during surgery and steps to be taken in the postoperative period to reduce morbidity and mortality?

The cardiac complications after noncardiac surgery depend on three things:

1. Procedure-related risk
2. Patient-related risk
3. Functional capacity (FC).

Procedure-related risk: The surgical risk for cardiac events depends on the type of procedure carried out. High-risk procedures have a mortality of 5%, intermediate-risk 1–5%, and low-risk less than 1% (Table 1).

Patient-related risk: The patient-related risk depends on the underlying disease as shown in table 2.

Functional capacity: It is an important test in preoperative cardiac risk assessment and is measured in metabolic equivalents (METs). Exercise testing provides an objective assessment of FC but without this it can be estimated from the ability to perform activities in daily life (Table 3).

Poor FC is associated with an increased incidence of postoperative cardiac events. When FC is good, the prognosis is excellent even in presence of stable ischemic heart disease (IHD) or risk factors.

TABLE 1: Procedure-related risk

High (5%)	Intermediate (1–5%)	Low (<1%)
Emergent major operations (elderly)	Carotid endarterectomy	Endoscopic procedures
Aortic and other major vascular surgery	Head and neck surgery	Superficial procedure
Peripheral vascular surgery	Intraperitoneal, Intrathoracic surgery	Cataract surgery
Anticipated prolonged surgical procedures	• Orthopedic surgery • Prostate surgery • Pulmonary, renal/ liver transplant	• Breast surgery • Dental • Gynecology, urologic–minor

TABLE 2: Patient-related risk

Major	Intermediate	Minor
ACS	Prior Myocardial infarction	Advanced age
Decompensated HF	Mild angina	Abnormal ECG
Significant arrhythmias	Compensated HF	Rhythm other than sinus
Severe VHD* stenotic lesions like AS, MS	Diabetes Mellitus	Past stroke
Poor FC	Renal insufficiency	Uncontrolled hypertension

ACS, acute coronary syndrome; AS, aortic stenosis; ECG, electrocardiogram; FC, functional capacity; HF, heart failure; MS, mitral stenosis; *VHD, valvular heart disease.

TABLE 3: Assessment of functional capacity

Severity	Assessment
Poor	Unable to climb a flight of stairs (<4 METs)
Moderate	Climbing flight of stairs (4–7 METs)
Good	Participation in moderate recreational activities (>7 METs)
Very good	Participation in strenuous sports swimming (>10 METs)

METs, metabolic equivalents.

TABLE 4: Revised cardiac risk index variables

Variables	Pts
Hx of IHD	1
Hx of CHF	1
Hx of CVD	1
Insulin for diabetes	1
Serum creatinine >2.0 mg/dL	1
High-risk surgery	1

CHF, congestive heart failure; CVD, cardiovascular disease; Hx, history; IHD, ischemic heart disease.

TABLE 5: Assessment of cardiac events in preoperative period based on RCRI points

Total RCRI points	Risk of MI, cardiac arrest, or death 30 days after surgery
0	0.4% (95% CI: 0.1–0.8)
1	1.0% (95% CI: 0.5–1.4)
2	2.4% (95% CI: 1.3–3.5)
≥3	5.4% (95% CI:2.8–7.9)

CI, confidence interval; MI, myocardial infarction; RCRI, revised cardiac risk index.

Perioperative cardiac morbidity risk evaluation: This is commonly assessed by revised cardiac risk index.

Revised cardiac risk index: The revised cardiac risk index[4,5] is a simple tool that has been validated to assess the perioperative risk of major cardiac events. The variables of this score are shown in table 4 and single point is assigned to every risk factor present. The risk of cardiac arrest or death 30 days after surgery is shown in table 5. Patients having zero or only one risk factor have a low-risk of major adverse cardiac events (MACE), whereas those with two or more risk factors have elevated risk.

ANCILLARY PREOPERATIVE CARDIAC TESTING: RECOMMENDATIONS

Electrocardiogram

A 12-lead electrocardiogram (ECG) preoperatively is useful in patients with atherosclerotic cardiovascular disease (ASCVD), structural heart diseases or arrhythmias. Low-risk patients going for surgery do not require ECG preoperatively.

Left Ventricular Function

Patients with HF or with documented left ventricular (LV) dysfunction in past or unexplained dyspnea should be subjected to echocardiography for assessment of LV function. Evaluation of all patients going for surgery is not required.[6] Decrease LV systolic function with ejection fraction less than 35% may be associated with adverse outcome. Further, in patients with LV systolic dysfunction, a restrictive pattern of mitral inflow on echocardiography is associated with increased morbidity and mortality because advanced diastolic dysfunction implies marked elevation of left ventricular enddiastolic pressure and this predisposes to precipitation of HF. In such patients surgery should be postponed and treatment optimized. Only when their LV function improves they should be submitted for surgery.

Stress Testing and Cardiopulmonary Testing

All patients undergoing noncardiac surgery do not require stress testing.[7] Only in patients with poor FC (4 METS), stress test is required. Patients with good FC can be directly submitted for surgery. In cardiopulmonary testing, a low anaerobic threshold of 9–11 mL/O_2/kg/min is a bad prognostic sign and condition of such patients should be improved prior to submission for surgery.

Pharmacological Testing

The use of pharmacological testing with stress dobutamine or myocardial perfusion imaging is restricted to patients who have poor FC and ECG changes like LV hypertrophy (LVH), left bundle branch block (LBBB), etc. which interferes with ECG evaluation of myocardial ischemia. All patients should not be submitted for these tests prior to surgery.[3] Presence of large areas of myocardial ischemia is associated with adverse CV outcome.

Coronary Angiography

Routine angiography is not indicated preoperatively except for patients who are candidates for organ transplantation like liver, kidney, etc. Calcium scoring on computed tomography is also not recommended.[9]

Therapeutic Strategies

Percutaneous Coronary Intervention or Coronary Artery Bypass Graft

Percutaneous coronary intervention or coronary artery bypass graft (PCI or CABG) is not recommended prior to noncardiac surgery as no benefit has been demonstrated.[10]

If patient develops ACS prior to surgery, then treatment is offered as per guidelines.

ELECTIVE NONCARDIAC SURGERY IN PATIENTS WITH PRIOR PERCUTANEOUS CORONARY INTERVENTION: TIMING AND RECOMMENDATIONS

Patient with bare-metal stent (BMS) or drug-eluting stent (DES) implantation, if they require noncardiac surgery in the early postimplantation period, i.e., less than 4 weeks for BMS and 6–12 months for DES[11,12] one should carefully assess the risk of stent thrombosis after withdrawal of antiplatelet drugs versus the bleeding risk during surgery due to continuation of dual antiplatelet therapy (DAPT) and then take decision.

The period during which noncardiac surgery should be avoided after balloon angioplasty/BMS/DES implantation is outlined in table 6.

If surgery is to be performed in BMS implantation before 30 days or DES implantation before 6–12 months, then the strategy for using antiplatelet drugs depends on the bleeding risk of the patient as outlined in table 7.

In such subset of patients, the surgeon should be encouraged to operate on aspirin at least in patients with low or intermediate bleeding risk.

ANTICOAGULANT THERAPY

Vitamin K Antagonists

The decision to continue anticoagulants or bridging with low molecular weight heparin (LMWH) or unfractionated heparin (UFH) depends on the thromboembolism risk of the patient and the bleeding risk of surgery. If the surgery is a low-bleeding risk like cataract surgery bridging is not required and surgery can be done without stopping anticoagulant.[13]

Prosthetic Valves

Patients of prosthetic valves on warfarin even in absence of risk factors for thromboembolism like atrial fibrillation (AF), past history of embolic episodes, LV dysfunction will require cessation of anticoagulant therapy and bridging with UFH/LMWH in the perioperative period.[13]

Atrial Fibrillation on Vitamin K Antagonists

Patients of AF with high thromboembolism risk, i.e., CHA_2DS_2-VASc score of 2 in males and 3 in females or more will require bridging with UFH/LMWH in perioperative period for surgery. If the thromboembolism risk is low with CHA_2DS_2-VASc score of 1 in males and 2 in females, anticoagulants can be stopped and when international normalized ratio (INR) is less than 2, surgery can be performed. Vitamin K antagonists (VKAs) can be restarted after homeostatic is achieved.[14,15]

Direct Oral Anticoagulants

The half-life of novel oral anticoagulants (NOACs) is about 12 hours. If the bleeding risk is mild-to-moderate, NOACs are discontinued for a period of 2–3 half-life but if the bleeding risk is high, they are discontinued for five times the half-life.

The renal function must always be assessed by estimated glomerular filtration rate (eGFR). This is particularly important for dabigatran because 80% is excreted through kidneys.[16] Apixaban, only 25% is excreted through kidneys and may be preferable in patients with chronic kidney disease. For reinitiating NOACs, the bleeding and embolic risk must be taken into consideration. For low-bleeding risk and high-embolic risk, NOACs can be resumed as early as 12–24 hours. If bleeding risk is high and embolic risk is low, one may wait

TABLE 6: Decision policy for noncardiac surgery in patients who have undergone prior coronary interventions

Recommendations	COR	LOE
Elective noncardiac surgery should not be performed within 14 days of balloon angioplasty in patients in whom aspirin will need to be discontinued perioperatively	III Harm	C
Elective noncardiac surgery should not be performed within 30 days after BMS implantation or within 6–12 months after DES implantation in patients in whom DAPT will need to be discontinued perioperatively	III Harm	B
Elective noncardiac surgery after DES implantation may be considered after 180 days if the risk of further delay is greater than the expected risks of ischemia and stent thrombosis	IIb	B

BMS, bare-metal stent; COR, class of recommendation; DAPT, dual antiplatelet therapy; DES, drug-eluting stent; LOE, level of evidence.

TABLE 7: Use of antiplatelet drugs in patients requiring early surgery after coronary intervention

Bleeding risk		
Low	Intermediate	High
Cataract, oral dental surgery	GI surgeries, cholecystectomy, appendectomy, etc.	Intracranial, prostate, aortic, ENT, posterior segment surgery
Continue aspirin and clopidogrel	Stop clopidogrel continue aspirin	Stop aspirin and clopidogrel and bridge with cangrelor: 0.75 µg/kg/min or tirofiban: 0.1 µg/kg/min. If renal dysfunction, decrease dose to 0.05 µg/kg and start 24–48 hours. After last dose and continue till 4–8 hours before surgery (ESC DAPT update 2017)

DAPT, dual antiplatelet therapy; ENT, ear, nose, and throat; ESC, European Society of Cardiology; GI, gastrointestinal.

for upto 72 hours. It must be ensured that homeostasis has been achieved before initiating NOACs. Periprocedural bridging with LMWH is not required because of short half-life of NOACs.

Reversal of Vitamin K Antagonist

Vitamin K is not preferred for reversal of VKAs because even after intravenous administration it takes 8–12 hours to act. Fresh frozen plasma or prothrombin complex concentrates are utilized for this purpose as their onset of action is immediate.[13]

Beta-blocker Therapy

The use of β-blocker in perioperative period[17] is outlined in table 8.

Statin Therapy

If patient is already on statins, this should be continued. Statins should be started in patients undergoing vascular surgery or they are indicated otherwise.[18]

Alpha-2 Agonist

Alpha-2 agonists are not useful in prevention of cardiac events in perioperative period.

Calcium-channel Blockers

Verapamil or diltiazem can precipitate HF in patients with reduced ejection fraction and they should be avoided in this subset of patients.

Angiotensin-converting Enzyme Inhibitors or Angiotensin Receptor Blockers

If the patient is already on angiotensin-converting enzyme (ACE) inhibitors or angiotensin II receptor blockers (ARBs) perioperatively they should be continued. If the patient is not on these drugs, it is desirable to restart as soon as possible postoperatively.[19]

PREOPERATIVE EVALUATION IN SPECIFIC PATIENTS POPULATION: GENERAL CONSIDERATIONS

Age

Noncardiac surgery in elderly patients is associated with increased morbidity and mortality because of associated diabetes, kidney disease, stroke, and other medical conditions.

Coronary Artery Disease

Coronary artery disease (CAD) is an important determinant of postoperative CV outcomes. Noncardiac surgery should not be performed for at least 3 months after acute myocardial infarction (AMI).[20] Perioperative AMI is associated with very-high morbidity and mortality and should be prevented as far as possible by appropriate pre-op check-up and treatment. Even mere elevation of serum markers without AMI is also associated with adverse outcomes.

Heart Failure

Patients with HF or even history of HF in past are associated with increased morbidity and mortality after noncardiac surgery Systolic dysfunction with an ejection fraction less than 35% even if it is asymptomatic is associated with increased morbidity and mortality.[21] In patients with LV systolic dysfunction, if there associated diastolic dysfunction with a restrictive pattern, surgery should be postponed and treatment optimized to improve LV function before submitting for surgery. Data suggest that mortality in HF is higher (9.3% ischemic and 9.2% nonischemic) compared to CAD mortality of 2.9%.[21]

PERIOPERATIVE ARRHYTHMIAS

The development of arrhythmias in perioperative period is multifactorial like ischemia, disturbed internal mileau, drug toxicity, underlying cardiopulmonary disease, etc.

TABLE 8: Perioperative beta-blocker therapy

Recommendations	COR	LOE
Beta-blocker should be continued in patients undergoing surgery who have been on it chronically	I	B[SR]
It is reasonable for the management of β-blocker after surgery to be guided by clinical circumstances, independent of when the agent was started	IIa	B[SR]
In patients with intermediate or high-risk myocardial ischemia noted in preoperative risk stratification tests, it may be reasonable to begin perioperative β-blocker	IIb	C[SR]
In patients with three or more RCRI risk factors (e.g., diabetes mellitus, HF, CAD, renal insufficiency, cerebrovascular accident), it may be reasonable to begin β-blocker before surgery	IIb	B[SR]
In patients with a compelling long-term indication for β-blocker therapy but no other RCRI risk factors, initiating β-blockers in the periopreative setting as an approach to reduce periopreative risk is of uncertain benefit	IIb	B[SR]
In patients in whom β-blocker therapy is initiated, it may be reasonable to begin perioperative β-blockers long enough in advance to assess safety and tolerability, preferably more than 1-day before surgery	IIb	B[SR]
Beta-blocker therapy should not be started on the day of surgery	III	B[SR]

CAD, coronary artery disease; COR, class of recommendation; HF, heart failure; LOE, level of evidence; RCRI, revised cardiac risk index.

Very few studies are available in this context. Patients with supraventricular or ventricular ectopics or nonsustained ventricular tachycardia are not of serious concern.[22,23] Patients with AF with CHA_2DS_2-VASc score of more than 2 in males and 3 in females should receive anticoagulation to prevent stroke. Routine use of antiarrhythmic drug prophylaxis is not recommended for postoperative AF as this would subject all patients to their potential side effects, while only a minority of the patients actually develops this problem postoperatively. Withdrawal of β-blockers in the postoperative period has been implicated as one of the major causes of postoperative atrial fibrillation (POAF). β-blockers and amiodarone are mainstays of pharmacological and treatment of POAF.

CONCLUSION

Clearing a cardiac patient for noncardiac surgery is a common issue in our day-to-day practice. CV complications like HF and ACS are the most common cause of death in first 48 hours while mortality from 48 hours to 6 weeks is usually due to a noncardiac complication like pneumonia, sepsis, pulmonary embolism, renal failure, etc. A careful evaluation of the patient taking into consideration the procedure-related risk, the patient-related risk, and FC coupled with use of appropriate drugs and necessary precautions paves the way for minimizing CV morbidity and mortality in the perioperative period and also shorten the hospital stay.

REFERENCES

1. Lee TH, Marcantonio ER, Mangione CM, et al. Derivation and prospective validation of a simple index for prediction of cardiac risk of major noncardiac surgery. Circulation. 1999;100:1043-9.
2. Weiser TG, Regenbogen SE, Thompson KD, et al. An estimation of the global volume of surgery: A modelling strategy based on available data. Lancet. 2008;372:139-44.
3. Bakker EJ, Ravensbergen NJ, Poldermans D. Peri-operative cardiac evaluation, monitoring, and risk reduction strategies in noncardiac surgery patients. Curr Opin Crit Care. 2011;17:409-15.
4. Fleisher LA, Fleischmann KE, Auerbach AD, et al. 2014 ACC/AHA guideline on peri-operative cardiovascular evaluation and management of patients undergoing noncardiac surgery: A report of the American College of Cardiology/American Heart Association Task Force on practice guidelines. J Am Coll Cardiol. 2014;64:e77-137.
5. Ford MK, Beattie WS, Wijeysundera DN. Systematic review: Prediction of peri-operative cardiac complications and mortality by the revised cardiac risk index. Ann Intern Med. 2010;152:26-35.
6. Rohde LE, Polanczyk CA, Goldman L, et al. Usefulness of transthoracic echocardiography as a tool for risk stratification of patients undergoing major noncardiac surgery. Am J Cardiol. 2001;87:505-9.
7. Eagle KA, Coley CM, Newell JB, et al. Combining clinical and thallium data optimizes preoperative assessment of cardiac risk before major vascular surgery. Ann Intern Med. 1989;110:859-66.
8. Das MK, Pellikka PA, Mahoney DW, et al. Assessment of cardiac risk before nonvascular surgery: Dobutamine stress echocardiography in 530 patients. J Am Coll Cardiol. 2000;35:1647-53.
9. Ahn JH, Park JR, Min JH, et al. Risk stratification using computed tomography coronary angiography in patients undergoing intermediate-risk noncardiac surgery. J Am Coll Cardiol. 2013;61:661-8.
10. McFalls EO, Ward HB, Moritz TE, et al. Coronary-artery revascularization before elective major vascular surgery. N Engl J Med. 2004;351:2795-804.
11. Kaluza GL, Joseph J, Lee JR, et al. Catastrophic outcomes of noncardiac surgery soon after coronary stenting. J Am Coll Cardiol. 2000;35:1288-94.
12. Tokushige A, Shiomi H, Morimoto T, et al. Incidence and outcome of surgical procedures after coronary bare-metal and drug-eluting stent implantation: A report from the CREDO-Kyoto PCI/CABG registry cohort-2. Circ Cardiovasc Interv. 2012;5:237-46.
13. Nishimura RA, Otto CM, Bonow RO, et al. 2014 AHA/ACC guideline for the management of patients with valvular heart disease: a report of the American College of Cardiology/American Heart Association Task Force on Practice Guidelines. J Am Coll Cardiol. 2014;63:e57-185.
14. January CT, Wann LS, Alpert JS, et al. 2014 AHA/ACC/HRS guideline for the management of patients with atrial fibrillation: A report of the American College of Cardiology/American Heart Association Task Force on practice guidelines and the Heart Rhythm Society. Circulation. 2014;130:e199-267.
15. Douketis JD, Spyropoulos AC, Kaatz S, et al. Peri-operative bridging anticoagulation in patients with atrial fibrillation. N Engl J Med. 2015;373:823-33.
16. Schulman S, Carrier M, Lee AY, et al. Peri-operative management of dabigatran: A prospective cohort study. Circulation. 2015;132:167-73.
17. Wijeysundera DN, Duncan D, Nkonde-Price C, et al. Peri-operative beta blockade in noncardiac surgery: A systematic review for the 2014 ACC/AHA guideline on peri-operative cardiovascular evaluation and management of patients undergoing noncardiac surgery: A report of the American College of Cardiology/American Heart Association Task Force on practice guidelines. J Am Coll Cardiol. 2014;64:2406-25.
18. Lindenauer PK, Pekow P, Wang K, et al. Lipid-lowering therapy and in-hospital mortality following major noncardiac surgery. JAMA. 2004;291:2092-9.
19. Rosenman DJ, McDonald FS, Ebbert JO, et al. Clinical consequences of withholding versus administering renin-angiotensin-aldosterone system antagonists in the preoperative period. J Hosp Med. 2008;3:319-25.
20. Livhits M, Ko CY, Leonardi MJ, et al. Risk of surgery following recent myocardial infarction. Ann Surg. 2011;253:857-64.
21. Healy KO, Waksmonski CA, Altman RK, et al. Peri-operative outcome and long-term mortality for heart failure patients undergoing intermediate- and high-risk noncardiac surgery: Impact of left ventricular ejection fraction. Congest Heart Fail. 2010;16:45-9.
22. Mahla E, Rotman B, Rehak P, et al. Peri-operative ventricular dysrhythmias in patients with structural heart disease undergoing noncardiac surgery. Anesth Analg. 1998;86:16-21.
23. O'Kelly B, Browner WS, Massie B, et al. Ventricular arrhythmias in patients undergoing noncardiac surgery. The study of peri-operative Ischemia Research Group. JAMA. 1992;268:217-21.

CHAPTER 153

How to Defend a Complaint in Cardiology

KK Aggarwal

Facing a lawsuit can be a traumatic and stressful experience for any person, more so for a doctor, who is dedicated to taking care of this patients. Lawsuits are not only expensive, they are also time-consuming as it may take a few years before the case goes to trial and a judgment is delivered. Recently, there has been an unprecedented increase in the number of malpractice claims being filed against doctors. Doctors are, more often than not, ignorant of the various nuances of the law as it relates to the practice of medicine because law as a subject is not a part of our medical curriculum.

There have been several landmark judgments of the Supreme Court of India on medical negligence in India. Defenses are available in these Supreme Court judgments, including those of the National Consumer Disputes Redressal Commission (NCDRC). It is very important that doctors are knowledgeable about these judgments and identify those defenses, which can be applied to their lawsuit, should such a situation arise. However, prevention is still the best defense. Follow all required guidelines and self-regulate to maintain professional standards and avoid litigation.

DEFENSE ARGUMENT NO. 1

"I have done nothing that any reasonable prudent doctor would not have done (act of commission) nor I have refrained from doing anything, which a reasonable prudent doctor would do (act of omission)."

"While a doctor cannot be forced to treat any person, he/she has certain responsibilities for those whom he/she accepts as patients. Some of these responsibilities may be recapitulated, in brief:

(c) to exhibit reasonable skill: The degree of skill a doctor undertakes is the average degree of skill possessed by his professional brethren of the same standing as himself. The best form of treatment may differ when different choices are available. There is an implied contract between the doctor and patient where the patient is told, in effect, "Medicine is not an exact science. I shall use my experience and best judgment and you take the risk that I may be wrong. I guarantee nothing" **(PB Desai versus State of Maharashtra, AIR 2014 SC 795)**.

DEFENSE ARGUMENT NO. 2

"I acted as per my thinking and at the most it can be a case of difference of opinion and or error of diagnosis and the same is not negligence. An error of diagnosis can never be labeled as deficiency in services."

"In the realm of diagnosis and treatment there is scope for genuine difference of opinion and one professional doctor is clearly not negligent merely because his conclusion differs from that of other professional doctor (v)" **[Kusum Sharma and Others versus Batra Hospital and Medical Research Centre, 2010 (3) SCC 480]**.

DEFENSE ARGUMENT NO. 3

"I have taken all the care that was expected from any reasonable prudent medical practitioner and therefore there cannot be any element of negligence or rashness in the services rendered by me."

"...Failure to act in accordance with the standard, reasonable, competent medical means at the time would not constitute a negligence. However, a medical practitioner must exercise the reasonable degree of care and skill and knowledge which he possesses. Failure to use due skill in diagnosis with the result that wrong treatment is given would be negligence (iv)" **(Malay Kumar Ganguly versus Sukumar Mukherjee & Ors. AIR 2010 SC 1162)**.

DEFENSE ARGUMENT NO. 4

"I am a qualified doctor (....degrees), have received many honors (.................), have over ...... years of experience and have been updating my knowledge regularly (......state CME hours)."

"76. The basic principle relating to the law of medical negligence is the Bolam Rule which has been quoted above.

The test in fixing negligence is the standard of the ordinary skilled doctor exercising and professing to have that special skill, but a doctor need not possess the highest expert skill" **[Martin F. D'Souza versus Mohd. Ishfaq, 2009 (3) SCC 1]**.

DEFENSE ARGUMENT NO. 5

"When I treated the patient, the line of treatment adopted by me was the best option thought by me."

"In case, the doctor brings in his task of providing medicine, a reasonable degree of skill and knowledge and exercise the same to a reasonable degree, then, the medical practitioner cannot be held guilty for the medical negligence only because someone else of better skill and knowledge had prescribed different treatment or operated in a different way. Petitioner failed to produce any evidence to show that the line of treatment adopted by the respondent was not in line with the reasonable body of medical practitioners. Mere difference of opinion in adopting different line of treatment than the one adopted by the medical practitioner does not prove that the medical practitioner was guilty of medical negligence. Respondent-doctor had taken due care and caution. The doctor cannot be held negligent simply because something went wrong. He also cannot be held liable for making one choice out of two or for favoring one school rather than another. He can be held guilt only where his conduct fell below that of the standards of a reasonably competent practitioner in his field, so much so, that his conduct might be deserving of censure or inexcusable" **[Prabha Shankar Ojha versus Neelmani Rai, 2009 (4) CPR 307]**.

DEFENSE ARGUMENT NO. 6

"There are .... number of diagnosis or treatment of .... medical problem and I have adopted this .... diagnosis or treatment for the same."

"Para 11: The duties which a doctor owes to his patient are clear. A person who holds himself out ready to give medical advice and treatment impliedly undertakes that he is possessed of skill and knowledge for the purpose. Such a person when consulted by a patient owes him certain duties, viz., a duty of care in deciding whether to undertake the case, a duty of care in deciding what treatment to give or a duty of care in the administration of that treatment. A breach of any of those duties gives a right of action for negligence to the patient. The practitioner must bring to his task a reasonable degree of skill and knowledge and must exercise a reasonable degree of care. Neither the very highest nor a very low degree of care and competence judged in the light of the particular circumstances of each case is what the law requires. The doctor no doubt has a discretion in choosing treatment which he proposes to give to the patient and such discretion is relatively ampler in cases of emergency" [Laxman Balkrishna Joshi v. Trimbak Bapu Godbole and Anr AIR 1969 SC 128].

DEFENSE ARGUMENT NO. 7

"Though the procedure/diagnosis/treatment adopted by me involves higher risk, it has greater chances of success in comparison to the other procedure, which involves less risk but has greater chances of failure."

"The medical professional is often called upon to adopt a procedure which involves higher element of risk, but which he honestly believes as providing greater chances of success for the patient rather than a procedure involving lesser risk but higher chances of failure. Just because a professional looking to the gravity of illness has taken higher element of risk to redeem the patient out of his/her suffering which did not yield the desired result may not amount to negligence (vi)" **[Kusum Sharma & Others versus Batra Hospital & Medical Research Centre, 2010 (3) SCC 480]**.

DEFENSE ARGUMENT NO. 8

"I have treated the patient as per general and approved practice. Expert opinions have been taken by me/us from other eminent doctors of the city and they too have agreed with the line of management adopted and found no negligence or deficiency in services."

"Negligence cannot be attributed to a doctor, so long as he performs his duties with reasonable skill and competence. Merely because the doctor chooses one course of action in preference to another available, he would not be liable if the course of action chosen by him was acceptable to the medical profession (vii)" **[Kusum Sharma & Others versus Batra Hospital & Medical Research Centre, 2010 (3) SCC 480]**.

DEFENSE ARGUMENT NO. 9

"I have added the opinion of experts, who have agreed with my line of treatment. Even if the experts about by the Council differ with the opinion of my experts, I must get the benefit of doubt."

"Thus in large majority of cases, it has been demonstrated that a doctor will be liable for negligence in respect of diagnosis and treatment in spite of a body of professional opinion approving his conduct where it has not been established to the courts satisfaction that such opinion relied on is reasonable or responsible. If it can be demonstrated that the professional opinion is not capable of withstanding the logical analysis, the court would be entitled to hold that the body of opinion is not reasonable or responsible" **[Vinitha Ashok versus Lakshmi Hospital, AIR 2001 SC 3914]**.

DEFENSE ARGUMENT NO. 10

"The complication, which occurred in this case has been well-described in literature (quote a reference) and cannot amount to negligence. Whatever happened during treatment in this case was a pure accident. Accidents are not actionable."

"Para 27: A mere deviation from normal professional practice is not necessarily evidence of negligence. Let it also be noted that a mere accident is not evidence of negligence. So also an error of judgment on the part of a professional is not negligence per se. Higher the acuteness in emergency and higher the complication, more are the chances of error of judgment. At times, the professional is confronted with making a choice between the devil and the deep sea and he has to choose the lesser evil. The medical professional is often called upon to adopt a procedure which involves higher element of risk, but which he honestly believes as providing greater chances of success for the patient rather than a procedure involving lesser risk but higher chances of failure. Which course is more appropriate to follow, would depend on the facts and circumstances of a given case. The usual practice prevalent nowadays is to obtain the consent of the patient or of the person in-charge of the patient if the patient is not in a position to give consent before adopting a given procedure. So long as it can be found that the procedure which was in fact adopted was one which was acceptable to medical science as on that date, the medical practitioner cannot be held negligent merely because he chose to follow one procedure and not another and the result was a failure" **[Jacob Mathew v. State of Punjab & Anr. 2005 (3) CPR 70]**.

DEFENSE ARGUMENT NO. 11

"I treated the patient in emergent situations and am likely to make errors. The standard expected from any medical practitioner in an emergency are always lower than the standards expected from him in an ideal setting is the law."

"The higher the acuteness in an emergency and the higher the complication, the more are the chances of error of judgment. At times, the professional is confronted with making a choice between the devil and the deep sea and has to choose the lesser evil. The doctor is often called upon to adopt a procedure which involves higher element of risk, but which he honestly believes as providing greater chances of success for the patient rather than a procedure involving lesser risk but higher chances of failure. Which course is more appropriate to follow, would depend on the facts and circumstances of a given case but a doctor cannot be penalized if he adopts the former procedure, even if it results in a failure. The usual practice prevalent nowadays is to obtain the consent of the patient or of the person in-charge of the patient if the patient is not in a position to give consent before adopting a given procedure (45)" **[Martin F. D'Souza versus Mohd. Ishfaq, 2009 (3) SCC 1]**.

DEFENSE ARGUMENT NO. 12

"The death did not occur due to negligence but was due to the consequence of ailments suffered. Because the patient died, it does not necessarily mean negligence."

"It must be remembered that sometimes despite their best efforts the treatment of a doctor fails. For instance, sometimes despite the best effort of a surgeon, the patient dies. That does not mean that the doctor or the surgeon must be held to be guilty of medical negligence, unless there is some strong evidence to suggest that he is (para 124)" **[Martin F. D'Souza versus Mohd. Ishfaq, 2009(3) SCC 1]**.

DEFENSE ARGUMENT NO. 13

"The respondent has come to the Council or Commission with unclean hands: (i) Deliberate nondisclosure of relevant information (suppressio veri) and (ii) Deliberately resorting to falsehood to obtain a favorable order (suggestio falsi)."

"Dismissal of frivolous or vexatious complaints - Where a complaint instituted before the District Forum, the State Commission or, as the case may be, the National Commission is found to be frivolous or vexatious, it shall, for reasons to be recorded in writing, dismiss the complaint and make an order that the complainant shall pay to the opposite party such cost, not exceeding ten thousand rupees, as may be specified in the order" (Section 26 of the Consumer Protection Act was amended by the Amendment Act of 1993 w.e.f. 18-6-1993.

"A litigant, who approaches the court, is bound to produce all the documents executed by him which are relevant to the litigation if he withholds a vital document in order to gain advantage on the other side than he would be guilty of playing fraud on the court as well as on the opposite party (para 8)" **[SP Chengalvaraya Naidu (dead) by LRs Appellants versus Jagannath (dead) by LRs and Ors. AIR, 1994 SC 853]**.

DEFENSE ARGUMENT NO. 14

"The law does not require professionals to give guarantee and warranty with respect to the end results of their services. I never gave any assurance or a guarantee to the patient/family about the treatment outcome."

"Negligence by professionals: In the law of negligence, professionals such as lawyers, doctors, architects and others are included in the category of persons professing some special skill or skilled persons generally. Any task which is required to be performed with a special skill would generally be admitted or undertaken to be performed only if the person possesses the requisite skill for performing that task. Any reasonable man entering into a profession which requires a particular level of learning to be called a professional of that branch, impliedly assures the person dealing with him that the skill which he professes to possess shall be exercised and exercised with reasonable degree of care and caution. He does not assure his client of the result. A lawyer does not tell his client that the client shall win the case in all circumstances. A physician would not assure the patient of full recovery in every case. A surgeon cannot and does not guarantee that the result of surgery would invariably be beneficial, much less to the extent of 100% for the person operated on. The only assurance which such a professional can give or can be understood to have given by implication is that he is possessed of the requisite skill in that branch of profession which he is practicing and while undertaking the performance of the task entrusted to him he would be exercising his skill with reasonable competence. This is all what the person approaching the professional can expect (para 20)" **[Jacob Mathew versus State of Punjab & Anr, 2005 (3) CPR 70]**.

DEFENSE ARGUMENT NO. 15

"No medical treatment or surgical operation is risk free."

"Some relevant decisions on the issue of medical negligence: It is to be accepted that every surgical operation involves risk. When a person who is ill and is going to be treated in a hospital no matter what care is taken, there always exists some risk. Simply because a mishap had occurred, neither the hospital nor the doctors cannot be made liable. A doctor is not guilty of negligence if he has acted in accordance with the practice accepted as proper by a responsible body of medical men skilled in that particular art. A doctor or a hospital is expected to take reasonable care in administration of the treatment. They cannot be condemned in case of misadventure.

It is also to be remembered that medical negligence is a complicated subject and the liability of doctor always depends upon the circumstances of a particular case.

Hence, in view of the aforesaid discussion and the law on the subject as the doctors have performed their duties to the best of their ability and with due care and caution, it cannot be held that there is deficiency in service. Admittedly, the deceased was a high-risk case and such accidental eventuality cannot be controlled or avoided. Further, as stated above, every surgical operation is attended by risk. And, therefore, simply because something goes wrong, conclusion of deficiency cannot be drawn" **[Mrs Shantaben Muljibhai Patel and Ors. versus Breach Candy Hospital and Research Centre and Ors, I (2005) CPJ 10]**.

DEFENSE ARGUMENT NO. 16

"Standard of care is the care, which the law expects from a doctor. Law does not expect the highest standard nor does it expect low standards. The standard of care expected is the standard of any reasonable medical practitioner. Circumstances in which a medical practitioner is placed always determines the standard expected from him. I have treated the patient with the best of my skill and knowledge."

"The medical professional is expected to bring a reasonable degree of skill and knowledge and must exercise a reasonable degree of care. Neither the very highest nor a very low degree of care and competence judged in the light of the particular circumstances of each case is what the law requires (iii).

A medical practitioner would be liable only where his conduct fell below that of the standards of a reasonably competent practitioner in his field (iv)" **[Kusum Sharma & Others versus Batra Hospital & Medical Research Centre, 2010 (3) SCC 480]**.

DEFENSE ARGUMENT NO. 17

"Whatever treatment I gave was the right thing to do; done by the right technique; done by the right person; done in the right place; done with all care and caution and an informed consent was taken which also included all the possible complications. Such an accident and/or complication is well-described in literature and can occur in spite of best of care."

Section 80 of the Indian Penal Code (IPC) has defined the word "accident". It states as follows: "Nothing is an offence which is done by accident or misfortune and without any criminal intention or knowledge in the doing of a lawful act in a lawful manner by lawful means and with proper care and caution".

"...At times, the professional is confronted with making a choice between the devil and the deep sea and he has to choose the lesser evil. The medical professional is often called upon to adopt a procedure which involves higher element of risk, but which he honestly believes as providing greater chances of success for the patient rather than a procedure involving lesser risk but higher chances of failure. Which course is more appropriate to follow, would depend on the facts and circumstances of a given case. The usual practice prevalent now-a-days is to obtain the consent of the patient or of the person in-charge of the patient if the patient is not be in a position to give consent before adopting a given procedure. So long as it can be found that the procedure which was in fact adopted was one which was acceptable to medical science as on that date, the medical practitioner cannot be held negligent merely because he chose to follow one procedure and not another and the result was a failure (para 27)."

No sensible professional would intentionally commit an act or omission which would result in loss or injury to the patient as the professional reputation of the person is at stake. A single failure may cost him dear in his career. Simply, because a patient has not favorably responded to a treatment given by a physician or a surgery has failed, the doctor cannot be held liable per se by applying the doctrine of *res ipsa loquitur* (para 28)" **[Jacob Mathew versus State of Punjab & Anr., 2005 (3) CPR 70]**.

DEFENSE ARGUMENT NO. 18

"I acted as per standard practice."

"While a doctor cannot be forced to treat any person, he or she has certain responsibilities for those whom he/she accepts as patients. Some of these responsibilities may be recapitulated, in brief:

- To continue to treat, except under certain circumstances when doctor can abandon his patient
- To take reasonable care of his patient
- To exhibit reasonable skill: The degree of skill a doctor undertakes is the average degree of skill possessed by his professional brethren of the same standing as himself. The best form of treatment may differ when different choices are available" **(PB Desai versus State of Maharashtra, AIR 2014 SC 795)**.

DEFENSE ARGUMENT NO. 19

"Just because things have gone wrong, it does not mean medical negligence."

"49. When a patient dies or suffers some mishap, there is a tendency to blame the doctor for this. Things have gone wrong and, therefore, somebody must be punished for it. However, it is well known that even the best professionals, what to say of the average professional, sometimes have failures. A lawyer cannot win every case in his professional career but surely he cannot be penalized for losing a case provided he appeared in it and made his submissions.

76. The basic principle relating to the law of medical negligence is the Bolam Rule which has been quoted above. The test in fixing negligence is the standard of the ordinary skilled doctor exercising and professing to have that special skill, but a doctor need not possess the highest expert skill" **[Martin F. D'Souza versus Mohd. Ishfaq, 2009 (3) SCC 1]**.

DEFENSE ARGUMENT NO. 20

"It was a complicated case and in such a situation, the doctor must get the benefit of doubt."

"The skill of medical practitioners differs from doctor to doctor. The very nature of the profession is such that there may be more than one course of treatment which may be advisable for treating a patient. Courts would indeed be slow in attributing negligence on the part of a doctor if he has performed his duties to the best of his ability and with due care and caution. Medical opinion may differ with regard to the course of action to be taken by a doctor treating a patient, but as long as a doctor acts in a manner which is acceptable to the medical profession, and the court finds that he has attended on the patient with due care skill and diligence and if the patient still does not survive or suffers a permanent ailment, it would be difficult to hold the doctor to be guilty of negligence" **[Achutrao Haribhau Khodwa versus State of Maharashtra, 1996 SCC (2) 634]**.

DEFENSE ARGUMENT NO. 21

"I observed all the precautions and adhered to all guidelines, which had also been verified by an expert I had consulted with as mentioned in the judgment of the Supreme Court in Martin D'Souza versus Mohd Ishfaq case."

The Supreme Court of India has laid down guidelines regarding precautions taken by doctors and hospitals in **Martin F. D'Souza versus Mohd. Ishfaq, 2009 (3) SCC 1** as follows:

- Current practices, infrastructure, paramedical, and other staff, hygiene and sterility should be observed strictly
- No prescription should ordinarily be given without actual examination. The tendency to give prescription over the telephone, except in an acute emergency, should be avoided
- A doctor should not merely go by the version of the patient regarding his symptoms, but should also make his own analysis including tests and investigations where necessary
- A doctor should not experiment unless necessary and even then he should ordinarily get a written consent from the patient
- An expert should be consulted in case of any doubt.

DEFENSE ARGUMENT NO. 22

"I cannot be liable for a service, which was not available in the hospital."

"We must bear in mind that negligence is attributed when existing facilities are not availed of. Medical negligence cannot be attributed for not rendering a facility which was not available. In our opinion, if hospitals knowingly fail to provide some amenities that are fundamental for the patients, it would certainly amount to medical malpractice. As it has been held in Smt Savita Garg (supra), that a hospital not having basic facilities like oxygen cylinders would not be excusable. Therein, this court has opined that even the so-called humanitarian approach of the hospital authorities in no way can be considered to be a factor in denying the compensation for mental agony suffered by the parents. The aforementioned principle applies to this case also in so far as it answers the contentions raised before us that the three senior doctors did not charge any professional fees" **[Malay Kumar Ganguly versus Sukumar Mukherjee & Ors. AIR, 2010 SC 1162]**.

DEFENSE ARGUMENT NO. 23

"I did not waive off the fee as the same was my right to charge."

"Where services are provided against charges including the charges for consumables, charges for ward, service charges, etc. by the government hospitals/health centers/ dispensaries, these services fall within the ambit of service for the purpose of section 2(1)(o) of the Act and the patient availing such service falls within the definition of consumer as defined by section 2(1)(d) of the Act. It is immaterial whether these charges are not charged from poor sections. If such charges are charged from any other patient, poor patients can avail the benefit as a consumer (iii) (26)" **[ESI Hospital versus Amresh Kumar dated 15-03-2007]**.

DEFENSE ARGUMENT NO. 24

"I did nothing that overruled the manufacturer's instructions. The dose prescribed by me was as recommended by the manufacturer."

A doctor may be liable for medical negligence if he/she fails to properly adhere to the instructions of the manufacturer given on the package of the medicine (or any medical equipment) including dosage and administration.

"The necessity of following the instructions given in the packet insert cannot be underestimated. Admittedly, the instructions in the said packet insert had not been followed in the instant case. EFFECT OF EXCESS DOSAGE There is, thus, a near unanimity that the doses of glucocorticosteroid and in particular Depomedrol were excessive. From the prescription of Dr Mukherjee, it is evident that he not only prescribed Depomedrol injection twice daily, but had also prescribed Wysolone which is also a steroid having the composition of Methyl Predinosolone.

We enumerate heretobelow the duty of care which ought to have been taken and the deficiency whereof is being complained of in the criminal case and the civil case, respectively, so far as respondent Nos. 1 to 3 are concerned.

When Dr Mukherjee examined Anuradha, she had rashes all over her body and this being the case of dermatology, he should have referred her to a dermatologist. Instead, he prescribed "Depomedrol" for the next 3 days on his assumption that it was a case of "vasculitis". The dosage of 120 mg Depomedrol per day is certainly a higher dose in case of a TEN Patient or for that matter any patient suffering from any other bypass of skin disease and the maximum recommended usage by the drug manufacturer has also been exceeded by Dr Mukherjee. On 11th May, 1998, the further prescription of Depomedrol without diagnosing the nature of the disease is a wrongful act on his part." **[Malay Kumar Ganguly versus Sukumar Mukherjee & Ors. AIR, 2010 SC 1162]**.

DEFENSE ARGUMENT NO. 25

"It is not a case of gross mistake."

"Adoption of one of the modes of treatment, if there are many, and treating the patient with due care and caution would not constitute any negligence (iii).

Failure to act in accordance with the standard, reasonable, and competent medical means at the time would not constitute a negligence. However, a medical practitioner must exercise the reasonable degree of care and skill and knowledge which he possesses. Failure to use due skill in diagnosis with the result that wrong treatment is given would be negligence (iv).

In a complicated case, the court would be slow in contributing negligence on the part of the doctor, if he is performing his duties to be best of his ability (v).

Bearing in mind the aforementioned principles, the individual liability of the doctors and hospital must be judged. **[Malay Kumar Ganguly versus Sukumar Mukherjee & Ors. AIR, 2010 SC 1162]**.

DEFENSE ARGUMENT NO. 26

"My junior was also competent."

"Gross medical mistake will always result in a finding of negligence. Use of wrong drug or wrong gas during the course of anesthetic will frequently lead to the imposition of liability and in some situations even the principle of *res ipsa loquitur* can be applied. Even delegation of responsibility to another may amount to negligence in certain circumstances. A consultant could be negligent where he delegates the responsibility to his junior with the knowledge that the junior was incapable of performing of his duties properly" **[Spring Meadows Hospital versus Harjol Ahluwalia, (1998) 4 SCC 39]**.

CONCLUSION

Facing a malpractice complaint is a serious matter for a physician because of the implications on their professional reputation as competent doctors. In medical colleges, doctors are taught clinical skills and not legal skills. Going through the process of defending a complaint therefore can be unnerving for them as they are ill-prepared and ill-equipped to handle such a situation. Being ignorant of the law can now be no more an excuse. While the best way to defend oneself in such situations is maintaining meticulous case records, knowledge about Court decisions supported by high-quality published evidence will also help shape the defense strategy. This can challenge even an expert opinion. Hence, all doctors should be vigilant about protecting themselves and read the judgements delivered by Courts in medical malpractice claims. Its time they become well-versed with the nuances of law as it applies to clinical practice.

CHAPTER 154

Sports and Heart Diseases

Kewal C Goswami, Vikash Kumar, Nagendra Boopathy Senguttuvan

INTRODUCTION

Athletes are the epitome of health, owing to their unique lifestyle and physical achievements. Numerous physiological changes occur in the heart, autonomic system, musculoskeleton, etc., when individuals perform repetitive activity and this enhances endurance and fitness. However, in a small proportion of individuals sports has been associated with sudden cardiac death (SCD) due to unmasking of silent cardiovascular (CV) abnormalities. In others it may lead to brady and tachyarrhythmias as well as structural changes that may be constituted as abnormal. In adult athletes, even recreational sports has been associated with sudden death due to coronary artery disease.

For this reason it is important for cardiologists to have a thorough knowledge of exercise physiology, benefits and risks of exercise, and adaptation of heart to exercise training as they are often confronted by athletes for advice on exercise, decide whether abnormal symptoms or findings in athletes represent disease or a physiologic response to exercise training.

DEFINITION OF TERMS

Athlete

While there are many definitions for an athlete, an athlete, in layman's terms is an individual proficient in a particular exercise, game, or sport that enhances strength, stamina, or endurance as well as participates in competitive sports. In order to have a uniform definition for medical professionals, an athlete is defined as a person who trains in sports to enhance his/her performance, participates in competitive events, is formally enrolled in a program (local/national), and spends most of his/her time in sports often making it a way of life.[1] All of these criteria must be met to define an athlete. The limitation of this definition is that it would necessarily exclude the recreational athlete who may achieve nearly the same level of fitness, stamina, and endurance, but would not be included as he would not meet the remaining criteria However, for clinical purposes his CV physiology would mimic that of a well-trained athlete. A young athlete is generally considered to be below 35 years of age while an adult athlete is anyone older.

Physical Activity

Physical activity refers literally to any body movement producing substantial increase in oxygen consumption. Physical activity designed to improve health or obtain performance benefits is called exercise.

TYPES OF EXERCISE

Exercise requiring increase in oxygen transport is called endurance or aerobic exercise, whereas exercise primarily stressing skeletal muscle is called strength or resistance exercise. Endurance or aerobic exercise helps improve overall stamina and the ability of the heart to pump oxygenated blood in those with and without prior CV disease. Strength or resistance exercise increases the muscle strength.

CARDIOVASCULAR RESPONSE TO EXERCISE

Aerobic or endurance exercise imposes a volume overload state on the CV system that affects all the four chambers of the heart. In response to aerobic exercise, the body reacts by increased oxygen uptake (VO_2), heart rate (HR), and cardiac output (Q). There will also be an initial peak and then plateau in stroke volume (SV). Each 1 liter increase in oxygen consumption causes increase in cardiac output by 5–6 liters.[2] Systolic blood pressure (SBP) progressively increases along with a drop in peripheral vascular resistance resulting in decreased diastolic blood pressure and the result is widened pulse pressure and a mild increase in mean pressure. Active exercising muscle selectively gets more blood, bypassing the less active ones. Arteriovenous oxygen difference (A-VO_2)

widens as the duration of exercise increases due to more and more oxygen being extracted by the exercising muscle.

If the exercise performed statically or isometrically, the contraction of muscles occurs in a fixed or stationary position (i.e., without movement). There are several daily activities which incorporate a static component, as do many sports (e.g., rowing, cycling, weightlifting, and wrestling). Most important difference in the CV response to static compared with dynamic exercise resides in its effect on the active muscle blood flow.

During an isometric contraction, there is a decrease in muscle blood flow in response to the stiffening of active muscle fibers, which increases intramuscular pressure causing a mechanical constriction of the vessels. Though a similar constriction occurs during dynamic exercise, there is rhythmic alternation between contraction and relaxation, such as in running which encourages blood flow through the muscle pump.

Intense and prolonged endurance exercise training produces wide spectrum of CV adaptations, resulting in a condition referred to as "athlete's heart".[3] Such changes include an increase in resting SV and a decrease in resting HR. Reduced HR in athletes is likely due to increased vagal tone and decreased sympathetic tone. Bradyarrhythmias that might be observed in athletes include significant sinus arrhythmia, first-degree heart block, second-degree atrioventricular (AV) block (type-1), or very rarely third-degree AV block during sleep. Such reduced AV conduction may unmask conduction through accessory pathways. One of the frequently observed patterns in athletes is early repolarization variant, which is also likely attributed to increased vagal tone.[4]

BENEFITS OF EXERCISE

Multiple cross-sectional studies examining the frequency of CV events in healthy individuals demonstrate that the more active participants have lower CV risk than their more sedentary counterparts.[5] The reduction in risk in the most active versus the least active individuals is approximately 40%.[5] It has recently shown that exercise causes mortality reduction in patients. The quantity of benefit is higher in high-risk patients. Beneficial effects of exercise attain a plateau at 9.1 hours of exercise per week.[5] After this level of exertion, there appears to be little additional benefit and, possibly diminution, of the beneficial effects.[5] Habitual physical activity has multiple, potentially beneficial affects on atherosclerotic risk factors. Specifically, habitual physical activity reduces SBP, body weight, blood glucose, and triglycerides and increases high-density lipoprotein cholesterol.[6]

RISKS OF EXERCISE

Evidence has shown that vigorous physical activity, generally defined as greater than six metabolic equivalents (METS) transiently increases the risk for SCD and acute myocardial infarction (AMI).[7,8] The pathologic substrate associated with these acute cardiac events varies by age, primarily because the prevalence of the pathologic cardiac conditions responsible for SCD also varies by age (Box 1).

Most of the exercise related SCD in young individuals has been attributed to congenital and inherited conditions, including hypertrophic cardiomyopathy (HCM) and anomalous coronary artery (ACA), although acquired conditions such as pericarditis, myocarditis, and cardiomyopathy can also cause exercise-related SCD in young individuals.[9]

However, recent studies have noted that up to 40% of SCDs in young athletes remain unexplained even after an autopsy suggesting that other conditions, such as inherited channelopathies, may be the cause.[10] HCM was responsible only for 6% of the deaths.[10]

Atherosclerotic cardiovascular disease (ASCVD) causes most exercise-related AMI and SCD in adults.[7] AMI occurring in a previously asymptomatic adult during exercise is usually associated with acute coronary arterial plaque disruption.[11] Higher flexing and more bending of coronary arteries might be associated with plaque rupture leading to AMI after exercise.[7] Approximately 33% of SCDs in adults caused by ASCVD are associated with clinical and pathologic findings of an acute coronary syndrome (ACS), whereas the remainder show evidence of nonacute ASCVD.[12]

CLINICAL PROBLEMS IN SPORTS CARDIOLOGY

Decreased Exercise Capacity

Exercise capacity is defined as the maximum amount of physical exertion that an athlete can sustain. Athletes who have decreased exercise capacity are frequently referred to cardiologists for evaluation. Unlike cardiac output which

BOX 1 Common cardiovascular conditions associated with sudden death in athletes

- HCM
- Congenital coronary anomalies
- Genetic channelopathies (Brugada, early repolarization syndrome, LQTS, SQTS, CPVT)
- Blunt trauma
- Commotio cordis
- Coronary artery disease
- ARVC
- Myocarditis
- Bicuspid aortic valve with stenosis or dilated aortic root
- WPW syndrome
- Heat stroke

ARVC, arrhythmogenic right ventricular cardiomyopathy; CPVT, catecholaminergic polymorphic ventricular tachyarrhythmias; HCM, hypertrophic cardiomyopathy; LQTS, long QT syndrome; SQTS, short QT syndrome; WPW, Wolff-Parkinson-White.

is critically dependent on SV, maximum oxygen uptake (VO_2max) requires HR and A-VO_2 difference other than SV. It is also dependent on signals from the central nervous system, skeletal muscle, and lungs. Decrements in any of these components can compromise exercise performance. Conditions resulting in inappropriately fast HR at low levels of exertion such as hyperthyroidism can decrease exercise performance, as can exercise-induced asthma, diseases of skeletal muscle, and reduced O_2-carrying capacity from anemia. Atrial fibrillation or frequent premature contractions during exercise can reduce exercise capacity.

These same issues can reduce exercise performance in older athletes, but occult coronary disease with atypical symptoms always requires consideration first in older patients. Psychological factors and overtraining also can cause decreased exercise capacity in athletes.

Unlike regular patients, athletes are very sensitive to their performance-related symptoms. A careful history-taking will reveal history of decreased underperformance in athletes. As compared to general public, the attributable risk of health-related problems in athletes for a given problem is high as they do high METs requiring exercise. Exercise echocardiography and oxygen pulse curve obtained from cardiopulmonary exercise testing are very useful measures in assessing their symptoms.

Arrhythmic issues in athletes can be addressed by long-term implantable loop recorders. Once all possible workup are done and have been found to be normal, psychological or emotional issues or overtraining in athletes need to be considered.

Cardiac Complaints in Athletes

It is common to see athletes underplaying and overplaying their symptoms. As they are very sensitive to their performance, most of the diseases could be diagnosed early in them, but sometimes their presentation might be fatal.

Chest pain is a common complaint seen in young and old athletes and should not be dismissed callously. Exertional chest pain may be the first sign of important cardiac diseases, including HCM, aortic stenosis, ACA, or coronary artery atherosclerosis. Very momentary chest pain might be due to ectopic atrial or ventricular beats. Few athletes who have died with ACA had normal exercise stress test results,[13] indicating the importance of pursuing workups that include coronary imaging in athletes if the symptoms are worrisome, even when exercise testing yields normal results.

Due to resting bradycardia and large venous capacity which permits sequestration of large quantity of blood, well-trained athletes often have vasovagal syncope, also known as "neurally-mediated syncope" when the athlete is upright and motionless.[14]

Athletes also often have positive tilt table tests as a result of the same physiologic changes. Neurally-mediated syncope most often occurs in athletes immediately following exercise, particularly with abrupt termination of exercise. This common entity called as "postexertional syncope", is benign and can frequently be managed by teaching the athlete avoidance techniques. The most important avoidance technique advised to the athlete is to keep moving after effort and to gradually slow down so that the muscle pump in the calf continues to return blood to the systemic circulation.

The key issue that needs to be evaluated for syncope in athletes is to determine whether the syncope occurred during exertion. Syncope at rest or immediately after exercise under conditions consistent with vasovagal syncope or postural syncope is usually benign. In contrast, syncope during exercise should prompt a careful search for more serious problems, including HCM, aortic stenosis, cardiac arrhythmia, or ACA.

Atrial fibrillation is now being described in long distance runners, cross country cyclists, and skiers.[15] Why such athletes are prone to atrial fibrillation as well as atrial flutter is still unclear, but an association is increasingly being recognized. Autonomic changes, cardiac remodeling, atrial ectopy, gastroesophageal reflux, food supplements, anabolic steroids, and other mechanisms are variously believed to be responsible for these arrhythmias.

SCREENING ABNORMALITIES

Both the American Heart Association (AHA) and the American College of Cardiology (ACC),[16] as well as the European Society of Cardiology (ESC),[17] recommend preparticipation screening (PPS) for athletes. The ESC also recommends a resting electrocardiogram (ECG) as a part of PPS, which is not recommended by AHA.

Regardless of the benefit, most of the athletes undergo screening with an ECG, and abnormalities are seen. Screening athletes with or without an ECG can detect a multitude of CV "problems."

Athletes can also have ECG evidence of biatrial hypertrophy, left ventricular hypertrophy (LVH),[18] incomplete or complete right bundle branch block (RBBB), ST-T wave abnormalities, and conduction abnormalities (Tables 1 and 2, Box 2). Most of these abnormalities occur in endurance athletes undergoing intense training. Such changes in strength-trained athletes or in endurance athletes with low training volumes should raise suspicion of a cardiac problem.

Most of the CV abnormalities found on screening may be normal, and can be dismissed by a simple clinical examination and review of the ECG or with cardiac imaging procedures to remove any doubt. Even then some athletes and families may have on going concern once a screening abnormality is identified. So it is advisable to make them return in 3–6 months even when no abnormalities are found, to provide them with additional reassurance.

Common problem that will be found in athletes with a screening abnormality is diagnostic creep which can be defined as the finding of a minor abnormality on screening such as early repolarization, sinus bradycardia or incomplete RBBB which may prompt for a second diagnostic test such as echocardiography, which reveals another borderline finding such as mild LVH, which may prompt for another diagnostic test like cardiac magnetic resonance imaging (MRI).

Sometimes, because of the extensive CV adaptations that may occur due to exercise training, each diagnostic study

TABLE 1: Classification of abnormalities of the athlete's electrocardiogram[17]

Group 1: Common and training-related ECG changes	Group 2: Uncommon and training-unrelated ECG changes
• Sinus bradycardia • First-degree AV block • Incomplete RBBB • Early repolarization • Isolated QRS voltage criteria for left ventricular hypertrophy	• T wave inversion • ST segment depression • Pathological Q waves • Left atrial enlargement • Left axis deviation/left anterior hemiblock • Right axis deviation/left posterior hemiblock • Right ventricular hypertrophy • Ventricular pre-excitation • Complete LBBB or RBBB • Long or short QT interval • Brugada-like early repolarization

AV, atrioventricular; LBBB, left bundle branch block; RBBB, right bundle branch block.

TABLE 2: Seattle criteria: Abnormal findings in athletes[19]

Abnormal ECG	Definition
T-wave inversion	>1 mm in depth in two or more leads V2–V6, II and aVF, or I and aVL (excludes III, aVR, and V1)
ST segment depression	≥0.5 mm in depth in two or more leads
Pathological Q waves	>3 mm in depth or >40 ms in duration in two or more leads (except for III and aVR)
Complete left bundle branch block	QRS ≥120 ms, predominantly negative QRS complex in lead V1 (QS or rS), and upright monophasic R wave in leads I and V6
Intraventricular conduction delay	Any QRS duration ≥140 ms
Left axis deviation	−30–90°
Left atrial enlargement	Prolonged P wave duration of >120 ms in leads I or II with negative portion of the P wave ≥1 mm in depth and ≥40 ms in duration in lead V1
Right ventricular hypertrophy pattern	R–V1+S–V5 >10.5 mm and right axis deviation >120°
Ventricular pre-excitation	PR interval <120 ms with a delta wave (slurred upstroke in the QRS complex) and wide QRS (>120 ms)
Long QT interval	QTc ≥470 ms (male) QTc ≥480 ms (female) QTc ≥500 ms (marked QT prolongation)
Short QT interval	QTc ≤320 ms
Brugada-like ECG pattern	High take-off and downsloping ST segment elevation followed by a negative T wave in ≥2 leads in V1–V3
Profound sinus bradycardia	<30 beats per minute or sinus pauses ≥3 s
Atrial tachyarrhythmias	Supraventricular tachycardia, atrial fibrillation, atrial flutter
Premature ventricular contractions (PVCs)	≥2 PVCs per 10 s tracing
Ventricular arrhythmias	Couplets, triplets and non-sustained ventricular tachycardia

BOX 2 Seattle criteria: Normal ECG variants in athletes[19]

- Sinus bradycardia (≥30 beats/min)
- Sinus arrhythmia
- Ectopic atrial rhythm
- Junctional escape rhythm
- 1° AV block (PR interval >200 ms)
- Mobitz type 1 (Wenckebach) 2° AV block
- Incomplete RBBB
- Isolated QRS voltage for LVH

Except: QRS voltage criteria for LVH occurring with any nonvoltage criteria for LVH such as left atrial enlargement, left axis deviation, ST segment depression, T-wave inversion, or pathological Q waves

- Early repolarization (ST elevation, J-point elevation, J-waves, or terminal QRS slurring)
- Convex ("domed") ST segment elevation combined with T-wave inversion in leads V1–V4 in Black/African athletes.

AV, atrioventricular; ECG, electrocardiogram; LVH, left ventricular hypertrophy; RBBB, right bundle branch block.

reveals an additional borderline abnormality, which will make it difficult for a clinician to declare the athlete is fit.

Hence, it is advisable to judge the screening abnormalities with less concern, especially if they are borderline abnormal than definite abnormalities that are seen in symptomatic athletes, because those screening abnormalities will mostly represent normal variants.

It must be recognized that some athletes are more likely to express extreme hypertrophy when they engage in intensive training programs. In these athletes left ventricular wall thickness may reach 16 mm in males. To distinguish this from HCM ECG, echo and tissue Doppler criteria have been evolved along with use of MRI.

Preparticipation Screening for Eligibility

In light of beneficial effects of screening first documented from Italy,[20] the ESC made it mandatory to undergo national PPS strategy with routine ECGs.[13] The International Olympic Committee (IOC) also recommends PPS with routine ECGs.

American Heart Association is conservative regarding usage of ECGs as a routine part of screening mainly due to cost-effectiveness and beneficial effects. It recommends thorough personal, family, and physical examination comprising of 14 elements as a part of PPS (Box 3).

The AHA and ACC had also developed eligibility and disqualification recommendations for cardiac conditions according with the advice of 15 task forces who created the guidelines based on the type of sports that the athlete is involved.[15] These guidelines may appear restrictive, but at present these are the best available resource to guide the athlete regarding the risk involved with sports participation.

The conditions for which eligibility and disqualification are advised are HCM, myocarditis, pericarditis, arrhythmogenic right ventricular cardiomyopathy, left ventricular noncompaction, congenital heart diseases, hypertension, valvular heart disease, ASCVD, arrhythmias, etc.

BOX 3 The 14 elements American Heart Association (AHA) recommendations for preparticipation cardiovascular screening of competitive athletes

Medical history

- Personal history
  - Chest pain/discomfort/tightness/pressure related to exertion
  - Unexplained syncope/near-syncope
  - Excessive and unexplained dyspnea/fatigue or palpitations, associated with exercise
  - Prior recognition of a heart murmur
  - Elevated systemic blood pressure
  - Prior restriction from participation in sports
  - Prior testing for the heart, ordered by a physician
- Family history
  - Premature death (sudden and unexpected, or otherwise) before 50 years of age attributable to heart disease in ≥1 relative
  - Disability from heart disease in close relative <50 years of age
  - Hypertrophic or dilated cardiomyopathy, long QT syndrome, or other ion channelopathies, Marfan syndrome, or clinically significant arrhythmias; specific knowledge of genetic cardiac conditions in family members
- Physical examination
  - Heart murmur
  - Femoral pulses to exclude aortic coarctation
  - Physical stigmata of Marfan syndrome
  - Brachial artery blood pressure (sitting positions)

CONCLUSION

Even though sports cardiology is evolving as a subspecialty of cardiology, general cardiologists should have a working knowledge of exercise physiology, the cardiovascular adaptations to exercise training, and also the risks and benefits of exercise to advise and evaluate athletes appropriately.

REFERENCES

1. Araujo CG, Scharhag J. Athlete: a working definition for medical and health sciences research. Scand J. Med Sci Sport. 2016;26:4-7.
2. Sue DY, Hansen JE. Normal values in adults during exercise testing. Clin Chest Med. 1984;5:89.
3. La Gerche A, Taylor AJ, Prior DL. Athlete's heart : the potential for multimodality imaging to address the critical remaining questions. JACC Cardiovasc Imaging. 2009;2(3):350-63.
4. Prior DL, La Gerche A. The athlete's heart. Heart. 2012;98(12):947-55
5. Joyner MJ, Green DJ. Exercise protects the cardiovascular system: effects beyond traditional risk factors. J Physiol. 2009;587:5551.
6. Hambrecht R, Wolf A, Gielen S, et al. Effect of exercise on coronary endothelial function in patients with coronary artery disease. N Engl J Med. 2000;342:454.
7. Siscovick DS, Weiss NS, Fletcher RH, et al. The incidence of primary cardiac arrest during vigorous exercise. N Engl J Med. 1984;311(14):874-7.
8. Maron BJ, Thompson PD, Ackerman MJ, et al. Recommendations and considerations related to preparticipation screening for cardiovascular abnormalities in competitive athletes: 2007 update: a scientific statement from the American Heart Association Council on Nutrition, Physical Activity, and Metabolism: endorsed by the American College of Cardiology Foundation. Circulation. 2007;115:1643-55.
9. Maron BJ, Thompson PD, Puffer JC, et al. Cardiovascular preparticipation screening of competitive athletes. A statement for health professionals from the Sudden Death Committee (clinical cardiology) and Congenital Cardiac Defects Committee (cardiovascular disease in the young), American Heart Association. Circulation. 1996;94:850-6.
10. Corrado D, Basso C, Schiavon M, et al. Screening for hypertrophic cardiomyopathy in young athletes. N Engl J Med. 1998;339:364-9.
11. Maron BJ, Shirani J, Poliac LC, et al. Sudden death in young competitive athletes. Clinical, demographic, and pathological profiles. JAMA. 1996;276:199-204.
12. Corrado D, Basso C, Pavei A, et al. Trends in sudden cardiovascular death in young competitive athletes after implementation of a preparticipation screening program. JAMA. 2006;296:1593-601.
13. Harmon KG, Zigman M, Drezner JA. The effectiveness of screening history, physical exam, and ECG to detect potentially lethal cardiac disorders in athletes: a systematic review/meta-analysis. J Electrocardiol. 2015;48:329-38.
14. O'Connor FG, Levine B. Syncope in athletes of cardiac origin: 2B. From personal history and physical examination sections. Curr Sports Med Rep. 2015;14:254-6.
15. Turagam Mohit K, Velagapudi Poonam, Kocheril Abraham G. Atrial fibrillation in athletes. Am J Cardiol. 2012;109(2):296-302.

16. Maron BJ, Levine BD, Washington RL, et al. Eligibility and disqualification recommendations for competitive athletes with cardiovascular abnormalities: Task force 2: Preparticipation screening for cardiovascular disease in competitive athletes: A scientific statement from the American Heart Association and American College of Cardiology. Circulation. 2015;132(22):e267-72.
17. Mont L, Pelliccia A, Sharma S, et al. Pre-participation cardiovascular evaluation for athletic participants to prevent sudden death: Position paper from the EHRA and the EACPR, branches of the ESC. Endorsed by APHRS, HRS, and SOLAECE. Europace. 2017;19:139-63.
18. Caselli S, Maron MS, Urbano-Moral JA, et al. Differentiating left ventricular hypertrophy in athletes from that in patients with hypertrophic cardiomyopathy. Am J Cardiol. 2014;114:1383-9.
19. Drezner JA, Ackerman MJ, Anderson J, et al. Electrocardiographic interpretation in athletes: the 'Seattle Criteria'. Br J Sports Med. 2013;47:122-4.
20. Pelliccia A, Di Paolo FM, Corrado D, et al. Evidence for efficacy of the Italian national pre-participation screening programme for identification of hypertrophic cardiomyopathy in competitive athletes. Eur Heart J. 2006;27:2196-200.

INDEX

Page numbers followed by *b* refer to box, *f* refer to figure, *fc* refer to flowchart, and *t* refer to table.

A

Abciximab 224, 241, 242, 336, 937
Abdomen 650
  computed tomography of 402
Ablation catheter, tip of 774
Academic research consortium 322
Acebutolol 189
Acetate-free biofiltration 1000
Acetyl CoA carboxylase 596
Acetylcholine 764
Acetylsalicylic acid 307, 311, 315
Achilles heel 809
Acid-base balance, correction of 743
Acidosis 763
  intracellular 786
Acquired immunodeficiency syndrome 700
Activated partial thromboplastin time 883
Activated prothrombin complex concentrate 340
Active muscle fibers, stiffening of 1062
Acute atrial fibrillation, immediate cardioversion of 981
Acute coronary events score, global registry of 236, 282
Acute coronary syndrome 37, 39, 57, 198, 201, 211, 235, 240, 241, 241*t*, 268, 276, 281, 283, 298, 305, 305*f*, 307, 307*t*, 308, 310, 311, 315, 315*t*, 316*f*, 317*f*, 38, 322, 324, 325, 328, 332, 351, 356, 379, 401, 412, 421, 570, 593, 656-658, 674, 721, 747, 749, 831, 926, 960, 1018, 1050, 1062
  assessment 785
  current status 235
  diagnosis of 240
  evaluation 239
  immediate post 749
  management of 243*f*
  risk stratification post 750
Acute heart failure
  different stages of 662
  factors triggering 657*b*
Adenoma, adrenal 139
Adenosine 412
  diphosphate 305, 306, 321, 328, 723
  effects of 615
  triphosphate 183, 187, 221, 321, 559, 723, 833
    activation of 584
Adipose derived regenerative cells 428, 429
Adjunctive reperfusion therapy 306
Adjuvant medical therapy 936
Ado-trastuzumab emtansine 621
Adrenomedullin 999
Adrenoreceptor stimulants 142
Adult cardiac surgery database 841
Advanced cardiac life support 742
  monitoring 784
  pharmacotherapy 784
Advanced echocardiographic techniques 794
Advanced heart failure 664
  therapies 664, 669
  treatment strategies 664
Adventitial cysts 942
Adverse cardiac event 173, 191, 193, 265, 419, 575, 1051
Adverse cardiovascular event 169, 328, 563
Adverse coronary events 413
Adverse drug reactions 612
Aerobic exercise 1061
Agents, newer 666
Air embolism 901
Airway disease, chronic obstructive 631, 821
Alanine aminotransferase 37, 58
Albuminuria 53
Alcohol 8, 9, 700, 1005
  ablation 455
  and cardiovascular disease, genetics of 10
  and coronary artery disease 8
  cardiovascular effects of 9
  consumption 115
    moderate 116
  dehydrogenase 10
  intake, detrimental effects of 11
Aldehyde dehydrogenase-2 10
Aldosterone
  antagonists 606, 635, 638, 639
  receptor antagonists 242
  receptor blockade 644
  secreting adenoma 146
  secretion 923
  synthase inhibitor 590
Aldosteronism, primary 146*t*
Alemtuzumab 621
Alirocumab 595
Allopurinol 182, 586
Alpha-blockers 615
Alpha-linolenic acid 47

Alpha-methyldopa 966, 1048
Alteplase, low-dose 888
Alzheimer's disease 80
Ambulatory blood pressure
  measurement 144*t*
  monitor 137, 143, 153, 160
    device 154
    record 157*f*
American Academy of Sleep Medicine 1008
American and European Hypertension Guidelines 127
American College of Cardiology 32, 74, 103, 120, 123, 124, 154, 181, 230, 282, 338, 664, 665*fc*, 831, 1025, 1063
American College of Cardiology Foundation 86, 383, 923
American College of Cardiology Meeting 391
American College of Chest Physicians 919
American College of Physicians 120
American College of Radiology 176, 919
American Diabetes Association 74, 79, 83
American Diabetes Association classification of diabetes 79*t*
American Heart Association 32, 74, 103, 120, 123, 124, 154, 176, 181, 187, 211, 338, 383, 457, 641, 664, 831, 854, 888, 919, 932, 1025, 1030, 1065, 1065, 1065*b*
  classification 665*fc*
  guideline 282, 923
American Society of Echocardiography 490, 511, 522
  guidelines 503
Aminopeptidase A 590
Aminopeptidase inhibitor 590
Amiodarone 614, 623, 693, 716, 734, 744, 747, 748, 764, 994
  drug interactions of 616*t*
Amiovirt 693
Amisulpride 623
Amitriptyline 623
Amlodipine 182
Amniotic fluid embolism 984
Amphetamine-like drugs 614
Amplatzer cardiac plug 470
Amplatzer muscular ventricular septal defect 465*f*
Amplatzer patent ductus arteriosus 535
Amplatzer septal occluder 465*f*
Amputation 950
Amyloid beta, catabolism of 589
Amyloidosis 577, 700, 1000
Analgesics 622
Anchoring wire 385, 388
Ancillary preoperative cardiac testing 1051
Anderson-Fabry disease 578
Anecdotal data 58
Anecdotal medicine 402
Anemia 142, 281, 636, 645, 878, 973, 1002
  consequences of 1002
  development of 1003*fc*
  epidemiology of 1002
  pathogenesis of 1002
  severe 658
  treatment of 1003
Anesthetic medications 622
Aneurysms 574
Angina 455
  mild 1050
  pectoris 189*t*, 583
  pharmacotherapy for 180, 182
Angiodysplasias 857
Angiogram 928*f*
Angiography 272, 839, 933
  conventional 566, 928
  invasive 175
Angioplasty 145, 925
  catheters 436
  primary 223, 265
Angiopoietin-like proteins inhibitors 598
Angiosome concept 946, 948*f*
Angiotensin 590
Angiotensin-converting enzyme 129, 282, 614, 648, 674, 841, 854, 933, 998, 1044
  inhibitor 125, 127, 129, 137, 143, 180, 181, 187, 242, 252, 606, 615, 618, 635, 636, 643, 661, 665, 690, 691, 698, 733, 791, 924, 961, 968, 974, 985, 1002, 1003, 1048, 1053
Angiotensin-receptor blockers 121, 125-127, 129, 137, 145, 180, 181, 242, 252, 606, 615, 635, 637, 643, 648, 665, 674, 690, 691, 698, 733, 791, 854, 925, 968, 974, 999, 1002, 1003, 1053
Angiotensin-receptor neprilysin inhibitor 628, 632, 637, 643, 644, 690, 691, 806, 854, 986
Ankle
  brachial index, assessment of 943*f*
  swelling 908
Ankle-brachial index 176, 943
Annual sudden cardiac death rate 802*f*
Annular tissue velocities 493*f*
Anomalous coronary artery 1062
Antegrade wiring 393
Anterior thoracotomy, small 837*f*
Anthracycline 620
Anthracycline
  cardiotoxicity 620
  cytotoxic action of 620
Antianginal drugs
  classification of 182*b*
  first-line 182
  second-line 183, 183*t*
Antianginals, newer 583*t*
Antiarrhythmic agent 994
Antiarrhythmic defibrillators 748
Antiarrhythmic drugs 615, 616, 710, 717, 747, 748, 1022
  therapy 710, 711
Antiarrhythmic medication 622, 764

Anticoagulant 139, 282, 601, 615, 616, 980
drugs, mechanism action of 726*f*
patients on long-term 718
therapy 240, 1052
in atrial fibrillation, risk for 706
Anticoagulation 718, 737, 920, 1022
after intracerebral hemorrhage, resuming 882
after ischemic stroke, initiation of 882
duration of 919
failure 919
postoperative 719
therapy 921
long-term 877
type of 919
Antidepressant 699
Antidiabetic therapies 96
Antiepileptic 623
Antifungal 616, 700
medicines 623
Antihyperkalemic drugs, newer 606
Antihypertensive drug 591, 699, 1048
classes of 588
first-line 135
Antihypertensive medications 622
Antihypertensive therapy 152, 934
effect of 933
Anti-inflammatory drugs 636
Anti-ischemic therapy 230
Antimetabolites 621
Antimicrobial medications 764
Antimuscarinics 614
Antioxidant 42, 182
effects 9
phytochemicals 42
vitamins 717
Antiplatelet 241, 336*t*, 612, 737, 945
and anticoagulant agents 728*t*
and anticoagulation treatment 231*t*
doses of 271
drug 615
therapy 311, 337, 706, 933, 934
optimal duration of dual 311
single 338, 340
subsequent dual 317
switching 324
Antiproliferative drug 405
Antipsychotic 614
drugs 699
medications 764
Antiretroviral drugs, cardiac effects of 623
Antisense oligonucleotide 596
Antithrombotic benefit 728
Antithrombotic combinations 729*f*
risk and benefits of 729*t*
Antithrombotic drugs, effect of 339
Antithrombotic effects 9
Antithrombotic medications 86
Antithrombotic therapy 230, 231, 278, 294, 708, 897
Anxiolytics 661
Aorta 449
aortoarteritis of 1034
ascending 450
coarctation of 142, 147, 1034
Aortic aneurysm, abdominal 947
Aortic annulus 450
Aortic arch 938
atheroma 938
disease 896
tortuosity, excessive 926
type II 937
Aortic atherosclerosis 845
Aortic coarctation 139, 942, 1065
Aortic disease, inflammatory 384
Aortic dissection 978
Aortic paravalvular leak closure 466
Aortic pressure 412*f*
Aortic regurgitation 451, 452, 452*f*, 532
significant 856
Aortic root 984
basic anatomy of 449*f*
dilated 985, 1062
Aortic sinus 388*f*
Aortic stenosis 531, 897, 903, 1034, 1050, 1063
quantification of 531
severe 443, 448, 449*f*, 938
Aortic valve 464, 530
disease 142
gradients, elevated 446*f*
interventions 545
replacement 463
surgical 443, 448
Aortic vascular surgery 338
Aortocaval compression 981
Aortocoronary grafts 387
Aortogram 451*f*
abdominal 928*f*
Aorto-ostial
landing zone 387
lesion 384, 386*f*, 388, 388*f*
Aortorenal dissection 923
Apical ballooning syndrome, typical of 516*f*
Apixaban 468, 601, 603, 708, 880, 881, 895
dose of 602
Apnea 1005
hypopnea index 144, 1005
Apolipoprotein B 91, 596, 597
Appropriate cells, selection of 427
Arch atheroma 937

Arginine vasopressin 656, 998
Armodafinil 1009
Arrhythmia 686, 688, 732, 748, 804, 986, 995, 1021, 1065
  atrial 715
  diagnosis 1017, 1022
  malignant 295
  observation of less 800
  perioperative 1053
  perpetuation of 1035
  rapid 658
  significant 1050
Arrhythmogenic right ventricular
  cardiomyopathy 570, 578, 751, 751*b*, 763, 1062, 1065
  dysplasia 577, 756-758, 984
    electrocardiography of 758*f*
Arterial conduits
  spasm of 822
  types of 820
Arterial disease
  prevention of progression of 86
  severe 912
Arterial graft 823, 837, 845
  configurations 826*f*
  disconnection of 822
  multiple 825
  patency of 822
  spasm, prevention of 822
  total 828*f*
Arterial line insertion 294
Arterial oxygen saturation 230
Arterial revascularization 820
  total 819, 837, 839
Arterial stenosis, iliofemoral 1034
Arterial stiffness 15
Arterial ventricular dyssynchrony, correction of 290
Arterial wall 370
  structure 419
Arteriovenous fistula 1034
Arteriovenous oxygen difference 1061
Artery disease
  lower-extremity 314
  peripheral 942*t*
Artery graft, left anterior descending 819
Artery
  hypothesis, open 277
  infarct related 253, 265
  left anterior descending 384, 387, 391, 396, 398, 411, 414, 415, 823, 825*fc*, 826, 846, 847
  size hypothesis 1045*f*
Arthritis 281
Asia Pacific Heart Rhythm Society 761
Aspirin 181, 241, 306, 313, 315, 336, 379, 617, 723, 728, 1052
  comprising of 320
  dose 322
  high doses of 616
  low-dose 313, 615
  mechanism action of 722, 722*b*, 722*fc*
  resistance 317
    mechanism of 723*b*
Astemizole 623
Asthma 1005
  exercise induced 1063
Asymptomatic carotid stenosis, clinical impact of 932
Asymptomatic patients, secondary prevention in 933
Atenolol 189, 241, 933
Atherectomy, directional 349, 949
Atheroablation, performance of 373
Atherogenic dyslipidemia, treatment of 593
Atheromatous plaque 227
Atherosclerosis 142, 143, 145, 151, 942, 1043, 1048
  accelerated 993
  diffuse
    coronary 828
    distal 849
  eradicating 29
  etiology of 1043
  in arterial conduits, low 819
  multi-ethnic study of 175, 960
  noninvasive imaging of 960
  premature 623, 1046
  reduces 21
  theories of 28
Atherosclerotic cardiovascular disease 32, 35, 35*t*, 36*t*, 41, 53, 55, 57, 83, 121, 593, 1025, 1025*f*, 1051, 1062
Atherosclerotic coronary artery disease 959
Atherosclerotic disease 145
Atherosclerotic ostioproximal stenosis, severe 927*f*
Atherosclerotic plaques, quantification of 568
Atherosclerotic renal artery 923
  stenosis 145, 923, 925-927
  stenosis, medical management of 924
Atherosclerotic risk factors 1062
Atherosclerotic vein graft, diffusely 843
Athlete 1061
  avoidance techniques 1063
  electrocardiogram 1064*t*
  heart 1062
  left ventricular wall thickness 1065
  represent disease 1061
Atomoxetine 702
Atonic bladder 698
Atorvastatin 617, 618, 724
Atrial and pulmonary vein potentials, left 713*f*
Atrial appendage
  closure device, left 468
  closure, left 545*f*, 1035

left 435, 464, 542, 735, 874, 879
occlusion, left 435
risk factors for left 898
Atrial assessment, left 525
Atrial cardiopathy, concept of 874
Atrial enlargement, left 1064
Atrial fibrillation 181, 435, 468, 601, 602, 628, 640, 641, 648, 654, 703, 705, 708, 710, 711, 715, 716, 721, 722, 724, 725, 727, 732, 732*fc*, 733-736, 763, 765, 873, 875, 878*t*, 879, 881, 882, 883, 892*f*, 893, 959, 978, 987, 991, 1006, 1035, 1052, 1063
ablation 711, 714
complications of 713
procedure for 712*f*
acute rate control 736*t*
and complications, prevention of 716
and stroke 873
anticoagulation 725
antithrombotic management of 706
catheter ablation of 710, 711*t*
complication of 705
detection 874
in stroke 875
device detected 735
in acute myocardial infarction, management of 736
in heart failure
management of 733*fc*
treatment of 732
managing 736
pathophysiology of 710
postoperative 715, 1054
predictors of 736
prevent stroke in patient with 724
prevention of 716
complications of 717
rate control 732
recent conversion from 764
risk stratification tools in 705
symptom control 732
treatment in 579, 732
trial 710
type of 876
Atrial fibrosis 874, 877
Atrial natriuretic peptide 206
Atrial pacing 717
Atrial premature beats 875
Atrial septal defect 1034
closure 544*f*
small 543
Atrial septum 577
Atrial systole 483
Atrial tachyarrhythmias 1064
Atrial thrombus, left 898
Atrial tissue properties 874
Atrial volume
index, left 641
left 488
Atrial wall, right 809
Atrioventricular block, second-degree 1062
Atrioventricular nodal blockers 718
Atrioventricular pressure gradients 482*f*
Atrium, left 732, 854
Atrophic kidneys 927
Atropine 981
Attenuation corrected images 550, 552-554, 556, 557
Attenuation corrected stress 550, 554
myocardial perfusion imaging examination 554*f*
Augmented vector foot 673, 757-760, 772, 773, 793
Australian National Blood Pressure study, second 134
Austrian mobile phone-based telemonitoring 1019
Autoimmune disease 958, 984,
Autologous stem cell implantation 948
Automated cardioverter defibrillator 749
Automated external defibrillator 784
Automatic implantable cardioverter defibrillator 805
implantation 804, 1035
Automatic power-generating system 809
Autonomic dysfunction, causes of 698
Autonomic failure 698
primary 698, 699
pure 698
Autonomic modulation 645
Autonomic nervous system 696, 744
Autonomic neuropathies, hereditary 700
Autonomic system 1061
Axillary artery 845
preferably 845
Axitinib 621
Ayushman bharat 839
Azilsartan medoxomil 589
Azole antifungals 617

B

Balloon angioplasty 371*t*, 927
subsequent to 349
Balloon dilatation, simple 390
Balloon expandable valve system 445
Balloon indentation technique 389*f*
Balloon mitral valvuloplasty 980, 1034
Bare-metal stent 315, 310, 339, 363, 396, 404, 406, 927, 947, 1052
Bariatric surgery 86
Baroreceptor reflex 697*fc*
Baroreflex 696
sensitivity 694
Basal ganglia, glial cells of 698
Baseline coronary angiography 456*f*
Basic fibroblast growth factor 206

Bazett's formula 752
Beating heart 833
  surgery 834
Beats per minute 485, 488
Belinostat 622
Bempedoic acid 62, 596
Bench research 1037
Bendavia 645
Berlin questionnaire 1006
Beta-adrenergic
  antagonists 607
  receptors, physiological actions of 189*t*
Beta-agonist bronchodilators 614
Beta-blocker 125, 182, 230, 241, 252, 279, 616, 628, 635, 644, 690, 716, 736, 744, 747, 772, 785, 979, 985, 1048
  administration 716
  adverse effects of 189
  pharmacotherapeutics of 188
  side effects to 182*t*
  therapy 242, 744, 1053
    perioperative 1053*t*
Beta-cell function, homeostatic model assessment for 80
Bevacizumab 620, 621
Bezold-Jarisch reflex 701
Biatrial hypertrophy 1063
Bicuspid aortic valve 1062
Bifurcation angle, anatomy of 354*f*
Bifurcation lesion 353, 354
  Medina classification of 354*f*
  true 359
Bifurcation stenting 353
Bile acid sequestrants 62, 593
Bile duct surgery 338
Bilevel positive airway pressure 659
Binary restenosis 408
Binswanger's disease 142
Bioabsorbable stent implantation 424
Biodegradable drug-eluting stents 408
Biolimus-eluting stent 407
Bioprosthetic mitral valve, paravalvular defects around 535*f*
Bioprosthetic valve 534*f*
Biopsy, endomyocardial 973
Bioresorbable drug-eluting stents 408
Bioresorbable vascular scaffolds 409, 948
Biotransformation 613
Biphasic mitral flow 491*f*
Bisoprolol 189, 635, 690
Black-blood spin-echo sequences 572
Bleeding 603, 706, 857, 878, 894
  complications, predicting 317
  high risk of 603, 895
  intracranial 726
  management of 336, 339, 340*fc*
  prevention of 337
  risk 230, 728
    assessment of 337, 878
  treatment of 339
Bleomycin 620, 910
Blood 591
  cell count, complete 972
  component prohemostatic measures 340*b*
  dyscrasias 1003
  flow, collateral 927
  test 972
  urea nitrogen 637
  volume 978
Blood glucose 1062
  control 75
Blood pressure 5, 113, 114, 123, 129, 130, 137, 138, 139, 139*b*, 153, 155*f*, 160, 180, 188, 621, 636, 684*f*, 925, 927, 928*f*, 933, 974, 1017
  average 250
  categories 123*t*
  control 85, 124*f*, 126, 945
    diastolic 151
  diastolic 120, 121, 123, 133, 959, 966, 994, 1061
  digital 119
  for different stages 120*t*
  goals and targets 133
  high 59, 103, 1043, 1047, 1048
  higher pretreatment 925
  levels, new goal for 124*t*
  load 156
  management of 73
  mean 856
  monitoring 144, 160
    out-of-office 137
  postoperatively 927
  reduction 116*f*, 127*f*, 696
  stage 1 of 121*f*
  stage 2 of 121*f*
  stages, treatment for 120*t*
  systolic 116, 116*t*, 120, 121, 123, 124, 133, 184, 229, 505, 656, 943, 959, 966, 978, 1061
  variability 156
Blood sugar
  levels 1046
  lowers 598
Blunt trauma 682, 1062
Body
  frames, small 43
  surface mapping 1018
  mass index 22, 44, 74, 59, 80, 110, 958, 967, 1005, 1007, 1014, 1046
Bone marrow
  derived mesenchymal cells 428, 429

laser revascularization 838
mononuclear cells 428, 429
Bortezomib 621
Bovine arch 937
Brachial artery blood pressure 1065
Brachytherapy 349
Bradbury-Eggleston syndrome 698
Bradyarrhythmia 809, 1061, 1062
toxic substances 657
Bradycardia 189, 487*f*, 764, 1063
anticipated 937
progressive 684*f*
Brain
natriuretic peptide 76, 206, 643, 651, 972
N-terminal prohormone of 651
stem death, notifying 868
Branch morphologies, threatened side 355
Branch ostial lesions 388
Breast
cancer 11, 958
diseases of 957
surgery 1050
British Hypertension Society 135
Bromocriptine 142, 974, 986
Bronchospasm 189
Brugada syndrome 751, 757, 758, 760*f*, 763
electrocardiography of 759*f*
genetic background 758
Brugada-like early repolarization 1064
Bruising 911
B-type natriuretic peptide 631, 641, 658, 999
Buffalo hump 146
Bulky lesions 349
Bull's eye map of global myocardial strain 512*f*
Bundle branch block 679, 687
left 628, 667, 772, 791, 792, 1051, 1064
right 758, 772, 773, 1063, 1064
Bupropion 623
Burning sensation 908
Buspirone 142
Butyrophenone neuroleptics 764
Bypass graft
anatomy 843
evaluation of 568
Bypass surgery 363
trials of 842

C

Cabozantinib 621
Calcific aortic stenosis, severe 857
Calcification, classification of 370
Calcified lesions, treatment of 370
Calcineurin inhibitors 139
Calcium 115
channel 764
blocker 124, 125, 127, 133, 139, 182, 184, 187, 230, 588, 615-618, 622, 698, 717, 724, 772, 933, 1053
gluconate 607
influx postischemic reperfusion 559
superficial 370
Calf swelling 908
Canadian Cardiovascular Society 179, 205, 585
Canagliflozin 589
cardiovascular assessment study 96
Cancer 916
in unprovoked deep vein thrombosis, screening for 921
therapy, complications of 620
Candesartan 635, 649, 974
Cangrelor 330, 336
to clopidogrel, transition from 329
to prasugrel, transition from 330
to ticagrelor, transition from 330
Captopril 635, 974
Carbamazapine 142, 623
Carbon dioxide 1008
Carcinoid syndrome 700
Cardiac amyloidosis 514*f*, 577*f*
Cardiac arrest 252, 296, 783, 785, 786
episodes 786
out-of-hospital 749
study Hamburg 748
victims 784*f*
Cardiac arrhythmia 786, 1000, 1005, 1063
suppression trial 748, 1039
Cardiac artery bypass grafting 480
Cardiac biomarkers 999
Cardiac cachexia 650
Cardiac catheterization 346, 448
Cardiac chamber 778
Cardiac computed tomography 542
angiography 960
Cardiac cycle, phase of 572
Cardiac death rates 179*t*
Cardiac defibrillator, wearable 744
Cardiac destabilization syndromes 926
Cardiac disease 572, 756, 756*f*, 983, 985
detectable 687
therapy for 664
Cardiac disorders 1028
Cardiac dysfunction 997
Cardiac dyspnea 484
Cardiac electrophysiology 1029
Cardiac embolism 892, 932
Cardiac enzymes 972
Cardiac events, acute 1062
Cardiac failure 515
congestive 183, 876, 1005

Cardiac function 569
evaluation of 573
heart failure, treatment of preserved 644
Cardiac glycosides 1048
Cardiac implantable electronic devices 651, 654, 789
Cardiac index 292, 573, 657
reduced 852
Cardiac innervation 746
Cardiac insufficiency bisoprolol study 189, 691
Cardiac magnetic resonance 228, 562, 564, 573-579
imaging 175, 228, 428, 429, 464, 524, 572, 672, 746, 972, 1063
additional role of 643
Cardiac masses 578
Cardiac motion quantification 518
Cardiac output 380, 382, 573, 856
Cardiac pacemakers, current leadless 810
Cardiac perfusion-imaging 568
Cardiac power output 856
Cardiac protection 620
Cardiac rehabilitation 210, 210*f*, 213, 283
indications of 211
Cardiac remodeling 1063
Cardiac resynchronization 800
Cardiac resynchronization therapy 480, 515, 526, 666, 667, 690, 791, 792, 797, 799, 800, 802, 811, 854, 856, 975, 1020
defibrillator 654, 748, 800, 807
pacemaker 654
Cardiac risk index, revised 1051, 1051*t*, 1053
Cardiac stem cells 430
Cardiac stenosis for cardiac surgery, screening of 938*t*
Cardiac stress testing 238
Cardiac surgery 316*t*, 719, 817, 836, 863
complications of 228
high-risk 666
Cardiac synchrony 382
Cardiac syncope 681
Cardiac tamponade 287, 749, 774
Cardiac toxicity 621
prevention of 621
symptoms of 621
Cardiac transplantation 669, 858
Cardiac troponin 235, 999
Cardiac tumors 898
primary 898
Cardiac valves, diseases of 973
Cardioembolic stroke
acute 874
causes of 893*b*
Cardioembolism, etiology of 893
Cardiogenic shock 251, 268, 273, 292, 293, 293*f*, 295, 296, 831, 832
complicating myocardial infarction, management of 296*t*
diagnosis 294
management of 661
Cardiological Society of India 300
Cardiology Society of India 1030
Cardiology
non-ischemic 693
subspecialty of 1065
telemonitoring in 1017
Cardiomyocyte apoptosis, prevention of 971
Cardiomyopathy 973, 1062
apical hypertrophic 517*f*
dilated 475, 575, 897, 972
hereditary 984
hypertrophic 455, 515, 516*f*, 552, 575, 576*f*, 711, 750, 751, 757, 775, 1062
obstructive 455, 684, 756
idiopathic dilated 627
inflammatory 643
ischemic 430, 514, 560, 573*f*, 574*f*, 775, 800
nonischemic 574, 576*f*, 690, 747, 750, 775, 776, 776*f*
dilated 431
reversible dilated 993
trial 691, 693
Cardioplegia 833
retrograde 846
Cardiopulmonary
bypass 397, 833, 980
collapse 910
disease, underlying 1053
exercise testing 1063
resuscitation 783, 785, 786
practice of 783
testing 1051
Cardiorenal anemia syndrome 998
Cardiorenal syndrome 997-1000
acute 997
chronic 997
current update 997
secondary 997
Cardioselective beta-blockers 125, 979
Cardiosphere derived cells 428, 429
Cardiotoxic drugs 623
Cardiotoxicity 620, 622, 623
acute 620
chronic 621
types of 620
Cardiovascular abnormalities 1061
Cardiovascular adaptations 1065
Cardiovascular care, emergency 783
Cardiovascular complications, risk of 81
Cardiovascular death 309, 583
Cardiovascular disease 4, 9, 13–18, 20, 32, 38, 39, 42, 43, 46, 58, 66, 67, 83, 86, 89, 95, 113, 120, 123, 129, 134, 173, 180, 204, 211, 226, 249, 251, 281, 298, 306, 426, 427, 588, 593, 606, 612, 648, 957, 983, 999, 1013, 1024, 1043, 1044, 1046, 1051
accelerated 923

burden of 249, 250
control of 74
determinants of 250
elevated risk of 994
large variety of 1035
management of 1047
pathophysiologic basis of 1043
prevention of 35, 150
risk of 73
Cardiovascular disorders 73, 74
Cardiovascular drugs, selection of proper 1048
Cardiovascular events
higher risk of 120
prevention of 130, 314
Cardiovascular functions 20
Cardiovascular intensive care unit 230
Cardiovascular intervention 345
Cardiovascular magnetic resonance 223, 289, 506
Cardiovascular management program, simplified 1014
Cardiovascular medications 9
Cardiovascular medicine 320
Cardiovascular mortality 8
risk of 95
Cardiovascular outcomes 925
Cardiovascular pharmacology 581
Cardiovascular structures to sternum, proximity of 844*f*
Cardiovascular system 345, 991, 998
effects on 995
functioning of 991
Cardioverter defibrillator
implantable 456, 651, 666, 667, 688, 690, 734, 742, 744, 748, 752, 760, 761, 765, 791, 792, 800, 801, 804, 805, 975, 1020
wearable 749
Carfilzomib 620, 621
Carotid artery
disease 933, 938
asymptomatic 934*t*, 939
management of 932
external 937
internal 819, 824, 825, 827, 843, 883, 927, 932
occlusion, contralateral 935
stenosis 935
severity 933
stenting 338, 932, 934-937, 937*t*, 938*t*, 1034
technique 936, 937*t*
timing of 935
Carotid atherosclerosis study, asymptomatic 932
Carotid baroreceptor stimulation 140
Carotid bifurcation 933
Carotid bulbs, dilated 933
Carotid emboli study, asymptomatic 933
Carotid endarterectomy 338, 932, 934, 935, 935*t*, 936, 936*t*, 938*t*, 1050
Carotid femoral pulse wave velocity 17, 138
Carotid interventions, timing of 935
Carotid intima media thickness 176, 994
regression of 933
Carotid stenosis 938, 1034
asymptomatic 934
symptomatic 934
Carotid surgery trial, asymptomatic 932
Carotid territory symptoms 934
Carvedilol 189, 241, 635, 690, 974
prospective randomized cumulative survival trial 189
Cataplexy 682
Cataract 1052
surgery 1050, 1052
Catastrophic health expenditure 251
Catecholaminergic polymorphic ventricular tachyarrhythmias 1062
Catheter ablation 710, 733, 734, 743, 749
reduces mortality 749
Catheter engages ostium 385
Catheter selection 272
Catheterization, acute 230
Celiprolol 618
Cell 591
administration, determining optimum timing of 427
based therapies 838
donors, selection of 427
doses of 427
membrane 613
depolarization of 606
recipient, selection of 427
therapy 426, 427, 838
types and mechanisms 427
Cellular proliferation, induction of 91
Central aortic
blood pressure measurement 158
cannulation 845
pulse pressure 589
systolic pressure 589
Central nervous system 614, 1063
Central venous pressure 412*f*
elevated 998
Cephalosporins 616
Cerebral autonomic nervous system 874
Cerebral embolic events, symptomatic 897
Cerebral embolization of thrombus 1035
Cerebral ischemia, focal temporary 932
Cerebral protection device 937
Cerebral vascular
accident 310
disease 121
Cerebral veins 916
Cerebrovascular accident 58

Cerebrovascular bleeding 983
Cerebrovascular complications 858
Cerebrovascular disease 123
Cerebrovascular events 396
Cerivastatin 617
Cervical sympathetic denervation 744
Cesarean section, lower segment 980
Chagas disease 700, 775
Characterized transporter protein 613
Chemicals arsenic trioxide 622
Chemotherapy agents 621, 622
Chest
- compression 783
  - mechanical devices for 784
- pain 235, 287, 972, 1063, 1065
  - acute 570
  - exertional 1063
- radiograph 972
- X-ray 642, 658, 843, 979, 1024

Chloroquine 623
Chlorpromazine 614, 623, 764
Chlorthalidone 125, 134, 637
Chlorzoxazone 617
Cholecystectomy 338
Cholesterol 27, 29, 32, 48, 84
- absorption inhibitors 62
- and diet 40
- combined 67
- functions of 28
- hypothesis 27
- particles 901
- remnant 67
- total 46, 66
- treatment trialists 36, 58, 84

Cholesteryl ester 54
- transfer protein 53, 54, 62, 85, 597
  - inhibitors 62, 597

Cholestyramine 62
Chronic kidney disease, moderate-to-severe 37
Chronic total occlusion 267, 391, 393, 394, 401, 949, 1034
- lesions 392
- management of 391
- percutaneous coronary intervention 393, 394*fc*
  - complications of 394

Chronic venous
- disease 908
- disorders 908, 908*t*
- insufficiency 907

Chronotropic incompetence 645
Cilostazol 336, 616, 945
Cinacalcet hydrochloride therapy, evaluation of 407
Circulatory failure 656
Circumflex artery, left 387, 415
Cirrhosis 700
Citalopram 623
Clarithromycin 764
Clarivein mechanochemical ablation 913
Claudication
- mild 942
- moderate 942
- severe 942

Clevidipine 589
Clinical syntax score 170
Clonidine 1048
Clopidogrel 241, 306-308, 312, 314, 315, 321, 323-325, 329, 330, 336, 612, 617, 618, 724, 728, 933, 1052
- active metabolite 312
- allergy 309
- low antiplatelet effect 317
- resistance 317
- treatment 307
- uses 618

Clot dislodgement 901
Coat hanger pain 700
Cobalt-chromium 405
Coenzyme A 586
- derivative 596

Coherent, shortage of 1038
Colchicine 717
Colesevelam 62
Colestipol 62
Collaborative atorvastatin diabetes study 84
Color Doppler 476
- jet area 479

Combination therapy 748
Common drug-drug interactions 615
Commotio cordis 1062
Community health
- centers 1013
- workers 1014

Co-morbidities, treatment of 645
Complete revascularization
- advantages of 265
- disadvantages of 265

Compression therapy 918
Computed tomographic angiography, multi-detector 844
Computed tomography 219, 428, 429, 464, 548, 570, 843, 883, 903, 1024
- angiogram 139, 567*f*, 844*f*
- angiography 175, 218, 568*f*, 569f, 882, 923, 933, 944, 944*f*
  - multi-detector row 174
- coronary angiography 385, 566, 570, 570*b*, 960
  - applications of 567
  - diagnostic performance of 566
- coronary calcium scoring 1025
- fractional flow reserve 568

imaging protocol 449
imaging, multidetector 450*f*
multiple-detector 920
of pelvis 402
scan 449
Concomitant cardiac pathology 450
Concomitant therapies 724
Congenital heart disease, pre-existing 973
Congestion 656*f*
Congestive heart failure, symptoms of 560
Conn's syndrome 142, 145, 147
Consciousness
classification of transient loss of 680
loss of 679
transient loss of 680
classification of 680
electrocardiogram 681
high-risk features 681
low-risk features 681
past medical history 681
physical examination 681
Constipation 146, 698
Contraceptives 139
hormonal 142
Conventional guideline directed medical therapy 661
Conventional pacing system, potential complications with 309
Cool shock study 296
Copeptin 999
Copernicus trial 691*f*
Copolymer 406
Cor pulmonale 145
Coronary angiogram 779*f*
Coronary angiography 192, 194*t*, 238, 252, 289, 345, 392, 419, 672, 785, 844, 957, 1034, 1051
arrival of 347
invasive 167
left 457
Coronary anomalies, congenital 1062
Coronary artery 175*f*, 350, 567*f*, 671, 826, 842
angiography 173
atherosclerosis 1063
bending of 1062
bifurcations 353
bypass 398
conduits, patency of 824*t*
bypass grafting 179, 192, 194, 195, 198, 199, 232, 251, 252, 266, 309, 310, 316, 316*t*, 328, 364, 364*t*, 396-398, 805, 825, 831, 836, 841, 843, 961, 1034, 1051
emergency 391
guideline for 195*t*
indications of 843*t*
over percutaneous coronary intervention, benefits of 396
recent advances in 836
robotic-assisted 397
surgery 230, 294, 347, 349, 372, 715
surgery, history of 370
syntax score 170
bypass surgery 204, 332, 363, 396, 583, 831, 832, 1028
evolution of 836*f*
calcium 35, 175, 566, 960, 1025
score 174, 175, 567, 1025*f*
dentification of 845
diagnosis of 347
disease 8, 15, 16*f*, 16*t*, 21*b*, 27, 35, 30, 39, 47, 53, 83, 89, 90*f*, 121, 123, 127, 130, 145, 167, 179, 187, 193, 195, 198, 204, 207*t*, 249, 271, 286, 307, 311, 320*f*, 321, 332, 419, 570, 379, 411, 513*f*, 514*f*, 548, 560, 566, 567, 575, 583, 601, 603, 604, 622, 628, 648, 674, 721, 746, 749, 765, 771, 804, 805, 814, 828, 836, 838, 841, 852, 893, 932, 935, 957, 993, 1005, 1022, 1028, 1029, 1044, 1044*f*, 1048, 1053, 1061, 1062
advanced 396
angiographic 179
chronic 165
consequence of 831
controversy 27
different extents of 179*t*
evaluation of 567
in asymptomatic adults, screening for 173
left main 363, 364*t*, 819
management of 370
pathophysiology of 187
prevalence of 89, 90*t*
prevention of 83
protection 9
proximal left anterior descending 195
risk of 1043
significant left main 363
symptomatic 363
three-vessel 195
two-vessel 195
injury 774
ischemia, detecting asymptomatic 174*t*
left 412
anterior descending 841
main 364, 387, 401
lesions, left main 401
lumen 569
right 272, 286, 386, 387, 412, 823, 845
role of 1025*f*
spasm 961, 962
stent 570
left main 365
surgery 315
Coronary atherectomy, directional 349

Coronary atherosclerosis
  noninvasive visualization of 566
  risk of 958
Coronary balloon angioplasty, development of 347
Coronary bifurcation
  anatomy of 353*f*
  lesion 353
  stenting 355
Coronary blood flow 559
  linear relationship of 412*f*
  restoration of 289
Coronary bypass surgery 820
Coronary calcification 15
  diagnosis of 370
Coronary calcium score 168
  assessment 167
Coronary care unit 294, 299, 659, 661, 662
Coronary catheter angiography 566
Coronary computed tomography 563
  angiogram 168
  angiography 167, 228
Coronary dissection, risk of 385
Coronary flow reserve 411, 994
  calculation of 556
  diminished 173
Coronary heart
  disease 9, 20, 21, 32, 34*f*, 39, 40, 42, 46, 90, 114, 133, 173, 599, 1043
    management of 962
    premature 958
  disorders 73, 74
Coronary injury 570
Coronary intervention 343
  evolution of 345
  history of 345
  study 401
Coronary ischemia
  consequences of 805
  preventing 722*b*
Coronary lithoplasty 437
Coronary microvascular dysfunction 959
Coronary occlusion, acute 559
Coronary ostia 774
Coronary ostium, height of 450
Coronary perfusion 382
Coronary reoperations 843, 845
  mortality of 849
Coronary revascularization 593
  hybrid 396-398
Coronary risk factors, management of 180
Coronary sinus
  lead implantation 797
  pacing from 713*f*
  reducer 437
Coronary stent 349
  contemporary 404
  evaluation of 569
  implantation 341
Coronary vasomotor, invasive 961
Coronary vasospasm, catheter induced 384
Coronary veins 774
Coronary venous bypass grafting 838, 839*f*
Cost-benefit ratio 1028
Cost-effective care 1036
Cough 786, 972
Coumarin derivatives 618
Coumarins, actions of 616
Craniofacial abnormalities 1008
C-reactive protein 9, 90, 1044
Creatine kinase 58, 59, 61
Creatinine 972, 998
  clearance 241, 312, 337
Critical limb ischemia 941, 943*t*, 952
  current management 941
  evaluation of 943
  pathophysiology of 941
Crush techniques 366
Crushing syndrome 139
Cryoablation balloon 712, 712*f*
Cryoplasty 948
Cryoprecipitate 340
Cryosclerosis 913
C-type natriuretic peptide 1044
Culotte technique 366
Culprit-only percutaneous coronary intervention 293
Culprit-shock trial 293
Cushing's syndrome 146
Cutting balloon 387
  angioplasty 371, 947
Cyanobacterium 62
Cyclic adenosine monophosphate 723
Cyclic guanosine monophosphate 206, 585, 641, 643
Cyclic guanylate monophosphate stimulators 644
Cyclooxygenase 336, 722, 723
  inhibiting nitric oxide donating 591
  inhibitor of 306
Cyclopentyl triazolopyrimidine 307, 321
Cyclophosphamide 620
Cyclosporine 139, 616, 617, 864
Cyclosporine-A 224
Cystatin C 999
Cystectomy, total 338
Cytochrome p450 591
Cytotoxic drugs 620, 622
  cardiotoxicity of 620

D

Dabigatran 468, 601, 603, 707, 880, 881, 894
    low-dose 603
Dabrafenib 622
Daily activities 1062
Dapagliflozin 589
Dasatinib 622
Death
    dominant cause of 298
    prevention of 191
DeBakey heart assist device 855*f*
Debulking devices 948, 949
Deceleration time 485
Decitabine 621
Decompensation, acute 636*b*
Decompression cardiopulmonary resuscitation 786
Deep sternal wound infection 847
Deep vein thrombosis 208, 908, 912, 916, 916*fc*, 918, 919
    acute proximal 918
    controversies and consensus 916
    evaluation of 916
    isolated distal 918*t*
    management of 916
        isolated distal 917
    treatment of 917*t*
Deflection index, maximum 776
Degenerative bioprosthetic aortic valves 444
Dehydroepiandrosterone 40
Dementia 123
Deoxyribonucleic acid 998
Depolarization, abnormalities of 766
Depression 1043
Descending artery, posterior 286
Desflurane 622
Desipramine 623
Desmopressin 340
Device implantation 470
Device migration 452
Device motion and ablation speed 375
Dewoods landmark demonstration 273
Dextrose 607
Dhadkan app 629*f*
Diabetes 53, 73, 211, 640, 698, 814, 876, 893, 901, 958, 1043, 1047, 1048
    and cardiovascular disease 73
    and coronary artery disease 89, 90
    classification 79, 80*t*
        new dimensions 79
    control and complications trial 74
    duration of 201
    history of 79
    management of 95, 934
    mellitus 16, 35, 46, 58, 73, 73*f*, 79, 83, 89, 90*f*, 95, 121, 145, 155, 181, 191, 194, 198, 233, 242, 250, 408, 636, 706, 724, 879, 935, 945, 958, 1000, 1050
        development of 84
        gestational 79
        insulin-dependent 79
        management of 181
        medication 622
        noninsulin-dependent 79, 90
        type 1 53, 79, 81
        type 2 42, 47, 53, 79, 81, 95, 95*t*, 606, 1015
    mild age-related 80
    prevalence of 89
    type of 79, 201
Diabetic interventions and complications, epidemiology of 74
Diabetic nephropathy 74, 590
Diacylglycerol, production of 92
Diagonal artery 826, 846
Dialysis 607, 812
Diaphoresis 287
Diarrhea 306, 607, 698
Diastasis 484, 486
Diastole, physiology of 482
Diastolic blood pressure, low 150, 151
Diastolic dysfunction 286, 481, 482, 494*f*, 577, 640, 923, 994
    advanced 494
    classification of 642*f*
    grading of 501*t*
Diastolic function 487, 496
    significance of 483
Diastolic heart failure, pure 483*f*
Diastolic hypertension, mild 993
Diastolic stress testing 500, 643
Diffusion fluid-attenuated inversion recovery 888
Digital stethoscope 1018*f*
Digital subtraction angiography 944
Digoxin 613, 616, 617, 661, 717, 736, 974, 985, 1048
    absorption 613
    bioavailability of 613
Dihydropyridine 127, 182, 184
Dilated cardiomyopathy
    nonischemic 799, 800, 800*t*, 801
    pathophysiology of 690
    pre-existing 973
Diltiazem 182
Dimethylarginine, asymmetrical 1044
Diode laser therapy, low-dose 946
Dipeptidyl peptidase-4 inhibitors 75, 76, 97, 589
Diphenhydramine 623
Dipyridamole 336
    interferes 722
Direct oral anticoagulant 734, 892, 1052

Direct thrombin inhibitor 601, 707, 881
Disability-adjusted life years 892
Disodium ethylenediaminetetraacetic acid 374
Disopyramide 614, 623, 748, 764
Displacement, degree of 613
Disseminated intravascular coagulation 898
Distal chronic total occlusion 272
Diuretic 125, 133, 289, 607, 638, 644, 658, 980, 985, 999
  low doses of 144
  optimization strategies evaluation trial 999
  therapy 985
Dizziness 700
DK crush technique 360*f*
Dobutamine 294, 659-661, 764, 974, 999
  stress 564
    echocardiography 561
    imaging 561
    low-dose 560
    magnetic resonance 561
Docosahexaenoic acid 47, 62
Donor heart 866
Dopamine 294, 659, 660, 1000
Doppler tissue imaging 490
Doppler wave 479
  continuous 479
Dorsalis pedis artery 951
Double kissing and crush 366
Doxazosin 140, 588, 615
Doxepin 623
Doxorubicin 620
Doxycycline 910
Dragonfly imaging catheter 420
Droperidol 623
Droxidopa 702
Drug 657, 984, 998
  absorption of 612, 613
  administration 894
  causing prolong QT 623*t*
  coated balloon 315, 947, 948
  combinations 184*t*
  distribution 612, 613
  drug interaction 321, 612
    actual incidence of 612
    mechanism of 612
  eluting stent 274, 310, 315, 339, 405, 406*t*, 407, 423, 927, 948, 1052
    platform, cross-section of 405*f*
    safety 198, 232, 278, 353, 363, 384, 408, 409
  excretion interaction 613
  food interactions 618
  induced torsade de pointes, risk factors for 764*b*
  interactions 613, 880
    in cardiology 612
  metabolism 612, 613
  monitoring 859
  newer 610
  of P2Y12 inhibitor 316
  provocation 684*f*
  therapy 734
  toxicity 1053
  transport proteins 613
Dual antiplatelet therapy 241, 251, 303, 305, 310-312, 313*t*, 315-317, 320, 322, 336-340, 360, 408, 470, 604, 706, 729, 737, 933, 1052
  duration of 318
  history of 320*f*
  reimplementation of 338
  score 311
Dual drug combinations 127
Duodenopancreatic surgery 338
Duration of therapy 919
Dyslipidemia 32, 37, 167, 593, 724, 945, 958, 1048
  development of 995
  drug for management of 36
  inadequate management of 34
  management of 34, 53, 181, 598, 599
  pathophysiology of 53
  prevalence of 33*f*
  treatment of 1047
Dyspepsia 881, 895
Dyspnea 455, 961, 962
Dysrhythmias 620, 757, 794
Dyssynchrony, intraventricular 494

E

Ecchymoses 911
Echocardiogram 1021
Echocardiography 228, 428, 429, 463, 481, 503, 521, 560, 564, 642, 658, 672, 960, 973
  intracardiac 980
  two-dimensional 524, 1024
Echolucent plaque 938
Eclampsia 973
  severe 973
Ectopic atrial rhythm 1064
Ectopy, atrial 1063
Edema
  chronic tissue 918
  high attitude pulmonary 1033
  interstitial 942
Edoxaban 601, 603, 708, 880, 895
Eicosapentaenoic acid 47
Eighth Joint National Committee 133
Ejection fraction 18, 194, 195, 205, 428, 429, 506, 513, 522, 573, 627, 641, 792, 800, 802, 805, 856
  determination of 572

midrange 647, 648
normal 640
preserved 436, 641, 641*f*, 643*f*
reduced 97, 650, 665, 732, 733*fc*, 804
Elastic compression therapy, duration of 919
Elastic lamina, external 420
Elective double stent strategy 359
Electrical cardioversion 657, 734
Electrical storm, catheter ablation of 744
Electrocardiogram 29, 173, 182, 235, 240, 484, 548, 570, 572, 642, 658, 772, 972, 979, 1024, 1046, 1050, 1051, 1063, 1064
artifact 476
gated stress imaging 550-552, 554, 556, 557
monitoring, prolong 687*t*
Electrocardiography 89, 204, 287, 300, 672, 756, 843, 960, 973, 1017
diagnosis 761
Electrocardiography-based tests 765, 765*t*
Electroencephalogram 1008
Electrolytes 972
Electromyography 61
Electronic batch record 811
Electronic clinical decision support system 1013
Electronic decision support system 1013
Electronic health record 1013
Electrophysiological device therapy 666
Electrophysiological studies-guided pacemaker implantation 679
Electrophysiology
interventional 1035
study 694
Embolic protection device 926, 938
Emergency department, management in 679
Emerging molecules 590, 590*t*
Empagliflozin 589
Enalapril 589, 635, 974
Encainide 623
End diastolic
velocity 923
volume 428, 429, 522, 573
wall thickness 561
End stage disease 664
End systolic volume 428, 429, 522, 573
Endocardial pacing 797
Endocardial radiofrequency catheter, failure of 775
Endocarditis 452, 1021
active 465
infective 533, 893, 898
risk of 465
Endocardium 746
Endogenous catecholamine levels 683
Endogenous tissue restoration 437
Endomyocardium, apical 577
Endoscopic bypass grafting 397
Endoscopic coronary artery bypass
grafting, total 397
total 836
Endoscopic procedures 1050
Endothelial cells 92
Endothelial dysfunction 91, 942, 959, 1043, 1047
Endothelin 586, 923, 998
receptor blockers 586
secretion 631
Endovascular aneurysm repair 338
Endovascular revascularization 946
techniques for 946
Endovascular therapy 889, 890
intracranial 935
Endovascular treatment, primary 890
Endovenous cyanoacrylate closure 913
Endovenous laser ablation 909, 911-914
catheter and laser fiber 912*f*
machine 911*f*
mechanism action of 912*f*
Endovenous laser treatment 912
Endovenous steam ablation 913
Endovenous therapies
advantages of 914*t*
disadvantages of 914*t*
Endurance exercise 1061
Energy 559
Enflurane 622
Enhanced external counterpulsation therapy 206, 206*fc*
acute hemodynamic effects of 206*f*
Enoximone 660
Enzyme 613, 725
Eosinophilic neoplasm 577
Epicardial ablation 775
Epicardial access, posterior approach for 777*t*
Epicardial space 774
Epicardial stenosis, assessment of hemodynamic severity of 192
Epicardial ventricular tachycardia 775, 781
Epicardium 746
Epidemiology 941, 983
Epigastric artery, inferior 820
Epinephrine 294, 660, 785
Epirubicin 620
Epithelial sodium channel 589
Eplerenone 635
Epoxide hydrolases 613
Eptifibatide 241, 336
Epworth sleepiness scale 1006
Erectile dysfunction 698, 1008, 1043, 1044*f*, 1046, 1047, 1047*t*, 1048
management of 1047
Erythrocyte fluidity 942
Erythromycin 623, 764

Erythropoietin 139, 998, 1002, 1003
Escalation 323, 324
Escitalopram 623
Esmolol 736
Esophageal cancer 11
Esophagectomy 338
Estrogens, cardiovascular benefits of 21, 21*b*
Ethanol 910
  abuse 878
Ethanolamine oleate 910
Ethylhexanoic acid 40
European Association for Cardiothoracic Surgery 831
European Association of Cardiovascular Imaging 501
European Association of Echocardiography Guidelines 490
European Atherosclerosis Society 57, 58
European Carotid Surgery Trial 932
European Collaborative Acute Stroke Study III 887
European Heart Rhythm Association 761
European Lacidipine Study on Atherosclerosis 933
European Medicines Agency 183, 894
European Society of Cardiology 34, 35, 96, 124, 134, 154, 176, 190, 236, 262, 279*f*, 338, 468, 603, 641, 659, 679, 736, 799, 831, 875, 1003, 1052, 1063
  guidelines 271, 682, 923, 934*t*
  recommendations 935*t*
European Society of Hypertension 124, 134, 154
European Thyroid Association Guidelines 994
Everolimus 621
  eluting stents 406, 407
Evolocumab 595
Excess salt consumption 970
Excimer laser coronary angioplasty 371
Exenatide plus dapagliflozin 589
Exercise
  benefits of 1062
  capacity 1062
  echocardiography 1063
  risks of 1062
  stress testing 960, 1046
  treadmill test , 167, 168
  types of 1061
External iliac artery, endofibrosis of 942
Extracardiac diseases 208
Extracellular fluid volume 998
Extracorporeal life support 381
  advantages 381
  disadvantages 381
Extracorporeal membrane oxygenator 742, 743, 784
Extracorporeal techniques 784
Extracranial carotid artery stenosis 932
Extravascular tissue pressure 188
Extremity veins, lower 907
Extrinsic compression 923
Eyes 747
Ezetimibe 593

F

Facial plethora 146
Familial chylomicronemia syndrome 597
Fatal bleeding 309
Fatal coronary heart disease 6
Fatigue 146, 908, 972, 993, 1065
Fats, composition of 46
Fatty acid 40, 42, 46
  binding protein 60
  fraction of 41*f*
  hydrogenated 47
  nonesterfied 53, 54, 54*f*
  transport 598
Femoral arterial access 926
Femoral artery 845
  common 947
  size 382
  stenosis of superficial 944*f*
  superficial 947
Femoral pulses 1065
Femoral vascular ultrasound 402
Femoral vein 907, 912
Femoropopliteal segment endovascular revascularization, technique for 950
Ferric carboxymaltose 1003
Ferric gluconate 1004
Ferric hydroxide sucrose 1004
Fetal antigen autoimmunity 970
Fetal biophysical profile, abnormal 969
Fetal microchimerism 970
Fetal myocardium 559
Fever 142
Fibrates 62, 617
Fibrin specificity 258, 889
Fibrinogen 20, 942
  concentrate 340
  depletion 258, 889
Fibrinolysis 256, 261, 737, 786
Fibrinolytic 257*t*
  drugs, classification 257
  therapy 242, 261
  treatment 256
Fibroatheroma, thin-cap 421
Fibroblast growth factor 426
Fibrocalcific pancreatic diabetes 79
Fibromuscular dysplasia 139, 142, 923, 927, 928*f*, 942, 963
Fibroplasia 842
FIbrosis 874, 1047
  endocardial 577*f*
  endomyocardial 577, 577*f*
Fibrotic plaques 387, 421*f*
Filling pressure, right-sided 287
Filtered back projection images 551, 552, 557
Final kissing balloon inflation 357, 360, 365
Finet's law 355

Finger plethysmogram 206*f*
First human heart transplant 863
Fixed dose combination 126
Flash pulmonary edema 145, 926
Floating wire technique 388, 388*f*
Flow-mediated dilatation 16, 17, 1046
Fluconazole 616
Fludrocortisone acetate 702
Fluid, intravenous 289
Fluorodeoxyglucose 175
  positron emission tomography 561
Fluoroquinolones 764
Fluoroscopy 451, 464, 1021
Foam sclerotherapy 914
  ultrasound-guided 909
Folate deficiency 1003
Fondaparinux 241, 279
Food-drug interaction 618*t*
Foot infection 942
Formation of blood clot, mechanism of 727*f*
Fractional flow reserve 167, 180, 193, 198, 265, 266, 272, 350, 372, 397, 411, 412-414, 416, 422, 436
  advantages of 412
  clinical utility of 413
  history of 350
Framingham heart study 95, 114
Free fatty acid 586
Freedom trial 199
Frequent ventricular extrasystole 476
Fresh frozen plasma 340
Functional mitral regurgitation, ultrasound assessment of 475
Functional syntax score 170, 413
Functional tricuspid regurgitation, significance of 434
Furosemide 637, 974
Fused single-photon emission computed tomography 555*f*
Fusidic acid 617
Fusion echocardiography 542
Fusion imaging, understanding 542

G

Gadolinium
  concentration 563, 802
  enhancement, late 561, 693, 751
  postadministration of 577
Galectin-3 633
Gastroepiploic artery 820, 825
  right 824, 847
Gastroesophageal reflux 1008, 1063
Gastrointestinal bleeding 857, 881, 895
GEA grafts, patency of 823
Gemcabene 596
Gene therapy 941, 948
Genome-wide association study 972
Gestational hypertension, treatment of 966
Giant cell arteritis 942
Gianturco-Roubin stent 404*f*
Glitazones, cardiac effects of 622
Global burden of disease study 39, 109, 226
Glomerular filtration rate 84, 139, 241, 606, 998
  estimated 876, 925, 926, 1052
Glomerulonephritis 997
  chronic 997
Glucagon-like peptide 1 75, 583, 587
  analogs 77
  receptor agonists 97
Glucocorticoid 139, 717
  remediable aldosteronism 139, 142
Gluconate 1004
Glucose
  advantages of 29
  disadvantages of 29
  insulin-potassium, combine administration of 224
  metabolism 559
  modulators 224
Glue 913, 914
Glutamic acid decarboxylase 80
Glutathione, reduced 93
Gluten-free diet 43
Glycation end products, advanced 90, 91, 91*b*
Glycemia control 85, 96
Glycemic control, worsening of 189
Glycemic status, management of 73
Glyceryl trinitrate 182
Glycogen
  accumulation 874
  storage 559
    disease 942
Glycoprotein IIB/IIIA inhibitor, selective 937
Glycosuria 76
Glycoxidation 93
Gordon syndrome 139
Gorlin's equation 531
Grace risk score 229
Grafting vessels with stenosis 414
Great saphenous vein 907, 912
Greater antithrombotic molecules 819
Growth differentiation factor-15 633
Growth factor, transforming 426
Guide catheter 359
Guide wire exchange 357
Guiding catheter 388
  maneuvers 385
  selection 385
  tendency 385

H

Hair loss 942
Haloperidol 614, 623, 764
Halothane 622
Handling saphenous vein grafts 847
Hardwares, selection of 385
Harmonize trial 609*f*
Harvesting technique 822
Head and neck surgery 338, 1050
Headache 700
Head-up tilt test 682, 683*f*, 684
  response to 683
Health professional's follow-up study 42
Health survey, district level 110
Healthcare quality index 110
Heart 669, 777, 1061
  and renal protection trial 1000
  block 189
  catheterization, right 973
  murmur 1065
  rhythm
    disorders, detection of 652
    irregular 892*f*
  structurally normal 746
  transplantation 668, 853, 858, 863, 864, 854*f*
  utilization 864
Heart disease 33, 1028
  chronic rheumatic 978
  congenital 570, 1021, 1065
  cyanotic 984, 985
  effect of 994
  hypertensive 973
  ischemic 6, 34, 39, 49, 66, 87, 195*t*, 221, 226, 249, 249*f*, 513, 569, 573, 583, 593, 627, 648, 684, 749, 756, 758, 853, 958, 959, 961, 973, 984, 1050, 1051
  patients with structural 763
  treatment of 1029
Heart failure 15, 18, 95, 95*t*, 96, 121, 130, 133, 151, 182, 204, 207*t*, 251, 426, 436, 483, 570, 584, 588, 615, 627, 628, 631, 635, 636, 640, 641, 647-651, 651*t*, 654, 656*f*, 664, 665, 665*fc*, 691, 710, 711, 732, 732*fc*, 735, 799, 800, 802, 804, 852, 853, 854*fc*, 856, 896, 901, 984, 993, 998, 1002, 1003*f*, 1005, 1015, 1017, 1019, 1050, 1053
  acute 233, 620, 656, 659, 659*fc*, 660, 661, 998
    decompensated 628, 656, 657*f*, 660*t*, 997
  biomarkers in 631
  burden 631
  cases 647
  causes 627
  chronic 17, 635*t*, 636*b*, 637*t*, 1000, 1003, 1019
    congestive 638
  clinical syndrome of 483
  coexistence of 95
  compensated 211
  congestive 1-51, 96, 123, 127, 189, 311, 312, 337, 462, 606, 647, 691, 692, 706, 763, 764, 791, 792, 853, 876, 879, 890, 893, 997
  diagnosis of 631, 641*t*, 650
  diastolic 644
  discharge acute decompensated 662
  disease-wise 852
  end stage 858
  etiologies of 853*f*
  in pregnancy 983
  in type 2 diabetes mellitus, screening for 95
  incidence of 852
  indication of 983
  interventions, mHealth-based 1015
  ischemic 560, 565
  management of 650, 791, 853
    acute 660*fc*, 662
    strategies 1020
  managing 732
  monitoring therapy in 650
  pathophysiology of 641*f*
  progression of 732
  remote monitoring of 651
  risk of 75
  sign of 645, 656
  symptomatic 970
  symptoms of 465, 645, 656
  systolic 483, 498
  telemonitoring of 651
  treatment 204, 579, 643*f*, 650
    in acute decompensated 662*b*
    modalities, end-stage 859*t*
    acute 658
  trial 993
    total annual mortality in large 802*f*
  with midrange ejection fraction 647
  with preserved ejection fraction 643
  with recovered ejection fraction 648
  with reduced ejection fraction 733
  worsening 692*f*
    in hemodynamics 653
Heart rate 5, 182, 184, 185, 229, 488, 522, 1061
  control, acute 736
  detection 765
  reducing 584, 636
  reduction of 188
  resting 766
  turbulence 694, 765
  variability 694, 765, 805
Heart Rhythm Society 761
Heart transplant
  centers, number of 864
  number of 866*f*

Heartmate 667*f*
  left ventricular assist device 855*f*
Heartware system 855*f*
Heat stroke 1062
Heavy calcification 938
HELLP syndrome 968
Hematopoietic stem cells 428
Hemimotor deficits 934
Hemochromatosis 576
Hemodialysis, discontinue 927
Hemodynamic instability, absence of 265
Hemodynamic monitoring device, implantable 1020*f*
Hemodynamic support devices 380
Hemofiltration 244
Hemoglobin 1002, 1014
  glycated 584
Hemoglobinuria 910
Hemorrhage
  gastrointestinal 603
  intracranial 258, 468, 469
Hemorrhagic stroke, risk factor for 901*b*
Heparin 252, 612
  unfractionated 241, 279, 305, 1052
Hepatic disease 878
Hepatic lipase 54
Hepatocyte growth factor 206
Hepatotoxicity 58
Hiatal hernia 281
  repair 338
Hibernating myocardium 559
High arginine vasopressin 638
High-density lipoprotein 15, 20, 21, 27, 33, 36, 40, 47, 53, 54, 74, 83, 90, 958
  cholesterol 5, 9, 41, 42, 593, 597, 1062
    infusion therapy 597
Highly active antiretroviral therapy 623
High-resolution epicardial coronary ultrasonography 839
High-sensitivity cardiac troponin 236, 237, 237*t*
  assays 236*fc*
High-sensitivity C-reactive protein 176, 206
High-sensitivity troponin 632
Hip surgery 338
Hirsutism 146
His bundle pacing 796, 797
Histone deacetylase inhibitors 622
Home blood pressure monitoring 153
  current status 160
  diagnostic performance of 160*t*
Home sleep apnea testing 1008
Hormone
  replacement therapy 20, 21*b*
    clinical studies of 21
    effects of 21
  trials, large 957
Household survey, district level 103, 109
Hriday card 629*f*
Human development index 110
Human immunodeficiency virus 700, 856
Hybrid cell design 937*f*
Hybrid revascularization, goals of 398*b*
Hydralazine 974
  isosorbide dinitrate 986
Hydrochlorothiazide 637, 974
Hydrogen peroxide 93
Hydroxychloroquine 623
Hyperaldosteronism
  idiopathic 146
  primary 139, 142, 145
  secondary 139, 145
Hyperbaric oxygen therapy 941, 946
Hypercalcemia 763
Hypercholesterolemia 33*f*, 35*f*, 1043
  familial 27, 33, 35, 37, 60
  primary 595
Hypercontractile basal segment 673*f*
Hyperemic pressure gradient, mean 924
Hyperemic systolic pressure gradient 924
Hypereosinophilic syndrome 576, 577
Hyperglycemia 53, 92, 93
  treatment of 86
Hyperhomocysteinemia 993
Hyperkalemia 606, 607, 609, 763
  clinical manifestations of 606
  electrocardiography changes of 607*f*
  history of 610
  incidence of 588
  moderate 609
  moderate-to-severe 609
  newer drugs for 607
  old drugs for 607*t*
  therapy for 607
Hyperlipidemia 211, 593, 1047
Hypernatremia 786
Hyperparathyroidism 142
Hyperpigmentation 909
Hyperplasia
  adrenal 147
  bilateral adrenal 139
  congenital adrenal 139, 142
  idiopathic adrenal 146
Hyperprolactinemia 1043
Hypertension 46, 58, 101, 104*t*, 105, 111, 116, 121, 123, 125, 129, 133, 134, 146, 147, 151, 152, 154*t*, 156, 160, 180, 181, 184, 211, 588, 603, 620, 621*t*, 627, 636, 640, 648, 690, 706, 814, 853, 876, 878, 879, 893, 894, 901, 925, 927, 958, 983, 993, 995, 1007
  acute 259
  and preeclampsia intervention trial 968

anticancer drugs causing 620
chronic 966, 968
classification of 113
coat 137, 142, 143
cutoff for 119
daytime 154
diagnosis of 119
enhanced control of 888
epidemiology of 103
essential 142
gestational 958, 966
grading of 966
high attitude pulmonary 1033
in pregnancy 966
incidence of 113
intra-abdominal 998
isolated systolic 133, 150, 152
lower prevalence of 103
malignant 926
management of 933
newer drugs for 588
pattern 143
perioperative 142
pharmacological treatment of 123
pregnancy-induced 970
prevalence 104*t*, 106*t*, 108*t*, 109*f*, 110
correlation of 110, 110*t*, 111*f*
recent multisite studies of 105*f*
prevention of 115*t*, 117
primary
drugs for 125*t*
prevention of 113, 114, 116
resistant 137
rule out secondary 137
secondary 137, 139*t*, 142, 142*b*, 143, 143*b*, 144, 144*fc*, 146, 147
causes of 121
severe 146, 926
sustained 156
treatment of 933, 934
treatment-resistant 139
uncomplicated 123
Hypertensive disorders, classification of 966
Hyperthyroidism 139, 142, 147, 991
Hypertriglyceridemia 33*f*, 598
drug for management of 36
Hypertrophic cardiomyopathy
electrocardiographic features of 757
electrocardiography of 757*f*
symptom-free 984
Hypertrophy 1047
express extreme 1065
Hypoglossal nerves 936
Hypoglycemia 616
Hypoglycemic drugs 75
Hypogonadism 1043
Hypokalemia 135, 764
significant 144
Hypokalemic symptoms 146
Hypomagnesemia 135
severe 764
Hypoosmolar contrast media 243
Hypopneas 1005, 1009
Hypotension 287
ambulatory 157
anticipated 937
classical triad of 287
isolated diastolic 151
symptomatic 659
Hypothalamus 874
Hypothermia 763
moderate 296
Hypothesis, two-hit 972
Hypothyroidism 60, 139, 142, 147, 993, 994, 1005
and heart, treatment of 994
cases of 993
include bradycardia, symptoms of 993
subclinical 994
Hypovolemia 701
Hypoxia 763, 981
intermittent 1006
Hysterectomy 959

I

Ibritumomab 621
Ibrutinib 621
Ibutilide 764
Idarubicin 620
Idioventricular rhythm, accelerated 743
Iliac artery
common 947
external 947
Imipramine 623
Immunosuppressive drugs, standard 864
Immunosuppressive therapy 930
Impella 381, 667*f*
advantages 381
disadvantages 381
Implantable cardioverter defibrillator
meta-analysis of 801*t*
primary prevention 800*t*
role of 691
Implanted monitoring-only devices, remote monitoring with 654
Implanted therapeutic devices, remote monitoring with 651, 652
In vitro interactions 613
Inaccessible lesions, surgically 935

Incidental cancer-related pulmonary embolism, treatment of 920
Indapamide 125, 637
Indian Heart Rhythm Society 873
Infection 657
Inflammation 222
Infusion of dobutamine, low-dose 574
Inherited primary arrhythmia syndromes
  diagnosis of 760*f*
  management of 760*f*
Inotropes 666, 999
  empirical use of 669
Inotropic action, negative 188
In-stent restenosis 405, 948
Insulin 98, 607
  hormone 98
  resistance 958
    homeostatic model assessment for 80
Intensive care unit 659, 662, 866, 998
Intercellular adhesion molecule 874, 1044
Internal mammary artery
  bilateral 826
  right 823, 826
Internal thoracic artery, right 846, 847
International Carotid Stenting Study 937
International Congestive Heart Failure 627
International Index of Erectile Function Score 1046
International Lipid Expert Panel 57
International normalized ratio 618, 706, 883
International Olympic Committee 1065
International Society for Heart and Lung Transplantation 864
International Society on Thrombosis and Haemostasis Registry 920
International stroke, third 887
Interstitial fibrosis, idiopathic 1005
Interstitial plus replacement 576
Intervention cardiology, practitioner of 345
Interventional cardiology 1029, 1033, 1035
  Research Incooperation Society 193
Intima-media thickness 15, 176
Intra-aortic balloon
  counterpulsation 290
  pump 293, 295, 296, 372, 380, 382, 661, 667*f*, 674, 833, 1000
    advantages 381
    disadvantages 381
Intracardiac defibrillator implantation 211
Intracellular calcium 747
  overload 221
Intracerebral bleed 969
Intracranial small vessel disease 932
Intrapartum hypertension, management of severe 968*b*
Intraprocedural pain ratings, mean 913
Intrathoracic lesions 932
Intrauterine growth
  restriction 979
  retardation 978
Intravascular ultrasound 218, 240, 278, 350, 354, 366, 370, 372, 385, 411, 419
Intravenous iron complexes
  administration of 1004*t*
  dosage of 1004*t*
Intravenous p2y12 receptor inhibitor 322
Intravenous tissue plasminogen activator 903
Intraventricular dyssynchrony, evaluation of 484
Ion channel polymorphism 764
Ionizing radiation exposure 944
Iron
  binding capacity, total 1003
  carbohydrate nanoparticles 1004
  deficiency 1000, 1002, 1003
    functional 645
  hydroxide dextran 1004
  intravenous 1003
Ischemia 559, 932, 942, 959, 998, 1053
  detection of 175
  reperfusion injury 221
Ischemia-mediated ventricular tachycardia, presumed 195
Ischemic cardiomyopathy, management of 563
Ischemic heart disease
  assessment of 960
  clinical spectrum of 961
  electrocardiography of 759*f*
  evaluation of 573
Ischemic injury, therapy to reduce 223
Ischemic myocardium, protection of 188*b*
Ischemic stroke
  management of acute 887
  risk factor for 901*t*
  thrombolysis in acute 887
Ischemic syndromes study 89
Isoflurane 622
Isosorbide
  5-mononitrate 182
  dinitrate 182, 660
  mononitrate, use of 644
Isovolumic contraction 483
  phase 484
  time 483-485
Isovolumic relaxation 483, 484, 486*f*
  phase 484
  time 483, 484, 485*f*
Itching 908
Ivabradine 182, 183, 584, 586, 986

J

J-wave syndrome 762, 763
Jailed guide wire 360
Jaipur heart watch 33
 studies 32
Japanese Association for Thoracic Surgery 841
J-curve
 concept 150*f*
 pathophysiology of 150
Joint National Committee 113, 123
Judkin's transfemoral approach 400
Jugular venous pressure 95, 287, 650, 985
Juxtalesional skin necrosis 909

K

Kaplan-Meier survival curve 849*f*
Ketamine 981
Ketosis-prone diabetes 79
Kidney disease 243, 1053
 chronic 18, 35, 36, 95, 121, 181, 241, 243*f*, 370, 408, 603, 606, 609, 627, 631, 648, 938, 997, 1002, 1036, 1052
 intraventricular 637
Kidney injury
 acute 243, 296, 997
 molecule-1 999
Kissing balloon inflation 355
Korotkoff sounds 153

L

Labetalol 189, 967, 968*b*
Lacidipine 933
Lactate dehydrogenase 967
Lange-Nielsen syndrome 761
Lapatinib 622
L-arginine 182, 587
Laryngeal nerves 936
Laryngeal palsy 935
Laser 948
 angioplasty 349
Lead
 fracture 810*f*
 implantation 795
Leadless pacemaker 809, 811*t*, 813
Leaflet thrombosis 452
Lecithin-cholesterol acyltransferase 62
Left atrial appendage
 occlude, role of 735
 role of 881
Left main bifurcation stenting strategy, selection of 365
Left renal angiogram, postintervention selective 927*f*
Left ventricle 575, 751
 analysis results 573*t*
 dyssynchrony analysis 526
 ejection fraction 575
 mass 523
 morphology of 673*f*
 regional wall motion abnormalities 523
 systolic function of 511
 takotsubo cardiomyopathy 673*f*
Left ventricular
 assist device 743, 853, 854, 855*f*, 856, 858
  therapy 211
 diastolic pressure 481
 dysfunction 195, 706, 747, 849, 896
 ejection fraction 181, 242, 278, 311, 312, 337, 372, 380, 391, 427-429, 465, 479, 480, 560, 751, 765, 805, 812, 897, 970, 1046
 end-diastolic
  diameter 477, 975
  pressure 382, 672
  volume 391
 endomyocardial fibrosis 515, 515*f*
 end-systolic
  diameter 477
  volume 477, 477
 function 771, 841, 1051
 global longitudinal strain 794
 hypertrophy 121, 127, 143, 145, 146, 665, 757, 764, 1063, 1064
 myocardial infarction 286
 noncompaction 577, 1065
 outflow tract 450, 463, 531, 751
  gradient 456
 pressure-volume loop 483*f*
 systolic function 185, 277
Leg
 cramps 908
 pain, differential diagnosis of 942
 warmth 908
Lenient rate control 733
Leptin resistance 1006
Lesion revascularization, target 358, 384, 407, 948
Lethal arrhythmia 664
Leukocyte migration 959
Leukoencephalopathy, posterior 902
Levosimendan 659, 660
Licorice 142
Liddle syndrome 139
Lidocaine 785
 intravenous 748
Life-threatening ventricular arrhythmias 831
Limb ischemia, treatment of critical 945
Linoleic acid 47
Linum usitatissimum 50
Lipid

lowering therapy 84, 933
modification trial 597
profile 29, 66, 1046
status, monitoring of 54
rich plaque 420
Lipodermatosclerosis 907
Lipoprotein 20, 21, 28, 67
cholesterol
low-density 5, 42, 46, 61, 83, 593, 594, 1015, 1047
safety of low-density 599
intermediate density 596
lipase 54
lipids, abnormal values of 32
low-density 9, 21, 27, 32, 33, 35, 36, 54, 55, 57, 74, 90, 91, 180, 187, 262, 595, 596, 958, 993
metabolism 593
modifications 91
non-high-density 250
receptor, low-density 594
synthesis, very-low-density 28
very low density 28, 32, 596
Lisinopril 635
Liver 747
cirrhosis 183, 606
function 603, 878
abnormal 706, 893, 894
test 972
microsomal enzymes 613
resection 338
specific thyroid hormone 993
transplant 1050
Loeffler's syndrome 577
Logistic clinical syntax score 170
Lomitapide 596
Loratadine 623
Losartan 635
Lovastatin 617, 618
Low cholesterol diet 27
benefits of 31
Low fat, benefits of 31
Lower limb revascularization, open 338
Low-molecular weight heparin 241, 279, 617, 917, 920, 980
Luminal diameter, minimal 422
Lung 669, 747, 1063
diseases, chronic 1005
fluid accumulation 1021
ventilation 848

M

Macrolide 764
antibiotics 617
Macrovascular disorders 83
Magnesium
intravenous 717, 748
sulfate 786
supplementation 115
Magnetic resonance
angiography 139, 882, 923, 933, 944, 944*f*
imaging 174, 446, 448, 463, 751, 888, 973, 1046
Mammary artery
left internal 195, 396, 398, 819, 823, 824, 826, 837
right internal 820
Mandibular advancement devices 1008
Marfan syndrome 985
physical stigmata of 1065
Mass, adrenal 147
Mastocytosis 700
Maternal sepsis 973
Mechanical circulatory support 295, 375, 661, 667, 857
devices, types of 668*b*
Mechanically assisted circulatory support 856
Mechanochemical ablation 914
Medical services, emergency 298
Medical therapy 179, 467, 665, 800, 801, 896, 925, 933, 934
guideline directed 799
requirements for 791
Medication compliance problems 895
Medroxyprogesterone acetate 21
Membrane attack complex 91
Meperidine 981
MERIT heart failure 691*f*
Metabolic
acidosis 606
alkalosis 786
disturbances 682
syndrome 37, 958, 1043
treatment of 606
vasodilators 187
Metformin 96
Methodological hierarchies
emergence of 1039
top of 1039
Methotrexate 614
Methyltransferases 613
Metolazone 637
Metoprolol 189, 224, 241, 306, 974
myocardial infarction trial 724
succinate, sustained-release 690
tartrate 736
Mevastatin 618
Mianserin 623
Miconazole significantly potentiates 616
Micra device 811*f*
Microalbuminuria 998
Microsomal triglyceride transfer protein 596
inhibitor 596

Microvascular thrombosis 942
Midodrine 702
Milrinone 660, 974
Mineralocorticoid receptor antagonist 588, 590, 644, 665, 691, 974
Minimally invasive
  cardiac surgery 837
  coronary artery bypass grafting 837
  direct coronary artery bypass 837
    grafting 837*f*
    surgery 397
Mipomersen 596
Mitochondria, redistribution of 874
Mitochondrial permeability transition pore 222
Mitraclip 480*t*, 535
  implantation 543
  procedure 545*f*
Mitral annular
  calcification 897
  motion with atrial contraction, velocity of 642
  velocities 492
Mitral annulus 476
Mitral filling assessment 478
Mitral flow propagation 499
Mitral inflow 491
  measurements 491
  velocities 490
Mitral regurgitation 293, 448, 475, 477, 480, 527, 732
  diastolic 666
  echocardiographic impact of 479
  etiology of 475
  functional 479*t*, 529*f*
  management of functional 475
  mechanism of 475
  quantification of 476
  replacement in secondary 480*t*
  severe 433
  severity, assessment of 529
Mitral replacement 980
Mitral stenosis 478, 530, 978, 1050
  in pregnancy 978
    pathophysiology of 979
  severity 530
Mitral stroke volume 478
Mitral transcatheter paravalvular leak closure 465
Mitral valve 449, 450, 462, 464, 477, 480, 504, 527
  analysis software 529*f*
  deformation 477
  disease 897
  en face view of 528*f*
  function 452
  interventions 545
  morphology, assessment of 528
  pathologies 528*f*
  prolapse 897, 985
  repair 477*b*
  replacement 463
  stenosis 897
  surgical repair of 433
Mitral valvoplasty, surgical 980
Modafinil 1009
Molecular weight heparin, low 305, 1052
Molsidomine 182, 587
  dilates venous 587
Monascus purpureus 61
Monoamine oxidase 613
  inhibitors 139, 142
Monoclonal antibody 621
  based tyrosine kinase inhibitors 621
Monocyte
  chemoattractant protein 1044
  chemotactic protein-1 206
  derived macrophages 92
Monomorphic ventricular tachycardia, sustained 743
Monophasic transmitral flow pattern 492*f*
Monounsaturated fatty acids 41, 42, 46, 47
Motion artifacts 550
Motor vehicle accidents 144
Mountain sickness, acute 1033
Multicenter automatic defibrillator implantation trial 804, 805
Multicenter chronic total occlusion registry of Japan 379
Multiorgan dysfunction 296
Multiple scoring systems 296
Multipotent cardiac stem cells 426
Multislice computed tomography 175, 542
  angiography 175
Multivessel coronary artery disease 265, 266
  trial 396
Multivessel percutaneous coronary intervention
  advantages of 266*t*
  disadvantages of 266*t*
Multivessel sternotomy 836
Murray's law 355
Muscle
  atrophy 942
  blood flow 1062
  exercising 1062
  hypertrophied 515
  pump 698, 1062
  weakness 146
Muscular artery 820
Myalgia 58
Mycophenolate mofetil 864
Myeloid 577

Myeloperoxidase 999
Myocardial biopsy 859
Myocardial blood flow, restoration of 831
Myocardial contraction 512*f*
Myocardial contrast echocardiography 561
Myocardial delayed-enhancement 574
Myocardial disorders 576
  heterogeneous 690
Myocardial dysfunction 575
Myocardial edema 576
Myocardial fibrosis 146, 575
Myocardial glucose metabolism 561
Myocardial hypertrophy 579
Myocardial infarction 9, 14, 33, 35, 16*f*, 58, 74, 81, 115, 133, 173, 179, 187, 191, 204, 221, 261, 271, 278, 286, 292, 293, 307, 309, 312, 314-317, 323, 337, 364, 383, 401, 405, 414, 514, 570, 573*f*, 574, 574*f*, 583, 665, 706, 741, 746, 804, 842, 843, 876, 893, 896, 916, 934, 962, 1018, 1050, 1051
  acute 167, 222*f*, 236, 238, 249, 257, 260, 266*t*, 278*t*, 293*f*, 379, 408, 426, 428, 428*t*, 429, 721, 736, 737, 741, 742*fc*. 748, 765, 804, 809, 831, 832, 957, 1053
  anterior wall 492*f*
  evaluation of 573
  inferior wall 287
  long-term evaluation 279
  perioperative 833
  recurrent 198
  risk of 604
  secondary prevention after 314
  surgery in acute 831
  thrombolysis in 237, 256, 332
  trial 261, 306
  uncomplicated 994
Myocardial injury 207*f*
Myocardial iron deposition 576
Myocardial ischemia 995
  acute regional 763
Myocardial necrosis 239
Myocardial oxygen 188
  consumption 991
Myocardial performance index 288, 506
Myocardial perfusion 560, 568
  imaging 174, 555*f*
  positron emission tomography 277
  scintigraphy 549*f*, 553, 557*f*
  scores 271
  single-photon emission computed tomography 167, 168, 548
Myocardial protection 845, 846
Myocardial reperfusion 222
  injury 223*f*
    mediators of 221
Myocardial revascularization, hybrid 838
Myocardial siderosis 577
Myocardial strain
  imaging 564
  of myocardial segment 512*f*
Myocardial viability
  assessment of 559, 565
  diagnosis of 561*t*
Myocarditis 515, 574, 575, 1062, 1065
  acute 575*f*, 973
  pericarditis like syndrome 620
Myocardium 564*t*
  dysfunctional 559
Myolysis 874
Myonecrosis 58
Myopathy 58
Myosin light chain 60
Myositis 58, 942

N

N-acetyl D glucosaminidase 999
N-acetylcysteine 243, 717, 1000
N-acetyltransferases 613
Nadolol 189
Naftidrofuryl 945
Nanostim device 811*f*
Naproxen 717
Narcotics 1005
Narrowed pulse pressure 993
Nasal congestion 1008
National Cholesterol Education Program 89
National Consumer Disputes Redressal Commission 1055
National Diabetes Data Group 79
National Family Health Survey 103, 105, 106*t*, 107, 250
National Heart, Lung, and Blood Institute 32, 177
National Informatics Center 305
National Institute for Health and Care Excellence 966, 967
  guidelines 66
National Institute of Health 30
  Stroke Scale 888, 890, 902, 903
National Institute of Neurological Disorders and Stroke 887, 902
National Interventional Council 191
National Lipid Association 57
National Organ and Tissue Transplant Organization 866
National Program for Prevention and Control of Cancer, Diabetes, Cardiovascular Diseases, and Stroke 1013
Native coronary artery stenosis 822
Natriuretic peptide 235, 631, 641, 658, 1000
  receptor agonist 590
Nausea 287, 306, 700, 961
N-butyl cyanoacrylate 909
Near-field communication technology 1019
Nebivolol 189, 1048

Neck irradiation, ipsilateral 935
Necrotic myocardial cells 561
Nefazodone 617
Neodymium-doped yttrium aluminum garnet 1034
Neonatal diabetes 79
Nephropathy
  contrast-induced 243
  ischemic 923, 926
  prevention of 130
Nephrotoxic drugs 637
Nephrotoxins 998
Neprilysin inhibitor 589
Nerve 747
Neurofibromatosis 142
Neurogenic hypertension 142
Neurohormonal blockade 610
Neurohumoral control 188
Neurologic
  disorders 142
  dysfunction, episode of 932
  prognostication 785
Neurological function, loss of 932
Neurosurgical procedures 785
Neurotoxic drugs 700
Neurotransmitter uptake reactions 614
Neutrophil gelatinase-associated lipocalin 998
New York Heart Association 98, 428, 429, 434, 462, 480, 526, 644, 651, 666, 747, 791, 792, 807, 842, 856, 857, 935, 979, 1003, 1020
Newer oral anticoagulants 881
Niacin 62, 617
Nicorandil 182, 183, 184, 230, 584, 586
  effect of 584
  mechanism action of 585*fc*
Nicotiana rustica 3
Nicotiana tabacum 3
Nicotinamide adenine dinucleotide 833
  phosphate 998
Nielsen syndrome 752
Nifedipine 967, 968*b*
Nilotinib 621, 622
Nitinol 947
  feet, self-expanding 389
Nitrates 182, 230, 279, 289
Nitric oxide 188, 290, 998, 1044
  donors 1047
Nitroglycerin 660, 684*f*, 961, 974, 999
Nitroprusside 660
Nitrous oxide 41
Nocturnal hypertension 154, 156
Nonacute chest pain 570
Nonadherence with salt 657
Nonantithrombotic therapies 279
Nonarrhythmic mortality 804
Nonbacterial thrombotic endocarditis 897
Noncardiac diseases 658
Noncardiac dyspnea 484
Noncardiac surgery 330, 1050, 1052
  timing of 338
  undergo 1050
Noncommunicable diseases 39, 1013, 1014
Noncontrast computed tomography 882, 903
Noncoronary aortic cusp 774
Noncoronary artery bypass graft 323, 401
Noncoronary sinus left ventricular pacing 795
Nondiabetic chronic kidney disease 17
Nondihydropyridine 182, 772
Nonfasting lipid levels 66
Nonfatal
  myocardial infarction 120, 593
  stroke 120
Nonhealing ulcer 942
Noninvasive functional syntax score 169
Nonischemic cardiomyopathy
  care in 799
  natural history of 806
  recent onset 806
Nonischemic dilated cardiomyopathy, primary prevention in 801*t*
Non-obstructive coronary arteries 962
Nonpharmacological treatment 645, 701
Nonrandomized well-designed controlled trials 1037
Nonreceptor-mediated mechanisms 91
Nonshockable rhythm 785
Non-ST elevation
  acute coronary syndrome 226, 231*t*, 236*fc*, 243, 252*f*
    management of 230*b*
  acute myocardial infarction 306
  myocardial infarction 211, 237, 237*f*, 240, 262, 328, 413, 961
Non-sternotomy coronary artery bypass 836
Nonsteroidal anti-inflammatory drugs 126, 139, 142, 614, 636, 999
Nonstructural heart disease 758, 764
Non-ST-segment elevation
  acute coronary syndromes 308
  myocardial infarction 308, 383, 832
Nonsustained ventricular tachycardia 743, 751, 805
Nonthienopyridine 308
Nonvalvular atrial fibrillation 232*f*, 468, 601, 1035
Nonvasoactive pharmacologic therapy 294
Nonviable myocardium 563
Non-vitamin K antagonist oral anticoagulants 601-603, 728, 729
Norepinephrine 660
  preferable over dopamine 661
  uptake inhibitors, selective 139

Normal myocardial perfusion
scan and variants 548
single-photon emission computed tomography 548*f*, 549*f*
Normal pregnancy, physiology of 970
Normotension 156
North American Paradox 308
North American Symptomatic Carotid Endarterectomy Trial 932
Nortriptyline 623
No-touch technique 926
Novel oral anticoagulants 1052
Novel therapy 645
N-terminal pro-B-type natriuretic peptide 631, 658
Nuclear
chromatin 874
medicine 564
equipment 556
stress test, interpretation of 548
Nurses
health study 42
telephone support 1019

O

Obesity 46, 146, 181, 958, 1043, 1047
education initiative 74
related diabetes, mild 80
Obstructive coronary artery disease 391, 1046
Obstructive pulmonary disease 379
Obstructive sleep apnea 137, 139, 142, 144, 874, 1005, 1007*t*
complications of 1006
consequences of 1006
diagnosis of 1008
management of 1009
screening tools for 1006
Occlutech paravalvular leak device 465*f*
Occult blood loss 1003
Occult coronary disease 1063
Off-pump coronary artery bypass 836, 837
grafting 833, 848
Olanzapine 623
Omega-3 fatty acids 47
Omeprazole 724
OPAL-HK trial 609*f*
OPAL-K trial 609*f*
Opiates relieve dyspnea 661
Opioid overdose 785
Optical coherence tomography 350, 351, 372, 385, 419, 421, 423
correlation of 422
disadvantages of 422
future of 351
imaging, clinical utility of 422
interpretation 420
intracoronary 419
principles of 419
role of 367
Optimal medical
management 179
therapy 179, 180, 191, 193, 204, 266, 843, 945
treatment 933, 945
Optimal replacement fatty acid 41
Optimizing platelet inhibition 309
Oral acetylsalicylic acid 278
Oral anticoagulant 468, 448*t*, 469, 879, 882, 883, 894
chronic 721
Drugs Act 601
new 468, 705, 707, 880, 881, 883, 895, 895*t*
Oral anticoagulation therapy 879
Oral antiplatelet agents 307*t*
Oral cavity 11
Oral contraceptive 918
Oral dental surgery 1052
Oral glucose 561
Oral soluble guanylate cyclase stimulators 644
Orbital atherectomy 371, 372, 373*t*, 376
Oregon-sudden unexpected death 766
Organ
damage, target 143
donation 864
states in 867*f*
protection, target 125
supply 859
Orthopedic surgery 916, 1050
Orthopnea 972
Orthostatic hypotension 681, 696, 700-702
causes of 698, 699*t*
clinical presentation 700
differential diagnosis 701
leading to syncope 680
management 701
nonpharmacological treatment 701
pharmacological treatment 701
prevalence of 696
testing for 700
treatment 701
Orthostatic
intolerance 701
response, physiology of normal 696
testing 700, 701
Oslo Diet-Heart study 27
Osteoarthritis
hip 942
knee 942
Ostial coronary lesions 384
Ostial disease, evaluation of 384
Ostial dissection 386*f*

Ostial internal iliac artery, stenosis of right 944*f*
Ostial lesions 384, 390
Ostial stent 390*b*
  placement, techniques for 388
Ostial superficial femoral artery 949*f*
Oxidative stress 90, 92, 93, 221, 923
  injury 923
Oxygen
  consumption, substantial increase in 1061
  peak volume of 644
  pulse curve 1063
  support 658
  uptake, maximum 1063

P

Pace mapping 773
Pacemaker implantation, permanent 445
Paclitaxel-eluting stents 406
Pain 700, 908
  abdominal 306
  prevention of 981
Painful gynecomastia 639
Palatine tonsils, enlargement of 1008
Pallor 147
Palmaz Schatz coronary stent 347, 404*f*
Pancuronium 981
Pansystolic murmur 985
Papaverine 412
Papillary muscle rupture 295, 831
Paraneoplastic autonomic neuropathies 700
Parasternal long-axis 505
Parasympathetic nervous system 997
Paravalvular leak 450, 463, 543
  closure 465, 467, 535, 543
    devices 465*f*
  etiology of 462
  percutaneous management of 462
Parenteral direct thrombin inhibitor 279
Paresthesia 911, 913
Parkinson's disease 698, 1043
Paroxysmal
  arrhythmias, diagnosis of 1022
  atrial fibrillation 814, 1022
  hypertension 147
  nocturnal dyspnea 961, 972, 985
  supraventricular tachycardia, ablation of 1035
Paroxysms 873
Patent bilateral internal mammary artery 823*f*
Patent ductus arteriosus 505, 985, 1034
Patent foramen ovale 435, 856, 893, 895, 896
  occluder device 290
  occlusion 435
Patent vein 845
Pathak trial 263
Patiromer
  adverse effects of 610*b*
  sorbitex calcium 607, 610
    adverse effects of patiromer 610
    dosage and administration 610
    OPAL-K trials 609
Pazopanib 621
Peak plasma concentration, time to 880
Peak systolic velocity 923
Pedal edema 145
Pediatric
  cardiology 1029
  heart transplant 865
Pemafibrate 598
Penbutolol 189
Penicillins 616
Penile artery 1045
Pentoxifylline 945
Percutaneous balloon mitral valvuloplasty 980
Percutaneous closure, program of 1034
Percutaneous coronary intervention 37, 95, 167, 179, 180, 191, 192, 194, 195, 195*t*, 199, 221, 230, 232, 242, 243, 252, 262, 266, 268, 271, 276, 279*f*, 282, 283, 289, 294, 296, 300, 310, 312, 313, 315*f*, 332, 336, 337, 339, 353, 363, 364, 364*t*, 370, 372, 380, 384, 391, 393, 396, 398, 400, 404, 411, 413-415, 419, 433, 448, 583, 603, 604, 721, 721*f*, 722, 722*b*, 727, 783, 831, 842, 843*t*, 961, 1018, 1051, 1052
  benefits of 1028
  high-risk 383*t*
  in atrial fibrillation 721
  primary 223, 242, 256, 261, 271, 298, 305, 265, 283, 283*f*, 737
  procedural planning of 422
  techniques 393
Percutaneous mitral valve
  repair 545
  therapies 433
Percutaneous paravalvular leak closure 465
Percutaneous robotically enhanced coronary intervention trial 436
Percutaneous septal ablation, historical development of 455
Percutaneous transluminal
  balloon angioplasty 946, 948
  coronary angioplasty 191, 243, 278, 347, 385, 415, 1034
  renal angioplasty 925
  septal myocardial ablation 455, 456*f*
Percutaneous tricuspid valve therapies 434
Percutaneous valve implantation 437
Percutaneous ventricular restoration 437
Percutaneous ventriculoplasty devices 434
Perfusion pressure, preserved 294
Periarteriolar autoregulation 187

Pericardial disease 484, 578
Pericardial mass 228
Pericarditis 1062, 1065
  constrictive 228, 287, 519*f*, 578*f*
Perimedial fibroplasia 928, 928*f*
Peripartum cardiomyopathy 970, 971, 971*f*, 972*b*, 974*t*, 978, 983, 984
  Association 984
  differential diagnoses of 973*b*
  etiopathogenesis of 970
  medications 974*t*
Peripheral angiography 944, 945*f*
Peripheral angioplasty 1034
Peripheral arterial
  angioplasty 338
  disease 893
Peripheral artery 1034
  disease 317, 318, 941
    management of 946, 947*f*
Peripheral health centers 669
Peripheral ischemic complications 295
Peripheral vascular
  disease 83, 123, 145, 211, 636, 819, 905
  resistance 1061
  surgery 1050
Periprocedural myocardial infarction 391
Periprocedural stroke 713, 937
Permeability glycoprotein 602
P-glycoprotein 601, 602, 613
Pharmacoinvasive strategy 256, 262
Pharmacokinetic interaction 612, 616
Pharmacological testing 1051
Pharmacological therapy 658
Pharmacological treatment 701
Pharmacology therapy 734
Pharyngeal cancers 11
Phenothiazine 614
  neuroleptics 764
Pheochromocytoma 139, 142, 147
Phillips volcano system 416*f*
Phone-based systems 1019
Phosphodiesterase
  inhibitor 999
  type 5 inhibitor 644
    agents 1047
Phosphorylcholine 405, 406
Photodynamic therapy 948
Photon emission computed tomography, single 277, 548
Phrenic nerve 712
Phytosterolemia 593
Pickering syndrome 145
Pickwickian syndrome 1005
Pindolol 189
Piroxicam 617
Placenta, hypoperfusion of 967
Placental abruption 969
Plain balloon angioplasty 947
Plain old balloon angioplasty 833
Plaque progression, reduce 181
Plasma
  aldosterone
    concentration 146
    renin ratio 137
  cholesterol profile 68*t*
Plasminogen activator
  inhibitor 20, 90, 889
  type 9
Platelet
  aggregation 21, 336, 942, 959
    assessment of 316
    inhibition of 317
  count 882
  dependent enzyme cyclooxygenase 722
  derived growth factor 999
  function
    inhibitors of 722
    testing of 316, 332
  inhibition 308
    and patient outcomes 309
    management of 329
  rich
    clot 258
    thrombus 889
  transfusion 340
    timing of 336
Platinum-chromium 405
Pneumatic compression, intermittent 941
Pneumonectomy 338
Pneumonia 658, 973, 1050, 1054
Pneumothorax 809
Polidocanol 910
Polycystic kidney disease 142
Polycystic ovarian
  disease 958
  syndrome 1005
Polydipsia 146
Polylactic acid 407
Polymer coating 405
Polymorphic ventricular tachycardia 743
Polysomnography 1005
Polytetrafluoroethylene 433
Polytrauma 919
Polyunsaturated fatty acid 40, 41, 47
Polyuria 146
Polyvinyl chloride 347
Ponatinib 621

Positive airway pressure, continuous 658, 659, 1006
Positive exercise stress test 549*f*
Positive pressure ventilation 658
Positron emission tomography 174, 416, 417, 561, 694, 960
Postatheroablation angioplasty 376
Postcardiac resynchronization therapy 793*f*
Postcardiac surgery 211
Postcardiac transplantation 579
Postcardioversion anticoagulation 737
Postcoronary angioplasty 211
Postcoronary artery bypass graft 569
Postdilatation 273
Postdischarge period 212
Posterior descending artery 824, 826, 846, 847
Postexertional syncope 1063
Postgadolinium administration 576
Postheart transplantation 579
Post-myocardial infarction 242
Postpartum hypertension 966
Postprandial hypotension 154, 157
Postprandial lipemia 53
Postprandial metabolic issues 43
Poststenting hypotension 937
Post-stress ejection fraction 552
Post-thrombotic syndrome 916, 918
Post-transcatheter aortic valve 453*f*
Postural orthostatic tachycardia syndrome 701
Postventricular assist device implantation management 856
Pot technique 356
Potassium
 channel blockers 748
 depleting drugs 614
 intake 115
 supplementation 115
Potential cardiac recipients, categorization of 668
Pot-side-pot technique 359*f*
Prasugrel 241, 282, 308, 312, 314, 321, 323-325, 330, 336, 728
 to ticagrelor, switch from 326
Pravastatin 617
Precordial thump 786
Preeclampsia 966, 967, 967*t*, 973, 983
 clinical symptoms of 967
 prevention of 967
 risk factors for developing 967*t*
 severe 967
Pregnancy 142, 983, 984
 hormonal milieu of 971
 hypertensive disorders of 966
Premature ventricular complexes, ablation of 774
Preparticipation screening 1063, 1065
Pressure
 half-time 463
  measurement 530
 ratio, resting 924
Pro-adrenomedullin, mid-regional 999
Proatrial natriuretic peptide, mid-regional 633
Procainamide 623, 764
Procalcitonin 633
Progenitor cells, circulating 428, 429
Proinflammatory markers and mediators, production of 1047
Prolactin 970
Proliferator-activated receptors gamma 590
Promotility medications 764
Prone cardiopulmonary resuscitation 785
Prone free-breathing stress imaging 553
Prophylactic hemodialysis 244
Propranolol 189, 241, 618
Proprotein convertase subtilisin/kexin inhibitors 55, 61, 62, 594, 595
Prostaglandin 615, 1048
 therapy 1048
Prostate
 carcinoma of 1043
 surgery 1050
Prosthetic cardiac valves 897
Prosthetic heart valves 985
 dysfunction, assessment of 534*f*
Prosthetic valve 534, 893, 1017, 1021, 1052
 annulus 465
 endocarditis 534
 rocking motion of 465
Proteasome inhibitors 620, 621
Protein
 activated 707
 from plant sources, role of 42*t*
 kinase C 90, 92
  activation 93
 source 42
Proteolysis 874
Prothrombin
 complex concentrate 339, 340
 time 616
Proton pump inhibitors 616
 interaction of 618
Provisional one-stent technique 365
Provisional side branch stenting strategy 356
Proximal isovelocity surface area 477
 method 477
Proximal right coronary artery 289*f*
Proximal veins 918*t*
 of legs 916
Pseudoaneurysms 574
Pseudo-delta wave 775, 776
Pseudohypertension 143
Pseudomonas aeruginosa 857
Psychogenic pseudosyncope 682
Psychosocial stress 1043
Pubic symphysis 980

Pulmonary arterial
hypertension 644, 1006
systolic pressure 979
Pulmonary artery 438, 1020, 1047
catheterization 890
denervation 438
pressure 438
diastolic 504, 505
mean 504, 505
Pulmonary capillary wedge pressure 379, 436, 489, 643, 657
Pulmonary disease, chronic obstructive 174, 636, 814, 935, 1005, 1008
Pulmonary edema 927, 927*ff*, 969, 978, 983
mild 984
Pulmonary embolism 657, 763, 910, 916, 919, 1050, 1054
acute 287, 658, 973
treatment of 601
Pulmonary hypertension 145, 576, 648, 984, 1017
severe 287, 863
sustained 910
telemonitoring in 1021
Pulmonary stenosis, mild 985
Pulmonary thromboembolism 208, 973
Pulmonary tuberculosis, streptomycin treatment of 1039
Pulmonary vascular resistance 504, 505
Pulmonary vein 479, 642, 874
flow 496, 497*f*, 498*f*
parameters 499
pattern 497*f*
signals, acquisition of 498
isolation 713
ostia 713*f*
Pulmonary venous return 286
Pulse 1017
Pulsed Doppler wave 478
Pulsed wave Doppler mitral flow 487*f*
Pump
failure, progressive 664
inhibitors 724
thrombosis 857
Purkinje fibers 749
Pursuit risk score 229

Q

QT interval, short 1064
QT syndrome
diagnosis short 762
diagnostic scoring scheme, short 763*t*
long 752, 757, 761, 763, 763*t*, 1062
short 757, 762, 763, 1062
subclinical long 764
Quantitative flow ratio 417, 436
Quetiapine 623
Quinidine 623, 748, 764
Quinine 623
Quinolones 616
Q-wave myocardial infarction 363

R

RADAR systems 1022
Radial artery 819, 820, 824-826, 846, 847
bilateral 820
unilateral 820
Radiation
injury 391
therapy 932
Radio detection and ranging 1017
Radiofrequency ablation 909, 910, 913, 914
Radionuclide
myocardial perfusion imaging 174
single proton emission computed tomography 174
ventriculography 288
Radiopaque contrast media 243
Ramipril 635, 974
Ramucirumab 621
Randomized clinical trials 443, 932
Randomized controlled trial 21, 43, 162, 211, 443, 604, 710, 733, 801, 875, 890, 1003, 1015, 1036, 1038-1041
Ranolazine 182, 183, 230, 583, 586, 623
mechanism action of 584*fc*
RAO cranial projection 416*f*
Rapamycin, mammalian target of 621
Rapid onset of dyspnea 972
Raynaud's phenomena 189
Reactive oxygen species 221, 222, 971, 998
Receptor neprilysin inhibitor 638
Recombinant tissue plasminogen activator 902
Recurrent sustained ventricular tachycardia, catheter ablation of 744
Red blood cell 462, 1003
deformability, reduced 942
Reflex syncope 680, 681
Reflux 908
Refractory angina 430, 437
Refractory ventricular
fibrillation, management of 744
tachycardia, management of 744
Regional wall motion abnormality 671
Regorafenib 621
Regurgitant fraction 463
Regurgitant orifice 477
effective 463, 479
Regurgitant volume 463, 479
Rehabilitation 233
Remote monitoring in heart failure, role of 652*t*
Renal angioplasty 928*f*

Renal artery
- chronic total occlusion, bilateral 927
- lesion 925
- occlusions 927
- stenosis 139, 145, 923, 924, 924*b*, 929, 1034
  - atheromatous 142
  - detection of 923
  - evaluation 924*t*
- stenting 925
  - no touch technique of 927*f*

Renal atherosclerotic lesion 925
Renal biomarker 998
Renal cell carcinoma 142
Renal denervation 140, 438
- catheter based 140

Renal disease 60, 603*t*, 878
- end-stage 123, 242, 876, 881, 1005

Renal double curve 927
Renal dysfunction 240, 241*t*, 281, 603, 881
Renal failure 133, 658, 901, 969, 1054
Renal flow reserve 924
Renal fractional flow reserve 924
Renal function 145, 637
- abnormal 706, 893, 894
- significant deterioration of 143
- tests 1046

Renal injury 391
Renal insufficiency 966, 1050
Renal parenchymal disease 146
Renal replacement therapy 243, 661
Renal segmental hypoplasia 142
Renal sympathetic activity 631
Renal tumors 142
Renin inhibitor 590
Renin promotes 698
Renin-angiotensin
- aldosterone 636
  - axis 923
  - system 15, 85, 96, 125-127, 139, 144, 207, 279, 606, 609, 643, 656, 698, 997, 1002, 1003
- system 129, 631, 923
  - local 691

Renocardiac syndrome
- acute 997
- chronic 997

Renovascular hypertension 142, 923
Reperfusion
- injury, reduce 224
- therapy 276, 283, 293

Repolarization, abnormalities of 766
Reproductive system 957
Rescue percutaneous coronary intervention 261
Research study designs, types of 1038
Reserpine 1048
Residual aortic regurgitation 444
Residual cholesterol risk 599
Residual syntax score 170
Resins 607
Resistant hypertension 137, 138*fc*, 926
- treating 137

Respiratory disturbance index 1009
Respiratory failure 656
Rest pain, ischemic 942
Restenosis 927, 938
Resting pressure gradient, mean 924
Restless legs 908
Restrictive cardiomyopathy 287, 576
Reticuloendothelial system 240, 241, 1003
Retinopathy 74, 121
- hypertensive 143

Revascularization 191, 560, 925, 945, 946
- modality 926
- surgical 950

Revascularizing nonculprit artery 265
Rhabdomyolysis 58
Rheumatic
- disease 475
- heart disease 627, 710, 852, 873
- mitral stenosis 530*f*

Rheumatoid arthritis 958
Rhythm control 718, 733, 736, 878
Ridaforolimus-eluting stent 407
Rifamycins 616
Right ventricle 791
- assessment 524
- Takotsubo cardiomyopathy 673*f*

Right ventricular
- assist device 290, 296
- chamber dimensions
  - and volumes 505*t*
  - assessment 503
- echocardiography 503
- ejection fraction, reduced 750
- fractional area change 506
- function 506*t*
- hypertrophy 979, 1064
  - pattern 1064
- infarction 296
- ischemia 286
- myocardial
  - infarction 286, 288*f*
  - performance index 506
- outflow tract 504, 505, 752, 773*f*, 814
- perforation of 809
- strain imaging 507
- wall motion assessment 509

Rituximab 621
Rivaroxaban 468, 601, 603, 708, 880, 881, 894, 895
  bioavailability 601
  dose of 602
  plus aspirin 318
Robotic percutaneous coronary intervention 436
Romano-Ward syndrome 761
Rotablation 948
Rotational atherectomy 349, 371, 372, 373*t*, 376
Rutherford classification of peripheral artery disease, modified 942*t*

S

Sacubitril 589
Safe pressure resistant cylindrical balloons 347
Salpingo-oophorectomy, bilateral 959
Saphenofemoral junction 907, 912, 912*f*
Saphenopopliteal junction 907
Saphenous vein
  graft 397, 819, 824, 825, 841, 843, 844, 846
  short 907
Sapheon 913
Sapien 3 valve 445
Sarcoidosis 576, 643
Sarcopenic adiposity 43
Sarcoplasmic reticulum 222, 874
Saroglitazar 598
Saturated fatty acid 41, 46
Scar ventricular tachycardia 758
Scientifically trustworthy empirical evidence 1036
Scleroderma 142
Sclerosing agents 909, 910*t*
Sclerosis, multiple 1043
Sclerotherapy 909
  efficacy of 910
  technique 910*f*
Scoring balloon 387, 947
  angioplasty 371
Screening abnormalities 1063
Screening tests 173
  safety of 176
Seagull's sign 475
Second-generation drug-eluting stents 200
Sedative drugs 1005
Sedentary counterparts 1062
Seizure disorder 682
Selenium deficiency 970
Sensitive inversion recovery 574, 575
Sepsis 1050, 1054
Septal
  ablation 455, 459
    technique of 456
  defect closure, interatrial 543
  hypertrophy, asymmetrical 758
  puncture 544*f*
  wall thinning 573*f*
Septum
  interatrial 504, 544
  intraventricular 457
  wall 550
Serotonin reuptake inhibitor, selective 139
Serum 25-hydroxy vitamin D level 16
Serum amyloid 90
Serum biomarkers 877
Serum creatinine 637
Serum ferritin 1003
Serum lactate dehydrogenase 462
Serum potassium 609, 637
Serum vitamin D levels
  after supplementation 18
  before supplementation 18
Sevoflurane 622
Sexual function 698
Sheath size 382
Shock 735
  trial 294
    registry 293
Shunting, right to left 896*f*
Shy-Drager syndrome 698
Side branch ostial disease 356
Siesta dipping 154
Sildenafil 614, 616
Simcard trial 1014
Simultaneous kissing stent 366
  technique 366
Simvastatin 616-618
Single-chamber pacemakers 813
Single-photon emission computed tomography 428, 429, 550*f*, 551*f*, 554*f*-557*f*, 561, 694
Sinotubular junction 449*f*, 450
Sinus
  arrhythmia 1062, 1064
  bradycardia 494, 496*f*, 1063, 1064
  rhythm, restoration of 718
Sirolimus-eluting stent 406, 407, 927
Sitosterolemia, homozygous 593
Six-minute walk distance 434
Sjögren's syndrome, primary 700
Skeletal muscle 1063
  diseases of 1063
Skeletonized harvesting 822
Skin 747
  atrophy 942
  fissures 942
  necrosis 914

Sleep
- disorders in heart failure by remote monitoring 652
- disruption, arousals 1006

Small dense low density lipoprotein 53
Small diameter vessels 349
Small molecule tyrosine kinase 622
- inhibitors 621

Smokeless cardiovascular
- disease 3, 6
- risk factors 5

Smokeless tobacco
- disease 3, 6
- risk factors 5
- types of 3*t*

Smoking 145, 958, 1048
- cessation 945
  - meta-analysis 1015

Snoring 144
Snuff 4
Sodium 589
- bicarbonate 607, 786
- channel 764
  - blockers 748
- chloride 1004
- current inhibition, late 645
- fecal contents of 607
- glucose co-transporter 2 75, 76, 86
  - inhibitors 76, 96
- intake 115
- polystyrene sulfonate 606, 607
- reduction 115, 923
- tetradecyl sulfate 909, 910
- zirconium cyclosilicate 607, 608, 608*f*

Soft tissue attenuation, artifacts of 549
Sole therapy 838
Solitary 927
Soluble nutrients 28
Soluble vascular endothelial growth factor receptor-1 999
Sorafenib 620, 621
Sotalol 189, 623, 716, 734, 748, 764
Speckle tracking 794
- echocardiography 561
- imaging method 507

Spinal cord
- disorders 1043
- injury 919
- stimulation 941
  - ultrasound therapy 945

Spinal immobility of neck 935
Spinal stenosis 942
Spine surgery 338
Spironolactone 635, 974, 985, 1048
Splanchnic veins 916
Splenectomy 338
Spontaneous coronary artery 963
- dissection 959, 961, 963, 978

Spontaneous echocardiographic contrasts 877
Sports
- and heart diseases 1061
- cardiology 1062

Stabilization, ischemic 306
Stable angina 184, 185, 192
- chronic 179, 191, 204, 211

Stable coronary artery disease 58, 179, 187, 191, 1028
Stable ischemic heart disease 179, 194, 194*t*, 195, 200
- guideline 204

Stamina 1061
Standalone instantaneous wave-free ratio approach 417
Standard-dose alteplase 888
Staphylococcus aureus 857
Stasis 916
State hypothesis, low-flow 997
Statin 53, 84, 182, 241, 242, 280, 618, 717, 945, 1048
- alternatives, second-line 62*b*
- associated muscle symptoms 57-59
- during carotid artery stenting 934
- induced muscle disease 61*f*
- intensity of 55*t*
- intolerance 57
  - evaluation of 59
  - management of 62*t*
  - types of 57
- therapy 934, 1048, 1053
  - initiation of 54

Status epilepticus 469
Stearic acid 49
ST-elevation
- in takotsubo cardiomyopathy 673*f*
- myocardial infarction 211, 223, 243, 256, 258, 265, 266, 268, 276, 281, 282, 295, 298, 306, 321, 379, 400, 657, 958, 1017
  - India project 299
  - treated 308

Stem cell 426
- cardiopoietic 430
- retention of 427
- therapy 579, 941, 946
- trials 428*t*
  - in ischemic cardiomyopathy 428*t*
  - in nonischemic cardiomyopathy 429*t*

Stenosed aortic valve 1034
Stenosis 925
- angiographic 932
- degree of 568, 822
- iliofemoral 1034
- left main 842

progression 933
severity, reliable measurement of 933
tubular areas of 928
Stenotic vein graft 847
multiple 843
Stent
choice of 274
deployment 387
diameter 423
expansion 423
length selection 423
malapposition 423
platforms, contemporary 406*f*
positioning 387
pull back technique 389, 389*f*
related complication 391
restenosis 843
selection 387, 423
and deployment 360
self-expandable 947
strut malapposition 422*f*
thrombosis 322, 405, 721
risk of 721
six 930
Stenting strategy in bifurcation lesions 356
Sterility 1059
Sternal wires, lifting of anterior 845*f*
Sternotomy
and dissection 845
lifting 845*f*
Steroid 142
anabolic 139, 1063
Sterol regulatory element-binding protein 2 595
Stitching artifact 421*f*
Stop-bang questionnaire 1006
Strain curves, velocities of 514*f*
Strain imaging, speckle tracking for 512
Streptokinase 257
fibrinolytic property of 256
global utilization of 282
Stress
cardiomyopathy 578
cardiovascular magnetic resonance 960
echocardiogram 168
echocardiography 167, 174, 574, 960
management 115
myocardial perfusion
positron emission tomography 960
single-photon emission computed tomography 960
positron emission tomography myocardial perfusion scintigraphy 548
testing 277, 1051
transthoracic echocardiogram 479
Stroke 74, 83, 133, 251, 309, 401, 446, 603, 706, 871, 873, 874, 878, 892, 894, 901, 903, 916, 933, 1005
acute ischemic 875, 882, 887, 888
algorithm 903*fc*
and transient ischemic attack 874
cardioembolic 892
cryptogenic 875
ischemic 435
definition of 932
evolution, understanding 889
hemorrhagic 249*f*, 902
high risk of 895
in atrial fibrillation 879*fc*
epidemiology of 705
primary prevention of 879, 881
in cardiac patients, prevention of 892
in cath lab 901, 902
differential diagnosis 902
evaluation 902
incidence 901
mechanism and risk factors 901
treatment 902
incidence of 901
index 573
ischemic 18, 902
mechanism in atrial fibrillation 874
perioperative 937
physicians 932
predictors in atrial fibrillation 877
prevention 37, 601, 705, 732, 734, 879
existing options of 468
in atrial fibrillation 705, 706, 725, 881, 893
primary 880*t*
secondary 880*t*
previous 895, 901
remains 892
risk 705, 722, 873
episodes predictive of 876
estimation of 705
in atrial fibrillation 877
stratification scores 876
thrombolysis 903
recent advances in 888
treatment of 937
volume 573, 852, 1061
Structural heart disease 542, 687, 757, 772, 775
Strut thickness in drug-eluting stents, significance of 407
ST-segment
depression 1064
elevation acute coronary syndrome 401
elevation myocardial infarction 226, 235, 247, 249, 260, 262, 311, 832
acute 261*t*, 271, 276

guidelines 262*t*
treatment delay in 260
Stump morphology 393
Stunning myocardium 560
phenomenon of 560
Subacute cardiotoxicity 620
Subarachnoid hemorrhage 763
Subclavian thrombosis 812
Subclinical hypothyroidism, treatment of 994
Subcutaneous cardioverter defibrillator 749
Subcutaneous fibrosis 918
Subcutaneous tissue 942
Subdiaphragmatic radiotracer activity, artifacts of 550
Subintimal angioplasty 949
Substance abuse 1005
Sucrose 1004
Sudden cardiac arrest, history of 763
Sudden cardiac death 690, 744, 746, 748, 749, 751, 756, 756*f*, 760, 801, 805, 993, 1061
burden of 799
electrocardiography in 756*t*
in heart failure 799
prevention of 799
risk of 804
drug therapy in 690
survivors of 195, 756
therapies for 747
Sudden death in dilated cardiomyopathy 690
Sudden infant death syndrome 763, 1022
Sulfonylureas 97
Summation reaction 614*t*
Sunflower oil 49
Sunitinib 620, 621
Superficial venous system, anatomy of 907*f*
Superoxide dismutase 971
Supine electrocardiogram-gated stress imaging 553, 555
Supra-aortic trunks 933
Supraventricular tachycardia, lower incidence of 583
Surgery
bleeding risk of 1052
types of 337, 338*t*
Swelling 909
Sympathetic nervous system 126, 139, 997, 998
Synchronous bilateral carotid interventions 936
Syncope 677, 679, 682, 687, 700, 962, 985
diagnosis of 680
during exercise 1063
exercise-related 455
patients with 686
severity 680
tilt table testing in 682
unexplained 687, 763
Synergistic reaction 614*t*
Syntax score 169, 170, 368
prognostic value of 169
Syntax trial 199
Systemic arterial vasodilation 1047
Systemic blood pressure 142, 1009
elevated 1065
Systemic diseases and heart 989
Systemic hypertension 123, 153
Systemic lupus erythematosus 958, 967, 1000
Systemic vascular resistance 978, 991
fall of 983
Systemic ventricular dysfunction 979
Systolic blood pressure reduction of 150
Systolic dysfunction 628, 970
Systolic dyssynchrony index 526
Systolic heart failure, nonischemic 692, 693
Systolic hypertension 151
Systolic pressure gradient
peak hyperemic 924
peak resting 924
resting 924
Systolic pulmonary artery pressure 504, 505
Systolic volume 522
Szabo's technique 388, 388*f*, 389*f*

T

T wave inversion 1064
Tachyarrhythmia 657, 1061
treatment of 994
Tachy-Brady syndrome 711, 812
Tachycardia 656, 981
focal ventricular 780*f*
incessant ventricular 807
Tacrolimus 139, 617, 864
Tail wire technique 388, 388*f*, 389*f*
Takayasu arteritis 384, 923, 929
Takotsubo cardiomyopathy 578, 671, 962
management of 674*t*
Tamil Nadu Health Systems Project 299
Tamponade 809
TandemHeart 295, 381, 667*f*
advantages 381
disadvantages 382
percutaneous ventricular assist device 290
Tapered stents, self-expanding 937
Technetium-99m 561
labeled tracer 550, 551, 553, 554-556
Technological advancements 809
Telangiectatic matting 909
Tele-echocardiography 1021
services 1017
Tele-electrocardiography 1018
Telehealthcare 1017

Telemonitoring systems 1022
Temporary pacemakers 786
Temporary pacing 374
Temsirolimus 621
Tenecteplase 257
Terfenadine 623
Termination of pregnancy, timing of 968
Tessari technique 910
Testosterone 586
  deficiency 1048
  replacement therapy 1048
  role of 1048
Tetralogy of Fallot, repaired 985
Thallium-201 561
Therapeutic implications 648
Therapeutic range 603
  time in 602
Thermal coronary angiography 839
Thiazide
  diuretic 135, 637, 1048
  like diuretic 134
  type diuretic 125, 135
Thiazolidinediones 98, 622
Thienopyridine 278, 307, 314, 321
Thioridazine 623, 764
Thiothixene 614
Thoracic artery, left internal 820, 844*f*, 845*f*, 846, 847
Thoracic epidural anesthesia 744
Thoracotomy 848
Three-dimensional echocardiography 521, 530
Thrombectomy
  solitaire with intention for 890
  standard 882
Thrombocytopenia 920, 920*f*, 966
Thromboembolism 874, 1021
  prevention of 737
  prophylaxis 661
Thrombolysis 298, 918
  catheter directed 918
  in myocardial infarction, risk of 313
  in wake-up stroke 888
  role of 888
  stroke study 888
Thrombolytic agent
  activates plasminogen 887
  next generation 888
Thrombolytic therapy, effects of 918
Thrombophilia 916
Thrombophlebitis 909
Thromboplastin time, partial 617
Thromboprophylactic and therapeutic realm 882
Thrombosis 942
  cancer-associated 919
  endovenous heat-induced 911
  prevention of 601
  risk of 336, 721
Thrombosuction 273
Thromboxane 257, 722, 723
Thrombus 901
  direct imaging of 917
Thyroid 747
  disorders 146
  dysfunction, amiodarone induced 994
  function 994
  hormone 991, 992*f*
    effects of 991
    metabolism 994
    response elements 991
  receptors 991
  replacement therapy 994
  stimulating hormone 147, 972, 991
Thyrotoxicosis 973
Ticagrelor 241, 282, 308, 312, 322, 330, 336, 728
  to prasugrel, switch from 326
Ticlopidine 306, 321, 616, 617
Timolol 189
Timothy syndrome 752
Tirofiban 241, 336
Tissue
  Doppler imaging 503, 561
    of right ventricular 507
  factor pathway inhibitor 707
  inhibitor of metalloproteinases 643
  loss, minor 942
  motion 487
  plasminogen activator 20, 278, 889, 903
  prolapse 424
Tobacco
  control policy 4
  use of 115, 1043
Toe-brachial index 943
Torasemide 140, 612, 637
Torsade de pointes 764*t*
Tortuous carotid artery 937
Total arterial revascularization 820, 825*fc*
Total ischemic time, function of 276*f*
Toxic substances 657
Toxicity, mechanism of 620
Tracheostoma 935
Tractus solitaries, nucleus of 697
Traditional syntax score, limitations of 170
Trametinib 621
Tranexamic acid 315, 340
Trans fatty acids 47
Transcatheter aortic valve 445
  implantation 443, 448, 451, 465, 531, 545
  replacement 443, 444, 444*t*, 445, 448, 467, 535, 542, 903, 1029

limitations of 445
procedure 546*t*
Transcatheter heart valve 450
Transcatheter mitral valve replacement 536, 545
Transcatheter paravalvular leak closure, technique of 465
Transcriptase inhibitors, reverse 623
Transcutaneous energy transmission 854
Transendocardial stem cell injection 428, 429
Transesophageal echocardiogram 476
three-dimentional 476*f*
Transesophageal echocardiography 434, 449, 451, 463, 469, 509, 533, 542, 893
role of 451
Transferrin saturation 1003
Transfusion dependent 576
Transient ischemic
attack 307, 682, 705, 706, 876, 879, 882, 892, 932, 935, 1045
dilation 175, 552
Transluminal extraction catheter 349
Transmitral flow 482, 498*f*
velocity with atrial contraction 642
Transmyocardial laser revascularization 838
Transoesophageal echocardiogram 476
Transradial interventions 400
Transthoracic echocardiogram 476, 972
two-dimensional 476
Transthoracic echocardiography 434, 448, 449*f*, 973
Trauma 916, 923, 941
Treadmill test 1024
Trendelenburg position, reverse 912
Tricuspid annular planar systolic excursion 288, 503, 506, 506*f*
Tricuspid regurgitation 286, 288, 505, 532
severe 809
velocity 503
Tricuspid stenosis 533
Tricuspid valve 434, 504, 532
closure 507*f*
en face view of 532*f*
Triglyceride 33, 46, 53, 66, 596, 958, 1062
high 59
reduction 597
rich lipoproteins 54*f*
transport protein 596
Trimetazidine 182, 183, 230, 585, 586
Triple drug combination 127
Triple vessel disease 842, 938
Trivandrum heart failure registry 95
Trophoblast invasion 967
Troponin 972
True bifurcation lesions, treatment of 359
Tumescent anesthesia 909, 911, 914
Tumor necrosis factor 9, 206, 636, 874, 967
alpha 91
T-wave alternans 765
Twiddler's syndrome 810*f*, 812
Two-catheter technique 389, 389*f*
Tyrosine kinase inhibitors 139

U

Ulcers 918
Ultrasonography 917, 967
Ultrasound, duplex 933, 943
Ultra-thin drug-eluting stents, clinical efficacy of 408
Umbilical cord derived mesenchymal stem cells 428
United States Food and Drug Administration 183, 910
Unsaturated fatty acids 46
Unscientific pathophysiologic rationale 1036
Unstable angina 211, 226, 235, 243, 251, 315, 413, 383
Upper limb 916
Urea 972

V

Valsalva maneuver 493*f*
end of 493*f*
Valsartan 589, 635, 974
Valve
assessment 527
durability 447
gradient 452
implantable 1034
in-valve international data registry 444
morphology 450
perforation 774
replacement or repair 290
thrombosis 446, 1021
Valvular disease 578
Valvular heart disease 534, 690, 893, 897, 973, 1050, 1065
pre-existing 973
Valvular injury 918
Valvular lesions 984
Valvular stenosis 973
Valvular surgery 211
Vandetanib 621, 622
Varicose vein 907, 914*t*
management of 909
sealing system 913
treatment for 908
Vascular access
approach, selection of 373
complication 391
Vascular cell adhesion molecule 92, 1044
Vascular disease 879
causes of 916
noninflammatory 927
Vascular endothelial growth factor 139, 207, 426, 971, 999

Vascular function 994
Vascular injury 916, 918
Vascular lesions 92
Vascular psychiatry 839
Vascular rarefaction 923
Vascular resistance, elevated 985
Vascular surgeons 932
Vascular surgery 338
Vascular thrombosis, risk of 722*b*
Vasoactive drugs 294
Vasoconstriction, excessive 942
Vasoconstrictor prostaglandins 923
Vasodilatory kinins, functions of 125
Vasopressin 294, 784
    use of 784
Vasopressors 661
Vasospastic angina 763
Vasovagal syncope 682, 1063
    pathophysiology of 682
Vein grafts 846
Vein thrombus, target 912
Veins of leg, superficial 907*f*
Velocity time integral 505
Vemurafenib 622
Vena cava
    filter
        retrievable 919
        role of inferior 919
    inferior 434, 919, 920, 978
    superior 434, 544
Vena contracta 477, 529
    width of 477
Venlafaxine 623
Venoarterial extracorporeal membrane oxygenation 295, 382
Venous cannulation 845
Venous thromboembolism 601, 916, 918, 918*t*, 919, 920
    despite anticoagulation, recurrent 920
    treatment of 601
Venous ulcers 907
Ventricular arrhythmias 221, 739, 741, 744, 746, 761, 1064
    and sudden death 746
    malignant 858
    management of 743
    mechanisms of 746
    pathogenesis of 741
    risk factors for 763*t*
    sustained 741
    therapies for 747
    treatment of 747, 748
    types of 741
Ventricular assist device 853, 856*fc*, 859, 860
    classification of 854
    implantation 858
    pros and cons of 860*t*
Ventricular cavities, dilatation of 636
Ventricular complex
    ablation, technique of premature 772
    premature 751, 771-773, 773*f*, 774, 778
Ventricular contractions, premature 1064
Ventricular dysfunction 805
Ventricular dyssynchrony 666
Ventricular ectopy 1035
Ventricular fibrillation 694, 741-743, 746, 751, 758, 760, 761, 763
    incidence of 741
    management of sustained 743
    syndromes 763*t*
    therapy 1021
Ventricular hypertrophy 923
Ventricular pre-excitation 1064
Ventricular premature beats 743, 746
Ventricular pseudoaneurysm 831
Ventricular rate, rapid 736
Ventricular septal
    defect 505, 831, 1034
    rupture 293
Ventricular single-chamber rate-modulated 811
Ventricular structure and systolic function, evaluation of 570
Ventricular tachyarrhythmias 690
Ventricular tachycardia 498, 672, 742, 751, 760, 763, 775, 776*f*, 805, 1035
    management of sustained 743
    predictors of sustained 741
    storm 742*fc*
        management of 742*fc*
Ventricular thrombus 893
Verapamil 182
Vessel
    failure, target 359
    last surviving 379
    occlusion, large 882, 888
    revascularization, target 169
    tortuosity 938
Viable myocardium, types of 559
Vinca alkaloids 620
Vincristine 700
Vinylidene fluoride-co-hexafluoropropylene 406
Viral and bacterial assays 973
Viral myocarditis 518*f*
Virchow's triad 916*fc*
Visceral obesity 1048
Vitamin
    B_{12} 30
        deficiency 700
    C 93
    D 13-15, 16*t*, 17
        deficiency 13
        mechanism of 15

nutritional status 13
receptors 13
supplementation 18, 18*t*
synthesis 14*f*
E 42, 93
K
antagonist 601, 707, 725, 725*f*, 726, 728, 729, 734, 879, 883, 893, 894, 920, 980, 1052, 1053
anticoagulants 602
dependent coagulation factor proteins 601
drugs 601
epoxide 725
K2 substances 616
Vomiting 287
Vorapaxar 336
Vorinostat 622
Vulnerable coronary plaques 217
Vulnerable plaque 217
assessment 421

W

Warfarin 612, 616, 617, 618
arm 603
indications 616
superior to 602
therapy, long term 881
Weightlifting 1062
White blood cells 312, 337
White coat hypertension 156
White thrombus 421
WICS-LV system 813
Wilms tumor 142
Window endovascular trials, late 889
Window paradox, late 890
Wireless cardiac stimulation system for left ventricle 812*f*
Wireless health care delivery systems 1013
Wolff-Parkinson-White syndrome 757, 1062
World Health Organization 103, 249, 932, 1002, 1018, 1024
Worsen angina 180
Wound care 945
Wrestling 1062

Y

Yttrium-aluminum-garnet 838

Z

Ziv-aflibercept 621
Z-offset drift 421
Zotarolimus-eluting stent 406, 407